Critical Care Pharmacotherapy

AMERICAN COLLEGE OF CLINICAL PHARMACY

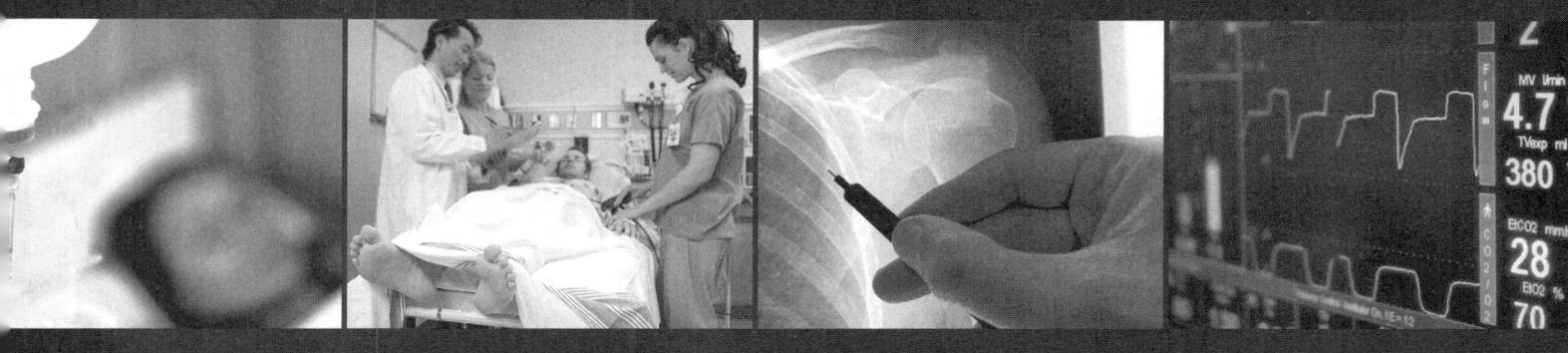

CRITICAL CARE
PHARMACOTHERAPY

BRIAN ERSTAD, PHARM.D., FCCP, BCPS, EDITOR

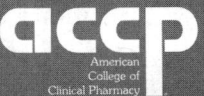

Director of Professional Development: Nancy M. Perrin, M.A., CAE
Associate Director of Professional Development: Wafa Dahdal, Pharm.D., BCPS
Publications Project Manager: David Shaw, M.B.A.
Desktop Publisher/Graphic Designer: Mary Ann Kuchta; Steve Brooker
Medical Editor: Kimma Sheldon, Ph.D., M.A.

For order information or questions, contact:
American College of Clinical Pharmacy
13000 W. 87th Street Parkway, Suite 100
Lenexa, KS 66215
(913) 492-3311
(913) 492-0088 (fax)
accp@accp.com

Copyright © 2016 by the American College of Clinical Pharmacy. No part of this publication may be reproduced, stored in a retrieval system, or transmitted, in any form or by any means, electronic or mechanical, including photocopy, without prior written permission of the American College of Clinical Pharmacy.

16 17 18 EBM 10 9 8 7 6 5 4 3 2 1

Printed in the United States of America.

ISBN: 978-1-939862-20-4
Library of Congress Control Number: 2015953696

DEDICATION

To my son, Alex, my wife, Sue,
and my mother, Donna, for their unwavering support.

B. Erstad

CONTENTS

Preface xiii
Brian L. Erstad, Pharm.D., FCCP, BCPS

Foreword xv
Joseph F. Dasta, M.S., FCCP; Curtis N. Sessler, M.D., FCCP, FCCM; Ashlee Dauenhauer, Pharm.D.; and Ohoud A. Aljuhani, Pharm.D.

Letter from ACCP xxi
Judith Jacobi, FCCP, MCCM, BCPS, BCCCP, ACCP President 2014–2015

SECTION 1: SUPPORTIVE CARE

Chapter 1: Acid-Base Disorders 3
Curtis E. Haas, Pharm.D.; David C. Kaufman, M.D.; and Brian L. Erstad, Pharm.D., FCCP, BCPS

Chapter 2: Fluid Therapy in the Critically Ill Patient 29
Brian L. Erstad, Pharm.D., FCCP, BCPS

Chapter 3: Electrolyte Disorders in the Critically Ill Population 58
Jeffrey J. Bruno, Pharm.D., BCPS, BCNSP; and Todd W. Canada, Pharm.D., FASHP, FTSHP, BCNSP

Chapter 4: Nutrition Support Therapy in Critically Ill Patients 98
Amber Verdell, Pharm.D., BCPS, BCNSP; and Carol J. Rollins, M.S., RD, Pharm.D., FASHP, FASPEN, BCNSP

Chapter 5: Glucose Management in the Critically Ill Population 128
Paul M. Szumita, Pharm.D., FCCM, BCCCP, BCPS; and James F. Gilmore, Pharm.D., BCCCP, BCPS

Chapter 6: Analgesia 147
Asad E. Patanwala, Pharm.D.

Chapter 7: Agitation and Comfort in the Intensive Care Unit 161
David J. Gagnon, Pharm.D.; Nicole Kovacic, Pharm.D.; and Gilles L. Fraser, Pharm.D., MCCM

Chapter 8: Delirium in Critically Ill Adults 186
John W. Devlin, Pharm.D., FCCP, FCCM

Chapter 9: Neuromuscular Blocking Agents 198
M. Claire McManus, Pharm.D., BS(Pharm)

Chapter 10: Shock Syndromes 225
Ishaq Lat, Pharm.D., FCCP, FCCM, BCPS; and Sajni Patel, Pharm.D., BCPS

Section 2: Infectious Diseases

Chapter 11: Appropriate Use of Antimicrobials 241
Scott T. Micek, Pharm.D.; and Marin H. Kollef, M.D.

Chapter 12: Pharmacokinetic and Pharmacodynamic Considerations
for Antimicrobial Use in Critically Ill Patients..252
Douglas N. Fish, Pharm.D., FCCP, FCCM, BCPS-AQ ID

Chapter 13: Laboratory Testing Considerations 283
Kali Martin, Pharm.D.; Shanna Cole, Pharm.D.; and Michael Klepser, Pharm.D.

Chapter 14: Antimicrobial Resistance in the Critical Care Environment..289
Andrew M. Roecker, Pharm.D.; and Steven J. Martin, Pharm.D.

Chapter 15: Severe Sepsis and Septic Shock...298
*Seth R. Bauer, Pharm.D., FCCM, BCPS; Simon W. Lam, Pharm.D., FCCM, BCPS; and
Lance J. Oyen, Pharm.D., FCCM, FCCP, BCPS*

Chapter 16: Invasive Fungal Infections...319
Kathryn R. Matthias, Pharm.D., BCPS-AQ ID

Chapter 17: Invasive Viral Infections in the Intensive Care Unit 331
*P. Brandon Bookstaver, Pharm.D., FCCP, BCPS-AQ ID, AAHIVP; and Caroline B. Derrick,
Pharm.D., BCPS*

Chapter 18: Antimicrobial Prophylaxis 351
Keith M. Olsen, Pharm.D., FCCP, FCCM; and Gregory Peitz, Pharm.D., BCPS

Section 3: Neurocritical Care

Chapter 19: Status Epilepticus and Acute Seizure Management...371
*Eljim P. Tesoro, Pharm.D., BCPS; Karen Berger, Pharm.D., BCPS; and Gretchen M. Brophy,
Pharm.D., FCCP, FCCM, FNCS, BCPS*

Chapter 20: Traumatic Brain Injury and Acute Spinal Cord Injury..388
A. Shaun Rowe, Pharm.D., BCPS; and Bradley A. Boucher, Pharm.D., BCPS

Chapter 21: Acute Management of Stroke 403
Martina Holder, Pharm.D., BCPS; and Stacy Voils, Pharm.D., M.Sc., BCPS

Chapter 22: Critical Care Management of Aneurysmal Subarachnoid Hemorrhage 416
*Denise H. Rhoney, Pharm.D., FCCP, FCCM, FNCS; Kathryn Morbitzer, Pharm.D.; and
J. Dedrick Jordan, M.D., Ph.D.*

SECTION 4: HEMATOLOGY

Chapter 23: Prevention and Treatment of Venous Thromboembolism..449
*William E. Dager, Pharm.D., FCCP, FCCM, FCSHP, FASHP, MCCM, BCPS; and
A. Josh Roberts, Pharm.D., BCPS*

Chapter 24: Hemostatic Agents for the Prevention and Management of Hemorrhage in the ICU 468
*Robert MacLaren, Pharm.D., MPH, FCCP, FCCM; Bradley A. Boucher, Pharm.D.,
FCCP, FCCM; and Laura Baumgartner, Pharm.D.*

Chapter 25: Laboratory Testing with Anticoagulation 499
Tyree H. Kiser, Pharm.D., FCCP, FCCM, BCPS

SECTION 5: ACUTE KIDNEY INJURY

Chapter 26: Acute Kidney Injury—Prevention and Management..523
Curtis L. Smith, Pharm.D., BCPS; and Thomas C. Dowling, Pharm.D., Ph.D., FCCP, FCP

Chapter 27: Drug Dosing in Acute Kidney Injury and Extracorporeal Therapies 538
*Melanie S. Joy, Pharm.D., Ph.D., FCCP, FASN; Michael L. Bentley, Pharm.D.; and
Katja M. Gist, D.O., M.A., MSCS*

SECTION 6: LIVER/GASTROINTESTINAL

Chapter 28: Management and Drug Dosing in Acute Liver Failure 573
Andrew C. Fritschle Hilliard, Pharm.D., BCPS, BCCCP; and David R. Foster, Pharm.D., FCCP

Chapter 29: Acute Gastrointestinal Bleeding: Prophylaxis and Treatment 591
Salmaan Kanji, Bsc. Pharm, Pharm.D.; and David Williamson, B. Pharm, M.Sc., Ph.D., BCPS

SECTION 7: ACUTE PULMONARY DISEASE

Chapter 30: Pulmonary Arterial Hypertension...609
Steven E. Pass, Pharm.D., FCCP, FCCM, FASHP, BCPS; and Joseph E. Mazur, Pharm.D., BCPS

Chapter 31: Critical Care Management of Asthma and Chronic Obstructive Pulmonary Disease................626
*Amanda Zomp, Pharm.D., BCPS; Katherine Bidwell, Pharm.D., BCPS; and
Stephanie Mallow Corbett, Pharm.D., FCCM*

Section 8: Cardiovascular Critical Care

Chapter 32: Acute Decompensated Heart Failure 645
Jo E. Rodgers, Pharm.D., FCCP, BCPS-AQ Cardiology; and Brent N. Reed, Pharm.D., FAHA, BCPS-AQ Cardiology

Chapter 33: Management of Acute Coronary Syndrome 660
Zachary A. Stacy, Pharm.D., M.S., FCCP, BCPS; and Paul P. Dobesh, Pharm.D., FCCP, BCPS-AQ Cardiology

Chapter 34: Management of Cardiac Arrest 688
Toby C. Trujillo, Pharm.D., FCCP, FAHA, BCPS-AQ Cardiology

Chapter 35: Acute Management of Arrhythmias 707
James E. Tisdale, Pharm.D., FCCP, FAPhA, FAHA, BCPS

Chapter 36: Pharmacologic Challenges During Mechanical Circulatory Support in Adults 735
Amy L. Dzierba, Pharm.D., FCCM, BCPS; and Erik Abel, Pharm.D., BCPS

Section 9: Other Urgencies and Emergencies

Chapter 37: Hypertensive Crisis 757
Jeremy Flynn, Pharm.D., FCCP, FCCM; Melissa Nestor, Pharm.D., BCPS; and Komal Pandya, Pharm.D., BCPS

Chapter 38: Medication Withdrawal in the Intensive Care Unit 781
Colgan T. Sloan, Pharm.D., BCPS; Robert French, M.D., MPH; Nicholas B. Hurst, M.D., M.S.; Stephen R. Karpen, Pharm.D.; and Mazda Shirazi, M.D., Ph.D.

Chapter 39: Endocrine Disorders 793
Robert L. Talbert, Pharm.D.

Chapter 40: Oncologic Emergencies 803
Ali McBride, Pharm.D., M.S., BCPS, BCOP; Michelle Nadeau, Pharm.D., BCPS; and Cory M. Vela, Pharm.D.

Section 10: Miscellaneous

Chapter 41: Drug Dosing in Special Intensive Care Unit Populations 821
Jeffrey F. Barletta, Pharm.D., FCCM

Chapter 42: Management of the Critically Ill Burn Patient 842
Claire V. Murphy, Pharm.D., BCPS; and Kate Oltrogge Pape, Pharm.D., BCPS

Chapter 43: The Role of Pharmacotherapy in the Treatment of the Multiple Trauma Patient 862
Rita Gayed, Pharm.D.; Prasad Abraham, Pharm.D., FCCM, BCPS; and David V. Feliciano, M.D., FACS

Chapter 44: Pediatric Critical Care 895
Elizabeth Farrington, Pharm.D., FCCP, FCCM, FPPAG, BCPS

Chapter 45: Drug Shortages: An Overview of Causes, Impact, and Management Strategies 925
Samuel E. Culli, Pharm.D., MPH; and John J. Lewin III, Pharm.D., MBA, FASHP, FCCM, FNCS

Chapter 46: Drug Interactions in the Intensive Care Unit 930
Cristian Merchan, Pharm.D.; and John Papadopoulos, Pharm.D., B.S., FCCM, BCNSP

Chapter 47: Acute Illness Scoring Systems 951
Thomas J. Johnson, Pharm.D., MBA, FASHP, FCCM, BCPS

Chapter 48: Leading and Managing Intensive Care Unit Pharmacy Services 960
Robert J. Weber, Pharm.D., M.S., FASHP, BCPS

Chapter 49: Medication Safety and Active Surveillance 971
Sandra L. Kane-Gill, Pharm.D., M.Sc., FCCP, FCCM; and Mitchell S. Buckley, Pharm.D., FCCP, FASHP, FCCM, BCPS

Chapter 50: Care of the Immunocompromised Patient 983
Heather Personett, Pharm.D., BCPS; and Simon W. Lam, Pharm.D., FCCM, BCPS

Chapter 51: Clinically Applied Pharmacogenomics in Critical Care Settings 999
Samuel G. Johnson, Pharm.D., FCCP; and Christina L. Aquilante, Pharm.D., FCCP

Contributors 1013

Reviewers 1017

Index 1019

Disclosure of Potential Conflicts of Interest 1047

PREFACE

Brian L. Erstad, Pharm.D., FCCP, BCPS

The origin of critical care as a specialty is open to debate. Critically ill patients have received care in groups near battlefields ever since organized large-scale fighting first occurred. In hospital settings, isolated postoperative units dedicated to critically ill patients have been reported since the early 1900s. However, the widespread need for mechanical ventilation (commonly called respirators at the time) of patients with polio during the epidemics of the 1940s and 1950s led to a tipping point in the formation of critical care specialization. One of the first papers describing the care of patients with polio referred to care "by a team" of clinicians, although pharmacists were not among the health professionals listed.[1] In addition to ventilators, other technologies that began to have more widespread use in critically ill patients by the 1950s included rudimentary dialysis machines, AC electrical defibrillators, and transvenous cardiac pacing equipment.[2] More invasive respiratory and hemodynamic monitoring tools were also increasingly used in the early intensive care units (ICUs) of the 1950s and 1960s. These developments in the care of critically ill patients necessitated specialization by physicians in areas such as internal medicine, trauma, and anesthesiology. Other specialized personnel such as nurses, respiratory therapists, and eventually pharmacists (circa 1970s–1980s) were needed to complement the increasing number of critical care physicians in more modern critical care units. Today, a multidisciplinary or interdisciplinary patient care team that includes pharmacists has become the practice mantra and is now the norm in many ICU settings.

The term *intensivist* is now used to describe physicians with critical care specialty training following primary residency training in areas like internal medicine, surgery, anesthesiology, emergency medicine, pediatrics, and obstetrics and gynecology. The first certification examination for critical care specialization by physicians was offered within internal medicine in 1987 by the American Board of Medical Specialties. Board certification for intensivists is now available from several specialty boards. For pharmacists, critical care has been recognized as a unique specialty by the Board of Pharmacy Specialties, with the first examination offered in the fall of 2015; widespread support for this certification within the profession of pharmacy is evidenced by the petition for specialty recognition that was jointly submitted by the American College of Clinical Pharmacy (ACCP), the American Pharmacists Association, and the American Society of Health-System Pharmacists.

In addition to specialty recognition, there are many other indicators of the growth and advancement of critical care pharmacy practice. The number of unit-based (i.e., clinical) critical care pharmacists increases in each new survey of critical care pharmacy practice. Similarly, the number of accredited PGY2 critical care residencies continues to increase. Fellowships in critical care have been developed, albeit in smaller numbers. Critical care pharmacists have their own recognized specialty groups in professional pharmacy organizations, such as the ACCP Critical Care Practice-Related Network (PRN). Position and opinion papers have been published that discuss the scope, level (i.e., fundamental, desirable, optimal), and justification of critical care pharmacy services and the credentialing of critical care pharmacists.[3,4] But perhaps the best testimonial to the advancement and success of critical care pharmacists is their own substantial involvement in interprofessional critical care societies, organizations, and associations.

The four largest professional groups in the United States with critical care practitioner membership are the American Thoracic Society, the American College of Chest Physicians, the American Association of Critical-Care Nurses, and the Society of Critical Care Medicine (SCCM). Together, these groups formed a loose association known as the Critical Care Societies Collaborative (CCSC), which was established in 2009 to work on common core critical issues. Of the organizations that constitute the CCSC, the first to recognize critical care pharmacists in a meaningful way was SCCM, established in 1970—as evidenced by its involvement in governance and committee work. Since 1998, critical care pharmacists have had a recognized section (Clinical Pharmacy and

Pharmacology) within the administrative structure of SCCM. Furthermore, critical care pharmacists have widespread involvement in governance and other aspects of SCCM, as evidenced by the pharmacists who have served in numerous high-level positions (including president), the highly respected awards and honors bestowed on critical care pharmacist members (e.g., Fellow of the American College of Critical Care Medicine, Master Critical Care Medicine, Shubin-Weil Master Clinician/Teacher: Excellence in Bedside Teaching Award), the number of pharmacists involved in SCCM educational programming and guideline development efforts, and the long-standing practice models that have recognized pharmacists as integral members of the critical care team.[5] Moreover, pharmacists continue to make inroads in other national critical care organizations that have traditionally been more physician-centric; for example, the Neurocritical Care Society recently placed a pharmacist in the governance line leading to the presidency.

The preceding overview of the evolution of critical care pharmacy practice serves as the backdrop for this first edition of *Critical Care Pharmacotherapy*. A cursory look at the authors of the chapters in this textbook reveals many of the pioneers and thought leaders in critical care pharmacy practice. Several of these authors were the first pharmacists to establish decentralized, unit-based critical care pharmacy services in their institutions. Many of the authors have held high-level positions in organizations with critical care membership, and most have active educational training and research programs. I am honored to be part of this collective effort.

The choice of chapters for this text was not an easy one, and I am indebted to many colleagues for their helpful suggestions. Chapters in general medical and pharmacy textbooks are often compiled on the basis of disease states or organ systems, but neither of these approaches was deemed appropriate for a critical care text focusing on pharmacotherapy. A pharmacologic approach to the chapters based on drug class was excluded because it would not integrate the disease-medication decision-making process that is reflective of actual practice. Ultimately, a combination approach was decided on. Many of the chapters are listed under an organ system section, but most of the specific chapters in each section use a medication-focused approach. Another large section of chapters pertains to supportive care because this reflects so many of the medications that are used in critical care practice. Finally, several miscellaneous topics, some of which involve special ICU populations, did not fit neatly into either the organ system or supportive care sections but were deemed necessary to present a complete picture of critical care pharmacy practice.

Although this text is primarily aimed at a critical care pharmacist audience, we hope that it will provide valuable information for other pharmacists who must periodically care for critically ill patients, as well as for other health professionals who care for critically ill patients and desire a pharmacotherapy-focused resource. Ultimately, the intent of this text is to better educate pharmacists and other health professionals on issues pertaining to critical care pharmacotherapy so that they can provide optimal care for our patients in an efficient and cost-effective manner.

References

1. Ibsen B. The anaesthetist's viewpoint on the treatment of respiratory complications in poliomyelitis during the epidemic in Copenhagen, 1952. Proc R Soc Med 1954;47:72-4.

2. Weil MH, Tang W. From intensive care to critical care medicine. Am J Respir Crit Care Med 2011;183:1451-3.

3. Rudis MI, Brandl KM. Society of Critical Care Medicine and American College of Clinical Pharmacy Task Force on Critical Care Pharmacy Services. Position paper on critical care pharmacy services. Crit Care Med 2000;28:3746-50.

4. Dager W, Bolesta S, Brophy G, et al. An opinion paper outlining recommendations for training, credentialing, and documenting and justifying critical care pharmacy services. Pharmacotherapy 2011;31:135e-175e.

5. Brilli RJ, Spevetz A, Branson RD, et al. Critical care delivery in the intensive care unit: defining clinical roles and the best practice mode. Crit Care Med 2001;29:2007-19.

FOREWORD

Joseph F. Dasta, M.S., FCCP

When I began to establish my clinical practice in 1979 in the medical intensive care unit (MICU) at The Ohio State University Hospital (now Wexner Medical Center), I knew of only two pharmacists in the United States who were critical care specialists. The first was David Angaran, M.S., at the University of Wisconsin trauma ICU. During my hospital pharmacy residency at Ohio State, we visited the University of Wisconsin in 1975 and toured the ICU, where I met David. He had been in that role since 1972. I was so impressed with his level of involvement in the care of the ICU patient that I recall saying to myself, "I want to be like him someday." The second was Thomas Majerus, Pharm.D., who had been practicing in the trauma ICU since 1977 at the Maryland Institute of Emergency Medical Services. He was also very involved with direct patient care. Clearly, both of these pharmacists filled an unmet need in pharmacotherapy, and they were practicing at a high level of clinical involvement, even in today's terms. They were the true pioneers of critical care pharmacy.[1]

My initial practice area in 1977 was pulmonary medicine, and my clinical responsibility at the college of pharmacy was to develop a practice site at the hospital for pharmacy students (B.S. program) to gain clinical experience. Please note that I was employed full-time by the college of pharmacy, not the hospital pharmacy, although I had a good relationship with the pharmacy department because I was a graduate of their residency. I decided to change my practice site in 1979 from pulmonary medicine to the MICU because the pulmonary medicine division became administratively responsible for establishing an ICU team with a pulmonologist as the attending physician. It sounded like an interesting area for a pharmacist. It may be of interest to know that I had no idea that critical care pharmacy would develop into what it is today. I had not considered the future potential of critical care; I was primarily interested in developing a site for pharmacy students to fulfill their clinical rotation requirements. As the adage goes, "I'd rather be lucky than good."

Even in 1979, Ohio State had a relatively well-established clinical pharmacy program whereby "floor pharmacists" were assigned to certain nursing units to evaluate the appropriateness of drug orders and to verify these orders before sending them to the central pharmacy for dispensing. As such, a floor pharmacist was assigned to the MICU; however, floor pharmacists usually did not attend daily ICU rounds because they had duties in other nursing units in the hospital. As such, I was the first pharmacist to consistently attend daily MICU rounds. I had not completed a formal training in the area of critical care pharmacy because no formal training programs yet existed; therefore, this practice setting posed many learning opportunities for me. I learned on my own by reading as much as I could and asking a lot of questions of the critical care nurses and physicians. During one visit to the health sciences library, I went to the stacks under the letter "C." I found several textbooks on critical care and a journal called Critical Care Medicine. I leafed through its pages and realized that it was the official journal of the Society of Critical Care Medicine (SCCM). I recall thinking "Wow, they even have a specialty society." A few days later, I called the society to inquire about membership. After I provided a brief explanation of my activities, a staff member said that it sounded like I was part of the critical care team and said, "Of course you can join … we'd love to have you as part of this society." I was flattered.…

It seemed to me that critical care would be a natural specialty for pharmacists. Patients are often hemodynamically unstable, they receive many drugs, and the data on therapies pertaining to the critically ill patient were scant to nonexistent. I hoped someday there would be many pharmacists specializing in critical care.

In 1981, I switched my practice to the surgical ICU (SICU). This unit was very different because there was no floor pharmacist. The pharmacy department sent drugs for the nurses to prepare (i.e., reconstitute vials and make an intravenous admixture) and administer. I heard rumors about this unit, which appeared in desperate need of a clinical pharmacist. I later discovered that the main interaction of the nurse with a pharmacist was for nurses to frequently call the pharmacy and say something like "my gentamicin was late." This was a ripe area for the total scope of pharmacy services, both distributional and clinical.

I decided to introduce myself to the physician director, Dr. Tom Reilley, an anesthesiologist. After I told him who I was, I'll never forget his words to me: "Where have you been ... I've been looking for a clinical pharmacologist since arriving here several years ago." He told me to meet him the next day at 9 a.m. in the SICU. Honestly, I was scared to death that someone would ask me a question that I could not answer. On rounds, one of the first patients we encountered was shaving his beard; of course, he did not have a razor. Apparently, this elderly man was hallucinating. A review of his medication list revealed that he was receiving intravenous cimetidine 300 mg every 6 hours, and his serum creatinine was about 3–4 mg/dL. I sheepishly pointed this out on rounds and suggested that his altered mental status could be from excess cimetidine. Dr. Reilley turned to me and asked me the dreaded question, "How do we fix this?" Although I was prepared to speculate and provide theories, it dawned on me that he wanted an action plan. I said to hold the dose for 24 hours and reinitiate cimetidine 300 mg every 12 hours. The order was changed according to my suggestion. A few days later, his mental status was better. Little did I know that, years later, I would be part of the SCCM clinical practice guideline on pain, agitation, and delirium!

The care of the critically ill patient in the early 1980s was much different from today. For example, most mechanically ventilated patients were heavily sedated. It was believed that ICU patients are best served if they don't participate in their care and have no memory of their critical illness. There is an observation made by Dr. Tom Petty at the University of Colorado, in mid-1998, where he reflects on seeing patients in the ICU motionless, sedated, paralyzed, and appearing to be dead, except for the monitors that told him otherwise.[2] I suspect that if I had suggested early mobility, it would have sounded like heresy.

Many patients in the ICU, particularly the SICU, had pulmonary artery catheters. As such, several hemodynamic monitoring variables were generated, often many times per day. All of this information plus laboratory results, drugs, and so forth was on paper-based flow sheets. It was difficult to make sense of the volume of data. Regarding the paper medication administration record, at least at Ohio State, the scheduled drugs were on the front page, and the as-needed drugs were on the reverse side. As I recall, we often ignored the as-needed drugs like analgesics and sedatives because that was considered a "nursing issue." Common orders included morphine 2–8 mg every 1–4 hours as needed, lorazepam 1–4 mg every 4–8 hours as needed, haloperidol 2.5–10 mg every 8–12 hours as needed, and diphenhydramine 25–50 mg intravenously every night at bedtime as needed for sleep. When I reviewed this page, I recall concluding that it appeared to be the nurse who was selecting the drug, the dose, how often to administer, and what parameter to monitor.

In addition to clinical practice and precepting B.S. pharmacy students, I initiated some clinical research studies. I quickly learned how difficult it was to conduct research in such an unstable population. After about 15 years of performing these functions, the pharmacy department opened an SICU/perioperative satellite pharmacy and later hired a Pharm.D. specifically for the SICU. My role changed to more of a clinical consultant, educator, and clinical researcher. My interaction with the SICU clinical pharmacist served as a model for optimal collaboration between hospital- and college-paid faculty. We co-precepted Pharm.D. students and collaborated on several clinical research studies.

During this time, I established one of the nation's first residencies in critical care pharmacy. My first resident was a woman who had just completed her Pharm.D. degree. She was passionate about the care of the critically ill patient. I soon realized that she was a very talented person; beyond being smart, hard-working, and an excellent communicator, she was able to step back and examine the big picture in ways that I could not have imagined. Of course, I'm referring to Judi Jacobi, Pharm.D., who became the first pharmacist president of SCCM in 2010 and is the 2015 president of ACCP.

During my tenure at Ohio State, I was fortunate to train 11 residents and 9 fellows. My first fellow was Robert Weber, whose program was funded by an ASHP grant in 1980. Bob is now administrator of pharmacy services at Ohio State. I am very proud of all the accomplishments of my 20 residents and fellows.

There have been many changes in pharmacy and health care since I first established my clinical practice in the late 1970s. The pharmacy department has evolved from a revenue-generating center to a cost center after capitated reimbursement was initiated. This generated numerous initiatives focused on cost reduction of pharmaceuticals. In the area of professional organizations, the Critical Care Practice Research Network of the American College of Clinical Pharmacy (ACCP) is consistently one of the largest PRNs within ACCP. Regarding SCCM, the Clinical Pharmacy and Pharmacy (CPP) section was formed in 1989 and currently has more than 2,000 members. It is a very active section, with pharmacists serving on key committees of the section and within the SCCM organization. Furthermore, there is a designed CPP seat on the council. There are usually four or five pharmacists on the editorial board of Critical Care Medicine, many pharmacists have been members of clinical practice guidelines and a few have been chair, and a pharmacist was recently selected as program co-chair for the annual congress. In 2015, the Board of Pharmacy Specialties (BPS) recognized critical care pharmacy as the seventh BPS specialty.

There usually are 70–80 critical care residencies, and many ICUs have pharmacist preceptors actively involved with direct patient care. However, the number of fellowships has dropped dramatically. It is of concern that so few critical care pharmacists are being trained for research-oriented academic positions. In addition, some critical care pharmacists are being diverted to other areas of the hospital, or they are being redirected to reduce drug costs. These changes are occurring despite data showing the important role of the critical care pharmacist.[3,4] Clearly, the critical care pharmacist should focus on providing cost-effective, quality care.

In summary, critical care pharmacy is a well-established specialty in the field of clinical pharmacy, which now has a board certification process. Thousands of ICU patients have benefited from critical care pharmacists providing excellence in patient care, leadership roles in professional societies, and clinical research resulting in improved outcomes. The future is bright. However, it will be important for pharmacists to be paid for their services and for organizations like the Joint Commission, Leapfrog, and the Centers for Medicare & Medicaid Services to endorse the critical care pharmacist as a crucial element in the provision of optimum care to the critically ill patient.

References

1. Dasta JF. Critical care. Ann Pharmacother 2006;40:736-7.
2. Petty T. Suspended life or extending death? Chest 1998;114:360-1.
3. Kane SL, Weber RJ, Dasta JF. The impact of critical care pharmacists on enhancing patient outcomes. Intensive Care Med 2003;29:691-8.
4. MacLaren R, Devlin JW, Martin SJ, et al. A national survey characterizing the practice of critical care pharmacists. Ann Pharmacother 2006;40:612-7.

Curtis N. Sessler, M.D., FCCP, FCCM

I recently celebrated my 30-year anniversary as an attending physician in the intensive care unit (ICU) setting and was thrilled when Brian Erstad invited me to reflect on the journey of critical care pharmacotherapy. I have long been an enthusiastic believer that by getting the right people with the right skills in the right seats on the bus, one can be confident of achieving the best possible outcomes. This is certainly true in critical care medicine, where the sickest patients have the most complex management, often proceeding at the fastest pace.

Although I am confident that we have been providing the best care possible for many years, I personally count the addition of the clinical pharmacist as a regular member of the ICU team as a sentinel moment in the quest to deliver high-quality patient care. I have had the very good fortune of working with some spectacular clinical pharmacists in a wide variety of settings—a reflection of the many roles that clinical pharmacists play and the different hats I've worn over the years. These roles have evolved to the point that, unquestionably, clinical pharmacists are essential for the optimal care of the individual ICU patient, as well as the safe, effective, and cost-conscious critical care delivered throughout hospitals around the world.

As is true for many clinicians, my most consistent appreciation for the clinical pharmacist is of the value added on a daily basis in their direct patient-centric role. The instances in which one of our clinical pharmacists has identified and corrected a potentially life-threatening drug interaction or adverse drug effect are too numerous to count. I recall one patient who had suffered a small stroke at another hospital but arrived to our ICU manifesting severe neurocognitive deficits. Our clinical pharmacist noted that the patient had been receiving an amiodarone infusion and recommended discontinuation as a potential cause of neurotoxicity. This patient rapidly improved and was eventually discharged home with good functional abilities.

Important roles our clinical pharmacists play in the daily management of ICU patients include participating in pharmacotherapy decision-making, providing pharmacokinetic consultation, identifying and mitigating potential drug interactions, taking steps to avoid or quickly recognize adverse drug effects, monitoring drug dosing and administration, and avoiding administration of costly or unnecessary medications. Widespread organ dysfunction, extensive lists of medications, and rapidly changing medical illnesses contribute to a fertile setting for the emergence of medication misadventure. In fact, among all patient groups, critically ill patients present perhaps the greatest challenges and therefore the greatest needs for the skills of a good clinical pharmacist. Although many ICU patients benefit from direct clinical pharmacist involvement, I consider the clinical pharmacist-physician partnership to be among the most powerful patient-care tools in the intensivist's armamentarium. In fact, one might consider this partnership to reflect the collective expertise as the therapeutic strategists who design and implement the pharmacologic therapeutic plan, as well as therapeutic tacticians who make fine adjustments to medications in the heat of medical battle. Together with ICU nurses, clinical pharmacists and physicians establish the core of the ICU team that provides patient-centered care.

My experiences as medical director for our medical ICU, as well as other leadership roles in the critical care community throughout our institution, have broadened my appreciation for the many important contributions by, and the unique expertise of, clinical pharmacists with respect to tackling important system-wide issues. Our clinical pharmacists are at the forefront of a wide variety of educational, administrative, and local policy-making activities. Many important activities focus on traditional pharmacy-based issues, but typically with an eye to educating and assisting other members of the health care team. For example, like many hospitals, we have experienced shortages of critical medications including vasopressors, sedative and opioid medications, and others. Our clinical pharmacists' action plans have included detailed and evidence-based guidelines for substitution medications with matching educational programs for all affected clinicians. In addition, our clinical pharmacists routinely serve as key members of multiprofessional taskforces that create order sets, checklists, treatment algorithms, and other tools and documents.

As an academician, I am delighted that we have a strong culture of scientific inquiry in our critical care community. Our clinical pharmacists are highly engaged and often lead the way in the process of addressing clinically relevant questions through clinical research and scholarly analysis. I'm proud of our clinical pharmacists who routinely present posters at national meetings and publish important original investigations and reviews. One of the more noteworthy accomplishments from the ICUs at our institution—developing and validating the Richmond Agitation-Sedation Scale (RASS)—initially emerged from a bedside conversation several clinical pharmacists and I were having about adjusting sedative medications. We concluded, let's make a better patient assessment tool and build one that includes the viewpoints of all the key stakeholders—nurses, pharmacists, and physicians—for this important and common problem.

For the past decade or so, I have had increasingly frequent collaboration with clinical pharmacy colleagues on several national projects, including serving on work groups addressing critical care workforce shortages, clinical practice guideline writing committees, and expert panels to address important problems like managing pain in the ICU. It is clear that clinical pharmacy is a discipline at the heart of critical care practice, research, and education and that clinical pharmacists provide the unique expertise that complements that of nurses, physicians, and other individuals, all striving to provide superlative patient care.

I conclude by applauding Dr. Erstad for leading a distinguished group of contributors in creating an outstanding textbook of critical care pharmacotherapy. I am grateful for the opportunity to contribute and, in doing so, to help celebrate the tremendous work performed by my clinical pharmacy colleagues.

Ashlee Dauenhauer, Pharm.D.

As a new practitioner in the field of critical care, I was ready to take my 8+ years of higher education and make a difference in patients' lives. What I quickly found is that the reality of daily patient care is much more complex than what is taught during those fruitful years of training. Even after a rigorous 2-year residency program, where I was seemingly exposed and prepared for every situation, I realized how much untapped knowledge exists in medicine. Nevertheless, some of the most indispensable information I have gained in the field of health care resulted from my daily experiences in the intensive care unit (ICU). As I reflect on my years of training and the first year of my career as an ICU pharmacist, I am exceptionally pleased with my decision to pursue the area of critical care.

I was first exposed to the acute care setting as a fourth-year pharmacy student during clinical rotations. At that time, I had a limited preconceived notion of what clinical pharmacists actually did on a daily basis. However, after observing my preceptors, I acknowledged the potential impact that pharmacists have on patient care through diligent patient and physician interaction. When I began my pharmacy residency, I was fortunate enough to train in a program that already had well-established clinical pharmacist positions. Pharmacists and pharmacy residents at the University of Arizona Medical Center have a recognized and respected relationship with other members of the health care profession. Training at an institution with a valued pharmacy presence has allowed me to grow exponentially in medical knowledge, workload efficiency, and team communication.

As a clinical pharmacy resident, I was much more involved with direct patient care than I had originally perceived. I was available at the patient's bedside to provide real-time medication-related recommendations and assistance for complex treatment plans. This decentralized pharmacy model allowed me to resolve medication-related issues immediately, creating more time for other health care professions such as physicians and nurses to provide excellent patient care. This pharmacist-physician collaboration also provided the patient with a multidisciplinary crafted treatment plan, consisting of the most evidence-based, cost-effective, and accessible medications. Although there has been substantial growth in clinical pharmacist positions among institutions, many are still without this multidisciplinary model. A focus of expanding this position to include a pharmacist on every unit is a current objective at my own institution, which will hopefully continue to improve health care collaboration and optimize patient care.

After accepting a position as a critical care pharmacist, I was placed mainly in the cardiothoracic ICU. Experiencing this specific unit made me recognize the importance of having specialty-trained pharmacists in all capacities of health care. Much like other areas of medicine, having the wealth of knowledge and experience with every single medication and interacting disease state is difficult because of the dynamic parameters that change with different patient populations. Being proficiently trained in medication pharmacodynamics, pharmacokinetics, and pharmacoeconomics specifically in the cardiothoracic population has given me comprehensive knowledge for the medications and disease states observed in this specialty area. This foundation includes acute decompensated heart failure requiring mechanical circulatory support and valve replacements as well as initiation, regulation, and monitoring of anticoagulation for cardiac device patients such as left ventricular assist devices, total artificial hearts, and extracorporeal membrane oxygenation.

After completing the first full year of my career, I find that being a new clinician has made me realize how far health care still needs to progress in the future. The proverb that "medicine is not black and white" could not be truer in the critical care setting. Many health care professionals practicing in this area can verify that the textbook patients included in medical studies simply do not exist in the ICU because of a perpetually aging population surrounded by many comorbidities. Therefore, providing optimal patient care established by evidence-based medicine becomes increasingly challenging in many cases. I believe that continuing to observe modern medical practice outcomes through research in every patient population will undoubtedly benefit the progression of health care. This past year, I have begun to direct my focus in clinical studies occurring at my institution, specifically in the cardiothoracic ICU setting. I hope to continue participating in research to further advance medical practice in cardiothoracic devices, all while providing my services to both patients and other health care professionals to make a difference in patients' lives.

Ohoud A. Aljuhani, Pharm.D.

Where I stand today is at the culmination of a journey that began 5 years ago when I took the first steps toward becoming a specialist in critical care pharmacy. As a pharmacist with a stable career at one of the largest universities and academic medical centers in Saudi Arabia, I found the decision to go back to school, travel to the United States, and start all over again to be a difficult one. I look back on my journey with no regrets.

In 2007, I began practicing as a clinical pharmacist in the medical intensive care unit (ICU) at King Abdul-Aziz University (KAU) Medical Center in Jeddah, Saudi Arabia. I remember my first day on the job seeing how excited the medical ICU team was to have a clinical pharmacist working with them. Even though the pharmacy profession had been well established in my country for more than 50 years, clinical pharmacy practice was still in its infancy. Although some specialty health care centers were practicing clinical pharmacy, most government-run hospitals, including KAU Medical Center, had yet to establish services, despite a growing patient population. A major step toward initiating these services was establishing the first Pharm.D.-granting institution in the country at KAU. Among the first group of graduates from this school, I was honored to participate in such a new and unique program.

After graduation, with the passion and energy of a young practitioner, I accepted a shared position with the School of Pharmacy and KAU Medical Center. This position provided mentors and guidance that helped me throughout my career. Initiating clinical pharmacy services in the ICU of a hospital with 500 beds was certainly a challenge. To meet this challenge, I sought advice from experienced clinical pharmacists, actively participated in the implementation of ICU pharmacotherapy protocols, participated in several hospital committees, made rounds with medical ICU teams, provided daily recommendations about therapies, and assisted with the training of pharmacy students at the hospital.

While practicing clinical pharmacy in the ICU's trauma/surgical and medical departments, I became aware of the need for well-trained clinical pharmacists in these areas. This moment of realization was the principal force driving me to make one of the important decisions in my life—to seek professional training in critical care pharmacotherapy. Unfortunately, the only available residency program in Saudi Arabia at that time was for general pharmacy training. Therefore, I made the decision to travel to the United States and receive specialized training in critical care pharmacotherapy at one of the country's top academic medical centers.

What I have learned and practiced in this program during the past few years has lit a candle of hope that I will carry back to my country. My postgraduate education has helped me become a well-trained and capable critical care pharmacist and researcher and will allow me to actively participate in the development of clinical pharmacy services in Saudi Arabia. If you are reading this book and hoping to play an active role in improving clinical pharmacy practice in your country, this foreword is dedicated for you.

LETTER FROM ACCP

Judith Jacobi, FCCP, MCCM, BCPS, BCCCP, ACCP President 2014–2015

When I consider the literature of critical care pharmacotherapy, I recall with fondness the text edited by Bart Chernow, M.D., FCCM, Master FCCP, initially published in 1983, titled *The Pharmacologic Approach to the Critically Ill Patient*. However, it was the third edition that embraced the role of the critical care team and included a large number of pharmacist authors.[1] This version blended pharmacology with the clinical nuance of critical care therapeutics. This "antique" remains in my library as an important reminder of both a simpler time and the tremendous progress we have made—and still how much we need to learn to optimally care for these patients. For those of us with long careers in critical care, books like this lend an important perspective on current practices and their foundation.

Much time has passed, and many other publications have come and gone from my critical care library. Critical care journals and other periodicals are generating data at a dizzying rate. One might ask how another textbook could contribute to the training and effectiveness of critical care clinicians. However, that is easy to answer with a publication of the quality of *Critical Care Pharmacotherapy*, which compiles key information in a format that illustrates our current understanding of pertinent therapeutic and pharmacologic topics. Indeed, this book will establish a new basis for future research and knowledge development and will hopefully become a foundational text for new practitioners and the growing number of Board Certified Critical Care Pharmacists.

Brian Erstad has assembled an impressive group of authors, many of whom are friends and colleagues in critical care pharmacy and have done the cutting-edge research that contributes to this expansive work. Many other talented and dedicated clinicians and researchers will be cited, but most contributors will remain in relative obscurity as our specialty continues to mature. As a past president of ACCP, I want to thank the efforts of the growing number of critical care clinicians who make such a difference in the care of our patients and who have contributed to the Critical Care Practice and Research Network and to this text. I anticipate that we will all use this text for our own education and as a teaching tool for future generations.

Reference

1. Chernow B. The Pharmacologic Approach to the Critically Ill Patient. Baltimore: Williams & Wilkins, 1994.

Critical Care Pharmacotherapy

Section 1

Supportive Care

Chapter 1

Acid-Base Disorders

Curtis E. Haas, Pharm.D.; David C. Kaufman, M.D.; and Brian L. Erstad, Pharm.D., FCCP, BCPS

LEARNING OBJECTIVES

1. Explain the common contributors to and potential clinical consequences of acid-base disorders in the critically ill patient.
2. Appreciate the differences between the traditional physiologic (carbonic acid-bicarbonate), standard base excess, and physiochemical (Stewart) models of acid-base physiology.
3. Complete the stepwise approach to assessment and reach a correct conclusion concerning the acid-base status of a critically ill patient.
4. Define the independent and dependent variables in acid-base physiology and their relevance to understanding the mechanisms and treatments for common acid-base disturbances.
5. Summarize the common causes, presentations, complications, and treatments for acid-base disorders commonly observed in critically ill patients.
6. Explain the relationship between fluid and electrolyte therapy and acid-base disturbances in critically ill patients, and explain how choice of fluids used during resuscitation can influence acid-base balance.

ABBREVIATIONS IN THIS CHAPTER

[x]	Denotes concentration of x	DKA	Diabetic ketoacidosis
ABG	Arterial blood gas	ICU	Intensive care unit
ACAG	Albumin-corrected anion gap	SBE	Standard base excess
ALCAG	Albumin and lactate corrected anion gap	SID	Strong ion difference
AG	Anion gap	SID_a	Apparent strong ion difference
A_{TOT}	Total weak acid concentration	SID_e	Effective strong ion difference
BE	Base excess	SIG	Strong ion gap
BE_{UA}	Base excess caused by unmeasured anions	UAG	Urinary anion gap

INTRODUCTION

Acid-base disorders are common findings in critically ill patients, are often complicated and multifactorial in nature, and are associated with significant morbidity and mortality. The diagnosis of the underlying causes of an acid-base disorder in critically ill patients is further complicated by concomitant and dynamic abnormalities in plasma protein concentrations, electrolyte profiles, free water or overall extracellular volume status, and ventilatory status. Given the often-complicated nature of the presentation, a simplistic or casual approach to evaluating acid-base disorders is inadequate for the intensive care unit (ICU) environment and may lead to a missed diagnosis or a complication that needs treatment. Although the mainstay for managing an acid-base disorder remains treatment of the underlying processes, a full understanding of the contributors to the acid-base status may identify a need for specific therapeutic interventions. This chapter is focused on an understandable and practical, but comprehensive, approach to assessing and managing the acid-base disorders commonly encountered in critically ill patients.

Several studies that have evaluated diagnostic approaches to metabolic acidosis provide some insights into the frequency of this disorder in different ICU settings. Cusack and coworkers reported on 100 consecutive adult patients admitted to a mixed medical-surgical ICU. Standard base excess (SBE) was abnormal in 57% of patients, corrected base excess (BE) was decreased in 86%, and corrected anion gap (AG) was elevated in 100%, indicating that laboratory evidence of metabolic acidosis was very common.[1] Of 427 patients admitted to an adult trauma ICU, hyperlactatemia was present in 18%, hyperchloremia in 21%, and an elevated strong ion gap (SIG) in 92%, consistent with evidence of metabolic acidosis.[2] Dubin et al. reported results from 935 patients admitted to a mixed medical-surgical ICU. The SIG and corrected AG were elevated in 71% and 74% of patients, respectively, and hyperlactatemia was evident in 34%, with 6% of patients having a lactate concentration greater than 5 mEq/L.[3] Chawla et al. reported on 143 patients admitted to a medical-surgical ICU. The mean albumin-corrected AG was 14.1 plus or minus 3.8 mEq/L, and 16.3% of patients had hyperlactatemia, despite the exclusion of patients with ketoacidosis, serum creatinine (SCr) greater than 6 mg/dL, or a history consistent with toxic ingestions.[4] Although most series have reported on evidence of metabolic acidosis, Liborio and coworkers evaluated serum bicarbonate concentrations from a database of 18,982 ICU patients for evidence of metabolic alkalosis, excluding patients with evidence of pure respiratory acidosis. During their ICU stay, 5,655 patients (29.3%) had a serum bicarbonate concentration greater than 30 mEq/L for at least 1 day, with most patients (86.6%) experiencing metabolic alkalosis within 72 hours of admission to the ICU. In addition, 17.9% of patients included in this database had evidence of a persistent metabolic acidosis. Most patients with an elevated serum bicarbonate concentration also had a metabolic acidosis at some point in their ICU stay. Only 11.4% had serum bicarbonate concentrations in the reference range throughout their ICU admission.[5] Although several of these reports may overestimate the overall prevalence of acid-base disorders in critically ill patients, because of the inclusion of only patients who underwent arterial blood gas (ABG) measurements, it is abundantly clear that metabolic acid-base abnormalities are common in the ICU. When the picture also includes all ICU patients with predominantly respiratory acid-base disorders, the argument is further strengthened that acid-base abnormalities are one of the most ubiquitous and heterogeneous disorders requiring assessment, monitoring, and treatment in critically ill patients.

The many potential contributing factors to acid-base abnormalities in critically ill patients will be discussed in much greater detail later. The major organ systems responsible for regulation of acid-base homeostasis are the respiratory and renal systems, with a lesser contribution from the liver.[6] Therefore, dysfunction or failure of any of these systems, not uncommon in the critically ill patient, is expected to be associated with acid-base disorders. Although the gastrointestinal (GI) system does not regulate acid-base balance, dysfunction or diseases of the GI tract including vomiting, high nasogastric tube output, diarrhea, ileostomy losses, villous adenoma of the colon, and high-volume pancreatic/biliary fluid drainage can contribute to metabolic acid-base imbalances.[7] Sepsis, shock, hypoxemia, trauma, microvascular dysfunction, dysregulation of cellular metabolism, hypoalbuminemia, renal replacement therapy, and many electrolyte disorders can also contribute to metabolic acid-base abnormalities. A variety of toxic ingestions may be associated with metabolic acidosis (e.g., alcohols, glycols, salicylates, iron). Iatrogenic factors in the ICU that can contribute to abnormal acid-base status include fluid resuscitation with high-chloride fluids (e.g., 0.9% sodium chloride solution), drugs (e.g., propofol, lorazepam, CNS depressants), over- or under-ventilation during mechanical ventilation, and total parenteral nutrition.[6,8,9] It is important to appreciate that acid-base disorders are not only a result of the underlying illness leading to ICU admission, but can also adversely be affected by the management of those illnesses and general supportive care.[10]

Although disorders of acid-base balance have been associated with increased ICU length of stay and increased mortality,[2,5,11,12] the findings are not universal.[1,13] The direct impact or attributable morbidity or mortality from metabolic acid-base disorders is controversial and difficult to separate from the contributions of the underlying illness.[8] Persistent severe acidemia (pH less than 7) or alkalemia (pH greater than 7.6) is considered incompatible with life; however, the cause-and-effect relationship with poor outcomes for more transient and moderate derangements of acid-base status is not conclusively shown.

Elevated blood lactate concentrations, regardless of the cause, have been associated with increased mortality, especially with sustained elevations or very high concentrations of lactate.[14] In a randomized, multicenter trial, early lactate-directed resuscitation led to a significant decline in risk-adjusted mortality (hazard ratio 0.61; 95% confidence interval, 0.43–0.87).[15] There is also growing evidence that using chloride-rich crystalloid therapy compared with a more balanced fluid after major surgery or after an ICU admission is associated with a greater frequency of acute kidney injury, more need for renal replacement therapy,[16,17] and higher in-hospital mortality.[16] Although these lines of evidence do not validate that treatment of acid-base disorders improves outcome independently of treating the underlying disease state, they do suggest that therapeutic approaches to the underlying problem that either improve or do not induce or exacerbate preexisting acid-base abnormalities are associated with better outcomes.

TERMINOLOGY AND CONCEPTS

In discussing acid-base analysis and the common abnormalities of acid-base status, the following terms and concepts are important to understand.

Acid and Base

For this chapter, we will use the definitions of an acid and base offered by Stewart.[18,19] An acid is a substance that increases the oxonium (formerly called hydronium ion) concentration ($[H_3O^+]$) of a solution, and a base is a substance that decreases the $[H_3O^+]$ of a solution. A decrease in $[H_3O^+]$ is equivalent to an increase in $[OH^-]$. Water is amphoteric and can therefore act as an acid or base. Remember that a solution is neutral when the $[H_3O^+]$ is equal to the hydroxyl ion concentration ($[OH^-]$).

Analysis of -emia vs. -osis

The usually accepted normal range for blood pH is 7.35–7.45, and throughout this chapter, we will use 7.4 as normal in all analyses. A blood pH of less than 7.35 represents an acidemia, whereas a blood pH of greater than 7.45 is an alkalemia. The terms *acidosis* and *alkalosis* define the underlying processes that lead to an acid-base disorder, but they should not be used to describe an abnormal blood pH value. For example, a patient may have a metabolic alkalosis and a respiratory acidosis or a metabolic acidosis and a respiratory alkalosis but a blood pH of 7.35–7.45.

Analysis of pH vs. [H$_3$O$^+$]

The pH value was adopted more than 100 years ago to express blood $[H_3O^+]$ in clinical medicine. The pH is the inverse $\log_{10} [H_3O^+]$ and is therefore an unfortunate, dimensionless, non-linear, and non-intuitive expression of the $[H_3O^+]$. Because of its nonlinear nature, a greater change in $[H_3O^+]$ is needed to decrease the pH to the acidemic range than the change in $[H_3O^+]$ resulting in an alkalemia. Although it is possible to manage acid-base disorders while working with the $[H_3O^+]$ in the physiologically and pathologically relevant pH range of 6.8–7.6 ($[H_3O^+]$ range of 160 nmol/L to 25 nmol/L, respectively), it is highly unlikely that $[H_3O^+]$ will supplant the use of pH in clinical medicine in the near future.

Strong vs. Weak Ions

Strong ions are essentially fully dissociated in solution; therefore, there is no dissociation equilibrium applicable to these electrolytes (e.g., Na$^+$ and Cl$^-$). Because they are fully dissociated at all times, they do not participate in any reactions within the solution. Weak ions, which are by definition only partly dissociated in solution, are defined by the following equilibrium expression:

$$[H^+] \times [A^-] = K_A \times [HA]$$

where *HA* is a weak acid, *H$^+$* and *A$^-$* are the dissociated proton and anion, and K_A is the weak acid dissociation constant.

Electroneutrality

In any aqueous solution, the sum of all positively charged and all negatively charged ions must be equal, resulting in an electrically neutral solution. It requires excess energy to maintain a charged solution, so an electrically neutral solution is naturally energetically favored. In vivo, any macroscopic fluid volume (e.g., plasma, extracellular fluid) will be electrically neutral, creating a link between the nonreactive strong ions and the equilibrating weak ions.

Conservation of Mass

The amount of substance in solution will change only if it is added, removed, generated, or destroyed. The relevance relative to clinical acid-base status is that strong ions like Na$^+$ and Cl$^-$ only change quantitatively if they are added or removed, whereas organic acids like lactate and pyruvate can be generated or metabolized. For partly dissociated substances, the total concentration is the sum of the dissociated and undissociated forms, which will equilibrate depending on the presence of other constituents in the solution.

Anion Gap

The AG is widely used in the diagnostic workup of metabolic acidosis. It represents the difference between the concentration of commonly measured and most abundant serum cations (Na$^+$ and K$^+$) and anions (Cl$^-$ and HCO$_3^-$). The equation for the AG is as follows:

$$AG = ([Na^+] + [K^+]) - ([Cl^-] + [HCO_3^-]) \quad (1)$$

where the concentration of each electrolyte is expressed as milliequivalents per liter. Because of the greater concentration of total unmeasured anions compared with unmeasured cations in equation 1, the normal range for the AG is usually quoted as 12 plus or minus 4 mEq/L. The actual value depends on the normal ranges for the reporting laboratory, which will vary depending on analytic methodology.[9,20,21] Because of the relatively narrow and tightly controlled range of serum [K$^+$], the equation is often simplified in clinical practice:

$$AG = [Na^+] - ([Cl^-] + [HCO_3^-]) \quad (2)$$

For this simplified equation, the normal range is 8 plus or minus 6 mEq/L. However, in the critically ill population, there is often greater variability in serum [K$^+$], and some authorities recommend not ignoring potassium's contribution to the AG.[9,22]

The major contributor (about 80%) to the serum AG is albumin, which is consistently low in critically ill patients. Hypoalbuminemia results in a falsely low serum AG and poor diagnostic performance; therefore, the AG must be corrected for the albumin concentration for all critically ill patients. For every 1-g/dL change in serum albumin, there is a directional change in the AG by 2.3–2.5

mEq/L.[21,22] A widely used equation for calculating the albumin-corrected AG (ACAG) is as follows:

$$ACAG = AG + 2.5([normal\ albumin] - [observed\ albumin])$$

The albumin concentrations are in grams per deciliter, and the normal albumin concentration should be the local laboratory normal value.

ACID-BASE MODELS: ANALYSIS AND INTERPRETATION

Traditional, Physiologic, or Bicarbonate-Centered Model

This model is based on the work of Henderson and Hasselbalch from more than 100 years ago and remains the most commonly used model for describing and interpreting acid-base disturbances.[23-25] This model is based on the assumption that the carbonic acid-bicarbonate buffer system is the major determinant of acid-base balance and is described by the Henderson-Hasselbalch equation:

$$pH = pK + \log_{10}\left(\frac{[HCO_3^-]}{(0.03 \times Paco_2)}\right)$$

where pK is the dissociation constant for carbonic acid (6.1), $Paco_2$ is the arterial blood partial pressure of carbon dioxide (CO_2) in millimeters of mercury, $[HCO_3^-]$ is the plasma bicarbonate concentration (measured as total CO_2 content) expressed as milliequivalents per liter, and 0.03 represents the solubility of CO_2 in plasma. From this model followed the concept that the major determinants of $[H_3O^+]$ are changes in $Paco_2$ and $[HCO_3^-]$ and that these parameters are adjusted in vivo as a control system to regulate alterations in acid-base balance. Disorders that are predominantly associated with alterations in $Paco_2$ are respiratory disorders, whereas those that are primarily associated with alterations in $[HCO_3^-]$ are metabolic disorders. This model is based on the equation describing CO_2/HCO_3^- equilibrium with carbonic acid:

$$CO_2 + H_2O \leftrightarrow H_2CO_3 \leftrightarrow H^+ + HCO_3^-$$

Assuming that this reaction will equilibrate (Le Châtelier's principle), metabolic acidosis has therefore been explained by either the addition of H^+ to the system, shifting the reaction to the left with a reduction in $[HCO_3^-]$, or the loss of bicarbonate from the body, shifting the reaction to the right to replace lost bicarbonate and increasing $[H^+]$.[25] It has also been taught that metabolic alkalosis is attributable to factors that can either increase the $[HCO_3^-]$ (e.g., bicarbonate generation and reabsorption by the kidney or contraction of the extracellular volume), which will shift the reaction to the left with a decrease in the $[H^+]$, or cause the loss of H^+ (e.g., vomiting), which will shift the reaction to the right, leading to an increase in $[HCO_3^-]$.

Carbon dioxide is the primary volatile acid produced through normal cellular metabolism, accounting for around 15,000 mmol/day of hydrogen ion equivalents for an average adult. The CO_2 is expired by the lungs. Sensitive receptors in the medulla and carotid and aortic bodies respond to alterations in $[CO_2]$ in the cerebrospinal fluid and the $Paco_2$ and $[H_3O^+]$ in plasma, respectively, leading to changes in minute ventilation to maintain $Paco_2$ and pH within tight ranges. Changes in ventilation to regulate acid-base disturbances are relatively rapid, with a new equilibrium achieved in minutes to hours, meaning that changes in minute ventilation and $Paco_2$ can rapidly compensate for a metabolic acid-base disorder. In contrast, with a persistent abnormality in ventilation leading to a chronic respiratory acid-base disorder, a metabolic compensation develops slowly over 2–5 days.[23,24]

Organic and inorganic non-volatile acids are produced to a lesser extent than the volatile acid CO_2. Organic acids are predominantly lactate and ketones, with about 1500 mmol/day being metabolized by the liver and kidney. The two most important inorganic acids are sulfate and phosphate, generated from dietary protein and amino acid metabolism and contributing about 1.5 mmol/kg/day. Most lactate undergoes hepatic metabolism either by an oxidative pathway to generate water and CO_2 (and subsequently HCO_3^-) or by gluconeogenesis to glucose, with both pathways consuming protons and therefore contributing to the maintenance of acid-base balance. The traditional teaching is that the free protons (H^+) from organic and inorganic acids are rapidly buffered by the bicarbonate-carbonate buffer system with consumption of HCO_3^-. The ability of the kidney to reclaim and regenerate HCO_3^- prevents the rapid depletion of the available buffer by continued acid production.[20,23,24]

In normal homeostasis, two major mechanisms have been implicated in the generation and reclamation of HCO_3^- by the kidney. The proximal tubular cell secretes free protons (by the NHE3 sodium-hydrogen exchanger) into the glomerular lumen, which combines with filtered HCO_3^- to form H_2CO_3. In the presence of luminal carbonic anhydrase, H_2CO_3 is converted to CO_2 and water, with the CO_2 freely back diffusing into the proximal tubular cell along its concentration gradient. Intracellular carbonic anhydrase then catalyzes the conversion of CO_2 and water to HCO_3^- and H^+ with the bicarbonate transported to the blood by the serosal NBC (sodium-bicarbonate) transporter, and the H^+ is secreted into the lumen to "reclaim" more bicarbonate. The regeneration of bicarbonate can also result from the conversion of CO_2 produced through normal tubular cell metabolism into HCO_3^- and H^+. The HCO_3^- is transported into the blood, and the H^+ passes into the tubular lumen, where it combines with a non-bicarbonate anion like ammonium or phosphate and is excreted in the urine, leading to a net increase in plasma HCO_3^- content and loss of H^+.[20,24,25] Given these mechanisms, it is estimated that the kidney filters and reabsorbs 4,500 mmol/day of bicarbonate.

The relationship between the liver and the kidney in renal ammoniagenesis and acid-base balance is also important to recognize. Nitrogen metabolism by the liver results in the production of glutamine, urea, and ammonium (NH_4^+). The liver normally releases only a very small amount of NH_4^+, but it incorporates this nitrogen into urea and glutamine, which are released into the systemic circulation. Renal ammoniagenesis involves the metabolism of glutamine to generate NH_4^+ and increases the renal excretion of H^+, leading to an alkalinizing effect on plasma. Acidosis stimulates hepatic glutaminogenesis and inhibits ureagenesis, therefore shifting the balance of nitrogen metabolism toward greater production of glutamine. This greater presentation of glutamine to the kidney increases renal ammoniagenesis, facilitating a greater renal alkalinizing effect.[6,24] This relationship between liver nitrogen metabolism and renal ammonium excretion appears to be an important mechanism in regulating the metabolic response to acid-base disorders.

Although the traditional physiologic model of acid-base analysis can be useful clinically to identify and diagnose acid-base disorders, viewing it as a mechanistic explanation for the underlying physiology of acid-base disturbances is problematic. The Henderson-Hasselbalch equation, although permitting a quantification of the severity of a respiratory disorder, cannot quantitatively represent the severity of a metabolic acid-base disturbance. It also tells the clinician nothing about the acids contributing to a metabolic disorder other than carbonic acid. Traditional teaching using the physiologic model implies that HCO_3^- is independently regulated in response to acid-base disorders; however, HCO_3^- cannot be regulated independently of $Paco_2$. The $[HCO_3^-]$ in plasma is always increased as the $Paco_2$ increases, but this does not represent a metabolic alkalosis. It is clear that bicarbonate is a dependent parameter in acid-base equilibrium and therefore cannot be presented as a variable that can be manipulated to independently regulate acid-base homeostasis. It is also important to recognize that at a normal plasma pH, the $[H_3O^+]$ is in the nanomolar range, whereas most acids and strong ions are in the millimolar range. That means that H_3O^+ values are about one-millionth the concentration of other contributors classically attributed to acid-base homeostasis, suggesting that something else must be primarily responsible for acid-base balance.[6,20] Stated another way, blaming the metabolic acidosis on the finding of a decreased $[HCO_3^-]$ is analogous to blaming the bacterial pneumonia on the abnormal chest radiograph. This may be a useful diagnostic test, but it is not the cause of the disorder.

BE Model

To overcome the inability of the Henderson-Hasselbalch equation to quantify the metabolic component of an acid-base disturbance, several methods have been developed, with BE being most widely used. Base excess is defined as the amount of acid or base that must be added to a sample of blood in vitro to restore the pH to 7.40 while the $Paco_2$ is held constant at 40 mm Hg at 37°C. Because of inaccuracies of this approach in vivo given the variability in $Paco_2$, the equation was empirically modified to account for an average hemoglobin content across extracellular fluid space, resulting in the SBE. An SBE less than −5 mmol/L is considered to represent a metabolic acidosis, whereas an SBE greater than 5 mmol/L represents a metabolic alkalosis. A negative SBE is often called a base deficit. Although the SBE is able to quantify the change in metabolic acid-base status in vivo, SBE is not regulated by the body and still does not tell the clinician anything about the underlying mechanism of a metabolic acid-base disturbance.[6,20] The SBE fails as a measure of metabolic acidosis in the patient with hypoalbuminemia, which is almost universal in critically ill patients.[4,26] The BE can be corrected for changes in albumin, chloride, free water, and $Paco_2$ to derive a calculation of the BE caused by unmeasured anions (BE_{UA}); however, the calculations are complex for use at the bedside. The BE_{UA} has been found to be superior at identifying lactic acidosis in critically ill patients compared with SBE or uncorrected AG[1,27,28] and is more closely associated with mortality in some studies.[2,27] However, the BE_{UA} is not superior to ACAG at detecting unmeasured anions or predicting mortality,[2,13] is more complex to apply, and is therefore not recommended for routine clinical use in the ICU.

The Physiochemical or Stewart Model

This model requires the application of two physical-chemical principles discussed previously in the analysis of acid-base physiology: electroneutrality and conservation of mass. In addition, all relevant biologic solutions are aqueous and alkaline ($[OH^-]$ is greater than $[H_3O^+]$). The physical-chemical properties of water that are relevant to acid-base physiology include a high dielectric constant, very slight dissociation into H^+ and OH^-, and extraordinarily high molar concentration (around 55.5 M). An aqueous solution provides an almost limitless supply of H^+, because of the dissociation of water, and electrolytes and CO_2 present in biologic solutions impart strong electrochemical forces that affect the dissociation of water. Stewart has hypothesized that three independent factors affect acid-base status in vivo: strong ion difference (SID), total weak acid concentration (A_{TOT}), and CO_2 content ($Paco_2$) of plasma. Changes in one or more of these three independent variables will result in changes in the dependent variables $[H_3O^+]$ (or pH) and $[HCO_3^-]$. That is, contrary to the physiologic or traditional model, alterations in acid-base status are not caused by changes in $[H_3O^+]$ or $[HCO_3^-]$, and these variables are not regulated to maintain homeostasis but are instead dependent on changes in SID, A_{TOT}, or $Paco_2$. In addition, acid-base homeostasis can be explained by mechanisms that regulate SID (metabolic disorders) and $Paco_2$ (respiratory disorders).[6,18,19]

Consistent with the traditional model, CO_2 content is an independent predictor of pH and is closely regulated by the respiratory center by influencing minute ventilation. In the ICU setting, fluctuations in minute ventilation may also result from the provision of mechanical ventilation with the possibility of iatrogenic respiratory acid-base disorders. Changes in CO_2 expiration that either exceed or fail to meet CO_2 production rates will result in a primary respiratory alkalosis or acidosis, respectively. A well-controlled and precise match of alveolar ventilation and metabolic CO_2 production will result in a normal $Paco_2$ of 40 mm Hg (35–45 mm Hg). Several signals may influence the respiratory center regulation of minute ventilation, including $Paco_2$, arterial pH, and arterial oxygenation. These variables may be influenced by exercise, anxiety, and wakefulness. This provides a relatively rapid regulatory mechanism for the regulation of acid-base balance in patients with adequate ventilatory reserve. In the setting of metabolic acidosis or alkalosis, the $Paco_2$ is adjusted in a predictable way, which is called respiratory compensation. In the setting of a persistent alteration in $Paco_2$ caused by an underlying respiratory, neurologic, or other disease process leading to a respiratory acidosis or alkalosis, the body will try to correct the acid-base disorder by regulating the independent variable SID, called metabolic compensation.[6,9,18,25]

The SID refers to the difference between the plasma concentrations of fully dissociated cations (Na^+, K^+, Mg^{2+}, Ca^{2+}) and anions (Cl^- and lactate). Plasma lactate is included because it is almost completely dissociated at a physiologically relevant pH range; it therefore acts as a strong anion. Urate plasma concentration has also been included in the SID calculation; however, it is often unavailable and is quantitatively a small contributor, so it is typically excluded from the calculation. This calculation of SID is also called the apparent SID (SID_a) because it does not consider weak acids, which are important physiologic buffers to SID:

$$SID_a = ([Na^+] + [K^+] + [Mg^{2+}] + [Ca^{2+}]) - ([Cl^-] + [lactate])$$

Concentrations are expressed as milliequivalents per liter, with calcium included as the ionized concentration (calculated or measured). Under normal conditions, the SID_a is about 40 mEq/L, the positive value consistent with the alkaline state of human plasma, which would be even more alkaline were it not for the presence of dissolved CO_2 in blood. The SID_a is often much lower than 40 mEq/L in critically ill patients because of alterations in albumin (reducing A_{TOT}).[6,9,18,29]

The SID has a strong effect on the dissociation of water and therefore the $[H_3O^+]$ and pH. An increasingly positive SID results in a progressive decrease in the weak cation H_3O^+ (increasing pH) to maintain electroneutrality. Likewise, a reduction in SID will lead to an increase in H_3O^+ (decreasing pH). The mechanisms underlying the regulation of SID are discussed in the paragraphs that follow.

A more complicated calculation developed by Figge et al.[30] incorporates the role of weak acids (albumin, phosphate) and $Paco_2$ to the electrical charge equilibrium to derive what is called the effective SID (SID_e). The SIG is the difference between SID_a and SID_e and represents the contribution of unmeasured anions to the SID (e.g., sulfates, ketones, citrate, pyruvate, acetate, and gluconate).[9,28-30] The recognition of the presence of unmeasured anions has diagnostic relevance for mixed acid-base disorders, and the presence of unmeasured anions has been correlated with increased mortality of critically ill patients.[2,11,27] The equations for SID_e and SIG are as follows:

$$SID_e = 1000 \times 2.46^{11} \times \frac{Paco_2}{(10^{-pH})} + [albumin] \times$$
$$(0.123 \times pH - 0.631) + [PO_4] \times (0.309 \times pH - 0.469)$$

In this equation, [albumin] is expressed in grams per deciliter, $Paco_2$ is expressed in millimeters of mercury, and $[PO_4]$ is the concentration of plasma phosphates in millimoles per liter.

$$SIG = SID_a - SID_e$$

Under normal conditions, the SIG is essentially zero. In the presence of unmeasured strong anions, the SIG is positive, and with accumulation of unmeasured strong cations, the value is negative. A positive SIG is analogous to an elevated ACAG or BE_{UA} because all three are affected by the presence of unmeasured strong anions like ketones, sulfates, and other exogenous acids associated with the ingestion of toxins.[6,24,28,29]

The SID is regulated by changes in the relative plasma concentrations of strong cations and strong anions, with the kidney being the primary organ responsible for adjustments in the SID through the regulation of Cl^- balance. A relative loss of Cl^- in the urine leads to an increase in the SID and alkalization of the plasma. Although renal regulation of Na^+ and K^+ could also affect SID and acid-base balance, Na^+ transport is prioritized to maintain intravascular volume and plasma osmolality, and K^+ homeostasis is essential to cardiac and neuromuscular function, so Cl^- regulation appears to be the predominant renal mechanism to alter SID and maintain acid-base balance without affecting other homeostatic mechanisms.[6,24] The traditional explanation of H^+ excretion being affected by renal ammoniagenesis may not be the true regulatory mechanism because water provides an unlimited source of H^+ on both sides of the renal tubular cell membrane through dissociation of water affected by the composition of the respective aqueous solutions. The importance of renal ammoniagenesis (and hepatic shift to glutaminogenesis described previously) is to increase the excretion of Cl⁻ without concomitant losses in Na⁺ and K⁺ by providing a weak cation (NH$_4^+$) to be excreted with Cl⁻, emphasizing the importance of electroneutrality as an explanation for many of the factors leading to normalcies and abnormalities in acid-base. The regulation of Cl⁻ excretion results in relatively small quantitative changes over time; therefore, subsequent changes in the plasma SID involves a slow process, consistent with the known delayed metabolic compensation in the presence of a persistent respiratory acid-base disorder.[6]

Several acid-base disorders that are common in the ICU can be used to show the important role of alterations of SID on [H$_3$O$^+$] and explain how the Stewart model provides a much more rational understanding of acid-base pathophysiology than the traditional, bicarbonate-based model. The infusion of a large volume of 0.9% sodium chloride for injection (normal saline) during the resuscitation of critically ill or injured patients can lead to a hyperchloremic metabolic acidosis. Under the traditional model, this has been called a *dilutional metabolic acidosis*, based on an explanation that dilution of bicarbonate in the extracellular fluid shifts the bicarbonate-carbonate equilibrium to the right, increasing [H$_3$O$^+$] and leading to an acidemia. According to the Stewart model, both [HCO$_3^-$] and [H$_3$O$^+$] are dependent variables in an aqueous biologic fluid; therefore, the dilutional mechanism is inadequate to explain the acid-base abnormality. Normal saline provides equal concentrations of Na⁺ and Cl⁻ (154 mEq/L); however, because of the higher concentration of Na⁺ relative to Cl⁻ in plasma, the infusion of normal saline leads to a greater relative accumulation of Cl⁻ and a reduction in the SID. The electrochemical force of a decreasing SID leads to an increase in [H$_3$O$^+$] to maintain electroneutrality and therefore the onset of acidemia. An alternative way to consider this is that for normal saline, the SID is zero (equal concentration of strong cations and strong anions). Therefore, infusing large volumes of a SID 0-mEq/L solution into moderately alkaline plasma (SID approximately equal to 40 mEq/L) will lead to a reduction in the plasma SID and a metabolic acidosis.[6]

Alterations in normal GI function are a common cause of metabolic acid-base disorders in critically ill patients. Under normal conditions, the stomach pumps out large amounts of Cl⁻, leading to a decrease of the SID in the lumen and reducing the pH of gastric contents. The loss of the Cl⁻ from plasma raises the plasma SID and is consistent with the alkaline tide observed at the start of a meal. The Cl⁻ is rapidly reabsorbed at the duodenum, quickly restoring plasma SID and pH. However, if the gastric secretions are lost because of either vomiting or nasogastric suctioning, the plasma SID is persistently increased, leading to a reduction in [H$_3$O$^+$] and a metabolic alkalosis. The traditional explanation of gastric H⁺ loss leading to a metabolic alkalosis is not plausible given that 1 L of gastric secretions with a pH between 1 and 2 would result in the loss of more total H⁺ content than is normally present in all of the extracellular fluid and should therefore lead to a profoundly fatal metabolic alkalosis. In actuality, this modest amount lost from 1 L of vomitus will have a mild effect on acid-base balance, showing that the loss of H⁺ cannot be the mechanistic explanation. In addition to the initial increase in SID secondary to Cl⁻ loss, the loss of intravascular volume leads to the need to conserve Na⁺ and water and maintain K⁺ balance. This combination of metabolic alkalosis and intravascular volume loss is commonly termed a *contraction alkalosis*. Activation of the renin-angiotensin-aldosterone axis increases sodium reabsorption at the proximal tubular Na-H exchanger (NHE3) and collecting duct Na channels, and activation of hydrogen-ATPase (type B intercalated cells) and K⁺-hydrogen ATPase (type A intercalated cells). The overall effect is to reduce urinary SID, leading to acidification of the urine and maintenance of the metabolic alkalosis. To correct the metabolic alkalosis, it is necessary to replace Na⁺ and Cl⁻ while restoring intravascular volume, replace lost K⁺, and decrease plasma SID. Administering normal saline with supplemental potassium chloride will achieve these goals. This example shows the important interaction between fluid and electrolyte balance and acid-base disorders. In traditional teaching, this is called a chloride-responsive metabolic alkalosis.[6,18,25]

The third independent variable determining acid-base status in the Stewart model is A_{TOT}, the total concentration of weak acids and their conjugate bases.

$$A_{TOT} = AH + A^-$$

The weak acids represented by A_{TOT} are mostly plasma proteins, with albumin being quantitatively most important, and phosphates. Some have suggested that given the independent role of A_{TOT} on acid-base balance, there should be six defined acid-base categories, adding proteinaceous alkalosis and acidosis to the traditional respiratory and metabolic disorders. Although the loss of albumin is associated with an alkalemia and the rapid infusion of albumin will cause a decrease in arterial pH,[31] there is no evidence that the active regulation of A_{TOT} is physiologically relevant in the maintenance of acid-base balance, so expanding the categories of acid-base disorders is not clinically relevant. Given that hypoalbuminemia is common in the critically ill patient, the A_{TOT} is reduced and is associated with a concomitant reduction in SID to maintain acid-base balance. This apparent compensatory SID response to hypoalbuminemia results in a new normal SID in critically ill patients of about 30–32 mEq/L.[6] From the perspective of the Stewart model, the regulation of Paco$_2$ and SID is the major determinant and therapeutic target of acid-base balance. The A_{TOT} should be considered an independent variable influencing acid-base status that is not actively regulated, or manipulated clinically to treat acid-base disorders.[18]

Although we believe that the physiochemical model provides a rational explanation of acid-base physiology and mechanistic explanations for common acid-base disorders and their treatments, other experts disagree that there is adequate evidence to accept Stewart's theories. Kurtz and colleagues provide a comprehensive and sophisticated critique of the issue and conclude that the Stewart and bicarbonate-based approaches provide quantitatively identical results and that the Stewart model provides no diagnostic or prognostic advantage to an approach using the Henderson-Hasselbalch equation. In addition, they argue that the underlying premise that the [H+] in any given fluid compartment is dependent on SID lacks an experimental basis.[32] Thus, although we favor the physiochemical model proposed by Stewart and others for teaching and clinical purposes, it is important to realize that it remains a controversial and unsettled area of debate.

DIAGNOSIS OF ACID-BASE DISORDERS (STEPWISE APPROACH)

The physiochemical or Stewart model provides a thorough diagnostic approach to acid-base balance that is also consistent with the mechanisms of acid-base abnormalities in clinical medicine. This understanding of the underlying mechanisms of metabolic disorders leads to a more rational therapeutic approach when intervention is warranted. However, the comprehensive analysis of acid-base status using the Figge-Stewart approach in a critically ill patient requires variables that are often not routinely measured in a simultaneous manner and requires rather complex computations that limit the practical utility of this approach at the bedside. The SBE approach, which accurately quantifies the extent of a metabolic acid-base abnormality, is routinely reported with blood gas results, but SBE is not effective at identifying mixed acid-base disorders without the use of complex corrections of the SBE, which are challenging during routine clinical care in the ICU. Several investigators have shown that the traditional bicarbonate approach with appropriate adjustment of the AG for hypoalbuminemia, with or without adjustment for lactate, has a diagnostic and prognostic value similar to that obtained with the more complex Figge-Stewart and corrected SBE methods[2-4,13,26,28,33] and may represent the most practical and easily performed diagnostic approach.[23,25,29]

An organized, consistent, stepwise approach to the diagnosis of acid-base disorders in critically ill patients is recommended to improve the identification of mixed acid-base disorders, reduce the potential for missing clinically important concomitant problems, and best inform the therapeutic approach to the patient. Although several stepwise approaches have been recommended,[23] the following approach is recommended for the critically ill patient with a suspected acid-base disturbance (also see Table 1.1).

Step 1 – Provide a careful clinical evaluation of the patient. Clinical assessment of the patient must include medical history, history of present illness, vital signs, level of consciousness, physical assessment, and medication history. Given this assessment, the expected acid-base abnormalities can be predicted (Table 1.2), and results of the stepwise approach that differ from these expected findings should be suspect and warrant reinvestigation of the patient history and presentation.

Step 2 – Determine the -emia. This is the easiest step in the process. For practical purposes, if the ABG pH is less than 7.38, the patient can be considered to have an acidemia. If the pH is greater than 7.42, the patient can be considered to have an alkalemia.

Step 3 – Determine the principal -osis. According to an evaluation of the ABG results, the principal or predominant disorder can normally be determined (Table 1.3). If the patient has a pH in the normal range of 7.35–7.45, the principal disorder will usually be associated with the relative direction of the pH above or below 7.40. An acidemia should be associated with either a decreased $[HCO_3^-]$ (metabolic acidosis) or an elevated $Paco_2$ (respiratory acidosis). An alkalemia will be associated with either an increased $[HCO_3^-]$ (metabolic alkalosis) or a decreased $Paco_2$ (respiratory alkalosis). The secondary or compensatory change in a simple acid-base disorder should be in the same direction as the principal change. For example, a principal metabolic acidosis should be associated with a decrease in $[HCO_3^-]$, and a compensatory decrease in $Paco_2$ (Table 1.3). In a complex ICU patient who may have an underlying chronic disorder (e.g., chronic obstructive lung disease), determining the principal disorder may be more challenging because the change from

Table 1.1 Stepwise Approach to Diagnosis of Acid-Base Status

Step 1	Careful clinical evaluation of the patient
Step 2	Determine the -emia
Step 3	Determine the primary -osis
Step 4	If the primary disorder is respiratory, is it acute or chronic?
Step 5	Is compensation for the primary disorder appropriate?
Step 6	Calculate the anion gap, corrected for albumin
Step 7	If corrected anion gap is elevated, calculate the delta ratio
Step 8	If normal anion gap and unknown cause, calculate the urinary anion gap

the patient's normal baseline values is what is relevant to diagnosing an acute change in acid-base status. Without specific data concerning the patient's baseline status, assumptions based on history and initial serum chemistry results will often need to be made.

Step 4 – If the principal disorder is respiratory, is it acute or chronic? The metabolic regulation of acid-base balance in response to a respiratory disorder takes 2–5 days to reach a new steady state; therefore, a respiratory disorder of less than 2–3 days' duration is considered an acute respiratory disorder, whereas a disorder of longer duration is considered chronic from the perspective of metabolic secondary response or compensation. Acute, smaller changes in metabolic status are considered primarily the result of cellular electrolyte shifts, whereas the later and quantitatively greater changes are the result of renal regulation of Cl^- excretion, leading to compensatory changes in plasma SID. Differentiating acute from chronic classification of respiratory acid-base disorders is necessary to determine whether the degree of compensation is appropriate and therefore determine the presence of simple or mixed acid-base disorders.

Step 5 – Is the secondary or compensatory response appropriate? There are highly conserved patterns between the changes that occur between $Paco_2$ and $[HCO_3^-]$ for various principal acid-base disorders that permit the creation of rules to define the secondary or compensatory response to a primary disorder.[6] These compensatory changes in either $Paco_2$ or $[HCO_3^-]$ should be considered the patient's new normal, and values that differ from the new normal are therefore abnormal and represent evidence of a second or concomitant acid-base disorder. Although several different estimations of appropriate compensation for the primary acid-base disorders have been published, Table 1.4 presents the estimations most commonly used in clinical medicine.[23]

Step 6 – Calculate the AG, corrected for albumin. See earlier text for the calculation of AG and ACAG. In critically ill patients, the AG is a poor estimate of unmeasured anions because of the very common presence of hypoalbuminemia; however, the correction for plasma [albumin] greatly improves the ability of the ACAG to detect the presence of "gap" anions.[2–4,26,33] Given the near-universal availability of plasma [lactate] in the diagnostic evaluation of metabolic acidosis, the AG can be further corrected for both albumin and lactate (ALCAG):

$$ALCAG = AG + 2.5([normal\ albumin] - [observed\ albumin]) - [lactate]$$

where albumin concentrations are expressed in grams per deciliter and lactate concentration in millimoles per liter or milliequivalents per liter. An elevated ALCAG provides evidence of unmeasured anions, which may include toxins (e.g., salicylate, toxic alcohol, and glycols), ketones, sulfates, phosphate, citrate, and d-lactate, among

Table 1.2 Acid-Base Disorders Associated with Common Clinical Findings

Metabolic Acidosis
Elevated Anion Gap
  Shock
  Hypoxia or ischemic injury
  Sepsis
  Type 1 diabetes
  Crush injury (rhabdomyolysis)
  Renal disease
  Liver failure
  Alcoholism
  Starvation/cachexia
  Toxic ingestions (salicylate, alcohols, glycols)
  Medications (metformin, propofol, NNRTI)
  Seizures
Normal Anion Gap
  Resuscitation with normal saline
  Diarrhea
  Biliary or pancreatic drainage
  History of renal tubular acidosis

Respiratory Acidosis
Chronic
  Chronic obstructive lung disease
  Neuromuscular diseases (hypoventilation)
  Restrictive lung diseases
Acute
  CNS depression – disease- or drug-induced
  Acute exacerbation of asthma
  Pneumonia
  Pulmonary edema
  Pulmonary embolism (massive)

Metabolic Alkalosis
  Diuretic use
  Vomiting
  NG tube losses
  Mineralocorticoid use
  Excessive alkali ingestion

Respiratory Alkalosis
Chronic
  Pregnancy
  Hyperthyroidism
  Liver disease
  Pulmonary embolism
Acute:
  Pain or anxiety
  Fever
  Neurologic injury (stroke, trauma, meningitis)
  Salicylate toxicity
  Pneumonia
  Pulmonary edema
  Pulmonary embolism
  Sepsis

NG = nasogastric; NNRTI = nonnucleoside reverse transcriptase inhibitor.

Table 1.3 Principal Acid-Base Disorders

Principal Disorder	Initial Laboratory Change	Compensatory Change
Metabolic acidosis	↓ [HCO_3^-]	↓ $Paco_2$
Metabolic alkalosis	↑ [HCO_3^-]	↑ $Paco_2$
Respiratory acidosis	↑ $Paco_2$	↑ [HCO_3^-]
Respiratory alkalosis	↓ $Paco_2$	↓ [HCO_3^-]

[HCO_3^-] = plasma bicarbonate concentration (mEq/L); $Paco_2$ = arterial partial pressure of carbon dioxide (mm Hg).

many others. This may provide diagnostic clues toward combined causes of a metabolic acidosis in a critically ill patient.[9] Unmeasured anions are important contributors to metabolic acidosis in critically ill patients and, in some studies, have been correlated with increased mortality.[2,11,27] Although some stepwise approaches recommend only calculating the AG when the principal disorder is a metabolic acidosis, failure to calculate the ACAG in the complex critically ill patient may lead to missing the presence of a concomitant elevated AG metabolic acidosis; therefore, routine calculation of the ACAG in critically ill patients is recommended regardless of the principal disorder.

Step 7 – If the ACAG is elevated, calculate the delta ratio. The delta ratio (also called the delta-delta) is a comparison of the magnitude of the abnormality of the ACAG (delta ACAG) with the change in the [HCO_3^-] (delta bicarbonate). When calculated as a ratio, the equation is as follows:

$$Delta\ Ratio = \frac{ACAG - normal\ AG}{Normal\ [HCO_3^-] - Measured\ [HCO_3^-]}$$

$$= \frac{(ACAG - 12)}{(24 - [HCO_3^-])}$$

where all variables have been previously defined and are expressed as milliequivalents per liter. A delta ratio of 1–2 is consistent with a pure elevated AG metabolic acidosis. A ratio less than 1 is predictive of a concomitant normal AG metabolic acidosis, and a ratio greater than 2 provides evidence of either a concomitant metabolic alkalosis or an appropriately compensated chronic respiratory acidosis. These estimates may be inaccurate in critically ill patients who may have abnormal baseline values because of other underlying processes, and some have raised serious concerns about the accuracy of relying on a single calculation to detect a mixed acid-base disorder. This should be used in the context of a complete understanding of the clinical presentation and history of the patient, together with continued monitoring of changes in the patient status. The delta ratio is just one piece of evidence that needs to be considered with other evidence in a complex ICU patient.[34]

Table 1.4 Normal Secondary or Compensatory Responses

Principal Disorder	Secondary Response Rule
Metabolic acidosis	$Paco_2 = 1.5 \times [HCO_3^-] + 8 \pm 2$
Metabolic alkalosis	$Paco_2 = 0.7 \times [HCO_3^-] + 20$
Respiratory acidosis	
Acute	[HCO_3^-] increases 1 mEq/L for each $Paco_2$ increase of 10 mm Hg above 40 mm Hg
Chronic	[HCO_3^-] increases 4–5 mEq/L for each $Paco_2$ increase of 10 mm Hg above 40 mm Hg
Respiratory alkalosis	
Acute	[HCO_3^-] decreases 2 mEq/L for each $Paco_2$ decrease of 10 mm Hg below 40 mm Hg
Chronic	[HCO_3^-] decreases 4–5 mEq/L for each $Paco_2$ decrease of 10 mm Hg below 40 mm Hg

Step 8 – If the ACAG is normal in the presence of a metabolic acidosis and the cause is unknown, calculate the urinary anion gap (UAG). Of note, it is uncommon for the critical care clinician to use the UAG or the urinary osmolal gap to evaluate a normal AG metabolic acidosis because the likely causes are typically already known. The UAG is calculated using measured urinary electrolytes:

$$UAG = [Na^+] + [K^+] - [Cl^-]$$

where all urinary electrolyte concentrations are expressed in milliequivalents per liter. The most common causes of normal AG metabolic acidosis with a negative UAG are infusion of large volumes of normal saline and diarrhea. Proximal renal tubular acidosis (RTA) is also associated with a negative UAG; however, new-onset proximal RTA is not a common cause of acidosis in critically ill patients with no history of RTA. A normal AG metabolic acidosis with a positive UAG may be seen with renal failure, distal RTA, and hypoaldosteronism because of an impaired ability to excrete NH_4^+ as NH_4Cl. When the UAG may be unreliable (polyuria, urine pH greater than 6.5, and the presence of other urinary anions [e.g., ketones]), the urinary osmolal gap may be used in place of the UAG. A urinary osmolal gap less than 40 mmol/L is equivalent to a positive UAG.[23]

Following this stepwise approach to evaluate an acid-base disturbance in the critically ill patient will normally result in an accurate and complete diagnosis of the acid-base disorders present. A more casual review of the blood gas and chemistry results will often lead to a missed concomitant disorder that may have important diagnostic and therapeutic implications. With practice, this stepwise approach will become routine and can be completed in just a few minutes using simple math and laboratory values commonly available at the bedside. Because of the inherent variability in the measurement of the relevant analytes and the dynamic status of critically ill patients, acid-base analysis is best conducted using results from samples obtained simultaneously.

CLINICAL SYNDROMES

The most common acid-base abnormality observed in critically ill patients is an acidosis (metabolic or respiratory). Common reasons for admission to an ICU including sepsis, shock, trauma, renal failure, toxic ingestion, surgical catastrophe, and endocrinologic emergency are associated with a metabolic acidosis, and initial resuscitation or intraoperative management of critically ill patients may lead to iatrogenic metabolic acidosis, predominantly because of large volumes of intravenous chloride-rich fluids. In addition, respiratory failure secondary to exacerbations of underlying lung disease, neurologic disorders, or toxic drug or substance exposures is associated with an acute respiratory acidosis. The complex nature of critically ill patients and their acute management commonly results in mixed acid-base disorders.[20] Although much of the critical care literature has focused on the recognition, risks, and management of an acidosis in the critically ill patient, recent evidence suggests that metabolic alkalosis is also a common finding during a critical care stay, with most episodes occurring within the first 72 hours of admission to the ICU.[5]

Metabolic Acidosis

As discussed previously, many of the medical and surgical reasons for admission to the ICU and treatments administered in the ICU can be associated with a metabolic acidosis. As shown in Table 1.3, the expected principal finding on an ABG result is a decreased $[HCO_3^-]$, with a secondary response of decreased $Paco_2$. Metabolic acidoses have historically been divided into those with an elevated AG and those with a normal AG. As discussed previously, it is critically important that the AG be corrected for serum albumin concentration (ACAG) in ICU patients to improve diagnostic value. An elevated ACAG is analogous to an elevated SIG or BE_{UA} for the Stewart and BE acid-base models, respectively. For diagnostic purposes, this is a valuable way to categorize metabolic acidosis, given that the elevated AG represents traditionally unmeasured anions that are weak or strong acids responsible for the acidosis and provides valuable clues to the underlying cause and therapeutic approach. Table 1.1 provides a list of common conditions associated with an elevated AG metabolic acidosis. Several acronyms have been used over the years to aid clinicians in remembering the common sources of unmeasured anions when presented with an elevated AG metabolic acidosis, with MUDPILES, GOLD MARRK, and the much simpler KULT being the most popular. Table 1.5 provides the detail of the components of these acronyms.

Lactic acidosis is one of the most common metabolic acidoses presenting in critically ill patients, with the most common causes being shock of any cause, sepsis, severe heart failure, and severe trauma.[14] The accumulation of lactate, which serves as a strong anion, leads to a reduction in the plasma SID, increasing $[H_3O^+]$, and resulting metabolic acidosis. An elevated lactate concentration has

Table 1.5 Elevated Anion Gap Metabolic Acidosis Acronyms

MUDPILES[a]:	GOLD MARRK
Methanol	**G**lycols (ethylene and propylene)
Uremia	**5-O**xoproline (pyroglutamic acid)
Diabetic ketoacidosis	
Paraldehyde (historically), or **P**ropylene Glycol	**L**-Lactate
Isoniazid (INH), or **I**ron, or **I**nfection	**D**-Lactate
	Methanol
Lactate	**A**spirin
Ethylene glycol	**R**enal Failure
Salicylate	**R**habdomyolysis
	Ketoacids
KULT	
Ketoacidosis	
Uremia	
Lactate	
Toxins	

[a]Revised by some to MUDPILERS, with the "R" representing rhabdomyolysis.

a quantitative relationship, both peak lactate and duration of hyperlactatemia, with the risk of mortality in critically ill patients,[14] and resuscitative measures leading to a reduction in blood lactate levels have been associated with improved clinical outcomes.[15] The L-isomer of lactate, as primarily the byproduct of anaerobic cellular metabolism, is the physiologically relevant form of lactate. However, D-lactate accumulation can be clinically important in the ICU setting after intravenous propylene glycol administration (e.g., lorazepam infusions), toxic ingestions of propylene glycol,[35,36] and ischemic bowel.[8] Routine clinical laboratory assays detect and report only L-lactate concentrations, so the presence of D-lactate represents an unmeasured anion that can contribute to a metabolic acidosis.

Pyruvate is generated primarily by cellular anaerobic glycolysis under hypoxic conditions and is reversibly converted to lactate by the following reaction:

$$Pyruvate + NADPH + H^+ \leftrightarrow Lactate + NAD^+$$

An adult human generates about 20 mmol/kg of lactate daily. Lactate is normally reconverted to pyruvate, which is then metabolized by mitochondrial oxidation within LDH-rich tissues including the liver (70%), kidneys, and skeletal muscle. Metabolism through the Cori cycle leads to the formation of glucose (gluconeogenesis). The tricarboxylic acid cycle and oxidative phosphorylation leads to the generation of CO_2 and water, which can lead to bicarbonate generation. Normal equilibrium of production and metabolism of lactate-pyruvate leads to low steady-state plasma concentrations of lactate; however, rapid increases in lactate production during various causes of tissue hypoxia can lead to sharp increases in blood lactate concentrations. The combination of decreased mitochondrial oxidative phosphorylation secondary to tissue hypoxia, microcirculatory failure, and tissue acidemia will also decrease lactate clearance, contributing to the increase in blood lactate. Other potential contributors to hyperlactatemia in critically ill patients may include underlying chronic liver disease, fulminant hepatic failure, renal failure, drugs that impair normal oxidative phosphorylation (e.g., antiretroviral agents, propofol, and metformin), and physiologic stress (e.g., severe trauma, pheochromocytoma) or drugs (e.g., epinephrine, albuterol) that cause β_2-adrenoceptor stimulation, leading to increased aerobic glycolysis independent of tissue hypoxia.[8,14] High-dose catecholamine infusions during treatment of shock can aggravate hyperlactatemia by β_2-adrenoceptor stimulation; this has especially been true with the use of epinephrine vasopressor therapy.[27,37-39]

Traditionally, lactic acidosis has been categorized into type A and type B; however, in a complex critically ill patient, differentiating type A from type B is difficult, artificial, and probably clinically irrelevant.[8,14]

An elevated serum AG, even with correction for plasma [albumin], lacks adequate sensitivity and specificity for the diagnosis of lactic acidosis.[4,33] In the setting of sepsis and other clinical conditions potentially associated with lactic acidosis, the current recommendation is to directly measure blood lactate concentrations rather than rely on a calculation of unmeasured anions like the AG or ACAG.[14,40] It is also important to recognize that in cases of metabolic acidosis with confirmed hyperlactatemia, there is often a significant contribution to the acidemia by other unmeasured anions, with studies showing that lactate contributes only a portion of the increased AG.[2,27,28,33] An elevation in unmeasured anions other than lactate has been associated with increased mortality,[11,27,28,33,41] but the finding has not been consistent.[1-3,13] Gunnerson et al.[41] reported the results of a retrospective study of 851 ICU patients, of which 584 had evidence of a metabolic acidosis. The patients were classified according to the primary anion contributing to metabolic acidosis as lactate, chloride, or other unmeasured anions (elevated SIG). To be classified as lactic or SIG acidosis, at least 50% of the contribution had to be from that factor, with many patients having a combined lactate and SIG contribution to the metabolic acidosis. The mortality rate for lactic acidosis was 56%, for hyperchloremic acidosis 29%, and for SIG acidosis 39% ($p<0.001$). Multivariate analysis found that independent predictors of mortality were serum lactate, SIG, serum phosphate, and age. Clearly, the contributors to metabolic acidosis in critically ill patients with hyperlactatemia can be complex, and the relevance of these combined contributors to metabolic acidosis on overall morbidity and mortality is uncertain.

Ketoacidosis is an elevated AG metabolic acidosis caused by the overproduction and accumulation of organic acids, most commonly secondary to diabetes mellitus. Other forms of ketoacidosis in critically ill patients are alcoholic and starvation ketoacidosis, although these are normally mild to moderate in severity. Although the overall attributable mortality to diabetic ketoacidosis (DKA) in adult patients is low (less than 1%), the mortality is greatest in older adults and patients with severe underlying illnesses. Although DKA is most common in patients with type 1 diabetes, about one-third of DKA episodes occur in type 2 diabetes with concomitant severe illness or injury caused by trauma, infection, or surgery.[42]

The combination of decreased effective insulin concentrations and increased counter-regulatory hormones (glucagon, cortisol, catecholamines, and growth hormone) results in hyperglycemia and ketosis. Lipolysis of adipose tissue leads to the release of free fatty acids into the circulation and hepatic fatty acid metabolism to ketones (β-hydroxybutyrate and acetoacetate).[42,43] This causes an increase in circulating ketones, which act as strong anions reducing the SID, leading to an increase in [H_3O^+] and an elevated AG metabolic acidosis. In addition to the acid-base disturbance, osmotic diuresis and natriuresis secondary to hyperglycemia leads to extracellular volume loss. An increase in plasma [albumin] secondary to the contraction of intravascular volume needs to be considered when evaluating the AG.[43] Administering normal saline to treat the hypovolemia associated with DKA may result in a concomitant hyperchloremic metabolic acidosis, as discussed in the text that follows.

The most common precipitating factor for DKA is infection. Other precipitants include discontinuation of insulin therapy, cerebrovascular accident, pancreatitis, myocardial infarction, and new-onset type 1 diabetes. Patients with DKA present with a history of polyuria, polydipsia, nausea and vomiting, dehydration, weakness, and mental status changes. Physical findings include skin and mucous membrane changes consistent with dehydration, Kussmaul respirations, diffuse abdominal pain, tachycardia, and hypotension. Metabolic acidosis, elevated AG, and the presence of circulating ketones in blood are diagnostic of DKA. A laboratory method that can detect both acetoacetate and β-hydroxybutyrate is preferred because the classic nitroprusside reaction does not detect β-hydroxybutyrate, which is the main ketone present in DKA.[42] Alcoholic and starvation ketoacidosis may be missed using the nitroprusside reaction for serum or urinary ketones because β-hydroxybutyrate is the relevant circulating ketone body for these forms of ketoacidosis.[8,23]

Acute and chronic renal failure are important causes of an elevated AG metabolic acidosis in critically ill patients. Unlike lactic acidosis and ketoacidosis, which are caused by increased production of organic acids, the acidosis caused by renal dysfunction is the result of decreased excretion of the inorganic sulfates and phosphates, primarily caused by the normal metabolism of dietary proteins and amino acids. In the setting of renal failure, an increase in unmeasured anions as reflected by a positive ALCAG or SIG is expected. Renal failure can also cause a normal AG acidosis as the kidneys lose the ability to secrete NH_4Cl. Metabolic acidosis is of greater concern as glomerular filtration rate decreases to less than 20 mL/minute. Acute renal failure may also contribute to lactic acidosis caused by decreased renal clearance of lactate.[8,20]

Toxic ingestions of ethylene glycol, methanol, acetone, and salicylate lead to an elevated AG metabolic acidosis. The presence of unmeasured anions in the setting of a metabolic acidosis in a recently admitted critically ill patient should raise concerns for a potential poisoning and trigger appropriate diagnostic testing. For suspected methanol or ethylene glycol ingestions, the osmolar gap (the difference between the measured and calculated osmolarity) is a useful screening tool. An osmolar gap greater than 10 mOsm/L, corrected for blood ethanol concentration, is considered abnormal.[8,9]

A normal AG, hyperchloremic metabolic acidosis is a common finding in the critically ill patient. The most common causes are resuscitation with chloride-rich, crystalloid intravenous solutions (primarily normal saline) and diarrhea. It is not uncommon that a hyperchloremic metabolic acidosis is concomitant with other acid-base disorders and is often the result of the treatment for the underlying cause of an initial elevated AG metabolic acidosis. As discussed previously, the metabolic acidosis secondary to the administration of normal saline is not mechanistically a dilutional acidosis caused by the expansion of extracellular fluid volume and the resulting dilution of a fixed quantity of bicarbonate, but is instead secondary to a reduction in the SID caused by the accumulation of chloride.[6,8,25,44,45]

Historically, the mechanistic explanation for hyperchloremic metabolic acidosis caused by severe or persistent diarrhea has been the loss of GI bicarbonate. However, it is the loss of strong cations (Na^+, K^+) in excess of strong anions (Cl^-) in the diarrheal fluids that decreases the plasma SID leading to an acidosis.[6,25] The changes in [HCO_3^-] and [H_3O^+] are secondary (dependent) to the primary (independent) change in the SID.

Hyperchloremic metabolic acidosis secondary to normal saline administration and diarrhea are both associated with a negative UAG because of an increased excretion of urinary ammonium chloride in response to the acidosis. Other, less common causes of a hyperchloremic acidosis with a negative UAG are proximal (type 2) renal tubular acidosis, ureteral diversion, loss of small bowel or pancreatic secretions, and some medications or toxins (e.g., toluene, ifosfamide, tenofovir, topiramate, and carbonic anhydrase inhibitors). Hyperchloremic metabolic acidosis with a positive UAG may be associated with renal dysfunction and distal (types 1 and 4) renal tubular acidosis.[23] Type 4 renal tubular acidosis caused by hypoaldosteronism may be observed with high-dose steroid therapy because of the mineralocorticoid effects of the drug.

The secondary response, often termed a *compensatory response*, to a metabolic acidosis is an increase in minute ventilation and a resulting decrease in $Paco_2$. The equation to describe this relatively well-preserved relationship is provided in Table 1.4, which assumes that the patient is able to mount and maintain a secondary respiratory response. Although this is often called a compensatory respiratory alkalosis, it is best to think of this secondary response as the new normal $Paco_2$ for the patient, given the extent of the primary metabolic disorder, and that a $Paco_2$ different from this new normal range is representative of a mixed metabolic-respiratory disorder. It is unusual that the degree of the secondary respiratory response is adequate to completely normalize or correct the acidemia caused by the metabolic disorder; therefore, the pH will typically remain in the lower end of the normal range with an appropriate secondary response. Patients with an underlying respiratory disorder (e.g., chronic obstructive lung disease) may have an abnormal $Paco_2$ at baseline, which needs to be considered when evaluating the appropriateness of the patient's response to a primary metabolic disorder, and will often limit the ability of the patient to maintain an adequate secondary response.

The treatment of the ICU patient with a metabolic acidosis should be primarily aimed at the treatment of the underlying disorder. Effective treatment of the predominant cause should lead to resolution of the metabolic acidosis. For patients presenting with sepsis, shock, severe heart failure, or other causes of tissue hypoxia leading to a predominantly lactic acidosis, the focus is on restoring hemodynamics with fluids, vasoactive and inotropic agents as indicated, treatment of any underlying infection, and other supportive measures as needed.[14] A reduction in lactate production and restoration of normal lactate-pyruvate equilibrium will lead to an increased SID because of the metabolism of excess lactate, reduction in [H_3O^+], and resolution of the elevated AG metabolic acidosis. As inferred previously, the choice of treatment for these complex ICU patients may contribute to worsening acidemia and increases in lactate, so the approach to restoring hemodynamic stability may be important. Overreliance on normal saline for fluid resuscitation may exacerbate the acidemia because of a superimposed hyperchloremic metabolic acidosis, and the use of epinephrine for vasopressor support may increase blood lactate concentrations because of a concomitant type B lactic acidosis secondary to an increase in aerobic glycolysis.[37-39]

The treatment of DKA requires the administration of insulin, restoration of intravascular volume, and careful management of electrolyte disturbances. In addition, underlying triggers for DKA (e.g., infection) require prompt management. The continuous intravenous administration of insulin is the cornerstone of the treatment of DKA, although recent studies have shown a potential role for subcutaneous rapid-acting insulin analogs. Insulin therapy will suppress the production of ketone bodies, and the metabolic clearance of circulating ketones will lead to an increase in the SID and resolution of the acidosis. Insulin therapy also leads to the resolution of hyperglycemia. A detailed discussion of the management of DKA is beyond the scope of this chapter, and the reader is referred to recent guidelines of the management of DKA in adult[42] and pediatric patients.[46]

An elevated AG metabolic acidosis secondary to toxins will require appropriate management to minimize continued absorption and enhance clearance of the toxin and administration of appropriate antidotes or metabolic blockers to minimize the impact of the toxic ingestion. A detailed discussion of the management of common drug overdoses and toxic exposures appears in chapter 39, "Medication Withdrawal in the ICU." An elevated AG metabolic acidosis secondary to severe renal dysfunction will typically require renal replacement therapy in the critically ill patient, and severe metabolic acidosis is one of the indications to acutely initiate renal replacement therapy (see Chapter 28, "Management and Drug Dosing in Acute Liver Failure").

The treatment of hyperchloremic metabolic acidosis secondary to the use of chloride-rich intravenous solutions usually involves discontinuing the implicated intravenous solution and, if continued fluid administration is indicated, switching to a balanced or more alkaline solution (e.g., lactated Ringer or Plasma-Lyte solutions). See the following text for a more detailed discussion of intravenous fluid choices and their potential influence on acid-base disorders. For patients with severe diarrhea or other GI fluid losses leading to hyperchloremic metabolic acidosis, treatment involves therapies aimed at the underlying diarrhea as well as restoration of fluid losses using a balanced or alkalinizing intravenous solution with careful monitoring and management of electrolyte disorders.

Severe metabolic acidosis characterized by a pH less than 7.2 or [HCO_3^-] less than 8 mEq/L may be associated with the direct adverse effects of decreased cardiac contractility, poor regulation of vascular tone with hypotension, cardiac arrhythmias, pulmonary hypertension, central nervous system (CNS) dysfunction, and other serious adverse metabolic consequences.[47,48] General treatment of severe metabolic acidosis has been advocated as a temporizing measure while specific treatment of the underlying condition is being pursued; however, strong evidence of the benefit of treatment is lacking.[48-50] For DKA, the current recommendation for the general treatment of acidosis is a pH less than 6.9.[42,46] Treatment goals should be partial correction of the acidosis to pH greater than 7.2, or [HCO_3^-] greater than 8–10 mEq/L, not normalization of the acidemia.[8,47,48] The goal in the treatment of DKA is a pH greater than 7.0.[42] The mainstay for the general treatment of metabolic acidosis in critically ill patients is sodium bicarbonate injection, available commercially as a 1-mEq/mL solution. The long-standing teaching under the physiologic or bicarbonate-centered model is that exogenous sodium bicarbonate replaces plasma bicarbonate, leading to improvement in the acidosis, and the recommended dose of sodium bicarbonate has been estimated using a calculation of the base deficit. However, the explanation from a physiochemical model perspective is that sodium bicarbonate provides a strong cation (Na^+) in the absence of a strong anion (HCO_3^- is a weak anion), leading to an increase in the SID and correction of the metabolic acidosis.[50] For example, an intravenous solution containing 75 mEq/L of sodium bicarbonate added to 0.45% sodium chloride for injection (½ normal saline; 77 mEq/L of sodium chloride) has a SID of 75 mEq/L and, when administered intravenously, will result in an increase in the plasma SID and therefore have an alkalinizing effect. In vivo, the [HCO_3^-] is dependent on the independent factors SID, A_{TOT}, and $Paco_2$, and not on the amount of exogenously administered HCO_3^-.

The dose of sodium bicarbonate has traditionally been calculated to determine the amount needed to raise the $[HCO_3^-]$ to some desired concentration according to an estimate of the bicarbonate space. Although the bicarbonate-centered approach to this estimate is physiologically incorrect, the estimation is likely still reasonable. To be conservative, the bicarbonate space is estimated to be 50% of the total body weight. The simplified equation is as follows:

$$\textit{Sodium Bicarbonate Dose} = [HCO_3^-]_{Desired} - [HCO_3^-]_{Actual} \times (BW \times 0.5)$$

where the sodium bicarbonate dose is in milliequivalents, $[HCO_3^-]$ values are in milliequivalents per liter, and BW is body weight in kilograms.[8,23,47,48] Although this equation has been widely recommended for many years, most ICU clinicians will empirically administer 50–100 mEq of sodium bicarbonate as a slow infusion while closely monitoring response. Additional sodium bicarbonate will be administered as indicated by pH response. Bolus administration should be reserved for severe, life-threatening acidosis, and most patients should be treated with a slow infusion over 2 hours or more. Common solutions are to add 75 mEq/L of sodium bicarbonate to 1 L of ½ normal saline or 150 mEq/L of sodium bicarbonate added to 1 L of sterile water for injection to provide an isotonic solution with a SID of 75 mEq/L or 150 mEq/L, respectively. Administering sodium bicarbonate as an infusion will reduce the risk of potential adverse effects.[48]

The potential adverse effects of treatment with sodium bicarbonate are hypernatremia and hyperosmolarity, extracellular fluid volume overload, overshoot alkalosis, worsening intracellular acidosis because of CO_2 production, reduction in ionized calcium leading to impaired cardiac contractility, hypokalemia, and increased risk of cerebral edema in children with DKA.[46–48] The risk of overshoot alkalosis is thought to be greatest in the treatment of metabolic acidosis secondary to organic acids (lactate and ketones) because of the metabolism of these anions leading to an increase in $[HCO_3^-]$.[47,48] However, if it is accepted that the $[HCO_3^-]$ is a dependent parameter, and not an independent determinant of acid-base status, this argument lacks rationale. Administering sodium bicarbonate to a target pH of 7.2 or less should avoid the risk of overtreatment leading to metabolic alkalosis. The aggravation of intracellular acidosis after the administration of sodium bicarbonate is believed to be the result of the formation of CO_2, which can readily permeate the cell and increase the intracellular CO_2 content leading to worsening acidosis. In theory, this is more likely to occur with rapid administration of sodium bicarbonate, a high hematocrit, and poor tissue clearance of CO_2 during low-flow states.[47,48,51,52] However, if 100 mEq of sodium bicarbonate were administered over 1 hour and led to a 100% formation of CO_2 (i.e., 100 mmol), this would represent about a 16% increase over normal CO_2 generation by an adult, which, unless there was severe impairment of pulmonary CO_2 excretion, or permissive hypercapnia for severe acute lung injury, should not have a significant effect on intracellular CO_2 content. One study of treating mild intraoperative hyperchloremic metabolic acidosis with 128 plus or minus 18 mEq of sodium bicarbonate administered over 20 minutes required a transient increase in minute ventilation by 40% to maintain end tidal Pco_2 at baseline, whereas after tris-hydroxymethyl aminomethane administration, the minute ventilation was decreased by 60%, suggesting that relatively rapid administration of sodium bicarbonate can lead to transient increases in CO_2 formation.[53] Administering low to moderate doses of sodium bicarbonate as a slow infusion over 1 hour or more is unlikely to have an important impact on CO_2 retention and intracellular acidosis in a patient with adequate ventilation and CO_2 excretion. Given the absence of a strong argument to routinely administer sodium bicarbonate and the potential for adverse effects, using sodium bicarbonate for severe acidosis is an individualized decision based on underlying cardiovascular disease, evidence of adverse effects of acidosis, ability to tolerate a fluid load from an isotonic infusion of sodium bicarbonate, and the theoretical risk of CO_2 retention and intracellular acidosis. During sodium bicarbonate treatment, careful monitoring of ionized calcium and potassium concentrations is recommended.

Tris-hydroxymethyl aminomethane is an alternative buffer that was developed to overcome some of the limitations of sodium bicarbonate. Tris-hydroxymethyl aminomethane is administered as a 0.3M solution and is proposed to act as a proton acceptor because of its ammonia moiety, leading to a decrease in $[H_3O^+]$ and an increase in pH in patients with metabolic acidosis. Because there is no production of CO_2 based on this mechanism and an un-ionized portion of the tris-hydroxymethyl aminomethane can penetrate intracellularly, a proposed advantage of tris-hydroxymethyl aminomethane is that it is does not worsen intracellular pH. When given in equivalent doses, tris-hydroxymethyl aminomethane appears to be as effective as sodium bicarbonate at improving extracellular acid-base parameters.[8,47,48,50,53] In a trial comparing tris-hydroxymethyl aminomethane and sodium bicarbonate for the treatment of intraoperative hyperchloremic metabolic acidosis, Rehm and Finsterer showed that the change in $[HCO_3^-]$ was correlated with a reduction in the SIG because of the increase in an unmeasured cation after the administration of tris-hydroxymethyl aminomethane, presumably the protonated form of tris-hydroxymethyl aminomethane.[53] Therefore, the mechanism of action of tris-hydroxymethyl aminomethane for correcting acidosis can be explained by the Stewart model, with protonated tris-hydroxymethyl aminomethane acting as a strong cation leading to an increase in the SID_e. The recommended dose of tris-hydroxymethyl aminomethane is based on a calculation incorporating the base deficit:

$$THAM\ dose\ (mL) = body\ dry\ weight \times ([HCO_3^-]_{desired} - [HCO_3^-]_{actual}) \times 1.1$$

where THAM is tris-hydroxymethyl aminomethane, dry body weight is in kilograms and $[HCO_3^-]$ values are in milliequivalents per liter.

Tris-hydroxymethyl aminomethane undergoes renal elimination; therefore, it is typically not recommended with a creatinine clearance of less than 30 mL/minute/1.73 m^2. Potential adverse effects associated with tris-hydroxymethyl aminomethane are extravasation injuries, hypoglycemia, respiratory depression, and hyperkalemia. Even though tris-hydroxymethyl aminomethane has been in clinical use since 1959, its role in managing metabolic acidosis remains uncertain and limited given its lack of demonstrated superiority to sodium bicarbonate, its major benefits being primarily theoretical, and its higher cost.[48]

Sodium acetate injection is an alternative to sodium bicarbonate that has been most widely used in parenteral nutrition, in balanced intravenous solutions (e.g., Plasma-Lyte), and during times of sodium bicarbonate shortages. To be an effective buffer by increasing SID, the acetate must be metabolized, which proceeds readily. In one comparative study of different buffer replacement solutions during continuous renal replacement therapy in critically ill patients, the use of a sodium acetate–based solution was less effective at improving acid-base status than either a lactate- or a bicarbonate-based replacement solution and was associated with less improvement in hemodynamic parameters, raising concerns that sodium acetate may be a less effective treatment for acidosis in critically ill patients with acute renal failure.[54] Comparative studies of sodium acetate and sodium bicarbonate as a general treatment for severe metabolic acidosis are unavailable; therefore, sodium acetate should not be considered a primary alternative unless sodium bicarbonate is unavailable.

Metabolic Alkalosis

Although metabolic alkalosis is less common and less well studied in critically ill patients, it is not rare and may often be present with, and masked by, a concomitant metabolic acidosis. In one large retrospective study, 29.3% of critically ill patients had at least one $[HCO_3^-]$ greater than 30 mEq/L during their ICU stay. An increased $[HCO_3^-]$ was associated with a longer ICU length of stay, more days on mechanical ventilation, and a greater hospital mortality rate.[5] The most common causes of a metabolic alkalosis in critically ill patients are chloride-wasting diuretic use and loss of upper GI fluids because of vomiting or nasogastric suctioning.[5] Less common causes are chloride diarrhea or mineralocorticoid excess. Metabolic alkalosis is characterized by an elevated $[HCO_3^-]$, with an increased $Paco_2$ as a secondary or compensatory response (see Table 1.3). Metabolic alkalosis is further subdivided into those that are chloride responsive and those that are chloride resistant. A chloride-responsive metabolic alkalosis is typically associated with a spot urinary chloride concentration less than 25 mEq/L (although this test is not usually necessary in the ICU to make the diagnosis given the clinical history) and is responsive to treatment with normal saline. However, in the face of continued loop diuretic use, the urinary chloride concentration may be elevated.[23] Most metabolic alkaloses in critically ill patients are chloride responsive. Usual causes of new-onset chloride-resistant metabolic alkaloses are uncommon in the ICU, with the possible exception of iatrogenic mineralocorticoid excess.

As described previously, the loss of upper GI secretions because of vomiting or nasogastric tube drainage leads to a loss of Cl$^-$, an increase in plasma SID, and the onset of metabolic alkalosis. The loss of intravascular volume and activation of the renin-angiotensin-aldosterone axis leads to further acidification of the urine and maintenance of the alkalotic state.[25] The frequent use of loop diuretics in the critically ill patient may also lead to the development of a metabolic alkalosis. Loop diuretics inhibit the sodium-potassium-chloride (NKCC) cotransporter in the thick ascending limb of the loop of Henle, leading to a greater net loss of Cl$^-$ than Na$^+$ in the urine. The greater loss of Cl$^-$ leads to an increase in plasma SID and the onset of metabolic alkalosis. Thiazide diuretics inhibit the sodium-chloride cotransporter of the distal convoluted tubular cells, with a relatively greater loss of Cl$^-$ than Na$^+$ from the extracellular fluid, leading to an increase in plasma SID and metabolic alkalosis.[25] Aggressive diuresis may lead to the loss of intravascular volume, and activation of the renin-angiotensin-aldosterone axis will serve to maintain the alkalosis as described previously.

The treatment of a metabolic alkalosis secondary to chloride loss is primarily aimed at treating the underlying process (e.g., vomiting), discontinuing diuretics, and replacing intravascular volume with normal saline. Potassium depletion can contribute to metabolic alkalosis[55]; therefore, correction of any potassium losses with potassium chloride is also required. There is a limited role for pharmacologic management of metabolic alkalosis.

Acetazolamide is a carbonic anhydrase inhibitor that can be administered intravenously for the treatment of metabolic alkalosis in critically ill patients.[56,57] Traditional teaching is that by inhibiting carbonic anhydrase, acetazolamide interferes with regeneration and recovery of urinary bicarbonate and increases urinary bicarbonate losses, leading to a decrease in plasma $[HCO_3^-]$ and resolution of the metabolic alkalosis. This is not consistent with the Stewart model, where HCO_3^- is a dependent parameter and does not have an independent role in regulating acid-base status. Moviat and coworkers showed that a single intravenous dose of acetazolamide 500 mg effectively corrected metabolic alkalosis in critically ill patients through a reduction in SID secondary to a significant increase in urinary Na^+ excretion without a concomitant Cl^- loss. For patients with a clinically significant metabolic alkalosis and no clinical evidence of intravascular volume depletion, acetazolamide is a reasonable and effective first treatment option when intravascular volume expansion is not indicated or wanted. The clinical evidence suggests that a single intravenous dose of 500 mg is as effective as repeated doses and, in the absence of ongoing chloride loss, has a persistent effect for at least 72 hours.[56,57] In our clinical experience, a repeat dose after 48–72 hours, if needed, may give additional response, but usually less than the initial dose. Routine, scheduled doses in critically ill patients are not recommended.

Chloride replacement is the preferred treatment for most patients with chloride-responsive metabolic alkalosis. Most commonly, ICU patients with metabolic alkalosis will have clinical evidence or history consistent with intravascular volume depletion; therefore, the treatment of choice is intravenous normal saline, often with supplemental potassium chloride. As discussed previously, normal saline provides 154 mEq/L of Na^+ and Cl^- with a SID of zero. Therefore, it provides relatively more Cl^- than Na^+ compared with plasma electrolyte concentrations, leading to a reduction in the plasma SID and resolution of the metabolic alkalosis. In the setting of a chloride-responsive metabolic alkalosis, normal saline is an effective chloride replacement solution. In addition, the reestablishment of an effective circulating volume will reverse the effects of the renin-angiotensin-aldosterone axis on sustaining urinary Cl^- losses.

Continuous infusion or regularly scheduled doses of loop diuretics to treat excessive extracellular volume in a stable ICU patient to facilitate weaning from mechanical ventilation and reduce edema will often result in a metabolic alkalosis that may be moderate to severe. In the absence of overt signs of intravascular volume depletion (e.g., hemodynamically stable and unchanged or improving renal function tests), it may be desired to continue aggressive diuresis; however, the metabolic alkalosis becomes the major barrier to continued treatment. Although administering normal saline would effectively treat the metabolic alkalosis, this would be counterproductive to the goals of removing excess extravascular fluids and reducing peripheral edema. Although acetazolamide may be an effective way to extend the duration of diuresis, the continued chloride loss caused by loop diuretics often leads to a limited and transient effect of the drug. Alternative chloride replacement options can be very useful to manage this clinical dilemma.

Dilute hydrochloric acid (0.1N or 0.2N) intravenous solutions have been used clinically for several decades to treat moderate to severe metabolic alkalosis.[58-63] These solutions have the advantage of providing a strong anion (Cl^-) in the absence of a strong cation, leading to a significant reduction in SID and improvement in the metabolic alkalosis without providing expansion of intravascular volume. Contrary to traditional teaching, the mechanism of action in the treatment of metabolic alkalosis is chloride replacement, not the provision of H^+. The SID of a 0.1N hydrochloric acid solution is –100 mEq/L, and the SID of the 0.2N solution is –200 mEq/L, so the volumes required to replace chloride are not excessive. There are no commercially available hydrochloric acid intravenous solutions, so they must be prepared extemporaneously from concentrated hydrochloric acid sterilized using cold filtration and added to sterile water for injection in glass containers. Because of the risk of severe extravasation injury with tissue necrosis,[64,65] it is strongly recommended that hydrochloric acid be infused through a central line using the distal port only after the position of the catheter has been confirmed radiographically. The dose can be estimated by calculating the chloride deficit or BE. The chloride deficit equation is as follows:

$$Cl^- \text{ Deficit} = (0.2 \text{ } L/kg \times BW) \times (103 - observed \text{ } serum \text{ } Cl^-)$$

where Cl^- deficit is milliequivalents, observed serum Cl^- is milliequivalents per liter, and BW is body weight in kilograms.[66] It is usually recommended to administer the calculated dose over 12–24 hours. However, if there are ongoing chloride losses, the calculation of the required dose will be inaccurate. In most cases, careful laboratory monitoring and adjustment of the dose to achieve the desired rate and extent of correction is usually adequate. The infusion can be started at 40–80 mEq/hour (40 mL/hour of the 0.1N or 0.2N solution, respectively) and adjusted as needed. If precautions are taken to minimize the risk of extravasation, hydrochloric acid infusions are well tolerated with very few reported adverse effects.[58-63]

Ammonium chloride is an alternative chloride replacement solution. It is available as a 100-mEq/20 mL solution for intravenous administration after further dilution in a compatible intravenous solution for the treatment of severe metabolic alkalosis. The dose is estimated by calculating the chloride deficit and replacing about one-half of the calculated dose over 12 hours, at a rate not to exceed 1 mEq/minute. Additional ammonium chloride can be administered as indicated. Ammonium chloride should be administered cautiously to patients with renal or hepatic dysfunction, and it is contraindicated in the presence of severe renal or hepatic impairment. Exacerbation of urea accumulation and uremic symptoms can be observed in the setting of renal failure. Hepatic dysfunction can lead to the accumulation of ammonia and CNS toxicity, including confusion, irritability, seizures, and coma.[66]

Respiratory Acidosis

An elevation in $Paco_2$ because of the failure to excrete CO_2 at a rate equivalent to production results in a respiratory acidosis. The $Paco_2$ is an independent variable in acid-base disorders, and the resulting change in $[H_3O^+]$ (or pH) depends on the overall changes in $Paco_2$ and SID, assuming that A_{TOT} is not altered to regulate acid-base status. The evaluation and management of respiratory acidosis is separated into acute versus chronic according to the clinical history. The secondary response is evidenced by a change in $[HCO_3^-]$ in the same direction as $Paco_2$ (Table 1.3) but is secondary to a positive change in SID.[67] The quantitative change in SID and $[HCO_3^-]$ is related to the acute versus chronic nature of the respiratory acidosis (see Table 1.4). The smaller change during an acute respiratory acidosis is believed to be secondary to a cellular shift of electrolytes, whereas the changes with a more prolonged respiratory acidosis (typically 3–5 days) are caused by the regulation of Cl^- by the kidney.[67] The secondary change is inadequate to fully correct the acidemia caused by the primary respiratory acidosis in most cases.

The causes of a respiratory acidosis can be divided into acute or chronic parenchymal lung or airway diseases, neuromuscular disorders, perfusion abnormalities, CNS-mediated respiratory failure, and iatrogenic ventilatory complications (see Table 1.6). Patients may present from being asymptomatic in the setting of stable, chronic hypercapnia to having serious neurologic signs including mental status changes, stupor, and seizures with an acute and significant rise in $Paco_2$. With acute, severe hypercapnia and acidemia, there may be a decline in cardiac output and hypotension because of reduced vascular resistance.[66]

Treatment of a respiratory acidosis is dependent on both the chronicity and the severity, with the management of acute changes from baseline being most clinically important. Acute hypoxemia is common in patients presenting with acute onset respiratory failure, and the treatment of hypoxemia with supplemental oxygen may be of greatest immediate concern. Establishing an airway, if necessary; providing adequate oxygen; and providing ventilatory support (mechanical ventilation or noninvasive ventilation) as indicated are the mainstays of acute management and stabilization of the patient with a severe acute or acute-on-chronic respiratory acidosis. In parallel, the underlying cause of the respiratory acidosis must be treated promptly and appropriately.

Oxygen therapy should be administered cautiously to patients with chronic hypercapnia who are breathing spontaneously because the primary driver of respiratory effort may be hypoxemia rather than hypercapnia. Supplemental oxygen may lead to a decrease in respiratory drive and a worsening of the respiratory acidosis. Careful monitoring after administering supplemental oxygen is necessary.

For a patient with chronic respiratory acidosis, most commonly because of chronic obstructive lung disease, who presents with acute respiratory failure requiring mechanical ventilation, it is important to target the patient's estimated baseline $Paco_2$. Overventilation of a patient with this presentation resulting in essentially normalization of the $Paco_2$ will lead to reversal of the patient's usual secondary metabolic alkalosis over several days. This will make it difficult to wean patients from mechanical ventilation when they are improved and physiologically ready for extubation. Patients will be unable to maintain an adequate minute ventilation and $Paco_2$ off the ventilator to avoid severe acidosis with their new $[HCO_3^-]$, resulting in rapid fatigue and respiratory failure after extubation. It may take several days of avoidable mechanical ventilation or the administration of exogenous alkali (sodium bicarbonate or oral sodium citrate) for patients to reconstitute their normal $[HCO_3^-]$ and permit them to be safely liberated from the ventilator, increasing the risk of complications and prolongation of their ICU stay. Attempts to keep patients close to their usual baseline blood gas results will reduce the likelihood of this iatrogenic complication, reduce time on mechanical ventilation, and potentially shorten ICU length of stay.

There are no specific drug treatments for managing a respiratory acidosis. Using several targeted drug therapies including bronchodilators, corticosteroids, antibiotics, anticoagulants, thrombolytics, opiate antagonists, and others is important in managing underlying causes of respiratory acidosis, but these have no direct effects on the acid-base disorder. Some have advocated for administering chloride replacement therapy in patients with a combined respiratory acidosis and metabolic alkalosis. The concomitant metabolic alkalosis further depresses respiratory drive, worsening the increase in $Paco_2$. The

Table 1.6 Respiratory Acidosis — Causes

Lung or Airway Abnormalities	CNS Abnormalities
Chronic obstructive lung disease	Stroke
Asthma	Seizure, status epilepticus
Airway obstruction (mechanical or edema)	Drug toxicity (e.g., opiates, sedatives)
Interstitial lung disease	Traumatic brain injury
Bronchiectasis	**Perfusion Abnormalities**
Severe pulmonary edema	Pulmonary embolism (massive)
Severe pneumonia	Cardiopulmonary arrest
Acute respiratory distress syndrome	
Neuromuscular Abnormalities	**Other**
Guillain-Barré syndrome	Iatrogenic hypoventilation
Myasthenia gravis	Restrictive lung disease
Spinal cord injury	

intravenous administration of dilute hydrochloric acid has resulted in resolution of the metabolic alkalosis and concomitant improvement in the respiratory acidosis.[58,59] Although this has been reported in the literature, it is an uncommon treatment approach in the setting of a severe respiratory acidosis.

Respiratory Alkalosis

Respiratory alkalosis is the least common of the acid-base disorders in critically ill patients. A persistent increase in minute ventilation leads to a reduction in $Paco_2$ and alkalemia. As with respiratory acidosis, the disorder is divided into acute and chronic respiratory alkalosis according to the clinical presentation and history. The secondary response is a reduction in SID and a resulting decline in $[HCO_3^-]$, with a greater quantitative response with a chronic respiratory alkalosis (see Table 1.3 and Table 1.4). The most common causes of respiratory alkalosis in critically ill patients are pain, anxiety, fever, and hypoxemia secondary to pneumonia, pulmonary edema, or pulmonary embolism. Central nervous system lesions secondary to traumatic brain injury or tumor are also potential causes of respiratory alkalosis. Salicylate overdose can stimulate respiratory drive, leading to a respiratory alkalosis, which is often associated with a concomitant elevated AG metabolic acidosis, although early in the presentation, the respiratory alkalosis may be predominant. Mild to moderate respiratory alkalosis is generally asymptomatic and does not typically require treatment; however, severe alkalosis (pH greater than 7.60) can be associated with light-headedness, confusion, syncope, and seizures, likely because of decreased cerebral blood flow. Patients may also be more prone to cardiac arrhythmias because of sensitization to circulating or exogenously administered catecholamines. Electrolyte abnormalities may include hypokalemia, decreased ionized calcium, and hypophosphatemia. For patients with traumatic brain injury, the reduction in cerebral blood flow associated with respiratory alkalosis may have a detrimental effect on maintaining adequate cerebral perfusion, especially in the presence of an elevated intracranial pressure.

Treatment is focused primarily on treating the underlying cause, including the administration of analgesics for pain, sedatives for anxiety, and antipyretics for fever, as appropriate. Treating the underlying cause of hypoxemia and providing supplemental oxygen can reduce minute ventilation and resolve the metabolic alkalosis. In patients with CNS-mediated increases in minute ventilation (e.g., traumatic brain injury or tumor), it is often difficult to lower minute ventilation because patients will often overbreathe the ventilator. Sedation, and in severe cases neuromuscular paralysis, may be needed to permit reductions in minute ventilation. Dead space can also be added to the ventilator circuit to increase the rebreathing of expired gases and increase $Paco_2$.[66]

Mixed Acid-Base Disorders

Mixed acid-base disorders are very common in critically ill patients because of the combination of acute illnesses, underlying chronic diseases, and the influence of treatments that are administered. Just about any combination of respiratory and metabolic acid-base abnormalities can coexist, depending on the clinical presentation, and it is therefore imperative that a full evaluation of the acid-base status using the stepwise approach discussed earlier be completed. It is not uncommon to have a patient with sepsis who has had significant vomiting or nasogastric tube losses who has been resuscitated with normal saline and administered vasopressors to support unstable hemodynamics. That combination of clinical events could lead to a mixed acid-base disorder, including elevated AG metabolic acidosis secondary to sepsis and shock, metabolic alkalosis owing to the loss of upper GI secretions, and hyperchloremic metabolic acidosis secondary to large volumes of normal saline. A patient with baseline chronic obstructive lung disease and a chronic respiratory acidosis presenting with severe diarrhea, hypovolemic shock secondary to intravascular volume loss, and acute respiratory failure could potentially have an acute-on-chronic respiratory acidosis, a hyperchloremic metabolic acidosis secondary to severe diarrhea, and an elevated AG metabolic acidosis owing to shock and poor tissue perfusion. These are just two examples to show the potential for mixed disorders as a result of the complexities of the presentation of acutely ill patients admitted to the adult ICU.

INTRAVENOUS FLUIDS AND ACID-BASE DISORDERS

As discussed previously, the choice of intravenous fluid therapy can have an important impact on acid-base status, and recent publications have raised concerns that fluid composition may also affect patient outcome.[16,17,68] The relative electrolyte content of the intravenous fluid compared with the patients' plasma concentrations and volume administered may have an important impact on SID and therefore acid-base status. A solution that has a SID lower than plasma $[HCO_3^-]$ will lead to a reduction in SID and the development of a hyperchloremic acidosis, whereas solutions with a SID greater than plasma $[HCO_3^-]$ will increase SID and lead to a metabolic alkalosis.[44,45,69]

As discussed previously, normal saline (0.9% sodium chloride for injection) has a SID of zero and, when administered in large volumes, will decrease plasma SID and lead to a hyperchloremic metabolic acidosis. Other intravenous fluids that are commercially available and considered more balanced electrolyte solutions are lactated

Ringer solution, Plasma-Lyte (available as Plasma-Lyte 148 and Plasma-Lyte A), and Normosol-R. Lactated Ringer solution has an effective SID of 28 mEq/L as long as the patient is able to clear the 28 mEq/L of lactate in the solution. In the setting of severe liver dysfunction, lactate clearance will be significantly decreased, and lactated Ringer solution will have an effective SID closer to zero. When lactate is adequately cleared, lactated Ringer solution is not expected to contribute to the development of a metabolic acidosis. Plasma-Lyte 148, Plasma-Lyte A, and Normosol-R solutions have an effective SID of 50 mEq/L because of the metabolic clearance of acetate and gluconate after administration of the fluid. Both Plasma-Lyte solutions have the same electrolyte composition; however, Plasma-Lyte A and Normosol-R have the solution pH adjusted to 7.4. This is not clinically relevant from an acid-base perspective, and the solutions can be used interchangeably. These balanced solutions have the added advantage of being able to be administered concomitantly with blood product transfusions, whereas lactated Ringer solution cannot because of the presence of lactate, which will cause the formation of a precipitant with the calcium contained in blood products. This is particularly relevant in the operating room, where fluids and blood products are often administered concomitantly through the same intravenous access. Because the SID of the balanced solutions is 50 mEq/L, large volumes of these solutions may lead to a metabolic alkalosis; therefore, careful monitoring is indicated.

Two extemporaneously prepared fluids that provide additional flexibility relative to managing acid-base status are ½ normal saline (0.45% sodium chloride for injection) with sodium bicarbonate 75 mEq/L and sterile water for injection with sodium bicarbonate 150 mEq/L. Both of these solutions are isotonic and have SIDs of 75 mEq/L and 150 mEq/L, respectively. It is recognized that it may not be practical in many clinical settings to routinely use these options, given the need to extemporaneously prepare the solutions. Combining these five intravenous fluid choices, the bedside ICU clinician has options that range from a SID of 0 mEq/L to 150 mEq/L, allowing an ability to carefully adjust and manage acid-base status during continued intravenous fluid resuscitation and maintenance therapy. If we include the options of 0.1N and 0.2N hydrochloric acid infusions, the range of SIDs available will be as low as –200 mEq/L.

Several recent clinical trials have shown that the choice of intravenous fluid in the resuscitation of critically ill patients does affect acid-base status. Chua et al. reported the results of a retrospective comparison of patients resuscitated with Plasma-Lyte 148 or normal saline in the treatment of DKA. Patients who received Plasma-Lyte had quicker resolution of their metabolic acidosis, less risk of developing hyperchloremia, improved urine output, and a higher mean arterial blood pressure at 2–4 hours than did the group of patients who received normal saline.[70] Young and coworkers conducted a randomized, double-blind trial comparing Plasma-Lyte A and normal saline for resuscitation during the first 24 hours after traumatic injury. All patients required blood transfusions and were intubated, and most went to surgery within 60 minutes of arrival. Patients receiving Plasma-Lyte A had a greater resolution of the baseline metabolic acidosis and a lower plasma [Cl–]. The volume of fluids administered and the urine output in the first 24 hours were not different, and there was no difference in mortality.[71] These studies are consistent with the expected effect of a balanced electrolyte solution on acid-base status compared with normal saline; however, they were inadequately powered to show an effect on important clinical outcomes.

A large observational study of patients undergoing major open abdominal surgery compared outcomes for patients receiving normal saline (n = 30,994) or a balanced electrolyte solution (n = 926) on the day of surgery. The saline-treated group had a greater mortality rate (5.6% vs. 2.9%; p<0.001) and more major complications (33.7% vs. 23%; p<0.001). In a propensity-matched sample, patients receiving the balanced electrolyte solution had significantly fewer complications, including postoperative infections, renal failure requiring dialysis, blood transfusions, and electrolyte disturbances. Patients receiving normal saline were also more likely to experience a metabolic acidosis requiring intervention.[16] Yunos and colleagues reported the results of a prospective, open-label, sequential study comparing patients who were treated with chloride-rich intravenous fluids (normal saline, 4% succinylated gelatin solution, or 4% albumin solution) during the control period (n = 760) and a chloride-restrictive fluid (Hartman solution, Plasma-Lyte 148, or chloride-poor 20% albumin) during the intervention period (n = 773). Patients receiving chloride-rich fluids had a significantly greater risk of experiencing acute kidney injury and requiring renal replacement therapy. There were no differences in hospital mortality, hospital or ICU length of stay, or need for renal replacement therapy after discharge.[17] These two studies suggest that resuscitation using chloride-rich intravenous fluids not only increases the risk of hyperchloremic metabolic acidosis, but also contributes to negative outcomes, including renal injury and the need for renal replacement therapy. A double-blind, randomized, crossover study of healthy volunteers receiving a 2-L volume of normal saline or Plasma-Lyte 148 over 1 hour showed that saline was associated with a significantly greater reduction in renal artery blood flow velocity and renal cortical tissue perfusion.[72] This experimental trial provides biologic plausibility that chloride-rich fluids adversely affect renal perfusion and consequently renal function in critically ill patients. However, it has been cautioned that well-controlled, adequately powered studies are needed to confirm or refute the benefits of a balanced electrolyte solution compared with normal saline. Critical care clinicians should treat resuscitation fluids like any other drug available in the ICU. The choice of fluid should be carefully considered in light of the indications, contraindications, and potential adverse effects and then reconsidered regularly according to the patient's metabolic and clinical response.[68]

EXAMPLE CASES

Case 1

The first case is a 57-year-old man with a history of poorly controlled type 2 diabetes, moderate obesity, peripheral vascular disease (after a left femoral-popliteal arterial bypass 2 years before admission), diabetic nephropathy (baseline SCr 1.8 mg/dL), hyperlipidemia, and hypertension. Medications before admission include glyburide, irbesartan, and atorvastatin.

He presents to the emergency department after a several-week history of a poorly healing wound on his left foot, for which he did not seek medical care. On admission, he is obtunded, hypotensive, tachycardic, and breathing rapidly and deeply. His initial blood pressure is reported as 89/43 mm Hg, his heart rate is 131 beats/minute, and his respiratory rate is 37 breaths/minute. He is diaphoretic, febrile to 39.2°C, and in clear respiratory distress. He is emergently intubated and placed on mechanical ventilation. His admission ABG was pH 7.16, $Paco_2$ 23 mm Hg, Pao_2 78 mm Hg, $[HCO_3^-]$ 8 mEq/L, and O_2 saturation 89%. His complete blood cell count showed a white blood cell count (WBC) of 26.7×10^3 cells/mm^3 with 21% bands on differential. His serum chemistries were as follows: Na^+ 138 mEq/L, K^+ 3.9 mEq/L, Cl^- 108 mEq/L, total CO_2 9 mEq/L, albumin 2.1 g/dL, blood glucose 479 mg/dL, SCr 6.2 mg/dL, and blood urea nitrogen (BUN) 64 mg/dL. Lactate was 5.2 mEq/L, and serum ketones were negative. He is oliguric with a urine output of less than 0.5 mL/kg/hour.

Physical examination reveals a necrotic, open, and draining left foot wound with cellulitic tissues surrounding areas of necrosis. The wound has significant surrounding crepitance, and there is concern that this represents early gangrene. There are no palpable pulses in the foot or lower leg. He is admitted with planned transfer to the surgical ICU for resuscitation, mechanical ventilation, and antibiotic therapy together with surgical evaluation. The admitting diagnosis is severe sepsis and septic shock secondary to necrotic, nonviable left foot.

Although a quick review of his laboratory data indicates that he has an elevated AG metabolic acidosis and elevated blood lactate concentration, a stepwise approach to his acid-base assessment is needed to fully understand his status. Taking the stepwise approach, the following results are found:

1. Given his clinical presentation, the following would be expected:

   Severe sepsis/shock – elevated AG metabolic acidosis

   Acute-on-chronic renal injury – elevated AG metabolic acidosis

2. pH = 7.16, consistent with acidemia
3. The $[HCO_3^-]$ = 8 mEq/L and $Paco_2$ = 23 mm Hg are consistent with a principal metabolic acidosis (see Table 1.3).
4. Not applicable. The principal disorder is not respiratory.
5. The secondary disorder equation for a principal metabolic acidosis is:

$$Pa_{co_2} = 1.5 \times [HCO_3^-] + 8 \pm 2$$

$$Paco_2 = 1.5 \times 8 \; mEq/L + 8 \pm 2 = 20 \pm 2 \; mEq/L$$

His actual $Paco_2$ is 23 mm Hg, which, within the limits of these estimates, is consistent with meeting his expected new normal $Paco_2$ for this degree of metabolic acidosis.

6. The equation for calculating the ACAG is (assuming a normal albumin of 4 g/dL):

$$ACAG = ([Na^+] + [K^+]) - ([Cl^-] + [HCO_3^-]) + 2.5([normal \; albumin] - [observed \; albumin])$$

$$ACAG = (138 + 3.9) - (108 + 8) + 2.5(4 - 2.1) = 30.7 \; mEq/L$$

7. The delta ratio equation is:

$$Delta \; Ratio = \frac{ACAG - normal \; AG}{Normal \; [HCO_3^-] - Measured \; [HCO_3^-]}$$

$$= \frac{(ACAG - 12)}{(24 - [HCO_3^-])}$$

$$Delta \; Ratio = \frac{30.7 - 12}{24 - 08} = \frac{18.7}{16} = 1.2$$

8. Not required

The final assessment from taking the stepwise approach is that the patient presented with an elevated AG metabolic acidosis with an appropriate secondary response and no evidence of a concomitant acid-base disorder. This is consistent with the clinical presentation. Of interest, the ALCAG can also be calculated to evaluate for other unmeasured anions contributing to the metabolic acidosis:

$$ALCAG = ACAG - [lactate] = 30.7 - 5.2 = 25.5 \; mEq/L$$

This indicates that there are unmeasured anions making a significant contribution to the metabolic acidosis in addition to lactate. This could be inorganic anions accumulating because of acute-on-chronic renal injury or other products of tissue necrosis and ischemia.

The treatment considerations in this case should be primarily focused on treating the septic shock with fluid resuscitation and vasopressors, if indicated; providing broad-spectrum antibiotics; and, as soon as stabilized, providing definitive surgical management of the source of infection. Fluid resuscitation should include either a bicarbonate-containing solution (e.g., ½ normal saline with 75 mEq/L of $NaHCO_3$) or a balanced electrolyte solution (e.g., Plasma-Lyte A). An initial bolus of 50–100 mEq of $NaHCO_3$ could be considered given his baseline pH of 7.16; however, giving prompt fluid resuscitation with an alkaline solution and providing mechanical ventilation will likely make this unnecessary. Targets are a central venous pressure of 8–12 mm Hg (if available) and a mean arterial pressure greater than 60–65 mm Hg.

His initial management in the emergency department consisted of fluid resuscitation with normal saline (about 70 mL/kg total), and, because of persistently low mean arterial pressure, an infusion of epinephrine was initiated and titrated to an infusion rate of 0.4 mcg/kg/hour. His mean arterial pressure is currently 65–68 mm Hg, and his urine output has improved to greater than 0.5 mL/kg/hour. Broad-spectrum antibiotics were initiated early. About 4 hours after presentation, laboratory testing was repeated, with ABG results of pH 7.31, $Paco_2$ 29 mm Hg, Pao_2 98 mm Hg, HCO_3^- 14 mEq/L, and O_2 saturation 96%. Lactate is improved but still elevated at 4.4 mEq/L. Serum chemistry results are Na^+ 141 mEq/L, K^+ 3.5 mEq/L, and Cl^- 116 mEq/L.

Using the stepwise approach, the results now show a principal metabolic acidosis and partial resolution of the elevated AG (ACAG is 19.3 mEq/L); however, the delta ratio is now 0.7 mEq/L, consistent with a concomitant normal AG, hyperchloremic metabolic acidosis presumably because of the large volume of normal saline administered. Despite the improvement in hemodynamics and urine output suggesting successful resuscitation, the lactate concentration remains elevated. Failure to clear lactate may be associated with a higher risk of mortality.[15] In this case, the persistently elevated lactate concentration may be a result of using epinephrine vasopressor therapy, which may increase aerobic glycolysis and contribute to a type B lactic acidosis.[37–39] At this point, the patient's fluid therapy should be changed to a bicarbonate-containing or balanced solution as initially recommended, and his epinephrine infusion should be transitioned to norepinephrine, which is less likely to increase lactate production. The stepwise approach showed a change in the acid-base status in this case secondary to iatrogenic factors that may not have been readily evident without a complete workup of the acid-base status. Fully understanding the acid-base disorder affected the therapeutic decisions for this patient.

Case 2

The second case is a 19-year-old man who was previously healthy. He was a non-restrained driver involved in a rollover motor vehicle accident and has sustained a significant traumatic brain injury (Glasgow Coma Scale score 8) together with many orthopedic injuries, including a significant crush injury to his right lower extremity with clinical evidence of compartment syndrome. The trauma team has opened the fascia of the anterior and posterior compartments of the right lower extremity. He was resuscitated with intravenous normal saline and is intubated, mechanically ventilated, and presently in the trauma ICU. His laboratory values include Na^+ 134 mEq/L, K^+ 4.6 mEq/L, Cl^- 114 mEq/L, and albumin 1.4 g/dL. His most recent ABG is pH 7.36, $Paco_2$ 22 mm Hg, Pao_2 97 mm Hg, HCO_3^- 12 mEq/L, and O_2 saturation 99%. He has evidence of rhabdomyolysis secondary to the crush injury with a creatine kinase of 12,540 U/L, SCr 1.4 mg/dL, and BUN 28 mg/dL, and he is relatively oliguric (urine output 25–50 mL/hour).

Using the stepwise approach to his acid-base status provides the following results:

1. The clinical presentation would suggest the following:
   Crush injury/rhabdomyolysis – elevated AG metabolic acidosis
   Resuscitation with normal saline – hyperchloremic metabolic acidosis
   Traumatic brain injury – respiratory alkalosis
2. pH = 7.36 is on the low end of the normal range.
3. $[HCO_3^-]$ = 12 mEq/L and $Paco_2$ = 22 mm Hg are consistent with a principal metabolic acidosis.
4. Not applicable
5.
$$Paco_2 = 1.5 \times [HCO_3^-] + 8 \pm 2$$
$$Paco_2 = 1.5 \times 12 \, mEq/L + 8 \pm 2 = 26 \pm 2 \, mEq/L$$

6. Calculation of the ACAG:
$$ACAG = ([Na^+] + [K^+]) - ([Cl^-] + [HCO_3^-]) + 2.5([normal\ albumin] - [observed\ albumin])$$
$$ACAG = (134 + 4.6) - (114 + 12) + 2.5(4 - 1.4) = 19.1 \, mEq/L$$

7. Calculation of the delta ratio:
$$Delta\ Ratio = \frac{ACAG - normal\ AG}{Normal\ [HCO_3^-] - Measured\ [HCO_3^-]}$$
$$= \frac{(ACAG - 12)}{(24 - [HCO_3^-])}$$
$$Delta\ Ratio = \frac{19.1 - 12}{24 - 12} = \frac{7.1}{12} = 0.6$$

8. Not applicable

The stepwise approach shows that the patient has a combined elevated AG metabolic acidosis, respiratory alkalosis, and normal AG, hyperchloremic metabolic acidosis. These are all consistent with the clinical presentation, but this would not be readily evident without using a stepwise approach because a quick review of the laboratory results would likely conclude that the patient had a compensated elevated AG metabolic acidosis secondary to his crush injury and rhabdomyolysis.

Although there is no urgency to treat the acid-base disorder, changing his current intravenous fluid therapy to a balanced electrolyte solution or a bicarbonate-containing intravenous solution is important to prevent worsening hyperchloremic metabolic acidosis. Performing a baseline and follow-up lactate concentration is recommended to monitor the effectiveness of treating the compartment syndrome, and the patient's acid-base status should be closely monitored, given that resolution of the AG and non-AG metabolic acidoses may lead to a significant alkalemia because of the concomitant respiratory alkalosis. Changes to minute ventilation should be tried to increase $Paco_2$; however, sedation may be needed if the patient has a persistent respiratory alkalosis despite ventilator setting changes. Additional dead space in the ventilator circuit could also be considered. A full understanding of this combined acid-base disorder permits the development of a comprehensive therapeutic plan relative to his acid-base status.

Case 3

The patient described in case 1 with the necrotic left foot and severe sepsis was stabilized and underwent left below-the-knee amputation. Early in the management of his severe sepsis, he required considerable fluid resuscitation to achieve and maintain goal hemodynamics, and his weight increased from a baseline 92 kg to 123 kg with evidence of significant peripheral edema. By day 5 of his hospital stay, he was hemodynamically stable and off all vasopressors, his SCr had decreased to 2.1 mg/dL, and he was making 30–50 mL/hour of urine. Because of a concern that the peripheral edema would impair his ability to wean from mechanical ventilation and increase his risk of skin breakdown, he was initiated on a continuous furosemide infusion at a rate of 4 mg/hour, resulting in a brisk diuresis. During the next 48 hours, he remained hemodynamically stable and had diuresed almost 16 L of fluid. His peripheral edema was markedly improved, and he was making progress weaning from mechanical ventilation. Morning laboratory results included an ABG with pH 7.52, $Paco_2$ 46 mm Hg, Pao_2 73 mm Hg, HCO_3^- 36 mEq/L, and O_2 saturation 92%. Serum chemistry results were Na^+ 138 mEq/L, K^+ 3.8 mEq/L, Cl^- 98 mEq/L, total CO_2 37 mEq/L, lactate 0.9 mEq/L, and albumin 2.1 g/dL. Given his stable hemodynamics, unchanged renal function tests, and continued need to remove excess fluids, the ICU team would like to continue diuresis with the goal of potentially shortening his time on mechanical ventilation and ICU length of stay.

The stepwise approach to his acid-base status results in the following analysis:
1. The clinical story since resolution of his initial severe sepsis is consistent with:
   Loop diuretic use – metabolic alkalosis
   Chronic renal disease – elevated AG metabolic acidosis, or possible normal AG metabolic acidosis
2. pH = 7.49 indicating alkalemia
3. $[HCO_3^-]$ = 36 mEq/L and $Paco_2$ = 46 mm Hg are consistent with a principal metabolic alkalosis.
4. Not indicated
5. The equation for the secondary change because of metabolic alkalosis is (see Table 1.4):
   The actual $Paco_2$ is 46 mm Hg, indicating that the secondary response is appropriate for his current $[HCO_3^-]$.
6. His ACAG is not elevated at 11.6 mEq/L.
7. Not indicated
8. Not indicated

The stepwise process shows that the patient has a metabolic alkalosis with an appropriate secondary respiratory response. Discontinuing the loop diuretic and administering normal saline adequate to replete the Cl^- deficit would be an effective treatment for this chloride-responsive metabolic alkalosis; however, that would be counterproductive to the goals of the ICU team to remove fluid and resolve his peripheral edema. The initial recommended treatment option is to administer acetazolamide (500 mg intravenously for one dose) to increase urinary Na^+ excretion and decrease SID. In our experience, this is adequate to lower $[HCO_3^-]$ with improvement in the metabolic alkalosis despite continuing diuresis; however, the effect is usually short-lived (24–36 hours). If, after that intervention, there is a continued need to diurese the patient, the chloride deficit can be replaced using an infusion of dilute 0.1N hydrochloric acid intravenous solution. Although the dose can be based on a calculation of the Cl^- deficit, we recommend starting at 40 mL/hour in an adult patient and adjusting the infusion according to the response, using the safety precautions discussed previously. A hydrochloric acid infusion can also be used as an initial treatment option in lieu of acetazolamide.

Case 4

The fourth case is a 76-year-old woman admitted to the hospital with a small bowel obstruction and 3 days of vomiting. Her medical history is significant for chronic obstructive lung disease (home O_2-dependent), hypertension, and hypercholesterolemia. She had a nasogastric tube inserted and placed to wall suction and was draining about 1 L per day. Her abdominal examination was considered benign, and she was admitted to the medical service for conservative management. On the second day of her hospitalization, she developed a temperature to 39.5°C, her WBC was elevated to 28.2 × 10³ cells/mm³, and she developed hypotension and tachycardia. She was tachypneic, diaphoretic, and clearly in respiratory distress. Just before intubation, her ABG results were pH 7.23, $Paco_2$ 36 mm Hg, Pao_2 74 mm Hg, HCO_3^- 15 mEq/L, and O_2 saturation 90%. Her chemistries showed the following: Na^+ 141 mEq/L, K^+ 3.9 mEq/L, Cl^- 105 mEq/L, and albumin 1.9 g/dL. Lactate was 5.8 mEq/L. She was initiated on broad-spectrum antibiotics, and resuscitative efforts were initiated. Surgery was consulted for evaluation and potential surgical management.

From the perspective of her acid-base status, the stepwise approach provides the following analysis:

1. Given the clinical presentation, the following would be expected:
   Chronic obstructive lung disease – chronic respiratory acidosis
   Respiratory failure – acute-on-chronic respiratory acidosis
   Sepsis/shock – elevated AG metabolic acidosis
   Vomiting/nasogastric tube losses – chloride-responsive metabolic alkalosis
2. pH = 7.23, indicating acidemia
3. $[HCO_3^-]$ = 15 mEq/L and $Paco_2$ = 36 mm Hg are consistent with a principal metabolic acidosis.
4. Given the principal disorder, this step could be skipped; however, given the history, it is likely this patient has a chronic respiratory acidosis. Her admission laboratory results included $[HCO_3^-]$ 38 mEq/L. Although that could represent a metabolic alkalosis secondary to her 3-day history of vomiting, it is also consistent with a chronic respiratory acidosis. Her acute respiratory failure may result in an acute-on-chronic respiratory acidosis that may confuse the interpretation of her secondary response to the metabolic acidosis.
5.
$$Paco_2 = 1.5 \times [HCO_3^-] + 8 \pm 2$$
$$Paco_2 = 1.5 \times 15 \ mEq/L + 8 \pm 2 = 30.5 \pm 2 \ mEq/L$$

   The actual $Paco_2$ is 36 mm Hg, consistent with a concomitant respiratory acidosis.
6.
$$ACAG = ([Na^+] + [K^+]) - ([Cl^-] + [HCO_3^-]) + 2.5([normal\ albumin] - [observed\ albumin])$$

$$ACAG = (141 + 3.9) - (108 + 15) + 2.5(4 - 1.9) = 33.2 \ mEq/L$$

7.
$$Delta\ Ratio = \frac{ACAG - normal\ AG}{Normal\ [HCO_3^-] - Measured\ [HCO_3^-]}$$
$$= \frac{(ACAG - 12)}{(24 - [HCO_3^-])}$$

$$Delta\ Ratio = \frac{33.2 - 12}{24 - 15} = \frac{21.2}{9} = 2.4$$

8. Not indicated

This patient has a triple acid-base disorder with concomitant elevated AG metabolic acidosis, respiratory acidosis, and metabolic alkalosis. This is consistent with the clinical presentation, and the metabolic alkalosis component is likely a combination of upper GI secretory losses and underlying chronic respiratory acidosis.

As with case 1, treatment of this patient must be focused on managing her severe sepsis, including fluid resuscitation with a balanced solution (e.g., Plasma-Lyte A), vasopressors as indicated according to response to fluids, broad-spectrum antibiotics, ventilator support, and appropriate surgical source control. Her presumed chronic respiratory acidosis will need to be considered in her treatment. Although reducing $Paco_2$ during mechanical ventilation may have some short-term benefit in the acute management of her metabolic acidosis, the goal longer term will need to be achieving a $Paco_2$ closer to her suspected baseline and administering bicarbonate-containing intravenous fluids to keep her $[HCO_3^-]$ close to her admission value. This will prepare this patient for the best chance of successfully weaning from mechanical ventilation when her condition improves. The metabolic alkalosis from upper nasogastric tube losses should improve with fluid resuscitation.

CONCLUSION

Acid-base disorders are common in critically ill patients, are often complex mixed disorders, and are associated with significant morbidity and mortality. A thorough stepwise approach to evaluating the acid-base status of an ICU patient is required to fully understand all contributors to the status of the patient and best inform the therapeutic approach and necessary monitoring plan. Although we acknowledge the practicality of taking a traditional bicarbonate-based approach to the diagnostic evaluation of acid-base status, this model is inadequate to explain the underlying physiology and therefore the most appropriate approach to treating the patient. The physiochemical model with its emphasis on the independent parameters that affect acid-base status, namely $Paco_2$, SID, and A_{TOT}, provides a clearer understanding of the causes and subsequent treatment approaches to complex acid-base disturbances. With advances in technology and automation and integrated electronic medical records, a bedside diagnostic approach using the Figge-Stewart model may be readily available in all ICUs and could become the routine diagnostic approach to acid-base disorders; however, this will require changes to how we teach students and trainees relative to the diagnosis and management of acid-base disturbances.

REFERENCES

1. Cusack RJ, Rhodes A, Lochhead P, et al. The strong ion gap does not have prognostic value in critically ill patients in a mixed medical/surgical adult ICU. Intensive Care Med 2002;28:864–9.
2. Martin M, Murray J, Berne T, et al. Diagnosis of acid-base derangements and mortality prediction in the trauma intensive care unit: the physiochemical approach. J Trauma 2005;58:238–43.
3. Dubin A, Menises MM, Masevicius FD, et al. Comparison of three different methods of evaluation of metabolic acid-base disorders. Crit Care Med 2007;35:1264–70.
4. Chawla LS, Shih S, Davison D, et al. Anion gap, anion gap corrected for albumin, base deficit and unmeasured anions in critically ill patients: implications on the assessment of metabolic acidosis and the diagnosis of hyperlactatemia. BMC Emerg Med 2008;8:18.
5. Liborio AB, Noritomi DT, Leite TT, et al. Increased serum bicarbonate in critically ill patients: a retrospective analysis. Intensive Care Med 2015;41:479–86.
6. Kellum JA. Determinants of blood pH in health and disesase. Crit Care 2000;4:6–14.
7. Gennari FJ, Weise WJ. Acid-base disturbances in gastrointestinal disease. Clin J Am Soc Nephr 2008;3:1861–8.
8. Morris CG, Low J. Metabolic acidosis in the critically ill. Part 2. Causes and treatment. Anaesthesia 2008;63:396–411.
9. Kellum JA. Disorders of acid-base balance. Crit Care Med 2007;35:2630–6.
10. Kellum JA. Metabolic acidosis in patients with sepsis: epiphenomenon or part of the pathophysiology? Crit Care Resusc 2004;6:197–203.
11. Kaplan LJ, Kellum JA. Initial pH, base deficit, lactate, anion gap, strong ion difference, and strong ion gap predict outcome from major vascular surgery. Crit Care Med 2004;32:1120–4.
12. Noritomi DT, Soriano FG, Kellum JA, et al. Metabolic acidosis in patients with severe sepsis and septic shock: a longitudinal quantitative study. Crit Care Med 2009;37:2733–9.
13. Rocktaeschel J, Morimatsu H, Uchino S, et al. Unmeasured anions in critically ill patients: can they predict mortality? Crit Care Med 2003;31:2131–6.
14. Kraut JA, Madias NE. Disorders of fluids and electrolytes: lactic acidosis. N Engl J Med 2014;371:2309–19.
15. Jansen TC, van Bommel J, Schoonderbeek FJ, et al. Early lactate-guided therapy in intensive care unit patients. Am J Respir Crit Care Med 2010;182:752–61.
16. Shaw AD, Bagshaw SM, Goldstein SL, et al. Major complications, mortality, and resource utilization after open abdominal surgery. 0.9% saline compared to Plasma-Lyte. Ann Surg 2012;255:821–9.
17. Yunos NM, Bellomo R, Hegarty C, et al. Association between a chloride-liberal vs chloride-restricted intravenous fluid administration strategy and kidney injury in critically ill adults. JAMA 2012;308:1566–72.
18. Stewart PA. Modern quantitative acid-base chemistry. Can J Physiol Pharmacol 1983;61:1444–61.
19. Stewart PA. How to Understand Acid-Base: A Quantitative Acid-Base Primer for Biology and Medicine. New York: Elsevier, 1981.
20. Morris CG, Low J. Metabolic acidosis in the critically ill. Part 1. Classification and pathophysiology. Anaesthesia 2008;63:294–301.
21. Kraut JA, Madias NE. Serum anion gap: its uses and limitations in clinical medicine. Clin J Am Soc Nephr 2007;2:162–74.
22. Figge J, Jabor A, Kazda A, et al. Anion gap and hypoalbuminemia. Crit Care Med 1998;26:1807–10.
23. Berend K, de Vries APJ, Gans ROB. Disorder of fluids and electrolytes: physiological approach to assessment of acid-base disturbances. N Engl J Med 2014;371:1434–45.
24. Sirker AA, Rhodes A, Grounds RM, et al. Acid-base physiology: the "traditional" and the "modern" approaches. Anaesthesia 2002;57:348–56.
25. Seifter JL. Disorders of fluids and electrolytes: integration of acid-base and electrolyte disorders. N Engl J Med 2014;371:1821–31.
26. Fencl V, Jabor A, Kazda A, et al. Diagnosis of metabolic acid-base distrubances in critically ill patients. Am J Respir Crit Care Med 2000;162:2246–51.
27. Balasubramanyan N, Havens PL, Hoffman GM. Unmeasured anions identified by the Fencl-Stewart method predicts mortality better than base excess, anion gap, and lactate in patients in the pediatric intensive care unit. Crit Care Med 1999;27:1577–81.
28. Kellum JA, Kramer DJ, Pinsky MR. Strong ion gap: a methodology for exploring unexplained anions. J Crit Care 1995;10:51–5.
29. Rinaldi S, De Gaudio AR. Strong ion difference and strong anion gap: the Stewart approach to acid base disturbances. Curr Anaesth Crit Care 2005;16:395–402.
30. Figge J, Rossing TH, Fencl V. The role of serum proteins in acid-base equilibria. J Lab Clin Med 1991;117:453–67.
31. Bruegger D, Jacob M, Scheingraber S, et al. Changes in acid-base balance following bolus infusion of 20% albumin solution in humans. Intensive Care Med 2005;31:1123–7.
32. Kurtz I, Kraut J, Ornekian V, et al. Acid-base analysis: a critique of the Stewart and bicarbonate-centered approaches. Am J Physiol Renal Physiol 2008;294:F1009-F31.
33. Moviat M, van Haren F, van der Hoeven H. Conventional or physiochemical approach in intensive care unit patients with metabolic acidosis. Crit Care 2003;7:R41-R5.
34. Rastegar A. Use of the $\Delta AG/\Delta HCO_3^-$ ratio in the diagnosis of mixed acid-base disorders. J Am Soc Nephrol 2007;18:2429–31.
35. Christopher MM, Eckfeldt JH, W EJ. Propylene glycol ingestion causes D-lactic acidosis. Lab Invest 1990;62:114–8.
36. Nelsen JL, Haas CE, Habtemariam B, et al. A prospective evaluation of propylene glycol clearance and accumulation during continuous-infusion lorazepam in critically ill patients. J Intensive Care Med 2008;23:184–94.
37. Levy B, Bollaert PE, Charpentier C, et al. Comparison of norepinephrine and dobutamine to epinephrine for hemodynamics, lactate metabolism, and gastric tonometric variables in septic shock: a prospective, randomized study. Intensive Care Med 1997;23:282–7.

38. Levy B, Desebbe O, Montemont C, et al. Increased aerobic glycolysis through β2 stimulation is a common mechanism involved in lactate formation during shock states. Shock 2008;30:417–21.
39. Myburgh JA, Higgins A, Jovanovska A, et al. A comparison of epinephrine and norepinephrine in critically ill patients. Intensive Care Med 2008;34:2226–34.
40. Dellinger RP, Levy MM, Rhodes A, et al. Surviving sepsis campaign: international guidelines for management of severe sepsis and septic shock: 2012. Crit Care Med 2013;41:580–637.
41. Gunnerson KJ, Saul M, He S, et al. Lactate versus non-lactate metabolic acidosis: a retrospective outcome evaluation of critically ill patients. Crit Care 2006;10:R22.
42. Kitabchi AE, Umpierrez GE, Miles JM, et al. Hyperglycemic crises in adult patients with diabetes. Diabetes Care 2009;32:1335–43.
43. Kamel KS, Halperin ML. Disorders of fluids and electrolytes: acid-base problems in diabetic ketoacidosis. N Engl J Med 2015;372:546–54.
44. Carlesso E, Maiocchi G, Tallarini F, et al. The rule regulating pH changes during crystalloid infusion. Intensive Care Med 2011;37:461–8.
45. Gattinoni L, Carlesso E, Maiocchi G, et al. Dilutional acidosis: where do the protons come from? Intensive Care Med 2009;35:2033–43.
46. Wolfsdorf J, Craig ME, Daneman D, et al. ISPAD clinical practice consensus guidelines 2009 compendium: diabetic ketoacidosis in children and adolescents with diabetes. Pediatr Diabetes 2009;10:118–33.
47. Adrogue HJ, Madias NE. Management of life-threatening acid-base disorders. N Engl J Med 1998;338:26–34.
48. Kraut JA, Madias NE. Treatment of acute metabolic acidosis: a pathophysiologic approach. Nat Rev Nephrol 2012;8:589–601.
49. Kraut JA, Kurtz I. Use of base in the treatment of severe acidemic states. Am J Kid Dis 2001;38:703–27.
50. Gehlbach BK, Schmidt GA. Bench-to-bedside review: treating acid-base abnormalities in the intensive care unit – the role of buffers. Crit Care 2004;8:259–65.
51. Levraut J, Garcia P, Giunti C, et al. The increase in CO2 production induced by NaHCO3 depends on blood albumin and hemoglobin concentrations. Intensive Care Med 2000;26:558–64.
52. Levraut J, Giunti C, Ciebiera JP, et al. Initial effect of sodium bicarbonate on intracellular pH depends on the extracellular nonbicarbonate buffering capacity. Crit Care Med 2001;29:1033–9.
53. Rehm M, Finsterer U. Treating intraoperative hyperchloremic acidosis with sodium bicarbonate or tris-hydroxymethyl aminomethane: a randomized prospective study. Anesth Analg 2003;96:1201–8.
54. Heering P, Ivens K, Thumer O, et al. The use of different buffers during continuous hemofiltration in critically ill patients with acute renal failure. Intensive Care Med 1999;25:1244–51.
55. Gennari FJ. Pathophysiology of metabolic alkalosis: a new classification based on the centrality of stimulated collecting duct ion transport. Am J Kidney Dis 2011;58:626–36.
56. Mazur JE, Devlin JW, Peters MJ, et al. Single versus multiple doses for acetazolamide for metabolic alkalosis in critically ill medical patients: a randomized, double-blind trial. Crit Care Med 1999;27:1257–61.
57. Moviat M, Pickkers P, van der Voort PHJ, et al. Acetazolamide-mediated decrease in strong ion difference accounts for the correction of metabolic alkalosis in critically ill patients. Crit Care 2006;10:R14.
58. Brimioulle S, Berre J, Dufaye P, et al. Hydrochloric acid infusion for treatment of metabolic alkalosis associated with respiratory acidosis. Crit Care Med 1989;17:232–6.
59. Brimioulle S, Vincent JL, Dufaye P, et al. Hydrochloric acid infusion for treatment of metabolic alkalosis: effects on acid-base balance and oxygenation. Crit Care Med 1985;13:738–42.
60. Kwun KB, Boucherlt T, Wong J, et al. Treatment of metabolic alkalosis wiht intravenous infusion of concentrated hydrochloric acid. Am J Surg 1983;146:328–30.
61. Reisman RI, Puri VK. Prolonged intravenous hydrochloric acid infusion for severe metabolic alkalosis. Intensive Care Med 1982;8:301–3.
62. Wagner CW, Nesbit RR, Mansberger AR. The use of intravenous hydrochloric acid in the treatment of thirty-four patients with metabolic alkalosis. Am Surgeon 1980;46:140–6.
63. Worthley LI. The ratinoal use of i.v. hydrochloric acid in the treatment of metabolic alkalosis. Br J Anaesth 1977;49:811–7.
64. Buchanan IB, Campbell BT, Peck MD, et al. Chest wall necrosis and death secondary to hydrochloric acid infusion for metabolic alkalosis. South Med J 2005;98:822–4.
65. Jankauskas SJ, Gursel E, Antonenko DR. Chest wall necrosis secondary to hydrochloric acid use in the treatment of metabolic alkalosis. Crit Care Med 1989;17:963–4.
66. Devlin JW, Matzke GR. Acid-base disorders. In: DiPiro JT, Talbert RL, Yee GC, et al., eds. Pharmacotherapy A Pathophysiologic Approach, 8th ed. New York: McGraw Hill, 2011:923–42.
67. Alfaro V, Torras R, Ibanez J, et al. A physical-chemical analysis of the acid-base response to chronic obstructive pulmonary disease. Can J Physiol Pharmacol 1996;74:1229–35.
68. Myburgh JA, Mythen MG. Resuscitation fluids. N Engl J Med 2013;369:1243–51.
69. Omron EM, Omron RM. A physiochemical model of crystalloid infusion on acid-base status. J Intensive Care Med 2010;25:271–80.
70. Chua HR, Venkatesh B, Stachowski E, et al. Plasma-lyte 148 vs 0.9% saline for fluid resuscitation in diabetic ketoacidosis. J Crit Care 2012;27:138–45.
71. Young JB, Utter GH, Schermer CR, et al. Saline versus Plasma-lyte A in initial resuscitation of trauma patients. A randomized trial. Ann Surg 2014;259:255–62.
72. Chowdhury AH, Cox EF, Francis ST, et al. A randomized, controlled, double-blind crossover study on the effects of 2-L infusions of 0.9% saline and Plasma-lyte 148 on renal blood flow velocity and renal cortical tissue perfusion in healthy volunteers. Ann Surg 2012;256:18–24.

Chapter 2

Fluid Therapy in the Critically Ill Patient

Brian L. Erstad, Pharm.D., FCCP, BCPS

LEARNING OBJECTIVES

1. Discriminate between the concepts of osmolality, osmolarity, and tonicity.
2. Compute the osmolarity of monovalent ions and albumin in an intravenous solution.
3. Explain the upper and lower limits of osmolarity for fluids or medications being administered by peripheral veins.
4. Describe the concept of a balanced intravenous crystalloid solution.
5. Compare the efficacy and adverse effect profiles of commercially available intravenous colloid solutions.
6. Characterize the properties of albumin that distinguish it from other colloids.
7. Summarize the findings of the large randomized controlled trials that have involved intravenous crystalloid and colloid comparisons.
8. Describe treatment considerations that are unique to the following subsets of critically ill patients requiring fluid resuscitation: trauma, severe sepsis/septic shock, and burns.
9. Explain the concerns of overly aggressive intravenous fluid administration for resuscitating patients in shock.
10. Appraise the benefits and limitations of invasive monitoring techniques that have been used for patients undergoing resuscitation.
11. Summarize the appropriate uses of colloids and crystalloids for resuscitating critically ill patients.

ABBREVIATIONS IN THIS CHAPTER

ARDS	Acute respiratory distress syndrome
CVP	Central venous pressure
ICU	Intensive care unit
RCT	Randomized controlled trial
ROC	Resuscitation Outcomes Consortium
TTE	Transthoracic echocardiography

Groups and Organizations

ALBIOS study	Albumin Italian Outcome Sepsis
ANZICS group	Australian and New Zealand Intensive Care Society
ARISE study	Australasian Resuscitation in Sepsis Evaluation
CHEST study	Crystalloid versus Hydroxyethyl Starch Trial
CRISTAL study	Colloids versus Crystalloids for the Resuscitation of the Critically Ill
CRYSTMAS study	Crystalloids Morbidity Associated with Severe Sepsis
EARSS study	Early Albumin Resuscitation for Sepsis and Septic Shock
EGDT group	Early Goal-Directed Therapy
FACTT	Fluid and Catheter Treatment Trial
FACTT Lite	Fluid and Catheter Treatment Trial Lite
FEAST study	Fluid Expansion as Supportive Therapy
ProCESS study	Protocolized Care for Early Septic Shock
ProMISe study	Protocolised Management in Sepsis
SAFE study	Saline versus Albumin Fluid Evaluation
6S study	Scandinavian Starch for Severe Sepsis/Septic Shock
VISEP study	Efficacy of Volume Substitution and Insulin Therapy in Severe Sepsis

INTRODUCTION

Discussions of fluid therapy in critically ill patients often devolve into a debate of colloid versus crystalloid administration. This is an oversimplification as well as an inappropriately restrictive dialogue of the important considerations associated with choosing and administering fluids to critically ill patients. The primary purpose of this chapter is to discuss important considerations when using intravenous crystalloid and colloid solutions for acute resuscitation. This first major section of this chapter will cover the general properties of these intravenous solutions, beginning with a discussion of the concepts of osmolality, osmolarity, and tonicity and whether central line access is indicated for fluid administration. A historical perspective for each of the more common intravenous fluids will be provided that leads into a discussion of more recent investigations. Albumin will be a major focus of the colloid discussion because it was the first colloid to receive widespread use in the clinical setting, has been the subject of much research, and is the standard of comparison for other colloids. The next two sections will review the most important and influential studies involving crystalloids and colloids in critically ill patients and major subsets of critically ill patients. This will be followed by sections on dosing and assessment issues related to fluid administration, with an abbreviated discussion of maintenance fluids post-resuscitation. The final section is devoted to general recommendations for the use of intravenous crystalloids and colloids in critically ill patients.

OVERVIEW OF CRYSTALLOIDS AND COLLOIDS USED IN CRITICALLY ILL PATIENTS

General Considerations

Disruptions in normal gastrointestinal and circulatory homeostasis in critically ill patients commonly necessitate the administration of intravenous fluid solutions to maintain oxygen delivery and associated cellular processes. From a macrocirculation standpoint, oxygen delivery is a function of three parameters: cardiac output, hemoglobin, and oxygen content (more specifically oxygen saturation). Under normal circulatory conditions, oxygen delivery greatly exceeds the amount of oxygen uptake needed by tissues (i.e., delivery-independent), but during more severe forms of shock, oxygen consumption by tissues is directly linked to oxygen delivery (i.e., delivery-dependent). Therefore, in patients undergoing resuscitation for shock, intravenous crystalloid and colloid solutions are given to increase plasma volume and optimize cardiac output. Regardless of the specific type of shock (e.g., hypovolemic, distributive, obstructive, cardiogenic), adequate intravascular expansion with fluids must be ensured. This includes patients with septic shock, who usually must receive at least 20 mL/kg of fluids to be classified as having refractory hypotension and be enrolled in randomized controlled trials (RCTs). Of the patients with septic shock who have met the criteria for study entry in large RCTs, around 25%–35% respond to intravenous fluids in conjunction with infection control and do not require additional vasoactive support. From a regional circulation or microcirculation standpoint, maintenance and monitoring of circulatory homeostasis is more complicated and depends on the type and severity of shock. For example, in the early hyperdynamic phase of sepsis, cardiac output typically increases to above-normal values in patients without preexisting cardiac disease, but local or regional shunting prevents selected tissues from benefiting from this enhanced global oxygen delivery. Together with the increased recognition of the importance of microcirculatory changes associated with states of impaired perfusion and the implications for fluid administration, there has been an increased appreciation of the pharmacologic actions of intravenous resuscitation fluids beyond simple plasma expansion. There is now a better understanding of how the electrolyte composition of intravenous fluids influences acid-base status (see Chapter 1 for a more in-depth discussion), how particular electrolytes such as chloride may have adverse effects beyond acid-base disturbances, and how certain colloidal products (particularly albumin) have physicochemical properties that may improve or worsen patient outcomes, depending on the specific clinical scenario.

Oncotic Pressure, Osmolality, Osmolarity, and Tonicity

From 1994 to 1998, the U.S. Food and Drug Administration (FDA) received 10 reports of patients who developed hemolysis after being administered an inappropriately diluted albumin solution. The details surrounding the hospital course of two of these patients (one who died) were discussed in an issue of *Morbidity and Mortality Weekly Report* published in 1999.[1] The hemolytic events occurred when a shortage of 5% albumin led hospital pharmacists to prepare a 5% albumin solution by diluting 25% albumin with sterile water for injection. This resulted in an albumin solution that was about one-fifth the osmolarity of normal plasma. In five of the reported cases, the pharmacists had used a reference handbook on injectable drugs for instructions on the albumin dilution process, but the version of the text being used contained erroneous information. Instead of using sterile water for injection for the dilution procedure, the pharmacists should have used a fluid such as normal saline or 5% dextrose in water to dilute the 25% albumin. These were preventable adverse events that would not have occurred had the involved pharmacists had an appreciation of osmolarity. The purpose of this section of the chapter is to provide definitions for the terms *oncotic pressure*, *osmolality*, *osmolarity*, and *tonicity*. Examples will be used to show how osmolarity is calculated for common intravenous fluids, and practical recommendations will be provided to help the clinician determine when low- and high-osmolarity intravenous solutions should be given by central versus peripheral intravenous lines.

Albumin is a plasma protein responsible for around 75% of *oncotic* pressure, but less than 1% of total osmotic pressure, in the blood. For this discussion, the term *colloid osmotic pressure* as an alternative to oncotic pressure will not be used because the former term causes confusion with respect to the measurement or estimation of osmotic pressure in the blood. Under physiological conditions, albumin does not readily pass through the semipermeable capillary membrane, so it is one of the main factors affecting transcapillary fluid movement through its oncotic activity. It is possible to measure oncotic activity with an oncometer, but this testing is not routinely available in the clinical setting. Because it is the number, not the size, of particles that determines osmolality/osmolarity, albumin exerts only a small amount of the total osmotic pressure in blood compared with other solutes like electrolytes. Osmolality is the measure of solute expressed in milliosmoles per kilogram (mOsm/kg) of solvent. The denominator of the units is expressed in kilograms because osmolality is reported by an osmometer in a clinical laboratory using methods such as freezing point depression (the gold standard) or vapor pressure and is not altered by changes in pressure or temperature. Osmolarity is the measure of solute expressed in milliosmoles per liter (mOsm/L) of solvent It is usually estimated from calculations made in serum laboratory indices (e.g., 2 × serum sodium + BUN/2.8 + glucose/18). From an intravenous medication or fluid administration standpoint, differences in the definitions of osmolality or osmolarity based on the denominator of each have little clinical importance because blood has a relatively constant temperature and pressure. For the remainder of this discussion, *osmole* or *osmolarity* will be used for simplicity.

Although osmolarity is a property irrespective of a membrane, osmolarity is referenced to fluid movement across the red blood cell membrane when referring to intravenous fluid administration. A hypo-osmolar solution will *tend* to move water into red blood cells, and a hyperosmolar solution will *tend* to move water out of red blood cells. The word *tend* is italicized because some osmoles such as urea equilibrate across cell membranes and cause no net fluid movement in or out of cells, although a high BUN would elevate blood osmolality as measured by a clinical laboratory. The fluid shifts associated with osmolarity differences are considered to occur during or within 1–2 hours after intravenous medication or fluid infusion. The calculated osmolarity of monovalent electrolytes in solution are straightforward if the usual assumption of complete dissociation is made. Using the example of an intravenous sodium chloride solution in which a milliequivalent per liter (mEq/L) equals a milliosmole per liter (mOsm/L), a 0.45% saline solution has 77 mEq/L (i.e., 77 mOsm/L) of sodium and 77 mEq/L (i.e., 77 mOsm/L) of chloride for a total osmolarity of 154 mOsm/L. This hypo-osmolar solution represents the lower limit of osmolarity usually tolerated by peripheral veins compared with the reference standard of normal blood osmolarity of around 300 mOsm/L. Normal saline with an osmolarity of 308 mOsm/L is considered iso-osmolar.

Tonicity is often called "effective osmolality" because it equals the sum of concentrations of *effective* solutes (not ineffective solutes such as urea) that exert osmotic activity after an intravenous solution has been administered and subsequently distributed into body fluid compartments, resulting in a state of final equilibrium. In the body, tonicity is referenced with respect to the cell membrane, so *isotonic* refers to no net fluid shift between the intracellular and the extracellular compartments. *Hypotonic* refers to expansion of intracellular fluid, and *hypertonic* refers to contraction or shrinkage of intracellular fluid, each with respect to the extracellular fluid compartment; as with osmolarity, extremes of tonicity cause cell damage. Taken together, osmolarity and tonicity can be used to describe common intravenous solutions. For example, normal saline is iso-osmolar and isotonic. A 5% dextrose solution is relatively iso-osmolar (252 mOsm/L) but hypotonic (two-thirds of the volume after final distribution is contained by the intracellular compartment and one-third by the extracellular compartment). A 25% dextrose solution (assuming adequate endogenous or exogenous insulin) would be hyperosmolar but hypotonic. However, a 25% dextrose solution administered to a patient with insulin deficiency likely would be considered both hyperosmolar and hypertonic, because the dextrose would not cross the cell membrane to be oxidized as it would under normal conditions.

Of note, ex vivo experiments of potential red blood cell lysis is a unique situation from a terminology perspective. In such experiments, red blood cells are added to various solutions to see whether the integrity of the red cell membrane is maintained. If hemolysis occurs, a solution is considered hypotonic or hypertonic, depending on the mechanism of cell damage.

Osmolarity is a function of the number of particles in solution and is independent of size or weight of particles. If 8 albumin molecules (MW 67,000) and 16 glucose molecules (MW 180.16) were separated by a semipermeable membrane in sterile water for injection, the water would move toward the glucose molecules because osmolarity is independent of size and weight. Thus, although the molecular weight and size of albumin are much greater compared with ions such as sodium or chloride, commercially available albumin solutions would have unacceptably low osmolarity if the solutions did not contain other additives with osmotic activity (usually sodium and chloride). See

Appendix 2.1 for an example of osmolarity calculations involving albumin.

Peripheral vs. Central Line Administration

Osmolarity is one of the main factors that determines whether fluids (or medications) should be given by intravenous peripheral or central line administration. The toxicity associated with hypo- or hyperosmolar solutions is a function of both the rate and the volume of the infusate administered and the duration of administration in addition to the peripheral or central route of access. Most studies that have evaluated potential osmolarity concerns have used continuous intravenous infusions of solutions for administration periods of at least 10 minutes. About 150 mOsm/L is generally considered the lower limit of osmolarity when infusing products through peripheral veins such as those in the antecubital fossa. Even a 0.45% sodium chloride solution with 154 mOsm/L will cause irritation and burning when infused through peripheral veins in some patients. In addition to causing a patient pain, administering hypo-osmolar solutions by peripheral veins may cause vein destruction, local tissue irritation caused by extravasation, and loss of access for fluid or medication administration. Although the latter local problems are unlikely to occur when central veins are used for infusing hypo-osmolar solutions, hemolysis caused by hypo-osmolarity is a concern regardless of central or peripheral access. Deaths caused by hemolysis and renal failure have been reported with the inadvertent administration of sterile water for injection (0 mOsm/L) in the intensive care unit (ICU) setting.[2]

The upper end of the acceptable range of osmolarity is controversial and often based on hemolysis in animal models, which may not be directly applicable to humans. For example, dog red blood cells are deficient in ATPase, and their permeability to positively charged cations is influenced by cell volume, so they are more fragile than human red blood cells.[3] In one ex vivo study of dog and human red blood cells, no hemolysis occurred when cells were mixed with sodium chloride in dextran solutions to yield osmolarity values of up to 600 mOsm/L (based on detection of free hemoglobin), but increasing hemolysis was noted over a range of 900–2400 mOsm/L.[4] These values of 600 mOsm/L and 900 mOsm/L are the upper limits of osmolarity often used in nursing and pharmacy guidelines or protocols, but another aspect of this study provided more information on osmolarity concerns. In the other part of the study, severely bled dogs were resuscitated with hyperosmolar solutions administered over 10 minutes by peripheral vein or into the right atrium. As defined by plasma-free hemoglobin concentrations, hemolysis was more than 2-fold greater when two hyperosmolar solutions (1.5 mL/kg of 25% sodium chloride in 24% dextran [around 8600 mOsm/L] or 2.5 mL/kg of 15% sodium chloride in 14.4% dextran [around 5200 mOsm/L]) were administered by peripheral vein versus the right atrium. No hemolysis was noted when 5 mL/kg of a 7.5% sodium chloride in a 6% dextran solution (around 2600 mOsm/L) was administered by peripheral vein. The findings of this and related earlier studies served as the basis for the upper limits of osmolarity used in subsequent studies involving the use of hypertonic saline solutions in trauma patients.

Much of the human data relating osmolarity to peripheral vein phlebitis have been derived from studies involving parenteral nutrition solutions, although the methods of assessing phlebitis in these studies varied. In one study, phlebitis occurred in 100% of patients when osmolarity was greater than 600 mOsm/L in those given either parenteral nutrition or crystalloid solutions.[5] In this same study, adding heparin (1000 units/L) to various solutions increased the risk of phlebitis over non–heparin-containing solutions ($p<0.05$). Although this finding seems counterintuitive given the known antiphlebitic actions of heparin, it appeared to be attributable to the increased osmolarity of solutions containing heparin (634 ± 153 vs. 477 ± 100 mOsm/L, $p<0.001$). Other studies have been unable to confirm an association between the osmolarity of parenteral nutrition solutions and the rate of phlebitis. For example, one study found no difference in tolerance using radioactive fibrinogen to assess thrombophlebitis when solutions of 280–1100 mOsm/L were administered.[6] In another study, parenteral nutrition solutions above 600 mOsm/L (630–983 mOsm/L) were well tolerated, and fat emulsion did not influence the rate or degree of phlebitis.[7] Similarly, there was no difference in phlebitis between the parenteral nutrition solutions of 1200 mOsm/L and 1700 mOsm/L when administered by peripheral lines.[8] The apparent lack of correlation between osmolarity and phlebitis when the solutions are less than around 1000 mOsm/L is at least partly explained by the results of one study involving peripheral vein tolerance of parenteral nutrition solutions of varying macronutrients, osmolarity, volume, and rate of administration.[9] In this study, there was poor correlation between rates of phlebitis, as determined by two observers and by factors such as macronutrient composition or osmolarity. But there was a high correlation ($r=0.95$) between phlebitis and osmolarity rate (osmolarity in mOsm/L times infusion rate in L/hour). The rate of phlebitis after 48 hours was 4%–27% with an osmolarity rate of 84–99 mOsm/hour. The time to onset of phlebitis was not related to the osmolarity rate.

Apart from parenteral nutrition solutions, the most studied high-osmolarity fluid given by peripheral vein in clinical trials has been hypertonic sodium chloride. Hypertonic sodium chloride of up to around 250 mL of a 7.5% solution (2566 mOsm/L) has been remarkably free of apparent complications such as phlebitis or hemolysis when given by one-time or intermittent bolus administration.[10] One of the first reports of the clinical use of 7.5% sodium chloride solutions in patients, not human volunteers, was published in 1989. Patients with penetrating trauma in a prehospital setting were randomized to receive a single 250-mL bolus of either an isotonic crystalloid solution or a 7.5% sodium chloride in 6% dextran 70 solution, each administered by a 14-gauge peripheral catheter. As with the 25 patients in the isotonic crystalloid group, none of the 23 patients randomized to the hypertonic sodium chloride group developed obvious infusion-related complications.[11] In a publication the following year, the potential risks of 7.5% sodium chloride with (n=23) or without (n=32) dextran were compared with lactated Ringer's (n=51) using data collected from two randomized double-blind investigations. There were no significant differences in measured osmolalities between the hypertonic sodium chloride and the lactated Ringer's groups at any time point. Nor was there any evidence of central pontine myelinolysis in the 52 patients who died, including 20 patients with serum osmolality measurements (obtained within 15 minutes in 75% of patients) greater than 350 mOsm/kg.[12] In 14 patients with repeated osmolality measurements, values were less than 350 mOsm/kg within 4–8 hours. There were no significant differences in serum sodium concentrations (a surrogate indicator of osmolality) between hypertonic sodium chloride (with or without dextran) and lactated Ringer's groups. Severe hypernatremia, as defined by a sodium of 160 mEq/L or greater, occurred in 1 of 32 patients administered hypertonic sodium chloride without dextran and in 1 of 24 patients receiving lactated Ringer's (this patient received 7.5% sodium bicarbonate as part of CPR 3–5 minutes before measurement) in one of the randomized trials and in 1 of 23 patients administered hypertonic sodium chloride plus dextran and 0 of 24 patients receiving lactated Ringer's in the other randomized trial. Although the findings from this evaluation of hypertonic sodium chloride solutions must be interpreted in light of the relatively small numbers of patients and potential confounders (e.g., elevated ethanol concentrations), the study is important because it has been cited as a proof-of-safety concept for subsequent investigations, including the two landmark Resuscitation Outcomes Consortium (ROC) trials. The ROC trials did not detail serum osmolality values related to hypertonic sodium chloride administration, but they did report on serum sodium values that can be used to estimate osmolality. In the first ROC trial, sodium concentrations greater than 160 mEq/L necessitating intervention occurred in 2.2% of patients receiving hypertonic sodium chloride, 1% of patients receiving hypertonic sodium chloride plus dextran, and 1.4% of patients receiving normal saline (no significant difference).[13] In the second trial, sodium concentrations greater than 160 mEq/L necessitating intervention occurred in 4.2% of patients receiving hypertonic sodium chloride, 2.9% of patients receiving hypertonic sodium chloride plus dextran, and 2.3% of patients receiving normal saline (no significant difference).[14] Other studies involving single doses of hypertonic sodium chloride have found sodium and chloride concentrations to be about 8–10 mEq/L higher than the values in isotonic crystalloid control groups, but usually less than 155 mEq/L for sodium and less than 120 mEq/L for chloride with no mention of phlebitis.[15,16] Although hypertonic sodium chloride causes acute increases in serum sodium concentrations that correspond with increases in serum osmolality measurements, correlation with other outcomes such as intracranial pressure is poor.[17]

Many of the studies looking at osmolarity issues of peripheral veins are difficult to interpret because they did not control for pH while investigating osmolarity issues. Intravenous solutions need to have a lower pH limit of about 6.5 to exclude acidity as a cause of phlebitis, based on histopathologic evaluations of infused solutions in rabbit ear veins.[18] A pH of 9 seems to be the upper limit of alkaline tolerability according to indirect evidence from infusions of medications such as THAM (tris-hydroxymethyl aminomethane).[19] Even if pH is controlled, osmolarity tolerance is a function of other patient-specific factors such as blood flow, diameter, and integrity of the vein being infused and duration of fluid administration. Histopathologic evaluations after infusions into rabbit ear veins with controlled pH (i.e., greater than 6.5) show that in vessels with poor flow, tolerance decreases as osmolarity increases from 550 mOsm/kg to 820 mOsm/kg; furthermore, tolerance with the 820-mOsm/kg solution is better with a higher infusion rate (i.e., 15 mL/kg/hour vs. 5–10 mL/kg/hour) when given as a 120-mL/kg total dose.[20] As mentioned earlier, the increased tolerance of higher-osmolarity solutions when given as one-time injections at a more rapid rate of administration over a relatively short period may explain how hypertonic sodium chloride solutions with osmolarity values above 2000 mOsm/L were apparently tolerated in studies of trauma patients.[21]

In light of these data, a conservative upper limit of osmolarity for fluids given as continuous infusions into peripheral veins would be 600 mOsm/L. An upper limit of 900 mOsm/L would be more practical for the macronutrient components of total nutrient admixture solutions (dextrose, protein, and fat) given by the peripheral intravenous route, particularly when fluid overload is a concern; however, it should be realized that adding micronutrients is likely to bring the final osmolarity closer to 1000–1100 mOsm/L, which may not be tolerated by patients with fragile vessels, including older adult patients. Similarly, although one-time doses of hypertonic sodium chloride solutions with osmolarities up to 2600 mOsm/L have been given by the peripheral route in clinical studies, a solution osmolarity of 900 mOsm/L is a conservative upper value that should limit the risk of hemolysis when solutions are administered by the peripheral route on a one-time or intermittent basis.[22] Although central veins can tolerate continuous infusions of high-osmolarity solutions because of their larger vessel size and more rapid blood flow rate, hemolysis is still a concern, especially as the infused solutions exceed 2600 mOsm/L. Finally, it is of note that osmolarity is not the only reason for giving intravenous solutions through central veins. Other factors include solutions with extremes of pH or potential for tissue damage if extravasation occurs (e.g., vasopressors).

Sodium Chloride Solutions

Although one of the first electrolyte solutions resembling the sodium, chloride, and bicarbonate content of blood was described in 1832,[23] it was not until 1896 that Hartog Hamburger was given credit for developing a 0.9% sodium chloride solution that was similar in osmolarity to human and animal blood.[24] When "normal saline" became synonymous with 0.9% sodium chloride and common parlance in the scientific community is unclear; furthermore, the terminology is misleading because the fluid does not resemble the amounts or composition of electrolytes in the intravascular compartment or any other fluid compartment of the body.[25]

When given rapidly in large amounts, "normal" saline will cause a hyperchloremic metabolic acidosis compared with other solutions more reflective of usual blood electrolyte composition.[26] Such pH changes, as occur with other intravenous solutions, assume a system that is open to carbon dioxide (i.e., an in vivo system). In an in vitro closed system, the regulators of acid-base status (i.e., carbon dioxide, weak acids, and the strong ion difference) are all diluted to the same degree by common intravenous solutions, resulting in no net pH change regardless of the particular solution being administered.[27] In addition to the metabolic acidosis associated with the high chloride content of normal saline–containing solutions, there is increasing evidence that excess chloride ion is associated with acute kidney injury and possibly increased mortality. The mechanism by which chloride might cause acute kidney injury is not clear, although studies of healthy volunteers have found better renal cortical perfusion with more balanced chloride intravenous solutions. Among other functions, the renal cortex is important for urine concentration, filtration, and metabolic waste regulation. In general, studies investigating the association between chloride and the various clinical outcomes fall into two general categories: studies involving intravenous solutions with more balanced (i.e., closer to normal serum chloride concentrations) versus high chloride concentrations and studies evaluating normal versus high serum chloride concentrations. Early studies investigating this association appeared in the surgery literature, but more recently, a similar concern has been raised in critically ill patients. In one prospective open-label trial, crystalloid and colloid fluids containing at least 128 mmol/L of chloride in a historical control period were compared with crystalloid and colloid fluids containing less than around 110 mmol/L of chloride (which includes the 20% albumin product manufactured in Australia where the study was conducted) during an intervention period in the year after high chloride-containing fluids had been phased out.[28] For the primary end points, the increase in creatinine and incidence of acute kidney injury as defined by RIFLE criteria (injury and failure class) were significantly greater (p=0.03 and p<0.001, respectively) in the historical control (i.e., high chloride fluids) compared with the intervention period; also, the need for renal replacement therapy was greater in the historical control group (p=0.005), although there were no significant differences in mortality or length of stay. Other cohort studies involving critically ill patients have found a relationship between high chloride concentrations in serum or intravenous fluids and increased mortality. Large randomized studies are needed to confirm this association between higher chloride concentrations and adverse outcomes, but the weight of the evidence to date is clearly cause for concern and has raised questions about the use of high chloride solutions as first-line resuscitation fluids.

Hypertonic Sodium Chloride Solutions

In addition to the potential for rapid extracellular expansion with smaller amounts of fluid, mechanistic arguments in favor of hypertonic sodium chloride products have been made. For example, hypertonic sodium chloride solution suppresses, whereas lactated Ringer's solution activates neutrophils in ex vivo models, and there is a concern that neutrophil activation may promote organ injury such as acute respiratory distress syndrome (ARDS).[29]

Of note, there is always the potential for adverse effects with any concentrated electrolyte solution, but there are also nomenclature concerns associated with the use of hypertonic sodium chloride (or hypertonic saline) solutions. In the past, hypertonic saline was often considered synonymous with 3% sodium chloride solution. In reality, any sodium chloride solution above isotonic saline of 0.9% is hypertonic, and commercially available solutions are available up to 23.4%. Therefore, the term *hypertonic saline* is at best misleading and is not sufficient to indicate the prescription of any particular product.

Other Crystalloid Solutions

Normal saline is often called unbalanced because its electrolyte composition does not resemble that of human blood. Attempts have been made to produce so-called balanced electrolyte solutions, although the term *balanced* implies a level of simplicity that does not exist in the clinical setting. Typically, *balanced* refers to congruence of the electrolyte composition of a fluid compared with that of blood in a healthy subject, although the terminology has not been standardized. This makes some sense for electrolytes like sodium and chloride that are primarily distributed into the extracellular compartment, but it makes less sense for electrolytes like potassium that are largely contained in the intracellular compartment. The issue is further complicated by electrolytes such as lactate, acetate, and gluconate that are metabolized over time to bicarbonate equivalents. Depending on the specific composition of electrolytes, the pH of blood might change as a solution is being administered because of strong ion differences and alterations in nonvolatile weak acids (e.g., albumin, phosphate). After fluid and electrolyte administration, blood pH might be further altered by weak acid metabolism, shifts or losses of albumin, or changes in carbon dioxide as might occur with mechanical ventilation. Few critically ill patients consistently have fluid and electrolyte compositions in the normal laboratory ranges for blood, so the amount and type of desired fluid depends on the specific patient. Of importance, because the term *balanced* has not been standardized, some researchers have considered a balanced solution primarily with respect to sodium and chloride concentrations that are less than that of normal saline (but in some cases, still higher than normal concentrations of blood). Perhaps it is more appropriate to refer to these more complex electrolyte solutions as *more* balanced than normal saline.

Arguably, the first solution to be studied as a more balanced alternative to normal saline was Ringer's solution. The origin of Ringer's solution can be traced to experiments by Sydney Ringer in the late 1800s in which he investigated the influence of various electrolytes on frog heart muscle contraction.[30,31] Ringer's solution containing potassium chloride, magnesium chloride, and calcium chloride was subsequently modified by Alexis Hartmann (i.e., Hartmann's solution) by adding sodium lactate.[32] Compared with normal saline, the electrolyte concentrations in Hartmann's solution and lactated Ringer's are more reflective of physiologic blood electrolyte composition. Of importance, there may be differences in the specific concentrations of electrolytes in lactated Ringer's, depending on the manufacturer and country of origin. In the United States, Lactated Ringer's Injection USP contains sodium 130 mmol/L, potassium 4 mmol/L, calcium 1.5 mmol/L, chloride 110 mmol/L, and lactate 28 mmol/L. For comparison, Hartmann's has 0.5 mmol/L more calcium and 1 mmol/L more of the remaining electrolytes. Of note, there are commercially available electrolyte solutions with concentrations of ions that are closer to normal physiologic blood concentrations (particularly with respect to sodium and chloride) than those in lactated Ringer's injection. For example, Plasma-Lyte A and Normosol-R each has the following additives: sodium 140 mmol/L, chloride 98 mmol/L, potassium 5 mmol/L, magnesium 1.5 mmol/L, acetate 27 mmol/L, and gluconate 23 mmol/L. In addition, in contrast to lactated Ringer's, Plasma-Lyte A–like normal saline is compatible with blood products. There is increasing support for these more balanced fluids. For example, a position statement by the Faculty of Intensive Care Medicine, the Royal College of Anaesthesia, the Intensive Care Society, and the College of Emergency Medicine states that balanced solutions "such as Hartmann's injection, Ringer's lactate or Plasma-Lyte 148® may be preferred to 0.9% sodium chloride" for fluid resuscitation in all forms of hypovolemic shock, including sepsis, burns, and trauma.[33] But as alluded to earlier, "normal" concentrations relative to blood may not be the appropriate goal for many patients, particularly in the post-resuscitation phase of hospitalization. For example, hyponatremia is common in many hospitalized patients, but it is far more likely to be caused by fluid overload than by sodium deficiency. In such patients, excess sodium may worsen the fluid overload state, and the appropriate intervention is to reduce fluid provision.

Except under extreme metabolic derangements (e.g., hepatic failure), the amount of lactate in lactated Ringer's injection (United States Pharmacopeia products) maintains a blood pH of around 7.4 soon after administration through its metabolism into bicarbonate in a 1:1 ratio. This is because an administered crystalloid solution such as a lactated Ringer's injection must have a strong ion difference of around 24 mEq/L to maintain normal blood pH.[34] Box 2.1 lists the common adverse effects of three of the more commonly used intravenous crystalloid solutions.

Box 2.1. Adverse Effects of Crystalloid Solutions

Normal saline

Primarily extensions of pharmacologic actions (e.g., fluid overload, dilutional coagulopathy)

Hyperchloremic metabolic acidosis (has 154 mEq/L [154 mmol/L] of chloride)

Hypernatremia (has 154 mEq/L [154 mmol/L] of sodium)

Lactated Ringer's

Primarily extensions of pharmacologic actions (e.g., fluid overload, dilutional coagulopathy)

Hyponatremia (has 130 mEq/L [130 mmol/L] of sodium)

Aggravation of preexisting hyperkalemia (has 4 mEq/L [4 mmol/L] of potassium)

Hypertonic sodium chloride

Primarily extensions of pharmacologic actions (e.g., fluid overload, dilutional coagulopathy; intracellular volume depletion)

Hypernatremia (has 513 mEq/L [513 mmol/L] of sodium)

Hyperchloremia (has 513 mEq/L [513 mmol/L] of chloride)

Adapted with permission from: Erstad BL. Hypovolemic shock. In: DiPiro JT, Talbert RL, Yee GC, Matzke GR, Wells BG, Posey LM, eds. Pharmacotherapy: A Pathophysiologic Approach, 9th ed. New York: McGraw-Hill, 2014;351-68.

Colloids

Four major classes of colloids have been used for fluid resuscitation in critically ill patients: gelatins, dextrans, hydroxyethyl starches, and albumin. Gelatins are not available in the United States and have not been investigated in any of the larger randomized blinded investigations sufficiently powered for a mortality end point. Furthermore, data from observational trials suggest an increased risk of acute kidney injury with gelatin products, so there is little justification for their use in the clinical setting. Similarly, although dextran products are commercially available, their use has been largely supplanted by other colloids, and they have not been investigated in adequately powered studies, with one exception. The exception is research investigations involving trauma patients (particularly those with head injuries) when dextrans have been used in combination with hypertonic sodium chloride products in an attempt to extend the duration of the plasma expansion of the crystalloid solutions. This use of dextrans is primarily based on their molecular mass (e.g., 6% dextran 70 has a relative molecular mass of 70,000) because the endothelial glycocalyx is impermeable to molecules greater than around 70,000 Da. Of importance, in contrast to albumin, which is a monodisperse molecule with a molecular mass of 67,000 Da, other colloid products are composed of polydisperse molecules, so their mass is relative (i.e., a range of molecular masses). Molecular mass has implications not only for intravascular retention, but also for potential adverse effects such as kidney injury. Furthermore, although often not considered in trial designs, colloid products such as the dextrans and starches have anticoagulation effects beyond those attributable to the hemodilution associated with the administration of any crystalloid or colloid plasma expander that does not contain red blood cells. Because of their infrequent use in the clinical setting (at least in the United States), neither the gelatins nor the dextrans will be discussed in more detail in this chapter.

As with the previous discussion of intravenous crystalloid products, each of the following sections covering albumin and hydroxyethyl starch products will begin with a historical perspective to give a context to the current controversies regarding their use. Because albumin has several properties with theoretical clinical benefits beyond plasma expansion, these properties will be reviewed. Box 2.2 lists the adverse effects of most concern with albumin, starch, and dextran products.

Box 2.2. Adverse Effects of Colloid Solutions

Albumin

- Primarily extensions of pharmacologic actions (e.g., fluid overload; dilutional coagulopathy)
- Amino acid profile and catabolism alterations (clinical significance?); potential protein overload if given with exogenous protein (e.g., parenteral nutrition)
- Anaphylactoid/anaphylactic reactions (life-threatening reactions rare; higher in patients with immunoglobulin A deficiency)
- Infectious complications (all reported cases have been associated with improper handling by manufacturer or institution; no reported cases of human immunodeficiency virus or hepatitis transmission)
- Interactions with medications and nutrients (clinical significance varies)
- Metal loading, particularly aluminum (long-term administration in patients with renal failure)
- Negative inotropic effect; reductions in ionized calcium concentrations (not well documented)
- Pyrogenic reactions (not well documented)
- Renal dysfunction with hyperoncotic albumin

Hydroxyethyl starch

- Primarily extensions of pharmacologic actions (e.g., fluid overload, dilutional coagulopathy)
- Bleeding; not recommended in critically ill patients or in patients with bleeding conditions such as subarachnoid hemorrhage)
- Macroamylase formation may cause an elevation in blood amylase that leads to an inaccurate diagnosis of pancreatitis
- Anaphylactoid/anaphylactic reactions
- Pruritus (particularly when large amounts are given; may take months to resolve)
- Renal dysfunction; not recommended in critically ill patients, patients at risk of renal dysfunction, or patients with preexisting renal dysfunction

Dextrans

- Primarily extensions of pharmacologic actions (e.g., fluid overload, dilutional coagulopathy)
- Anaphylactoid/anaphylactic reactions (increased incidence of anaphylaxis with increased molecular weight)
- Bleeding (sometimes used for anticoagulant activity, so not recommended for patients with or at risk of severe bleeding)
- Renal dysfunction

Adapted with permission from: Erstad BL. Hypovolemic shock. In: DiPiro JT, Talbert RL, Yee GC, Matzke GR, Wells BG, Posey LM, eds. Pharmacotherapy: A Pathophysiologic Approach, 9th ed. New York: McGraw-Hill, 2014:351-68.

Albumin

Although some of the first experiments of the oncotic actions of albumin were conducted by Lazarus-Barlow and Starling in the late 1890s,[35,36] clinical investigations of albumin did not begin until albumin was separated from plasma through a fractionation process developed by the protein chemist Edwin Cohn of Harvard Medical School at the request of the armed forces in 1940 in preparation for World War II. Bovine-derived albumin was the initial focus of plasma substitution efforts, but serum sickness reactions associated with the product further shifted efforts to studies with human plasma and albumin. The bovine albumin program officially ended near the end of 1943. A

25% human serum albumin product was developed that met the armed services request for a product that was not only safe and effective, but also concentrated, stable, and easy to transport and administer. Cohn was instrumental in developing the procedures for the commercial production of albumin. The small amount of albumin that had been produced by 1941 was given to casualties of Pearl Harbor and deemed effective, so in January 1942, the National Research Council recommended that albumin be used by all the armed forces.[37] In conjunction with its use on the battlefield, albumin continued to be studied for its clinical effects in normal volunteers (mainly medical students) and patients with shock.[38–40]

Many of the physicochemical properties (e.g., molecular weight, oncotic activity), clinical benefits (e.g., ease of administration, efficacy for shock), and risks (e.g., venous and pulmonary edema) of albumin were elucidated soon after the fractionation process was developed.[41–43] Part of the research on albumin involved ways to improve its stability and clinical efficacy through the addition of various additives, including sodium chloride. Consideration was even given to albumin in dry powder form with a diluent that contained glucose. Sodium chloride concentrations as high as 0.3 molar were considered and tested as dispersion mediums for albumin, but eventually, a "salt-poor" 0.15 molar sodium chloride concentration (i.e., 0.9%) was used. By 1950 (the year in which albumin was included in the United States Pharmacopeia), research on albumin had provided several findings that were subsequently confirmed in later investigations with more advanced techniques. Examples include:

- Concentrated 25% albumin draws fluid from the extravascular to the intravascular space, so concomitant isotonic fluid administration is needed to optimize plasma expansion and prevent potential adverse effects in patients with preexisting extravascular depletion.
- The major adverse effect of albumin is fluid overload resulting from excessive administration; other serious adverse reactions are rare.
- Albumin begins to leak into the extravascular space soon after administration, particularly in patients with increased vascular permeability (e.g., cirrhosis, nephrosis, burns).
- Albumin is not a substitute for whole blood in patients with hemorrhagic shock.
- Denaturation of albumin occurs with production and storage.

By the earlier 1970s, there was a widespread perception that the clinical use of albumin had increased substantially. There were concerns that some of the widespread use of albumin might be inappropriate, especially in light of the cost of the product. This led to a workshop on albumin that was sponsored by the Division of Blood and Blood Products, the Bureau of Biologics, the FDA, and the Division of Blood Diseases and Resources, National Heart and Lung Institute, NIH.[44] In preparation for the workshop, a survey of 1.4% of hospitals registered by the American Hospital Association showed that 25% albumin was most prescribed on a unit basis (18,845 units of 50 mL), followed by plasma protein fraction (9956 units of 250 mL) and 5% albumin (1650 of 250 mL).[45] The 2-day workshop convened sessions on the history of albumin, the biochemistry and physiology of albumin, the physiology of body fluid compartments, and the clinical uses and safety of albumin. In addition to the publication of the proceedings by the Division of Blood Diseases and the Resources of the National Heart and Lung Institute, a summary of the findings of the proceedings was published in two parts in the Journal of the American Medical Association (*JAMA*) in 1977.[46,47] The uses for albumin defined as "appropriate" were shock, adult respiratory distress syndrome, and cardiopulmonary bypass. "Occasional use" was deemed appropriate for acute liver failure, red blood cell suspension media, ascites, after surgery, acute nephrosis, and renal dialysis. The only uses considered "unjustified" were undernutrition, chronic nephrosis, and chronic cirrhosis. Of note, not a single RCT involving albumin had been published when the workshop took place. The recommendations were mainly based on mechanistic and experimental models, and observational studies. Although it was clear that albumin had several biological functions, the importance of these functions was not always clear. For example, by the early 1970s, the condition of analbuminemia was recognized in which patients lived well into adulthood, despite a lack of detectable albumin concentrations in the blood. Although it was difficult to try to limit albumin use in the absence of randomized trials and when general indications such as shock were considered appropriate, many clinicians developed institutional guidelines and protocols for albumin use using the results of the conference proceedings. One could argue that the publication of the *JAMA* paper was the beginning of the so-called *colloid versus crystalloid debate* that still rages. No other attempts were made to define the appropriate uses of albumin on a widespread basis until the early 1990s, when the University Hospital Consortium (now known as the University HealthSystem Consortium) compiled recommendations for the appropriate uses of albumin and other nonprotein colloids, published in 1995.[48] These recommendations were based largely on evidence from RCTs that had been conducted since the first trials in the mid to late 1970s. Using the University HealthSystem Consortium recommendations to define appropriate albumin use, an observational study was conducted at 15 academic medical centers in the United States. Almost two-thirds of albumin use in this study was found to be inappropriate, with an associated institutional cost of about $125,000.[49] By the late 1990s, when recombinant albumin was successfully produced (but not economically viable by large-scale production), the crystalloid-colloid debate was reignited by several factors, including increasing use of albumin substitutes for cost containment, increased use of systematic reviews and/or meta-analyses to evaluate crystalloid-colloid efficacy and safety in critically ill patients, and the publication of RCTs of sufficient sample size to assess mortality as an end point in critically ill patients receiving crystalloids and colloids.

Properties of Albumin

The plasma expansion by albumin was previously thought to be caused by its oncotic actions in a simple physiological model in which transcapillary fluid transport was determined by intravascular and interstitial oncotic and hydrostatic forces in conjunction with membrane permeability coefficients for protein and water. Fluid transport across the endothelium is now known to be a function of the oncotic and hydrostatic forces of blood and the subglyceal (not the interstitial) space.[50] The oncotic pressure of the subglyceal space is determined by albumin. When the glycocalyx is damaged, as may occur during critical illness, fluid leaks into the interstitial space. This leak, together with the increased rate of catabolism of albumin, accounts for the hypoalbuminemia that commonly occurs in critically ill patients. Other colloids such as hydroxyethyl starch may help maintain glycocalyx integrity, but not to the same degree as albumin.[51]

Albumin has a variety of other properties not shared by other colloid or crystalloid solutions (see Box 2.3).[52] These properties have been used to support mechanistic explanations for the clinical benefits of exogenous albumin administration, even though most comparative studies with other colloids or crystalloids have found no advantage to albumin on clinically relevant patient outcomes. Some have argued that the apparent lack of benefit of albumin over other fluid products is that it has not been studied using the appropriate methodology in specific subsets of critically ill patients. There are other explanations as well. One alternative explanation is that other proteins take over the functions of albumin during states of albumin deficiency, and another explanation is that exogenous albumin does not have the same physicochemical properties of endogenous albumin. Each of these alternative explanations will be discussed.

Albumin does provide a source of amino acids, but it is a poor source of essential amino acids, and albumin deficiency is unlikely to be a rate-limiting step in protein synthesis except in cases of prolonged malnutrition. Albumin is considered an antioxidant, but depending on other clinical conditions such as iron overload, it may have no significant antioxidant activity and may even have pro-oxidant effects. Albumin serves as a reversible binding protein for several endogenous and exogenous ligands, but the clinical importance of this binding has not been well established. For those who argue for albumin's beneficial mechanistic actions, perhaps the most cogent counterargument is based on cases of analbuminemia in which patients lived well into adulthood without obvious consequences. Obviously, the functions of albumin in such cases were taken over by other proteins, so the important questions from a clinical standpoint are whether this compensatory process occurs in the setting of critical illness and, if so, how long it takes other proteins to perform the more important functions of albumin.

Endogenous albumin has both positive and negative charges on different parts of the molecule, although there is an overall net negative charge. This accounts not only for the binding of endogenous substances such as bilirubin, but also for some of the medications commonly used in critically ill patients such as midazolam, phenytoin, and valproate. The binding properties may be impaired during the manufacturing and storage of albumin products. Denatured albumin has decreased oncotic activity and may dispose patients to sensitivity reactions. For these reasons, commercially available albumin products are not biologically similar to endogenous albumin.

Hydroxyethyl Starch

The first hydroxyethyl starch solution licensed in the United States was Hespan (1972) formulated in normal saline, followed by Hextend (1999) formulated in Ringer's lactate, and finally, Voluven (2007) formulated in normal saline. Hespan approval was based on small randomized comparisons with albumin in a variety of surgical and critically ill patient populations, whereas the Hextend and Voluven approval studies used other starch products such as Hespan as the control. All of these products had upper dose limits in the labeling (20 mL/kg for Hespan and Hextend, 50 mL/kg for Voluven). Bleeding concerns beyond dilutional effects were noted in early studies of Hespan and Hextend, but renal adverse effects did not become a significant concern until larger head-to-head comparisons with other colloids or crystalloids began to appear in

---

Box 2.3. Properties of Albumin Beyond Plasma Expansion and Glycocalyx Integrity

- Suppresses effects of cytokines (TNF neutrophil burst)
- Anticoagulant actions possibly caused by nitric oxide inactivation
- No neutrophil activation and decreased neutrophil sequestration in lung
- Transport/binding to endogenous substances (bilirubin, steroids, fatty acids, nitric oxide) and drugs
- Scavenger for reactive oxygen species
- Source of amino acids

TNF = tumor necrosis factor.

Table 2.1 Electrolyte Compositions of Colloids and Crystalloids Used in Large Randomized Trials of ICU Patients

	Finfer[53] Albumex 4 Albumin	Brunkhorst[54] Sterofundin Ringer's Lactate	Brunkhorst[54] Hemohes 10% HES 0.45–0.55	Perner[55] Tetraspan 6% HES 130/0.4	Perner[55] Ringerfundin Ringer's acetate	Myburgh[56] Voluven 6% HES 130/0.4
Sodium	140 mmol/L	140 mmol/L	154 mol/L	140 mmol/L	145 mmol/L	154 mmol/L
Chloride	128 mmol/L	106 mmol/L	154 mmol/L	118 mmol/L	127 mmol/L	154 mmol/L
Potassium	-	4 mmol/L	-	4 mmol/L	4 mmol/L	-
Magnesium	-	1 mmol/L	-	1 mmol/L	1 mmol/L	-
Calcium	-	2.5 mmol/L	-	2.5 mmol/L	2.5 mmol/L	-
Lactate	-	45 mmol/L	-	-	-	-
Acetate	-	-	-	24 mmol/L	24 mmol/L	-
Octanoate	6.4 mmol/L	-	-	-	-	-
Malate	-	-	-	5 mmol/L	5 mmol/L	-

HES = hydroxyethyl starch.

the literature in the early part of this century. Overarching conclusions about evaluations of starch efficacy, as well as adverse effect concerns such as bleeding, have been complicated by the variety of products that have been studied in the United States and other countries. In contrast to albumin, starch products are not monodisperse. Each starch product has a range of molecular weights, a degree of hydroxyethyl starch molar substitution on glucose subunits, and a degree of hydroxyethyl starch molar substitution on glucose subunits typically expressed as the ratio of hydroxyethyl groups at C2 versus C6. For example, Voluven is described as 6% hydroxyethyl starch 130/0.4, where 6% indicates the weight, 130 is the molar substitution, and 0.4 is the ratio of hydroxyethyl groups. It was previously thought that higher molecular weight and degree of starch substitution were the primary causes of the adverse effects of the hydroxyethyl starch products because of prolonged retention in reticuloendothelial tissues and alterations in coagulation. Therefore, more recent promotional materials and research has focused on products like Voluven.

CRYSTALLOID AND COLLOID STUDIES IN CRITICALLY ILL PATIENTS

Potential differences in the electrolyte composition of intravenous solutions that may influence the efficacy and safety end points in clinical studies are an issue not only for crystalloid products but also for colloid products. This point needs to be considered as the following results of important crystalloid and colloid trials are discussed. Table 2.1 lists the electrolyte compositions of the crystalloids and colloids administered in some of the larger RCTs involving critically ill patients.[53–56] It is currently unknown how these electrolyte differences may have influenced the results of these trials, but it should serve as a cautionary note in the design of future clinical trials.

In 1998, a systematic review conducted by the respected Cochrane group found a 6% excess mortality with albumin compared with isotonic crystalloid solutions.[57] The authors of the analysis recommended that albumin not be used in critically ill patients outside the confines of RCTs. This publication led to a series of pro-con albumin letters to the editor of the journal, with some pointing out the various flaws of the systematic review and others recommending that albumin use be discontinued because of the findings of the review. The Cochrane analysis prompted the FDA to issue a "Dear Doctor" letter in August 1998 that urged discretion in the use of albumin and recommended that clinicians be aware of current guidelines; the specific guideline referenced was the 1995 publication by the University HealthSystem Consortium. The next year, in 1999, a well-respected group of Canadian critical care researchers published a systematic review that found no difference in clinically relevant end points between isotonic crystalloid solutions and colloids such as albumin for fluid resuscitation, with one exception. Lower mortality was noted in trauma patients who received crystalloid solutions (relative risk [RR] 0.39; 95% CI, 0.17–0.89). However, the authors of the systematic review noted that methodological limitations precluded high-level evidence-based recommendations and called for more randomized trials.[58] Many other systematic reviews and meta-analyses comparing crystalloids and colloids were published within a few years of the Canadian systematic review, most of which had similar findings—no important differences in clinically relevant end points with the notable exception of trauma subgroups, which had worse outcomes with albumin.

In 2004, the results of a randomized study were published that compared 4% albumin with normal saline for fluid resuscitation of critically ill patients.[53] This trial, known as SAFE, was a landmark investigation not only for its size (n=6997 patients), but also for the rigor of methodology. There were no significant differences between the albumin and saline groups for the primary end point (all-cause death at 28 days) or any of the secondary end points (duration of mechanical ventilation, length of stay, or days of renal replacement therapy). However, there was a trend toward reduced mortality with albumin in patients with severe sepsis (RR 0.87; 95% CI, 0.74–1.02), and consistent with previous meta-analyses, there was a trend toward increased mortality in patients with trauma (RR 1.36; 95% CI, 0.99–1.86). In May 2005, the FDA issued a follow-up "Dear Health Care Providers" letter stating that the SAFE study had resolved the safety concerns related to albumin raised by the 1998 Cochrane systematic review.

In 2012, the CHEST study was published in which 7000 patients admitted to ICUs with a need for fluid resuscitation were randomized in a blinded manner to receive a 6% hydroxyethyl starch (130/0.4) in normal saline or normal saline.[56] The study was modeled after the SAFE study—both had mixed medical and surgical ICU patients, and both used a pragmatic design with interventions apart from study fluids left to the discretion of the treating physicians. This type of design necessitates the large patient enrollment in both the CHEST and the SAFE trials but allows for increased generalizability of the findings. There was no significant difference in the primary end point of 90-day mortality between the starch and the saline solutions (RR 1.06; 95% CI, 0.96–1.18), but the starch solution was associated with more overall adverse effects (5.3% vs. 2.8%, p<0.001). Furthermore, there was increased acute kidney injury (34.6% vs. 38.0%, p=0.005) and increased need for renal replacement therapy (RR 1.21; 95% CI, 1.00–1.45) in patients receiving the starch solution.

Most RCTs involving crystalloid-colloid comparisons in critically ill patients have used one crystalloid solution and one colloid solution, usually in specific subsets of patients, to limit heterogeneity and sample size. An exception to this was the CRISTAL trial published in 2013.[59] This multicenter trial randomized critically ill patients in an open-label fashion to receive colloids (gelatins, dextrans, starches, and albumin products not limited by type or concentration of colloid) or crystalloids (normal saline, hypertonic sodium chloride, and Ringer's lactate) for fluid maintenance; patients were stratified by trauma, sepsis, or shock without sepsis or trauma. No difference was found for the primary end point of 28-day mortality between the colloid group and the crystalloid group (RR 0.96; 95% CI, 0.88–1.04). However, at 90 days, mortality was reduced in the colloid group (RR 0.92; 95% CI, 0.86–0.99). Although a few other secondary end points had significant findings in favor of colloids, most other comparisons stratified by type of specific fluid or shock revealed no significant differences. It is very difficult to draw conclusions from this study, given the many potential confounders and statistical concerns with the results that were mentioned in letters to the editor by leading researchers in fluid resuscitation. Although the 2857 patients evaluated in this study seems like a large number, consider that the SAFE trial had 6997 patients, and only two fluids were compared.

CRYSTALLOID AND COLLOID STUDIES IN SUBSETS OF CRITICALLY ILL PATIENTS

Trauma

In a post hoc follow-up trial of SAFE, 460 patients with traumatic brain injury and a Glasgow Coma Scale (GCS) score of 13 or less from the original SAFE investigation were followed for 24 months.[60] Mortality was higher in the albumin group than in the saline group (RR 1.63; 95% CI, 1.17–2.26), particularly in patients with more severe injury, as defined by a GCS score of 3–8 (RR 1.88; 95% CI, 1.31–2.70). So, although albumin appears to be safe in a general ICU population, saline is recommended for resuscitating patients with traumatic brain injury.

Hypertonic sodium chloride products have been studied as resuscitation fluids for trauma, and particularly for traumatic brain injury, for decades. In May 2006, enrollment began in two randomized blinded studies conducted under the auspices of ROC, a research network with studies that include evaluations of prehospital resuscitation interventions. One of the studies investigated the efficacy and safety of prehospital administration of hypertonic sodium chloride solutions for shock caused by traumatic hemorrhage, and a parallel study investigated these solutions and end points specifically for patients with traumatic brain injury. The fluids under study were single 250-mL boluses of 7.5% sodium chloride in 6% dextran, 7.5% sodium chloride, or 0.9% isotonic saline. This dose of hypertonic sodium chloride solution was chosen because of its frequent use and safety in previous trials. Enrollment in the shock trial was suspended early (n=853) when the study monitoring board found no significant difference (p=0.91) between groups for the primary outcome of 28-day mortality.[13] Higher mortality was associated with hypertonic sodium chloride administration in a subgroup of patients not undergoing transfusion in the first 24 hours (p<0.01). Enrollment was also terminated early (n=1331) in the second study involving patients with traumatic brain injury when no significant difference (p=0.67) was found in the primary end point of 6-month neurologic outcome (based on the Extended Glasgow Outcome Scale) between the hypertonic solution and the isotonic sodium chloride solution.[14] Furthermore, there was no significant difference between groups for 28-day survival (p=0.88). In both trials, there were few statistically significant differences for a wide range of other outcome and adverse effect measures. Although the hypertonic sodium chloride groups had more sodium concentrations above the normal range, there were similar small numbers of patients in each group (less than 2.5% in the groups in the shock trial with numbers too small to estimate significance and less than 5% in each group in the brain injury trial with a p=0.25) with sodium concentrations greater than 160 mmol/L requiring intervention.

Severe Sepsis and Septic Shock

Patients with severe sepsis was one of the predefined subgroups of the SAFE study.[61] Although the unadjusted risk of death with albumin was lower and trended toward statistical significance, the risk of death with albumin after adjustment for other dependent variables was significantly lower (odds ratio [OR] 0.71; 95% CI, 0.52–0.97). There were no significant differences between the albumin group and the saline group for safety outcomes such as need for renal replacement therapy. In contrast to the SAFE trial, which used a 4% albumin product with relatively standard resuscitation end points, a subsequent large (n=1818) multicenter trial (ALBIOS) involving patients with severe sepsis or septic shock used 20% albumin targeted to achieve a serum albumin concentration of at least 30 g/L.[62] Patients randomized to both the albumin and the no-albumin groups received crystalloids for fluid replacement. Although patients in the albumin group had higher mean arterial pressure (MAP) values (p=0.03) and lower net fluid balance (p<0.001), there were no significant differences in 28-day or 90-day mortality or any secondary outcome measures. There was a significant difference in favor of albumin in a subset of patients with septic shock (43.6% with albumin vs. 49.9% with crystalloid, p=0.03), but this finding should be considered hypothesis generating, given that this was a post hoc rather than a prespecified subgroup analysis. A systematic review that included the ALBIOS trial, as well as another multicenter trial involving 20% albumin that was unpublished at the time (Early Albumin Resuscitation in Septic Shock or EARSS), found no difference in the primary end point of 28-day mortality or any secondary end points, including 90-day mortality, regardless of the degree of sepsis severity or whether serum albumin concentration was changed.[63]

There is a concern that unbalanced high chloride solutions such as normal saline are more likely than balanced solutions to cause acute kidney injury. This is a potential confounding factor in randomized trials and systematic reviews comparing colloids with crystalloids in patients with sepsis when balanced and unbalanced (e.g., normal saline) solutions are combined to form a crystalloid group. In one systematic review of patients with sepsis that had separate balanced and unbalanced crystalloid groups, the balanced crystalloid group had lower mortality than the saline or starch product groups.[64] It is worth noting that this systematic review used a complicated, non-standard meta-analytic methodology, and there was significant trial heterogeneity with low confidence in most of the findings. Furthermore, the albumin arm of the analysis also showed lower mortality than the saline or starch solution arms, but the implications of this finding are hindered by the use of low and high chloride-containing albumin and starch products.

The concerns with hydroxyethyl starch solutions in patients with sepsis are not limited to products with high chloride concentrations. Large randomized studies have shown safety issues with high and low chloride-containing starch solutions in patients with sepsis. One of the first large investigations to raise concerns with starch products was known as the VISEP trial.[54] In the fluid resuscitation part of this 2 × 2 factorial trial, a lower-molecular-weight starch (i.e., 200/0.5 pentastarch) formulated in a normal saline solution was compared with Ringer's lactate. At 90 days, there was a trend toward increased mortality in the starch group compared with the Ringer's lactate group (p=0.09), as well as an increased rate of acute renal failure (34.9% vs. 22.8%, p=0.002) and need for renal replacement therapy (p=0.001). In another multicenter randomized blinded study known as the 6S trial, 6% hydroxyethyl starch 130/0.4 in Ringer's acetate (118 mEq/L chloride, 24 mEq/L acetate) was compared with Ringer's acetate, each in a dose of 33 mL/kg/day, for resuscitating 804 patients with severe sepsis.[55] Despite the use of a low-molecular-weight hydroxyethyl starch solution that was more balanced with respect to chloride concentration, there was increased 90-day mortality (RR 1.17; 95% CI, 1.01–1.36), an increased need for renal replacement therapy (RR 1.35; 95% CI, 1.01–1.80), and a trend toward increased bleeding (RR 1.52; 95% CI, 0.94–2.48) in the starch group. In light of these findings, the FDA has required hydroxyethyl starch product information to contain a black box warning on the increased mortality and renal injury requiring renal replacement therapy associated with these solutions.

Burns

There is surprisingly little evidence to support the use of albumin in patients with burns, despite research of its efficacy and safety that dates back to the 1970s. The few randomized studies conducted have been inadequately powered to investigate clinically meaningful end points, even though albumin or fresh frozen plasma is often part of resuscitation protocols. Guidelines by the American Burn Association recognize the limitations of the literature in this area and begin by recognizing that data are insufficient to support a treatment standard.[65] In the guidelines, colloid therapy such as albumin is simply listed as an option that may reduce fluid requirements if given at least 12–24 hours after injury. Nevertheless, the theoretical benefit of albumin is appealing, particularly in patients with large burns who require substantial fluid administration. In one investigation with a before-after design (n=98 before, n=61 after), 5% albumin was used to replace lactated Ringer's solution at 12 hours post-burn when estimated fluid requirements at 12 hours suggested that a patient would need at least 6 mL/kg per percent burn at 24 hours.[66] Ventilator-associated pneumonia (p<0.01), number of days on the ventilator (p<0.05), and mortality (p<0.01) were lower in the after (i.e., albumin) phase of the study. In addition to the possibility of a type I statistical error, given the substantial difference in mortality between groups, the results are confounded by the use of a historical control (with use of colloids per physician discretion after 24 hours in the before phase) and the implementation of a protocol that included standardization beyond the addition of albumin in the after phase. Larger randomized trials are needed to confirm the findings of this study.

Miscellaneous

Albumin in particular has been studied for several specific disease states and in conjunction with a variety of surgical and nonsurgical procedures in critically ill patients. Apart from fluid resuscitation studies that typically have involved isotonic crystalloid versus relatively iso-oncotic colloids such as albumin 4% or 5%, the hyperoncotic albumin products (20% and 25%) have been studied for conditions in which interstitial to intravascular fluid movement is thought to be desirable and conditions that would appear to benefit from the properties of albumin beyond plasma expansion. However, the trial by Sort et al. involving patients with spontaneous bacterial peritonitis is the only adequately powered RCT to date to find a significant reduction in unadjusted mortality with hyperoncotic albumin (20%) compared with no albumin with mortality being a primary end point of the study.[67] With patients in both groups receiving cefotaxime, the mortality rates with and without albumin were 41% and 22% (p=0.03), respectively, and the rates of renal impairment were 33% and 10% (p=0.002), respectively. Other areas of investigation of albumin, particularly hyperoncotic albumin, include nephrosis, cirrhosis, cardiopulmonary bypass surgery, and the adult respiratory distress syndrome. There is no high-level evidence to support the routine use of albumin in these areas. An in-depth discussion of each of these uses is beyond the scope of this chapter, but Table 2.2 provides an example of some of the more common purported indications for albumin, together with possible dosing regimens and evidence to support each use.[68-74] This protocol adapted from the author's institution is not intended to contain the definitive or sole uses of albumin that might be considered for a critically ill patient. Rather, the table is intended to serve as an example of how a protocol for albumin use might be configured.

DOSING OF FLUID ADMINISTRATION

Since the 1940s and until the 1990s, the traditional dosing of intravenous fluids in a patient with shock was administration of a bolus of isotonic crystalloid solution of around 1500–3000 mL (or an equivalent amount of colloid). A paradigm shift occurred, at least with respect to the resuscitation of trauma patients, with the publication of a landmark study in 1994 that showed increased mortality in patients receiving aggressive preoperative fluids.[75] Delayed resuscitation of fluids until the operating room was associated with increased survival (p=0.04) in patients with gunshot or stab wound injuries to the torso who had systolic blood pressure recordings less than 90 mm Hg. It was postulated that the aggressive fluid administration led to increased bleeding by dilution of clotting factors and by clot destabilization. This led to the concept of permissive hypotension for patients with traumatic hemorrhage in which mini-boluses of fluid (250–500 mL) are given to achieve a palpable pulse or central arterial pressure recordings, just sufficient to maintain vital organ perfusion. In patients without obvious exsanguination, a fluid bolus may help differentiate simple extracellular depletion (i.e., an appropriate and relatively sustained response) from ongoing blood loss (relatively rapid recurrence of hypotension). The most appropriate dose of fluids for patients with blunt trauma may be a function of the presence or absence of hypotension before resuscitation, according to the analysis of a subset of data obtained from a multicenter prospective study of prehospital fluid administration.[76] When more severely injured (defined as an ISS [injury severity score] greater than 15) patients with blunt trauma were divided into low-volume (less than 500 mL) or high-volume (greater than 500 mL) crystalloid administration, patients with hypotension (systolic blood pressure of at least 90 mm Hg on presentation to the emergency department) had increased mortality (HR 2.5; 95% CI, 1.3–4.9) when given high-volume crystalloids. In the patients with blunt trauma having hypotension, each 1-mm Hg increase in systolic blood pressure was associated with a 2% increase in survival (OR 1.02; 95% CI, 1.01–1.03).

The concept of permissive hypotension in fluid resuscitation traditionally has not been applied to the resuscitation of patients with nonhemorrhagic forms of shock when aggravation of blood loss was not a factor. For example, in the Surviving Sepsis Campaign guidelines published in 2013, crystalloid boluses up to 20 mL/kg (or an equivalent amount of albumin) given over 5–10 minutes were recommended for the initial resuscitation of shock; further, the authors stated that larger fluid deficits might

Table 2.2 Miscellaneous Uses of Albumin and Supportive Evidence[a]

Use	Dosing Regimen	Evidence
Indications where widespread consensus occurs		
Spontaneous bacterial peritonitis (SBP) (ascitic fluid PMN ≥ 250 cells/mm³)	Albumin 25% (1.5 g/kg [max 150 g] within 6 hr of diagnosis of SBP; then 1 g/kg [max 100 g] on day 3) in conjunction with broad-spectrum antibiotics	Single RCT showing mortality benefit[67]
Plasmapheresis with large-volume exchanges	Albumin 5% for exchanges > 20 mL/kg in one session or > 20 mL/kg/wk in repeated sessions	No large RCTs but widespread consensus[68,69]
Large-volume paracentesis (LVP) in patients with large ascites	Albumin 25% (8 g/L of fluid removed) in conjunction with LVP (> 5 L of ascetic fluid removed in adults or > 20 mL/kg in children)	Small RCTs primarily looking at benefits on surrogate markers such as serum sodium but recommended in guidelines[69–73]
Indications where use may be considered when specific criteria met		
Hepatorenal syndrome type 1 (doubling of baseline SCr to a final level > 2.5 mg/dL in 2 wk)	Albumin 25% (1 g/kg [max 100] on day 1, followed by 50 g/day) may be considered when used in combination with a vasoactive medication. The goal is to decrease serum creatinine to < 1.5 mg/dL (complete response)	Small RCTs with limitations, but syndrome is associated with high mortality, so benefits thought to exceed risks[69–72]
Hepatic resection (> 40%) or liver transplantation	Albumin 25% may be considered in the presence of clinically important edema OR when large amounts of crystalloids have failed to produce an adequate cardiovascular response in patients with hypoalbuminemia and hematocrit > 30%	Observational and retrospective studies[69]
Nephrotic syndrome	Albumin 25% may be considered when MAXIMIZED diuretic therapy fails in the presence of clinically important edema AND hypoalbuminemia	Data primarily from retrospective and observational trials; benefit, if any, is short term[69]
Cardiac surgery	Albumin 5% may be considered when it is important to avoid clinically important edema OR when large amounts of crystalloids have failed to produce an adequate cardiovascular response	Data from retrospective studies[69,74]

[a]Definitions:
- Clinically important edema (e.g., massive ascites and pulmonary edema)
- Large amounts of crystalloid (0.9 NaCl, lactated Ringer's injection, etc.): > 4 L for adults or > 40 mL/kg in children
- Maximized diuretic therapy or diuretic resistance or development of adverse drug events: furosemide equivalent 200 mg intravenously as a single bolus, 20 mg/hr as an intravenous infusion, or 500 mg/day intravenously as a total
- Hypoalbuminemia: < 1.5 g/dL in neonates < 2 wk of age OR < 2.5 g/dL for children ≥ 2 wk and adults

PMN = polymorphonuclear leukocyte; RCT = randomized controlled trial

necessitate fluid doses up to 60 mL/kg. Vasopressors were recommended in the guidelines when response to this initial fluid resuscitation was insufficient.[77] Until recently, the use of an initial bolus dose of fluids during resuscitation was relatively unquestioned. In a study investigating African children with infection and impaired perfusion (known as the FEAST study), increased 48-hour mortality was found with bolus administration (20–40 mL/kg over 1 hour) compared with no-bolus fluid administration, regardless of whether the fluid bolus was 5% albumin or normal saline (10.6% and 10.5%, respectively, vs. 7.3% with no bolus, p=0.003).[78] Because the main cause of death was cardiovascular collapse, there is a suggestion that somehow fluid boluses alter normal homeostatic mechanisms in a negative way. This study was remarkable, not only for its findings but also for the methodologic problems that had to be overcome to conduct a randomized trial outside the confines of sophisticated critical care facilities. Whether the findings should change the initial fluid management of nonhemorrhagic shock in adult patients in more industrialized countries with well-equipped health care facilities is open to debate, but at a minimum, it has raised an important question that needs to be answered in future investigations.

The amount of fluid compartment expansion for many crystalloids and colloids as determined in clinical investigations is often far different from the expansion predicted for these fluids using traditional factors such as hydrostatic and colloid osmotic pressure with membrane permeability coefficients (Table 2.3). Estimates of fluid distribution that do not consider leakage of colloid over time suggest that 3 or 4 times as much as normal saline are required to give the equivalent plasma expansion of albumin (4% or 5%) or 6% hydroxyethyl starch. But plasma expansion is time sensitive, with a peak usually occurring within 2 hours of fluid administration, followed by a decline phase associated with albumin (or starch) and accompanying fluid leakage to the interstitial compartment. For example, in normal volunteers administered 4 mL/kg (average 260 mL) of 7.5% sodium chloride solution over 30 minutes, plasma volume as measured by the dilution of iodine-125 (^{125}I)-labeled albumin increased 442 ± 167 mL during the infusion to 465 ± 83 mL at the end of the monitoring period, 90 minutes from baseline.[79] In a study of patients undergoing elective surgery, plasma expansion with 50 g of albumin given over 90 minutes as solutions of 5% (145 mmol/L sodium), 20% (100 mmol/L), or 25% albumin (100 mmol/L sodium) was compared using ^{131}I-labeled albumin.[80] The plasma volume increased by an estimated 500 mL in all groups, suggesting that albumin dose, not concentration, was the determining factor for intravascular expansion. This translated to about an 11-mL increase in plasma volume for each 1 g of infused albumin. Albumin has also been studied in patients with sepsis. In one study using ^{125}I-labeled albumin, transcapillary escape of albumin was measured after the infusion of 200 mL of

Table 2.3 Theoretical Fluid Distribution by Body Compartment[a]

Fluid	Intracellular	Interstitial	Intravascular	Major Indication
Normal saline or lactated Ringer's	None	750 mL	250 mL	Intravascular repletion in symptomatic patients
3% sodium chloride	→	750 mL+	250 mL+	Small amounts (e.g., 250 mL) by intermittent infusion have been used in conjunction with normal saline or lactated Ringer's for intravascular depletion in patients with head trauma
5% dextrose/0.45% sodium chloride	333 mL	500 mL	167 mL	Maintenance fluid in euvolemic or dehydrated (sodium and water loss) patients with mild signs/symptoms of volume depletion
5% dextrose	667 mL	250 mL	83 mL	Dehydration (primarily water loss) in patients with mild signs/symptoms of volume depletion
5% albumin	None	None	1000 mL[b]	Intravascular repletion in symptomatic patients
25% albumin	→	→	1000 mL+++[b]	Usually given by intermittent infusion of small volumes (e.g., 50–100 mL) or by continuous infusion titrated to response in hypovolemic patients with excess interstitial fluid accumulation

[a]Based on administration of 1 L of each solution *for comparative purposes only*. This amount of fluid, particularly for 3% saline and 25% albumin, would be inappropriate and likely harmful if given over a short period. Numbers are approximations and likely not reflective of actual fluid distribution in critically ill patients; arrows indicate direction of fluid shift, and plus signs indicate fluid pulled from other compartments.

[b]After distribution and attainment of steady-state conditions, 60% of albumin (and associated fluid) is in the interstitial compartment, and 40% is in the intravascular compartment.

Adapted with permission from: Erstad BL. Hypovolemic shock. In: DiPiro JT, Talbert RL, Yee GC, Matzke GR, Wells BG, Posey LM, eds. Pharmacotherapy: A Pathophysiologic Approach, 9th ed. New York: McGraw-Hill, 2014:351-68.

20% albumin.[81] Despite a near-doubling of serum albumin concentrations, transcapillary fluid escape was unchanged (p=0.55), suggesting no effect of albumin on vessel permeability. Furthermore, colloid osmotic pressure, which had increased quickly after albumin infusion, decreased to 50% of peak concentrations by 240 minutes. In another study, 200 mL of 20% albumin was given by rapid infusion to patients with septic shock or controls. Albumin concentrations increased by almost 100% in the patients with sepsis receiving this dose. The estimated plasma expansion, as noted by changes in hematocrit corrected for dilution by the infused volume, was maximal at 30 minutes, which was 430 mL and 500 mL (not significantly different) in patients with sepsis and controls, respectively.[82] However, by 15 minutes, more albumin was being lost from the intravascular compartment in patients with sepsis, and by 4 hours, 32% of the increased albumin in the patients with sepsis and 21% of the albumin in the controls (p<0.001) had shifted to the interstitial compartment, consistent with increased capillary permeability in patients with sepsis. These studies should be interpreted in light of animal studies that suggest that plasma expansion by colloids (but not normal saline) is affected by infusion rate, with greater expansion when colloids are given at a slower rate.[83]

These single-dose studies of plasma expansion with crystalloids and colloids suggest that the actual volume expansion associated with these fluids in critically ill patients can be substantially different from the expansion estimated by body compartment size or studies of normal healthy volunteers. This impression is further reinforced by clinical investigations that used fluid dosing regimens similar to those used in actual clinical practice. For example, in one double-blind RCT comparing 6% hydroxyethyl starch 130/0.4 with normal saline in patients with severe sepsis (CRYSTMAS trial), the amount of normal saline required to achieve initial fluid resuscitation end points was only 24% higher than that needed for starch resuscitation.[84] Similarly, in the landmark SAFE trial involving 6997 mixed medical-surgical ICU patients, the amount of 4% albumin required for fluid resuscitation was only 32% higher than for normal saline on study day 1, and by study day 4, there was no significant difference in study fluid needed in each group. In addition to the smaller-than-expected increases in plasma expansion with colloids in the CRYSTMAS and SAFE trials, there were no significant differences in other measures of efficacy between the crystalloid group and the colloid group.

The dosing of fluids in critically ill patients with ARDS has been evaluated in a large RCT (known as FACCT) undertaken by the National Heart, Lung, and Blood Institute Acute Respiratory Distress Syndrome (ARDS) Clinical Trials Network.[85] The study randomized 1000 patients (66% medical) with acute lung injury (now considered to have adult respiratory distress syndrome) to a conservative or liberal fluid management strategy with a primary end point of 60-day mortality. A 2 × 2 factorial design was used that allowed for a comparison of right heart catheter with central venous pressure (CVP) monitoring to guide conservative versus liberal fluid management. Other primary monitoring values were MAP (focus on fluids or vasopressors only if less than 60 mm Hg), urine output (decreased if less than 0.5 mL/kg/hour or normal if 0.5 mL/kg/hour or more), and physical examination findings (inadequate circulation if cold mottled skin with capillary refill time greater than 2 seconds) for the CVP monitoring group or cardiac index (inadequate circulation if less than 2.5 L/kg/minute) for the right heart catheter group. The study should be considered a post-resuscitation study in the sense that the mean time from ICU admission to protocol implementation averaged about 41–44 hours in both groups. The type of catheter used to guide fluid management did not influence the study findings, so all results were reported, irrespective of catheter assignment. Net fluid balance was negative in the conservative group and positive in the liberal group (p<0.001), which was associated with more ventilator-free days and non–ICU-stay days in the conservative group (p<0.001 for both). Although minor adverse effects (e.g., metabolic alkalosis and electrolyte abnormalities) were more common with the conservative fluid strategy, the percentage of patients requiring renal replacement therapy was actually lower (p=0.06) with the conservative approach. The study findings would appear to be relatively robust for general medical-surgical ICU patients who develop adult respiratory distress syndrome within the first 2 days of ICU admission, regardless of the fluids administered during the initial resuscitation for shock. The findings strongly suggest that lung function can be improved without sacrificing renal function using a conservative fluid administration approach. One concern with applying the results of the FACCT investigation to the clinical setting is the complicated protocol that was used for monitoring and interventions. Fortunately, a follow-up study known as FACTT Lite has suggested that a less complicated protocol based on CVP and urine output recordings yields similar beneficial results.[86]

MONITORING OF RESUSCITATION

Many patients with shock are first seen in the emergency department, and the appropriate monitoring parameters depend on factors such as type and severity of shock. For a patient with traumatic hemorrhage, the monitoring may be limited to an assessment of heart rate and mental status as indicators of more severe blood loss necessitating immediate transfer to the operating room for definitive control of bleeding. For a patient with possible septic shock, the monitoring should include blood collections for lactate concentration and cultures in addition to vital signs, oxygen saturation, and urine output (by urine catheter) determinations. The challenge is early identification of hypovolemia and fluid responsiveness after compensatory changes have begun to fail, as indicated by parameters such as hypotension and decreased urine output. For patients in the ICU setting with impending or overt shock, there is general consensus on the need for an appropriate physical examination in conjunction with assessments of mental status, temperature, blood pressure, heart rate, respiratory rate, fluid balance, urine output, weight, and basic laboratory monitoring that includes electrolytes, complete blood cell count, glucose, lactate, serum BUN, and creatinine. No single parameter in isolation is sufficient, some parameters are not immediately available (e.g., laboratory values), and consensus begins to fade as the type of monitoring technique becomes more invasive and more expensive (Table 2.4 and Table 2.5). Some of the skepticism associated with more invasive monitoring tools originates in previous widespread use of the right heart catheter in many ICU settings, given the perceived advantages of titrating fluids and cardiovascular medications to hemodynamic indices (e.g., cardiac index) using this technique. Subsequently, large-scale studies were unable to find a clinically important outcome benefit with using right heart catheters.[87-89] Nevertheless, some still argue that the lack of outcome improvement in some of these studies occurred because of a lack of appropriate patient selection and a lack of training and expertise by many of the physicians using the catheters. In addition, it can be argued that the use of right heart catheters is appropriate in selected critically ill populations (e.g., cardiac surgery patients), which were not the focus of the large randomized studies.

More Sophisticated and/or Invasive Monitoring Techniques

During episodes of hypovolemic shock, a decreasing output with increased systemic vascular resistance is noted by a reduced pulse pressure (systolic minus diastolic pressure is less than 25% of systolic) that should correct with appropriate resuscitation. In hypovolemic patients receiving conventional mechanical ventilation with tidal volumes of at least 8 mL/kg, it is possible to monitor the rise and fall in arterial pressure associated with the rise and fall in intrathoracic pressure, a condition known as reverse pulsus paradoxus (to contrast it with the pulsus paradoxus that occurs in a spontaneously breathing patient). Maximum minus minimum systolic pressure variations or pulse pressure variations greater

Table 2.4 Adequacy of Resuscitation Using Upstream and Downstream Markers[a]

Upstream (or Leading) Markers	Downstream (or Lagging) Markers
Blood pressure	Lactate
Heart rate	Base deficit
Oxygen tension	Urine output
Hemoglobin	Mixed venous oxygen saturation
Central venous pressure (CVP)	Tissue oxygenation
Pulmonary artery occlusive pressure (PAOP/PCWP)	Gastric tonometry
Cardiac output (CO)	Level of consciousness

[a]Upstream markers may help determine the form of shock (e.g., hypovolemic vs. distributive), but they tend to be isolated static indicators of global hemodynamics or oxygenation. Downstream markers tend to be more reflective of effective tissue perfusion.
PAOP = pulmonary artery occlusive pressure; PCWP = pulmonary capillary wedge pressure.

Table 2.5 Adequacy of Resuscitation Using Invasive Assessment

Static Measures	Dynamic Measures
Central venous pressure (CVP)	Systolic pressure variation or pulse pressure variation as surrogates for stroke volume variation
Pulmonary artery occlusion pressure	
Right ventricular end-diastolic volume by thermodilution	Stroke volume variation (also known as pulse contour or waveform analysis)
Left ventricular end-diastolic volume by thermodilution	Echocardiography to assess variation in inferior vena cava diameter, transaortic stroke volume variation with passive leg raising, or transaortic stroke volume variation with respiration

than 10% are considered dynamic indicators of fluid responsiveness. More sophisticated technologies have used stroke volume variation (also known as pulse contour or waveform analysis) for cardiac output determinations.

Central venous pressure is often recommended as one of the more important parameters used to assess intravascular volume status during fluid challenges, but it has important limitations as an indicator of fluid responsiveness because it is influenced by abdominal pressure, pleural pressure, and different forms of mechanical ventilation. Vincent and Weil have reviewed issues related to fluid challenges in critically ill patients with hypovolemia and stated what they considered misconceptions regarding monitoring parameters such as CVP:[90]

- "Fluid administration should be withheld because the central venous pressure is high."
- "Fluid administration should be withheld because there is evidence of lung edema on the chest roentgenogram."
- "Fluid administration should be withheld because the patient has already received a large volume in a short time interval."
- "Tachycardia is due to fluid deficit and should prompt increases in fluid administration."
- "I gave fluids to increase the central venous pressure to 12 mm Hg to exclude an underlying hypovolemia."

Vincent and Weil expressed concern with using filling pressures as indices of effective resuscitation but stated that monitoring of CVP is "acceptable" as a safety limit for fluid challenge, assuming no preexisting heart or lung disease. They proposed a modified "2–5 rule" (modified from previous technique) in which a fluid challenge (e.g., 500 mL of isotonic crystalloid over 30 minutes) is administered in conjunction with an ongoing monitoring of efficacy and safety end points, including CVP. If the efficacy end points are reached, or if CVP at any point increases to greater than 5 mm Hg above baseline or reaches a predefined safety limit such as 15 mm Hg, fluid administration should be discontinued.

In addition to a catheter to monitor CVP, various types of peripheral venous, central venous, and arterial catheters have been placed to assess components of oxygen delivery and oxygen consumption in conjunction with fluid and drug administration in critically ill patients. The prototype central catheter was the right heart catheter (a.k.a. pulmonary artery or Swan-Ganz catheter) that used indicator dilution to assess several cardiorespiratory variables, including cardiac output. An indicator is injected and monitored for dilution (y-axis) by time (x-axis) that allows the calculation of area under the curve (AUC). The usual indicator is fluid temperature, so the technique is known as thermodilution, but other dyes or markers have been used for the same purpose. The cardiac output is subsequently calculated by the dose of indicator administered (times a constant) divided by the AUC. Modern catheters can provide continuous monitoring (Box 2.4). In addition, less invasive peripheral artery catheters have been used to estimate stroke volume or cardiac output through a technique called waveform analysis, in which algorithms are used to relate peripheral to central pressures.

Apart from a general consensus (albeit without much evidence) that allows for catheter placement to monitor blood pressure and possibly CVP in patients with shock, there is little evidence from a cost-effective standpoint to justify the routine use of other catheters for the hemodynamic monitoring of critically ill patients undergoing resuscitation. The risks associated with monitoring catheters varies by degree of invasiveness, but neither the older, more invasive central catheters (e.g., right heart catheter) nor the newer, less invasive central (e.g., internal jugular or femoral vein) or peripheral catheters have been shown to improve clinically important end points in a general critical care population in adequately powered randomized studies. Some would argue that the catheter used in the trial by Rivers et al. and the Early Goal-Directed Therapy (EGDT) Collaborative Group is an exception to the latter statement, because there was a statistically significant reduction in mortality in the EGDT group with the use of a special catheter capable of continuous central venous oxygen saturation monitoring ($Scvo_2$).[91] In contrast to Svo_2, which requires placement of a right heart catheter, $Scvo_2$ measurements can be obtained through a special catheter inserted as a probe through a lumen of a traditional central venous catheter or as an integrated system placed at the same site as a traditional central venous line (i.e., internal jugular, femoral, or subclavian vein). However, the applicability of this study to the ICU setting is unclear because of the following: the study was limited to patients with severe sepsis or septic shock who were treated in an emergency department, patients received several other interventions by protocol in

---

Box 2.4. Catheters Based on Indicator Dilution

Right heart catheter with thermistor for intermittent thermodilution

Cold fluid injected near right atrium with detection in pulmonary artery

Right heart catheter with thermistor for continuous (actually averaged values) thermodilution: Vigilance®

Heat energy by random off/on pattern with detection in pulmonary artery

Transpulmonary intermittent thermodilution: PiCCO®

Cold fluid injected near right atrium (internal jugular or right subclavian) with detection by thermistor tip in femoral/axillary artery

Transpulmonary lithium dilution: LiDCO®

Same principle as PiCCO® but uses lithium solution, not cold fluid

the EGDT group (so was it the protocol, not the catheter per se?), and monitoring with the catheter was discontinued before ICU admission. Furthermore, the mortality rate in the control group was unexpectedly high compared with the EGDT group (46.5% vs. 30.5%, respectively, p=0.009), which raised questions about the single study site and/or randomization process. However, the strongest argument against any unique benefit associated with Scvo$_2$ monitoring is based on more recent randomized multicenter trials of EGDT monitoring by the ProCESS investigators from the United States,[92] the ARISE investigators from the Australian and New Zealand Intensive Care Society (ANZICS) Clinical Trials Group,[93] and the ProMISe investigators from the United Kingdom.[94] In the ProCESS (n=1341), ARISE (n=1600), and ProMISe (n=1260) studies, the investigators tried to follow the EGDT protocol from the original study by Rivers et al. with continuous Scvo$_2$ monitoring during the first 6 hours after patient presentation to the emergency department. In ProCESS and ProMISe, Scvo$_2$ and CVP monitoring were required in the EGDT group, and continuous arterial pressure monitoring was recommended but not required. The usual care groups in ProCESS, but not ProMISe, received protocol-based care. In ARISE, Scvo$_2$, CVP, and continuous arterial pressure monitoring were required in the EGDT group, but the usual care group did not receive protocol-based care; thus, CVP and arterial pressure monitoring were allowed if deemed appropriate by the treating clinicians. Otherwise, the EGDT protocols were similar, as were the study results. There was no significant difference between the EGDT and the usual therapy groups for the primary end points of 60-day mortality in ProCESS (p=0.83) and 90-day mortality in ARISE and ProMISe (p=0.90 for both studies). Similarly, there were no significant differences in any of the major secondary end points, including length of stay. As with the right heart catheter, central venous catheters placed for continuous monitoring have yet to show an evidence-based indication.

An alternative to both CVP and other forms of invasive hemodynamic monitoring used to assess fluid responsiveness is ultrasonography or echocardiography, usually transthoracic echocardiography (TTE). Not only is TTE monitoring noninvasive and performable by non-cardiologists, but it can also be considered a dynamic (albeit not continuous) rather than static form of monitoring that estimates fluid responsiveness by evaluating the collapsibility of the inferior vena cava. The most clear-cut indicator of fluid responsiveness is complete vessel collapse, although less obvious collapse may be detected by having the patient sniff (rapidly and audibly drawing in air through the nose) and assessing the percent collapse because this maneuver causes a negative inspiratory pressure. In addition to providing an assessment of volume status, TTE can be used by critical care practitioners to assess cardiac function and determine whether a patient with shock has a component of left ventricular dysfunction that might be amenable to a form of therapy other than fluids (e.g., inotropes), or determine whether a patient has pericardial effusion or tamponade. Other forms of TTE evaluation include transaortic stroke volume variation with passive leg raising or with respiration. One systematic review found that all three of these forms of TTE (i.e., inferior vena cava diameter and transaortic stroke volume variation with passive leg raising or with respiration) had very good predictive ability (receiver operating curve greater than 0.9) and could be used in patients with spontaneous breathing efforts and arrhythmias.[95] Transesophageal echocardiography has potential advantages with respect to image quality but requires more specialized training for appropriate use, and patients must be sedated. As with invasive forms of hemodynamic monitoring for shock or impending shock, there is little evidence and few data on cost-effectiveness to support the routine use of more specialized monitoring techniques like TTE.

General Recommendations for Monitoring

A task force of the European Society of Intensive Care Medicine has produced a series of statements relevant to the monitoring of all forms of circulatory shock.[96] Most recommendations are based on either ungraded or the lowest level of evidence; nevertheless, they provide a useful consensus guidance to the clinician. Some of the more salient points include:

- Individualizing target blood pressure (initial target MAP of 65 mm Hg or more) on the basis of factors such as uncontrolled bleeding in the absence of brain injury (lower MAP target) or in patients with sepsis with a history of hypertension (higher MAP target if evidence of clinical improvement)
- Use of several variables (monitoring of heart rate, blood pressure, temperature, physical examination, urine output, and mental status considered best practice; lactate in all cases of suspected shock) for assessment, with dynamic preferred to static measurements
- Use of arterial and central venous catheter monitoring when shock is not responsive to initial therapies or when vasopressors are required
- Use of echocardiography preferred when more advanced monitoring is needed; reserving more invasive forms of monitoring, such as right heart catheterization, to complex patients with severe or refractory shock

MAINTENANCE FLUID ADMINISTRATION

The National Institute for Health and Care Excellence of the United Kingdom has published guidelines for intravenous fluid administration in hospitalized adults.[97]

Although the guidelines were not specific to critically ill patients, they contain a useful algorithm of factors to consider during maintenance fluid administration (Figure 2.1) and a useful figure for estimating electrolyte losses from the body (Figure 2.2). Assuming relatively normal electrolyte and glucose panels without organ dysfunction (e.g., renal failure) that might dramatically alter maintenance requirements, an example of a typical initial intravenous maintenance fluid would be 5% dextrose in 0.22% sodium chloride with 30 mEq/L of potassium chloride at a rate usually not exceeding 25–30 mL/kg/day (using an ideal or lean body weight for dosing patients with obesity because plasma volume does not increase proportionally with excess weight gain), with lower rates for patients with, or predisposed to, fluid-related complications such as ARDS. In patients with complications such as ARDS, a simplified version (based on MAP, CVP, and need for vasopressors) of the monitoring protocol used for conservative fluid administration in the FACTT trial resulted in more fluid accumulation but similar clinical outcomes (FACTT Lite trial).[98]

APPROPRIATE USE OF CRYSTALLOIDS AND COLLOIDS IN CRITICALLY ILL PATIENTS

Of the various crystalloids and colloids that have been studied in critically ill patients, the hydroxyethyl starch products have no substantial evidence of superior efficacy compared with other commonly used intravenous fluids. Furthermore, safety concerns have been raised in every large randomized study with single fluid-to-fluid comparisons. Therefore, as with gelatin and dextran products, the routine use of hydroxyethyl starch products as a resuscitation fluid for critically ill patients cannot be justified. Indeed, leading researchers in the field have even raised ethical issues about informed consent when hydroxyethyl starch solutions are used in ongoing and future research investigations, and they have recommended that the products be withdrawn from the market.[99]

The proper role of albumin in critically ill patients is becoming better defined, given studies of the properties of exogenous albumin and the efficacy and safety findings in large randomized investigations. With respect to fluid resuscitation in general mixed medical-surgical ICU populations, albumin has no convincing evidence of superiority over less expensive isotonic crystalloid solutions, so it should be considered a second-line agent, if used at all. Similarly, there is little justification for albumin use in trauma patients, and it should be avoided in patients with traumatic brain injury. Isotonic crystalloid solutions remain the resuscitation fluid of choice in patients with traumatic brain injury. In patients with severe sepsis and septic shock, albumin or isotonic crystalloids are options for resuscitation according to current practice guidelines, but evidence of albumin superiority over crystalloids is weak at best, so clinicians should feel no compulsion to consider albumin a first-line option, given its higher cost. Albumin use is recommended in consensus-based guidelines for other subsets of ICU populations; however, with the notable exception of spontaneous bacterial peritonitis, these uses are based on low-level evidence and should be considered on a patient-specific basis.

In the not-too-distant past, the choice of fluid in the ICU setting was largely framed in terms of isotonic crystalloid versus colloid solutions. More recently, the specific composition of electrolytes in crystalloid and colloid solutions has received attention by the medical community. There is increasing concern about excessive administration of certain electrolytes, most notably chloride. This concern is reflected in changes in some resuscitation guidelines that now recommend more balanced isotonic crystalloid solutions over normal saline. Table 2.6 lists some of the more applicable systematic reviews and guidelines that pertain to resuscitation and that are likely to undergo periodic updating as new evidence arises.[65,100-105] Finally, Box 2.5 provides some overarching considerations concerning fluid administration in critically ill patients.

The focus of this chapter has been on fluid resuscitation, but vasoactive medications are also used in the hypotensive patient. The appropriate use of vasoactive agents will be discussed in other chapters, but in all forms of shock, proper attention must be paid to maintaining intravascular volume by fluid administration, particularly during the early stages of resuscitation. This is true even for septic shock that is defined as persistent hypotension after adequate fluid resuscitation. In a recent retrospective evaluation of a large observational database, there was a significant (p<0.0001) interaction between fluids and use of vasoactive agents. Mortality rates were lowest in patients who received delayed use (1–6 hours after shock onset) of vasoactive agents.[106]

FUTURE DIRECTIONS

Ideally, future large RCTs will be conducted that provide evidence for or against the use of specific fluids and monitoring tools in critically ill patients. Unfortunately, the design of these trials is fraught with challenges beyond usual issues, such sample size and blinding. As discussed earlier, both colloid fluids and crystalloid fluids vary in electrolyte composition, and it has been established that some commercially available exogenous albumin preparations do not have the same physicochemical characteristics as endogenous albumin. Table 2.7 shows some of these challenges using landmark studies involving albumin as an example, but the comments are applicable to studies using other fluids such as high-chloride-containing crystalloid solutions.[107,108] One challenge is deciding which patients to study and with which study design. The three large,

continued on page 53

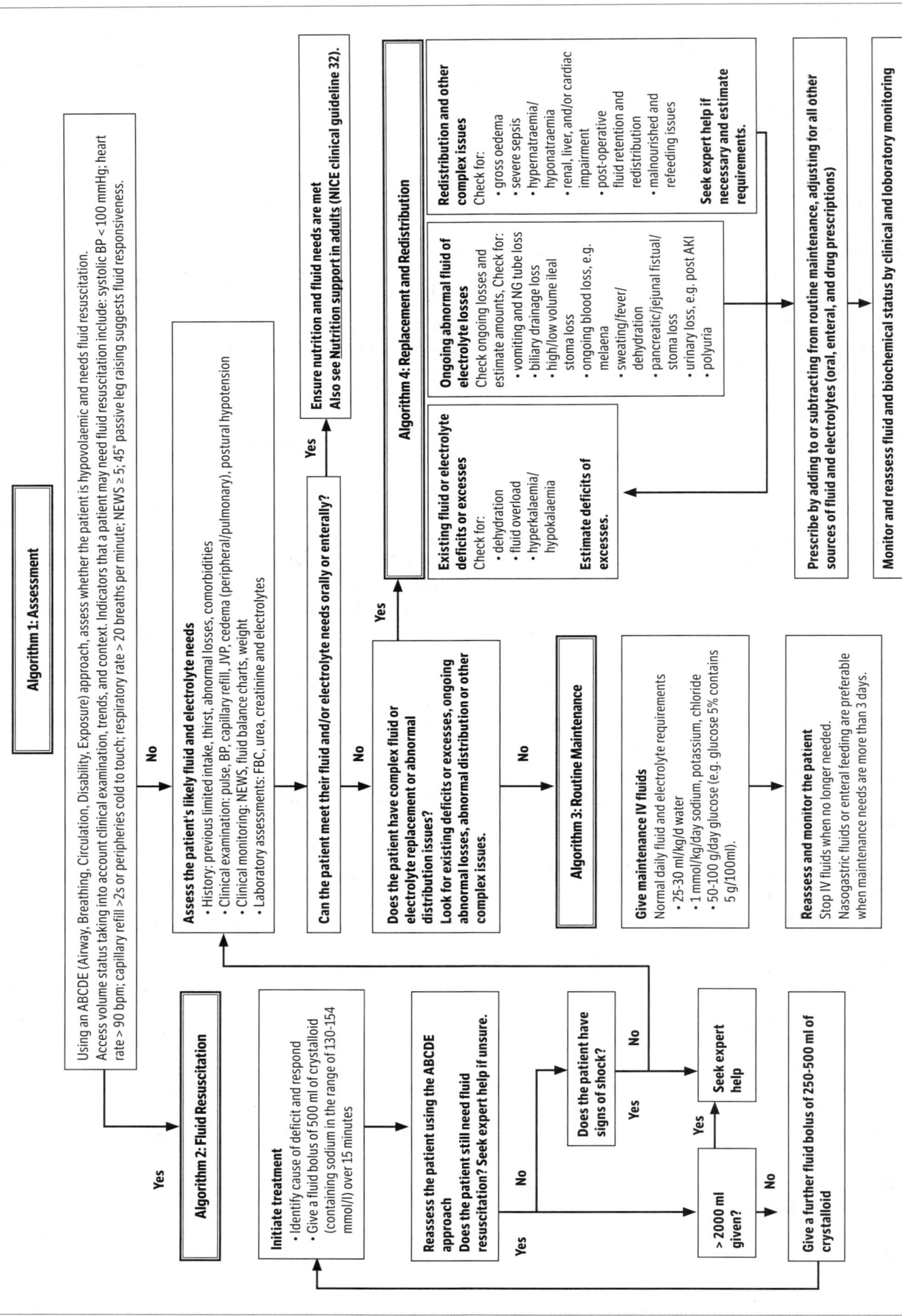

Figure 2.1 Algorithms for intravenous fluid therapy from NICE clinical guideline.

Reproduced with permission from: National Institute for Health and Care Excellence (NICE) Clinical Guideline 174. Intravenous Fluid Therapy in Adults in Hospital. December 2013. Available at https://www.nice.org.uk/guidance/cg174/resources/guidance-intravenous-fluid-therapy-in-adults-in-hospital-pdf. Accessed June 10, 2015.

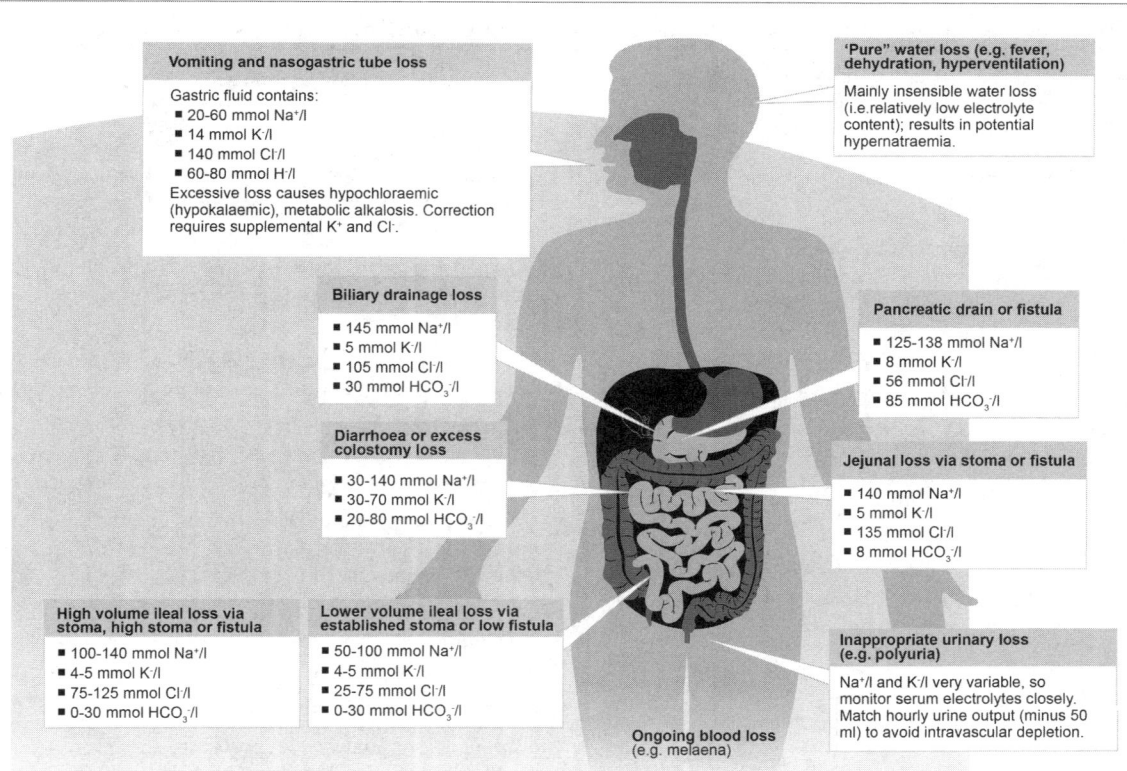

Figure 2.2 Electrolyte losses from the body from National Institute for Health and Care Excellence (NICE) clinical guideline.

Reproduced with permission from: National Institute for Health and Care Excellence (NICE) Clinical Guideline 174. Intravenous Fluid Therapy in Adults in Hospital. December 2013. Available at https://www.nice.org.uk/guidance/cg174/resources/guidance-intravenous-fluid-therapy-in-adults-in-hospital-pdf. Accessed June 10, 2015.

Table 2.6 Systematic Reviews and Guidelines Pertaining to Fluid Resuscitation

Source	Type of Evidence	Recommendation/Conclusion
ATLS recommendations[100]	Evidence-based consensus recommendations of fluids in trauma patients with shock	Warmed isotonic crystalloid solutions such as normal saline or lactated Ringer's should be used (LOE3); hypertonic sodium chloride is an alternative with no mortality advantage (LOE4)
EAST guideline[101]	Evidence-based consensus recommendations for prehospital fluids in trauma patients	Insufficient data to recommend one fluid over another when comparing normal saline, lactated Ringer's, 3% sodium chloride, or 7.5% sodium chloride (level I)
Cochrane collaboration[102]	Systematic review of colloids vs. crystalloids in critically ill patients	No evidence that colloids reduce mortality compared with crystalloids in patients with trauma or burns, or after surgery; hydroxyethyl starch products may increase mortality
Cochrane collaboration[103]	Systematic review of different colloids for fluid resuscitation	No evidence that one colloid is more effective than another in efficacy or safety; could not exclude clinically important differences because of wide confidence intervals; did not include trials after December 1, 2011
Cochrane collaboration[104]	Systematic review of albumin solutions vs. no albumin or crystalloids for fluid resuscitation in critically ill patients	No evidence that albumin reduces mortality compared with crystalloid solutions such as normal saline but cannot exclude benefit in specific subsets of critically ill patients
British consensus guidelines[105]	Guidelines for perioperative fluid prescribing	Balanced salt solutions such as lactated Ringer's are preferred to normal saline for crystalloid resuscitation unless hypochloremia is present (level 1b); balanced salt solutions or colloids until packed red blood cells are available for hypovolemia with blood loss (level 1b)
American Burn Association[65]	Guidelines for burn shock resuscitation that include fluid recommendations	Near-isotonic crystalloid recommended for initial resuscitation (grade C); hypertonic sodium chloride reserved for clinicians experienced with use (grade B); adding colloid 12–24 hr postburn may decrease fluid requirements (grade A)

ATLS = advanced trauma life support; EAST = Eastern Association for the Surgery of Trauma; grade A, at least one large prospective trial with clear-cut results; grade B, several small prospective trials with similar results; grade C, single small prospective trial, retrospective studies, or expert opinion; level 1b, randomized controlled trial with narrow confidence interval, or quality cohort studies (specific definitions); level I = convincingly justifiable; LOE3, level of evidence based on case-control or retrospective cohort studies, or a systematic review with at least three studies; LOE4 = level of evidence based on case series.

Adapted with permission from: Erstad BL. Hypovolemic shock. In: DiPiro JT, Talbert RL, Yee GC, Matzke GR, Wells BG, Posey LM, eds. Pharmacotherapy: A Pathophysiologic Approach, 9th ed. New York: McGraw-Hill, 2014:351-68.

Box 2.5. Overarching Considerations for Fluid Administration in Critically Ill Patients

Have established policies and protocols for fluids (and medications) that should be given by central rather than peripheral intravenous lines.

For dilution of fluids such as 25% albumin, osmolarity and tonicity issues must be considered.

Appreciate that much of the terminology of fluids is not standardized (e.g., hypertonic saline is not synonymous with 3% sodium chloride solution but is any sodium chloride solution above 0.9%; a *balanced* electrolyte solution does not refer to a specific fluid).

Electrolyte composition differences of crystalloid and colloid solutions must be considered in clinical investigations.

Clinical trials that combine disparate fluids into one group (e.g., colloids vs. crystalloids) will have results that are difficult to interpret.

For intravenous gelatin, dextran, and starch products, the benefits do not outweigh the risks in most, if not all, critically ill patients.

Spontaneous bacterial peritonitis is the only disease state in which albumin has been shown to reduce unadjusted mortality (evidence from only one randomized controlled trial).

Albumin is more likely to cause harm than benefit in the resuscitation of patients with traumatic brain injury.

Commercially available albumin does not have the same physicochemical characteristics as endogenous albumin, so mechanistic arguments for exogenous albumin administration based on endogenous albumin properties are not a substitute for randomized trials.

Hypertonic sodium chloride has no benefit over isotonic crystalloid solutions for fluid resuscitation and is a concentrated electrolyte solution with the potential for medication errors and adverse drug events.

In patients with severe traumatic hemorrhage, the definitive intervention is surgery for bleeding control, not plasma expansion.

Colloids do not provide the expected plasma expansion suggested by models of fluid distribution in body compartments.

There is increasing concern that administering large bolus doses of fluids during the initial phase of resuscitation of shock may negatively affect normal adaptive homeostatic responses.

There is increasing evidence to suggest that fluids more balanced in electrolytes, particularly chloride, are preferable for the initial resuscitation of patients with shock.

Fluid administration post-resuscitation must be individualized according to patient-specific conditions.

For most patients who develop ARDS in the post-resuscitation phase of management, fluid restriction is indicated.

No high-level evidence supports the use of more invasive, costly catheters as part of routine monitoring of shock.

No single monitoring parameter in isolation is adequate for assessing the adequacy of resuscitation.

ARDS = acute respiratory distress syndrome.

Table 2.7 Examples of Design Considerations in Landmark Randomized Trials Involving Albumin

Trial	SAFE[53]	ALBIOS[62]	EARSS[109]	Sort et al.[67]
Type of critically ill patients	Multidisciplinary medical and surgical	Multidisciplinary medical and surgical with severe sepsis	Multidisciplinary medical and surgical with septic shock	Patients with cirrhosis and spontaneous bacterial peritonitis
Eligibility/time of study entry	Enrolled if need for fluid administration for intravascular replacement so variable time of study entry	Enrolled anytime during ICU stay if severe sepsis within 24 hr	Diagnosis of septic shock within 6 hr after initiation of catecholamines	Diagnosis of spontaneous bacterial peritonitis with stringent enrollment criteria
Traditional vs. pragmatic	Pragmatic (all fluids except study fluid left to clinician discretion); albumin titrated to resuscitation end points	Pragmatic (all fluids except albumin left to clinician discretion but no colloids allowed); albumin titrated to albumin concentration	Pragmatic	Traditional (although details of non-study fluid not mentioned)
Duration of study fluid administration	Death, ICU discharge, or 28 days (sample size based on 28-day mortality)	Death, ICU discharge, or 28 days (sample size based on 28-day mortality)	Albumin administered as fixed dose every 8 hr for 3 days (sample size based on 28-day mortality)	Two doses of 20% albumin on days 1 and 3 (sample size based on renal impairment)

continued from page 49

pragmatic studies involving albumin enrolled patients in multidisciplinary medical and surgical ICU settings and left all decisions regarding concomitant crystalloid fluids to the clinicians caring for the patients.[53,62,107] With a large sample size, the advantage to this approach is that the findings are more likely to be generalizable. A disadvantage to this approach is that a potential beneficial effect in a particular subset of patients cannot be ruled out, as exemplified by the reductions in mortality found when albumin was administered to patients with spontaneous bacterial peritonitis.[66] Patient eligibility requirements and time to study entry are other factors that may complicate study conclusions. For example, arguments can be made for administering albumin earlier (e.g., early stage of shock before multiple organ dysfunction) or later (e.g., ARDS or burn injury after capillary permeability is restored) during ICU stay. If administered later during ICU stay, investigators must consider how pre-study (prehospital, emergency department, operating room, ward if transfer, and/or ICU stay before albumin administration) colloid or crystalloid administration might influence study end points. The appropriate dose, duration, and end points of albumin administration are other questions open to debate, particularly if the presumed beneficial mechanism of action of albumin being tested is something other than its oncotic and plasma expansion properties. There is no single right or wrong approach to any of these considerations, but the important point is that they must be considered during study design and later when interpreting study results.

REFERENCES

1. Centers for Disease Control and Prevention (CDC). Hemolysis associated with 25% human albumin diluted with sterile water—United States, 1994-1998. Morb Mortal Wkly Repo 1999;48:157-9.
2. Anonymous. Sterile water should not be given "freely." Pa Patient Saf Advis 2008;5:53-6.
3. Parker JC. Dog red blood cells. J Gen Physiol 1973;62:147-56.
4. Rocha e Silva MR, Velasco IT, Porfirio MF. Hypertonic saline resuscitation: saturated salt-dextran solutions are equally effective, but induce hemolysis in dogs. Crit Care Med 1990;18:203-7.
5. Gazitua R, Wilson K, Bistrian BR, et al. Factors determining peripheral vein tolerance to amino acid infusions. Arch Surg 1979;114:897-900.
6. Bodoky A, Zbinden A, Muller J, et al. Peripher-venose vertraglichkeit hyperosmalarer infusionslosungen. Helv Chir Acta 1980;47:151-6.
7. Daly JM, Masser E, Hansen L, et al. Peripheral vein infusion of dextrose/amino acid solutions ± 20% fat emulsion. JPEN 1985;9:296-9.
8. Kane KF, Cologiovanni L, McKiernan J, et al. High osmolality feedings do not increase the incidence of thrombophlebitis as defined by subjective/objective (observer) factors during peripheral IV nutrition. JPEN 1996;20:194-7.
9. Timmer JG, Schipper HG. Peripheral venous nutrition: the equal relevance of volume load and osmolarity in relation to phlebitis. Clin Nutr 1991;10:71-5.
10. Marko NF. Hyperosmolar therapy for intracranial hypertension: time to dispel antiquated myths. Am J Respir Crit Care Med 2012;185:467-78.
11. Maningas PA, Mattox KL, Pepe PE, et al. Hypertonic saline-dextran solutions for the prehospital management of traumatic hypotension. Am J Surg 1989;157:528-35.
12. Vassar MJ, Perry CA, Holcroft JW. Analysis of potential risks associated with 7.5% sodium chloride resuscitation of traumatic shock. Arch Surg 1990;125:1309-15.
13. Bulger EM, May S, Kerby JD, et al. Out-of-hospital hypertonic resuscitation after traumatic hypovolemic shock. Ann Surg 2011;253:431-41.
14. Bulger EM, May S, Brasel KJ, et al. Out-of-hospital hypertonic resuscitation following severe traumatic brain injury. JAMA 2010;304:1455-64.
15. Cooper DJ, Myles PS, McDermott FT, et al. Prehospital hypertonic saline resuscitation of patients with hypotension and severe traumatic brain injury. JAMA 2004;291:1350-7.
16. Bulger EM, Jurkovich GJ, Nathens AB, et al. Hypertonic resuscitation of hypovolemic shock after blunt trauma. Arch Surg 2008;143:139-48.
17. White H, Cook D, Venkatesh B. The use of hypertonic saline for treating intracranial hypertension after traumatic brain injury. Anesth Analg 2006;102:1836-46.
18. Kuwahara T, Asanami S, Kawauchi Y, et al. Experimental infusion phlebitis: tolerance pH of peripheral vein. J Toxicol Sci 1999;24:113-21.
19. Nahas GG, Sutin KM, Fermon C, et al. Guidelines for the treatment of acidaemia with THAM. Drugs 1998;55:191-224.
20. Kuwahara T, Asanami S, Kubo S. Experimental infusion phlebitis: tolerance osmolality of peripheral venous endothelial cells. Nutrition 1998;14:496-501.
21. Patanwala AE, Amini A, Erstad BL. Use of hypertonic saline injection in trauma. Am J Health Syst Pharm 2010;67:1920-8.
22. Torre-Healy A, Marko NF, Weil RJ. Hyperosmolar therapy for intracranial hypertension. Neurocrit Care 2012;17:117-30.
23. Latta T. Saline venous injections in cases of malignant cholera performed while in the vapour-bath. Part 1. Lancet 1832;19:173-6.
24. Lazarus-Barlow WS. On the initial rate of osmosis of blood-serum with reference to the composition of "physiological saline solution" in mammals. J Physiol 1896;20:145-57.
25. Awad S, Allison SP, Lobo DN. The history of 0.9% saline. Clin Nutr 2008;27:179-88.
26. Scheingraber S, Rehm M, Sehmisch C, et al. Rapid saline infusion produces hyperchloremic acidosis in patients undergoing gynecologic surgery. Anesthesiology 1999;90:1265-70.
27. Gattinoni L, Carlesso E, Maiocchi G, et al. Dilutional acidosis: where do the protons come from? Intensive Care Med 2009;35:2033-43.
28. Yunos NM, Bellomo R, Hegarty C, et al. Association between a chloride-liberal vs chloride-restrictive IV fluid administration strategy and kidney injury in critically ill patients. JAMA 2012;308:1566-72.

29. Alam HB, Rhee P. New developments in fluid resuscitation. Surg Clin North Am 2007;87:55-72.

30. Ringer S. Concerning the influence exerted by each of the constituents of the blood on the contraction of the ventricle. J Physiol 1882;3:380-93.

31. Ringer S. A further contribution regarding the influence of the different constituents of the blood on the contraction of the heart. J Physiol 1883;4:29-42.

32. Hartmann AF. Theory and practice of parenteral fluid administration. JAMA 1934;103:1349-54.

33. Risk Benefit of HES solutions Questioned by EMA. Position Statement by the Faculty of Intensive Care Medicine, the Royal College of Anaesthesia, the Intensive Care Society and the College of Emergency Medicine. Available at www.rcoa.ac.uk/news-and-bulletin/rcoa-news-and-statements/risk-benefit-of-hes-solutions-questioned-ema. Accessed September 30, 2014.

34. Carlesso E, Maiocchi G, Tallarini F, et al. The rule regulating pH changes during crystalloid infusion. Intensive Care Med 2011;37:461-8.

35. Lazarus-Barlow WS. Observations upon the initial rates of osmosis of certain substances in water and in fluids containing albumen. J Physiol 1895;19:140-66.

36. Starling EH. On the absorption of fluids from the connective tissue spaces. J Physiol 1896;19:312-26.

37. Janeway CA. Human serum albumin: historical review. In: Sgouris JT, Rene A, eds. Proceedings of the Workshop on Albumin. DHEW Publication (NIH) 76-925. Washington, DC: U.S. Government Printing Office, 1976:3-21.

38. Cohn EJ, Oncley JL, Strong LE, et al. Chemical, clinical, and immunological studies on the products of human plasma fractionation. I. The characterization of the protein fractions of human plasma. J Clin Invest 1944;23:417-32.

39. Heyl JT, Gibson JG, Janeway CA, et al. Studies of the plasma proteins. V. The effect of concentrated solutions of human and bovine serum albumin on blood volume after acute blood loss in man. J Clin Invest 1943;22:763-73.

40. Cournand A, Noble RP, Breed ES, et al. Chemical, clinical, and immunological studies on the products of human plasma fractionation. VIII. Clinical use of concentrated human serum albumin in shock, and comparison with whole blood and with rapid saline infusion. J Clin Invest 1944;23:491-505.

41. Scatchard G, Batchelder AC, Brown A. Chemical, clinical, and immunological studies on the products of human plasma fractionation. VI. The osmotic pressure of plasma and serum albumin. J Clin Invest 1944;23:458-64.

42. Janeway CA, Gibson ST, Woodruff LM, et al. Chemical, clinical, and immunological studies on the products of human plasma fractionation. VII. Concentrated human serum albumin. J Clin Invest 1944;23:465-90.

43. Warren JV, Stead EA, Merrill AJ, et al. Chemical, clinical, and immunological studies on the products of human plasma fractionation. IX. The treatment of shock with concentrated human serum albumin: a preliminary report. J Clin Invest 1944;23:506-9.

44. Sgouris JT, Rene A, eds. Proceedings of the Workshop on Albumin. DHEW Publication (NIH) 76-925. Washington, DC: U.S. Government Printing Office, 1976:1-358.

45. Sgouris JT, Dorsey HW. Survey of the use of plasma expanders in the United States. Proceedings of the Workshop on Albumin. In: Sgouris JT, Rene A, eds. DHEW Publication (NIH) 76-925. Washington, DC: U.S. Government Printing Office, 1976:137-48.

46. Tullis JL. Albumin: 1. Background and use. JAMA 1977;237:355-60.

47. Tullis JL. Albumin: 2. Guidelines for clinical use. JAMA 1977;237:460-3.

48. Vermeulen LC, Ratko TA, Erstad BL, et al. A paradigm for consensus: the University Hospital Consortium guidelines for the use of albumin, nonprotein colloid, and crystalloid solutions. Arch Intern Med 1995;155:373-9.

49. Yim JM, Vermeulen LC, Erstad BL, et al. Albumin and nonprotein colloid solution use in U.S. academic health centers Arch Intern Med 1995;155:2450-5.

50. Chappell D, Jacob M, Hofman-Kiefer K, et al. A rational approach to perioperative fluid management. Anesthesiology 2008;109:723-40.

51. Jacob M, Bruegger D, Rehm M, et al. Contrasting effects of colloid and crystalloid resuscitation fluids on cardiac vascular permeability. Anesthesiology 2006;104:1223-31.

52. Quinlan GJ, Martin GS, Evans TW. Albumin: biochemical properties and therapeutic potential. Hepatology 2006;41:1211-19.

53. Finfer S, Bellomo R, Boyce N, et al. A comparison of albumin and saline for fluid resuscitation in the intensive care unit. N Engl J Med 2004;350:2247-56.

54. Brunkhorst FM, Engel C, Bloos F, et al. Intensive insulin therapy and pentastarch resuscitation in severe sepsis. N Engl J Med 2008;358:125-39.

55. Perner A, Haase N, Guttormsen AB, et al. Hydroxyethyl starch 130/0.4 versus Ringer's acetate in severe sepsis. N Engl J Med 2012;367:124-34.

56. Myburgh JA, Finfer S, Bellomo R, et al. Hydroxyethyl starch or saline for fluid resuscitation in intensive care. N Engl J Med 2012;367:1901-11.

57. Cochrane Injuries Group Albumin Reviewers. Human albumin administration in critically ill patients: systematic review of randomised controlled trials. BMJ 1998;317:235-40.

58. Choi P, Yip G, Quinonez LG, et al. Crystalloids vs. colloids in fluid resuscitation: a systematic review. Crit Care Med 1999;27:200-10.

59. Annane D, Siami S, Jaber S, et al. Effects of fluid resuscitation with colloids vs crystalloids on mortality in critically ill patients presenting with hypovolemic shock. JAMA 2013;310:1809-17.

60. The SAFE Study Investigators. Saline or albumin for fluid resuscitation in patients with traumatic brain injury. N Engl J Med 2007;357:874-84.

61. The SAFE Investigators. Impact of albumin compared to saline on organ function and mortality of patients with severe sepsis. Intensive Care Med 2011;37:86-96.

62. Caironi P, Tognoni G, Masson S, et al. Albumin replacement in patients with severe sepsis or septic shock. N Engl J Med 2014;370:1412-21.

63. Patel A, Laffan MA, Waheed U, et al. Randomised trials of human albumin for adults with sepsis: systematic review and

63. meta-analysis with trial sequential analysis of all-cause mortality. BMJ 2014;349:g4561.
64. Rochwerg B, Alhazzani W, Sindl A, et al. Fluid resuscitation in sepsis: a systematic review and network meta-analysis. Ann Intern Med 2014;161:347-55.
65. Pham TN, Cancio LC, Gibran NS. American Burn Association practice guidelines burn shock resuscitation. J Burn Care Res 2008;29:257-66.
66. Park SH, Hemmila MR, Wahl WL. Early albumin use improves mortality in difficult to resuscitate burn patients. J Trauma Acute Care Surg 2012;73:1294-7.
67. Sort P, Navasa M, Arroyo V, et al. Effect of IV albumin on renal impairment and mortality in patients with cirrhosis and spontaneous bacterial peritonitis. N Engl J Med 1999;34:403-9.
68. McLeod BC. Plasma and plasma derivatives in therapeutic plasmapheresis. Transfusion 2012;52:38s-44s.
69. Liumbruno G, Bennardello F, Latannzio A, et al. Recommendations for the use of albumin and immunoglobulin. Blood Tranfus 2009;7:216-34.
70. Runyon BA. Management of adult patients with ascites due to cirrhosis: update 2012. Hepatology 2013;53:1-27.
71. European Association for the Study of the Liver. EASL clinical practice guidelines on the management of ascites, spontaneous bacterial peritonitis, and hepatorenal syndrome in cirrhosis. J Hepatol 2010;53:397-417.
72. Brochard L, Abroug F, Brenner M, et al. An official ATS/ERS/ESICM/SCCM/SRLF statement: prevention and management of acute renal failure in the ICU patient. Am J Respir Crit Care Med 2010;181:1128-55.
73. Bernardi M, Caraceni P, Navickes RJ, et al. Albumin infusion in patients undergoing large-volume paracentesis: a meta-analysis of randomized trials. Hepatology 2012;55:1172-81.
74. Reinhart K, Perner A, Sprung CL, et al. Consensus statement of the ESICM task force on colloid volume therapy in critically ill patients. Intensive Care Med 2012;38:368-83.
75. Bickell WH, Wall MJ, Pepe PE, et al. Immediate versus delayed fluid resuscitation for hypotensive patients with penetrating torso injuries. N Engl J Med 1994;331:1105-9.
76. Brown JB, Cohen MJ, Minei JP, et al. Goal-directed resuscitation in the prehospital setting: a propensity-adjusted analysis. J Trauma Acute Care Surg 2013;74:1207-14.
77. Dellinger RP, Levy MM, Rhodes A, et al. Surviving Sepsis Campaign: international guidelines for management of severe sepsis and septic shock: 2012. Crit Care Med 2013;41:580-637.
78. Maitland K, Kiguli S, Opoka RO, et al. Mortality after fluid bolus in African children with severe infection. N Engl J Med 2011;364:2483-95.
79. Jarvela K, Koskinen M, Koobi T. Effects of hypertonic saline (7.5%) on extracellular fluid volumes in healthy volunteers. Anaesthesia 2003;58:874-910.
80. Lamke LO, Liljedahl SO. Plasma volume expansion after infusion of 5%, 20% and 25% albumin solutions in patients. Resuscitation 1976;5:85-92.
81. Margarson MP, Soni NC. Effects of albumin supplementation on microvascular permeability in septic patients. J Appl Physiol 2002;92:2139-45.
82. Margarson MP, Soni NC. Changes in serum albumin concentration and volume expanding effects following a bolus of albumin 20% in septic patients. Br J Anaesth 2004;92:821-6.
83. Bark BP, Persson J, Grande PO. Importance of the infusion rate for the plasma expanding effect of 5% albumin, 6% HES 130/04, 4% gelatin, and 0.9% NaCl in the septic rate. Crit Care Med 2013;41:857-66.
84. Guidet B, Martinet O, Boulain T, et al. Assessment of hemodynamic efficacy and safety of 6% hydroxyethyl starch 130/0.4 versus 0.9% NaCl fluid replacement in patients with severe sepsis: the CRYSTMAS study. Crit Care 2012;16:R94.
85. National Heart, Lung, and Blood Institute Acute Respiratory Distress Syndrome (ARDS) Clinical Trials Network. Comparison of two fluid-management strategies in acute lung injury. N Engl J Med 2006;354:2564-75.
86. Grisson CK, Hirshberg EL, Dickerson JB, et al. Fluid management with a simplified conservative protocol for the acute respiratory distress syndrome. Crit Care Med 2015;43:288-95.
87. Sandham JD, Hull RD, Brant RF, et al. Canadian Critical Care Trials Group: a randomized, controlled trial of the use of pulmonary artery catheters in high-risk surgical patients. N Engl J Med 2003;348:5-14.
88. Harvey S, Harrison DA, Singer M, et al.; PAC-Man Study Collaboration: assessment of the clinical effectiveness of pulmonary artery catheters in management of patients in intensive care (PAC-Man): a randomized controlled trial. Lancet 2005;366:472-7.
89. Wheeler AP, Bernard GR, Thompson BT, et al. Pulmonary-artery versus central venous catheter to guide treatment of acute lung injury. N Engl J Med 2006;354:2213-24.
90. Vincent JL, Weil MH. Fluid challenge revisited. Crit Care Med 2006;34:1333-7.
91. Rivers E, Nguyen B, Havstad S, et al. Early goal-directed therapy in the treatment of severe sepsis and septic shock. N Engl J Med 2001;345:1368-77.
92. The ProCESS Investigators. A randomized trial of protocol-based care for early septic shock. N Engl J Med 2014;370:1683-93.
93. The ARISE Investigators and the ANZICS Clinical Trials Group. Goal-directed resuscitation for patients with early septic shock. N Engl J Med 2014;371:1496-506.
94. Mouncey PR, Osborn TM, Power S, et al. Trial of early, goal-directed resuscitation for septic shock. N Engl J Med 2015;372:1301-11.
95. Mandeville JC, Colebourn CL. Can transthoracic echocardiography be used to predict fluid responsiveness in the critically ill patient? A systematic review. Crit Care Res Pract 2012;2012:513480.
96. Ceccnoi M, De Backer D, Antonelli M, et al. Consensus on circulatory shock and hemodynamic monitoring. Task force of the European Society of Intensive Care Medicine. Intensive Care Med 2014;40:1795-815.
97. National Institute for Health and Care Excellence (NICE) Clinical Guideline 174. Intravenous Fluid Therapy in Adults in Hospital. December 2013. Available at https://www.nice.org.uk/guidance/cg174/resources/guidance-intravenous-fluid-therapy-in-adults-in-hospital-pdf. Accessed June 10, 2015.

98. Grissom CK, Hirshberg EL, Dickerson JB, et al. Fluid management with a simplified conservative protocol for the acute respiratory distress syndrome. Crit Care Med 2015;43:288-95.

99. Bion J, Bellomo R, Myburgh J, et al. Hydroxyethyl starch: putting patient safety first. Intensive Care Med 2014;40:256-9.

100. Kortbeek JB, Al Turki SA, Ali J, et al. Advanced trauma life support, 8th edition, the evidence for change. J Trauma 2008;64:1638-50.

101. Cotton BA, Jerome R, Collier BR, et al. Guidelines for prehospital fluid resuscitation in the injured patient. J Trauma 2009;67:389-402.

102. Perel P, Roberts I, Ker K. Colloids versus crystalloids for fluid resuscitation in critically ill patients. Cochrane Database Syst Rev 2013;2:CD000567.

103. Bunn F, Trivedi D. Colloid solutions for fluid resuscitation. Cochrane Database Syst Rev 2012;7:CD001319.

104. Roberts I, Blackhall K, Alderson P, et al. Human albumin solution for resuscitation and volume expansion in critically ill patients. Cochrane Database Syst Rev 2011;11:CD001208.

105. Soni N. British consensus guidelines on IV fluid therapy for adult surgical patients – Cassandra's view. Anesthesia 2009;64:235-8.

106. Waechter J, Kumar A, Lapinsky SE, et al. Interaction between fluids and vasoactive agents on mortality in septic shock: a multicenter, observational study. Crit Care Med 2014;42:2158-68.

107. Young P, Bailey M, Beasley R, et al. Effect of a buffered cyrstalloid solution vs saline on acute kidney injury among patients in the intensive care unit: The SPLIT randomized clinical trial. JAMA 2015; 314(16):1701-10.

108. Kellum JA, Shaw AD. Assessing toxicity of intravenous crystalloids in critically ill patients. JAMA 2015;314(editorial):1695-97.

109. Charpentier J, Mira JP; EARSS Study Group. Efficacy and tolerance of hyperoncotic albumin administration in septic shock patients: the EARSS study. Intensive Care Med 2011;37 (suppl 1):S115.

Appendix 2.1. Examples of Osmolarity Calculations

Here is an example that shows the concept of osmolarity using an albumin solution that is presumed to be formulated in a normal saline solution. Assume we have 50 mL of a 25% (i.e., 12.5 g per 50 mL or 25 g per 100 mL) albumin solution in 0.9% sodium chloride; the osmolarity using albumin is calculated as follows:

1 mole of albumin = 1 eq wt of albumin = 70,000 g
1 mmol of albumin = 1 mEq wt of albumin = 70 g

So,

$$\frac{1 \text{ mEq wt}}{70 \text{ g}} = \frac{X}{12.5 \text{ g}} \qquad X = 0.17857 \text{ mEq of albumin in 50 mL of 25\%}$$

$$\frac{0.17857 \text{ mEq}}{50 \text{ mL}} = \frac{X}{1000 \text{ mL}} \qquad X = 3.57 \text{ mEq or mOsm of albumin in 1000 mL}$$

Or an easier way,

There is 250 g/L of albumin in this solution, so:

$$\frac{1 \text{ mEq}}{70 \text{ g}} = \frac{X}{250 \text{ g}} \qquad X = 3.57 \text{ mEq or mOsm of albumin in 1000 mL}$$

For the sodium chloride component, there is 0.45 g in the 50-mL (or 0.9 g per 100 mL) solution:

1 mole of sodium chloride = 1 eq wt of sodium (23 g) + 1 eq wt of chloride (35.5 g) = 58.5 g
1 mmol of sodium chloride = 1 mEq wt of sodium + 1 mEq wt of chloride = 0.0585 g

So,

$$\frac{2 \text{ mEq wt}}{0.0585 \text{ g}} = \frac{X}{0.45 \text{ g}} \qquad X = 15.4 \text{ mEq of sodium and chloride in 50 mL}$$

$$\frac{15.4 \text{ mEq}}{50 \text{ mL}} = \frac{X}{1000 \text{ mL}} \qquad X = 308 \text{ mEq or mOsm of sodium and chloride in 1000 mL}$$

Or an easier way,

There is 9 g/L of sodium chloride in this solution, so:

$$\frac{2 \text{ mEq}}{0.0585 \text{ g}} = \frac{X}{9 \text{ g}} \qquad X = 308 \text{ mEq or mOsm of sodium and chloride in 1000 mL}$$

Because 1 mEq = 1 mOsm for albumin (not ionized), albumin contributes 3.57 mOsm/L to the total osmolarity of the commercially available 25% solution. Assuming complete ionization, the 154 mEq/L of sodium chloride in this same solution contributes 308 mOsm/L for a total osmolarity of 311.57 mOsm/L.

A variety of online calculators are available on the Internet for determining the osmolarity of various electrolytes, and some calculators are available that determine the osmole content of complex admixtures (e.g., www.globalrph.com), but any calculation should be verified by at least one other method.

Chapter 3: Electrolyte Disorders in the Critically Ill Population

Jeffrey J. Bruno, Pharm.D., BCPS, BCNSP; and Todd W. Canada, Pharm.D., FASHP, FTSHP, BCNSP

LEARNING OBJECTIVES

1. Distinguish the homeostatic mechanisms responsible for normal sodium, potassium, magnesium, phosphorus, and calcium balance in critically ill patients.
2. Provide the most common etiologies of hypo- and hypernatremia, hypo- and hyperkalemia, hypo- and hypermagnesemia, hypo- and hyperphosphatemia, and hypo- and hypercalcemia in critically ill patients.
3. Determine clinical estimates of replacement therapy involving sodium, potassium, magnesium, phosphate, and calcium in the critically ill population.

ABBREVIATIONS IN THIS CHAPTER

ADH	Antidiuretic hormone	ICU	Intensive care unit
AMI	Acute myocardial infarction	ODS	Osmotic demyelination syndrome
ATP	Adenosine triphosphate	PTH	Parathyroid hormone
CNS	Central nervous system	RBC	Red blood cell
ECF	Extracellular fluid	SIADH	Syndrome of inappropriate antidiuretic hormone
ECG	Electrocardiogram		
ICF	Intracellular fluid	TBW	Total body water

INTRODUCTION

This chapter provides a concise and clinically oriented overview of sodium, potassium, magnesium, phosphorus, and calcium derangements. Emphasis is placed on the clinical management of such disorders at the bedside, and when available, pertinent primary literature is discussed. Areas for which primary literature does not exist are clearly delineated, with guidance provided by published expert opinion and sound clinical judgment.

SODIUM AND WATER HOMEOSTASIS

Before discussing sodium disorders, it is important to have a firm understanding of total body water (TBW) and serum osmolality, given the relationship among these three entities. Overall, about 50% of body weight in females and elderly males and 60% in non-elderly males consists of water.[1] Most TBW is located in the intracellular space (60%). The remaining 40% of TBW is found in the extracellular space, with 25% intravascular and 75% interstitial.[2]

Under normal physiologic conditions, water moves between the extracellular fluid (ECF) and the intracellular fluid (ICF) in response to osmotic gradients. Osmotic gradients are generated by differences in the concentration of effective osmoles (i.e., solutes than cannot freely cross cell membranes) between the ECF and the ICF. Sodium and chloride are the primary effective osmoles responsible for ECF osmolality, whereas potassium and phosphate primarily drive ICF osmolality.[2] Water can freely or passively move across cell membranes and will move from areas of low to high osmolality in an attempt to maintain a normal serum osmolality (i.e., 275–290 mOsm/kg). Serum osmolality can either be directly measured by laboratory analysis or estimated using equation 3.1.[2] Discrepancies can arise between the measured and the calculated serum osmolality when effective osmoles not accounted for in the equation are administered exogenously and accumulate (e.g., propylene glycol from lorazepam or ethylene glycol toxicity), resulting in the development of an osmolar gap.[3]

$$\text{serum osmolality (mOsm/kg)} = 2 \times \text{serum sodium (mEq/L)} + \text{serum glucose (mg/dL)}/18 + \text{blood urea nitrogen (mg/dL)}/2.8 \text{ (equation 3.1)}[2]$$

Mechanisms exist to facilitate sodium and water homeostasis, thereby maintaining a normal serum osmolality.[1,2] The hypothalamus plays an integral role, with as little as a 1% change in serum osmolality triggering homeostatic mechanisms.[1] In the setting of increased serum osmolality, the hypothalamus stimulates the thirst mechanism as well as the release of arginine vasopressin (AVP), or antidiuretic hormone (ADH), from the posterior pituitary gland. Unfortunately, in many critically ill patients, the thirst mechanism may be of little utility given the limitations imposed by acute illness on the self-administration of fluids, leaving both fluid administration and fluid composition at the discretion of the clinician(s). Antidiuretic hormone works by binding to vasopressin 2 (V_2) receptors on renal tubular epithelial cells. This results in the insertion and opening of aquaporin 2 channels, facilitating reabsorption of water back into the systemic circulation and thereby decreasing serum osmolality.[1,2] However, a change in serum osmolality is not the only trigger for mediators of sodium and water homeostasis. For example, hypotension triggers arterial baroreceptors in the carotid sinus and glomerular afferent arterioles, subsequently activating the renin-angiotensin-aldosterone system. Activation of the renin-angiotensin-aldosterone system will induce sodium and water retention as well as ADH release, irrespective of serum osmolality.[2] In addition, ADH release can be triggered by pain and stress, such as during the immediate postoperative period.[4-6]

HYPONATREMIA

Hyponatremia is defined as a serum sodium concentration less than 135 mEq/L. Retrospective studies indicate that hyponatremia affects 20%–38% of hospitalized patients[7-9] and 11%–38% of critically ill patients.[7,10-12] Prevalence variations are likely associated with differences in diagnostic threshold, patient populations, and reporting of intensive care unit (ICU)-admission, ICU-acquired, or spot check hyponatremia.

Pathophysiology and Classification of Hyponatremia: Isotonic, Hypertonic, and Hypotonic

Hyponatremia is usually associated with a hypotonic state and is much less commonly observed in a hypertonic or isotonic setting. In the past, serum sodium concentrations were determined using flame photometry. With such practice, elevated concentrations of lipids (e.g., hypertriglyceridemia) and proteins (e.g., hyperproteinemia in multiple myeloma) led to falsely low serum sodium concentrations or pseudohyponatremia. Measurement of serum sodium by ion-specific electrodes has made pseudohyponatremia nonexistent.[1] Isotonic hyponatremia is characterized by a serum osmolality of 275–290 mOsm/kg and a serum sodium less than 135 mEq/L. Systemic absorption of irrigation solutions, such as dextrose or 1.5% glycine, can result in isotonic hyponatremia, as seen after transurethral resection of the prostate.[1]

Hypertonic hyponatremia is characterized by a serum osmolality greater than 305 mOsm/kg and a serum sodium less than 135 mEq/L. Common causes of hypertonic hyponatremia include hyperglycemia and infusion of glycerin- or mannitol-containing solutions.[1,2] Essentially, the increase in or introduction of effective osmoles other than sodium to the ECF leads to a rise in serum osmolality, movement of free water from the ICF to the ECF, and subsequent hyponatremia. Management of hypertonic hyponatremia involves correcting the underlying cause (i.e., minimizing or removing the non-sodium effective osmole). Traditionally, for each 100 mg/dL increase in serum glucose above 100 mg/dL, serum sodium was expected to fall by 1.6 mEq/L[13]; however, others have shown a correction factor of 2.4 mEq/L to be more appropriate.[14] Equation 3.2 can be used to determine a corrected serum sodium in the presence of hyperglycemia. Clinicians should be cognizant that the fall in serum sodium with hyperglycemia is nonlinear and can be as high as 4 mEq/L when the blood glucose is greater than 400 mg/dL.[14]

$$\text{corrected serum sodium (mEq/L)} = \text{serum sodium (mEq/L)} + 0.024 \, [\text{serum glucose (mg/dL)} - 100] \text{ (equation 3.2)}[14]$$

Hypotonic hyponatremia, characterized by a serum osmolality less than 275 mOsm/kg and a serum sodium less than 135 mEq/L, is the most common type of hyponatremia and therefore the most clinically relevant. Hypotonic hyponatremia is further classified into hypovolemic, euvolemic, or hypervolemic depending on the patient's fluid status.[1,4] The differential diagnosis for hypotonic hyponatremia is discussed later in this chapter.

Clinical Manifestations

Clinical manifestations of hyponatremia predominantly include disorders of the central nervous system (CNS) and vary widely among patients depending on the degree of hyponatremia and duration of development. Overall, it is safe to assume that the greater the decrease in serum sodium from baseline and the more rapid the decline, the greater the shift of water from the ECF to the ICF, the greater the degree of cerebral edema, and the greater the probability for symptom development. Within minutes of hyponatremia development, brain cells try to accommodate by the efflux of sodium and potassium ions to the extracellular space (rapid adaptation); however, movement of organic osmolytes to the extracellular space (slow adaptation) does not occur until 48 hours or more.[4] Thus, patients with acute hyponatremia (onset less than 48 hours) are at the highest risk of severe neurological sequelae associated with cerebral edema, including vomiting, somnolence, neurogenic pulmonary edema, seizures, coma, and potential fatal brain herniation. The risk of herniation is greatest when acute hyponatremia develops over several hours.[15] Other potential neurological symptoms include nausea without vomiting, confusion, and headache. In contrast, patients in whom hyponatremia is chronic (i.e., develops over 48 hours or more) are less prone to cerebral edema and herniation.[4,15] These patients typically have minimal brain swelling and present with malaise, fatigue, cramps, confusion, and/or falls. A 10% incidence of seizures has been reported when the serum sodium concentration falls below 110 mEq/L in this population.[16] Osteoporosis and fractures can also be seen with chronic hyponatremia.[16]

Morbidity and Mortality

Hyponatremia has been associated with an increased risk of hospital mortality in several retrospective evaluations[8-10,17] and in a meta-analysis.[18] Of interest, some reports show a significantly increased risk of death among patients with mild or moderate, but not severe, hyponatremia compared with patients who are normonatremic.[8,19] In a single-center retrospective review of almost 46,000 episodes of hyponatremia (less than 135 mEq/L), Chawla and colleagues showed a bell-shaped curve between the severity of hyponatremia and mortality, with the following specific rates: 4% (less than 110 mEq/L), 8% (110–114 mEq/L), 11% (115–119 mEq/L), 11% (120–124 mEq/L), 10%, (125–129 mEq/L), 5% (130–134 mEq/L), and 2% (greater than 135 mEq/L).[19] Furthermore, in an evaluation of patients who died with a serum sodium less than 120 mEq/L (n=53), the average Charlson comorbidity index was 5.5 (i.e., high severity of illness); 66% of patients had correction in serum sodium to 128 mEq/L or more, and only 4% presented with hyponatremia-related seizures with one case of brain herniation. In contrast, the authors' review of 32 survivors with a serum sodium concentration less than 110 mEq/L showed a low severity of illness (Charlson comorbidity index of 1.8), serum sodium less than 120 mEq/L 24 hours after the lowest serum sodium in 75%, a 9% incidence of hyponatremia-related seizures, and medications (e.g., thiazide diuretics, selective serotonin reuptake inhibitors) as the predominant etiology. Although limited information was provided regarding the actual rate of sodium correction from hyponatremia, it may be speculated that patients die with (i.e., as a concomitant factor of their underlying illness), in contrast to die from hyponatremia.[19] In a retrospective review of more than 13,000 serum sodium measurements from critically ill patients included in the Extended Prevalence of Infection in Intensive Care (EPIC II) study, logistic regression revealed an overall increased risk of death among patients with mild (130–134 mEq/L), moderate (125–129 mEq/L), and severe hyponatremia (less than 125 mEq/L). However, among patients with severe hyponatremia, a significantly increased risk of death was only observed among the subset of patients admitted with this disorder (odds ratio [OR] 3.79; 95% confidence interval [CI], 1.66–8.61) in contrast to those who were in the ICU at the time of evaluation (OR 1.62; 95% CI, 0.86–3.05).[11] Of note, resolution of hyponatremia during hospitalization may help mitigate the increased mortality risk.[8]

Assessment

Once hyponatremia is identified, the first step in assessment is to determine whether the patient is symptomatic or asymptomatic. Patients with severe neurological sequelae (e.g., vomiting, seizures, coma) should promptly receive treatment without delaying for further assessment (see Severely Symptomatic Hyponatremia section).[15] Next, it should be determined whether the hyponatremia is acute or chronic. This can be done by a simple trending of the patient's serum sodium concentration for a given period (e.g., 2–14 days), if available. If the duration is unclear (i.e., no prior laboratory results and no signs of an acute etiology), hyponatremia should be presumed as chronic to avoid the adverse consequences associated with too rapid of a correction, most notably osmotic demyelination syndrome (ODS).[15] Chronic hyponatremia should trigger consideration of etiologies that are persistent versus episodic in nature, such as syndrome of inappropriate antidiuretic hormone (SIADH) from malignancy or long-term thiazide therapy in contrast to acute vomiting. A thorough physical examination should be performed together with a review of the patient's history and fluid balance (if available, a minimum of 2 days) before hyponatremia development. These steps may be sufficient for rather obvious etiologies of hyponatremia (e.g., dry mucus membranes in the setting of increased nasogastric [NG] tube output, consistent with hypovolemic hypotonic hyponatremia), and treatment can be instituted accordingly.

If the hyponatremia classification and etiology are not apparent from the previous steps alone, serum osmolality, urine osmolality, and urine sodium concentrations should be ordered. Serum osmolality will allow the clinician to distinguish between hypertonic (greater than 290 mOsm/kg), isotonic (275–290 mOsm/kg) and hypotonic (less than 275 mOsm/kg) hyponatremia. In hypotonic hyponatremia, the urine osmolality and urine sodium results should be coupled with the physical examination findings indicative of the patient's fluid status (i.e., hypovolemic, euvolemic, or hypervolemic) to determine the potential etiology and subsequent intervention. Of interest, although fluid status should routinely be assessed, misjudgment is common.[20] In addition, clinicians should be cautioned regarding the interpretation of urine sodium concentrations because many medications administered in the critically ill population can influence these results, rendering them unreliable. Some of these medications include diuretics (thiazide and loop diuretics),[21] sodium chloride tablets, mannitol, and corticosteroids. According to the results of these urine studies, other laboratory tests (e.g., serum cortisol, thyroid stimulating hormone) may be needed to assist with the differential diagnosis. A diagnostic algorithm for hypotonic hyponatremia is provided in Figure 3.1.[2,20] Clinicians should note that many hyponatremia algorithms have been published and that slight variations in the threshold values for hyponatremia, urine sodium, and/or urine osmolality exist. Of interest, use of an algorithm versus non-guided senior physician evaluation of hyponatremia resulted in an increased ability to properly diagnose and categorize hypotonic hyponatremia.[20]

Management

The treatment goals for hyponatremia are to prevent or provide relief of symptoms while avoiding complications associated with overcorrecting or correcting too rapidly (i.e., ODS). Unfortunately, data are limited regarding the acute management of hyponatremia, with most studies retrospective in nature and, for the most part, of low-quality methodology. Nevertheless, clinicians must provide therapeutic interventions at the bedside to care for these patients. This section will summarize the available data for the treatment of hypotonic hyponatremia, including treatment of the severely symptomatic patient; recommended serum sodium correction rates; and a brief discussion on addressing the underlying etiology. Osmotic demyelination syndrome will be discussed first, given the concern for iatrogenic development while treating hyponatremia and avoidance of ODS when determining serum sodium correction rates.

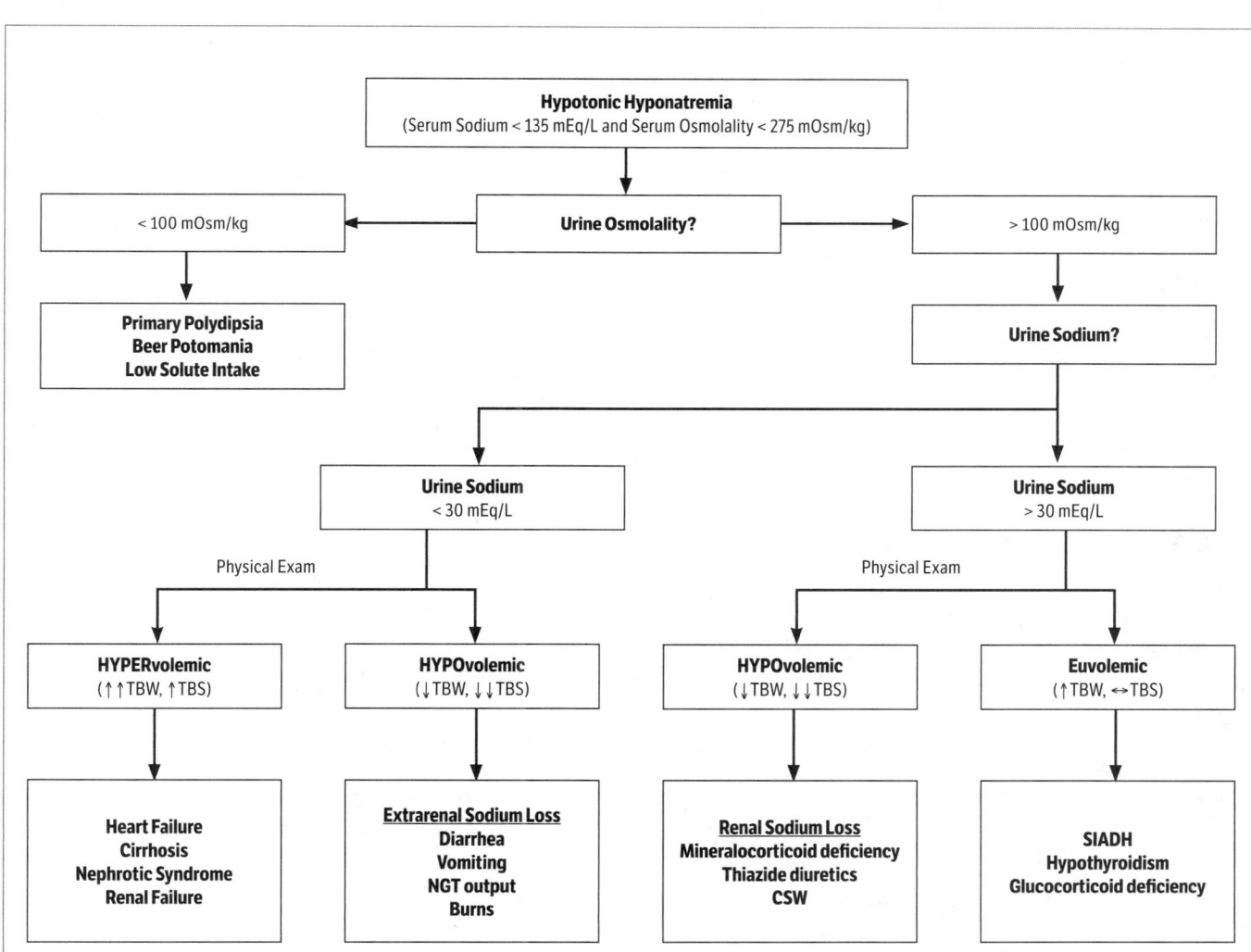

Figure 3.1 Diagnostic algorithm for hypotonic hyponatremia.[2,20]

CSW = Cerebral salt wasting; NGT = Nasogastric tube; SIADH = Syndrome of inappropriate antidiuretic hormone; TBS = Total body sodium; TBW = Total body water
Information adapted from Fenske W, et al. Am J Med 2010;123:652-657; and Coyle JD, et al. In: Dipiro JT (ed.) Pharmacotherapy: A Pathophysiologic Approach, 8th ed., New York: McGraw-Hill, 2011:873-90.

Prevention of Osmotic Demyelination Syndrome

In 1976, Tomlinson and colleagues described the development of central pontine and extrapontine myelinolysis in two women with profound hyponatremia after treatment with 3% sodium chloride and a subsequent rise in serum sodium of 25 mEq/L and 32 mEq/L by 48 hours.[22] This observation was later confirmed in experimental animal models of chronic hyponatremia after rapid serum sodium correction. Overall, demyelination occurs secondary to shrinkage of brain cells. As explained earlier, the brain adapts to the presence of hyponatremia through the loss of organic osmolytes in an attempt to minimize cerebral edema. Upon rapid correction of hyponatremia, the brain is unable to reclaim the lost organic osmolytes at a rate sufficient to keep up with the rise in serum sodium; thus, water shifts from the ICF to the ECF, leading to brain cell shrinkage and ultimately demyelination.[15] Demyelination is characterized by a biphasic illness, termed ODS, that can occur 1–7 days after serum sodium correction. Initially, patients experience recovery of symptoms associated with hyponatremia only to later have other neurological sequelae, even in the presence of normonatremia, including seizures, behavioral abnormalities, movement disorders, and/or a "locked-in" phenomenon characterized by the inability to move, speak, or swallow. Patients may recover, have permanent disability, or even die.[16] Osmotic demyelination syndrome is predominantly a concern for patients presenting with chronic hyponatremia.

The absolute rise in serum sodium that will induce demyelination and the development of ODS is unknown, and recommended serum sodium correction thresholds are predominantly based on case reports and case series that show avoidance of ODS. In 1986, a review of 51 patients with hyponatremia revealed no cases of ODS in those with a correction of serum sodium less than 12 mEq/L/day (n=13), whereas 37% of patients (n=38) in whom sodium was corrected by greater than 12 mEq/L/day developed or were suspected to have developed ODS.[23] Current serum sodium correction thresholds for patients with chronic hyponatremia follow these observations. Even though ODS is most likely to occur in patients with chronic hyponatremia, concern still exists, and caution must be exercised, in patients with acute hyponatremia. Finally, patients who are malnourished, have a history of alcoholism and/or liver disease, are hypokalemic, or have a serum sodium less than 105 mEq/L are considered at high risk of ODS.[15,16]

Severely Symptomatic Hyponatremia

Hyponatremia associated with severe neurological symptoms (e.g., vomiting, seizures, coma) is a medical emergency that requires prompt intervention, regardless of whether the development is acute or chronic.[15] In addition to the morbidity associated with these symptoms directly, their development is indicative of increased intracranial pressure, which may result in brain herniation if the serum sodium concentration is not adequately raised, particularly in the setting of acute hyponatremia. Thus, the goal of therapy is to halt neurological injury and prevent progression. Increasing the serum sodium concentration by 4–6 mEq/L has been suggested to be sufficient to halt hyponatremia-related seizure activity and prevent impending brain herniation.[15] This is primarily derived from a review of 13 case reports (individually published) of patients with severely symptomatic hyponatremia (initial serum sodium of 99–117 mEq/L with seizures [n=12] or known cerebral edema [n=2; 1 patient had cerebral edema

Table 3.1 Summary of Interventions for the Management of Hyponatremia

Symptom Severity	Hypovolemic Hyponatremia	Euvolemic Hyponatremia (i.e., SIADH)	Hypervolemic Hyponatremia
Severe	3% NaCl	3% NaCl	3% NaCl
• Seizures		+	+
• Respiratory distress		Loop diuretic	Loop diuretic
• Coma		+	+
• Vomiting		Fluid restriction	Fluid restriction
Moderate	0.9% NaCl	Fluid restriction (primary modality)	Loop diuretics (primary modality)
• Nausea			
• Confusion		±	+
• Headache		Loop diuretic	Fluid restriction
• Lethargy			
Or			
Asymptomatic		Consider: Demeclocycline NaCl tablets	Uncertainty: V_2 receptor antagonists
		Uncertainty: V_2 receptor antagonists	

NaCl = sodium chloride; SIADH = syndrome of inappropriate antidiuretic hormone; V_2 = vasopressin type 2.

and seizure activity]). Administration of intravenous hypertonic saline (i.e., 3% sodium chloride) resulted in an increase in serum sodium by 3–9 mEq/L within 0.5–4 hours. Eleven patients recovered, and only one patient developed ODS after a serum sodium rise of 6 mEq/L over 3.6 hours, but the patient recovered. An additional patient who had an overall increase in serum sodium of 31 mEq/L over 8 hours was disabled.[15] Targeting absolute values for serum sodium correction (e.g., 8 mEq/L/day) is recommended, in contrast to hourly rates (e.g., 1–2 mEq/L/hour), which may obscure the rise needed within the first few critical hours of management.[24]

Administration of intravenous hypertonic saline, usually 3% sodium chloride (513 mEq sodium per liter), is considered the definitive therapy for elevating serum sodium concentrations in severely symptomatic hyponatremia (Table 3.1). Unfortunately, no randomized trials have evaluated this intervention, and limited data are available to guide clinicians. In prior reviews, bolus intravenous administration of 3% sodium chloride (2 mL/kg or maximum 100 mL) administered over 10 minutes, with repeat administration twice if needed, was recommended to halt severe symptoms in patients with hyponatremia.[1,15,16,25] Such recommendations are based on the assumption that in the absence of free water loss in the urine, 1 mL/kg of 3% sodium chloride will increase serum sodium by about 1 mEq/L (e.g., if a patient weighing 70 kg receives the recommended maximum amount of 3% sodium chloride, 300 mL, serum sodium should increase by about 4 mEq/L).[16] The 2014 European clinical practice guidelines for the diagnosis and treatment of hyponatremia (representing a joint effort on behalf of three European societies inclusive of intensive care, endocrinology, and nephrology) recommend a similar approach with intravenous administration of 3% sodium chloride as a 2-mL/kg bolus (maximum 150 mL) over 20 minutes, with repeat doses as needed until the symptoms improve or a rise in serum sodium of 5 mEq/L is attained, whichever comes first.[26] Rapid (10–20 minutes) bolus intravenous administration of 3% sodium chloride has also been suggested for patients with acute hyponatremia and less severe symptoms (e.g., nausea, confusion, headache)[25,26] in an attempt to prevent progression as well as for those who are relatively asymptomatic but have neurological or neurosurgical conditions (because of limited tolerance to changes in intracranial pressure).[15] Overall, rapid bolus intravenous therapy is to provide a controlled and immediate rise in serum sodium with little risk of inadvertent overcorrection compared with administration by continuous intravenous infusion.[25] In addition, it is suggested that this method can safely assist clinicians in ruling out hyponatremia as the cause for such symptoms (i.e., if symptoms do not resolve after a 4- to 6-mEq/L rise in serum sodium, hyponatremia is likely not the etiology).[25,26] Clinicians should be aware that recommendations to administer 3% sodium chloride by small rapid intravenous infusions are primarily based on brief reports and consensus recommendations for the management of exercise-associated hyponatremic encephalopathy.[27,28] A review of the literature did not identify any trials specifically evaluating the efficacy and safety of this approach in hospitalized patients. In a retrospective review of patients with severe hyponatremia (treated with 3% sodium chloride in conjunction with desmopressin [n=25]), use of an initial intravenous bolus of 50–100 mL was reported in five patients with "more severe symptoms," but outcomes specifically related to the bolus intravenous infusion (i.e., resolution of symptoms) were not provided.[29] Therefore, the utility of this approach remains unknown. If clinicians choose to use rapid bolus intravenous administration of 3% sodium chloride, serum sodium concentrations must be monitored post-administration of each dose in order to guide subsequent steps in management and avoid potential complications.

Administration of 3% sodium chloride by continuous intravenous infusion is another option for managing symptomatic hyponatremia. Data analyses documenting the utility of this administration method are primarily based on retrospective case series, with most analyses including patients with both moderate and severe symptoms of hyponatremia.[29-33] Ayus and colleagues conducted a recent, retrospective review of 64 adult patients with hyponatremia (less than 130 mEq/L) treated with a uniform protocol of 500 mL of 3% sodium chloride administered intravenously over 6 hours (i.e., 83 mL/hour) after presentation to the emergency department with hyponatremic encephalopathy.[33] Of the 64 patients, 46 had severe symptoms (seizures, n=29; stupor, n=10; coma, n=5; neurogenic pulmonary edema, n=2); specifics regarding other symptoms were not provided. The median symptom duration before treatment was 48 hours (range 4 hours to 15 days). The baseline serum sodium was 114 ± 0.8 mEq/L, which rose by about 4 mEq/L, 8 mEq/L, 10 mEq/L, and 14 mEq/L at 3 hours (mid-infusion), 12 hours (6 hours post-infusion), 24 hours (18 hours post-infusion), and 48 hours (42 hours post-infusion), respectively. Of interest, within a "few hours" of initiating 3% sodium chloride intravenously, there was a marked improvement in 97% of hyponatremia cases and complete neurological recovery by 48 hours. Two patients who presented with seizures had permanent neurological injury after having only a 2- and 3-mEq/L rise, respectively, in serum sodium. Five patients experienced a rise in serum sodium by 25 mEq/L or more at 48 hours, but no cases of ODS were reported. This strategy provides a relatively prompt and safe response to a 6-hour intravenous infusion of 3% sodium chloride in most patients with hyponatremia with moderate to severe symptoms, but frequent monitoring and adjustment of therapy may be needed to promptly identify patients needing more aggressive intervention.[33] The only prospective trial evaluating 3% sodium chloride intravenously for the acute management of hyponatremia was conducted by Bhaskar and colleagues.[34] A total of 58 adult patients with euvolemic hyponatremia (mean serum sodium 114 mEq/L) and moderate to severe symptoms (coma 14%) for less than 24 hours were included. The initial management protocol entailed an intravenous infusion of 3% sodium chloride 100 mL over 4 hours (i.e., 25 mL/hour) targeting a rise in serum sodium by 1 mEq/L or more post-infusion, with protocol adjustments for non-responders. Overall, 78% of patients had a rise in serum sodium of 1 mEq/L or more post-infusion with a mean of 2 mEq/L (range 0–6 mEq/L), but 22% required an additional 100–200 mL of 3% sodium chloride administered intravenously over 1–2 hours, respectively, to attain any change in serum sodium.[34] Symptom improvement was only reported at the 24-hour mark (in contrast to post-infusion), and patients with seizure activity were excluded from the study, thus limiting the ability to determine the efficacy of this approach in severely ill patients. Accordingly, this approach may only be suitable for patients with moderate symptoms. Overall, although 3% sodium chloride intravenously can be considered a standard of clinical care for symptomatic hyponatremia, future research is needed to determine how best to deliver such therapy. Specifically, a prospective randomized trial evaluating the safety and efficacy of intravenous bolus (i.e., over 10–20 minutes) versus rapid intravenous infusion (i.e., 500 mL over 4–6 hours) of 3% sodium chloride is needed for severely symptomatic patients.

Given that 3% sodium chloride represents the primary management strategy for severely symptomatic hyponatremia, some practical considerations deserve mentioning. First, infusion by a central venous access device is recommended to minimize the development of phlebitis because of the hypertonic nature of the solution (513 mEq of sodium per liter and 1,026 mOsm/L). In patients with severe symptoms or impending herniation, 3% sodium chloride may be administered through a large peripheral vein (i.e., antecubital) if a central venous access device is not available in order to avoid delays in administration. A recent report did not show phlebitis or extravasation injuries with peripheral administration,[29] yet the risk still exists. Second, serum sodium concentrations must be monitored a minimum of every 4 hours in all patients receiving 3% sodium chloride intravenously. This will help identify unforeseen elevations (or lack thereof) while treating the patient with hyponatremia, allowing prompt intervention. Finally, institution-specific policies must be present regarding the intravenous administration of 3% sodium chloride, and clinicians should investigate such details to prevent delays in the provision of care to symptomatic patients. In acute care settings such as an ICU, intravenous sodium chloride concentrations greater than 0.9% are currently listed as a high-alert medication (i.e., categorized with a heightened risk of causing significant patient harm when used in error) from the Institute of Safe Medication Practices (www.ismp.org/Tools/institutionalhighAlert.asp).[35]

After initial stabilization of severely symptomatic patients, it is essential to differentiate acute from chronic hyponatremia because this will determine the next steps of treatment (see Table 3.2). For chronic hyponatremia, treatment guidelines recommend the following maximum limits of sodium correction: 10 mEq/L in 24 hours and 18 mEq/L in 48 hours.[36] Some experts suggest more modest goals of a 6- to 8-mEq/L rise in serum sodium in 24 hours, 12–14 mEq/L in 48 hours, and 14–16 mEq/L in 72 hours because patients with chronic hyponatremia are considered at the highest risk of ODS with serum sodium overcorrection.[15] Thus, depending on the serum concentration and symptoms post-initial intervention, a further rise in serum sodium may not be indicated. In patients who develop acute hyponatremia over 24–48 hours, the goal serum sodium correction should be 10 mEq/L/day or less to minimize the probability of developing ODS. In contrast, for patients who develop acute hyponatremia over "several hours," limits on the maximum amount of sodium correction within a 24-hour period have not been determined, and in general, excessive correction is not known to be harmful (i.e., no known risk of ODS).[16] Use of 3% sodium chloride by continuous intravenous infusion may be needed to facilitate continued sodium correction and prevent redevelopment of symptoms. Use of other interventions in conjunction with 3% sodium chloride intravenously should be considered depending on the fluid status of the patient (e.g., loop diuretics for hypervolemic or euvolemic hyponatremia).[30,37]

Determining Intravenous Infusion Rates for Hyponatremia Correction

The Adrogue-Madias equation (equation 3.3) can be used to determine the infusion rate of 3% sodium chloride required to facilitate the desired absolute rise in serum sodium.[4] Essentially, this equation estimates the change in serum sodium after the infusion of 1 L of any infusate. The targeted rise in serum sodium (e.g., 8 mEq/L in a 24-hour period) is then divided by the estimated change in serum sodium per liter of infusate to determine the total number of liters needed, and ultimately the infusion rate per hour.

$$\text{Change in serum sodium (mEq/L)} = \frac{\text{infusate sodium + potassium content (mEq/L)} - \text{measured serum sodium (mEq/L)}}{\text{TBW} + 1} \quad \text{(equation 3.3)}^{4}$$

Infusate sodium content is as follows: 3% NaCl = 513 mEq/L, 0.9% NaCl = 154 mEq/L, 0.45% NaCl = 77 mEq/L, 0.225% NaCl = 38 mEq/L, where NaCl is sodium chloride.

In a single-center retrospective review of adult patients with hyponatremia treated with 3% sodium chloride

Table 3.2 Suggested Serum Sodium Correction for Hypo- and Hypernatremia[15,16,36]

Duration	Severe Symptoms	Moderate Symptoms or Asymptomatic	Risk with Inadvertent Overcorrection
HYPOnatremia			
Acute (minutes to hours)	↑ Serum sodium by 4–6 mEq/L within 1–4 hr; no daily threshold	Consider ↑ serum sodium by 4–6 mEq/L within 6 hr for prevention of severe symptoms; no daily threshold	No known risk
Acute (24–48 hr)	↑ Serum sodium by 4–6 mEq/L within 1–4 hr, max correction 10 mEq/L/day	Max ↑ serum sodium by 10 mEq/L/day	ODS (relatively, risk << than with chronic hyponatremia)
Chronic (> 48 hr) or uncertain	↑ Serum sodium by <u>lowest</u> amount needed for symptom resolution (max 4–6 mEq/L within first 6 hr, 10 mEq/L in 24 hr, and 18 mEq/L in 48 hr)	Max ↑ serum sodium by 8 mEq/L in 24 hr, 14 mEq/L in 48 hr, and 16 mEq/L in 72 hr	ODS
HYPERnatremia			
Acute (minutes to hours)	↓ Serum sodium by 2–3 mEq/L/hr; no daily threshold	Consider ↓ serum sodium by 2–3 mEq/L/hr for prevention of severe symptoms; no daily threshold	No known risk
Acute (24–48 hr)	↓ Serum sodium by 2–3 mEq/L/hr until 145 mEq/L; no daily threshold	Consider ↓ serum sodium by 2–3 mEq/L/hr until 145 mEq/L; no daily threshold	No known risk of cerebral edema, but recommend caution with ↓ serum sodium by > 10 mEq/L/day
Chronic (> 48 hr) or uncertain	↓ Serum sodium by 0.5 mEq/L/hr; max reduction of 10 mEq/L/day[a]	↓ Serum sodium by 0.25–0.5 mEq/L/hr, max reduction of 10 mEq/L/day[a]	Cerebral edema/herniation

[a]Serum sodium reduction by < 0.25 mEq/L/hr within the first 24 hours of presentation may be associated with increased 30-day mortality[56]
ODS = osmotic demyelination syndrome.

intravenously, the observed increase in serum sodium concentration was compared with that predicted by the Adrogue-Madias formula (i.e., equation 3.3). Among 31 patients with severe hyponatremia (less than 120 mEq/L), use of the formula underestimated serum sodium correction in 74%. The average rate of serum sodium correction was 1.66 times that predicted with the formula.[31] This implies that intravenous prescribing of 3% sodium chloride using the Adrogue-Madias formula alone can result in frequent overcorrection among patients, particularly concerning with chronic hyponatremia given a higher risk of ODS.

Clinicians should note that the Adrogue-Madias formula (equation 3.3) provides only an estimate, is derived from the perspective that the body is a closed system (i.e., without losses), and does not account for other factors (i.e., water diuresis mid-infusion). Overall, it is recommended that this equation be used only in determining an initial infusion rate. Frequent serum sodium concentration monitoring (e.g., every 2–6 hours) should ultimately guide therapy.

Inadvertent Overcorrection of Hyponatremia

Inadvertent overcorrection of serum sodium can occur while managing hyponatremia, and such results may confer a higher risk of ODS. Overcorrection can develop during mid-treatment for several reasons; however, the primary reason is rapid resolution of the underlying hyponatremia etiology in conjunction with inadequate serum sodium concentration monitoring. Inadvertent overcorrection of serum sodium can be managed by the provision of free water enterally, intravenous infusion of 5% dextrose in water, and/or administration of intravenous desmopressin. Commercially available sterile water for injection should not be administered intravenously because of the risk of hemolysis. Desmopressin, available as an intravenous, subcutaneous, or intranasal dosage form, is a synthetic analog of ADH that inhibits free water excretion, thereby reducing serum sodium concentrations. Using desmopressin without consulting clinicians skilled in using it is not recommended because there is a potential for redevelopment of hyponatremia and associated neurological sequelae.

Addressing the Underlying Etiology of Hyponatremia

Determining the underlying etiology for hyponatremia is of vital importance for instituting methods to elevate the serum sodium concentration (i.e., aside from 3% sodium chloride). As mentioned previously, this requires examining the patient's fluid status in conjunction with measuring serum osmolality, as well as urine sodium and osmolality (see Figure 3.1). Included in the following text are general considerations regarding the management of hypovolemic, euvolemic, and hypervolemic hyponatremia.

Proper management of hypovolemic hypotonic hyponatremia depends on whether the insult is caused by extrarenal or renal sodium losses. In the setting of extrarenal sodium loss (e.g., NG tube output, diarrhea), intravenous 0.9% sodium chloride (with or without potassium chloride) should be administered to replace both sodium and fluid losses. Hypotonic fluids (e.g., 0.45% sodium chloride) should be avoided because this may worsen hyponatremia. In the absence of other concomitant factors, the specific infusion rate should be dictated by the volume lost and maintenance fluid requirements. In the setting of acute hypovolemia causing hemodynamic compromise, bolus and/or aggressive intravenous infusion rates are needed immediately. Hyponatremia should resolve with proper intravenous fluid supplementation and/or after resolution of the underlying insult (i.e., removal of the NG tube and resolution of diarrhea). In the setting of renal sodium loss, intravenous 0.9% sodium chloride should be administered with attention focused on the workup and treatment of the underlying etiology. For example, if adrenal insufficiency is identified, management should focus on glucocorticoid and mineralocorticoid supplementation. In cerebral salt wasting, intravenous fluid supplementation with 0.9% sodium chloride is typically sufficient until spontaneous resolution occurs, usually within 2–3 weeks of cerebral injury.[38]

Euvolemic hypotonic hyponatremia is most often associated with SIADH,[2] and in fact, SIADH is the most common cause of hyponatremia.[37] A complete discussion of causes of SIADH (or syndrome of inappropriate antidiuresis) can be found elsewhere.[37] Particularly of concern in critically ill patients is the potential for transient development of SIADH postoperatively,[5,6] in response to pain,[4] in conjunction with pneumonia,[39] or secondary to neurological insult such as subarachnoid hemorrhage.[40] Free water restriction is the mainstay of therapy for managing mild symptomatic hyponatremia associated with SIADH.[4] Unfortunately, enteral free water restriction may be of little utility in critically ill patients because this population is often unable to drink by mouth. However, in patients receiving enteral nutrition and/or medications by enteral tube, consideration should be given to reducing the volume of free water flushes to the minimum required to prevent enteral tube occlusion.[41] Intravenous fluid should be restricted by discontinuing all hypotonic fluids (e.g., 0.45% sodium chloride or 5% dextrose in water by maintenance intravenous fluids or intravenous medication diluents) and replacing them with 0.9% sodium chloride, if feasible or compatible. This will likely be insufficient to fully correct hyponatremia associated with SIADH, and other therapies may be necessary such as loop diuretics, oral or enteral sodium chloride tablets (i.e., salt tablets), and/or demeclocycline. With respect to oral sodium chloride, each 1 g tablet contains about 18 mEq of sodium and 18 mEq of chloride. The intent behind sodium chloride tablet administration is to increase urine osmolality, helping create an osmolar gradient within the renal tubules to counteract the effect of elevated ADH concentrations and allow greater free water excretion.[2] Unfortunately, sodium chloride tablet administration is limited by the need for enteral access and the risk of adverse sequelae from sodium loading, including pulmonary edema. Demeclocycline is a tetracycline antibiotic that blocks ADH activity at the renal tubules and facilitates free water excretion. In addition to requiring enteral access, this agent has a delayed onset of action (3–6 days) and should be avoided in the setting of renal and/or hepatic impairment (common complications of critical illness).[1,2] In light of this information, clinicians are often left with loop diuretics as the only viable treatment option for managing SIADH in critically ill patients (in addition to intravenous fluid restriction). Diuresis with loop diuretics is typically equivalent to 0.45% sodium chloride[1]; hence, more free water than sodium is excreted, helping raise serum sodium concentrations.

Management of hypervolemic hypotonic hyponatremia targets the elevated ECF volume characteristic of disease states commonly associated with this condition (e.g., heart failure, cirrhosis, nephrotic syndrome). Disorders of the cardiovascular, renal, and hepatic systems are common in critically ill patients, and as such, hypervolemic hyponatremia should be of concern. Essentially, the goals are to achieve a negative fluid balance (by diuresis) and to minimize sodium intake. To manage this type of hyponatremia, the clinician must focus on improving the status of the underlying comorbidity. For example, in the setting of heart failure–induced hyponatremia, loop diuretic therapy is often escalated to promote aggressive diuresis. However, this is often a temporary measure because improvement in cardiac contractility is needed in order to avoid further release in ADH and activation of the renin-angiotensin-aldosterone system in response to a decreased effective circulating volume. Thus, agents such as angiotensin-converting enzyme inhibitors or angiotensin receptor blockers can be implemented, if feasible.[4] Cirrhosis is another condition marked by the non-osmotic release of ADH in response to decreased effective circulating volume.

Vasopressin Receptor Antagonists in Hyponatremia

Vasopressin receptor antagonists, also known as aquaretics, result in increased electrolyte-free water excretion by competitive antagonism of ADH at V_2 receptors on the renal tubule collecting ducts.[2] Currently, two agents are U.S. Food and Drug Administration (FDA) approved, conivaptan and tolvaptan, and both are indicated for euvolemic and/or hypervolemic hyponatremia.[42,43] Conivaptan is only available as an intravenous formulation, and tolvaptan is only available as an oral tablet. Neither agent has proven to provide symptomatic relief to patients with acute hyponatremia.

Limited data exist with use of these agents in the management of acute hyponatremia in critically ill patients. Only one publication documenting two case reports of tolvaptan use in critically ill patients with euvolemic hypotonic hyponatremia from SIADH is available.[44] With respect to conivaptan, two small pilot trials of neuro-ICU patients have been published (n=19 and n=6).[45,46] Although the second trial was terminated early because of difficulties with enrollment,[46] both studies showed conivaptan's ability to raise serum sodium concentrations in neuro-ICU patients, providing merit for a larger, randomized controlled trial. Overall, the paucity of data with use of aquaretics in the critically ill population is not of great concern given similar deficits of well-designed controlled trials with the other interventions mentioned previously. However, given the lack of clinical symptomatic hyponatremia experience in the ICU, inability to titrate, and highly dynamic nature of critically ill patients, the role of aquaretics in the critically ill population remains to be determined.

HYPERNATREMIA

Hypernatremia is defined as a serum sodium concentration greater than 145 mEq/L. Given that sodium is a functionally impermeable solute, hypernatremia always denotes a hypertonic state, representing a deficit in TBW in relation to total body sodium.[47,48] In most cases, hypernatremia is iatrogenic, developing during the hospital or ICU stay.[11,49] The published incidence varies in the literature depending on the patient population studied (e.g., medical vs. surgical ICU) and the serum sodium diagnostic threshold (i.e., greater than 145 vs. greater than 150 mEq/L). Reports show an incidence of ICU-acquired hypernatremia of 4%–11%, with one evaluation in a mixed ICU population showing an incidence of 26%.[48] Critically ill patients who are unconscious or have an altered mental status as well as those who are intubated or receiving non-invasive mechanical ventilation are considered at highest risk of hypernatremia.

In such scenarios, patients cannot regulate their own fluid intake and are completely reliant on the medical team to ensure adequate fluid provision while avoiding excessive sodium administration. Overall, ICU-acquired hypernatremia (i.e., development during ICU stay) has been proposed to be indicative of poor quality care.[50]

Pathophysiology and Classification

A combination of net water loss and net sodium gain is often the driving force for hypernatremia in the critically ill population.[48,51] Free water loss can occur by extrarenal or renal mechanisms. Extrarenal water loss contributes to the development of ICU-acquired hypernatremia in more than 50% of patients, primarily by way of fever.[51] Insensible losses, typically 10 mL/kg/day, should be considered when evaluating fluid balance.[52] In addition, with each 1 degree increase in temperature above 37°C, insensible losses increase by 25% (i.e., 2.5 mL/kg/day).[52] Other sources of extrarenal loss include, but are not limited to, diarrhea or ostomy output (i.e., ileostomy or colostomy), NG tube output, vomiting, surgical drain output, and losses by wounds/wound management devices. Although output is difficult to ascertain at times, clinicians should measure it from such sources in order to best assess daily fluid balance. Potential causes of renal free water loss in the critically ill population include osmotic diuresis (e.g., from hyperglycemia, protein supplementation, or mannitol), loop diuretic administration (i.e., diuresis approximates 0.45% sodium chloride),[1] and diabetes insipidus (central or nephrogenic).

Sodium gain (i.e., a positive solute balance) is seldom the sole cause of hypernatremia in the critically ill population, but it often plays a role because of the frequent administration of sodium-containing fluids.[51] For example, 0.9% sodium chloride is often considered the standard for fluid resuscitation, such as in patients with sepsis. However, given that the sodium content (154 mEq/L) exceeds the sodium concentration of the ECF (135–145 mEq/L), hypernatremia may develop with continued or excessive administration, particularly in the setting of extrarenal and/or renal water losses. In addition, 0.9% sodium chloride is commonly used as the diluent for medications administered by intravenous piggyback, the impact of which varies depending on the total fluid intake per day attributable to such medications. Intravenous push administration of sodium bicarbonate 8.4% (i.e., 1,000 mEq of sodium per liter) for correction of acidosis may also contribute to the development of hypernatremia in the critically ill population. Sodium is also a structural component of many antimicrobial agents, an often overlooked but important source of intake.[53] Finally, the sodium content of enteral and parenteral nutrition should be considered. Determining daily sodium balance is not feasible because of the inability to determine sodium loss (e.g., by stool, urine, and other sources); however, clinicians should remain cognizant of the many common avenues by which sodium is both intentionally and unintentionally provided to critically ill patients.

Given the fluid status of the patient, hypernatremia may be classified as hypovolemic, hypervolemic, or euvolemic hypernatremia, which also provides insight into the potential etiology.[2,48] Hypovolemic hypernatremia is marked by a decrease in total body sodium, but an even greater decrease in TBW, giving rise to hypernatremia. This is often a result of fluid losses by the gastrointestinal (GI) tract, excessive diuresis with loop diuretics, or insensible losses by the skin and lungs. Hypervolemic hypernatremia is marked by an increase in TBW, but an even greater increase in total body sodium. This is associated with excessive sodium supplementation (i.e., hypertonic saline or sodium bicarbonate) and/or hyperaldosteronism/corticosteroid supplementation. Euvolemic hypernatremia is marked by a loss of water with a relatively stable total body sodium content. In patients who have access to free water, euvolemic hypernatremia can be seen with diabetes insipidus. In critically ill patients who often lack access to free water, diabetes insipidus will likely manifest as hypovolemic hypernatremia. Many conditions can lead to central diabetes insipidus, including, but not limited to, neurological trauma, neurosurgical intervention, and infections (e.g., meningitis) or malignancies of the CNS. Nephrogenic diabetes insipidus can be associated with several ICU medications, including aminoglycosides, foscarnet, and amphotericin B.[54,55]

Clinical Manifestations

Clinical manifestations directly related to hypernatremia primarily involve the CNS. The development of hypernatremia results in the movement of free water from within brain cells to the extracellular space, leading to brain cell shrinkage. Brain cell shrinkage can lead to vascular rupture, hemorrhage, ODS, and potentially permanent neurological damage or death in severe cases.[47,48] During rapid adaptation, brain cell volume is partly restored by the movement of electrolytes intracellularly; however, normalization of brain volume does not occur rapidly because the movement of organic osmolytes intracellularly takes several days (essentially, the adaptive process for hypernatremia is the opposite of that for hyponatremia).[47] In general, patients who have a rapid rise (i.e., within hours) or large absolute rise in serum sodium are at high risk of developing severe neurological symptoms.[47] In addition to neurological manifestations, hypernatremia has been associated with muscle weakness or cramps, rhabdomyolysis, impaired gluconeogenesis, impaired glucose use, impaired lactate clearance, and decreased left ventricular contractility.[48]

Morbidity and Mortality

Several retrospective studies evaluating the incidence of ICU-acquired hypernatremia have shown significantly longer ICU lengths of stay and higher mortality rates among patients who developed hypernatremia than among those who did not.[48] In the retrospective review of more than 13,000 patients included in the EPIC II trial (mentioned earlier in the Hyponatremia section), a significantly increased risk of death was seen among all patients with hypernatremia, which increased in a stepwise fashion as the degree of hypernatremia progressed from mild (146–150 mEq/L; OR 1.97 [95% CI 1.74–2.23]) to moderate (151–155 mEq/L; OR 2.03 [95% CI 1.60–2.57]) to severe (greater than 155 mEq/L; OR 2.62 [95% CI, 1.90–3.61]). Of interest, these findings were primarily driven by patients who were already in the ICU at the time of hypernatremia diagnosis in contrast to those with hypernatremia at the time of admission.[11] Given the retrospective nature of this information, causality cannot be confirmed between hypernatremia, timing of hypernatremia development, and mortality; nevertheless, the potential association should be of great concern for critical care clinicians.

Management

In general, the correction rate for hypernatremia depends on the presence or risk of severe neurological symptoms and the duration over which hypernatremia developed. Unfortunately, there are no prospective trials comparing treatment options or rate of correction for hypernatremia. As a result, treatment recommendations are primarily based on retrospective studies and expert opinion.

Patients who develop acute hypernatremia (i.e., within 48 hours or less) are at a higher risk of developing severe neurological symptoms, such as seizures, coma, and intracranial hemorrhage, if not already present.[16,48] This is particularly true for hypernatremia that develops over minutes to hours, such as in the case of salt poisoning or inadvertent administration of hypertonic saline.[16] With acute hypernatremia, excessive correction of serum sodium is not known to be harmful (i.e., minimal to no risk of cerebral edema) because of insufficient time for the brain to adapt to the hypertonic state.[16,48] As such, it is recommended to correct serum sodium at a rate of 2–3 mEq/L/hour until a serum sodium of 145 mEq/L is attained; then treatment should stop.[16] Other experts recommend a more modest correction rate of 1 mEq/L/hour.[47] For patients with chronic hypernatremia or hypernatremia of unknown duration, particularly in the absence of severe neurological symptoms, it is recommended to lower the serum by 0.5 mEq/L/hour or less.[16,47,48] In addition, the total daily correction should be limited to 8–10 mEq/L/day.[47,48] This is because brain cells have already adapted to the hypernatremic state, and cerebral edema may develop with rapid serum sodium correction.

A single-center, retrospective study evaluated serum sodium correction rates and mortality in 117 adult patients with hypernatremia (serum sodium greater than 155 mEq/L).[56] Overall, the mean baseline serum sodium was 159 mEq/L; 20% of patients had acute and 80% had chronic (or unknown duration) hypernatremia, and 30% were admitted to the ICU. Minimal information was provided regarding symptomatology, only mentioning that 49% had impaired neurological status, and there was no standardized protocol at the institution for hypernatremia correction (i.e., according to physician discretion). The mean serum sodium correction rate was 0.15 ± 0.3 mEq/L/hour and 0.13 ± 0.1 mEq/L/hour within 24 and 72 hours, respectively. Multivariate analysis showed a significantly increased risk of 30-day mortality among patients with a serum sodium correction of less than 0.25 mEq/L/hour in the first 24 hours. The 30-day mortality rate was 46% (36 of 78) with a serum sodium correction of less than 0.25 mEq/L/hour compared with 18% (7 of 39) among those with a serum sodium correction of 0.25 mEq/L/hour or more (p=0.0029). In patients with acute hypernatremia, the overall rate of serum sodium correction was faster (0.36 ± 0.48 mEq/L/hour vs. 0.09 ± 0.21 mEq/L/hour) and mortality was lower (21% vs. 41%; p=0.0962) than in those with chronic hypernatremia.[56] This study suggests that overly conservative serum sodium correction within 72 hours of presentation may be detrimental in patients with chronic hypernatremia. Overall, evaluation of serum sodium correction rates and correlation with outcomes in both acute and chronic hypernatremia deserve prospective evaluation.

Fluid administration is the cornerstone of therapy for hypernatremia. The previously recommended corrections in serum sodium for both acute and chronic hypernatremia can be accomplished by intravenous administration of 5% dextrose in water (emergent dialysis can also be considered, depending on the clinical presentation of the patient).[48] The initial intravenous infusion rate for 5% dextrose in water can be determined using the Adrogue-Madias formula (equation 3.3) provided earlier in this chapter; however, the intravenous infusion rate should be adjusted according to serial sodium measurements (e.g., every 2–6 hours).[47] In uncontrolled hyperglycemia, 0.45% sodium chloride can be used, but concomitant use of loop diuretics should be considered to induce natriuresis.[48] Use of 0.9% sodium chloride or other isotonic solutions (e.g., Ringer lactate) is not recommended except in hemodynamic instability.[48]

Once symptoms are controlled, the route of fluid administration can be changed to enteral, if feasible (i.e., orally or per feeding tube). If the enteral route is not feasible, continuation of 5% dextrose in water or use of 0.45% sodium chloride is appropriate. At this time, clinicians should also focus on determining the underlying etiology of hypernatremia (e.g., excessive insensible losses, overuse of loop diuretics, diabetes insipidus) and intervene accordingly. In addition, sources of sodium intake should be minimized.

POTASSIUM

Potassium is the most abundant intracellular cation in the body, with 98% of total body stores located in the intracellular space and only 2% in the extracellular space.[57] Skeletal muscle houses most intracellular potassium (about 75%), with the remaining potassium located within the liver and red blood cells (RBCs). The sodium-potassium adenosine triphosphatase (Na-K-ATPase) pump regulates potassium's distribution between the ICF and the ECF by pumping potassium inside cells in exchange for sodium, maintaining ECF (i.e., serum) potassium concentrations within a normal range of 3.5–5 mEq/L in drastic contrast to an ICF potassium concentration of about 150 mEq/L.[57] Although potassium plays several vital roles within the body (e.g., protein and glycogen synthesis), the function of most concern for critical care clinicians is maintenance of cardiac muscle resting membrane potential. Variations in serum potassium concentrations resulting in either hyperkalemia or hypokalemia can result in significant and life-threatening arrhythmias.

Potassium homeostasis is mediated by several key factors, most importantly aldosterone, insulin, and catecholamines, and is highly dependent on renal function. Around 90% of potassium excretion occurs by renal elimination (with the remaining 10% from GI loss by feces), and aldosterone is the primary mediator for this process.[58,59] A feedback loop exists whereby aldosterone production is stimulated, and thereby, renal excretion of potassium is increased in the presence of hyperkalemia and suppressed by hypokalemia.[59] As such, aldosterone is the main regulator of total body stores of potassium. Insulin is the most important mediator of the transcellular gradient of potassium, facilitating the movement of potassium intracellularly by stimulation of the Na-K-ATPase pump. Similar to aldosterone, a feedback loops exist for insulin release.[59] Given the heightened focus on glycemic control in the critically ill population,[60] many ICU patients currently receive exogenous intravenous insulin infusions. In addition to facilitating the cellular uptake of potassium, a prospective cohort involving 178 surgical ICU patients showed that intravenous insulin administration is independently and positively associated with renal potassium excretion (r^2 = 0.52, p<0.001).[61] Catecholamines lower serum potassium by stimulating the Na-K-ATPase pump, as well as promoting glycogenolysis and subsequent endogenous insulin release. In addition to hormonal mediation, serum potassium concentrations are affected by acute acid-base disorders. Overall, acidosis results in an increase in serum potassium, whereas alkalosis results in a decrease. Some experts report that a 0.1-unit change in serum pH results in a change in serum potassium by about 0.6 mEq/L in the opposite direction; however, the magnitude of change in serum potassium appears to vary depending on the type of acid-base disorder and cannot reliably be predicted by this generalization.[62]

The primary route of potassium intake is by the diet, which in critically ill patients is often administered as enteral or parenteral nutrition. The recommended dietary allowance (RDA) of potassium is about 50 mEq/day.[63] Accordingly, adult enteral nutrition formulas typically contain 40–60 mEq/L of potassium in an attempt to meet the RDA, unless specifically formulated for patients with chronic kidney disease (e.g., Novasource Renal, 24 mEq/L). Potassium supplementation may be also administered through maintenance intravenous fluids. Of note, hypokalemia can be sustained with inadequate potassium supplementation and depletion of total body stores regardless of appropriate hormonal feedback and renal function; however, hyperkalemia typically resolves quickly unless one or more regulatory mechanisms are impaired.[58]

HYPOKALEMIA

Hypokalemia is defined as a serum potassium less than 3.5 mEq/L, with severe hypokalemia typically marked by a serum potassium less than 2.5 mEq/L.[59] Few studies have evaluated the prevalence of hypokalemia in the critically ill population. A single-center investigation of more than 10,000 ICU patients revealed about a 19% incidence of mild hypokalemia (3–3.49 mEq/L) and 3%–4% of severe hypokalemia.[64]

Pathophysiology

Hypokalemia can be the result of abnormal losses of potassium, imbalance of the transcellular gradient by intracellular shifting of potassium, inadequate intake or supplementation, or a combination of these three mechanisms.[58,59] In most cases, hypokalemia is a result of abnormal losses of potassium, and diuretics (loop and/or thiazide diuretics) are the primary culprit.[58,63] Abnormal losses by the GI tract should also be considered from the patient's history. Factors associated with the development of hypokalemia are listed in Table 3.3.[58,59]

Clinical Manifestations

Clinical manifestations of hypokalemia vary widely among patients and are primarily neuromuscular, GI, or cardiac related. Neuromuscular changes are often considered mild or nonspecific and include cramping, myalgia, and weakness. Even if these manifestations are present, critically ill patients are often unable to communicate such symptoms, which often go unnoticed until attempts are made to ambulate the patient. Severe neuromuscular symptoms, such as rhabdomyolysis and paralysis, may occur at serum potassium concentrations of less than 2.5 mEq/L and 2 mEq/L, respectively. Hypokalemia may also manifest as constipation or development of an ileus.[58] Cardiac abnormalities represent a primary concern for clinicians but are considered unusual in the absence of underlying heart disease (e.g., heart failure, left ventricular hypertrophy, or cardiac ischemia).[58,63] Electrocardiogram (ECG) changes may include flattening or inversion of the T wave, ST-segment depression, or prominent U waves.[63] Because of alterations in the resting membrane potential of cardiac cells, hypokalemia can trigger arrhythmias such as heart block, atrial flutter or fibrillation, ventricular tachycardia, ventricular fibrillation, or torsades de pointes. In addition, the risk of hypokalemia-induced arrhythmia may be increased in the setting of digoxin toxicity.[63]

Morbidity and Mortality

A prospective, single-center observational trial (n=60) of patients with acute myocardial infarction (AMI) showed an inverse relationship with serum potassium and the development of ventricular tachycardia. The lowest probability for ventricular tachycardia was seen with serum potassium concentrations of 4–5 mEq/L.[65] A subsequent, larger prospective observational study (n=482) of patients with AMI showed a significantly lower mean serum potassium concentration among 17 patients who developed ventricular fibrillation compared with 417 who did not (3.58 vs. 3.89 mEq/L, p<0.05).[66] These studies together with others led to guideline recommendations to maintain a serum potassium concentration of at least 4 mEq/L (i.e., 4–5 mEq/L) in patients with a history of cardiac arrhythmias, hypertension, heart failure, or coronary ischemia.[63] The association of serum potassium concentrations with the development of arrhythmias, as well as the incidence of mortality, has been revisited since these prior recommendations were published. In 2012, a retrospective cohort study of 38,689 patients with biomarker-confirmed AMI across 67 hospitals was published.[67] Overall, a U-shaped relationship between mean post-admission serum potassium and in-hospital mortality was identified. A 4.8% and 5% incidence of death was observed among patients in the 3.5 to less than 4 mEq/L and 4 to less than 4.5 mEq/L serum potassium groups, respectively; however, mortality significantly increased in the presence of progressive hypokalemia and hyperkalemia. Of interest, the incidence of ventricular fibrillation was relatively similar among patients with a serum potassium concentration of 3 mEq/L to less than 4.9 mEq/L.[67] This study suggests that maintaining serum potassium concentrations of 3.5–4.5 mEq/L may be sufficient in patients with AMI. Similarly, a minimum serum potassium threshold of 3.5 mEq/L has also been suggested to be sufficient to prevent peri- and intraoperative arrhythmias,

Table 3.3 Causes of Hypokalemia and Hyperkalemia Encountered in the Critically Ill Patient[58,59]

HYPOkalemia

Abnormal Loss
- GI
  - Vomiting, NG tube drainage
  - Diarrhea
  - High-output ileostomy or colostomy
  - Fistulas (e.g., enterocutaneous)
  - Medication-induced fecal elimination: sodium polystyrene sulfonate or sorbitol-containing enteral medications
- Renal
  - Loop diuretics
  - Thiazide diuretics
  - Amphotericin B
  - Fludrocortisone > hydrocortisone
  - Hypomagnesemia
  - Renal tubular damage (e.g., cisplatin)
  - Type 1 renal tubular acidosis

Intracellular Shift (ECF → ICF)
- Metabolic or respiratory alkalosis
- Sodium bicarbonate
- Insulin
- Nebulized β_2-agonists (e.g., albuterol, levalbuterol)
- Catecholamines (e.g., norepinephrine)
- Theophylline
- Refeeding syndrome

Inadequate Supplementation
- Prolonged NPO or potassium-free IV fluids

HYPERkalemia

Pseudohyperkalemia
- Extravascular hemolysis (i.e., inappropriate handling of laboratory specimen)

Impaired Renal Elimination
- Renal failure (chronic > acute)
- Adrenal insufficiency/hypoaldosteronism
- Aldosterone blockade/reduced synthesis
  - ACE inhibitors
  - Angiotensin receptor blockers
  - Spironolactone, eplerenone
  - Heparin
  - NSAIDs (also reduce GFR)
- Other medications
  - Potassium-sparing diuretics
  - Trimethoprim
  - Tacrolimus
  - Cyclosporine

Extracellular Shift (ICF → ECF)
- Metabolic or respiratory acidosis
- Cell lysis
  - Tumor lysis syndrome
  - Rhabdomyolysis
- Insulin deficiency/resistance (e.g., diabetes mellitus)
- Medications
  - β_2-Antagonists
  - Succinylcholine
  - Digoxin

Increased Intake/Supplementation
- Iatrogenic (e.g., potassium-containing IV fluids)
- Nonadherence to diet or potassium salt substitutes in chronic kidney disease

ACE = angiotensin-converting enzyme; ECF = extracellular fluid; GI = gastrointestinal; GFR = glomerular filtration rate; ICF = intracellular fluid; IV = intravenous; NG = nasogastric; NPO = nothing by mouth; NSAID = nonsteroidal anti-inflammatory drug.

---

as well as postoperative atrial fibrillation or flutter in patients undergoing coronary artery bypass grafting.[68]

The ideal serum potassium concentration for "critically ill" patients in general remains a conundrum, given the variety of patients cared for in the ICU. Recently, Hessels and colleagues evaluated the relationship between serum potassium, concentration variability, and outcomes among 10,451 adult ICU patients in a single-center, retrospective, observational cohort study.[64] The study population consisted of predominantly surgical (73%) as well as medical (27%) ICU patients with a median Acute Physiology and Chronic Health Evaluation (APACHE) II score of 16, a 33% incidence of acute kidney injury, and mean serum potassium concentrations of 4.1 mEq/L and 4.2 mEq/L on admission and during their ICU stay, respectively. A U-shaped relationship between serum potassium concentrations and in-hospital mortality was identified (regardless of whether serum potassium on ICU day 1 or throughout the ICU stay was evaluated), with the lowest incidence of death among patients with a serum potassium concentration of 3.5–5 mEq/L. In addition, greater variability in serum potassium concentrations was independently associated with in-hospital mortality, even for patients with a serum potassium concentration of 3.5–5 mEq/L. Overall, potassium derangements (hypo- or hyperkalemia) and potassium variability remained independently associated with in-hospital mortality when controlling for APACHE II, presence of acute kidney injury, and other confounders.[64] This publication suggests that a serum potassium concentration of 3.5–5 mEq/L is safe for most critically ill patients.

Management

For the treatment of hypokalemia, potassium supplementation may be administered orally or parenterally. Unfortunately, there is no one-size-fits-all approach, and the route of administration should be influenced by the urgency of the situation (i.e., presence of symptoms, degree of hypokalemia) and the feasibility (i.e., presence of enteral feeding tube or central vs. peripheral venous access). Overall, enteral potassium replacement is recommended in critically ill patients who are asymptomatic (both clinically and by ECG), have a serum potassium concentration of 3 mEq/L or more, and have shown tolerance to other enterally administered substances (e.g., enteral nutrition or medications). Some of the available enteral potassium replacement products and specific considerations with such therapies are listed in Table 3.4. Various potassium salts are available for enteral administration including, but not limited to, chloride, bicarbonate, citrate, gluconate, and phosphate. Potassium chloride should be the standard potassium salt used for supplementation in most cases. If hypokalemia is caused by loop or thiazide diuretic use, concomitant use of a potassium-sparing diuretic (e.g., triamterene) or spironolactone can be considered. Serum potassium concentrations should be reevaluated daily in patients receiving oral or enteral supplementation.

Intravenous administration of potassium may be required in critically ill patients because of the lack of enteral access or patient intolerance to enteral potassium or for acute treatment of symptomatic patients. Unfortunately, recommendations vary regarding the specifics of intravenous potassium therapy, including maximum concentrations for peripheral versus central venous access device administration and maximum infusion rates. In 1990, Kruse et al. published a retrospective trial including 190 medical ICU patients who received a total of 1,351 potassium chloride intravenous infusions.[69] A severity of illness score was not provided, but 61% of patients had respiratory failure, 42% sepsis, and 11% oliguric renal failure. Potassium supplementation consisted of 20 mEq of potassium chloride in 100 mL of 0.9% sodium chloride (200 mEq/L) administered intravenously over 1 hour through a central vein (77%) or peripheral vein (23%), with most patients receiving two or three consecutive doses (range of one to eight doses). Overall, the average change in serum potassium 1 hour post-infusion per 20 mEq administered intravenously was 0.25 mEq/L. The mean change in serum potassium per amount of potassium received is depicted in Figure 3.2. Phlebitis and/or pain during the intravenous infusion occurred in 2.6% of cases of peripheral administration; however, this could be underreported because of limitations in the ability of patients to communicate (particularly if comatose or mechanically ventilated) and the retrospective study design. There were no instances of ventricular arrhythmias or cardiac arrest.[69] Kruse and colleagues conducted a smaller, single-center prospective study using the same intravenous potassium chloride regimen in 40 ICU patients with a baseline serum potassium of 2.9 mEq/L (central venous access device administration in 65% of patients).[70] In this trial, the mean change in serum potassium 1 hour post-infusion per 20 mEq administered intravenously was also 0.25 ± 0.08 mEq/L. Continuous ECG monitoring revealed a significant reduction in the incidence of premature ventricular contractions during potassium infusion.[70] Hamill and colleagues conducted a prospective cohort study evaluating potassium chloride 20 mEq, 30 mEq, or 40 mEq in 100 mL 0.9% sodium chloride administered intravenously over 1 hour (maximum concentration 400 mEq/L; maximum infusion rate 40 mEq/hour).[71] The small sample size (n=48) in the context of a three-arm analysis (i.e., 20-, 30-, and 40-mEq doses), subgrouping of each study group into those with and without an elevated serum creatinine, and significant variations in pretreatment serum potassium concentrations limit the ability to analyze the effects of each intervention.[71] Collectively, the literature supports a change in serum potassium of about 0.1 mEq/L for each 10 mEq of potassium chloride intravenously administered, as well as the safety of an infusion rate up to 40 mEq/hour with concentrations of 200–400 mEq/L by a central venous access device. Unfortunately, because of low patient numbers, recommendations cannot be provided regarding potassium concentrations and maximum infusion rates by peripheral administration in the critically ill population.

Table 3.5 provides an overview of the specifics regarding intravenous potassium administration as derived from available literature. In addition, all critically ill patients with a serum potassium below 3 mEq/L, regardless of symptom presence or absence, should receive intravenous supplementation, given the risk of cardiac arrhythmias. It is also recommended that serum potassium concentrations be rechecked within 2 hours after completion of each intravenous dose, with further supplementation as needed.

Table 3.4 Enteral Electrolyte Replacement and Considerations

Electrolyte	Select Formulations	Typical Starting Dose	Considerations
Potassium	Potassium chloride • Tablet ER: 8, 10, 15, or 20 mEq • Capsule ER: 8 or 10 mEq • Solution: 20 mEq or 40 mEq/15 mL • Powder for solution: 20 mEq or 25 mEq/packet	Highly variable • 40–80 mEq/day divided into four equal doses of 20 mEq	• Recommended to limit single doses to 20–25 mEq to minimize GI upset (N/V, diarrhea, and/or abdominal pain) • Reports of GI ulceration and bleeding; would avoid use in patients with active or history of peptic ulcer disease • Powder for solution should be reconstituted with ≥ 120 mL of water per dose • Tablets and capsules are ER and should not be crushed; certain products may be dissolved in water • For enteral tube administration, solution is recommended
Magnesium	Magnesium oxide 400 mg tablet (240 mg of elemental magnesium) Magnesium citrate solution (48 mg of elemental magnesium/5 mL) Magnesium hydroxide suspension (167–333 mg of elemental magnesium/5 mL) Magnesium gluconate • Tablet: 500 mg (27 mg of elemental magnesium) • Liquid: 54 mg of elemental magnesium/5 mL	Elemental magnesium 500–1000 mg per day in two or three divided doses Examples: • Magnesium oxide 400 mg, 2 tablets BID • Magnesium citrate 30 mL per feeding tube BID	• Magnesium is a cathartic, and development of diarrhea may impair absorption; divided doses are recommended to minimize cathartic effect • For enteral tube administration, solution is recommended • Separate magnesium administration from oral fluoroquinolone and tetracycline antibiotics by ≥ 2 hr
Phosphorus	Sodium phosphate • Tablet: 10.8 mmol of phosphate/tablet Potassium phosphate/sodium phosphate • Powder for solution: 8 mmol of phosphate/packet • Tablet: 8 mmol of phosphate/tablet	Phosphate 24–48 mmol per day in two or three divided doses Examples: • Potassium phosphate/sodium phosphate 2 packets or tablets BID – TID	• Phosphate is a cathartic, and development of diarrhea may impair absorption; divided doses are recommended to minimize cathartic effect • Use of potassium phosphate/sodium phosphate is recommended in patients needing both phosphate and potassium supplementation • Each packet of potassium phosphate/sodium phosphate (Phos-NaK) contains 7 mEq of potassium and 7 mEq of sodium • Various formulations of potassium phosphate/sodium phosphate tablets are available with different amounts of potassium and sodium; specify product when ordering
Calcium	Calcium carbonate • Many formulations including tablets and suspension Calcium citrate • Tablet or capsule • 180–250 mg of elemental calcium Calcium gluconate suspension (115 mg of elemental calcium/5 mL)	Elemental calcium 1,200–1,500 mg/day in two or three divided doses Examples: • Calcium carbonate (200 mg of elemental calcium/tablet), 2 tablets PO TID • Calcium carbonate suspension (500 mg of elemental calcium/5 mL) 5 mL PO TID	• Calcium may cause constipation • Caution in patients with hyperphosphatemia; risk of calcium-phosphate precipitation • Separate administration from oral fluoroquinolone and tetracycline antibiotics by ≥ 2 hr • Calcium is not commercially available as a solution; use caution with administration of suspensions by feeding tube (not recommended with enteral tubes 10 French or smaller).

BID = twice daily; ER = extended release; N/V = nausea and vomiting; TID = three times daily. PO = orally.

If frequent potassium administration intravenously is required, consideration should be given to adding potassium to the maintenance intravenous fluids (i.e., to provide 20–80 mEq/day), as feasible, given the renal function and acid-base status of the patient. This may assist in preventing hypokalemia[72] as well as minimize serum potassium variability and associated negative outcomes.[64] In general, ECG monitoring is recommended with intravenous potassium infusion rates of greater than 10 mEq/hour or with lower infusion rates according to individual patient risk factor assessment.

Finally, clinicians should be cognizant that concomitant hypomagnesemia may result in refractory hypokalemia.[73] Hypomagnesemia appears to promote renal potassium wasting as well as impair the Na-K-ATPase pump. In a single-center, prospective, double-blind, randomized, placebo-controlled trial including 30 surgical ICU patients with hypokalemia (serum potassium less than 3.5 mEq/L), potassium retention after intravenous supplementation was significantly greater among patients maintained with a mean serum magnesium concentration of about 2.8–3 mg/dL versus about 2 mg/dL. Despite similar baseline serum potassium concentrations (3.3–3.4 mEq/L) and attainment of similar serum potassium concentrations (3.7–3.8 mEq/L) throughout the 48-hour study, patients who maintained a serum magnesium concentration of 2.8–3 mg/dL had a net potassium balance (i.e., intake minus urinary losses) of +72 mEq vs. -74 mEq (p<0.05) in the lower serum magnesium group and also required an average of about 100 mEq less potassium.[74] These results highlight renal retention of potassium by intravenous magnesium supplementation. According to this study, it is prudent in the setting of concomitant hypokalemia and hypomagnesemia that intravenous magnesium be supplemented before intravenous potassium unless severe hypokalemia-related symptoms (i.e., cardiac arrhythmias) are present. In addition, if hypokalemia fails to resolve after conventional potassium replacement, consideration should be given to targeting a serum magnesium concentration of about 3 mg/dL with intravenous magnesium supplementation.

HYPERKALEMIA

Hyperkalemia is defined as a serum potassium concentration greater than 5 mEq/L, with greater than 6.5 mEq/L indicative of severe hyperkalemia.[59] A large, two-center retrospective observational study involving more than 39,000 critically ill patients showed a 22% prevalence of hyperkalemia on ICU admission.[75] A subsequent single-center investigation of 10,451 critically ill patients showed a 15% prevalence of mild hyperkalemia (5–6 mEq/L) and a 3.6% prevalence of severe hyperkalemia (greater than 6 mEq/L) during their ICU stay.[64] Thus, hyperkalemia appears to be a problem confronting clinicians both at the time of admission and throughout critical illness.

Pathophysiology

Hyperkalemia typically occurs in response to reduced potassium excretion, a shift from the intracellular to the extracellular space, or a combination of the two. Factors associated with the development of hyperkalemia are listed in Table 3.3. Impaired renal excretion is responsible for more than 80% of episodes of hyperkalemia,[59] which should be of concern for critical care clinicians given that acute kidney injury can develop in up to 60% of critically ill patients.[76]

Clinical Manifestations

Clinical manifestations of hyperkalemia are typically cardiac related and can be life threatening. An early ECG finding is peaked T waves (in contrast to inverted T waves associated with hypokalemia).[59] Typically, as the serum potassium concentration continues to rise, conduction delays occur, characterized by widening of the PR interval, loss of the P wave, and then widening of the QRS complex. Patients may develop atrioventricular conduction blockade and ultimately ventricular fibrillation or asystole.[59] As such, focus should be placed on prevention of hyperkalemia and prompt intervention, should it develop.

Morbidity and Mortality

As mentioned earlier in this chapter, studies of both patients with AMI[67] and critically ill patients in general[64] showed a U-shaped relationship between serum potassium and ventricular fibrillation[67] as well as in-hospital mortality. In the study by Hessels and colleagues, the incidence of mortality increased from about 15% with a mean ICU serum potassium concentration of 3.5–5 mEq/L to upward of about 45%, about 60%, and about 70% with mean serum potassium concentrations of 5.6–6 mEq/L, 6.1–6.5 mEq/L, and greater than 6.5 mEq/L, respectively.[64] In addition, hyperkalemia on ICU admission has been associated with 30-day mortality. In a two-center, retrospective study of 39,705 critically ill patients (46% medical, 54% surgical) who were normokalemic

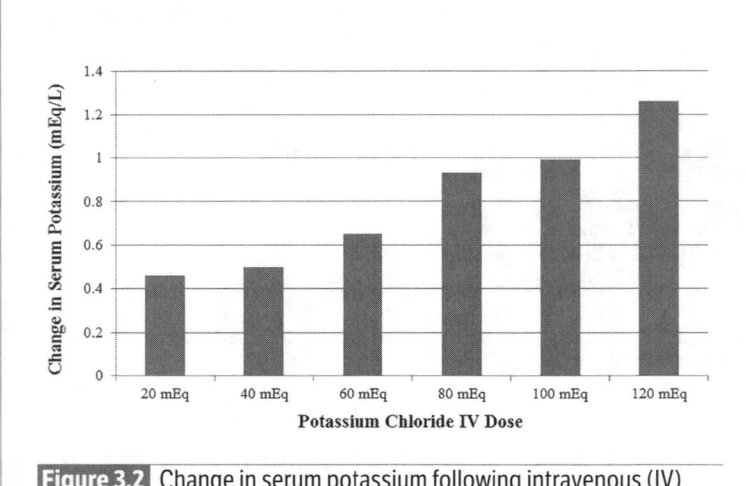

Figure 3.2 Change in serum potassium following intravenous (IV) potassium supplementation.

Overall, the average change in serum potassium 1 hour post-infusion per 20 mEq IV potassium chloride administered was 0.25 mEq/L.

Information obtained from: Kruse JA and Carlson RW. *Arch Intern Med* 1990;150:613-617.

Table 3.5 Intravenous Electrolyte Replacement and Considerations

Electrolyte	Standard Infusion Rate	Concentrations Commercially Available for Central Line	Considerations
Potassium	10 mEq/hr (max 40 mEq/hr)	Potassium chloride • 40 mEq/100 mL Premixed solutions are not commercially available for potassium acetate or potassium phosphate	Available potassium salts • Potassium chloride (agent of choice) • Potassium acetate (reserve for patients w/uncompensated metabolic acidosis) • Potassium phosphate (reserve for patients w/concomitant hypophosphatemia) IV potassium is a vesicant • Central line administration preferred • Maximum concentration for peripheral administration is not known; monitor for phlebitis/intolerance Do <u>not</u> administer IV potassium undiluted or by IV push ECG monitoring recommended with potassium infusion rate > 10 mEq/hr
Magnesium	8 mEq/hr (max 16 mEq/hr)	Magnesium sulfate • 32 mEq/100 mL	Magnesium sulfate and chloride are the only parenteral formulations available in the United States IV magnesium is not a vesicant; concentration does not have to be reduced for peripheral IV administration Renal elimination of magnesium is directly correlated with serum concentrations; slow infusion (i.e., 8 mEq/hr) recommended in asymptomatic patients
Phosphorus	7.5 mmol/hr (max 15 mmol/hr)	Premixed solutions are not commercially available Suggested concentrations: • Sodium phosphate 30 mmol/250 mL D_5W • Potassium phosphate 30 mmol/100 mL NS or D_5W	Available products • <u>Sodium</u> phosphate: 3 mmol phosphate/4 mEq sodium per 1 mL • <u>Potassium</u> phosphate: 3 mmol phosphate/4.4 mEq potassium per 1 mL Maximum concentration of sodium phosphate suggested is 160 mEq sodium per liter Standard infusion rate of 7.5 mmol/hr recommended to minimize renal elimination of phosphate Do not administer in same lumen as calcium (risk of calcium-phosphate precipitation)
Calcium	1 g/hr	Calcium gluconate • 2 g/50 mL Calcium chloride • 1 g/50 mL	Calcium is a vesicant • Central line administration preferred • Maximum concentration for peripheral administration is not known; monitor for phlebitis/intolerance • Risk of tissue necrosis theoretically greater with equal doses of calcium chloride vs. gluconate because of higher elemental calcium content (13.6 mEq vs. 4.65 mEq of calcium/gram) Do not administer in same lumen as phosphate (risk of calcium-phosphate precipitation)

D_5W = 5% dextrose in water; IV = intravenous; NS = normal saline (0.9% NaCl).

Table 3.6 Treatment Options for Hyperkalemia[57,59,77]

Class/Agent	Mechanism of Action	Typical Dose	Adverse Effects	Comments
Calcium • Gluconate • Chloride	Stabilizes the cardiac membrane	1 g IVPB over 5–10 min	Hypertension Arrhythmias	Does not lower serum potassium; only stabilizes the cardiac membrane Onset of action within minutes; duration of action 15–60 min Caution: Calcium is a vesicant and central line administration is preferred; lack of central access should not delay administration in acutely symptomatic patients (risk vs. benefit) Risk of tissue necrosis theoretically greater with equal doses of calcium chloride vs. gluconate because of higher calcium content Caution: Risk of calcium-phosphate precipitation in the setting of hyperphosphatemia or when both infused through the same lumen
Regular insulin/dextrose	Causes shift of potassium from ECF to ICF by activating the Na-K-ATPase pump	Regular insulin: 10 units IV push Dextrose 50%: 25 g IV push	Hypoglycemia	First-line agent in symptomatic patients because of predictability and utility regardless of underlying etiology Lowers serum potassium by ~0.5–1.5 mEq/L; onset of action ~15 min and duration of action 2–3 hr Consider withholding dextrose if BG > 250 mg/dL Caution: Obtain BG within 30 min or sooner if patient becomes unresponsive
Inhaled β_2-agonists • Albuterol	Causes shift of potassium from ECF to ICF primarily by activating the Na-K-ATPase pump (may also stimulate pancreatic β receptors to ↑ insulin)	10–20 mg nebulized over 10 min	Tachycardia Angina CNS stimulation (hyperactivity)	Lowers serum potassium by ~0.5–1 mEq/L (dose-dependent); in some reports, as effective as insulin/dextrose; some reports also document synergy Onset of action 15–30 min and duration of action up to 2 hr Despite efficacy, not recommended as first-line for hyperkalemia because of potential for development/worsening of tachycardia Note: Dose of nebulized albuterol is 4 times standard dose used for bronchoconstriction Levalbuterol 2.5 mg is also an option[78]
Alkalinizing agents • Sodium bicarbonate	Causes shift of potassium from ECF to ICF by activating the H-K-ATPase pump	50–100 mEq IV push over 5 min	Hypernatremia Edema Metabolic alkalosis	Reserve for patients with hyperkalemia in the setting of suspected or confirmed metabolic acidosis Unproven benefit as monotherapy (potential ~0.5 mEq/L reduction in serum potassium); some reports document synergy with insulin/dextrose Cautious use in patients with heart failure and chronic kidney disease (because of sodium load) Hypertonic solution – central line administration is preferred if available; lack of central access should not delay administration in acutely symptomatic patients (risk vs. benefit)

Table 3.6 Treatment Options for Hyperkalemia[57,59,77] (continued)

Class/Agent	Mechanism of Action	Typical Dose	Adverse Effects	Comments
Loop diuretics • Furosemide • Torsemide • Bumetanide • Ethacrynic acid	Increases renal excretion of potassium	Furosemide 20–40 mg IV push	Hypotension Hypomagnesemia Hypocalcemia	Only applicable in patients who are not anuric Consider concomitant IV fluids unless patient is fluid overloaded Onset: ~15 min; duration of action up to 6 hr; if no response within 30 min, consider doubling dose (i.e., 40–80 mg IV push) May repeat every 6 hr if needed
Sodium polystyrene sulfonate	Resin that exchanges sodium for potassium ions in the GI tract, preventing potassium absorption	PO: 15–30 g Rectal: 30–60 g	Hypernatremia Hypomagnesemia Constipation Alkalemia	Slow onset with enteral administration (4–6 hr), faster onset per rectum (1 hr); only appropriate for asymptomatic patients Bowel movement needed for elimination of resin bound potassium Caution: Reports of colonic necrosis led to an FDA advisory in 2009/2011 recommending to avoid use in patients with or at risk of constipation/impaction and in postoperative patients who have not had a bowel movement[79,80]
Hemodialysis	Removal of potassium from the ECF	N/A	Hypotension	Most effective and predictable method of decreasing serum potassium Use reserved for symptomatic patients unless other indications present for dialysis initiation Intervention requires coordination of critical care and nephrology teams (in most cases), physical setup, and placement of dialysis catheter; delays in initiation possible without proper communication Continuous dialysis modes effective for managing conditions associated with persistent hyperkalemia, such as tumor lysis syndrome

BG = blood glucose; FDA = Food and Drug Administration; GI = gastrointestinal; H-K-ATPase = hydrogen-potassium adenosine triphosphatase; IV = intravenous; IVPB = intravenous piggyback; N/A = not applicable; Na-K-ATPase = sodium-potassium adenosine triphosphatase; PO = by mouth.

(i.e., 4 mEq/L or more) on ICU admission, a statistically significant increased risk of death was identified among patients with a serum potassium concentration of 4.5 mEq/L or more compared with those with a concentration of 4–4.5 mEq/L, even after adjusting for several covariates.[75] This was observed in each 0.5-mEq/L incremental category of serum potassium from 4.5–5 mEq/L to greater than 6.5 mEq/L (e.g., 5–5.5 mEq/L, 5.5–6 mEq/L). Although none of the previously mentioned studies can prove causality between hyperkalemia and mortality, the association is plausible.

Management

Treatment of hyperkalemia consists of the following: provision of cardioprotection, shifting of potassium from the ECF to the ICF, and enhancing potassium excretion. In addition to these interventions, exogenous sources of potassium must be removed, and as feasible, medications that may indirectly contribute to potassium retention should be held. An overview of treatments used in the management of hyperkalemia is presented in Table 3.6.[57,59,77-80] Patients presenting with cardiac symptoms must be treated promptly to prevent progression to a life-threatening event. No treatment algorithms for symptomatic or asymptomatic patients with hyperkalemia have been validated in the literature, particularly in the care of critically ill patients. A suggested algorithm for the management of hyperkalemia in the critically ill population is presented in Figure 3.3. In general, asymptomatic patients whose serum potassium concentration is less than 5.5 mEq/L may need no medical intervention other than source control (i.e., remove all exogenous potassium and intervene depending on the underlying etiology, as feasible). Patients with a serum

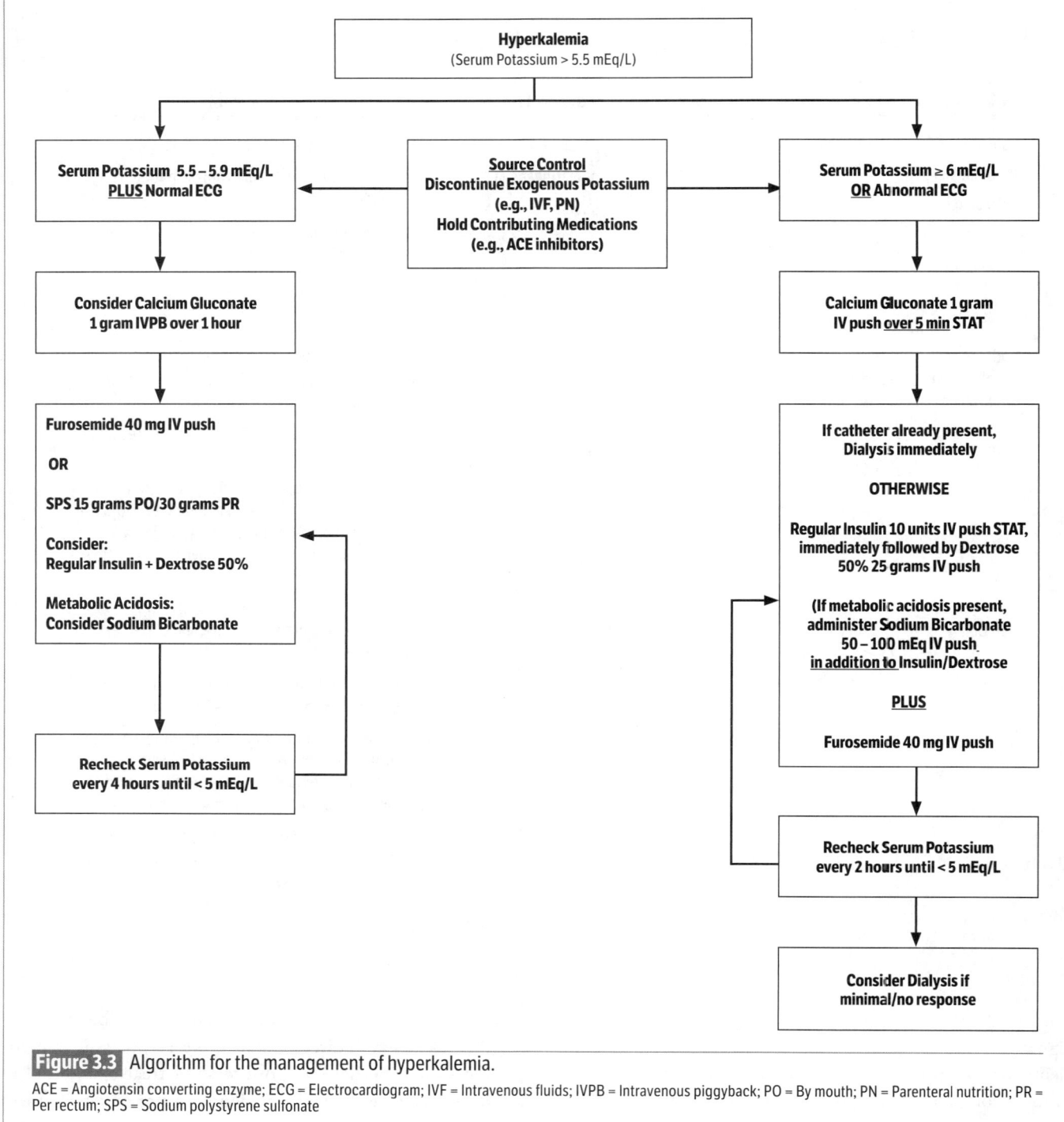

Figure 3.3 Algorithm for the management of hyperkalemia.

ACE = Angiotensin converting enzyme; ECG = Electrocardiogram; IVF = Intravenous fluids; IVPB = Intravenous piggyback; PO = By mouth; PN = Parenteral nutrition; PR = Per rectum; SPS = Sodium polystyrene sulfonate

potassium concentration of 5.5–5.9 mEq/L require prompt evaluation with a 12-lead ECG. In addition to source control, at a minimum, such patients may benefit from pharmacologic therapy to eliminate excess potassium.

Symptomatic patients (i.e., those with ECG abnormalities) regardless of the degree of hyperkalemia require emergent intervention. Intravenous calcium should be administered to stabilize the cardiac membrane (i.e., to restore resting membrane potential and thereby increase the threshold for generating a cardiac action potential). The amount of calcium necessary to achieve this goal is unknown, but use of either calcium gluconate 1–2 g intravenously or calcium chloride 1 g intravenously is acceptable. Calcium chloride may be preferred because of a theorized faster dissociation of calcium from the chloride salt and thus more immediate impact, but superiority has never been shown. Overall, calcium should be administered to all symptomatic patients with the exception of hyperkalemia in the setting of digoxin toxicity because calcium can propagate such toxicity.[59] In addition, regular insulin (10 units) and dextrose (25–50 g) should be administered because this intervention has been shown to rapidly (within 15 minutes) and reliably shift potassium intracellularly (0.5- to 1.5-mEq/L reduction in serum potassium that can last 2–3 hours).[77] Intravenous sodium bicarbonate (e.g., 50 mEq by intravenous push) can also cause modest intracellular shifts in potassium (about 0.5 mEq/L reduction in serum potassium), but this is only effective in the setting of a non-anion gap metabolic acidosis and should be reserved as adjunctive therapy in such cases.[57,77] Granted that shifting of potassium intracellularly is a temporizing measure, interventions to eliminate excess potassium should be implemented as well, such as administration of loop diuretics (e.g., furosemide 20–40 mg intravenously). Hemodialysis is the most predictable and effective method for rapidly reducing serum potassium; however, in the absence of an existing dialysis catheter, this intervention may not be the most practical or efficient. Regardless, a nephrologist should be contacted early, should the patient not respond to pharmacologic methods.

MAGNESIUM

Magnesium is the second most abundant intracellular cation. Normal body stores of magnesium are 23–25 g with about 99% in the intracellular space, located predominantly in bone (50%–60%), skeletal muscle (20%–30%), and soft tissues (20%). Only about 0.3% of total body magnesium is located in the serum.[81,82] As such, normal serum magnesium concentrations range from 1.8 to 2.4 mg/dL (1.5–2 mEq/L) and are not reflective of total body stores.[81]

Most magnesium in the ECF is in the ionized (active) form, with 20% bound to serum proteins.[83] Results vary regarding whether total and ionized serum magnesium concentrations correlate in critically ill patients, with some studies showing a strong[84] and others a poor correlation.[85,86] There have also been investigations regarding whether ionized serum magnesium concentrations are better predictors of clinical outcomes and response to magnesium supplementation, but similarly, conflicting results exist.[82] The magnesium tolerance test may be the most accurate method of determining magnesium deficiency[87]; however, the requirement for "normal" renal function, influence of diuretic therapy, and cumbersome procedure lead to little utility in critically ill patients.[82] At this time, assessment of total serum magnesium concentrations remains the most widely available and accepted method of evaluation in critically ill patients.

Magnesium is an essential cofactor in hundreds of enzymatic reactions, including the formation of ATP, replication and transcription of DNA, and translation of messenger RNA.[81,82] Magnesium is essential to mitochondrial function, cell membrane function, neuromuscular transmission, parathyroid hormone (PTH) secretion, and glucose metabolism.[83] As mentioned earlier under hypokalemia, the Na-K-ATPase enzyme is dependent on magnesium for proper functioning; thus, magnesium helps regulate the transcellular gradient as well as renal excretion of potassium. Magnesium also plays a role in smooth muscle tone by regulating intracellular calcium concentrations.[82] Specifically, magnesium decreases activation of inositol triphosphate, decreasing calcium release from the sarcoplasmic reticulum, and also activates calcium ATPase, facilitating the movement of calcium back into the sarcoplasmic reticulum and from the ICF to the ECF. Magnesium deficiency has been proposed to cause coronary vasospasm, hypertension, bronchial airway constriction, and seizures.[82]

Magnesium homeostasis is regulated by the small bowel and the kidneys.[81-83] Overall, 30%–50% of dietary magnesium is absorbed under normal conditions, primarily in the jejunum and ileum. Gastrointestinal absorption of magnesium is saturable and inversely proportional to intake. The kidneys play the most important role in magnesium homeostasis, with about 95% of all filtered magnesium reabsorbed into the systemic circulation. Most reabsorption occurs in the thick ascending limb of the loop of Henle (65%–75%), followed by the proximal tubule (15%–20%) and the distal tubule (5%–10%).[83] The serum magnesium concentration is the primary regulator of magnesium reabsorption because calcium and magnesium receptors located on the capillary side of the thick ascending limb of the loop of Henle sense serum magnesium concentrations and enhance or reduce reabsorption accordingly.[81] There are no hormonal mediators of magnesium homeostasis; thus, serum magnesium concentrations can profoundly be affected by changes in intake and/or renal function (including use of diuretics).

HYPOMAGNESEMIA

Hypomagnesemia is defined as a serum magnesium concentration less than 1.8 mg/dL (less than 1.5 mEq/L). The incidence of hypomagnesemia on ICU admission ranges from 20% to 61%,[87-92] with the large variation likely attributable to different diagnostic thresholds and patient populations. The incidence of ICU-acquired hypomagnesemia is not well reported.

Pathophysiology

The predominant causes of hypomagnesemia can be divided into two categories: GI and renal-related losses. The content of magnesium in upper GI fluids (i.e., stomach) is about 1 mEq/L, which is in contrast to the 15 mEq/L found in the lower intestines.[82] Hypomagnesemia from GI loss of magnesium can be observed with frequent vomiting, high NG tube output, diarrhea (including excessive use of cathartic agents), high ileostomy or colostomy output, and enterocutaneous fistulae. Damage to the bowel can lead to decreased magnesium absorption (i.e., increased output by feces) such as that seen with radiation enteritis, Crohn disease, or ulcerative colitis. In addition, physical manipulation of the bowel may limit the surface area for magnesium absorption, such as that seen with extensive small bowel resections.[81,82]

Renal loss of magnesium in critically ill patients may often be iatrogenic and associated with medications provided to treat their acute illness. Loop diuretics are a prominent cause, given their activity at the thick ascending limb of the loop of Henle.[82] Aminoglycosides, amphotericin B products, and foscarnet have been associated with renal magnesium wasting, as have cyclosporine and tacrolimus. For critically ill oncology patients, prior use of a platinum-based chemotherapeutic agent (e.g., cisplatin, carboplatin, oxaliplatin) will predictably result in renal magnesium wasting.[81,82] Renal magnesium wasting can also be seen with hyperglycemia (secondary to an osmotic diuresis), in the diuretic phase of acute kidney injury, and in those with chronic alcohol abuse.[81,82] Other less common causes of hypomagnesemia (e.g., hungry bone syndrome) have also been reported in the literature.[81]

Clinical Manifestations

Hypomagnesemia can be considered an "excitatory" state, and potential clinical manifestations are listed in Table 3.7. Cardiac complications are a prominent concern for clinicians, particularly development of atrial fibrillation, supraventricular tachycardia, or ventricular arrhythmias, such as torsades de pointes.[82] Electrocardiographic abnormalities that can be seen include a prolonged PR interval, widening of the QRS complex, and peaked (mild hypomagnesemia) or flattened (severe hypomagnesemia) T waves.[82,83] Given that hypomagnesemia and hypokalemia often coexist,[93] it is difficult to attribute such cardiac abnormalities to hypomagnesemia alone. Neuromuscular hyperexcitability, including spontaneous carpal-pedal spasms and seizures, may develop.[82] Seizures should be of particular concern in patients with hypomagnesemia and a history of epilepsy or those considered at high risk (e.g., neurosurgical intervention, alcoholism). Refractory hypokalemia can be observed in the presence of hypomagnesemia for reasons mentioned earlier. Finally, through inhibition of PTH release and/or activity, hypomagnesemia can also contribute to the development of hypocalcemia, which may exacerbate neuromuscular excitability.[82]

Morbidity and Mortality

With respect to clinical outcomes, observational trials have shown a significantly higher mortality among patients with versus without hypomagnesemia on ICU admission.[88-90,94] In addition, reports have associated hypomagnesemia with increased ICU and hospital length of stay,[94] lack of recovery from acute kidney injury,[91] and lactic acidosis.[92] Of note, in none of these reports can causality be determined.

Management

Overall, there are few data regarding the treatment of patients with severely symptomatic hypomagnesemia. Intravenous administration of magnesium is plausible for the treatment of such patients, and magnesium sulfate or chloride are the only intravenous formulations currently available in the United States. For patients with torsades de pointes, magnesium sulfate is the drug of choice according to the American Heart Association guidelines, with a recommended dose of 2 g administered by intravenous push over 1–2 minutes (with 10–20 mL of 0.9% sodium chloride flush to ensure systemic delivery).[95] If the response is inadequate, a second intravenous bolus of 2 g can be administered within 5 minutes.[96] This recommendation is primarily based on a case series of 12 patients with torsades de pointes successfully treated with this regimen.[96] It is unclear whether this dosing regimen for magnesium sulfate could also be considered in patients who are hypomagnesemic presenting with other atrial or ventricular arrhythmias, as well as those with refractory status epilepticus. After the initial bolus, a continuous intravenous infusion should be provided to sustain the serum magnesium concentrations, yet data are lacking for the specifics of such therapy in these clinical scenarios. When reviewing the protocols for magnesium sulfate evaluated in clinical trials for AMI and stroke,

Table 3.7 Clinical Manifestations of Magnesium Disorders[a,83]

Organ System	Hypomagnesemia (serum < 1.8 mg/dL)	Hypermagnesemia (serum > 3.5 mg/dL)
Neurologic	Nystagmus	Sedation (> 6 mg/dL)
	Ataxia	Coma (> 12 mg/dL)
	Seizures	
Cardiac	Atrial fibrillation	Hypotension (> 3.5 mg/dL)
	Ventricular arrhythmias	Bradycardia (> 4.5–5 mg/dL)
	Torsades de pointes	Bundle branch block (> 6 mg/dL)
	Digitalis toxicity	Asystole (> 18 mg/dL)
Neuromuscular	Hyperreflexia	Hyporeflexia (> 8 mg/dL)
	Muscle twitching/tremors	Muscle paralysis (> 13 mg/dL)
	(+) Chvostek/Trousseau sign	Respiratory depression (> 14.5 mg/dL)
Electrolyte disorders	Refractory hypokalemia	N/A
	Refractory hypocalcemia	

[a]To convert magnesium in mg/dL to mEq/L, divide by 1.2.

dosages of up to 160 mEq have been infused intravenously over 24 hours and safely used in patients with a serum creatinine concentration of less than 2.3 mg/dL.[97-101] Intravenous recommendations for continuous magnesium sulfate in the treatment of symptomatic patients are provided in Table 3.8. As a safety measure with such high doses, patients' respiratory rate, deep tendon reflexes, and urine output should be monitored often. Clinicians should expect serum magnesium concentrations to be elevated during the infusion, but concentrations up to 3.5 mg/dL may be tolerated. After the first 24 hours of magnesium treatment, an additional 0.5 mEq/kg/day intravenously is recommended on days 2–5 to account for potential total body magnesium deficits.[102] Magnesium replacement should be continued until hypocalcemia or hypokalemia unresponsive to conventional supplementation resolves. Administration of large doses of magnesium sulfate as described in Table 3.8 should be avoided in patients with hypotension, bradycardia, or heart block because hypermagnesemia may exacerbate these conditions.

In asymptomatic patients, magnesium supplementation is often provided in a preventive manner to maintain normal serum concentrations. As mentioned earlier, poor outcomes have been observed in patients admitted to the ICU with hypomagnesemia; however, the ability of magnesium supplementation to prevent such outcomes remains unknown, as does the ideal serum magnesium concentration in asymptomatic critically ill patients. Conventionally, many ICU clinicians target a serum magnesium concentration of about 2 mg/dL; however, no data support that this practice is more beneficial than simply maintaining normomagnesemia (i.e., 1.8 mg/dL or more). Table 3.4 lists some of the available enteral magnesium products. These products can be considered for maintenance therapy, but they often have a limited role because of their low bioavailability and potential cathartic effect. As a result, intravenous magnesium is often used. In general, for every 1 g of magnesium sulfate administered, the serum magnesium concentration is expected to increase by 0.1 mg/dL.[98,99] Considerations regarding intravenous magnesium sulfate administration are provided in Table 3.5, including a recommended infusion rate. Although an infusion rate of 32 mEq/hour has been reported in the literature, using conservative infusion rates of 4–16 mEq/hour is recommended because renal elimination of magnesium is directly correlated with serum concentrations. In the presence of normal serum magnesium concentrations, renal elimination of magnesium is increased[103]; therefore, an unnecessarily rapid rise in serum magnesium concentration may lead to a greater portion of the administered dose being eliminated by the kidneys, ultimately impairing the ability to replete total body stores. In addition, a minimum of 2 g of intravenous magnesium sulfate is recommended in order to observe any significant change in the serum magnesium concentration. Serum magnesium concentrations should be rechecked 2 hours after completion of each intravenous infusion. If consistent replacement is needed, clinicians are encouraged to add magnesium to the patient's maintenance intravenous fluids to avoid serum concentration oscillations (similar to that recommended for potassium).

HYPERMAGNESEMIA

Technically, hypermagnesemia is defined as a serum magnesium concentration greater than 2.4 mg/dL (2 mEq/L); however, symptoms of hypermagnesemia typically do not develop until serum concentrations reach or surpass 3.5 mg/dL.[83] The incidence of hypermagnesemia on ICU admission is relatively low (5%–7%),[88-90] and no data are available regarding ICU-acquired hypermagnesemia.

Hypotension is usually the first clinical manifestation of hypermagnesemia, followed by bradycardia, sedation, and hyporeflexia. If serum magnesium concentrations rise drastically (8.5 mg/dL or higher), patients can have somnolence, coma, respiratory depression, and even asystole (Table 3.7).[83] In critically ill patients, hypermagnesemia can be iatrogenic (i.e., overcorrection of hypomagnesemia) or a result of acute renal failure. Other potential, less likely causes of hypermagnesemia in the critically ill population include drug induced (i.e., magnesium-containing cathartics), hypothyroidism, Addison disease, and diabetic ketoacidosis.[83]

Management of hypermagnesemia revolves around reversing the symptoms (if present) and lowering the serum magnesium concentration in addition to correcting

Table 3.8 Suggestions for the Treatment of Symptomatic Hypomagnesemia[a,b]

Degree of Deficiency	Serum Magnesium Range (mg/dL)	Treatment in First 24 hr (IV infusion) (mEq/kg)[c]
Mild hypomagnesemia	1.6–1.8	0.5
Moderate hypomagnesemia	1.2–1.5	1
Severe hypomagnesemia	<1.2	2

[a]Subsequent therapy after 2 g (16 mEq) IV push of magnesium sulfate for patients with severe symptoms.

[b]To convert magnesium in mg/dL to mEq/L, divide by 1.2.

[c]Based on ideal body weight and provided as a continuous infusion over 24 hr; only suggested for use in patients with urine output > 0.5 mL/kg/hr and estimated creatinine clearance > 50 mL/minute/1.73 m²; in the setting of renal insufficiency, consider 25%–50% of suggested dose and reevaluate serum magnesium concentration every 12 hr.

the underlying etiology. In the presence of cardiac or neuromuscular symptoms, administration of 100–200 mg of intravenous elemental calcium (i.e., calcium gluconate 1–2 g or calcium chloride 500 mg to 1 g) is recommended because calcium antagonizes the activity of magnesium. In addition, cardiac support (e.g., vasopressor therapy, transcutaneous pacing) and/or respiratory support (e.g., endotracheal intubation) may be needed for severe hypermagnesemia. In patients with preserved renal function, serum magnesium concentrations may be lowered using loop diuretics (e.g., furosemide 20–40 mg intravenous push) in addition to intravenous hydration with an isotonic fluid.[83] Finally, immediate hemodialysis may be needed, particularly in patients with chronic kidney disease or those who are acutely oliguric or anuric.[81,83]

PHOSPHORUS

Phosphorus is the body's primary intracellular anion and is present as both organic (i.e., bound) and inorganic (i.e., free) phosphate. Most intracellular phosphate consists of organic phosphate esters, including 2,3-diphosphoglycerate, adenosine, and guanosine triphosphate. Most inorganic phosphate is contained within the ECF.[104]

Phosphate is essential in the development of phospholipid cell membranes, nucleic acids, phosphoproteins, and ATP, the main energy source for most cellular functions.[104] On average, the human body contains only 250 g of ATP and turns over its own body weight equivalent in ATP each day. Phosphate also regulates several enzymatic reactions, including glycolysis, ammoniagenesis, and the 1-hydroxylation of 25-hydroxyvitamin D. In addition, phosphate is required for the production of 2,3-diphosphoglycerate in RBCs, a compound necessary for proper oxygen delivery to tissues.[104] Finally, phosphate serves as the primary buffer in the urine.

The normal serum phosphorus concentration in adults is 2.5–4.5 mg/dL.[81,104] During the day, serum phosphorus concentrations can oscillate by as much as 2 mg/dL, reflecting acute changes in transcellular distribution secondary to carbohydrate intake and insulin secretion.[104] 1,25-Dihydroxycholecalciferol (i.e., activated vitamin D) and PTH are the primary mediators of phosphorus homeostasis (Figure 3.4). Around 60%–80% of ingested phosphorus is absorbed in the GI tract, primarily in the jejunum, through both active and passive processes. Gastrointestinal absorption of phosphorus by active transport is directly facilitated by 1,25-dihydroxycholecalciferol and indirectly by PTH (through activation of vitamin D).[104,105] Parathyroid hormone also increases serum phosphorus concentrations by stimulating the release of phosphorus from bones.[105] However, PTH prevents renal tubular reabsorption of phosphorus after glomerular filtration, ultimately reducing serum phosphorus concentrations

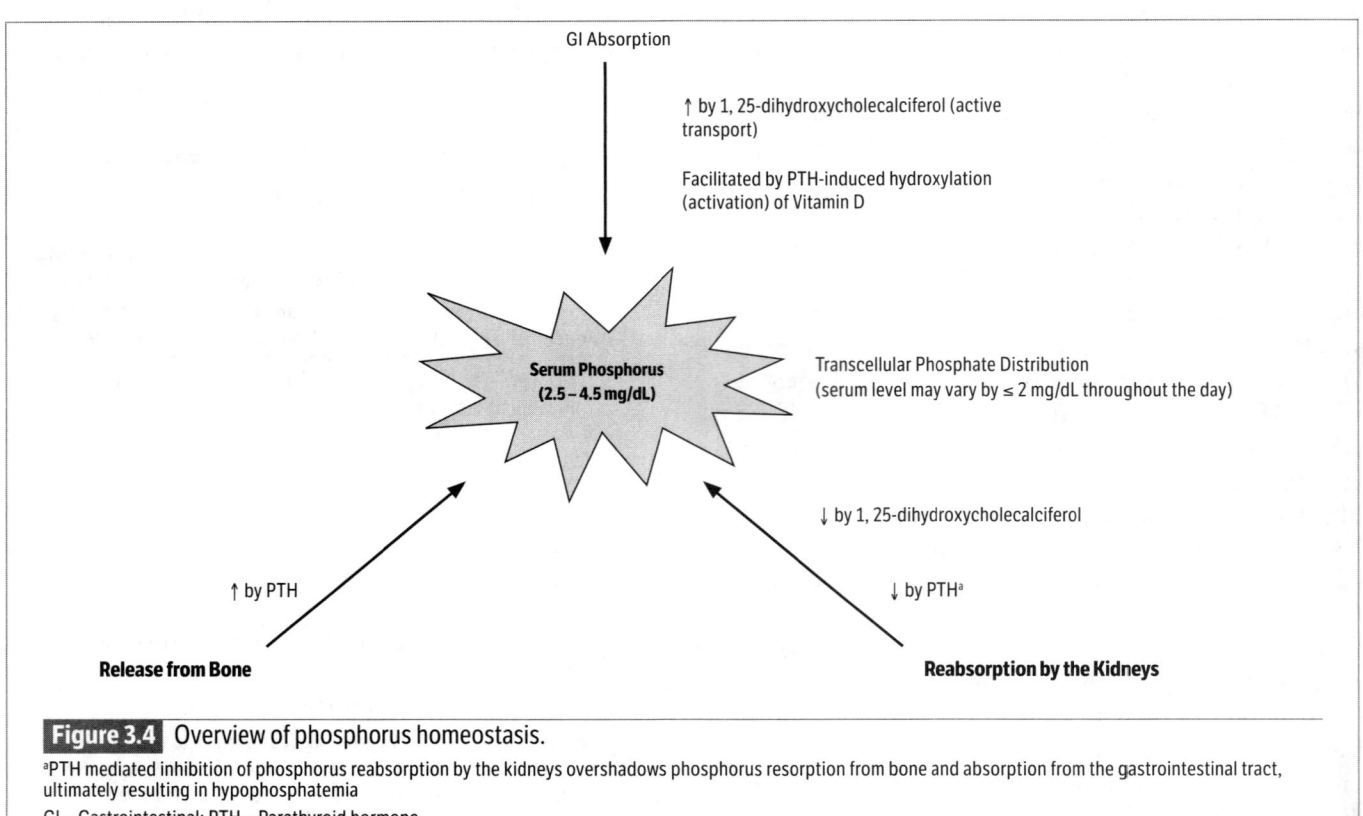

Figure 3.4 Overview of phosphorus homeostasis.

[a]PTH mediated inhibition of phosphorus reabsorption by the kidneys overshadows phosphorus resorption from bone and absorption from the gastrointestinal tract, ultimately resulting in hypophosphatemia
GI = Gastrointestinal; PTH = Parathyroid hormone
Information obtained from: Kelly A, et al. *J Intensive Care Med* 2013;28:166-177

because this effect overshadows PTH-mediated GI absorption and release from bone.[105]

HYPOPHOSPHATEMIA

Hypophosphatemia is defined as a serum phosphorus concentration less than 2.5 mg/dL, with severe hypophosphatemia characterized by a concentration of less than 1 mg/dL. The prevalence of hypophosphatemia in critically ill patients varies widely (10%–80%).[106] A recent large, single-center retrospective study involving 2,730 adult critically ill patients showed a 20% prevalence of hypophosphatemia.[107]

Pathophysiology

Hypophosphatemia can develop as a result of decreased intake/absorption, increased renal excretion, and/or internal redistribution. Internal redistribution of phosphorus (i.e., from the ECF to the ICF) is considered the most common cause of hypophosphatemia and can be seen with hyperventilation/respiratory alkalosis, insulin secretion/provision (e.g., management of diabetic ketoacidosis), hungry bone syndrome after parathyroidectomy, and refeeding syndrome.[81] Refeeding syndrome is typically observed when glucose (either enterally or parenterally) is provided to patients after periods of prolonged (e.g., 7–10 days) starvation or inadequate nutrition, resulting in rapid intracellular shifts of potassium, magnesium, and phosphorus.[108] Patients who have insufficient phosphorus stores because of preexisting malnutrition, such as in those who abuse alcohol and patients with cancer cachexia, may be particularly prone to refeeding-induced hypophosphatemia. In addition, in the setting of extensive burns and prolonged hyperventilation, phosphate stores may be quickly exhausted through the building of new cells and maintenance of ATP quantities sufficient for diaphragmatic contractions.[104] Decreased GI absorption of phosphate may occur as a result of vitamin D deficiency, excessive administration of phosphate-binding agents (e.g., sevelamer, calcium carbonate), or use of other enteral medications that inadvertently bind phosphate in the GI tract (e.g., sucralfate). Increased urinary excretion of phosphate can be seen with primary and secondary hyperparathyroidism, osmotic diuresis, volume resuscitation, and Fanconi syndrome.[81]

Clinical Manifestations

Given the many roles of phosphate in the body, it is not surprising that hypophosphatemia can affect many organ systems. Clinical manifestations of hypophosphatemia are thought to be primarily related to the depletion of ATP (e.g., myalgia, respiratory failure, heart failure) and reduced RBC concentrations of 2,3-diphosphoglycerate (e.g., metabolic encephalopathy syndrome from tissue hypoxia).[104] Significant neuromuscular and cardiac sequelae can be seen with severe hypophosphatemia (i.e., less than 1 mg/dL).[109] However, moderate hypophosphatemia (i.e., 1–2 mg/dL) can also result in significant clinical manifestations, including impaired diaphragmatic contractility, intermittent ventricular tachycardia, and insulin resistance.[109]

Morbidity and Mortality

Despite the wide array of organ systems affected, hypophosphatemia does not appear to be associated with an overall increased risk of mortality. In a recent single-center observational study including 2,730 adult critically ill patients (34% surgical, baseline APACHE II of 18), multivariate logistic regression failed to reveal an independent association of hypophosphatemia with ICU mortality (OR 0.86; 95% CI, 0.66–1.10) or hospital mortality (OR 0.89; 95% CI, 0.73–1.07).[107] The lack of statistical significance was observed regardless of the hypophosphatemia threshold evaluated (1.9 or less, 1.5 or less, 1.2 or less, 0.9 or less, 0.6 mg/dL or less), although the small number of patients with a serum phosphorus concentration of 0.9 mg/dL or less (n=55) may have influenced the results for this subset.[107] In contrast, critically ill patients undergoing intermittent hemodialysis and experiencing hypophosphatemia had an increased incidence of in-hospital and 1-year mortality, as well as prolonged dialysis dependency, delayed recovery of complete renal function, and a higher prevalence of chronic kidney disease at 1 year.[110] Overall, the impact of hypophosphatemia on mortality in critically ill patients, irrespective of renal function, deserves evaluation in prospective trials. The potential impact of hypophosphatemia on vital organ function (e.g., reduced cardiac contractility and impaired diaphragmatic contraction) demands daily serum phosphorus evaluation and prompt supplementation in the critically ill population.

Management

Hypophosphatemia can be corrected with oral or intravenous phosphate supplementation. In general, oral phosphate replacement should be reserved for patients who are asymptomatic and may be considered when the serum phosphorus concentration is greater than or equal to 2 mg/dL. Some of the more commonly used enteral replacement options for phosphate are presented in Table 3.4. Clinicians must be cognizant that oral phosphate administration can result in a cathartic effect, and some preparations contain significant amounts of potassium.

Intravenous administration of phosphate is the recommended route for managing symptomatic hypophosphatemia and is typically recommended for critically ill patients with a serum phosphorus concentration less than 2 mg/dL, even in the absence of symptoms. Intravenous phosphate is available as both a sodium and potassium salt. The management of hypophosphatemia may be the most widely studied electrolyte derangement in the critically ill population other than hyponatremia. Table 3.9 provides a summary of the available data regarding intravenous

continued on page 87

Table 3.9 Trials Evaluating Intravenous Phosphate Replacement[106,109,111-118]

Citation/Design	Study Population	Intervention/Infusion Rate	Outcomes	Comments
Vannatta J, et al. 1981[111] SC, P, OL trial	Adult patients (n=10) • Serum phosphorus ≤ 1 mg/dL • Urine output > 30 mL/hr	**Potassium phosphate 9 mmol IV over 12 hr** • Could repeat as needed every 12 hr for 48 hr Diluent • 0.45% NaCl (volume not provided) Infusion rate • 0.75 mmol/hr	**Mean Serum Phosphorus Concentration**[a] • Baseline: 0.81 mg/dL • At 12 hr: 1.27 mg/dL **Phosphorus > 1 mg/dL at 12 hr:** 60% **Phosphorus 2.5–4.5 mg/dL at 48 hr:** 60%	• Overall, supplementation dose inadequate for severe hypophosphatemia, as evidenced by 40% with peak conc < 1 mg/dL and 100% with peak conc < 2 mg/dL after first dose • According to body weight, phosphorus dose range = 0.1–0.17 mmol/kg • No mention of number of repeat doses • Limited information regarding study population; 60% with alcoholism • No incident of hyperkalemia • Serum calcium 6.3 mg/dL (n=1), asymptomatic • Serum phosphorus 5.2 mg/dL (n=1), asymptomatic
Vannatta J, et al. 1983[112] SC, P, OL trial	Adult patients (n=10) • Serum phosphorus ≤ 1 mg/dL • Urine output > 30 mL/hr • Two or more reasons for hypophosphatemia	Potassium phosphate 0.32 mmol/kg IV over 12 hr • Criteria for escalation mid-infusion to 0.48 mmol/kg • Repeat dose until serum phosphorus ≥ 2 mg/dL Diluent • 0.45% NaCl ("volume determined for each patient individually") Infusion rate • 0.03–0.04 mmol/kg/hr	**Patients with Serum Phosphorus > 2 mg/dL** By 6 hr: 1 of 10 By 12 hr: 4 of 10 By 24 hr: 7 of 10 By 36 hr: 9 of 10 By 48 hr: 10 of 10 **Patients Needing Repeat Doses of Phosphorus** At 12 hr: 6 of 9 At 24 hr: 3 of 6 At 36 hr: 1 of 3 At 48 hr: 0 of 1	• Follow-up study to that published in 1981 • Increased dose appears more adequate • Dose escalation to 0.48 mmol/kg conducted in one patient (although two met the criteria for escalation) • Body weight not provided; unable to determine absolute dose or infusion rate (estimate for 70-kg patient, 22–34 mmol and 2.1–2.8 mmol/hr) • No patients with serum calcium < 7 mg/dL • No patients had hyperphosphatemia; however, monitoring stopped on attainment of phosphorus ≥ 2 mg/dL • Limited information regarding study population; 60% with alcoholism
Kingston M, et al. 1985[113] SC, P, OL trial	Adult, "seriously ill" patients with hypophosphatemia (n=31)	Sodium phosphate (n=17) or potassium phosphate (n=14) • Dose not standardized • Most (28/31) received 10–15 mmol Diluent (250 mL each) • 0.9% NaCl or 5% dextrose Infusion rate • Over 4 hr (2.5–3.75 mmol/hr)	**Mean Serum Phosphorus**[a] Baseline: 0.88 ± 0.4 mg/dL End infusion: 2.3 ± 0.9 mg/dL **Correlation Between Delta Phosphorus and mg/kg Dose** r = 0.74	• 16 patients (52%) malnourished • One patient with hyperphosphatemia (peak conc of 5.3 mg/dL) • No change in mean serum calcium

Table 3.9 Trials Evaluating Intravenous Phosphate Replacement[106,109,111-118] (continued)

Citation/Design	Study Population	Intervention/Infusion Rate	Outcomes	Comments
Rosen G, et al. 1995[109]	Adult, surgical and trauma patients with phosphorus < 2 mg/dL (n=11) • Baseline 1.6–1.9 mg/dL	Sodium phosphate 15 mmol (or potassium phosphate if serum potassium ≤ 3.5 mEq/L) Diluent • 0.9% NaCl 100 mL Infusion rate • 7.5 mmol/hr If phosphorus remained < 2 mg/dL at 6 hr post-infusion or on routine follow-up, administration of 15 mmol was repeated (max 45 mmol/24 hr)	**Serum Phosphorus ≥ 2 mg/dL 6 hr Post-infusion:** 9 of 10 Total of three patients required additional doses to achieve/maintain serum phosphorus ≥ 2 mg/dL within 24 hr	• All patients critically ill, but severity of illness not provided • PN patients (n=3) received 12 mmol of phosphorus/L in addition to study amount • Incidence of peak (immediately post-infusion) serum phosphorus > 6 mg/dL: 0% • Corrected calcium: 8.5–9.7 mg/dL during study • One patient with serum potassium of 5.1 mEq/L • Given baseline serum phosphorus of 1.6–1.9 mg/dL, high success of achieving ≥ 2 mg/dL can be expected
Clark C, et al. 1995[114] SC, P, OL trial	Consecutive, adult patients co-managed by nutrition support service with serum phosphorus < 3 mg/dL, divided into three groups (n=67) • Mild (2.3–3 mg/dL); n=31 • Moderate (1.6–2.2 mg/dL); n=22 • Severe (≤ 1.5 mg/dL); n=14	One dose of sodium phosphate (or potassium phosphate if serum potassium < 4 mEq/L) per graduated dosing scheme • Mild (0.16 mmol/kg) • Moderate (0.32 mmol/kg) • Severe (0.64 mmol/kg) Diluent • 0.9% NaCl or 5% dextrose • 100 mL (mild/moderate) • 150 mL (severe) Infusion rate • 4–6 hr (mild/moderate group) • 8–12 hr (severe group)	**Mean Rise in Serum Phosphorus from Baseline** • Mild: 0.7 ± 0.6 mg/dL[b] • Moderate: 0.8 ± 0.6 mg/dL[b] • Severe: 1 ± 0.8 mg/dL[b] **Phosphorus (> 2.5 mg/dL) on day 1 or 2** Mild: 81%/97% Moderate: 68%/73% Severe: 21%/50%	• Patient population: trauma (73%); general surgery (12%), burn (10.5%), medicine (4.5%) • Excluded patients > 130% IBW • Patients received EN (76%; 23 mmol of phosphate/L), PN (18%; 15 mmol of phosphate/L), or a combination (6%) • Patients followed for 48 hr after study dose • Additional doses of phosphate could be provided as needed; percentage of patients given additional doses • Mild – Day 1 (32%)/day 2 (13%) • Moderate – Day 1 (50%)/day 2 (45%) • Severe – Day 1 (50%)/day 2 (64%) • No decrease in mean serum calcium
Perreault M, et al. 1997[115] SC, P, OL trial	Adult surgical, trauma, or medical ICU patients with serum phosphorus < 2.48 mg/dL and central line Hypophosphatemia episodes (n=37) • Group 1 (1.27–2.48 mg/dL; n=27) • Group 2 (≤ 1.24 mg/dL; n=10)	Potassium phosphate • Group 1: 15 mmol • Group 2: 30 mmol Diluent (both groups) • 0.9% NaCl, 5% dextrose, or 5% dextrose-0.9% NaCl • 250 mL Infusion rate (both groups) • Over 3 hr (5–10 mmol/hr) If phosphorus < 2.48 mg/dL after initial dose, repeat IV dose per protocol or oral supplementation per physician	**Serum Phosphorus (2.48–4.19 mg/dL) 3 hr Post-infusion** • Group 1: 81.5% • Group 2: 30% **Mean Rise in Phosphorus (mg/dL) from Baseline** Group 1[a] • Baseline 2.02 ± 0.28 • Post-infusion: 2.82 ± 0.50 Group 2[a] • Baseline 0.83 ± 0.40 • Post-infusion: 2.17 ± 0.81	• Total of 27 patients with 37 episodes of hypophosphatemia; reenrollment possible if episodes separated by ≥ 72 hr • Excluded patients with serum potassium > 4.8 mEq/L • Baseline APACHE II ~20; 85% MV • Nutrition: EN (63%), PN (22%), both (8%); none (8%). PN with 15 mmol of phosphate/L • No significant decrease in serum calcium • Maximum serum potassium increase of 0.6 and 1.1 mEq/L in groups 1 and 2, respectively; no episodes of hyperkalemia • Recurrent hypophosphatemia seen in 47% of patients in group 1 on study days 2–3 • In group 2, mean total dose of phosphate on day 1 was 38 ± 11 mmol (30–60 mmol)

Table 3.9 Trials Evaluating Intravenous Phosphate Replacement[106,109,111-118] (continued)

Citation/Design	Study Population	Intervention/Infusion Rate	Outcomes	Comments
Charron T, et al. 2003[116] SC, R	Adult medical and surgical ICU patients with serum phosphorus ≤ 0.64 mmol/L (n=47) • Moderate (0.4–0.64 mmol/L); n=37 • Severe (< 0.4 mmol/L) n=10 Patients in each category of hypophosphatemia were randomized to one of two arms	Potassium phosphate Moderate (0.4–0.64 mmol/L) • Group 1: 30 mmol in 50 mL over 2 hr (n=19) • Group 2: 30 mmol in 100 mL over 4 hr (n=18) Severe (< 0.4 mmol/L) • Group 3: 45 mmol in 100 mL over 3 hr (n=5) • Group 2: 45 mmol in 100 mL over 6 hr (n=5) Diluent (both groups) • 0.9% NaCl, 50–100 mL Infusion rate • 7.5–15 mmol/hr	**Serum Phosphorus > 0.65 mmol/L at End of Infusion:** 98% (all except 1 patient in group 2) **Mean Serum Phosphate at End of Infusion/at 24 hr** Group 1: 1.28/0.86 mmol/L Group 2: 1.20/0.89 mmol/L Group 3: 1.32/0.83 mmol/L Group 4: 1.07/0.61 mmol/L **Urinary Fractional Excretion of Phosphate (FePO$_4$)** Group 1: 46 ± 18% Group 2: 36 ± 29% Group 3: 54 ± 31% Group 4: 22 ± 26%	• Intervention effective at achieving serum phosphorus > 0.65 mmol/L (> 2 mg/dL) • 15 mmol/hr infusion (groups 1 and 3) resulted in absolute increase in FePO$_4$ compared with 7.5 mmol/hr • Maximum study drug concentration (potassium 900 mEq/L) not recommended in clinical practice • Transient (mid-infusion) hyperphosphatemia and hyperkalemia seen in five and eight patients, respectively
Taylor B, et al. 2004[117] SC, 2-phase	Adult, surgical ICU patients with serum phosphorus ≤ 2.2 mg/dL or who received phosphate despite normal concentrations (n=158) • Pre-intervention (n=47) • Post-intervention (n=111)	Intervention Period • Graduated dosing scheme (three tier) based on both phosphorus concentration and patient weight • Sodium phosphate (or potassium phosphate if serum potassium < 4 mEq/L), range 10–50 mmol Diluent • 250 mL, 5% dextrose Infusion rate: • Over 6 hr (1.7–8.3 mmol/hr)	**Treatment Success (i.e., serum phosphorus > 2.2 mg/dL within 18–24 hr)^a** • Pre: 47% • Post: 76%	• Excluded patients: > 120 kg, < 40 kg, receiving phosphate-containing PN • 39% trauma patients • Dosing tier essentially 0.16–0.25 mmol/kg (for phosphorus 1.8–2.2 mg/dL), 0.3–0.5 mmol/kg (for phosphorus 1–1.7 mg/dL), and 0.42–0.75 mmol/kg (for phosphorus < 1 mg/dL) • Protocol improved successful supplementation in patients with moderate (1.5–2.2 mg/dL) and severe hypophosphatemia (< 1.5 mg/dL) • No patients had hyperphosphatemia in either pre- or post-intervention groups • Protocol implementation reduced percentage of patients not receiving supplementation when indicated
Brown KA, et al. 2006[118] SC, R, OL trial	Adult trauma patients, followed by the nutrition support service with a serum phosphorus ≤ 3 mg/dL (n=79) • Mild (2.3–3 mg/dL); n=34 • Moderate (1.6–2.2 mg/dL); n=30 • Severe (≤ 1.5 mg/dL); n=15	Graduated dosing scheme • Mild (0.32 mmol/kg) • Moderate (0.64 mmol/kg) • Severe (1 mmol/kg) Diluent • 0.9% NaCl or 5% dextrose • 100 mL (mild/moderate group) • 250 mL (severe group) Infusion rate • 7.5 mmol/hr	**Mean Serum Phosphorus (mg/dL) on Study Days 1/2/3** • Mild: 2.57/2.66/2.97 • Moderate: 1.98/2.38^a/2.88^a • Severe: 1.18/2.88^a/2.66^a **Normal Serum Phosphorus (> 2.5 mg/dL) on Day 2/3** • Mild: 59%/59% • Moderate: 50%/70% • Severe: 53%/60%	• 78% of patients with traumatic brain injury, likely contributing to high phosphate requirements • Adjusted BW used if > 130% IBW; patients with BMI > 40 kg/m^2 excluded • All patients received EN (93.5%; 26–39 mmol phosphate/L), PN (2.5%; 15 mmol phosphate/L), or a combination (4%) • If indicated, additional doses could be provided on days 2 or 3 according to the protocol or according to the discretion of the trauma team; percentage of patients given additional doses on study day 2: mild 71%, moderate 80%, severe 73% • 3.4% incidence of serum phosphorus > 4.5 mg/dL • 5% of patients with hypocalcemia

Table 3.9 Trials Evaluating Intravenous Phosphate Replacement[106,109,111-118] (continued)

Citation/ Design	Study Population	Intervention/ Infusion Rate	Outcomes	Comments
Bech A, et al. 2013[106] SC, R, OL trial	Adult general medical-surgical ICU patients with serum phosphorus < 1.8 mg/dL (n=50)	Calculated phosphate dose • BW (kg) × 0.5 L/kg (1.25 mmol/L – serum phosphate mmol/L) • Sodium-potassium-phosphate (NaKP; Netherlands) Standard preparation • 30 mL of 0.9% NaCl + 20 mL NaKP Infusion rate • 17 mL/hr (10 mmol/hr) by syringe pump	**Mean Serum Phosphorus**[a] • Baseline: 0.46 ± 0.01 mmol/L • End infusion: 1.08 ± 0.03 mmol/L • Next morning: 0.78 ± 0.04 mmol/L **Tubular Maximum Phosphate Reabsorption per GFR (n=7)** • < 0.6 mmol/L in 6 of 7	• Only two patients with severe hypophosphatemia, limiting applicability to this subset • Phosphate replacement based on Vd of 0.5 L/kg • NaKP – Sodium-potassium-phosphate contains 1.5 mmol/mL phosphate, 0.75 mEq/mL sodium, 1.25 mEq/mL potassium • Study drug concentration (potassium 0.5 mEq/mL) not recommended • Infusion rate of 10 mmol/hr led to phosphaturia

[a] $p<0.05$.
[b] $p>0.05$ between study groups.
APACHE = Acute Physiology and Chronic Health Evaluation; BMI = body mass index; BW = body weight; conc = concentration; EN = enteral nutrition; GFR = glomerular filtration rate; IBW = ideal body weight; MV = mechanical ventilation; OL = open label; P = prospective; PN = parenteral nutrition; R = randomized; SC = single center; Vd = volume of distribution.

continued from page 83

phosphate replacement.[106,109,111-118] Overall, studies vary widely in many respects including, but not limited to, the patient population (e.g., trauma, mixed medical-surgical), classification of hypophosphatemia, phosphate replacement regimen (e.g., fixed vs. weight-based dosing), infusion rate, and assessment of efficacy. In general, patients with renal dysfunction (e.g., urine output less than 30 mL/hour), hypo- or hypercalcemia, and conditions associated with phosphaturia (e.g., Fanconi syndrome) were excluded from most trials. When the larger and more recent trials evaluating intravenous phosphate replacement are viewed together,[114,117,118] it appears that doses of 0.16–0.32 mmol/kg, 0.32–0.64 mmol/kg, and 0.64–1 mmol/kg are required to correct mild (i.e., 2.2–2.9 mg/dL), moderate (1.6–2.2 mg/dL), and severe (1.5 mg/dL or less) hypophosphatemia, respectively, in most critically ill patients. As shown by Brown and colleagues, it may be prudent to use the upper limit of such recommendations in trauma patients, particularly those with traumatic brain injury.[118] The dose of intravenous phosphate should be rounded to the nearest 3-mmol interval (e.g., 21 mmol vs. 20 mmol) to ease compounding because both intravenous sodium and potassium phosphate include 3 mmol of phosphate per milliliter. In addition, it is imperative to repeat serum phosphate concentrations 2–6 hours post-infusion and daily because serum phosphorus may undergo rapid redistribution, and additional supplementation may be necessary in the setting of a total body deficit. Serum calcium and magnesium should be monitored concurrently.

With respect to the ideal infusion rate of intravenous phosphate, a study that compared 7.5 mmol/hour with 15 mmol/hour showed a greater urinary fractional excretion of phosphorus with 15 mmol/hour and no difference in serum phosphorus concentrations between the groups at the end of infusion.[116] This suggests that 15 mmol/hour exceeds the renal threshold for phosphorus reabsorption (and may also contribute to hyperkalemia if potassium phosphate is administered). Bech and colleagues showed impaired tubular reabsorption of phosphorus with an infusion rate of 10 mmol/hour.[106] Accordingly, a standard infusion rate for intravenous phosphate of 7.5 mmol/hour is recommended, with a maximum of 15 mmol/hour in patients having severe symptoms (i.e., respiratory failure) for which rapid correction is needed.

HYPERPHOSPHATEMIA

Hyperphosphatemia is defined as a serum phosphorus concentration greater than 4.5 mg/dL. In one report of 2,730 critically ill patients and more than 10,000 serum phosphorus measurements, 45% of all serum phosphorus measurements were indicative of hyperphosphatemia[107]; however, the prevalence of hyperphosphatemia in the critically ill population is not well defined. Hyperphosphatemia is predominantly an electrolyte derangement of those who are dialysis-dependent and has been associated with an increased risk of all-cause[119,120] and cardiovascular[120] mortality in this population.

Pathophysiology

Hyperphosphatemia is usually a complication of renal dysfunction in which filtration of phosphorus is impaired.[81] This can be seen in both acute kidney injury and chronic kidney disease, often leading to the use of phosphate-binding agents in patients with dialysis dependence.[104]

Other causes of hyperphosphatemia in the critically ill population include iatrogenic administration of large phosphate loads, cell destruction (e.g., tumor lysis syndrome, trauma, rhabdomyolysis, hemolysis), lactic or diabetic ketoacidosis, and hypoparathyroidism.[81,104] Clinicians should be cognizant of the large amounts of phosphorus contained in rectal cathartic products. For example, adult phosphate cathartic enemas contain about 180 mmol per dose. Caution should be exercised with use of these products in older adults, patients with impaired renal function, and patients taking other medications that may affect renal function (e.g., ketorolac). Tumor lysis syndrome is of concern in the critically ill oncologic population, particularly those with a highly proliferative malignancy (e.g., non-Hodgkin lymphoma) or severe leukocytosis, especially in the presence of concomitant chronic kidney disease. Spontaneous or treatment-induced cell lysis will result in the release of intracellular phosphate stores into the ECF compartment.[121,122] Cellular damage and release of intracellular phosphorus is also the pathophysiology of hyperphosphatemia in the setting of trauma, rhabdomyolysis, and hemolysis.[81] Lactic and diabetic ketoacidosis can result in the shifting of phosphorus from the ICF to the ECF, raising serum phosphorus concentrations. This shift is temporary, and clinicians should be aware of the potential for hypophosphatemia after correction of the underlying acidosis.[104] Finally, in the setting of hypoparathyroidism, serum phosphorus concentrations will increase primarily because of decreased renal elimination (i.e., increased renal tubular reabsorption from decreased PTH).

Clinical Manifestations

Serum phosphorus can complex with serum calcium, leading to the development of calcium-phosphate precipitates. These precipitates can deposit in the lungs (impairing respiratory function possibly resulting in death),[123] kidneys (impairing filtration), bladder (resulting in nephrolithiasis), and/or ureters (causing obstructive uropathy). Other potential acute manifestations include nausea, vomiting, diarrhea, lethargy, and/or seizures. Long-term complications include accumulation of calcium-phosphate precipitates in the soft tissues and vasculature of the body, as well as complications from associated hypocalcemia.[104]

Management

In general, emergency treatment of hyperphosphatemia is only needed if a patient is having severe symptoms from associated hypocalcemia (e.g., tetany). In such cases, intravenous calcium gluconate or calcium chloride may be administered cautiously until symptoms resolve at the lowest possible dose of calcium. Although this increases the risk of calcium-phosphate precipitation, correction of tetany is of primary importance.[104] Dialysis could be considered first to correct severe hyperphosphatemia. Continuous dialysis may be needed in cases of continued release of intracellular phosphorus from ongoing damage (e.g., tumor lysis syndrome).[124] For non-emergent hyperphosphatemia, reduction in phosphate administration (e.g., phosphate-restricted diet or use of enteral nutrition appropriate for chronic kidney disease) should occur. In addition, use of phosphate-binding agents, such as calcium carbonate or sevelamer, can be considered, particularly in patients with chronic kidney disease. Chronic administration of aluminum-containing antacids to facilitate phosphate binding is not recommended because of the potential to elicit anemia, bone disease, and altered mental status from aluminum accumulation.[104]

CALCIUM

Calcium is predominantly an extracellular cation, with an extracellular to intracellular gradient of about 10,000:1 mmol.[125] Most (99%) total body calcium is stored in the bones.[105] In the serum, calcium circulates in three forms: ionized (50% of total serum calcium), protein bound (40%, predominantly to albumin), and as a complex with organic and inorganic acids, such as citrate and phosphate (about 10%).[105] Ionized calcium is the only biologically active form and has several vital roles within the body.[105,125] These include the propagation of neuromuscular activity, mediation of action potential in cardiac and smooth muscles, excitation/contraction coupling in skeletal muscle, regulation of endocrine and exocrine secretory functions, blood coagulation and platelet adhesion, cell membrane stability and for the structural integrity of bones.[104,105,125] Thus, alterations in serum calcium can result in several clinical manifestations including muscle weakness, tetany, convulsions, hypotension, systolic dysfunction, and potentially cardiac arrest.

Calcium homeostasis is primarily maintained through the activity of PTH and vitamin D, with other hormones (e.g., calcitonin) playing only a minor role (Figure 3.5).[105,125] In general, PTH secretion is stimulated by low serum ionized calcium concentrations and inhibited by elevated concentrations. Parathyroid hormone increases serum ionized calcium by directly stimulating the release of calcium from bone and reabsorption by the kidneys. Parathyroid hormone also stimulates 1-β-hydroxylase, the enzyme responsible for the rate-limiting step of vitamin D activation (i.e., conversion of 25-hydroxyvitamin D to 1,25-dihydroxyvitamin D or calcitriol). Calcitriol directly increases ionized calcium concentrations by facilitating the absorption of ingested calcium in the small intestine by active transport.[105,125] Under normal conditions, 30%–35% of dietary calcium is absorbed by both passive and vitamin D–mediated active transport.[125] As calcitriol concentrations rise with subsequent elevations in ionized calcium, PTH secretion is suppressed. Calcitonin works the opposite of PTH, impairing calcium release from bone and reabsorption in the renal tubules, ultimately decreasing serum calcium. However, endogenous production of calcitonin has little overall impact on serum calcium homeostasis because PTH activity predominates.[105]

Reference ranges for total serum calcium and ionized calcium are 8.5–10.5 mg/dL and 1.12–1.33 mmol/L, respectively.[125] In critically ill patients, it is recommended to evaluate ionized in contrast to total serum calcium. This recommendation is made because of the following: (1) ionized calcium is the biologically active form (as mentioned previously); (2) changes in serum albumin are commonly seen in critically ill patients, and such changes can profoundly affect total calcium concentrations; and (3) use of equations to adjust total serum calcium for changes in serum albumin do not correlate well with measured ionized calcium. In general, as serum albumin falls, so does the measured total calcium. The modified Orrell method (equation 3.4) is commonly used for adjusting total serum calcium concentrations.[126,127]

$$\text{corrected serum calcium (mg/dL)} = \text{measured serum calcium (mg/dL)} + 0.8[4 - \text{albumin (g/dL)}]$$
(equation 3.4)[127]

Trials evaluating the utility of the modified Orrell equation against measured ionized calcium show that the formula overestimates hypercalcemia[128] or normocalcemia[129] and underestimates[129] or fails to identify hypocalcemia.[128] In a study of 100 critically ill trauma patients receiving nutrition support, 22 different formulas (7 to estimate ionized calcium and 15 to correct total calcium) were evaluated against measured ionized calcium.[130] In this trial, 21% of patients were hypocalcemic (measured ionized calcium of 1.12 mmol/L or less), and 6% were hypercalcemic (measured ionized calcium of 1.33 mmol/L or greater). Overall, for the 22 methods, the mean sensitivity for predicting hypocalcemia was 25%, specificity 90%, false-positive rate 10%, and false-negative rate 75%; for predicting hypercalcemia, the sensitivity was 15%, specificity 83%, false-positive rate 17%, and false-negative rate 85%. Although some formulas performed better than others, none of the formulas had a sensitivity and specificity above 80% for predicting both hypo- and hypercalcemia.[130] If only a total serum calcium concentration is available, a concentration less than 7 mg/dL has been associated with a higher rate of ionized hypocalcemia, whereas concentrations of 7–7.9 mg/dL have not.[131]

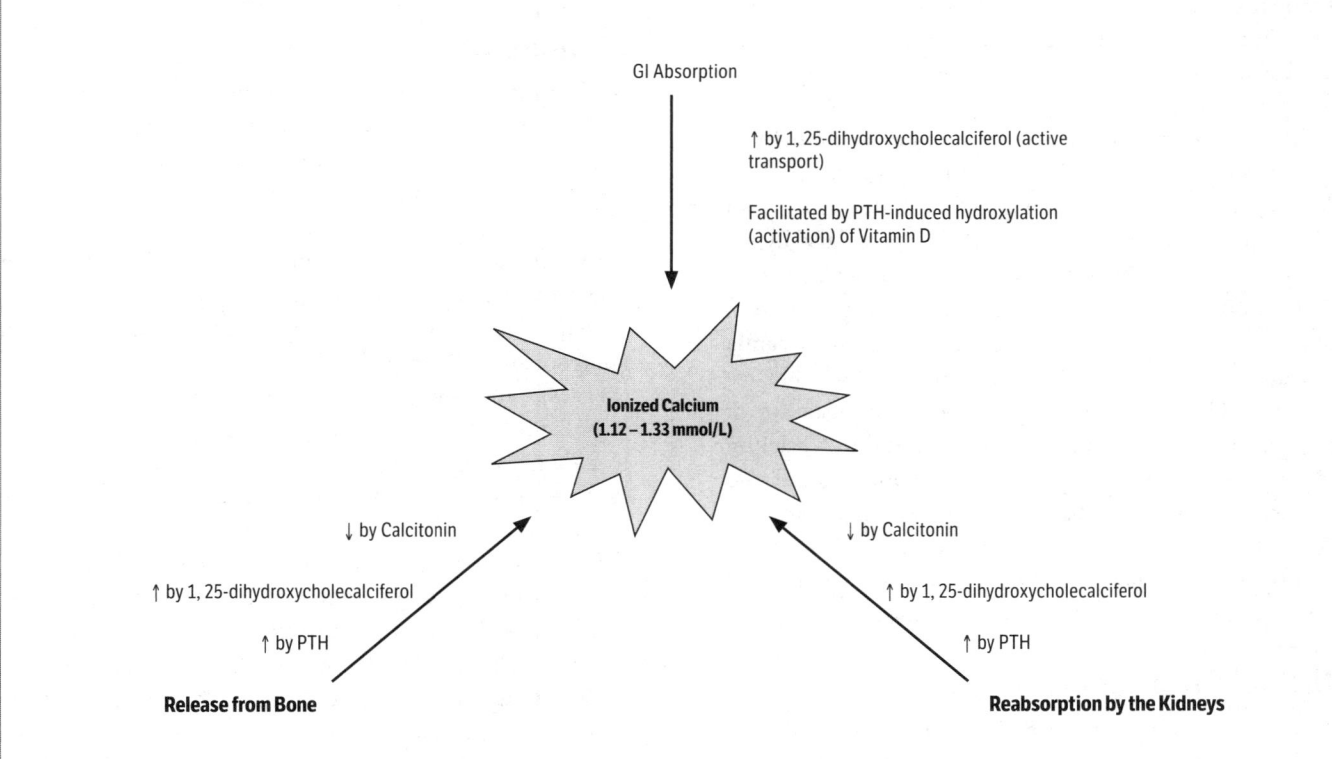

Figure 3.5 Overview of calcium homeostasis.

Essentially, serum calcium levels are increased by parathyroid hormone and activated Vitamin D (1, 25-dihydroxycholecalciferol); whereas calcitonin reduces serum calcium levels. GI = gastrointestinal; PTH = parathyroid hormone.

Information obtained from: Zaloga G. *Crit Care Med* 1992;20:251-262 and Kelly A, et al. *J Intensive Care Med* 2013;28:166-177

HYPOCALCEMIA

Hypocalcemia is defined as an ionized calcium concentration of 1.12 mmol/L or less (or total serum calcium less than 8.5 mg/dL, although this method of assessment is not recommended because of the reasons discussed previously). The incidence of hypocalcemia in the critically ill population varies widely secondary to differences in definition (i.e., use of ionized vs. total calcium, variations in threshold) and study population (e.g., trauma, surgical). Ionized hypocalcemia is reported to occur in 15%–88% of critically ill patients.[125,129,131-134]

Pathophysiology

The etiology of hypocalcemia in critically ill patients is likely multifactorial. Proposed factors include secondary hypoparathyroidism or relative PTH deficiency, impaired activation of vitamin D, calcium chelation, acid-base abnormalities, hyperphosphatemia, and iatrogenic causes.[125,131] Patients with liver and/or renal dysfunction may be predisposed to hypocalcemia because of impaired hydroxylation of vitamin D to 25-hydroxyvitamin D and subsequently to 1,25-dihydroxyvitamin, respectively.[125] In addition, frequent packed RBC transfusion may contribute to hypocalcemia by chelation of calcium by citrate.[135] Citrate-mediated chelation is also of concern with continuous renal replacement therapy, necessitating frequent assessment of ionized calcium.[136] Development of alkalosis facilitates protein binding of calcium and can therefore decrease ionized calcium concentrations. In general, for every 0.1-unit increase in serum pH above 7.4, ionized calcium is expected to decrease by about 0.05 mmol/L.[131] In the setting of chronic kidney disease, hyperphosphatemia can cause hypocalcemia by the complexing of calcium and phosphate, as mentioned earlier. Secondary hypoparathyroidism can be seen after head and neck surgical intervention with excision or damage to the parathyroid gland (e.g., thyroidectomy). In addition, hypomagnesemia can lead to both decreased PTH secretion and PTH resistance.[125] Hypocalcemia can also be a complication of acute pancreatitis secondary to saponification of calcium with free fatty acids.[125,131] Finally, medications should also be considered in the differential diagnosis that result in unintended calcium wasting in the urine, such as foscarnet and loop diuretics, as well as therapeutic measures to treat hypercalcemia, such as calcitonin or bisphosphonates.[125]

Clinical Manifestations

Clinical findings of hypocalcemia are associated with the neuromuscular, cardiovascular, respiratory, and central nervous systems. Some experts consider neuromuscular irritability the hallmark of hypocalcemia, manifesting as tetany (characterized by circumoral numbness, distal extremity paresthesia, and muscle cramps). Other potential neuromuscular findings include Trousseau sign, Chvostek sign, and hyperactive reflexes. Such findings are a result of a lower resting membrane potential, allowing more frequent nerve signal generation.[105] Cardiovascular compromise, including decreased systolic function, hypotension, and arrhythmias, can be seen with hypocalcemia.[125] In critically ill patients, cardiovascular findings are likely the most often seen because of continuous telemetry monitoring. Central nervous system manifestations of hypocalcemia are usually vague and include symptoms such as anxiety, irritability, depression, psychosis, and confusion.[105,125]

Morbidity and Mortality

Many reports detail increased mortality among critically ill patients with hypocalcemia.[132,133,137-139] A multicenter retrospective epidemiological study of 7,024 critically ill patients with 177,578 ionized calcium measurements (corrected to a pH of 7.4) showed a progressive increase in hospital and ICU mortality with worsening degrees of hypocalcemia. Multivariate logistic regression revealed that an ionized calcium concentration of 0.8 mmol/L or less using the lowest recorded value during the ICU stay was significantly associated with ICU and hospital mortality (similar findings were observed for a maximum ionized calcium concentration greater than 1.4 mmol/L).[134] The potential influence of hypocalcemia on mortality deserves further investigation in prospective studies.

Management

Management of hypocalcemia in the critically ill population has not been well studied. In fact, no trials have evaluated the impact of parenteral calcium supplementation on outcomes or complications in critically ill patients.[140] This is of particular concern, given that animal models with sepsis and trauma show increased mortality and end-organ dysfunction with calcium administration and potential protective effects of hypocalcemia and/or calcium antagonism.[140] Regardless, clinicians must make decisions every day regarding calcium supplementation. Although an agreement that intravenous calcium should be provided to patients who are hypocalcemic with symptoms can be assumed, particularly in cardiovascular compromise, many other questions remain. These include the proper threshold for supplementation among asymptomatic patients, method of calcium replacement (i.e., intermittent vs. continuous intravenous infusion), choice of calcium salt (gluconate vs. chloride), and amount of calcium to administer.

With respect to treatment threshold in asymptomatic patients, some experts recommend reserving treatment unless the ionized calcium is 0.8 mmol/L[125] or less, whereas others suggest a more conservative threshold of 1 mmol/L[131,141] or less in an attempt to prevent the development of cardiac sequelae. Trials have not been conducted to compare these two recommended thresholds. However, one small trial evaluating hemodynamic changes associated with calcium supplementation in hemodynamically compromised patients with hypocalcemia may assist clinicians in identifying a treatment threshold.[142] In a prospective observational trial, Vincent and colleagues administered calcium chloride 1 g intravenously over 10 minutes to 17 consecutive ICU patients with hypocalcemia (ionized serum calcium less than 1.05 mmol/L) who were undergoing invasive cardiac monitoring. The mean baseline ionized calcium was 0.91 ± 0.12 mmol/L, which rose to 1.11 and 1.09 mmol/L at 30 and 60 minutes post-infusion. In addition, at 30 and 60 minutes post-infusion, a statistically significant rise in mean arterial pressure (from 77.2 mm Hg to 89.9 and 88 mm Hg, respectively) and left ventricular stroke work index was observed, showing improved vascular tone and myocardial contractility compared with baseline. A non-significant rise in cardiac index was observed as well, whereas no other changes were made in hemodynamic management (i.e., vasopressor escalation) during the time of intravenous calcium administration and evaluation.[142] In light of these findings, and those of select case reports, an ionized calcium target of greater than 1 mmol/L may be considered in patients who are hypocalcemic with systolic dysfunction and/or hypotension. Currently, no data are available to suggest that targeting a normal ionized calcium concentration (1.12–1.33 mmol/L) is more beneficial than a concentration greater than 1 mmol/L.[131]

Two intravenous calcium products are currently available in the United States, calcium gluconate and calcium chloride, both 10% solutions (i.e., 1 g per 10 mL). Calcium gluconate contains 4.65 mEq of elemental calcium per gram, whereas calcium chloride contains 13.6 mEq of elemental calcium per gram. Therefore, calcium chloride is about 3 times more potent than calcium gluconate, and there are no direct trials comparing these two agents for calcium supplementation. Because calcium is a vesicant, both agents should be administered by a central venous access device. Dosing recommendations for intravenous calcium supplementation have been provided in several publications,[105,143-145] but such recommendations appear to be based primarily on opinion rather than available data. In many cases, calcium administration by continuous or prolonged intravenous infusion is recommended. However, continuous administration may not be practical in most critically ill patients because of incompatibility with other infusions (e.g., medications, phosphate replacement, parenteral nutrition) and subsequent need for a dedicated or additional central venous access device. In the absence of data confirming the superiority of continuous to intermittent intravenous infusion, no ideal strategy is recommended for critically ill patients. Intermittent intravenous calcium administration appears to be the most practical; limited available data to support this strategy are provided in Table 3.10.[146,147]

In accordance with targeting an ionized calcium concentration of 1 mmol/L or greater (in contrast to normalization), supplementation with 2 g of calcium gluconate intravenously over 2 hours through a central venous access device for critically ill patients with an ionized calcium of less than 1 mmol/L, regardless of the presence or absence of symptoms, appears safe. In patients who are hypertensive, it is recommended to withhold calcium supplementation unless the ionized calcium is less than 0.8 mmol/L or the patient is symptomatic. Repeat laboratory assessment should be conducted 2–12 hours post-infusion, with further supplementation if indicated. In addition, management should include interventions for correctable underlying etiologies, such as hyperphosphatemia. Further research is needed to delineate the impact of intravenous calcium administration on outcomes in critically ill patients.

HYPERCALCEMIA

Hypercalcemia is defined as an ionized calcium concentration greater than 1.33 mmol/L (or a total serum calcium greater than 10.5 mg/dL). In general, hypercalcemia is not a disorder commonly associated with critical illness, and thus, the incidence among critically ill patients is relatively low (3.4–15%),[129,130,133,148] although one large study showed an incidence of 23%.[134] Clinical manifestations vary widely, are associated with reduced activity or slowing of the affected organ systems (in contrast to an excitatory state associated with hypocalcemia), and progress in severity as the calcium concentration rises. Hypercalcemia can affect the CNS (resulting in apathy, somnolence, and/or coma), cardiovascular system (hypertension, bradycardia, and cardiac arrest), GI system (nausea/vomiting, constipation, and ileus), muscular system (fatigue, bone pain, and/or fractures), and genitourinary system (polyuria, nephrolithiasis, and oliguria). As mentioned earlier, an ionized calcium greater than 1.4 mmol/L was independently associated with increased ICU and hospital mortality in a large, multicenter retrospective study; however, this has yet to be confirmed prospectively.[134]

Hypercalcemia may be a result of excessive vitamin D or calcium intake, may be medication-induced (e.g., thiazide diuretics), or may be the result of granulomatous diseases (e.g., tuberculosis), excessive immobility, Paget disease, or familial hypocalciuric hypercalcemia. Most often, hypercalcemia is a result of malignancy and/or primary hyperparathyroidism. As such, readers are encouraged to visit the chapters related to oncologic and endocrine emergencies for details regarding the management of hypercalcemia.

ELECTROLYTE PROTOCOLS

Protocol-driven, in contrast to prescriber-driven, electrolyte replacement appears to have become rather common in daily practice. Although variations exist, protocol-driven electrolyte replacement entails the use of a standing order-set executed by a prescriber that provides the bedside nurse the authority to administer electrolyte replacement doses as needed on the basis of observed laboratory results (and may also provide standing orders for follow-up monitoring post-replacement). The utility of protocol-driven electrolyte replacement has been evaluated in several single-center before-and-after investigations.[149-152] Overall, protocol-driven electrolyte replacement has been shown to reduce the time to electrolyte administration[149,150] as well as the number of missed electrolyte replacement doses.[149-151] Certain studies also report increased efficacy by way of a higher percentage of "normalized" serum concentrations post-replacement with protocol versus prescriber-driven dosing, particularly with respect to potassium.[151,152] In addition, physicians and nurses report high satisfaction with protocol-driven electrolyte replacement.[150] Figure 3.6 provides an example of protocol-driven electrolyte replacement for a critically ill patient with a central venous access device.

CONCLUSION

Electrolyte disorders are prevalent among critically ill patients and confer the risk of adverse sequelae. Patients with severe symptoms require prompt evaluation and intervention. Unfortunately, limited primary literature exists to guide decisions regarding the management of electrolyte disorders in the critically ill population, and as such, clinicians are often left with only their clinical judgment and little formal training. In particular, well-designed, prospective trials are needed to determine the ideal management strategy for severely symptomatic hyponatremia.

Table 3.10 Trials Evaluating Intermittent Intravenous Calcium Replacement in the Critically Ill Patient[146,147]

Citation	Study Population	Intervention/ Infusion Rate	Outcomes	Comments
Dickerson R, et al. 2005[146] SC, P, OL trial	Adult trauma ICU patients, followed by the nutrition support service with an iCa ≤ 1.12 mmol/L (n=37) Exclusion criteria • PRBC, calcium, vitamin D, furosemide, therapeutic heparin within 24 hr of iCa laboratory value obtained • Phosphorus > 6 mg/dL, magnesium ≤ 1.5 mg/dL • Dialysis or pancreatitis • History of cancer, PTH abnormality, and/or bone disease	Calcium gluconate (all patients) iCa 1–1.12 mmol/L (mild; n=29) • 1–2 g IV • Baseline iCa 1.08 ± 0.03 mmol/L iCa < 1 mmol/L (moderate-severe; n=8) • 2–4 g IV • Baseline iCa 0.93 ± 0.09 mmol/L Infusion rate • 1 g/hr	**Post-dose iCa > 1.12 mmol/L** Mild (baseline iCa 1–1.12 mmol/L) • 1 g (100%; 8/8) • 2 g (71%; 15/21) Moderate-severe (baseline iCa < 1 mmol/L) • 2 g (40%; 2/5) • 3 g (0%; 0/2) • 4 g (100%; 1/1)	• Overall, 1–2 g of calcium gluconate effective for mild hypocalcemia; 2 g may be insufficient with moderate to severe hypocalcemia (limited sample size) • All patients received enteral (76%; 40 mEq Ca/L), PN (22%; 5–10 mEq Ca/L), or a combination (2%) • Post-dose iCa concentration obtained 14 ± 6 hr after infusion • Only one patient developed hypercalcemia (iCa 1.34 mmol/L) • Investigators noted no clinically relevant adverse events, but details were not provided (e.g., hemodynamic changes)
Dickerson R, et al. 2007[147] SC, P, OL trial	Adult trauma ICU patients, followed by the nutrition support service with an iCa ≤ 1 mmol/L (n=20) • Baseline iCa 0.9 ± 0.08 mmol/L Exclusion criteria similar to those in 2005 trial	Calcium gluconate • 4 g IV by central line Infusion rate • 1 g/hr	**Efficacy** • Post-dose iCa > 1.12 mmol/L: 70% • Post-dose iCa > 1 mmol/L: 95%	• Follow-up to 2005 study • Post-dose iCa concentration obtained 12 ± 4 hr after infusion • Two patients developed hypercalcemia (iCa > 1.32 mmol/L) • Four patients required calcium gluconate on day 2 • Investigators noted no clinically relevant adverse events, but details were not provided (e.g., hemodynamic changes)

Ca = calcium; iCa = ionized calcium; OL = open label; P = prospective; PRBC = packed red blood cell; PTH = parathyroid hormone; SC = single center.

ICU Adult Electrolyte Replacement Protocol
via CVC or PICC (For Use in Critical Care Unit Only)

Attending Physician: _____

Allergies: _____ Height: _____ cm Weight: _____ Kg

Notify physician if:
1. Patient initiated on dialysis (IHD or CRRT).
2. Serum creatinine greater than 1.5 mg/dL or increased by 0.3 mg/dL since last value reported.
3. Urine output less than 500 mL in past 24 hrs.
4. Patient's body weight is less than 30 kg.
5. No CVC or PICC access.

LABS
Recheck serum electrolyte(s) **2 hours** after the end of an electrolyte replacement infusion and with **AM labs**.
- Only recheck serum electrolyte(s) that were replaced per protocol.
- If potassium phosphate is administered, both serum phosphate and potassium levels must be rechecked.

MAGNESIUM
Serum magnesium 1.8 – 2 mg/dL
- Magnesium Sulfate 16 mEq (2 grams) in 50 mL of sterile water IVPB (PYXIS premix) infused over 4 hours.

Serum magnesium less than 1.8 mg/dL
- Magnesium Sulfate 32 mEq (4 grams) in 100 mL of sterile water IVPB (PYXIS premix) infused over 6 hours.

Contact ICU physician if serum magnesium is less than 1.5 mg/dL.

POTASSIUM
Serum potassium 3.3 – 4 mEq/L
- Potassium Chloride 40 mEq in 100 mL of sterile water IVPB (PYXIS premix) infused via CVC or PICC over 4 hours.

Serum potassium less than 3.3 mEq/L
- Potassium Chloride 40 mEq in 100 mL of sterile water IVPB (PYXIS premix) infused via CVC or PICC over 2 hours for 2 doses (total dose 80 mEq over 4 hours).

Contact ICU physician if serum potassium is less than 2.5 mEq/L.

PHOSPHATE
Serum phosphate less than 2.5 mg/dL (replacement is dependent on serum potassium and/or sodium levels)

If phosphate less than 2.5 mg/dL, potassium less than or equal to 4 mEq/L, and Potassium Chloride not administered:
- Potassium Phosphate 30 mmol in 100 mL of 0.9% NaCl IVPB infused via CVC or PICC over 6 hours
  (Thirty mmol of potassium phosphate equals 45 mEq of potassium)

If phosphate less than 2.5 mg/dL, potassium greater than 4 mEq/L and sodium less than 145 mEq/L:
- Sodium Phosphate 30 mmol in 250 ml of D5W IVPB infused over 6 hours

Contact ICU physician if serum phosphorus is less than 1 mg/dL.

ELECTROLYTE GUIDELINE REMINDERS
- **All electrolytes must be infused via pump.**
- When both serum magnesium and serum potassium are low, replace magnesium unless otherwise instructed.
- Calcium replacement to be determined per ICU physician based on ionized calcium results.
- Do **NOT** infuse calcium (including Lactated Ringers) and phosphate together.

Figure 3.6 Example of protocol-driven electrolyte replacement.

Finally, and perhaps of greatest importance, critical care clinicians should focus their efforts on identifying risk factors and appropriately intervening before development of electrolyte disorders or associated clinical manifestations. Use of protocol-directed electrolyte replacement appears to be a step in the right direction.

REFERENCES

1. Pokaharel M, Block CA. Dysnatremia in the ICU. Curr Opin Crit Care 2011;17:581-93.
2. Coyle JD, Matzke GR. Disorders of sodium and water homeostasis. In: DiPiro JT, Talbert RL, Yee GC, et al., eds. Pharmacotherapy: A Pathophysiologic Approach, 8th ed. New York: McGraw-Hill, 2011:873-90.
3. Arroliga AC, Shehab N, McCarthy K, et al. Relationship of continuous infusion lorazepam to serum propylene glycol concentration in critically ill adults. Crit Care Med 2004;32:1709-14.

4. Adrogue HJ, Madias NE. Hyponatremia. N Engl J Med 2000;342:1581-9.

5. Moran WH, Miltenberger FW, Shuayb WA, et al. The relationship of antidiuretic hormone secretion to surgical stress. Surgery 1964;56:99-108.

6. Cornforth BM. SIADH following laparoscopic cholecystectomy. Can J Anaesth 1998;45:223-5.

7. Hoorn EJ, Lindemans J, Zietse R. Development of severe hyponatremia in hospitalized patients: treatment-related risk factors and inadequate management. Nephrol Dial Transplant 2006;21:70-6.

8. Waikar SS, Mount DB, Curhan GC. Mortality after hospitalization with mild, moderate, and severe hyponatremia. Am J Med 2009;122:857-65.

9. Wald R, Jaber BL, Price LL, et al. Impact of hospital-associated hyponatremia on selected outcomes. Arch Intern Med 2010;170:294-302.

10. Stelfox HT, Ahmed SB, Zygun D, et al. Characterization of intensive care unit acquired hyponatremia and hypernatremia following cardiac surgery. Can J Anaesth 2010;57:650-8.

11. Vandergheynst F, Sakr Y, Felleiter P, et al. Incidence and prognosis of dysnatremia in critically ill patients: analysis of a large prevalence study. Eur J Clin Invest 2013;43:933-48.

12. Spatenkova V, Bradac O, Skrabalek P. Outcome and frequency of sodium disturbances in neurocritically ill patients. Acta Neurol Belg 2013;113:139-45.

13. Katz MA. Hyperglycemia-induced hyponatremia: calculation of expected serum sodium depression. N Engl J Med 1973;289:843-4.

14. Hillier TA, Abbott RD, Barrett EJ. Hyponatremia: evaluating the correction factor for hyperglycemia. Am J Med 1999;106:399-403.

15. Sterns RH, Nigwekar SU, Hix JK. The treatment of hyponatremia. Semin Nephrol 2009;29:282-99.

16. Sterns RH. Disorders of plasma sodium – causes, consequences, and correction. N Engl J Med 2015;372:55-65.

17. Funk GC, Lindner G, Druml W, et al. Incidence and prognosis of dysnatremias present on ICU admission. Intensive Care Med 2010;36:304-11.

18. Corona G, Giulani C, Parenti G, et al. Moderate hyponatremia is associated with increased risk of mortality: evidence from a meta-analysis. PLoS One 2013;8:1-11.

19. Chawla A, Sterns RH, Nigwekar SU, et al. Mortality and serum sodium: do patients die from or with hyponatremia. Clin J Am Soc Nephrol 2011;6:960-5.

20. Fenske W, Maier SKG, Blechschmidt A, et al. Utility and limitations of the traditional diagnostic approach to hyponatremia: a diagnostic study. Am J Med 2010;123:652-7.

21. Fenske W, Stork S, Koschker AC, et al. Value of fractional uric acid excretion in differential diagnosis of hyponatremic patients on diuretics. J Clin Endocrinol Metab 2008;93:2991-7.

22. Tomlinson BE, Pierides AM, Bradley WG. Central pontine myelinolysis: two cases with associated electrolyte disturbance. Q J Med 1976;45:373-86.

23. Sterns RH, Riggs JE, Schochet SS. Osmotic demyelination syndrome following correction of hyponatremia. N Engl J Med 1986;314:1535-42.

24. Sterns RH. The treatment of hyponatremia: first, do no harm. Am J Med 1990;88:557-60.

25. Moritz ML, Ayus JC. 100cc 3% sodium chloride bolus: a novel treatment for hyponatremic encephalopathy. Metab Brain Dis 2010;25:91-6.

26. Spasovski G, Vanholder R, Allolio B, et al. Clinical practice guideline on diagnosis and treatment of hyponatremia. Nephrol Dial Transplant 2014;29(suppl 2):ii1-ii39.

27. Hew-Butler T, Anley C, Schwartz P, et al. The treatment of symptomatic hyponatremia with hypertonic saline in an ironman triathlete. Clin J Sport Med 2007;17:68-9.

28. Hew-Butler T, Ayus JC, Kipps C, et al. Statement of the second international exercise-associated hyponatremia consensus development conference, New Zealand, 2007. Clin J Sport Med 2008;18:111-21.

29. Sood L, Sterns RH, Hix JK, et al. Hypertonic saline and desmopressin: a simple strategy for safe correction of severe hyponatremia. Am J Kidney Dis 2013;61:571-8.

30. Forssell G, Nordlander R, Orinius E. Treatment of dilutional hyponatremia in congestive heart failure. Acta Med Scand 1980;207:279-81.

31. Mohmand HK, Issa D, Ahmad Z, et al. Hypertonic saline for hyponatremia: risk of inadvertent overcorrection. Clin J Am Soc Nephrol 2007;2:1110-7.

32. Woo CH, Rao VA, Sheridan W, et al. Performance characteristics of a sliding-scale hypertonic saline infusion protocol for the treatment of acute neurologic hyponatremia. Neurocrit Care 2009;11:228-34.

33. Ayus JC, Caputo D, Bazerque F, et al. Treatment of hyponatremic encephalopathy with a 3% sodium chloride protocol: a case series. Am J Kidney Dis 2015;65:435-42.

34. Bhaskar E, Kumar B, Ramalakshmi S. Evaluation of a protocol for hypertonic saline administration in acute euvolemic symptomatic hyponatremia: a prospective observational trial. Indian J Crit Care Med 2014;14:170-4.

35. Institute for Safe Medication Practices. ISMP List of High-Alert Medications in Acute Care Settings. Available at www.ismp.org/tools/institutionalhighalert.asp. Accessed August 30, 2015.

36. Verbalis JG, Goldsmith SR, Greenburg A, et al. Hyponatremia treatment guidelines 2007: expert panel recommendations. Am J Med 2007;120:S1-S21.

37. Ellison DH, Berl T. The syndrome of inappropriate antidiuresis. N Engl J Med 2007;356:2064-72.

38. Vachharajani TJ, Zamon F, Abreo KD. Hyponatremia in critically ill patients. J Intensive Care Med 2003;18:3-8.

39. Dreyfuss D, Leviel F, Paillard M, et al. Acute infectious pneumonia is accompanied by a latent vasopressin-dependent impairment of renal water excretion. Am Rev Respir Dis 1988;138:583-9.

40. Hannon MJ, Behan LA, O'Brien MM, et al. Hyponatremia following mild/moderate subarachnoid hemorrhage is due to SIAD and glucocorticoid deficiency and not cerebral salt wasting. J Clin Endocrinol Metab 2014;99:291-8.

41. Bankhead R, Boullata J, Brantley S, et al. A.S.P.E.N. Enteral nutrition practice recommendations. JPEN J Parenter Enteral Nutr 2009;33:122-67.

42. Samsca® [package insert]. Tokyo: Otsuka Pharmaceuticals, 2014.

43. Vaprisol® [package insert]. Nashville: Cumberland Pharmaceuticals, 2004.

44. Friedman B, Cirulli J. Hyponatremia in critical care patients: frequency, outcome, characteristics, and treatment with the vasopressin V2-receptor antagonist tolvaptan. J Crit Care 2013;285:219.e1-219.e12.

45. Murphy T, Dhar R, Diriginer M. Conivaptan bolus dosing for the correction of hyponatremia in the neurointensive care unit. Neurocrit Care 2009;11:14-9.

46. Naidech AM, Paparello J, Leibling SM, et al. Use of conivaptan (Vaprisol) for hyponatremia neuro-ICU patients. Neurocrit Care 2010;13:57-61.

47. Adrogue HJ, Madias NE. Hypernatremia. N Engl J Med 2000;342:1493-9.

48. Lindner G, Funk G. Hypernatremia in critically ill patients. J Crit Care 2013;28:216.e11-216.e20.

49. Lindner G, Funk G, Schwarz C, et al. Hypernatremia in the critically ill is an independent risk factor for mortality. Am J Kidney Dis 2007;50:952-7.

50. Polderman KH, Schreuder WO, Strack van Schijndel RJ, et al. Hypernatremia in the intensive care unit: an indicator of quality of care? Crit Care Med 1999;27:1105-8.

51. Lindner G, Kneidinger N, Holzinger U, et al. Tonicity balance in patients with hypernatremia acquired in the intensive care unit. Am J Kidney Dis 2009;54:674-9.

52. Cox P. Insensible water loss and its assessment in adult patients: a review. Acta Anaesthesiol Scand 1987;31:771-6.

53. Szarfman A, Kuchenberg T, Soreth J, et al. Declaring the sodium content of drug products. N Engl J Med 1995;333:1291.

54. Bendz H, Aurell M. Drug-induced diabetes insipidus: incidence, prevention and management. Drug Saf 1999;21:449-56.

55. Canada TW, Weavind LM, Augustin KM. Possible liposomal amphotericin B-induced nephrogenic diabetes insipidus. Ann Pharmacother 2003;37:70-3.

56. Alshayeb HM, Showkat A, Babar F, et al. Severe hypernatremia correction rate and mortality in hospitalized patients. Am J Med Sci 2011;341:356-60.

57. Medford-Davis L, Rafique Z. Derangements of potassium. Emerg Med Clin North Am 2014;32:329-47.

58. Gennari FJ. Hypokalemia. N Engl J Med 1998;339:451-8.

59. Gennari FJ. Disorders of potassium homeostasis, hypokalemia and hyperkalemia. Crit Care Clin 2002;18:273-88.

60. van den Berghe G, Wouters P, Weekers F, et al. Intensive insulin therapy in critically ill patients. N Engl J Med 2001;345:1359-67.

61. Hoekstra M, Yeh L, Lansink AO, et al. Determinants of renal potassium excretion in critically ill patients: the role of insulin therapy. Crit Care Med 2012;40:762-5.

62. Adrogue HJ, Madias NE. Changes in plasma potassium concentrations during acute acid-base disturbances. Am J Med 1981;71:456-67.

63. Cohn JN, Kowey PR, Whelton PK, et al. New guidelines for potassium replacement in clinical practice. Arch Intern Med 2000;160:2429-36.

64. Hessels L, Hoekstra M, Mijzen LJ, et al. The relationship between serum potassium, potassium variability and in-hospital mortality in critically ill patients and a before-after analysis of the impact of computer-assisted potassium control. Crit Care 2015;19:4.

65. Nordrehaug JE, Johannessen K, Von Der Lippe G. Serum potassium concentrations as a risk factor of ventricular arrhythmias early in acute myocardial infarction. Circulation 1985;71:645-9.

66. Higham PD, Adams PC, Murray A, et al. Plasma potassium, serum magnesium and ventricular fibrillation: a prospective study. Q J Med 1993;86:609-17.

67. Goyal A, Spertus JA, Gosch K, et al. Serum potassium levels and mortality in acute myocardial infarction. JAMA 2012;307:157-64.

68. Wahr JA, Parks R, Boisvert D, et al. Preoperative serum potassium levels and perioperative outcomes in cardiac surgery patients. JAMA 1999;281:2203-10.

69. Kruse JA, Carlson RW. Rapid correction of hypokalemia using concentrated intravenous potassium chloride infusions. Arch Intern Med 1990;150:613-7.

70. Kruse JA, Clark V, Carlson RW, et al. Concentrated potassium chloride infusions in critically ill patients with hypokalemia. J Clin Pharmacol 1994;34:1077-82.

71. Hamill RJ, Robinson LM, Wexler R, et al. Efficacy and safety of potassium infusion therapy in hypokalemic critically ill patients. Crit Care Med 1991;19:694-9.

72. Scotto CJ, Fridline M, Menhart CJ, et al. Preventing hypokalemia in critically ill patients. Am J Crit Care 2014;23:145-9.

73. Whang R, Whang DD, Ryan MP. Refractory potassium repletion. A consequence of magnesium deficiency. Arch Intern Med 1992;152:40-5.

74. Hamill-Ruth R, McGory R. Magnesium repletion and its effect on potassium homeostasis in critically ill adults: results of a double-blind, randomized, controlled trial. Crit Care Med 1996;24:38-45.

75. McMahon GM, Mendu ML, Gibbons FK, et al. Association between hyperkalemia at critical care initiation and mortality. Intensive Care Med 2012;38:1834-42.

76. Valette X, du Cheyron D. A critical appraisal of the accuracy of the RIFLE and AKIN classifications in defining "acute kidney insufficiency" in critically ill patients. J Crit Care 2013;28:116-25.

77. Mahoney BA, Smith WA, Lo DS, et al. Emergency interventions for hyperkalemia. Cochrane Database Syst Rev 2005;2:CD003235.

78. Pancu D, LaFlamme M, Evans E, et al. Levalbuterol is as effective as racemic albuterol in lowering serum potassium. J Emerg Med 2003;25:13-6.

79. Watson M, Abbott KC, Yuan CM. Damned if you do, damned if you don't: potassium binding resins in hyperkalemia. Clin J Am Soc Nephrol 2010;5:1723-6.

80. U.S. Food and Drug Administration. Kayexalate® (sodium polystyrene sulfonate) Powder [prescribing information]. January 2011. Available at www.fda.gov/Safety/MedWatch/SafetyInformation/ucm186845.htm. Accessed March 5, 2015.

81. Weisinger JR, Bellorin-Font E. Magnesium and phosphorus. Lancet 1998;352:391-6.

82. Tong GM, Rude RK. Magnesium deficiency in critical illness. Intensive Care Med 2005;20:3-17.

83. Brophy DF, Frumin J. Disorders of potassium and magnesium homeostasis. In: DiPiro JT, Talbert RL, Yee GC, et al., eds. Pharmacotherapy: A Pathophysiologic Approach, 8th ed. New York: McGraw-Hill, 2011:909-22.

84. Koch SM, Warters RD, Mehlhorn U. The simultaneous measurement of ionized and total calcium and ionized and total magnesium in intensive care unit patients. J Crit Care 2002;17:203-5.

85. Huijgen HG, Soesan M, Sanders R, et al. Magnesium levels in critically ill patients: what should we measure? Am J Clin Pathol 2000;114:688-95.

86. Barrera R, Fleischer M, Miletic J, et al. Ionized magnesium supplementation in critically ill patients: comparing ionized and total magnesium. J Crit Care 2000;15:36-40.

87. Ryzen E, Wagers PW, Singer FR, et al. Magnesium deficiency in a medical ICU population. Crit Care Med 1985;13:19-21.

88. Rubeiz GJ, Thill-Baharozian M, Hardie D, et al. Association of hypomagnesemia and mortality in acutely ill medical patients. Crit Care Med 1993;21:203-9.

89. Chernow B, Bamberger S, Stolko M, et al. Hypomagnesemia in patients in postoperative intensive care. Chest 1989;95:391-7.

90. Limaye CS, Londhey VA, Nadkar MY, et al. Hypomagnesemia in critically ill medical patients. J Assoc Physicians India 2011;59:19-22.

91. Alves SC, Tomasi CD, Constantino L, et al. Hypomagnesemia as a risk factor for the non-recovery of the renal function in critically ill patients with acute kidney injury. Nephrol Dial Transplant 2013;28:910-6.

92. Moskowitz A, Lee J, Donnino MW, et al. The association between admission magnesium concentrations and lactic acidosis in critical illness. J Intensive Care Med 2014 Apr 14. [Epub ahead of print]

93. Whang R, Oei TO, Aikawa JK, et al. Predictors of clinical hypomagnesemia. Hypokalemia, hypophosphatemia, hyponatremia, and hypocalcemia. Arch Intern Med 1984;144:1794-6.

94. Safavi M, Honarmand A. Admission hypomagnesemia – impact on mortality or morbidity in critically ill patients. Middle East J Anaesthesiol 2007;19:645-60.

95. American Heart Association. Advanced cardiovascular life support: algorithm approach to ACLS emergencies. Circulation 2000;102:I-136-65.

96. Tzivoni D, Banai S, Schuger C, et al. Treatment of torsade de pointes with magnesium sulfate. Circulation 1988;77:392-7.

97. Woods KL, Fletcher S, Roffe C, et al. Intravenous magnesium sulphate in suspected acute myocardial infarction: results of the second Leicester intravenous magnesium intervention trial (LIMIT-2). Lancet 1992;339:1553-8.

98. Shechter M, Hod H, Chouraqui P, et al. Magnesium therapy in acute myocardial infarction when patients are not candidates for thrombolytic therapy. Am J Cardiol 1995;321-3.

99. Raghu C, Rao P, Rao D. Protective effect of intravenous magnesium in acute myocardial infarction following thrombolytic therapy. Int J Cardiol 1999;71:209-15.

100. Muir KW, Lees KR, Ford I, et al. Magnesium for acute stroke (intravenous magnesium efficacy in stroke trial). Lancet 2004;363:439-45.

101. Saver JL, Starkman S, Eckstein M, et al. Prehospital use of magnesium sulfate as neuroprotection in acute stroke. N Engl J Med 2015;372:528-36.

102. Flink EB. Therapy of magnesium deficiency. Ann N Y Acad Sci 1969;162:901-5.

103. Rude RK, Ryzen E. TmMg and renal Mg threshold in normal man and in certain pathophysiologic conditions. Magnesium 1986;5:273-81.

104. Barton Pai A. Disorders of calcium and phosphorus homeostasis. In: DiPiro JT, Talbert RL, Yee GC, et al., eds. Pharmacotherapy: A Pathophysiologic Approach, 8th ed. New York: McGraw-Hill, 2011:891-907.

105. Kelly A, Levine MA. Hypocalcemia in the critically ill patient. J Intensive Care Med 2013;28:166-77.

106. Bech A, Blans M, Raaijmakers M, et al. Hypophosphatemia on the intensive care unit: individualized phosphate replacement based on serum levels and distribution volume. J Crit Care 2013;28:838-43.

107. Suzuki S, Egi M, Schneider AG, et al. Hypophosphatemia in critically ill patients. J Crit Care 2013;28:536.e9-536.e19.

108. Boateng AA, Sriram K, Mequid MM, et al. Refeeding syndrome: treatment considerations based on collective analysis of literature case reports. Nutrition 2010;26:156-67.

109. Rosen GH, Boullata JL, O'Rangers EA, et al. Intravenous phosphate repletion regimen for critically ill patients with moderate hypophosphatemia. Crit Care Med 1995;23:1204-10.

110. Schiffl H, Lang SM. Severe acute hypophosphatemia during renal replacement therapy adversely affects outcome of critically ill patients with acute kidney injury. Int Urol Nephrol 2013;45:191-7.

111. Vannatta JB, Whang R, Papper S. Efficacy of intravenous phosphate therapy in the severely hypophosphatemic patient. Arch Intern Med 1981;141:885-7.

112. Vannatta JB, Andress DL, Whang R, et al. High-dose intravenous phosphate therapy for severe complicated hypophosphatemia. South Med J 1983;76:1424-6.

113. Kingston M, Al-Siba'i MB. Treatment of severe hypophosphatemia. Crit Care Med 1985;13:16-8.

114. Clark C, Sacks G, Dickerson R, et al. Treatment of hypophosphatemia in patients receiving specialized nutrition support using a graduated dosing scheme: results from a prospective clinical trial. Crit Care Med 1995;23:1504-11.

115. Perreault MM, Ostrop NJ, Tierney MG. Efficacy and safety of intravenous phosphate replacement in critically ill patients. Ann Pharmacother 1997;31:683-8.

116. Charron T, Bernard F, Skrobik Y, et al. Intravenous phosphate in the intensive care unit: more aggressive repletion regimens for moderate and severe hypophosphatemia. Intensive Care Med 2003;29:1273-8.

117. Taylor BE, Huey W, Buchman TG, et al. Treatment of hypophosphatemia using a protocol based on patient weight and serum phosphorus level in a surgical intensive care unit. J Am Coll Surg 2004;198:198-204.

118. Brown KA, Dickerson RN, Morgan LM, et al. A new graduated dosing regimen for phosphorus replacement in patients receiving nutrition support. JPEN 2006;30:209-14.

119. Block GA, Klassen PS, Lazarus JM, et al. Mineral metabolism, mortality, and morbidity in maintenance hemodialysis. J Am Soc Nephrol 2004;15:2208-18.

120. Young EW, Albert JM, Satayathum S, et al. Predictors and consequences of altered mineral metabolism: the dialysis outcomes and practice patterns study. Kidney Int 2005;67:1179-87.

121. Davidson MB, Thakkar S, Hix JK, et al. Pathophysiology, clinical consequences, and treatment of tumor lysis syndrome. Am J Med 2004;116:546-54.

122. Cairo MS, Bishop M. Tumor lysis syndrome: new therapeutic strategies and classification. Br J Haematol 2004;127:3-11.

123. Shay DK, Fann LM, Jarvis WR. Respiratory distress and sudden death associated with receipt of a peripheral parenteral nutrition admixture. Infect Control Hosp Epidemiol 1997;18:814-7.

124. Howard SC, Jones DP, Pui CH. The tumor lysis syndrome. N Engl J Med 2011;364:1844-54.

125. Zaloga G. Hypocalcemia in critically ill patients. Crit Care Med 1992;20:251-62.

126. Orrell DH. Albumin as an aid to the interpretation of serum calcium. Clin Chim Acta 1971;35:483-9.

127. Endres DB, Rude RK. Mineral and bone metabolism. In: Burtis CA, Ashwood ER, eds. Tietz Textbook of Clinical Chemistry, 3rd ed. Philadelphia: WB Saunders, 1999:1395-406.

128. Slomp J, van der Voort P, Gerritsen R, et al. Albumin-adjusted calcium is not suitable for diagnosis of hyper- and hypocalcemia in the critically ill. Crit Care Med 2003;31:1389-93.

129. Byrnes MC, Huynh K, Helmer SD, et al. A comparison of corrected serum calcium levels to ionized calcium levels among critically ill surgical patients. Am J Surg 2005;189:310-4.

130. Dickerson RN, Alexander KH, Minard G, et al. Accuracy of methods to estimate ionized and corrected serum calcium concentrations in critically ill multiple trauma patients receiving specialized nutrition support. JPEN 2004;28:133-41.

131. Dickerson RN. Treatment of hypocalcemia in critical illness – part 1. Nutrition 2007;23:358-61.

132. Zivin JR, Gooley T, Zager RA, et al. Hypocalcemia: a pervasive metabolic abnormality in the critically ill. Am J Kidney Dis 2001;37:689-98.

133. Hastbacka J, Pettila V. Prevalence and predictive value of ionized hypocalcemia among critically ill patients. Acta Anaesthesiol Scand 2003;47:1264-9.

134. Egi M, Kim I, Nichol A, et al. Ionized calcium concentration and outcome in critical illness. Crit Care Med 2011;39:314-21.

135. Wilson RF, Binkley LE, Sabo FM, et al. Electrolyte and acid-base changes with massive blood transfusion. Am Surg 1992;58:535-44.

136. Salahudeen AK, Kumar V, Madan N, et al. Sustained low efficiency dialysis in the continuous mode (C-SLED): dialysis efficacy, clinical outcomes, and survival predictors in critically ill cancer patients. Clin J Am Soc Nephrol 2009;4:1338-46.

137. Carlstedt F, Lind L, Rastad J, et al. Parathyroid hormone and ionized calcium levels are related to the severity of illness and survival in critically ill patients. Eur J Clin Invest 1998;28:898-903.

138. Burchard KW, Gann DS, Colliton J, et al. Ionized calcium, parathormone, and mortality in critically ill surgical patients. Ann Surg 1990;212:543-9.

139. Ward RT, Colton DM, Meade PC, et al. Serum levels of calcium and albumin in survivors versus nonsurvivors after critical injury. J Crit Care 2004;19:54-64.

140. Forsythe RM, Wessel CB, Billiar TR, et al. Parenteral calcium for intensive care unit patients. Cochrane Database Syst Rev 2008;4:CD006163.

141. Dickerson RN. Treatment of hypocalcemia in critical illness – part 2. Nutrition 2007;23:436-7.

142. Vincent JL, Bredas P, Jankowski S, et al. Correction of hypocalcemia in the critically ill: what is the hemodynamic benefit? Intensive Care Med 1995;21:838-41.

143. Zaloga GP. Hypocalcemic crisis. Crit Care Clin 1991;7:191-200.

144. Body JJ, Bouillon R. Emergencies of calcium homeostasis. Rev Endocr Metab Disord 2003;4:167-75.

145. Reber PM, Heath H. Hypocalcemic emergencies. Med Clin North Am 1995;79:93-106.

146. Dickerson RN, Morgan LM, Cauthen AD, et al. Treatment of acute hypocalcemia in critically ill multiple-trauma patients. JPEN 2005;29:436-41.

147. Dickerson RN, Morgan LM, Croce MA, et al. Treatment of moderate to severe acute hypocalcemia in critically ill trauma patients. JPEN 2007;31:228-33.

148. Forster J, Querusio L, Burchard KW, et al. Hypercalcemia in critically ill surgical patients. Ann Surg 1985;202:512-8.

149. Hijazi M, Al-Ansari M. Protocol-driven vs. physician-driven electrolyte replacement in adult critically ill patients. Ann Saudi Med 2005;25:105-10.

150. Kanji Z, Jung K. Evaluation of an electrolyte replacement protocol in an adult intensive care unit: a retrospective before and after analysis. Intensive Crit Care Nurs 2009;25:181-9.

151. Todd SR, Sucher JF, Moore LJ, et al. A multidisciplinary protocol improves electrolyte replacement and its effectiveness. Am J Surg 2009;198:911-15.

152. Couture J, Letourneau A, Dubuc A, et al. Evaluation of an electrolyte repletion protocol for cardiac surgery intensive care patients. Can J Hosp Pharm 2013;66:96-103.

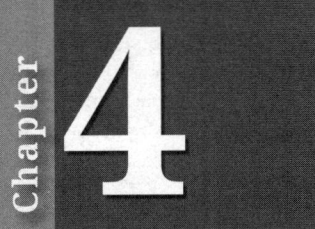

Nutrition Support Therapy in Critically Ill Patients

Amber Verdell, Pharm.D., BCPS, BCNSP; and Carol J. Rollins, M.S., RD, Pharm.D., FASHP, FASPEN, BCNSP

LEARNING OBJECTIVES

1. Evaluate the applicability of a given predictive equation for determining caloric requirements in a critical care population based on factors such as age and weight.
2. Discuss the appropriateness of permissive underfeeding in a given patient scenario based on the route of feeding and patient characteristics, including malnutrition.
3. Evaluate the role of individual nutrients, such as glutamine, arginine, antioxidants, and omega-3 fatty acids, in the nutritional regimen for critically ill patients.
4. Discuss the impact of various dialysis procedures (hemodialysis, continuous venovenous hemofiltration, continuous venovenous hemodialysis, hemodiafiltration) on nutritional goals of the critically ill patient.
5. Evaluate a protocol for pancreatic enzyme administration with enteral nutrition.

ABBREVIATIONS IN THIS CHAPTER

AKI	Acute kidney injury	EN	Enteral nutrition
ALI	Acute lung injury	ESPEN	European Society for Parenteral and Enteral Nutrition
ARDS	Acute respiratory distress syndrome		
ASPEN	American Society for Parenteral and Enteral Nutrition	ICU	Intensive care unit
		LOS	Length of stay
BCAA	Brained chain amino acid	PN	Parenteral nutrition
BMI	Body mass index	RDA	Recommended dietary allowance
CKD	Chronic kidney disease	SCCM	Society of Critical Care Medicine
CRRT	Continuous renal replacement therapy	SGA	Subjective global assessment
DRI	Dietary reference intake		

INTRODUCTION

Depriving the human body of adequate calories and nutrients results in death within 6–12 weeks in young, healthy men only consuming water to avoid dehydration.[1] Altered metabolism in critically ill patients is associated with more rapid nutritional deterioration than expected from reports in healthy individuals or those having famine, and poor outcomes are correlated with malnutrition in the critically ill patient.[2] Providing full nutrient requirements to the critically ill patient as soon as possible would, therefore, seem rational. Unfortunately, despite ongoing research and many randomized controlled trials during the past 2 decades, there are no decisive answers regarding the best time to feed, where or how to feed, and what to feed the critically ill patient. What seems like an answer from early studies is often of no benefit—or worse, is harmful to some patients—after further data analysis or more rigorous studies. This chapter explores available information and the many controversies related to nutrition support for critically ill patients in intensive care unit (ICU) settings.

MALNUTRITION IN THE ICU

Malnutrition has a prevalence of 20%–60% in hospitalized patients, depending on the criteria used.[3-5] Most studies do not use rigorous criteria to define malnutrition, do not clearly delineate criteria for critical illness, and often depend on parameters negatively influenced by non-nutritional factors. Simply defined, malnutrition is abnormal nutrition related to macronutrients or micronutrients. As commonly used, malnutrition refers to undernutrition, although obesity also presents nutritional challenges, especially when metabolic alterations associated with critical illness are present. Critically ill patients are at particular risk of malnutrition because of increased nutritional demands and altered metabolism that result in far different clinical consequences than simple starvation.

The hallmark of the stress response in critical illness as related to nutrition is failure to adapt energy and protein use to restore homeostasis, which would otherwise occur in simple starvation. Neuroendocrine and inflammatory components of the stress response culminate in hyperglycemia, insulin resistance, accelerated protein catabolism, diminished efficiency of protein use, loss of skeletal muscle, and reduced lean muscle tissue.[6-10] Activation of the sympathetic nervous system occurs within minutes of a stress event, followed within hours by activation of the hypothalamus-pituitary axis and release of thyroid-stimulating hormone, growth hormone, adrenocorticotropic hormone, and others. Growth hormone, catecholamines, and cortisol serve as cell mediators acting in conjunction with various hormones to drive the inflammatory response and increase the conversion of protein to glucose through the process of gluconeogenesis. Excessive glucose production by the liver is a major contributor to stress hyperglycemia. Peripheral resistance to the effects of insulin, thyroid hormone, growth hormone, and cortisol affects the metabolism of glucose, protein, and fat through the post-injury phase. Cytokines released as part of the inflammatory component cause weight loss, protein breakdown, and lipolysis, in addition to triggering anorexia.

Assessment of Nutritional Status

Longer length of stay (LOS), increased complications, and higher mortality have been associated with hospitalized patients identified as being at nutrition risk or malnourished.[11] Nutrition screening is intended to identify patients who would benefit from a more comprehensive nutrition evaluation, yet some nutrition factors are used in both screening and assessment. Nutrition assessment, as defined by the American Society for Parenteral and Enteral Nutrition (ASPEN), is "a comprehensive approach to diagnosing nutrition problems that uses a combination of the following: medical, nutrition, and medication histories; physical examination; anthropometric measurements; and laboratory data."[12] In addition, from a practice or research perspective, nutrition assessment results should correlate with outcomes. In a systematic review of studies including construct or criterion validity versus a reference method, or predictive validity related to outcomes such as mortality, LOS, or complications, 32 nutrition screening or assessment tools used in hospitalized patients were identified.[13] The tools included individual parameters and scoring systems using a combination of factors. A few tools performed fair to good for determining nutrition status or predicting outcomes in specific non-ICU patient populations; however, none performed well across all populations, and none was designed specifically to assess critically ill patients.

Most anthropometric, biochemical (laboratory), and clinical parameters used for nutrition screening and assessment have significant limitations in the critical care setting because of fluid changes, effects of inflammation, sedation, and loss of consciousness, limiting ability to obtain data requiring patient participation (weight and dietary histories, previous gastrointestinal [GI] symptoms, functional parameters), and effects of medications commonly used in ICUs. Recorded weight has been found in less than 20% of charts during quality audits of hospitalized patients.[14] Acute-phase proteins, including serum albumin, transthyretin (prealbumin), and transferrin, are not valid in critically ill patients as markers of nutritional status and do not predict outcome in this population.[15,16]

Physical assessment and anthropometric measures commonly used to evaluate critically ill patients enrolled in clinical research should be applicable in the non-research setting and show clinical utility to allow better alignment of practice with research results. An analytic observational study evaluated the performance of individual bedside measures used in clinical research to determine clinical usefulness for identifying malnourished critically ill patients and ability to predict outcomes, primarily increased risk of mortality.[17] Measures evaluated did not require patient participation and were collected by trained assessors for 1,363 patients in 31 hospitals from 31 ICUs in Australia and New Zealand. Five measures, including mid-upper-arm circumference, mid-arm muscle circumference, subcutaneous muscle wasting and fat loss (both assessed by physical assessment using subjective global assessment [SGA] criteria[18]), and body mass index (BMI) analyzed as a continuous variable, showed statistically significant clinical usefulness and predictive ability. However, the strength of clinical utility was poor for any individual measurement. The area under the receiver operating characteristic curves (aROCs) ranged from 0.52 to 0.56, and the 95% confidence interval (CI) did not exceed 0.60. An aROC under 0.70 is considered a poor test; acceptable performance in sensitivity and specificity is typically based on a minimum performance threshold of 0.70 (aROC 0.70).[19] Multivariate analysis identified the best combination of factors showing independent clinical usefulness and predictive ability to be mid-arm-muscle-circumference and subcutaneous fat loss assessed by SGA criteria.[17,18] Triceps skinfold thickness and BMI categorized by World Health Organization (WHO)[20] breakpoints failed to show a significant predictive ability for mortality at hospital discharge.

The statement on malnutrition by the Academy of Nutrition and Dietetics and ASPEN, called the Consensus Statement on Malnutrition, uses an etiology-based construct incorporating inflammation as a primary factor distinguishing starvation-related malnutrition (inflammation not present) from disease- or injury-related malnutrition with inflammation present.[21] Chronic disease–related malnutrition is characterized by mild to moderate inflammation, as occurs in organ failure and sarcopenic obesity; acute disease– or injury-related malnutrition is associated with marked inflammation, as noted with major infections, trauma, and burns. Critically ill patients may develop acute on top of chronic disease–related or starvation-related malnutrition; however, pure starvation-related malnutrition is rare in this population. Recognizing the importance of inflammation in disease- or injury-related malnutrition is a starting point for assessing nutrition status in critically ill patients; however, other measures or combinations of factors are also necessary. The Consensus Statement on Malnutrition requires two of six characteristics—weight loss, reduced nutrition intake, edema, muscle wasting, fat loss, and impaired functional status—to be present for the diagnosis of malnutrition.[21]

Assessment of muscle wasting and fat loss is required when using either the Consensus Statement on Malnutrition or SGA.[18,21] Conducting a nutrition-focused physical examination to assess muscle and fat can be difficult in critically ill patients because of the effects of edema, fluid overload, presence of lines and tubes, distortion of facial tissue from oxygen masks or mechanical ventilation tubes, and body tissue alterations related to lying in bed and fluid redistribution. The quadriceps region is an area where skeletal muscle wasting can be identified in critically ill patients.[22,23] The deltoids and temporalis muscles are other important areas to assess for muscle wasting, although guidelines for evaluating and rating of seven muscle regions (temple, clavicle bone, shoulder and acromion bone, scapula and upper back, anterior thigh, patella, and posterior calf) and 12 muscle groups typically included in a complete nutrition-focused physical examination are available.[18,22] Loss of subcutaneous fat can be assessed by physical examination in three regions using guidelines for nutrition-focused physical examination; however, the upper arm region overlying the triceps may be the most readily assessed and least likely to be altered by non-nutritional factors in critically ill patients. Promising areas of research for assessing muscle and fat changes in critically ill patients include use of computed tomography (CT) and ultrasound techniques.[23,24] A small study of 56 mechanically ventilated patients suggests that CT also detects sarcopenia more readily than SGA.[25] Patients classified as normal nourished by SGA were misclassified 50% or more of the time according to detection of sarcopenia using CT. Patients more likely to be misclassified in this study were male, minority, and overweight or obese. Despite its apparent limitations in identifying sarcopenia and need for patient participation, SGA has been shown to be an independent predictor of length of hospital stay in several patient populations and for LOS, readmission to the ICU, and probability of death in critically ill patients.[5,11,26-28]

The Nutrition Risk in the Critically Ill (NUTRIC) score was developed specifically to identify the critically ill patients most likely to benefit from nutritional therapy and is calculated from age, Acute Physiology and Chronic Health Evaluation II (APACHE II), Sequential Organ Failure Assessment (SOFA), number of comorbidities, and days from hospital to ICU admission.[29] Interleukin-6 is included in the NUTRIC calculation when available. A modified NUTRIC score without interleukin-6 has been validated in 1,199 critically ill patients with multi-organ failure.[30] Nutritional adequacy has a high positive association with 28-day and 6-month survival in patients with high modified NUTRIC scores. The modified NUTRIC score, however, identifies different patients than does SGA.[31] Calculation of the modified NUTRIC score and SGA in the same patients identified 26% (36 of 139) and 80% (111 of 139), respectively, as candidates for nutrition support or as malnourished. Using these two methods plus the institution's routine screening method, only 6.7% of patients were determined to be at nutrition risk and malnourished by all three methods. In this small study of 294 patients admitted to the ICU with 139 deemed at nutrition risk or malnourished by at least one of the three methods, the modified NUTRIC score identified patients with the longest hospital and ICU LOSs, whereas SGA identified patients more likely to be discharged to a rehabilitation facility.

Determining nutrition status in critically ill patients is difficult; limitations exist for all available assessment methods. However, assessing nutrition status is necessary to appropriately apply available research results and clinical guidelines. Using a combination of methods may therefore be rational. The modified NUTRIC score should be considered as one of the combination of methods because it was specifically developed and validated for critically ill patients.[29,30] However, compared with other assessment methods, modified NUTRIC identifies a relatively small percentage of patients as most likely to benefit from nutritional therapy; other patients who would conceivably benefit are not identified.[31] The Consensus Statement on Malnutrition is a second method to consider as part of a combination of assessment methods because it is one of the few methods to incorporate inflammation as a factor in defining the type and severity of malnutrition.[21] Use of SGA in combination with the other two methods could also be considered. It is unclear whether combining assessment using the Consensus Statement on Malnutrition criteria and SGA would provide any added benefit for clinical utility or predictive ability regarding outcomes in critically ill patients compared with one of the methods alone. Several components of SGA are incorporated into the Consensus Statement on Malnutrition; however, SGA includes specific areas for assessment of fat and muscle, as well as assessment of GI symptoms and metabolic stress.[18] Patients likely to require discharge to a rehabilitation facility are identified by SGA; the Consensus Statement on Malnutrition has not been evaluated in this context, although inclusion of functional status makes it reasonable to expect the Consensus Statement on Malnutrition to perform similarly to SGA in this respect.[21,31] No studies comparing the Consensus Statement on Malnutrition criteria and SGA are available, including none in critically ill patients and none evaluating the ability to predict patient outcomes. Nor has routine use of both the NUTRIC or modified NUTRIC score and the Consensus Statement on Malnutrition criteria in critically ill patients been evaluated, despite an apparent rationale for the combination.

Timing and Route of Nutrition Support

When to feed critically ill patients remains controversial. The route of feeding (enteral vs. parenteral), volume of feeding (trophic or partial feeding vs. full goal), and patient characteristics, including disease severity, comorbidities, and degree of malnutrition, all influence when to feed. The debate over when feeding should start is significantly influenced by the route of feeding. Four major clinical guidelines addressing the care of critically ill patients, including joint guidelines of the Society of Critical Care Medicine (SCCM) and ASPEN, Canadian Clinical Practice Guidelines, European Society for Parenteral and Enteral Nutrition (ESPEN) guidelines on enteral nutrition (EN), and the Surviving Sepsis Campaign, recommend initiating EN within 24 or 48 hours of ICU admission when patients cannot tolerate oral intake and are expected to remain in the ICU.[32-35] The recommendation for early EN is repeated in the ESPEN guidelines on parenteral nutrition (PN).[36] No new studies with significantly different results were available for the 2015 update to the Canadian Clinical Practice Guidelines, and the recommendation was continued without change.[37] The strength of the recommendation is not strong; the Canadian Clinical Practice Guidelines reported only a trend toward a reduction in mortality and infectious complications with early EN.

There are no randomized studies showing a survival benefit with early EN in critically ill patients, with or without sepsis. Statistically significant reductions in mortality (odds ratio [OR] 0.34; 95% confidence interval [CI], 0.14–0.85) and pneumonia (OR 0.31; 95% CI, 0.12–0.78) were noted with EN initiated within 24 hours of ICU admission in a meta-analysis of six randomized controlled trials.[38] A total of 234 patients were analyzed for the meta-analysis; 117 were trauma patients, and only 28 patients were mechanically ventilated. Despite inclusion criteria intended to select only trials with sound methodology, several risks of bias were present.[39] Benefits in secondary outcomes attributed to early EN include preservation of GI integrity, decreased LOS in the hospital and ICU, lower risk of infection, and reduced time on mechanical ventilation.[40-43] When randomized trials reporting clinical outcomes with early EN versus delayed EN or no nutrition were evaluated for the presence of methodological bias, all 15 trials meeting rigorous inclusion criteria showed substantial heterogeneity, and none were low risk of bias.[39] An early review of 111 studies also found substantial methodologic limitations in trials evaluating nutrition support in critically ill patients.[44] Two trials encompassing 87 total patients were classified as "more robust" and assessed alone versus 10 "less robust" trials with 632 total patients evaluated for mortality and 11 trials with 580 total patients for infectious morbidity; neither mortality nor infectious morbidity was significantly different.[39] Only one of the trials identified as more robust was of critically ill patients.[45] Overall, less robust trials were the only ones to show a clinically significant mortality benefit for early EN. The same is true for infectious morbidity; however, there was little difference in the size of the estimated effect of bias between more robust and less robust studies in this group. Pneumonia, days on mechanical ventilation, and ICU LOS were not different between more and less robust trials in this evaluation, and no data were reported for non-infectious morbidity, adverse events, hospital LOS, and cost in more robust trials. The authors concluded that randomized controlled trials with low bias are needed before early EN can be considered beneficial compared with late EN or no nutrition. Conversely, there is no evidence that early EN is harmful when initiated in appropriate patients, defined as after adequate fluid resuscitation has been completed and the patient is hemodynamically stable with no contraindication to EN.[32,33]

Guidance for early EN in patients who require vasoactive agents is limited because of a lack of adequate studies. The Canadian Clinical Practice Guidelines and the ESPEN guidelines indicate uncertainty regarding this patient population.[33,34] The SCCM/ASPEN guidelines clearly state that small bowel EN should be held in patients with a mean arterial blood pressure under 60 mm Hg and when high doses or escalating doses of vasoactive agents are required to maintain perfusion.[32] Cautious use of EN with close clinical monitoring for any signs of intolerance is supported at that lowest level of evidence for patients receiving "stable low doses of vasopressor agents," but low dose is not defined.

Reports of nonocclusive mesenteric ischemia and bowel necrosis in hemodynamically unstable patients receiving EN fuel the caution and uncertainty of early EN in this population.[46-48] Administration of EN is postulated to cause inadequate intestinal perfusion resulting in necrosis as further compromise of splanchnic blood flow on top of that caused by hypotension and the underlying disease process occurs. Although cases of ischemia and necrosis have occurred in hemodynamically unstable patients receiving EN, no studies have adequately evaluated the premise related to perfusion and EN administration. In addition, individual vasoactive agents, and sometimes different doses of the same agent, exert different GI effects and may produce different responses with early EN.[47]

Changes in hemodynamic parameters, including decreased mean arterial pressure and systemic vascular resistance in addition to increased cardiac index and stoke volume, have been shown with early EN in patients receiving vasopressor agents after cardiac surgery.[49] Patients in this prospective study required cardiopulmonary bypass during surgery the previous day and were receiving stable doses of dobutamine or dobutamine plus norepinephrine; EN was administered by a postpyloric tube. The study collected baseline data during 2 hours of fasting, followed by data collection during 3 hours of EN. Study limitations, including an extremely small sample size of only nine patients, none with evidence of bowel ischemia, and the short duration of EN make it problematic to extrapolate the data to patient care. Another small prospective study of patients who were post-cardiac surgery compared 23 patients receiving dopamine, dobutamine, norepinephrine, or a combination of these medications at doses well below maximum clinical doses with 16 patients not requiring vasoactive therapy.[50] Splanchnic blood flow increased with EN, as indicated by increased indocyanine green clearance after EN compared with before EN. Patients receiving vasopressor support tolerated EN but averaged about half of the 25-calorie/kg/day goal. A larger retrospective study using information in a multi-institution ICU database evaluated 1,174 patients requiring mechanical ventilation for over 2 days and requiring vasopressor agents (norepinephrine, epinephrine, dopamine, or phenylephrine).[51] The early enteral group was composed of 707 patients receiving EN within 48 hours of starting mechanical ventilation; the remaining 467 patients constituted the late enteral group. Results showed a benefit of early EN on both ICU and hospital mortality, with the patients receiving several vasopressor agents during the first 2 days of ventilatory support benefiting the most (OR 0.36; 95% CI, 0.15–0.85). Patients requiring vasopressor support for more than 2 days also had greater benefit with early EN (OR 0.59; 95% CI, 0.39–0.90). After correcting for confounders, early EN was associated with a 30%–35% decreased risk of death according to Cox proportional hazards analyses. Ventilator-associated pneumonia, ICU LOS, and ventilator-free days were not statistically different, and no evidence of harm was found with early EN. Assessment at 28 days indicated no significant change in results. Slight differences did exist between groups, with patients in the early EN group being slightly older but also having a lower severity of illness with two of the three methods assessed. A respiratory diagnosis was also more likely at ICU admission in the early EN group. These results support the cautious use of early EN in patients requiring vasopressor agents. A large randomized trial is now needed to confirm the retrospective data.

Until more definitive answers are available, several factors should be considered when deciding whether a patient requiring vasopressor support is appropriate for a trial of early EN. Patients already at risk of nonocclusive mesenteric ischemia are likely to be at higher risk when starting EN. This includes patients with a history of sepsis, major infection, diabetes mellitus, smoking, or critical stenosis in the mesenteric vasculature, and older adult patients with cardiovascular disease or arrhythmia.[48,52] Conditions present at the time of evaluation that suggest not proceeding with EN include low mean arterial blood pressure (consistently less than 60 mm Hg), increasing doses of vasoactive agents, cardiac failure resulting in a low flow state, active bleeding requiring ongoing transfusions, and requirement for massive fluid resuscitation. The vasoactive agent being administered and its dose also need to be considered. One recommended classification of a high-dose vasopressor agent indicating greater caution for initiation of EN is as follows: dopamine over 10 mcg/kg/minute, epinephrine or norepinephrine over 5 mcg/minute, vasopressin above 0.04 unit/minute, and milrinone above 0.375 mcg/kg/minute.[48] Phenylephrine has been associated with nonocclusive mesenteric ischemia and may be more risky than other pharmacologic agents when EN is provided.[52] In addition, partial enteral support may be more appropriate than full support, at least when EN is first initiated. Close clinical monitoring for any signs of intolerance is essential.[32,48]

Optimal timing for initiation of PN has not been determined; research has produced mixed results. From a practice standpoint, knowing the most appropriate time to initiate PN often becomes a question of nutrition versus no nutrition in the first few days of ICU admission because early EN is often not achievable in patients either with or without prior malnutrition. In a retrospective observational study evaluating actual practices for early EN in critically ill patients, 60.8% of patients met a goal of EN within 48 hours of ICU admission; 13.3% received EN within 24 hours.[53] The study was international in scope and included 2,946 patients from 158 ICUs, indicating that the problem of delay in initiating EN is widespread in ICUs.

Initiating PN within 24–48 hours of ICU admission if the GI tract cannot be used within 3 days is recommended by the ESPEN guidelines, whereas the SCCM/ASPEN guidelines recommend not initiating PN until after 7 days.[32,36] The initial 2003 Canadian Clinical Practice Guidelines recommended against the routine use of PN in patients with an intact GI tract, and subsequent updates, including the 2015 update, have continued this recommendation.[33,37] However, the 2015 update included an additional statement to consider PN when a relative contraindication to early EN existed in patients with high nutritional risk.[37] The American Thoracic Society, together with four other professional societies, included not using PN within the first 7 days of ICU admission in adequately nourished patients as the third of five recommendations for its Choosing Wisely Top 5 list in critical care medicine.[54] All recommendations or guidelines assume no preexisting malnutrition.

The SCCM/ASPEN guidelines rely heavily on two meta-analyses comparing no nutrition support with use of PN for their recommendations. The first meta-analysis reported significantly lower infectious morbidity with no nutrition support (relative risk [RR] 0.77; 95% CI, 0.65–0.91) in critically ill patients without preexisting malnutrition than in patients receiving PN.[55] The difference in complications was not statistically significant, although a trend toward lower overall complications was reported. A significant increase in mortality with PN (RR 1.78; 95% CI, 1.11–2.85) was noted in the second meta-analysis.[56] A trend toward more complications was found with PN compared with no nutrition support. The impact of adequate glucose management on outcome was not yet recognized when the studies in these two meta-analyses were completed; therefore, it is unclear whether inadequate glucose control contributed to worse outcomes with PN. The eventual risk of harm from not feeding was recognized when determining the point at which PN would be better than no nutrition in the guidelines. Data indicated that after 14 days with no nutrition compared with providing PN, mortality and hospital LOS increased in hospitalized patients.[57] The SCCM/ASPEN guidelines selected over 7 days as their recommendation for initiating PN.[32] Guidelines from ESPEN were swayed by a meta-analysis of 11 trials, which included both elective surgery and critically ill patients when early EN was not feasible.[36,58] Better survival was shown when PN was initiated within 24 hours of ICU admission than when EN was initiated late (OR 0.29; 95% CI, 0.12–0.70). No subanalysis was conducted to separate effects on critically ill patients compared with elective surgery patients, despite the heterogeneity between these two populations.

Studies available after both the ESPEN and the SCCM/ASPEN guidelines were published in 2009 have shown variable outcomes related to initiating PN in ICU patients, as shown in Table 4.1. Trials as a whole define early nutrition support, either EN or PN, as starting within 48 hours of ICU admission and late as starting after 48 hours. The term *delayed PN* is sometimes used to define the initiation of PN specifically after ICU day 7. These definitions are used here unless otherwise specified.

An observational study of 703 critically ill patients with a medical diagnosis and remaining in the ICU over 72 hours found that early PN better met goals for calories (74.1% ± 21.2%) and protein (71.5% ± 24.9%) than either late PN (57.4% ± 22.7% calories, 53.2% ± 22.7% protein) or late EN (42.9% ± 21.2% calories, 38.7% ± 21.6% protein).[59] Although the 83 patients initiated on early PN received more of their goal calories and protein than the 79 patients receiving late PN or the 541 patients receiving late EN, there was no statistically significant difference in mortality or hospital and ICU LOS.

The trial known as Early Parenteral Nutrition Completing Enteral Nutrition in Adult Critically Ill Patients, or EPaNIC, compared early PN, as recommended by ESPEN, with PN initiated after 7 days in the ICU (delayed PN), as recommended in the SCCM/ASPEN guidelines.[32,60] The early PN group had 2,312 patients, and the delayed PN group had 2,328 patients; all patients were at nutritional risk. Hospital, ICU, and 90-day mortality did not differ between early and delayed PN. Overall, delayed initiation of PN was associated with better outcomes than was early PN, including a greater likelihood of live discharge from the ICU at day 8, earlier ICU discharge by a median of 1 day (HR 1.06; 95% CI, 1.00–1.13), earlier hospital discharge by a median of 2 days (HR 1.06; 95% CI, 1.00–1.13), fewer new infections, a lower percentage of patients requiring mechanical ventilation for more than 2 days, and a shorter duration of renal replacement therapy. Inflammation measured by C-reactive protein was higher, and more patients had hypoglycemia with delayed PN. Functional status was not different at discharge.

The EPaNIC study design was different from that of previous studies evaluating the timing for PN initiation because patients were randomized to early versus late PN as a supplement to inadequate EN initiated early; the goal for PN was to meet calorie requirements with PN plus EN.[60] Patient demographics were different from those in many studies evaluating nutrition support in ICU patients; enrolled patients were about 90% surgery patients, and more than 50% appeared to be elective admissions. Cardiac surgery patients represented about 60% of each group. However, outcomes in cardiac surgery patients were no different from those in the entire study population. Severity of illness appeared to be relatively low, given that most patients had a short ICU LOS and under 10% ICU mortality. A predefined post hoc subgroup analysis was performed in the 517 patients at high nutritional risk, based on complex surgery with a contraindication to early EN and no nutrition by ICU day 7. In the high-risk group, patients receiving delayed PN had a lower infection rate (29.9% vs. 40.2%) and were more likely to be discharged alive from the ICU sooner (HR 1.20; 95% CI, 1.00–1.44) than were patients in the early PN group. Early PN, with or without concomitant EN, was detrimental compared with delayed PN in the patient population studied, including patients at nutritional risk.

Table 4.1 Studies on Initiating PN in Critically Ill Patients Published Since ESPEN and SCCM/ASPEN Guidelines in 2009

Study	Type of Study	Patient Number and Characteristics	Comments	Outcome: Infection	Outcome: LOS	Outcome: Mortality	Outcome: Overall
Cahill et al.[59] Early PN vs. late PN or late EN	Observational	703, medical diagnosis			ND ICU or hospital	ND	Early PN better at meeting calorie and protein goals
Casaer et al.[60] EPaNIC, early PN vs. delayed PN	Prospective RCT, multicenter; predefined post hoc analysis	2,312 early PN; 2,328 delayed PN; 90% surgery patients with >50% elective admissions; about 60% cardiac patients	EN initiated in all patients without contraindication (4,123)	More new infections with early PN (26.2% vs. 22.8%, p=0.008)	ND ICU or hospital	ND, ICU, hospital, 90 day	Early PN ± concomitant EN, was detrimental, including less likelihood of live discharge by ICU day 8 and MV > 2 days was required in more patients
Casaer et al.[61] EPaNIC post hoc analysis	Post hoc analysis for severity of illness	Post hoc analysis of 517	Contraindication to early EN and no nutrition by ICU day 7				Detrimental effect of early PN ± concomitant EN, was not related to severity of illness
Kutsogiannis et al.[63] Addition of PN to EN vs. EN alone	Observational, multicenter	Total EPaNIC population (4,640) divided into quartiles by APACHE II score	Subgroup analysis of patients with early or persistent GI intolerance and GI admitting diagnosis		Increased for both ICU and hospital with PN. Later discharge alive with PN	Increased	Worse outcomes with addition of PN, either early or late, to EN. Longer MV Did not change for subgroup analysis
		2,920 total, 188 with early PN and 170 with late PN					
Heidegger et al.[64] Supplemental PN or SPN PN added to supplement EN on ICU days 4–8 vs. EN alone	RCT, two centers	305, mixed medical and surgical; patients receiving <60% goal calories by EN enrolled on ICU day 3	Calories by indirect calorimetry or set at 25/kg for women, 30/kg for men using IBW Achieved 103% goal with PN vs. 77% with EN only Evaluated days 9–28 and full 28 days	Fewer patients developed nosocomial infection with PN vs. EN alone (27% vs. 38%, p=0.0338) days 9–28; ND full 28 days			ND for full 28 days but statistical difference in nosocomial infection for day 9–28 evaluation; difference in "other" infection, not typical ICU (pneumonia, bloodstream, urogenital, or abdominal) infections
Doig et al.[65] Early PN vs. standard care (EN, PN, no nutrition per attending physician)	RCT	1,372, relative contraindication to EN	40.8% in standard care arm received no nutrition, 43.7% received EN at some time in ICU	ND		ND, 60 day	ND, including organ failure
Harvey et al.[66] CALORIES, early PN vs. early EN	RCT, multicenter	2,388, >90% well-nourished before ICU based on BMI and weight loss; moderate severity of illness	No contraindication to either PN or EN; fed for 5 days in ICU Protein < 1 g/kg/day, calorie goals not reached in either group	ND in treated infections	ND	ND, 30 and 90 day	ND

APACHE = Acute Physiology and Chronic Health Evaluation; ASPEN = American Society for Parenteral and Enteral Nutrition; EN = enteral nutrition; ESPEN = European Society for Parenteral and Enteral Nutrition; IBW = ideal body weight; ICU = intensive care unit; LOS = length of stay; MV = mechanical ventilation; ND = no difference; PN = parenteral nutrition; RCT = randomized controlled trial; SCCM = Society of Critical Care Medicine.

Because of criticism of the original EPaNIC trial, a post hoc analysis was conducted to determine whether severity of illness influences the results.[61] The total EPaNIC population was divided into quartiles according to severity of illness as defined by the Acute Physiology and Chronic Health Evaluation II (APACHE II) score. The APACHE II quartiles in order of increasing severity of illness were 10–13, 16–18, 22–30, and 35–41. No quartile showed a benefit from early PN with respect to live discharge from the ICU at day 8. Delayed PN remained a benefit across all quartiles when evaluating the percentage of patients developing a new infection; quartiles for APACHE II of 16–18 and 22–39 showed a decrease in the percentage of patients developing new infection. Adverse effects of early PN initiation were not related to the severity of illness in this post hoc analysis.

A small preplanned substudy of EPaNIC evaluated changes in muscle and adipose tissue in 15 patients admitted to the ICU with intracranial bleed, isolated brain trauma, or subarachnoid hemorrhage.[62] Inclusion criteria required a clinical indication for CT scanning within 48 hours of ICU admission and repeat CT scanning scheduled at ICU admission for 1 week later. Six demographically matched healthy volunteers served as controls and underwent repeat CT scanning at an interval of 7 days. Repeat quantitative CT images, both mid-femur and abdominal, were used to estimate muscle and adipose tissue volume. Ten patients were in the early PN group of EPaNIC and five in the delayed PN group. Muscle wasting occurred with both early and delayed PN. Early PN was associated with increased lipid and water content of muscles. According to this small study, early PN does not prevent muscle wasting better than delayed initiation of PN and may result in more accumulation of water and fat in the muscles.

The EPaNIC study primarily evaluated the addition of PN, either early or late, in patients receiving early EN to bring the total caloric intake to 100% of estimated requirements. An observational study of 2,920 patients from 226 ICUs compared both early and late addition of PN to EN with early EN alone.[63] This study design allows a better comparison of PN effects with EN than does the EPaNIC design because there was a group randomly assigned to early EN alone. A diligent attempt to use the GI tract in study patients is suggested by only a small percentage of the total study population in the two PN groups: 188 patients (6.4%) with PN added early and 170 patients (5.8%) with PN added late. Both PN groups of patients were more likely to have early and persistent GI dysfunction than were patients receiving only early EN, and the late PN group of patients had more persistent GI dysfunction than did patients with PN added early. Outcomes were worse with the addition of PN than with EN alone. Either early or late PN was associated with higher mortality and longer time on mechanical ventilation, and both ICU and hospital LOS were longer. Patients receiving early PN had a later discharge alive (HR 0.75; 95% CI, 0.59–0.96), as did patients receiving late PN (HR 0.64; 95% CI, 0.51–0.81). Subgroup analysis was conducted on high nutritional risk categories, including patients with EN intolerance, either early (258 patients) or persistent (379 patients), and those with a GI admitting diagnosis (178 patients). No benefit to early or late addition of PN was found in patients with either early or late GI intolerance. Compared with patients in the subgroup receiving EN alone, time to discharge alive was longer for patients with an admitting GI diagnosis for either early PN (HR 0.35; 95% CI, 0.19–0.63) or late PN (HR 0.62; 95% CI, 0.41–0.94).

In contrast to these and EPaNIC's results, a much smaller study reported better outcomes when PN was added to inadequate EN for critically ill patients.[64] The trial, often called the Supplemental Parenteral Nutrition trial, included 305 ICU patients from two centers and enrolled patients on ICU day 3. By default, this relatively late enrollment indicated that patients were at higher risk nutritionally, as did attention to patients with GI intolerance. Patients receiving less than 60% of goal calories from EN were randomized to supplemental PN (153 patients) on ICU days 4–8 or continued EN alone (152 patients). Calorie requirements were determined on ICU day 3 by indirect calorimetry or, if not available, set at 25 or 30 calories per kilogram per day using ideal body weight for women and men, respectively. Between days 4 and 8, patients receiving supplemental PN achieved their calorie goal; the EN group received 77% ± 27% of goal. The primary outcome was nosocomial infection rate after the intervention and was measured from day 9 to day 28. The supplemental PN group had a reduced nosocomial infection rate (HR 0.65; 95% CI, 0.43–0.97) together with fewer total infections per patient. The major discrepancy was in "other" infections post-intervention (4% in supplemental PN; 18% in EN group); most infections typically identified as problematic in critically ill patients (pneumonia, bloodstream, urogenital, and abdominal infections) appeared in a similar percentage of patients in the two groups. There was no definition of "other" infections.

Evaluation of 1,372 critically ill patients with a relative contraindication to EN showed no difference in the primary outcome of 60-day mortality between the half randomized to PN starting within 24 hours of ICU admission and those receiving standard care, including EN, PN, or no nutrition as determined by the attending physician.[65] Nutrition support was initiated in standard care patients at a mean of 2.8 days after study randomization, which occurred within the first 24 hours of ICU stay. Neither EN nor PN was administered to 40.8% of standard care patients; at some time during their ICU stay, 43.7% received EN. Mechanical ventilation was required for about 1 less day with early PN, and coagulation failure averaged about

½ day less. Infection rates did not differ between groups, nor did organ failure (renal, pulmonary, hepatic, cardiovascular, and multisystem failure).

A randomized comparison of early PN with early EN, called the CALORIES trial, was conducted in 2,388 patients admitted to one of 33 participating ICUs.[66] Inclusion criteria required no contraindications to either PN or EN. Nutrition was administered by the assigned route for 5 days (120 hours) unless the patient transitioned to a complete oral diet, was discharged from the ICU, or died before this time. No difference between PN and EN was found in the primary outcome of 30-day mortality (RR for PN 0.97; 95% CI, 0.86–1.08) or secondary outcome of mean number of treated infectious complications (0.22 vs. 0.21). Rates of hypoglycemia and vomiting were significantly less with PN, and increased liver function tests occurred more commonly. Other secondary outcomes did not differ between EN and PN, including days alive and free of organ support at 30 days, abdominal distention, ICU and hospital LOS, and death in the ICU, hospital, or at 90 days.

The CALORIES trial showed that early PN was not associated with worse outcomes than early EN.[65] Mortality was not increased, nor was morbidity, including infectious risk. However, the patient population studied must be considered before widely extrapolating these data to critically ill patients, especially those at nutritional risk. Given the BMI and percentage of weight loss in the previous 6 months, more than 90% of the patients in the CALORIES trial were well nourished before ICU admission. Severity-of-illness scores were moderately high; the APACHE II score was slightly under 20, and the SOFA score was slightly below 10 in both groups. Vasoactive agents were required in 80%–85% and mechanical ventilation in 83%–84% of patients in both groups. Protein provision was very low at 0.6–0.7 g/kg/day in both groups, and the calorie goal of 25 calories per kilogram per day was not reached in either group.

Taken as a whole, trials published since the ESPEN and SCCM/ASPEN guidelines became available in 2009 have added to the controversy regarding the best practice for nutrition support in critically ill patients. Early EN continues to be recognized as the best practice; however, many patients do not meet the goal of early EN.[32-36,53] A concerted effort to initiate early EN should be made; however, PN now appears to be a more viable option for some patients than continued inadequate nutrition. Studies must be evaluated carefully to determine the study population, including severity of illness and nutritional status, and applicability of results to an individual patient. Patients with the greatest severity of illness and high nutritional risk are most likely to benefit from, and not be harmed by, early PN. The 2015 Canadian Clinical Practice Guidelines recommend consideration of early PN in patients at high nutritional risk with a relative contraindication to EN.[37]

NUTRITIONAL GOALS—MACRONUTRIENTS

Paralleling the question of timing for nutrition support is the question of how much to feed the critically ill patient. Various methods are used to determine calorie goals, including measurement of metabolic substrates and products, predictive equations ranging from simple to complex, and fixed caloric targets based on weight. The doubly labeled water method is the gold standard for establishing caloric requirements, although clinical use is limited by the 1-week or more delay in obtaining results.[67] Indirect calorimetry is the standard to which other methods for determining the resting energy expenditure are compared in the clinical setting. Nonetheless, the Canadian Clinical Practice Guidelines committee found insufficient data to make a recommendation on the use of indirect calorimetry compared with predictive equations during its initial guidelines development or for any subsequent updates.[33,37,68,69] Limitations to indirect calorimetry include availability, cost, and decreased accuracy in the presence of several commonly encountered ICU conditions including high oxygen requirements; leaks in the airway circuit from endotracheal cuffs, chest tubes, or bronchial-pleural fistulas; and removal of carbon dioxide by renal replacement therapy or extracorporeal systems. Determining an activity factor to account for energy expenditure above the resting state can also be problematic in the critical care setting, especially when patients are not comatose or heavily sedated.

Predictive equations use anthropometric data and other variables developed from regression analysis to predict caloric requirements of a specified population. Only a few predictive equations among the hundreds published were designed for use in critically ill patients. Many predictive equations used in the ICU were not developed or validated in this setting and are not accurate across the full range of ages and body habitus encountered in the critically ill population. Compared with indirect calorimetry in 202 ventilated patients, overall accuracy of various predictive equations ranged from 18% to 67%.[70] Among the predictive equations tested, the Penn State equations incorporating Mifflin equations to account for demographic data (weight, height, age, sex) were the most accurate, had the lowest percentage of estimates over 15% different from measured, and were not biased overall or in any subgroups (young nonobese or obese, older adult nonobese or obese).[70,71] The Mifflin equations themselves are supported by considerable evidence and widely used; however, in the critically ill population, the equations lack precision, have a 25% accuracy rate, and are consistently biased toward underestimating energy requirements.[70-73] Harris-Benedict equations are widely used in the original form and various permutations; however, they are not recommended for use in critical care.[73] Because of inaccuracies in the older adult group with obesity using almost all predictive equations, modified Penn State equations were developed for this population.[74] Table 4.2 summarizes guideline recommendations for calorie goals and predictive equations commonly in use or designed specifically to estimate the resting energy expenditure for critically ill patients.[32,33,34,37,68,69,72,74-79]

The question of how much to feed the critically ill patient is not answered by determining energy expenditure. The effect of underfeeding versus full feeding on outcomes remains an area of investigation and ongoing discussion. Major guidelines do not agree on the best strategy, especially regarding the dose for PN, as shown in Table 4.3.[32-34,37,68,69] As with the timing of nutrition support, the answer may depend on many factors, including the route of nutrition support and patient characteristics.

The Canadian Clinical Practice Guidelines show the progression in recommendations for underfeeding versus full feeding as well as some of the uncertainties in definitions and need for clarifications. When the initial Canadian Clinical Practice Guidelines were developed, data were insufficient to make a recommendation on achieving the target dose of EN except in patients with severe head injuries, where one trial indicated less infections and more rapid recovery but no difference in mortality when closer to goal calories and protein were fed.[33] At the same time, the guidelines indicated that hypocaloric PN should be considered in specific patients, but there was no consensus on the definition of hypocaloric because of the inconsistency among studies. By the 2009 Canadian Clinical Practice Guidelines, the recommendation for EN implied that the target dose of EN should be considered for all critically ill patients rather than any specific subgroup.[68] Starting in 2013, patients with acute lung injury (ALI) were identified as a group in whom trophic feeds should not be considered.[37,69] Guidelines have not changed regarding hypocaloric PN since the 2007 clarification regarding insufficient data in specific populations (malnourished, obese patients, PN more than 10 days).[37,68,69]

Studies evaluating hypocaloric feeding versus full nutrition have produced varied results. *Hypocaloric feeding* is not a standardized term with a defined caloric intake but varies from study to study and encompasses other terms used to categorize the degree of underfeeding. Trickle feeding is often defined by a rate of 10 or 15 mL per hour and trophic feeding as 25% or less of estimated requirements. These feeding amounts are intended to maintain gut integrity. The term *permissive underfeeding* is sometimes used to signify about one-half of estimated requirements with a range of one-third to two-thirds of requirements typically used. Table 4.4 summarizes studies evaluating hypocaloric feeding versus goal or full feeding published after the guidelines from SCCM/ASPEN, ESPEN, and the Canadian Clinical Practice Guidelines committee in 2009.[32,34,41,68,80-89]

Interpretation and comparison of these studies is difficult because of differences in patient populations and nutrient provision. Inadequate differences between underfeeding and full feeding may confound the results in some studies (e.g., 59% vs. 71% of goal calories).[87] Severity of illness appeared to vary between studies when assessing several parameters, such as the percentage of patients with sepsis enrolled, time on the ventilator, and average ICU LOS. In several studies, the average age was in the low to mid-50s range, a relatively young critically ill population, whereas the average age was in the lower 60s for other studies. Nutritional status was not always clarified or considered for study enrollment; thus, it is unclear whether patients at lower nutritional risk may have skewed results in some studies.

Most studies included BMI when comparing patient characteristics, which provides some indication of adequate calorie stores. The BMI could also signal the likelihood of response to varied nutrient provision. In an observational cohort study including 167 ICUs and 2,772 patients, mortality was unaffected by increased calorie provision in patients with a BMI of 25 kg/m^2 to less than 35 kg/m^2, whereas mortality was lower with increased calories on either side of this BMI range.[90] Two studies with lower average BMI (26–28 kg/m^2) and higher average age (61–63 years) showed a benefit to increased calorie and protein provision.[41,82] However, in a study comparing early EN alone with the addition of either early or late PN, the early EN plus early PN group had a low BMI (24.5 kg/m^2) and average age of 62.3 years versus 27.2 kg/m^2 and 58.4 years for the group receiving early EN alone.[63] The early EN plus early PN group received the most adequate calories (81.2% of goal) and protein (80.1%) but had worse outcomes than the early EN alone group, where calorie and protein provision were considerably less (63.4% and 59.3%, respectively). The percentage of patients in either group with a respiratory diagnosis or sepsis (33.2% and 9.3% EN; 28.2% and 3.7% EN plus early PN, respectively) at ICU admission was much lower than in the study by Elke et al., where all patients had either sepsis (45%) or pneumonia (55%).[41,63]

Two striking features when evaluating studies comparing underfeeding with full feeding are the nutrition goals and the actual nutrition provided with full feeding. Caloric goals are determined by various methods in the studies; none of the studies uses indirect calorimetry exclusively; some studies use methods with poor performance in critically ill patients, such as Harris-Benedict equations. This raises the question of whether appropriate calorie goals were established. Most studies were conducted during the acute phase of illness when exogenous calorie requirements are lower because of endogenous glucose production, which again raises the question of appropriate calorie goals. With calorie goals set at 30 calories per kilogram per day, or 25–30 nonprotein calories per kilogram per day, it is probable that full feeding was actually overfeeding and may have contributed to worse outcomes.[84,85]

Table 4.2 Guidelines and Predictive Equations for Determining Energy Expenditure in Critically Ill Patients

Source	Critical Care Subgroup	Recommended Calorie Goal	Grade or Accuracy and Errors[a]	Overall Bias[b]	Specific Bias[b]
SCCM/ASPEN Guidelines	Critically ill patients	EN: Calculate energy requirements using indirect calorimetry, published predictive equations, or simplistic formulas (25–30 kcal/kg/day). For individual patients, predictive equations are less accurate than indirect calorimetry	Grade E		
		PN: 80% of calculated energy requirement	Grade C		
		After patient stabilizes, increase to meet energy requirement	Grade E		
SCCM/ASPEN Guidelines	Patients with obesity (BMI ≥ 30 kg/m²)	EN and PN: Do not exceed 60%–70% of goal kcal or 11–14 kcal/kg actual BW/day or 22–25 kcal/kg IBW/day	Grade D		
Canadian Clinical Practice Guidelines	Critically ill patients	No recommendation is made for calorie goals or the use of indirect calorimetry vs. predictive equations because of insufficient evidence			
ESPEN	Patients in acute or initial phase of illness	EN: No more than 20–25 kcal/kg BW/day	Grade C		
		PN: 25 kcal/kg BW/day when indirect calorimetry is not available	Grade C		
ESPEN	Patients in recovery (anabolic) phase of illness	EN or PN: 25–30 kcal/kg BW/day	Grade C		
ESPEN	Severely undernourished patients	EN: Up to 25–30 kcal/kg BW/day	Grade C		
American College of Chest Physicians (ACCP) Consensus statement	Critically ill patients	25 kcal/kg usual BW/day	35% overall accuracy; range 12% in older adult obese to 50% in older adult nonobese Errors: 51%, highest in older adult obese (78%)	Over-estimate	Under-estimates in young nonobese Over-estimates in other groups (young obese, older adult obese or nonobese)
Penn State equations, original Harris-Benedict equations modified with addition of Tmax and Ve factors plus a new constant	Ventilated patients, mixed ICU population; developed from 169 patients	Men: [13.75 (Wt) + 5 (Ht) – 6.8 (A) + 66] (0.85) + [175 (Tmax) + 33 (Ve)] – 6344 Women: [9.6 (Wt) + 1.8 (Ht) – 4.7 (A) + 655] (0.85) + [175 (Tmax) + 33 (Ve)] – 6344	64% overall accuracy; range 46% in older adult obese to 77% in older adult nonobese Errors: 20%, highest in older adult obese (37%)	Not biased	Not biased in obese, young, and older adult or nonobese older adult Under-estimates in young nonobese
Penn State equations, modified Mifflin St. Jeor equations modified by addition of Tmax and Ve factors plus a new constant	Ventilated patients	Men: [10 (Wt) + 6.25 (Ht) – 5 (A) + 5] (0.96) + [167 (Tmax) + 31 (Ve)] – 6212 Women: [10 (Wt) + 6.25 (Ht) – 5 (A) – 161] (0.96) + [167 (Tmax) + 31 (Ve)] – 6212	67% overall accuracy; range 53% older adult obese to 77% older adult nonobese Errors: 19%, highest in older adult obese (33%)	Not biased	Not biased in any group (young, older adult, obese, nonobese)
Penn State equations, modified for obesity and age	Ventilated, 51 patients with BMI ≥ 30 kg/m² and age ≥ 60 yr	Men: [10 (Wt) + 6.25 (Ht) – 5 (A) + 5] (0.71) + [85 (Tmax) + 64 (Ve)] – 3085 Women: [10 (Wt) + 6.25 (Ht) – 5 (A) – 161] (0.71) + [85 (Tmax) + 64 (Ve)] – 3085	74% accuracy in obese older adult		

Table 4.2 Guidelines and Predictive Equations for Determining Energy Expenditure in Critically Ill Patients
(continued)

Source	Critical Care Subgroup	Recommended Calorie Goal	Grade or Accuracy and Errors[a]	Overall Bias[b]	Specific Bias[b]
Ireton-Jones	Spontaneous breathing, acutely ill patients; developed from 65 patients, half being patients with burns	5 (Wt) – 10 (A) + 281 (Male) + 292 (Trauma) + 851 (Burn) Male, trauma, and burn are replaced by 1 if present, 0 if absent	46% overall accuracy; range 33% young nonobese to 51% older adult obese Errors: 39%, highest in young obese (58%)	Not biased	Not biased in older adult obese Under-estimation in young obese Over-estimation in nonobese, young, and older adult
Swinamer	Critically ill patients, mixed medical-surgical ICU population; developed from 112 patients	941 (BSA) – 6.3 (A) + 104 (T) + 24 (RR) + 804 (tidal volume in liters) – 4243	54% overall accuracy; range 43% older adult obese to 61% young nonobese Errors: 30%, highest in older adult obese (47%)	Over-estimate	Over-estimates in all groups (young, older adult, obese, nonobese)
Mifflin St. Jeor	Developed from 498 healthy people	Men: 10 (Wt) + 6.25 (Ht) – 5 (A) + 5 Women: 10 (Wt) + 6.25 (Ht) – 5 (A) – 161	25% overall accuracy; range 21% young obese and older adult nonobese to 35% older adult obese Errors: 60%, highest in nonobese, young, and older adult (67%)	Under-estimate	Under-estimates in all groups
Brandi Modified Harris-Benedict equations with addition of HR and Ve factors plus a new constant	Critically ill trauma patients; developed from 26 patients	Men: [13.75 (Wt) + 5 (Ht) – 6.8 (A) + 66](0.96) + [7 (HR) + 48 (Ve)] – 702 Women: [9.6 (Wt) + 1.8 (Ht) – 4.7 (A) + 655] (0.96) + [7 (HR) + 48 (Ve)] – 702	55% overall accuracy; range 41% older adult obese to 61% nonobese, older adult, and young Errors: 33%, highest in older adult obese (51%)	Not biased	Over-estimates in obese, young, and older adult Not biased in nonobese, young, or older adult
Faisy	Critically ill medical patients; developed from 70 patients	8 (Wt) + 14 (Ht) + 32 (Ve) + 94 (T) – 4834	53% overall accuracy; range 37% older adult nonobese to 72% young obese Errors: 36%, highest in older adult nonobese (56%)	Not biased	Over-estimates in older adult, obese and nonobese Not biased in young, obese, or nonobese

[a]Grade is based on the level of evidence as described in McClave SA, Martindale RG, Vanek VW, et al. Guidelines for the provision and assessment of nutrition support therapy in the adult critically ill patient: Society of Critical Care Medicine (SCCM) and American Society for Parenteral and Enteral Nutrition (A.S.P.E.N.). JPEN J Parenter Enteral Nutr 2009;33:277-316; and Dellinger RP, Levy MM, Rhodes A, et al. Surviving Sepsis Campaign: international guidelines for management of severe sepsis and septic shock, 2012. Intensive Care Med 2013;39:165-228. Accuracy based on percentage of calculated energy expenditure estimates with 10% of measured by indirect calorimetry. Errors based on overall incidence of estimates more than 15% different between calculated and measured energy expenditure.

[b]Bias based on difference between resting energy expenditure calculated from the equation and measured by indirect calorimetry, 95% coefficient of variation.

A = age in years; BSA = body surface area in m²; BW = body weight; HR = heart rate in beats/minute; Ht = height in cm; IC = indirect calorimetry; RR = respiratory rate in breaths/minute; T = temperature in degrees Celsius; Tmax = maximum body temperature in previous 24 hours in degrees Celsius; Wt = weight in kg; Ve = minute ventilation read from ventilator at time of measurement.

The low amount of nutrients actually provided with full feeding is alarming in some studies and raises the question of whether both groups were being underfed.[41,80] A retrospective analysis of prospectively collected data for 475 patients requiring mechanical ventilation indicated that almost 40% of patients received no more than 50% of estimated nutritional requirements during the first 8 days in the ICU, and less than 15% received 80% or more of estimated requirements.[81] In a study with 523 patients analyzing data for up to 7 days in the ICU, almost 33% of the patients received

Table 4.3	Recommendations of Major Nutrition Guidelines for Underfeeding vs. Full Nutrition	
Guideline	**EN Goal**	**PN Goal**
SCCM/ASPEN[32]	Advance toward goal (100%) over 2–3 days after initiating early EN in ICU	Mild underfeeding with 80% of estimated requirements initially. Expert opinion suggests calories can be increased to goal at some point when the patient is stable
	Minimum of 50%–65% of goal calories required to gain clinical benefits of EN	
Canadian Clinical Practice Guidelines[33,37,68,69]	2003: Insufficient data except in severe head injury, where EN should be optimized to meet target dose	Hypocaloric feeding in patients who are not malnourished, receive some EN, or require PN < 10 days
	2009: Upgrade to indicate achieving the target dose of EN should be considered in critically ill patients	2007: Added insufficient data to make recommendation for hypocaloric PN in malnourished or obese patients, or when PN was needed > 10 days
	2013: Same as 2009 with the addition of patients with acute lung injury should NOT be considered for trophic feeds	
ESPEN[34,36]	100% measured or estimated calories	100% measured or estimated calories

less than 33% of estimated requirements, and 67% received no more than 65%.[89] Protein delivery, when evaluated, also tends to be poor; average protein intake of 0.7 g/kg/day has been reported.[41,80] This is less than the 0.8 g/kg/day recommended for healthy adults and may be a contributing factor to poor outcomes.[82,91] However, a 12-month follow-up of 510 surviving patients from the EDEN study found no difference in functional status for those receiving trophic feeding versus those receiving full feeding.[85,92] All survivors showed significant impairments in physical, cognitive, and psychosocial functioning compared with population norms matched for age and sex; the physical function score at 12 months was 55 compared with 82 ($p<0.001$) but had improved from the 6-month assessment.

Poor performance in meeting nutritional goals with EN alone resulted in attempts to meet nutritional goals by adding supplemental PN when EN alone was inadequate. As reviewed earlier in this chapter, the benefit of added PN versus the risks does not have a definitive answer. It is unclear whether adding PN has adverse effects that counter the positive effects of more adequate nutrition in some patients but not others. There is almost certainly a complex interplay between several factors that determines which patients benefit from increased calorie provision and which do not. Unfortunately, available data are insufficient to devise a predictive algorithm or equation to assist the practitioner in identifying the patients who will benefit from aggressive nutrition.

NUTRITION SUPPORT—MICRONUTRIENTS

Vitamins and Trace Elements

There are no current guidelines for vitamin or mineral requirements in critically ill patients. Although evidence suggests that some vitamins and minerals have increased requirements in critical illness because of increased metabolic demands, evidence is lacking to suggest that vitamins and minerals should be supplemented above physiologic amounts in critically ill patients. Enteral formulas supply the dietary reference intakes (DRIs), which includes recommended dietary allowances (RDAs) where these have been determined, at a certain volume, typically 1,000 mL.[91] The DRI/RDA applies only to oral or enteral vitamins and minerals. If less than this amount is delivered to a patient daily, the patient will require additional vitamin and mineral supplementation. The parenteral multivitamins that are available in the United States provide fat-soluble vitamins at about the same dose as the DRI/RDA, even though there is a difference in oral and parenteral bioavailability. Water-soluble vitamins are provided at about 2.5–5 times the RDA in these multivitamin products. These doses have been used for 3 decades without reports of toxicity and allow for adequate dosing despite limited stability of some vitamins in PN. The increased doses provided parenterally will be enough to replete deficiencies or accommodate increased metabolic demands.[93]

Vitamin D

Vitamin D deficiency is an emerging area of research in the ICU. Observational studies of non-ICU patients suggest that vitamin D has pleiotropic effects; hypovitaminosis D is implicated in musculoskeletal disorders, falls, altered immunity, infections, glucose intolerance, and cardiovascular disease.[94] Serum 25-hydroxyvitamin D (25(OH)D) is typically ordered to assess vitamin D status, although specific guidelines for monitoring are still controversial. Although some sources recommend thresholds for vitamin D deficiency and insufficiency as less than 50 and 75 nmol/L, respectively,[94]

continued on page 113

Table 4.4 Studies Published After 2009 Comparing Underfeeding with Full Feeding

Study	Study Design	Patient Population	Feeding Characteristics	Outcomes
PERMIT trial[80] Permissive underfeeding or standard EN with same protein	RCT, non-blinded with data collection up to 14 days; seven centers enrolled patients	894 patients, 75% medical and 21% nonoperative trauma admissions, 35% severe sepsis Mean age 51 yr, BMI about 29 kg/m²	Permissive underfeeding: averaged 46% of calculated requirements Standard EN averaged 71% of goal calories Similar protein intake for both groups (averaged 0.7 g/kg/day)	No difference in 90-day all-cause mortality, ICU or hospital LOS, or nosocomial ICU infections There was no difference in diarrhea or feeding intolerance
Wei et al.[81] Nutritional adequacy and long-term outcomes	Retrospective analysis of prospectively collected data, observational cohort study; multicenter	475 patients on MV > 8 days and having at least two organ failures Mean age 62 yr, BMI 30 kg/m²	Low (< 50%) or moderate (50% to < 80%) nutritional adequacy vs. close to goal (80% to < 110%)	Higher mortality at 6 mo with low (HR 1.7; 95% CI, 1.1–2.6) and moderate (HR 1.3; 95% CI, 0.7–2.3) vs. near-goal nutrition Improved function at 3 mo with each 25% increase in nutritional adequacy but no longer significant at 6 mo
Yeh et al.[82] Adequate nutrition may get you home	Prospective observational cohort study; single center	213 patients, surgical ICU receiving EN > 72 hr; data collected up to 14 days Mean age 63 yr; BMI 26.5 kg/m²	Categorized by cumulative nutrient deficit in the ICU: Low if < 6,000 calories or < 300 g of protein (averaged 80% of goal calories and protein) High if ≥ 6,000 calories or ≥ 300 g of protein (averaged 54% and 60% of goal calories and protein, respectively) Goals set using actual body weight (IBW when BMI was > 30 kg/m²); 25–30 calories/kg/day and protein 1.5–2 g/kg/day	More ventilator-free days, lower ICU and hospital LOS, and lower hospital and 30-day mortality in low deficit group (i.e., more adequate nutrition). Discharge home was more likely in the low deficit group
Elke et al.[41] Close to goal calorie and protein by EN	Secondary analysis of pooled data, collected prospectively from international nutrition studies for up to 12 days (351 ICUs)	2,270 patients, MV with diagnosis of sepsis (45%) or pneumonia (55%) Mean age 61.7 yr; BMI 27.6 kg/m²	Goal calories set by each site, most commonly with weight-based calculation (53.7%), rarely with IC (0.6%); overall 61% of prescribed EN was received Mean calories 14.5 calories/kg/day; mean protein intake 0.7 g/kg/day	60-day mortality was decreased with each additional 1,000 calories/day (OR 0.61; 95% CI, 0.48–0.77, p<0.001) and with a 30-g increase in protein (OR 0.76; 95% CI, 0.65–0.87, p<0.001) Ventilator-free days increased with each additional 1,000 calories/day (2.81 days; 95% CI, 0.53–5.08; p=0.02) and with a 30-g increase in protein (1.92 days; 95% CI, 0.58–3.27, p=0.005)
Nicolo et al.[83] Clinical outcomes related to protein delivery	Retrospective analysis of data from an international pragmatic observational study	2,828 patients in the ≥ 4-day analysis; 1,584 in the ≥ 12-day analysis Mean age 60 yr, BMI 27 kg/m²	Goal calories and protein set by each site Mean energy in 4-day group was 1,100 calories (64% of goal) and protein 51 g (61% of goal); 1,200 calories (70.7% of goal) and 57 g (66.7% of goal) for the 12-day group	60-day mortality was decreased with receiving at least 80% of goal energy (OR 0.73; 95% CI, 0.58–0.91) and protein (OR 0.63; 95% CI, 0.47–0.84) for an ICU stay of ≥ 4 days and for an ICU stay of ≥ 12 days for energy (OR 0.72; 95% CI, 0.51–0.997) and protein (OR 0.58; 95% CI, 0.38–0.86)
INTACT study[84] Intensive medical nutrition therapy vs. standard nutrition therapy	Prospective RCT; single center	78 patients, medical and surgical ICU; ALI diagnosis Mean age 52–59 yr; BMI about 30 kg/m²	Intensive therapy provided 84.7% of estimated energy requirements vs. 55.4% for standard therapy Goal calories set at 30 calories/kg admission weight or adjusted for obesity. The overall percentage of calories from PN was < 10% in each group	No difference in infectious complications (primary end point), time on ventilator, or hospital LOS. Study was terminated early because of higher deaths in intensive therapy group (40% vs. 16%, p=0.02)

Table 4.4 Studies Published After 2009 Comparing Underfeeding with Full Feeding (continued)

Study	Study Design	Patient Population	Feeding Characteristics	Outcomes
Heidegger et al.[64] Supplemental PN added to EN on ICU days 4–8 vs. EN alone	RCT, two centers	305 patients, mixed medical and surgical; enrolled on ICU day 3 if receiving < 60% goal calories by EN	Calories by IC or set at 25/kg/day for women, 30/kg/day for men using IBW Achieved 103% goal with PN added vs. 77% with EN only Evaluated days 9–28 and full 28 days	No difference for full 28 days but statistically fewer nosocomial infections in evaluation for days 9–28 with PN added vs. EN alone (27% vs. 38%, p=0.0338); difference in "other" infection, not in typical ICU (pneumonia, bloodstream, urogenital, or abdominal) infections
EDEN trial[85] Trophic feeding vs. full feeding for the first 6 days of MV	Prospective RCT, non-blinded study; 44 centers enrolled patients	1,000 patients, about 60% medical ICU; ALI diagnoses: 13%–16% sepsis, 63%–67% pneumonia Mean age 52 yr, BMI near 30 kg/m²	Trophic feeding was about 25% of full requirements Goal calories set as 25–30 nonprotein calories/kg/day	No difference in ventilator-free days to day 28, ICU-free days, organ failure–free days, LOS, 60-day mortality, or infectious complications Less GI intolerance with trophic feeds
Rice et al.[86] Initial trophic vs. full-energy EN for first 6 days of MV	RCT, open-label; single center	200 patients, acute respiratory failure; diagnoses: about 20% ALI, 11% sepsis, 15%–19% pneumonia Mean age 53–54 years, BMI 28–29 kg/m²	Trophic feeding averaged 15% of goal calories vs. 74.8% for full feeding Goal calories set by Harris-Benedict equations or 25 calories/kg IBW	No difference in ventilator-free days to day 28, ICU-free days, organ failure–free days, all-cause hospital mortality Less GI intolerance with trophic feeds
Arabi et al.[87] Permissive underfeeding and intensive insulin	Prospective RCT, 2 × 2 factorial design; single center	240 patients, medical-surgical ICU; about 30% with sepsis	Permissive underfeeding averaged 59% of goal calories vs. 71% average for full feeds Goal calories set by Harris-Benedict equations with stress factors	No difference in 23-day all-cause mortality, hospital or ICU LOS, or days on ventilator
TICACOS[88] Tight calorie control study using supplemental PN to achieve goal	Prospective RCT, open-label; single center	130 patients enrolled, 112 randomized, general ICU	Calorie administration based on repeated IC or 25 calories/kg/day. PN used to supplement EN if goal not reached	Increased ICU LOS (17.2 vs. 11.7 days, p=0.02) and days on ventilator (16.1 vs. 10.5 days, p=0.03) with increased calorie intake
Kutsogiannis et al.[63] EN alone vs. early or late PN supplementation	Pooled data from two prospective observational studies; multicenter (260 ICUs)	2,920 patients, 73% medical and 27% surgical admissions. All received EN within first 48 hr in ICU; 188 early PN and 170 late PN supplementation Mean age (years); % with BMI 30–40 kg/m²: Early EN 58 yr, 19.4% EN + early PN 62 yr, 10.6% EN + late PN 56 yr, 19.7%	Calorie and protein goals set by each participating ICU PN accounted for about 50% of total calories and protein in both PN groups	Caloric adequacy was highest with EN + early PN (81.2%) and lowest with EN alone (63.4%). Protein adequacy was highest with EN + early PN (80.1%) and lowest with EN alone (59.3%) 60-day mortality was decreased with EN alone (27.8%) vs. EN + early PN (34.6%) or EN + late PN (35.3%), as were days on MV, ICU LOS, and hospital LOS

Table 4.4 Studies Published After 2009 Comparing Underfeeding with Full Feeding *(continued)*

Study	Study Design	Patient Population	Feeding Characteristics	Outcomes
Arabi et al.[89] Near-target calories associated with adverse outcomes	Nested cohort study of patients enrolled in an RCT	523 patients, 83% medical admissions. Divided into tertiles, with almost equal numbers of patients, based on percentage of goal caloric intake: I. < 33.4% II. 33.4%–64.6% III. > 64.6% Overall mean age 52.4 yr, BMI 27.3 kg/m²	Calorie goal set using Harris-Benedict equations with stress factors Protein goals calculated as 0.8–1.5 g/kg/day (effect of protein intake was not evaluated separately from total calories)	Tertile III had the worst outcomes for hospital mortality (OR 1.99; 95% CI, 1.31–3.50, p=0.02) and ICU nosocomial infections (OR 2.45; 95% CI, 1.30–4.63, p=0.006) Days on MV, ICU LOS, and hospital LOS increased significantly (p<0.0001 for each) with increasing caloric intake

ALI = acute lung injury; HR = hazard ratio

continued from page 110

the IOM defines vitamin D deficiency and insufficiency as 30 and 50 nmol/L, respectively.[95] The difficulty in monitoring vitamin D status during critical illness is caused by the effect of the systemic inflammatory response on serum or plasma concentrations. A prospective study from 2012 evaluated baseline vitamin D concentrations and followed subsequent daily vitamin D concentrations through 10 days after ICU admission. The authors found that baseline levels decreased 3 days after admission and remained low while patients were in the ICU.[96] Index of suspicion for deficiency is likely as good as 25(OH)D serum concentrations and more cost-effective when determining the need for supplemental vitamin D in critically ill patients.

Although 25(OH)D is measured to determine vitamin D status, 1,25-dihydroxyvitamin D is the compound that has physiologic activity. Vitamin D refers to either ergocalciferol (vitamin D_2), which is consumed in the diet, or cholecalciferol (vitamin D_3), which is synthesized in the skin. The RDA for vitamin D was increased in 2010 from 200 international units to 400–800 international units, depending on age.[93] Cholecalciferol and ergocalciferol are generally considered interchangeable, and oral supplements are available in both forms. However, some evidence suggests that cholecalciferol better increases vitamin D serum concentrations.[93] No individual parenteral vitamin D product is available in the United States, and the adult parenteral multivitamin products contain only 200 international units. However, pediatric parenteral multivitamin products contain 400 international units per standard dose. With diligent attention to total amounts of all vitamins provided, use of a pediatric parenteral multivitamin could be considered for patients at high risk of complications from a true vitamin D deficiency (i.e., concentrations not influenced by systemic inflammatory response) when oral supplementation of vitamin D will not be possible for weeks to months.

Prospective studies evaluating vitamin D supplementation and patient outcomes in critically ill patients are rare. The VITdAL-ICU study evaluated 475 critically ill patients with 25(OH)D concentrations less than 20 ng/mL (50 nmol/L).[97] This single-center double-blind study randomized patients to either placebo or vitamin D_3 orally or by nasogastric tube at a dose of 540,000 international units once, followed by monthly doses of 90,000 international units for 5 months. There was no difference in the primary outcome of hospital LOS, nor was there any difference in secondary outcomes. The authors found a statistically significant decrease in hospital mortality among the subgroup of patients with 25(OH)D concentrations less than 12 ng/mL (30 nmol/L), but this disappeared at 6 months.

Data are insufficient to recommend vitamin D supplementation in critically ill patients.

Vitamins C and E

Decreased concentrations of vitamins C and E have been found in patients with burns, sepsis, trauma, and major surgery.[98,99] With many vitamins, systemic inflammation is known to decrease vitamin concentrations, but unfortunately, few studies on vitamins C and E evaluate the presence of inflammation concomitantly. Supplementation of vitamins C and E is most often delivered as part of an antioxidant "cocktail" with selenium, or included in an immune-modulating enteral formula. However, the 2015 update of the Canadian Clinical Practice Guidelines added a new section regarding intravenous vitamin C, although evidence was insufficient to make a recommendation on supplementation of vitamin C in critically ill patients.[37] The supplementation of antioxidants in critical illness is discussed later.

Selenium

Selenium is a trace element that is essential in many metabolic processes, including the enzymes glutathione peroxidase and selenoprotein P.[94] Both enzymes are necessary for oxidative defense. Because selenium is classified as an essential trace element, it is added to enteral formulas and is included in five-ingredient multitrace additives for PN. Because of selenium's role in antioxidant defense, it has also been studied at a suprapysiologic dose to improve outcomes in critically ill patients. Patients with sepsis and systemic inflammatory response have high selenium-dependent glutathione peroxidase activity and low selenium concentrations.[100] Older guidelines recommend intravenous selenium, primarily because of a small study published in 2007 and a meta-analysis from 2005, which showed potential benefit from doses of 500–1,000 mcg/day.[32,37,69] The SIC (Selenium in Intensive Care) trial evaluated 249 patients with systemic inflammatory response, sepsis, and septic shock. Patients were randomized to receive 1,000 mcg intravenously of sodium selenite followed by 14 daily infusions of 1,000 mcg or placebo.[100] The intention-to-treat analysis showed no significant difference in the primary outcome of 28-day mortality; however, the 92 per-protocol patients showed reduced mortality (p=0.49; OR 0.56; CI, 0.32–1.0). A meta-analysis published in 2005 aggregated seven studies with 186 patients and reported that selenium supplementation (alone and in combination with other antioxidants) was associated with a trend toward lower mortality (RR 0.59; 95% CI, 0.32, 1.08 p=0.09).[101] For higher doses of selenium, one trial evaluating 60 patients with septic shock found no benefit in time to vasopressor withdrawal when 4,000 mcg was given on the first day and 1,000 mcg was given daily afterward for 9 days.[102] A meta-analysis from 2012 aggregated 16 studies of critically ill patients and compared different dosing schemes used for selenium supplementation. Overall, the analysis found no mortality benefit to selenium in critically ill patients. When comparing selenium dosed at greater than 500 mcg, equal to 500 mcg, and less than 500 mcg daily, no dose achieved a statistically significant improvement in mortality.[103] A separate meta-analysis from 2013 evaluated nine trials with 792 patients with sepsis only and found lower mortality (OR 0.73; 95% CI, 0.54, 0.98; p=0.03; I^2 = 0%) with selenium supplementation than with placebo.[104] In conclusion, given the available data, there appears to be no consistent benefit to supplementing suprapysiologic doses of selenium, and it cannot be recommended to routinely supplement selenium in critically ill patients.

Other Substances

Glutamine

Glutamine is an amino acid that has been studied in critically ill patients for more than 20 years. It is classified as conditionally essential in catabolic states. In critically ill patients, the main consumers of glutamine are macrophages and lymphocytes, which deplete glutamine stores in muscle tissues.[105,106] Consequently, plasma glutamine concentrations fall.[80,82] When this occurs, glutamine may be unavailable for immune cells and other rapidly dividing cells or the synthesis of glutathione, renal ammonia, and glycogen.[105,107]

The practice of supplementing glutamine in critically ill patients has changed substantially as new studies have been published, which may serve as a cautionary tale for interpreting small studies. A small prospective cohort trial associated low plasma glutamine concentrations at ICU admission with increased hospital mortality in 2001.[105] As a result, some clinicians began supplementing glutamine in critically ill patients. This was done either enterally (in doses of 0.16–0.5 g/kg of body weight per day) or parenterally (in doses of 0.18–0.57 g/kg/day), usually in combination with nutrition support.

A meta-analysis of smaller studies from 2002 found that critically ill patients given glutamine supplementation had a reduction in complication and mortality rates; the greatest benefit occurred in patients receiving high-dose, parenteral glutamine.[108] The initial Canadian Clinical Practice Guidelines published in 2003 recommended supplementation of PN with parenteral glutamine, when available, but data were inadequate to make a recommendation on intravenous supplementation for patients receiving EN.[33] Enteral glutamine was regarded as appropriate to consider in burn and trauma patients, but data were inadequate in other critically ill patients to suggest routine use. The nutrition guidelines for critically ill patients from SCCM/ASPEN, published in 2009, give a grade B and C recommendation to consider enteral and parenteral glutamine supplementation.[32]

However, two subsequent larger trials failed to find a benefit to intravenous glutamine supplementation.[109,110] The most recent and largest trials to date, the REDOXs[111] and the METAPLUS[112] trials, have actually found a signal of harm in supplementing glutamine to the most critically ill patients. The REDOXs trial supplemented glutamine as 0.35 g/kg of ideal body weight per day intravenously and 30 g enterally per day. Patients enrolled in this trial were required to receive mechanical ventilation and have at least two organ system failures. The patients who received glutamine had a statistically significant increase in in-hospital and 6-month mortality.[111] The METAPLUS study, in contrast, used enteral glutamine at a dose of 0.3–0.5 g/kg/day as part of an immune-modulating enteral product that also contained omega-3 fatty acids and antioxidants. These patients were mechanically ventilated with a maximum SOFA score of 12. In this trial, there was also a statistically significant increase in 6-month mortality for the patients who received glutamine supplementation.[112]

These two studies differed in the route of administration and the dose of glutamine supplemented, but both found evidence of harm. The benefit seen previously was present in small single-center trials that were underpowered to detect an increase in mortality.[113] After these studies were published, the Canadian Clinical Practice

Guidelines 2013 updates added a caution for use of any glutamine in patients with shock or multiorgan failure.[69] By the 2015 Canadian Clinical Practice Guidelines update, use of enteral glutamine was not recommended in critically ill patients.[37] In conclusion, given the available evidence, it cannot be recommended to routinely supplement glutamine in critically ill patients.

Arginine

Arginine is another amino acid that has been studied for supplementation in critically ill patients. Soon after trauma or surgery, plasma arginine concentrations drop and remain low for days to weeks after the injury.[114] Arginine is a substrate for nitric oxide production in several cell types, including T lymphocytes and myeloid cells. Physical injury causes myeloid-derived suppressor cells to appear; these cells express arginase-1, which leads to arginine deficiency and T-lymphocyte dysfunction.[114-116] A recent meta-analysis that included about 3,000 patients found a treatment effect of arginine therapy, at doses delivered in immune-modulating enteral formulas of around 12 g/day, after major surgery; arginine treatment reduced risk of infection by 40% and overall LOS versus standard EN.[115] However, the same may not be true in patients with sepsis. Most trials show very little benefit or, more commonly, harm when arginine is supplemented in patients with sepsis.[117-119] The explanation for this effect may be the supraphysiologic supplement dose (8–20 g/day vs. 3–5 g/day normally ingested) promotes excessive nitric oxide, which worsens hypotension and may increase mortality.[114,119,120] The 2009 SCCM/ASPEN guidelines recommended arginine supplementation as part of an immune-modulating enteral formula for patients with major GI surgery, trauma, burns, and head and neck cancers and for critically ill patients who were not severely septic.[32] However, the Canadian Clinical Practice Guidelines have never recommended the use of arginine for critically ill mechanically ventilated patients.[33,37,69,121] Because of the lack of high-quality studies supporting the use of arginine and the potential harm, it is not recommended to supplement arginine in critically ill patients.

Antioxidants

Antioxidants have been studied together with glutamine and/or arginine as part of an immune-modulating or immune-enhancing diet, but they have also been studied separately. Under normal physiologic conditions and inspiration of 21% oxygen, there are adequate defenses against reactive oxygen species and reactive nitrogen-oxygen species, commonly known as free radicals.[122] Cellular injury occurs when the overproduction of free radicals overwhelms endogenous antioxidant defenses such as glutathione, superoxide dismutase, and antioxidant vitamins. Data have shown that in surgery, trauma, and sepsis, antioxidant levels are decreased and that the more severe the injury, the more depleted the antioxidant defenses become.[101]

The body's antioxidant defense mechanisms depend on selenium, zinc, manganese, and iron, which are cofactors for antioxidant enzymes and the vitamins C, E, and beta-carotene. A recent meta-analysis pooled 21 randomized controlled trials with around 2,500 patients that evaluated antioxidant supplementation in critically ill patients.[123] Of note, this analysis excluded trials that also combined glutamine or arginine with antioxidant vitamins and trace elements. The authors found a decrease in overall mortality of 18% in the antioxidant-treated group (RR 0.82; 95% CI, 0.72–0.93; p=0.002). The analysis also noted a decrease in ventilator-days from a small group of included studies, and in the subgroup analysis of enterally versus parenterally supplied antioxidants, only the enteral route achieved a statistically significant benefit. Many of the studies performed with antioxidant supplementation have used slightly different doses of each antioxidant, though most include vitamins C and E and selenium, and the therapy ranges from 7 to 28 days, which should be considered when making a recommendation. Previous guidelines have recommended supplemental antioxidants for critically ill patients.[32,37,69] Although the results from smaller studies and aggregated results from meta-analyses are promising, we do not yet know the optimal composition, dose, or route for supplementing antioxidants. Because of these unknowns, routine supplementation of antioxidants in critically ill patients cannot be recommended.

Omega-3 Fatty Acids

Another nutrient with the potential to affect immune function is the omega-3 fatty acids. Omega-6 fatty acids are metabolized into eicosanoids that tend to be proinflammatory; omega-3 fatty acids are metabolized into a different series of prostaglandins, leukotrienes, and thromboxanes that do not promote inflammation and thrombosis, and may be referred to as anti-inflammatory. In addition, when omega-3 fatty acids are incorporated into membrane phospholipids of immune cells, they alter membrane fluidity, which affects secondary messengers, transporters, receptors, and enzymes.[124,172] Many studies have found a benefit with an omega-3–supplemented enteral formula (Oxepa) in patients with ALI or acute respiratory distress syndrome (ARDS) when compared to high-fat formulas, not typical ICU formulas.[125-127] Use of omega-3–supplemented formulas will be discussed in greater detail later. In addition, a recent meta-analysis concluded that critically ill patients who received enteral formulas with a high percentage of omega-3 fatty acids had decreased infectious rates, hospital LOS, and mortality.[128] Although data suggest that parenteral omega-3 fatty acids are also beneficial, no products are currently approved for use in the United States. However, European intravenous omega-3 products can be obtained if an Investigational New Drug (IND) application is authorized for each patient by the U.S. Food and Drug Administration (FDA). Omega-3–containing enteral formulas are recommended for patients with ALI/ARDS, and recommendations for omega-3 fatty acid in other forms will change as products become available in the United States.

Probiotics

Probiotics have the potential to treat gut and immune disturbances in the critically ill population through competitively inhibiting the growth of pathogenic organisms, enhancing the mucosal barrier, and modulating the host inflammatory response. Understanding and modifying the human gut microbiome is still a developing area of research, and unfortunately, trials of probiotics in the critically ill population have not shown comprehensive benefit. Some studies have shown benefit, whereas others have shown no difference, likely because of differences between ICU populations and strains of probiotics used. The 2009 SCCM/ASPEN guidelines do not recommend providing probiotics to the general ICU population, but they do recommend probiotics for patients with transplantation, major abdominal surgery, and severe trauma (grade C).[32] However, in light of conflicting evidence, the potential for harm, and the legal issues of providing non–FDA-approved products to hospitalized patients, use of probiotics in the critically ill population remains controversial.

ORGAN-SPECIFIC CONSIDERATIONS

Renal

Renal dysfunction is a common diagnosis in the ICU. Both acute kidney injury (AKI) and chronic kidney disease (CKD) affect a patient's nutritional requirements and tolerance. To assess nutritional status, it is recommended to evaluate a patient's weight and inflammatory status in setting nutritional goals.[129] Indirect calorimetry is preferred to determine caloric needs in renal dysfunction. Protein goals, electrolyte provision, and vitamin/mineral needs depend on whether the patient is receiving renal replacement therapy and the type of therapy.

Acute Kidney Injury

Patients with AKI are both hypermetabolic and hypercatabolic as a result of the inflammatory response associated with acute injury.[130] Metabolic complications that may occur in AKI include loss of glucose homeostasis, muscle wasting, protein catabolism, electrolyte imbalance, and development of metabolic acidosis.[130] Protein catabolism causes accumulation of protein metabolism byproducts resulting in azotemia. Tissue catabolism also releases intracellular electrolytes such as potassium, phosphorus, magnesium, and protein-bound acids such as sulfuric acid and hydrochloric acid.[131] This, combined with decreased renal clearance, leads to electrolyte imbalance and metabolic acidosis.

Continuous Renal Replacement Therapy

Continuous renal replacement therapy (CRRT) uses specialized filtration membranes that are highly permeable and that remove solutes by convection with or without diffusion. To discuss the implications of fluids used during CRRT, we will first discuss CRRT modalities. Continuous venovenous hemofiltration (CVVH), the most commonly used modality, uses convection to remove solutes and water. To prevent hypovolemia, water removed during hemofiltration must be returned to the patient as replacement fluid in the CRRT circuit. Conversely, continuous venovenous hemodialysis (CVVHD) uses dialysate to remove solutes. If the concentration in the dialysate is lower than the blood concentration, the solute is removed by diffusion; if the opposite is true, the solute will be delivered to the patient. Continuous venovenous hemodialysis does not use replacement fluids in the circuit. Finally, continuous venovenous hemodiafiltration (CVVHDF) uses both dialysate and replacement fluids. Depending on the modality, CRRT dialysate fluids contain dextrose and either bicarbonate or lactate, and they may contain additional electrolytes. Dextrose amounts can vary in commercial CRRT dialysate solutions. Using a dialysate that contains just 1.5% dextrose at a flow rate of 1 L/hour can result in the patient's receiving 500 dextrose calories from the CRRT alone.[132] There are also disadvantages to using a dialysate with very low dextrose. Glucose losses may occur in the ultrafiltrate fluid removed during CRRT. Glucose losses into the dialysate are dependent on and are equal to the serum blood glucose concentration they are dialyzed against.[133] Another source of calories from CRRT solutions is citrate, which is being used more commonly for anticoagulation during CRRT. In one study, a mean caloric load of citrate anticoagulation during CRRT was 1,323 calories per day.[134] At a CVVHDF flow rate of 2 L/hour, another study found a caloric load of 63 calories/hour with a 2.2% citrate solution, 20 calories/hour with a 4% trisodium citrate solution, and 60 calories/hour with heparin anticoagulation.[135]

Continuous renal replacement therapy dialysate solutions may contain electrolytes, and all replacement fluids should contain dextrose, sodium, chloride, potassium, calcium, and magnesium. Occasionally, dialysate fluids are also used as replacement fluids. Of special note, phosphorus cannot be added to a calcium-containing CRRT solution, so frequent monitoring and replacement of phosphorus is prudent.

Protein needs are elevated for patients with AKI receiving CRRT, largely because of the severity of their illness and the accompanying inflammatory response. In addition, small proteins and amino acids are lost through CRRT. Studies have shown that at least 1.5 g/kg/day of protein is needed daily, and up to 2.5 g/kg/day may be required for positive nitrogen balance.[129] An amino acid solution is available for use in PN formulas for patients with AKI; however, evidence is insufficient to support its use, and current guidelines recommend a standard amino acid solution.[129] Patients receiving CRRT do not usually require fluid restriction, so concentrated enteral or parenteral formulas are not necessary.

If a patient receiving CRRT requires enteral feeding, the recommendation is to start with a standard enteral formula and to follow standard ICU calorie and protein requirements. If significant electrolyte disturbances occur, a formula designed for renal failure with lower electrolyte provision may be considered.[129] However, high hemofiltration rates increase the removal rate for small molecules like electrolytes, so patients receiving CRRT do not typically require lower amounts of electrolytes while the CRRT is being used. If a patient is receiving PN while on CRRT, electrolytes may require frequent adjustment, so clinicians may prefer to minimize electrolytes in the PN solution and adjust by CRRT fluids or replace outside the PN.

Chronic Kidney Disease

Patients with preexisting CKD may require nutrition support in the ICU. Patients with CKD develop protein energy wasting as a result of neuroendocrine factors that include reduced protein synthesis and increased protein breakdown. Many patients also have glucose intolerance and hypertriglyceridemia. Altered calcium/phosphorus metabolism and anemia should be considered when prescribing nutrition. Finally, because of decreased renal clearance, patients with CKD will also have impaired clearance of electrolytes, metabolic acidosis, and altered fluid status.

Restricted protein diets have long been used and advocated for delaying the progression to dialysis.[133,136-138] These studies typically targeted a protein goal of 0.6 g/kg/day or less of protein. However, while these patients are acutely ill and hospitalized, catabolism will increase protein requirements, and patients may require dialysis to aid in removal of metabolic wastes.[129] Patients should be prescribed protein that meets their needs according to degree of critical illness.

Hemodialysis

Energy requirements for patients receiving hemodialysis are similar to those for patients without renal failure. The current protein recommendation for patients with CKD on maintenance hemodialysis is 1.2 g/kg/day; however, in critical illness, protein should be provided according to critical care guidelines, 1.0–2.5 g/kg/day, to meet increased metabolic demands.[129] Vitamin status is an additional concern. Hemodialysis removes water-soluble vitamins, including vitamin C, pyridoxine (B_6), cyanocobalamin (B_{12}), thiamine (B_1), and folic acid, as well as vitamin D.[129] A standard oral renal vitamin may be used to replace these if the patient has oral or enteral access.

Peritoneal Dialysis

Calories from the dextrose-containing peritoneal dialysis solutions may be as high as 500–1,000 calories per day and should be accounted for when designing the nutrition prescription.[130] Wideroe et al. have developed a system to estimate the amount of absorbed glucose from the peritoneal dialysis solution.[139] As with other CRRT modalities, calorie and protein goals in critical illness should be set to goals according to the patient's level of catabolism.

Respiratory

In the past, high lipid feedings were recommended for patients with respiratory compromise. The theory behind this practice was that using lipids for calories produces less carbon dioxide than carbohydrates or protein and therefore will aid in weaning from the ventilator or improving respiratory status. This is represented as a respiratory quotient (RQ) equal to carbon dioxide production (Vco_2) divided by oxygen consumption (Vo_2), with an RQ from lipid oxidation being 0.85, protein 0.82, and carbohydrates 1. However, early reports of respiratory dysfunction and failure with high-carbohydrate feedings provided excessive calories overall.[140] A study by Talpers et al. shows this; 20 mechanically ventilated patients received a low, medium, or high proportion of carbohydrates in enteral feeding or 1.0, 1.5, or 2.0 times their basal energy expenditure in total calories. There was no difference in Vco_2 between the different carbohydrate feedings, but the Vco_2 significantly increased as total calories increased.[141] This classic study supports the argument, and current practice, that limiting total calories will do more to prevent ventilatory adverse effects than limiting carbohydrates or increasing lipids.

Both ALI and ARDS have an inflammatory component. In both conditions, eicosanoid-mediated neutrophil migration into the alveolar space causes lung damage.[127,142] The type and activity of eicosanoids can be modified by omega-6 or omega-3 fatty acids. In addition, γ-linolenic acid (GLA) decreases neutrophil leukotriene synthesis and increase prostaglandin E_1, which may be beneficial in ALI/ARDS.[141] Table 4.5 compares studies evaluating omega-3–supplemented EN in patients with ALI/ARDS.

Many clinical trials using an enteral formula supplemented with omega-3 fatty acids, GLA, and antioxidants (Oxepa) have shown benefit in patients with ALI/ARDS.[125-127,143] One study found a mortality benefit in the supplemented group compared with the group receiving the high-fat control formula.[143] Limitations of these studies include small patient numbers, use of a high-fat comparator, and heterogeneous etiology/severity of ALI/

ARDS in included patients, although patients with a diagnosis of ALI/ARDS are inherently heterogeneous. The largest study to date found no benefit to supplementing with omega-3s, GLA, and antioxidants; this study used a twice-daily enteral supplement (not the commercially available Oxepa formula) to bolus the nutrients and used a high-carbohydrate control formula, unlike previous studies.[142] Further large studies using typical ICU formulas rather than high-fat formulas are needed to determine whether these nutrients can be bloused separately from the enteral formula or whether they need to be given continuously to be beneficial. No studies have shown increased adverse events with omega-3–supplemented EN compared with the control formula.[125-127,142,143] With the mixed data available, some clinicians choose to recommend an enteral formula supplemented with omega-3 fatty acids, GLA, and antioxidants Oxepa for patients with ALI/ARDS, whereas others do not.

Hepatic

Patients with advanced hepatic failure represent a challenge in nutritional assessment and delivery. Many patients with chronic liver disease are malnourished, but available tools for assessment may be inaccurate. Malnutrition occurs in most patients with alcoholic liver disease, but it may be less common in patients with non-alcoholic steatohepatitis.[144] Body weight and fluid distribution is altered in patients with cirrhosis, and many patients have

Table 4.5 Comparison of Studies Evaluating Omega-3–Supplemented EN in Patients with ALI/ARDS

Study; Patient Population (baseline Pao_2/Fio_2 study, control)	Study Diet and Control Diet	Results – Primary Outcome(s)	Limitations
Gadek et al., 1999[125] 146 ARDS (165.2, 177.4)	Oxepa vs. high-fat control (Pulmocare)	MV days: ITT: 9.6 vs. 13.2 (p=0.27)/PP: 11 vs. 16.3 (p=0.011); ICU days: ITT: 11 vs. 14.8 (p=0.16)/PP: 12.8 vs. 17.5 (p=0.16); Supplemental oxygen days: ITT: 13.6 vs. 17.1 (p=0.78)/PP: 15.8 vs. 20.2 (p=0.053)	Excluded patients with severe ARDS (Pao_2/Fio_2 < 100), industry-sponsored
Singer et al., 2006[126] 100 ALI/ARDS (207.7, 230.5)	Oxepa vs. Pulmocare	Pao_2/Fio_2 on day 4, 317.4 vs. 214.3 (p<0.05); day 7, 296.5 vs. 236.3 (p<0.05); Tidal volumes and PEEP not significantly different	PP, open-label, industry-sponsored
Pontes-Arruda et al., 2006[143] 165 severe sepsis/septic shock (156.1, 158.4)	Oxepa vs. Pulmocare	All-cause mortality: 18 vs. 25 RR = 0.63 (p=0.037 [95% CI, 0.39–1.00])	PP, industry-sponsored
Grau-Carmona et al., 2011[173] 160 sepsis (71% with ARDS, 20% with septic shock) (205, 192)	Oxepa vs. Ensure Plus HN	New organ dysfunction: SOFA change: 2 vs. -2 (p=0.4)	Open-label, study terminated early because of being underpowered, industry-sponsored
Rice et al., 2011[86] 272 ALI (159.9, 172.5)	BID EPA 6.8-g, DHA 3.4-g, GLA 5.92-g bolus (480 kcal/day) vs. carbohydrate-rich control bolus (474 kcal/day)	Ventilator-free days: 14.0 vs. 17.2 (p=0.02 [95% CI, -5.8 to -0.7])	Only study to use bolus delivery independently of EN; composition of study supplement did not match Oxepa product; futility and efficacy values asymmetric, so cannot conclude n-3 supplement caused harm
Elamin et al., 2012[127] 22 ARDS (157, 138)	Oxepa vs. Pulmocare	Oxygenation and modified LIS: Lower ventilation variables: (p<0.001), decrease in lung injury score: (p<0.003)	PP, small patient number, not powered to detect mortality difference

ARDS = acute respiratory distress syndrome; BID = twice daily; DHA = docosahexaenoic acid; EPA = eicosapentaenoic acid; Fio_2 = fraction of inspired oxygen; ITT = intention-to-treat analysis; LIS = lung injury score; PEEP = positive end-expiratory volume; PP = per-protocol analysis; RR = relative risk; SOFA = Sequential Organ Failure Assessment (score).

hypoalbuminemia and decreased concentrations of other blood proteins. Providing nutrition support to patients with liver disease is challenging. The liver is responsible for the metabolism of proteins, carbohydrates, and lipids. Altered protein metabolism is a well-known sign of advanced liver disease. These patients have low plasma concentrations of the branched-chain amino acids (BCAAs); leucine, valine, and isoleucine; and high concentrations of aromatic amino acids. In healthy patients, BCAAs are taken up by skeletal muscle to create glutamine, a carrier for ammonia, or are transported to the liver for gluconeogenesis. In patients with cirrhosis, excessive glutamine is produced in the muscle while the liver is unable to convert ammonia to urea, resulting in increased concentrations of ammonia.[145] Patients with cirrhosis also have glucose intolerance and insulin resistance. This is associated with the early use of protein and lipid for fuel.[145] Finally, patients with advanced liver disease also have impaired lipid metabolism. Altered absorption is caused by decreased concentrations of intraluminal bile salts, concurrent pancreatic or intestinal disease, and mucosal edema. In addition, there is an imbalance between triglyceride synthesis and catabolism, which depletes lipid stores.[145]

Caloric requirements for these patients may be difficult to ascertain. The Harris-Benedict equation is inaccurate in patients with cirrhosis.[146] Anthropometry, 24-hour urinary creatinine collection, and SGA will yield more accurate information about the patient's nutritional status.[147] Although there may be a theoretical basis to consider restricting protein in patients with liver disease, this is not necessary. A study by Cordoba et al. showed that hepatic encephalopathy developed at a similar rate in patients given either a low-protein or a standard-protein formula.[148] In addition, Gheorghe et al. found that when patients with cirrhosis were given an oral diet with standard calories and protein, their hepatic encephalopathy improved, with the greatest improvement occurring in the most severe patients.[149] Critically ill patients should receive the amount of protein that meets their catabolic needs (1.5–2.0 g/kg/day). Stable or less critically ill patients with liver disease require 1–1.5 g/kg/day of protein.

The preferred route for nutrition support in patients with liver disease is the enteral route. Enteral supplementation in these patients improves nutritional status and, in some cases, markers of hepatic function.[149-152] The enteral route is preferred because of the infection risk with a central vascular line and preservation of gut mucosa and accompanying decreased risk of bacterial translocation.[145] In addition, PN can cause liver damage in the long term and, in some cases, with short-term use. Fear of bleeding in patients with esophageal varices may delay placement of nasoenteric feeding tubes. However, small-bore soft-tipped nasally or orally placed tubes have a low risk of causing bleeding in non-bleeding varices, and placement should not be delayed or deferred.[153] After variceal hemorrhage, however, it may be advisable to wait 48 hours after bleeding has been stopped before resuming feeding.[153]

Standard enteral formulas should be used for critically ill patients with liver disease. Some outpatient studies suggest that oral supplementation with BCAAs delays progression of liver disease. No studies show that short-term supplementation has any benefit in the critically ill population. The current guidelines recommend reserving formulas with BCAAs for the rare patient with hepatic encephalopathy who is refractory to medical treatment.[32]

Other nutritional considerations for patients with liver disease include vitamins and electrolytes. Vitamin D deficiency is common in patients with liver disease, especially cholestatic liver disease, so monitoring and replacement is important in these patients.[145] Thiamine deficiency and refeeding syndrome may be common in patients with liver disease who continue to consume alcohol.[145,154] Another important consideration is to restrict sodium to 2 g daily in patients with ascites.

In summary, it may be difficult to assess critically ill patients with acute or chronic liver disease for malnutrition, but malnutrition is common in these patients. Calorie and protein goals should be provided to meet the catabolic needs of critical illness, with care not to restrict protein. Special amino acid preparations containing high amounts of branched chain amino acids are not necessary, except for patients with hepatic encephalopathy refractory to lactulose and luminal antibiotics. Vitamin D and electrolytes should be monitored.

Pancreatic

Nutrition support may be required for patients who have either acute pancreatitis or a history of chronic pancreatitis. The main nutritional considerations in acute pancreatitis are hypermetabolic/hypercatabolic state, hyperglycemia, hypertriglyceridemia, and hypocalcemia. Nutritional considerations for chronic pancreatitis include anorexia, weight loss, exocrine insufficiency, and malabsorption. We will discuss the primary issues in patients with pancreatic disease, including timing and type of nutrition support initiation and pancreatic enzyme replacement.

Route and Type of Feeding

The discussion of pancreatic rest in acute pancreatitis and its implications for nutrition support has changed dramatically in the past 20 years. In the past, many clinicians considered pancreatic rest synonymous with bowel rest, and patients were placed on PN in an effort to decrease complications. Providing pancreatic rest as a sole management strategy does not improve patient outcome.[155] Enteral nutrition is superior to PN, especially in patients with severe acute pancreatitis.[156-159] In one study where 100% of the enrolled patients had severe acute pancreatitis, overall and septic complications were significantly reduced.[159]

Evidence is still insufficient to show the superiority of EN to a standard oral diet, although smaller studies suggest it.[160] Many trials evaluating the safety of EN in severe acute pancreatitis used jejunal tube placement to avoid gastric stimulation.[161] Although fewer studies support gastric feeding over jejunal feeding, the American College of Gastroenterology and SCCM/ASPEN guidelines recommend gastric and jejunal feeding equally.[32,162] Standard polymeric formulas should be the first choice for enteral feeding.[155] If the patient has increased nausea or increased abdominal pain, the tube position should be checked or advanced distally to the jejunum, the patient switched to continuous enteral feeding, or the feeding changed to a semi-elemental or elemental formula.[32] Increased nausea is not a contraindication to continuing EN.

If a patient develops persistent ileus or bowel obstruction, PN may be considered after 5 days of admission. Because intravenous lipids do not worsen symptoms of pancreatitis, they can be safely used when serum triglyceride is below 400 mg/dL.[155] Standard guidelines apply to formulating PN for patients with acute pancreatitis.

Enzyme Replacement

Pancreatic enzyme replacement will be necessary for many patients with chronic pancreatitis. Recently, the FDA required all manufacturers of pancreatic enzyme supplements to submit an NDA by April 2010 or to stop distributing their products. Before this, there were around 25 pancreatic enzyme products, and because this deadline has passed, there are six pancreatic enzymes on the U.S. market: Creon, Zenpep, Pancreaze, Ultresa, Viokace, and Pertzye. Each product has several strengths with differing amounts of amylase, lipase, and protease. Viokace is the only product without an enteric coating and is labeled to take with a proton pump inhibitor. Labeled dosing for all products recommends dosing according to the Cystic Fibrosis Foundation, beginning with 500 units of lipase per kilogram per meal and titrating to a maximum of 2,500 lipase units per kilogram per meal. Many other dosing schemes are available.[155] Although none of the available products are labeled for administration through gastrostomy or distal feeding tubes, dosing and administration methods have been reported in the literature. One method is to provide 1,000 lipase units for each gram of fat provided by the enteral feed and dose this every 3 hours for continuous feeding.[163] For gastric tubes, it is recommended to suspend enteric-coated microspheres (all products except Viokace) in a nectar thick acidic liquid and administer by syringe into the feeding tube.[163] For distal feeding tubes, the enteric-coated spheres must be mixed with sodium bicarbonate to activate the enzymes, which may take more than 30 minutes.[163,164] The only products found to dissolve completely in sodium bicarbonate within 30 minutes, dosed in lipase units, are Creon 24,000, Ultresa 23,000, and Zenpep 20,000 and 40,000.[164] Water, carbonated beverages, or sweetened beverages should not be used to dilute pancreatic enzymes because this increases the adhesiveness of the enteric coating, which can cause tube obstruction. Crushing the microspheres is not recommended because this causes coagulation of the formula, and the powder can potentially be inhaled or come into contact with the eyes. It is not recommended to add pancreatic enzymes directly to the enteral feeding because this may compromise sterility and will cause coagulation of the formula, which may cause clogging. Table 4.6 summarizes information on pancreatic enzyme administration with EN.

In conclusion, patients with severe acute pancreatitis should receive nutrition support by the enteral route whenever possible. Enteral feeding is associated with not only an improvement in nutritional status but also a reduction in complication rates. Patients with acute pancreatitis may be fed by either the gastric or the jejunal route. If a critically ill patient requires pancreatic enzyme replacement, the pharmacist should be aware of new formulations and dosing strategies.

DISEASE-SPECIFIC CONSIDERATIONS

Diabetes/Glucose Control

A recent survey of U.S. hospitals reported that hyperglycemia occurred in 46% of critically ill patients.[165] Hyperglycemia has been associated with many poor outcomes in critically ill patients, including infections, septic shock, poor wound healing, and increased ICU stay.[166] Both hyper- and hypoglycemia should be avoided in critically ill patients. Current ASPEN guidelines recommend a blood glucose target of 140–180 mg/dL in adult critically ill patients receiving nutrition support.[165] This recommendation is in line with the current AACE/ADA (American Association of Clinical Endocrinologists/American Diabetes Association) recommendations for critically ill patients. Avoiding overfeeding is critical in patients with hyperglycemia; excess calories can contribute to hyperglycemia and associated poor outcomes. All sources of calories should be included in the nutritional assessment, including propofol and dextrose-containing intravenous fluids.

Either standard or specialized diabetes/hyperglycemia enteral formulas are appropriate for critically ill patients with hyperglycemia.[165] Many clinicians choose specialized formulas because of a lower provision of glucose and a relatively high provision of protein, which is needed for critical illness. Continuous enteral feeding is more commonly tolerated with less variation in serum glucose. Serum glucose should be monitored as enteral feeding is advanced to goal rate, and intravenous insulin infusions may be necessary.

If PN is necessary in a patient with hyperglycemia, it is prudent to begin insulin therapy before or concurrently with PN and/or to reduce dextrose in the PN. Parenteral

Table 4.6 Pancreatic Enzyme Administration with EN			
Feeding Tube Access	Pancreatic Enzyme Product (dose in units of lipase)	Dose (in units of lipase per g of fat in enteral formula)	Administration Procedure
Gastrostomy 10 Fr and larger	Creon, Zenpep, Pancreaze, Ultresa, Pertzye	500 units of lipase/g of fat up to 2,500 units/g of fat; suggested starting dose of 1,000 units of lipase/g of fat. For bolus feeds, give dose for each bolus no more than 30 min before or after initiation of feed. For cyclic (overnight) feeds, give 50%–75% of dose at initiation of feeding and may give remainder of dose if patient awakes during the night. For continuous feeds, give the total daily dose of lipase divided q2–3hr	Open capsule and suspend microspheres in 50–100 mL of nectar-thick fruit juice or acidic liquid; administer by syringe
Small bowel feeding tube	Zenpep 40,000 dissolves most efficiently; alternatively, Creon 24,000, Ultresa 23,000, or Zenpep 20,000		Open capsule and dissolve in 20 mL of sodium bicarbonate 8.4% injection, let stand for 30 min; administer by syringe

Fr = French; q = every.

nutrition is associated with greater hyperglycemia than EN.[166] Initially, intravenous insulin infusion that may be titrated separately from the PN infusion is recommended; if the infusion is to be discontinued, 80% of the daily dose from the infusion may be added to the PN. Another strategy for estimating the insulin requirements to be added to PN is to add 0.05–0.1 unit of regular human insulin per gram of dextrose in the PN. It is best to be conservative when estimating insulin requirements in PN because most facilities prepare PN solutions 12–24 hours before they are administered, and changing insulin requirements can be difficult to predict. Additional subcutaneous insulin may be needed for unexpected hyperglycemia.

Thermal Injury

Burn injuries result in a hypermetabolic state similar to trauma or sepsis. The degree to which patients with severe burns are hypermetabolic and hypercatabolic is much greater, however. Because of the hypermetabolic nature of burn injuries, the resting energy expenditures of pediatric patients with severe burns have been reported to be up to 150% greater than expected and up to 160% greater in adults.[167] In addition, patients with burns may oxidize amino acids at a rate 50% higher than fasting controls, leading to a significant protein deficit.[168] This significant calorie and protein hypermetabolism may continue for up to 2 years post-injury.[166] If nutritional interventions are not made, significant weight loss can occur. A 10% loss of total body mass in patients with burns leads to immune dysfunction; 20%, to impaired wound healing; 30%, to severe infections; and 40%, eventually to death.[167] Time to receipt of EN is critical to lessen the impact of the hypermetabolic state through modulation of catecholamine concentrations and maintaining gut mucosal integrity. Early enteral feeding initiated less than 24 hours after injury is recommended.[167] Parenteral nutrition should only be used if the patient has a non-functional GI tract; it is unclear whether PN should be used in addition to EN when calorie and protein goals cannot be met with EN alone.

Indirect calorimetry is the most reliable way to measure caloric needs in patients with severe burns. If indirect calorimetry is not available, predictive equations may be used. Some authors suggest the Galveston, Curreri, or Toronto equations,[167] whereas others suggest that the Milner and Carlson equations are most accurate.[169] Overall, it can be expected that the caloric requirements of these patients will be higher than in patients without burns. The next nutritional consideration is the balance of substrates to provide.

Patients with severe burns will have high caloric requirements, so it is important to provide glucose at less than the maximum glucose oxidation rate (7 mg/kg/hour). High-carbohydrate formulas are typically provided to patients with burns because this has been associated with improved outcomes.[168] Conversely, insulin therapy is used at some burn centers for purposes other than glucose control. Typically, this is done with continuous infusions of insulin and dextrose titrated to euglycemia. Insulin therapy in patients with burns stimulates muscle protein synthesis, increases lean body mass, and is associated with improved wound healing, without increasing hepatic triglyceride production.[167]

Immediately after burn injury, fat metabolism and use are altered. There is an increase in peripheral fat breakdown and use by the liver. About 30% of the available free fatty acids are used for fuel through beta-oxidation; the rest undergoes reesterification and potential accumulation in the liver.[167] Some centers may therefore limit fat administration to the minimal amount needed to prevent essential fatty acid deficiency.

Increased proteolysis is an important metabolic implication of burns. Protein requirements are estimated at 1.5–2 g/kg/day in adults with burns and at 2.5–4.0 g/kg/day in children with burns.[32,167] Some clinicians advocate the use of the amino acid glutamine for patients with burns. The 2009 SCCM/ASPEN guidelines recommend immune-modulating enteral formulas that contain glutamine for patients with burns, as well as enteral supplementation.[32]

Certain vitamins and minerals are also recommended for patients with burns. Decreased vitamin and mineral concentrations are associated with poor outcome; however, further research is needed to determine the dosages for these micronutrients. An older study recommends the following daily for patients with greater than 20% total body surface area burns: one multivitamin, 500 mg of ascorbic acid twice daily, 10,000 international units of vitamin A, and 45–50 mg of zinc.[170] European guidelines recommend supplementation of vitamin C, copper, selenium, and zinc.[171] Recently, low vitamin D concentrations were reported in children with burns despite supplementation, but the significance of this is not yet known.

In summary, patients with severe burns are highly catabolic. These patients will have high caloric and protein needs immediately post-burn and potentially long after the initial injury. Protein requirements are estimated at up to 2 g/kg/day for adults and up to 4 g/kg/day for children with severe burns. Early enteral feeding is preferred; a formula with a high carbohydrate to fat proportion is a reasonable choice. Patients with severe burns should receive the RDA of necessary vitamins and minerals at a minimum and may require additional supplementation.

SUMMARY

Critically ill patients are characterized by an inflammatory response that results in a failure to adapt energy and protein use to restore homeostasis, as occurs in simple starvation. The complexities of nutrition support are many in this population, and there are several controversies with few definitive answers regarding the optimal nutrition therapy for best outcomes. However, nutrition support therapy in critically ill patients is a rapidly evolving aspect of patient care with many new studies being conducted. Practitioners must remain cognizant of emerging data, and studies must be evaluated carefully to determine the study population, including severity of illness and nutritional status, and applicability of results to an individual patient. Until more robust data are available, clinical practice guidelines will continue to guide clinicians in their selection of nutrition support therapy but cannot determine the most appropriate therapy for any individual patient.

REFERENCES

1. The Hunger Strike of 1981 – A Chronology of Main Events. Hunger Strike: [Dead]. Available at cain.ulst.ac.uk/events/hstrike/chronology.htm. Accessed June 15, 2015.
2. Giner M, Laviano A, Meguid MM, et al. In 1995 a correlation between malnutrition and poor outcome in critically ill patients still exists. Nutrition 1996;12:23-9.
3. Norman K, Pichard C, Pirlich M. Prognostic impact of disease-related malnutrition. Clin Nutr 2008;27:5-15.
4. Baccaro F, Moreno JB, Borlenghi C, et al. Subjective global assessment in the clinical setting. JPEN J Parenter Enteral Nutr 2007;31:406-9.
5. Fontes D, Generoso S, Correia MITD. Subjective global assessment: a reliable nutrition assessment tool to predict outcomes in critically ill patients. Clin Nutr 2014;33:291-5.
6. Hoffer IJ. Metabolic consequences of starvation. In: Ross AC, Caballaero B, Cousins RJ, et al., eds. Modern Nutrition in Health and Disease, 11th ed. Philadelphia: Lippincott Williams & Wilkins, 2012:660-77.
7. Winkler MF, Malone AM. Medical nutrition therapy for metabolic stress: sepsis, trauma, burns, and surgery. In: Mahan KL, Escott-Stump S, eds. Krause's Food and Nutrition Therapy, 12th ed. St. Louis: Saunders Elsevier, 2008:1022-26.
8. Preiser JC, Ichai C, Orban JC, et al. Metabolic response to the stress of critical illness. Br J Anaesth 2014;113:945-54.
9. Jensen GL, Bistrian B, Roubenoff R, et al. Malnutrition syndromes: a conundrum vs continuum. JPEN J Parenter Enteral Nutr 2009;33:710-6.
10. Hoffer LJ, Bistrian BR. Why critically ill patients are protein deprived. JPEN J Parenter Enteral Nutr 2013;37:300-9.
11. Mueller C, Compher C, Druyan ME; the American Society for Parenteral and Enteral Nutrition (A.S.P.E.N.) Board of Directors. A.S.P.E.N. clinical guidelines. Nutrition screening, assessment, and intervention in adults. JPEN J Parenter Enteral Nutr 2011;35:16-24.
12. American Society for Parenteral and Enteral Nutrition (A.S.P.E.N.) Board of Directors and Clinical Practice Committee. July 2010. Definition of Terms, Style and Conventions Used in A.S.P.E.N. Board of Directors-Approved Documents. American Society for Parenteral and Enteral Nutrition. Available at www.nutritioncare.org/Library.aspx. Accessed May 10, 2015.
13. van Bokhorst-de van der Schueren MAE, Guaitoli PR, Jansma EP, et al. Nutrition screening tools: does one size fit all? A systematic review of screening tools for the hospital setting. Clin Nutr 2014;33:39-58.
14. Evans A. Positive patient outcomes in acute care: does obtaining and recording accurate weight make a difference? Aust J Adv Nurs 2012;29:62-9.
15. Fuhrman MP, Charney P, Mueller CM. Hepatic proteins and nutrition assessment. J Am Diet Assoc 2004;104:128-64.
16. Ferrie S, Allman-Farinelli M. Commonly used "nutrition" indicators do not predict outcomes in the critically ill: a systematic review. Nutr Clin Pract 2013;28:463-84.
17. Simpson F, Doig GS (for the Early PN Trial Investigator Group). Physical assessment and anthropometric measures for use in clinical research conducted in critically ill patient populations:

18. Detsky AS, McLaughlin JR, Baker JP, et al. What is subjective global assessment of nutritional status? JPEN J Parenter Enteral Nutr 1987;11:8-13.
19. Hanley JA, McNeil BJ. The meaning and use of the area under a receiver operating characteristic (ROC) curve. Radiology 1982;143:29-36.
20. World Health Organization (WHO). Physical Status: The Use and Interpretation of Anthropometry. A Report of the WHO Expert Committee. Geneva: WHO, 1995.
21. White JV, Guenter P, Jensen G, et al. Consensus statement of the Academy of Nutrition and Dietetics/American Society for Parenteral and Enteral Nutrition: characteristics recommended for the identification and documentation of adult malnutrition (undernutrition). J Acad Nutr Diet 2012;112:730-8.
22. Fisher M, JeVenn A, Hipskind P. Evaluation of muscle and fat loss as diagnostic criteria for malnutrition. Nutr Clin Pract 2015;30:239-48.
23. Puthucheary ZA, Rawal J, McPhail M, et al. Acute skeletal muscle wasting in critical illness. JAMA 2013;310:1591-600.
24. Braunschweig CA, Sheean PM, Peterson SJ, et al. Exploitation of diagnostic computed tomography scans to assess the impact of nutritional supplementation on body composition changes in respiratory failure patients. JPEN J Parenter Enteral Nutr 2014;38:880-5.
25. Sheean PM, Peterson SJ, Perez SG, et al. The prevalence of sarcopenia in patients with respiratory failure classified as normally nourished using computed tomography and subjective global assessment. JPEN J Parenter Enteral Nutr 2014;38:873-9.
26. Sungurtekin H, Sungurtekin U, Oner O, et al. Nutrition assessment in critically ill patients. Nutr Clin Pract 2008;23:635-41.
27. Sheehan PM, Peterson SJ, Gurka DP, et al. Nutrition assessment: the reproducibility of subjective global assessment in patients requiring mechanical ventilation. Eur J Clin Nutr 201;64:1358-64.
28. Jeejeebhoy KN, Keller H, Gramlich L, et al. Nutritional assessment: comparison of clinical assessment and objective variables for the prediction of length of hospital stay and readmission. Am J Clin Nutr 2015;101:956-65.
29. Heyland DK, Dhaliwal R, Jiang X, et al. Identifying critically ill patients who benefit the most from nutrition therapy: the development and initial validation of a novel risk assessment tool. Crit Care 2011;15:R268. (Score variables and scoring system available at www.criticalcarenutrition.com/docs/qi_tools/NUTRIC%20Score%201%20page%20summary-19March2013.pdf. Accessed July 4, 2015.)
30. Rahman A, Hasan R, Agarwala R, et al. Identifying critically-ill patients who will benefit most from nutritional therapy: further validation of the "modified NUTRIC" nutritional risk tool. Clin Nutr 2015 Jan 28. [Epub ahead of print]
31. Coltman A, Peterson S, Roehl K, et al. Use of 3 tools to assess nutrition risk in the intensive care unit. JPEN J Parenter Enteral Nutr 2015;39:28-33.
32. McClave SA, Martindale RG, Vanek VW, et al. Guidelines for the provision and assessment of nutrition support therapy in the adult critically ill patient: Society of Critical Care Medicine (SCCM) and American Society for Parenteral and Enteral Nutrition (A.S.P.E.N.). JPEN J Parenter Enteral Nutr 2009;33:277-316.
33. Heyland DK, Dhaliwal R, Drover JW, et al.; Canadian Critical Care Clinical Practice Guidelines Committee. Canadian clinical practice guidelines for nutrition support in mechanically ventilated, critically ill adult patients. JPEN J Parenter Enteral Nutr 2003;27:355-73.
34. Kreymanna KG, Bergerb MM, Deutzc NEP, et al. ESPEN guidelines on enteral nutrition: intensive care. Clin Nutr 2006;25:210-23.
35. Dellinger RP, Levy MM, Rhodes A, et al. Surviving Sepsis Campaign: international guidelines for management of severe sepsis and septic shock, 2012. Intensive Care Med 2013;39:165-228.
36. Singer P, Berger MM, Van den Berghe G, et al. ESPEN guidelines on parenteral nutrition: intensive care. Clin Nutr 2009;28:387-400.
37. Canadian Critical Care Clinical Practice Guidelines Committee. Canadian Clinical Practice Guidelines 2015. Summary of Revisions to the Recommendations. May 25, 2015. Available at www.criticalcarenutrition.com/docs/CPG%202015/Summary%20CPG%202015%20vs%202013.pdf. Accessed July 10, 2015.
38. Doig GS, Heighes PT, Simpson F, et al. Early enteral nutrition, provided within 24 h of injury or intensive care unit admission, significantly reduces mortality in critically ill patients: a meta-analysis of randomised controlled trials. Intensive Care Med 2009;35:2018-27.
39. Koretz RL, Lipman TO. The presence and effect of bias in trials of early enteral nutrition. Clin Nutr 2014;33:240-5.
40. Marik PE, Zaloga GP. Early enteral nutrition in acutely ill patients: a systematic review. Crit Care Med 2001;29:2264-70.
41. Elke G, Wang M, Weiler N, et al. Close to recommended caloric and protein intake by enteral nutrition is associated with better clinical outcome of critically ill septic patients: secondary analysis of a large international nutrition database. Crit Care 2014;18:R29.
42. McClave SA, Heyland DK. The physiologic response and associated clinical benefits from provision of early enteral nutrition. Nutr Clin Pract 2009;24:305-15.
43. Fremont RD, Rice TW. Pros and cons of feeding the septic intensive care unit patient. Nutr Clin Pract 2015;30:344-50.
44. Doing GS, Simpson F, Delaney A. Review of the true methodological quality of nutrition support trials conducted in the critically ill: time for improvement. Anesth Analg 2005;100:527-33.
45. Nguyen NQ, Fraser RJ, Bryant LK, et al. Delayed enteral feeding impairs intestinal carbohydrate absorption in critically ill patients. Crit Care Med 2012;40:50-4.
46. Yang S, Wu X, Yu W, et al. Early enteral nutrition in critically ill patients with hemodynamic instability: an evidence-based review and practical advice. Nutr Clin Pract 2014;29:90-6.
47. Allen JM. Vasoactive substances and their effects on nutrition in the critically ill patient. Nutr Clin Pract 2012;27:335-9.
48. Turza KC, Krenistsky J, Sawyer RG. Enteral feeding and vasoactive agents: suggested guidelines for clinicians. Pract

49. Revelly JP, Tappy L, Berger MM, et al. Early metabolic and splanchnic responses to enteral nutrition in post-operative cardiac surgery patients with circulatory compromise. Intensive Care Med 2001;27:540-9.

50. Berger MM, Berger-Gryllaki M, Wiesel PH, et al. Intestinal absorption in patients after cardiac surgery. Crit Care Med 2000;28:2217-23.

51. Khalid I, Doshi P, DiGiovine B. Early enteral nutrition and outcomes of critically ill patients treated with vasopressors and mechanical ventilation. AJCC Am J Crit Care 2010;19:261-8.

52. McClave SA, Chang WK. Feeding the hypotensive patient: does enteral feeding precipitate or protect against ischemic bowel? Nutr Clin Pract 2003;18:279-84.

53. Cahill NE, Dhaliwal R, Day AG, et al. Nutrition therapy in the critical care setting: what is "best achievable" practice? An international multicenter observational study. Crit Care Med 2010;38:395-401.

54. Halpern SD, Becker D, Curtis JR, et al. An official American Thoracic Society/American Association of Critical-Care Nurses/American College of Chest Physicians/Society of Critical Care Medicine policy statement: the choosing wisely top 5 list in critical care medicine. Am J Respir Crit Care Med 2014;190:818-26.

55. Braunschweig CL, Levy P, Sheean PM, et al. Enteral compared to parenteral nutrition: a meta-analysis. Am J Clin Nutr 2001;74:534-42.

56. Heyland DK, MacDonald S, Keefe L, et al. Total parenteral nutrition in the critically ill patient: a meta-analysis. JAMA 1998;280:2013-19.

57. Sanderstrom R, Drott C, Hyltander A, et al. The effect of post-operative intravenous feeding (TPN) on outcome following major surgery evaluated in a randomized study. Ann Surg 1993;217:185-95.

58. Simpson F, Doig GS. Parenteral vs. enteral nutrition in the critically ill patient: a meta-analysis of trials using the intention to treat principle. Intensive Care Med 2005;31:12-23.

59. Cahill NE, Murch L, Jeejeebhoy K, et al. When early enteral feeding is not possible in critically ill patients: results of a multicenter observational study. JPEN J Parenter Enteral Nutr 2011;35:160-8.

60. Casaer MP, Mesotten D, Hermans G, et al. Early versus late parenteral nutrition in critically ill adults. N Engl J Med 2011;365:506-17.

61. Casaer MP, Wilmer A, Hermans G, et al. Role of disease and macronutrient dose in the randomized controlled EPaNIC trial. Am J Respir Crit Care Med 2013;187:247-55.

62. Casaer MP, Langouche L, Coudyzer W, et al. Impact of early parenteral nutrition on muscle and adipose tissue compartments during critical illness. Crit Care Med 2013;41:2298-309.

63. Kutsogiannis J, Alberda C, Gramlich L, et al. Early use of supplemental parenteral nutrition in critically ill patients: results of an international multicenter observational study. Crit Care Med 2011;39:2691-9.

64. Heidegger CP, Berger MM, Graf S, et al. Optimisation of energy provision with supplemental parenteral nutrition in critically ill patients: a randomized controlled clinical trial. Lancet 2013;381:385-93.

65. Doig GS, Simpson F, Sweetman EA, et al. Early parenteral nutrition in critically ill patients with short-term relative contraindications to early enteral nutrition. JAMA 2013;309:2130-8.

66. Harvey SE, Parrott F, Harrison DA, et al. Trial of the route of early nutritional support in critically ill adults. N Engl J Med 2014;371:1673-84.

67. Fraipont V, Preiser JC. Energy estimation and measurement in critically ill patients. JPEN 2013;37:705-13.

68. Canadian Clinical Practice Guidelines Committee. Canadian Clinical Practice Guidelines. Summary of Topics and Recommendations. May 28, 2009. Available at www.criticalcarenutrition.com/docs/cpg/srrev.pdf. Accessed October 6, 2015.

69. Dhaliwal K, Cahill N, Lemieux H, et al. The Canadian critical care nutrition guidelines in 2013: an update on current recommendations and implementation strategies. Nutr Clin Pract 2014;29:29-43.

70. Frankenfield DC, Coleman A, Alam S, et al. Analysis of estimation methods for resting metabolic rate in critically ill adults. JPEN J Parenter Enteral Nutr 2009;33:27-36.

71. Mifflin MD, St. Jeor ST, Hill LA, et al. A new predictive equation for resting energy expenditure in healthy individuals. Am J Clin Nutr 1990;51:241-7.

72. Frankenfield DC, Rowe WA, Smith JS, et al. Validation of several established equations for resting metabolic rate in obese and nonobese people. J Am Diet Assoc 2003;103:1152-9.

73. Frankenfield DC, Hise M, Malone A, et al. Evidence Analysis Working Group. Prediction of resting metabolic rate in critically ill adult patients: results of a systematic review of evidence. J Am Diet Assoc 2007;107:1552-61.

74. Frankenfield D. Validation of an equation for resting metabolic rate in older obese, critically ill patients. JPEN J Parenter Enteral Nutr 2011;35:264-9.

75. Cerra FB, Benitez MR, Blackburn GL, et al. Applied nutrition in ICU patients. A consensus statement of the American College of Chest Physicians. Chest 1997;111:769-78.

76. Frankenfield DC, Smith JS, Cooney RN. Validation of two approaches to predicting resting metabolic rate in critically ill patients. JPEN J Parenter Enteral Nutr 2004;28:259-64.

77. Ireton-Jones CS, Turner WW, Liepa GU, et al. Equations for estimation of energy expenditure of patients with burns with special reference to ventilator status. J Burn Care Rehabil 1992;13:330-3.

78. Swinamer DL, Grace MG, Hamilton SM, et al. Predictive equations for assessing energy expenditure in mechanically ventilated critically ill patients. Crit Care Med 1990;18:657-61.

79. Faisy C, Guerot E, Diehl JL, et al. Assessment of energy expenditure in mechanically ventilated patients. Am J Clin Nutr 2003;78:241-9.

80. Arabi YM, Aldawood AS, Haddad SH, et al. Permissive underfeeding or standard enteral feeding in critically ill adults. N Engl J Med 2015;372:2398-408.

81. Wei X, Day AG, Ouellette-Kuntz H, et al. The association between nutritional adequacy and long-term outcomes in critically ill patients requiring prolonged mechanical ventilation:

82. Yeh DD, Fuentes E, Quraishi SA, et al. Adequate nutrition may get you home: effect of caloric/protein deficits on the discharge destination of critically ill surgical patients. JPEN 2015 Apr 29. [Epub ahead of print]

83. Nicolo M, Heyland DK, Chittams J, et al. Clinical outcomes related to protein delivery in a critically ill population: a multicenter, multinational observational study. JPEN J Parenter Enteral Nutr 2015 Apr 21. [Epub ahead of print]

84. Braunschweig CA, Sheean PM, Peterson SJ, et al. Intensive nutrition in acute lung injury: a clinical trial (INTACT). JPEN J Parenter Enteral Nutr 2015;39:13-20.

85. The National Heart, Lung, and Blood Institute Acute Respiratory Distress Syndrome (ARDS) Clinical Trials Network. Initial trophic vs full enteral feeding in patients with acute lung injury. The EDEN randomized trial. JAMA 2012;307:795-803.

86. Rice TW, Mogan S, Hays MA, et al. A randomized trial of initial trophic versus full-energy enteral nutrition in mechanically ventilated patients with acute respiratory failure. Crit Care Med 2011;39:967-74.

87. Arabi YM, Tamim HM, Dhar GS, et al. Permissive underfeeding and intensive insulin therapy in critically ill patients: a randomized controlled trial. Am J Clin Nutr 2011;93:569-77.

88. Singer P, Anbar R, Cohen J, et al. The Tight Calorie Control Study (TICACOS): a prospective, randomized, controlled pilot study of nutritional support in critically ill patients. Intensive Care Med 2011;37:601-9.

89. Arabi YM, Haddad SH, Tamim HM, et al. Near-target caloric intake in critically ill medical-surgical patients is associated with adverse outcomes. JPEN J Parenter Enteral Nutr 2010;34:280-8.

90. Alberda C, Gramlich L, Jones N, et al. The relationship between nutritional intake and clinical outcomes in critically ill patients: results of an international multicenter observational study. Intensive Care Med 2009;35:1728-37.

91. Institute of Medicine of the National Academies. Dietary Reference Intakes Tables. National Agricultural Library, U.S. Department of Agriculture. Available at http://fnic.nal.usda.gov/dietary-guidance/dietary-reference-intakes/dri-tables-and-application-reports. Accessed July 26, 2015.

92. Needham DM, Dinglas VD, Bienvenu OJ, et al. One year outcomes in patients with acute lung injury randomized to initial trophic or full enteral feeding: prospective follow-up of EDEN randomized trial. BMJ 2013;346:f1532-44.

93. Vanek VW, Borum P, Buchman A, et al. A.S.P.E.N. position paper: recommendations for changes in commercially available parenteral multivitamin and multi-trace element products. Nutr Clin Pract 2012;27:440.

94. Clark SF. Vitamins and trace elements. In: Mueller CM, Kovacevich DS, McClave SA, et al., eds. The A.S.P.E.N. Adult Nutrition Support Core Curriculum: A.S.P.E.N., 2012:121-51.

95. Institute of Medicine. Dietary Reference Intakes for Calcium and Vitamin D. Washington, DC: National Academies Press, 2011.

96. Higgins DM, Wischmeyer PE, Queensland KM, et al. Relationship of vitamin D deficiency to clinical outcomes in critically ill patients. J Parenter Enteral Nutr 2012;36:713-20.

97. Amrein K, Schnedl C, Holl A, et al. Effect of high-dose vitamin D3 on hospital length of stay in critically ill patients with vitamin D deficiency. The VITdAL-ICU Randomized Clinical Trial. JAMA 2014;312:1520-30.

98. Louw JA, Werbeck A, Louw ME, et al. Blood vitamin concentrations during the acute phase response. Crit Care Med 1992;20:934-41.

99. Schorah CJ, Downing C, Piripitsi A, et al. Total vitamin C, ascorbic acid, and dehydroascorbic acid concentrations in plasma of critically ill patients. Am J Clin Nutr 1996;63:760-5.

100. Angstwurm MW, Engelmann L, Zimmermann T, et al. Selenium in intensive care (SIC): results of a prospective, randomized, placebo controlled, multiple-center study in patients with severe systemic inflammatory response syndrome, sepsis, and septic shock. Crit Care Med 2007;35:118-26.

101. Heyland DK, Dhaliwal R, Suchner U, et al. Antioxidant nutrients: a systematic review of trace elements and vitamins in the critically ill patient. Intensive Care Med 2005;31:327-37.

102. Forceville X, Laviolle B, Annane D, et al. Effects of high doses of selenium, as sodium selenite, in septic shock: a placebo-controlled, randomized, double-blind, phase II study. Crit Care 2007;11:R73.

103. Manzanares W, Dhaliwal R, Jiang X, et al. Antioxidant micronutrients in the critically ill: a systematic review and meta-analysis. Crit Care 2012;16:R66.

104. Alhazzani W, Jacobi J, Sindi A, et al. The effect of selenium therapy on mortality in patients with sepsis syndrome: a systematic review and meta-analysis of randomized controlled trials. Crit Care Med 2013;41:1555-64.

105. Oudemans-van Straaten HM, Bosman RJ, Treskes M, et al. Plasma glutamine depletion and patient outcome in acute ICU admissions. Intensive Care Med 2001;27:84-90.

106. Coeffier M, Dechelotte P. The role of glutamine in intensive care unit patients: mechanisms of action and clinical outcome. Nutr Rev 2005;63:65-9.

107. Souba WW. Nutritional support. N Engl J Med 1997;336:41-8.

108. Novak F, Heyland DK, Avenell A, et al. Glutamine supplementation in serious illness: a systematic review of the evidence. Crit Care Med 2002;30:2022-9.

109. Andrews PJ, Avenell A, Noble DW, et al. Randomised trial of glutamine, selenium, or both, to supplement parenteral nutrition for critically ill patients. BMJ 2011;17:1542.

110. Wernerman J, Kirketieg T, Andersson B, et al. Scandinavian glutamine trial: a pragmatic multi-centre randomized clinical trial of intensive care unit patients. Acta Anaesthesiol Scand 2011;55:812-8.

111. Heyland D, Muscedere J, Wischmeyer PE, et al. A randomized trial of glutamine and antioxidants in critically ill patients. N Engl J Med 2013;368:1489-97.

112. van Zanten AR, Sztark F, Kaisers UX, et al. High-protein enteral nutrition enriched with immune-modulating nutrients vs standard high-protein enteral nutrition and nosocomial infections in the ICU: a randomized clinical trial. JAMA 2014;312:514-24.

113. van Zanten AR, Hofman Z, Heyland DK. Consequences of the REDOXs and METAPLUS trials: the end of an era for glutamine and antioxidant supplementation for critically ill patients? JPEN J Parenter Enteral Nutr 2015;39:890-2.

114. Zhu X, Herrera G, Ochoa JB. Immunosuppression and infection after major surgery: a nutritional deficiency. Crit Care Clin 2010;26:491-500, ix.

115. Drover JW, Dhaliwal R, Weitzel L, et al. Perioperative use of arginine supplemented diets: a systematic review of the evidence. J Am Coll Surg 2011;212:385-99; e381.

116. Liuking YC, Poeze M, Ramsay G, et al. Reduced citrulline production in sepsis is related to diminished de novo arginine and nitric oxide production. Am J Clin Nutr 2009;89:142-52.

117. Bertolini G, Iapichino G, Radrizzani D, et al. Early enteral immunonutrition in patients with severe sepsis: results of an interim analysis of a randomized multicenter clinical trial. Intensive Care Med 2003;29:834-40.

118. Kalil AC, Danner RL. L-Arginine supplementation in sepsis: beneficial or harmful? Curr Opin Crit Care 2006;12:303-8.

119. Heyland DK, Samis A. Does immunonutrition in patients with sepsis do more harm than good? Intensive Care Med 2003;29:669-71.

120. Boher RH. The pharmacodynamics of L-arginine. 6th Amino Acid Assessment Workshop. J Nutr 2007;137:1650-5S.

121. Canadian Clinical Practice Guidelines Committee. Canadian Clinical Practice Guidelines. Summary of Topics and Recommendations. May 28, 2009. Available at www.criticalcarenutrition.com/docs/cpg/srrev.pdf. Accessed August 16, 2015.

122. Macdonald J, Galley HF, Webster NR. Oxidative stress and gene expression in sepsis. Br J Anaesth 2003;90:221-32.

123. Manzanares W, Dhaliwal R, Jiang X, et al. Antioxidant micronutrients in the critically ill: a systematic review and meta-analysis. Crit Care 2012;16:R66.

124. Collier BR, Cherry-Burkoweic JR, Mills ME. Trauma, surgery, and burns. In: Mueller CM, Kovacevich DS, McClave SA, et al., eds. The A.S.P.E.N. Adult Nutrition Support Core Curriculum: A.S.P.E.N., 2012:392-411.

125. Gadek JE, DeMichele SJ, Karlstad MD, et al. Effect of enteral feeding with eicosapentaenoic acid, gamma-linolenic acid, and antioxidants in patients with acute respiratory distress syndrome. Crit Care Med 1999;27:1409-20.

126. Singer P, Theilla M, Fisher H, et al. Benefit of an enteral diet enriched with eicosapentaenoic acid and gamma-linolenic acid in ventilated patients with acute lung injury. Crit Care Med 2006;34:1033-8.

127. Elamin E, Miller A, Ziad S. Immune enteral nutrition can improve outcomes in medical-surgical patients with ARDS: a prospective randomized controlled trial. J Nutr Disord Ther 2012;2:109.

128. Marik PE, Zaloga GP. Immunonutrition in critically ill patients: a systematic review and analysis of the literature. Intensive Care Med 2008;34:1980-90.

129. Brown RO, Compher C. A.S.P.E.N. clinical guidelines: nutrition support in acute and chronic renal failure. J Parenter Enter Nutr 2010;34:366-77.

130. Wolk R, Foulks CJ. Renal disease. In: Mueller CM, Kovacevich DS, McClave SA, et al., eds. The A.S.P.E.N. Adult Nutrition Support Core Curriculum: A.S.P.E.N., 2012:491-510.

131. Kopple JD. Nutritional therapy in kidney failure. Nutr Rev 1981;39:193-206.

132. Wooley JA, Btaiche IF, Good KL. Metabolic and nutritional aspects of acute kidney injury in critically ill patients requiring continuous renal replacement therapy. Nutr Clin Pract 2005;20:176-91.

133. Scheinkestel CD, Adams F, Mahony L, et al. Impact of increasing parenteral protein loads on amino acid levels and balance in critically ill anuric patients on continuous renal replacement therapy. Nutrition 2003;19:733-40.

134. Balik M, Zakharchenko M, Otahal M, et al. Quantification of systemic delivery of substrates for intermediate metabolism during citrate anticoagulation of continuous renal replacement therapy. Blood Purif 2012;33:80-7.

135. Balik M, Zakharchenko M, Leden P, et al. Bioenergetic gain of citrate anticoagulated continuous hemodiafiltration—a comparison between 2 citrate modalities and unfractionated heparin. J Crit Care 2013;28:87-95.

136. Klahr S, Levey AS, Beck GJ, et al. The effects of dietary protein restriction and blood-pressure control on the progression of chronic renal disease. N Engl J Med 1994;330:877-84.

137. Levey AS, Adler S, Caggiula AW, et al. Effects of dietary protein restriction on the progression of advanced renal disease in the Modification of Diet in Renal Disease study. Am J Kidney Dis 1996;27:652-63.

138. Locatelli F, Alberti D, Graziani G, et al. Prospective, randomized, multi-center trial of effect of protein restriction on progression of chronic renal insufficiency. Lancet 1991;337:1299-304.

139. Wideroe TE, Sneby LC, Berg KJ, et al. Intraperitoneal insulin absorption during intermittent and continuous peritoneal dialysis. Kidney Int 1983;23:22-8.

140. Malone A. Enteral formula selection: a review of selected product categories. Pract Gastroenterol 2005;28:44-74.

141. Talpers SS, Romberger DJ, Bunce SB, et al. Nutritionally associated increased carbon dioxide production: excess total calories vs. high proportion of carbohydrate calories. Chest 1992;102:551-5.

142. Rice TW, Wheeler AP, Thompson BT, et al. Enteral omega-3 fatty acid, gamma-linolenic acid, and antioxidant supplementation in acute lung injury. JAMA 2011;306:1574-81.

143. Pontes-Arruda A, Aragao AM, Albuquerque JD. Effects of enteral feeding with eicosapentaenoic acid, gamma-linolenic acid, and antioxidants in mechanically ventilated patients with severe sepsis and septic shock. Crit Care Med 2006;34:2325-33.

144. Mendenhall CL, Anderson S, Weesner RE, et al. Protein-calorie malnutrition associated with alcoholic hepatitis. Veterans Administration Cooperative Study Group on Alcoholic Hepatitis. Am J Med 1984;76:211-22.

145. Frazier TH, Wheeler BE, McClain CJ, et al. Liver disease. In: Mueller CM, Kovacevich DS, McClave SA, et al., eds. The A.S.P.E.N. Adult Nutrition Support Core Curriculum: A.S.P.E.N., 2012:454-71.

146. Shanbhouge RL, Bistrian BR, Jenkins RL, et al. Resting energy expenditure in patients with end-stage liver disease and in normal population. JPEN J Parenter Enteral Nutr 1987;11:305-8.

147. Lieber CS. Relationships between nutrition, alcohol use, and liver disease. Alcohol Res Health 2003;27:220-31.

148. Cordoba J, Lopez-Hellin J, Planas M, et al. Normal protein diet for episodic hepatic encephalopathy: results of a randomized study. J Hepatol 2004;41:38-43.

149. Gheorge L, Iacob R, Vadan R, et al. Improvement of hepatic encephalopathy using a modified high-calorie high-protein diet. Rom J Gastroenterol 2005;14:231-8.

150. Hirsch S, de la Maza MP, Gattas V, et al. Nutritional support in alcoholic cirrhotic patients improves host defenses. J Am Coll Nutr 1999;18:434-41.

151. Kearns PJ, Young H, Garcia G, et al. Accelerated improvement of alcoholic liver disease with enteral nutrition. Gastroenterology 1992;102:200-5.

152. Cabre E, Rodriguez-Iglesias P, Caballeria J, et al. Short- and long-term outcome of severe alcohol-induced hepatitis treated with steroids or enteral nutrition: a multicenter randomized trial. Hepatology 2000;32:36-42.

153. Hebuterne X, Vanbiervliet G. Feeding the patients with upper gastrointestinal bleeding. Curr Opin Clin Nutr Metab Care 2011;14:197-201.

154. Khan LU, Ahmed J, Khan S, et al. Refeeding syndrome: a literature review. Gastroenterol Res Pract 2011;2011.

155. Parrish CR, Krenitsky J, McClave SA. Pancreatitis. In: Mueller CM, Kovacevich DS, McClave SA, et al., eds. The A.S.P.E.N. Adult Nutrition Support Core Curriculum: A.S.P.E.N., 2012:472-90.

156. Windsor AC, Kanwar S, Li AG, et al. Compared with parenteral nutrition, enteral feeding attenuates the acute phase response and improves disease severity in acute pancreatitis. Gut 1998;42:431-5.

157. Abou-Assi S, Craig K, O'Keefe SJ. Hypocaloric jejunal feeding is better than total parenteral nutrition in acute pancreatitis: results of a randomized comparative study. Am J Gastroenterol 2002;97:2255-62.

158. McClave SA, Greene LM, Snider HL, et al. Comparison of the safety of early enteral vs parenteral nutrition in mild acute pancreatitis. J Parenter Enteral Nutr 1997;21:14-20.

159. Powell JJ, Murchison JT, Fearon KC, et al. Randomized controlled trial of the effect of early enteral nutrition on markers of the inflammatory response in predicted severe acute pancreatitis. Br J Surg 2000;87:1375-81.

160. Kalfarentzos F, Kehagias J, Mead N, et al. Enteral nutrition is superior to parenteral nutrition in severe acute pancreatitis: results of a randomized prospective trial. Br J Surg 1997;84:1665-9.

161. McClave SA, Chang WK, Dhaliwal R, et al. Nutrition support in acute pancreatitis: a systematic review of the literature. J Parenter Enteral Nutr 2006;30:143-56.

162. Tenner S, Baillie J, DeWitt J, et al. Management of acute pancreatitis. Am J Gastroenterol 2013;108:1400-15.

163. Ferrie S, Graham C, Hoyle M. Pancreatic enzyme supplementation for patients receiving enteral feeds. Nutr Clin Pract 2011;26:349-51.

164. Boullata AM, Boullata JI. Pancreatic enzymes prepared in bicarbonate solution for administration through enteral feeding tubes. Am J Health Syst Pharm 2015;72:1210-4.

165. McMahon MM, Nystrom E, Braunschweig C, et al. A.S.P.E.N. clinical guidelines: nutrition support of adult patients with hyperglycemia. J Parenter Enteral Nutr 2013;27:23-6.

166. Newton L, Garvey WT. Nutritional and medical management of diabetes mellitus in hospitalized patients. In: Mueller CM, Kovacevich DS, McClave SA, et al., eds. The A.S.P.E.N. Adult Nutrition Support Core Curriculum: A.S.P.E.N., 2012:580-602.

167. Rodriguez NA, Jeschke MG, Williams FN, et al. Nutrition in burns: Galveston contributions. J Parenter Enteral Nutr 2011;35:704-14.

168. Abdullahi A, Jeschke MG. Nutrition and anabolic pharmacotherapies in the care of burn patients. Nutr Clin Pract 2014;29:621-30.

169. Shields BA, Doty KA, Chung KK, et al. Determination of resting energy expenditure after severe burn. J Burn Care Res 2013;34:22-8.

170. Gottschlich MM, Warden GD. Vitamin supplementation in the patient with burns. J Burn Care Rehabil 1990;11:275-9.

171. Rousseau A, Losser M, Ichai C, et al. ESPEN endorsed recommendations: nutritional therapy in major burns. Clin Nutr 2013;32:497-502.

172. Stapleton RD, Martin JM, Mayer K. Fish oil in critical illness: mechanisms and clinical applications. Crit Care Clin 2010;26(3):501-514, ix.

173. Grau-Carmona T, Morán-García V, García-de-Lorenzo A, et al. Effect of an enteral diet enriched with eicosapentaenoic acid, gamma-linolenic acid and anti-oxidants on the outcome of mechanically ventilated, critically ill, septic patients. Clin Nutr 2011;30(5):578-84.

Chapter 5: Glucose Management in the Critically Ill Population

Paul M. Szumita, Pharm.D., FCCM, BCCCP, BCPS;
and James F. Gilmore, Pharm.D., BCCCP, BCPS

LEARNING OBJECTIVES

1. Describe sources of hyperglycemia in critically ill patients.
2. Critique primary literature and multidisciplinary guidelines on glucose management in the intensive care unit.
3. Analyze medication therapy options for glucose management in a critically ill patient.
4. Categorize and construct treatment plans for patients with hyperglycemic emergencies (diabetic ketoacidosis and hyperglycemic hyperosmolar state).
5. Formulate a plan for an institution-wide multidisciplinary approach to glucose management.

ABBREVIATIONS IN THIS CHAPTER

BG	Blood glucose	POCT	Point-of-care testing
DKA	Diabetic ketoacidosis	RCT	Randomized controlled trial
HHS	Hyperglycemic hyperosmolar state	SICU	Surgical intensive care unit
ICU	Intensive care unit	STS	Society of Thoracic Surgeons
MICU	Medical intensive care unit	TPN	Total parenteral nutrition

INTRODUCTION

Management of blood glucose (BG) in critically ill patients is one of the key facets of supportive care. Retrospective analyses have shown increased mortality and morbidity with dysglycemia.[1-5] In this chapter, we will review the causes of hyperglycemia in the critically ill population as well as in the primary literature focused on glucose management in the intensive care unit (ICU) population. We will also evaluate medication therapy options for patients with hyperglycemia, as well as for patients undergoing a hyperglycemic emergency such as diabetic ketoacidosis (DKA) or hyperglycemic hyperosmolar state (HHS).

PATHOPHYSIOLOGY/CAUSES OF HYPERGLYCEMIA

Several mechanisms are responsible for acute hyperglycemia in ICU patients. These include insufficient antihyperglycemic therapy in patients with a known history of diabetes because many patients with diabetes on oral agents have their oral agents discontinued on admission, which are not replaced with an effective inpatient antihyperglycemic regimen.[6] Critically ill patients also commonly have increased insulin resistance among peripheral tissue, and increases in both hepatic and renal gluconeogenesis.[7] Acute hyperglycemia related to critical illness, also called stress hyperglycemia, is caused by release of the hormones norepinephrine, epinephrine, cortisol, and growth hormone and increases in the inflammatory mediators that lead to insulin resistance.[8] Hyperglycemia can increase proinflammatory cytokines, prothrombotic mediators, and oxidative stress.[9] External factors potentially contributing to hyperglycemia are the use of dextrose-containing intravenous admixtures and maintenance fluids as well as nutrition with high-carbohydrate tube feedings.[6] Hyperglycemia can also impair blood flow and cause decreased perfusion in patients with acute coronary syndromes.[10]

The deleterious effects of hyperglycemia are well documented in many organ systems throughout the body, and as such, it is important to address glucose status in all ICU patients. We will discuss the benefits to glucose management shown in the primary literature later in this chapter.

RANDOMIZED CONTROLLED TRIALS: TIGHT VS. MODERATE GLUCOSE MANAGEMENT

Ideal goal BG concentrations for critically ill patients remain a topic of controversy. In this section, we will review the primary literature comparing "tight" BG control with "moderate" BG control in the ICU.

Leuven SICU

A 2001 Belgian single-center, nonblinded, randomized controlled trial (RCT) of 1,548 patients, known as the Leuven SICU trial by Van den Berghe et al., compared treatment of surgical intensive care unit (SICU) patients with intensive or conventional glycemic control.[11] Most patients in this analysis were post-cardiac surgery (63% in the conventional arm and 62% in the intensive arm). This was the first large trial to show a decrease in morbidity and mortality associated with tight glycemic control in the ICU. The intensive arm aimed for a goal glucose of 80–110 mg/dL, whereas the conventional glycemic control arm treated patients to a goal glucose of 180–200 mg/dL. For the primary end point of mortality, a significant reduction was noted in the intensive arm (4.6% vs. 8%; p<0.04). Secondary outcomes that improved in the intensive glycemic control arm included in-hospital death (7.2% vs. 10.9%; p=0.01) and in-hospital death among those in the ICU for more than 5 days (16.8% vs. 26.3%; p=0.01). The increased mortality in the conventional arm can likely be attributed to the increased morbidity in several categories compared with the intensive glycemic control arm: need for renal replacement (8.2% vs. 4.8%; p=0.007), septicemia (7.8% vs. 4.2%; p=0.003), median number of red blood cell transfusions per patient (2 vs. 1; p<0.001), and polyneuropathy (51.9% vs. 28.7%; p<0.001). Hypoglycemia defined as a glucose value less than 40 mg/dL was increased in the intensive arm (5.1% vs. 0.8%; p<0.001).

Leuven MICU

Investigators tried to replicate the results of the SICU trial in the medical intensive care unit (MICU) at the same center.[12] Twelve hundred MICU patients were randomized to either intensive or conventional arms with identical goals. There was no significant difference in the primary end point of in-hospital mortality, which was 40.0% in the conventional treatment group versus 37.3% in the intensive treatment group (p=0.33). However, for patients who stayed in the ICU for 3 days or more, in-hospital mortality was reduced in the intensive insulin therapy arm (52.5% vs. 43%; p=0.009).

Significant differences in morbidity occurred in all patients receiving intensive insulin therapy (newly acquired kidney injury: 5.9% vs. 8.9%; p=0.04; earlier weaning from mechanical ventilation with intensive insulin therapy: hazard ratio 1.21; 95% confidence interval [CI], 1.02–1.44; p=0.03), with earlier discharge from the ICU (p=0.04) and the hospital (p=0.05). In the subgroup of patients in the ICU for more than 3 days, intensive insulin therapy compared with conventional therapy had a similar morbidity benefit between arms in accelerated weaning from mechanical ventilation (p<0.001), discharge from the ICU (p=0.002), and discharge from the hospital (p<0.001).

There was no difference in the need for new renal replacement therapy between arms, though fewer patients in the intensive treatment arm acquired kidney injury, defined as a serum creatinine doubling that at presentation (12.6% vs. 8.3%; p=0.05), and fewer patients in the intensive arm reached a peak serum creatinine concentration greater than 2.5 mg/dL (39.4% vs. 32.5%; p=0.04). Hyperbilirubinemia was also reduced in the intensive treatment group (55.2% vs. 47.3%; p=0.04). Hypoglycemia (less than 40 mg/dL) occurred more often in the intensive treatment arm (18.7% vs. 3.1%; p<0.001).

VISEP Trial

Brunkhorst et al. assessed intensive insulin therapy compared with conventional insulin therapy in severe sepsis in a multicenter, open-label, 2 × 2 factorial design that also randomized patients to receive 10% pentastarch or modified Ringer lactate.[13] The Efficacy of Volume Substitution and Insulin Therapy in Severe Sepsis (VISEP) trial recruited patients in 18 academic medical center ICUs within 24 hours of ICU admission. The intensive insulin therapy arm was suspended prematurely after a safety analysis of 537 patients showed an increase in hypoglycemia (less than 40 mg/dL) in the intensive insulin therapy group (17% vs. 4.1%; p<0.001). No significant difference between mortality and SOFA (Sequential Organ Failure Assessment) scores was noted between the intensive and conventional insulin therapy arms.

Glucontrol

In an attempt to replicate the results of the Leuven trials in a multicenter study, Preiser et al. published the Glucontrol study in 2009.[14] Glucontrol was initially designed to enroll 3,500 patients at 19 MICUs and SICUs into either an intensive (80–100 mg/dL) or a conventional (140–180 mg/dL) glycemic control arm. The trial was terminated early after randomizing only 1,101 patients after a high rate of unexpected protocol violations were detected. The intention-to-treat population that was evaluated for ICU mortality showed no significant difference, though the study was underpowered. As in previous trials, intensive insulin therapy was associated with significantly higher hypoglycemia (8.7% vs. 2.7%, p<0.001).

A post hoc analysis of the Glucontrol trial showed an increased odds ratio of survival in patients who had achieved at least 50% of cumulative time with BG at a goal of 80–100 mg/dL, though no significant differences in rate or severity of organ dysfunction were seen.[15] Given the methodological flaws of the study and the lack of protocol adherence, these findings should be hypothesis generating for future analyses of tight glucose control.

NICE-SUGAR Trial

The largest randomized trial to date comparing glycemic targets was the Normoglycemia in Intensive Care Evaluation-Survival Using Glucose Algorithm Regulation (NICE-SUGAR) trial.[16] In this study, 6,104 MICU and SICU patients with an expected ICU length of stay of 3 or more days were randomized to intensive (81–108 mg/dL) or conventional (140–180 mg/dL) glycemic control arms. No difference in mortality occurred at 28 days; however, at 90 days, mortality was increased in the intensive treatment arm (27.5% vs. 24.9%; p=0.02).

Unlike the prior two Leuven trials from Van den Berghe and colleagues, no notable differences in morbidity were seen despite the increase in mortality in the NICE-SUGAR analysis. No significant differences between arms were seen when comparing days on mechanical ventilation, positive blood culture, use of renal replacement therapy, or red blood cell transfusion.

A BG value of 40 mg/dL or less was seen more often in the intensive insulin therapy arm (6.8% vs. 0.5%; p<0.001). A post hoc analysis found an increased incidence of death in either arm (in patients whose death was not attributable to respiratory, arrhythmia, or neurologic causes) associated with severe (less than 40 mg/dL) hypoglycemia (p=0.002).[17] In the subgroup of patients with death from distributive shock, a significant correlation was seen with both moderate hypoglycemia (40–70 mg/dL) and severe hypoglycemia (p<0.001). Because the analysis was conducted post hoc, a causal relationship with hypoglycemia and mortality cannot be established.

Meta-analyses

Griesdale and colleagues published a meta-analysis that included 26 trials and 13,567 patients.[18] Although 26 studies were included, the five studies discussed in detail earlier accounted for 10,406 (76.7%) of the evaluated patients.

No significant difference in mortality was seen in any of the patients. When evaluating specific cohorts, patients in SICUs had decreased mortality when treated with intensive insulin therapy compared with standard therapy (7.4% vs. 11.8%; relative risk [RR] 0.93; 95% CI, 0.83–1.04); however, no mortality difference was seen in other ICUs. Rates of hypoglycemia were significantly increased in patients treated with intensive insulin therapy compared with the control arms (10.7% vs. 1.6%; RR 5.99; 95% CI, 4.47–8.03).

The authors concluded that intensive insulin therapy increased the risk of hypoglycemia without a benefit in mortality in the critically ill population; however, patients treated in SICUs may benefit from intensive insulin therapy.

Summary of the Primary Literature in Critically Ill Glucose Management

Randomized assessments of intensive versus conventional glucose management in critically ill populations provided mixed results. The most polarizing result, which remains under debate, is whether either an increase or a decrease in mortality is seen with intensive insulin therapy to a BG of 80–110 mg/dL, or whether any difference between the two interventions exists. The most likely cause for the variability in results is the heterogeneity of the patients, interventions, and statistical analysis of the trials. Table 5.1 highlights notable differences that may have affected the investigators' findings. The Leuven SICU trial's sample size was about one-fourth that of the NICE-SUGAR analysis, though the Leuven SICU enrolled more than 99% of the patients screened, whereas NICE-SUGAR's analysis ultimately excluded 85% of the patients screened. The patients in the Leuven SICU were predictably less sick than the patients in the Leuven MICU trial as well as in the analyses conducted in mixed ICUs, as evidenced by their lower Acute Physiology and Chronic Health Evaluation II (APACHE II) scores and mortality rates.

Nutritional support was provided parenterally in 85% of patients in both Leuven trials, compared with only 25% of patients in the NICE-SUGAR analysis, not only serving as a distinct display of different national standards of care, but also calling into question whether there was a difference in the amount of glucose in the form of nutrition supplied to patients who were treated without total parenteral nutrition (TPN).

The many protocol violations in the Glucontrol analysis that led to its premature end make it difficult to thoroughly evaluate the results' applicability to practice. Protocol violations, however, are a logistic problem in all of the previously mentioned trials, as well as in clinical practice. Adherence to institutional insulin protocols is variable to low, with many trials reporting adherence in the 61%–72% range.[19-22] Protocol violations of either correct frequency of monitoring or correct dose adjustment calculation can lead to hypoglycemic episodes or decreased time in therapeutic range. Protocol adherence of greater than 90% has been positively associated with greater time in therapeutic range.[22]

Hypoglycemia (less than 40 mg/dL) was significantly increased in the intensive insulin therapy arm in all five of the discussed trials (p<0.001 for all) (Figure 5.1). Of interest, the hypoglycemia that led to the early suspension of the intensive insulin therapy arm in the VISEP trial occurred less often than in the Leuven MICU study, which detected a mortality benefit in patients who were in the MICU for more than 3 days. That hypoglycemia was

Table 5.1 Randomized Controlled Trials of Glucose Control in the ICU					
	Leuven I	Leuven II	VISEP	Glucontrol	NICE-SUGAR
Population	SICU	MICU	Sepsis in mixed ICU	Mixed	Mixed
Centers	1	1	18	19	42
Sample size	1,548	1,200	488/537	1,101	~6,030
Excluded	14	863	1,612	?	34,067
Stopped early	No	No	Yes	Yes	No
Primary diet	TPN 85%	TPN 85%	60% TPN	27% TPN	25% TPN
Diagnosis of diabetes	13%	16.9%	30.4%	18.8%	20.1%
APACHE II	~9	~23	~20	~15	~21
Mortality	ICU: ~7% Hospital: ~10%	ICU: ~25% Hospital: ~40%	28 days: ~27%	ICU: ~16% Hospital: ~22%	28 days: ~21%
Protocol	Leuven	Leuven	Leuven	Variable	NICE
Target	80–110	80–110	80–110	80–110	81–108
Control	<180	<180	<180	140–180	144–180
Timing	ICU admit	ICU admit	<12 hr	Unknown	<24 hr
Duration	Entire ICU	Entire ICU	ICU/21 days	ICU or 56 days	Eating or 90 days

ICU = intensive care unit; MICU = medical intensive care unit; SICU = surgical intensive care unit; TPN = total parenteral nutrition.

significantly increased in all the intensive insulin therapy arms suggests a failure of the protocols and guidelines used by the study investigators.

Further suggesting a failure of the interventions used in the primary literature is the "glycemic separation" between the different analyses (Figure 5.2). Glycemic separation is defined as the difference between the mean BG values achieved in the intensive therapy arm and those achieved in the conventional therapy arm. Investigating this shows that of the five trials discussed, only the Leuven SICU analysis was able to reach a mean BG value within the specified goal range of 80–110 mg/dL, with a glycemic separation of 50 mg/dL between interventions. Patients in the NICE-SUGAR analysis in the conventional therapy arm had a mean BG of less than 150 mg/dL, and only a 27 mg/dL glycemic separation was shown between arms.

GUIDELINES FOR GLUCOSE MANAGEMENT IN THE ICU

Given the controversy in the results found in the primary literature for glucose management in the ICU, multidisciplinary guidelines play an important role in guiding therapy for health professionals. Recommendations on glucose management in the critically ill population are made by several professional organizations.

Society of Thoracic Surgeons

The first and most specific guideline with respect to target populations is the Society of Thoracic Surgeons (STS) practice guideline for blood glucose management during adult cardiac surgery.[23] The STS lists the following advantages to targeting BG values less than 180 mg/dL: reduced mortality, reduced morbidity, lowered incidence of wound infections, reduced hospital length of stay, and enhanced long-term survival. The STS thus recommends that cardiac surgery patients with BG values greater than 180 mg/dL receive intravenous insulin to maintain BG values below 180 mg/dL for the duration of their ICU stay (level A recommendation). The STS also recommends that patients requiring 3 or more days in the ICU have a continuous insulin infusion to keep BG values at 150 mg/dL or less (level B recommendation).

The Surgical Care Improvement Project (SCIP) as overseen by the Joint Commission made glucose management in cardiac surgery patients a reportable quality measure, citing the recommendations made in the STS guidelines. The SCIP recommendations allowed the incidence of cardiac surgery patients with a controlled postoperative BG (180 mg/dL or less) in the 18–24 hours after anesthesia to be a reportable inpatient quality measure until January 2015, when the Joint Commission announced that reporting of this measure is to be indefinitely suspended.[24] The Joint Commission cited the requirement not reflecting current clinical guidelines as the reason for the suspension.

ADA/AACE Consensus Statement

In 2009, the most recent consensus statement from the American Diabetes Association (ADA) and the American Association of Clinical Endocrinologists (AACE) on inpatient glycemic control was released.[25] For the subset of critically ill patients, it is recommended to initiate insulin therapy at a BG threshold of no more than 180 mg/dL, and a goal BG value of 140–180 mg/dL is recommended for most critically ill patients. They recommend using intravenous infusions as the preferred method of delivering insulin, as well as a validated intravenous insulin protocol with demonstrated efficacy and low rates of hypoglycemia.

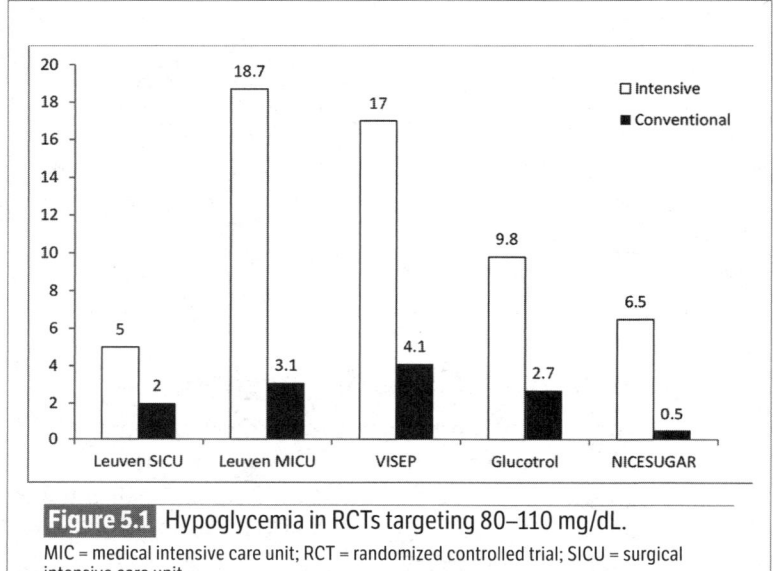

Figure 5.1 Hypoglycemia in RCTs targeting 80–110 mg/dL.

MIC = medical intensive care unit; RCT = randomized controlled trial; SICU = surgical intensive care unit.

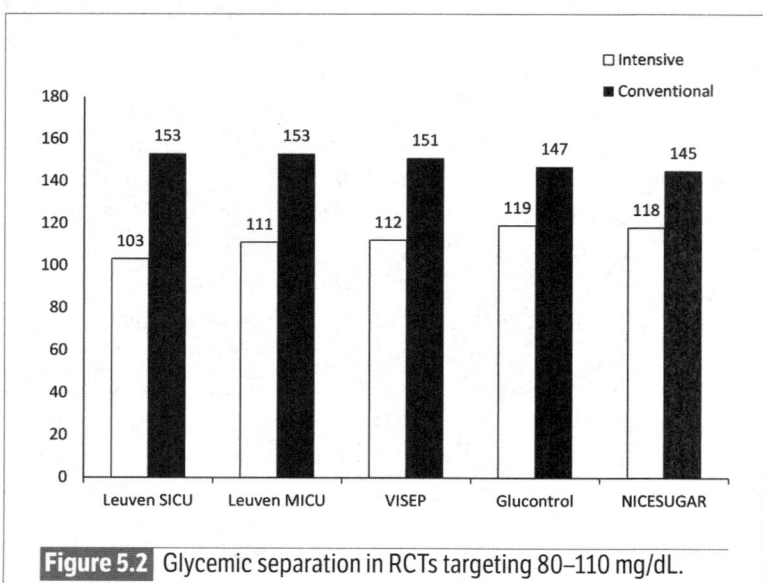

Figure 5.2 Glycemic separation in RCTs targeting 80–110 mg/dL.

American Diabetes Association

In the 2015 recommendations for critically ill patients, the ADA recommends initiating insulin therapy at a BG concentration of no more than 180 mg/dL, with a goal BG range of 140–180 mg/dL for most critically ill patients[26] (grade A recommendation). The guidelines concede, however, that tighter BG goals may be appropriate for selected patients if the intervention used to achieve them does not lead to increases in hypoglycemia (grade C recommendation). The guidelines recognize the failure of insulin protocols in RCTs, recommending that providers use an intravenous insulin protocol with demonstrated efficacy in achieving the desired glucose values without increasing the risk of severe hypoglycemia (grade E recommendation). The guidelines also strongly recommend against using sliding-scale insulin alone for hyperglycemia management in the hospital setting because of the reactive nature of sliding-scale insulin (grade A recommendation).

ACCM/SCCM

Further guidelines on using intravenous insulin in the critically ill population are offered from the American College of Critical Care Medicine/Society of Critical Care Medicine (ACCM/SCCM) guidelines published in 2012.[27] These guidelines recommend initiating insulin therapy when BG values are 150 mg/dL or greater (level of evidence: low) and state that most ICU patients should be treated to a BG goal of less than 150 mg/dL and absolutely less than 180 mg/dL using a protocol that shows low rates of hypoglycemia, suggesting that BG values of 70 mg/dL or less are associated with increased mortality and that even brief BG values of 40 mg/dL or less are independently associated with a greater risk of mortality (quality of evidence: low). Blood glucose less than 100 mg/dL should be avoided during insulin infusion for brain injury patients (quality of evidence: very low).

The guidelines offer no example of an intravenous insulin protocol, though they suggest that BG be monitored routinely every 1–2 hours for most patients receiving an insulin infusion (quality of evidence: very low). Monitoring for most patients on insulin infusion can be done using most point-of-care glucose meters, even though they are not optimal, cautioning clinicians to be aware of potential limitations in accuracy for patients with anemia, hypoxia, and interfering drugs (quality of evidence: very low). Patients in shock, on vasopressor therapy, or with severe peripheral edema, and for any patient on a prolonged insulin infusion, these guidelines suggest arterial or venous whole blood sampling instead of fingerstick capillary BG testing (quality of evidence: moderate).

Surviving Sepsis Campaign

Again, different recommendations are put forth in the 2012 Surviving Sepsis Campaign (SSC) guideline for initiation of therapy and BG target.[28] The 2012 guidelines recommend initiating a protocol for glucose management when two consecutive BG concentrations are greater than 180 mg/dL in patients with severe sepsis, targeting a BG concentration of 180 mg/dL or less (grade 1A). These guidelines, like the ACCM/SCCM guidelines, offer no recommended insulin infusion protocol, though they do recommend a monitoring regimen of every 1–2 hours until glucose values and insulin infusion rates are stable, followed by every 4 hours (grade 1C). The SSC guidelines also recommend caution with BG tests obtained by point-of-care testing (POCT) (ungraded recommendation).

American Society for Parenteral and Enteral Nutrition

Because nutritional support is not only an important ICU issue but also a major contributor to hyperglycemia in critically ill patients, official recommendations from nutritional support and organizations have also been put forth. The American Society for Parenteral and Enteral Nutrition (ASPEN) recommends a goal BG range of 140–180 mg/dL (strong recommendation), noting no clinical trial has established outcomes for different BG targets in patients receiving nutritional support.[29]

There is no clear consensus among professional organizations for the goal BG in critically ill patients, or recommendations on intravenous insulin protocols to achieve specific BG targets. The recommendations put forth in these guidelines are summarized in Table 5.2. This increases the need for vigilance at the institutional level to implement and rigorously evaluate glucose management in the ICU population using the multidisciplinary team approach.

Table 5.2 Summary of Recommendations of National/International Guidelines

	Goal BG in ICU	Definition of Hypoglycemia	Goal BG in Severe Sepsis	Guidance on Insulin Therapy
STS	< 180 mg/dL for cardiac surgery patients	None provided	None provided	Before intravenous insulin infusions are discontinued, patients should be transitioned to a subcutaneous insulin schedule using institutional protocols
ADA/AACE consensus statement	140–180 mg/dL	None provided	None provided	Use of validated insulin infusion protocols showed safety and efficacy, with low rates of hypoglycemia
ADA	< 150 mg/dL	< 70 mg/dL, severe: < 40 mg/dL	None provided	Avoid hypoglycemia
ACCM/SCCM	< 150 mg, absolutely < 180 mg/dL	< 70 mg/dL	None provided	Avoid hypoglycemia, monitor BG every 1–2 hr
SSC	None provided	Severe: < 40 mg/dL	< 180 mg/dL	Avoid hypoglycemia, monitor BG every 1–2 hr until glucose values and insulin infusion rates are stable, followed by every 4 hr
ASPEN	140–180 mg/dL	< 70 mg/dL	None provided	None provided

BG = blood glucose.

AREAS FOR FUTURE RESEARCH IN RCTS

Given the contradictory results of the RCTs, a more targeted approach to glucose management research in the ICU is necessary in future studies to fully understand the role of intensive insulin therapy and to best identify patients who may benefit from the intervention. In this section, we will briefly review end points that have yet to be rigorously studied prospectively.

Diagnosis of Diabetes vs. Non-diabetes

The question remains whether there should be different goal BG values for patients depending on prior to admission diabetes status. The question is based on the theory that in patients with diabetes, adaptation to a chronic hyperglycemic state may occur, and thus patients with diabetes do not benefit from glucose values of 80–110 mg/dL because a normoglycemic range for these patients may be higher.

A retrospective cohort analysis conducted by Lanspa et al. evaluated 3,529 patients using the same protocol, allowing providers to choose between 80–110 mg/dL and 90–140 mg/dL for a goal BG concentration, in 12 ICUs across eight hospitals.[30] After multivariate analysis, there was no significant difference in 30-day mortality between the groups with respect to glucose target. When stratified according to diabetic status, the multivariate analysis showed that the 90- to 140-mg/dL glucose target was independently associated with increased risk of mortality in patients without diabetes (p<0.05) but with decreased risk of mortality in patients with diabetes (p<0.01).

Similar to previous trials, significantly higher rates of severe hypoglycemia (less than 40 mg/dL) occurred in the cohort of patients who were treated to a goal of 80–110 mg/dL (3.6% vs. 2.0%; p<0.01). Mortality was increased in patients with at least one documented episode of severe hypoglycemia (17.3% vs. 10.3%; p<0.01). No difference in mortality was shown between goal glucose values for patients with a documented episode of severe hypoglycemia. The rate of severe hypoglycemia in this analysis was much lower than in the previously published analysis, suggesting an improvement in insulin intervention in this analysis compared with those in the RCTs described previously.

Glycemic Variability

Glycemic variability, introduced as a metric with which to monitor outpatients with type 2 diabetes mellitus, has yielded compelling results retrospectively in the critically ill population.[31] A pooled analysis of the Leuven MICU and SICU studies examined in depth some more specific glucometrics of the patients in the RCT, including a mean daily delta BG (mean of daily [maximum-minimum] BG) as a measure of glycemic variability and a standard deviation (SD) of all glucose values that were obtained electronically.[32]

Glycemic variability had a strong independent effect on mortality. Mean daily delta BG was significantly lower in survivors compared with non-survivors and, on multivariate analysis, was confirmed to be independently associated with mortality. The mean daily delta BG was lower in the SICU subgroup than in the MICU subgroup, raising questions regarding whether the mortality benefit in the SICU analysis may have been enhanced by the decreased glycemic variability in all patients. In the patients in the MICU subgroup, the SD of BG was lower in survivors than in non-survivors (p<0.001) and was an independent predictor of mortality using a multivariate analysis.

The ideal metric for studying glycemic variability is also a matter for debate.[33] In addition to those discussed previously, variables assessed retrospectively across analyses include the MGL (mean glucose level), an SD of MGL, and use of a coefficient of variation (SD/MGL). It is not yet clear which, if any, of these metrics, if targeted, will lead to a decrease in mortality. Although these variables continue to provide interesting data for retrospective analysis, accurate continuous glucose monitoring will need to be used for an analysis to prospectively optimize these metrics without creating excess risk of hypoglycemia.

Time in Target Range

As discussed previously, the gaps showed that goal BG values and BG values achieved in clinical trials are profound. Several factors play a role in this disparity, first of which is the method by which intravenous insulin is administered and titrated, which we will discuss further in the Medications section. Frequency and method of monitoring of BG may play the largest role in detecting BG values outside the goal range. For patients on intravenous insulin, previously published analyses show variability in the recommended monitoring intervals to as often as every 30 minutes for up to 4 hours in other published data sets. If BG values are out of a specified goal range and not detected and rectified in a timely manner, the benefits of the goal glucose range may not be fully realized.

New developments in medical technology will allow for continuous monitoring of whole BG to eliminate the need for capillary BG monitoring in the future, as well as allow real-time titration for medical providers.[34] Continuous BG monitoring could also decrease the occurrence of severe hypoglycemia. Challenges in implementing continuous BG monitoring will include the cost to institutions, both in equipment and in staff training. Although proprietary continuous BG monitoring systems have shown success in reaching BG values of 80–110 mg/dL with very small rates of severe hypoglycemia, these systems should next be evaluated in a randomized fashion against a conventional glucose management protocol cohort to evaluate for differences in morbidity and mortality as well as the development of hypoglycemia.

Monitoring in Critically Ill Patients

Because specific BG values are so closely linked with the treatment selected, it is important for members of the multidisciplinary team to understand the methods available for BG monitoring and the advantages and disadvantages of each method.

Frequency of BG Monitoring in the ICU

There is no primary literature showing the optimal BG monitoring regimen for patients in the ICU. Most ICU patients should have BG checks at least every 6 hours to screen for hyperglycemia.[35] Patients in the ICU on intravenous insulin should have BG testing hourly on initiation and whenever a rate change to the infusion takes place. More frequent BG testing should occur on any changes in their source of glucose such as held tube feeds. If aggressive monitoring is not done in patients on insulin infusions, episodes of hypoglycemia and hyperglycemia may be missed. Only when insulin rates are stable for several hours should less BG monitoring occur. Patients who can be treated subcutaneously and eat discrete meals can be tested preprandially and at bedtime.

Methods of Monitoring BG in the ICU

The most common methods for BG monitoring are bedside or POCT devices and laboratory determination using a sample obtained by venipuncture. Point-of-care testing devices usually use capillary blood obtained by fingerstick. Although the results are available within minutes, use of these devices requires training of nursing staff to ensure proper technique for adequate results. The convenience of use and fast result times with POCT devices remain their major benefits of use. Unfortunately, accuracy with using POCT devices is decreased compared with methods used in a central laboratory.[36] There is demonstrated variability between glucose meters as well as test trips that can vary from lot to lot. This is a fundamental issue with POCT BG monitoring systems because the U.S. Food and Drug Administration (FDA) requirement for accuracy is that displayed values be within 20% of the actual BG for all readings greater than 75 mg/dL.[37]

Point-of-care testing devices can measure blood samples from arterial, venous, or capillary blood, depending on the patient's available access points for nursing staff. Because reasonable variability is expected between each of these sites, patients should be consistently assessed at the same site. Comparing POCT results from different sites concurrently could lead to erroneous intervention, potentially leading to hypoglycemia or hyperglycemia.

Samples collected by venipuncture and sent to a central laboratory are usually processed with a whole blood analyzer or an arterial blood gas analyzer. These methods produce the most accurate results; however, using them takes considerably more time to collect the results, which may not be appropriate for the frequency of BG monitoring required for critically ill patients.[38]

To summarize, the risks and benefits of POCT compared with laboratory BG testing include many pros and cons. Starting with a cost consideration, using capillary whole blood is the least expensive method; however, it allows for the largest possibility of inaccurate results. Using an arterial catheter increases the cost and requires catheter changes every several days, depending on institutional standards. In an attempt to decrease the variability of BG readings from POCT devices, a formal internal training program should be implemented for use with all POCT devices for BG. This policy should dictate the use of only a single brand and model of POCT devices and the routine use of quality control solutions on all devices.

Controversies with POCT in Critically Ill Patients

The convenience of POCT for BG in the critically ill population has made it a standard of care in many ICUs. However, there is controversy about the appropriateness of this practice. In January 2014, an FDA memorandum stated that there was not yet a POCT device with labeled use in the critically ill population, and a guidance was released for what the FDA would request to label devices for use in the critically ill population.[39] This included an evaluation of meter precision so that 99% of all values achieved are within 10% of the reference method for BG values greater than 70 mg/dL. In April 2014, the American Association for Clinical Chemistry provided a rebuttal to the requirements put forth by the FDA, suggesting that they unnecessarily increase the regulatory burden and health care system costs without a demonstrable benefit in patient care.

In September 2014, the FDA approved the Nova Stat-Strip glucose hospital meter system for use in critically ill patients, making it the first POCT device for BG monitoring approved by the FDA.[40] Of note, the device is only meant to be used with arterial and venous blood samples, so the convenience of POCT devices using capillary blood samples is still an obstacle to overcome. It is anticipated that in the coming years, the Joint Commission, the accrediting body for Centers for Medicare & Medicaid Services reimbursement, will begin issuing citations to institutions using unapproved POCT for BG measurement in critically ill patients.

In March 2015, the FDA temporarily withdrew its initial memorandum and reissued it in draft form only.[41] The FDA stated that although off-label use of meters is not prohibited, additional safeguards should be in place when this practice is used. The FDA is currently obtaining more information on using POCT glucose monitoring systems from manufacturers and hospitals, as well as trying to promote education regarding requirements put forth under the Clinical Laboratory Improvement Amendments. This controversy has not yet been resolved and will continue to unfold and shape clinical practice for the next several years.

MEDICATIONS

In this section, we will discuss available medications and review their role in the treatment of the critically ill population.

Oral Antidiabetic Medications

Oral antidiabetic medications are generally not preferred in the acute setting for critically ill patients who may be experiencing decreased absorption from their gastrointestinal tract. Many oral antidiabetic medications rely on hepatic or renal metabolism or excretion. Because end-organ function may be fluctuating or impaired in critical illness, clearance of oral agents may be impaired. This can lead to increased adverse effects such as hypoglycemia with sulfonylureas or lactic acidosis with metformin. The 2009 ADA consensus statement states that noninsulin agents are inappropriate in most hospitalized patients.[25]

Insulin

Insulin therapy is usually the treatment of choice when managing hyperglycemia in the critically ill population. Insulin is versatile, considering the many available formulations and their ability to be administered by several routes. When deciding whether to treat a patient by the intravenous or subcutaneous route, many factors should be considered. In the acute phases of critical illness, patients may require vasopressor support and have rapidly changing insulin requirements, generalized edema, impaired subcutaneous perfusion, and/or variable nutritional support, all of which make the subcutaneous route nonideal for administering insulin in the critically ill patient.

Intravenous insulin infusions provide advantages over the subcutaneous route in critically ill patients with respect to rapidity of onset of effect and overall ability to achieve glycemic targets. With intravenous insulin, hypoglycemia occurs for shorter periods, whereas in the same patient receiving repeated subcutaneous doses of insulin, it may result in a "stacking" of the insulin's effect, causing protracted hypoglycemia, given that the pharmacologic effect of subcutaneous insulin is longer than that of intravenous insulin.

Intravenous Infusions

As discussed in the previous section on guidelines for glucose management in the ICU, intravenous infusions often require the use of an intravenous insulin protocol with demonstrated efficacy and safety in achieving desired glucose goals without increasing the risk of severe hypoglycemia.[27] A standardized trigger point should be set for initiating intravenous insulin in the critically ill patient. We recommend initiating an insulin infusion in ICU patients with at least one of the following:

- Critically ill with a BG greater than 180 mg/dL and an expected ICU stay greater than 3 days
- All with type 1 diabetes mellitus
- With an unstable clinical condition (e.g., steroids, pressors, variable nutrition) and at a high risk of hyperglycemia
- With BG persistently elevated and not controlled with subcutaneous insulin therapy

Intravenous insulin protocols may be initiated with or without a bolus dose. If electing to use a bolus dose, the bolus and initial rate of insulin should be based on the patient's BG concentration (Table 5.3). If not using a bolus dose, the initial rate of insulin should still be based on the patient's initial BG concentration (Table 5.4).

After initiating an insulin infusion, providers have options. We will compare two commonly used types of intravenous insulin titration protocols: the "fixed" insulin titration protocol and protocols that use an adjustment factor.

Fixed Protocol

A fixed insulin titration protocol refers to a protocol that recommends a change to the infusion rate only according to the current glucose concentration.[42] An example of a fixed insulin titration protocol can be found in Table 5.5.

The primary advantage of a fixed-dose titration is ease of use by the end user. Titrations of 1 unit/hour are unlikely to lead to

Table 5.3 Initiation of Intravenous Insulin Using Insulin Bolus

Blood Glucose (mg/dL)	Regular Insulin IV Push (units)	Insulin Infusion Rate (units/hr)
< 150	0	0.5
150–179	2	1
180–240	4	2
241–300	6	3
301–360	8	4
> 360	10	5

IV = intravenous.

errors in the administered amount. A primary disadvantage of using the fixed titration protocols is the lack of accounting for the rate of change in the patient's BG. For example, a patient with a BG value of 130 mg/dL would continue on the same rate of insulin currently being administered, regardless of whether the previous hour's BG value was 140 mg/dL or 300 mg/dL. For a patient who is changing more than 100 mg/dL over 1 hour, there is an increased likelihood that the BG value will continue to fall, placing the patient at a higher risk of hypoglycemia on the next BG check. These changes in glucose may not always be so dramatic because a downward trend in BG values could be seen for hours and not recognized until hypoglycemia occurs. Fixed intravenous insulin protocols typically do not differentiate between patients' variable levels of insulin sensitivity or resistance, which causes delays in achieving goal BG concentrations.

Adjustment Factor Protocols

Intravenous insulin titration protocols that account for the rate of change between hourly BG values are called adjustment factor protocols.[43] An example of an adjustment factor protocol can be seen in Table 5.6. On receipt of the current BG value, the bedside practitioner can examine the relationship with the previous hour's BG and the rate of change between the two. The bedside practitioner then multiplies the infusion rate according to the protocol.

Continuous titrations with an adjustment factor protocol require frequent calculations by bedside providers. This introduces a potential source for errors to be made in calculation, decreasing compliance with the protocol. To aid in calculation, institutions can have the continuous calculation done using a paper chart or electronic software.[44] Paper-based protocols may be more labor-intensive to bedside providers, though an evaluation of the example protocol provided earlier as a paper-based insulin titration was effective at achieving an average BG of 145 mg/dL with minimal hypoglycemic events.[20,45]

Software-based protocols provide an advantage to paper-based protocols in many ways. First, an electronic titration protocol removes the potential for human error with calculations on rate adjustments. An electronic protocol also provides the ICU team with an avenue to potentially change the glucose targets for a specific patient and to calculate

Table 5.4 Initiation of Intravenous Insulin Without Insulin Bolus

Blood Glucose (mg/dL)	Regular Insulin IV Push (units)	Insulin Infusion Rate (units/hr)
< 150	0	0.5
150–179	0	1
180–240	0	2
241–300	0	3
301–360	0	4
< 360	0	5

Table 5.5 "Fixed-Dose" Insulin Titration Protocol

BBG Value (mg/dL)	Action to Be Taken
< 50	• Stop insulin; give 25 mL of 50% dextrose; recheck BG in 30 min • When BG > 75 mg/dL, reinitiate with 50% of previous rate
50–75	• Stop insulin; if previous BG > 100 mg/dL, give 25 mL of 50% dextrose; recheck BG in 30 min • When BG > 75 mg/dL, reinitiate with 50% of previous rate
76–100	• If < 10 mg/dL lower than last test, decrease rate by 0.5 unit/hr • If > 10 mg/dL lower than last test, decrease rate by 50% • If ≥ last test result, maintain same rate
101–150	• Same rate
151–200	• If 20 mg/dL lower than previous test, maintain same rate • If higher than previous test, increase by 0.5 unit/hr

BBG = bedside blood glucose.

infusion rates using a rate of change to try to achieve a different glycemic target. Electronic protocols can account for insulin sensitivity across different patients and recommend more aggressive rate changes in resistant patients and less aggressive adjustments in sensitive patients, such as patients with type 1 diabetes mellitus. Electronic protocols also provide prompts for continued glucose monitoring at intervals that can be specified by the protocol, rather than have changes initiated by the bedside provider, as is done with the paper-based protocol.

Subcutaneous Basal/Bolus

Given the high-risk nature of insulin and the many available products, it is imperative that the ICU pharmacist be familiar with the different profiles of available insulin products. Table 5.7 summarizes these profiles.

When initiating a subcutaneous regimen, it is recommended to initiate a weight-based dosing regimen (0.3–0.5 unit/kg). The weight-based amount should be distributed to be administered to the patient throughout the day. Usual recommendations are for basal insulin to be 40%–50% of the total daily dose (TDD) and for nutritional insulin to be 50%–60%. When choosing to manage hyperglycemia in the critically ill patient by the subcutaneous route, it is important that each patient's regimen consist of three insulin types: basal, nutritional/prandial, and correctional.[35,46-48]

Basal

Basal insulin refers to the patient's insulin requirements that exist regardless of the patient's caloric intake. Basal insulin should be given to patients regardless of whether they are eating or not eating. Options for basal insulin can be either a once-daily dose of a long-acting insulin such as insulin glargine or insulin detemir or a twice-daily intermediate-acting insulin such as neutral protamine Hagedorn (NPH).

Nutritional

Critically ill patient situations are often unstable, and patients' caloric intake can fluctuate for several reasons such as nothing by mouth (NPO) for procedure, loss of nasogastric tube access, and emesis. For these reasons, it is important to separate out nutritional insulin administration from the previously mentioned basal insulin administration. It is also important that orders be written correctly to allow for acute changes in carbohydrate intake; in such instances, prandial insulin doses can be held to avoid causing episodes of hypoglycemia.

When choosing a nutritional or prandial insulin product, it is of utmost importance to distinguish the source of a patient's glucose intake. For patients who are on a continuous hourly rate of tube feeding or receiving TPN, providing a fixed dose of regular insulin every 6 hours should provide consistent coverage and avoid the stacking of insulin doses. For patients eating discrete meals or receiving

Table 5.6 Adjustment Factor Insulin Titration Protocol[a]

Current Blood Glucose (mg/dL)	Change in Blood Glucose Since the Prior Reading (mg/dL)				
	Decreased –30	Decreased 11–30	No Change ± 10	Increased 11–30	Increased –30
< 70	Hold insulin infusion and evaluate patient for hypoglycemia				
70–110	× 0.25	× 0.50	× 0.75	Continue current rate	× 1.5
111–150	× 0.50	× 0.75	Continue current rate	× 1.25	× 1.5
151–180	× 0.75	Continue current rate	× 1.25	× 1.5	× 2.0
181–210	Continue current rate		× 1.5		× 2.0
> 210	Continue current rate	× 1.5		× 2.0	

[a]The above protocol can be used as a guide for the ICU team to account for the rate of change of BG between hourly BG checks. With each new BG result available, the prescriber, nurse, or ICU pharmacist can examine the relationship with the previous hour's BG and the rate of change between the two. This chart will titrate to a mean BG of 145 mg/dL. The chart will then instruct the ICU team on how to adjust the insulin infusion rate according to a multiplication factor. Because calculations are often made for patients treated according to a protocol like this one, it is important to have safety checks in place to ensure the calculations are done accurately, either electronic or human double-check.

Table 5.7 Subcutaneous Profiles of Available Insulin

	Type	Onset	Peak	Duration
Rapid acting	Insulin aspart (NovoLog)	5–15 min	30–90 min	< 5 hr
	Insulin Lispro (Humalog)			
	Insulin glulisine (Apidra)			
Short acting	Regular insulin	30–60 min	2–3 hr	5–8 hr
Intermediate acting	NPH insulin	2–4 hr	4–10 hr	10–16 hr
Long acting	Insulin detemir	3–8 hr	Relatively peakless	6–23 hr
	Insulin glargine (Lantus)	2–4 hr	Relatively peakless	20–24 hr

bolus tube feeding, using rapid-acting insulin such as insulin aspart or insulin lispro before meals to cover the carbohydrate intake is preferred because the insulin analogs offer a profile similar to the natural pancreatic insulin production in response to carbohydrate intake.

Correctional Insulin

The final piece to a successful subcutaneous insulin regimen is correctional insulin, to be administered on top of, and at the same time as, the patient's prandial insulin. Correctional insulin is usually seen in the form of sliding-scale insulin. There should be different levels of sliding-scale insulin, designed for the patient's level of insulin sensitivity, which can be determined by counting the patient's daily requirement of insulin units. An example of sliding-scale insulin delivered according to scheduled insulin requirement can be found in Table 5.8.

An important point in managing hyperglycemia is to avoid monotherapy with sliding-scale insulin. The monitoring provided with a sliding scale is important information; however, managing hyperglycemia with only a sliding scale is reactive, rather than proactive, in avoiding hyperglycemia.

Transition from Intravenous to Subcutaneous

For patients initially treated with an intravenous insulin infusion, transition to a subcutaneous regimen should be considered when one of the following criteria is met:

- The patient is ready for transfer from the ICU
- The patient has been on a stable dose of the insulin drip for more than 24 hours; the glucose is controlled, and the patient is no longer critically ill

To transition patients from intravenous to subcutaneous insulin safely, the critical care pharmacist should:

1. Determine the TDD of insulin according to the insulin infusion rate for past 6 hours.
2. TDD = (average insulin drip rate for past 6 hours) × 24 hours
3. Reduce the TDD to around 80% of the above; because insulin is a protein, about 20% of the hourly rate of intravenous insulin will bind to intravenous bags or intravenous tubing and, as such, will not reach the patient.[49]
4. Give 50% of the TDD as basal insulin and 50% as nutritional insulin. If the patient is NPO, give 100% of TDD as basal insulin.
5. Give supplemental insulin sliding scale according to the TDD.
6. Stop the insulin drip 1–2 hours after the first dose of prandial insulin or 2–3 hours after the first dose of basal insulin is administered.

Example Patient Cases

1. Conversion from intravenous to subcutaneous insulin in a patient receiving nutrition. If the average insulin infusion rate for the past 6 hours is 2.5 units/hour:

   - TDD is 2.5 units/hour × 24 hours = 60 units
   - 80% of 60 units = 48 units
   - Basal insulin = 24 units/day
     - Insulin NPH 12 units every morning and 12 units every evening

   OR

     - Insulin glargine 24 units every morning or every evening
   - Nutritional insulin = 24 units/day
     - If the patient is eating discrete meals: 8 units of insulin aspart three times daily with meals
     - If the patient is on continuous tube feeds or TPN: 6 units of regular insulin every 6 hours
   - Correctional insulin
     - Discrete meals: insulin aspart with meals
     - Continuous tube feeds, TPN: regular insulin every 6 hours

Table 5.8 Example of Correctional Insulin Scales Based on Scheduled Insulin Requirement			
Blood Glucose (mg/dL)	**< 40 Units/Day Scheduled Insulin "Low Scale" (units of correctional insulin)**	**40–80 Units/Day Scheduled Insulin "Medium Scale" (units of correctional insulin)**	**> 80 Units/Day Scheduled Insulin "High Scale" (units of correctional insulin)**
150–199	1	1	2
200–249	2	3	4
250–299	3	5	7
300–349	4	7	10
> 349	5	8	12

2. Conversion from intravenous to subcutaneous insulin in a patient NOT receiving nutrition (NPO). If the average insulin rate for the past 6 hours is 2.5 units/hour:
    - TDD is 2.5 units/hour × 24 hours = 60 units
    - 80% of 60 units = 48 units
    - Basal insulin = 48 units/day
        - Insulin NPH 24 units every morning and 24 units every evening

OR

        - Insulin glargine 48 units every morning or every evening
    - Nutritional insulin = none
    - Correctional insulin
        - NPO: regular insulin every 6 hours

Medication Reconciliation

Many patients with a diagnosis of diabetes before their hospitalization will be on existing pharmacotherapy for managing the disease. It is often suggested to continue patients on their outpatient regimen on admission to the ICU. It is important to recognize that critically ill patients are often unstable, and as such, continuing a patient's home regimen may not be appropriate when patients are in the ICU. Patients' home regimens may incorporate oral agents that may cause toxicities when organ function is compromised, or consist of products that are not carried on an institution's formulary such as combination insulin products. Sources of carbohydrate intake are also likely to be variable in the ICU compared with the patient's prehospital glucose intake.

Considering all of the previously mentioned variables, no single algorithm is suitable for use in all ICU patients. Some patients may benefit most from an intravenous insulin infusion, whereas others may benefit most from a subcutaneous regimen. Monitoring BG values closely when the patient in the ICU is of paramount importance, and when reassessing medications on discharge from the ICU to non-ICU floors, it may be appropriate to reinitiate elements of a patient's home antidiabetic regimen.

Management of Hypoglycemia

When patients have hypoglycemia, swift intervention is required to minimize the potential for lasting adverse events. Signs and symptoms of hypoglycemia include confusion, diaphoresis, irritability, slurred speech, fatigue, disorientation, and, in severe cases, loss of consciousness, seizures, and decreased response to noxious stimuli.[50]

When hypoglycemia is suspected, a POCT glucose measurement should be obtained as quickly as possible. If patients are determined to be hypoglycemic with a symptomatic BG of 70 mg/dL or less, they will require treatment. If the patient is NPO or unresponsive and intravenous access is available, 12.5–25 g of dextrose 50% should be administered. If the patient is NPO or unresponsive and intravenous access is not available, 1 mg of glucagon intramuscularly should be administered. If a patient is responsive and able to receive enteral glucose, institutions should have a protocol in place to guide practitioners in administering 15–20 g of oral carbohydrate. Examples of rapid-acting carbohydrates are 4 oz of fruit juice or a non-diet soda, or 3 to 4 glucose tablets. After supplementation, the patient's BG values should be reassessed every 15 minutes until the BG is greater than 70 mg/dL. Providers should be cautious of overcorrecting with treatment of hypoglycemia, which could potentially lead to hyperglycemia. One retrospective analysis of critically ill patients who received dextrose 50% while on an insulin infusion showed that the median increase in BG was 4 mg/dL per gram of dextrose 50% administered.[51]

After stabilizing the hypoglycemic episode, the ICU team should try to identify the cause of the episode. Once the cause has been identified, modifications should be made to the patient's current management regimen, including glucose source and insulin regimen.

HYPERGLYCEMIC EMERGENCY MANAGEMENT

The most serious acute complications of hyperglycemia are DKA and HHS. Diabetic ketoacidosis most often clinically manifests with uncontrolled hyperglycemia, metabolic acidosis, and an increase in ketone production. Patients with HHS often present with dehydration, hyperglycemia, and hyperosmolality, usually in the absence of a significant acidosis. Most patients presenting with DKA have type 1 diabetes mellitus; however, patients having type 2 diabetes mellitus with a precipitating illness such as infection are also at risk of progressing to DKA.

Pathophysiology

Diabetic ketoacidosis and HHS are caused by a complex metabolic process that results from the combination of absolute or relative insulin deficiency. Episodes of DKA and HHS usually develop secondary to an underlying cause. The most common cause of DKA and HHS is infection.[52] Other common causes are inadequate insulin therapy (including patient nonadherence), pancreatitis, myocardial infarction, and medications. Severe dehydration that progresses to HHS can occur in chronic illnesses with decreased water intake, potentially because patients are bedridden. Many patients who develop HHS have no previous diagnosis of diabetes, so the development of HHS is not recognized in a timely manner, and treatment is not initiated early.

Many medications have been implicated as precipitating factors for hyperglycemic emergencies, including corticosteroids, thiazide diuretics, and atypical antipsychotic agents.

The initiating factor can cause hyperglycemia because of increased gluconeogenesis and decreased glucose use by peripheral tissues.[53] The hyperglycemic process can progress to DKA or HHS because of a combination of absolute or relative insulin deficiency and an increase in counterregulatory hormones such as glucagon. The resulting insulin deficiency and increased hormone productions will also lead to lipolysis from adipose tissue and increased hepatic ketone production, ultimately causing a metabolic acidosis.

Management

The most recent consensus statement from the ADA on the management of DKA and HHS was published in 2009. The ADA put forth treatment strategies, including monitoring, correction of fluid and electrolyte status, and insulin therapy for patients with DKA and HHS. We will discuss these treatment strategies in this section.

Laboratory Values/Diagnosis

Classifying the severity of episodes of DKA and HHS can be important when determining optimal treatment strategies as well as when determining the level of care patients will require on admission to the hospital. Table 5.9 describes the classification of severity of episodes of DKA and HHS. Severity of DKA is classified into mild, moderate, and severe DKA according to laboratory findings. Some patients may present with a mixed picture of both DKA and HHS.

Although DKA is not a diagnosis of exclusion, several other disease states can produce some of the same laboratory abnormalities. Alternative causes of ketoacidosis include starvation ketosis and alcoholic ketoacidosis; however, these cases often also present with uncontrolled hyperglycemia. A severe anion gap metabolic acidosis can present from several toxic ingestions such as ethylene glycol, salicylates, and methanol. For these reasons, it is important to do a thorough history, including previous drug use, to ensure an adequate diagnosis.

Fluids

Initially, the goal of fluid therapy should be to expand the patient's intravascular and interstitial volume because both are reduced in a patient with a hyperglycemic emergency. The resuscitation fluid of choice in a hyperglycemic emergency is 0.9% sodium chloride, initially infused at a rate of 15–20 mL/kg/hour, or as 1–1.5 L during the first hour. Patient-specific adjustments should be considered in patients with known cardiac or renal dysfunction to avoid causing dramatic fluid overload. After the initial bolus, the maintenance fluid rate should be based on physiologic parameters to maintain hemodynamic stability as well as the intravascular and extravascular volume. Providers should also calculate a corrected sodium (corrected sodium = measured sodium + 0.016 × [serum glucose 100 mg/dL]). If the corrected sodium is high or normal, use of 0.45% sodium chloride at a rate of 250–500 mL/hour is appropriate. If the corrected sodium is low, maintenance fluid resuscitation should continue with 0.9% sodium chloride. Hyperglycemia will likely resolve before the ketoacidosis has resolved; as such, providers should consider adding dextrose 5% in water in patients with DKA having a BG less than 200 mg/dL or an anion gap less than 12 and in patients with HHS having a BG less than 300 mg/dL or until osmolality is less than 315 mOsm/kg and until patients are mentally alert or receiving carbohydrates in the form of nutrition. Monitoring of serum chloride is also important because large volumes of sodium chloride–containing resuscitation fluids are often given to patients undergoing a DKA/HHS episode. Excessive chloride administration can lead to a prematurely closed anion gap, complicating assessment of the patient's acid-base status. In these patients, it may be appropriate to change to a non–chloride-containing resuscitation fluid.

Table 5.9 Classification of Severity of DKA and HHS

	Diabetic Ketoacidosis			Hyperglycemic Hyperosmolar State
	Mild (BG > 250 mg/dL)	Moderate (BG > 250 mg/dL)	Severe (BG > 250 mg/dL)	BG > 600 mg/dL
Arterial pH	< 7.30	7.00–7.24	< 7.0	> 7.3
Serum bicarbonate	15–18	10–14	< 10	> 18
Urine ketone	1–3+	1–3+	1–3+	Trace
B-hydroxybutyrate (mmol/L)	> 1	> 1	> 1	Trace
Serum osmolality	Normal to elevated	Normal to elevated	Normal to elevated	> 320 mOsm/kg
Anion gap	> 10	> 12	> 12	Variable

Electrolytes

In addition to monitoring sodium concentrations when determining the fluid and rate of resuscitation, other electrolyte abnormalities that need to be managed in patients having a hyperglycemic emergency include potassium, bicarbonate, and phosphate.

Potassium management in a patient with DKA/HHS can prove the most complicated. Many patients have a mild-moderate hyperkalemia on presentation. On initiation of fluid resuscitation, insulin therapy, and correction of the ketoacidosis, a shift toward decreased serum potassium concentration occurs. To prevent the occurrence of severe hypokalemia, it is recommended to initiate potassium supplementation when serum potassium concentrations fall below 5 mEq/L. This can be achieved using a potassium chloride–containing maintenance fluid. If severe hypokalemia occurs, patients may require placement of a central venous catheter to allow infusion of concentrated potassium chloride. If patients require greater than 10 mEq of potassium chloride per hour, cardiac monitoring should be initiated. In the rare case that patients having a hyperglycemic emergency are severely hypokalemic (potassium value less than 3.3 mEq/L) on presentation, insulin therapy should be delayed until a potassium value greater than 3.3 mEq is obtained.

Using sodium bicarbonate in DKA is controversial; current recommendations favor adding intravenous sodium bicarbonate only in patients with a severe acidosis (pH less than 6.9) who are hypotensive and not responsive to intravenous fluids.

Similar to potassium, serum phosphate concentrations also decrease after initiating insulin therapy. Currently, no benefit on clinical outcomes has been shown with phosphate supplementation of patients in DKA. Because of concern for excess phosphate supplementation causing hypocalcemia, routine phosphate supplementation is not recommended for patients with a phosphate concentration greater than 1.0 mmol/dL.

Insulin

Intravenous insulin therapy is the mainstay of therapy in patients with DKA and HHS in the ICU, though patients with an uncomplicated mild-moderate episode of DKA and HHS can be treated safely and effectively by a subcutaneous regimen. Patient-specific factors such as hemodynamic status and etiology of DKA/HHS should be considered when selecting the route of administration for insulin because severely ill patients may have decreased subcutaneous absorption.

An example of a weight-based intravenous insulin regimen is described in Table 5.10. Currently, debate exists about whether to initiate therapy using an intravenous bolus of insulin. If using an intravenous insulin bolus, the dose recommended is 0.1 unit/kg of actual body weight, and the initial rate of insulin should be 0.1 unit/kg/hour. If therapy is not initiated using an insulin bolus, it is recommended to initiate therapy at 0.14 unit/kg/hour. Hourly monitoring of BG is recommended, and strategies for adjusting the rate of insulin infusion can be found in Table 5.10.

The transition from intravenous insulin to subcutaneous insulin should take place once the DKA/HHS episode has resolved. Resolution of DKA is described as a BG less than 200 mg/dL and two of the following: serum bicarbonate greater than 15 mEq/L, venous pH greater than 7.3, and anion gap less than 12. Resolution of HHS is described as a BG less than 300 mg/dL, a plasma osmolality less than 315 mOsm/kg, and a patient who is mentally alert. It is critical to overlap the first dose of subcutaneous insulin with the infusion by 1–2 hours before discontinuing the infusion. Patients who were on a stable regimen of insulin before the DKA/HHS episode may be reinitiated on their previous regimen if the underlying cause of the emergency has been resolved. Patients who are insulin naive can be initiated on a weight-based subcutaneous regimen of 0.5–0.8 unit per day, split between a basal insulin and a nutritional insulin. A correctional component (sliding scale) of BG monitoring several times daily is also critical for a complete subcutaneous regimen.

Table 5.10 Intravenous Regular Insulin Management of Hyperglycemic Emergencies

Initial bolus dose (optional)	0.1 unit/kg
Initial rate	0.1 unit/kg/hr in patients who receive bolus
	0.14 unit/kg/hr in patients who do not receive bolus
If BG decreases < 10% in first hour	Administer intravenous bolus of 0.14 unit/kg and continue previous rate
If BG decreases > 75 mg/dL per hour	Decrease infusion rate to 0.05 unit/kg/hr
DKA: If BG is < 250 mg/dL	0.05 unit/kg/hr until anion gap is < 12
HHS: if BG is < 300 mg/dL	0.05 unit/kg/hr until osmolality is < 315 mOsm/kg

For patients determined to be appropriate candidates for subcutaneously administered insulin, recommendations for dosing can be found in Table 5.11. A similar rate of ketone reduction should be expected between patients who are treated with intravenous or subcutaneous insulin; however, until further research is available, subcutaneous insulin may not be ideal for patients with severe DKA, anasarca, or hemodynamic instability.

Follow-up and Diabetes Education

Although it may not be required while patients are in the ICU, consultation with an available local clinical management team such as endocrine or a diabetes management service should be considered for patients with complicated DKA/HHS or for patients with a new diagnosis of diabetes to provide a continuity of care when the patients go to the general ward and are eventually discharged. Diabetes education to enforce medication adherence, as well as to show how to recognize the signs and symptoms of hypoglycemia and hyperglycemia, may also be appropriate for patients who may be able to avoid progression to DKA/HHS in the future. Follow-up with existing or new diabetes outpatient providers should be ensured before discharge to prevent readmission.

TEAM APPROACH

Because insulin is a high-risk medication and the primary medication for inpatient management of hyperglycemia, implementing a safe and effective environment for glucose management in the ICU requires resources across several disciplines.[54] When implementing treatment protocols to optimize patient care outcomes and minimize adverse events, a standardized, multidisciplinary team approach should be used.

In this section, we will describe two main types of glucose teams: (1) the "multidisciplinary steering committee" with a focus on global oversight of glucose management for an institution and (2) the best practice "clinical management team" with a focus on bedside clinical management of a patient's glucose.[55]

Table 5.11 Management of Hyperglycemic Emergencies with Subcutaneous Insulin

	Subcutaneous rapid-acting insulin (aspart or lispro)
Initial dose	0.3 unit/kg
Subsequent dose	0.2 unit/kg every 2 hr
When BG is < 250 mg/dL	0.1 unit/kg every 2 hr

Multidisciplinary Steering Committee

The multidisciplinary steering committee's role is to provide global oversight of its institution's development and implementation of policies, order sets, protocols, and guidelines. The goals of the multidisciplinary committee should be individualized to the needs of the institution; these goals should be established and agreed on at the time of formation and maintained through future works. The multidisciplinary steering committee should focus on protocol development, implementation, and performance improvement. When forming committee goals, optimizing patient outcomes put forth by nationally established performance metrics should be primary points of interest for quality improvement projects and new initiatives.

Implementing a new guideline or protocol, or changing the current culture, should address a few key principles. A new directive or initiative should help simplify providers' ability to treat their patients while being highly reliable to ensure long-term compliance. Current workflow and patient care demands should be considered before implementing change because it will potentially have both a positive and a negative impact on current daily practice.

Metrics that can be assessed by the multidisciplinary committee include, but are not limited to, instances of BG less than 70 mg/dL stratified per patient-days, recurrent hypoglycemia, and percentage of BG readings per stay in the therapeutic range. The committee can also conduct medication use evaluations to evaluate hypoglycemia evaluation and treatment, intravenous-to-subcutaneous transitions, and efficacy and safety of insulin infusions.

Once a steering committee or task force team has been formed and subsequent committees and task forces have been identified, key stakeholders need to be informed of the intentions of this team. This is to ensure early adoption of the steering committee's or task force team's goals and directives and help plan educational efforts.[56] Stakeholders to consider are physicians from different patient care areas, particularly medical directors, the chief medical officer, the pharmacy and therapeutics committee, departmental committees, nursing leadership, nutrition services, and information and technology services, as well as all other parties involved in direct patient care. Sustained feedback from stakeholders is necessary to revise the goals and directives continually to ensure that the most current needs of the institution are being met.

Designated champions from each involved discipline may be necessary to implement the initiatives put forth by the multidisciplinary team on a departmental basis. Disciplines that should be involved in glucose management teams include pharmacists, physicians, nurses, data analysts, and nutritionists, among others. Because members of the steering committee often serve as liaisons to other institutional bodies, designated representatives of each discipline must be familiar with the principles of managing hyperglycemia and hypoglycemia in the critically ill population.

Once an area for improvement has been identified, the committee determines the best course of action for implementing change according to the expertise of its members and institutional support with resources. Guidelines and protocols are essential because they improve outcomes in BG management. A new policy, order set, protocol, or guideline may not always be the best option if existing guidance exists at the institution; however, existing protocols often need to be revised as more information becomes available from internal analyses. The goal of a committee should be to provide encompassing direction without overburdening staff with excess policies and guidelines.

The steering committee should anticipate and plan for barriers to successful implementation and have a system in place to monitor for success or opportunities for improvement once the change has been implemented.

For critically ill patients, the focus should be placed on identifying the causes of hypoglycemia and developing protocols for intravenous insulin infusions and transitioning patients from infusions to subcutaneous insulin regimens during the transition to general wards. Administering intravenous insulin requires trained nurses with explicit instructions for use. Because of the increased workload on ICU nurses administering intravenous insulin, it is critical to address nursing concerns when implementing changes as well as to have extensive educational sessions surrounding implementation. A key part of this education should be focused on how the proposed change works and the impact the change will have on nurses' daily lives. Describing the rationale to bedside staff will create allies for future changes and will often increase awareness of why changes are needed once the efforts have begun. Example guidelines for intravenous insulin protocols and converting a patient from an intravenous insulin infusion to a subcutaneous regimen can be found in the Medications section of this chapter.

Other specialized guidelines or protocols pertinent to patient care include those regarding DKA or HHS. Creating and adhering to these protocols improve clinical outcomes without increasing the incidence of adverse events such as hypoglycemia.[57]

Clinical Management Team

In addition to the steering committee, some health care systems may have a "clinical management team" doing consultative services for individual patients. The order sets, protocols, and guidelines developed by the steering committee should assist multidisciplinary providers in treating most patients. Complex patient cases in the acute care setting may require assistance beyond what is offered by these guidelines, and in these cases, the clinical management team serves to offer expert guidance. Clinical management teams can include endocrinologists, endocrine fellows, hospitalists, nurse practitioners, physician assistants, and clinical pharmacists. In addition to bedside practice, the clinical management team can be involved in staff education, discharge planning and counseling, and facilitating change in culture.

One example of a clinical management service consisted of a nurse practitioner, physician assistant, endocrine fellow, and attending endocrinologist who provided consults to surgical patients.[56] The team used hospital glucose treatment protocols, with a clinically acceptable BG range of 80–180 mg/dL, to treat patients as they transitioned from intravenous to subcutaneous insulin therapy while minimizing significant hypoglycemia (less than 60 mg/dL) and hyperglycemia (greater than 400 mg/dL). The management service achieved clinically acceptable BG concentrations in 74.3% of the glycemic values with low rates of hypoglycemia and hyperglycemia, which was accepted by the surgical staff. An observational analysis of a clinical management team using a designated group of pharmacists yielded similar results. The team worked on a consultation basis using a protocol to manage perioperative dysglycemia during hospitalization with goal point-of-care BG values of 70–180 mg/dL.[58] The main aims of the protocol used in this analysis targeted appropriate use of intravenous and subcutaneous insulin, including titration and how to transition to a subcutaneous regimen. A total of 1,294 patients in the preintervention group were compared with 4,842 patients in the postintervention. The analysis showed a 12.9% increase in patient-days with goal glycemic control (90.3% vs. 77.4%) with a decrease in hypoglycemia, defined as a point-of-care BG less than 70 mg/dL, of 4% (4.6% vs. 8.6%). Using this protocol and the glycemic control team improved both the efficacy and the safety of glucose management in a perioperative patient population.

In addition to improved patient care, the clinical management service model may generate revenue if advanced practice clinicians are able to bill for consultation services.[59] An unfortunate potential cultural shift to instituting a clinical management team for glucose management is the perception that interns and residents may be less engaged in managing glucose therapy and may start to refer uncomplicated patients to the clinical management team.

Glucose management in the inpatient setting requires a multidisciplinary team approach. Creating a steering committee or task force focused on development, oversight, implementation, and quality assessment and improvement can standardize and coordinate glucose management measures within an institution. Clinical glucose management teams with a focus on direct patient care may also help improve patient outcomes.

CONCLUSION

Glucose management is an important issue in the treatment of all critically patients. Episodes of hypoglycemia and hyperglycemia alike can increase morbidity, length of stay, and mortality. Many aspects of glucose management in the critically ill population remain controversial, including monitoring, treatment goals, and the ideal intravenous insulin protocol. These challenges have led to glucose management as a popular area for research as well as a quality measure for accrediting bodies. Because of the high-risk nature of the medications involved in glucose management, the ICU pharmacist can play a significant role in ensuring the safe and effective management of their patients' BG values.

REFERENCES

1. Krinsely JS. Association between hyperglycemia and increased hospital mortality in a heterogeneous population of critically ill patients. Mayo Clin Proc 2003;78:1471-8.
2. Estrada CA, Young JA, Nifong LW, et al. Outcomes and perioperative hyperglycemia in patients with or without diabetes mellitus undergoing coronary artery bypass grafting. Ann Thorac Surg 2003;75:1392-9.
3. Bagshaw SM, Egi M, George C, et al.; Australia New Zealand Intensive Care Society Database Management Committee. Early blood glucose control and mortality in critically ill patients in Australia. Crit Care Med 2009;37:463-70.
4. Pasquel FJ, Spiegelman R, McCauley M, et al. Hyperglycemia during total parenteral nutrition: an important marker of poor outcome and mortality in hospitalized patients. Diabetes Care 2010;33:739-41.
5. Schlenk F, Vajkoczy P, Sarrafzadeh A. Inpatient hyperglycemia following aneurysmal subarachnoid hemorrhage: relation to cerebral metabolism and outcome. Neurocrit Care 2009;11:56-63.
6. Smith WD, Winterstein AG, Johns T, et al. Causes of hyperglycemia and hypoglycemia in adult inpatients. Am J Health Syst Pharm 2005;62:714-9.
7. Turina M, Fry DE, Polk HC. Acute hyperglycemia and the innate immune system: clinical, cellular, and molecular aspects. Crit Care Med 2005;33:1624-33.
8. Mizock BA. Alterations in carbohydrate metabolism during stress: a review of the literature. Am J Med 1995;98:75-84.
9. McCowen KC, Malhotra A, Bistrian BR. Stress-induced hyperglycemia. Crit Care Clin 2001;17:107-24.
10. Kosiborod M, Inzucchi SE, Krumholz HM, et al. Glucometrics in patients hospitalized with acute myocardial infarction. Circulation 2008;117:1018-27.
11. Van den Berghe G, Wouters P, Weekers F, et al. Intensive insulin therapy in critically ill patients. N Engl J Med 2001;345:1359-67.
12. Van den Berghe G, Wilmer A, Hermans G, et al. Intensive insulin therapy in the medical ICU. N Engl J Med 2006;354:449-61.
13. Brunkhorst FM, Engel C, Bloos F, et al. Intensive insulin therapy and pentastarch resuscitation in severe sepsis. N Engl J Med 2008;358:125-39.
14. Preiser JC, Devos P, Ruiz-Santana S, et al. A prospective randomised multi-centre controlled trial on tight glucose control by intensive insulin therapy in adult intensive care units: the Glucontrol study. Intensive Care Med 2009;35:1738-48.
15. Penning S, Chase JG, Preiser JC, et al. Does the achievement of an intermediate glycemic target reduce organ failure and mortality? A post hoc analysis of the Glucontrol trial. J Crit Care 2014;29:374-9.
16. Finfer S, Chittock DR, Su SY, et al. Intensive versus conventional glucose control in critically ill patients. N Engl J Med 2009;360:1283-97.
17. Finfer S, Liu B, Chittock DR, et al. Hypoglycemia and risk of death in critically ill patients. N Engl J Med 2012;367:1108-18.
18. Griesdale DE, de Souza RJ, van Dam RM, et al. Intensive insulin therapy and mortality among critically ill patients: a meta-analysis including NICE-SUGAR study data. CMAJ 2009;180:821-7.
19. Malesker MA, Foral PA, McPhillips AC, et al. An efficiency evaluation of protocols for tight glycemic control in intensive care units. Am J Crit Care 2007;16:589-98.
20. Cyrus RM, Szumita PM, Greenwood BC, et al. Evaluation of compliance with a paper-based, multiplication-factor, intravenous insulin protocol. Ann Pharmacother 2009;43:1413-8.
21. Oeyen SG, Hoste EA, Roosens CD, et al. Adherence to and efficacy and safety of an insulin protocol in the critically ill: a prospective observational study. Am J Crit Care 2007;16:599-608.
22. Dickerson RN, Johnson JL, Maish GO III, et al. Evaluation of nursing adherence to a paper-based graduated continuous intravenous regular human insulin infusion algorithm. Nutrition 2012;28:1008-11.
23. Lazar HL, McDonnell M, Chipkin SR, et al. The Society of Thoracic Surgeons practice guideline series: blood glucose management during adult cardiac surgery. Ann Thorac Surg 2009;87:663-9.
24. Joint Commission Online. January 28, 2015. Available at www.jointcommission.org/assets/1/23/jconline_January_28_15.pdf. Accessed February 24, 2015.
25. Moghissi ES, Korytkowski MT, DiNardo M, et al. American Associate of Clinical Endocrinologists and American Diabetic Association consensus statement on inpatient glycemic control. Endocr Pract 2009;15:353-69.
26. American Diabetes Association (ADA). Diabetes care in the hospital, nursing home, and skilled nursing facility. Diabetes Care 2015;38(suppl):S80-5.
27. Jacobi J, Bircher N, Krinsley J, et al. Guidelines for the use of an insulin infusion for the management of hyperglycemia in critically ill patients. Crit Care Med 2012;40:3251-76.
28. Dellinger RP, Levy MM, Rhodes A, et al. Surviving Sepsis Campaign: international guidelines for management of severe sepsis and septic shock: 2012. Crit Care Med 2013;41:580-637.
29. McMahon MM, Nystrom E, Braunschweig C, et al. A.S.P.E.N. clinical guidelines: nutrition support of adult patients with hyperglycemia. JPEN J Parenter Enteral Nutr 2013;37:23-36.
30. Lanspa MJ, Hirshberg EL, Phillips GD, et al. Moderate glucose control is associated with increased mortality compared with tight glucose control in critically ill patients without diabetes. Chest 2013;143:1226-34.
31. Monnier L, Mas E, Ginet C, et al. Activation of oxidative stress by acute glucose fluctuations compared with sustained chronic hyperglycemia in patients with type 2 diabetes. JAMA 2006;295:1681-7.

32. Meyfroidt G, Keenan DM, Wang X, et al. Dynamic characteristics of blood glucose time series during the course of critical illness: effects of intensive insulin therapy and relative association with mortality. Crit Care Med 2010;38:1021-9.

33. Krinsley JS. Glycemic variability in critical illness and the end of chapter 1. Crit Care Med 2010;38:1206-8.

34. Joseph JI, Hipszer B, Mraovic B, et al. Clinical need for continuous glucose monitoring in the hospital. J Diabetes Sci Technol 2009;3:1309-18.

35. Clement S, Braithwaite SS, Magee MF, et al. Management of diabetes and hyperglycemia in hospitals. Diabetes Care 2004;27:553-91.

36. Atkin SH, Dasmahapatra A, Jaker M, et al. Fingerstick glucose determination in shock. Ann Intern Med 1991;114:1020-4.

37. U.S. Food and Drug Administration (FDA). Blood Glucose Monitoring Test Systems for Prescription Point-of-Care Use Draft Guidance for Industry and Food and Drug Administration Staff. Available at www.fda.gov/downloads/MedicalDevices/DeviceRegulationandGuidance/GuidanceDocuments/UCM380325.pdf. Accessed February 23, 2015.

38. Inoue S, Egi M, Kotani J, et al. Accuracy of blood-glucose measurements using glucose meters and arterial blood gas analyzers in critically ill adult patients: systematic review. Crit Care 2013;17:R48.

39. The American Association for Clinical Chemistry (AACC) Comment on the Food and Drug Administration's (FDA's) January 7, 2014 draft guidance, "Blood Glucose Monitoring Test Systems for Prescription Point-of Care Use." Available at www.aacc.org/~/media/files/legislative-issues/2014/aaccbgmscomments-429.pdf?la=en. Accessed February 23, 2015.

40. FDA Clears Glucose Monitoring System for Use in Hospital Critical Care Units. FDA News Release. Available at www.fda.gov/NewsEvents/Newsroom/PressAnnouncements/ucm416144.htm. Accessed February 23, 2015.

41. Centers for Medicare & Medicaid Services. Reissuance of S&C 15-11 As DRAFT ONLY – FOR COMMENT. Off-Label/Modified Use of Waived Blood Glucose Monitoring Systems (BGMS). Available at www.cms.gov/Medicare/Provider-Enrollment-and-Certification/SurveyCertificationGenInfo/Downloads/Survey-and-Cert-Letter-15-11.PDF. Accessed June 23, 2015.

42. Furnary AP, Wu Y, Bookin SO. Effect of hyperglycemia and continuous intravenous insulin infusions on outcomes of cardiac surgical procedures: the Portland Diabetic Project. Endocr Pract 2004;10(suppl 2):21-33.

43. Osburne RC, Cook CB, Stockton L, et al. Improving hyperglycemia management in the intensive care unit: preliminary report of a nurse-driven quality improvement project using a redesigned insulin infusion algorithm. Diabetes Educ 2006;32:394-403.

44. Davidson PC, Steed RD, Bode BW. Glucommander: a computer-directed intravenous insulin system shown to be safe, simple, and effective in 120,618 h of operation. Diabetes Care 2005;28:2418-23.

45. Wong S, Anger KE, Frawley B, et al. Glucometric assessment of a moderate versus intensive paper-based intravenous insulin protocol at a tertiary academic medical center. Crit Care Med 2010;38(suppl):70.

46. Hirsch IB. Insulin analogues. N Engl J Med 2005;352:174-83.

47. American Diabetes Association (ADA). Standards of medical care in diabetes—2010. Diabetes Care 2010;33(suppl 1):S11-S61.

48. Rodbard HW, Blonde L, Braithwaite SS, et al. American Association of Clinical Endocrinologists medical guidelines for clinical practice for the management of diabetes mellitus. Endocr Pract 2007;13(suppl 1):1-68.

49. Rocchio MA, Belisle CD, Greenwood BC, et al. Evaluation of the maximum beyond-use-date stability of regular human insulin extemporaneously prepared in 0.9% sodium chloride in a polyvinyl chloride bag. Diabetes Metab Syndr Obes 2013;6:389-92.

50. Tomky D. Detection, prevention, and treatment of hypoglycemia in the hospital. Diabetes Spectr 2005;18:39-44.

51. Murthy MS, Duby JJ, Parker PL, et al. Blood glucose response to rescue dextrose in hypoglycemic, critically ill patients receiving an insulin infusion. Ann Pharmacother 2015;49:892-6.

52. Kitabchi AE, Umpierrez GE, Miles JM, et al. Hyperglycemic crises in adult patients with diabetes. Diabetes Care 2009;32:1335-43.

53. Delaney MF, Zisman A, Kettyle WM. Diabetic ketoacidosis and hyperglycemic hyperosmolar nonketotic syndrome. Endocrinol Metab Clin North Am 2000;29:683-705.

54. Anger KE, Szumita PM. Barriers to glucose control in the intensive care unit. Pharmacotherapy 2006;26:214-28.

55. Szumita PM, Reardon DP. Team approach for glucose management. In: Garg R, Hudson M, eds. Hyperglycemia in the Hospital Setting. Philadelphia: Jaypee Brothers, 2014:100-8.

56. DeSantis AJ, Schmeltz LR, Schmidt K, et al. Inpatient management of hyperglycemia: the northwestern experience. Endocr Pract 2006;12:491-505.

57. Beik N, Anger KE, Forni AA, et al. Evaluation of an institution-wide guideline for hyperglycemic emergencies at a tertiary academic medical center. Ann Pharmacother 2013;47:1260-5.

58. Mularski KS, Yeh CP, Bains JK, et al. Pharmacist glycemic control team improves quality of glycemic control in surgical patients with perioperative dysglycemia. Perm J 2012;16:28-33.

59. Magee MF, Beck A. Practical strategies for developing the business case for hospital glycemic control teams. J Hosp Med 2008;3:76-83.

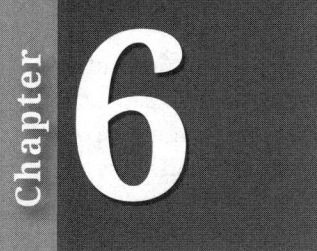

Chapter 6: Analgesia

Asad E. Patanwala, Pharm.D.

LEARNING OBJECTIVES

1. Describe the incidence of pain, consequences of inadequate treatment, and unique challenges pertinent to analgesia in the critically ill.
2. Design a plan for the assessment of pain in communicative and noncommunicative patients.
3. Construct an analgosedation approach for the management of patient comfort.
4. Compare and contrast commonly used opioids in the intensive care unit (ICU).
5. Explain the role of non-opioids as part of a multimodal plan for the management of pain.
6. Describe evidence to support nonpharmacologic therapy for the provision of analgesia.
7. Discuss the evidence to support the use of ketamine in the critically ill.
8. Develop a strategy to optimize pain management during procedures.
9. Explain concepts pertaining to opioid conversions in the ICU.
10. Design an approach to optimize pain control during transition from the ICU to the general ward.

ABBREVIATIONS IN THIS CHAPTER

BPS	Behavioral Pain Scale	NSAID	Nonsteroidal anti-inflammatory agent
CPOT	Critical-Care Pain Observation Tool	VAS-H	Visual Analog Scale-Horizontal
ICU	Intensive care unit	VAS-V	Visual Analog Scale-Vertical
NRS-O	Numeric rating scale-oral	VDS	Verbal descriptor scale
NRS-V	Numeric rating scale-visual		

INTRODUCTION

Most patients who are admitted to the intensive care unit (ICU) will experience pain, and the optimal management of pain is humane, necessary, and a basic human right.[1,2] The definition of pain according to the International Association for the Study of Pain is an "unpleasant sensory and emotional experience associated with actual or potential tissue damage, or described in terms of such damage."[3] This definition is not unique to the critically ill population, but it highlights the fact that pain is subjective, and the best assessment is one that is self-reported. Thus, good communication between patients and providers is crucial for optimizing patient comfort. However, self-reported pain in the ICU is only possible in a subset of patients who can communicate, either verbally or nonverbally. But the absence of self-report, which is the norm in most critically ill patients, should not be construed as a lack of pain. Thus, additional precautions need to be taken in these patients.[4]

Critically ill patients usually have several sources of pain, including injury, surgery, acute illness, and comorbidities. Some patients may have chronic pain conditions before ICU admission, amplifying the pain experienced during critical illness. In addition, diagnostic and therapeutic procedures commonly done in the critically ill population such as turning, endotracheal suction, wound dressing changes and drain removal, incision and drainage, chest tube placement and removal, and central line placement, among others, are a great source of pain and discomfort.[5] Prolonged mechanical ventilation itself can be a very bothersome and stressful experience for patients.[6] The inadequate management of pain can have long-term physiological and psychological consequences. Stressors such as pain in the ICU have been associated with negative effects on health-related quality of life and posttraumatic stress syndrome.[7,8] This occurs to a greater extent as the severity of illness increases.[9]

In this chapter, the appropriate assessment of pain in communicative and noncommunicative patients is discussed because this serves as the foundation for optimizing drug therapy use for the treatment of pain. Analgesia and sedation are interrelated, and both need to be optimized for patient comfort. This chapter focuses on analgesics and their role in the provision of analgesia-based sedation. Therapeutic options are discussed, including the commonly used opioids, and non-opioids, for somatic and neuropathic pain. The role of nonpharmacologic therapy is also briefly examined. Finally, special situations that commonly occur in the ICU such as pain management during procedures, concepts pertaining to opioid conversions, and optimizing the transition from the ICU to the general ward are reviewed to provide a comprehensive understanding of all aspects of analgesia in the ICU.

PAIN ASSESSMENT

Adequate pain assessment that incorporates the unique characteristics of the critically ill population serves as a foundation for optimal pain management. The systematic evaluation of pain and agitation, together with an effective management plan, not only decreases the incidence of pain and agitation, but also results in a decreased duration of mechanical ventilation, lower incidence of nosocomial infections, and shorter ICU length of stay.[10,11] This was shown in a two-phase prospective study in which a systematic evaluation plan was implemented that included a routine assessment of pain at rest, during and after any procedures, and several other times during the day by bedside nurses.[10] This was then promptly communicated to physicians, which led to many therapeutic changes. The incidence of pain decreased significantly in the intervention group (63% vs. 42%, p=0.002). The duration of mechanical ventilation was greatly reduced (120 vs. 65 hours, p=0.01); similarly, the incidence of nosocomial infections decreased from 17% to 8% (p<0.05). This was confirmed in a subsequent propensity-adjusted cohort study in which pain assessment on day 2 of hospitalization was associated with a shorter duration of mechanical ventilation (8 vs. 11 days, p<0.01) and shorter duration of stay in the ICU (13 vs. 18 days, p<0.01).[11]

The ideal pain scale for assessment should be valid, reliable, and feasible. Given that there is currently no known or readily available objective biological measure to assess pain, the gold standard for assessment is patient self-report. In the ICU, some patients are communicative and able to report pain, even if they are unable to verbalize because of the presence of an endotracheal tube. In these patients, common self-report pain scales can be used. However, the self-report scale used must consider the method of nonverbal communication and the patient's motor skills (e.g., ability to write or gesture). In most patients, communication is not possible; thus, pain must be assessed by observing patient behavior. According to the Society of Critical Care Medicine guidelines, pain should typically be assessed at least four times every nursing shift (e.g., every 3 hours) and as needed such as before, during, and after procedures, as well as before and after the provision of analgesics.[1] Note that vital signs can only serve as a cue to further assessment using a validated scale and should not be used as the sole assessment to base treatment decisions. This is because hemodynamic measures such as blood pressure and heart rate are nonspecific to pain and are unreliable measures in the ICU.[12]

Communicative Patients

Before choosing the correct pain assessment tool, critically ill patients should be evaluated for their ability to interact using verbal or nonverbal communication. The pain scale chosen may need to change in the course of hospitalization. Early during ICU care, patients may be unable to communicate at all; however, as they progress, nonverbal communication may be possible, and after extubation, patients may be able to verbalize their pain. Commonly used self-report scales in the ICU setting include the Visual Analog Scale, which is available in a horizontal or vertical orientation (VAS-H or VAS-V); the verbal descriptor scale (VDS); and the numeric rating scale, which can be administered orally or visually (NRS-O or NRS-V). The VAS is a 10-cm line that is anchored at the ends with the words "no pain" and "extreme pain." Patients then choose a point on the line that best represents their pain. Drawbacks of using this scale in the ICU include the need to measure distance on the line to calculate pain severity, ability to write with manual dexterity, and appropriate vision, which can often be impractical from a nursing perspective and challenging for patients. The VDS was derived from the Present Pain Index component of the McGill Pain Questionnaire.[13] Although the number of verbal descriptors can vary, a 5-descriptor scale has been suggested as adequate.[14] Patients are asked to choose from the phrase that best describes their pain, which includes "no pain," "mild pain," "moderate pain," "severe pain," and "extreme pain." The NRS-O is perhaps the most common pain scale used in adult hospitalized patients. Patients verbalize a number from 0 to 10, which best represents their pain severity, with 0 being "no pain" and 10 being the "worst possible pain." It is important that the clinician administering the NRS-O use consistent wording for the anchors to the scale because using different descriptions provided to patients has the potential to affect pain scores. Both the VDS and the NRS-O require verbal input from patients and thus may not be possible in many critically ill patients. One alternative in patients who are unable to verbalize is a visual scale such as the NRS-V. This is an enlarged plastic laminated scale (e.g., 4 × 12 inches) anchored at opposite ends with 0 "no pain" and 10 "extreme pain" (Figure 6.1). Patients can then point to numbers directly on the scale or hold up the appropriate number of fingers indicative of their pain score with one or both hands. One study compared the use of these scales in 111 ICU patients who were communicative.[15] The response rate measured before and after analgesic use or painful procedure was highest for the NRS-V (91%), followed by the NRS-O (83%), VDS (78%), VAS-H (68%), and VAS-V (66%). The authors concluded that the NRS-V should be the self-report tool of choice for assessing pain in ICU patients.

Noncommunicative Patients

In patients unable to communicate, observation of patient behaviors using a structured scale is possible with behavioral pain scales. Several scales have been developed for this purpose, including the Behavioral Pain Scale (BPS), BPS-Non-intubated (BPS-NI), Critical-Care Pain Observation Tool (CPOT), Nonverbal Pain Scale (initial or revised), Pain Behavioral Assessment Tool, and Pain Assessment Intervention and Notation. Of these scales, the BPS and the CPOT are considered the most valid and reliable for use in the ICU (Figure 6.1). Both scales include similar components of facial expression, body movements, and ventilator compliance. In addition, the CPOT includes an evaluation of muscle tension. One advantage of the CPOT is that it can be used in patients who are not intubated by including an assessment of vocalization. The BPS was adapted to the BPS-NI for this purpose, but it has been evaluated in only 30 patients; thus, more evidence is needed for the BPS-NI before widespread implementation.[16] These scales can be successfully implemented in nursing practice[17]; however, the routine use of behavioral pain scales in noncommunicative patients remains lower than anticipated. In one investigation that included a survey of more than 800 nurses, the use of self-report pain scales was 89%, but in patients who could not communicate, the use of an assessment tool was only 33%.[18] Thus, a concerted effort is needed to increase the adoption of behavioral pain scales into clinical practice. In addition, it is important to emphasize that in some patients, such as those with motor function impairments (e.g., pharmacologic paralysis), these scales cannot be used because scoring depends on facial expressions such as grimacing, patient movement, and ventilator compliance, which require intact motor function. In these patients, deep sedation and aggressive analgesia should be provided. In addition, these scales have not been validated in patients with brain injury. Behavioral responses that may be atypical and an altered level of consciousness complicate pain assessment in these patients. However, studies suggest that even patients in an apparent vegetative state are able to perceive pain.[19] Thus, it is reasonable to err on the side of treatment when routine assessment methods may be unreliable.

TREATMENT APPROACH AND ANALGOSEDATION

The management of pain and agitation are interrelated. Traditionally, agitation has been primarily managed with the use of sedatives such as propofol, dexmedetomidine, and benzodiazepines. Recent guidelines recommend that, in most patients, a light level of sedation be

Behavioral Pain Scale

Facial Expression
- Relaxed = 1
- Partly tightened = 2
- (e.g., brow lowering)
- Fully tightened = 3
- (e.g., eyelid closing)
- Grimacing = 4

Upper Limb Movement
- No movement = 1
- Partly bent = 2
- Fully bent with finger flexion = 3
- Permanently retracted = 4

Adherence to Ventilator
- Tolerating = 1
- Coughing but tolerating = 2
- Fighting ventilator = 3
- Unable to control ventilation = 4

Significant pain = score > 5

Critical-Care Pain Observation Tool

Facial Expression
- Relaxed = 0
- Tense = 1
- Grimacing = 2

Body Movements
- Normal = 0
- Protection = 1
- Restlessness = 2

Muscle Tension
- Relaxed = 0
- Tense, rigid = 1
- Very tense or rigid = 2

Intubation Status

Intubated Patients
- Tolerating ventilator = 0
- Coughing but tolerating = 1
- Fighting ventilator = 2

OR

Extubated Patients
- Talking normal or no sound = 0
- Sighing, moaning = 1
- Crying out, sobbing = 2

Significant pain = score > 5

Numeric Rating Scale - Visual

0 1 2 3 4 5 6 7 8 9 10

Figure 6.1 Pain assessment scales.

maintained and titrated to an appropriate sedation scale (see the chapter on sedation for more details).[1] However, this agitation is often the result of underlying pain and discomfort. Although most sedatives can decrease consciousness, they have no analgesic effects (except for ketamine and dexmedetomidine); however, at high doses, central nervous system (CNS) depression may suppress the response to pain and the resulting agitation. This approach leads to more sedative use than necessary and contributes to producing a deep level of sedation. But sedative use may be associated with a greater risk of adverse effects such as hypotension with higher doses of propofol.[20] It is also known that use of sedatives, especially benzodiazepines, may increase the risk of delirium and result in poor patient outcomes, including increased length of mechanical ventilation and duration of stay.[21] An alternative approach, called analgesia-first or analgosedation, is used when agitated patients are given an analgesic first, and the sedative is used as a rescue agent. International guidelines from the Society of Critical Care Medicine suggest that analgesia-first sedation is preferred to traditional sedation in mechanically ventilated patients.[1] However, this was given a weak recommendation because of moderate-quality evidence, suggesting that although this method can be considered, more evidence is needed before routine implementation.

Some open-label trials, most of which have been conducted in Europe, have compared an analgesia-first approach with a traditional sedation-based approach.[22] Advantages of the analgesia-first sedation included decreased days of mechanical ventilation, decreased ICU length of stay, and improved sedation-agitation scores.[23-26] However, there was more agitated delirium in one study.[26] Most studies evaluating analgosedation have been conducted using remifentanil. However, in one trial, fentanyl was comparable to remifentanil using this approach.[27] In this trial, patients in the remifentanil group had greater pain after opioid discontinuation, which may have occurred because of the quick offset of effect from this agent. Currently, given the high cost of remifentanil in the United States, the use of fentanyl is an acceptable alternative in the ICU. Other concerns also remain with this approach because higher doses of opioids affect bowel motility and respiratory function. In addition, the risk of opioid withdrawal on discontinuation of higher prolonged doses should be anticipated. A logistical issue with this approach is also a greater effect on nursing resources. In one study, a 1:1 nurse/patient ratio was used to keep patients calm and avoid sedative provision until necessary.[26] One suggested approach using an analgosedation technique is provided in Figure 6.2. There is no consensus regarding certain parameters such as bolus doses to be used, trigger doses to

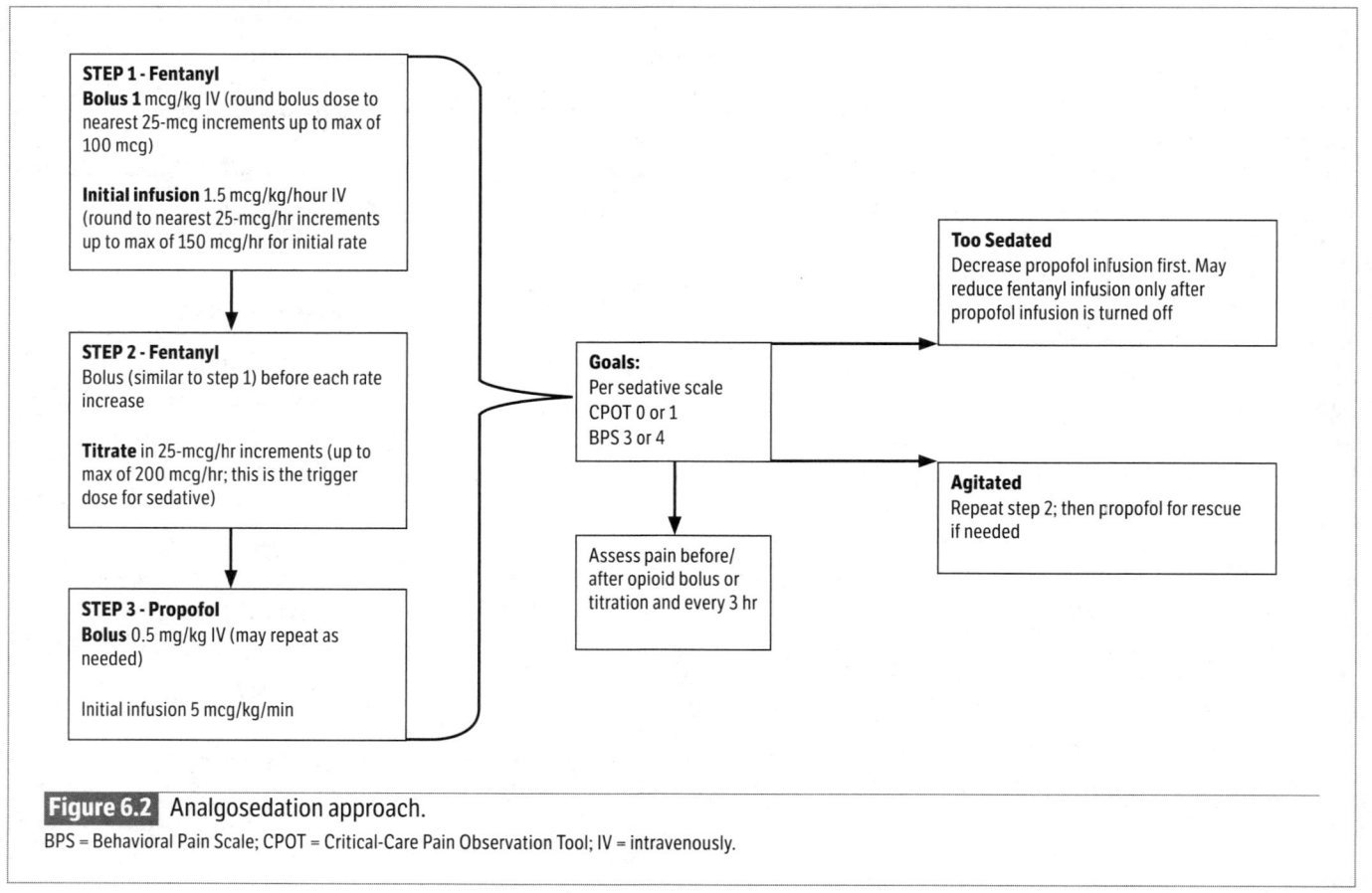

Figure 6.2 Analgosedation approach.
BPS = Behavioral Pain Scale; CPOT = Critical-Care Pain Observation Tool; IV = intravenously.

Table 6.1: Opioid Pharmacokinetics and Pharmacodynamics

Opioid	Equianalgesic Dose (mg) (IV)	Bolus/Intermittent Dose	Infusion Rate	Onset (IV) (min)	Peak Effect (min)	Duration of Effect	Elimination Half-life	Metabolism	Metabolites	Renal Elimination
Fentanyl	0.1	0.5–1.5 mcg/kg	0.7–10 mcg/kg/hr	1–3	10	30–60 min	3–12 hr	N-dealkylation CYP3A4 (liver and intestinal mucosa)	Norfentanyl (inactive)	<10% unchanged
Hydromorphone	1.5	0.2–1 mg	0.5–3 mg/hr	5	10–20	2–4 hr	2–3 hr	Glucuronidation	Hydromorphone-3-glucuronide (inactive)	7% unchanged
Morphine	10	2–10 mg	2–30 mg/hr	5	20	2–4 hr (extended in renal insufficiency)	2–4 hr	Glucuronidation	Morphine-3-glucuronide (inactive) Morphine-6-glucuronide (active)	2%–12% unchanged
Remifentanil	0.6	N/A	0.1–0.4 mcg/kg/min	1–3	3–5	3–10 min	3–10 min	Hydrolysis by plasma and tissue esterases	Carboxylic acid (inactive)	<10% unchanged

IV = intravenous(ly); N/A = not applicable.

provide sedation, or maximum infusion rates. Figure 6.2 is based on the trial protocol used in the study by Muellejans et al.,[27] but it can be adapted to suit institutional requirements and provider preferences.

THERAPEUTIC OPTIONS

Opioids

Given the severity of pain experienced by the critically ill population, opioids remain the analgesic agents of choice in the ICU. At this time, no comparative studies show that any one opioid is preferred to the others. Thus, therapy is selected according to the pharmacokinetic and pharmacodynamic characteristics of the opioid, patient history, comorbidities, adverse event profile, cost, and availability. Characteristics of commonly used opioids are listed in Table 6.1, and common adverse effects are listed in Figure 6.3. The most appropriate route for administering opioids in the critically ill population is the intravenous route.[28] This is because of unpredictable and inadequate absorption by the gastrointestinal (GI) tract when mesenteric perfusion may be suboptimal.[29] In addition, the intravenous route allows for the most rapid onset of effect and drug titration. This is crucial because severe pain should be treated as quickly as possible. The difficulty of predicting analgesic requirements in these patients necessitates the ability to respond rapidly by altering or providing additional doses. Typically, pain is first controlled by the repeated use of bolus doses to achieve adequate serum and CNS concentrations while initiating a continuous infusion as maintenance therapy. This strategy has been used in trials comparing analgesia-based regimens in the ICU.[27,30] Because of the shift in care toward analgosedation, intubated patients should receive a continuous opioid infusion, with few exceptions.

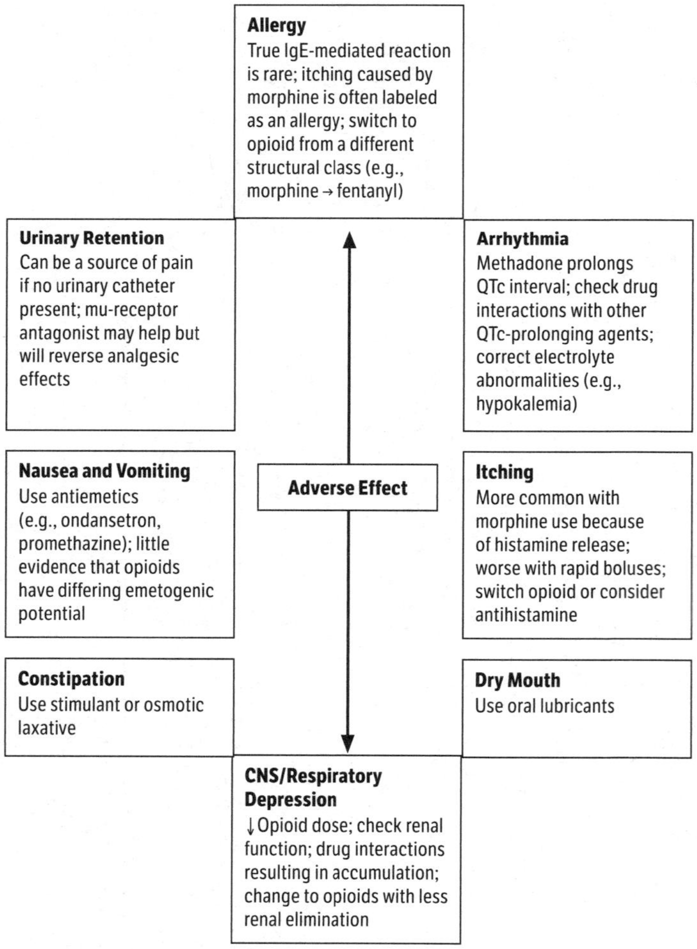

Some unique issues pertaining to commonly used opioids are important to discuss because they are commonly encountered during clinical care. For instance, morphine has always been the gold standard to which other opioids have been compared. However, it requires renal elimination and has active metabolites, which can lead to drug accumulation in patients with renal dysfunction. Renal function often fluctuates in the critically ill population, and some degree of impairment is common, especially in older adult patients or those receiving concurrent nephrotoxic therapies. Thus, continuous infusions may lead to prolonged effects even after drug discontinuation.[31] This has the potential to increase time on mechanical ventilation and ICU length of stay. On the contrary, isolated bolus doses of morphine are unlikely to be problematic in this regard. The duration of effect of opioids is a function of several factors that include hepatic metabolism, presence of active metabolites, distribution and accumulation within deep tissue, and renal elimination. Hence, even more lipophilic opioids such hydromorphone and fentanyl may have prolonged effects after sustained use because of accumulation within fatty tissue or organ dysfunction. Another disadvantage of morphine is its histamine-related effect on blood pressure, which is of concern in patients with hemodynamic instability. But this is more likely to occur when large doses are given as a rapid infusion. Hence, using a continuous infusion of morphine is still considered appropriate in patients who are hypotensive. Using synthetic opioids such as fentanyl has become more popular among ICU clinicians because of their rapid onset of effect, lack of effect on blood pressure, few adverse effects,

Figure 6.3 Opioid adverse effects.
IgE = immunoglobulin E.

and relatively low accumulation with organ dysfunction. However, high bolus doses of fentanyl (e.g., 3–5 mcg/kg) have been associated with chest wall rigidity, particularly during anesthesia. Fortunately, this risk is minimal in the ICU, where bolus doses are usually 1–2 mcg/kg. Other common adverse effects of opioids include central nervous and respiratory depression, constipation, and nausea and vomiting. Tolerance to constipation does not develop, and most patients in the ICU should be given a stimulant or osmotic laxative on a scheduled basis. Given the high incidence of constipation, it is better to err on the side of treatment, holding the laxative only if the patient develops diarrhea.[32] Unless patient-specific circumstances warrant an alternative approach, it is reasonable to use fentanyl as the first-line opioid analgesic infusion in most patients.

Non-opioids and Multimodal Therapy

A multimodal analgesia approach involves the simultaneous use of two or more analgesic agents with different therapeutic mechanisms such that the effect is synergic.[33] This also has the potential to minimize dose-related adverse effects by reducing the extent of exposure to any one agent. Opioids serve as the mainstay of treatment in this patient population, but use of opioids alone targets only mu-opioid receptors, allowing nociceptive transmission by other pain pathways. In the critically ill population, this approach usually incorporates non-opioids such as acetaminophen and nonsteroidal anti-inflammatory agents (NSAIDs). Adding agents such as gabapentin and carbamazepine can be beneficial when neuropathic pain is

Table 6.2 Non-opioid Characteristics

Non-opioid	Dose	Onset	Duration of Effect	Metabolism	Elimination	Comments
Acetaminophen	Oral: 325–650 mg every 4–6 hr or 1000 mg every 6–8 hr IV: 650 mg every 4 hr or 1000 mg every 6 hr (maximum < 4000 mg/24 hr)	Oral: < 1 hr IV: 5–10 min	4–6 hr (half-life 2–3 hr)	Hepatic conjugation with glucuronide or sulfate; or oxidation	< 5% unchanged in the urine	Hepatotoxicity possible; drug interactions with other hepatic metabolized medications
Carbamazepine	Oral: 50–100 mg every 12 hr; then increase to 100–200 mg every 4–6 hr (maximum 1200 mg/24 hr)	4–5 hr	Effect may last several days after therapeutic concentration attained (half-life initial 25–65 hr; then 12–17 hr)	Hepatic by CYP3A4 (98%); induces own metabolism after a few weeks; has an active metabolite (carbamazepine-10,11-epoxide)	72% renal, 28% feces	Studies in the ICU started at 100 mg every 8 hr; consider initiating at this dose; potential for drug interactions; many adverse effects with neurologic, hematologic, and cardiovascular systems
Gabapentin	Oral: 100 mg every 8 hr; may increase to 300–1200 mg every 8 hr	2–4 hr	Varies according to renal function (half-life 5–7 hr)	No appreciable metabolism	76%–81% urine, 10%–23% feces	Studies in the ICU started at 300 mg every 8 hr; adverse effects include sedation, ataxia, dizziness, fatigue, nystagmus, hypotension
Ibuprofen	Oral: 200–600 every 4–6 hr (maximum 2,400/24 hr) IV: 400–800 every 6 hr (maximum 3,200 mg/24 hr); infuse each dose over at least 30 min	30–60 min	4–6 hr (half-life 2–3 hr)	Primarily hepatic by CYP2C9 to inactive metabolites	Primarily urine	Potential for GI bleeding, acute renal failure, and cardiovascular adverse effects; patients should be well hydrated before IV use
Ketamine	IV: 0.5–1 mg/kg bolus for procedures; 2 mcg/kg/min or 0.1–0.2 mg/kg/hr as a continuous infusion and titrated as needed	< 1 min	10 min (half-life 2–3 hr)	Primarily hepatic N-demethylation by the CYP system to form norketamine, which is hydroxylated and conjugated to water-soluble compounds	Primarily urine (< 5% feces)	Potential for hallucinations and psychosis; increases catecholamine release, leading to higher blood pressure and heart rate
Ketorolac	IV: 30 mg once; then 15–30 mg every 6 hr ´ 5 days (use up to maximum of 5 days); use 15-mg dose in older adult patients	30 min	4–6 hr (half-life 5–6 hr)	Hepatic by hydroxylation and conjugation to inactive metabolites	Primarily urine (6% feces)	Same adverse effects but more potent than ibuprofen. May have greater pain relief and higher risk of adverse effects than oral NSAIDs

present. Regional blocks, local anesthetics, and epidural analgesia can also complement systemic opioid therapy when indicated. Pharmacologic characteristics of commonly used non-opioids are listed in Table 6.2.

Much of the evidence for multimodal analgesia is from studies conducted in non–critically ill postoperative patients or those with chronic pain.[34] Benefits include reduced postoperative pain, decreased opioid consumption, and improved participation in physical therapy. The American Pain Society suggests this approach for managing acute and chronic pain, but there is a relative lack of evidence in the critically ill population.[35] However, there are challenges to using a multimodal approach in the ICU because some non-opioid adjunctive agents must be given by the oral route because of dosage form availability. Some non-opioid agents also have unique adverse effects and drug interactions that need to be considered.

Acetaminophen used for this purpose is appealing and may be administered by the enteral or rectal route, but drug absorption may be unpredictable. In some situations, enteral administration is not possible, in which case rectal suppositories may be used. But the patient needs to be turned for rectal administration; this is a procedure that itself is painful, mitigating some of the benefit of the analgesic. In addition, the drug dose is lost with bowel movements, precluding this route in patients with diarrhea. The availability of an intravenous formulation has made this a suitable option in patients for whom these former routes are not feasible. In one randomized controlled trial conducted in Turkey, using intravenous paracetamol 1 g every 6 hours in postoperative ICU patients was associated with decreased pain, decreased opioid consumption, shorter time to extubation, and less nausea and vomiting.[36] But this was a small study of only 40 patients, and the opioid used was meperidine; this agent, which is no longer recommended for analgesia in the critically ill population, may have accentuated the differences between groups. Thus, this study limits extrapolation to common practice in the United States, especially when using an analgosedation approach with an opioid such as fentanyl. Also of concern is that, in one study in Europe, an intravenous paracetamol product was associated with a clinically relevant decrease in systolic blood pressure in 33% of the patients, and 16% overall required some intervention such as a fluid bolus or vasopressor administration to correct hypotension.[37] The mechanism for this effect on blood pressure is unknown.

Nonsteroidal anti-inflammatory drugs are also readily available in a variety of dosage forms that can be given by the oral, rectal, or intravenous route (e.g., ibuprofen, ketorolac). In postoperative patients after coronary artery bypass, using diclofenac given rectally was associated with decreased time to extubation, inotropic use, and rescue analgesic use.[38] However, the method of opioid provision between the treatment arms was different, making it difficult to ascertain the effect of the NSAID alone.[38] Of note, NSAIDs may be associated with adverse effects such as renal failure, GI bleeding, and interference with bone healing.[28] This may be particularly problematic in patients who are already on concurrent nephrotoxic therapies or medications such as antiplatelets and anticoagulants, which can predispose them to bleeding. The occurrence of organ failure is multifactorial and related to the underlying diagnosis (e.g., sepsis); using NSAIDs in these circumstances can exacerbate an already tenuous situation. Thus, adding NSAIDs needs to be individualized, weighing the individual risks versus the benefits. As a rule, if a non-opioid analgesic is being considered for multimodal therapy in the ICU, it is reasonable to consider oral acetaminophen first in most patients before NSAIDs.

Agents for Neuropathic Pain

Neuropathic pain originates from pathology of the nervous system. Although neuropathy is commonly associated with conditions such as diabetes and shingles, it can occur with nerve damage caused by trauma or surgery.[39] All patients with injuries or surgery likely have some neuropathic component to their pain. Voltage-gated sodium channels play an important role in pain transmission, leading to the effectiveness of certain drug therapies such as carbamazepine and gabapentin, which stabilize these channels. Studies in the ICU have been conducted in patients with Guillain-Barré syndrome.[40,41] In one trial, 12 critically ill patients with Guillain-Barré syndrome were given carbamazepine 100 mg every 8 hours or placebo by nasogastric tube in a randomized, double-blind, crossover design. Carbamazepine use was associated with lower pain scores and opioid requirements.[41] This is a relatively old study, and the breakthrough opioid used was pethidine, which is no longer used. In another randomized three-arm trial in a similar population, patients were given carbamazepine 100 mg, gabapentin 300 mg, or placebo every 8 hours for 7 days.[40] In this study, pain scores and opioid requirements were lowest in the gabapentin group during the study period. This trial more closely reflects clinical practice because fentanyl was used for breakthrough pain. This suggests that gabapentin is more suitable in the critically ill population. Carbamazepine is metabolized by cytochrome P450 (CYP) 3A4 and is susceptible to drug interactions with medications commonly used in the ICU. In addition, carbamazepine is associated with serious dermatologic reactions such as toxic epidermal necrosis and Stevens-Johnson syndrome, requiring immediate discontinuation if a rash occurs. Patients with Chinese ancestry are at high risk of these serious dermatological conditions if they carry the genetic variant of the *HLA-B* gene, *HLA-B*1502*. Because of its reduced efficacy compared with gabapentin and its potential for drug interactions and serious adverse effects, carbamazepine should not be used first line. An important consideration is that in both of these studies, pain scores were self-reported; thus, the results pertain to a subset of patients who were able to communicate. Ideally, a larger study in the ICU that includes a broader population of postoperative patients would help establish the role of gabapentin and other anticonvulsant therapies in the critically ill population. Studies evaluating the use of gabapentin for postoperative pain have shown benefits, but this can depend on the type and extent of surgery done.[42] In most of these studies, gabapentin was used preoperatively and continued for a few postoperative days. At this time, it is reasonable to consider the use of gabapentin 300 mg every 8 hours in patients at risk of neuropathic pain, particularly in those who have escalating opioid requirements.

Ketamine

Ketamine is an *N*-methyl-D-aspartate (NMDA) antagonist with analgesic and dissociative properties. It is most commonly used in the emergency department setting for procedural sedation, induction for rapid sequence intubation, and refractory bronchospasm. For procedural sedation, it is provided as a bolus dose of 1 mg/kg and may be repeated in increments of 0.5 mg/kg to achieve a dissociative state.[43] Ketamine is particularly appealing because it enables the provision of analgosedation with minimal risk of respiratory depression. In addition, in contrast to other commonly used anesthetics (e.g., propofol), ketamine use is associated with an increase in blood pressure and heart rate because of increased endogenous catecholamine release. Thus, it is suitable in patients with tenuous blood pressure readings who require a procedure in the ICU. Ketamine should be reserved for more invasive procedures that require a state of dissociation. However, lower doses such as 0.2–0.3 mg/kg intravenously are less likely to cause dissociation and are opioid sparing, especially in trauma patients.[44]

There is great interest in the sustained use of ketamine as a continuous infusion for analgosedation in the ICU. However, there is very little evidence to guide clinicians regarding the risks, benefits, and strategies for implementing this approach. Case reports using continuous infusions of ketamine in the ICU have shown it to be effective in patients with refractory pain with escalating sedative and opioid requirements. The doses used in these cases varied greatly, ranging more than 10-fold. Only one randomized trial is available that evaluated ketamine for postoperative pain after abdominal surgery.[45] In this study, patients were given a bolus of 0.5 mg/kg, followed by an infusion of 2 mcg/kg/minute for 24 hours; this was reduced to 1 mcg/kg/minute for the next 24 hours. Morphine consumption was lower in the ketamine group than in the control group (58 vs. 80 mg, p<0.05), but pain scores were similar. At this time, ketamine may be considered in patients with refractory pain and escalating opioid and sedative requirements. Once initiated, the duration of use should be kept to a minimum and reevaluated each day. Ketamine is known to be associated with hallucinations and psychosis, which usually occur after awakening from procedural sedation in adults—a term coined "emergence phenomenon." Prolonged use may predispose patients to delirium; thus, prolonged infusions should be avoided for routine use until more evidence is available. When ketamine is used for refractory pain as a sustained infusion, it is reasonable to start at a dose similar to that used in the randomized trial described previously (2 mcg/kg/minute or 0.1–0.2 mg/kg/hour), titrated as needed. Although a maximum dose has not been established, a rate of 2 mg/kg/hour (10-fold higher) would be consistent with the high doses in case reports.

Nonpharmacologic Therapy

Melzack and Wall proposed the gate control theory of pain in 1965.[46] They theorized that the substantia gelatinosa in the dorsal horn of the spinal cord acted as a gate, modulating noxious stimuli from peripheral nerves. This serves as the basis for nonpharmacologic cutaneous interventions such as massage therapy in the critically ill population. For instance, using massage stimulates large-diameter nerve fibers that can potentially decrease pain by inhibiting the conduction of nociceptive stimuli from smaller nerve fibers. Stimulating higher brain centers that are associated with cognition and affect can prevent the transmission of pain from the periphery by descending inhibition. Thus, nonpharmacologic interventions such as music and relaxation can help alleviate pain by facilitating inhibitory neural pathways from the brain to the spinal cord.

Nonpharmacologic therapies for analgesia with the potential to be implemented in the ICU include massage, music, relaxation, and the provision of sensory and procedural information.[28] Only a few studies evaluate the use of massage in the critically ill population.[47-50] Massage interventions in trials have varied by anatomic site (e.g., hands, feet, limbs, back, shoulders, scalp), duration of massage, and number of episodes. In one pilot study in the ICU, the use of hand massage was considered feasible and was well accepted by patients.[49] The intervention consisted of a 5-minute massage on the palm and back of the hand, repeated for each hand, and conducted three times within 24 hours of ICU admission. Alternatively, 30-minute periods have been used on specific locations such as the feet or according to areas of concern for the patient. This latter approach requires communication from the patient. For instance, although some of these trials were conducted in the ICU, they were done after extubation.[47,51] Thus, extrapolation to those who are intubated or noncommunicative is difficult. The focus of these studies is not specific to pain and includes effect on anxiety and sleep. Interventions often include combination approaches that incorporate music and relaxation. Hence, the effect of massage alone is difficult to interpret. Most studies have small sample sizes and are hypothesis generating, but they generally support an effect on pain reduction and relaxation.[52] Questions remain regarding whether nurses can do this because qualified therapists or investigators did interventions in the trials. Although touch is known to be a form of communication for caring and comfort, personal interpretations can vary depending on cultural background, previous experience, and attitude of family and friends. It is unknown whether this would be harmful in patients with psychosis or delirium, who were excluded in studies. Caution should be exercised in those with injuries or wounds, which would be contraindications to massage depending on the anatomic area affected. Lubricants and aromatics (e.g., lavender oil) used during the massage can be problematic because of the possibility for dermatologic allergies. Although guidelines from the Society of Critical Care Medicine suggest that nonpharmacologic interventions are relatively benign, easy to conduct, and low in cost, this particular intervention has potential for harm if not conducted appropriately and is an additional task requiring nursing resources. If certified massage therapists are used, this intervention will indeed have an additional cost.

Studies evaluating the effect of music therapy on pain and opioid consumption are heterogeneous and are considerably varied in the effect of the intervention.[53] In the subset of studies of postoperative patients, the pain reduction attributed to music therapy was modest (i.e., 0.5 points on a 0–10 scale), and there was no greater benefit when patients were able to select their own music. Postoperative morphine consumption was 1 mg less at 2 hours and 5.7 mg less at 24 hours after surgery in the intervention groups.[53] It is difficult to extrapolate these findings to critically ill patients. Important questions remain regarding how and when music therapy can be incorporated. Another intervention evaluated in postoperative patients is the use of muscle relaxation techniques that were taught preoperatively.[54] Relaxation decreases anxiety and muscle tension and distracts from pain. Relaxation interventions have focused on one anatomic location such as the jaw (e.g., letting the lower drop slightly, resting the tongue and lips, breathing slowly, without thinking about speaking) or using a systematic technique.[55,56] In a systematic technique, the patient is asked to lie in a comfortable position in the bed with closed eyes, followed by sequential relaxation of each body part, starting from the feet and moving to the head. The process lasts 5 minutes and is repeated three times.[56] Both of these relaxation techniques were associated with better pain control. The challenge of incorporating this process in the ICU is that it would probably have to be taught after ICU admission, rather than preoperatively, given the often-emergent nature of critical illness. Both of these studies were conducted in non–critically ill postoperative patients.

Finally, it is important to communicate information related to future procedures, and the pain likely to be associated with them, to critically ill patients. This is possible depending on the cognitive ability and level of sedation of patients. In one meta-analysis, providing information before procedures was beneficial for pain and distress, but the effect was highly variable.[57] It is uncertain how this can be extrapolated to patients in the ICU. However, communicating information to patients is ethical and considered the standard of care. This can enable patients to anticipate and cope with the procedure. However, some patients may amplify negative cognitive and emotional processes; this phenomenon, known as catastrophizing, may lead to a more painful experience and heightened anxiety.[58] At this time, given the uncertainty of the evidence, it is reasonable to err on the side of providing patients with the appropriate information. Future studies are needed to determine whether patients with certain traits such as catastrophizing will benefit if they are provided with limited rather than complete information before procedures. Overall, nonpharmacologic therapy for pain in the ICU may be provided in addition to standard pharmacologic therapies such as opioids and non-opioid adjuncts. High-level evidence to support these interventions is lacking, but most of these interventions are relatively benign, are feasible, and have low cost if implemented in a manner that augments rather than disrupts nursing care. Ideally, a combination of therapies can be used that incorporates the use of touch, music, and relaxation.

PROCEDURAL PAIN

Procedures done in the ICU include chest tube removal, wound drain removal, endotracheal and tracheal suctioning, line insertion (arterial, peripheral venous, and central venous), peripheral blood draw, turning, respiratory exercises, positioning, wound care, and mobilization. Most recently, a large prospective cross-sectional study included data from 4,812 procedures done in 3,851 patients from 192 ICUs in 28 countries.[59] The study found that chest tube removal, wound drain removal, and arterial line insertion were associated with the highest pain intensity; median pain intensities measured on a 0–10 NRS were 5, 4.5, and 4, respectively, during these three procedures. The change from baseline pain was about a 2- or 3-point increase. However, less than 50% of patients routinely receive analgesia before procedures.[60] In addition, it is important that the timing of the analgesic be such that its peak effect occurs during the procedure. For instance, morphine has a peak effect occurring at 20 minutes or longer. Thus, patients will not benefit from morphine if the procedure is done too soon after drug administration. Fentanyl intravenous has a more rapid onset of effect within 1 minute and may be more suitable when the procedure is emergent. Of the common procedures previously listed, endotracheal suctioning may need to be done emergently. Moreover, in some situations, such as placement of arterial lines, physician availability can lead to logistical challenges. Waiting 20 minutes for morphine to have peak effect may not be feasible when the physician is ready at the bedside. In these circumstances, an analgesic with a very rapid onset of effect (e.g., fentanyl) is preferred. Clinical trials have not shown the superiority of one analgesic over another. In fact, an NSAID such as ketorolac 30 mg intravenously was comparable with morphine 4 mg intravenously when given before chest tube removal in cardiac surgery patients.[61] Ketorolac was administered 60 minutes before the procedure, which is consistent with its peak effect. Even the most appropriate opioid dose to be used is unclear. For instance, one trial showed that morphine 2.5 mg intravenously was similar to 7.5 mg intravenously during painful procedures.[62] It is reasonable to use a bolus dose of morphine 4 mg intravenously or fentanyl 50 mcg intravenously for most adult patients. This dose can be increased for those with prior pain conditions or those who are opioid tolerant. The dose may be repeated if proven insufficient during the procedure. More-invasive procedures such as wound debridement, abscess drainage, and endoscopy should be treated differently because these require a state of unconsciousness. These patients require a deeper level of sedation in addition to analgesia. Ketamine is a valuable option in these circumstances, as described in the previous section. Alternatively, the level of sedation can be temporarily increased in those already receiving sedative infusions. This can be accomplished by giving a sedative bolus with an increase in the infusion rate. Patients may have several procedures during a day, and analgesic provision before each procedure may lead to several additional doses provided. If possible, it is beneficial to cluster procedures so that repeated doses are not needed.

OPIOID CONVERSIONS

Converting from one opioid to another may be necessary because of drug-related adverse effects, lack of effectiveness, changes in the route of administration, drug availability, and transfer to the general medical ward. The equianalgesic potency of commonly used intravenous opioids is provided in Table 6.1. It is widely accepted that fentanyl intravenous is 100 times more potent than morphine intravenous, whereas hydromorphone intravenous is 6–7 times more potent than morphine intravenous.[63] Newer agents such as remifentanil have no available potency ratios in product labeling information.[64] According to a study comparing fentanyl with remifentanil, the initial doses used and the mean doses required provide justification that fentanyl is 5–6 times more potent than remifentanil.[27] Oral options in the ICU most commonly include morphine, hydromorphone, and oxycodone. Hydromorphone oral is 4 times more potent than morphine oral. This is different from the intravenous ratio between these agents, which is attributable to differences in bioavailability. Oxycodone oral is considered 1.5 times more potent than morphine oral, although it may be equivalent to morphine in some patients. Methadone is another option, which is considered in patients with refractory pain or to prevent opioid withdrawal. However, conversion ratios with methadone are not constant but change, depending on the previous opioid dose used.[65] In general, conversions to methadone should not occur in the ICU. Rather methadone is used as add-on therapy, and most adults can be initiated at a dose of 5–10 mg every 8 hours. This strategy will help minimize errors and will be acceptable for most patients in whom this agent is deemed essential.

When considering these ratios, it is important to understand where the evidence for these values came from. Most studies were conducted in patients with chronic pain conditions such as cancer pain or were single-dose trials.[63] This was necessary for study designs because the validity and calculation of a ratio depended on a stable pain condition. In the ICU, pain is dynamic and changes during the course of critical illness. Pain and opioid requirements are anticipated to decrease as patients recover; thus, opioid use trends are more important than absolute values. Moreover, the ratios represent the mean values from studies. On closer inspection, opioid conversion studies show a considerable range around these mean values.[63] Thus, there is likely to be great interpatient variability during the switching process. It is imperative that the risk of undertreatment be weighed against the risk of dose-related toxicity. In an intubated patient, higher calculated infusion rates may be acceptable because the risk of respiratory depression is mitigated by the fact that the patient is mechanically ventilated. However, after extubation, the risk-benefit ratio changes, so it is safer to err on the conservative side. Equianalgesic conversion ratios serve as a starting point for dose selection. Appropriate and timely drug titration to patient comfort is more important than the initial dose selected.

TRANSITION FROM ICU TO WARD

Typically, continuous opioid infusions are not permitted outside the ICU setting. This is because of fewer resources on general medical wards such as monitoring equipment and an increase in nurse/patient ratios. Moreover, after extubation, using continuous opioid infusions is risky. Thus, although bolus doses of opioids can be used for breakthrough pain during this transition, patients must be converted to oral or enteral opioids and other adjunctive analgesics to meet baseline requirements as they are transferred to a general ward. One strategy is to use enteral opioids, when feasible, during the ICU stay (e.g., oxycodone immediate release) at scheduled intervals while decreasing opioid infusions each day. Sustained-release products cannot be crushed or given by feeding tubes, and the dynamic and fluctuating course of pain and analgesic requirements in the critically ill population makes this dosage form less desirable. There is little evidence regarding the best practice for this approach, and selection of the opioid, dose, and titration has not been formally evaluated. It is reasonable to start by providing 10%–20% of the total daily dose by the enteral route (divided and administered every

4–6 hours) using an equianalgesic ratio. The opioid infusion can simultaneously be decreased by a similar amount. An important consideration is that pain is anticipated to decrease over time; hence, opioid requirements should decrease rather than increase during the ICU stay. As the daily opioid provision is reduced, it is important to monitor for withdrawal, which is more likely to occur with rapid de-escalation in patients who received higher doses of opioids for extended durations. An additional opioid bolus may be needed, or the drip rate may have to be temporarily increased. Patients may be eligible for a trial off the opioid drip when the rate is tapered to a minimum of 25 mcg/hour of fentanyl intravenous equivalents, with adequate pain control and no signs of withdrawal.

In patients with or at risk of withdrawal, one strategy is to use enteral methadone. Methadone is an NMDA antagonist and may benefit opioid-tolerant patients. Hence, even small doses may have profound effects on opioid requirements. Using methadone for this purpose has primarily been evaluated in the pediatric patient population. In one prospective cohort study, most pediatric patients with symptoms of withdrawal successfully completed a 10-day methadone weaning protocol.[66] The protocol involved converting previous 24-hour fentanyl use to an equivalent oral morphine dose and then converting the patient to methadone. However, these patients did not require mechanical ventilation at the time of enrollment, limiting extrapolation to this patient subset. Using oral morphine as an intermediate step may be unnecessary, and the complexity of the calculations may result in medication errors. In a randomized controlled trial involving 78 pediatric patients who were on prolonged fentanyl infusions, patients were randomized to a low-dose methadone strategy or a high-dose strategy.[67] Patients in the low-dose group were given a 0.1-mg/kg/dose (e.g., a 10-kg patient would receive a 1-mg/dose irrespective of fentanyl infusion rate).[67] The high-dose group was given a 0.1-mg/kg/dose multiplied by weight and fentanyl infusion rate (e.g., a 10-kg patient receiving fentanyl 3 mcg/kg/hour would receive a dose of 3 mg). Methadone was given every 6 hours for the first 24 hours, followed by every 12 hours for the second 24 hours, followed by daily use for the next 10 days, during which the dose was decreased by 10% each day. The fentanyl infusion was tapered off within 72 hours of the first dose of methadone. There was no significant difference in the proportion of patients who completed the methadone taper successfully in the low- and high-dose groups (56% vs. 62%, p=0.79; respectively). Because of these results, complexity of the protocol, and feasibility of implementation, it is reasonable to use a low-dose strategy when methadone use is being considered in the pediatric patient population. Although similar studies have not been conducted in adults, a similar taper using 5–10 mg of methadone given every 8 hours as a starting dose is a reasonable approach for most patients. Given that the ratio between methadone and morphine changes according to the amount of previous morphine use, the methadone dose required varies very little, and a fixed-dose strategy (e.g., starting at 10 mg every 6 hours; then taper) is acceptable. Methadone use has been associated with corrected QT (QTc) interval prolongation. This can be particularly problematic in patients with a high baseline QTc or those on concurrent medications that prolong the QTc. Thus, methadone use should be avoided unless necessary, and if used, electrocardiogram monitoring is required during therapy.

It is also important to optimize the use of non-opioid adjunctive analgesics as described in the previous section during transition to the ward. This will reduce opioid requirements and work synergistically for pain control. Although no evidence suggests which patients are likely to have poor pain control during transition to the ward, patient history and ICU course will likely help target patients at risk. Specific variables to consider include pain control in the ICU, opioid requirements, rate of opioid de-escalation, time between when opioid infusion was terminated and transfer, surgical procedures, injuries, chronic pain conditions, and psychiatric illness.

SUMMARY

Pain is ubiquitous in the ICU, and treatment of pain is essential and humane. Appropriate and routine pain assessment using validated scales such as the NRS-V for communicative patients or the BPS and CPOT for noncommunicative patients is the first step toward better pain management and improved patient outcomes. Opioid analgesia is the mainstay of treatment given the severity of pain experienced in the ICU; however, non-opioid adjuncts and nonpharmacologic therapy may be used as part of a multimodal approach. Although more evidence is needed, an analgosedation strategy is preferred to the traditional sedative-based approach to managing patient comfort. Clinicians should be mindful of the important pharmacologic considerations during procedures, opioid conversions, and transitions of care that occur when patients are transferred from the ICU to the general ward.

REFERENCES

1. Barr J, Fraser GL, Puntillo K, et al. Clinical practice guidelines for the management of pain, agitation, and delirium in adult patients in the intensive care unit. Crit Care Med 2013;41:263-306.

2. Brennan F, Carr DB, Cousins M. Pain management: a fundamental human right. Anesth Analg 2007;105:205-21.

3. Pain terms: a list with definitions and notes on usage. Recommended by the IASP Subcommittee on Taxonomy. Pain 1979;6:249.

4. Shannon K, Bucknall T. Pain assessment in critical care: what have we learnt from research. Intensive Crit Care Nurs 2003;19:154-62.

5. Puntillo KA, White C, Morris AB, et al. Patients' perceptions and responses to procedural pain: results from Thunder Project II. Am J Crit Care 2001;10:238-51.

6. Rotondi AJ, Chelluri L, Sirio C, et al. Patients' recollections of stressful experiences while receiving prolonged mechanical ventilation in an intensive care unit. Crit Care Med 2002;30:746-52.

7. Schelling G, Richter M, Roozendaal B, et al. Exposure to high stress in the intensive care unit may have negative effects on health-related quality-of-life outcomes after cardiac surgery. Crit Care Med 2003;31:1971-80.

8. Schelling G, Stoll C, Haller M, et al. Health-related quality of life and posttraumatic stress disorder in survivors of the acute respiratory distress syndrome. Crit Care Med 1998;26:651-9.

9. Granja C, Gomes E, Amaro A, et al. Understanding posttraumatic stress disorder-related symptoms after critical care: the early illness amnesia hypothesis. Crit Care Med 2008;36:2801-9.

10. Chanques G, Jaber S, Barbotte E, et al. Impact of systematic evaluation of pain and agitation in an intensive care unit. Crit Care Med 2006;34:1691-9.

11. Payen JF, Bosson JL, Chanques G, et al. Pain assessment is associated with decreased duration of mechanical ventilation in the intensive care unit: a post hoc analysis of the DOLOREA study. Anesthesiology 2009;111:1308-16.

12. Gelinas C, Tousignant-Laflamme Y, Tanguay A, et al. Exploring the validity of the bispectral index, the Critical-Care Pain Observation Tool and vital signs for the detection of pain in sedated and mechanically ventilated critically ill adults: a pilot study. Intensive Crit Care Nurs 2011;27:46-52.

13. Melzack R. The McGill Pain Questionnaire: major properties and scoring methods. Pain 1975;1:277-99.

14. Hamill-Ruth RJ, Marohn ML. Evaluation of pain in the critically ill patient. Crit Care Clin 1999;15:35-54, v-vi.

15. Chanques G, Viel E, Constantin JM, et al. The measurement of pain in intensive care unit: comparison of 5 self-report intensity scales. Pain 2010;151:711-21.

16. Chanques G, Payen JF, Mercier G, et al. Assessing pain in non-intubated critically ill patients unable to self report: an adaptation of the Behavioral Pain Scale. Intensive Care Med 2009;35:2060-7.

17. Gelinas C, Arbour C, Michaud C, et al. Implementation of the Critical-Care Pain Observation Tool on pain assessment/management nursing practices in an intensive care unit with nonverbal critically ill adults: a before and after study. Int J Nurs Stud 2011;48:1495-504.

18. Rose L, Smith O, Gelinas C, et al. Critical care nurses' pain assessment and management practices: a survey in Canada. Am J Crit Care 2012;21:251-9.

19. Roulin MJ, Ramelet AS. Pain indicators in brain-injured critical care adults: an integrative review. Aust Crit Care 2012;25:110-8.

20. Shearin AE, Patanwala AE, Tang A, et al. Predictors of hypotension associated with propofol in trauma patients. J Trauma Nurs 2014;21:4-8.

21. Riker RR, Shehabi Y, Bokesch PM, et al. Dexmedetomidine vs midazolam for sedation of critically ill patients: a randomized trial. JAMA 2009;301:489-99.

22. Devabhakthuni S, Armahizer MJ, Dasta JF, et al. Analgosedation: a paradigm shift in intensive care unit sedation practice. Ann Pharmacother 2012;46:530-40.

23. Breen D, Karabinis A, Malbrain M, et al. Decreased duration of mechanical ventilation when comparing analgesia-based sedation using remifentanil with standard hypnotic-based sedation for up to 10 days in intensive care unit patients: a randomised trial [ISRCTN47583497]. Crit Care 2005;9:R200-10.

24. Park G, Lane M, Rogers S, et al. A comparison of hypnotic and analgesic based sedation in a general intensive care unit. Br J Anaesth 2007;98:76-82.

25. Rozendaal FW, Spronk PE, Snellen FF, et al. Remifentanil-propofol analgo-sedation shortens duration of ventilation and length of ICU stay compared to a conventional regimen: a centre randomised, cross-over, open-label study in the Netherlands. Intensive Care Med 2009;35:291-8.

26. Strom T, Martinussen T, Toft P. A protocol of no sedation for critically ill patients receiving mechanical ventilation: a randomised trial. Lancet 2010;375:475-80.

27. Muellejans B, Lopez A, Cross MH, et al. Remifentanil versus fentanyl for analgesia based sedation to provide patient comfort in the intensive care unit: a randomized, double-blind controlled trial [ISRCTN43755713]. Crit Care 2004;8:R1-R11.

28. Erstad BL, Puntillo K, Gilbert HC, et al. Pain management principles in the critically ill. Chest 2009;135:1075-86.

29. Smith BS, Yogaratnam D, Levasseur-Franklin KE, et al. Introduction to drug pharmacokinetics in the critically ill patient. Chest 2012;141:1327-36.

30. Dahaba AA, Grabner T, Rehak PH, et al. Remifentanil versus morphine analgesia and sedation for mechanically ventilated critically ill patients: a randomized double blind study. Anesthesiology 2004;101:640-6.

31. Chauvin M, Sandouk P, Scherrmann JM, et al. Morphine pharmacokinetics in renal failure. Anesthesiology 1987;66:327-31.

32. Patanwala AE, Abarca J, Huckleberry Y, et al. Pharmacologic management of constipation in the critically ill patient. Pharmacotherapy 2006;26:896-902.

33. White PF. Multimodal analgesia: its role in preventing postoperative pain. Curr Opin Invest Drugs 2008;9:76-82.

34. American Society of Anesthesiologists Task Force on Acute Pain M. Practice guidelines for acute pain management in the perioperative setting: an updated report by the American Society of Anesthesiologists Task Force on Acute Pain Management. Anesthesiology 2012;116:248-73.

35. American Pain Society (APS). Principles of Analgesic Use in the Treatment of Acute Pain and Cancer Pain, 6th ed. Chicago, IL: APS, 2008.

36. Memis D, Inal MT, Kavalci G, et al. Intravenous paracetamol reduced the use of opioids, extubation time, and opioid-related adverse effects after major surgery in intensive care unit. J Crit Care 2010;25:458-62.

37. de Maat MM, Tijssen TA, Bruggemann RJ, et al. Paracetamol for intravenous use in medium- and intensive care patients: pharmacokinetics and tolerance. Eur J Clin Pharmacol 2010;66:713-9.

38. Maddali MM, Kurian E, Fahr J. Extubation time, hemodynamic stability, and postoperative pain control in patients undergoing

38. coronary artery bypass surgery: an evaluation of fentanyl, remifentanil, and nonsteroidal antiinflammatory drugs with propofol for perioperative and postoperative management. J Clin Anesth 2006;18:605-10.

39. Campbell JN, Meyer RA. Mechanisms of neuropathic pain. Neuron 2006;52:77-92.

40. Pandey CK, Raza M, Tripathi M, et al. The comparative evaluation of gabapentin and carbamazepine for pain management in Guillain-Barré syndrome patients in the intensive care unit. Anesth Analg 2005;101:220-5, table of contents.

41. Tripathi M, Kaushik S. Carbamezapine for pain management in Guillain-Barré syndrome patients in the intensive care unit. Crit Care Med 2000;28:655-8.

42. Chang CY, Challa CK, Shah J, et al. Gabapentin in acute postoperative pain management. Biomed Res Int 2014;2014:631756.

43. Green SM, Roback MG, Kennedy RM, et al. Clinical practice guideline for emergency department ketamine dissociative sedation: 2011 update. Ann Emerg Med 2011;57:449-61.

44. Galinski M, Dolveck F, Combes X, et al. Management of severe acute pain in emergency settings: ketamine reduces morphine consumption. Am J Emerg Med 2007;25:385-90.

45. Guillou N, Tanguy M, Seguin P, et al. The effects of small-dose ketamine on morphine consumption in surgical intensive care unit patients after major abdominal surgery. Anesth Analg 2003;97:843-7.

46. Melzack R, Wall PD. Pain mechanisms: a new theory. Science 1965;150:971-9.

47. Dunn C, Sleep J, Collett D. Sensing an improvement: an experimental study to evaluate the use of aromatherapy, massage and periods of rest in an intensive care unit. J Adv Nurs 1995;21:34-40.

48. Gunnarsdottir TJ, Jonsdottir H. Does the experimental design capture the effects of complementary therapy? A study using reflexology for patients undergoing coronary artery bypass graft surgery. J Clin Nurs 2007;16:777-85.

49. Martorella G, Boitor M, Michaud C, et al. Feasibility and acceptability of hand massage therapy for pain management of postoperative cardiac surgery patients in the intensive care unit. Heart Lung 2014;43:437-44.

50. Richards KC. Effect of a back massage and relaxation intervention on sleep in critically ill patients. Am J Crit Care 1998;7:288-99.

51. Bauer BA, Cutshall SM, Wentworth LJ, et al. Effect of massage therapy on pain, anxiety, and tension after cardiac surgery: a randomized study. Complement Ther Clin Pract 2010;16:70-5.

52. Richards KC, Gibson R, Overton-McCoy AL. Effects of massage in acute and critical care. AACN Clin Issues 2000;11:77-96.

53. Cepeda MS, Carr DB, Lau J, et al. Music for pain relief. Cochrane Database Syst Rev 2006;2:CD004843.

54. Kwekkeboom KL, Gretarsdottir E. Systematic review of relaxation interventions for pain. J Nurs Scholarsh 2006;38:269-77.

55. Good M, Stanton-Hicks M, Grass JA, et al. Relief of postoperative pain with jaw relaxation, music and their combination. Pain 1999;81:163-72.

56. Roykulcharoen V, Good M. Systematic relaxation to relieve postoperative pain. J Adv Nurs 2004;48:140-8.

57. Suls J, Wan CK. Effects of sensory and procedural information on coping with stressful medical procedures and pain: a meta-analysis. J Consult Clin Psychol 1989;57:372-9.

58. Pavlin DJ, Sullivan MJ, Freund PR, et al. Catastrophizing: a risk factor for postsurgical pain. Clin J Pain 2005;21:83-90.

59. Puntillo KA, Max A, Timsit JF, et al. Determinants of procedural pain intensity in the intensive care unit. The Europain study. Am J Respir Crit Care Med. 2014;189:39-47.

60. Siffleet J, Young J, Nikoletti S, et al. Patients' self-report of procedural pain in the intensive care unit. J Clin Nurs 2007;16:2142-8.

61. Puntillo K, Ley SJ. Appropriately timed analgesics control pain due to chest tube removal. Am J Crit Care 2004;13:292-301; discussion 2; quiz 3-4.

62. Ahlers SJ, van Gulik L, van Dongen EP, et al. Efficacy of an intravenous bolus of morphine 2.5 versus morphine 7.5 mg for procedural pain relief in postoperative cardiothoracic patients in the intensive care unit: a randomised double-blind controlled trial. Anaesth Intensive Care 2012;40:417-26.

63. Patanwala AE, Duby J, Waters D, et al. Opioid conversions in acute care. Ann Pharmacother 2007;41:255-66.

64. Ultiva (Remifenantil hydrochloride injection, powder, lyophilized, for solution). Rockford, IL: Mylan Institutional, July 2011.

65. Ripamonti C, Groff L, Brunelli C, et al. Switching from morphine to oral methadone in treating cancer pain: what is the equianalgesic dose ratio? J Clin Oncol 1998;16:3216-21.

66. Meyer MM, Berens RJ. Efficacy of an enteral 10-day methadone wean to prevent opioid withdrawal in fentanyl-tolerant pediatric intensive care unit patients. Pediatr Crit Care Med 2001;2:329-33.

67. Bowens CD, Thompson JA, Thompson MT, et al. A trial of methadone tapering schedules in pediatric intensive care unit patients exposed to prolonged sedative infusions. Pediatr Crit Care Med 2011;12:504-11.

Chapter 7

Agitation and Comfort in the Intensive Care Unit

David J. Gagnon, Pharm.D.; Nicole Kovacic, Pharm.D.; and Gilles L. Fraser, Pharm.D., MCCM

LEARNING OBJECTIVES

1. Define and characterize agitation in critically ill patients.
2. State the estimated incidence of agitation in the intensive care unit.
3. Identify the etiology of agitation, including patient-related, illness-related, and environmental factors.
4. Describe the clinical significance of agitation.
5. Discuss the importance of routinely assessing comfort, and compare subjective and objective monitoring techniques.
6. Summarize nonpharmacologic interventions used to treat and prevent agitation.
7. Compare and contrast the pharmacologic agents used to provide comfort.
8. Develop an evidence-based, patient-specific approach to providing comfort.

ABBREVIATIONS IN THIS CHAPTER

BIS	Bispectral index	LOS	Length of stay
CAM-ICU	Confusion assessment method for the intensive care unit	NMDA	N-methyl-D-aspartate
		PAD	Pain, agitation, and delirium
EEG	Electroencephalography	RASS	Richmond Agitation-Sedation Scale
GABA	γ-Aminobutyric acid	SAS	Sedation-Agitation Scale
ICU	Intensive care unit	SCCM	Society of Critical Care Medicine
ICP	Intracranial pressure		

INTRODUCTION

Agitation in the intensive care unit (ICU) is common and distressful for patients, families, and caregivers. It is often precipitated by instrumentation, unfamiliar surroundings, hemodynamic or metabolic derangements, pain, or the inability to communicate. Provision of evidence-based, humane care should include regular assessments of comfort, liberal treatment of pain, titration of sedation to a patient-specific goal, use of sedation protocols, and avoidance of coma. A multidisciplinary team is best suited to meet these ends. This chapter will provide a pragmatic review of agitation in the ICU with a focus on its incidence, etiology, significance, assessment, and management.

DEFINING AGITATION

There is no unanimously accepted definition for agitation. Definitions typically include its psychomotor manifestations, which are often an expression of immense inner tension. Agitated patients generally have inappropriate, irrational, and counterproductive behaviors that are out of proportion to the situation.[1,2] Nonpurposeful behaviors are common (e.g., thrashing), but so are purposeful ones (e.g., deliberate attempts to remove an endotracheal tube). Agitation caused by delirium (i.e., hyperactive delirium) is a distinct diagnosis and is examined in detail in the Delirium chapter.

Agitation may be best defined using bedside descriptors. Commonly used terms include restlessness, pulling at medical devices, overbreathing the mechanical ventilator, moving from side-to-side, rambling, shouting, or moaning.[3,4] Many of these descriptors have been incorporated into subjective sedation scales, which will be examined in greater detail later. Although most experienced caregivers can identify agitation, a universally accepted definition would be helpful.

INCIDENCE

Agitation may occur in 16%–71% of critically ill patients.[4-8] Variability in the reported incidence is because of heterogeneity in descriptive studies. Differences include the patient population, definition of agitation, study design, and methods of assessing and providing comfort. Regardless of its exact incidence, agitation is an important source of discomfort for patients, families, and caregivers.[9]

Agitation typically begins within 4 days of ICU admission and is most severe within the first few days.[4,6,8] About 43% of agitated patients will be so on admission, and 40%–86% will be agitated within the first 24 hours.[5-8] Early-onset agitation may be a result of acute illness, pain, instrumentation, or an unfamiliar environment. About 75% of patients will be agitated for several days.[4,6,8] Agitation occurs at a similar rate at night and during the day, which may be because of sundowning or disturbances in the sleep-wake cycle.[6,8] Overall, it can arise throughout an ICU admission and is typically because of several interrelated factors.

ETIOLOGY

Identifying the cause of agitation can help guide corrective efforts. No study has used self-report to elucidate its etiology because patients are often too encephalopathic to provide usable information. In addition, they are often unable to communicate because of medication effect or the presence of an endotracheal tube. Pathophysiologically, agitation may be caused by excessive sympathetic neurotransmission, dopaminergic hyperactivity, changes in pain sensation, or hypothalamic-pituitary-adrenal axis dysfunction.[10] The etiology is often multifactorial with contributions from patient-related, illness-related, or environmental factors.

Patient-Related Factors

Medical comorbidities often cause agitation or predispose patients to developing it. Pain may be present in more than 50% of ICU patients and has been identified as a considerable cause of anxiety.[11-13] Psychiatric illness and psychoactive drug use have also been associated with agitation.[5,8] Cognitive impairment, present in 6%–42% of ICU patients, has been implicated, and more than half of physicians are unaware that patients have this deficit at baseline.[14-16] Kidney and liver failure can cause metabolic encephalopathy with associated restlessness.[17,18] Nicotine dependence, present in 22%–46% of ICU patients, may increase the risk of agitation by 3-fold.[19-21] Alcohol and substance abuse disorders can be found in 39% of ICU patients and are associated with greater sedative and analgesic requirements.[5,7,8,22] The association between age and agitation remains unclear.[4,7,8]

Home medications and those initiated in the ICU can also cause agitation. Reinitiation of home psychoactive medications, when clinically appropriate, can prevent withdrawal-induced discomfort. On the other hand, drug-induced agitation may occur with agents initiated in the ICU, including central nervous system (CNS) stimulants (amphetamines or modafinil), glucocorticosteroids, anticholinergics, serotonergics, opioids, antimicrobials (cefepime or fluoroquinolones), histamine-1 (H_1)- or H_2-receptor antagonists (famotidine, ranitidine, or diphenhydramine), dopaminergics (amantadine or bromocriptine), sedatives (ketamine, benzodiazepines, or propofol), and volatile anesthetics.[23-26] Readers are encouraged to review more comprehensive sources on drug-induced agitation.[27,28]

Illness-Related Factors

Acute illnesses can increase the risk of developing agitation. Respiratory failure and hypoxemia (Pao_2/Fio_2 ratio less than 200) have been implicated.[4,5] Acidosis has also been correlated with agitation.[5,7,29] Febrile patients may be 4.5 times more likely to develop agitation.[4,6,29] Sepsis-associated brain dysfunction, present in up to 70% of patients with sepsis, can manifest as agitation.[4,8,30] Meningitis, encephalitis, and urinary tract infections can do so as well. Neurological insults including strokes, brain abscesses, cerebral malignancies, and seizures can provoke agitation.[3] Delirium, especially the hyperactive or mixed variant, can cause periodic aggression.[31] Electrolyte abnormalities (hypernatremia, hyponatremia, hypokalemia, or hypermagnesemia) may also play a role.[8,29]

Environmental Factors

Routine aspects of care to providers are far from the norm for ICU patients. Mechanical ventilation and the endotracheal tube are one of the most common causes of distress.[32] About one-half of mechanically ventilated patients recollect anxiety, fear, pain, and the inability to talk.[32,33] Likewise, about one-third report discomfort associated with secretions, difficulty sleeping, panic, choking, and not getting enough air.[32,33] In addition, ventilator dyssynchrony can cause insecurity, fear, and lack of sleep.[33] Vascular access and feeding tubes are other notable causes of apprehension.[12,13]

Patients report that the following are the most prominent stressors in the ICU: pain, sleep deprivation, instrumentation, loss of control, restraints, receiving no explanations of treatments, not knowing when things will be done, thirst, and having the lights on constantly.[9,12,13,34] Caregivers should remember that pain can occur at rest and during routine procedures like dressing changes, turning, suctioning, and chest tube removal.[35-37] Accordingly, liberal treatment of pain is imperative.[38]

Excessive noise is also a stressor in the ICU.[9,12,13] Sound levels almost always exceed the 35 average A-weighted energy-equivalent sound pressure in decibels (dBA L_{Aeq}) limit set by the World Health Organization.[39,40] Peak levels are similar to that of heavy traffic (85 dBA), and they continue to rise each year.[40,41] Excessive sound can cause sleep deprivation and altered sleep-wake cycles, which are common causes of stress and delirium.[42] Systematically assessing patient-related, illness-related, and environmental precipitants of agitation is the first step in providing comfort in the ICU.

CLINICAL SIGNIFICANCE

The clinical impact of agitation reportedly ranges from minor discomfort to increased mortality.[43,44] Most reports fail to capture the potential psychological impact of agitation on patients, families, and caregivers and its post-ICU implications. An appreciation for its significance may serve as an impetus to better understand its causes, treatment, and prevention.

The outcome most commonly associated with agitation is medical device removal. Removal of minimally invasive devices such as oxygen masks, wound dressings, or cardiac monitors increases nursing workload, whereas the removal of invasive devices such as peripherally inserted or central catheters, arterial catheters, endotracheal tubes, or surgical drains may lead to significant morbidity.[45,46] Agitation may be present in 58%–74% of patients preceding device removal, and inadequate analgesia and sedation has been implicated in about 30% of cases.[45,46]

Self-extubation is the most well-known form of medical device removal.[47-52] Restless or agitated patients may be 5.5 times more likely to self-extubate than those who are calm.[50] It may occur more commonly in patients receiving no sedation (opioids only) compared with those receiving intermittent or continuous sedation, although data are conflicting.[52,53] Reintubation may be required in 22%–78% of these patients.[51,52] Unplanned extubation has been associated with longer ICU and hospital length of stay (LOS), prolonged mechanical ventilation, and a greater likelihood of being transferred to a long-term care facility.[50,51,54] Negative sequela are largely driven by patients who require reintubation.[51,54]

Agitation can also cause maladaptive physiologic effects. Catecholamine concentrations, which are typically elevated in critically ill patients, are further increased by agitation.[55-58] Resultant tachycardia can exacerbate myocardial ischemia and, when sustained, is associated with longer ICU LOS and major cardiac events.[55,59] Blood pressure elevations can be catastrophic in patients with intracerebral hemorrhages or aortic dissections. Agitation may also lead to clenching and excessive peripheral muscle metabolism and lactate production.[10] Similarly, systemic and myocardial oxygen consumption increases when sedation is withdrawn or when weaning from mechanical ventilation fails.[60,61]

Many other negative outcomes have been associated with agitation. An increase in nosocomial infections may occur because of the immunosuppressant effects of sedatives, but it is more likely the result of an increase in ICU LOS and mechanical ventilator duration that accompanies oversedation.[8,62,63] The influence of agitation on ICU LOS and duration of ventilation varies, but they are probably prolonged because of increased sedation administration, greater infection risk, and the need to taper pharmacotherapy before transferring to a non-ICU bed.[5,7,8] It may also lead to a greater workload for caregivers.[8] Ameliorating agitation's negative physical and psychological responses can improve outcomes and help patients and families adapt to the ICU environment.

ASSESSING AGITATION AND SEDATION

The value of systematically monitoring patient comfort cannot be overstated. Regular assessments may reduce the incidence of severe agitation by 59%; decrease the amount of sedatives, analgesics, or vasoactive drugs administered; and reduce nosocomial infections and duration of mechanical ventilation.[64-66] Monitoring can be accomplished with subjective sedation scales (e.g., Sedation-Agitation Scale [SAS] or Richmond Agitation-Sedation Scale [RASS]) or objective measures (e.g., bispectral index [BIS] or continuous electroencephalography [EEG]). Large-scale implementation of comfort monitoring is feasible and highly encouraged.[67] The 2013 Society of Critical Care Medicine (SCCM) pain, agitation, and delirium (PAD) guidelines suggest that comfort should be assessed at least four times per shift and as needed thereafter.[11]

Subjective Sedation Scales

Subjective sedation scales help facilitate communication between caregivers, establish goals for sedation, and guide therapeutic options. Most can be completed in less than 2 minutes.[68,69] Unfortunately, only half of caregivers routinely use them.[70] Arousal is the central domain assessed by these scales. Because agitation and sedation are part of a continuum, subjective assessment scales should encompass coma to dangerous agitation.[71]

Subjective sedation scales are evaluated according to their psychometric properties, which includes item selection, content validation, reliability, construct validity, feasibility, and impact on patient outcomes.[11,72] Because no "gold standard" exists, validity (i.e., ability of the scale to accurately assess agitation and sedation) has been established with content validation and construct validity.[72] In general, subjective sedation scales were developed using a variety of methods and are necessarily subjective in nature.

The 2013 SCCM PAD guidelines examined 10 subjective sedation scales.[11] A subsequent study identified one more, bringing the total to 11: Adaptation to the Intensive

Care Environment, Motor Activity Assessment Scale, Minnesota Sedation Assessment Tool, Observer's Assessment of Alertness/Sedation, SAS, Sedation Intensive Care Score, New Sheffield Sedation Scale, Ramsay Sedation Scale, RASS, Vancouver Interaction and Calmness Scale, and Nursing Instrument for the Communication of Sedation.[72] Several other scales have been developed, but most lack the methodological quality for formal evaluation.[73] The RASS and SAS have consistently performed well in studies that have evaluated their psychometric properties, and they are endorsed by the 2013 SCCM PAD guidelines.[11,72]

Ramsay Sedation Scale

Before the SAS and RASS were conceived, caregivers and researchers used the Ramsay scale. Originally named the controlled sedation scale, the Ramsay scale was developed in 1974 to assess various depths of sedation (Table 7.1).[74,75] Its biggest drawback is that it contains only one level of agitation, which makes it difficult to distinguish mild, moderate, or severe distress. Regardless, the Ramsay scale remains one of the most widely used subjective sedation scales worldwide.[76]

Sedation-Agitation Scale

The SAS was developed in 1992 while evaluating continuous infusion haloperidol for ICU agitation.[77] Riker and colleagues realized that there was no way to comprehensively describe agitation and sedation, so they developed a graded scale using bedside descriptors.[75] A subsequent editorial urging the creation of subjective sedation scales prompted the investigators to revisit the SAS, and a revised iteration was published in 1999 (Table 7.2).[68,78]

The SAS is centered around a score of 4 (calm and cooperative) and has seven tiers that range from 1 (unarousable) to 7 (dangerous agitation). It was initially validated against the Ramsay and Harris scales and later against the BIS and Visual Analog Scale.[68,79,80] It has been studied in more than 1,500 patients and has been published in several languages.[72] The salient feature of the SAS is that sedated patients (SAS score of 3) should be able to follow

Table 7.1 Ramsay Scale

Score	Description
1	Patient anxious and agitated
2	Patient cooperative, oriented, and tranquil
3	Patient responds to commands only
4	Patient asleep and has a brisk response to a glabellar tap
5	Patient asleep and has a sluggish response to a glabellar tap
6	Patient asleep and has no response to a glabellar tap

Information from: Ramsay MA, Savege TM, Simpson BR, et al. Controlled sedation with alphaxalone-alphadolone. Br Med J 1974;2:656-9.

Table 7.2 Sedation-Agitation Scale[a]

Score	Term	Description
7	Dangerous agitation	Pulling at the endotracheal tube, trying to remove catheters, climbing over bed rail, striking at staff, thrashing side-to-side
6	Very agitated	Does not calm despite frequent verbal reminding of limits, requires physical restraints, biting endotracheal tube
5	Agitated	Anxious or mildly agitated, trying to sit up, calms down to verbal instructions
4	Calm and cooperative	Calm, awakens easily, follows commands
3	Sedated	Difficult to arouse, awakens to verbal stimuli or gentle shaking but drifts off again, follows simple commands
2	Very sedated	Arouses to physical stimuli but does not communicate or follow commands, may move spontaneously
1	Unarousable	Minimal or no response to noxious stimuli, does not communicate or follow commands

[a]Patients who are a SAS 1 or 2 should not be assessed for delirium. The scale should not be used for patients receiving paralytics. The SAS has not been validated in patients with neurological injury or those requiring medically induced coma (i.e., intracranial pressure elevations or status epilepticus).

Adapted from: Riker RR, Picard JT, Fraser GL. Prospective Evaluation of the Sedation-Agitation Scale for adult critically ill patients. Crit Care Med 1999;27:1325.

simple commands (e.g., open eyes, maintain eye contact, squeeze hand, stick out tongue, and wiggle toes).

Richmond Agitation-Sedation Scale

The RASS was developed in 1999 in an effort to create a scale that offered more distinction between levels of agitation and sedation (Table 7.3).[75,81] The RASS is centered around zero (alert and calm) and has four levels of agitation (restless to combative) and five levels of sedation (drowsy to unarousable). It was originally validated against the Ramsay scale, Glasgow Coma Scale, Visual Analog Scale, and SAS.[81] It was later validated against a geriatric psychiatrist and geriatric neuropsychologist and the BIS.[69] The RASS has been studied in more than 3,400 patients and has been translated into several languages.[72]

The RASS uses eye contact as a surrogate for arousal, content of thought, and ultimately consciousness.[69] The biggest drawback of the RASS is that it does not examine patients' ability to interact with their environment (i.e., wakefulness), which should be present when assessing pain, evaluating delirium, and determining whether a patient is a candidate for mobilization. Although there is no validated definition of wakefulness, following simple commands may be the most appropriate way to identify it.[11]

Objective Monitoring

Objective measures of sedation can supplement subjective scales, make up for subjective scale shortcomings (e.g., need for motor responsiveness or patient cooperation), and partly address variations in sedation practices.[82] Objective measures include vital signs, auditory evoked potentials, BIS, Narcotrend Index, patient state index, and state entropy. Use of vital signs should be avoided because they can nonspecifically fluctuate, and studies detailing their appropriateness are conflicting.[83,84] Data describing the use of auditory evoked potentials, Narcotrend Index, patient state index, or state entropy are in their infancy.[11] Of all the objective measures, the BIS is the most advanced.

The BIS interprets raw EEG signals by a proprietary algorithm to create a single number for level of consciousness ranging from 0 to 100.[85] A major assumption is that cortical activity is reflective of consciousness.[75] Other data analyzed include power spectral information, degree of EEG suppression, beta frequency activation, and

Table 7.3 Richmond Agitation-Sedation Scale[a]

Score	Term	Description
+4	Combative	Overtly combative or violent; immediate danger to staff
+3	Very agitated	Pulls on or removes tube(s) or catheter(s) or has aggressive behavior toward staff
+2	Agitated	Frequent nonpurposeful movement or patient-ventilator dyssynchrony
+1	Restless	Anxious or apprehensive but movements not aggressive or vigorous
0	Alert and calm	
-1	Drowsy	Not fully alert, but has sustained (> 10 seconds) awakening, with eye contact, to voice
-2	Light sedation	Briefly (< 10 seconds) awakens with eye contact to voice
-3	Moderate sedation	Any movement (but no eye contact) to voice
-4	Deep sedation	No response to voice, but any movement to physical stimulation
-5	Unarousable	No response to voice or physical stimulation

[a]Patients who are a RASS -3 to -5 should not be assessed for delirium. The scale should not be used for patients receiving paralytics. The RASS has been validated in patients in a medical respiratory, neuroscience, coronary, surgical trauma, and cardiac surgery ICU. RASS should not be used in those requiring medically induced coma (i.e., intracranial pressure elevations or status epilepticus) or in those with severe auditory or visual impairments.

Adapted with permission from: American Thoracic Society. Copyright © 2015 American Thoracic Society. Sessler CN, Gosnell MS, Grap MJ, et al. Am J Respir Crit Care Med 2002;166:1338.

synchronization with lower frequencies.[86] Bispectral index scores can be interpreted as follows: 0 is complete EEG suppression, 1–40 is deep sedation, 41–60 is moderate sedation, 61–70 is light sedation, and 71–100 is light sedation to fully awake.[71] Caregivers should be cognizant that the BIS is influenced by sleep, neurological disease, encephalopathy, cerebral ischemia, electromyography, hypothermia, genetically determined low-voltage patterns, placement of the leads, drugs, and sound.[85,87,88]

The BIS has been compared with several subjective sedation scales, but a consistent linear relationship between them has been elusive.[75,85,87,89] Discrepancies may occur because the BIS tops out, whereas subjective scales bottom out (Figure 7.1).[85] A BIS value less than 60 may be appropriate for deeper sedation, according to studies showing that surgical patients rarely recall their experience when values are less than 60.[85] Overall, the BIS should be reserved for select ICU patients such as those requiring prognostication during targeted temperature management, burst suppression to control intracranial pressure (ICP), neuromuscular blockade, or deep sedation for any other reason.[90,91]

NONPHARMACOLOGIC INTERVENTIONS

Nonpharmacologic comfort measures can be used alone or in addition to pharmacologic agents.[43] Data supporting their use are limited, but their benefits likely outweigh the risks. Intensive care unit survivors have reported that caregiver support, explanations, and a personal approach are vital to psychological well-being.[92] Encouragement, allowing patients to write, and explaining care plans are viewed as stress-relieving. Responding slowly to call bells imparts feelings of helplessness and dependency.[92] Caregivers are encouraged to explain what they are doing, even when they perceive patients as comatose.

Noise is a stressor that can be obviated with nonpharmacologic interventions.[9,12,13] Noise-reducing strategies such as ear plugs, sound masking, and acoustic absorption have been evaluated with favorable results.[93,94] Reducing noise with behavioral modification and source control may circumvent the need for other modalities.[95] Patient-directed music therapy represents another potential way to reduce the burden of unpleasant sounds.[96]

Several other nonpharmacologic strategies can be employed. Eye masks, light dimming, and rooms with windows represent ways of reducing bothersome artificial lighting. Manipulative medicine and physical therapy can be used to relieve pain.[2,97] Routine procedures like bladder emptying and repositioning are also crucial. Physical restraints should be reserved for severe agitation (e.g., imminent harm to the patient or caregiver) because of ethical considerations, psychological distress (including the development posttraumatic stress disorder), and risk of delirium.[98-101] Although

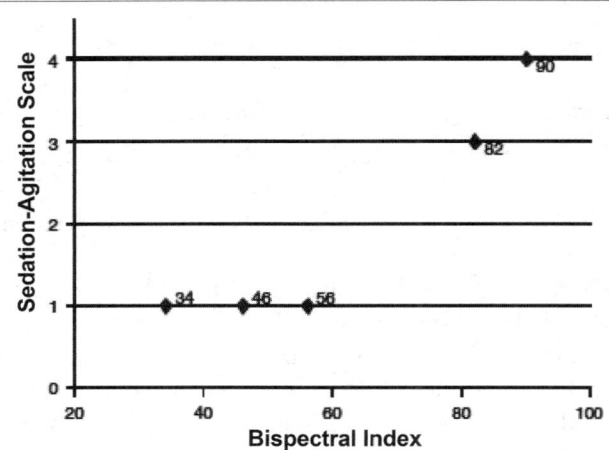

Figure 7.1 Sedation-agitation scale vs. bispectral index.

Once unresponsiveness is achieved, subjective assessment tools like the SAS can no longer quantify sedation depth. Processed electroencephalographic monitors like the BIS can continue to quantify sedation depth all the way down to an isoelectric state. For example, when a patient has a SAS score of 1, providers cannot describe deeper sedation; however, the BIS can assess brain activity down to an isoelectric state.

Adapted with permission from: Fraser GL, Riker RR. Bispectral index monitoring in the intensive care unit providers more signal than noise. Pharmacotherapy 2005;25(5 pt 2):19S-27S.

nonpharmacologic interventions are sometimes successful, pharmacologic therapy will be needed more often than not.

PHARMACOLOGIC AGENTS

More than 50% of mechanically ventilated patients require sedation.[102-104] Nonventilated patients occupy 60%–80% of ICU beds and often require sedation as well.[105] Unfortunately, no ideal sedative agent exists, and no agent has been found to be universally superior to the rest.[106] This section will review the pharmacology, pharmacokinetics, and appropriate clinical context for using opioids, traditional sedatives, and alternative agents.

Opioids

Opioids (fentanyl, hydromorphone, morphine, remifentanil, and methadone) are commonly used in the ICU for relief of pain and analgosedation.[107] Analgosedation is a sedation strategy that targets pain and discomfort with analgesics before more traditional sedatives are introduced.[108] All opioids are equally effective when titrated to patient-specific goals (Table 7.4).[11] Opioids predominantly agonize mu-receptors, which results in analgesia, euphoria, and serenity.[109] Class-wide adverse effects include tolerance, constipation, suppression of cough reflexes, respiratory depression, and hypotension; these effects occur especially with morphine, which induces histamine release and venodilation.[110] The opioids are briefly discussed with a focus on analgosedation, and more information can be found in the Pain chapter.

Fentanyl

Fentanyl is a synthetic phenylpiperidine derivative and is one of the most commonly prescribed opioids in ICUs worldwide.[102,104,109,111,112] It is about 100 times more potent than morphine.[113] In general, it is given as an intermittent injection or continuous infusion. Transdermal patches should not be used for acute treatment of pain because of delayed onset and sporadic absorption; however, they may find utility when de-escalating care.[114]

Only 10% of fentanyl is excreted unchanged by the kidneys, and data supporting dosing adjustments with impared renal function are low quality[115,116] Fentanyl is lipophilic and can accumulate in adipose tissue, resulting in a prolonged duration of action with long-term use.[110,117] As a substrate for cytochrome P450 (CYP) 3A4, fentanyl may interact with enzyme system inhibitors (e.g., azole antifungals, macrolides, protease inhibitors, or non-dihydropyridine calcium channel blockers) and inducers (barbiturates, phenytoin, rifampin, or carbamazepine). Some cases of fentanyl-induced serotonin syndrome have been described when combined with selective serotonin reuptake inhibitors.[118,119] Fentanyl infrequently causes chest wall rigidity when large doses are administered rapidly.[110] Overall, its favorable pharmacokinetics/pharmacodynamics and cost profiles make it an attractive analgosedative.

Hydromorphone

Hydromorphone is a semisynthetic phenanthrene that is derived from morphine and is about 6.5 times more potent.[109,113] Because of its relatively long half-life (2–3 hours) and prolonged time to steady state, bolus dosing is encouraged when initiating or titrating an infusion.[11] Hydromorphone is metabolized to hydromorphone-3-glucuronide, which has been implicated in neurotoxic events in patients who receive high doses or have renal impairment.[120,121]

Hydromorphone is an option for opioid rotation because it may restore analgesia and sedation in patients who no longer respond to high doses of other opioids. The mechanism by which opioid rotation restores analgesia is unknown, but it may be because of incomplete cross-tolerance, genetic polymorphisms, and interindividual differences in opioid receptor types, interactions, density, or binding.[122] Data supporting this strategy are extrapolated from the oncology literature, where intravenous hydromorphone has been used to manage intractable cancer pain in patients whose other opioids have failed.[123,124] A

Table 7.4 Pharmacologic Properties of Opioids

Opioid	Equianalgesic Dose (IV)[a]	Intermittent Dosing[a]	Infusion Rates[a]	Onset (IV)[a,b]	Metabolism	Elimination	Active Metabolites	Half-life[a,b]	Cost
Fentanyl	0.1 mg	0.35–0.5 mcg/kg IV q0.5–1 hr	0.7–10 mcg/kg/hr	1–2 min	N-dealkylation, CYP3A4[a,b]	Renal[d]	No[d]	2–4 hr	$
Hydromorphone	1.5 mg	0.2–0.6 mg IV q1–2 hr	0.5–3 mg/hr	5–15 min	Glucuronidation[a,b]	Renal[d]	No[b,d]	2–3 hr	$
Morphine	10 mg	2–4 mg IV q1–2 hr	2–30 mg/hr	5–10 min	Demethylation and glucuronidation[c]	Renal[d]	Morphine-3-glucuronide, morphine-6-glucuronide[d]	3–4 hr	$
Remifentanil	N/A	N/A	Loading dose: 1.5 mcg/kg/hr; Maintenance dose: 0.5–15 mcg/kg/hr	1–3 min	Tissue and plasma esterases[a,b]	Renal[e]	No[e]	3–10 min	$$$
Methadone	N/A	5–15 mg IV/PO q6–12 hr	N/A	30 min	Demethylation, CYP 3A4/5, 2D6, 2B6, 1A2[a,b]	Renal[d]	No[b,c,d]	15–60 hr	$

IBW = ideal body weight; IV = intravenous(ly); N/A = not applicable; PO = oral(ly); q = every.

[a]Barr J, Fraser GL, Puntillo K, et al. Clinical practice guidelines for the management of pain, agitation, and delirium in adult patients in the intensive care unit. Crit Care Med 2013;41:263-306.
[b]Devlin JW, Roberts RJ. Pharmacology of commonly used analgesics and sedatives in the ICU: benzodiazepines, propofol, and opioids. Anesthesiol Clin 2011;29:567-585.
[c]Trescot AM, Datta S, Lee M, et al. Opioid pharmacology. Pain Physician 2008;11(2 suppl):S133-S153.
[d]Davies G, Kingswood C, Street M. Pharmacokinetics of opioids in renal dysfunction. Clin Pharmacokinet 1996;31:410-322.
[e]Bürkle H, Dunbar S, Van Aken H. Remifentanil: a novel, short-acting, mu-opioid. Anesth Analg 1996;83:646-651.

1- or 2-mg intravenous test dose can be given, and if a patient responds favorably, it can be scheduled, or an infusion can be initiated.

Morphine

Morphine is the prototypical phenanthrene.[109] Its use has steadily declined for several reasons.[102,111,125,126] First, it is hepatically metabolized to the active metabolites morphine-3-glucuronide and morphine-6-glucuronide. The former can cause neurotoxicity and hyperalgesia, whereas the latter can cause oversedation.[127,128] Second, morphine is hydrophilic, which results in a slow onset of action.[129] Third, its metabolism and active metabolite elimination are reduced in the setting of renal or hepatic impairment.[115,130] Fourth, it is poorly titratable because of its long-half-life compared with other opioids. Finally, it induces histamine release, which can cause bronchospasm and venodilation.[129] In general, other opioids may be safer analgosedatives.

Remifentanil

Remifentanil is a synthetic phenylpiperidine derivate with potency similar to fentanyl.[109] Remifentanil contains an ester linkage, which is rapidly metabolized by nonspecific tissue and plasma esterases to inactive metabolites.[117] Because of this, it has a short half-life (3–10 minutes) and duration of action regardless of infusion duration and end-organ function.[131] This represents an advantage if frequent neurological evaluations are necessary, but it can be problematic as well.[132] Withdrawal or resurgence of pain can occur if the infusion is abruptly or inadvertently discontinued.[133] Rescue opioids should be immediately available. Despite many interesting characteristics, its use remains low across the globe.[102,111,112,134]

Remifentanil is the most studied analgosedative and is an attractive option in brain-injured patients because of its predictable pharmacokinetics.[132,135-141] It acts synergistically with propofol, inhaled anesthetics, and benzodiazepines.[142] Hyperalgesia and withdrawal symptoms should be monitored for and can be diminished by administering longer-acting opioids during tapering.[88,143] Ultimately, its safety and efficacy are similar to that of fentanyl, making the latter more used on the basis of cost, ease of use, and familiarity.[138]

Methadone

Methadone is a synthetic diphenylheptane derivative that is unique from other opioids because it antagonizes N-methyl-D-aspartate (NMDA) receptors.[109,144] Methadone's relative potency compared with morphine is contingent on the duration of administration and tolerance.[145] Its long half-life and tendency to prolong the QTc interval limit its usefulness in the ICU.[144,146] Total daily dose of methadone is the most established risk factor for QTc prolongation, but patients taking as little as 30–40 mg/day have developed torsades de pointes.[146,147] Pharmacists should monitor for other risk factors for QTc prolongation, including electrolyte abnormalities (hypokalemia or hypomagnesaemia) and QTc-prolonging medications (e.g., fluoroquinolones, antipsychotics, amiodarone, or erythromycin).[148]

Methadone can be used to facilitate the discontinuation of opioid infusions. A reasonable starting dose is 10 mg every 6–8 hours. It may reduce ventilator weaning time and obviate the need for continuously infused opioids, but its impact on ICU LOS, total opioid exposure, and duration of mechanical ventilation remains unclear.[149,150] Methadone has also shown promise in the setting of opioid tolerance and hyperalgesia, which may be because of excessive NMDA receptor stimulation.[151] Rotating to methadone from other opioids has been studied in the setting of intractable or cancer-related pain, but it has yet to be studied in the ICU for this indication.[122]

Traditional Sedatives

Benzodiazepines

Benzodiazepines (midazolam and lorazepam) potentiate the activity of γ-aminobutyric acid (GABA) at $GABA_A$ receptors, which increases chloride influx leading to neuronal hyperpolarization (Table 7.5).[152] Collectively, benzodiazepines produce anxiolytic, amnestic, sedative, hypnotic, and anticonvulsant effects, but no analgesia.[11] Class-wide adverse effects include cardiorespiratory depression, altered sensorium, and paradoxical excitatory reactions.[152] Hemodynamic instability can occur with an etiology that is uncertain, but likely the result of blunting the stress response rather than direct vasodilation. Tolerance and withdrawal can develop with prolonged use and is addressed later.[153]

The use of benzodiazepines has been scrutinized recently. They are associated with prolonged mechanical ventilation duration and ICU LOS compared with nonbenzodiazepines (i.e., dexmedetomidine or propofol).[11,154] These findings are probably the result of drug accumulation with long-term use and inappropriate sedation titration. In addition, the benzodiazepines have been inconsistently associated with the development of delirium.[155-159] A causal relationship has yet to be established, and the association may stem from confounding of delirium assessments during sedation.[160] This topic is further examined later. Despite these concerns, the benzodiazepines should continue to be viewed as first-line agents for acute agitation or alcohol withdrawal.

Midazolam

Midazolam is the most commonly used benzodiazepine in ICUs.[102] It is about half as potent as lorazepam, and because it is highly lipophilic, it can accumulate in adipose

Table 7.5 Pharmacologic Properties of Traditional Sedatives

Drug	Dose Range	Onset[b] (IV)	Mechanism[b]	Metabolism	Elimination	Active Metabolites	Half-life[b]	Cost
Midazolam[a]	Bolus: 0.01–0.05 mg/kg q1hr PRN	2–5 min	$GABA_A$ receptor agonist	CYP3A4[d]	Renal[d]	α-Hydroxymidazolam (60% potency of parent)	3–11 hr	$
	Infusion: 0.02–0.1 mg/kg/hr[b]					α-Hydroxymidazolam glucuronide (10% potency of parent)[c]		
Lorazepam[a]	0.02–0.04 mg/kg q2–6 hr PRN[b]	15–20 min	$GABA_A$ receptor agonist	Glucuronidation[d]	Renal[d]	No[d]	8–15 hr	$
Propofol[a]	5–50 mcg/kg/min[b]	1–2 min	$GABA_A$ receptor agonist	CYP2B6, 3A4, and extrahepatic[e]	Renal[e]	No[e]	3–12 hr Extended use: 24–30 hr	$$
Dexmedetomidine	0.2–1.4 mcg/kg/hr[c]	5–10 min	Selective central $α_2$-receptor agonist	Hydroxylation by CYP2A6 and glucuronidation[f]	Renal[f]	No[f]	2–2.5 hr	$$$

[a]Continuous infusion requires mechanical ventilation.
PRN = as needed.
[b]Barr J, Fraser GL, Puntillo K, et al. Clinical practice guidelines for the management of pain, agitation, and delirium in adult patients in the intensive care unit. Crit Care Med 2013;41:263-306.
[c]Jakob SM, Ruokonen E, Grounds RM, et al. Dexmedetomidine vs midazolam or propofol for sedation during prolonged mechanical ventilation: two randomized controlled trials. JAMA 2012;307:1151-1160.
[d]Young CC, Prielipp RC. Benzodiazepines in the intensive care unit. Crit Care Clin 2001;17:843-862.
[e]Devlin JW, Roberts RJ. Pharmacology of commonly used analgesics and sedatives in the ICU: benzodiazepines, propofol, and opioids. Anesthesiol Clin 2011;29:567-585.
[f]Gertler R, Brown HC, Mitchell DH, et al. Dexmedetomidine: a novel sedative-analgesic agent. Proc (Bayl Univ Med Cent) 2001;14:13-21.

tissue. Midazolam is metabolized by CYP3A4 to active metabolites, α-hydroxymidazolam (60% potency of midazolam), and α-hydroxymidazolam glucuronide (10% potency of midazolam), which are renally cleared.[152] It works synergistically with propofol because of a CYP-mediated drug-drug interaction leading to increased midazolam availability or enhanced GABA receptor agonism.[161,162] In general, it is most appropriate for acute agitation, inducing deep sedation for the treatment of refractory seizures or elevated ICP, as a premedication for procedures, or in the setting of hemodynamic instability that precludes the use of more readily titratable agents (propofol or dexmedetomidine).

Lorazepam

Lorazepam is the second most commonly used benzodiazepine in the ICU.[102] It should be used as an intermittent injection because of its long half-life and propensity to accumulate in adipose tissue or in the setting of hepatic impairment.[11] Lorazepam (high-performance liquid chromatography index relative to diazepam = 0.48) is less lipophilic than midazolam (high-performance liquid chromatography index relative to diazepam = 1.54), which results in a slower onset of action and slower egress from the CNS.[11,129,163]

Propylene glycol toxicity, which can occur with high-dose lorazepam therapy, has hampered its use. Each 2-mg/mL vial contains 830 mg of propylene glycol. An infusion of 2 mg/hour to a patient weighing 70 kg would deliver 20 g of propylene glycol in 24 hours, which is about 11 times the allowable dose set forth by the World Health Organization.[164] Propylene glycol toxicity manifests as metabolic acidosis (as a result of the production of pyruvate and lactic acid), renal impairment, and hyperosmolality. Because most centers cannot assay propylene glycol concentrations in a timely fashion, an osmolar gap of greater than 15 mOsm/kg can serve as a surrogate for accumulation of this toxin.[165] Ultimately, lorazepam should be used judiciously as an intermittent injection to calm acutely agitated patients and to abort seizures.

Propofol

Propofol has recently become the most popular ICU sedative (Table 7.5).[102,166] Its mechanism of action is uncertain and likely involves GABA, glycine, nicotinic, and muscarinic receptors. Stimulation of these receptors produces sedative, hypnotic, anxiolytic, amnestic, antiemetic, and anticonvulsant effects, but no analgesia.[11] Propofol is readily titratable during short-term use, especially when titrated to light levels of sedation, because of rapid redistribution and high hepatic and extrahepatic clearance.[167,168] However, it can accumulate in adipose tissue and slowly redistribute during prolonged infusions, resulting in a terminal half-life in excess of 24–30 hours.[169,170]

Propofol is generally safe, but certain aspects of its administration can be problematic. Propofol induces dose-dependent respiratory depression and can cause hypotension because of systemic vasodilation.[11] It is dissolved in a

10% lipid emulsion that contains egg lecithin and soybean oil, which can lead to allergic reactions, adds considerable calories (1.1 kcal/mL), and may lead to hypertriglyceridemia in as many as 18% of patients.[106,171,172] Pancreatitis has also been described during propofol therapy.[173] Although hypertriglyceridemia is a likely cause, reports of pancreatitis in the absence of hypertriglyceridemia suggest other mechanisms are at play.[174] Serum triglycerides and lipase should be monitored regularly and infusions discontinued when triglyceride concentrations exceed 500 mg/dL. Rare reports of propofol-induced myoclonus exist.[175] Of interest, propofol can turn urine green because of phenolic metabolites excreted in the urine.[176]

Propofol-related infusion syndrome (PRIS) may occur in 1%–10% of patients, depending on the patient population studied.[177,178] It has been associated with a mortality rate from 30% to greater than 80%.[177] The pathophysiology is unknown, but it may occur because of mitochondrial toxicity.[179] Propofol should be discontinued if unexpected metabolic acidosis, acute renal failure, rhabdomyolysis, transaminitis, hypotension, bradycardia, or Brugada-like coved ST-segments manifest.[180-182] Doses should be capped at 80 mcg/kg/minute because of a possible link between propofol exposure and PRIS, but this has been challenged in a study that found 82% of patients who developed PRIS were receiving doses of less than 83 mcg/kg/minute.[177] Despite potentially profound adverse effects, propofol should be considered a first-line sedative in hemodynamically stable patients.

Central α_2-Receptor Agonists

Centrally acting α_2-receptor agonists (dexmedetomidine and clonidine) reduce sympathetic outflow to produce cooperative levels of sedation without respiratory depression (Table 7.5).[183-185] Their primary site of action may be presynaptic neurons in the locus coeruleus, which regulates arousal, wakefulness, and sleep-wake cycles.[186,187] Analgesic-sparing activity has been well described with α_2-receptor agonists, which may be due to antinociceptive effects in the CNS and spinal cord.[188,189] Their adverse effects include bradycardia, heart block, and hypotension.[11] The α_2-receptor agonists are rapidly becoming popular ICU sedatives.[102,166]

Dexmedetomidine

Dexmedetomidine is the dextro enantiomer of medetomidine.[25] Its use has steadily increased during the past 15 years.[102] A α_2/α_1 selectivity ratio of 1620:1 is often cited, but medetomidine was used to establish it.[190] Loading doses should be avoided because of the risk of hypotension (α_{2A}-receptor agonism) or hypertension (α_{2B}- or α_1-receptor agonism).[191] Dexmedetomidine is readily titratable despite a long half-life (2–2.5 hours), which may be prolonged in older adult patients and those with liver disease.[25,192] Despite a relatively long half-life, the sedative effects of dexmedetomidine tend to wear off quickly after infusion discontinuation.[193]

Dexmedetomidine offers many advantages over other sedatives. Maintenance of respiratory drive allows for administration to non-intubated patients and may facilitate mechanical ventilator weaning. Cooperative levels of sedation allow for self-reporting of pain, mobilization, and accurate delirium screening. Dexmedetomidine has typically been shown to reduce the incidence of delirium, duration of mechanical ventilation, and ICU LOS compared with benzodiazepines.[11,154,194-196] It has also been used as an adjunctive agent in the management of alcohol withdrawal.[197] Variability in response and drug acquisition cost are its most significant drawbacks.[198] Drug acquisition cost may be offset by reduced ICU LOS, by shorter duration of ventilation, or with transition to enteral clonidine.[199-201]

Clonidine

Clonidine is the prototypical α_2-receptor agonist.[202] It is much less selective for α_2-receptors than medetomidine, with an α_2/α_1 selectivity ratio of 220:1.[190] Clonidine is highly lipophilic and produces dose-dependent sedation within 1–2 hours after an enteral dose, which coincides with peak plasma concentrations.[203-205] Clonidine is routinely used internationally as an intravenous sedative.[202,206-209] Enteral clonidine represents an emerging stand-alone sedative or alternative to dexmedetomidine in the United States.

Until recently, data supporting the use of enteral clonidine as an ICU sedative were limited to case reports and pediatric studies.[210-212] A recent single-center study showed that transitioning from dexmedetomidine to enteral clonidine (0.2–0.5 mg every 6–8 hours) may be a safe, effective, and less-costly way of providing α_2-receptor agonist therapy.[200] Similarly, a randomized trial found that enteral clonidine (0.1–0.2 mg three times daily) reduced morphine and midazolam requirements.[213] Withdrawal, which may occur in 13%–86% of patients receiving it for hypertension, is usually mild (e.g., palpitations, insomnia, or tremor) and can be avoided by tapering the dose on discontinuation.[214-216] Clonidine patches should be avoided because peak and steady-state concentrations are not reached until 4 days after the transdermal system is applied.[205] Ultimately, more robust data on clonidine as an ICU sedative are needed.

Alternative Sedatives

Valproic Acid

Valproic acid is a simple, branched-chain carboxylic acid that was first isolated in 1882 (Table 7.6).[217] Mechanistically, it blocks voltage-dependent sodium and calcium channels, increases GABA synthesis, potentiates GABA release, blocks GABA degradation, and attenuates the activation of NMDA receptors.[218] These actions culminate in anticonvulsant and mood-stabilizing effects. Recently, valproic acid has been used to treat alcohol withdrawal, agitation in dementia, and schizophrenia.[219-221]

Data describing valproic acid's safety and efficacy in critically ill patients are limited to two abstracts and a case series.[222-224] A loading dose of 30 mg/kg followed by 30 mg/kg/day may be appropriate according to bipolar disorder guidelines and anecdotal evidence.[225] Serum concentrations can be monitored and maintained between 50 mcg/mL and 125 mcg/mL because exposure may play a role in its efficacy.[226]

Patients receiving valproic acid should be monitored for several adverse effects. Ammonia concentrations should be obtained to monitor for hyperammonemia, which is because of valproic acid's interference with the urea cycle.[227] Levocarnitine therapy should be reserved for severe situations because the serum ammonia concentration will often return to normal after discontinuation.[228] Thrombocytopenia can occur and may be immune mediated in the acute setting or because of marrow suppression in the chronic setting.[229,230] Hepatotoxicity and pancreatitis are well described and require periodic liver function and serum lipase monitoring.[231,232] Valproic acid should be discontinued if a rash develops because of the risk of Stevens-Johnson syndrome.

Drug-drug interactions should also be monitored for during valproic acid therapy. Carbapenem antibiotics

Table 7.6 Pharmacologic Properties of Alternative Sedatives

Drug	Dose	Mechanism	Metabolism	Elimination	Active Metabolites	Half-life	Cost
Clonidine	0.2–0.5 mg PO or SL q6–8hr[a]	α_2-receptor agonist[a]	CYP2D6, 1A2, 3A4/5, and 1A1[k]	Renal[n]	No[n]	6–25 hr[n]	$
Valproic acid	Bolus: 30 mg/kg IV Maintenance: 30 mg/kg/day in three or four divided doses IV or PO[b]	Potentiates GABA and reduces NMDA receptor activation[h]	Mitochondrial beta-oxidation and hepatic by CYP (2C9, 2C19, 2B6, and 2A6), glucuronidation[h]	Renal[h]	2-en-valproate, 4-en-valproate[h]	9–16 hr[h]	$
Phenobarbital	Bolus: 7.5 mg/kg IV Maintenance: 1–2 mg/kg IV in two divided doses Rescue: 65–130 mg IV q1hr PRN[c]	Prolongs GABA channel opening[i]	CYP2C9, 2C19, and 2E1[l]	Renal[l]	No[l]	70–145 hr[l]	$
Ketamine	0.05–0.4 mg/kg/hr[d]	NMDA receptor antagonist[j]	CYP 3A4, 2B6, and 2C9[m]	Renal[j]	Norketamine (~30% potency of parent)[d,m]	2.5 hr[d]	$
Hydroxyzine	12.5–25 mg PO q6–8 hr Max = 100 mg/d[e,f,g]	H_1 receptor antagonist[e,f]	CYP3A4/5	Renal[f]	Yes	20–25 hr	$

SL = sublingual(ly).

[a]Gagnon DJ, Riker RR, Glisic EK, et al. Transition from dexmedetomidine to enteral clonidine for ICU sedation: an observational pilot study. Pharmacotherapy 2015;35:251-259.
[b]American Psychiatric Association: Practice guideline for the treatment of patients with bipolar disorder (revision). Am J Psychiatry 2002; 159:1–50.
[c]Fraser GL, Riker RR. Phenobarbital provides effective sedation for a select cohort of adult ICU patients intolerant of standard treatment: a brief report. Hosp Pharm 2006;41:17-23.
[d]Barr J, Fraser GL, Puntillo K, et al. Clinical practice guidelines for the management of pain, agitation, and delirium in adult patients in the intensive care unit. Crit Care Med 2013;41:263-306.
[e]Mistraletti G, Mantovani ES, Cadringher P, et al. Enteral vs. intravenous ICU sedation management: study protocol for a randomized controlled trial. Trials 2013;14:92.
[f]Cigada M, Pezzi A, Di Mauro P, et al. Sedation in the critically ill ventilated patient: possible role of enteral drugs. Intensive Care Med 2005;31:482-6.
[g]New restrictions to minimise the risks of effects on heart rhythm with hydroxyzine-containing medicines. European Medicines Agency. Available at www.ema.europa.eu/ema/index.jsp?curl=pages/medicines/human/referrals/Hydroxyzine/human_referral_prac_000043.jsp&mid=WC0b01ac05805c516f. Accessed July 1, 2015
[h]Perucca E. Pharmacological and therapeutic properties of valproate: a summary after 35 years of clinical experience. CNS Drugs 2002;16:695-714.
[i]Smith MC, Riskin BJ. The clinical use of barbiturates in neurological disorders. Drugs 1991;42:365-78.
[j]Panzer O, Moitra V, Sladen RN. Pharmacology of sedative-analgesic agents: dexmedetomidine, remifentanil, ketamine, volatile anesthetics, and the role of peripheral mu antagonists. Crit Care Clin 2009;25:451-69, vii.
[k]Claessens AJ1, Risler LJ, Eyal S, Shen DD, Easterling TR, Hebert MF. CYP2D6 mediates 4-hydroxylation of clonidine in vitro: implication for pregnancy-induced changes in clonidine clearance. Drug Metab Dispos 2010;38(9):1393-6.
[l]Kwan P, Brodie MJ Phenobarbital. for the treatment of epilepsy in the 21st century: a critical review. Epilepsia 2004;45:1141-9.
[m]Wolff K, Winstock AR. Ketamine: from medicine to misuse. CNS Drugs 2006;20:199-218.
[n]Lowenthal DT, Matzek KM, MacGregor TR. Clinical pharmacokinetics of clonidine. Clin Pharmacokinet 1988;14:287-310.

reduce valproic acid serum concentrations by more than 50%.[233,234] Proposed mechanisms include repression of valproic acid absorption from the intestinal lumen, reduced enterohepatic recirculation because of decreased β-glucuronidase activity, increased hepatic glucuronidation because of increases in uridine diphosphate glucuronic acid concentrations, and increased distribution of valproic acid into red blood cells.[234] In addition, valproic acid is a CYP2C9 inhibitor, which may reduce the metabolism of CYP2C9 substrates (e.g., phenobarbital, phenytoin, or carbamazepine). However, valproic acid's metabolism can be increased by CYP2C9 inducers (e.g., phenobarbital, phenytoin, carbamazepine, or rifampin) or decreased by CYP2C19 inhibitors (e.g., felbamate or topiramate).[235]

Phenobarbital

Phenobarbital is a barbiturate that was first developed in 1911 (Table 7.6).[236] The barbiturates prolong GABA channel opening, which increases chloride ion influx and hyperpolarizes neuronal membranes.[237] This action results in anticonvulsant, anesthetic, anxiolytic, and sedating effects. Phenobarbital use is limited because of its long half-life (70 to 145 hours), which results in poor titratability.[236] Interest in phenobarbital has increased because it does not require mechanical ventilation for administration and can be given enterally.

Phenobarbital is predominantly used to treat alcohol withdrawal and refractory seizures.[236,238] Only one case series has described its safety and tolerability for ICU sedation.[239] In that study, an intravenous loading dose of 7.5 mg/kg was followed by a maintenance regimen of 1–2 mg/kg intravenously divided twice daily with 65- to 130-mg rescue doses as needed. Phenobarbital was well tolerated and was not associated with hemodynamic derangements.

Other than sedation, adverse effects associated with phenobarbital are relatively uncommon. Patients receiving intravenous loading doses should be monitored for cardiorespiratory depression. Clinically significant drug interactions may occur during phenobarbital therapy because it is a potent inducer of CYP3A4 and the CYP2C subfamily.[235] Serum concentration monitoring is not necessary unless toxicity is suspected. Phenobarbital can be considered in severe agitation or alcohol withdrawal, but more data are needed to define its role in the ICU.

Ketamine

Ketamine is a dissociative anesthetic and phencyclidine derivative that gained popularity on the battlefield during the Vietnam War (Table 7.6).[25] Its mechanism of action includes NMDA receptor antagonism and mu and kappa opioid receptor agonism.[240] These actions produce dissociative, sedative, analgesic, and amnestic effects. Interest in ketamine to provide comfort in the ICU has increased because it does not depress cardiorespiratory function.[106]

Few studies have described the use of ketamine as a continuous infusion to manage agitation in the ICU.[241,242] Because of this and unfamiliarity with its use, it is typically reserved for severe agitation or intractable pain. Of interest, ketamine has been shown to attenuate delirium after cardiac surgery.[243] In addition, it has been used to manage alcohol withdrawal.[244]

Patients receiving ketamine should be monitored for a hyperadrenergic state, exacerbation of coronary ischemia, psychiatric disturbances, and emergence phenomena (confusion, nightmares, or hallucinations).[25] Although earlier data suggested it increases ICP, recent studies have refuted this.[245] Until more robust data are available, ketamine should be reserved for select patients who do not respond to more traditional agents.

Antipsychotics

Antipsychotics antagonize dopamine, serotonin, histamine, α-adrenergic, and muscarinic receptors, resulting in mood-stabilizing effects.[246] They are characterized as typical (chlorpromazine, perphenazine, prochlorperazine, and haloperidol) or atypical (aripiprazole, clozapine, olanzapine, quetiapine, and risperidone). Each antipsychotic has a unique affinity for the receptors it interacts with, which leads to varying degrees of response.[247] Most studies describe antipsychotic use for hyperactive delirium.[248] Data supporting their use for primary agitation have not been developed. Nonetheless, they are commonly used.[249-252]

Haloperidol is the most commonly used antipsychotic because of the availability of a parenteral formulation, although this route of administration has not been approved by the U.S. Food and Drug Administration. Intermittent boluses of 0.5–10 mg intravenously as needed are reasonable. Quetiapine (12.5–100 mg given every 6–12 hours) and olanzapine (2.5–30 mg/day) may also be used.[253,254] Patients receiving antipsychotics should be closely monitored for extrapyramidal symptoms (akathisia, parkinsonism, or dystonias), QTc interval prolongation, and neuroleptic malignant syndrome.[164,255,256] In addition, these agents can lower the seizure threshold.[257] More information on the antipsychotics can be found in the Delirium chapter.

Volatile Anesthetics

The introduction of an anesthetic-conserving device to reduce atmospheric pollution has led to renewed interest in volatile anesthetics (isoflurane, sevoflurane, and desflurane) as ICU sedatives.[258] These agents may interfere with GABA activity or interact with cell membrane lipids, proteins, or ion channels. These mechanisms result in rapid loss of consciousness, immobility, analgesia, anterograde amnesia, and respiratory depression.[25,259] Volatile anesthetics are predominantly eliminated by the lungs, but small amounts are cleared hepatically by CYP2E1.[260] Adverse effects include hemodynamic instability, malignant hyperthermia, and renal or hepatic toxicity.[261]

In addition, sevoflurane-induced sedation in patients with stroke or subarachnoid hemorrhage has been associated with transient elevations in ICP.[262] Volatile anesthetics have been included in international ICU comfort guidelines because of their titratability, tolerability, favorable pharmacokinetic profiles, and potential post-conditioning effects.[209,263]

Data describing the safety and efficacy of volatile anesthetics are limited. Isoflurane has been the most studied agent, followed by sevoflurane and desflurane. Most investigations have shown that they shorten awakening time after sedative discontinuation compared with traditional agents (midazolam or propofol)[258,264-267]; however, results are conflicting.[268] They may also shorten time to extubation after sedation discontinuation and be associated with better survival and psychological outcomes.[258,265,267,269,270] Interpreting these studies is difficult because of variations in the patients studied, duration of sedation, anesthetic used, control group treatment, outcomes reported, and use of validated sedation scales. Concerns about the use of these agents include the short- and long-term impact of atmospheric pollution on caregivers, use by non-anesthesiologists, costs, and operational issues.[25,271] Routine use should be reserved until these shortcomings are addressed.

Hydroxyzine

Hydroxyzine is a first-generation antihistamine that antagonizes H$_1$ receptors. It also has anticholinergic, antiserotonergic, antiemetic, and gastric antisecretory properties.[272] Hydroxyzine has been used for several decades for generalized anxiety and as an anesthesia premedication.[273-275] It has been evaluated as an enteral ICU sedative in adults at a dose 6–12 mg/kg/day in divided doses.[276] More recent data suggest that doses should not exceed 100 mg/day in adults or 50 mg/day in older adult patients because of the risk of QT interval prolongation and cardiac arrhythmias.[277] In addition, hydroxyzine should be avoided in patients with acquired or congenital QT interval prolongation, electrolyte abnormalities (hypokalemia or hypomagnesemia), family history of sudden cardiac death, significant bradycardia, or concomitant use of drugs known to prolong the QT interval.

IATROGENIC WITHDRAWAL FROM SEDATION

Caregivers should closely monitor patients for signs and symptoms of withdrawal after extended exposure to sedatives. Withdrawal may occur in 32% of patients who received at least 7 days of sedation.[278] Risk factors may include higher daily and peak exposures and abrupt weaning of these agents.[278,279] Acute opioid withdrawal may occur because of hyperactivity within the nociceptive system, which is supported by studies that have shown β-endorphins and met-enkephalins are elevated during withdrawal.[280] Symptoms are often the opposite of the drug's pharmacologic effect and include agitation, tachycardia, hypertension, tachypnea, insomnia, delirium, nausea, diarrhea, diaphoresis, and fever.[281] Diagnosing iatrogenic withdrawal can be accomplished by replenishing the drug in question and observing the patient's response.

To avoid precipitating withdrawal, slow tapering of sedation is encouraged. Reducing infusion rates by 25%–50% per day is a reasonable approach. Methadone or other longer-acting enteral opioids (e.g., hydromorphone or oxycodone) can be used to facilitate the discontinuation of opioid infusions.[149,150] Longer-acting benzodiazepines like clonazepam can be used to taper off benzodiazepine infusions. Although withdrawal from dexmedetomidine rarely occurs in routine practice, clonidine can be used to transition off dexmedetomidine.[200,282] Pharmacists are well situated to identify patients at risk of withdrawal and to develop sedation-tapering strategies.

TRANSITIONS OF CARE AND SEDATION

Pharmacists are in an excellent position to improve transitions of care. It is not uncommon for patients to be transferred from the ICU or discharged home on a new psychoactive medication. Confounding the situation is the fact that 36% of medications are used off-label in the ICU, which can create confusion during de-escalation of care.[283] One study found that 47% of patients prescribed an atypical antipsychotic in the ICU have them continued on ICU discharge.[284] In a recent systematic review of ICU discharge literature, only 2% of studies focused on medication reconciliation.[285] Strategies to improve transitions of care are desperately needed and should be a focus of future research efforts.

SEDATION CONFOUNDING OF DELIRIUM ASSESSMENTS

The introduction of valid and reliable delirium screening tools in 2001 represented a monumental advancement in ICU care. These tools allowed for a more rigorous assessment of risk factors for ICU delirium and significant advances in our understanding of this complex process. Preexisting dementia, hypertension, alcoholism, and coma have consistently been identified as risk factors, whereas an association between sedative use and ICU delirium has been less clear.[11] The benzodiazepines have been the most implicated agents, but the issue may be broader than a single agent or drug class.[155-159]

Level of consciousness is a central component of both the confusion assessment method for the intensive care unit (CAM-ICU) and the Intensive Care Delirium Screening Checklist (ICDSC).[286,287] Sedatives, from any drug class, have the ability to interfere with level of consciousness and therefore delirium assessments. One study has shown that the frequency of positive CAM-ICU assessments increased by 20% if the RASS score went from -2 to -3.[288] Although the original studies of the ICDSC did not address the potential for sedatives to confound assessments, subsequent studies have suggested that components of the ICDSC that are influenced by sedation should not be assessed in the presence of sedatives.[158] No such clarification has been made regarding the CAM-ICU.

Recent data have begun to elucidate the differences between persistent and rapidly reversible sedation-related delirium.[288,289] In the study by Patel et al., CAM-ICU assessments were completed before and after sedation interruption, and patients were classified as never delirious, as persistently delirious (positive CAM-ICU scores 2 hours after sedation discontinuation), or as having rapidly reversible sedation-related delirium (positive CAM-ICU scores before sedation interruption but negative scores after). Patients with rapidly reversible sedation-related delirium had long-term outcomes similar to those who were never delirious. Of importance, only 54% of patients were exposed to midazolam in that trial for a median duration of 1 hour, whereas more than 95% received propofol and fentanyl. In the study by Haenggi et al., just 20% of patients received continuously infused benzodiazepines. These data suggest that rapidly reversible sedation-related delirium can occur with any sedative and that its impact on outcomes is unclear. Accordingly, the 2013 SCCM PAD guidelines suggest that delirium assessments be completed when patients are wakeful (i.e., SAS 3 to 4 or RASS −2 to 0 or ability to follow simple commands).[11]

SEDATION STRATEGIES

One of the most important discoveries in ICU sedation during the past 2 decades has been that the method by which sedatives and analgesics are administered is just as important as the drugs themselves. Titration of sedatives to comfort and wakefulness allows patients to participate in their care. It also allows a more accurate rendering of analgesic need and the presence of delirium. Beyond this, light sedation may affect long-term outcomes by facilitating early mobilization and its associated beneficial effect on functional outcomes and the formation of factual memories, which may limit the risk of posttraumatic stress disorder.[290-293]

Deep sedation, by contrast, may be associated with delayed liberation for mechanical ventilation; higher in-hospital, 180-day, and 2-year follow-up mortality; and a greater need for tracheostomy.[294-298] In addition, deep sedation has been associated with lack of ICU recall and delusional memories, which may increase the risk of posttraumatic stress disorder.[299-301] Deep sedation may be appropriate in certain situations (e.g., neuromuscular blockade, ventilator dyssynchrony, status epilepticus, open abdomen, or elevated ICP). Despite the availability of a large amount of consistent data suggesting that light sedation confers outcomes benefits, 40%–50% of patients remain oversedated, and 32% of patients continue to be sedated to the point of coma.[250,251]

Protocolized Sedation

A protocolized approach to comfort is endorsed in the 2013 SCCM PAD guidelines. Although daily sedation interruption is often a component of a sedation protocol, it will be discussed separately in this chapter. Protocols emphasize the identification of underlying etiologies of discomfort, selection of a patient-specific sedation goal, liberal treatment of pain, and the choice of sedative or analgesic depending on sedation goal and end-organ function. Protocols are often managed autonomously by bedside nurses. The benefits of a sedation protocol largely stem from thoughtful titration of sedation. Despite clear advantages, about 30% of ICUs do not use sedation protocols.[302]

Until the late 1990s, most studies on ICU comfort focused on comparing one sedative with another. A landmark trial changed that by evaluating a nurse-driven sedation protocol.[303] The protocol encouraged nurses to identify and address possible etiologies for agitation, treat pain with intermittent boluses of opioids, and treat agitation with intermittent boluses of benzodiazepines. Continuous infusions were reserved for persistent agitation. The nurse-driven protocol shortened the duration of continuously infused sedation, mechanical ventilation, ICU and hospital LOS, and tracheostomy rate compared with the standard of care (i.e., physician order only). Those findings ignited a wave of studies that evaluated sedation protocols.

Most studies have shown that a protocolized approach to comfort reduces duration of mechanical ventilation.[53,303-312] This is usually associated with a shorter hospital and ICU LOS.[53,303-305,307-311] These benefits are probably because of reduced exposure to sedatives and the avoidance of coma.[53,303-305,307-313] No increases in self-extubation, physical restraints, nurse workload, or psychological distress have been noted in these studies.[53,304-307,310,314,315] Although most trials have shown that protocolized sedation improves outcomes, a select few have questioned its benefits.[316-318] Most conflicting data have their genesis in ICU health care models that use 1:1 nurse/patient ratios, closed units, nurse ventilator management, and shorter-acting sedatives like propofol. Nonetheless, a recent meta-analysis found that protocolized sedation improves outcomes compared with usual care.[319]

The ideal protocol should be developed by a multidisciplinary team. First, it should mandate systematic assessments of sedation and agitation at least four times per nursing shift. Second, it should encourage the identification and correction of the underlying etiology. Third, it should emphasize the establishment of a patient-specific sedation goal. In the absence of an indication for deep sedation, targeting wakefulness is encouraged. Fourth, it should stress routine pain assessment and treatment. Fifth, it should advocate for intermittent boluses of sedatives and analgesics. If it is ineffective, continuous infusions of short-acting agents (dexmedetomidine or propofol) should be encouraged. Titration and taper instructions should be present. Finally, it should incorporate spontaneous breathing trials and delirium assessments when patients are wakeful (i.e., SAS 3 to 4 or RASS −2 to 0 or ability to follow simple commands).

Sedation Interruption

Daily sedation interruption involves the discontinuation of continuously infused sedatives until patients are wakeful. Interruption allows for more productive neurological examinations, spontaneous breathing trials, delirium screening, mobilization attempts, and self-reporting of pain. Indications to forego interruption include active seizures, alcohol withdrawal, neuromuscular blockade, hemodynamic instability, elevated ICP greater than 20 mm Hg, extracorporeal membrane oxygenation, myocardial ischemia in the past 24 hours, and dangerous agitation.[290,320,321] Interruption in patients with neurological injury should be done with caution because dangerous elevations of ICP, cerebral perfusion pressure, and catecholamine concentrations; hemodynamic instability; and reductions in brain tissue oxygen tension may occur.[58,322,323]

Daily sedation interruption was evaluated in a sentinel trial in 2000.[324] It reduced the duration of mechanical ventilation, ICU LOS, sedatives and analgesics administered, and need for diagnostic tests to evaluate neurological status. Conversely, it increased the number of days that patients were wakeful and improved discharge disposition. A subsequent analysis found that ICU complications (e.g., ventilator-associated pneumonia, gastrointestinal bleeding, or bacteremia) were reduced by 50%.[325] Initial concerns about psychological distress and cardiovascular compromise were later thwarted.[55,56,326,327] Although more recent trials and a meta-analysis have questioned the utility of sedation interruption, its benefits likely outweigh the risks.[328-330]

Only one study has compared protocolized sedation with protocolized sedation with a daily interruption.[331] The protocol maximized the use of opioids, minimized benzodiazepines, and targeted light levels of sedation (SAS 3 or 4 or RASS −3 to 0). Of interest, clinical outcomes were similar between groups. These findings could have been because of higher benzodiazepine and opioid use in the intervention group, the low rate of sedation interruption (72%), not pairing spontaneous breathing trials with sedation interruption, or the fact that sedation was titrated by bedside versus research nurses.[320] The 2013 SCCM PAD guidelines recommend that either daily sedation interruption or a protocolized approach to comfort be used.[11]

Interruption of sedation has rapidly become a component of ICU care bundles, which incorporate evidence-based, multicomponent, and multidisciplinary strategies into everyday practice.[290] Pairing sedation interruption with spontaneous breathing trials has been shown to increase ventilator-free days and reduce ICU and hospital LOS, 1-year mortality, days with coma, and benzodiazepine doses.[332] Long-term cognitive and psychological outcomes were similar between groups at 12 months.[333] Combining sedation interruption with spontaneous breathing trials and early mobilization increases ventilator-free days and mobilization while decreasing delirium, hospital mortality, and benzodiazepine use.[290] Unfortunately, daily sedation interruption is at best used in 78% of eligible patients because of concerns about medical device removal, respiratory compromise, patient discomfort, and lack of adequate patient care resources.[76,334-338] Education and quality improvement initiatives can address this.

SUMMARY AND FUTURE DIRECTIONS

Despite more attention than ever before, agitation is still common in critically ill patients. It is often because of a combination of patient-related, illness-related, and environmental factors. Discomfort in the ICU can be distressful for patients, families, and caregivers. In addition, it is closely linked to negative clinical outcomes and maladaptive physiologic responses. Routine assessment of comfort with subjective sedation scales or objective measures is imperative. Nonpharmacologic interventions should used in all ICU patients with the understanding that pharmacologic therapy will often be necessary. Sedation protocols should guide the administration of sedatives and analgesics and should focus on treating pain first and targeting wakefulness, when clinically appropriate.

Several gaps remain in how best to provide comfort in the ICU. The role of pharmacists as sedation stewards needs to be further evaluated. Strategies to reduce inappropriate continuation of psychoactive medications initiated in the ICU during transitions of care need to be developed. Sedation strategies in non-intubated patients or those with neurological injuries, end-organ dysfunction, or hemodynamic instability need to be better established. The short- and long-term impact of sedation-related delirium is only beginning to be elucidated. In addition, more robust data are needed in respect to alternative sedatives. Although these questions and many others remain unanswered, a systematic and multidisciplinary approach to ICU comfort can improve outcomes during a hospitalization and beyond.

REFERENCES

1. Szokol JW, Vender JS. Anxiety, delirium, and pain in the intensive care unit. Crit Care Clin 2001;17:821-42.
2. Sessler CN, Grap MJ, Brophy GM. Multidisciplinary management of sedation and analgesia in critical care. Semin Respir Crit Care Med 2001;22:211-26.

3. The management of the agitated ICU patient. Crit Care Med 2002;30:S97-S123.
4. Fraser GL, Prato BS, Riker RR, et al. Frequency, severity, and treatment of agitation in young versus elderly patients in the ICU. Pharmacotherapy 2000;20:75-82.
5. Burk RS, Grap MJ, Munro CL, et al. Predictors of agitation in critically ill adults. Am J Crit Care 2014;23:414-23.
6. Burk RS, Grap MJ, Munro CL, et al. Agitation onset, frequency, and associated temporal factors in critically ill adults. Am J Crit Care 2014;23:296-304.
7. Woods JC, Mion LC, Connor JT, et al. Severe agitation among ventilated medical intensive care unit patients: frequency, characteristics and outcomes. Intensive Care Med 2004;30:1066-72.
8. Jaber S, Chanques G, Altairac C, et al. A prospective study of agitation in a medical-surgical ICU: incidence, risk factors, and outcomes. Chest 2005;128:2749-57.
9. Novaes MA, Knobel E, Bork AM, et al. Stressors in ICU: perception of the patient, relatives and health care team. Intensive Care Med 1999;25:1421-6.
10. Crippen D. Agitation in the ICU: part one. Anatomical and physiologic basis for the agitated state. Crit Care 1999;3:R35-R46.
11. Barr J, Fraser GL, Puntillo K, et al. Clinical practice guidelines for the management of pain, agitation, and delirium in adult patients in the intensive care unit. Crit Care Med 2013;41:263-306.
12. Novaes MA, Aronovich A, Ferraz MB, et al. Stressors in ICU: patients' evaluation. Intensive Care Med 1997;23:1282-5.
13. van de Leur JP, van der Schans CP, Loef BG, et al. Discomfort and factual recollection in intensive care unit patients. Crit Care 2004;8:R467-R473.
14. Pandharipande PP, Girard TD, Jackson JC, et al. Long-term cognitive impairment after critical illness. N Engl J Med 2013;369:1306-16.
15. McNicoll L, Pisani MA, Zhang Y, et al. Delirium in the intensive care unit: occurrence and clinical course in older patients. J Am Geriatr Soc 2003;51:591-8.
16. Pisani MA, Redlich C, McNicoll L, et al. Underrecognition of preexisting cognitive impairment by physicians in older ICU patients. Chest 2003;124:2267-74.
17. Seifter JL, Samuels MA. Uremic encephalopathy and other brain disorders associated with renal failure. Semin Neurol 2011;31:139-43.
18. Blei AT, Córdoba J; Practice Parameters Committee of the American College of Gastroenterology. Hepatic encephalopathy. Am J Gastroenterol 2001;96:1968-76.
19. Clark BJ, Moss M. Secondary prevention in the intensive care unit: does intensive care unit admission represent a "teachable moment?" Crit Care Med 2011;39:1500-6.
20. Lucidarme O, Seguin A, Daubin C, et al. Nicotine withdrawal and agitation in ventilated critically ill patients. Crit Care 2010;14:R58.
21. Awissi DK, Lebrun G, Fagnan M, et al.; Regroupement de Soins Critiques, Réseau de Soins Respiratoires, Québec. Alcohol, nicotine, and iatrogenic withdrawals in the ICU. Crit Care Med 2013;41(9 suppl 1):S57-S68.
22. de Wit M, Wan SY, Gill S, et al. Prevalence and impact of alcohol and other drug use disorders on sedation and mechanical ventilation: a retrospective study. BMC Anesthesiol 2007;7:3.
23. Boyer EW, Shannon M. The serotonin syndrome. N Engl J Med 2005;352:1112-20.
24. Fugate JE, Kalimullah EA, Hocker SE, et al. Cefepime neurotoxicity in the intensive care unit: a cause of severe, underappreciated encephalopathy. Crit Care 2013;17:R264.
25. Panzer O, Moitra V, Sladen RN. Pharmacology of sedative-analgesic agents: dexmedetomidine, remifentanil, ketamine, volatile anesthetics, and the role of peripheral mu antagonists. Crit Care Clin 2009;25:451-69, vii.
26. Eger EI II. Characteristics of anesthetic agents used for induction and maintenance of general anesthesia. Am J Health Syst Pharm 2004;61(suppl 4):S3-10.
27. Devlin JW, Fraser GL, Riker RR. Drug-induced delirium and coma. In: Papadopoulos J, ed. Drug-Induced Complications in the Critically Ill Patient: A Guide for Recognition and Treatment. Mount Prospect, IL: Society of Critical Care Medicine, 2012:107-16.
28. Fuller MA, Borovicka MC. Delirium. In: Tisdale JE, Miller DA, eds. Drug-Induced Diseases: Prevention, Detection, and Management, 2nd ed. Bethesda, MD: American Society of Health-System Pharmacists, 2010:275-92.
29. Kiekkas P, Samios A, Skartsani C, et al. Fever and agitation in elderly ICU patients: a descriptive study. Intensive Crit Care Nurs 2010;26:169-74.
30. Hosokawa K, Gaspard N, Su F, et al. Clinical neurophysiological assessment of sepsis-associated brain dysfunction: a systematic review. Crit Care 2014;18:674.
31. Micek ST, Anand NJ, Laible BR, et al. Delirium as detected by the CAM-ICU predicts restraint use among mechanically ventilated medical patients. Crit Care Med 2005;33:1260-5.
32. Rotondi AJ, Chelluri L, Sirio C, et al. Patients' recollections of stressful experiences while receiving prolonged mechanical ventilation in an intensive care unit. Crit Care Med 2002;30:746-52.
33. Bergbom-Engberg I, Haljamäe H. Assessment of patients' experience of discomforts during respirator therapy. Crit Care Med 1989;17:1068-72.
34. Abuatiq A, Burkard J, Clark MJ. Literature review: patients' and health care providers' perceptions of stressors in critical care units. Dimens Crit Care Nurs 2013;32:22-7.
35. Chanques G, Sebbane M, Barbotte E, et al. A prospective study of pain at rest: incidence and characteristics of an unrecognized symptom in surgical and trauma versus medical intensive care unit patients. Anesthesiology 2007;107:858-60.
36. Arroyo-Novoa CM, Figueroa-Ramos MI, Puntillo KA, et al. Pain related to tracheal suctioning in awake acutely and critically ill adults: a descriptive study. Intensive Crit Care Nurs 2008;24:20-7.
37. Puntillo KA, Max A, Timsit JF, et al. Determinants of procedural pain intensity in the intensive care unit. The Europain® study. Am J Respir Crit Care Med 2014;189:39-47.
38. Puntillo K, Ley SJ. Appropriately timed analgesics control pain due to chest tube removal. Am J Crit Care 2004;13:292-301.

39. Akansel N, Kaymakçi S. Effects of intensive care unit noise on patients: a study on coronary artery bypass graft surgery patients. J Clin Nurs 2008;17:1581-90.

40. Darbyshire JL, Young JD. An investigation of sound levels on intensive care units with reference to the WHO guidelines. Crit Care 2013;17:R187.

41. Busch-Vishniac IJ, West JE, Barnhill C, et al. Noise levels in Johns Hopkins Hospital. J Acoust Soc Am 2005;118:3629-45.

42. Freedman NS, Gazendam J, Levan L, et al. Abnormal sleep/wake cycles and the effect of environmental noise on sleep disruption in the intensive care unit. Am J Respir Crit Care Med 2001;163:451-7.

43. Siegel MD. Management of agitation in the intensive care unit. Clin Chest Med 2003;24:713-25.

44. Marquis F, Ouimet S, Riker R, et al. Individual delirium symptoms: do they matter? Crit Care Med 2007;35:2533-7.

45. Fraser GL, Riker RR, Prato BS, et al. The frequency and cost of patient-initiated device removal in the ICU. Pharmacotherapy 2001;21:1-6.

46. Mion LC, Minnick AF, Leipzig R, et al. Patient-initiated device removal in intensive care units: a national prevalence study. Crit Care Med 2007;35:2714-20.

47. Coppolo DP, May JJ. Self-extubations. A 12-month experience. Chest 1990;98:165-9.

48. Boulain T. Unplanned extubations in the adult intensive care unit: a prospective multicenter study. Association des Réanimateurs du Centre-Ouest. Am J Respir Crit Care Med 1998;157(4 pt 1):1131-7.

49. Betbesé AJ, Pérez M, Bak E, et al. A prospective study of unplanned endotracheal extubation in intensive care unit patients. Crit Care Med 1998;26:1180-6.

50. Atkins PM, Mion LC, Mendelson W, et al. Characteristics and outcomes of patients who self-extubate from ventilatory support: a case-control study. Chest 1997;112:1317-23.

51. Krinsley JS, Barone JE. The drive to survive: unplanned extubation in the ICU. Chest 2005;128:560-6.

52. Tanios M, Epstein S, Grzeskowiak M, et al. Influence of sedation strategies on unplanned extubation in a mixed intensive care unit. Am J Crit Care 2014;23:306-14.

53. Strøm T, Martinussen T, Toft P. A protocol of no sedation for critically ill patients receiving mechanical ventilation: a randomised trial. Lancet 2010;375:475-80.

54. Epstein SK, Nevins ML, Chung J. Effect of unplanned extubation on outcome of mechanical ventilation. Am J Respir Crit Care Med 2000;161:1912-6.

55. Kress JP, Vinayak AG, Levitt J, et al. Daily sedative interruption in mechanically ventilated patients at risk for coronary artery disease. Crit Care Med 2007;35:365-71.

56. Kong KL, Willatts SM, Prys-Roberts C, et al. Plasma catecholamine concentration during sedation in ventilated patients requiring intensive therapy. Intensive Care Med 1990;16:171-4.

57. Dünser MW, Hasibeder WR. Sympathetic overstimulation during critical illness: adverse effects of adrenergic stress. J Intensive Care Med 2009;24:293-316.

58. Skoglund K, Enblad P, Hillered L, et al. The neurological wake-up test increases stress hormone levels in patients with severe traumatic brain injury. Crit Care Med 2012;40:216-22.

59. Sander O, Welters ID, Foëx P, et al. Impact of prolonged elevated heart rate on incidence of major cardiac events in critically ill patients with a high risk of cardiac complications. Crit Care Med 2005;33:81-8.

60. Bruder N, Lassegue D, Pelissier D, et al. Energy expenditure and withdrawal of sedation in severe head-injured patients. Crit Care Med 1994;22:1114-9.

61. Srivastava S, Chatila W, Amoateng-Adjepong Y, et al. Myocardial ischemia and weaning failure in patients with coronary artery disease: an update. Crit Care Med 1999;27:2109-12.

62. Smith MA, Hibino M, Falcione BA, et al. Immunosuppressive aspects of analgesics and sedatives used in mechanically ventilated patients: an underappreciated risk factor for the development of ventilator-associated pneumonia in critically ill patients. Ann Pharmacother 2014;48:77-85.

63. Nseir S, Makris D, Mathieu D, et al. Intensive care unit-acquired infection as a side effect of sedation. Crit Care 2010;14:R30.

64. Chanques G, Jaber S, Barbotte E, et al. Impact of systematic evaluation of pain and agitation in an intensive care unit. Crit Care Med 2006;34:1691-9.

65. Botha JA, Mudholkar P. The effect of a sedation scale on ventilation hours, sedative, analgesic and inotropic use in an intensive care unit. Crit Care Resusc 2004;6:253-7.

66. Brattebø G, Hofoss D, Flaatten H, et al. Effect of a scoring system and protocol for sedation on duration of patients' need for ventilator support in a surgical intensive care unit. BMJ 2002;324:1386-9.

67. Pun BT, Gordon SM, Peterson JF, et al. Large-scale implementation of sedation and delirium monitoring in the intensive care unit: a report from two medical centers. Crit Care Med 2005;33:1199-205.

68. Riker RR, Picard JT, Fraser GL. Prospective evaluation of the Sedation-Agitation Scale for adult critically ill patients. Crit Care Med 1999;27:1325-9.

69. Ely EW, Truman B, Shintani A, et al. Monitoring sedation status over time in ICU patients: reliability and validity of the Richmond Agitation-Sedation Scale (RASS). JAMA 2003;289:2983-91.

70. Mehta S, Burry L, Fischer S, et al. Canadian survey of the use of sedatives, analgesics, and neuromuscular blocking agents in critically ill patients. Crit Care Med 2006;34:374-80.

71. Riker RR, Fraser GL. Monitoring sedation, agitation, analgesia, neuromuscular blockade, and delirium in adult ICU patients. Semin Respir Crit Care Med 2001;22:189-98.

72. Robinson BR, Berube M, Barr J, et al. Psychometric analysis of subjective sedation scales in critically ill adults. Crit Care Med 2013;41(9 suppl 1):S16-S29.

73. De Jonghe B, Cook D, Appere-De-Vecchi C, et al. Using and understanding sedation scoring systems: a systematic review. Intensive Care Med 2000;26:275-85.

74. Ramsay MA, Savege TM, Simpson BR, et al. Controlled sedation with alphaxalone-alphadolone. Br Med J 1974;2:656-9.

75. Sessler CN, Riker RR, Ramsay MA. Evaluating and monitoring sedation, arousal, and agitation in the ICU. Semin Respir Crit Care Med 2013;34:169-78.

76. Mehta S, McCullagh I, Burry L. Current sedation practices: lessons learned from international surveys. Crit Care Clin 2009;25:471-88, vii-viii.

77. Riker RR, Fraser GL, Cox PM. Continuous infusion of haloperidol controls agitation in critically ill patients. Crit Care Med 1994;22:433-40.

78. Hansen-Flaschen J, Cowen J, Polomano RC. Beyond the Ramsay scale: need for a validated measure of sedating drug efficacy in the intensive care unit [editorial]. Crit Care Med 1994;22:732-3.

79. Riker RR, Fraser GL, Simmons LE, et al. Validating the Sedation-Agitation Scale with the Bispectral Index and Visual Analog Scale in adult ICU patients after cardiac surgery. Intensive Care Med 2001;27:853-8.

80. Simmons LE, Riker RR, Prato BS, et al. Assessing sedation during intensive care unit mechanical ventilation with the Bispectral Index and the Sedation-Agitation Scale. Crit Care Med 1999;27:1499-504.

81. Sessler CN, Gosnell MS, Grap MJ, et al. The Richmond Agitation-Sedation Scale: validity and reliability in adult intensive care unit patients. Am J Respir Crit Care Med 2002;166:1338-44.

82. Weinert CR, Chlan L, Gross C. Sedating critically ill patients: factors affecting nurses' delivery of sedative therapy. Am J Crit Care 2001;10:156-65.

83. Struys MM, Jensen EW, Smith W, et al. Performance of the ARX-derived auditory evoked potential index as an indicator of anesthetic depth: a comparison with bispectral index and hemodynamic measures during propofol administration. Anesthesiology 2002;96:803-16.

84. Haberthür C, Lehmann F, Ritz R. Assessment of depth of midazolam sedation using objective parameters. Intensive Care Med 1996;22:1385-90.

85. Fraser GL, Riker RR. Bispectral index monitoring in the intensive care unit provides more signal than noise. Pharmacotherapy 2005;25(5 pt 2):19S-27S.

86. Rampil IJ. A primer for EEG signal processing in anesthesia. Anesthesiology 1998;89:980-1002.

87. LeBlanc JM, Dasta JF, Kane-Gill SL. Role of the bispectral index in sedation monitoring in the ICU. Ann Pharmacother 2006;40:490-500.

88. Sessler CN, Varney K. Patient-focused sedation and analgesia in the ICU. Chest 2008;133:552-65.

89. Yaman F, Ozcan N, Ozcan A, et al. Assessment of correlation between bispectral index and four common sedation scales used in mechanically ventilated patients in ICU. Eur Rev Med Pharmacol Sci 2012;16:660-6.

90. Riker RR, Fraser GL, Wilkins ML. Comparing the bispectral index and suppression ratio with burst suppression of the electroencephalogram during pentobarbital infusions in adult intensive care patients. Pharmacotherapy 2003;23:1087-93.

91. Seder DB, Fraser GL, Robbins T, et al. The bispectral index and suppression ratio are very early predictors of neurological outcome during therapeutic hypothermia after cardiac arrest. Intensive Care Med 2010;36:281-8.

92. Hofhuis JG, Spronk PE, van Stel HF, et al. Experiences of critically ill patients in the ICU. Intensive Crit Care Nurs 2008;24:300-13.

93. Hu RF, Jiang XY, Hegadoren KM, et al. Effects of earplugs and eye masks combined with relaxing music on sleep, melatonin and cortisol levels in ICU patients: a randomized controlled trial. Crit Care 2015;19:115.

94. Xie H, Kang J, Mills GH. Clinical review: the impact of noise on patients' sleep and the effectiveness of noise reduction strategies in intensive care units. Crit Care 2009;13:208.

95. Kahn DM, Cook TE, Carlisle CC, et al. Identification and modification of environmental noise in an ICU setting. Chest 1998;114:535-40.

96. Chlan LL, Weinert CR, Heiderscheit A, et al. Effects of patient-directed music intervention on anxiety and sedative exposure in critically ill patients receiving mechanical ventilatory support: a randomized clinical trial. JAMA 2013;309:2335-44.

97. Gélinas C, Arbour C, Michaud C, et al. Patients and ICU nurses' perspectives of non-pharmacological interventions for pain management. Nurs Crit Care 2013;18:307-18.

98. Maccioli GA, Dorman T, Brown BR, et al. Clinical practice guidelines for the maintenance of patient physical safety in the intensive care unit: use of restraining therapies—American College of Critical Care Medicine Task Force 2001-2002. Crit Care Med 2003;31:2665-76.

99. Luk E, Sneyers B, Rose L, et al. Predictors of physical restraint use in Canadian intensive care units. Crit Care 2014;18:R46.

100. McPherson JA, Wagner CE, Boehm LM, et al. Delirium in the cardiovascular ICU: exploring modifiable risk factors. Crit Care Med 2013;41:405-13.

101. Strout TD. Perspectives on the experience of being physically restrained: an integrative review of the qualitative literature. Int J Ment Health Nurs 2010;19:416-27.

102. Wunsch H, Kahn JM, Kramer AA, et al. Use of intravenous infusion sedation among mechanically ventilated patients in the United States. Crit Care Med 2009;37:3031-9.

103. Arroliga AC, Thompson BT, Ancukiewicz M, et al. Use of sedatives, opioids, and neuromuscular blocking agents in patients with acute lung injury and acute respiratory distress syndrome. Crit Care Med 2008;36:1083-8.

104. Arroliga A, Frutos-Vivar F, Hall J, et al. Use of sedatives and neuromuscular blockers in a cohort of patients receiving mechanical ventilation. Chest 2005;128:496-506.

105. Wunsch H, Wagner J, Herlim M, et al. ICU occupancy and mechanical ventilator use in the United States. Crit Care Med 2013;41:2712-9.

106. Roberts DJ, Haroon B, Hall RI. Sedation for critically ill or injured adults in the intensive care unit: a shifting paradigm. Drugs 2012;72:1881-916.

107. Devabhakthuni S, Armahizer MJ, Dasta JF, et al. Analgosedation: a paradigm shift in intensive care unit sedation practice. Ann Pharmacother 2012;46:530-40.

108. Mattia C, Savoia G, Paoletti F, et al. SIAARTI recommendations for analgo-sedation in intensive care unit. Minerva Anestesiol 2006;72:769-805.

109. Trescot AM, Datta S, Lee M, et al. Opioid pharmacology. Pain Physician 2008;11(2 suppl):S133-S153.

110. Erstad BL, Puntillo K, Gilbert HC, et al. Pain management principles in the critically ill. Chest 2009;135:1075-86.

111. Martin J, Parsch A, Franck M, et al. Practice of sedation and analgesia in German intensive care units: results of a national survey. Crit Care 2005;9:R117-R123.

112. Wøien H, Stubhaug A, Bjørk IT. Analgesia and sedation of mechanically ventilated patients - a national survey of clinical practice. Acta Anaesthesiol Scand 2012;56:23-9.

113. McPherson ML. Demystifying Opioid Conversion Calculations: A Guide for Effective Dosing. Bethesda, MD: American Society of Health-System Pharmacists, 2009.

114. Smith BS, Yogaratnam D, Levasseur-Franklin KE, et al. Introduction to drug pharmacokinetics in the critically ill patient. Chest 2012;141:1327-36.

115. Davies G, Kingswood C, Street M. Pharmacokinetics of opioids in renal dysfunction. Clin Pharmacokinet 1996;31:410-22.

116. Koehntop DE, Rodman JH. Fentanyl pharmacokinetics in patients undergoing renal transplantation. Pharmacotherapy 1997;17:746-52.

117. Egan TD, Lemmens HJ, Fiset P, et al. The pharmacokinetics of the new short-acting opioid remifentanil (GI87084B) in healthy adult male volunteers. Anesthesiology 1993;79:881-92.

118. Kirschner R, Donovan JW. Serotonin syndrome precipitated by fentanyl during procedural sedation. J Emerg Med 2010;38:477-80.

119. Ailawadhi S, Sung KW, Carlson LA, et al. Serotonin syndrome caused by interaction between citalopram and fentanyl. J Clin Pharm Ther 2007;32:199-202.

120. Gagnon DJ, Jwo K. Tremors and agitation following low-dose intravenous hydromorphone administration in a patient with kidney dysfunction. Ann Pharmacother 2013;47:e34.

121. Thwaites D, McCann S, Broderick P. Hydromorphone neuroexcitation. J Palliat Med 2004;7:545-50.

122. McLean S, Twomey F. Methods of rotation from another strong opioid to methadone for the management of cancer pain: a systematic review of the available evidence. J Pain Symptom Manage. 2015 Apr 18. [Epub ahead of print]

123. Fine PG, Portenoy RK; Ad Hoc Expert Panel on Evidence Review and Guidelines for Opioid Rotation. Establishing "best practices" for opioid rotation: conclusions of an expert panel. J Pain Symptom Manage 2009;38:418-25.

124. Oldenmenger WH, Lieverse PJ, Janssen PJ, et al. Efficacy of opioid rotation to continuous parenteral hydromorphone in advanced cancer patients failing on other opioids. Support Care Cancer 2012;20:1639-47.

125. Hansen-Flaschen JH, Brazinsky S, Basile C, et al. Use of sedating drugs and neuromuscular blocking agents in patients requiring mechanical ventilation for respiratory failure. A national survey. JAMA 1991;266:2870-5.

126. Soliman HM, Mélot C, Vincent JL. Sedative and analgesic practice in the intensive care unit: the results of a European survey. Br J Anaesth 2001;87:186-92.

127. Smith MT. Neuroexcitatory effects of morphine and hydromorphone: evidence implicating the 3-glucuronide metabolites. Clin Exp Pharmacol Physiol 2000;27:524-8.

128. Lee M, Silverman SM, Hansen H, et al. A comprehensive review of opioid-induced hyperalgesia. Pain Physician 2011;14:145-61.

129. Devlin JW, Roberts RJ. Pharmacology of commonly used analgesics and sedatives in the ICU: benzodiazepines, propofol, and opioids. Anesthesiol Clin 2011;29:567-85.

130. Bosilkovska M, Walder B, Besson M, et al. Analgesics in patients with hepatic impairment: pharmacology and clinical implications. Drugs 2012;72:1645-69.

131. Battershill AJ, Keating GM. Remifentanil: a review of its analgesic and sedative use in the intensive care unit. Drugs 2006;66:365-85.

132. Karabinis A, Mandragos K, Stergiopoulos S, et al. Safety and efficacy of analgesia-based sedation with remifentanil versus standard hypnotic-based regimens in intensive care unit patients with brain injuries: a randomized, controlled trial. Crit Care 2004;8:R268-R280.

133. Kim SH, Stoicea N, Soghomonyan S, et al. Remifentanil-acute opioid tolerance and opioid-induced hyperalgesia: a systematic review. Am J Ther 2015;22:e62-74.

134. Martin J, Franck M, Fischer M, et al. Sedation and analgesia in German intensive care units: how is it done in reality? Results of a patient-based survey of analgesia and sedation. Intensive Care Med 2006;32:1137-42.

135. Muellejans B, López A, Cross MH, et al. Remifentanil versus fentanyl for analgesia based sedation to provide patient comfort in the intensive care unit: a randomized, double-blind controlled trial [ISRCTN43755713]. Crit Care 2004;8:R1-R11.

136. Breen D, Karabinis A, Malbrain M, et al. Decreased duration of mechanical ventilation when comparing analgesia-based sedation using remifentanil with standard hypnotic-based sedation for up to 10 days in intensive care unit patients: a randomised trial [ISRCTN47583497]. Crit Care 2005;9:R200-R210.

137. Dahaba AA, Grabner T, Rehak PH, et al. Remifentanil versus morphine analgesia and sedation for mechanically ventilated critically ill patients: a randomized double blind study. Anesthesiology 2004;101:640-6.

138. Spies C, Macguill M, Heymann A, et al. A prospective, randomized, double-blind, multicenter study comparing remifentanil with fentanyl in mechanically ventilated patients. Intensive Care Med 2011;37:469-76.

139. Tan JA, Ho KM. Use of remifentanil as a sedative agent in critically ill adult patients: a meta-analysis. Anaesthesia 2009;64:1342-52.

140. Bjelland TW, Dale O, Kaisen K, et al. Propofol and remifentanil versus midazolam and fentanyl for sedation during therapeutic hypothermia after cardiac arrest: a randomized trial. Intensive Care Med 2012;38:959-67.

141. Samaniego EA, Mlynash M, Caulfield AF, et al. Sedation confounds outcome prediction in cardiac arrest survivors treated with hypothermia. Neurocrit Care 2011;15:113-9.

142. Bürkle H, Dunbar S, Van Aken H. Remifentanil: a novel, short-acting, mu-opioid. Anesth Analg 1996;83:646-51.

143. Guignard B, Bossard AE, Coste C, et al. Acute opioid tolerance: intraoperative remifentanil increases postoperative pain and morphine requirement. Anesthesiology 2000;93:409-17.

144. Fredheim OM, Moksnes K, Borchgrevink PC, et al. Clinical pharmacology of methadone for pain. Acta Anaesthesiol Scand 2008;52:879-89.

145. Patanwala AE, Duby J, Waters D, et al. Opioid conversions in acute care. Ann Pharmacother 2007;41:255-66.

146. Krantz MJ, Kutinsky IB, Robertson AD, et al. Dose-related effects of methadone on QT prolongation in a series of patients with torsade de pointes. Pharmacotherapy 2003;23:802-5.

147. Stringer J, Welsh C, Tommasello A. Methadone-associated Q-T interval prolongation and torsades de pointes. Am J Health Syst Pharm 2009;66:825-33.

148. Ng TM, Bell AM, Hong C, et al. Pharmacist monitoring of QTc interval-prolonging medications in critically ill medical patients: a pilot study. Ann Pharmacother 2008;42:475-82.

149. Wanzuita R, Poli-de-Figueiredo LF, Pfuetzenreiter F, et al. Replacement of fentanyl infusion by enteral methadone decreases the weaning time from mechanical ventilation: a randomized controlled trial. Crit Care 2012;16:R49.

150. Al-Qadheeb NS, Roberts RJ, Griffin R, et al. Impact of enteral methadone on the ability to wean off continuously infused opioids in critically ill, mechanically ventilated adults: a case-control study. Ann Pharmacother 2012;46:1160-6.

151. Price DD, Mayer DJ, Mao J, et al. NMDA-receptor antagonists and opioid receptor interactions as related to analgesia and tolerance. J Pain Symptom Manage 2000;19(1 suppl):S7-S11.

152. Young CC, Prielipp RC. Benzodiazepines in the intensive care unit. Crit Care Clin 2001;17:843-62.

153. Tobias JD. Tolerance, withdrawal, and physical dependency after long-term sedation and analgesia of children in the pediatric intensive care unit. Crit Care Med 2000;28:2122-32.

154. Fraser GL, Devlin JW, Worby CP, et al. Benzodiazepine versus nonbenzodiazepine-based sedation for mechanically ventilated, critically ill adults: a systematic review and meta-analysis of randomized trials. Crit Care Med 2013;41(9 suppl 1):S30-S38.

155. Pandharipande P, Shintani A, Peterson J, et al. Lorazepam is an independent risk factor for transitioning to delirium in intensive care unit patients. Anesthesiology 2006;104:21-6.

156. Pandharipande P, Cotton BA, Shintani A, et al. Prevalence and risk factors for development of delirium in surgical and trauma intensive care unit patients. J Trauma 2008;65:34-41.

157. Mehta S, Cook D, Devlin JW, et al. Prevalence, risk factors, and outcomes of delirium in mechanically ventilated adults. Crit Care Med 2015;43:557-66.

158. Ouimet S, Kavanagh BP, Gottfried SB, et al. Incidence, risk factors and consequences of ICU delirium. Intensive Care Med 2007;33:66-73.

159. Pisani MA, Murphy TE, Araujo KL, et al. Benzodiazepine and opioid use and the duration of intensive care unit delirium in an older population. Crit Care Med 2009;37:177-83.

160. Fraser GL, Gagnon DJ, Riker RR. SLEAP: a wake-up call to question the oversimplification of ICU delirium. Crit Care Med 2015;43:703-5.

161. Hamaoka N, Oda Y, Hase I, et al. Propofol decreases the clearance of midazolam by inhibiting CYP3A4: an in vivo and in vitro study. Clin Pharmacol Ther 1999;66:110-7.

162. Carrasco G, Cabré L, Sobrepere G, et al. Synergistic sedation with propofol and midazolam in intensive care patients after coronary artery bypass grafting. Crit Care Med 1998;26:844-51.

163. Greenblatt DJ, Miller LG, Shader RI. Clonazepam pharmacokinetics, brain uptake, and receptor interactions. J Clin Psychiatry 1987;48(suppl):4-11.

164. Riker RR, Fraser GL. Adverse events associated with sedatives, analgesics, and other drugs that provide patient comfort in the intensive care unit. Pharmacotherapy 2005;25(5 pt 2):8S-18S.

165. Yahwak JA, Riker RR, Fraser GL, et al. Determination of a lorazepam dose threshold for using the osmol gap to monitor for propylene glycol toxicity. Pharmacotherapy 2008;28:984-91.

166. Yassin SM, Terblanche M, Yassin J, et al. A web-based survey of United Kingdom sedation practice in the intensive care unit. J Crit Care 2015;30:436.e1-6.

167. McKeage K, Perry CM. Propofol: a review of its use in intensive care sedation of adults. CNS Drugs 2003;17:235-72.

168. Barr J, Egan TD, Sandoval NF, et al. Propofol dosing regimens for ICU sedation based upon an integrated pharmacokinetic-pharmacodynamic model. Anesthesiology 2001;95:324-33.

169. Albanese J, Martin C, Lacarelle B, et al. Pharmacokinetics of long-term propofol infusion used for sedation in ICU patients. Anesthesiology 1990;73:214-7.

170. Bailie GR, Cockshott ID, Douglas EJ, et al. Pharmacokinetics of propofol during and after long-term continuous infusion for maintenance of sedation in ICU patients. Br J Anaesth 1992;68:486-91.

171. Murphy A, Campbell DE, Baines D, et al. Allergic reactions to propofol in egg-allergic children. Anesth Analg 2011;113:140-4.

172. Devlin JW, Lau AK, Tanios MA. Propofol-associated hypertriglyceridemia and pancreatitis in the intensive care unit: an analysis of frequency and risk factors. Pharmacotherapy 2005;25:1348-52.

173. Leisure GS, O'Flaherty J, Green L, et al. Propofol and postoperative pancreatitis. Anesthesiology 1996;84:224-7.

174. Kumar AN, Schwartz DE, Lim KG. Propofol-induced pancreatitis: recurrence of pancreatitis after rechallenge. Chest 1999;115:1198-9.

175. Walder B, Tramèr MR, Seeck M. Seizure-like phenomena and propofol: a systematic review. Neurology 2002;58:1327-32.

176. Blakey SA, Hixson-Wallace JA. Clinical significance of rare and benign side effects: propofol and green urine. Pharmacotherapy 2000;20:1120-2.

177. Roberts RJ, Barletta JF, Fong JJ, et al. Incidence of propofol-related infusion syndrome in critically ill adults: a prospective, multicenter study. Crit Care 2009;13:R169.

178. Iyer VN, Hoel R, Rabinstein AA. Propofol infusion syndrome in patients with refractory status epilepticus: an 11-year clinical experience. Crit Care Med 2009;37:3024-30.

179. Vasile B, Rasulo F, Candiani A, et al. The pathophysiology of propofol infusion syndrome: a simple name for a complex syndrome. Intensive Care Med 2003;29:1417-25.

180. Orsini J, Nadkarni A, Chen J, et al. Propofol infusion syndrome: case report and literature review. Am J Health Syst Pharm 2009;66:908-15.

181. Vernooy K, Delhaas T, Cremer OL, et al. Electrocardiographic changes predicting sudden death in propofol-related infusion syndrome. Heart Rhythm 2006;3:131-7.

182. Fong JJ, Sylvia L, Ruthazer R, et al. Predictors of mortality in patients with suspected propofol infusion syndrome. Crit Care Med 2008;36:2281-7.

183. Kamibayashi T, Maze M. Clinical uses of alpha2-adrenergic agonists. Anesthesiology 2000;93:1345-9.

184. Belleville JP, Ward DS, Bloor BC, et al. Effects of intravenous dexmedetomidine in humans. I. Sedation, ventilation, and metabolic rate. Anesthesiology 1992;77:1125-33.

185. Bailey PL, Sperry RJ, Johnson GK, et al. Respiratory effects of clonidine alone and combined with morphine, in humans. Anesthesiology 1991;74:43-84.

186. Correa-Sales C, Rabin BC, Maze M. A hypnotic response to dexmedetomidine, an alpha 2 agonist, is mediated in the locus coeruleus in rats. Anesthesiology 1992;76:948-52.

187. Sakamoto H, Fukuda S, Minakawa Y, et al. Clonidine induces sedation through acting on the perifornical area and the locus coeruleus in rats. J Neurosurg Anesthesiol 2013;25:399-407.

188. Schnabel A, Meyer-Frießem CH, Reichl SU, et al. Is intraoperative dexmedetomidine a new option for postoperative pain treatment? A meta-analysis of randomized controlled trials. Pain 2013;154:1140-9.

189. Blaudszun G, Lysakowski C, Elia N, et al. Effect of perioperative systemic α2 agonists on postoperative morphine consumption and pain intensity: systematic review and meta-analysis of randomized controlled trials. Anesthesiology 2012;116:1312-22.

190. Virtanen R, Savola JM, Saano V, et al. Characterization of the selectivity, specificity and potency of medetomidine as an alpha 2-adrenoceptor agonist. Eur J Pharmacol 1988;150:9-14.

191. Knaus AE, Muthig V, Schickinger S, et al. Alpha2-adrenoceptor subtypes—unexpected functions for receptors and ligands derived from gene-targeted mouse models. Neurochem Int 2007;51:277-81.

192. Iirola T, Ihmsen H, Laitio R, et al. Population pharmacokinetics of dexmedetomidine during long-term sedation in intensive care patients. Br J Anaesth 2012;108:460-8.

193. Venn RM, Karol MD, Grounds RM. Pharmacokinetics of dexmedetomidine infusions for sedation of postoperative patients requiring intensive care. Br J Anaesth 2002;88:669-75.

194. Riker RR, Shehabi Y, Bokesch PM, et al. Dexmedetomidine vs midazolam for sedation of critically ill patients: a randomized trial. JAMA 2009;301:489-99.

195. Jakob SM, Ruokonen E, Grounds RM, et al. Dexmedetomidine vs midazolam or propofol for sedation during prolonged mechanical ventilation: two randomized controlled trials. JAMA 2012;307:1151-60.

196. Pandharipande PP, Pun BT, Herr DL, et al. Effect of sedation with dexmedetomidine vs lorazepam on acute brain dysfunction in mechanically ventilated patients: the MENDS randomized controlled trial. JAMA 2007;298:2644-53.

197. Mueller SW, Preslaski CR, Kiser TH, et al. A randomized, double-blind, placebo-controlled dose range study of dexmedetomidine as adjunctive therapy for alcohol withdrawal. Crit Care Med 2014;42:1131-9.

198. Holliday SF, Kane-Gill SL, Empey PE, et al. Interpatient variability in dexmedetomidine response: a survey of the literature. ScientificWorldJournal 2014;2014:805013.

199. Bioc JJ, Magee C, Cucchi J, et al. Cost effectiveness of a benzodiazepine vs a nonbenzodiazepine-based sedation regimen for mechanically ventilated, critically ill adults. J Crit Care 2014;29:753-7.

200. Gagnon DJ, Riker RR, Glisic EK, et al. Transition from dexmedetomidine to enteral clonidine for ICU sedation: an observational pilot study. Pharmacotherapy 2015;35:251-9.

201. Turunen H, Jakob SM, Ruokonen E, et al. Dexmedetomidine versus standard care sedation with propofol or midazolam in intensive care: an economic evaluation. Crit Care 2015;19:67.

202. Jamadarkhana S, Gopal S. Clonidine in adults as a sedative agent in the intensive care unit. J Anaesthesiol Clin Pharmacol 2010;26:439-45.

203. Ahmed I, Takeshita J. Clonidine a critical review of its role in the treatment of psychiatric disorders. CNS Drugs 1996;6:53-70.

204. Eisenach JC, De Kock M, Klimscha W. Alpha(2)-adrenergic agonists for regional anesthesia. A clinical review of clonidine (1984-1995). Anesthesiology 1996;85:655-74.

205. Lowenthal DT, Matzek KM, MacGregor TR. Clinical pharmacokinetics of clonidine. Clin Pharmacokinet 1988;14:287-310.

206. Pichot C, Ghignone M, Quintin L. Dexmedetomidine and clonidine: from second- to first-line sedative agents in the critical care setting? J Intensive Care Med 2012;27:219-37.

207. Playfor S, Jenkins I, Boyles C, et al. Consensus guidelines on sedation and analgesia in critically ill children. Intensive Care Med 2006;32:1125-36.

208. Chen K, Lu Z, Xin YC, et al. Alpha-2 agonists for long-term sedation during mechanical ventilation in critically ill patients. Cochrane Database Syst Rev 2015;1:CD010269.

209. Martin J, Heymann A, Bäsell K, et al. Evidence and consensus-based German guidelines for the management of analgesia, sedation and delirium in intensive care—short version. Ger Med Sci 2010;8:Doc02.

210. Kariya N, Shindoh M, Nishi S, et al. Oral clonidine for sedation and analgesia in a burn patient. J Clin Anesth 1998;10:514-7.

211. Arenas-Lopez S, Riphagen S, Tibby SM, et al. Use of oral clonidine for sedation in ventilated paediatric intensive care patients. Intensive Care Med 2004;30:1625-9.

212. Duffett M, Choong K, Foster J, et al. Clonidine in the sedation of mechanically ventilated children: a pilot randomized trial. J Crit Care 2014;29:758-63.

213. Farasatinasab M, Kouchek M, Sistanizad M, et al. A randomized placebo-controlled trial of clonidine impact on sedation of mechanically ventilated ICU patients. Iran J Pharm Res 2015;14:167-75.

214. Whitsett TL, Chrysant SG, Dillard BL, et al. Abrupt cessation of clonidine administration: a prospective study. Am J Cardiol 1978;41:1285-90.

215. Weber MA. Discontinuation syndrome following cessation of treatment with clonidine and other antihypertensive agents. J Cardiovasc Pharmacol 1980;2(suppl 1):S73-S89.

216. Geyskes GG, Boer P, Dorhout Mees EJ. Clonidine withdrawal. Mechanism and frequency of rebound hypertension. Br J Clin Pharmacol 1979;7:55-62.

217. Löscher W. Basic pharmacology of valproate: a review after 35 years of clinical use for the treatment of epilepsy. CNS Drugs 2002;16:669-94.

218. Perucca E. Pharmacological and therapeutic properties of valproate: a summary after 35 years of clinical experience. CNS Drugs 2002;16:695-714.

219. Lum E, Gorman SK, Slavik RS. Valproic acid management of acute alcohol withdrawal. Ann Pharmacother 2006;40:441-8.

220. Gallagher D, Herrmann N. Antiepileptic drugs for the treatment of agitation and aggression in dementia: do they have a place in therapy? Drugs 2014;74:1747-55.

221. Schwarz C, Volz A, Li C, et al. Valproate for schizophrenia. Cochrane Database Syst Rev 2008;3:CD004028.

222. Sher YI, Miller AC, Lolak S, et al. Valproic acid as an adjunct treatment for hyperactive delirium: Postulated mechanisms of deliriolytic action and case series [abstract]. Psychosom Med 2014;76:3(A-39).

223. Fitz K, Harding A. Safety and efficacy of valproic acid for treatment of delirium in critically ill patients [abstract]. Crit Care Med 2011;39(12 suppl):239.

224. Bourgeois JA, Koike AK, Simmons JE, et al. Adjunctive valproic acid for delirium and/or agitation on a consultation-liaison service: a report of six cases. J Neuropsychiatry Clin Neurosci 2005;17:232-8.

225. American Psychiatric Association. Practice guideline for the treatment of patients with bipolar disorder (revision). Am J Psychiatry 2002; 159:1–50.

226. Allen MH, Hirschfeld RM, Wozniak PJ, et al. Linear relationship of valproate serum concentration to response and optimal serum levels for acute mania. Am J Psychiatry 2006;163:272-5.

227. Carr RB, Shrewsbury K. Hyperammonemia due to valproic acid in the psychiatric setting. Am J Psychiatry 2007;164:1020-7.

228. Perrott J, Murphy NG, Zed PJ. L-carnitine for acute valproic acid overdose: a systematic review of published cases. Ann Pharmacother 2010;44:1287-93.

229. Nasreddine W, Beydoun A. Valproate-induced thrombocytopenia: a prospective monotherapy study. Epilepsia 2008;49:438-45.

230. Proulle V, Masnou P, Cartron J, et al. GPIaIIa as a candidate target for anti-platelet autoantibody occurring during valproate therapy and associated with perioperative bleeding. Thromb Haemost 2000;83:175-6.

231. Gerstner T, Büsing D, Bell N, et al. Valproic acid-induced pancreatitis: 16 new cases and a review of the literature. J Gastroenterol 2007;42:39-48.

232. Powell-Jackson PR, Tredger JM, Williams R. Hepatotoxicity to sodium valproate: a review. Gut 1984;25:673-81.

233. Spriet I, Goyens J, Meersseman W, et al. Interaction between valproate and meropenem: a retrospective study. Ann Pharmacother 2007;41:1130-6.

234. Park MK, Lim KS, Kim TE, et al. Reduced valproic acid serum concentrations due to drug interactions with carbapenem antibiotics: overview of 6 cases. Ther Drug Monit 2012;34:599-603.

235. Anderson GD. A mechanistic approach to antiepileptic drug interactions. Ann Pharmacother 1998;32:554-63.

236. Kwan P, Brodie MJ Phenobarbital. for the treatment of epilepsy in the 21st century: a critical review. Epilepsia 2004;45:1141-9.

237. Smith MC, Riskin BJ. The clinical use of barbiturates in neurological disorders. Drugs 1991;42:365-78.

238. Rosenson J, Clements C, Simon B, et al. Phenobarbital for acute alcohol withdrawal: a prospective randomized double-blind placebo-controlled study. J Emerg Med 2013;44:592-598.e2.

239. Fraser GL, Riker RR. Phenobarbital provides effective sedation for a select cohort of adult ICU patients intolerant of standard treatment: a brief report. Hosp Pharm 2006;41:17-23.

240. Wolff K, Winstock AR. Ketamine: from medicine to misuse. CNS Drugs 2006;20:199-218.

241. Mohrien KM, Jones GM, MacDermott JR, et al. Remifentanil, ketamine, and fospropofol: a review of alterative continuous infusion agents for sedation in the critically ill. Crit Care Nurs Q 2014;37:137-51.

242. Miller AC, Jamin CT, Elamin EM. Continuous intravenous infusion of ketamine for maintenance sedation. Minerva Anestesiol 2011;77:812-20.

243. Hudetz JA, Patterson KM, Iqbal Z, et al. Ketamine attenuates delirium after cardiac surgery with cardiopulmonary bypass. J Cardiothorac Vasc Anesth 2009;23:651-7.

244. Wong A, Benedict NJ, Armahizer MJ, et al. Evaluation of adjunctive ketamine to benzodiazepines for management of alcohol withdrawal syndrome. Ann Pharmacother 2015;49:14-9.

245. Zeiler FA, Teitelbaum J, West M, et al. The ketamine effect on ICP in traumatic brain injury. Neurocrit Care 2014;21:163-73.

246. Howard P, Twycross R, Shuster J, et al. Antipsychotics. J Pain Symptom Manage 2011;41:956-65.

247. Correll CU. From receptor pharmacology to improved outcomes: individualising the selection, dosing, and switching of antipsychotics. Eur Psychiatry 2010;25(suppl 2):S12-S21.

248. Serafim RB, Bozza FA, Soares M, et al. Pharmacologic prevention and treatment of delirium in intensive care patients: a systematic review. J Crit Care 2015;30:799-807.

249. Sedation in French intensive care units: a survey of clinical practice. Ann Intensive Care 2013;3:24.

250. Weinert CR, Calvin AD. Epidemiology of sedation and sedation adequacy for mechanically ventilated patients in a medical and surgical intensive care unit. Crit Care Med 2007;35:393-401.

251. Payen JF, Chanques G, Mantz J, et al. Current practices in sedation and analgesia for mechanically ventilated critically ill patients: a prospective multicenter patient-based study. Anesthesiology 2007;106:687-95.

252. Burry LD, Williamson DR, Perreault MM, et al. Analgesic, sedative, antipsychotic, and neuromuscular blocker use in Canadian intensive care units: a prospective, multicentre, observational study. Can J Anaesth 2014;61:619-30.

253. Skrobik YK, Bergeron N, Dumont M, et al. Olanzapine vs haloperidol: treating delirium in a critical care setting. Intensive Care Med 2004;30:444-9.

254. Rea RS, Battistone S, Fong JJ, et al. Atypical antipsychotics versus haloperidol for treatment of delirium in acutely ill patients. Pharmacotherapy 2007;27:588-94.

255. Devlin JW, Mallow-Corbett S, Riker RR. Adverse drug events associated with the use of analgesics, sedatives, and antipsychotics in the intensive care unit. Crit Care Med 2010;38(6 suppl):S231-S243.

256. Hale GM, Kane-Gill SL, Groetzinger L, et al. An evaluation of adverse drug reactions associated with antipsychotic use for the treatment of delirium in the intensive care unit. J Pharm Pract 2015 Jan 20. [Epub ahead of print]

257. Alper K, Schwartz KA, Kolts RL, et al. Seizure incidence in psychopharmacological clinical trials: an analysis of Food and

Drug Administration (FDA) summary basis of approval reports. Biol Psychiatry 2007;62:345-54.

258. Sackey PV, Martling CR, Granath F, et al. Prolonged isoflurane sedation of intensive care unit patients with the Anesthetic Conserving Device. Crit Care Med 2004;32:2241-6.

259. Perouansky M, Pearce RA, Hemmings HC. Inhaled anesthetics: mechanisms of action. In: Miller RD, Cohen NH, Eriksson LI, et al., eds. Miller's Anesthesia, 8th ed. Philadelphia: Elsevier, 2015:614-37.

260. Forman SA, Ishizawa Y. Inhaled anesthetic pharmacokinetics: uptake, distribution, metabolism and, toxicity. In: Miller RD, Cohen NH, Eriksson LI, et al., eds. Miller's Anesthesia, 8th ed. Philadelphia: Elsevier, 2015:638-69.

261. Torri G. Inhalation anesthetics: a review. Minerva Anestesiol 2010;76:215-28.

262. Purrucker JC, Renzland J, Uhlmann L, et al. Volatile sedation with sevoflurane in intensive care patients with acute stroke or subarachnoid haemorrhage using AnaConDa®: an observational study. Br J Anaesth 2015;114:934-43.

263. Lee JJ, Li L, Jung HH, et al. Postconditioning with isoflurane reduced ischemia-induced brain injury in rats. Anesthesiology 2008;108:1055-62.

264. Kong KL, Willatts SM, Prys-Roberts C. Isoflurane compared with midazolam for sedation in the intensive care unit. BMJ 1989;298:1277-80.

265. Spencer EM, Willatts SM. Isoflurane for prolonged sedation in the intensive care unit; efficacy and safety. Intensive Care Med 1992;18:415-21.

266. Meiser A, Sirtl C, Bellgardt M, et al. Desflurane compared with propofol for postoperative sedation in the intensive care unit. Br J Anaesth 2003;90:273-80.

267. Mesnil M, Capdevila X, Bringuier S, et al. Long-term sedation in intensive care unit: a randomized comparison between inhaled sevoflurane and intravenous propofol or midazolam. Intensive Care Med 2011;37:933-41.

268. Migliari M, Bellani G, Rona R, et al. Short-term evaluation of sedation with sevoflurane administered by the anesthetic conserving device in critically ill patients. Intensive Care Med 2009;35:1240-6.

269. Sackey PV, Martling CR, Carlswärd C, et al. Short- and long-term follow-up of intensive care unit patients after sedation with isoflurane and midazolam—a pilot study. Crit Care Med 2008;36:801-6.

270. Bellgardt M, Bomberg H, Herzog-Niescery J, et al. Survival after long-term isoflurane sedation as opposed to intravenous sedation in critically ill surgical patients. Eur J Anaesthesiol. 2015 Mar 19. [Epub ahead of print]

271. Maccioli GA, Cohen NH. General anesthesia in the intensive care unit: Is it ready for "prime time"? [editorial]. Crit Care Med 2005;33:687-8.

272. Mistraletti G, Mantovani ES, Cadringher P, et al. Enteral vs. intravenous ICU sedation management: study protocol for a randomized controlled trial. Trials 2013;14:92.

273. Mixon BM Jr, Pittinger CB. Hydroxyzine as an adjunct to preanesthetic medication. Anesth Analg 1968;47:330-3.

274. Franssen C, Hans P, Brichant JF, et al. Comparison between alprazolam and hydroxyzine for oral premedication. Can J Anaesth 1993;40:13-7.

275. Guaiana G, Barbui C, Cipriani A. Hydroxyzine for generalised anxiety disorder. Cochrane Database Syst Rev 2010;12:CD006815.

276. Cigada M, Pezzi A, Di Mauro P, et al. Sedation in the critically ill ventilated patient: possible role of enteral drugs. Intensive Care Med 2005;31:482-6.

277. New restrictions to Minimise the Risks of Effects on Heart Rhythm with Hydroxyzine-Containing Medicines. European Medicines Agency. Available at www.ema.europa.eu/ema/index.jsp?curl=pages/medicines/human/referrals/Hydroxyzine/human_referral_prac_000043.jsp&mid=WC0b01ac05805c516f. Accessed July 1, 2015.

278. Cammarano WB, Pittet JF, Weitz S, et al. Acute withdrawal syndrome related to the administration of analgesic and sedative medications in adult intensive care unit patients. Crit Care Med 1998;26:676-84.

279. Katz R, Kelly HW, Hsi A. Prospective study on the occurrence of withdrawal in critically ill children who receive fentanyl by continuous infusion. Crit Care Med 1994;22:763-7.

280. Korak-Leiter M, Likar R, Oher M, et al. Withdrawal following sufentanil/propofol and sufentanil/midazolam. Sedation in surgical ICU patients: correlation with central nervous parameters and endogenous opioids. Intensive Care Med 2005;31:380-7.

281. Zapantis A, Leung S. Tolerance and withdrawal issues with sedation. Crit Care Nurs Clin North Am 2005;17:211-23.

282. Kukoyi A, Coker S, Lewis L, et al. Two cases of acute dexmedetomidine withdrawal syndrome following prolonged infusion in the intensive care unit: report of cases and review of the literature. Hum Exp Toxicol 2013;32:107-10.

283. Lat I, Micek S, Janzen J, et al. Off-label medication use in adult critical care patients. J Crit Care 2011;26:89-94.

284. Jasiak KD, Middleton EA, Camamo JM, et al. Evaluation of discontinuation of atypical antipsychotics prescribed for ICU delirium. J Pharm Pract 2013;26:253-6.

285. Stelfox HT, Lane D, Boyd JM, et al. A scoping review of patient discharge from intensive care: opportunities and tools to improve care. Chest 2015;147:317-27.

286. Ely EW, Inouye SK, Bernard GR, et al. Delirium in mechanically ventilated patients: validity and reliability of the confusion assessment method for the intensive care unit (CAM-ICU). JAMA 2001;286:2703-10.

287. Bergeron N, Dubois MJ, Dumont M, et al. Intensive Care Delirium Screening Checklist: evaluation of a new screening tool. Intensive Care Med 2001;27:859-64.

288. Haenggi M, Blum S, Brechbuehl R, et al. Effect of sedation level on the prevalence of delirium when assessed with CAM-ICU and ICDSC. Intensive Care Med 2013;39:2171-9.

289. Patel SB, Poston JT, Pohlman A, et al. Rapidly reversible, sedation-related delirium versus persistent delirium in the intensive care unit. Am J Respir Crit Care Med 2014;189:658-65.

290. Balas MC, Vasilevskis EE, Olsen KM, et al. Effectiveness and safety of the awakening and breathing coordination, delirium monitoring/management, and early exercise/mobility bundle. Crit Care Med 2014;42:1024-36.

291. TEAM Study Investigators, Hodgson C, Bellomo R, et al. Early mobilization and recovery in mechanically ventilated patients in

292. Patel BK, Pohlman AS, Hall JB, et al. Impact of early mobilization on glycemic control and ICU-acquired weakness in critically ill patients who are mechanically ventilated. Chest 2014;146:583-9.

293. Schweickert WD, Pohlman MC, Pohlman AS, et al. Early physical and occupational therapy in mechanically ventilated, critically ill patients: a randomised controlled trial. Lancet 2009;373:1874-82.

294. Balzer F, Weiß B, Kumpf O, et al. Early deep sedation is associated with decreased in-hospital and two-year follow-up survival. Crit Care 2015;19:197.

295. Shehabi Y, Bellomo R, Reade MC, et al. Early intensive care sedation predicts long-term mortality in ventilated critically ill patients. Am J Respir Crit Care Med 2012;186:724-31.

296. Shehabi Y, Chan L, Kadiman S, et al. Sedation depth and long-term mortality in mechanically ventilated critically ill adults: a prospective longitudinal multicentre cohort study. Intensive Care Med 2013;39:910-8.

297. Tanaka LM, Azevedo LC, Park M, et al. Early sedation and clinical outcomes of mechanically ventilated patients: a prospective multicenter cohort study. Crit Care 2014;18:R156.

298. Fraser GL, Riker RR. Comfort without coma: changing sedation practices [editorial]. Crit Care Med 2007;35:635-7.

299. Samuelson K, Lundberg D, Fridlund B. Memory in relation to depth of sedation in adult mechanically ventilated intensive care patients. Intensive Care Med 2006;32:660-7.

300. Jones C, Griffiths RD, Humphris G, et al. Memory, delusions, and the development of acute posttraumatic stress disorder-related symptoms after intensive care. Crit Care Med 2001;29:573-80.

301. Jones C, Bäckman C, Capuzzo M, et al. Precipitants of post-traumatic stress disorder following intensive care: a hypothesis generating study of diversity in care. Intensive Care Med 2007;33:978-85.

302. Patel RP, Gambrell M, Speroff T, et al. Delirium and sedation in the intensive care unit: survey of behaviors and attitudes of 1384 healthcare professionals. Crit Care Med 2009;37:825-32.

303. Brook AD, Ahrens TS, Schaiff R, et al. Effect of a nursing-implemented sedation protocol on the duration of mechanical ventilation. Crit Care Med 1999;27:2609-15.

304. De Jonghe B, Bastuji-Garin S, Fangio P, et al. Sedation algorithm in critically ill patients without acute brain injury. Crit Care Med 2005;33:120-7.

305. Quenot JP, Ladoire S, Devoucoux F, et al. Effect of a nurse-implemented sedation protocol on the incidence of ventilator-associated pneumonia. Crit Care Med 2007;35:2031-6.

306. Arias-Rivera S, Sánchez-Sánchez Mdel M, Santos-Díaz R, et al. Effect of a nursing-implemented sedation protocol on weaning outcome. Crit Care Med 2008;36:2054-60.

307. Marshall J, Finn CA, Theodore AC. Impact of a clinical pharmacist-enforced intensive care unit sedation protocol on duration of mechanical ventilation and hospital stay. Crit Care Med 2008;36:427-33.

308. Robinson BR, Mueller EW, Henson K, et al. An analgesia-delirium-sedation protocol for critically ill trauma patients reduces ventilator days and hospital length of stay. J Trauma 2008;65:517-26.

309. Skrobik Y, Ahern S, Leblanc M, et al. Protocolized intensive care unit management of analgesia, sedation, and delirium improves analgesia and subsyndromal delirium rates. Anesth Analg 2010;111:451-63.

310. Mansouri P, Javadpour S, Zand F, et al. Implementation of a protocol for integrated management of pain, agitation, and delirium can improve clinical outcomes in the intensive care unit: a randomized clinical trial. J Crit Care 2013;28:918-22.

311. Dale CR, Kannas DA, Fan VS, et al. Improved analgesia, sedation, and delirium protocol associated with decreased duration of delirium and mechanical ventilation. Ann Am Thorac Soc 2014;11:367-74.

312. Ranzani OT, Simpson ES, Augusto TB, et al.; AMIL Critical Care Group. Evaluation of a minimal sedation protocol using ICU sedative consumption as a monitoring tool: a quality improvement multicenter project. Crit Care 2014;18:580.

313. MacLaren R, Plamondon JM, Ramsay KB, et al. A prospective evaluation of empiric versus protocol-based sedation and analgesia. Pharmacotherapy 2000;20:662-72.

314. Strøm T, Stylsvig M, Toft P. Long-term psychological effects of a no-sedation protocol in critically ill patients. Crit Care 2011;15:R293.

315. Shehabi Y, Bellomo R, Reade MC, et al. Early goal-directed sedation versus standard sedation in mechanically ventilated critically ill patients: a pilot study*. Crit Care Med 2013;41:1983-91.

316. Bucknall TK, Manias E, Presneill JJ. A randomized trial of protocol-directed sedation management for mechanical ventilation in an Australian intensive care unit. Crit Care Med 2008;36:1444-50.

317. Elliott R, McKinley S, Aitken LM, et al. The effect of an algorithm-based sedation guideline on the duration of mechanical ventilation in an Australian intensive care unit. Intensive Care Med 2006;32:1506-14.

318. Aitken LM, Bucknall T, Kent B, et al. Protocol-directed sedation versus non-protocol-directed sedation to reduce duration of mechanical ventilation in mechanically ventilated intensive care patients. Cochrane Database Syst Rev 2015;1:CD009771.

319. Minhas MA, Velasquez AG, Kaul A, et al. Effect of protocolized sedation on clinical outcomes in mechanically ventilated intensive care unit patients: a systematic review and meta-analysis of randomized controlled trials. Mayo Clin Proc 2015;90:613-23.

320. Hughes CG, Girard TD, Pandharipande PP. Daily sedation interruption versus targeted light sedation strategies in ICU patients. Crit Care Med 2013;41(9 suppl 1):S39-S45.

321. de Wit M, Gennings C, Jenvey WI, et al. Randomized trial comparing daily interruption of sedation and nursing-implemented sedation algorithm in medical intensive care unit patients. Crit Care 2008;12:R70.

322. Helbok R, Kurtz P, Schmidt MJ, et al. Effects of the neurological wake-up test on clinical examination, intracranial pressure, brain metabolism and brain tissue oxygenation in severely brain-injured patients. Crit Care 2012;16:R226.

323. Skoglund K, Enblad P, Marklund N. Effects of the neurological wake-up test on intracranial pressure and cerebral

323. perfusion pressure in brain-injured patients. Neurocrit Care 2009;11:135-42.

324. Kress JP, Pohlman AS, O'Connor MF, et al. Daily interruption of sedative infusions in critically ill patients undergoing mechanical ventilation. N Engl J Med 2000;342:1471-7.

325. Schweickert WD, Gehlbach BK, Pohlman AS, et al. Daily interruption of sedative infusions and complications of critical illness in mechanically ventilated patients. Crit Care Med 2004;32:1272-6.

326. Heffner JE. A wake-up call in the intensive care unit [abstract]. N Engl J Med 2000;342:1520-2.

327. Kress JP, Gehlbach B, Lacy M, et al. The long-term psychological effects of daily sedative interruption on critically ill patients. Am J Respir Crit Care Med 2003;168:1457-61.

328. Anifantaki S, Prinianakis G, Vitsaksaki E, et al. Daily interruption of sedative infusions in an adult medical-surgical intensive care unit: randomized controlled trial. J Adv Nurs 2009;65:1054-60.

329. Augustes R, Ho KM. Meta-analysis of randomised controlled trials on daily sedation interruption for critically ill adult patients. Anaesth Intensive Care 2011;39:401-9.

330. Burry L, Rose L, McCullagh IJ, et al. Daily sedation interruption versus no daily sedation interruption for critically ill adult patients requiring invasive mechanical ventilation. Cochrane Database Syst Rev 2014;7:CD009176.

331. Mehta S, Burry L, Cook D, et al. Daily sedation interruption in mechanically ventilated critically ill patients cared for with a sedation protocol: a randomized controlled trial. JAMA 2012;308:1985-92.

332. Girard TD, Kress JP, Fuchs BD, et al. Efficacy and safety of a paired sedation and ventilator weaning protocol for mechanically ventilated patients in intensive care (Awakening and Breathing Controlled trial): a randomised controlled trial. Lancet 2008;371:126-34.

333. Jackson JC, Girard TD, Gordon SM, et al. Long-term cognitive and psychological outcomes in the awakening and breathing controlled trial. Am J Respir Crit Care Med 2010;182:183-91.

334. Gill KV, Voils SA, Chenault GA, et al. Perceived versus actual sedation practices in adult intensive care unit patients receiving mechanical ventilation. Ann Pharmacother 2012;46:1331-9.

335. Tanios MA, de Wit M, Epstein SK, et al. Perceived barriers to the use of sedation protocols and daily sedation interruption: a multidisciplinary survey. J Crit Care 2009;24:66-73.

336. Carrothers KM, Barr J, Spurlock B, et al. Contextual issues influencing implementation and outcomes associated with an integrated approach to managing pain, agitation, and delirium in adult ICUs. Crit Care Med 2013;41(9 suppl 1):S128-S135.

337. Devlin JW, Pohlman AS. Everybody, every day: an "awakening and breathing coordination, delirium monitoring/management, and early exercise/mobility" culture is feasible in your ICU [abstract]. Crit Care Med 2014;42:1280-1.

338. Rose L, Fitzgerald E, Cook D, et al. Clinician perspectives on protocols designed to minimize sedation. J Crit Care 2015;30:348-52.

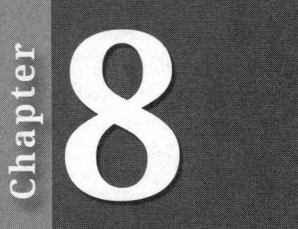

Delirium in Critically Ill Adults

John W. Devlin, Pharm.D., FCCP, FCCM

LEARNING OBJECTIVES

1. Describe the outcomes of delirium in critically ill adults.
2. Recognize the importance of routine delirium screening in the intensive care unit (ICU) using the CAM-ICU (Confusion Assessment Method for the Intensive Care Unit) or the ICDSC (Intensive Care Delirium Screening Checklist).
3. Identify modifiable risk factors for delirium in critically ill adults.
4. Apply nonpharmacologic strategies to reduce the burden of delirium in critically ill adults.
5. Understand the current limited role of medication when treating delirium in the ICU.

ABBREVIATIONS IN THIS CHAPTER

ABCDEF	**A**ssessment, prevention, and management of pain, **B**oth spontaneous awakening trials and spontaneous breathing trials, **C**hoice of analgesia and sedation, **D**elirium assessment, prevention, and management, **E**arly mobility and exercise, and **F**amily engagement and empowerment	CAM-ICU	Confusion Assessment Method for the Intensive Care Unit
		ICDSC	Intensive Care Delirium Screening Checklist
		ICU	Intensive care unit
		RASS	Richmond Agitation-Sedation Scale
		SAS	Sedation-Agitation scale
		SAT	Spontaneous awakening trial

INTRODUCTION

Delirium is often encountered in the intensive care unit (ICU) and is associated with significant adverse outcomes. The increasingly recognized consequences of ICU delirium should enhance efforts to improve recognition and management of this serious sequelae of critical illness. We aim to review the recent literature on ICU delirium, including risk factors, detection, management, and the long-term impact of this disease.

DESCRIPTION OF DELIRIUM

Delirium is a syndrome characterized by the acute onset of cerebral dysfunction with a change or fluctuation in baseline mental status, inattention, and either disorganized thinking or an altered level of consciousness.[1] The cardinal features of delirium are (1) a disturbed level of consciousness (i.e., a reduced clarity of awareness of the environment), with a reduced ability to focus, sustain, or shift attention; and (2) either a change in cognition (i.e., memory deficit, disorientation, language disturbance) or the development of a perceptual disturbance (i.e., hallucinations, delusions).

Although the recent fifth edition of the *Diagnostic and Statistical Manual of Mental Disorders* of the American Psychiatric Association now operationalizes "consciousness" as "changes in attention," this minor change does not influence the validity of instruments developed for delirium recognition in the ICU, given that level of arousal, a key part of attention, corresponds directly with level of consciousness, and all patients must have an adequate level of arousal before the presence of inattention can be evaluated.[2]

Other symptoms commonly associated with delirium include sleep disturbances, abnormal psychomotor activity, hallucinations/delusions, and emotional disturbances (i.e., fear, anxiety, anger, depression, apathy, and euphoria).[3] These symptoms are often those that are of most concern to patients, family members, and caregivers and thus often require treatment. Patients with delirium may be agitated (hyperactive delirium), calm, or lethargic (hypoactive delirium), or they may fluctuate between the two subtypes (mixed).[4] Among patients with delirium, 75% have delirium that is either hypoactive or mixed. Patients with only some of the characteristics of delirium have subsyndromal delirium, a condition that may result in outcomes almost as bad as those with delirium.[5]

Although epidemiologic studies from more than a decade ago reported delirium to occur in up to 80% of mechanically ventilated, critically ill adults, more recent investigations of ICU patients who are less likely to be deeply sedated and more likely to have been mobilized report a delirium incidence rate closer to 40%.[6,7] The likelihood that delirium will occur in any ICU patient is dependent on the patient's baseline risk of delirium and the number of delirium-precipitating causes the patient is exposed to during the ICU stay.[8] Critically ill medical patients have a higher incidence of delirium than do surgical patients, particularly patients undergoing cardiac surgery. Up to 30% of ICU patients are admitted to the ICU with delirium.[6,7]

During their ICU stay, critically ill patients may develop a subcategory of delirium related to either drug withdrawal or alcohol withdrawal, which usually manifests as a hyperactive type of delirium. The pathophysiology, diagnosis, and treatment of delirium related to drug and alcohol withdrawal is distinct from delirium related to other causes and thus will not be reviewed in this chapter.[9]

IMPACT OF DELIRIUM ON PATIENT OUTCOME

Delirium, as a manifestation of acute brain dysfunction, is an important independent predictor of negative clinical outcomes in the ICU, including self-extubation, duration of mechanical ventilation, length of ICU stay, and ICU mortality.[7] Delirium increases both hospital and longer-term (e.g., 6 months) mortality. The trajectory of a patient's severity of illness during the ICU admission influences the relationship between delirium occurrence and mortality.[10] Given that the number of ICU days spent with delirium is associated with both 6- and 12- month mortality, optimizing the use of strategies shown to reduce the number of ICU days spent with delirium is an important goal of therapy.[7]

At hospital discharge, patients who developed delirium in the ICU are more likely to transition to a skilled nursing facility (e.g., nursing home) than to a rehabilitation facility or home.[7] Delirium may lead to long-term cognitive impairment that is not unlike that seen in patients with dementia or a traumatic brain injury.[11] These cognitive deficits often persist for weeks or months (or never resolve at all) and often delay a return to work and the ability to resume pre-critical illness activities and function. Patients who experience ICU delirium have a greater incidence of depression and often experience prolonged sleep abnormalities. This burden of delirium can have profound effects on spouses and family members, particularly if they are required to assume a caregiver role on a persistent basis. Given that the effects of delirium often persist long after ICU discharge, delirium is now recognized as a major public health problem that costs the United States up to $16 billion each year.[9]

PATHOPHYSIOLOGY OF DELIRIUM IN THE ICU

Although the study of delirium in critically ill patients has expanded tremendously during the past 15 years, the underlying pathophysiology of delirium in this population remains poorly understood. Although several different metabolic pathways have been postulated to cause delirium, including inflammation, neurotransmitter dysfunction, ischemia, glucose dysregulation, disruption of the hypothalamic-pituitary axis, and tryptophan metabolism, our understanding of how these various mechanisms interact to cause delirium state remains limited (Figure 8.1).[12]

It should be emphasized that this is a complex area of research, given that delirium likely occurs through a complex interplay of different systems and mechanisms and that critical illness itself is a dynamic, ever-changing process. A valid animal model for delirium has yet to be developed. Finally, neither imaging techniques nor biomarkers have been shown as valid methods to either predict or identify delirium in the ICU; thus, all mechanistic-focused delirium studies in this setting still rely on a diagnosis of delirium that is based on a symptom-based assessment at the patient bedside.[13]

RECOGNITION OF DELIRIUM IN THE ICU

Given the multifactorial and fluctuating nature of delirium, a cursory "one-time only" evaluation of delirium at the ICU bedside, without the use of a validated screening tool, is often ineffectual and is thus a poor strategy to identify delirium in critically ill adults.[14] Delirium is challenging to recognize in the ICU setting: most patients are intubated and cannot verbally communicate, the use of medications that reduce level of consciousness is prevalent, hypoactive delirium is common, and patients may be too unstable to participate in lengthy assessments.[15] The ability to accurately evaluate for delirium is a key component when developing ICU strategies focused on reducing reversible causes for delirium and promoting the regular interprofessional discussion of the cognitive status of patients.[9]

The ideal delirium screening tool combines high sensitivity (i.e., will be positive when delirium is present)

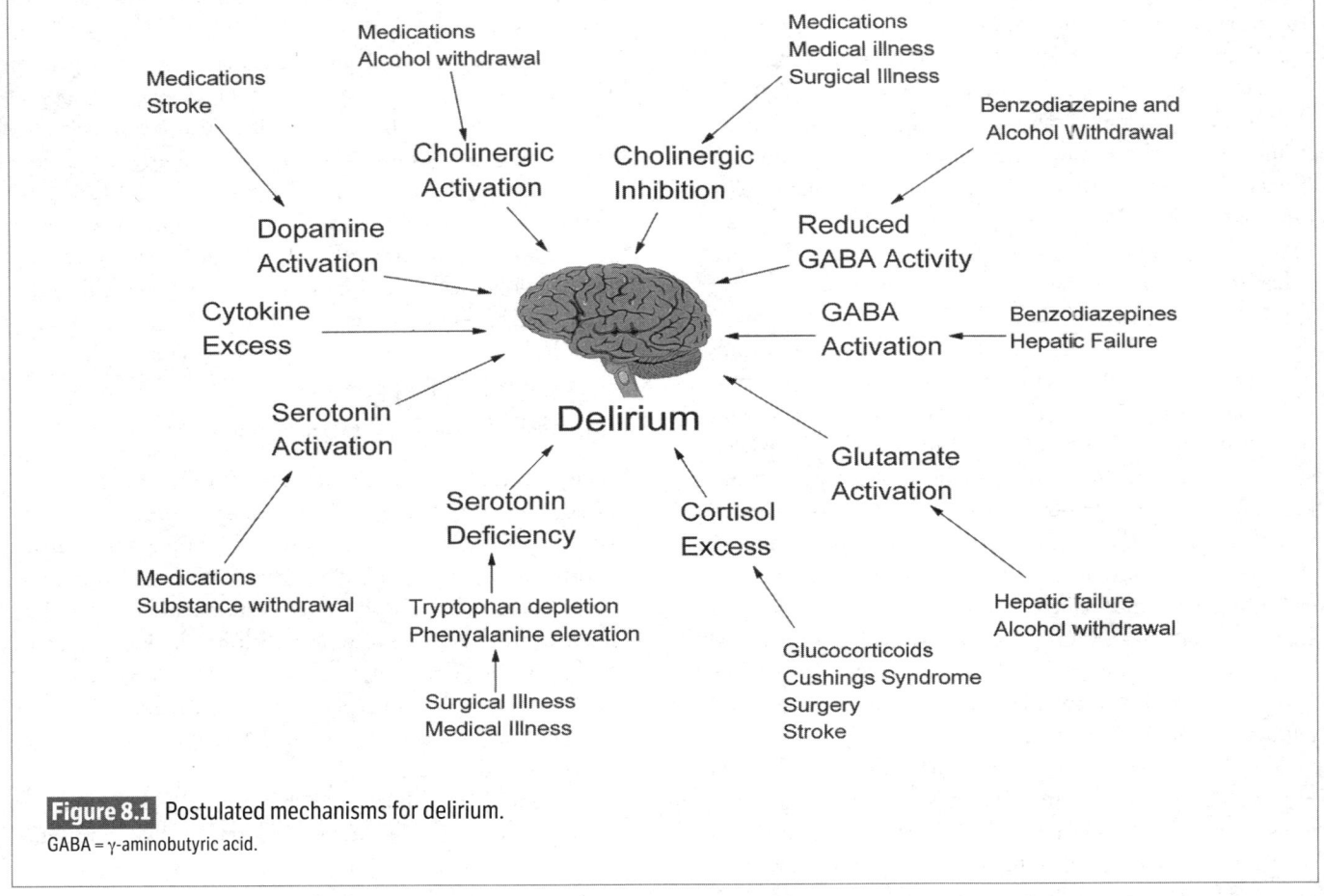

Figure 8.1 Postulated mechanisms for delirium. GABA = γ-aminobutyric acid.

and high specificity (i.e., will be negative when delirium is not present). Among the ICU delirium screening tools developed, the Confusion Assessment Method for the ICU (CAM-ICU) and the Intensive Care Delirium Screening Checklist (ICDSC) have the greatest psychometric strength.[9,16,17] A comprehensive discussion of the psychometric properties of the CAM-ICU and ICDSC is beyond the scope of this chapter. Nevertheless, two recent meta-analyses highlight the robust data that support the use of the CAM-ICU or the ICDSC in clinical practice.[18,19]

The Confusion Assessment Method for the ICU

The CAM-ICU is derived from the confusion assessment method and accounts for the nonverbal nature of most ICU patients by substituting the Attention Screening Exam for the Mini-Mental State Examination.[2] This instrument evaluates the four key diagnostic features of delirium: (1) acute change or fluctuation in mental status from baseline, (2) inattention, (3) altered level of consciousness, and (4) disorganized thinking (Figure 8.2).[16]

Feature 1 uses clinical information to assess the patient's mental status and is positive if the patient has a change in mental status from his or her prehospital baseline or has a fluctuation in mental status during the preceding 24 hours. Feature 2 asks the patient to complete a test of attention (e.g., asking the patient to squeeze the examiner's hand every time the patient hears the letter "A" as the examiner spells out S-A-V-E-A-H-A-A-R-T). Feature 3 evaluates level of consciousness with the use of a sedation scale (e.g., Richmond Agitation-Sedation Scale [RASS]) and is positive if the patient's level of consciousness is anything but alert and calm. Finally, feature 8.4 evaluates for disorganized thinking by asking the patient to perform a multistep task (e.g., holding up two fingers and then adding a third) and by answering four "yes/no" questions (e.g., Do fish live in the sea?). The CAM-ICU is considered positive if features 1 and 2 and either feature 3 or feature 4 is present.

Of note, patients who are deeply sedated (RASS of -4 or less) cannot be evaluated with the CAM-ICU until they are more awake.[14] Although the RASS is the standard sedation scale used in conjunction with the CAM-ICU, other validated sedation scales like the sedation-agitation scale (SAS) can be used. Patients receiving continuous sedation should be evaluated for delirium with the CAM-ICU after a spontaneous awakening trial (SAT) given that delirium that is recognized before the SAT is likely to be rapidly reversible and not clinically significant.[20] It is recommended to perform CAM-ICU screening several times per day (at a minimum twice) given the fluctuating nature of delirium. Additional assessments are recommended when changes in mental status occur.[14]

The Intensive Care Delirium Screening Checklist

The Intensive Care Delirium Screening Checklist (ICDSC) is an eight-item instrument based on criteria of the fourth edition of *Diagnostic and Statistical Manual of Mental Disorders* and other features of delirium that evaluates eight different delirium domains (Table 8.1).[17] The ICDSC was developed to provide ICU providers with an easy-to-use bedside screening tool that circumvents the communication limitations of ICU patients, incorporates data that are gathered during routine patient care and can be completed quickly by the patients' nurse, physician, or pharmacist. Patients who are not heavily sedated (i.e., RASS of -4 or less or SAS of 2 or less) are evaluated for domains 1–4 using a focused bedside assessment, for domains 5 and 6 over the course of the shift and domains 7 and 8 over the current and previous shift (i.e., during the prior 24 hours). At the end of each nursing shift, 1 point is given for each domain that is present, with a score of 4 or higher denoting the presence of delirium.

Although the ICDSC evaluates more symptoms of delirium than the CAM-ICU, the symptoms that each share in common (i.e., inattention, disorientation and agitation) are the delirium symptoms that are most commonly detected during ICDSC use and that have the best ability to discriminate between patients with delirium and those without.[3,14,17] The ICDSC can identify patients with subsyndromal delirium (i.e., an ICDSC score of 1–3). Emerging data also suggest that the CAM-ICU can be used to detect subsyndromal delirium.[5]

Implementing and Sustaining Delirium Screening Efforts

Because of the many limitations associated with use of a subjective approach, new consensus guidelines from the

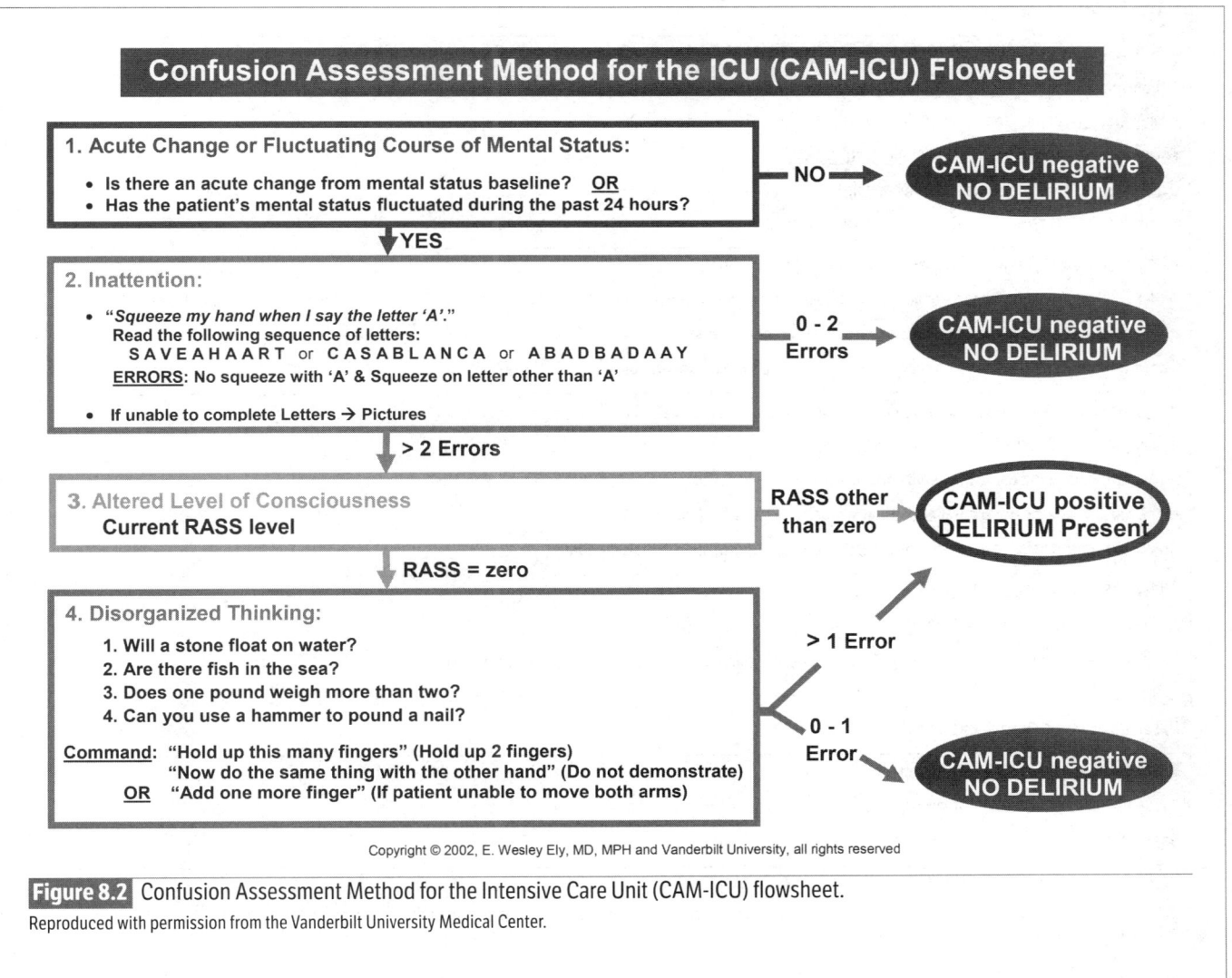

Figure 8.2 Confusion Assessment Method for the Intensive Care Unit (CAM-ICU) flowsheet.
Reproduced with permission from the Vanderbilt University Medical Center.

Table 8.1 The Intensive Care Delirium Screening Checklist

1. Altered level of consciousness Choose ONE from A–E.		
Note: May need to reassess patient if current or recent administration of sedation therapy		
A. Exaggerated response to normal stimulation	Riker/SAS = 5, 6, or 7	Score 1 point
B. Normal wakefulness	Riker/SAS = 4	Score 0 point
C. Response to mild or moderate stimulation (follows commands)	Riker/SAS = 3	Score 1 point *Score 0 if LOC related to recent sedation/analgesia
D. Response only to intense and repeated stimulation (e.g., loud voice and pain)	Riker/SAS = 2	*Stop assessment
E. No response	Riker/SAS = 1	*Stop assessment

2. Inattention Score 1 point for any of the following abnormalities:

A. Difficulty in following commands OR

B. Easily distracted by external stimuli OR

C. Difficulty in shifting focus

Does the patient follow you with his/her eyes?

3. Disorientation Score 1 point for any one obvious abnormality:

A. Mistake in time, place, or person

Does the patient recognize ICU caregivers who have cared for him/her and not recognize those who have not? What kind of place are you in? (list examples)

4. Hallucinations or Delusions Score 1 point for either:

A. Equivocal evidence of hallucinations or a behavior caused by hallucinations

(Hallucination = perception of something that is not there with NO stimulus) OR

B. Delusions or gross impairment of reality testing

(Delusion = false belief that is fixed/unchanging)

Any hallucinations now or during past 24 hr? Are you afraid of the people or things around you? [fear that is inappropriate to the clinical situation]

5. Psychomotor Agitation or Retardation Score 1 point for either:

A. Hyperactivity requiring the use of additional sedative drugs or restraints in order to control potential danger (e.g., pulling out IV lines or hitting staff) OR

B. Hypoactive or clinically noticeable psychomotor slowing or retardation

Based on documentation and observation over shift by primary caregiver

6. Inappropriate Speech or Mood Score 1 point for either:

A. Inappropriate, disorganized, or incoherent speech OR

B. Inappropriate mood related to events or situation

Is the patient apathetic to current clinical situation (i.e., lack of emotion)?

Any gross abnormalities in speech or mood? Is patient inappropriately demanding?

7. Sleep/Wake Cycle Disturbance Score 1 point for:

A. Sleeping less than 4 hours at night OR

B. Waking frequently at night (do not include wakefulness initiated by medical staff or loud environment) OR

C. Sleep ≥ 4 hours during day

Based on primary caregiver assessment

8. Symptom Fluctuation Score 1 point for:

fluctuation of any of the above items (i.e., 1–7) over 24 hours (e.g., from one shift to another)

Based on primary caregiver assessment

TOTAL ICDSC SCORE (Add 1–8)

IV = intravenous; LOC = level of consciousness.

Society of Critical Care Medicine advocate that critically ill patients should be routinely screened for delirium using either the CAM-ICU or the ICDSC.[9] More information about each tool may be found at www.icudelirium.org. Many studies have shown that large-score implementation of a delirium screening tool in the ICU is both feasible and sustainable.[14] Education regarding delirium assessment should be provided both didactically and at the bedside to all members of the ICU team and on a regular basis.[14] The results of delirium screening efforts should be presented during morning report and/or bedside rounds.[21] All ICU clinicians, including pharmacists and physicians, should be trained to screen for delirium in their patients. Routine delirium screening plays an integral role in the "ABCDEF" approach to managing sedation, delirium, early mobilization, and mechanical ventilation.[22] The ABCDEF is a standard bundle of ICU measures that includes routine Assessment for and management of pain, Both SATs and spontaneous breathing trials (SBTs), attention to the Choice of sedation and analgesia, Delirium monitoring and management, Early mobility, and Family engagement.

RISK FACTORS FOR DELIRIUM

During the past decade, a vast amount of research has focused on better understanding those aspects of ICU delirium that are predictable, preventable, detectable, and treatable.[17] Any critically ill patient's risk of delirium depends on a complex interplay between predisposing and precipitating risk factors. Given the current paucity of effective treatment options for delirium in the ICU, clinicians should focus their efforts on preventing delirium as soon as the patient is admitted to the ICU given that many risk factors for delirium in this setting are potentially modifiable.[9,21] Early recognition of these potentially reversible risk factors should constitute the foundation of all ICU delirium prevention programs.

Although the number of published ICU delirium risk factor papers has expanded considerably during the past few years, the methodological rigor of many of these studies is poor, the patient case-mix is variable, and both the method and the intensity of delirium evaluation are less than ideal.[8] Although cohort studies evaluate association, only randomized controlled studies define causality.[23]

A recent ICU delirium risk factor systematic review is instructive.[8] Although almost more than 1,000 studies were initially identified, only 25 high-quality studies, each incorporating appropriate multivariate modeling, were able to be included. Among the 90 potential ICU risk factors for delirium evaluated in these studies, only 18 factors were deemed to have a level of evidence that was adequate to define them as risk factors. Strong risk factors included age, a history of dementia, the need for pre-ICU emergency surgery or trauma, a greater severity of illness (as defined by the admission APACHE II [Acute Physiology and Chronic Health Evaluation II] score), need for mechanical ventilation, presence of sepsis, metabolic acidosis, or iatrogenic coma and benzodiazepine use. Risk factors classified as moderate were alcohol consumption, hypertension, moderate cognitive impairment, admission with infection or respiratory insufficiency, medical admission and opioid use. One recent evaluation of the SLEAP randomized study found the following modifiable antecedent factors to be independently associated with delirium onset: restraint use, antipsychotic administration, and the midazolam dose administered.[23]

Modifiable Risk Factors

Although baseline risks for delirium (i.e., those factors present at the time of ICU admission) are usually not modifiable, several environmental and medication-related factors shown to increase the risk of delirium in critically ill adults are often reversible.[8,9] The nonpharmacologic delirium risk factors of greatest importance include patient immobilization, application of patient restraints, excessive ambient noise, and admission to an ICU room without windows, clocks, and other features conducive to the maintenance of orientation and circadian normalcy.

Drug-Associated Delirium

Several medications used in the ICU may cause or worsen delirium (Table 8.2).[24] Factors that have been shown to predispose patients to drug-induced delirium include (1) the number of agents administered (greater than three); (2) pharmacokinetic derangements, whether associated with aging, organ dysfunction, or drug interactions; (3) medical comorbidities such as dementia or stroke, which are associated with impaired integrity of the blood-brain barrier; and (4) the use of psychoactive medications. Suggested mechanisms for drug-induced delirium include an excess of dopamine, norepinephrine, and glutamate release together with both increased and decreased serotonergic and γ-aminobutyric acid (GABA) activity. The diagnosis of drug-induced delirium is challenging and is generally one of exclusion based on temporal onset and offset relationships. Heightened awareness of the potential for a deliriogenic effect is required for drugs in which a clear temporal relationship is not seen.

Given that medication exposure, many of the non-medication delirium risk factors, and the presence of delirium itself vary over each day that a patient spends in the ICU, complex, time-dependent models are needed to evaluate the association between medication exposure and delirium occurrence in critically ill adults.[25] Thus, an increasing number of time-dependent, multivariate analyses focused on evaluating the association between medication exposure (including benzodiazepines, corticosteroids, and anticholinergics) and the daily odds of transitioning from

Table 8.2 ICU Medications Commonly Associated with Delirium

Category of Medication	Examples	Mechanism
Analgesics	Fentanyl	GABA antagonism
	Hydromorphone	GABA antagonism
	Morphine	GABA antagonism
	NSAIDs	Anticholinergic activity
Anti-infectives	Acyclovir	Unknown
	Amphotericin	Unknown
	Cefepime	GABA antagonism
	Linezolid	Serotonergic dysfunction
	Macrolides	
	Quinolones	Unknown
	Voriconazole	GABA antagonism
		Unknown
Anticholinergics	Atropine	Anticholinergic activity
	Benztropine	Anticholinergic activity
Anticonvulsants	Levetiracetam	Unknown
Antidepressants	Serotonin release inhibitors	Serotonergic dysfunction
Antihistamines	Diphenhydramine	Anticholinergic activity
Cardiac medications	α-Blockers	Anticholinergic activity
	Amiodarone	Anticholinergic activity
Antipsychotics	Haloperidol	Anticholinergic activity
	Olanzapine	Anticholinergic activity
Corticosteroids	Dexamethasone	Anticholinergic activity
	Hydrocortisone	Anticholinergic activity
	Methylprednisolone	Anticholinergic activity
Dopaminergics	Amantadine	Excess dopaminergic activity
	Bromocriptine	Excess dopaminergic activity
Prokinetics	Metoclopramide	Excess glucocorticoid activity
Sedatives	Ketamine	NMDA antagonism
	Lorazepam	GABA antagonism
	Midazolam	GABA antagonism
	Propofol	GABA antagonism

GABA = γ-aminobutyric acid; NMDA = N-methyl-D-aspartate; NSAID = nonsteroidal anti-inflammatory drug.

an awake and non-delirious state to delirium the next day have been published.[26-31] Although a dose-related association between benzodiazepine exposure and a daily transition to delirium has been reported in several investigations,[26-28] one recent analysis failed to show an association between anticholinergic drug exposure and a daily transition to delirium.[30] Although one analysis of patients with acute lung injury (ALI) found that exposure to corticosteroid therapy was associated with a greater odds of transitioning to delirium,[29] a much larger analysis of critically ill adults both with and without ALI was unable to show such an association.[31] Although the results of negative association studies like these suggest that the association between a medication class and delirium is likely very low, they cannot rule out that an association does not exist.

Medications remain an important cause of delirium in the critically ill population. If the use of an "at-risk" medication cannot be avoided, the lowest dose of the medication should be prescribed, and the duration of therapy should be as short as possible.[24] Common strategies that can be used to reduce medication-associated delirium are presented in Box 8.1.

DELIRIUM PREVENTION

Given that risk factors for ICU delirium may be modifiable, a careful preemptive evaluation of environmental and medication-related risk factors associated with delirium should be made, and active prevention strategies should also be considered for all patients.[9,21]

Nonpharmacologic Strategies

The evidence to use nonpharmacologic delirium prevention strategies in critically ill adults is far stronger than that available to support the use of a pharmacologic prevention strategy.[9] With sedative-induced coma being an important risk factor for delirium, strategies focused on maintaining patients in an awake (or lightly sedated) state such as SAT or the use of a sedation protocol are critical to use.[9] Early patient mobilization (which can only be completed in a patient who is awake) reduces both the incidence and the duration of delirium and significantly increases the likelihood that patients after hospital discharge will return to their pre-ICU functional state.[32] Frequent reorientation and daytime environmental stimulation reduce delirium incidence.[33] Sleep deprivation and fragmentation is an important risk factor for delirium; thus, protocols focused on improving sleep quality (e.g., reduced nighttime stimulation/procedures, use of earplugs, prevention of daytime napping, opening of window shades during the day) have been shown to reduce delirium but, of interest, not to improve sleep quality.[27,34]

Pharmacologic Strategies

The 2013 Society of Critical Care Medicine pain, agitation, and delirium guidelines do not advocate that a pharmacologic intervention be used to prevent delirium in critically ill adults.[9] Currently, no medication has been approved by the U.S. Food and Drug Administration for the prevention of delirium in the ICU. One recent randomized, placebo-controlled pilot study of 68 critically ill, mechanically ventilated adults with subsyndromal delirium in the first 48 hours of ICU admission found that administering haloperidol 1 mg intravenously every 6 hours did not prevent a transition to delirium and was associated with important safety concerns.[35] A well-designed, but underpowered, multicenter, randomized controlled trial of delirium prophylaxis with either haloperidol or ziprasidone, versus placebo, showed no benefit with either treatment group compared with placebo.[36]

Other randomized studies have evaluated a medication-based delirium prophylaxis strategy but only in patients undergoing a surgical procedure, primarily elective, who generally have a short duration of postsurgical ICU care.[37] There is no evidence to suggest that the perioperative use of dexmedetomidine prevents delirium in the ICU. In the largest ICU delirium pharmacologic prophylaxis study published to date, Wang et al. found that a low-dose infusion of haloperidol administered for 12 hours after major abdominal surgery reduced the incidence of delirium from 23% to 15% (p=0.03).[38] Of note, however, the severity of illness of these patients was low, and most spent less than 24 hours in the ICU. Further research to better define the safety and efficacy of dexmedetomidine and both typical and atypical antipsychotics is currently under way.

DELIRIUM TREATMENT

Removal or reduction of delirium risk factors is the most important strategy when resolving delirium and the symptoms and burden associated with it.[9,21] Mnemonics such as "I-C-U-D-E-L-I-R-I-U-M-S" can be used by clinicians to help remember the common risk factors and causes for delirium in the ICU when evaluating a patient who has developed delirium in an effort to identify potentially reversible causes (Table 8.3). To date, seven prospective, randomized studies have evaluated various drugs to treat delirium in critically ill patients (Table 8.4).[36,39-44] The impact of each potential delirium-reducing intervention was reported in one or more of four different ways: presence of delirium at the end of treatment period (n=4), time to delirium resolution (n=2), duration (or time patients had delirium) (n=3), and severity of delirium (n=1).

Antipsychotics

Of the four studies evaluating the efficacy of an antipsychotic for the treatment of delirium,[36,39,43,44] only one showed a difference in any of these outcomes.[43] In this small pilot study, patients with delirium who were being treated with haloperidol were randomized to additionally receive either quetiapine 50 mg or placebo every 12 hours. The quetiapine dose was increased by 50 mg if more than one dose of haloperidol was given in the previous 24 hours. All patients were allowed to receive haloperidol 1–10 mg every 2 hours as needed. Delirium resolved faster in patients administered quetiapine and resulted in patients spending less time with delirium. This study has many limitations, including its small size and the fact that all patients in the placebo group received one or more intravenous doses of haloperidol. Evidence therefore remains weak to support the routine use of antipsychotic therapy for the treatment of delirium in any ICU patient population, particularly for ICU patients with delirium who are not acutely agitated.[9,37]

Despite a relative lack of evidence to support the use of an antipsychotic agent to manage delirium and recent ICU practice guidelines that do not recommend their use, antipsychotics are commonly administered in the ICU to patients with either proven or suspected delirium.[45,46] This persistent high use is likely the result of a belief among clinicians that delirium is predominantly a neurotransmitter-mediated process, a greater familiarity with older delirium guidelines that advocate for antipsychotic use, the challenge of managing agitation in a patient with delirium, and a dramatic underappreciation of the risks associated with these agents.

Cholinesterase Inhibitors

One multicenter, randomized, placebo-controlled study that evaluated rivastigmine for the treatment of delirium was

---

Box 8.1. Strategies to Reduce Medication-Related Delirium in the ICU

- Avoid polypharmacy and ensure that medication dosing is appropriate
- Consider medication withdrawal
- Avoid anticholinergic medications when possible
- Avoid benzodiazepines when possible (including sleep aids)
- Use the lowest effective corticosteroid dose
- Use the lowest effective opioid dose to control pain/optimize non-opioid analgesics
- Avoid metoclopramide when possible
- If delirium occurs with levetiracetam (Keppra), consider other anticonvulsant options
- Reassess need for continued antibiotic therapy
- Monitor diuretic therapy for signs of dehydration and/or electrolyte abnormalities

Table 8.3 Mnemonic for Risk Factors and Causes of ICU Delirium: "I-C-U-D-E-L-I-R-I-U-M-S"

Iatrogenic exposure	Consider any diagnostic procedure or therapeutic intervention or any harmful occurrence that was not a natural consequence of the patient's illness
Cognitive impairment	Preexisting dementia, or MCI or depression
Use of restraints and catheters	Reevaluate the use of restraints and bladder catheters daily
Drugs	Evaluate the use of sedatives (e.g., benzodiazepines or opiates) and medications with anticholinergic activity. Consider the abrupt cessation of smoking or alcohol. Consider withdrawal from chronically used sedatives
Elderly	Evaluate patients older than 65 years with greater attention
Laboratory abnormalities	Especially hyponatremia, azotemia, hyperbilirubinemia, hypocalcemia, and metabolic acidosis
Infection	Sepsis and severe sepsis. Especially urinary, respiratory tract infections
Respiratory	Consider respiratory failure (Pco_2 greater than 45 mm Hg or Po_2 less than 55 mm Hg or oxygen saturation less than 88%). Consider causes such as COPD, ARDS, PE
Intracranial perfusion	Consider presence of hypertension or hypotension. Consider hemorrhage, stroke, tumor
Urinary/faecal retention	Consider urinary retention or fecal impaction, especially in older adults and postoperative patients
Myocardial	Consider myocardial causes: myocardial infarction, acute heart failure, arrhythmia
Sleep and **S**ensory deprivation	Consider the alterations of the sleep cycle and sleep deprivation. Consider the non-availability of glasses (poor vision). Consider the non-availability of hearing devices (poor hearing)

ARDS = acute respiratory distress syndrome; COPD = chronic obstructive pulmonary disease; MCI = mild cognitive impairment; PE = pulmonary embolism.

terminated early because rivastigmine was associated with greater mortality.[47] In addition, there was a trend for a longer duration of delirium with the use of rivastigmine. Cholinesterase inhibitors should never be used to prevent or treat delirium in any ICU patient population.[9]

Dexmedetomidine

Among four large, randomized studies comparing dexmedetomidine and benzodiazepine sedation strategies,[40-42,48] two of the studies that evaluated the presence of delirium each day found that patients receiving dexmedetomidine were less likely to continue to have delirium at the end of therapy.[41,42] However, these data analyses are inconclusive about whether benzodiazepine use raised the risk of delirium, or dexmedetomidine use reduced the risk, and thus, further investigations are needed to address this question. In one small study of mechanically ventilated patients with agitated delirium, the use of dexmedetomidine, rather than a haloperidol infusion, did not help resolve delirium more rapidly.[49] Once clinicians address the underlying other potential causes for agitation (e.g., pain, withdrawal) and the modifiable causes for delirium, the proportion of patients with delirium in any ICU who require dexmedetomidine therapy is anticipated to be low.

Future Research

Sufficiently powered, carefully designed, multicenter trials that incorporate a true placebo arm are needed to address the hypothesis that antipsychotics are beneficial in the treatment of delirium in critically ill patients. More recently, it has been suggested that delirium treatment studies should focus on evaluating the effect of antipsychotic therapy on the outcomes that are of greatest importance to patients such as duration of mechanical ventilation, length of hospitalization, or functional status after discharge.[50]

Practice Recommendations

The 2013 guidelines of the Society of Critical Care Medicine on pain, agitation, and delirium make several important statements and recommendations surrounding delirium in critically ill adults (Box 8.2).[9] In ICU patients who develop delirium, the presence of underlying risk factors for delirium should be removed or reversed whenever possible.[9,37] Among ICU patients with delirium who are agitated, ensure that the patient is not in pain or experiencing opioid or sedative withdrawal. In a patient with delirium who is agitated enough to require continuous sedative therapy, institute dexmedetomidine, particularly if the patient is currently receiving continuous benzodiazepine therapy. For patients who have milder agitation or who have other symptoms of delirium bothersome to the patient (e.g., fear, delusions), low-dose intravenous haloperidol (8 mg/day or less) should be considered. In a patient who can tolerate an oral or enteral medication or who has corrected QT (QTc) interval prolongation that precludes haloperidol administration, quetiapine should be considered.[9,37,50] In a patient who cannot tolerate oral or enteral therapy, particularly in one who has QTc interval prolongation, intravenous valproic acid (i.e., 500 mg intravenously × 1; then 50–100 mg intravenously every 6 hours) has been reported in a small case series to reduce delirium-associated agitation.[51]

QUALITY IMPROVEMENT CONSIDERATIONS

Use of a Protocolized ABCDEF Approach

A multidisciplinary, ICU bundled approach (e.g., the ABCDEF bundle) should be used to recognize and reduce delirium in the ICU.[9,22] This requires that all patients be evaluated for delirium by a member of the ICU team at least once per shift and that the results of these evaluations be documented in the patient record.[9,14] The ICU team should discuss the results of delirium assessments, strategies to reduce potential modifiable ICU delirium risk factors, and the use of nonpharmacologic strategies to reduce delirium incidence and burden at least daily on patient care rounds.

A protocolized, integrated management approach that also includes the assessment of pain (in addition to sedation and delirium), automatic sedation-minimizing strategies (such as daily interruption), and an early mobilization strategy has been shown to significantly improve patient outcomes by reducing the duration of mechanical ventilation and ICU length of stay; avoiding the complications associated with inadequate or inappropriate management of pain, agitation, and delirium; and decreasing health care costs.[9,22]

Role of Pharmacists

Pharmacists play an important role in helping to boost delirium recognition efforts, recognize risk factors for delirium that may be present (particularly medications), and educate the ICU team on the general lack of evidence supporting pharmacologic interventions to either prevent or treat delirium.[9,37,46] For patients who are initiated on antipsychotic therapy, a plan to either decrease or discontinue these agents should be made before the patient leaves the ICU.

Table 8.4 Randomized Studies Evaluating an Antipsychotic or Dexmedetomidine Delirium Treatment Strategy in the Critically Ill[a]

Author (Year)	Skrobik (2004)[39]	Pandharipande (2007)[40]	Ruokonen (2009)[41]	Riker (2009)[42]	Devlin (2010)[43]	Girard (2010)[36]	Page (2013)[44]
Baseline delirium (%)	100	61	NR	60	100	49	NR
Patient population	Surgical = 95% Intubated = 0%	Medical = 70% Intubated = 100%	Medical = 53% Intubated = 100%	Medical = 86% Intubated = 100%	Medical = 75% Intubated = 81%	Medical = 62% Intubated = 100%	Medical = 65% Intubated = 100%
Intervention	Olanzapine 5 mg/day (n=28)	Dexmed up to 1.5 mcg/kg/hr (n=52)	Dexmed to 1.4 mcg/kg/hr (n=41)	Dexmed to 1.4 mcg/kg/hr (n=244)	Quetiapine NG BID (n=18)	Ziprasidone up to q6hr (n=30)	Haloperidol 2.5 mg IV q8hr (n=71)
Control	Haloperidol PO q8hr (n=45)	Lorazepam IV infusion (n=51)	Midazolam / propofol per protocol (n=44)	Midazolam IV (n=122) infusion	Placebo NG (n=18)	C1 Haloperidol 5 mg q6hr (n=35) C2 Placebo (n=36)	Placebo IV (n=70)
Delirium present at end of study period (%)	NR	79 vs. 82; p=0.65	44 vs. 25; p=0.035	54 vs. 77; p<0.001	NR	69 vs. 77; p=0.28	NR
Duration of delirium	NR	Delirium-free days 9 (5–11) vs. 7 (5–11); p=0.09	NR	NR	36 (12–87) vs. 120 (60–195) hr; p=0.006	4 (2–7) vs. 4 (2–8) [C1] vs. 2 (0-5) [C2] days; p=0.93	5 (2–8) vs. 5 (1–8)

[a]Data presented as median (interquartile range).

BID = twice daily; Dexmed = dexmedetomidine; IV = intravenous(ly); NG = nasogastric (tube); NR = not reported; PO = orally; q = every.

Box 8.2. Recommendations Related to Delirium in the 2013 SCCM Pain, Agitation, and Delirium Guidelines[9]

Delirium outcomes

Delirium is associated with increased mortality in adult ICU patients (A).

Delirium is associated with prolonged ICU and hospital lengths of stay in adult ICU patients (A).

Delirium is associated with the development of post-ICU cognitive impairment in adult ICU patients (B).

Detecting and monitoring delirium

We recommend routine monitoring for delirium in adult ICU patients (+1B).

The Confusion Assessment Method for the ICU (CAM-ICU) and the Intensive Care Delirium Screening Checklist (ICDSC) are the most valid and reliable delirium monitoring tools in adult ICU patients (A).

Routine monitoring of delirium in adult ICU patients is feasible in clinical practice (B).

Delirium risk factors

Four baseline risk factors are positively and significantly associated with the development of delirium in the ICU: pre-existing dementia, history of hypertension, history of alcoholism, and a high severity of illness on admission (B).

Coma is an independent risk factor for the development of delirium in ICU patients (B).

Conflicting data surround the relationship between opioid use and the development of delirium in adult ICU patients (B).

Benzodiazepines may be a risk factor for the development of delirium in adult ICU patients (B).

There are insufficient data to determine the relationship between propofol use and the development of delirium in adult ICU patients (C).

Delirium prevention

We provide no recommendation for using a pharmacological delirium prevention protocol in adult ICU patients, as no compelling data demonstrate that this reduces the incidence or duration of delirium in these patients (0,C).

We do not suggest that either haloperidol or atypical antipsychotics be administered to prevent delirium in adult ICU patients (-2C).

We provide no recommendation for the use of dexmedetomidine to prevent delirium in adult ICU patients, as there is no compelling evidence regarding its effectiveness in these patients (0,C).

Delirium treatment

There is no published evidence that treatment with haloperidol reduces the duration of delirium in adult ICU patients (No Evidence).

Atypical antipsychotics may reduce the duration of delirium in adult ICU patients (C).

We do not recommend administering rivastigmine to reduce the duration of delirium in ICU patients (-1B).

We do not suggest using antipsychotics in patients at significant risk for torsades de pointes (i.e., patients with baseline prolongation of QT interval, patients receiving concomitant medications known to prolong the QT interval, or patients with a history of this arrhythmia) (-2C).

We suggest that in adult ICU patients with delirium unrelated to alcohol or benzodiazepine withdrawal, that continuous IV infusions of dexmedetomidine rather than benzodiazepine infusions be administered for sedation to reduce the duration of delirium in these patients (+2B).

REFERENCES

1. American Psychiatric Association (APA). Diagnostic and Statistical Manual of Mental Disorders, 4th ed. Washington, DC: APA, 1994.
2. European Delirium Association; American Delirium Society. The DSM-5 criteria, level of arousal and delirium diagnosis: inclusiveness is safer. BMC Med 2014;12:141.
3. Marquis F, Ouimet S, Riker R, et al. Individual delirium symptoms: do they matter? Crit Care Med 2007;35:2533-7.
4. Peterson JF, Pun BT, Dittus RS, et al. Delirium and its motoric subtypes: a study of 614 critically ill patients. J Am Geriatr Soc 2006;54:479-84.
5. Ouimet S, Riker R, Bergeron N, et al. Subsyndromal delirium in the ICU: evidence for a disease spectrum. Intensive Care Med 2007;33:1007-13.
6. Ely EW, Shintani A, Truman B, et al. Delirium as a predictor of mortality in mechanically ventilated patients in the intensive care unit. JAMA 2004;291:1753-62.
7. Salluh JI, Wang H, Scheider EB, et al. Outcome of delirium in critically ill patients: systematic review and meta-analysis. BMJ 2015;350:h2538.
8. Zaal IJ, Devlin JW, Peelen LM, et al. A systematic review of risk factors for delirium in the intensive care unit. Crit Care Med 2015;41:40-7.
9. Barr J, Fraser GL, Puntillo K, et al. Clinical practice guidelines for the management of pain, agitation and delirium in adult ICU patients. Crit Care Med 2013;41:263-306.
10. Klein Klouwenberg PM, Zaal IJ, Spitoni C, et al. The attributable mortality of delirium in critically ill patients: prospective cohort study. BMJ 2014;349:g6652.
11. Pandharipande PP, Girard TD, Jackson JC, et al. Long-term cognitive impairment after critical illness. BRAIN-ICU Study Investigators. N Engl J Med 2013;369:1306-16.
12. Flacker JM, Lipsitz LA Neural mechanisms of delirium: current hypotheses and evolving concepts. J Gerontol A Biol Sci Med Sci 1999;54:B239-46.
13. AGS/NIA Delirium Conference Writing Group, Planning Committee and Faculty; The American Geriatrics Society/National Institute on Aging Bedside-to-Bench Conference: research agenda on delirium in older adults. J Am Geriatr Soc 2015;63:843-52.
14. Pun B, Devlin JW. Delirium assessment tools in critical care. Semin Respir Crit Care Med 2013;34:179-88.
15. Devlin JW, Fong J, Fraser G, et al. Delirium assessment in the critically Ill. Intensive Care Med 2007;33:929-40.
16. Ely EW, Inouye SK, Bernard GR, et al. Delirium in mechanically ventilated patients: validity and reliability of the confusion assessment method for the intensive care unit (CAM-ICU). JAMA 2001;286:2703-10.
17. Bergeron N, Dubois MJ, Dumont M, et al. Intensive Care Delirium Screening Checklist: evaluation of a new screening tool. Intensive Care Med 2001;27:859-64.
18. Neto AS, Nassar AP Jr, Cardoso SO, et al. Delirium screening in critically ill patients: a systematic review and meta-analysis. Crit Care Med 2012;40:1946-51.
19. Gusmao-Flores D, Salluh JI, Chalhub RA, et al. The Confusion Assessment Method for the Intensive Care Unit (CAM-ICU)

and Intensive Care Delirium Screening Checklist (ICDSC) for the diagnosis of delirium: a systematic review and meta-analysis of clinical studies. Crit Care 2012;16:R115.

20. Patel SB, Poston JT, Pohlman A, et al. Rapidly reversible, sedation-related delirium versus persistent delirium in the intensive care unit. Am J Respir Crit Care Med 2014;189:658-65.

21. Trogrlić Z, van der Jagt M, Bakker J, et al. A systematic review of implementation strategies for assessment, prevention, and management of ICU delirium and their effect on clinical outcomes. Crit Care 2015;19:157.

22. Balas MC, Vasilevskis EE, Olsen KM, et al. Effectiveness and safety of the awakening and breathing coordination, delirium monitoring/management, and early exercise/mobility bundle. Crit Care Med 2014;42:1024-36.

23. Mehta S, Cook D, Devlin JW, et al. Prevalence, risk factors, and outcomes of delirium in mechanically ventilated adults. Crit Care Med 2015;43:557-66.

24. Devlin JW, Fraser GL, Riker RR. Drug-induced coma and delirium. In: Papadopoulos J, Cooper B, Kane-Gill S, et al., eds. Drug-Induced Complications in the Critically Ill Patient: A Guide for Recognition and Treatment. Chicago: Society of Critical Care Medicine, 2011.

25. Devlin JW, Zaal IJ, Slooter AJ. Clarifying the confusion surrounding drug-associated delirium in the ICU. Crit Care Med 2014;42:1565-6.

26. Pandharipande P, Shintani A, Peterson J, et al. Lorazepam is an independent risk factor for transitioning to delirium in intensive care unit patients. Anesthesiology 2006;104:21-6.

27. Kamdar BB, Niessen T, Colantuoni E, et al. Delirium transitions in the medical ICU: exploring the role of sleep quality and other factors. Crit Care Med 2015;43:135-41.

28. Zaal IJ, Devlin JW, Hazelbag M, et al. Benzodiazepine-associated delirium in critically ill adults. Intensive Care Med 2015;41:2130-7.

29. Schreiber MP, Colantuoni E, Bienvenu OJ, et al. Corticosteroids and transition to delirium in patients with acute lung injury. Crit Care Med 2014;42:1480-6.

30. Wolters AE, Zaal IJ, Veldhuijzen DS, et al. Anticholinergic drugs and the daily transition to delirium in critically ill patients: a prospective cohort study. Crit Care Med 2015;43:1846-52.

31. Wolters AE, Veldhuijzen DS, Zaal IJ, et al. Systemic corticosteroids and transition to delirium in critically ill patients. Crit Care Med 2015 (ahead of press September 30).

32. Schweickert WD, Pohlman MC, Pohlman AS, et al. Early physical and occupational therapy in mechanically ventilated, critically ill patients: a randomised controlled trial. Lancet 2009;373:1874-82.

33. Colombo R, Corona A, Praga F, et al. A reorientation strategy for reducing delirium in the critically ill. Results of an interventional study. Minerva Anestesiol 2012;78:1026-35.

34. Kamdar BB, King LM, Collop NA, et al. The effect of a quality improvement intervention on perceived sleep quality and cognition in a medical ICU. Crit Care Med 2013;41:800-9.

35. Al-Qadheeb NS, Skrobik Y, Schumaker G, et al. Preventing ICU subsyndromal delirium conversion to delirium with low-dose IV haloperidol: a double-blind, placebo-controlled, pilot study. Crit Care Med 2015 (ahead of press November 4).

36. Girard TD, Pandharipande PP, Carson SS, et al. Feasibility, efficacy, and safety of antipsychotics for intensive care unit delirium: the MIND randomized, placebo-controlled trial. Crit Care Med 2010;38:428-37.

37. Serafim RB, Bozza FA, Soares M, et al. Pharmacologic prevention and treatment of delirium in intensive care patients: a systematic review. J Crit Care 2015;30:799-807.

38. Wang W, Li HL, Wang DX, et al. Haloperidol prophylaxis decreases delirium incidence in elderly patients after noncardiac surgery: a randomized controlled trial. Crit Care Med 2012;40:1-9.

39. Skrobik YK, Bergeron N, Dumont M, et al. Olanzapine vs haloperidol: treating delirium in a critical care setting. Intensive Care Med 2004;30:444-9.

40. Pandharipande PP, Pun BT, Herr DL, et al. Effect of sedation with dexmedetomidine vs lorazepam on acute brain dysfunction in mechanically ventilated patients: the MENDS randomized controlled trial. JAMA 2007;298:2644-53.

41. Ruokonen E, Parviainen I, Jakob S, et al. Dexmedetomidine versus propofol/midazolam for long-term sedation during mechanical ventilation. Intensive Care Med 2009;35:282-90.

42. Riker RR, Shehabi Y, Bokesch PM, et al. Dexmedetomidine vs midazolam for sedation of critically ill patients: a randomized trial. JAMA 2009;301:489-99.

43. Devlin JW, Roberts R, Fong JJ, et al. Efficacy and safety of quetiapine for delirium in the ICU: a randomized, double-blind, placebo-controlled pilot study. Crit Care Med 2010;38:419-27.

44. Page VJ, Ely EW, Gates S, et al. Effect of intravenous haloperidol on the duration of delirium and coma in critically ill patients (Hope-ICU): a randomised, double-blind, placebo-controlled trial. Lancet Respir Med 2013;1:515-23.

45. Patel RL, Gambrell MA, Speroff T, et al. Delirium and sedation in the intensive care unit (ICU): survey of behaviors and attitudes of 1,384 healthcare professionals. Crit Care Med 2009;37:825-32.

46. Devlin JW, Bhat S, Roberts R, et al. Current critical care pharmacists' perceptions and practices surrounding the treatment of delirium in the intensive care unit. Ann Pharmacother 2011;45:1217-29.

47. van Eijk MM, Roes KC, Honing ML, et al. Effect of rivastigmine as an adjunct to usual care with haloperidol on duration of delirium and mortality in critically ill patients: a multicentre, double-blind, placebo-controlled randomised trial. Lancet 2010;376:1829-37.

48. Jakob SM, Ruokonen E, Grounds RM, et al. Dexmedetomidine vs. midazolam or propofol for sedation during prolonged mechanical ventilation: two randomized controlled trials. JAMA 2012;307:1151-60.

49. Reade MC, O'Sullivan K, Bates S, et al. Dexmedetomidine vs. haloperidol in delirious, agitated, intubated patients: a randomised open-label trial. Crit Care 2009;13:R75.

50. Devlin JW, Fraser GL, Ely EW, et al. Pharmacological management of sedation and delirium in mechanically ventilated ICU patients. Semin Respir Crit Care Med 2013;34:201-15.

51. Sher Y, Miller AC, Lolak S, et al. Adjunctive valproic acid in management-refractory hyperactive delirium: a case series and rationale. J Neuropsychiatry Clin Neurosci 2015;27:365-70.

Chapter 9
Neuromuscular Blocking Agents

M. Claire McManus, Pharm.D., BS(Pharm)

LEARNING OBJECTIVES

1. Understand the pharmacokinetics of neuromuscular blocking agents (NMBAs) and important drug interactions associated with their use, and appreciate their pharmacologic characteristics when used in the critical care and surgical settings.
2. Know the evidence for use of NMBAs for various clinical indications in critical care and surgery.
3. Understand how to monitor these agents in the critical care and surgical settings.
4. Be aware of special populations that require caution in relation to dosage and unpredictable response when administering NMBAs.
5. Appreciate the controversy surrounding the association between NMBAs and intensive care unit–acquired weakness.
6. Know when to reverse NMBAs, know which NMBAs can be reversed, and understand how to choose a reversal agent.

ABBREVIATIONS IN THIS CHAPTER

ARDS	Acute respiratory distress syndrome	NMBA	Neuromuscular blocking agent
CIP/M	Critical illness polyneuropathy/myopathy	NMJ	Neuromuscular junction
CS	Corticosteroids	PNS	Peripheral nerve stimulation
ICU	Intensive care unit	RCT	Randomized controlled trial
ICUAW	Intensive care unit–acquired weakness	TOF	Train-of-four
MV	Mechanical ventilation		
ND	Nondepolarizing		

INTRODUCTION

Curare is a generic term for various poisons applied for centuries by South American Indians to the tips of their arrows when hunting animals. Reports of its use spread to Europe during the Spanish conquest of South America and were relayed in the book *De Orbe Novo* by Peter Martyr d'Anghiera of the Spanish Court in 1516. New World explorers noted how the Indians ate the meat of the poisoned animals and remained unaffected, because "the poison only kills if it enters the blood," an oblique reference to the drug's lack of oral absorption. The modern clinical use of curare apparently dates from 1932 when Ranyard West used highly purified fractions in patients with tetanus and spastic disorders. In the 1930s, Squibb isolated, purified, and marketed curare as Intocostrin, releasing some samples for research purposes early in 1940. Around this time, Lewis H. Wright, an anesthesiologist, suggested its use as a relaxant during surgery, and in 1942, Harold Griffith of Montreal used it successfully, launching the drug in, and firmly establishing its role as an important adjunct to, anesthesia.[1-4]

Despite its unfavorable cardiac effects, tubocurarine was popular for years in the practice of anesthesia. In 1952, succinylcholine, the sole depolarizing agent in use today, was introduced, and it is still used because of its desirable pharmacokinetic profile (rapid onset and short duration). However, it can cause severe, although uncommon adverse drug events such as malignant hyperthermia, masseter muscle rigidity, bradycardia and hyperkalemia, and, more commonly, myalgia. The focus of attention has been to find an agent with a pharmacokinetic profile similar to that of succinylcholine without the adverse effects.

In that endeavor, pancuronium, an aminosteroid, was synthesized, and it became available in the later 1960s. It has a pharmacokinetic profile similar to that of tubocurarine but with less histamine-releasing and ganglionic-blocking properties and with mild vagolytic properties; the accompanying cardiac stability was appealing. The search for a drug with a profile ideal for surgery continued—short onset and duration, safety in renal and hepatic impairment, minimal cardiac adverse effects—leading to agents such as vecuronium, atracurium, cisatracurium, and rocuronium, all of which are currently in use today.[1,5]

Apart from a shorter duration of action, the newer agents have greatly diminished the incidence of adverse effects, chief of which are ganglionic blockade, block of vagal responses, and histamine release. Mivacurium, no longer widely used in the United States, is extremely sensitive to catalysis by acetylcholinesterase or other plasma hydrolases, therein accounting for its short duration of action.[1] Although the adverse effects of these agents are considerably less than those of their predecessors, their pharmacokinetic characteristics still fall well short of "ideal" for use in surgery, and the quest for the ideal agent continues. The clinical use of neuromuscular blocking agents (NMBAs) has expanded beyond the domains of surgery and emergency medicine to the intensive care unit (ICU), where, in addition to management of patient-ventilator dyssynchrony, they may show promise in areas such as acute respiratory distress syndrome (ARDS), increased intracranial and abdominal pressures, and the targeted temperature management of post-cardiac arrest patients.

BACKGROUND

Anatomy of the Neuromuscular Junction

A somatic lower motor neuron and the skeletal muscle fibers it innervates form a motor unit. A single motor unit may innervate hundreds or, as in the case of large muscles, thousands of muscle fibers. The efferent neuron of the motor unit originates in the ventral horn of the spinal cord and ends at the synaptic bouton, where it loses its myelin sheath and branches out in a terminal arborization in apposition to a specialized area on the muscle cell known as the muscle endplate. The nerve terminal and muscle endplate constitute the neuromuscular junction (NMJ). The terminal neural bouton contains the neurotransmitter acetylcholine stored internally in vesicles docked at the presynaptic membrane. Each vesicle stores a quantum of acetylcholine, in the range of 1,000–50,000 molecules, and each terminal has 300,000 or more vesicles. Across the synaptic cleft, the nicotinic receptors are largely confined to the endplate on the muscle cell; rarely are they expressed extrajunctionally except in denervation, a condition characterized by increased muscle responses. Acetylcholinesterase is concentrated near the synaptic folds close to the nicotinic receptors, strategically placed so that it can inactivate free acetylcholine immediately, preventing it from recombining with the receptor. Butyrylcholinesterase (pseudocholinesterase or plasma cholinesterase), present in low amounts in glial or satellite cells and responsible for the metabolism of succinylcholine, is virtually absent from the NMJ. In the resting state, there is a continual slow release of isolated quanta of acetylcholine, seen as small depolarizations (i.e., miniature endplate potentials that maintain low-level activity, particularly important because skeletal muscle lacks any inherent tone).[6-8]

Physiology

For muscle contraction to occur, the impulse is conducted from the somatic cell body in the ventral horn along the length of the axon in rapid saltatory fashion to the NMJ, where it is transmitted chemically across the synaptic cleft.[7] Very few pharmacologic agents block axonal conduction in therapeutic doses except for local anesthetics; it is also blocked by puffer fish toxin. When the action potential invades the nerve terminal, it causes local depolarization, increasing calcium permeability through presynaptic voltage-gated calcium channels. Increased intracellular calcium stimulates fusion of vesicles to the membrane and exocytosis of acetylcholine into the synapse. Several hundred quanta are released synchronously, representing several million acetylcholine molecules. Calcium is crucial for release; it forms a complex with a protein, synaptotagmin, which in turn promotes exocytosis of the docked vesicles and formation of a pore through which the acetylcholine can egress. A lack of calcium and an increased magnesium will inhibit this process, magnesium presumably by competing with calcium at the presynaptic site. In addition, magnesium decreases the sensitivity of the postsynaptic nicotinic receptor to acetylcholine.[6-10] It appears that a small proportion of vesicles are immediately releasable, whereas a much larger reserve pool can be mobilized more slowly. With repetitive stimulation, the amount of acetylcholine released decreases rapidly because immediate stores are exhausted quickly; to sustain release during high-frequency stimulation, vesicles must be mobilized from the reserve pool. Although not in the release process directly, secretion of acetylcholine is enhanced by positive feedback stimulation of homologous presynaptic nicotinic receptors at the NMJ. This serves to maintain the availability of acetylcholine when demand for it is high (e.g., during tetany). Botulinum toxin and some *Clostridium* toxins block this release process. From 1 to 4 million acetylcholine molecules are released at a time, but only a small fraction of the nicotinic receptors, between 1 and 10 million, require activation for muscular contraction, showing the large margin of safety for successful neurotransmission.[1,7,8,11-13] Certain medications interfere with transmission at the NMJ (see Figure 9.1; Table 9.1).

The Nicotinic Receptor

The nicotinic receptor belongs to a superfamily of ionotropic receptors that conduct primarily sodium, cause depolarization, and are excitatory. They are found in specific regions of the brain, autonomic ganglia, and skeletal muscle fibers. The nicotinic receptor is the prototype for pentameric ligand-gated ion channels and is composed of four distinct transmembrane spanning subunits ($2\alpha:1\beta:1\gamma:1\delta$) that surround an ion channel. Acetylcholine binds to only two of the five subunit interfaces, $\alpha\gamma$ and $\alpha\delta$. The acetylcholine binding site on the receptor is intimately coupled with an ion channel; simultaneous binding of two agonist molecules is necessary for activation and results in a rapid conformational change that opens the channel. At the motor endplate in skeletal muscle, the receptor is present at high densities in a regular packing order and is virtually absent from the adjacent extrajunctional sites.[1,6,7,9]

On receptor activation by acetylcholine, the intrinsic channel opens for about 1 millisecond, permitting around 50,000 sodium ions to traverse inward and a smaller amount of potassium ions outward. A localized depolarization or miniature endplate potential ensues; each miniature endplate potential reflects stimulation of a defined number of nicotinic receptors activated by one quantum of acetylcholine. After nerve stimulation, several miniature endplate potentials result and can summate to produce an

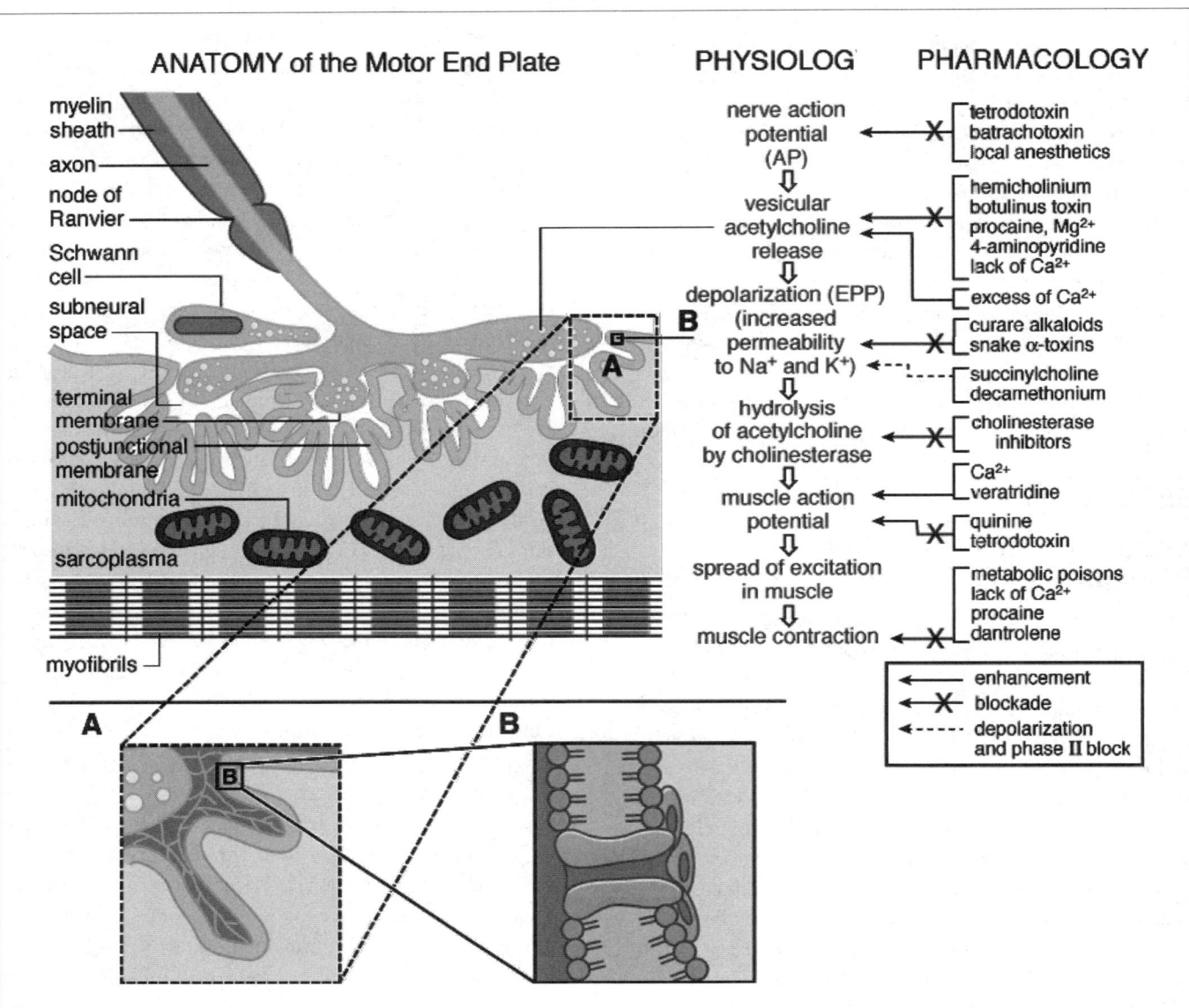

Figure 9.1 Sites of action of pharmacologic agents at the neuromuscular junction and adjacent structures.

The sequence of events leading to voluntary muscle contraction are depicted, and the agents that modify the process are shown on the right. An arrow marked with an X indicates inhibition or block; an unmarked arrow indicates enhancement or activation. The insets are enlargements of the indicated structures, where B depicts the nicotinic receptor.

Reprinted with permission from: Goodman and Gilman's The Pharmacological Basis of Therapeutics, 12th ed. New York: McGraw-Hill, 2011.

endplate potential, which, when it reaches threshold, will trigger the muscle action potential by stimulating voltage-gated sodium channels located perijunctionally. The action potential is generated by a rapid influx of sodium ions, but the channels are inactivated quickly, resulting in termination and repolarization. Because of their all-or-none nature and refractory periods, action potentials, unlike endplate potentials, cannot summate, and a stronger stimulus cannot produce an action potential of greater amplitude. The muscle action potential propagates along the membrane and, in turn, stimulates voltage-gated, calcium dihydropyridine channels, which are coupled to ryanodine receptors on the apposing sarcoplasmic reticulum. This increases intracellular calcium, culminating in contraction of the muscle.[6,7]

MECHANISM OF ACTION AND PHARMACOLOGIC EFFECTS

Neuromuscular blocking agents are divided into depolarizing and nondepolarizing (ND) or competitive agents. The competitive or ND NMBAs include pancuronium, vecuronium, rocuronium, mivacurium, atracurium, and cisatracurium; succinylcholine is the only depolarizing agent in use. The development of NMBAs has been driven by their use in surgery, and in this case, the ideal agent should have minimal cardiac and other adverse effects, a rapid onset, a duration of action sufficiently long to last the procedure, and a predictable and quick offset. Select pharmacologic characteristics of currently available NMBAs are summarized in Table 9.2.

Mechanism of Action

ND NMBAs

At the NMJ, the nicotinic receptor is functionally closed in the resting state and opens when two acetylcholine molecules bind to the α sites to elicit an excitatory miniature endplate potential. Competitive antagonists bind to the receptor and block acetylcholine, and this will progressively diminish the amplitude of the endplate potential, which may fall to 70% or less before it is insufficient to initiate a muscle action potential and subsequent contraction. This, together with the fact that only a few receptors are required for activation despite the large amount of acetylcholine released, demonstrates the aforementioned safety factor in neurotransmission. The redundancy is reflected further in animal studies, which have shown that the threshold is around 75% and 95% receptor occupancy for onset of clinically evident and complete block, respectively.[1,8] Binding is mutually exclusive, and unlike agonists, only one antagonist molecule is required for effect. Acetylcholine is metabolized quickly by acetylcholinesterase in the synapse and does not have the opportunity to rebind with the receptor and compete with the ND NMBA. Nondepolarizing NMBAs also act at presynaptic nicotinic receptors to decrease further release of neuronal acetylcholine, and this is thought to contribute to the phenomenon of fade seen with the competitive agents during repetitive and tetanic stimulation. The mechanism of fade, a gradual and diminished response with repetitive stimulation, has not been fully elucidated, but ND NMBAs are thought to prevent mobilization of vesicles to the presynaptic membrane for docking and thus acetylcholine from being made available fast enough to support tetanic or train-of-four (TOF) stimulation. At higher concentrations, competitive antagonists block the channel directly in a fashion that is noncompetitive with agonists and dependent on membrane potential.[1,11,14] Fade and post-tetanic stimulation are notable characteristics of competitive block. The mechanism underlying the latter, where a TOF applied after titanic stimulation results in an augmented response,

Table 9.1 Factors That Interact with Neuromuscular Blocking Agents[a]	
Potentiating Factors	**Antagonizing Factors**
Inhalation anesthetics[1]	Carbamazepine (chronic use)[5,7]
Hypermagnesemia[1,2]	Phenytoin (chronic use)[5,7]
Hypocalcemia[1]	Corticosteroids[2]
Aminoglycosides[1,2]	Demyelinating lesions[7]
Clindamycin[1,2]	Peripheral neuropathies[7]
Colistin[1,2]	Diabetes[7]
Vancomycin[1]	ACHEI[8]
Succinylcholine before ND NMBAs[1]	Hypercalcemia[2,3]
Corticosteroids[1]	ND NMBAs before succinylcholine[1]
Calcium channel blockers[2,3]	
Phenytoin[2]	
Lithium[2]	
Procainamide[2]	
Furosemide[2]	
Tetracyclines[4]	
Acidosis[5]	
Hypothermia[5]	
Local anesthetics[6]	
Dantrolene[3]	
Myasthenia gravis[1]	

[a]Mechanisms of action: 1= decreased sensitivity/block at post-synaptic receptors/endplate; 2 = presynaptic acetylcholine release; 3 = decreased excitation – contraction coupling; 4 = calcium chelation; 5 = decreased NMBA clearance; 6 = depressed axonal conduction; 7 = up-regulation of postsynaptic receptors; 8 = acetylcholinesterase inhibition.

ND = nondepolarizing; NMBA = neuromuscular blocking agent.

is presumably because after the tetanic stimulation, more of the stored acetylcholine is mobilized to the docking area and is available for release with subsequent stimulation—in this case, TOF—so that the competitive block can be overcome. Moreover, in contrast to depolarized block, competitive block can be reversed using acetylcholinesterase inhibitors.[8,9]

Depolarizing NMBAs

Succinylcholine, the only depolarizing agent currently in use, operates in a different fashion that is less well understood. Like acetylcholine, it depolarizes the membrane and activates sodium channels in the muscle, which is manifested as a brief initial period of fasciculation. Unlike acetylcholine, succinylcholine persists at the NMJ for a longer period because it is metabolized by butyrylcholinesterase, which is virtually absent at the NMJ, leading to a longer-lasting depolarization. Block ensues because the desensitized state of the nicotinic receptor is promoted as a self-regulatory mechanism after prolonged exposure to the agonist, which in turn and for similar reasons, inactivates the perijunctional voltage-gated sodium channels. After succinylcholine administration, a sequence of repetitive stimulations (fasciculations), followed by block of transmission and neuromuscular paralysis, is elicited and has been called *phase 1* block. Any agonist, including acetylcholine, if permitted to activate the membrane for an extended period, can initiate this series of events culminating in block. Acetylcholine is metabolized so rapidly by acetylcholinesterase, however, that it is not normally relevant. Competitive and depolarizing blocks are distinguishable. In contrast to competitive agents, there is no additive blocking effect for depolarizing agents with ND NMBAs; acetylcholinesterase inhibitors do not reverse it, initial fasciculations are seen, and there is a well-sustained contraction after tetanic stimulation during partial block. In some animals and occasionally in humans, depolarizing agents produce a blockade with unique features, some of which combine characteristics of competitive and depolarizing agents, which is thus termed *dual mechanism block*. Under clinical circumstances in humans, with increasing concentrations of succinylcholine and over time, the block may slowly convert from a depolarizing to an ND type, termed *phase 1* and *phase 2* blocks, respectively. Characteristics of ND block described earlier emerge in phase 2, such as the phenomenon of fade and antagonism by acetylcholinesterase inhibitors.[1,6,9,11,15]

Pharmacologic Effects

Extra-NMJ Actions

Most extra-NMJ actions associated with the NMBAs occur because of cross-reactivity and histamine release resulting in adverse effects, most notably those of a cardiac nature.[9]

Cross-reactivity

All of the NMBAs can potentially cross-react with extrajunctional nicotinic and muscarinic receptors in the body. Apart from pre- and postjunctional sites, nicotinic receptors are also present in autonomic ganglia and prejunctional effector sites of the sympathetic nervous system, in which they increase norepinephrine release. Muscarinic receptors are found in postjunctional parasympathetic nervous system effector sites, autonomic ganglia, presynaptic sympathetic effector sites in which they decrease norepinephrine release, and blood vessels.

Agent/ Characteristic	Bolus Dose (mg/kg)	Continuous Infusion (mcg/kg/min)	Onset (min)	Duration (min) (to 25% recovery)	Mode of Elimination (%)
Succinylcholine	0.3–1.5	N/A	1–1.5	5–8	Plasma cholinesterase, 100
Mivacurium	0.15–0.25	6–10	2.5–5	13–20	Plasma cholinesterase, 100
Atracurium	0.4–0.5	4–20	2–4	35–45	Hofmann; plasma esterase; renal < 5
Cisatracurium	0.15–0.2	0.5–10	5–7	35–45	Hofmann, renal + hepatic < 20
Pancuronium	0.02–0.1	0.8–1.7	4–6	60–120	Renal 60–80; liver 15–40
Rocuronium	0.6–1.2	0.48–0.72	1.5–3	30–40	Liver 70; renal 30
Vecuronium	0.1–0.1	0.8–1.7	3–4	35–45	Liver < 20, renal 20–30

Table 9.2 Pharmacology of Neuromuscular Blocking Agents

N/A = not applicable.

Muscarinic type 2 (M_2)-receptors promote bronchodilation and bradycardia, whereas muscarinic type 3 (M_3)-receptors produce bronchospasm.

The older agent, tubocurarine, has the greatest affinity for ganglionic nicotinic receptors. Pancuronium has significant blockade at muscarinic M_2-receptors in the parasympathetic nervous system and at presynaptic muscarinic receptors in the peripheral sympathetic nervous system, with the former resulting in vagolytic action and the latter increasing norepinephrine release, both of which cause tachycardia. Rocuronium has affinity for the vagus and other peripheral muscarinic receptors in the parasympathetic nervous system, more so than vecuronium. The remaining ND agents have even weaker affinities for the muscarinic receptor. The most significant manifestation of these extrajunctional actions is tachycardia; bronchoconstriction is not reported with any frequency, probably because of the equal antagonism of pulmonary M_2- and M_3-receptors. The depolarizing agent, succinylcholine, has affinity for nicotinic and muscarinic receptors at ganglionic and vagal sites, respectively; see Cardiac Effects below.[16-21]

Cardiac Effects

Cardiac effects are the major adverse events associated with the older agents curare and succinylcholine and are related to histamine release and cross-reactivity at extrajunctional cholinergic receptors, causing peripheral autonomic and ganglionic effects.[16,22] The capacity to cause these effects is found with all available agents, although it varies considerably among them and may not be seen at clinical doses. Among ND NMBAs, pancuronium and atracurium have the greatest potential to cause adverse cardiac effects. The following mechanisms may apply:

1. Histamine release. Originally seen with curare, histamine release is predominantly found with the use of atracurium, mivacurium, and succinylcholine. Pancuronium use releases minimal amounts of histamine and cisatracurium, virtually none. Histamine release has not been seen with rocuronium. Isolated reports of vecuronium-induced histamine release have not been confirmed, even with high doses, although hypotension and flushing have been reported after vecuronium administration and may be related to decreased histamine catabolism through inhibition of histamine *N*-methyltransferase. The phenomenon is associated with large doses and rapid administration of NMBAs; therefore, it is less likely to occur with the doses administered in ICU regimens. It can be prevented by slowly injecting the agent over 1–3 minutes or by pretreating with histamine-1 (H_1)- and histamine-2 (H_2)-receptor antagonists. Histamine release typically is a direct action of the muscle relaxant on the mast cell rather than immunoglobulin E (IgE)-mediated anaphylaxis.[8,16,23-33]

2. Vagolytic actions. Vagolytic actions are most prominent with pancuronium use and result in mild and dose-dependent tachycardia. However, this is a significant enough adverse effect to recommend avoiding its use in patients with coronary artery disease because of the risk of increased myocardial ischemia, ventricular extrasystoles, and, as reported in one case, cardiovascular collapse. Rocuronium also has affinity for vagal receptors, which manifests as tachycardia. Theoretically, this is also true of vecuronium, but to a much lesser degree, and there is little reference to it in the literature. Clinically, vecuronium has relatively little effect on the heart. Curiously, bradycardia has been reported with its use, although a causal relationship is not always evident. The mechanism for this is unclear but may be related to vagal stimulation (see mechanism 5 in this section). Cisatracurium may also block M_2 vagal receptors, but clinical tachycardia does not appear to be important. Atracurium and mivacurium lack any appreciable vagolytic effects.[8,16-18,34-48]

3. Ganglionic blockade. Ganglionic blockade is seen with curare, and all agents will demonstrate it if given in large enough doses; pancuronium has weak ganglionic activity at recommended doses. Atracurium, vecuronium, rocuronium, mivacurium, and cisatracurium are even more selective and, in recommended doses, cause minimal, if any, ganglionic blockade. The effect on heart rate depends on the patient's dominant tone, which at rest is generally vagal (M_2 muscarinic), thus resulting in tachycardia.[1,16,47,49-51]

4. Sympathetic stimulation. Sympathetic stimulation is seen with pancuronium. The mechanism is not entirely clear but is probably related to the blockade of various presynaptic muscarinic and nicotinic receptors, which have opposing activities. The net effect is the increased release of norepinephrine causing tachycardia.[8,52]

5. Ganglionic or muscarinic stimulation. Succinylcholine may cause bradycardia through ganglionic or muscarinic stimulation at the vagus,[8,22] and it has been suggested that vecuronium is also vagotonic when administered concurrently with potent opioids.[53-56]

Malignant Hyperthermia

Malignant hyperthermia, a channelopathy, is a rare genetic disorder triggered by exposure to depolarizing NMBAs (succinylcholine) and inhalation anesthetics containing halogenated hydrocarbons, and it has a mortality rate of 80% if left untreated. The offending agent superimposes a change in the host's genetically altered ryanodine receptor, resulting in an uncontrolled efflux of calcium from the sarcoplasmic reticulum with subsequent tetany, increased skeletal metabolism, and heat production. Onset usually occurs within 1 hour of, and rarely up to 11 hours after, administration. Early features of malignant hyperthermia are tachycardia, cyanosis, and muscle rigidity, which is most prominent in the masseter muscle. Marked hyperthermia occurs hours later, commonly accompanied by hypotension, dysrhythmias, rhabdomyolysis, electrolyte abnormalities, disseminated intravascular coagulation, and mixed acidosis. Rarely, patients have rhabdomyolysis without hyperthermia.[1,57-69] Conventionally, it is diagnosed using the classical caffeine halothane contracture test (in North America) and in vitro contracture test (in Europe), but these are expensive and invasive. Curiously, a recent pilot study (n=24) suggested that lymphocyte adenosine levels present a diagnostic alternative. Evidently, lymphocytes contain the same ryanodine receptor as muscle cells and, in the presence of high amounts of intracellular calcium, lead to activation of ATP-dependent calcium pumps, producing free adenosine as a by-product. Compared with controls, there was marked accumulation of adenosine in lymphocytes from susceptible individuals, providing a potential diagnostic marker for malignant hyperthermia in affected individuals.[70]

Treatment, which should dissipate heat quickly to prevent death, involves rapid cooling, giving 100% oxygen, controlling acidosis, and administering intravenous dantrolene, which blocks calcium release from the sarcoplasmic reticulum and decreases myoplasmic free calcium concentration, culminating in decreased muscle tone and heat production. With early diagnosis and treatment, recovery occurs in virtually 100% of patients.[65,71-73]

Histamine Release and Immediate Hypersensitivity Reactions

Immediate hypersensitivity reactions are classified as immune- or nonimmune-mediated, the most severe appearing as anaphylaxis. Allergic anaphylaxis is commonly mediated by IgE binding to the FCeRI receptor on mast and other immune cells, culminating in the release of inflammatory mediators such as histamine, tryptase, prostaglandins, leukotrienes, and several chemokines and cytokines. Non-immune anaphylaxis is thought to be caused by direct stimulation of mast cells and basophils releasing inflammatory mediators as a result; it does not entail the immune system, and thus, previous exposure is not required. Although previous sensitization is a prerequisite for allergic anaphylaxis to occur, it is not obligatory, and sensitization may occur through cross-reactivity. Specific IgE assays and skin testing are available to test for NMBA sensitivity. Intraoperative anaphylaxis is a rare but significant event, and NMBAs are the drugs most commonly implicated. It is usually IgE mediated, and quaternary and tertiary ammonium ions are considered the epitopes. However, other chemical characteristics such as hydrophobicity as well as flexibility of the molecule may be involved. More-flexible molecules like succinylcholine are considered more antigenic than the aminosteroids, which are quite rigid and bulky. Cross-reactivity occurs between the NMBAs themselves and with unrelated drugs and foods that possess the common ammonium ion structure. There are reports that pholcodine, a cough suppressant with a structure similar to the quaternary ammonium ion in NMBAs, and used in Europe but not in the United States, may be incriminated in the sensitization process. This offers one explanation for the differing prevalence of rocuronium-induced reactions according to geographic location: some European countries where pholcodine use is high have higher rates of sensitivity; in contrast, the reported rates are extremely low in the United States, where the drug is not available.[74,75]

Histamine release per se, most evident with succinylcholine, atracurium, and mivacurium, can be reduced by slowing the rate of NMBA administration and giving smaller doses. Histamine-induced cutaneous reactions occur in 5%–10% of patients receiving atracurium and do not necessarily indicate that more-serious effects will follow. Pretreating with H_1- and H_2-antagonists may also reduce histamine release.[31,32] Rapid injection of 0.6 mg/kg or greater of atracurium besylate causes clinically significant hypotension, tachycardia, bronchospasm, and flushing. Cisatracurium causes less histamine release than atracurium, and the effect is insignificant in recommended doses.[76-80]

The pertinent questions for the clinician are (1) which NMBA is least likely to cause anaphylaxis in routine practice and (2) what is the likelihood of cross-reactivity to other NMBAs. These questions were addressed in a recent study[75] from Australia, in which the investigators confirmed similar reports[74] from France that anaphylaxis to rocuronium is emerging and relatively prevalent. In this retrospective study (n=80), investigators analyzed patients who had a documented immediate-type sensitivity reaction during surgery and who underwent subsequent skin testing to the NMBA used and other possible triggering agents. Strict criteria needed to be fulfilled before applying the diagnosis of NMBA anaphylaxis. Cross-reactivity testing to other agents was also done. Investigators reviewed patients over a 10-year period from 2002 to 2011 and calculated exposure rates from purchasing data, which were available for the second 5-year period of the study and extrapolated to the full 10-year span. Their results showed that NMBAs are common triggers of anaphylaxis in anesthesia in Western Australia; rocuronium may be associated with a higher incidence compared with other NMBAs and had a 3-fold increased risk of IgE-mediated anaphylaxis compared with vecuronium. Although a rate could not be computed for succinylcholine—purchasing data were not reliable in determining exposure rates because of the common practice of wasting half-used vials—cross-reactivity results suggested that it also has a high incidence of triggering anaphylaxis. As regards cross-reactivity, cisatracurium had the lowest incidence in patients with previous anaphylaxis to rocuronium or vecuronium, and the authors suggested its consideration in such cases. Although the study was well designed, there were some limitations, including retrospective nature, small numbers, extrapolation of exposure rates from purchasing data and from a 5-year period, and possible referral bias.

ICU-Acquired Muscle Weakness

A group of neuromuscular disorders that is now recognized in critically ill patients with multiple organ dysfunction syndrome commonly occurs and is characterized by generalized muscle weakness and failure to wean from mechanical ventilation (MV). The muscular weakness previously attributed to starvation-induced or disuse atrophy is now ascribed to the adversely affected functions of peripheral nerves, NMJs, and skeletal muscles in the critically ill and has been collectively called critical illness polyneuropathy and myopathy (CIP/M). Neuromuscular blocking agents, especially if used in combination with corticosteroids (CS), may contribute to the development of CIP/M, though the evidence is conflicting. Neuromuscular blocking agents may alternatively cause intensive care unit–acquired weakness (ICUAW) because of prolonged neuromuscular blockade as a result of reduced drug clearance. The latter, a protracted therapeutic effect secondary to impaired elimination of the NMBA as a result of either organ dysfunction or drug interactions, can manifest as weakness but is without overt pathology.

Critical Illness Polyneuropathy and Myopathy

Critical illness polyneuropathy (CIP) and critical illness myopathy are major complications of severe critical illness and its management and may significantly prolong weaning from MV and patient rehabilitation. The pathophysiology is complex and unclear. It has been hypothesized that a disturbance in the microcirculation caused by sepsis, cytokines, and/or hyperglycemia, or a combination of these, is central to its etiology (see Figure 9.2).[81] As mentioned, CIP/M encompasses weakness caused by polyneuropathy, a motor and sensory axonal neuropathy,

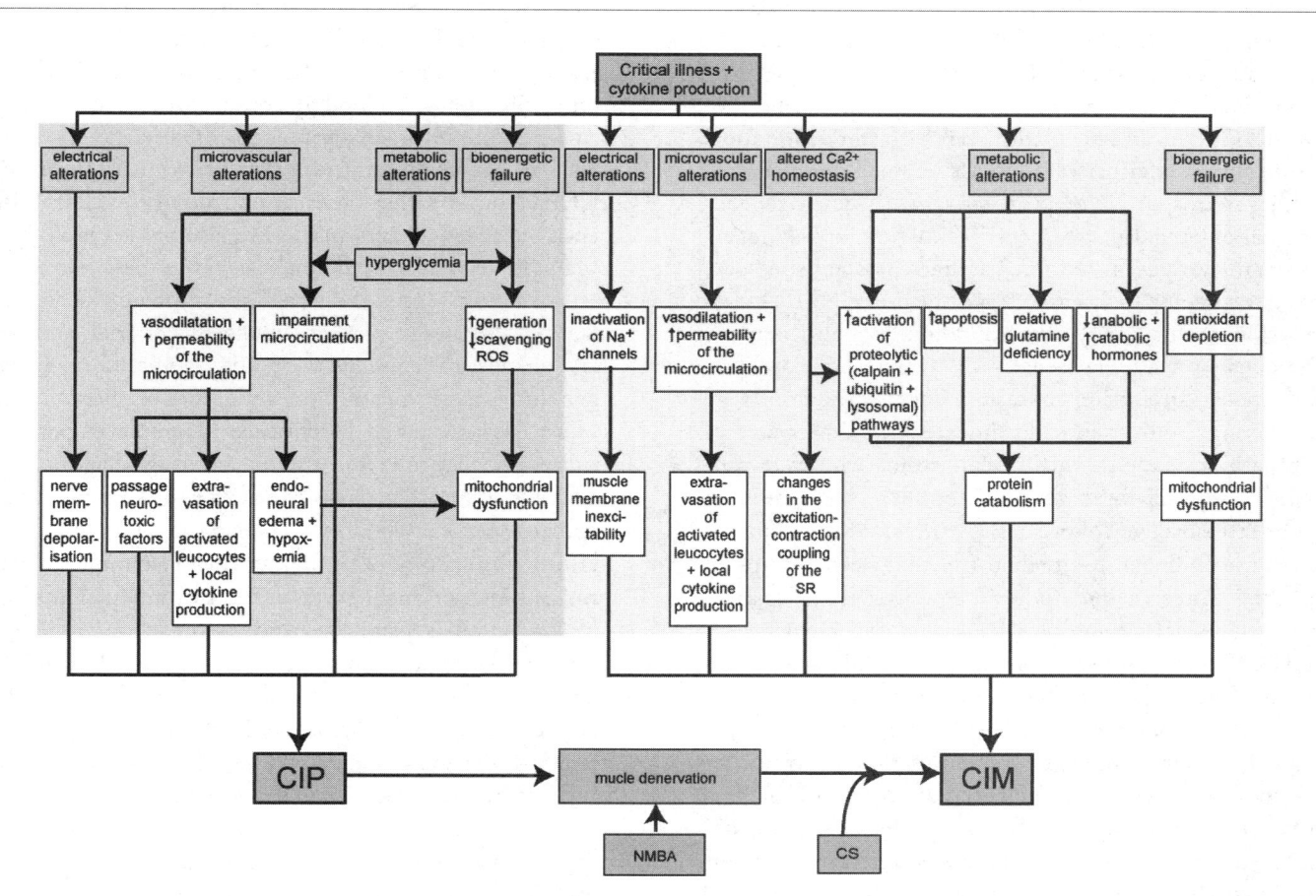

Figure 9.2 Presumed pathophysiologic mechanisms and their interactions involved in the development of critical illness polyneuropathy/myopathy.

CIM = critical illness myopathy; CIP = critical illness polyneuropathy; CS = corticosteroids; NMBA = neuromuscular blocking agents; ROS = reactive oxygen species; SR = sarcoplasmic reticulum.

Reprinted with permission from: Hermans G, De Jonghe B, Bruynickx F, et al. Clinical review: critical illness polyneuropathy and myopathy. Crit Care 2008;12:238.

and a common complication of severe sepsis, by myopathy, which has been reported with the use of CS and NMBA and by NMJ dysfunction. Histologically, CIP is primarily distal axonal degeneration with no evidence of demyelination or inflammation and typically presents as sensorimotor polyneuropathy. Critical illness myopathy, in contrast, encompasses a spectrum of pathologies including acute necrosis, regeneration, type 2 fiber atrophy, and selective but patchy loss of thick filament/myosin.[82-85] Thick-filament myopathy and myonecrosis with sensory function remaining intact has been described in patients receiving NMBAs in combination with CS. Although it is unclear whether NMBAs are associated with weakness when not coadministered with steroids, Bolton and others[83] suggested that such an entity, manifesting as polyneuropathy, exists when NMBAs are given in the presence of sepsis. In general, the aminosteroids, pancuronium and vecuronium, were implicated; whether this reflects a prevalence in their use at the time or is related to their similarity in structure to steroids is unclear. This notwithstanding, sepsis was thought by the authors to be the main etiologic event, with the role of NMBAs being merely contributory. Other reports identifying NMBA-associated weakness do not always clarify whether CS were coadministered.[84,86-100]

Several studies have investigated the relationship between NMBAs and myopathy, each with some limitation. All of these are either case reports or small observational studies, retrospective or prospective, with heterogeneous populations and drug regimens. Techniques for diagnosing myopathy varied; in addition, baseline characteristics were not always compared, and in some, the use of NMBAs was very low or for a very short duration.[97,101] Furthermore, the details on CS and sedative use are not always clear, potentially introducing confusion. Overall, the results are conflicting. Four studies documented the emergence of myopathy in patients with severe asthma who were ventilated and receiving high-dose steroids.[102-105] These were all of retrospective cohort design; three did not compare severity of illness comprehensively between groups at baseline. Three of the studies[103-105] found an association between NMBA duration of use and the incidence of ICUAW. Atracurium was implicated equally as often as the aminosteroids, pancuronium and vecuronium. Patients were sicker at baseline in the NMBA group in one study[104] (n=101), and in another, the respiratory illness severity between groups was not illuminated at all (n=86), making interpretation difficult.[105] The fourth study[102] (n=96) did not find an association, but there was a trend toward less weakness with restriction of paralysis, which, according to the authors, could have reached statistical significance if the numbers had been larger; as it was, the study was underpowered to detect it. They concluded, however, that the use of NMBAs is not considered a prerequisite for weakness in patients with asthma on MV; rather it is immobilization that, whatever the cause, most likely constitutes the final common pathway.[102] Two case reports of near-fatal patients with asthma on MV and high-dose CS merit mention.[84,95] One of these treated three such patients, all of whom received NMBAs for at least 7 days.[84] Biopsy revealed necrosis. All three had previous admissions where they received MV and CS in the absence of NMBAs and had no sign of weakness, implicating NMBAs in the index visit. The details of sedative administration were lacking, however, for previous admissions, thus limiting the comparison. In a prospective case series of 44 critically ill patients, Coakley et al. found that weakness occurred in patients regardless of NMBA administration.[106] Some patients received both CS and NMBAs (11 of 44). Numbers were too small to draw a definite conclusion, but the authors believed that if used judiciously, NMBAs could be used safely. Much of the published literature accounting for NMBA-associated myopathy involves patients with asthma, but there are also, albeit limited, data in patients with sepsis receiving NMBAs alone. Witt et al. (n=43) evaluated the risk factors associated with CIP/M in patients with sepsis and found no association with NMBAs, but these agents were only rarely used in this study, rendering any inference invalid.[97] Instead, the authors found a clear correlation between CIP/M and ICU length of stay, serum albumin, and blood glucose in patients with sepsis having multiple organ dysfunction. Garnacho-Montero et al. (n=73) found an association between NMBAs and ICUAW in an earlier observation study of patients with sepsis but failed to confirm this in a later study (n=64).[99,101] Again, there were several confounders in these two studies, including sepsis and coadministration of sedatives; also, NMBA usage was low in the earlier trial, and details on dosage regimens were not elaborated on in either study. Segredo et al.,[96] in a prospective observational cohort design, studied 16 critically ill ventilated patients with pulmonary infection and/or sepsis who had received at least 2 consecutive days of vecuronium. They identified weakness clinically and by peripheral nerve stimulation/train-of-four (PNS/TOF) monitoring; electrophysiologic studies were not done. Seven of the 16 study patients had "prolonged block," and the incidence of renal failure was higher in that group of patients. However, bicarbonate and pH were significantly lower, magnesium was reduced, and renal failure was more common in the weak group, confounding the picture and rendering interpretation difficult. Furthermore, sedative doses were not revealed, which could be influential. The authors suggested that it was prolonged blockade, but they could not rule out CIP/M as a cause because they did not test for it.

Finally, in three relatively recent, well-conducted, large, randomized controlled trials (RCTs), a short course of cisatracurium, less than 48 hours, in patients with ARDS was not associated with ICUAW.[107-109] In summary, in small observational studies, NMBAs in conjunction with CS have commonly been implicated in the development of ICUAW, manifesting as a quadriparesis, the underlying pathology generally being a myopathy with sensory function intact. Intensive care unit–acquired weakness is purportedly related to the dose and duration of NMBAs. However, study results on this issue of association with ICUAW are not unanimous in their affirmation. Thus, although a common perception, the evidence that NMBAs cause ICUAW is not conclusive, and more standardized large prospective trials are needed to identify the risk factors.[106,110,111] In the interim, it is prudent to use these agents for a short duration in critically ill patients in the ICU and to monitor them closely.

Other Pharmacologic Effects

Succinylcholine increases intragastric pressure; however, it increases lower esophageal sphincter pressure even more, such that aspiration is unlikely unless the esophageal sphincter is incompetent. Succinylcholine can also increase intraocular and intracranial pressures. Fasciculations and hyperkalemia may develop after succinylcholine, especially in sensitive patients with up-regulation of NMJ receptors. The risk is increased during prolonged depolarization with succinylcholine, where muscle cells may lose significant quantities of potassium and gain sodium, chloride, and calcium. The loss of potassium can be critical in patients receiving continued administration of succinylcholine who have had extensive soft tissue injuries. Succinylcholine-induced hyperkalemia can be life threatening in patients with congestive heart failure receiving digoxin or diuretics, and its use is contraindicated or should be done with great caution in patients with nontraumatic rhabdomyolysis, ocular lacerations, spinal cord injuries with paraplegia or quadriplegia, or muscular dystrophies.[1,8,9,112]

PHARMACOKINETICS

Relative efficacy of these agents is measured quantitatively as the ED95. The ED95 is the average dose needed to produce 95% suppression of the adductor pollicis twitch response to ulnar stimulation; the intubation dose ranges from 1 to 3 times the ED95, depending on the NMBA. The dose range reflects a difference in sensitivities between muscle groups. However, the dose, as well as other pharmacokinetic parameters such as onset and duration, also depends on cardiac output and muscle blood flow, indicating that a muscle's response is not always a reflection of its sensitivity alone. Various pharmacokinetic values are shown in Table 9.2; onset and duration are dose-dependent. Duration of effect is organ-dependent for pancuronium; for vecuronium and rocuronium, it is also related to redistribution; and for atracurium, cisatracurium, succinylcholine, and mivacurium, it is governed by metabolism in the plasma.[8,9,11,113,114]

A critical number of receptors must be occupied before a drug can elicit an initial response. Thus, less-potent agents tend to have a faster onset than more-potent ones because a greater concentration is available to block spare receptors—the comparison between rocuronium and cisatracurium can be made. The duration of action is defined as the time from drug administration to the time when the evoked neuromuscular function of the thumb returns to 25% baseline, and the recovery time index is the time from 25%–75% twitch recovery of the adductor pollicis muscles.[8,9,114] Pharmacokinetic activity for NMBAs may vary in older adults, which may be related to age-related differences in cardiac output resulting in decreased clearance. Succinylcholine, which is metabolized by liver and plasma butyrylcholinesterase, may have modest prolongation of action in hepatic failure, in patients who have an atypical plasma cholinesterase or a deficiency of the enzyme owing to allelic variations or pregnancy, and with high doses (e.g., greater than 2 mg/kg of succinylcholine) because of slow diffusion from the NMJ.[1,8,11,115,116] Cisatracurium and atracurium are metabolized by ester and Hofmann elimination to laudanosine and to a mono-quaternary acrylate, both of which may be toxic, although the levels associated with cisatracurium may be 1/10th those with atracurium.[8,11,117] There have been rare reports of seizures after prolonged infusions of atracurium,[8,11,117-121] presumably because of laudanosines's activity at the γ-aminobutyric acid receptors, although evidence is scant. Clinically, laudanosine concentrations may not reach adequate levels to produce this effect. In general, atracurium and cisatracurium are better suited for patients with organ dysfunction. Hypothermia and acidosis decrease the clearance of atracurium and cisatracurium because Hofmann elimination is pH- and temperature-dependent. Accumulation in renal failure is seen with pancuronium, vecuronium, and possibly, albeit to a lesser degree, rocuronium after several doses. Vecuronium and rocuronium may accumulate in patients with hepatic failure and severe disease, respectively, because of decreased biliary uptake. Moreover, rocuronium's volume of distribution may be increased in hepatic disease, further prolonging its duration and onset of action.[8,9,11,122,123]

INDICATIONS FOR THE ICU

Whereas the ideal NMBA in surgery should have a rapid onset and duration of action as well as minimal cardiac adverse effects, such characteristics are not as critical for use in the ICU. In fact, a longer duration may be preferred if a prolonged effect is desired, and in such cases, the aminosteroids may be administered (i.e., pancuronium or vecuronium). The benzylisoquinoline agents, atracurium and cisatracurium, offer the unique advantage of being independent of kidney and liver function for clearance, an important consideration and thus a popular choice in critically ill patients.

Proposed adjunctive applications for NMBAs in the ICU include the following: improving chest wall compliance, eliminating ventilator dyssynchrony, reducing intra-abdominal pressures,[124,125] preventing and treating shivering during therapeutic hypothermia, and preventing elevations in intracranial pressure from airway stimulation. Select indications are discussed in the sections that follow (see Table 9.3 for summary of studies discussed).

Acute Respiratory Distress Syndrome

Acute respiratory distress syndrome is characterized by intense lung inflammation, consolidation, and progressive microatelectasis and is associated with severe hypoxemia, ventilator dyssynchrony, barotrauma, and ventilator-induced lung injury. Low tidal volume ventilation has been shown to improve survival in ARDS, and other strategies such as high positive end-expiratory pressure, prone ventilation, and the use of NMBAs may have merits.[126-129] There is interest in elucidating the role NMBAs may play, if at all, in the management of ARDS. In this capacity, several trials, varying in quality of design, have evaluated the use of NMBAs.[107-109,130-132] Three noteworthy RCTs, all from the same authors (n=431), addressed the use of cisatracurium in mechanically ventilated patients with early ARDS for a 48-hour duration in several ICUs in France.[107-109] Cisatracurium administration was weight based and guided by TOF in two studies,[108,109] and in the third,[107] it was given as a fixed, high dose of 37.5 mg per hour without adaptation to PNS. A subsequent meta-analysis of these studies was done by a separate group, but they collaborated with the original authors to gain further clarification and access to unpublished data.[133] Combining the three trials, they deemed the quality of evidence related to mortality as moderate and limited because of nonblinded caregivers, and the evidence related to ICUAW weak because it relied solely on clinical diagnosis.[133] Otherwise, the results were large, precise and consistent across studies. In this meta-analysis, a 48-hour infusion of cisatracurium consistently reduced mortality at 28 days, in addition to mortality at ICU discharge and at hospital discharge. The incidence of barotrauma was similarly reduced, with the duration of MV and the risk of ICUAW not being affected. The mortality reduction findings associated with NMBA therapy were large and robust; the authors determined that for every nine adults with ARDS treated with cisatracurium, one life was saved in the first 90 days of hospital admission. Duration of MV was not significantly different between groups; however, in those receiving NMBAs, ventilator-free days were increased, the latter of which was thought to be because of competing risks of death and duration of MV. Mechanisms responsible for this improvement may be related to improved oxygenation; reduced inflammation (whether indirect or direct remains to be elucidated); and improved synchrony.[108,109,126,133] These results are somewhat echoed in a study[134] published in the Chinese literature comparing vecuronium for 24–48 hours in patients with ARDS and severe sepsis with controls (n=48), where the authors found decreased mortality and improvement in morbidity with the treatment group. For this chapter, the source for these results was confined to the abstract because it was the only section translated into English, thus restricting the interpretation. In summary, early short-term use of cisatracurium for the treatment of ARDS shows promise; more RCTs are needed to substantiate existing findings.

Status Asthmaticus

Many small studies and case reports have been published evaluating various aspects of treating patients with asthma when an NMBA is included in the regimen. The mortality rate may be too low in patients with severe asthma receiving MV for it to serve as an end point, however, because a very large sample size would be required to assess an effect on survival.[102-104] Therefore, other outcomes or composite outcomes were sought to assess efficacy or risk-benefit relationships in this population. Four studies, including the aforementioned three,[102-105] evaluated NMBA therapy in patients with severe asthma on MV; however, only one was designed to address mortality[104] as part of a composite outcome, and the remaining three examined the association of NMBA with ICUAW. In addition, these patients were all deeply sedated and receiving CS, which could have misguided data interpretation. In the study by Adnet et al.[104] (n=101), NMBA use was the strongest independent factor for the composite outcome of ICU death, multiple organ failure, pneumonia, and paresis. Three studies[103-105] showed increased ICUAW with prolonged duration of administration. Atracurium held no advantage over the aminosteroids. Kessler et al.[102] (n=96) compared patients receiving NMBA regimens of much shorter duration with those on long-duration therapy and did not find a significant decrease in weakness with therapy of short duration, although an association with NMBA therapy of longer duration was the trend, and the authors believed it would have reached significance had the study population been sufficiently large. Nevertheless, they opined that in patients who are deeply sedated and mechanically ventilated, immobilization is inevitable and is itself an important contributor to the etiology. Overall, because of the paucity of information in this population, it is recommended that NMBAs be reserved for those with severe gas-trapping and lung hyperinflation that is life threatening and refractory to other therapies.[122]

Increased Intracranial Pressure

Control of increased intracranial pressure is fundamental to the treatment of patients with head injury, and sedatives and analgesics play an important pharmacologic role. In a retrospective review of data from the National Traumatic Coma Data Bank (n=514), early, routine, long-term use of NMBAs in patients with severe head injuries to manage

Table 9.3 Select Studies Evaluating Neuromuscular Blockers for Use in ARDS, Asthma, and Sepsis

Study	Design	Patients, Regimen	Goal/Comparison vs. NMBA	Results	Notes
Segredo 1992[96]	Prospective observational cohort	n=16; 15/16 ALI/ARDS Vecuronium boluses	Incidence of weakness in patients on NMBA	7/16 had weakness because of "prolonged block." The etiology could potentially have been CIP/M as did not test for it	Unclear if taking CS. No baseline severity-of-illness comparison
Kupfer 1987[95]	Case report	n=1; asthma Pancuronium boluses, high-dose CS	Observe weakness	Clinical examination and EMG supported disuse atrophy	
Griffin 1992[84]	Case reports	n=3; asthma. Pancuronium/vecuronium x 9 days. High-dose CS	Index visit compared with previous admissions when on high CS but no NMBA	All three had biopsy revealing degenerating type 1 and type 2 muscle fibers as well as necrotic cells. All had profound weakness	No history of weakness in previous admissions
Garnacho-Montero 2001[99]	Prospective observational cohort	n=73; severe sepsis on MV. Vecuronium and atracurium for several days in 11/73 (total dose translates to about 2–7 days of therapy)	Impact of CIP on MV, LOS, and hospital mortality	CIP associated with an increase in hospital mortality and MV duration. After multivariate analysis, independent risk factors for CIP included hyperosmolarity (OR 4.8), parenteral nutrition (OR 5.11), neurologic failure (OR 24.02), and NMBA (OR 16.32; CI, 1.34–199; p=0.0008)	Severity scores not compared for NMBA and non-NMBA groups. Paucity of patients on NMBA makes valid comparison difficult
Coakley 1998[106]	Prospective case series	n=44. In ICU > 7 days; sepsis MODS included	Identify risk factors for CIP	No correlation between CIP and use of NMBA	Heterogeneous populations; many confounders; CS regimens unknown
Garnacho-Montero 2005[101]	Prospective cohort	n=64 severe sepsis and on MV > 7 days. Vecuronium, atracurium	Impact of CIP, on LOS, MV duration	CIP increases duration of MV (p<0.001) 10/34 with CIP got NMBA vs. 3/30 without CIP were on NMBA (p=0.055) NMBA not associated with the development of CIP	Confounders: sepsis and sedatives. A trend toward significance. Earlier study (2001) found an association
Steingrub 2014[100]	Retrospective cohort	n=7864 from 339 centers. On MV by day 2 in ICU. Severe sepsis	Hospital MR for patients on NMBA with severe sepsis and on MV. Matched to non-NMBA patients with similar propensity	NMBA use associated with decrease in mortality, p<0.001. No difference in incidence of ICUAW	Younger patients (62yo vs 68yo) in NMBA group; diagnoses of ICUAW, etc., based on ICD-9-CM billing codes; unknown if NMBAs given for intubations because indication not investigated

Study	Design	Patients, Regimen	Goal/Comparison vs. NMBA	Results	Notes
Kessler 2009[102]	Retrospective cohort; historic controls	n=96 from 1983 to 1995; n=74 1995–2004 Pts with asthma on CS	NMBA association with ICUAW (NMBA use much less in second phase [1995–2004])	No decline in ICUAW with diminished use of NMBAs	A trend toward more weakness in the higher-use NMBA group; underpowered to detect difference. Immobilization key causal element
Leatherman 1996[103]	Retrospective cohort	n=107 asthma episodes (94 pts) CS, MV. 69 pts on NMBA. Atracurium, pancuronium, vecuronium	Weakness in CS + NMBA vs. CS; atracurium vs. aminosteroids; association of MV with paresis	NMBA significantly associated with weakness: 20/69 pts on CS + NMBA were weak. No weak patients in CS-only group 0/38, p<0.001. Duration of NMBA was significantly longer in weak vs. non-weak patients 0.6 vs. 3.4 days, p<0.001. No difference in CS doses in weak vs. non-weak patients (post hoc) No difference in weakness between atracurium and aminosteroids	Steroid use was a confounder; illness severity at baseline not compared between NMBA and NMBA + CS groups. Functional definition may have excluded some patients; EP studies and biopsy done only when confirmed weak
Adnet 2001[104]	Retrospective cohort	n=101; asthma, MV and on CS. Pancuronium; vecuronium, atracurium	In-hospital mortality and composite outcome. NMBA use > 12 hr vs. NMBA < 12 hr	In-hospital mortality same; composite outcome (ICU death, MOF, PNA, paresis) increased in the NMBA > 12-hr group vs. the < 12-hr group, p=0.01. NMBA was the strongest independent factor for paresis, p=0.007	Respiratory severity values not compared between groups at baseline. NMBA > 12-hr group sicker at baseline
Behbehani 1999[105]	Retrospective cohort	n=86; asthma MV 30/86 on NMBA. Pancuronium, vecuronium, atracurium	Incidence of, and risk factors for, myopathy in pts with asthma on MV	Duration of NMBA only independent predictor for myopathy, p=0.001. The OR for developing myopathy with each additional day of NMBA was 2.1	No severity-of-illness comparison for NMBA vs. no-NMBA groups, especially respiratory illness severity
Gainnier 2004[109]	RCT	n=56; ARDS P/F ≤ 150	Cisatracurium early infusion for 48 hr vs. placebo. Evaluate oxygenation parameters	Improved oxygenation (p=0.021). Significant decrease in F_{IO_2} and PEEP requirements (p<0.001 and p=0.036, respectively)	Limitation: risk of bias; patient nurse not blinded
Forel 2006[108]	RCT	n=36; ARDS P/F < 200	Cisatracurium early infusion for 48 hr vs. placebo. Evaluate inflammation effects	Improved oxygenation (p<0.001) Reduced conc of pulmonary IL-β, p=0.005; IL-6, p=0.038; IL-8, p=0.017; and of systemic IL-β, p=0.037; IL-6, p=0.04	Limitation: risk of bias; patient nurse not blinded

Table 9.3 Select Studies Evaluating Neuromuscular Blockers for Use in ARDS, Asthma, and Sepsis
(continued)

Study	Design	Patients, Regimen	Goal/Comparison vs. NMBA	Results	Notes
Papazian 2010[107]	RCT	n=340; ARDS P/F < 150	Cisatracurium early infusion for 48 hr vs. placebo. Evaluate 90-day mortality (primary outcome)	Decrease in adjusted 90-day mortality, HR of 0.68, p=0.04. Secondary outcomes: no difference in 28-day mortality and ICUAW; increased ventilator-free days (p=0.03 at 90 days) and organ free-days (p=0.01), decreases incidence of barotrauma (p=0.03) with NMBA	Limitation: clinical diagnosis of paresis (MRC score); not supplemented with EP testing
Arroliga 2005[132]	Retrospective observational	n=5183 MV for ≥ 12 hr. NMBA in 13% of all pts and in 87/231 ARDS	Primary outcome: use of sedatives and NMBA. Impact on MV duration, ICU stay, and mortality	Increased duration of MV associated with NMBA (7 vs. 3 days, p<0.001), increased ICU stay (10 vs. 7 days, p<0.001). NMBA use independently associated with ICU mortality (OR 1.39, p<0.001)	Low usage. Illness severity not compared between NMBA and non-NMBA; diverse population; NMBA regimens unknown
Arroliga 2008[130]	Retrospective observational ALVEOLI Trial (Assessment of Low Tidal Volume and increased End-expiratory volume to Obviate Lung Injury)	n=549; ALI/ARDS P/F < 300, low vs. high PEEP groups	Impact of NMBAs, etc., on MV duration, 60-day mortality, and time to wean in first 28 days	No significant difference in adjusted 60-day mortality or duration of MV. The use of sedatives and opioids, but not NMBAs, was associated with a longer time to achieve important weaning landmarks, p<0.0001	NMBA use short; regimens unknown; sepsis, severity-of-illness sedative, and opioids confound. Severity of illness not compared between NMBA and non-NMBA. Application of two comparator groups to this study unclear

ALI = acute lung injury; ARDS = acute respiratory distress syndrome; CIP/M = critical illness polyneuropathy/myopathy; CS = corticosteroids; EMG = electromyogram; EP = electrophysiologic; FIO_2 = fraction of inspired oxygen; HR = hazard ratio; ICD-9-CM = International Classification of Diseases, ninth Revision, Clinical Modification; ICUAW = intensive care unit acquired weakness; IL = interleukin; LOS = length of stay; MODS = multiple organ dysfunction syndrome; MOF = multiple organ failure; MRC = Medical Research Council; MV = mechanical ventilation; NMBA = neuromuscular blocking agent; OR = odds ratio; PEEP = positive end expiratory pressure; P/F = ratio of arterial oxygen partial pressure to fractional inspired oxygen; PNA = pneumonia; pts = patients; RCT = randomized controlled trial; TOF = train-of-four.

increased intracranial pressure did not improve overall outcome and may actually have prolonged ICU stay and increased extracranial complications.[135] Although NMBA use was associated with fewer deaths (p<0.001), the group receiving them had a higher incidence of sepsis, pneumonia, and more vegetative or severely disabled survivors. A second large retrospective study (n=326)[136] found no difference in mortality or length of stay between patients with traumatic brain injury, whether they received NMBAs or not. Other smaller studies focusing on physiologic changes have shown that, in general, NMBAs do not affect hemodynamic parameters such as intracranial, mean arterial, and cerebral perfusion pressures but may attenuate acute changes in these variables during suctioning.[137-140] Because of design limitations, the current body of evidence does not provide a conclusive answer, and a recommendation for their use in increased intracranial pressure cannot be made. In general, NMBAs in this population should be selective and considered only when deep sedation is insufficient to prevent dangerous elevations in intracranial pressure (e.g., during suctioning or with sudden cough or shivering).[122,141,142]

Targeted Temperature Management After Cardiac Arrest

In the early 2000s, two clinical trials evaluated mild hypothermia for 12–24 hours in which body temperature was reduced to 32°C–34°C in comatose survivors of cardiac arrest, and pancuronium or vecuronium was part of the protocol to reduce shivering. Neurological outcomes and mortality were improved.[143,144] Several years later when Chamorro et al.[145] investigated ICU protocols for targeted temperature management of post-cardiac arrest patients worldwide, the authors found that NMBAs were commonly used for preventing and/or treating shivering. There was considerable variation with respect to the type of NMBA used, regimens, and monitoring habits. Pancuronium was the most commonly used, with usage in 24 of 68 participating ICUs. Cisatracurium was second, being included in 14 of the 68 ICU protocols. Train-of-four monitoring was used in three of the ICUs and continuous monitoring of cerebral activity in only three. Status epilepticus is a recognized risk in postanoxic injury, and diagnoses may be difficult when the patient is paralysed; indeed, status epilepticus occurred in 25 of 68 ICUs with an incidence of 0%–44%. Still, the value of continuous electroencephalogram monitoring in predicting prognosis and guiding management has yet to be confirmed in this population.[146]

However, there are no prospective controlled studies comparing the efficacy of NMBAs in this population (i.e., a direct comparison between an NMBA group and a non-NMBA group or between various NMBAs). Salciccioli et al.[147] (n=111) did a post hoc analysis of a prospective observational trial of comatose patients after cardiac arrest where the primary exposure of interest was neuromuscular blockade for 24 hours, and primary outcomes were in-hospital survival and functional status at discharge. They showed an increased probability of survival and improvement in lactate clearance, a secondary outcome. There was a trend toward improved functional outcome. Limitations included small size, observational design, post hoc analysis, and potential for bias. In a retrospective study comparing vecuronium with cisatracurium use in cardiac arrest patients, Baker et al.[148] (n=201) examined the association between NMBA use and neurological outcome. After multivariable regression analysis, computation of the adjusted odds ratio for good neurological outcome showed that cisatracurium was the only independent variable with positive association (p=0.014). Similarly, limitations applied to this study because it was retrospective in nature, and the groups were not prespecified so that baseline characteristics could have differed between them. Multivariable regression analysis was done to minimize such inherent bias. Moreover, the numbers were small and unequal between groups (60 received cisatracurium, and 36 received vecuronium), and details of regimens, including total dose administered, were not explicit. The authors suggested that pharmacokinetic differences accounted for these variances because vecuronium relies on organ function for clearance, which may be impaired in these patients, whereas cisatracurium does not. It could be argued, however, that the clearance of cisatracurium, which is achieved by Hofmann elimination and in itself is temperature-dependent, would be expected to be impaired in the hypothermic condition, thus challenging this notion. In general, it is acknowledged that hypothermia to this degree per se may reduce the clearance of all NMBAs; however, the comparative order of magnitude is unknown in this population because most of the data are derived from cardiopulmonary bypass patients.[148] Further studies are required to evaluate the role and choice of NMBAs in targeted temperature management before a definite recommendation can be given.[122]

Otherwise, if using NMBAs for this indication, the impact of hypothermia on pharmacodynamics and pharmacokinetics must be considered. As mentioned earlier, the effects of NMBAs may be amplified during hypothermia,[123] and doses may typically be 20%–25% less, although other authors have described resistance to NMBAs as well as differing pharmacologic results.[123,145,148,149] For example, Heier et al.[150] found no difference in the pharmacodynamic effects of vecuronium in hypothermic versus normothermic intraoperative patients. It must be stated, however, that first, the temperature difference was relatively small between groups in this study (34.4°C vs. 36.8°C), and second, the degree of hypothermia attained was not as low as the convention (i.e., to 32°C–33°C, a common range). The authors did not investigate pharmacokinetic changes in this study, so we cannot comment. However, Cammu et al.[151] (n=17) found a reduction in cisatracurium, but not rocuronium, infusion rates in mildly hypothermic intraoperative patients (33°C). Because the elimination of cisatracurium is known to be temperature-dependent, this may account for the difference. Because of the different underlying populations in these studies, however, it is probably imprecise to extrapolate these intraoperative findings to the hypothermic post-cardiac arrest patient. Further concerns arise when monitoring the hypothermic patient on NMBAs. For example, PNS may be less accurate because the twitch tension may be dampened and may correlate poorly with degree of blockade.[123,149] It is important to be aware of this blunting of response in cooled patients when using PNS and to supplement its use with clinical assessment such as elimination of shivering. As alluded to, the other consideration is that NMBAs may mask seizure activity. Although the emergence of seizure activity is a sign of worse outcomes in these patients, controlling them has not yet been shown to improve neurologic prognosis.[145,152]

Increased Intra-Abdominal Pressure

Intra-abdominal hypertension is defined as a repeated elevation in intra-abdominal pressure of at least 12 mm Hg. Acute compartment syndrome is defined as continued intra-abdominal pressure of greater than 20 mm Hg with end-organ dysfunction or failure. Reduced abdominal wall compliance caused by third-spaced fluids, tense abdominal closures, and pain or inadequate sedation can lead to further increases in intra-abdominal pressures and subsequent organ failure. Neuromuscular blocking agents have been reported to improve elevated intra-abdominal pressures by reducing abdominal muscle tone. Neuromuscular blockade may provide clinicians with more time to remove fluid or treat the underlying cause of intra-abdominal hypertension and avoid surgical decompression.[153,154] A small prospective trial (n=10) suggested that a bolus dose of cisatracurium was effective in significantly decreasing mild elevations in intra-abdominal pressure.[155] A recent case report describing a patient undergoing adrenalectomy who had acute compartmental syndrome reported that a prolonged NMBA infusion of 48 hours was effective in reducing intra-abdominal pressure and providing a good recovery.[156] It has been recommended (grade 2C) by the International Acute Compartment Syndrome Consensus Definitions Conference Committee that NMBAs be used in selected patients to reduce mild to moderate elevations in intra-abdominal pressure.[153,154]

Sepsis

Several studies evaluating the use of NMBAs in patients with sepsis examine adverse outcomes such as ICUAW as end points rather than clinical efficacy and mortality (see ICU-Acquired Muscle Weakness section).[96,99,101] In contrast, Steingrub et al.[100] reviewed the impact of NMBA administration in ICU patients with pulmonary sepsis on MV where the primary outcome was in-hospital mortality. This was observational in nature involving 339 centers (n=7,864), and the authors used robust methods to adjust for known and suspected confounders by sensitivity analysis, using regression and instrumental variable analyses and propensity matching. Secondary outcomes included the number of days on MV and hospital and ICU lengths of stay. Intensive care unit–acquired weakness was also assessed and was based on ICD-9-CM codes, which is a list of codes adapted by the U.S. healthcare system to describe diagnoses. Results showed a significant reduction in hospital mortality with NMBA use (risk ratio [RR] 0.88; 95% confidence interval [CI], 0.80–0.96). There was a low incidence of ICUAW. By nature of its design, the investigation suffers from bias and other limitations. First, because of confounding, the demonstrated improvement in mortality may have been related more to an overall center effect because of differing degrees of success in implementing evidence-based practices between hospitals (e.g., lung-protective ventilation and early goal-directed therapy) rather than NMBA use itself. Second, the study used detailed billing data and ICD-9-CM codes instead of chart review, a fact likely to influence the incidence of ICUAW as a result of undercoding. Third, it was difficult to separate NMBA administration used for procedures and NMBAs used for long-term treatment, prompting a sensitivity analysis restricted to those on NMBA treatment for at least 2 days or on a total daily dose suggestive of an infusion. In this case, the investigators found no difference; indeed, they even found a trend (nonsignificant) toward higher mortality associated with NMBA use (RR 1.10; 95% CI, 0.91–1.33), further highlighting the need for caution in interpreting and extrapolating the results in "causal" terms.[157] It must be declared, however, that the unanimity of results computed using several different analytic techniques lends greater credence to the mortality findings in the primary outcome of this study. Clearly, more prospective studies are needed to confirm these claims.

INDICATIONS FOR USE IN SURGERY

Neuromuscular blocking agents, which have rapid onset and offset and minimal cardiac effects, are ideal for surgical procedures. Apart from their use in the operating theater, NMBAs have other applications in the anesthesia/surgical setting such as rapid sequence intubation, priming doses, and defasciculation.

Rapid Sequence Intubation

Rapid sequence intubation is used to secure a definitive airway in uncooperative, unfasting, unstable, and/or critically ill patients who may be at risk of aspiration. The anesthetist needs to intubate quickly before the anesthetic takes effect and the gag reflex is lost.[158-160] It is important to have an NMBA with a fast onset, and succinylcholine is commonly used to accomplish this. However, some patients are excluded from receiving it because of undesirable adverse effects (see Introduction and Pharmacologic Effects), so it is important to have an alternative. In this endeavor, rocuronium has been compared with succinylcholine in several trials and in a subsequent meta-analysis of these trials. In one prospective RCT (n=401), no difference was noted in oxygen desaturations between succinylcholine and rocuronium in critically ill patients undergoing emergency rapid sequence intubation.[161] In the meta-analysis,[160] data from 37 controlled trials (n=2,690) were reviewed, comparing the quality of intubating conditions provided by rocuronium and succinylcholine. There was a dose effect: in the subgroup of patients receiving rocuronium 0.6–0.7 mg/kg, there was a relative risk favoring succinylcholine for excellent intubating conditions (RR 0.81; 95% CI, 0.73–0.90), and the number needed to harm was 6. There was significant heterogeneity between the studies in this subgroup. In the groups that received 0.9–1.0 mg/kg of rocuronium and 1.2 mg/kg of rocuronium, there were no statistical differences for excellent or acceptable intubation conditions; however, succinylcholine, which had the advantage of a shorter duration of action, was thus ultimately deemed superior. There was no significant heterogeneity between the studies in the 0.9- to

1.0-mg/kg or 1.2-mg/kg rocuronium subgroups. Overall, the results showed that succinylcholine was superior to rocuronium (RR 0.86; 95% CI, 0.8–0.97), and the authors concluded that rocuronium's role should be relegated to that of an alternative agent. Typical doses for succinylcholine in this capacity are 1 mg/kg but may be as high as 2 mg/kg, especially in children. The usual range for rocuronium is 0.6–1.2 mg/kg.[8]

An acetylcholinesterase inhibitor should be available if intubation is unsuccessful; this does not apply when succinylcholine is being used. With succinylcholine, a patient's history should be known so that the risks of hyperkalemia and malignant hyperthermia may be minimized. Dantrolene should also be available during short procedures if succinylcholine is the chosen agent.[159]

Priming Strategy

Nondepolarizing NMBAs can also be administered in "priming" doses in an effort to overcome their slow onset. Theoretically, by giving small priming doses, the spare receptors are blocked without the patient having clinical weakness. The priming dose is generally considered to be 10% of the ED95, although there is no exact consensus on this detail.[162-164] Ideally, the patient should be able to breathe spontaneously and maintain an open airway in order to avoid aspiration after a priming dose. After about 4 minutes, a large bolus is given, decreasing the time to paralysis from 3–5 minutes to 70–100 seconds, comparable to succinylcholine. The clinician needs to closely monitor the patient and be ready to intubate in an emergency when using priming doses. In a small randomized trial of female patients undergoing anesthesia induction (n=30), Schmidt et al.[164] compared the effect of a priming technique with a bolus application of rocuronium on the onset of NMBA at the laryngeal adductor and the adductor pollicis muscles. After transcutaneous stimulation of the recurrent laryngeal nerve and ulnar nerve, a bolus of rocuronium 0.6 mg/kg (bolus group) or a priming dose of rocuronium 0.06 mg/kg, followed by rocuronium 0.54 mg/kg 3 minutes later (priming group), were injected. Lag time, onset 90%, onset time, and peak effect of NMBA were recorded and compared. The onset 90% and onset time measured at the laryngeal adductor muscles (onset was 44.7 ± 7.4 vs. 74.0 ± 23.8 seconds) and at the adductor pollicis (onset was 105.4 ± 29.9 vs. 139.2 ± 51.5 seconds) were significantly shorter in the priming group than in the bolus group, indicating that a priming technique with rocuronium significantly accelerated the onset of NMBA at the laryngeal adductor muscles. Under clinical circumstances, however, the technique is limited because some patients become profoundly weak after the priming dose, necessitating prompt control of ventilation and giving concern for aspiration.[159,165] Just as some individuals will be quite sensitive to priming doses of ND NMBA, others will show resistance. Enthusiasm for the priming technique has been tempered with time, mainly because response is unpredictable.[162]

Defasciculation Strategy

Using ND NMBAs as agents to prevent fasciculations is another strategy in surgery. After administration of the depolarizing agent succinylcholine, muscle fasciculations occur briefly, particularly over the chest and abdomen; then, relaxation occurs within 1 minute, becomes maximal within 2 minutes when transient apnea may occur, and disappears, as a rule, within 5 minutes.[1] Severe muscle soreness may follow succinylcholine administration. Applications of small doses of competitive NMBAs before succinylcholine have been used to minimize such fasciculations with attendant muscle pain and possibly hyperkalemia, although the practice is controversial because it may increase requirements for succinylcholine.

The defasciculating dose is generally 10% of the ED95 and is given 3–5 minutes beforehand. Rocuronium has been administered in this capacity (0.03–0.04 mg/kg or 10% of the ED95) where it decreased the incidence of fasciculations from 90% to 10%.[8] A recent meta-analysis shows that adverse effects of weakness have commonly occurred in studies of defasciculating doses of ND NMBAs, but these adverse effects are probably related to higher doses (e.g., rocuronium 0.06 mg/kg).[8,166] After the defasciculating dose of ND NMBA, the succinylcholine dose must be increased from 1 mg/kg to 1.5 mg/kg, or even 2 mg/kg, because of antagonism between ND and depolarizing drugs. Administering small doses of succinylcholine (e.g., 10 mg 1 minute before the intubating dose) appears ineffective in this respect and has largely been abandoned.[8]

INTERACTIONS WITH NMBAS

Several conditions as well as many drugs interact with NMBAs, most importantly inhalation anesthetics, certain antimicrobials, calcium channel blockers, and acetylcholinesterase inhibitors.[1,8] The mechanisms are broadly outlined in Table 9.1. There may be additive interactions if two NMBAs of similar structure are given together (e.g., atracurium-cisatracurium),[11] or the effect can be potentiated if NMBAs of dissimilar structure are coadministered (e.g., rocuronium/cisatracurium).[167] Administering small doses of NMBAs before succinylcholine can prevent fasciculations caused by succinylcholine, a practice called administration of defasciculating doses (see Defasciculation Strategy section).[8,11] In contrast, administering succinylcholine before ND NMBAs has given conflicting results, some reporting potentiation of block[168-170] and others seeing no effect at all.[171-173]

Aminoglycosides interact by inhibiting acetylcholine release from the presynaptic terminal (through competition with calcium) and, to a lesser extent, by noncompetitively blocking the postsynaptic receptor. The blockade is antagonized by calcium salts but only inconsistently by acetylcholinesterase inhibitors. The tetracyclines cause blockade, possibly by chelation of calcium and polymyxin B; colistin and clindamycin do so by both pre- and postsynaptic actions. Calcium channel blockers enhance neuromuscular blockade produced by both competitive and depolarizing antagonists. It is unclear whether this is a result of a diminution of calcium-dependent release of transmitter from the nerve ending or whether it is a postsynaptic action. When co-administering these drugs with NMBAs, dose adjustments should be considered; if recovery of spontaneous respiration is delayed, calcium salts may facilitate. Magnesium interacts significantly probably only at doses used for treating preeclampsia.[1,11] Miscellaneous drugs that may have significant interactions with either competitive or depolarizing NMBAs include opioid analgesics, procaine, lidocaine, quinidine, phenelzine, phenytoin, propranolol, magnesium salts, CS, digitalis glycosides, chloroquine, catecholamines, and diuretics. Dantrolene blocks release of calcium from the sarcoplasmic reticulum and is used in the treatment of malignant hyperthermia (see Malignant Hyperthermia section). Acidosis and hypothermia may produce unpredictable effects with ND NMBAs. However, hypercalcemia, demyelinating lesions, peripheral neuropathies, and diabetes have been reported to antagonize ND NMBA because of up-regulation of extrajunctional receptors.[1,9,123,174-176]

MONITORING

Peripheral Nerve Stimulation

After administering an adequate dose of NMBA, motor weakness progresses to a rapid paralysis. Small rapidly moving muscles (e.g., eyes, jaw, and larynx) relax before those of the limbs and trunk. Eventually, the intercostals and finally the diaphragm are paralyzed, and respiration then ceases. Recovery of muscles usually occurs in the reverse order so that the diaphragm is ordinarily the first muscle to regain function. However, paralysis is affected not only by the differential sensitivity of muscles to block but also by the regional blood flow. Thus, even though the diaphragm is more resistant to blockade, it receives greater blood flow and drug delivery, permitting a quicker onset of paralysis than that of the adductor pollicis in the thumb. The orbicularis oculi muscle is less sensitive than the adductor pollicis, and its time to paralysis correlates more closely with that of the diaphragm.[1,9,11,177,178]

The margin of safety for these agents is small because there is little effect until most receptors (spare receptors) are occupied so that the therapeutic range exists over a very narrow range of receptor occupancy (see Figure 9.3).[1,8,9,11] Peripheral nerve stimulation is generally used to monitor for the potential toxicity of NMBAs in ICU patients, efficacy being better assessed using clinical parameters, such as respiratory variables, in patients with ventilator dyssynchrony. On the contrary, PNS is used to assess efficacy in the operating theater, the goal being to keep the sedated patient completely immobilized. With PNS, a stimulator is applied to a peripheral nerve, and the response of the muscle it innervates is observed. The response to PNS indicates the level of neurotransmission in the muscle of interest, usually the diaphragm, because it cannot be monitored directly. The nerve response to electrical stimulation depends on the current applied (maximum current 60–80 mA), duration for which the current is applied, and position of the electrodes (in that at least one electrode must be placed over the nerve).[179] The patterns of stimulation vary and elicit different characteristics of ND neuromuscular blockade. For example, when high-frequency stimulation is used, fade and post-tetanic facilitation occur. The use of these patterns applies mainly to ND NMBAs because such responses are not seen with the depolarizing agents. Fade appears to be caused by a decrease in acetylcholine release at the NMJ because the margin of safety for neurotransmission is compromised in

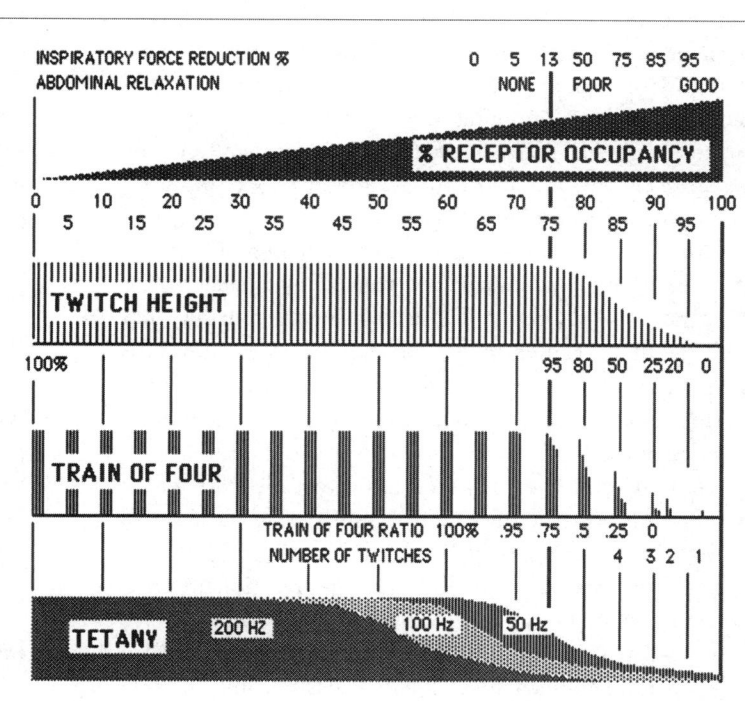

Figure 9.3 Receptor occupancy and clinical responses.

Receptor occupancy is at least 75% (top panel) before a reduction in response to peripheral nerve stimulation (lower panels) or a change in clinical examination (uppermost text) is evident.

Reprinted with permission from: University of Sydney. Monitoring the Neuromuscular Junction. www.anaesthesia.med.usyd.edu.au/resources/lectures/nmj_monitoring_clt/Resources/levelofblock.gif. Accessed July 22, 2015.

the presence of blockade. Although acetylcholine release decreases when high-frequency stimulation is used, even in the absence of blockade, fade is not detected because of the sufficiently wide margin of safety for neurotransmission. The TOF pattern is the most commonly used mode of stimulation in the ICU and surgical settings, where it is interpreted by visual or tactile perception and thus is prone to error. With TOF stimulation, a supramaximal stimulus is delivered by PNS at a frequency of 2 Hz for 0.2 millisecond; the stimuli are applied in trains of 2 seconds (500 milliseconds apart) at an interval of 10 seconds or greater. This low frequency permits tactile and visual measurement. In theory, the supramaximal stimulus is determined by increasing the current until there is no further increase in response. However, health care providers often obviate this in practice using a maximal current from the beginning. At least 10–15 seconds should pass between stimulations to allow for full repolarization of the nerve.[8,180-184] Conceptually, we think of muscular response to PNS stimulation in terms of receptor occupancy at the NMJ. Although this conceptualization describes the dose-response relationship as a whole, each muscle fiber in the group has an all-or-none response once a critical number of its receptors are blocked.[6] In other words, there is no gradual decline in individual fiber responses with increasing doses; rather, there is an all-or-none response, and depending on fiber sensitivity, some will succumb sooner than others to escalating doses. Therefore, although not an accurate representation, receptor occupancy serves a useful purpose in understanding the dose-response relationship. It is envisioned that 75% of receptors must be occupied before any clinical blockade is seen. Continuing from 75% to 95% receptor occupancy, a gradual blockade of transmission is manifested by a decrease in twitch height from 100% to 0%, resulting in total blockade of the muscle group.[185] Train-of-four can be interpreted as a count in which the absolute number of contractions is evaluated visually, manually, or by calculating the TOF ratio (T4 divided by T1), comparing the fourth twitch with the first for intensity and height. The TOF ratio must be quantified by tactile methods, which is difficult, and may require using a transducer for accuracy. Thus, it is not recommended in the ICU.

A TOF count of 1/4–2/4 indicates adequate block without undue risk of toxicity. Similarly, a TOF ratio of 0.25 indicates onset of block, and a ratio of 0.75 implies clinical recovery. The TOF ratio is traditionally used postoperatively to assess recovery, but some patients have weakness at 0.8, whereas others do not recover until a TOF ratio of 0.9 is achieved, which has become the reference for recovery of ventilatory function. Many clinicians fail to detect fade at a TOF ratio of 0.6 during the recovery phase, implying that significant weakness can go undetected. On the contrary, it may be missed by the PNS when a response is seen or felt clinically.[186,187] Therefore, it is important to do both clinical tests and TOF to assess recovery when patients leave the operating room.

Both methods have shortcomings, but if used in combination, they form a more powerful monitoring tool.[8] Finally, there are several sources of error in interpreting the TOF, including variation between operators, incorrect positioning of the electrode pads, improper attachment of wires to pads, insufficient time for nerve repolarization, inconsistent pressure, and visual versus tactile assessment. All can invalidate the results. Problems arise if the patient is hypothermic, has oily or hairy skin, or has edema on the area where the pads are applied or if the batteries are low and the current is inadequate.[9,123,134]

In the ICU, TOF monitoring was associated with decreased costs when used to monitor vecuronium, but this did not extrapolate to atracurium and cisatracurium, perhaps because the pharmacology of the latter agents is less affected by organ impairment in critical illness.[188-190] Because evidence is sparse, it is recommended that PNS monitoring not be relied on exclusively, rather, that clinical parameters be identified (ventilator synchrony, increased chest wall compliance, decreased O_2 consumption) to assess patients on NMBAs and to further guide therapy. Caution in interpreting the TOF is advised when used in hypothermic patients.[123,149]

REVERSAL

In contradistinction to ICU patients in whom reversal agents are rarely used, rapid recovery from neuromuscular blockade is important postoperatively where the rate of recovery is dictated by both the NMBA used (the spontaneous rate) and the reversal agent (the accelerated reversal rate). Residual blockade with a TOF ratio less than 0.9 may occur in up to 33% of patients arriving in the post-anesthesia care unit.[191,192] A study by Murphy et al. (n=7,459) suggests that a large proportion of cases of postoperative upper airway obstruction and/or hypoxemia can be attributed to residual neuromuscular blockade.[193] Prevention of residual paralysis depends on judicious neuromuscular blocker management, monitoring, and use of reversal agents. Replacing long-acting drugs with more protracted spontaneous rates of recovery by intermediate agents has been largely accomplished, and monitoring has been improved.[187,194,195] Moreover, acetylcholinesterase inhibitors are used to reverse competitive blockade in postoperative patients, further accelerating recovery.

The mechanism of action of acetylcholinesterase inhibitors involves acetylcholinesterase inhibition. Neostigmine and pyridostigmine attach at the esteratic and anionic sites of the acetylcholinesterase molecule and produce longer-lasting inhibition than edrophonium. Neostigmine and pyridostigmine are inactivated by acetylcholinesterase, whereas edrophonium is unaffected. The inhibition of acetylcholinesterase increases the amount of time that acetylcholine spends in the synaptic cleft, leading to the increased size and duration of the excitatory postsynaptic endplate potential. Neostigmine is the most commonly used agent because of the long onset of pyridostigmine and the limited availability of edrophonium. Neostigmine is the most potent of the acetylcholinesterase inhibitors. The dose-response curve reaches a ceiling effect for these drugs at a dose of 0.07 mg/kg of neostigmine or its equivalent for other agents. However, it may even be as low as 0.03–0.05 mg/kg so that neostigmine offers only partial recovery. Neostigmine is more efficacious during intense blockade than the other two agents, and it is effective against all ND NMBAs.[187,196-198] It is generally recommended to wait for four twitches on the TOF to appear before administering neostigmine because there is no advantage in the time it takes to gain full recovery by administering it early. In clinical doses, it may unexpectedly produce a degree of blockade, particularly if a second dose is given. This is unlikely with a single modest dose, and any effects are probably short-lived.[199-201] The mechanism for this effect is unknown, but a possible explanation may be that the muscle has fully recovered after the first dose and the second dose is acting on normal unblocked muscle, producing an acetylcholine-induced blockade.[202] Mivacurium poses a challenge for reversal. Like succinylcholine, its metabolism may be inhibited by neostigmine, introducing a risk of prolonging blockade. Edrophonium does not inhibit plasma cholinesterase, perhaps making it better suited for the reversal of mivacurium. Muscarinic effects such as bradycardia, increased salivation, and gastrointestinal motility as well bronchoconstriction are common with acetylcholinesterase inhibitors and can be prevented by coadministering anticholinergics. Confusion is also associated with acetylcholinesterase inhibitors. Less than 1% of patients have other central nervous system effects, including dysphoria, restlessness, agitation, seizures, headache, and drowsiness.[9,187]

Sugammadex, currently unavailable in the United States, is a modified A-cyclodextrin that binds tightly to steroid-based NMBAs such as vecuronium and rocuronium, permitting accelerated removal of the drugs from the plasma and subsequently from the NMJ through an increased concentration gradient. It is ineffective against atracurium and cisatracurium. Sugammadex has no muscarinic effects because it lacks affinity for the acetylcholine receptor. The dose required depends on the amount of NMBA present and thus the degree of block and when adequate doses are given, recovery to a TOF ratio greater than 0.9 is attained in 2–3 minutes.[187] It has few adverse effects and is expensive. Sugammadex has been studied postoperatively and in rapid sequence intubation, but it has not been evaluated in critical care patients.[203,204]

CONCOMITANT CARE

Awareness during surgery and in the ICU has been described in paralyzed patients.[153,205] Although there are no controlled studies evaluating the use of sedatives in critically ill patients receiving NMBAs, it is recommended to administer these drugs before commencing and throughout any paralytic regimen. The bispectral index monitor (BIS monitor-Aspect Medical Systems, Covidien, Mansfield, MA) is used to assess sedation, but it is unclear whether awareness can totally be avoided by its use because large doses of NMBAs can depress the bispectral index in certain circumstances.[11,153,205,206]

For completion, the following aspects of care should be attended to in the patient receiving NMBAs: frequent suctioning because the cough reflex is inhibited; light taping and lubrication of the eyes to prevent corneal drying and ulceration; regular turning to prevent decubitus ulcers; elevating the head of the bed to reduce the risk of aspiration, particularly during enteral feeding; and monitoring the pupillary reflexes to assess neurologic status (pancuronium is unreliable in this respect because of its relatively strong muscarinic effects); hyperglycemia should be managed with a target blood glucose of less than 180–200 mg/dL, and venous thrombus and stress ulcer prophylaxis should be instituted.[122] As alluded to previously, it is crucial to provide adequate sedation and pain relief with sedatives and analgesics because such properties are not within the pharmacologic spectrum of the NMBAs.

SPECIAL POPULATIONS

There is some controversy regarding the corresponding effects on recovery when NMBAs are dosed according to actual body weight versus ideal body weight. For atracurium, ideal body weight was considered more predictable with less variability by some authors but not by others.[207-209] Similarly, Meyhoff et al. and Leykin et al. showed more optimal recovery times when dosing atracurium according to ideal weight, but Puhringer found no statistical difference.[210-213] The patient population in Leykin's study was severely obese, however, whereas Puhringer's patient population was moderately so, which may have accounted for the difference.[211,214] For both vecuronium and cisatracurium, ideal body weight was more predictable than actual weight.[209,214] Thus, ideal body weight or some adjusted body weight that accounts for changes in body mass is recommended when dosing patients with obesity.[8,11]

Sensitivity, particularly to the hyperkalemic effects of succinylcholine, can occur in those with up-regulation and extrajunctional proliferation of nicotinic receptors beyond the endplate to the sarcolemma. Such up-regulation is seen in denervated muscle caused by acute upper and lower motor neuron disease (spinal cord injury, stroke, demyelinating disease, encephalitis, prolonged immobility with disease, chronic progressive neurologic disease, muscular dystrophies, amyotrophic lateral sclerosis paraplegia, and crush injuries) and in postburn and posttrauma patients.

Caution is advised.[1,6,8,215-217] Care should be exercised when administering succinylcholine to hypoxemic patients because this, together with potential hyperkalemia, introduces a second risk factor for arrhythmias. Succinylcholine administration is further confounded by the fact that the drug's effects may last 12–18 minutes and cannot be reversed. In patients with myasthenia gravis, there is enhanced sensitivity to the blockade caused by NMBAs because antibodies are directed to the host's NMJ nicotinic receptors, impairing baseline response. Therefore, reduced doses, together with individual assessment and PNS monitoring at the orbicularis oculi muscle, are recommended in patients with myasthenia gravis. Patients with abnormal or reduced plasma cholinesterase may have reduced capacity to metabolize succinylcholine. This category includes those with genetically determined reductions in or absence of the enzyme, pregnancy, liver disease, uremia, malnutrition, burns, plasmapheresis, and oral contraceptives. Plasma cholinesterase is also reduced by some acetylcholinesterase inhibitors such as neostigmine and pyridostigmine but not edrophonium, prolonging the duration of action of succinylcholine and mivacurium.[8,9]

CONCLUSION

Neuromuscular blocking agents, well established as important players in the surgical arena, are gaining recognition as adjuncts to care of patients in the ICU, particularly in ARDS and targeted temperature management. Guidelines for using these agents are currently being revised by the Society of Critical Care Medicine to offer guidance for use in the critical care setting.[112,218] These agents are administered by continuous infusion in the ICU, as opposed to bolus dosing, which is commonly practiced in surgery. Cisatracurium and atracurium do not depend on normal organ function for adequate elimination and thus are well suited for the critical care patient. Neuromuscular blocking agents carry their own complement of risks when administered to the critically ill population, including drug interactions, exaggerated and unpredictable responses when given to patients with certain conditions, and sundry adverse effects, most notably prolongation of neuromuscular blockade and ICUAW. Whether NMBAs directly cause CIP/M manifesting as ICUAW remains unresolved; nevertheless, prudence in using these agents should be exercised at all times. In this respect, clinical evaluation and PNS/TOF are recommended as monitoring aids, although both methods are prone to error. Competitive NMBAs, but not depolarizing agents, can be reversed by administering acetylcholinesterase inhibitors. The latter drugs have various shortcomings because they provide only partial reversal, and the effect can be delayed. Sugammadex, a newer agent and not yet unavailable in the United States, has a faster onset and more complete reversal of aminosteroid block and represents an important advance in postoperative recovery.

REFERENCES

1. Taylor P. Agents acting at the neuromuscular junction and autonomic ganglia. In: Brunton LL, Lazo JS, Parker KL, eds. Goodman & Gilman's The Pharmacological Basis of Therapeutics, 11th ed. New York: McGraw-Hill, 2006:217-36.
2. Nedergaard OA. Curare: the flying death. Pharmacol Toxicol 2003;92:154-5.
3. West R. The pharmacology and therapeutics of curare and its constituents (Section of Therapeutics and Pharmacology). Proc R Soc Med 1935;28:565-8.
4. Bechter AM. The civilizing of curare: a history of its development and introduction into anesthesiology. Anesth Analg 1977;56:305-19.
5. Foldes FF, McNall PG, Borrego-Hinojosa JM. Succinylcholine: a new approach to muscular relaxation in anaesthesiology. N Engl J Med 1952;247:596-600.
6. Fox SI. Muscle: mechanisms of contraction and neural control. In: Human Physiology, 11th ed. New York: McGraw-Hill, 2009:355-97.
7. Westfall TC, Westfall DP. Neurotransmission: the autonomic and somatic motor nervous systems. In: Brunton LL, Lazo JS, Parker KL, eds. Goodman & Gilman's The Pharmacological Basis of Therapeutics, 11th ed. New York: McGraw-Hill, 2006:137-82.
8. Donati F, Bevan DR. Neuromuscular blocking agents. In: Barash PG, Cullen BF, Stoelting RK, eds. Clinical Anesthesia, 5th ed. Philadelphia: Lippincott Williams & Wilkins, 2006:421-52.
9. McManus MC. Neuromuscular blockers in surgery and in the intensive care unit, part 1. Am J Health Syst Pharm 2001;58:2287-99.
10. Fisher DM. Clinical pharmacology of neuromuscular blocking agents. Am J Health Syst Pharm 1999;56(suppl):S4-9.
11. Naguib M, Lien C. Pharmacology of muscle relaxants and their antagonists. In: Miller RD, ed. Miller's Anesthesia, 7th ed. Philadelphia: Churchill Livingstone, 2010:859-912.
12. Bowman WC, Prior C, Marshall IG. Presynaptic receptors in the neuromuscular junction. Ann N Y Acad Sci 1990;604:69-81.
13. Wood SJ, Slater CR. Safety factor at the neuromuscular junction. Prog Neurobiol 2001;64:393-429.
14. Colquhoun D, Dreyer F, Sheridan RE. The actions of tubocurarine at the frog neuromuscular junction. J Physiol 1979;293:247-84.
15. Bahring R, Covarrubias M. Mechanisms of closed-state inactivation in voltage-gated ion channels. J Physiol 2011;589:461-79.
16. Hibbs RE, Zambon AC. Agents acting at the neuromuscular junction and autonomic ganglia. In: Brunton LL, Chabner BA, Knollmann BC, eds. Goodman & Gilman's The Pharmacological Basis of Therapeutics, 12th ed. New York: McGraw-Hill, 2011:chap 11. Available at www.accessmedicine.com/content.aspx?aID=16661089. Accessed January 11, 2015.
17. Hou VY, Emala CW. Neuromuscular relaxants as antagonists for M2 and M3 muscarinic receptors. Anesthesiology 1998;88:744-50.
18. Lee C. Conformation, action and mechanism of action of neuromuscular blocking muscle relaxants. Pharmacol Ther 2003;98:143-69.

19. Milchert M, Spassov A, Meissner K. Skeletal muscle relaxants inhibit rat tracheal smooth muscle tone in vitro. J Physiol Pharmacol 2009;60(suppl 8):5-11.

20. Martin L, Bratton SL, O'Rourke P. Clinical uses and controversies of neuromuscular blocking agents in infants and children. Crit Care Med 1999;27:1358-68.

21. O'Connor MF, Roizen MF. Use of muscle relaxants in the intensive care unit. J Intensive Care Med 1993;8:34-46.

22. Longnecker DE, Murphy FL. Muscle relaxants. In: Dripps/Eckenhoff/Vandam: Introduction to Anesthesia, 8th ed. Philadelphia: Saunders, 1992:110-24.

23. Naguib M, Samarkandi A, Bakhamees H, et al. Histamine-release haemodynamic changes produced by rocuronium, vecuronium, mivacurium, atracurium and tubocurarine. Br J Anaesth 1995;75:588-92.

24. Savarese JJ, Ali HH, Basta SJ, et al. The clinical neuromuscular pharmacology of mivacurium chloride (BW B1090U). A short-acting nondepolarizing ester neuromuscular blocking drug. Anesthesiology 1988;68:723-32.

25. Stoops CM, Curtis CA, Kovach DA, et al. Hemodynamic effects of mivacurium chloride administered to patients during oxygen-sufentanil anesthesia for coronary artery bypass grafting or valve replacement. Anesth Analg 1989;68:333-9.

26. Spence AG, Barnetson RS. Reaction to vecuronium bromide. Lancet 1985;1:979-80.

27. Hilgenberg JC. Comparison of the pharmacology of vecuronium and atracurium with that of other currently available muscle relaxants. Anesth Analg 1983;62:524-31.

28. Fahey MR, Morris RB, Miller RD, et al. Clinical pharmacology of ORG NC45 (Norcuron): a new nondepolarizing muscle relaxant. Anesthesiology 1981;55:6-11.

29. Futo J, Kupferberg JP, Moss J. Inhibition of histamine N-methyltransferase (HNMT) in vitro by neuromuscular relaxants. Biochem Pharmacol 1990;39:415-20.

30. Levy JH, Davis GK, Duggan J, et al. Determination of the hemodynamics and histamine release of rocuronium (Org 9426) when administered in increased doses under N20/O2-sufentanil anesthesia. Anesth Analg 1994;78:318-21.

31. Basta SJ, Savarese JJ, Ali HH, et al. Histamine releasing potencies of atracurium, dimethyl tubocurarine and tubocurarine. Br J Anaesth 1983;55:105S-6S.

32. Scott RPF, Savarese JJ, Basta SJ, et al. Atracurium: clinical strategies for preventing histamine release and attenuating the hemodynamic response. Br J Anaesth 1985;57:550-3.

33. Watkins J. Adverse reaction to neuromuscular blockers: frequency, investigation and epidemiology. Acta Anaesthesiol Scand 1994;102:6-10.

34. Gyrmek L, Cantley EM. Comparison of the onset, spontaneous recovery and train of four of the clinical neuromuscular block produced by pancuronium and pipecuronium. Int J Clin Pharmacol Ther 1994;32:600-5.

35. Cabal LA, Siassi B, Artal R, et al. Cardiovascular and catecholamine changes after administration of pancuronium in distressed neonates. Pediatrics 1985;75:284-7.

36. Orkin FK, Pegg JR. Cardiac effects of pancuronium bromide [letter]. JAMA 1973;224:630.

37. Brichard G. Arrhythmia inducing action of pancuronium in patients under halothane [in French]. Anesth Analg 1973;30:947-50.

38. Darwish AK, Challen PD. Unexplained death during anaesthesia. Br J Anaesth 1977;49:192-3.

39. Appiah-Ankam J, Hunter JM. Pharmacology of neuromuscular blocking drugs. Contin Educ Anaesth Crit Care Pain 2004;4:2-7.

40. Sugai Y, Sugai K, Hirata T, et al. The interaction of pancuronium and vecuronium with cardiac muscarinic receptors. Acta Anaesthesiol Scand 1987;31:224-6.

41. Futo J, Kupferberg JP, Moss J, et al. Vecuronium inhibits histamine N-methyltransferase. Anesthesiology. 1988;69:92-6.

42. Husby P, Gramstad L, Rosland J, et al. Haemodynamic effects of high-dose vecuronium compared with pancuronium in beta-blocked patients with coronary artery disease during fentanyl-diazepam-nitrous oxide anaesthesia. Acta Anaesthesiol Scand 1996;40:26-31.

43. Abel M, Book WJ, Eisenkraft JB. Adverse effects of nondepolarizing neuromuscular blocking agents: incidence, prevention and management. Drug Saf 1994;10:420-38.

44. Engbaek J, Ording H, Sorenson B, et al. Cardiac effects of vecuronium and pancuronium during halothane anaesthesia. Br J Anaesth 1983;55:501-5.

45. Lines D, Shipton EA. Severe bradycardia and sinus arrest after administration of vecuronium, fentanyl and halothane. South Afr Med J 1991;80:200-1.

46. Inoue K, el-Banayosy A, Stolarski L, et al. Vecuronium induced bradycardia following induction of anaesthesia with etomidate or thiopentone, with or without fentanyl. Br J Anaesth 1988;60:10-7.

47. Jooste E, Klafter F, Hirshman C, et al. A mechanism for rapacuronium-induced bronchospasm. M2 muscarinic receptor antagonism. Anesthesiology 2003;98:906-11.

48. Soukup J, Doenicke A Hoerneke R, et al. Cardiovascular effects after bolus administration of cisatracurium. A comparison with vecuronium [in German]. Anaesthesist 1996;45:1024-9.

49. Booij L. The use of rocuronium in various clinical situations. Asean J Anaesthesiol 2005;6(suppl 5):5-14.

50. Bevan DR. Newer neuromuscular blocking agents. Pharmacol Toxicol 1994;74:3-9.

51. Pollard BJ. Interactions involving relaxants. In: Pollard BJ, ed. Applied Neuromuscular Pharmacology. Oxford, UK: Oxford University Press, 1994:202-48.

52. Boehm S, Kubista H. Fine tuning of sympathetic transmitter release via ionotropic and metabotropic presynaptic receptors. Pharm Rev 2002;54:43-99.

53. Clayton D. Asystole associated with vecuronium. Br J Anaesth 1986;58:937.

54. Starr NJ, Sethna DH, Estafanous FG. Bradycardia and asystole following the rapid administration of sufentanil with vecuronium. Anesthesiology 1986;64:521.

55. Cozanitis DA, Erkola O. A clinical study into the possible intrinsic bradycardiac activity of vecuronium. Anaesthesia 1989;44:648.

56. Brown JH, Laiken N. Muscarinic receptor agonists and antagonists. In: Brunton LL, Chabner BA, Knollmann BC, eds. Goodman & Gilman's The Pharmacological

Basis of Therapeutics, 12th ed. New York: McGraw-Hill, 2011:chap 9. Available at www.accessmedicine.com/content.aspx?aID=16660596. Accessed December 14, 2014.

57. Rott J, Lerche H, Lehmann-Horn F. Skeletal muscle channelopathies. J Neurol 2002;249:1493-502.

58. Rosenberg H. Malignant hyperthermia. Perioper Pharm 1999;2:5-6.

59. Simon HB. Hyperthermia. N Engl J Med 1993;329:483-7.

60. MacLennan DH, Phillips MS. Malignant hyperthermia. Science 1992;256:789-94.

61. Lee-Chiong TL, Stitt JT. Disorders of temperature regulation. Compr Ther 1995;21:697-704.

62. Schneider SM. Neuroleptic malignant syndrome: controversies in treatment. Am J Emerg Med 1991;9:360-2.

63. Totten VY, Hirschenstein E, Hew P. Neuroleptic malignant syndrome presenting without initial fever: a case report. J Emerg Med 1994;12:43-7.

64. Otsu K, Nishida K, Kimura Y, et al. The point mutation Arg615-Cys in the Ca2+ release channel of skeletal sarcoplasmic reticulum is responsible for hypersensitivity to caffeine and halothane in malignant hyperthermia. J Biol Chem 1994;269:9413-5.

65. Bross MH, Nash BT, Carlton FB. Heat emergencies. Am Fam Physician 1994;50:389-96.

66. Sangal R, Dimitrijevic R. Neuroleptic malignant syndrome: successful treatment with pancuronium. JAMA 1985;254:2795-6.

67. Quane QA, Healy JM, Keating KE, et al. Mutations in the ryanodine receptor gene in central core disease and malignant hyperthermia. Nat Genet 1993;5:51-5.

68. Ellis FR, Heffron JJA. Clinical and biochemical aspects of malignant hyperthermia. In: Atkinson RS, Adams AP, eds. Recent Advances in Anaesthesia and Analgesia. New York: Churchill Livingstone, 1985:173-207.

69. Censier K, Urwyler A, Zorzato F, et al. Intracellular calcium homeostasis in human primary muscle cells from malignant hyperthermia- susceptible and normal individuals. J Clin Invest 1998;101:1233-42.

70. Bina S, Capacchione J, Munkhuu B, et al. Is lymphocyte adenosine a diagnostic marker of clinical malignant hyperthermia? A pilot study. Crit Care Med 2015;43:584-93.

71. Becker BN, Ismail N. The neuroleptic malignant syndrome and acute renal failure. J Am Soc Nephrol 1994;4:1406-12.

72. Ward A, Chaffman MO, Sorkin EM. Dantrolene. A review of its pharmacodynamic and pharmacokinetic properties and therapeutic use in malignant hyperthermia, the neuroleptic malignant syndrome and an update of its use in muscle spasticity. Drugs 1986;32:130-6.

73. Al-Mashhadani SA, Gader AG, al Harthi SS, et al. The coagulopathy of heat stroke: alterations in coagulation and fibrinolysis in heat stroke patients during the pilgrimage (Haj) to Makkah. Blood Coagul Fibrinolysis 1994;5:731-6.

74. Mertes PM, Tajima K, Regnier-Kimmoun MA, et al. Perioperative anaphylaxis. Med Clin North Am 2010;94:761-89.

75. Sadlier PHM, Clarke RC, Bunning DL, et al. Anaphylaxis to neuromuscular blocking agents: incidence and cross-reactivity in Western Australia from 2002 to 2011. Br J Anaesth 2013;110:981-7.

76. Jick H, Andrews EB, Tilson HH, et al. Atracurium—a post-marketing surveillance study: methods and US experience. Br J Anaesth 1989;62:590-5.

77. Mirakhur RK. Side effects of atracurium. Br J Anaesth 1990;64:124-5.

78. Siler JN, Mager JG Jr, Wyche MQ Jr. Atracurium: hypotension, tachycardia and bronchospasm. Anesthesiology 1985;62:645-6.

79. Mercer JD. A severe anaphylactoid reaction to atracurium. Anaesth Intensive Care 1984;12:262-3.

80. Lien CA, Belmont MR, Abalos A, et al. The cardiovascular effects and histamine-releasing properties of 51W89 in patients receiving nitrous oxide/opioid/barbiturate anesthesia. Anesthesiology 1995;82:1131-8.

81. Hermans G, De Jonghe B, Bruyninckx F, et al. Clinical review: critical illness polyneuropathy and myopathy. Crit Care 2008;12:238.

82. Stevens RD, Marshall SA, Cornblath DR, et al. A framework for diagnosing and classifying intensive care unit-acquired weakness. Crit Care Med 2009;37(suppl):S299-S308.

83. Bolton CF, Gilbert JJ, Hahn AF, et al. Polyneuropathy in critically ill patients. J Neurol Neurosurg Psychiatry 1984;47:1223-31.

84. Griffin D, Fairman N, Coursin D, et al. Acute myopathy during treatment of status asthmaticus with corticosteroids and steroidal muscle relaxants. Chest 1992;102:510-4.

85. Larsson L, Li X, Edstrom L, et al. Acute quadriplegia and loss of muscle myosin in patients treated with nondepolarizing neuromuscular blocking agents and corticosteroids: mechanisms at the cellular and molecular levels. Crit Care Med 2000;28:34-45.

86. Danon MJ, Carpenter S. Myopathy with thick filament (myosin) loss following prolonged paralysis with vecuronium during steroid treatment. Muscle Nerve 1991;14:1131-9.

87. Hirano M, Ott BR, Raps EC, et al. Acute quadriplegia myopathy: a complication of treatment with steroids, nondepolarizing blocking agents or both. Neurology 1992;42:2082-7.

88. Waclawik AJ, Sufit RL, Beinlich BR, et al. Acute myopathy with selective degeneration of myosin filaments following status asthmaticus. J Neurol Sci 1990;98(suppl):470.

89. Op de Coul AAW. Critical illness myopathy. Eur J Anaesthesiol 1998;15:92-3.

90. MacFarlane I, Rosenthal F. Severe myopathy after status asthmaticus. Lancet 1977;2:615.

91. Zochodne DW, Bolton CF, Wells GA, et al. Critical illness polyneuropathy. A complication of sepsis and multiple organ failure. Brain 1987;35:575-84.

92. Williams T, O'Hehir R, Czarny D, et al. Acute myopathy in severe acute asthma with intravenously administered corticosteroids. Am Rev Respir Dis 1988;137:460-3.

93. Sitwell L, Weinshenker B, Monpetit V, et al. Complete ophthalmoplegia as a complication of acute CS-and-pancuronium-associated myopathy. Neurology 1991;41:921-2.

94. Panaceak EA. Letter to the editor. Crit Care Med 1988;16:732.

95. Kupfer Y, Okrent DG, Twersky RA, et al. Disuse atrophy in a ventilated patient with status asthmaticus receiving neuromuscular blockade. Crit Care Med 1987;15:795-6.

96. Segredo V, Caldwell JE, Matthay MA, et al. Persistent paralysis in critically ill patients after long-term administration of vecuronium. N Engl J Med 1992;327:524-8.

97. Witt NJ, Zochodne DW, Bolton CF, et al. Peripheral nerve function in sepsis and multiple organ failure. Chest 1991;99:176-84.

98. Bolton CF. Neuromuscular complication of sepsis. Intensive Care Med 1993;19:S58-S63.

99. Garnacho-Montero J, Madrazo-Osuna J, Garcia-Gamendia JL, et al. Critical illness polyneuropathy: risk factors and clinical consequences. A cohort study in septic patients. Intensive Care Med 2001;27:1288-96.

100. Steingrub JS, Lagu T, Rothberg MB, et al. Treatment with neuromuscular blocking agents and the risk of in-hospital mortality among mechanically ventilated patients with severe sepsis. Br Care Med 2014;42:90-6.

101. Garnacho-Montero J, Amaya-Villar R, Garcia-Garmendia JL, et al. Effect of critical illness polyneuropathy on the withdrawal from mechanical ventilation. Crit Care Med 2005;33:349-54.

102. Kessler SM, Sprenkle MD, David WS, et al. Severe weakness complicating status asthmaticus despite minimal duration of neuromuscular paralysis. 2009;35:157-60.

103. Leatherman JW, Fluegel WL, David WS, et al. Muscle weakness in mechanically ventilated patients with severe asthma. Am J Respir Crit Care Med 1996;153:1686-90.

104. Adnet F, Dhissi G, Borron SW, et al. Complication profiles of adult asthmatics requiring paralysis during mechanical ventilation. Intensive Care Med 2001;27:1729-36.

105. Behbehani NA, Al-Mane F, D'yachkova Y, et al. Myopathy following mechanical ventilation for acute severe asthma. The role of muscle relaxants and corticosteroids. Chest 1999;115:1627-31.

106. Coakley JH, Nagendran K, Yarwood GD, et al. Patterns of neurophysiological abnormality in prolonged critical illness. Intensive Care Med 1998;24:801-7.

107. Papazian L, Forel JM, Gacouin A, et al. Neuromuscular blockers in early acute respiratory distress syndrome. N Engl J Med 2010;363:1108-16.

108. Forel JM, Roch A, Marin V, et al. Neuromuscular blocking agents decrease inflammatory response in patients with acute respiratory distress syndrome. Crit Care Med 2006;34:2749-57.

109. Gainnier M, Roch A, Forel JM, et al. Effect of neuromuscular blocking agents on gas exchange in patients with acute respiratory distress syndrome. Crit Care Med 2004;32:113-9.

110. Puthucheary Z, Rawal J, Ratnayake G, et al. Neuromuscular blockade and skeletal muscle weakness in critically ill patients. Time to rethink the evidence? Am J Respir Crit Care Med 2012;185:911-7.

111. Forel JM, Roch A, Papazian L. Paralytics in critical care: not always the bad guy. Curr Opin Crit Care 2009;15:59-66.

112. Murray MJ, Cowen J, DeBlock H, et al. Clinical practice guidelines for sustained neuromuscular blockade in the critically ill adult. Crit Care Med 2002;30:142-56.

113. Donati F, Meistelman C, Plaud B. Vecuronium neuromuscular blockade at the diaphragm, the orbicularis oculi and adductor pollicis muscles. Anesthesiology 1990;73:870-5.

114. Donati F. Neuromuscular blocking drugs for the new millennium: current practice, future trends— comparative pharmacology of neuromuscular blocking drugs. Anesth Analg 2000;90(5S):S2-S6.

115. Pantuck EJ. Plasma cholinesterase: gene and variations. Anesth Analg 1993;77:380-6.

116. Primo-Parmo SL, Bartels CF, Wiersema B, et al. Characterization of 12 silent alleles of the human butyrylcholinesterase (BCHE) gene. Am J Hum Genet 1996;58:52-64.

117. Chapple DJ, Miller AA, Ward JB, et al. Cardiovascular and neurological effects of laudanosine. Studies in mice and rats and in conscious and anesthetized dogs. Br J Anaesth 1987;59:218-25.

118. Manthous CA, Chatila W. Atracurium and status epilepticus? Crit Care Med 1995;23:1440-2.

119. Griffiths RB, Hunter JM, Jones RS. Atracurium infusions in patients with renal failure on ITU. Anaesthesia 1986;41:375-81.

120. Beemer GH, Dawson PJ, Bjorksten AR, et al. Early postoperative seizures in neurosurgical patients administered atracurium and isoflurane. Anaesth Intensive Care 1989;17:504-9.

121. Eddleston JM, Harper NJ, Pollard BJ, et al. Concentrations of atracurium and laudanosine in cerebrospinal fluid and plasma during intracranial surgery. Br J Anaesth 1989;63:525-30.

122. Warr J, Thiboutot Z, Rose L, et al. Current therapeutic uses, pharmacology and clinical considerations of neuromuscular blocking agents for critically ill adults. Ann Pharmacother 2011;45:1116-26.

123. Mueller SW, Winn R, Macht M, et al. Neuromuscular blockade resistance during therapeutic hypothermia. Ann Pharmacother 2011;45:e15

124. Morken J, West MA. Abdominal compartment syndrome in the intensive care unit. Curr Opin Crit Care 2001;7:268-74.

125. Cheatham ML, Malbrain ML, Kirkpatrick A, et al. Results from the International Conference of Experts on Intra-abdominal Hypertension and Abdominal Compartment Syndrome: II. Recommendations. Intensive Care Med 2007;33:951-62.

126. Acute Respiratory Distress Syndrome Network. Ventilation with lower tidal volumes as compared with traditional tidal volumes for acute lung injury and the acute respiratory distress syndrome. N Engl J Med 2000;342:1301-8.

127. Burns KE, Adhikari NK, Slutsky AS, et al. Pressure and volume limited ventilation for the ventilator management of patients with acute lung injury: a systematic review and meat-analysis. PLoS ONE 2011;6:e14623.

128. Briel M, Meade M, Mercat A, et al. Higher vs lower positive end-expiratory pressure in patients with acute lung injury and acute respiratory distress syndrome: systematic review and meta-analysis. JAMA 2010;303:865-73.

129. Sud S, Friedrich JO, Taccone P, et al. Prone ventilation reduces mortality in patients with acute respiratory failure and severe hypoxemia: systematic review and meta-analysis. Intensive Care Med 2010;36:585-99.

130. Arroliga AC, Thompson T, Ancukiewicz M, et al. Use of sedatives, opioids and neuromuscular blocking agents in patients with acute lung injury and acute respiratory distress syndrome. Crit Care Med 2008;36:1038-88.

131. Carlon GC, Combs A. Role of sedation and analgesia in mechanical ventilation. Crit Care Med 2008;36:1366-7.

132. Arroliga AC, Frutos-Vivar F, Hall J, et al. Use of sedatives and neuromuscular blocking agents in a cohort of patients receiving mechanical ventilation. Chest 2005;128:496-506.

133. Alhazzani W, Alshahrani M, Jaeschke R, et al. Neuromuscular blocking agents in acute respiratory distress syndrome: a systematic review and meta-analysis of randomized controlled trials. Crit Care 2013;17:R43.

134. Clinical study of early use of neuromuscular blocking agents in patients with severe sepsis and acute respiratory distress syndrome [in Chinese]. Zhonghua Wei Zhong Bing Ji Jiu Yi Xue 2014;26:325-9.

135. Hsiang JK, Chestnut RM, Crisp CB, et al. Early routine paralysis for intracranial pressure control in severe head injury: is it necessary? Crit Care Med 1994;22:1471-6.

136. Juul N, Morris GF, Marshall SB, et al. Neuromuscular blocking agents in neurointensive care. Acta Neurochir Suppl 2000;76:467-70.

137. Prielipp RC, Robinson JC, Wilson JA, et al. Dose response, recovery and cost of doxacurium as a continuous infusion in neurosurgical intensive care unit patients. Crit Care Med 1997;25:1236-41.

138. Schramm WM, Papousek A, Michalek-Sauberer A, et al. The cerebral and cardiovascular effects of cisatracurium and atracurium in neurosurgical patients. Anesth Analg 1998;86:123-7.

139. Schramm WM, Jesenko R, Bartunek A, et al. Effects of cisatracurium on cerebral and cardiovascular hemodynamics in patients with severe brain injury. Acta Anaesthesiol Scand 1997;41:1319-23

140. Kerr ME, Sereika SM, Orndoff P, et al. Effect of neuromuscular blockers and opiates on the cerebrovascular response to endotracheal suctioning in adults with severe head injuries. Am J Crit Care 1998;7:205-17.

141. Prough DS. Does early neuromuscular blockade contribute to adverse outcome after acute head injury. Crit Care Med 1994;22:1349-50.

142. Rangel-Castillo L, Gopinath S, Robertson CS. Management of intracranial hypertension. Neurol Clin 2008;26:521-41.

143. Bernard SA, Gray TW, Buist MD, et al. Treatment of comatose survivors of out-of-hospital cardiac arrest with induced hypothermia. N Engl J Med 2002;346:557-63.

144. The Hypothermia After Cardiac Arrest Study Group. Mild therapeutic hypothermia to improve the neurologic outcome after cardiac arrest. N Engl J Med 2002;346:549-56.

145. Chamorro C, Borrallo JM, Romera MA. Anesthesia and analgesia protocol during therapeutic hypothermia after cardiac arrest: a systematic review. Anesth Analg 2010;110:1328-35.

146. Rosetti AO, Urbano LA, Delodder F, et al. Prognostic value of continuous EEG monitoring during therapeutic hypothermia after cardiac arrest. Crit Care 2010;14:R173.

147. Salciccioli JD, Cocchi MN, Rittenberger JC, et al. Continuous neuromuscular blockade with decreased mortality in post-cardiac arrest patients. Resuscitation 2013;84:1728-33.

148. Baker WL, Geronila G, Kallur R, et al. Effect of neuromuscular blockers on outcomes in patients receiving therapeutic hypothermia following cardiac arrest. Analg Resusc Curr Res 2013, S1. Available at http://dx.doi.org/10.4172/2324-903X. Accessed July 22, 2015.

149. Heier T, Caldwell JE. Impact of hypothermia on the response to neuromuscular blocking drugs. Anesthesiology 2006;104:1070-80.

150. Heier T, Caldwell JE, Sharma ML, et al. Mild intraoperative hypothermia does not change the pharmacodynamics (concentration-effect relationship) of vecuronium in humans. Anesth Analg 1994;78:973-7.

151. Cammu G, Coddens J, Hendrickx J, et al. Dose requirements of infusions of cisatracurium or rocuronium during hypothermic cardiopulmonary bypass. Br J Anaesth 2000;84:587-90.

152. Crepeau AZ, Rabinstein AA, Fugate JE, et al. Continuous EEG in therapeutic hypothermia after cardiac arrest: prognostic and clinical value. Neurology 2013;80:339-44.

153. Greenberg SB, Vender J. The use of neuromuscular blocking agents in the ICU: where are we now? Crit Care Med 2013;41:1332-44.

154. Cheatham ML, Malbrain MLNG, Kirkpatrick A, et al. Results from the conference of experts on intra-abdominal hypertension and abdominal compartment syndrome. Part II: recommendations. Intensive Care Med 2007;33:951-62.

155. De Laet I, Hoste E, Verholen E, et al. The effect of neuromuscular blockers on intraabdominal pressure. Crit Care Med 2006;34:A70.

156. Davies J, Aghahoseini A, Crawford J, et al. To close or not to close? Treatment of abdominal compartment syndrome by neuromuscular blockade without laparostomy. Ann R Coll Surg Engl 2010;92:W8-W9.

157. Goddard S, Fan E. "Only few find the way, some don't recognize it when they do…" – can we "observe" causality? Crit Care Med 2014;42:208-9.

158. Stolling JL, Diedrich DA, Oven LJ, et al. Rapid sequence intubation: a review of the process and considerations when choosing medications. Ann Pharmacother 2014;48:62-76.

159. McManus MC. Neuromuscular blockers in surgery and intensive care, part 2. Am J Health Syst Pharm 2001;58:2381-99.

160. Perry JJ, Lee JS, Sillberg VAH, et al. Rocuronium versus succinylcholine for rapid sequence induction intubation (review). Cochrane Database Syst Rev 2008;2:CD002788.

161. Marsch SC, Steiner L, Bucher E, et al. Succinylcholine versus rocuronium for rapid sequence intubation in intensive care: a prospective, randomized controlled trial. Crit Care 2011;15:R1999.

162. Kopman AF, Khan NA, Neuman GC. Precurarization and priming: a theoretical analysis of safety and timing. Anesth Analg 2001;93:1253-6.

163. Donati F. The priming saga: where do we stand now [editorial]? Can J Anaesth 1988;35:1-4.

164. Schmidt J, Irouschek A, Muenster T, et al. A priming technique accelerates onset of neuromuscular blockade at the laryngeal adductor muscles. Can J Anesth 2005;52:50-4.

165. Engbaek J, Howardy-Hansen P, Ording J, et al. Precurarization with vecuronium and pancuronium in awake, healthy volunteers: the influence on neuromuscular transmission and pulmonary function. Acta Anaesthesiol Scand 1985;29:117-20.

166. Schreiber JU, Lysakowski C, Fuchs-Buder T, et al. Prevention of succinylcholine-induced fasciculation and myalgia: a meta-analysis of randomized trials. Anesthesiology 2005;103:877-84.

167. Naguib M, Samarkandi AH, Ammar A, et al. Comparative clinical pharmacology of rocuronium, cisatracurium and their combination. Anesthesiology 1998;89:1116-24.

168. Katz RL. Modification of the action of pancuronium by succinylcholine and halothane. Anesthesiology 1971;35:602-6.

169. Ono K, Manabe N, Ohta Y, et al. Influence of suxamethonium on the action of subsequently administered vecuronium or pancuronium. Br J Anaesth 1989;62:324-6.

170. Stirt JA, Katz RL, Murray AL, et al. Modification of atracurium blockade by halothane and suxamethonium: a review of clinical experience. Br J Anaesth 1983;55(suppl 1):71S-75S.

171. Naguib M, Abdulatif M, Selim M, et al. Dose-response studies of the interaction between mivacurium and suxamethonium. Br J Anaesth 1995;74:26-30.

172. Walts LF, Rusin WD. The influence of succinylcholine on the duration of pancuronium neuromuscular blockade. Anesth Analg 1977;56:22-5.

173. Cooper R, Mirakhur RK, Clarke RS, et al. Comparison of intubating conditions after administration of Org 9246 (rocuronium) and suxamethonium. Br J Anaesth 1992;69:269-73.

174. Tortorici MA, Tortorici MA, Kochanek PM, et al. Effects of hypothermia on drug disposition, metabolism and response: a focus of hypothermia-mediated alterations on the cytochrome P450 enzyme system. Crit Care Med 2007;35:2196-204.

175. Arpino PA, Greer DM. Practical pharmacologic aspects of therapeutic hypothermia after cardiac arrest. Pharmacotherapy 2008;28:102-11.

176. Van den Broeck MPH, Groenendaal F, Egberts ACG, et al. Effects of hypothermia on pharmacokinetics and pharmacodynamics. A systematic review of preclinical and clinical studies. Clin Pharmacokinet 2010;49:277-94.

177. Feldman SA, Fauvel N. Onset of neuromuscular block. In: Pollard BJ, ed. Applied Neuromuscular Pharmacology. Oxford, UK: Oxford University Press, 1994:69-84.

178. Donati F, Meistelman C, Plaud B. Vecuronium neuromuscular blockade at the diaphragm, the orbicularis oculi and adductor pollicis muscles. Anesthesiology 1990;73:870-5.

179. Kopman AF, Lawson D. Milliamperage requirements for supramaximal stimulation of the ulnar nerve with surface electrodes. Anesthesiology 1984;61:83-5.

180. Waud BE, Waud DR. The relation between the response to "train-of-four" stimulation and receptor occlusion during competitive neuromuscular block. Anesthesiology 1972;37:413-6.

181. Waud BE, Waud DR. The margin of safety of neuromuscular transmission in the muscle of the diaphragm. Anesthesiology 1972;37:417-22.

182. Lee C, Katz RL. Fade of neurally evoked compound electromyogram during neuromuscular block by d-tubocurarine. Anesth Analg 1977;56:271-5.

183. Dulin PG, Williams CJ. Monitoring and preventive care of the paralyzed patient in respiratory failure. Crit Care Clin 1994;10:815-27.

184. Rudis MI, Guslits BG, Zarowitz BJ. Technical and interpretive problems of peripheral nerve stimulation in monitoring neuromuscular blockade in the intensive care unit. Ann Pharmacother 1996;30:165-7.

185. Ali HH, Utting JE, Gray TC. Quantitative assessment of residual antidepolarizing block. Br J Anaesth 1971;43:473-7.

186. Dutton RP, Donati F. A twitch in time. Anesth Analg 2014;119:230-1.

187. Donati F. Residual paralysis: a real problem or did we invent a new disease? Can J Anesth 2013;60:714-29.

188. Rudis MI, Sikora CA, Angus E, et al. A prospective, randomized controlled evaluation of peripheral nerve stimulation versus standard clinical dosing of neuromuscular blocking agents in critically ill patients. Crit Care Med 1997;25:575-93.

189. Strange C, Vaughan L, Franklin C, et al. Comparison of train-of-four and best clinical assessment during continuous paralysis. Am J Respir Crit Care Med 1997;156:1556-61.

190. Baumann MH, McAlpin W, Brown K, et al. A prospective randomized comparison of train-of-four monitoring and clinical assessment during continuous ICU cisatracurium paralysis. Chest 2004;126:1267-73.

191. El-Orbany M, Ali HH, Baraka A, et al. Residual neuromuscular block should, and can be, a "never" event. Anesth Analg 2014;118:691.

192. Murphy GS, Szokol JW, Avram MJ, et al. Postoperative residual neuromuscular blockade is associated with impaired clinical recovery. Anesth Analg 2013;117:133-41.

193. Murphy GS, Szokol JW, Marymont JH, et al. Residual neuromuscular blockade and critical respiratory events in the postanesthesia care unit. Anesth Analg 2008;107:130-7.

194. Donati F, McCarroll SM, Antzaka C, et al. Dose-response curves for edrophonium, neostigmine, and pyridostigmine after pancuronium and d-tubocurarine. Anesthesiology 1987;66:471-6.

195. Smith CE, Donati F, Bevan DR. Dose response relationships for edrophonium and neostigmine as antagonists of atracurium and vecuronium neuromuscular blockade. Anesthesiology 1989;71:37-43.

196. Goldhill DR, Carter JA, Suresh D, et al. Antagonism of atracurium with neostigmine. Effect of dose on speed of recovery. Anaesthesia 1991;46:496-9.

197. McCourt KC, Mirakhur RK, Kerr CM. Dosage of neostigmine for reversal of rocuronium block from two levels of spontaneous recovery. Anaesthesia 1999;54:651-5.

198. Morita T, Kurosaki D, Tsukagoshi H, et al. Factors affecting neostigmine reversal of vecuronium block during sevoflurane anaesthesia. Anaesthesia 1997;52:538-43.

199. Bevan JC, Collins L, Fowler C, et al. Early and late reversal of rocuronium and vecuronium with neostigmine in adults and children. Anesth Analg 1999;89:333-9.

200. Goldhill DR, Wainwright AP, Stuart CS, et al. Neostigmine after spontaneous recovery from neuromuscular blockade. Effect on depth of blockade monitored with train-of-four and tetanic stimuli. Anaesthesia 1989;44:293-9.

201. Astley BA, Katz RL, Payne JP. Electrical and mechanical responses after neuromuscular blockade with vecuronium, and subsequent antagonism with neostigmine or edrophonium. Br J Anaesth 1987;59:983-8.

202. Payne JP, Hughes R, Al Azawi S. Neuromuscular blockade by neostigmine in anaesthetized man. Br J Anaesth 1980;52:69-76.

203. Srivastava A, Hunter JM. Reversal of neuromuscular block. Br J Anaesth 2009;103:115-29.

204. Caldwell JE. Clinical limitations of acetylcholinesterase antagonists. J Crit Care 2009;24:21-8.
205. Ballard N, Robley L, Barrett D, et al. Patients' recollections of therapeutic paralysis in the intensive care unit. Am J Crit Care 2006;15:86-94.
206. Ekman A, Stalberg E, Sundman E, et al. The effect of neuromuscular block and noxious stimulation on hypnosis monitoring during sevoflurane anesthesia. Anesth Analg 2007;105:688.
207. Van Kralingen SI, van de Garde EM, Knibbe CA, et al. Comparative evaluation of atracurium dosed on ideal body weight vs. total body weight in morbidly obese patients. Br J Clin Pharmacol 2011;71:34-40.
208. Kirkegaard-Nielsen H, Helbo-Hansen HS, Lindholm P, et al. Anthropometric variables as predictors for the duration of action of atracurium-induced neuromuscular block. Anesth Analg 1996;83:1076-80.
209. Weinstein JA, Matteo RS, Ornstein E, et al. Pharmacodynamics of vecuronium and Atracurium in the obese surgical patient. Anesth Analg 1988;67:1149-53.
210. Meyhoff CS, Lund J, Jenstrup MT, et al. Should dosing of rocuronium in obese patients be based on ideal or corrected body weight? Anesth Analg 2009;109:787-92.
211. Leykin Y, Pellis T, Lucca M, et al. The pharmacodynamic effects of rocuronium when dosed according to real body weight or ideal body weight in morbidly obese patients. Anesth Analg 2004;99:1086-9.
212. Puhringer FK, Khuenl-Brady KS, Mitterschiffthaler G. Rocuronium bromide: time course of action in underweight, normal weight, overweight and obese patients. Eur J Anaesthesiol 1995;12(suppl 11):107-10.
213. Puhringer FK, Keller C, Kleinsasser A, et al. Pharmacokinetics of rocuronium bromide in obese patients. Eur J Anaesthesiol 1999;16:507-10.
214. Leykin Y, Pellis T, Lucca M, et al. The effects of cisatracurium on morbidly obese women. Anesth Analg 2004;99:1090-4.
215. O'Connor MF, Roizen MF. Use of muscle relaxants in the intensive care unit. J Intensive Care Med 1993;8:34-46.30.
216. Mazze RI, Escue HM, Houston JB. Hyperkalemia and cardiovascular collapse following administration of succinylcholine to the traumatized patient. Anesthesiology 1969;31:540-7.
217. Tobey RE, Jacobsen PM, Kahle CT, et al. The serum potassium response to muscle relaxants in neural injury. Anesthesiology 1972;37:332-7.
218. Murray MJ, DeBlock H, Erstad B, et al. Clinical practice guidelines for the use of neuromuscular-blocking agents in the critically ill adult. Crit Care Med 2016. In press.

Chapter 10

Shock Syndromes

Ishaq Lat, Pharm.D., FCCP, FCCM, BCPS; and Sajni Patel, Pharm.D., BCPS

LEARNING OBJECTIVES

1. Distinguish between the various shock syndromes given a patient's clinical and hemodynamic parameters.
2. Identify critical determinants affecting oxygen delivery.
3. Construct a hemodynamic monitoring plan that incorporates data from monitoring devices and markers of perfusion.
4. Devise a treatment strategy for the treatment of a patient with hypovolemic or obstructive shock.

ABBREVIATIONS IN THIS CHAPTER

CO	Cardiac output	PCWP	Pulmonary capillary wedge pressure
CVC	Central venous catheter	PE	Pulmonary embolism
CVP	Central venous pressure	RV	Right ventricle/ventricular
DO_2	Oxygen delivery	SBP	Systolic blood pressure
LV	Left ventricle/ventricular	SV	Stroke volume
MAP	Mean arterial pressure	SVR	Systemic vascular resistance
PAC	Pulmonary arterial catheter	VO_2	Oxygen consumption
PCC	Prothrombin complex concentrate		

INTRODUCTION

Shock is a heterogeneous syndrome affecting about one-third of all patients requiring intensive care.[1] Best defined as circulatory failure, shock originates from a mismatch in oxygen delivery (DO_2) and oxygen consumption (VO_2). Shock is a heterogeneous syndrome spanning a wide spectrum, beginning with oxygen mismatch. Continued shock ultimately results in end-organ failure and death. The clinical presentation of shock can be subtle in many patients, and the diagnosis of shock is typically based on the interpretation of clinical, hemodynamic, and laboratory findings.[2] In many cases, shock becomes evident in the setting of arterial hypotension, with a systolic blood pressure (SBP) less than 90 mm Hg or a mean arterial pressure (MAP) less than 70 mm Hg. However, these values are arbitrary and population based, possibly leading to under-recognition of the syndrome in select patients. For example, a patient with persistent hypertension and a baseline SBP of 170 mm Hg may have a suboptimal DO_2 with an SBP of 110 mm Hg.

Clinical manifestation of shock can present in a variety of forms. Typically, shock can be identified in gross examination of three distinct end-organ systems: central nervous system (mentation, orientation), renal (urine output less than 0.5 mL/kg/hour), and skin (cold and clammy, reduced capillary refill, decreased skin turgor).[2]

Dysoxia is typified by the development of hyperlactatemia. The exact threshold by which to define hyperlactatemia is variable but is commonly described as greater than 1.5 or 2 mmol/L.[3,4] When insufficient oxygen is present at tissue beds, lactate and adenosine triphosphate production is promoted through the lactate dehydrogenase pathway.[5]

The circulatory system serves the vital need of delivering oxygen to promote homeostasis and end-organ function. End-organ function is dependent on a critical supply of DO_2. In healthy adults, oxygen is inspired and delivered by passive diffusion into the alveoli, where it reversibly binds to hemoglobin, and is taken to the myocardium. Oxygen transportation to the end organs is dependent on stable cardiac output (CO). On reaching the tissue beds, oxygen is taken up by the mitochondria for aerobic metabolism. In advanced shock syndromes, blood flow is redirected from extravital end organs (e.g., skin, gut, kidneys) to prioritize consistent DO_2 to vital organs (e.g., heart and brain). Oxygen delivery is dependent on several tightly regulated variables (Table 10.1).

HEMODYNAMIC MARKERS AND PERFUSION

Hemodynamic parameters can directly be measured from noninvasive monitoring devices or invasive monitoring devices, or they can be calculated using direct measurements (Table 10.2).

Mean arterial blood pressure is the driving pressure for peripheral blood flow and is used as a surrogate marker to estimate end-organ perfusion. Mean arterial pressure can be calculated by noninvasive measures using the following equation: MAP = [SBP + (2 × DBP)]/3. Blood pressure can be measured by auscultation using a sphygmomanometer or oscillometry, or it can be directly measured using an intra-arterial catheter. Noninvasive blood pressure is obtained by inflating the cuff above the patient's SBP, resulting in occlusion of blood flow and no audible sound on auscultation.[6,7] The first Korotkoff sound will be heard once the cuff pressure is incrementally reduced to the level of the patient's SBP. This sound is the result of vibration caused by the return of intermittent blood flow against the arterial wall. In conditions with high vascular resistance (e.g., cardiogenic shock), there is low venous compliance, resulting in diminished sound formation. Likewise, in conditions with low vascular resistance (e.g., septic shock), low flow results in diminished sound formation. In the setting of shock, blood pressures obtained from auscultation may underestimate the systolic and diastolic blood pressures and are often unreliable. Oscillometry measures the pulsation of the artery wall as a pressure vibration against an inflated cuff. It can be set to automatically cycle, allowing for dynamic monitoring of critically ill patients with shock. The accuracy of this modality largely depends on the appropriate size and fit of the cuff.

Intra-arterial Catheter

Arterial catheters provide a means for continuous blood pressure monitoring, and they are considered the gold standard monitoring modality for patients who are being treated for shock requiring the administration of vasoactive medications. Arterial catheters are also used for obtaining arterial blood samples to assess pulmonary gas exchange. They are placed under sterile conditions, usually in the radial artery, but they can be placed in the axillary, brachial, femoral, and dorsalis pedis arteries. Complications from arterial access include hemorrhage, access-site hematoma, arterial thrombosis, pseudoaneurysm, and infection.[8]

Central Venous Catheter

The central venous catheter (CVC) can be used to measure the central venous pressure (CVP), administer medications and fluids, procure venous blood gases, and perform other laboratory assays. Central venous catheters are placed under sterile conditions into the internal jugular vein, subclavian vein, axillary vein, or femoral vein. Complications from CVC access include pneumothorax, catheter-associated bloodstream infection, hemorrhage, and thrombosis.[9]

Central venous pressure is used interchangeably with *right atrial pressure*. The utility of CVP as a marker of fluid resuscitation and fluid responsiveness is limited by several variables. It is falsely elevated in patients with tricuspid regurgitation, isolated right ventricular (RV) dysfunction, high pulmonary arterial pressures, and mechanical ventilation because of increased intrathoracic pressure.[9-11] Central venous pressure is a poor quantitative measure of volume status because its utility in determining fluid responsiveness is lacking.[12-14] Central venous pressure should be used with caution to estimate left ventricular (LV) end-diastolic volume.[9] In one single-center study of 96 patients with severe sepsis or septic shock that looked at the relationship between pre-resuscitation CVP and fluid responsiveness, fluid responsiveness was defined as a rise in cardiac index greater than 15%.[14] The authors concluded that a pre-resuscitation CVP less than 8 mm Hg predicted fluid responsiveness with a sensitivity of 62%, specificity of 54%, and positive predictive value of only 51%. Given the data analyses suggesting mortality improvement in targeting a CVP greater than 8 mm Hg in the early management of sepsis, recent guidelines recommend that the use of CVP as a resuscitation parameter be limited to the brief initial resuscitation period in early sepsis management.[15,16] However, this

Table 10.1 Oxygen Delivery and Consumption

Variables	Equation
Cao_2, Cvo_2, VO_2, CO	CO = VO_2/(Cao_2 − Cvo_2)
DO_2, CO, Cao_2	DO_2 (mL/minute) = 10 × CO (L/minute) − (Cao_2)
Cao_2, Sao_2, Pao_2	(Cao_2 = (1.34 × Hgb × Sao_2) + (0.003 × Pao_2))
VO_2, CO, Cao_2, Cvo_2	VO_2 (mL/minute) = 10 × CO (L/minute) × (Cao_2 − Cvo_2)
Cvo_2, Svo_2, Pvo_2	Cvo_2 = (1.34 × Hgb × Svo_2) + (0.003 × Pvo_2)

Cao_2 = arterial oxygen content; Cvo_2 = venous oxygen content; DO_2 = oxygen delivery; Hgb = hemoglobin; Pvo_2 = mixed venous oxygen tension; Sao_2 = arterial oxygen saturation; Svo_2 = venous saturation; VO_2 = oxygen consumption.

recommendation may be reevaluated in light of recent findings inconclusive of previous findings.[17,18]

Pulmonary Arterial Catheter

The pulmonary arterial catheter (PAC; Swan-Ganz catheter) provides several useful hemodynamic parameters, including pulmonary artery systolic pressure; pulmonary artery diastolic pressure; pulmonary capillary wedge pressure (PCWP), also known as pulmonary artery occlusion pressure; and mixed venous oxygen saturation. In addition, CO and systemic vascular resistance (SVR) can be calculated using parameters measured from the PAC. The routine use of PACs to guide therapies has largely fallen out of favor in critically ill patients.[16] In clinical practice, most PAC use is reserved for patients with advanced heart failure requiring inotropic support, patients with mixed-picture shock to optimize hemodynamics, and patients undergoing cardiothoracic surgery.[19,20] Complications of PAC include arrhythmia, right bundle branch block, complete heart block in patients with left bundle branch block, pulmonary infarction, infection, thrombus, air embolus, and pulmonary artery rupture.[21]

Cardiac output is the product of heart rate and stroke volume (SV).[22] In the presence of normal electrical conduction, heart rate is largely mediated by the autonomic nervous system. In healthy patients, tachycardia does not result in hemodynamic compromise. Conversely, in the setting of shock or myocardial dysfunction, tachycardia results in increased myocardial oxygen demand, decreased diastolic filling time, reduced SV, decreased CO, and decreased coronary artery perfusion. Severe bradycardia can also precipitate a shock syndrome in patients with myocardial dysfunction. Slow heart rate can result in increased ventricular filling and derangement of the Frank-Starling curve in patients with myocardial dysfunction.[23]

Stroke volume is the volume of blood ejected during systole, calculated by subtracting the end-systolic volume from the end-diastolic volume. Stroke volume is primarily determined by preload, afterload, and contractility. Preload is the ventricular end-diastolic volume and is directly proportional to SV through the Frank-Starling mechanism. Increased venous return results in a stretch of the myocardial sarcomeres and increased force of contraction. Of note, the Frank-Starling mechanism can have significant derangements in

Table 10.2 Hemodynamic Parameters

Parameter	Equation (as applicable)	Normal Value
Systolic blood pressure (SBP)		90–140 mm Hg
Diastolic blood pressure (DBP)		60–90 mm Hg
Mean arterial pressure (MAP)	[SBP + (2 × DBP)]/3	70–100
Heart rate (HR)		60–80
Central venous pressure (CVP) or right atrial pressure (RAP)		2–6 mm Hg
Right ventricular systolic pressure (RVSP)		
Right ventricular diastolic pressure (RVDP)		
Pulmonary artery systolic pressure (PASP)		20–30 mm Hg
Pulmonary artery diastolic pressure (PADP)		8–12 mm Hg
Mean pulmonary arterial pressure (mPAP)	[PASP + (2 × PADP)]/3	12–15 mm Hg
Pulmonary capillary wedge pressure (PCWP) or pulmonary arterial occlusion pressure (PAOP)		5–12 mm Hg
Pulmonary vascular resistance (PVR)	80 × [(mPAP − PCWP)/CO] (divide by 80 for W units)	20–120 dynes·s·cm^{-5} (< 2 Wood units)
Mixed venous oxygen saturation (Svo$_2$)		70%–75%
Left ventricular end-diastolic pressure (LVEDP)		
Cardiac output (CO)	HR × SV	4–7 L/min
Cardiac index (CI)	CO/BSA	2.5–4.2 L/min/m^2
Stroke volume (SV)	CO/HR	60–130 mL/beat
Systemic vascular resistance (SVR)	80 × [(MAP − CVP)/CO]	800–1200 dynes·s·cm^{-5}
Arterial oxygen saturation (Sao$_2$)		95%–100%

the presence of heart failure with a reduced ejection fraction.[24-26] Preload is estimated in patients with a PAC using the PCWP. The PCWP requires inflation of a balloon at the distal tip of the PAC that wedges in the pulmonary artery capillary bed during diastole. This results in a static column of blood that connects the tip of the PAC to the left atrium while completely occluding the right heart and pulmonary artery diastolic pressures. Thus, PCWP estimates left atrial pressure and LV end-diastolic pressure (because the mitral valve is open during diastole). Afterload is the arterial resistance to systole. In a heart with normal systolic function, an increase in afterload has little impact on SV. Conversely, in heart failure with a reduced ejection fraction, increased afterload results in decreased SV and increased ventricular end-systolic pressure. The heart has two distinctly different afterloads to overcome. Pulmonary artery systolic pressure and pulmonary vascular resistance mediate RV afterload. Left ventricular afterload is mediated by SVR (also known as total peripheral resistance). Systemic vasoconstriction increases SVR, whereas vasodilation decreases SVR. Contractility is the intrinsic ability of the myocardium to contract. Activation of the sympathetic nervous system or the use of medications with inotropic properties can increase contractility. Heart failure with a reduced ejection, acute myocardial infarction, acidosis, and medications with negative inotropic properties can result in decreased contractility.

Cardiac output is the volume of blood ejected from the LV per minute.[22] Because CO is heart rate × SV, CO can be manipulated by altering either variable. Cardiac output can be determined by two means: through thermodilution or using the Fick equation. Thermodilution involves an injection of chilled intravenous fluid with a known temperature into the right atrial port of the PAC and the subsequent measurement of temperature change of the blood in the pulmonary artery.[27-29] In patients with a reduced CO, more time is required for the temperature to return to baseline, whereas in patients with normal or high CO, blood flow is carried quickly through the heart, and temperature rapidly returns to normal. Thermodilution is not accurate in patients with tricuspid regurgitation, patients with intracardiac shunting, mechanically ventilated patients with high positive end-expiratory pressure, and patients with severely reduced ventricular function. In these patients, the Fick CO is calculated using the equation CO = [(135 mL/minute O_2/m^2) × BSA]/[13.4 × hemoglobin × (Sao_2 − Svo_2)]. Fick is considered the gold standard in determining CO; however, it is sometimes not used because it requires the collection of several variables (expired air sample, hemoglobin, arterial oxygen saturation [Sao_2], central venous oxygen saturation [$Scvo_2$]).

Clinical Indices of Hypoperfusion

General indices of hypoperfusion include a MAP less than 60 mm Hg, oliguria (urine output less than 0.5 mL/kg/hour), altered mental status, delayed capillary refill, and cool skin.[9,30,31] Other measures include oxyhemoglobin saturation and serum lactate concentration.

The oxyhemoglobin saturation of venous blood drawn from a central vein ($Scvo_2$) or the pulmonary artery (Svo_2) is expressed as a percentage and is used as a surrogate marker for CO. The normal range for Svo_2 is 65%–75%. The $Scvo_2$ is drawn from a subclavian or internal jugular CVC where the catheter tip terminates in the superior vena cava. As such, $Scvo_2$ is a reflection of oxygen extraction in the brain and upper body more than systemic oxygen extraction. The $Scvo_2$ drawn from a femoral CVC reflects only oxygen extraction from the lower body and does not account for cerebral oxygen extraction. Therefore, a femoral $Scvo_2$ cannot be used interchangeably with an $Scvo_2$ drawn from a thoracic CVC.[32,33]

The Svo_2 value is drawn from a PAC and is a more accurate representation of systemic oxygen extraction because it represents the mixing of venous blood from the superior vena cava (upper extremity and cerebral oxygen extraction), inferior vena cava (lower extremity and abdominal organ oxygen extraction), and coronary sinus (myocardial oxygen extraction). Low Svo_2 is an indicator of a mismatch in the VO_2/DO_2 ratio, suggesting inadequate tissue perfusion. A low Svo_2 (less than 70%) is predictive of poor outcomes and has been associated with increased mortality.[32,34] Early reperfusion strategies targeting an Svo_2 greater than 70% in patients with septic shock showed improved survival.[15] However, more recent studies tested the value of using resuscitation protocols, targeting an Svo_2 greater than 70% in patients with septic shock, failed to show a survival benefit from this intervention.[17,18] Therefore, venous oxygen monitoring in septic shock should be used judiciously. In sepsis, microcirculatory shunting in the periphery can result in a lack of oxygen extraction. In addition, impaired mitochondrial oxygen use can result in normal or supranormal Svo_2, despite the presence of severe local tissue dysoxia.[35]

Strategies to improve Svo_2 include fluid resuscitation, transfusion of packed red blood cells when the hemoglobin is less than 7 (for most critically ill patients) to increase oxygen supply, or administration of inotropic medications to improve DO_2.[36]

Elevated blood lactate concentration (above 2 mmol/L) can also be used as a marker of tissue hypoperfusion. In the setting of dysoxia and shock, glycolysis transitions to anaerobic metabolism. Under these circumstances, lactate is the end product of glycolysis.[37-39] Elevated lactate concentrations may be the result of increased production (type A), decreased clearance (type B), or both. Type A lactic acidosis occurs in the setting of decreased DO_2 to tissues. Type B lactic acidosis occurs in the setting of impaired lactate clearance from the liver or kidneys or has medication-related causes that impair oxidative phosphorylation (e.g., metformin, epinephrine, linezolid, propylene glycol, cocaine, or toxic alcohols).[5] Serial lactate concentrations can be used as a resuscitation parameter, with the resolution of hyperlactatemia signifying the return of adequate systemic oxygenation.[40,41] However, the utility of lactate as a resuscitation parameter is limited in severe liver dysfunction because of the major role (60%–70%) of the liver in the clearance of lactate.[42] Severe liver dysfunction can lead to persistent or worsened lactate elevations in shock states.

DIFFERENTIATION OF SHOCK STATES

Classically, shock can be classified into one of four categories: (1) hypovolemic, (2) obstructive, (3) cardiogenic, and (4) distributive.[43] The various subtypes of shock are not mutually exclusive and can occur simultaneously. The estimated mortality increases with the co-occurrence of shock syndromes. Each of the shock categories is characterized by some mix of fluid loss, depressed CO, or maldistribution of oxygen because of the insufficiency of the peripheral uptake of oxygen (Table 10.3).

In a prospective, multicenter study of 1,679 intensive care unit patients, septic shock was the most common form of shock, accounting for greater than 60% of all patients with shock.[44] Septic shock is characterized as a form of distributive shock, representing a complex interplay of cardiac and peripheral components to dysoxia. Septic shock will be discussed in detail in another chapter.

Other forms of shock become apparent on physical examination and focused assessment of hemodynamic parameters. For example, cardiogenic shock is likely in advanced heart failure or after a massive myocardial infarction. In a multinational study of patients hospitalized with acute coronary syndrome between 1999 and 2007, the incidence of cardiogenic shock was 4.6%, with an in-hospital mortality rate of 59.4%.[45] Hypovolemic shock usually presents after acute loss of plasma (e.g., traumatic hemorrhage, surgical bleeding, gastrointestinal [GI] bleeding), burn injury, or sequestration of fluid within a body compartment (e.g., third spacing). Obstructive shock is apparent in impaired systolic contraction (e.g., pulmonary hypertension, massive pulmonary embolism [PE], or aortic dissection) or impaired diastolic filling (e.g., cardiac tamponade, tension pneumothorax, pericarditis).

Vasopressors and Inotropes

In most cases, vasopressors and inotropes are administered transiently to get patients through a critical period until the underlying etiology of shock is resolved. Vasopressors are initiated in patients who remain hypotensive despite adequate fluid resuscitation or in patients with severe hypotension during fluid resuscitation (see the Fluids, Electrolytes, and Nutrition section for further discussion of fluid components). Dynamic markers of resuscitation should be used to determine the efficacy of vasoactive agents; however, data are sparse regarding which resuscitation parameter is best.[46,47] Resuscitation goals should depend on a confluence of patient-specific factors and will evolve throughout the care of a patient with shock. The clinician should use the patient-specific hemodynamic parameters when choosing a vasoactive agent (Table 10.4).[48] Ultimately, the initiation and continuation of vasoactive agents are targeted to optimize the VO_2/DO_2 relationship. Of importance, it is critical to acknowledge that, for all vasopressors, doses and titration of therapy are unknown and based on collective experience. Dose suggestions provided in this chapter are taken from the primary literature.

The β_1-receptors are found primarily in the heart. Agonism at the β_1-receptor results in increased inotropy (contractility), increased chronotropy (heart heart), and increased dromotropy (conduction velocity). In general, agents with higher β_1-receptor affinity are used in patients with cardiogenic shock to improve contractility or in select patients with bradyarrhythmias to increase chronotropy. The most common adverse effects of β_1-receptor stimulation are atrial and ventricular tachyarrhythmias. The β_2-receptors are located in the vascular smooth muscle, and agonism results in systemic vasodilation.

The α_1-receptors are located throughout the body within the arteries, stomach, intestine, kidneys, and liver. The α_1-receptors are a primary mediator of arterial tone. Agonism at the α_1-receptors within the arteries results in vasoconstriction and an increase in SVR.

The dopamine 1 (D_1) receptors are located in the kidney, heart, and splanchnic vasculature. Agonism at the D_1-receptor results in vasodilation of the renal, coronary, and mesenteric beds.[48,49]

Table 10.3 Hemodynamic Profile of Shock States

Shock State	CVP	PCWP	CO	SVR
Hypovolemic	↓	↓	↑	↑
Cardiogenic	↑	↑	↓	↑
Distributive	↓	↓	↑	↓
Obstructive				
Impaired diastolic filling	↑	↑	↓	↑
Obstructive				
Impaired systolic contraction	↑	↓	↓	↑

Table 10.4	Vasoactive Pharmacology					
	α^1	β^1	β^2	Dopamine	Vasopressin	Dose
Phenylephrine	+++	-	-	-	-	0.25–9 mcg/kg/min
Norepinephrine	+++	++	-	-	-	2.5–40 mcg/kg/min
Epinephrine	+++	+++	+	-	-	1–20 mcg/kg/min
Dopamine	++	+++	+	+++	-	0.5–50 mcg/kg/min
Vasopressin	-	-	-	-	+++	0.01–0.04 unit/min

The vasopressin (V_1, V_2) receptor, also called antidiuretic hormone, is an endogenous substance secreted from the hypothalamus in response to hypotension and high serum osmolality. The V_1-receptors are located in the vascular smooth muscle; agonism at this receptor results in vasoconstriction. The V_2-receptors are located within the renal collecting duct; V_2 agonism results in water reabsorption from the distal tubules and collecting ducts of the nephron.[50,51]

Dopamine is an endogenous catecholamine with dose-dependent receptor activity at the D_1-, β_1-, and α_1-receptors. Dopamine dosing breakpoints listed in this section are generalizations and should therefore not be considered absolute rules because patients can have variable responses to this medication according to their clinical scenario. Low doses (less than 3 mcg/kg/minute) cause vasodilation in the renal and mesenteric beds.[52-54] However, studies have shown no renal protective effect from the use of low-dose dopamine in critically ill patients.[52,55,56] Furthermore, the use of low-dose dopamine can have deleterious effects on respiratory drive, can induce or aggravate euthyroid sick syndrome, and can cause visceral ischemia.[57] For this reason, this treatment modality is not recommended.[16] Moderate doses (3–10 mcg/kg/minute) are thought to primarily cause β_1-agonist activity and increased contractility and chronotropy. High doses (10–20 mcg/kg/minute) have mixed β_1 and α_1 activity resulting in increased SVR and contractility. Dopamine has many adverse effects including digital ischemia, tachyarrhythmias, and cardiac ischemia. In addition, there is evidence that dopamine can blunt hypoxic respiratory ventilator response, and it has been theorized that dopamine use in critically ill patients can delay liberation from mechanical ventilation.[58-60] Dopamine is no longer recommended as a first-line agent in the management of shock states as a result of a large, multicenter, randomized control trial comparing dopamine with norepinephrine in all-comers with shock. The study found no difference in mortality between the two groups at 28 days. However, dopamine use resulted in significantly higher rates of arrhythmic events (24.1% vs. 12.4%, p<0.001). In addition, in the subgroup analysis of patients with cardiogenic shock, dopamine administration resulted in a significantly higher rate of all-cause mortality.[44]

Norepinephrine is an endogenous catecholamine with a strong affinity for the α_1-receptor and a modest β_1-agonist effect. This results in increased SVR in patients with shock but has a moderate effect on cardiac contractility and chronotropy. Because norepinephrine has a reduced effect on chronotropy compared with dopamine, it is often used in patients with shock complicated by tachyarrhythmias. Prolonged exposure to norepinephrine can result in digital ischemia, visceral ischemia, and cardiotoxicity, causing myocardial chamber dilation, hypertrophy, and ultimately systolic dysfunction.[61,62]

Epinephrine is an endogenous catecholamine with agonist activity at the β_1-, β_2-, and α_1-receptors. At low doses of epinephrine, β_1 and β_2 activity predominates, resulting in increased inotropy, chronotropy, and CO. At higher doses, epinephrine has a strong affinity for the α_1-receptor, resulting in increased vascular tone and SVR.[61,63,64] Low-dose epinephrine is commonly used after cardiac surgery for inotropic effects or for chronotropic effect in patients with bradycardia associated with high-grade atrioventricular nodal block. Adverse effects of epinephrine include renal and splanchnic vasoconstriction, tachyarrhythmias, and digital ischemia. Prolonged infusions can result in myocardial dysfunction through myocyte apoptosis.[48,49,65]

Phenylephrine is a pure α_1-receptor agonist that increases MAP by increasing SVR. Phenylephrine is used as an adjunct to other vasopressors in refractory shock, to increase SVR in patients with severe aortic stenosis or to decrease LV outflow tract gradient in patients with hypertrophic obstructive cardiomyopathy. It is also used in patients with shock complicated by tachyarrhythmias. Adverse effects of phenylephrine include baroreceptor-mediated reflex bradycardia, digital ischemia, visceral ischemia, and tissue necrosis with extravasation.[48,64,66] See Figure 10.1 for selection of vasopressor therapy.

Hypovolemic Shock

Hypovolemic shock is primarily caused by hemorrhage and acute bleeding disorders. Occasionally, hypovolemic shock may be attributed to extensive volume loss (e.g.,

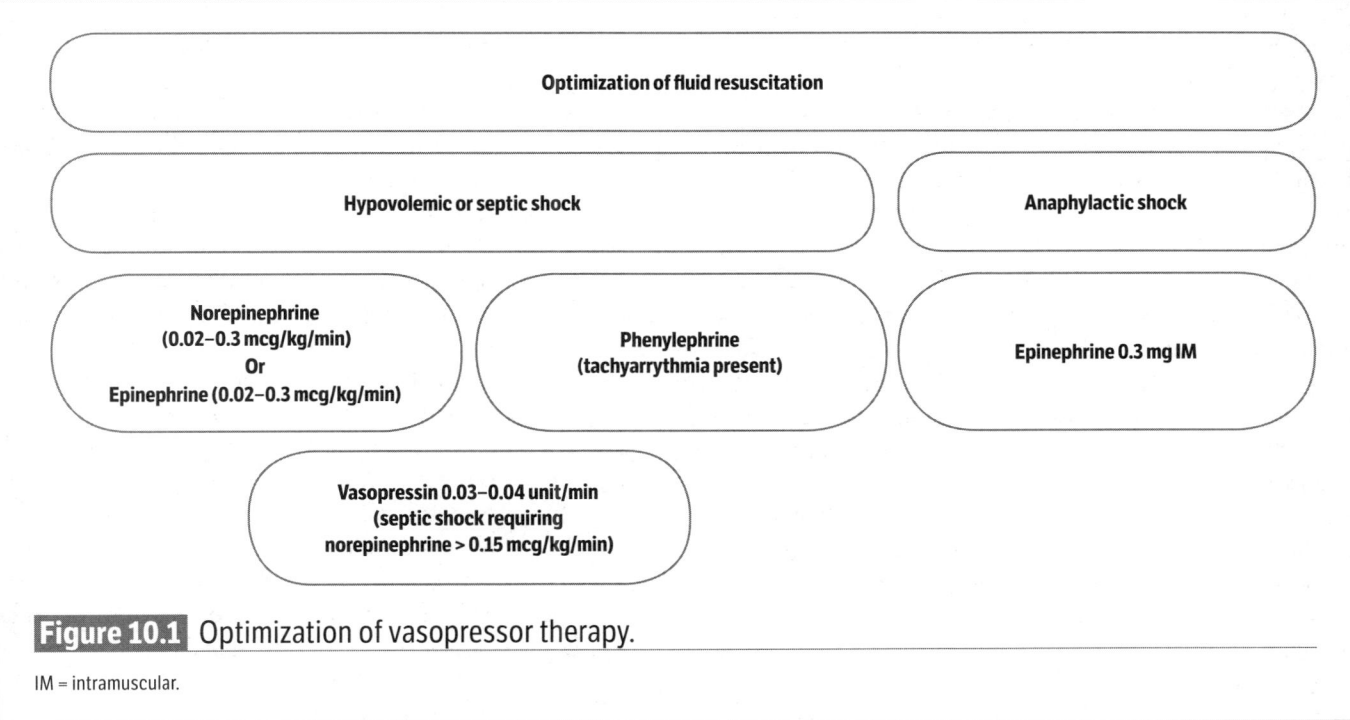

Figure 10.1 Optimization of vasopressor therapy.

IM = intramuscular.

hemodialysis, diabetes insipidus) or extensive third spacing of intravascular volume. In the setting of bleeding, the principal concern is the circulatory system's inability to tolerate loss of blood.

Fluids account for around 50%–60% of total body weight in normal adults. Of this total, blood accounts for 60–66 mL/kg of body weight, representing 7%–12% of total body fluid.[67,68] Acute blood loss activates rapid changes to maintain blood volume and perfusion.[69] The initial response will facilitate capillary fill from the interstitium.[70] However, this movement of fluid will result in a deficit in the interstitial compartment. Progressively, activation of the renin-angiotensin-aldosterone system (RAAS) leads to sodium retention and replenishment of the interstitial fluid deficit. Activation of the RAAS may begin 8–12 hours after acute blood loss. Collectively, this compensatory response will maintain effective blood volume in the case of mild volume loss (less than 15% of blood volume) while resulting in adaptation in the form of SV, heart rate, and SVR. Volume loss in excess of 15% will require intravascular repletion. Blood loss is classified in four categories (Table 10.5).

Specific to hemorrhagic shock, clotting factors and platelets will be lost in addition to blood. It is estimated that 25% of all trauma patients will have an established coagulopathy on presentation to the emergency department.[71] The loss of hemoglobin will compromise DO_2. In addition, crystalloid resuscitation will lead to a dilutional coagulopathy, further compromising the ability to cease bleeding.

Resuscitation Strategies for Hypovolemic Shock

In hypovolemic shock, mortality is directly related to the extent of organ hypoperfusion. Therefore, prompt and deliberate repletion of intravascular fluids is key to survival and restoration of end-organ function.[72] When possible, cessation of bleeding, or volume loss, is key.

The goals of resuscitation are to restore end-organ perfusion and improve DO_2, beginning with the administration of intravenous fluids. After establishing venous access, the essential questions to guide resuscitation are as follows: (1) what type of fluid, (2) how much, (3) over what period, and (4) when to stop (i.e., what are therapeutic end points?). Patients with severe bleeding will not have compromised tissue oxygenation as long as an effective intravascular volume is maintained, even at low hemoglobin concentrations.[73] Although there exists the debate of crystalloid versus colloid fluid choice, literature and many clinicians believe crystalloid resuscitation, in the form of lactated Ringer solution or normal saline, to be the primary means of intravenous resuscitation. However, many clinicians prefer lactated Ringer when large-volume resuscitation is needed because of the development of hyperchloremic metabolic acidosis with large volumes of normal saline.[67] Recognition of third-space losses has led to a "three-to-one" rule for resuscitation: 3 mL of crystalloid fluid for every 1 mL of blood loss.[73-75]

Hypertonic saline has held promise among many clinicians as a resuscitative fluid. Potential benefits of hypertonic saline include its lesser distribution in the interstitium, oncotic effects to expand the vascular space, and portability because of the lesser amount of fluid needed to exert the same therapeutic benefit as isotonic fluids (normal saline or lactated Ringer).[76,77] However, there is a lack of convincing data to date that shows the superiority of hypertonic saline.[78]

There has existed a long-standing debate regarding the utility of colloidal fluids for resuscitation. Commonly reported colloidal therapies include albumin, hetastarch, and dextran. The primary purported benefit of colloids is their ability to be retained in the vascular compartment to a greater degree than crystalloids. This would mainly be because of their greater molecular weight. However, clinical trials have no found no benefit of one fluid over another.[79-82]

Blood transfusions are indicated when the estimated blood loss exceeds 30%. However, estimating blood loss in the clinical setting is exceedingly difficult, and the decision to transfuse blood products is largely empirical. In practice, many clinicians transfuse blood products if the patient is hypotensive despite receiving 2 L of crystalloid fluid in the setting of an acute bleed. Practice guidelines recommend blood transfusion for a hemoglobin of 6–8 g/dL in critically ill patients.[83] A randomized controlled trial of a restrictive transfusion strategy (hemoglobin 7–9 g/dL) compared with a conventional transfusion strategy (hemoglobin 10–12 g/dL) showed similar survival outcomes (19% vs. 23%, p=0.11), and mortality during hospitalization was significantly lower in the conservative transfusion arm (22% vs. 28%, p=0.05). A conservative transfusion strategy (hemoglobin 7–9 g/dL) has since become a standard of care in many intensive care units.[36] Mortality during hospitalization was significantly lower in the conservative transfusion arm (22% vs. 28%, p=0.05). In the setting of GI hemorrhage, a conservative transfusion strategy (hemoglobin less than 7 g/dL) compared with a liberal transfusion strategy (hemoglobin less than 9 g/dL) was associated with reduced rates of further bleeding (10% vs. 16%, p=0.01), fewer adverse effects (40% vs. 48%, p=0.02), and improved survival at 6 weeks (95% vs. 91%, hazard ratio 0.55 [95% confidence interval, 0.33–0.92; p=0.02]). Both studies support the notion that maintaining a hemoglobin in excess of 10 g/dL, without the necessity of improving DO_2, is largely unnecessary and may be harmful. Transfusion of blood products is not innocuous and carries the risk of viral transmission (e.g., HIV, hepatitis). Other adverse effects related to transfusions include electrolyte abnormalities, transfusion-related reactions, and the concern for immunosuppression.

Currently, the timing and intensity of resuscitation in the patient with hypovolemic shock is largely unanswered. Although it may seem intuitive to initiate prompt and aggressive resuscitation, literature from the trauma setting suggests otherwise.[84] In a prospective study of 598 adult patients with penetrating torso trauma and an SBP less than 90 mm Hg, delayed resuscitation until operative intervention was associated with an improved survival and discharge from the hospital alive (70% vs. 62%, p=0.04). Urban location, time to hospital transfer, and time to operative intervention are factors that may challenge the external validity of the study findings. Nevertheless, there is a lack of evidence in other clinical scenarios of hypovolemic shock that warrant further study. Concerns with aggressive resuscitation include the risk of worsening bleeding injury through increased velocity through the bleeding diathesis, worsening coagulopathy, and oxidative injury.

COAGULOPATHY

The incidence of coagulopathy after acute hemorrhage is associated with increased mortality and acute lung injury, multiple organ failure, and infections.[85] In the wake of an acute hemorrhage, a combination of hypothermia, acidosis, and coagulopathy contribute to a maladaptive hemostatic response, further perpetuating the bleeding episode.[86-88] Hypothermia is of serious consequence in the setting of hypovolemic shock because oxygen is not as readily uncoupled from hemoglobin to facilitate O_2 delivery as in the normothermic patient. Hypothermia also potentiates coagulopathy by inhibiting full activation of the clotting cascade.[87,89] Passive and active warming methods to establish a core body temperature greater than 34°C are essential to reestablishing normal physiology and promoting hemostasis. In addition, prompt correction of acidosis to a pH greater than 7.20, through preload resuscitation, and coagulopathy, through blood product replacement, are essential to reversal of the triad. A typical approach to blood product replacement has been transfusion of packed red blood cells, fresh frozen plasma, cryoprecipitate, and platelets in a 1:1:1:1 ratio.[90]

Table 10.5 American College of Surgeons Hemorrhage Categories

Class	Blood Loss	Description
I	≤15%	Minor, clinical findings of shock absent
II	15%–30%	Mild tachycardia, postural hypotension, and reduced urine output
III	30%–40%	Moderate tachycardia, hypotension, oliguria, and marked confusion. Reduced response to vasopressor therapy
IV	≥40%	Exaggerated tachycardia, hypotension, anuria, and obtundation

Modified from: Committee on Trauma. Advanced Trauma Life Support Student Manual. Chicago: American College of Surgeons, 1997:103-12.

Systemic therapies to establish hemostasis in the patient with bleeding have been studied and reported. Recombinant activated factor VIIa (rFVIIa) works by activating the extrinsic pathway of the coagulation cascade by interacting with tissue factor to activate factor X to factor Xa and factor IX to factor IXa. Preliminary case reports and case reports have suggested that administering rFVIIa improved clinical outcomes. However, a multicenter, randomized, controlled trial of rFVIIa in trauma patients was terminated early because of futility in the primary end point of mortality, despite showing a reduction in transfusion of packed red blood cells.[91] Database reviews report an increased incidence of venous and arterial thromboembolic events with off-label rFVIIa use.[92,93] Currently, there is no consensus on how rFVIIa should be used for the treatment of acute bleeding and hypovolemic shock.

Four different forms of prothrombin complex concentrates (PCCs) are available in the United States (Table 10.6). Of the different types of PCCs, only FEIBA (factor eight inhibitor bypassing inhibitor activity) possesses activated clotting factors. Kcentra is the only PCC to be approved for the indication of reversal of warfarin-related bleeding. All other PCC products are approved for hemophilia-related bleeding disorders. Extrapolating the use of PCCs for the treatment of acute bleeding disorders not related to the approved indications is experimental, and thoughtful consideration should be given to pharmacology, time to administration in the acute setting, and potential harms.

Tranexamic acid is an antifibrinolytic agent that has its pharmacodynamic effect through binding plasminogen to prevent the dissolution of a fibrin clot. Tranexamic acid was studied in trauma patients with hypovolemic shock caused by acute bleeding in a multicenter, randomized, placebo-controlled trial that showed improvement in 28-day mortality and mortality attributable to bleeding.[94] In a subsequent analysis, the greatest benefit to the administration of tranexamic acid was noted when administered within the first 3 hours of injury. Tranexamic acid and α-aminocaproic acid have been studied for use in other settings, but with limited evidence.

OBSTRUCTIVE SHOCK

Obstructive shock is defined as the physical obstruction of the great vessels (pulmonary artery and aorta) or the heart itself. Therefore, obstructive shock is further broken into two distinct pathophysiologic mechanisms: impairment in diastolic filling (tension pneumothorax, cardiac tamponade, or constrictive pericarditis) and excessive afterload (severe pulmonary arterial hypertension, PE).

Cardiac tamponade occurs secondary to fluid accumulation within the intrapericardial space, resulting in alteration in the cardiac pressure-volume relationship, where the intrapericardial pressure exceeds that of the intracardiac pressure. This leads to diastolic collapse of the right atrial and ventricular free walls during expiration, a reduction in venous return, a subsequent reduction in CO, and ultimately shock.[95] The emergency drainage of pericardial effusions is typically reserved for patients with RV collapse, hemodynamic instability (SBP less than 110 mm Hg), and the presence of pulsus paradoxus (greater than a 10-mm Hg drop in SBP during inspiration). Pericardiocentesis can be performed under fluoroscopy in the cardiac catheterization laboratory, drained under echocardiography at the bedside, or surgically drained. The creation of a surgical pericardial window is typically reserved for the management of recurrent effusions. Given the RV dependence on preload, initial management strategies may also include the judicious administration of intravenous fluids to patients with hemodynamic instability. However, fluid administration is only transiently beneficial, and a definitive strategy is required in patients with signs of impending collapse. Mechanical ventilation should be initiated with caution in patients with tamponade physiology caused by increased intrathoracic pressure, which can further decrease diastolic filling and may result in hemodynamic collapse.

Tension pneumothorax is typically caused by blunt thoracic trauma. It results in the progressive accumulation of air within the pleural space and displacement of the mediastinum. Mediastinal displacement can obstruct venous return, resulting in shock. Treatment requires immediate tube thoracostomy or needle decompression. Similar to tamponade, positive pressure ventilation can exacerbate pneumothorax; therefore, pneumothorax should be treated before intubation.

Pulmonary embolism refers to the thrombotic occlusion of the pulmonary artery. The clinical presentation of PE can be heterogeneous, making diagnosis and the initiation of prompt treatment a challenge. Pulmonary embolism is a common etiology of obstructive shock caused by a severe increase in RV afterload resulting in RV overload (Table 10.7). Typically, the RV pumps blood into the low pressure pulmonary

Table 10.6 Comparison of Prothrombin Complex Concentrates

	Factor II	Factor VII	Factor IX	Factor X
Bebulin VH	X		X	X
FEIBA[a]	X	X	X	X
Kcentra[b]	X	X	X	X
Profilnine SD	X	X	X	X

[a]Contains mainly nonactivated factors II, IX, and X; factor VII is mainly in the activated form. Values expressed are for the FEIBA 500-unit vial, which also contains protein C 550 units.

[b]Values expressed are for the Kcentra 500-unit vial, which also contains protein C 420–820 units and protein S 240–680 units.

Table 10.7 Markers of RV Dysfunction in Pulmonary Embolism

Test	Findings
Cardiac biomarkers	Brain natriuretic peptide > 90 pg/mL
	N-terminal pro-brain natriuretic peptide (> 500 pg/mL)
	Troponin-I (> 0.4 ng/mL)
	Troponin-T (> 0.1 ng/mL)
Echocardiography	Septal bowing
	RV hypokinesis
	RV systolic pressure > 40 mm Hg
Computed tomography	RV diameter/LV diameter ratio > 0.9
Electrocardiogram	Right bundle branch block (incomplete or complete)
	T-wave inversions in V^1–V^4
	S1Q3T3: S wave in lead I, Q wave in lead III, and T-wave inversion in lead III

LV = left ventricular; RV = right ventricular.

Box 10.1. Contraindications for the Use of Fibrinolysis in Pulmonary Embolism

Absolute Contraindications
- Any prior intracranial hemorrhage
- Known structural cerebrovascular disease
- Known malignant intracranial neoplasm
- Ischemic stroke within the past 3 months
- Suspected aortic dissection
- Active bleeding or bleeding diathesis
- Recent surgery on the brain or spinal canal
- Recent significant closed-head or facial trauma with radiographic evidence of bony fracture or brain injury

Relative Contraindications
- Age > 75 years
- Current use of anticoagulation
- Pregnancy
- Noncompressible vascular punctures
- Traumatic or prolonged cardiopulmonary resuscitation (> 10 minutes)
- Recent internal bleeding (within 2–4 weeks)
- History of chronic, severe, and poorly controlled hypertension
- Severe uncontrolled hypertension on presentation (SBP > 180 mm Hg or DBP > 110 mm Hg)
- Dementia
- Remote (> 3 months) ischemic stroke
- Major surgery within 3 weeks

---

artery. However, in an acute PE, the RV must overcome a mechanical obstruction in addition to an acute rise in pulmonary arterial pressure secondary to hypoxic vasoconstriction. This results in RV overload and RV dilation, derangement of the Frank-Starling pressure-volume relationship, RV hypokinesis, intraventricular septal deviation toward the LV, reduction in LV size and preload, and reduction in systemic CO. The ensuing systemic hypotension and shock results in a decreased right coronary artery perfusion, RV ischemia and infarction, reduction in RV contractility, and further decrease in RV CO.

The initial management strategy for the management of a hemodynamically significant PE includes the judicious administration of fluids to maintain RV preload and CO; thrombolytic medications, when indicated; and anticoagulants (Box 10.1). Close monitoring of these patients must be used to ensure that over-resuscitation does not worsen RV dilation and contractility. (See chapter 23, "Prevention and Treatment of Venous Thromboembolism," for additional information.)

DISTRIBUTIVE SHOCK

Distributive shock is best characterized as an acute failure of the capacitance vessels, leading to a loss in perfusion and DO_2 to end organs. Most commonly, this occurs in the setting of acute infection and is called septic shock. Septic shock stems from an infection that leads to an imbalance in proinflammatory and anti-inflammatory cytokines, which also contributes to disorders of the coagulation system and the microcirculation. Septic shock will be described in detail in chapter 15, "Severe Sepsis and Septic Shock."

Anaphylactic shock is the most feared complication of allergic reactions. Patients with eczema, asthma, and allergic rhinitis are at greatest risk of having anaphylactic reactions. Primarily because of the release of inflammatory cytokines from mast cells and basophils in response to antigen exposure, a multisystem organ failure rapidly develops, leading to hives, flushing, diarrhea, stridor, angioedema, and hypotension. Antigens can include a variety of exposures, not limited to bee stings, eggs, nuts, and medications (e.g., β-lactams, aspirin, protamine). Antigen binding to immunoglobulin E (IgE) triggers a series of pathophysiologic processes resulting in bronchial smooth muscle contraction, vasodilation, and ventricular depression. Epinephrine administered intramuscularly is the primary treatment for an anaphylactic episode (0.01 mg/kg for children weighing less than 10 kg; 0.15 mg for children weighing 10–25 kg; 0.30 mg for children and adults weighing more than 25 kg). Although intuitive, evidence does not support the administration of antihistamines (histamine-1 and histamine-2 antagonists) for the treatment of anaphylactic reactions. Corticosteroids have no benefit in the immediate treatment, but they may mitigate the risk of a biphasic anaphylactic reaction.[96,97]

CONCLUSION

Shock represents a heterogeneous collection of syndromes. Effective treatment requires a thorough assessment of patient-specific factors, an understanding of pharmacologic agents, and a time-sensitive application of therapies.

REFERENCES

1. Sakr Y, Reinhart K, Vincent JL, et al. Does dopamine administration in shock influence outcome? Results of the sepsis occurrence in acutely ill patients (SOAP) study. Crit Care Med 2006;34:589-97.
2. Vincent JL, De Backer D. Circulatory shock. N Engl J Med 2013;369:1726-34.
3. Nichol AD, Egi M, Pettila V, et al. Research relative hyperlactatemia and hospital mortality in critically ill patients: a retrospective multi-centre study. Crit Care 2010;14:R25.
4. van Hall G. Lactate kinetics in human tissues at rest and during exercise. Acta Physiol 2010;199:499-508.
5. Kraut JA, Madias NE. Lactic acidosis. N Engl J Med 2014;371:2309-19.
6. Van Bergen FH, Weatherhead DS, Treloar AE, et al. Comparison of indirect and direct methods of measuring arterial blood pressure. Circulation 1954;10:481-90.
7. Bur A, Herkner H, Vlcek M, et al. Factors influencing the accuracy of oscillometric blood pressure measurement in critically ill patients. Crit Care Med 2003;31:793-9.
8. Montenij LJ, de Waal EE, Buhre WF. Arterial waveform analysis in anesthesia and critical care. Curr Opin Anaesthesiol 2011;24:651-6.
9. Hollenberg SM. Hemodynamic monitoring. Chest J 2013;14:1480-8.
10. Antonelli M, Levy M, Andrews PJ, et al. Hemodynamic monitoring in shock and implications for management. International Consensus Conference, Paris, France, 27-28 April 2006. Intensive Care Med 2007;33:575-90.
11. Fessler HE, Brower RG, Wise RA, et al. Effects of positive end-expiratory pressure on the canine venous return curve. Am Rev Respir Dis 1992;146:4-10.
12. Michard F, Teboul JL. Predicting fluid responsiveness in ICU patients: a critical analysis of the evidence. Chest 2002;121:2000-8.
13. Vincent JL, Weil MH. Fluid challenge revisited. Crit Care Med 2006;34:1333-7.
14. Osman D, Ridel C, Ray P, et al. Cardiac filling pressures are not appropriate to predict hemodynamic response to volume challenge. Crit Care Med 2007;35:64-8.
15. Rivers E, Nguyen B, Havstad S, et al. Early goal-directed therapy in the treatment of severe sepsis and septic shock. N Engl J Med 2001;345:1368-77.
16. Dellinger RP, Levy MM, Rhodes A, et al. Surviving Sepsis Campaign: international guidelines for management of severe sepsis and septic shock: 2012. Crit Care Med 2013;41:580-637.
17. ARISE Investigators, ANZICS Clinical Trials Group, Peake SL, et al. Goal-directed resuscitation for patients with early septic shock. N Engl J Med 2014;371:1496-506.
18. ProCESS Investigators, Yealy DM, Kellum JA, et al. A randomized trial of protocol-based care for early septic shock. N Engl J Med 2014;370:1683-93.
19. Valentine RJ, Duke ML, Inman MH, et al. Effectiveness of pulmonary artery catheters in aortic surgery: a randomized trial. J Vasc Surg 1998;27:203-11; discussion 211-2.
20. Bender JS, Smith-Meek MA, Jones CE. Routine pulmonary artery catheterization does not reduce morbidity and mortality of elective vascular surgery: results of a prospective, randomized trial. Ann Surg 1997;226:229-36; discussion 236-7.
21. Gidwani UK, Mohanty B, Chatterjee K. The pulmonary artery catheter: a critical reappraisal. Cardiol Clin 2013;31:545-65, viii.
22. Vincent JL. Understanding cardiac output. Crit Care 2008;12:174.
23. Magder SA. The ups and downs of heart rate. Crit Care Med 2012;40:239-45.
24. Bristow MR, Ginsburg R, Minobe W, et al. Decreased catecholamine sensitivity and beta-adrenergic-receptor density in failing human hearts. N Engl J Med 1982;307:205-11.
25. Bristow MR, Minobe W, Rasmussen R, et al. Beta-adrenergic neuroeffector abnormalities in the failing human heart are produced by local rather than systemic mechanisms. J Clin Invest 1992;89:803-15.
26. Schwinger RH, Bohm M, Koch A, et al. The failing human heart is unable to use the frank-starling mechanism. Circ Res 1994;74:959-69.
27. Horster S, Stemmler HJ, Sparrer J, et al. Mechanical ventilation with positive end-expiratory pressure in critically ill patients: comparison of CW-doppler ultrasound cardiac output monitoring (USCOM) and thermodilution (PiCCO). Acta Cardiol 2012;67:177-85.
28. Hillis LD, Firth BG, Winniford MD. Analysis of factors affecting the variability of fick versus indicator dilution measurements of cardiac output. Am J Cardiol 1985;56:764-8.
29. Moranville MP, Mieure KD, Santayana EM. Evaluation and management of shock states: hypovolemic, distributive, and cardiogenic shock. J Pharm Pract 2011;24:44-60.
30. Worthley LI. Shock: a review of pathophysiology and management. Part I. Crit Care Resusc 2000;2:55-65.
31. Hollenberg SM. Vasopressor support in septic shock. Chest 2007;132:1678-87.
32. Kandel G, Aberman A. Mixed venous oxygen saturation: its role in the assessment of the critically ill patient. Arch Intern Med 1983;143:1400-2.

33. van Beest P, Wietasch G, Scheeren T, et al. Clinical review: use of venous oxygen saturations as a goal – a yet unfinished puzzle. Crit Care 2011;15:232.

34. Varpula M, Karlsson S, Ruokonen E, et al. Mixed venous oxygen saturation cannot be estimated by central venous oxygen saturation in septic shock. Intensive Care Med 2006;32:1336-43.

35. Tyagi A, Sethi AK, Girotra G, et al. The microcirculation in sepsis. Indian J Anaesth 2009;53:281-93.

36. Hebert PC, Wells G, Blajchman MA, et al. A multicenter, randomized, controlled clinical trial of transfusion requirements in critical care. Transfusion requirements in critical care investigators, Canadian Critical Care Trials Group. N Engl J Med 1999;340:409-17.

37. Bakker J, Nijsten MW, Jansen TC. Clinical use of lactate monitoring in critically ill patients. Ann Intensive Care 2013;3:12.

38. Broder G, Weil MH. Excess lactate: an index of reversibility of shock in human patients. Science 1964;143:1457-9.

39. Howell MD, Donnino M, Clardy P, et al. Occult hypoperfusion and mortality in patients with suspected infection. Intensive Care Med 2007;33:1892-9.

40. Shapiro NI, Howell MD, Talmor D, et al. Serum lactate as a predictor of mortality in emergency department patients with infection. Ann Emerg Med 2005;45:524-8.

41. Jones AE, Shapiro NI, Trzeciak S, et al. Lactate clearance vs central venous oxygen saturation as goals of early sepsis therapy: a randomized clinical trial. JAMA 2010;303:739-46.

42. Bellomo R. Bench-to-bedside review: lactate and the kidney. Crit Care 2002;6:322-6.

43. Weil MH, Shubin H. Proposed reclassification of shock states with special reference to distributive defects. Adv Exp Med Biol 1971;23:13-23.

44. De Backer D, Biston P, Devriendt J, et al. Comparison of dopamine and norepinephrine in the treatment of shock. N Engl J Med 2010;362:779-89.

45. Awad HH, Anderson FA Jr, Gore JM, et al. Cardiogenic shock complicating acute coronary syndromes: insights from the global registry of acute coronary events. Am Heart J 2012;163:963-71.

46. Marik PE, Cavallazzi R, Vasu T, et al. Dynamic changes in arterial waveform derived variables and fluid responsiveness in mechanically ventilated patients: a systematic review of the literature. Crit Care Med 2009;37:2642-7.

47. De Backer D, Creteur J, Silva E, et al. Effects of dopamine, norepinephrine, and epinephrine on the splanchnic circulation in septic shock: which is best? Crit Care Med 2003;31:1659-67.

48. Overgaard CB, Dzavik V. Inotropes and vasopressors: review of physiology and clinical use in cardiovascular disease. Circulation 2008;118:1047-56.

49. Day NP, Phu NH, Mai NT, et al. Effects of dopamine and epinephrine infusions on renal hemodynamics in severe malaria and severe sepsis. Crit Care Med 2000;28:1353-62.

50. Holmes CL, Walley KR, Chittock DR, et al. The effects of vasopressin on hemodynamics and renal function in severe septic shock: a case series. Intensive Care Med 2001;27:1416-21.

51. Holmes CL, Patel BM, Russell JA, et al. Physiology of vasopressin relevant to management of septic shock. Chest 2001;120:989-1002.

52. Olson D, Pohlman A, Hall JB. Administration of low-dose dopamine to nonoliguric patients with sepsis syndrome does not raise intramucosal gastric pH nor improve creatinine clearance. Am J Respir Crit Care Med 1996;154(6 pt 1):1664-70.

53. Jakob SM, Ruokonen E, Takala J. Effects of dopamine on systemic and regional blood flow and metabolism in septic and cardiac surgery patients. Shock 2002;18:8-13.

54. Hoogenberg K, Smit AJ, Girbes AR. Effects of low-dose dopamine on renal and systemic hemodynamics during incremental norepinephrine infusion in healthy volunteers. Crit Care Med 1998;26:260-5.

55. Bellomo R, Chapman M, Finfer S, et al. Low-dose dopamine in patients with early renal dysfunction: a placebo-controlled randomised trial. Australian and New Zealand Intensive Care Society (ANZICS) clinical trials group. Lancet 2000;356:2139-43.

56. Marik PE, Iglesias J. Low-dose dopamine does not prevent acute renal failure in patients with septic shock and oliguria. NORASEPT II study investigators. Am J Med 1999;107:387-90.

57. Holmes CL, Walley KR. Bad medicine: low-dose dopamine in the ICU. Chest 2003;123:1266-75.

58. Weiss M, Schneider EM, Tarnow J, et al. Is inhibition of oxygen radical production of neutrophils by sympathomimetics mediated via beta-2 adrenoceptors? J Pharmacol Exp Ther 1996;278:1105-13.

59. Fortenberry JD, Huber AR, Owens ML. Inotropes inhibit endothelial cell surface adhesion molecules induced by interleukin-1beta. Crit Care Med 1997;25:303-8.

60. Dive A, Foret F, Jamart J, et al. Effect of dopamine on gastrointestinal motility during critical illness. Intensive Care Med 2000;26:901-7.

61. Duranteau J, Sitbon P, Teboul JL, et al. Effects of epinephrine, norepinephrine, or the combination of norepinephrine and dobutamine on gastric mucosa in septic shock. Crit Care Med 1999;27:893-900.

62. Reinelt H, Radermacher P, Fischer G, et al. Effects of a dobutamine-induced increase in splanchnic blood flow on hepatic metabolic activity in patients with septic shock. Anesthesiology 1997;86:818-24.

63. Martin C, Viviand X, Arnaud S, et al. Effects of norepinephrine plus dobutamine or norepinephrine alone on left ventricular performance of septic shock patients. Crit Care Med 1999;27:1708-13.

64. Uusaro A, Takala J. Vasoactive drugs and splanchnic perfusion in septic shock. Crit Care Med 1998;26:1458-60.

65. Woolsey CA, Coopersmith CM. Vasoactive drugs and the gut: is there anything new? Curr Opin Crit Care 2006;12:155-9.

66. Yamazaki T, Shimada Y, Taenaka N, et al. Circulatory responses to afterloading with phenylephrine in hyperdynamic sepsis. Crit Care Med 1982;10:432-5.

67. Shires T, Coln D, Carrico J, et al. Fluid therapy in hemorrhagic shock. Arch Surg 1964;88:688-93.

68. Kasuya H, Onda H, Yoneyama T, et al. Bedside monitoring of circulating blood volume after subarachnoid hemorrhage. Stroke 2003;34:956-60.

69. Moore FD. The effects of hemorrhage on body composition. N Engl J Med 1965;273:567-77.

70. Schadt JC, Ludbrook J. Hemodynamic and neurohumoral responses to acute hypovolemia in conscious mammals. Am J Physiol 1991;260(2 pt 2):H305-18.

71. Brohi K, Singh J, Heron M, et al. Acute traumatic coagulopathy. J Trauma 2003;54:1127-30.

72. Husain FA, Martin MJ, Mullenix PS, et al. Serum lactate and base deficit as predictors of mortality and morbidity. Am J Surg 2003;185:485-91.

73. Gutierrez G, Reines HD, Wulf-Gutierrez ME. Clinical review: hemorrhagic shock. Crit Care 2004;8:373-81.

74. Gutierrez G, Wulf-Gutierrez ME, Reines HD. Monitoring oxygen transport and tissue oxygenation. Curr Opin Anaesthesiol 2004;17:107-17.

75. Gutierrez G, Fuller SP. Of hemorrhagic shock, spherical cows and aloe vera. Crit Care 2004;8:406-7.

76. Kramer GC. Hypertonic resuscitation: physiologic mechanisms and recommendations for trauma care. J Trauma 2003;54(5 suppl):S89-99.

77. Rhee P, Koustova E, Alam HB. Searching for the optimal resuscitation method: recommendations for the initial fluid resuscitation of combat casualties. J Trauma 2003;54(5 suppl):S52-62.

78. Wade CE, Kramer GC, Grady JJ, et al. Efficacy of hypertonic 7.5% saline and 6% dextran-70 in treating trauma: a meta-analysis of controlled clinical studies. Surgery 1997;122:609-16.

79. Finfer S, Bellomo R, Boyce N, et al. A comparison of albumin and saline for fluid resuscitation in the intensive care unit. N Engl J Med 2004;350:2247-56.

80. Myburgh JA, Finfer S, Bellomo R, et al. Hydroxyethyl starch or saline for fluid resuscitation in intensive care. N Engl J Med 2012;367:1901-11.

81. Perner A, Haase N, Guttormsen AB, et al. Hydroxyethyl starch 130/0.42 versus ringer's acetate in severe sepsis. N Engl J Med 2012;367:124-34.

82. Brunkhorst FM, Engel C, Bloos F, et al. Intensive insulin therapy and pentastarch resuscitation in severe sepsis. N Engl J Med 2008;358:125-39.

83. Consensus conference. Perioperative red blood cell transfusion. JAMA 1988;260:2700-3.

84. Bickell WH, Wall MJ Jr, Pepe PE, et al. Immediate versus delayed fluid resuscitation for hypotensive patients with penetrating torso injuries. N Engl J Med 1994;331:1105-9.

85. Mitra B, Wasiak J, Cameron PA, et al. Early coagulopathy of major burns. Injury 2013;44:40-3.

86. Gruen RL, Brohi K, Schreiber M, et al. Haemorrhage control in severely injured patients. Lancet 2012;380:1099-108.

87. Cosgriff N, Moore EE, Sauaia A, et al. Predicting life-threatening coagulopathy in the massively transfused trauma patient: hypothermia and acidoses revisited. J Trauma 1997;42:857-61; discussion 861-2.

88. Dunham CM, Siegel JH, Weireter L, et al. Oxygen debt and metabolic acidemia as quantitative predictors of mortality and the severity of the ischemic insult in hemorrhagic shock. Crit Care Med 1991;19:231-43.

89. Counts RB, Haisch C, Simon TL, et al. Hemostasis in massively transfused trauma patients. Ann Surg 1979;190:91-9.

90. Holcomb JB, Tilley BC, Baraniuk S, et al. Transfusion of plasma, platelets, and red blood cells in a 1:1:1 vs a 1:1:2 ratio and mortality in patients with severe trauma: the PROPPR randomized clinical trial. JAMA 2015;313:471-82.

91. Hauser CJ, Boffard K, Dutton R, et al. Results of the CONTROL trial: efficacy and safety of recombinant activated factor VII in the management of refractory traumatic hemorrhage. J Trauma 2010;69:489-500.

92. Logan AC, Yank V, Stafford RS. Off-label use of recombinant factor VIIa in U.S. hospitals: analysis of hospital records. Ann Intern Med 2011;154:516-22.

93. Yank V, Tuohy CV, Logan AC, et al. Systematic review: benefits and harms of in-hospital use of recombinant factor VIIa for off-label indications. Ann Intern Med 2011;154:529-40.

94. CRASH-2 trial collaborators; Shakur H, Roberts I, et al. Effects of tranexamic acid on death, vascular occlusive events, and blood transfusion in trauma patients with significant haemorrhage (CRASH-2): a randomised, placebo-controlled trial. Lancet 2010;376:23-32.

95. Little WC, Freeman GL. Pericardial disease. Circulation 2006;113:1622-32.

96. Jarvinen KM, Amalanayagam S, Shreffler WG, et al. Epinephrine treatment is infrequent and biphasic reactions are rare in food-induced reactions during oral food challenges in children. J Allergy Clin Immunol 2009;124:1267-72.

97. Tedeschi A, Lorini M, Suli C, et al. Detection of serum histamine-releasing factors in a patient with idiopathic anaphylaxis and multiple drug allergy syndrome. J Investig Allergol Clin Immunol 2007;17:122-5.

Section 2

Infectious Diseases

Chapter 11
Appropriate Use of Antimicrobials

Scott T. Micek, Pharm.D.; and Marin H. Kollef, M.D.

LEARNING OBJECTIVES

1. Describe a strategy to deliver appropriate initial antibiotic regimen employing knowledge of local epidemiology, antibiotic resistance prediction tools and clinical decision support systems.
2. Identify possible pharmacokinetic abnormalities in critically ill patients and provide a method to optimize drug dosing given the specific alteration.
3. Describe an approach to antibiotic de-escalation based on negative and positive results of microbiological studies.
4. Provide justification for implementation of antimicrobial stewardship programs in the intensive care unit.

ABBREVIATIONS IN THIS CHAPTER

ARC	Augmented renal clearance	MDR	Multidrug resistant
ASP	Antimicrobial stewardship program	MRSA	Methicillin-resistant *Staphylococcus aureus*
GNB	Gram-negative bacilli	TDM	Therapeutic drug monitoring
HAP	Hospital-acquired pneumonia	VAP	Ventilator-associated pneumonia
ICU	Intensive care unit		

INTRODUCTION

Appropriate use of antimicrobials is an important concept that is pertinent to virtually every clinician. This practice is intended to ensure the optimal selection, dose, and duration of antimicrobials leading to the best clinical outcome for the treatment or prevention of infection while producing the fewest possible adverse effects and the lowest risk of subsequent resistance.[1,2] Although progress in achieving these goals has been realized through the implementation of stewardship programs,[3] there is considerable room for improvement.[4,5] Given the critical nature of patients admitted to the intensive care unit (ICU) setting, optimization of antimicrobial practices in the ICU is of paramount importance.[3,5-7]

Appropriate Antimicrobial Selection

Administering appropriate initial antibiotic therapy is the cornerstone of the management of septic shock as well as of any serious infection requiring ICU care. Appropriate initial antibiotic therapy is defined as an antimicrobial regimen that has in vitro activity against the isolated organism(s) responsible for the infection, whereas inappropriate initial antibiotic therapy is defined as an initial regimen showing a lack of in vitro activity against the causative pathogen(s).[8] The administration of inappropriate initial antibiotic therapy can lead to treatment failures and adverse outcomes.[9,10] It has been shown that patients with septic shock attributed to bacterial infection who received inappropriate initial antimicrobial therapy have an increased risk of mortality relative to patients treated with appropriate initial therapy (odds ratios [ORs] of 1.80–6.86).[11-15] Similar associations between the administration of inappropriate initial antimicrobial therapy and greater mortality have been shown for *Candida* bloodstream infections.[16-18] Moreover, the importance of treating pathogens associated with serious infection was further emphasized by a retrospective cohort analysis of patients with bloodstream infection complicated by severe sepsis and septic shock.[19] For the entire cohort, the number needed to treat (NNT) with appropriate initial antimicrobial therapy to prevent one patient death was 4.0 (95% confidence interval [CI], 3.7–4.3). The prevalence-adjusted pathogen-specific NNT with appropriate initial antimicrobial therapy to prevent one patient death was lowest for multidrug-resistant (MDR) bacteria (NNT = 20), followed by *Candida* spp. (NNT = 34), methicillin-resistant *Staphylococcus aureus* (MRSA; NNT = 38), *Pseudomonas aeruginosa* (NNT = 38), *Escherichia coli* (NNT = 40), and methicillin-susceptible *S. aureus* (NNT = 47).[19]

The importance of selecting appropriate initial antimicrobial therapy has been emphasized in the Surviving Sepsis Guidelines.[20] The guidelines recommend that initial empirical anti-infective therapy include one or more drugs with activity against all likely pathogens (bacterial and/or fungal or viral) and that the antibiotics penetrate in adequate concentrations into the tissues presumed to be the source of sepsis (grade 1B).[20] This guideline urges clinicians to use the patient's history, including drug intolerances, recent receipt of antibiotics, underlying disease, clinical syndrome, and susceptibility patterns of pathogens in the community and hospital that have been previously documented to colonize or infect the patient when making decisions regarding initial antimicrobial regimen selection. However, given the severity of illness for ICU patients with severe sepsis and septic shock, erring on the side of initial overtreatment may be preferable to administering an inappropriate initial antibiotic regimen. Balancing these competing interests is at the core of antimicrobial stewardship in the ICU, and methods for refining this balance are subsequently described.

Identifying Patients at Risk of MDR Pathogens

Knowledge of patient risk factors associated with the presence of infection caused by antibiotic-resistant pathogens should be a routine part of initial antibiotic decision-making (Box 11.1). For example, in patients presenting from the community with pneumonia, risk factors for antibiotic-resistant pathogens include prior hospitalization, immunosuppression, previous antibiotic use, use of gastric acid-suppressive therapy, tube feeding, and nonambulatory status.[21] Severity of illness is another risk factor that has been associated with a higher frequency of MDR pathogens in patients presenting to the hospital with pneumonia.[22] Scoring systems that assign points to individual patients on the basis of disease severity as well as other potential risk factors for MDR pathogens is an approach that can be used to improve the rates of appropriate initial therapy without excessive use of broad-spectrum antibiotic therapy. A retrospective study examined patients admitted with pneumonia and found four variables predictive of antibiotic-resistant pneumonia: recent hospitalization, nursing home residence, hemodialysis, and ICU admission.[23] A scoring system assigning 4, 3, 2,

---

Box 11.1. Risk Factors Associated with Antimicrobial Resistance

Prior antimicrobial exposure
Prolonged antimicrobial therapy
Subtherapeutic antimicrobial dosing
Previous hospitalization
Prolonged hospital stay
Intensive care unit admission or increasing severity of illness
Recent surgery
Insertion of an invasive device(s) (e.g., urinary catheter, central venous catheter, endotracheal tube)
Admission from a long-term care facility
Poor functional status before admission
Chronic comorbidities (heart, lung, liver, or kidney disease; diabetes, immunocompromised)

---

and 1 points, respectively, for each variable had moderate predictive power for segregating those with and without resistant bacteria. Among patients with fewer than 3 points, the prevalence of resistant pathogens was less than 20% compared with 55% and more than 75% in individuals with scores of 3–5 and more than 5 points, respectively. The same scoring system was validated in an independent population showing that it performed better at identifying patients infected with antibiotic-resistant bacteria than simply using the definition of health care–associated pneumonia (HCAP).[24] The risk score was statistically greater among patients with antibiotic-resistant infections (median score, 4 vs. 1; p<0.001). A recent meta-analysis also found that the current definition used for HCAP did not accurately identify infections attributed to antibiotic-resistant pathogens, providing further support for the use of more specific criteria to make this clinically important determination.[25] It is unclear, however, whether clinicians can effectively apply scoring systems prospectively in an effort to target the administration of broad-spectrum antibiotics in patients at greatest risk of infection with antibiotic-resistant infections. This has served as the impetus for developing clinical decision support systems to facilitate such decision-making at the patient's bedside.

Clinical Decision Support Systems

Clinical decision support systems represent a method of coupling patient-specific risk factors for antibiotic-resistant bacteria that is warehoused in local data repositories with historical culture and susceptibility reports to facilitate bedside decision-making. Use of such data at the point of antimicrobial prescription has resulted in a significant reduction in the proportion of patients prescribed broad-spectrum antibiotics after adjustment for risk factors including APACHE II (Acute Physiology and Chronic Health Evaluation II) score, suspected infection, positive microbiology, intubation, and length of stay.[26] In addition, the decision support tool was associated with a 10.5% reduction in both total antibiotic use and use of the highest-volume broad-spectrum antibiotics. Similarly, an automated decision support system with real-time access to patients' prior antibiotic exposures and microbiologic results, including those from prior hospitalizations at outside institutions, has shown that the use of inappropriate initial therapy can be reduced by almost 50% and that access to these data assist in the performance of timely de-escalation.[27] Other benefits derived from the use of computerized systems include improvements in the efficiency and costs of existing stewardship programs, improvements in clinicians' knowledge regarding the treatment of infectious diseases, and improvements in pathogen prediction.[28-33] These data suggest that an opportunity exists to use hospital informatics systems to improve the identification of patients at risk of, or infected with, antibiotic-resistant bacteria in order to prescribe more appropriate initial therapy.

Timing of Antibiotic Administration

In addition to selecting an appropriate initial antimicrobial regimen, the timing of antibiotic administration relative to the onset of symptoms or culture collection is an essential element in determining the outcome of critically ill patients with infection. In a prospective study of patients with ventilator-associated pneumonia (VAP), the administration of appropriate initial therapy that was delayed 24 hours or more after the patient met the diagnostic criteria was identified as a risk factor independently associated with hospital mortality by logistic regression analysis (adjusted OR 7.68; 95% CI, 4.50–13.09; p<0.001).[34] A retrospective study of 2,154 patients with septic shock who received effective antimicrobial therapy in conjunction with the onset of recurrent or persistent hypotension found a strong relationship between the delay in treatment and in-hospital mortality (adjusted OR for increased mortality 1.119 [per hour delay], 95% CI, 1.103–1.136, p<0.0001).[35] Administration of an antimicrobial regimen determined to be effective for the isolated or suspected pathogens within the first hour of documented hypotension was associated with a survival rate of 79.9%. Each hour of delay in antimicrobial administration over the ensuing 6 hours was associated with an average decrease in survival of 7.6% per hour.[35]

A meta-analysis of randomized and observational studies evaluating the impact of goal-directed bundles on the outcomes of patients with septic shock found that timely antibiotic administration was statistically more common among patients receiving protocolized management of septic shock than among those receiving non-protocolized care.[36] One study in this meta-analysis was a prospective observational study that evaluated adult patients with severe sepsis from 77 ICUs.[37] Using a propensity-adjusted multivariate analysis, the authors found that early broad-spectrum antibiotic treatment (treatment within 1 hour vs. no treatment within the first 6 hours of diagnosis) was associated with a significant reduction in hospital mortality (OR 0.67; 95% CI, 0.50–0.90; p=0.008). A retrospective analysis of a large data set collected prospectively from 165 ICUs in Europe, the United States, and South America found a statically significant increase in the probability of death associated with the number of hours of delay for first antibiotic administration.[38] Hospital mortality increased from 24.6% to 33.1% as the time to antibiotic administration increased from 0 to greater than 6 hours where 0–1 hour was the referent group.

Timely administration of effective antibiotics appears to be an important element in determining the outcome of critically ill patients. Emergency departments and ICUs should ensure that processes are in place to obtain and deliver antibiotic therapy expeditiously once the order for such therapy is received from the treating physicians.

Adequate Dosing of Antimicrobials

In addition to delivering timely appropriate antibiotic regimens, adequate drug concentrations at the site of infection are needed to optimize clinical outcomes. It is widely accepted that time-dependent antimicrobials show optimal bacterial killing when the duration of time of the free drug concentration exceeds the pathogen minimum inhibitory concentration (T_{FREE}/MIC). For example, a T_{FREE}/MIC of 100% of the dosage interval should be a theoretical target for β-lactams and carbapenems.[39] However, further improvement in the efficacy of β-lactams has been observed when concentrations 4- to 5-fold greater than the MIC are achieved for prolonged periods during each dosing interval.[40,41] An example of the need for proper antibiotic dosing and drug exposure at the site of infection in critically ill patients was shown in a multicenter trial designed to evaluate whether antibiotic concentrations affect patient outcomes.[42] Of the 248 patients treated with β-lactams for infection, 16% did not achieve a T_{FREE}/MIC greater than 1 at 50% of the dosing interval, and these patients were 32% less likely to have a positive clinical outcome. A positive clinical outcome was associated with a T_{FREE}/MIC ratio greater than 1 at both 50% and 100% of the dosing intervals (OR 1.02 and 1.56, respectively; p<0.03). These data suggest that many critically ill patients have adverse outcomes as a result of inadequate antibiotic exposure.

Several other studies have shown that the doses of antibiotics administered to critically ill patients may need to be augmented despite the clinician's having selected an appropriate initial regimen. Meta-analyses of tigecycline for the treatment of nosocomial infections have shown an increased mortality versus comparator agents, particularly in VAP caused by gram-negative pathogens.[43-45]

A randomized trial of patients with hospital-acquired pneumonia (HAP) found that tigecycline, with or without ceftazidime, had inferior cure rates to imipenem/cilastatin with or without vancomycin across all pathogens (cure rates for VAP were 48% vs. 70%).[46] Researchers hypothesized that the tigecycline dose (75 mg every 12 hours) was too low to achieve high enough concentrations above the MICs of pathogens, which prompted a higher-dose study (100 mg every 12 hours) compared with imipenem/cilastatin.[47] In this study, 85% of the patients in the high-dose tigecycline group achieved clinical cure compared with 75% in the imipenem group, suggesting that underdosing of tigecycline has contributed to the poor outcomes observed in prior trials, especially in VAP. Similarly, ceftobiprole, a cephalosporin with activity against MRSA and a gram-negative spectrum similar to that of ceftazidime or cefepime, was compared with linezolid and ceftazidime in patients with HAP/VAP.[48] Even though similar cure rates in HAP were achieved, ceftobiprole was inferior to linezolid and ceftazidime in patients with VAP (cure rates from intention to treat analysis: 23.1% vs. 36.8%). This finding was thought to be largely because of the underdosing of ceftobiprole in critically ill patients. The concern for underdosing in critically ill patients has led to a doubling of the dose of ceftolozane/tazobactam in the ongoing clinical registration trials of HAP/VAP compared with the dosing regimens used in the intra-abdominal and urinary tract infection registration trials.[49,50]

Pharmacokinetic Considerations

Many factors influence the pharmacokinetics of antimicrobials in critically ill patients and may contribute to the underdosing of antimicrobials. Hypoalbuminemia, large-volume crystalloid administration, large pleural effusions or abdominal ascites, catecholamines, and renal replacement therapies (see Table 11.1) can all significantly alter infection-site concentrations of administered antibiotics.[51,52] One factor worth specific mention is augmented renal clearance (ARC).

Augmented renal clearance is defined as an 8-hour creatinine clearance (CrCl) of 130 mL/minute/1.73 m² or more. At least one recent study suggests that more than 65% of ICU patients have an ARC on at least one occasion during the first 7 days of their critical illness.[53] Augmented renal clearance has been linked with subtherapeutic β-lactam[54] and glycopeptide concentrations[55] as well as increased therapeutic failures in patients receiving antimicrobial therapy, resulting in adverse patient outcomes.[56] In a study comparing 10 days of imipenem/cilastatin with 7 days of doripenem for VAP caused by gram-negative bacilli (GNB), the largest difference in clinical cure rates, which favored the longer-duration imipenem/cilastatin regimen, was in the subgroup of patients with a CrCl greater than 150 mL/minute/1.73 m².[57] This finding suggests that shorter therapy durations among patients with ARC, and thus lower circulating antibiotic concentrations, can contribute to excess mortality. One group of investigators has developed a scoring system to identify patients at high risk of ARC because of the following factors: age 50 years or younger (6 points), trauma (3 points), and Sequential Organ Failure Assessment (SOFA) score of 4 or less (1 point).[58] Higher summated scores were significantly associated with ARC. A subsequent study found that the ARC score was 100% sensitive and 71.4% specific for detecting ARC.[59]

Prolonged Infusions of Antibiotics

To adjust for altered pharmacokinetic parameters in critically ill patients and achieve greater Time>MIC for β-lactams, alternative antimicrobial dosing and administration strategies have been studied. The most common strategy studied has been prolonged or continuous infusions of time-dependent antimicrobials including β-lactams, carbapenems, and vancomycin. Although observational studies have shown better clinical cure rates with prolonged or continuous infusion of β-lactams, two meta-analyses have failed to confirm these findings.[60,61] However, a meta-analysis that included vancomycin and linezolid[62] and another focusing specifically on piperacillin/tazobactam or carbapenems[63] found improved clinical outcomes, including lower mortality, when antibiotics were administered by prolonged or continuous infusion compared with bolus injections. Of note, many of the trials included in these analyses were retrospective in design

Table 11.1 Factors Associated with Underdosing of Antimicrobials

Factor	Pharmacokinetic Effect
Increased cardiac index	Increased antimicrobial clearance
Volume expansion with intravenous fluid resuscitation	Increased volume of distribution
	Decreased maximal antimicrobial concentration
	Increased antimicrobial clearance
Hypoalbuminemia	Increased volume of distribution
	Decreased maximal antimicrobial concentration
	Increased antimicrobial clearance
Augmented renal clearance	Increased antimicrobial clearance in antimicrobials with renal elimination
Continuous renal replacement therapy	Increased antimicrobial clearance in antimicrobials with renal elimination

or of limited power because of small sample size. It is also important to recognize that prolonged infusion of antibiotics will not compensate for poor initial drug selection, inferior drug characteristics, or underdosing of these agents in critically ill patients, as suggested by the tigecycline experience[43-45] and the ceftobiprole study of HAP/VAP.[48] The largest (n=432) randomized, multicenter trial conducted to date of continuous β-lactam infusion compared with intermittent infusion in critically ill patients with severe sepsis found no difference in alive ICU-free days, 90-day survival, or clinical cure 14 days after antibiotic cessation.[64]

Therapeutic Drug Monitoring

The best method to ensure adequate drug concentrations in the serum is therapeutic drug monitoring (TDM).[65,66] However, the use of TDM for antibiotics other than vancomycin, aminoglycosides, and voriconazole has not become a routine or standard practice in most ICUs. Studies have shown the ability of TDM to identify the need for antibiotic dosing adjustments in the setting normal kidney function,[67] fluctuating kidney function,[68] and in the patients with acute kidney injury requiring continuous renal replacement therapy.[69] Unfortunately, large variations currently exist in the type of β-lactams tested, the patients selected for TDM, drug assay methodologies, pharmacokinetic/pharmacodynamic targets, and dose adjustment strategies used in critically ill patients, and further studies are thus needed.[70,71]

Rapid Microbiologic Diagnostics

Conventional microbiologic procedures typically require several days for isolation, identification, and antimicrobial susceptibility testing of isolated bacteria from clinical samples including blood, respiratory tract, urine, and sterile site specimens. Because of the time-consuming nature of these procedures, identification of resistant bacteria is often delayed, resulting in the administration of inappropriate initial antibiotic therapy. Rapid diagnostic methods offer the capability of influencing early antibiotic decision-making in order to allow for administration of appropriate therapy for antibiotic-resistant bacteria that is more prompt, as well as minimization of unnecessary use of broad-spectrum agents. Several molecular diagnostic platforms for the rapid diagnosis of bacterial species and their accompanying resistance genes have been introduced and evaluated, including the LightCycler SeptiFast Test (Roche, Basel, Switzerland), peptide nucleic acid fluorescence in situ hybridization (PNA-FISH) (AdvanDx, Woburn, MA), matrix-assisted laser desorption-ionization time of flight mass spectrometry (MALDI-TOF MS) (VITEK MS; bioMérieux, Inc., Durham, NC), and DNA-based microarray platforms (Prove-it sepsis assay [Mobidiag, Keilaranta, Finland] and the Verigene Gram-Positive Blood Culture assay [Nanosphere, Northbrook, IL]).[72] In addition, automated microscopy methods such as the ID/AST system (Accelerate Diagnostics, Tucson, AZ) are in development using both genomic and phenotypic technologies to provide pathogen identification and antimicrobial susceptibilities in a rapid manner.[73]

The potential impact of rapid diagnostic technology in the clinical setting has been reported. A quasi-experimental study evaluated MALDI-TOF MS in conjunction with an antimicrobial stewardship team intervention in patients with bloodstream infections.[74] In this study, the antimicrobial stewardship team provided antibiotic recommendations after receiving real-time notification following blood culture Gram stain, organism identification, and antimicrobial susceptibilities using conventional microbiology methods in the before-period and MALDI-TOF MS in the after-period. Use of MALDI-TOF MS significantly decreased time to organism identification and improved time to effective antibiotic therapy as well as optimal directed antibiotic therapy. Mortality, length of ICU stay, and recurrent bacteremia were significantly lower during the intervention period. Similarly, use of the PCR-based GeneXpert MRSA/SA diagnostic platform (Cepheid, Sunnyvale, CA) showed that for methicillin-susceptible *S. aureus* bacteremia, the mean time to initiation of appropriate therapy was reduced from 49.8 hours to 5.2 hours, and the duration of unnecessary MRSA drug therapy was reduced by 61 hours per patient.[75] It is expected that as rapid diagnostics further develop, their impact on antimicrobial stewardship will increase, given their enhanced ability to direct early appropriate treatment and avoid unnecessary antibiotic exposure.

De-escalation of Empirical Antibiotic Regimen

When risk factors for antibiotic resistance are identified in patients with a serious infection, broad-spectrum antimicrobials should be prescribed. This approach usually requires initial combination antimicrobial treatment targeting nonfermenting GNB (*P. aeruginosa*, *Acinetobacter* spp., *Stenotrophomonas maltophilia*) and MRSA.[76] However, depending on clinical presentation, patient risk factors, and local epidemiology, other pathogens such as *Candida* spp. and *Clostridium difficile*, especially when diarrhea is present, may also need to be covered. Once the microbiologic results are available and the patient's clinical response is observed, the antibiotic regimen can de-escalated or narrowed depending the susceptibilities of the identified pathogen(s). De-escalation (see Figure 11.1) usually refers to a reduction in the spectrum of administered antibiotics through the discontinuation of antibiotics providing activity against pathogens that were not identified, discontinuation of antibiotics with similar activity, or switching to an agent with a narrower spectrum.[77] Through the practice of de-escalation, clinicians limit unnecessary antimicrobial exposure in order to curtail the emergence of resistance.[78]

Intensivists should expect that a de-escalation approach to antimicrobial therapy in critically ill patients will optimize patient outcomes.[79,80] A prospective observational study evaluated the clinical outcomes of a de-escalation strategy compared with those of standard practices in 628 patients with severe sepsis or septic shock at ICU admission who were treated empirically with broad-spectrum antibiotics.[81] Antibiotic therapy was guided by written protocols advocating for de-escalation therapy once the microbiological results became available (day of culture results), although this decision was ultimately the responsibility of the physician in charge of the patient. By multivariate analysis, factors independently associated with in-hospital mortality were septic shock, SOFA score on the day of culture results, and inappropriate empirical antimicrobial therapy, whereas de-escalation of antimicrobial therapy was found to be an independent variable associated with significantly improved odds of hospital survival. In addition, among patients receiving appropriate therapy, the only factor independently associated with mortality was the SOFA score on the day of culture results, whereas de-escalation therapy was again found to be a protective factor. These investigators found that 57 of 628 patients (9.1%) received inappropriate empirical therapy and 246 of 628 patients (39.2%) had no change in their empirical antibiotic regimens, indicating further opportunity to improve their de-escalation practice.

Strategies described in the literature that promote antimicrobial de-escalation in critically ill patients include protocol-driven de-escalation, clinical pharmacist–led de-escalation,[82] and infection-specific treatment pathways (VAP[76] and skin and soft tissue infections[83,84]). Each method has shown significantly shorter durations of antimicrobial treatment than a standard, physician-led approach.

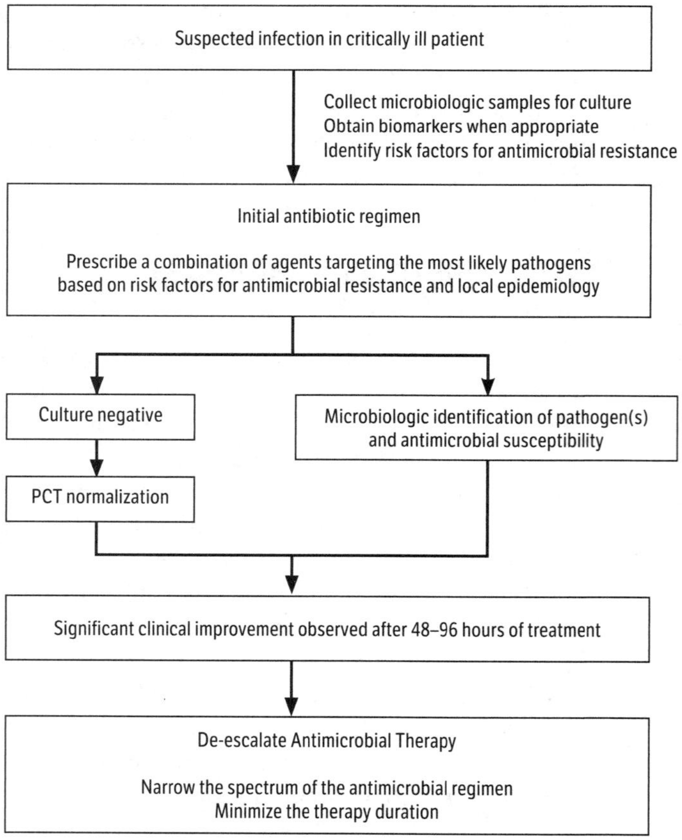

Biomarker Guidance of Antibiotic Therapy

The biomarker procalcitonin is a precursor of calcitonin that is released rapidly into the bloodstream in the presence of an infection. Serial measurements of procalcitonin have been evaluated as a method to guide decisions regarding the duration of antimicrobial therapy. In a randomized trial, 101 patients with VAP were assigned to a de-escalation strategy as recommended by the American Thoracic Society/Infectious Diseases Society of America guidelines, with active education regarding those guidelines, versus a procalcitonin-dictated de-escalation protocol.[85] At 72 hours into the treatment course, the discontinuation of antimicrobials was strongly encouraged if procalcitonin concentrations were less than 0.5 mcg/L or if procalcitonin concentrations had decreased by greater than 80%. When comparing these with treatment approaches, a 27% absolute reduction in the overall duration of antibiotics was achieved in the procalcitonin group compared with the group receiving guideline-driven therapy. Similar findings showing reduced antimicrobial use with a procalcitonin-directed approach to the duration of therapy have been observed in other studies.[86,87] In addition, two meta-analyses suggest that procalcitonin guidance can be used to shorten the duration of antimicrobial therapy in the ICU setting.[88,89]

However, not all experiences with procalcitonin-guided decision-making have shown reductions in duration of antibiotic exposure. A multicenter trial that enrolled 400 patients with suspected bacterial infection/sepsis found a similar number of antibiotic treatment days when comparing procalcitonin-guided antibiotic management with standard care.[90] Perhaps the discrepancy in findings related to the duration of therapy associated

Figure 11.1 De-escalation pathway.
PCT = procalcitonin.

with procalcitonin-guided antibiotic management in critically ill patients can be explained by the utility, or lack thereof, in procalcitonin's ability to discriminate between the various stages in the continuum of SIRS (systemic inflammatory response syndrome), sepsis, severe sepsis, and septic shock.[91] Although higher procalcitonin concentrations suggest the presence of a systemic bacterial infection as opposed to a viral, fungal, or inflammatory etiology of sepsis, serum procalcitonin concentrations have not been shown to correlate with the severity of sepsis or with mortality and therefore should not be used to dictate the timing and appropriateness of de-escalation (or escalation) of antimicrobial therapy in patients with sepsis.

Fungal infections often present a considerable diagnostic challenge to clinicians, and the mere suspicion of these infections often leads to liberal and prolonged antifungal use. The serum markers, (1,3)-β-D-glucan, a fungal wall component and galactomannan *Aspergillus* antigen, have been studied in conjunction with standard culture techniques to quickly identify patients with invasive fungal infections and assist in clinician decision-making regarding continued antifungal therapy. Because of their high negative predictive value in the appropriate clinical setting, the most suitable use of these markers seems to be in excluding the presence of invasive fungal infections and de-escalating antifungal therapy.[92-94] However, one study suggests that (1,3)-β-D-glucan is the most rapid method for identifying intra-abdominal candidiasis in order to provide timely therapy in such patients.[95] In addition, an investigation that measured galactomannan concentrations in bronchoalveolar lavage (BAL) fluid obtained from ICU patients lends support to its use in the identification of *Aspergillus* and early treatment of pulmonary infection.[96] Nonetheless, a more recent study showed only modest agreement between galactomannan in BAL fluid and validated clinical diagnostic criteria for invasive fungal disease.[97] These markers of infection have the potential to enhance stewardship—primarily through de-escalation once a fungal infection has been excluded—and future clinical experience with these markers will determine whether this potential can be fully realized.

Duration of Antibiotic Therapy

For most critically ill patients, empirical antibiotic courses of 7–8 treatment days should suffice unless specific infections are identified such as bacteremia, fungemia, endocarditis, osteomyelitis, and others that would require longer treatment durations. The data supporting the use of shorter courses of antibiotic therapy are probably strongest for VAP, depending on clinical severity, rapidity of clinical improvement, and, most importantly, the underlying microbiology.[98-100] The exceptions to shorter courses of antibiotic therapy in VAP are the difficult-to-treat pathogens like *P. aeruginosa* and other nonfermenting GNB such as *Acinetobacter* spp. that have a higher recurrence rate with shorter treatment regimens.[101] At least one randomized trial has found a greater mortality among patients with *P. aeruginosa* VAP receiving only 7 days of treatment.[57] This study, which compared 7 days of doripenem (4-hour infusion) and 10 days of imipenem/cilastatin (1-hour infusion) in patients with microbiologically confirmed VAP, was halted before completion because of excessive higher 28-day mortality in the doripenem group. Longer treatment durations for nonfermenting GNB may be most important when antibiotic exposure in the lung is limited by host factors such as increased volume of drug distribution and ARC.

In summary, clinicians should be aware that 7–8 days of therapy should suffice for empirical antibiotic treatment in most ICU patients. However, even shorter courses of empirical therapy should be used when the presence of infection is excluded, and longer treatment regimens may be required when dealing with specific sources of infection (i.e., endocarditis) and certain pathogens, including *P. aeruginosa*. It is most important to critically review all antibiotics on a daily basis to ensure that they are indeed necessary and, if so, that they are delivered in adequate concentrations.[82]

Formalized Antimicrobial Stewardship Programs

Hospitals are often seen as inflexible institutions when it comes to implementing practice changes. This has resulted in a call to have executive-level planning, local cooperation, sustained education, emphasis on de-escalation, and locally derived care bundles used singly or in combination in order to promote practice changes that are consistent with antimicrobial stewardship goals and aimed toward decreasing antimicrobial resistance.[102] Formally implemented antimicrobial stewardship programs (ASPs) have been associated not only with reduced infection rates but also significant cost savings associated with reductions in the defined daily doses of the antimicrobials targeted by the ASP.[103] Antimicrobial stewardship programs have been shown to increase the appropriateness of therapy for serious infections such as CAP as well as to increase the number of infectious diseases consultations, which might also dramatically improve patient outcomes including mortality, hospital lengths of stay, and readmission rates by providing more precise antibiotic prescription.[104-107] These attributes of ASPs account for why they are now recognized as mandatory components of hospital quality improvement efforts.

A meta-analysis of ASPs has solidified the benefits of these quality improvement initiatives.[108] This meta-analysis found that ASPs could significantly result in less antimicrobial use and that these programs were associated with reductions in *C. difficile* infections and colonization or infection with aminoglycoside- or cephalosporin-resistant GNB,

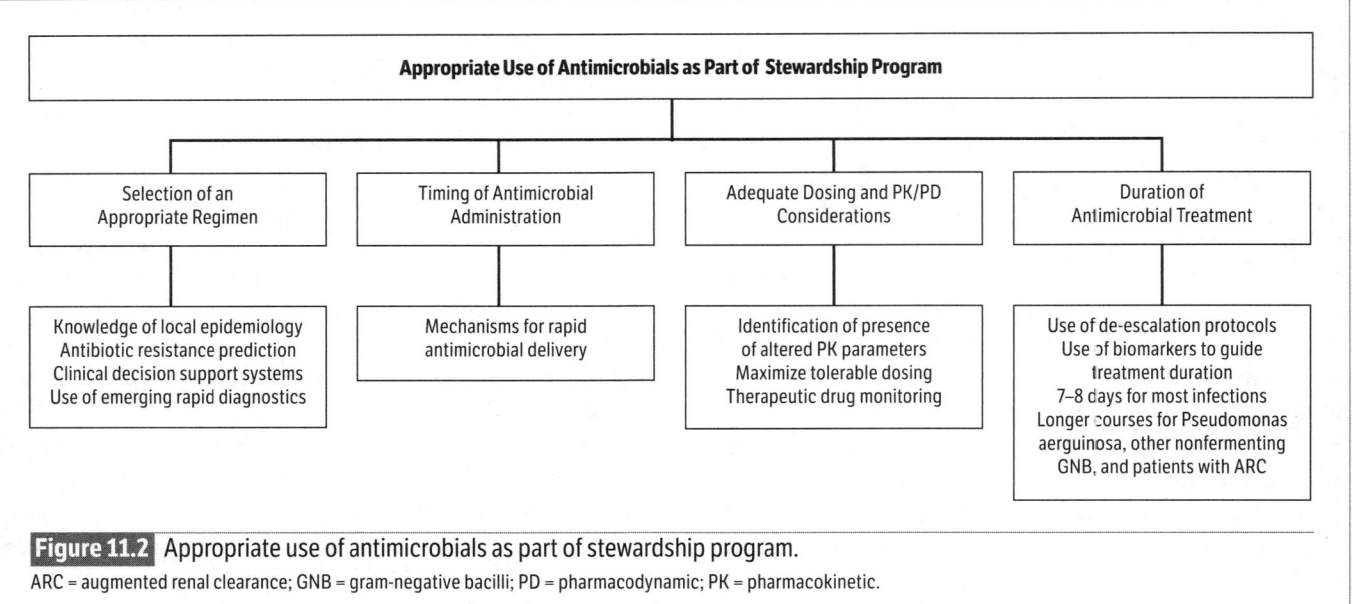

Figure 11.2 Appropriate use of antimicrobials as part of stewardship program.
ARC = augmented renal clearance; GNB = gram-negative bacilli; PD = pharmacodynamic; PK = pharmacokinetic.

MRSA, and vancomycin-resistant *Enterococcus faecalis*. In addition, antibiotic prescribing practices for pneumonia made more effective because of the presence of an ASP were associated with a significant reduction in mortality, whereas practices aimed at decreasing excessive antibiotic prescribing were not associated with any significant increase in mortality. This meta-analysis supports the role of formalized ASPs not only to restrict the use of unnecessary antibiotics but also to ensure that antimicrobials are used in an effective manner to optimize patient outcomes.

CONCLUSION

Although antimicrobial therapy is often prescribed, clinicians should realize that these important therapeutic agents should be used wisely. Judicious use of antibiotics serves to combat the emergence of resistance, improve clinical outcomes, and decrease costs (Figure 11.2). The challenge to ICU clinicians is how to use these agents most effectively in order to maximize patient benefits while minimizing the emergence of resistance. Intensive care unit clinicians must be the leaders in ensuring that their institutions have robust and effective ASPs.[109]

REFERENCES

1. Lawrence KL, Kollef MH. Antimicrobial stewardship in the intensive care unit: advances and obstacles. Am J Respir Crit Care Med 2009;179:434-8.
2. Patel D, Lawson W, Guglielmo BJ. Antimicrobial stewardship programs: interventions and associated outcomes. Expert Rev Anti Infect Ther 2008;6:209-22.
3. Kollef MH, Micek ST. Rational use of antibiotics in the ICU: balancing stewardship and clinical outcomes. JAMA 2014;312:1403-4.
4. Barlam TF, DiVall M. Antibiotic-stewardship practices at top academic centers throughout the United States and at hospitals throughout Massachusetts. Infect Control Hosp Epidemiol 2006;27:695-703.
5. Kollef MH. Antibiotics for the critically ill: more than just selecting appropriate initial therapy. Crit Care 2013;17:146.
6. Owens RC Jr. Antimicrobial stewardship: concepts and strategies in the 21st century. Diagn Microbiol Infect Dis 2008;61:110-28.
7. Paterson DL. The role of antimicrobial management programs in optimizing antibiotic prescribing within hospitals. Clin Infect Dis 2006;42(suppl 2):S90-5.
8. Kollef MH. Broad-spectrum antimicrobials and treatment of serious bacterial infections: getting it right up front. Clin Infect Dis 2008;47(suppl 1):S3-13.
9. Micek ST, Lang A, Fuller BM, et al. Clinical implications for patients treated inappropriately for community-acquired pneumonia in the emergency department. BMC Infect Dis 2014;14:61.
10. Shorr AF, Zilberberg MD, Micek ST, et al. Predictors of hospital mortality among septic ICU patients with *Acinetobacter* spp. bacteremia: a cohort study. BMC Infect Dis 2014;14:572.
11. Vardakas KZ, Rafailidis PI, Konstantelias AA, et al. Predictors of mortality in patients with infections due to multi-drug resistant gram negative bacteria: the study, the patient, the bug or the drug? J Infect 2013;66:401-14.
12. Harbarth S, Garbino J, Pugin J, et al. Inappropriate initial antimicrobial therapy and its effect on survival in a clinical trial of immunomodulating therapy for severe sepsis. Am J Med 2003;115:529-35.
13. Ibrahim EH, Sherman G, Ward S, et al. The influence of inadequate antimicrobial treatment of bloodstream infections on patient outcomes in the ICU setting. Chest 2000;118:146-55.
14. Kollef MH, Sherman G, Ward S, et al. Inadequate antimicrobial treatment of infections: a risk factor for hospital mortality among critically ill patients. Chest 1999;115:462-74.

15. Micek ST, Lloyd AE, Ritchie DJ, et al. *Pseudomonas aeruginosa* bloodstream infection: importance of appropriate initial antimicrobial treatment. Antimicrob Agents Chemother 2005;49:1306-11.
16. Labelle AJ, Micek ST, Roubinian N, et al. Treatment-related risk factors for hospital mortality in *Candida* bloodstream infections. Crit Care Med 2008;36:2967-72.
17. Kollef M, Micek S, Hampton N, et al. Septic shock attributed to *Candida* infection: importance of empiric therapy and source control. Clin Infect Dis 2012;54:1739-46.
18. Bassetti M, Righi E, Ansaldi F, et al. A multicenter study of septic shock due to candidemia: outcomes and predictors of mortality. Intensive Care Med 2014;40:839-45.
19. Vazquez-Guillamet C, Scolari M, Zilberberg MD, et al. Using the number needed to treat to assess appropriate antimicrobial therapy as a determinant of outcome in severe sepsis and septic shock. Crit Care Med 2014;42:2342-9.
20. Dellinger RP, Levy MM, Rhodes A, et al. Surviving Sepsis Campaign: international guidelines for management of severe sepsis and septic shock: 2012. Crit Care Med 2013;41:580-637.
21. Shindo Y, Ito R, Kobayashi D, et al. Risk factors for drug-resistant pathogens in community-acquired and healthcare-associated pneumonia. Am J Respir Crit Care Med 2013;188:985-95.
22. Maruyama T, Fujisawa T, Okuno M, et al. A new strategy for healthcare-associated pneumonia: a 2-year prospective multicenter cohort study using risk factors for multidrug-resistant pathogens to select initial empiric therapy. Clin Infect Dis 2013;57:1373-83.
23. Shorr AF, Zilberberg MD, Micek ST, et al. Prediction of infection due to antibiotic-resistant bacteria by select risk factors for health care-associated pneumonia. Arch Intern Med 2008;168:2205-10.
24. Shorr AF, Zilberberg MD, Reichley R, et al. Validation of a clinical score for assessing the risk of resistant pathogens in patients with pneumonia presenting to the emergency department. Clin Infect Dis 2012;54:193-8.
25. Chalmers JD, Rother C, Salih W, et al. Healthcare-associated pneumonia does not accurately identify potentially resistant pathogens: a systematic review and meta-analysis. Clin Infect Dis 2014;58:330-9.
26. Thursky KA, Buising KL, Bak N, et al. Reduction of broad-spectrum antibiotic use with computerized decision support in an intensive care unit. Int J Qual Health Care 2006;18:224-31.
27. Micek ST, Heard KM, Gowan M, et al. Identifying critically ill patients at risk for inappropriate antibiotic therapy: a pilot study of a point-of-care decision support alert. Crit Care Med 2014;42:1832-8.
28. Evans RS, Pestotnik SL, Classen DC, et al. A computer-assisted management program for antibiotics and other antiinfective agents. N Engl J Med 1998;338:232-8.
29. Pestotnik SL, Classen DC, Evans RS, et al. Implementing antibiotic practice guidelines through computer-assisted decision support: clinical and financial outcomes. Ann Intern Med 1996;124:884-90.
30. Paul M, Nielsen AD, Goldberg E, et al. Prediction of specific pathogens in patients with sepsis: evaluation of TREAT, a computerized decision support system. J Antimicrob Chemother 2007;59:1204-7.
31. McGregor JC, Weekes E, Forrest GN, et al. Impact of a computerized clinical decision support system on reducing inappropriate antimicrobial use: a randomized controlled trial. J Am Med Inform Assoc 2006;13:378-84.
32. Bochicchio GV, Smit PA, Moore R, et al. Pilot study of a web-based antibiotic decision management guide. J Am Coll Surg 2006;202:459-67.
33. Thiel SW, Asghar MF, Micek ST, et al. Hospital-wide impact of a standardized order set for the management of bacteremic severe sepsis. Crit Care Med 2009;37:819-24.
34. Iregui M, Ward S, Sherman G, et al. Clinical importance of delays in the initiation of appropriate antibiotic treatment for ventilator-associated pneumonia. Chest 2002;122:262-8.
35. Kumar A, Roberts D, Wood KE, et al. Duration of hypotension before initiation of effective antimicrobial therapy is the critical determinant of survival in human septic shock. Crit Care Med 2006;34:1589-96.
36. Chen C, Kollef MH. Conservative fluid therapy in septic shock: an example of targeted therapeutic minimization. Crit Care 2014;18:481.
37. Ferrer R, Artigas A, Suarez D, et al. Effectiveness of treatments for severe sepsis: a prospective, multicenter, observational study. Am J Respir Crit Care Med 2009;180:861-6.
38. Ferrer R, Martin-Loeches I, Phillips G, et al. Empiric antibiotic treatment reduces mortality in severe sepsis and septic shock from the first hour: results from a guideline-based performance improvement program. Crit Care Med 2014;42:1749-55.
39. Vitrat V, Hautefeuille S, Janssen C, et al. Optimizing antimicrobial therapy in critically ill patients. Infect Drug Resist 2014;7:261-71.
40. Tam VH, McKinnon PS, Akins RL, et al. Pharmacodynamics of cefepime in patients with gram-negative infections. J Antimicrob Chemother 2002;50:425-28.
41. Hengzhuang W, Ciofu O, Yang L, et al. High β-lactamase levels change the pharmacodynamics of β-lactam antibiotics in *Pseudomonas aeruginosa* biofilms. Antimicrob Agents Chemother 2013;57:196-204.
42. Roberts JA, Paul SK, Akova M, et al. DALI: defining antibiotic levels in intensive care unit patients: are current β-lactam antibiotic doses sufficient for critically ill patients? Clin Infect Dis 2014;58:1072-83.
43. Cai Y, Wang R, Liang B, et al. Systematic review and meta-analysis of the effectiveness and safety of tigecycline for treatment of infectious disease. Antimicrob Agents Chemother 2011;55:1162-72.
44. McGovern PC, Wible M, El-Tahtawy A, et al. All-cause mortality imbalance in the tigecycline phase 3 and 4 clinical trials. Int J Antimicrob Agents 2013;41:463-7.
45. Prasad P, Sun J, Danner RL, et al. Excess deaths associated with tigecycline after approval based on noninferiority trials. Clin Infect Dis 2012;54:1699-709.
46. Freire AT, Melnyk V, Kim MJ, et al. Comparison of tigecycline with imipenem/cilastatin for the treatment of hospital-acquired pneumonia. Diagn Microbiol Infect Dis 2010;68:140-51.
47. Ramirez J, Dartois N, Gandjini H, et al. Randomized phase 2 trial to evaluate the clinical efficacy of two high-dosage

48. Awad SS, Rodriguez AH, Chuang YC, et al. A phase 3 randomized double-blind comparison of ceftobiprole medocaril versus ceftazidime plus linezolid for the treatment of hospital-acquired pneumonia. Clin Infect Dis 2014;59:51-61.

49. Chandorkar G, Huntington JA, Gotfried MH, et al. Intrapulmonary penetration of ceftolozane/tazobactam and piperacillin/tazobactam in healthy adult subjects. J Antimicrob Chemother 2012;67:2463-9.

50. Xiao AJ, Miller BW, Huntington JA, et al. Ceftolozane/tazobactam pharmacokinetic/pharmacodynamic-derived dose justification for phase 3 studies in patients with nosocomial pneumonia. J Clin Pharmacol 2015 Jun 10. [Epub ahead of print]

51. Pea F. Plasma pharmacokinetics of antimicrobial agents in critically ill patients. Curr Clin Pharmacol 2013;8:5-12.

52. De Waele JJ, Carlier M. Beta-lactam antibiotic dosing during continuous renal replacement therapy: how can we optimize therapy? Crit Care 2014;18:158.

53. Udy AA, Baptista JP, Lim NL, et al. Augmented renal clearance in the ICU: results of a multicenter observational study of renal function in critically ill patients with normal plasma. Crit Care Med 2014;42:520-7.

54. Carlier M, Carrette S, Roberts JA, et al. Meropenem and piperacillin/tazobactam prescribing in critically ill patients: does augmented renal clearance affect pharmacokinetic/pharmacodynamic target attainment when extended infusions are used? Crit Care 2013;17:R84.

55. Baptista JP, Sousa E, Martins PJ, et al. Augmented renal clearance in septic patients and implications for vancomycin optimisation. Int J Antimicrob Agents 2012;39:420-3.

56. Claus BO, Hoste EA, Colpaert K, et al. Augmented renal clearance is a common finding with worse clinical outcome in critically ill patients receiving antimicrobial therapy. J Crit Care 2013;28:695-700.

57. Kollef MH, Chastre J, Clavel M, et al. A randomized trial of 7-day doripenem versus 10-day imipenem-cilastatin for ventilator-associated pneumonia. Crit Care 2012;16:R218.

58. Udy AA, Roberts JA, Shorr AF, et al. Augmented renal clearance in septic and traumatized patients with normal plasma creatinine concentrations: identifying at-risk patients. Crit Care 2013;17:R35.

59. Akers KS, Niece KL, Chung KK, et al. Modified augmented renal clearance score predicts rapid piperacillin and tazobactam clearance in critically ill surgery and trauma patients. J Trauma Acute Care Surg 2014;77(3 suppl 2):S163-70.

60. Roberts JA, Webb S, Paterson D, et al. A systematic review on clinical benefits of continuous administration of beta-lactam antibiotics. Crit Care Med 2009;37:2071-8.

61. Kasiakou SK, Sermaides GJ, Michalopoulos A, et al. Continuous versus intermittent intravenous administration of antibiotics: a meta-analysis of randomised controlled trials. Lancet Infect Dis 2005;5:581-9.

62. Chant C, Leung A, Friedrich JO. Optimal dosing of antibiotics in critically ill patients by using continuous/extended infusions: a systematic review and meta-analysis. Crit Care 2013;17:R279.

63. Falagas ME, Tansarli GS, Ikawa K, et al. Clinical outcomes with extended or continuous versus short-term intravenous infusion of carbapenems and piperacillin/tazobactam: a systematic review and meta-analysis. Clin Infect Dis 2013;56:272-82.

64. Dulhunty JM, Roberts JA, Davis JS, et al. A multicenter randomized trial of continuous versus intermittent β-lactam infusion in severe sepsis. Am J Respir Crit Care Med 2015 Jul 22. [Epub ahead of print]

65. Barco S, Bandettini R, Maffia A, et al. Quantification of piperacillin, tazobactam, meropenem, ceftazidime, and linezolid in human plasma by liquid chromatography/tandem mass spectrometry. J Chemother 2014. [Epub ahead of print]

66. Zander J, Maier B, Suhr A, et al. Quantification of piperacillin, tazobactam, cefepime, meropenem, ciprofloxacin and linezolid in serum using an isotope dilution UHPLC-MS/MS method with semi-automated sample preparation. Clin Chem Lab Med 2015;53:781-91.

67. DeWaele JJ, Carrette S, Carlier M, et al. Therapeutic drug monitoring-based dose optimization of piperacillin and meropenem: a randomized controlled trial. Intensive Care Med 2014;40:380-7.

68. Afaneh CI, Ho VP, McWhorter P, et al. Minor fluctuations in renal function may alter therapeutic drug concentrations substantially during high-dose, continuous-infusion beta-lactam therapy for multi-drug-resistant gram-negative bacilli. Surg Infect (Larchmt) 2012;13:415-7.

69. Beumier M, Casu GS, Hites M, et al. β-lactam antibiotic concentrations during continuous renal replacement therapy. Crit Care 2014;18:R105.

70. Wong G, Brinkman A, Benefield RJ, et al. An international, multicentre survey of β-lactam antibiotic therapeutic drug monitoring practice in intensive care units. J Antimicrob Chemother 2014;69:1416-23.

71. Carlier M, Stove V, Wallis SC, et al. Assays for therapeutic drug monitoring of β-lactam antibiotics: a structured review. Int J Antimicrob Agents 2015 Jul 28. [Epub ahead of print]

72. Tojo M, Fujita T, Ainoda Y, et al. Evaluation of an automated rapid diagnostic assay for detection of gram-negative bacteria and their drug-resistance genes in positive blood cultures. PLoS One 2014;9:e94064.

73. Burnham CA, Frobel RA, Herrera ML, et al. Rapid ertapenem susceptibility testing and Klebsiella pneumoniae carbapenemase phenotype detection in *Klebsiella pneumoniae* isolates by use of automated microscopy of immobilized live bacterial cells. J Clin Microbiol 2014;52:982-6.

74. Huang A, Newton D, Kunapuli A, et al. Impact of rapid organism identification via matrix-assisted laser desorption/ionization time-of-flight combined with antimicrobial stewardship team intervention in adult patients with bacteremia and candidemia. Clin Infect Dis 2013;57:1237-45.

75. Parta M, Goebel M, Thomas J, et al. Impact of an assay that enables rapid determination of *Staphylococcus* species and their drug susceptibility on the treatment of patients with positive blood culture results. Infect Control Hosp Epidemiol 2010;31:1043-48.

76. Ibrahim EH, Ward S, Sherman G, et al. Experience with a clinical guideline for the treatment of ventilator-associated pneumonia. Crit Care Med 2001;29:1109-15.

77. Garnacho-Montero J, Escoresca-Ortega A, Fernandez-Delgado E. Antibiotic de-escalation in the ICU: how is it best done? Curr Opin Infect Dis 2015;28:193-8.

78. Kollef MH, Micek ST. Strategies to prevent antimicrobial resistance in the intensive care unit. Crit Care Med 2005;33:1845-53.

79. Shorr AF, Micek ST, Welch EC, et al. Inappropriate antibiotic therapy in gram-negative sepsis increases hospital length of stay. Crit Care Med 2011;39:46-51.

80. Rello J, Vidaur L, Sandiumenge A, et al. De-escalation therapy in ventilator-associated pneumonia. Crit Care Med 2004;32:2183-90.

81. Garnacho-Montero J, Gutiérrez-Pizarraya A, Escoresca-Ortega A, et al. De-escalation of empirical therapy is associated with lower mortality in patients with severe sepsis and septic shock. Intensive Care Med 2014;40:32-40.

82. Micek ST, Ward S, Fraser VJ, et al. A randomized controlled trial of an antibiotic discontinuation policy for clinically suspected ventilator-associated pneumonia. Chest 2004;125:1791-9.

83. Jenkins TC, Sabel AL, Sarcone EE, et al. Skin and soft-tissue infections requiring hospitalization at an academic medical center: opportunities for antimicrobial stewardship. Clin Infect Dis 2010;51:895-903.

84. Jenkins TC, Knepper BC, Sabel AL, et al. Decreased antibiotic utilization after implementation of a guideline for inpatient cellulitis and cutaneous abscess. Arch Intern Med 2011;171:1072-9.

85. Stolz D, Smyrnios N, Eggimann P, et al. Procalcitonin for reduced antibiotic exposure in ventilator-associated pneumonia: a randomised study. Eur Respir J 2009;34:1364-75.

86. Bouadma L, Luyt CE, Tubach F, et al. PRORATA trial group. Use of procalcitonin to reduce patients' exposure to antibiotics in intensive care units (PRORATA trial): a multicentre randomised controlled trial. Lancet 2010;375:463-74.

87. Hochreiter M, Köhler T, Schweiger AM, et al. Procalcitonin to guide duration of antibiotic therapy in intensive care patients: a randomized prospective controlled trial. Crit Care 2009;13:R83.

88. Prkno A, Wacker C, Brunkhorst FM, et al. Procalcitonin-guided therapy in intensive care unit patients with severe sepsis and septic shock—a systematic review and meta-analysis Crit Care 2013;17:R291.

89. Soni NJ, Samson DJ, Galaydick JL, et al. Procalcitonin-guided antibiotic therapy: a systematic review and meta-analysis. J Hosp Med 2013;8:530-40.

90. Shehabi Y, Sterba M, Garrett PM, et al. Procalcitonin algorithm in critically ill adults with undifferentiated infection or suspected sepsis. A randomized controlled trial. Am J Respir Crit Care Med 2014;190:1102-10.

91. Sridharan P, Chamberlain RS. The efficacy of procalcitonin as a biomarker in the management of sepsis: slaying dragons or tilting at windmills? Surg Infect (Larchmt) 2013;14:489-511.

92. Maertens J, Deeren D, Dierickx D, et al. Preemptive antifungal therapy: still a way to go. Curr Opin Infect Dis 2006;19:551-6.

93. Pfeiffer CD, Fine JP, Safdar N. Diagnosis of invasive aspergillosis using a galactomannan assay: a meta-analysis. Clin Infect Dis 2006;42:1417-27.

94. Martinez-Jimenez MC, Munoz P, Valerio M, et al. Combination of Candida biomarkers in patients receiving empirical antifungal therapy in a Spanish tertiary hospital: a potential role in reducing duration of treatment. J Antimicrob Chemother 2015 Aug 25. [Epub ahead of print]

95. Tissot F, Lamoth F, Hauser PM, et al. β-glucan antigenemia anticipates diagnosis of blood culture-negative intraabdominal candidiasis. Am J Respir Crit Care Med 2013;188:1100-9.

96. Meersseman W, Lagrou K, Maertens J, et al. Galactomannan in bronchoalveolar lavage fluid: a tool for diagnosing aspergillosis in intensive care unit patients. Am J Respir Crit Care Med 2008;177:27-34.

97. Affolter K, Tamm M, Jahn K, et al. Galactomannan in bronchoalveolar lavage for diagnosing invasive fungal disease. Am J Respir Crit Care Med 2014;190:309-17.

98. Chastre J, Wolff M, Fagon JY, et al. Comparison of 8 vs 15 days of antibiotic therapy for ventilator-associated pneumonia in adults: a randomized trial. JAMA 2003;290:2588-98.

99. Capellier G, Mockly H, Charpentier C, et al. Early-onset ventilator-associated pneumonia in adults randomized clinical trial: comparison of 8 versus 15 days of antibiotic treatment. PLoS One 2012;7:e41290.

100. Dimopoulos G, Poulakou G, Pneumatikos IA, et al. Short- vs long-duration antibiotic regimens for ventilator-associated pneumonia: a systematic review and meta-analysis. Chest 2013;144:1759-67.

101. Pugh R, Grant C, Cooke RP, et al. Short-course versus prolonged-course antibiotic therapy for hospital-acquired pneumonia in critically ill adults. Cochrane Database Syst Rev 2011;10:CD007577.

102. Bal AM, Gould IM. Antibiotic stewardship: overcoming implementation barriers. Curr Opin Infect Dis 2011;24:357-62.

103. Malani AN, Richards PG, Kapila S, et al. Clinical and economic outcomes from a community hospital's antimicrobial stewardship program. Am J Infect Control 2013;41:145-8.

104. Ambroggio L, Thomson J, Murtagh Kurowski E, et al. Quality improvement methods increase appropriate antibiotic prescribing for childhood pneumonia. Pediatrics 2013;131:e1623-31.

105. Morrill HJ, Gaitanis MM, LaPlante KL. Antimicrobial stewardship program prompts increased and earlier infectious diseases consultation. Antimicrob Resist Infect Control 2014;3:12.

106. Pasquale TR, Trienski TL, Olexia DE, et al. Impact of an antimicrobial stewardship program on patients with acute bacterial skin and skin structure infections. Am J Health Syst Pharm 2014;71:1136-9.

107. Wenisch JM, Equiluz-Bruck S, Fudel M, et al. Decreasing Clostridium difficile infections by an antimicrobial stewardship program that reduces moxifloxacin use. Antimicrob Agents Chemother 2014;58:5079-83.

108. Davey P, Brown E, Charani E, et al. Interventions to improve antibiotic prescribing practices for hospital inpatients. Cochrane Database Syst Rev 2013;4:CD003543.

109. Kollef MH, Micek ST. Antimicrobial stewardship programs: mandatory for all ICUs. Crit Care 2012;16:179.

Chapter 12: Pharmacokinetic and Pharmacodynamic Considerations for Antimicrobial Use in Critically Ill Patients

Douglas N. Fish, Pharm.D., FCCP, FCCM, BCPS-AQ ID

LEARNING OBJECTIVES

1. Describe basic principles of antimicrobial pharmacodynamics (PD) and the specific parameters used to describe the properties of time- and concentration-dependent drugs.
2. Discuss the cause and significance of potential pharmacokinetic (PK) alterations in critically ill patients, including changes in drug absorption, distribution, clearance, protein binding, and half-life.
3. Discuss general strategies for antimicrobial dosing and dose adjustments in critically ill patients.
4. Describe specific PK/PD goals for dosing of time-dependent antibiotics, concentration-dependent antibiotics, and antifungal agents.
5. Discuss clinical applications of PD principles that are currently being used or investigated for dose optimization of antimicrobials.
6. Describe potential limitations to applying PK/PD principles of dose optimization in critically ill populations.
7. Given a critically ill patient requiring antimicrobial therapy, apply appropriate PK/PD principles to recommend an appropriate dosing regimen that incorporates consideration of potential PK alterations and desired PD targets.

ABBREVIATIONS IN THIS CHAPTER

ARC	Augmented renal clearance	ICU	Intensive care unit
AUC_{0-24}/MIC	Ratio of the 24-hour area under the serum concentration versus time curve to pathogen MIC	MCS	Monte Carlo simulation
		MIC	Minimum inhibitory concentration
		PK	Pharmacokinetic
Cmax/MIC	Ratio of maximum serum drug concentration to MIC	PD	Pharmacodynamic
		TDM	Therapeutic drug monitoring
$fT>MIC$	Time during which unbound/free drug concentration remains above the pathogen MIC	Vss	Volume of distribution at steady state

INTRODUCTION

Antibiotic treatment of critically ill patients remains a significant challenge to clinicians worldwide because of high infection-related mortality and morbidity rates. Patients are often admitted to the intensive care unit (ICU) for the treatment of community- or hospital-acquired infections, and many other patients require treatment for nosocomial infections acquired during their ICU stay. Although patients in ICUs represent only 8%–15% of hospital admissions in the United States,[1] these patients have a disproportionately high rate of infectious complications and are exposed to very high rates of antimicrobial use.[1-3] The importance of effective antimicrobial therapy is also underscored by the ever-increasing severity of illness of patients being admitted to the ICU.[4] The importance of antimicrobial drugs in the modern management of critically ill patients with a variety of bacterial, fungal, and viral infections can scarcely be understated. However, despite the availability of improved diagnostic techniques and a wide variety of potent, highly effective antimicrobials, the appropriate treatment of infections in ICU patients remains a formidable challenge to the clinician.

Optimization of antimicrobial therapy remains a high priority in the management of critically ill patients. Antimicrobials are often selected primarily because of their spectrum of antimicrobial activity against presumed or documented pathogens. However, because of the high risk of severe morbidity and mortality associated with infections in critically ill patients, particular consideration must also be given to other pharmacologic properties. Optimization of antimicrobial therapy requires that drugs be dosed in a manner that maximizes their pharmacologic activity while minimizing the risk of adverse effects and toxicities. Special consideration must therefore be given to antimicrobial pharmacokinetic (PK) and pharmacodynamic (PD) properties; indeed, the optimization of antimicrobial dosing regimens is almost as important as the actual choice of drug with respect to achieving favorable patient outcomes while minimizing the risk of antimicrobial resistance.[5-11]

An endless variety of physiological alterations may occur in critically ill patients, many of which have the ability to significantly affect the PK/PD properties of drugs used in this patient population. Pharmacokinetic changes often result from organ dysfunction, most importantly the kidneys and liver, but they may also be caused by therapeutic interventions including volume resuscitation and renal replacement therapy. Knowledge of potential PK alterations is important to the ICU clinician because these changes also have the ability to adversely affect antimicrobial concentrations at infection sites, cause alterations in the PK-dependent PD properties of the drugs, and further complicate antimicrobial dosing. Knowledge of potential PK alterations and resultant changes in the probability of achieving desired PD targets pertaining to the antimicrobials used for the treatment of critically ill patients is therefore essential for selecting appropriate antibiotic dosing regimens that will optimize patient outcomes. The purpose of this chapter is to review and discuss pathophysiological changes that are known to occur in critically ill patients, the effect of these changes on antimicrobial PK properties, and current applications of antimicrobial PK/PD properties that have the potential to optimize antimicrobial use in ICU patients.

BASIC PD PRINCIPLES

Pharmacodynamics is the discipline that tries to define and apply the relationships between concentrations of a drug and its pharmacologic effects (both desirable and undesirable).[5,7,9,11] Although both the pharmacologic activity of an agent and its PK disposition are important considerations in drug selection and dosing, it is the combination of these two properties that is critical to achieving optimal outcomes during treatment of infections. The pharmacologic activities of antibacterial drugs are commonly defined by their minimum inhibitory concentration (MIC) as determined by in vitro testing. The MIC is the minimal concentration required to inhibit the growth of a target organism; highly active agents are associated with low MICs (i.e., only low concentrations are required to inhibit bacterial growth), whereas agents with poor activity are associated with high MICs for the organism in question. It is logical that even extremely active agents with very low MICs will not be efficacious against a pathogen if the drug does not reach the infection site in sufficient quantity; likewise, agents with relatively poor activity and higher MICs may be just as clinically efficacious if they can achieve high drug concentrations at the infection site. Pharmacodynamic considerations combine MIC-defined pharmacologic activity and PK properties of a drug to make predictions regarding the drug's probable efficacy in the treatment of a given type of infection. Models of infection have allowed antibacterial drugs to be broadly classified into two major categories: concentration-dependent agents and time-dependent (concentration-independent) agents.[5,7,11]

Concentration-dependent agents exert bactericidal activities when drug concentrations are well above the MIC of the organism; the higher the ratio of drug concentration at the infection site to the MIC, the more rapid and/or complete the bacterial killing becomes. Previous studies have established that important PD predictors of the clinical efficacy of concentration-dependent agents include the ratio of maximum serum concentration divided by the MIC (C_{max}/MIC) and/or the ratio of the 24-hour area under the serum concentration versus time curve divided by the MIC (AUC_{0-24}/MIC).[5,7,11] Both C_{max}/MIC and AUC_{0-24}/MIC ratios appear to be important determinants of clinical and microbiological outcomes, although it is sometimes less clear which of these parameters is most predictive of drug efficacy because they are closely linked by the PK properties of the drugs.

Time-dependent agents exert antimicrobial effects only when their concentrations at the infection site are higher than the MIC of the pathogen; the time above MIC (T>MIC) thus becomes the PD parameter of interest for these drugs.[5,7,11] More specifically, the percentage of time (relative to the dosing interval or total 24-hour period) in which the concentration of free unbound drug remains above the MIC ($fT>MIC$) is the key PD parameter for time-dependent antimicrobials. Studies indicate that $fT>MIC$ should be at least 40%–50% of the dosing interval for β-lactam agents, although it has also been suggested that achieving $fT>MIC$ for 100% of the dosing interval is desirable for optimal outcome.[5,7,11] These studies have also suggested that both the AUC_{0-24}/MIC and the $fT>MIC$ are important predictors of clinical efficacy and the risk of developing microbial resistance.[5,7,8,10,11]

Because patients in the ICU are often infected with serious nosocomial pathogens that have decreased susceptibilities to antimicrobials and are prone to developing resistance with inadequate therapy, failure to properly dose antimicrobial agents predisposes patients to clinical and microbiological failure. The appropriate consideration of PD principles in the treatment of infection in critically ill patients enables clinicians to select dosing regimens that will maximize the potential effectiveness of the specific agent. However, the ability to adequately achieve desired PD targets for key parameters (Cmax/MIC, AUC_{0-24}/MIC, and fT>MIC) is obviously highly dependent on the PK properties of the drugs and the ability to anticipate or compensate for potential PK alterations in individual patients.

PK ALTERATIONS IN CRITICAL ILLNESS

Pharmacokinetic properties that should be specifically considered in critically ill patients include distribution to various tissues and fluids, and routes of metabolism and excretion.[12] The ability of a drug to penetrate to the infection site in sufficient quantities to have activity against a pathogen is crucial for achieving clinical and microbiological efficacy. Although the distributional characteristics of antimicrobials are often only specifically considered in the treatment of central nervous system or bone infections, good penetration to tissues and fluids present at the infection site is a necessary consideration when selecting agents for any infection in ICU patients. Routes of drug metabolism and elimination are also important PK properties because of the prevalence of acute and chronic organ failures in most critically ill populations. Antimicrobials are not titrated to a desired response in the same way as sedatives, analgesics, and vasopressors, and there is often a prolonged lag time between initiation of an antimicrobial regimen and occurrence of an observable or measurable response to therapy. Practitioners must therefore be familiar with the PK properties of commonly used antimicrobials as well as sources of potential PK alterations in order to use them in an efficacious and safe manner.[12]

Several studies have shown that the PK of antimicrobials is often significantly altered in critical illness and that a high degree of interpatient (and also intrapatient) variability exists in this population.[13-20] Alterations to the PK properties of antimicrobials in critically ill patients are driven by both drug- and disease-related factors. Physicochemical properties of the molecule such as hydrophilicity and lipophilicity, molecular weight, and protein binding will influence the types of PK alterations that may be seen in the presence of pathophysiological changes in critically ill patients. Table 12.1 summarizes the relationship between hydrophilicity and lipophilicity and general PK characteristics of commonly used antimicrobials. Although the relative hydrophilicity and lipophilicity of drugs is an often imprecise predictor of PK characteristics, such information is readily available to clinicians and does offer a useful starting point for predicting the significance of potential PK alterations within individual patients.

Changes in Drug Absorption

Although oral administration of antimicrobials is not as common as intravenous administration in critically ill patients, factors that may affect the absorption of orally administered drugs are nevertheless worth discussing. The rate and extent of drug absorption after oral administration is dependent on several physiochemical properties of the drug, including molecular weight; solubility in aqueous fluids; relative lipophilicity, which will govern the ability of the drug to cross membranes of the gastrointestinal (GI) tract; net ionization state of the drug; and chemical stability of the drug at pHs found in the GI tract. Physiological factors affecting drug absorption from the GI tract include pH, blood flow to organs and tissues of the GI tract, surface area of membranes across which the drug is absorbed, and GI motility. Because many of these physiological factors are disrupted during critical illness, especially early in ICU stays when patients are not yet stable, both the rate and the extent (bioavailability) of absorption of orally administered drugs may be significantly and adversely altered. Perfusion abnormalities in patients with shock states are associated with redistribution and shunting of blood to more vital organs at the frequent expense of the GI tract. The use of vasoactive drugs often results in further reductions in regional blood flow to abdominal organs.[21] This decreased perfusion of the GI tract and the attendant dysfunction adversely affect the absorption of drugs in shock states.[22] In addition to hypoperfusion of the gut, the use of opiates in patients requiring analgesia may contribute to decreased GI motility and impaired oral absorption.[23,24] Finally, patients in an unfed state (i.e., not receiving enterally administered nutrition) have been shown to rapidly develop intestinal atrophy, loss of intestinal surface area, and impaired cellular function.[25,26] In light of these many causes of GI dysfunction and impaired absorption, intravenous administration is often the preferred route of drug administration in critically ill patients. This is particularly true for antimicrobials in patients with severe infections where rapid, more reliable achievement of therapeutic drug concentrations is required.

Changes in Volume of Distribution at Steady State

The volume of distribution at steady state (Vss) of an antimicrobial can be mathematically expressed as C_0 = dose/Vss, where C_0 is the initial concentration of a drug after administration of an intravenous bolus dose and Vss is the volume of distribution. Distribution of drugs throughout various fluids and tissues is dependent on several factors including blood flow, lipid solubility of the drug, degree of protein binding, permeability of the tissues, and pH of the fluid or tissue in relation to the net ionization state of the drug. Drugs with relatively small Vss values (less than 0.1–0.8 L/kg) are assumed to have low passive diffusion through plasma membranes and to be primarily distributed into body water, particularly intravascular and interstitial fluids. Drugs with larger Vss values (greater than 0.8 L/kg) are assumed to more freely diffuse through cell membranes and to achieve relatively greater penetration into and concentration within tissues, including adipose tissue.

During critical illness, many factors related to disease states or therapeutic interventions can alter drug distribution. Distribution of antimicrobials to infected tissues may also be affected by hemodynamic instability and regional or local changes in perfusion of various organs and tissues. Hepatic disease, renal disease or injury, administration of large volumes of fluid such as during resuscitation regimens, and malnutrition are examples of factors that may lead to the increased Vss values of hydrophilic drugs through increased total body water and increased intravascular and interstitial

Table 12.1 Relationship Between Hydrophilicity and Lipophilicity of Antimicrobials and Potential for PK Alterations in Critically Ill Patients

	Hydrophilic Drugs	**Lipophilic Drugs**
Example antimicrobials	Penicillins	(Fluoroquinolones)[a]
	Cephalosporins	Macrolides
	Carbapenems	Clindamycin
	Monobactams	Tigecycline
	(Fluoroquinolones)[a]	Rifampin
	Aminoglycosides	Voriconazole
	Vancomycin	Posaconazole
	Daptomycin	Itraconazole
	Linezolid	Amphotericin B
	Colistin	
	Fluconazole	
	Acyclovir	
General PK characteristics	Low Vss (≤ 0.8 L/kg)	Higher Vss (> 0.8 L/kg)
	Low degree of intracellular penetration, primarily distributed to intravascular, interstitial, and other extracellular fluids	Higher degree of intracellular penetration, distributed into adipose tissues
	Primarily eliminated through renal clearance of unmetabolized drug	Primarily eliminated through hepatic metabolism and clearance followed by renal elimination of metabolites
Potential PK alterations in critically ill patients	Potential for highly variable PK disposition:	Usually less variability in PK disposition:
	↑↑ Vss associated with many factors	↔/↑ Vss, largely unchanged for most drugs
	↑ or ↓ clearance depending on renal function, presence of ARC, other factors	↑ or ↓ clearance depending on hepatic function
	↓ Protein binding in many patients, may affect both Vss and clearance	↓ Protein binding in many patients, not usually clinically relevant
	↑ or ↓ $T_{1/2}$ depending on relative changes in Vss and clearance	↔/↑ $t_{1/2}$ depending primarily on changes in clearance
General dosing considerations in critically ill patients	↑ Dose may be required for loading doses, intermittent doses of concentration-dependent drugs	↑ Doses may be required in obesity; otherwise, loading and intermittent doses not usually affected
	↑ or ↓ in total daily doses may be required depending on net changes in clearance, $t_{1/2}$	↑ or ↓ in total daily doses may be required depending on net changes in clearance, $t_{1/2}$

[a]Fluoroquinolones do not clearly fit into one specific category as being either hydrophilic or lipophilic. Fluoroquinolones are zwitterionic compounds; although often characterized as hydrophilic, they also have PK characteristics of more lipophilic compounds.

ARC = augmented renal clearance; PK = pharmacokinetic; $t_{1/2}$ = half-life; Vss = volume of distribution at steady state.

fluid volumes (Table 12.2). Infections themselves are also often associated with altered Vss values. Microbial endotoxins and proteins may stimulate the production of proinflammatory mediators that may affect the vascular endothelium, resulting in vasoconstriction or vasodilatation with maldistribution of blood flow, endothelial damage, increased capillary permeability, and decreased plasma oncotic pressure.[27-29] The resulting capillary leak syndrome results in fluid shifts from the intravascular compartment to the interstitial space and other anatomical spaces (i.e., third spacing)[30,31]; this in turn has the potential to increase the Vss of hydrophilic drugs and decrease tissue and plasma drug concentrations. The Vss of hydrophilic drugs may also be increased by the presence of other proinflammatory states such as trauma, burn injuries, mediastinitis, peritonitis, and mechanical ventilation.[13-17,19,20,32-34] Such shifts in body fluid as described previously have been implicated as a major cause of alterations in Vss in critical illness. Aggressive administration of crystalloids or colloids to maintain intravascular volumes in patients with sepsis, trauma, or burns also contributes to significant third spacing and alterations in Vss. Fluid collections such as pleural effusions, ascites, peritoneal exudates, mediastinitis, and edema serve as additional reservoirs where hydrophilic drugs such as the aminoglycosides and β-lactams may be distributed, further increasing their Vss.[13,14,16,32,35-47]

Decreased plasma albumin concentrations occur commonly in a wide variety of critically ill patients. Hypoalbuminemia may be the result of capillary leak syndrome, fluid overload, malnutrition, or hypercatabolic states.[13] Reductions in plasma oncotic pressure as a result of hypoalbuminemia may result in increased fluid extravasation and third spacing, which in turn contributes to increased Vss for hydrophilic antimicrobials. Protein binding of antimicrobials that bind primarily to albumin may also be significantly altered. In the setting of hypoalbuminemia, drugs that are normally highly bound to albumin have increased proportions of unbound drug (free fraction, or f_u); this unbound drug is free to distribute to tissues to which the albumin-bound drug was not previously accessible.[48,49] A notable example is ceftriaxone (95% bound to albumin), which has Vss values increased by as much as 90% in critically ill patients.[49] Several drugs have been shown to have increased Vss, and sometimes increased drug clearance as well, because of altered protein binding in patients with hypoalbuminemia and increased fluid extravasation.[13] Although antimicrobial f_u is often increased in hypoalbuminemia, the actual unbound concentration of drug (C_u) is not necessarily increased because the reduced protein binding also causes an increased clearance of this free drug. For hydrophilic drugs, this increased clearance is often because of increased renal elimination of unbound drug through the glomerulus; any increases in C_u are thus transient as the unbound drug is rapidly eliminated.

As a rule, the Vss of hydrophilic drugs is likely to be greater than normal in critically ill patients, and peak drug concentrations are likely to be correspondingly lower after any given dose. Thus, the ability of concentration-dependent antimicrobials to meet desired PK/PD targets such as the Cmax/MIC ratio is more likely to be adversely affected by changes in Vss. Lipophilic drugs tend to be less affected by these types of changes in body water and pathophysiological changes. However, changes in Vss are highly variable and may actually be decreased in certain patients. In addition, fluid shifts alone do not completely explain changes in antimicrobial Vss because other factors (e.g., protein binding) may also be responsible for Vss alterations in critically ill patients.

Obesity represents a major challenge for accurate drug dosing in the critically ill. The clinical significance of obesity in the dosing of antimicrobials is represented by data suggesting associations between obesity and subtherapeutic antibiotic concentrations or antibiotic treatment failure.[50-52] Because data are currently sparse, particularly in the critical care setting, it is difficult to make specific recommendations regarding the dosing of most antimicrobials in obesity. Obesity is known to increase the Vss of both hydrophilic and lipophilic drugs and may also be associated with increased clearance of certain drugs, particularly through enhanced clearance mechanisms.[53,54] The presence of obesity should be carefully evaluated in formulating antimicrobial dosing recommendations and potential PK changes accounted for as appropriate. Although beyond the scope of this chapter, useful recommendations for dosing of antimicrobials in obesity have been published elsewhere.[55-57]

Changes in Drug Clearance

Clearance, generally described as the intrinsic ability of the body to remove drug, is also significantly affected by the many disease processes that occur in critically ill patients. Although metabolism and excretion are two separate processes in a strictly PK sense, with respect to PK alterations in the critically ill, it is most useful to consider these processes together. Lipophilic drugs usually undergo clearance through hepatic metabolism followed by excretion of inactive metabolites through urine, bile, or feces. Although the formation of active metabolites through hepatic metabolic pathways is common for other classes of drugs, it is unusual and largely insignificant for most antimicrobials. Hydrophilic drugs, in contrast, do not usually undergo significant metabolism and are largely eliminated through renal excretion, with the kidneys serving as the organ of clearance. Changes in drug clearance are therefore usually because of either alterations in hepatic metabolism or alterations in renal function, or both.

Table 12.2 Selected Clinical Factors Associated with Alterations in Antimicrobial Pharmacokinetics in Critically Ill Patients

		Increased	Decreased
Absorption			Shock states
			Vasopressors
			Lack of enteral nutrition
			Drugs that decrease GI motility (e.g., opiates)
Volume of distribution	Hydrophilic drugs	Acid-base disturbances	Dehydration
		Aggressive volume resuscitation	
		Ascites	
		Cachexia, muscle mass depletion	
		Capillary leak syndromes	
		Chronic fluid overload	
		Edema	
		Heart failure	
		Hypoalbuminemia	
		Large TBSA burn injury	
		Large pleural effusions	
		Malnutrition	
		Mechanical ventilation	
		Mediastinitis	
		Peritonitis, peritoneal exudates	
		Third spacing	
		Trauma	
	Lipophilic drugs	Obesity	
Clearance	Renally eliminated drugs	Augmented renal clearance	Hepatic disease or injury
		Burn injuries (> 30%–40% TBSA)	Hemodynamic instability or failure
		Hypoalbuminemia	Protein malnutrition
		Postsurgical drains with high drainage volumes	Renal disease or injury
		Vasopressors[a]	Sepsis
			Shock states
			Vasopressors[a]
	Hepatically eliminated drugs	Drug-drug interactions (e.g., hepatic enzyme inducers)	Drug-drug interactions (e.g., hepatic enzyme inhibitors)
		Vasopressors[a]	Hepatic disease or injury
			Sepsis
			Shock states
			Vasopressors[a]
Protein binding		Burn injury	Hepatic disease
		Trauma	Hypoalbuminemia
			Malnutrition

[a]Effects are dependent on net effects on renal and hepatic perfusion.

TBSA = total body surface area.

Hepatic Metabolism and Hepatic Drug Clearance

Hepatic metabolism of drugs is primarily dependent on three separate physiological processes: hepatic blood flow, intrinsic activity of metabolic enzymes, and protein binding of drugs. Models of hepatic drug metabolism include an important factor, the hepatic extraction ratio (E_H), which generally describes the efficiency with which a particular drug is removed (i.e., cleared) from the blood during a single pass through the liver. Although detailed descriptions of hepatic extraction ratios are beyond the scope of this chapter, it is important to recognize that drugs may be broadly classified on the basis of their hepatic metabolism as either high extraction ratio or low extraction ratio. Drugs classified as high extraction ratio (E_H greater than 0.70) are metabolized by the liver with very high efficiency; their rate of metabolism and thus of drug clearance will be highly dependent on hepatic blood flow. Relatively minor changes in intrinsic enzyme activity (e.g., drug interactions involving weak to moderate inhibition of hepatic enzymes and protein binding alterations) are unlikely to cause significant changes in hepatic clearance. In contrast, the hepatic metabolism and clearance of low extraction ratio drugs (E_H less than 0.30) will be highly dependent on both protein binding and the intrinsic activity of specific enzymes involved in the metabolism of those drugs. Given known or predicted changes in blood flow, intrinsic enzyme activity, and/or protein binding in a critically ill patient, characterizing a particular drug as either high or low E_H is useful in predicting corresponding alterations in drug metabolism, clearance, and potential need for changes in dosing regimens.

Alterations in blood flow to the liver may commonly be seen in critically ill patients. Conditions in which significantly reduced hepatic perfusion may occur include severe sepsis and septic shock in which organ malperfusion is present, other shock states (hemorrhagic, hypovolemic, cardiogenic, anaphylactic), myocardial infarction, acute heart failure, thrombotic disorders involving the hepatic circulation, and therapeutic hypothermia. All of these various disorders are potentially associated with reduced clearance of drugs.[58,59] Mechanical ventilation with or without the administration of PEEP (positive end-expiratory pressure) has also been associated with decreased hepatic perfusion,[60] as well as the administration of α-adrenergic agents such as epinephrine, norepinephrine, phenylephrine, vasopressin, and high-dose dopamine.[61-63] Conversely, inotropic agents such as dobutamine and dopamine and vasodilators such as nitroglycerin may increase hepatic perfusion through improved hemodynamics and increasing cardiac output.

Regarding the intrinsic activity of metabolic enzymes, the induction or suppression of the metabolizing enzymes by disease state–related mechanisms or drug-drug interactions may also have significant effects on drug metabolism. Several mediators commonly present in critically ill patients have been associated with significant inhibition of both phase I oxidative metabolism involving the cytochrome P450 (CYP) system and phase II conjugative metabolism, which includes acetylation, glucuronidation, and sulfation pathways. These inhibitory mediators include stress hormones such as cortisol, epinephrine, and norepinephrine and proinflammatory cytokines including interleukin-1b, interleukin-6, and tumor necrosis factor-α.[58,64] Conversely, hepatic metabolism has been shown to increase for selected medications in patients with traumatic brain injury. Both phase I and phase II metabolism has been shown to be increased in this population, raising the potential for subtherapeutic concentrations of drugs that are dependent on these metabolic pathways.[65] Nutritional supplementation with increased amounts of dietary protein has also been shown to increase hepatic metabolism and drug clearance.[66]

Alterations in protein binding may have important effects on the hepatic metabolism of low extraction ratio drugs. Critically ill patients commonly have alterations in plasma proteins as a result of physiological stress, including decreased concentrations of plasma albumin and increased concentrations of $α_1$-acid glycoprotein (AAG). Albumin concentrations are often decreased in response to hepatic processes and catabolic states, whereas AAG concentrations are known to increase in many inflammatory processes such as severe thermal injuries. Albumin binds acidic drugs, and decreased albumin concentrations potentially result in increased f_u, whereas increased concentrations of AAG result in decreased f_u of basic drugs. Such changes in protein binding tend to produce temporary, offsetting changes in hepatic metabolism so that the net changes in free drug concentrations are minimal. The activity of CYP may be unchanged, increased, or decreased because of hepatocellular loss, enzyme induction, or inhibition.

The net effect of these many changes in protein binding, hepatic blood flow, effects of critical illness, or drug-drug interactions on liver function and drug clearance is extremely complex and difficult to predict in the clinical setting. Fortunately, the overall number of agents for which protein-binding alterations significantly affect drug exposure has been proposed to be relatively limited.[67] In addition, for most antimicrobials, hepatic metabolism is limited, and protein binding is low enough to make little difference to their effectiveness. Specific antimicrobials for which lowering of doses in patients with severe hepatic disease would be advisable include clindamycin, metronidazole, nafcillin, erythromycin, and certain antifungals such as voriconazole, posaconazole, and the echinocandins.

Renal Clearance of Drugs

Renal elimination of parent drugs or their metabolites is the primary route of excretion for most pharmacologic

Table 12.3 Selected Pharmacokinetic Parameters for Antimicrobials Commonly Used in Critically Ill Patients

Antimicrobial	Volume of Distribution at Steady State (L/kg)	Protein Binding (%)	Metabolism?	Renal Clearance (% as unchanged drug)	Plasma Half-life (hours)
Aminoglycosides (gentamicin, tobramycin, amikacin)	0.30	<10	None	95	2-3
Nafcillin	0.30	90	Hepatic	30	0.5-1
Piperacillin	0.25	26	Moderate hepatic	50-70	0.7-1.2
Cefazolin	0.30	75-85	Minimal hepatic	>80-90	2
Ceftriaxone	0.14	90	Moderate hepatic	60	6-9
Ceftazidime	0.25	17	None	90	1-2
Cefepime	0.30	20	Minimal	85	2
Imipenem/cilastatin	0.26	20	No hepatic	70	1
Meropenem	0.30	2	Minimal	75	1
Aztreonam	0.25	56	Minimal	60-70	1.5-2
Vancomycin	0.70	50	None	100	4-6
Linezolid	0.5-0.6	31	Hepatic	30	4-5
Daptomycin	0.10	90	Minor	80	9-10
Azithromycin	31.1	30-40	Biliary excretion	6	70-80
Ciprofloxacin	2.1-2.7	40	Moderate hepatic	50	3-4
Levofloxacin	1.0-1.5	30	None	60-80	6-10
Clindamycin	0.6-1.2	90	Hepatic	10	1.5-5
Metronidazole	0.80	20	Hepatic	20	8
Fluconazole	0.60	10	Minor hepatic	90	31
Amphotericin B deoxycholate	1.8-2.0	>95	Minimal hepatic	3-20	100-160
Liposomal amphotericin B	0.80	>95	Minimal hepatic	5	100-153
Caspofungin	0.40	97	Hepatic	<2	30
Anidulafungin	0.4-0.7	84	None	<2	26
Micafungin	0.40	99	Hepatic	<2	15
Voriconazole	4.6	58	Hepatic	<2	6
Posaconazole	4.1	99	Hepatic	<2	25
Acyclovir	0.70	10-30	None	>85	2.5-4
Ganciclovir	0.70	1-2	None	>95	4-6
Colistin	0.2-1.5	Unknown	Minimal	>80	2-4

agents, including most antimicrobial agents (Table 12.3). In critically ill patients, renal failure may occur because of several pathophysiological processes including severe sepsis and septic shock, multiple organ failure syndrome, extensive burns, trauma, hypovolemic shock, heart failure, and cardiogenic shock.[13] Acute kidney injury may also be caused by drug toxicities as well as therapeutic use of vasopressors, which may cause reduced renal blood flow and decreased renal clearance of drugs.[39] Because preexisting renal impairment related to underlying illnesses and acute kidney injury are common among critically ill patients of all types, decreased clearance of renally eliminated drugs is of major importance in the ICU setting. Severe renal impairment requiring renal replacement therapy is also common and presents special challenges to clinicians related to appropriate drug dosing. Although methods for assessing renal function such as the Cockcroft-Gault (CG) and MDRD (Modified Diet in Renal Disease) equations are commonly used in the ICU because they are familiar to clinicians and simple,[68,69] it must be remembered that they are also known to be relatively inaccurate in critically ill patients and do not always provide reliable measures of drug clearance.[70-76]

In the absence of significant organ dysfunction, critically ill patients often have increased renal perfusion, increased glomerular filtration rates and creatinine clearance, and subsequently increased clearance of hydrophilic antibiotics.[77-79] Further evidence suggests that critically ill patients have higher creatinine clearances even in the presence of normal plasma creatinine concentrations.[80-85] The recognition of *augmented renal clearance* (*ARC*), defined as a creatinine clearance greater than 130 mL/minute/1.73 m², in many critically ill patients adds yet another measure of uncertainty in the evaluation of renal function and drug clearance for purposes of antimicrobial dosing. Augmented renal clearance occurs at highly variable rates and has been reported to occur in 30%–86% of patients in ICUs.[80,83,84,86-88] Specific risk factors have not been identified, although several factors have consistently been reported among various studies; these include younger age (50 years or younger), male, trauma, traumatic brain injury, mechanical ventilation, and lesser severity of illness.[80,83,85] However, the occurrence of ARC is highly unpredictable and has also been reported among 40% of patients with sepsis, in older patients, and in patients with high severity of illness.[84-88] Although the timing of onset and duration of ARC have not been well characterized, it may already be present on ICU admission and last for 1 week or more.[84-88] The presence of ARC is a significant problem for antimicrobial dosing in critically ill patients because, if unrecognized, use of improperly adjusted drug doses may result in underdosing of antimicrobials, subtherapeutic drug concentrations, and therapeutic failure in the treatment of infections.[81,86-90]

Among specific types of patients, trauma patients have commonly been reported to have increased clearance of renally eliminated drugs. However, actual studies have provided mixed results with respect to renal clearance and dosing requirements of various antibiotics in this population.[14] Despite the apparently high incidence of ARC in this population, studies have nevertheless noted a high degree of variability in drug clearance among trauma patients.[14] Medical and surgical ICU patients are likewise highly variable with respect to alterations in renal clearance. A review of literature reporting antibiotic PK in medical and surgical patients concluded that, although some patients did in fact have increased renal clearance, a similar number of patients had no changes or even reduced renal clearance of antibiotics.[14] The high degree of variability in drug clearance among medical and surgical ICU patients likely mirrors the high degree of patient heterogeneity found among this population with respect to patient demographics, underlying comorbidities, and reason for admission to the ICU.[14]

Patients with burn injuries have also been often reported to have increased renal clearance of antibiotics. Similar to trauma patients, patients with burn injuries tend to be younger, have fewer baseline comorbidities, are initially hypermetabolic, and receive large volumes of resuscitation fluids.[14] Many studies of this population have shown increased renal clearance compared with normal patients not in ICUs, but patients with burn injuries also tended to have a high degree of variability with respect to both increased and decreased clearance. Antimicrobials such as aminoglycosides, vancomycin, ciprofloxacin, and fluconazole usually have increased clearance, whereas individual β-lactam agents are more variable in the effects of their injuries.[14,91-96] Clinicians should remember that patients with burn injuries often require higher daily doses of antimicrobials in order to meet desired PK/PD targets, but that such aggressive dosing may also place patients at greater risk of drug-related toxicities if patients do not actually have increased renal clearance.[14] This is a potentially problematic finding, because drug concentrations that are much more variable than in normal subjects could result in a higher incidence of subtherapeutic or toxic concentrations. Although toxic concentrations in a patient may be detected by adverse events that manifest as clinical or laboratory abnormalities, the risk of subtherapeutic drug concentrations from rapid clearance is largely undetectable at the bedside and is compounded by the increased volume of distribution commonly seen in these patients.

Changes in Plasma Protein Binding and Antibiotic Penetration to Tissues

The effects of altered protein binding on V_{ss} and hepatic drug clearance have already been described. Drugs with reduced binding to albumin or other plasma proteins may have increased f_u of antibiotic, which could potentially have therapeutic implications. Because time-dependent antibiotics rely on free drug concentrations to be consistently above the pathogen MIC ($fT>MIC$ being the key PD parameter for these agents), it is possible that increased f_u of these drugs may actually contribute to enhanced therapeutic efficacy. However, decreased protein binding produces mixed effects on PK parameters, including both V_{ss} and clearance, which may offset the theoretical advantages. As previously discussed, decreased protein binding is often associated with increased V_{ss} and may result in reduced concentrations of hydrophilic drugs in plasma, interstitial fluids, and other tissues through a dilutional effect. This alteration in V_{ss} may therefore have adverse effects on concentration-dependent drugs unless doses are correspondingly increased. Protein binding alterations are not usually clinically relevant for hepatically cleared drugs because clearance of high E_H drugs is not limited by protein binding and, for low E_H drugs, changes in f_u are often quickly offset by corresponding increases in hepatic clearance. The most relevant effect of decreased protein binding for most antimicrobials, particularly those that are renally cleared, is that increasing f_u values often result in more rapid renal drug elimination.[97] However, hypoalbuminemia and other causes for altered protein binding are only likely to significantly influence antibiotic clearance when the agent is highly protein bound (90% or greater) and has an intrinsically low Vss.[98] Protein binding is sufficiently low for most antimicrobials that alterations in f_u are not likely to pose a problem with respect to altered drug clearance (Table 12.3).

The foregoing discussion regarding the PK effects of altered protein binding largely assumes that patients have otherwise normal hepatic and renal function and will follow well-established models of PK disposition of drugs. This is obviously not the case for critically ill patients in whom significant renal and hepatic impairment is common, as well as hemodynamic changes that may alter normal processes related to Vss and clearance. Although the protein binding of antimicrobials in critically ill patients is known to be altered, the true clinical significance of these alterations is not well understood and likely varies considerably among individual patients.

Antimicrobial penetration into infection sites is also an important consideration related to the PK/PD properties of the drugs. The ability of antibiotics to penetrate to tissue sites is related to the type of antibiotic, protein binding, tissue characteristics, and method of antibiotic administration. The disposition of antibiotics has traditionally been studied by comparing tissue to serum concentration ratios in infected and non-infected tissues. However, these studies have also shown high variability in estimates of tissue distribution. In vitro and in vivo studies suggest that high intravascular protein binding restricts the penetration of antibiotics into extravascular tissue sites.[98-101] Microdialysis is an in vivo sampling technique that is being increasingly used to characterize antimicrobial tissue penetration, particularly in critically ill patients.[102-106] Several studies using microdialysis techniques have shown quite good correlations between degree of protein binding and drug concentrations in interstitial fluids. However, free drug concentrations in plasma are often not representative of drug concentrations being achieved at actual infection sites because of physiological shunting or otherwise impaired tissue perfusion. Data analyses suggest that antibiotic penetration into tissues of patients with septic shock is impaired because of hemodynamic instability and regional perfusion abnormalities. Antibiotic concentrations in tissues of patients with septic shock may be 5- to 10-fold lower than in healthy volunteers or patients with less severe sepsis.[102-106] Aggressive dosing of antibiotics is probably required to maximize antibiotic penetration into infected tissue, particularly in patients with shock states, although data to support this are currently lacking, and even administration of very high doses may be insufficient to overcome tissue perfusion abnormalities, which may be present in various pathophysiological processes. For highly bound antimicrobials that undergo primarily renal elimination, aggressive dosing may likewise be required to overcome potentially enhanced renal clearance in patients without renal impairment.

Changes in Antibiotic Half-Life

The elimination half-life of a drug is directly related to its clearance and Vss characteristics. The half-life is mathematically represented by the following equation:

$$t_{1/2} = \frac{0.693 \times V_{ss}}{\text{clearance}}$$

The half-life of a drug is directly related to changes in both Vss and clearance; increased Vss and/or decreased clearance will increase the half-life, whereas decreased Vss and/or increased clearance will decrease the half-life. An increase in Vss that prolongs the half-life might be therapeutically advantageous for time-dependent antimicrobials from a PK/PD perspective but a potential disadvantage for concentration-dependent agents that are dependent on achieving adequate Cmax concentrations. The same considerations could apply to reductions in drug clearance, which would also potentially be advantageous for time-dependent antimicrobials because of the reduced elimination rates and maintenance of drug concentrations over longer periods. However, such generalizations do not adequately represent the complexities of the many pathophysiological processes that influence Vss and clearance (often simultaneously), the dynamic nature of critically ill patients in whom PK properties of drugs may be changing on a daily (if not hourly) basis because of therapeutic interventions and evolving pathophysiological processes, or the significant difficulties in adequately assessing and characterizing the potential PK alterations that may be present in an individual patient. Although it is predictable that PK alterations are occurring in many critically ill patients, it is also extremely difficult for clinicians to make informed dosing decisions on the basis of accurate estimates of the magnitude of these changes.

General Strategies for Dosing Adjustments Based on PK Alterations

A general strategy for assessing the need for potential dose adjustments of antimicrobials in critically ill patients is first to determine whether the specific drug is primarily cleared through hepatic metabolism or renal excretion. As previously discussed, antimicrobials that are hepatically metabolized do not generally require dosage adjustments in ICU patients unless significant hepatic dysfunction is present. For drugs that are renally cleared, reduction in total daily doses may be considered in the presence of renal impairment, whereas the presence of certain other conditions (Table 12.2) should prompt clinicians to consider increasing total daily doses. Clinicians should also consider increasing doses of hydrophilic drugs in the presence of conditions that are associated with increased Vss values of these agents (Table 12.2). Beyond these simple considerations, determining if and how antimicrobial regimens should be appropriately adjusted in ICU patients becomes much more difficult.

Because of the severity of infections encountered in critically ill patients and because of the variability in PK, tissue penetration, presence of obesity, pathogen MICs, and other factors relating to the efficacy of antimicrobials, the general recommendation for antimicrobials in ICU patients is to use high, aggressive initial doses. Aggressive dosing of antimicrobials (at least during empiric therapy in high-risk patients) should be a standard practice in ICUs to optimize the PD performance of the drugs. Use of high initial doses (until pathogens and susceptibilities are determined and/or patients show favorable clinical response) potentially compensates for PK variability that may be present and helps ensure that patients are receiving enough drug to successfully achieve the PD goals of antimicrobial use. Reliable attainment of key PK/PD targets (AUC_{0-24}/MIC, Cmax/MIC, and fT>MIC) depends on being able to adequately estimate the PK disposition of antimicrobials in individual patients. Beyond PK considerations, the other important variable in PD targets is the pathogen MIC. As bacterial pathogens encountered in the ICU continue to become less susceptible with higher MICs,[107-112] the use of aggressive initial dosing regimens becomes even more important because the selected dosing regimens have to allow for the elevated MICs as well as variability in PK parameters.[107] Given the extreme variability of PK parameters such as Vss and clearance and the inability to precisely assess renal function, hepatic function, protein binding, and tissue penetration of antimicrobials in critically ill patients, clinicians should err on the side of aggressive dosing in order to avoid being too conservative with administered regimens.[16,20,76,113] However, use of high doses also places patients at higher risk of drug-related adverse effects and toxicities, again partly owing to PK variability in drug Vss and clearance. Although drug dosing should be aggressive, it must also be based on appropriate clinical considerations involving relevant issues such as appropriate PK/PD goals, careful clinical assessment for the presence of renal or hepatic dysfunction that may lead to drug accumulation, presence of obesity, the presumed infection site and the ability of the drug to achieve adequate concentrations in that site, susceptibilities of presumed or documented pathogens to the drugs in question, and potential drug toxicities.

Because achieving appropriate PK/PD targets for antimicrobials is an important predictor of clinical efficacy and the risk of developing microbial resistance, clinicians must take care not to underdose antimicrobials in critically ill patients. Given the known inaccuracies in estimating creatinine clearance on the basis of serum creatinine, clinicians should not rely on estimated creatinine clearance as a sole consideration for choosing drug dosing regimens in patients with renal impairment. Apparently, "proper" dosing adjustments on the basis of estimated creatinine and published recommendations for dose adjustment (e.g., product package inserts) may effectively reduce total drug use and drug cost and potentially also reduce adverse effects of some drugs. However, given the need to achieve PD targets in the setting of variable PK parameters and difficult pathogens, even high doses of many drugs are already marginal, and alternative dosing strategies are sometimes necessary.[113-117] Because serum creatinine–based methods of assessing renal function are notoriously inaccurate for predicting drug clearance in ICU patients,[70-76] clinicians should not try to "fine-tune" dose adjustments because doing so may place some patients at risk of treatment failure. For example, in a severely infected patient with a creatinine clearance estimated at 48 mL/minute by the CG method, antimicrobial doses should not necessarily be reduced just because the product labeling specifies dose reduction at calculated creatinine clearances less than 50 mL/minute. Rather, clinicians must consider potential risks to the patient (drug toxicities, etc.) versus the potential benefits to be gained by administering higher doses than those recommended, at least until the patient starts having a response to antimicrobial therapy.[20,116]

Given the apparently high prevalence of ARC and the potential for patients to be underdosed in this setting, clinicians should be alert to patients who fit the currently recognized risk factors for ARC (young, male, trauma, low severity of illness, etc.) and be prepared to administer higher-than-normal doses to such patients. Recognition of ARC also depends on accurate assessment of renal function. Because serum creatinine–based methods are not reliably accurate, including among patients with ARC,[71] the use of timed urinary creatinine measurements should be standard practice when more accurate assessment of renal function is needed.[15,84,118-120] Although timed urinary creatinine measurements are also not completely accurate, this method is generally recognized as providing somewhat more accurate estimates of GFR (glomerular filtration rate) in critically ill patients. Because U.S. Food and Drug Administration (FDA)-labeled dosing of antimicrobials does not specifically address recommended doses in patients with a creatinine clearance greater than 130–150 mL/minute and no other formal dosing recommendations exist for patients with ARC, clinicians will need to exercise their best judgment in determining appropriate doses. One recent study found that 55% of patients in a medical/surgical ICU receiving standard doses of meropenem (1 g every 8 hours) or piperacillin/tazobactam (4.5 g every 6 hours) did not meet the PK/PD targets intended to treat *Pseudomonas aeruginosa* infections, even when 3-hour extended infusions were used for drug administration.[90]

Therapeutic drug monitoring (TDM) of aminoglycosides and vancomycin is common in current practice and is considered a standard of care for patients receiving these agents. Because of the extreme PK variability of β-lactam agents in ICU patients, routine TDM has been suggested for these drugs as well.[121-123] The ability to routinely measure and adjust β-lactam concentrations could be very advantageous in detecting patients with significant alterations in PK parameters and adjusting doses to more effectively meet PD targets. Unfortunately, β-lactam assays are not routinely available to most hospital laboratories or clinicians, and TDM for β-lactam antibiotics is not currently feasible. Plasma concentrations of certain antifungal agents such as voriconazole and posaconazole are also occasionally measured, and a routine role for TDM has been advocated,[124-127] but routine TDM practices for antifungal agents have not yet been established. For most antimicrobials, reliance on population PK studies and close clinical monitoring for evidence of clinical response to therapy and drug toxicities remain the only available option.

In light of the many challenges in determining appropriate dosing of antimicrobials, newer dosing strategies (e.g., extended infusions for β-lactams) may play an important role in optimizing drug therapy in order to more reliably meet desired PK/PD goals. Such strategies have been purposely developed and studied in order to provide more reliable and effective dosing options for treatment of difficult pathogens in severely ill patients. Critically ill patients certainly have many risk factors for poor outcomes of antimicrobial therapy, and newer dosing options as discussed in later sections of this chapter should be considered for patients in the ICU.

PD CONSIDERATIONS FOR DRUG DOSING IN THE ICU

The rate and extent of the activity of an antimicrobial drug is dependent on many factors including the interaction between drug concentrations at the infection site and the MIC of the pathogen. A change in the PK properties of an antimicrobial agent may therefore affect the activity of the drug against a particular pathogen and may also affect the outcome of therapy. Conversely, developing dosing regimens that optimize the PK characteristics of the drug in relation to the MIC potentially improve clinical responses, accelerate the rate of clinical response with the potential for reducing durations of drug therapy, and minimize the risk of developing antibacterial resistance. An understanding of the PD properties of drugs, which describe the nature of such PK-MIC interactions, is necessary in order to make informed decisions regarding selection of an appropriate regimen for a given patient.

Given the potential for extreme variability of antimicrobial PK properties in critically ill patients, maximizing the PD "performance" of a drug is often very challenging. However, a working knowledge of the PD relationships of various drugs as well as an understanding of critical illness maximizes the potential for optimizing dosing regimens for individual critically ill patients. Clinicians also need to be familiar with MICs relevant to the chosen antibacterial agent for suspected or known pathogens in the ICU setting. The remainder of this chapter will review currently recommended PK/PD targets for common antimicrobials, discuss examples of clinical applications of PD principles, and describe potential limitations to the application of PK/PD in the clinical setting.

PD Goals

Pharmacodynamic parameters correlating with antimicrobial efficacy have been widely published and are summarized in Table 12.4.[5,7,8,117,128-135] These parameters have been determined from in vitro and in vivo studies and, for many drugs, also validated in humans through clinical data obtained either retrospectively or prospectively. It is important to recognize that these targets have sometimes been modified over time as additional studies are performed and our understanding of PK/PD relationships is increased. However, PD parameters summarized in Table 12.4 reflect our current understanding of the complex relationships governing antimicrobial actions and efficacy. Because plasma or tissue concentrations are not routinely measured for most of these agents, computer modeling techniques such as Monte Carlo simulation (MCS) form the basis for dosing recommendations that seek to maximize the attainment of PD goals in patients requiring antimicrobial therapy.

Antibacterials

Time-Dependent Drugs

In general, the goal of a dosage regimen for a time-dependent antibiotic is to optimize the duration of drug exposure above the MIC. Although meeting a minimum effective concentration of drug is also necessary, increasing the concentration beyond 4–6 times the MIC does not appear to result in enhanced killing but may instead require unnecessarily high doses of drug.[5,7,11] Once effective concentrations have been reached, extending the time those concentrations remain above the MIC should enhance antibacterial activity and presumably efficacy as well. The $fT>MIC$ is the PK/PD parameter considered most predictive of bactericidal activity of many time-dependent antimicrobials such as the β-lactams, although the AUC_{0-24}/MIC is a good predictor of efficacy for some time-dependent drugs such as vancomycin and linezolid.[5,7,8,11,131]

Table 12.4 PD Parameters and Goal Values Correlating with Efficacy of Antimicrobial Drugs

PD Characteristics	Antimicrobials	Specific PK/PD Goal
Time-dependent	Penicillins	50% $fT>MIC$
	Cephalosporins	60%–70% $fT>MIC$
	Monobactams	60%–70% $fT>MIC$
	Carbapenems	40% $fT>MIC$
	Vancomycin	$AUC_{0-24}/MIC \geq 350–400$
		(TDM: trough 15–20 mg/L for severe infections)
	Linezolid	> 85% $fT>MIC$
		$AUC_{0-24}/MIC > 85$
	Flucytosine	> 40% $fT>MIC$
		(TDM: peak < 100 mcg/mL, trough < 10–50 mcg/mL)
Concentration-dependent	Aminoglycosides	$Cmax/MIC > 8–10$
		AUC_{0-24}/MIC 80–125
	Fluoroquinolones	$Cmax/MIC > 10–12$
		$AUC_{0-24}/MIC > 125–250^a$
		$AUC_{0-24}/MIC > 30–50^b$
	Daptomycin	AUC_{0-24}/MIC^c
	Tigecycline	$fAUC_{0-24}/MIC > 0.9$
	Colistin	$AUC_{0-24}/MIC > 60$
	Metronidazole	$AUC_{0-24}/MIC > 70$
	Fluconazole	$fAUC_{0-24}/MIC > 25$
		(Dose in mg/MIC >50 has also been recommended as a surrogate PK/PD indicator)
	Itraconazole	$fAUC_{0-24}/MIC > 25$
		(TDM: trough > 1.0 mcg/mL for treatment)
	Voriconazole	$fAUC_{0-24}/MIC > 25$
		(TDM: trough > 2 for treatment efficacy, < 5.5 mcg/mL for ↓ toxicities)
	Posaconazole	$fAUC_{0-24}/MIC > 25$
		(TDM: trough > 0.7 mcg/mL for prophylaxis, > 1.5 mcg/mL for treatment)
	Echinocandins	$fAUC_{0-24}/MIC > 10^d$
		$fAUC_{0-24}/MIC > 10^e$
	Amphotericin B deoxycholate	$fCmax/MIC > 40$

[a]For gram-negative bacteria.
[b]For *Streptococcus pneumoniae*.
[c]Specific goal value not determined.
[d]For treatment of *Candida* infections.
[e]For treatment of *Aspergillus* infections.

AUC_{0-24}/MIC = ratio of the 24-hour area under the serum concentration versus time curve divided by the MIC; Cmax/MIC = ratio of maximum serum concentration divided by the MIC; $fAUC_{0-24}/MIC$ = ratio of the 24-hour area under the serum concentration versus time curve for unbound/free drug divided by the MIC; $fCmax/MIC$ = ratio of maximum serum concentration of unbound/free drug divided by the MIC; $fT>MIC$ = time during which unbound/free drug remains above the pathogen MIC. MIC = minimum inhibitory concentration; PD = pharmacodynamic; PK = pharmacokinetic; TDM = therapeutic drug monitoring.

For β-lactam antibiotics, in vitro and in vivo studies have shown that $fT>MIC$ is the best predictor of bacterial killing and microbiological response against gram-negative bacteria.[5,7,8,11] However, these studies have also shown that the specific $fT>MIC$ target is different for the various types of β-lactam antibiotics.[5,7,8,11] For penicillins, an $fT>MIC$ of 30% produces bacteriostatic effects on bacteria, whereas a 50% $fT>MIC$ is required for maximal bactericidal effects. Cephalosporins require somewhat greater $fT>MIC$ than do penicillins: 35%–40% for bacteriostatic activity and 60%–70% for bactericidal effects. For bacteriostatic and bactericidal effects, the carbapenems require $fT>MIC$ values of about 20%–30% and 40%, respectively.

The AUC_{0-24}/MIC ratio is the best PK/PD predictor of response to vancomycin therapy according to data from animal models and in vitro studies. Those studies suggest that an AUC_{0-24}/MIC ratio of at least 350–400 is essential for a good clinical outcome.[132,136-141] The current recommendations to target trough vancomycin concentrations of 15–20 mg/L for treatment of severe infections are based on the fact that these trough concentrations correlate with AUC_{0-24}/MIC values of 350–400 or greater in the treatment of *Staphylococcus aureus* infections caused by strains with MICs less than 1 mg/L.[136-140]

Linezolid is also a time-dependent antibiotic that has been associated with both $fT>MIC$ and AUC_{0-24}/MIC as the parameters that best describe its antibacterial activity.[131,142] Clinical efficacy of linezolid has been correlated with an $fT>MIC$ of 85% and greater and an AUC_{0-24}/MIC greater than 85.[131] Similar numbers have also been associated with high microbiological cure rates, which may in turn relate to reduced risk of selecting gram-positive resistance to linezolid.[131]

Concentration-Dependent Drugs

The PD parameters associated with bactericidal effects of concentration-dependent drugs include both Cmax/MIC and AUC_{0-24}/MIC ratios. Aminoglycosides and fluoroquinolones are among the antibiotics that have these PK-PD relationships. In vitro time-kill studies have shown that the rate and extent of bactericidal activity increases as antibiotic concentrations increase in relation to the bacterial MIC for these drugs.[5] Bactericidal activity and clinical efficacy of the aminoglycosides have been associated with a Cmax/MIC ratio of greater than 8–10.[143-146] The AUC_{0-24}/MIC has also been studied as a determinant of clinical efficacy, and it has been suggested that this parameter is a better indicator of total aminoglycoside exposure.[144,146-148] Several studies have evaluated the AUC_{0-24}/MIC and determined that a target of 80–125 is a good predictor of bactericidal killing and antibacterial efficacy in animal models. Although the exact AUC_{0-24}/MIC target is unknown and may in fact vary somewhat depending on bacterial organism and type of infection being treated, the range of 80–125 seems to provide the best combination of maximizing the probability of clinical efficacy while minimizing nephrotoxicity risk.[144,146-148]

Studies have clearly shown that the fluoroquinolones have concentration-dependent bacterial killing.[148-153] Many studies, including a prospectively developed model of the PD response to levofloxacin during treatment of respiratory tract, skin, and urinary tract infections, have provided evidence that achieving a Cmax/MIC ratio of greater than 10–12 appears to be predictive of clinical drug efficacy and successful bacterial eradication.[148-153] The AUC_{0-24}/MIC has also been shown in vitro and retrospectively in vivo to be predictive of favorable clinical response and reduced development of resistance.[148-153] Although the optimal AUC_{0-24}/MIC ratio breakpoints are still unclear, favorable AUC_{0-24}/MIC ratios appear to be 125–250 for gram-negative organisms and 30–50 for *S. pneumoniae*.[148-153] These PD targets are generally applied to all currently used fluoroquinolones including ciprofloxacin, levofloxacin, and moxifloxacin. Whether either the Cmax/MIC ratio or the AUC_{0-24}/MIC ratio is superior to the other parameter and which specific ratios are most predictive of drug efficacy remain somewhat controversial; however, the strong relationships between these PD parameters and the clinical and microbiological outcomes during fluoroquinolone therapy have been well established.

Daptomycin is important to note among other the other concentration-dependent drugs.[154-156] Although PK/PD parameters best associated with clinical and microbiological efficacy of daptomycin have not been well established, its concentration-dependent properties serve as the basis for use of doses larger than the 4- to 6-mg/kg (depending on indication) doses currently recommended in the manufacturer's approved labeling.[157] Clinical data definitively showing improved outcomes of these higher doses (e.g., 8–12 mg/kg) are not yet available, although daptomycin has been shown to be safe and well tolerated at these doses.[158,159]

Antifungals

Similar to antibacterial agents, antifungal drugs have different PK/PD properties in vivo. These patterns of activity may be correlated with drug dose and pathogen MIC to identify dosing strategies that maximize antifungal efficacy while reducing the risk of toxicity. Similar to antibacterial drugs, inadequate dosing of antifungals may contribute to both treatment failure and the emergence of resistance.[160,161] With the increasing prevalence of non-albicans *Candida* spp. and their reduced susceptibility to certain antifungal agents,[162] appropriate choice and dosing of antifungals is essential for optimizing clinical outcomes and minimizing resistance. Pharmacodynamic data may also be useful for predicting infection sites where antifungal drugs have a higher risk of treatment failure because of poor tissue penetration and resultant low drug concentrations.

Although for many years there was a paucity of data related to antifungal PK/PD properties, these characteristics have more recently been reasonably well characterized and are increasingly recognized as potentially important factors for drug selection in the treatment of invasive fungal infections. Although PD principles are best established for *Candida* bloodstream infections, PK/PD principles have more recently also been successfully applied to the treatment of molds including *Aspergillus* spp. Of interest, PD characteristics of antifungal agents can be described using the same PK/PD parameters as those used for antibacterial drugs: Cmax/MIC ratio, AUC_{0-24}/MIC ratio, and T>MIC. For the antifungal agents, these parameters all seem to be best correlated with free unbound concentrations of drug;[134] thus, the following terms will be used to describe the PK/PD properties of the antifungals as they relate to free drug concentrations: fCmax/MIC ratio, $fAUC_{0-24}$/MIC ratio, and fT>MIC. These descriptions of antifungal PK/PD goals will of necessity be very brief, but several excellent review articles are available that provide comprehensive overviews of how antifungal PK/PD goals were derived and how they should be applied clinically.[124,126,133-135,163,164]

Time-Dependent Drugs

Flucytosine appears to be the only antifungal agent that has time-dependent antimicrobial activity in a manner similar to time-dependent antibacterials such as the β-lactams. Flucytosine has fungistatic activity against *Candida* spp. with 40% fT>MIC being the apparently optimal measure of drug exposure. This fT>MIC of 40% has been associated with favorable clinical outcomes in several studies.[124,126,133-135,163,164]

Concentration-Dependent Drugs

Fluconazole and the other azole-type antifungals have concentration-dependent PD properties and are best characterized against *Candida* spp. by $fAUC_{0-24}$/MIC. An $fAUC_{0-24}$/MIC of 25 or greater (using the Clinical and Laboratory Standards Institute [CLSI] MIC method) has been reported to maximize the efficacy of fluconazole with improved clinical outcomes shown in in vitro, in vivo, and clinical studies.[124,126,133-135,163,164] This same PD target of $fAUC_{0-24}$/MIC of 25 or greater appears to also describe other azoles reasonably well; clinical trial data analyses from mucosal and systemic candidiasis have identified a similar PD target for voriconazole and itraconazole.[124,126,133-135,163-168] Clinical data analyses regarding PD targets in the treatment of *Aspergillus* spp or other invasive molds remain limited. However, in patients receiving voriconazole for invasive aspergillosis for whom drug monitoring and clinical outcome data were available, rates of clinical success and survival were significantly higher in patients who achieved serum trough concentrations of 1–2 mg/mL.[169,170] Factoring in protein binding characteristics and the MIC for *Aspergillus* isolates, the resulting value for $fAUC_{0-24}$/MIC was again around 25.[169,170]

In contrast to the azoles, amphotericin B deoxycholate has concentration-dependent fungicidal activity against *Candida* spp., and its efficacy is best correlated with an fCmax/MIC ratio of 2–4.[124,126,133-135,163,164] Unfortunately, few data exist for the lipid formulations of amphotericin B (LAMB). According to a study of children that included a small cohort with invasive aspergillosis, maximal antifungal efficacy of LAMB was observed with an fCmax/MIC greater than 40.[171]

Echinocandins also have concentration-dependent fungicidal activity against *Candida* spp., and both fCmax/MIC and $fAUC_{0-24}$/MIC have been associated with clinical efficacy.[124,126,133-135,163,164,172] Studies of both animal models and patients with invasive candidiasis have identified similar PD targets with maximal antifungal efficacy achieved at an $fAUC_{0-24}$/MIC near 10. Data analyses defining PK/PD targets for treatment of invasive aspergillosis with echinocandins are few. However, one study found an fCmax/MIC ratio of 10–20 to be associated with maximal efficacy.[173]

Antivirals and Antiprotozoals

Although antiviral agents such as acyclovir and ganciclovir are used with regularity in the ICU, the PD properties of antiviral agents are not well characterized, and no formal PK/PD-based dosing recommendations can be made. Aggressive dosing in seriously ill patients, thoughtful assessment of organ function with recommended dosage adjustments made as appropriate, and close monitoring of patients for evidence of clinical response and drug-related toxicities continue to be the mainstays of antiviral use in the ICU. Similarly, the PDs of antiprotozoal drugs have not been well described, and no formal recommendations for use in ICU patients can be made.

CLINICAL APPLICATIONS OF PD PRINCIPLES IN THE CRITICALLY ILL

Prolonged and Continuous Infusions of β-Lacam Antibiotics

Optimization of drug exposure for time-dependent antibiotics such as the β-lactams requires maintaining antibiotic concentrations above the MIC for prolonged periods. With an increased understanding of PK/PD characteristics of the β-lactams, there has also come a concern that the traditional method of administering antibiotics by intermittent short-infusion methods may not actually optimize drug use in many patients. As has been previously reviewed, significant alterations in β-lactam PK parameters may lead to significantly reduced total drug exposure in critically ill patients. Increases in Vss may reduce peak concentrations after intermittent dosing, whereas increases in clearance (as with ARC) may further significantly reduce the period during which antibiotic concentrations remain above the pathogen MIC. Intermittent dosing of β-lactams may therefore result in a concentration versus time profile that actually minimizes the chance of achieving an optimal PD profile and favorable clinical outcome, particularly in patients with potentially significant PK alterations. Intermittent dosing of β-lactams has historically produced excellent clinical efficacy in the treatment of infections caused by susceptible pathogens with very low MICs. However, as multidrug-resistant pathogens such as *P. aeruginosa* have become more common and even susceptible strains often have relatively high MICs (often at or near the susceptibility breakpoint), potentially suboptimal intermittent dosing of β-lactams has become of more concern.

There are several potential methods of increasing the time-dependent PD exposure of β-lactams antibiotics, including increasing the daily dose using higher doses or dosing more often, administering the drug by continuous infusion, and administering the drug by prolonged infusion (or extended infusions) (i.e., increasing administration time from 0.5–1.0 hour to 3–4 hours). Administering higher daily doses by increasing dose or frequency is usually less desirable because it is more expensive, may place patients at higher risk of drug-related adverse effects and toxicities, and increases workload of hospital personnel. Moreover, from a PK/PD standpoint, using higher daily doses is inefficient because doubling the dose of β-lactams leads to an increased $fT>MIC$ of only one additional half-life (only about 1 hour for most agents).[174]

There has been a renewed interest in administering β-lactam antibiotics by a 24-hour continuous infusion because this represents an efficient way of optimizing the PD to achieving a 100% $fT>MIC$ for even high-MIC pathogens while minimizing the risk of drug toxicities and using the least amount of total daily drug, drug supplies, and labor costs. Continuous infusion is also attractive for many β-lactam antibiotics because of their relatively short half-lives.[174] Continuous infusions of β-lactams consistently provide better PD parameters than does intermittent dosing in less susceptible bacteria, although the method of dosing is not as critical in highly sensitive strains.[106,175-180] Continuous infusions may also achieve higher tissue concentrations than intermittent dosing.[105]

Although administration of continuous infusions has many potential advantages, this administration strategy may not be practical in all patients. The use of continuous infusion medications generally requires a dedicated intravenous line to prevent potential incompatibilities and allow for concomitant administration of other intravenous medications. However, it is often not practical to dedicate a catheter line for an entire 24-hour period in critically ill patients who often require many other medications as well as fluids, blood products, and other reasons for intravenous access.[128] In addition, given that antibiotics administered by continuous infusion are ideally best prepared once daily and infused at room temperature over the full 24 hours, antibiotic stability may be insufficient under those conditions.[128] The carbapenems in particular are relatively unstable at room temperature and may require preparation of fresh doses several times daily in order to be infused throughout the 24-hour day.[181-183] Patients most likely to benefit from administration as continuous infusions are those infected with less susceptible bacteria with high MICs at or near their susceptibility breakpoints. As MICs potentially continue to increase, continuous infusion may become more beneficial because of the enhanced PD target attainment at higher MICs.[128,129,174,178] However, for antibiotics with short room-temperature stability (e.g., carbapenems) or for use in critically ill patients for whom dedicated line access is not feasible, continuous infusions may not be the most viable option for antibiotic administration.[128]

Clinicians must also recognize that achieving the potential benefits of a continuous infusion assumes that the proper dose is being administered and that the pathogen MIC is in fact being exceeded by concentrations achieved at a given infusion rate. Use of inadequate total daily doses, particularly in the management of infections caused by pathogens with high MICs at or near the susceptibility breakpoint, has the potential for producing subtherapeutic concentrations that inconsistently (or even never) exceed the MIC and therefore could increase the risk of treatment failure.

Extending β-lactam administration times over periods that are longer than intermittent infusions (0.5–1.0 hour) but shorter than 24-hour continuous infusions is another strategy that is becoming increasing popular in clinical practice, Administering β-lactams as a typically 3- to 4-hour prolonged infusion allows drug concentrations to remain in excess of the MIC for a longer period than would be possible after intermittent short infusions. This potential advantage also holds true against organisms with high MIC values where differences between prolonged infusion and intermittent infusion became more pronounced.[184-186] With respect to achieving desired $fT>MIC$ PD targets, continuous and prolonged infusion strategies often produce very similar profiles; modeling studies have generally shown little difference between continuous infusions and prolonged infusions in achieving desired $fT>MIC$ PD targets.[184-187] Finally, use of prolonged rather than continuous infusions may help resolve issues related to drug stability and intravenous line access. Maximizing carbapenem exposure through use of prolonged infusions may allow for more aggressive dosing in patients with severe infections and/or those infected with pathogens with high MICs while still providing cost-effective therapy.[128] Because there appear to be few clinically relevant differences in achieving $fT>MIC$ targets or proven clinical efficacy with prolonged infusions of carbapenems compared with continuous infusions, and because prolonged infusions avoid potential drug stability issues, it is recommended that carbapenems be administered over 3- or 4-hour infusion times.[128] Likewise, prolonged and continuous infusion regimens of piperacillin/tazobactam provide similar probabilities of meeting $fT>MIC$ targets when the same total daily doses are administered. Similar to carbapenems, administration of piperacillin/tazobactam by prolonged 4-hour infusions is recommended over continuous infusions.[128,185]

Of note, antibiotic therapy with continuous infusions should always be initiated with a loading dose. The ability to significantly improve the achievement of $fT>MIC$ targets also depends on rapidly attaining steady state–like concentrations of antibiotics that are at or near desired target concentrations. Although the β-lactam antibiotics that are most likely to be administered by continuous infusion have short half-lives (about 1 hour) in patients with normal renal function, it will still require 5 hours or more to reach steady state at desired concentrations; it will take even longer in patients with reduced drug clearance and longer half-life. For this reason, as a rule, antibiotic loading doses should always be administered at the initiation of continuous infusion regimens.

The β-lactam antibiotics that have been most extensively studied using alternative continuous and prolonged dosing regimens include piperacillin/tazobactam, cephalosporins (ceftazidime, cefepime), and the carbapenems (imipenem, meropenem, doripenem).[11,12,187] Perhaps the most significant of the early studies of the potential benefits of prolonged-infusion regimens was a retrospective pre-post trial evaluating implementation of prolonged-infusion piperacillin/tazobactam regimens in an academic medical center.[187] Clinical outcomes achieved with piperacillin/tazobactam 3.375 g administered as standard infusions every 4 or 6 hours were compared with those obtained after switching to 3.375 g every 8 hours administered as a 4-hour prolonged infusion. All patients included in the study were being treated for *P. aeruginosa* infections. Overall, no significant differences in either 14-day all-cause mortality or hospital length of stay were observed across the entire population of 194 patients. However, when patients were stratified according to severity of illness as determined by Acute Physiology and Chronic Health Evaluation II (APACHE II) scores, significant differences in both mortality (12.2% in the prolonged infusion group vs. 31.6% in the short infusion group; p<0.04) and hospital length of stay (median 21 vs. 38 days, respectively; p<0.02) were observed among the cohort of more severely ill patients with APACHE II scores of 17 or higher. The significance of this study was that it highlighted the importance of optimizing antibiotic dosing in the subset of patients who are most likely to see clinical benefit: high severity of illness, potential for significant PK alterations, and infection with difficult pathogens most likely to have higher MICs.[187]

The PD, clinical efficacy, and safety data for piperacillin/tazobactam, cephalosporins, and carbapenems when administered as continuous or prolonged infusion regimens have been extensively reviewed and at least four different meta-analyses conducted to determine whether these alternative dosing strategies can be recommended over traditional intermittent dosing (Table 12.5).[188-191] Two earlier meta-analyses addressing continuous infusion regimens compared with intermittent dosing regimens found that continuous antibiotic infusions were associated with statistically significant improvements in neither clinical cure rates nor mortality.[188,189] Although it was observed that patients with a higher acuity of illness had a greater response to the continuous infusion regimens,[189] echoing the results of the earlier study of piperacillin/tazobactam prolonged infusions,[187] no definitive recommendations could be made because of several limitations of the data at that time: limited numbers of randomized controlled trials, usually small patient numbers, inadequately powered, and designed as pilot studies or noninferiority studies.[128] However, two more recent meta-analyses concluded that continuous or prolonged β-lactam infusions were associated with statistically significant reductions in mortality.[190,191] Although these studies are more recent and had conclusions more favorable for alternative dosing strategies, both studies were beset by the same limitations as the two earlier meta-analyses and emphasized the need for well-designed, larger, multicenter, randomized controlled trials in order to clearly define the role of continuous or prolonged infusion regimens.[190,191] Indeed, the need for additional well-conducted studies is highlighted by a recent study that compared intermittent dosing with continuous infusions of various β-lactams including piperacillin/tazobactam, ticarcillin/clavulanate, and meropenem.[192] This was a prospective, double-blind, randomized, controlled, multicenter trial, apparently the first such trial ever to have been conducted for evaluation of this particular question. The study end points were trough unbound plasma antibiotic concentrations above the MIC of the isolated pathogens on days 3 and 4, clinical response 7–14 days after the last dose of study drug, ICU-free days at day 28, and hospital survival. Sixty patients were enrolled: 30 each in the intermittent and continuous infusion groups. Results of the study showed statistically significant differences in trough unbound plasma concentrations exceeding the MIC (82% continuous vs. 29% intermittent; p=0.001) and clinical response (70% continuous vs. 43% intermittent; p=0.037). However, no differences between groups were found with respect to ICU-free days (p=0.14) or hospital survival (p=0.47). Additional large, well-designed studies of this type are required to truly define the role of β-lactam administration by continuous or prolonged infusion and the clinical benefits to be expected.[192]

Table 12.5 Summary of Meta-analyses Evaluating Continuous and/or Prolonged Infusions vs. Intermittent infusions of β-Lactam Antibiotics

Reference	No. of Studies Included in Final Analysis	Infusion Method(s)	Antibiotics Evaluated (no. of studies)	Types of Infections	Results of Analysis
Kasiakou et al., 2005[188]	9 RCTs; total 769 patients	Continuous	Cefamandole (1) Ceftazidime (4) Cefepime (1); also Vancomycin (1) Aminoglycosides (2)	Primarily GNB; nosocomial pneumonia, bacteremia, sepsis, UTI, SSTI, miscellaneous other infections; five studies of ICU patients	No significant difference in clinical failure rates (OR 0.73; 95% CI, 0.53–1.01) Significantly reduced clinical failure rates in subset of studies where patients in both groups received same total daily antibiotic dose (OR 0.70; 95% CI, 0.50–0.98) No significant differences in mortality (OR 0.89; 95% CI, 0.48–1.64) or nephrotoxicity (OR 0.91; 95% CI, 0.56–1.47)
Roberts et al., 2009[189]	14: 8 retrospective, 3 prospective, 3 RCTs; total 1,229 patients	Continuous and prolonged	Piperacillin/tazobactam (3) Piperacillin (1) Cefamandole (1) Cefoperazone (1) Cefotaxime (1) Ceftriaxone (1) Ceftazidime (3) Cefepime (1) Meropenem (1) Imipenem/cilastatin (1)	Primarily GNB, but also GPO or not specified; HAP, VAP, CAP, bacteremia, sepsis, UTI, SSTI, cIAI, miscellaneous other infections; most studies of ICU patients	Significantly reduced mortality with pooled CAI/PI (RR 0.59; 95% CI, 0.41–0.83) Significantly reduced mortality with CAI alone (RR 0.50; 95% CI, 0.26–0.96) or PI alone (RR 0.63; 95% CI, 0.41–0.95) Significantly reduced mortality with piperacillin/tazobactam CAI/PI (RR 0.55; 95% CI, 0.34–0.89) but not carbapenem CAI/PI (RR 0.66; 95% CI, 0.34–1.30) Significantly reduced mortality with CAI/PI in patients with pneumonia (RR 0.50; 95% CI, 0.26–0.96)
Falagas et al., 2013[190]	14 RCTs; total 846 patients	Continuous and prolonged	Piperacillin/tazobactam (3) Piperacillin (1) Cefamandole (1) Cefoperazone (1) Cefotaxime (1) Ceftriaxone (1) Ceftazidime (3) Cefepime (1) Meropenem (1) Imipenem/cilastatin (1)	Primarily GNB; HAP, VAP, CAP, bacteremia, sepsis, UTI, SSTI, cIAI, miscellaneous other infections; most studies of ICU patients	No significant improvement in clinical cure with CAI/PI (OR 1.04; 95% CI, 0.74–1.46; p=0.83) No significant difference in mortality with CAI/PI (OR 1.00; 95% CI, 0.48–2.06; p=1.00)

Table 12.5 Summary of Meta-analyses Evaluating Continuous and/or Prolonged Infusions vs. Intermittent infusions of β-Lactam Antibiotics *(continued)*

Reference	No. of Studies Included in Final Analysis	Infusion Method(s)	Antibiotics Evaluated (no. of studies)	Types of Infections	Results of Analysis
Teo et al., 2014[191]	29: 18 RCTs, 11 observational; total 2,206 patients	Continuous and prolonged	Piperacillin/tazobactam (9) ticarcillin/clavulanate (1) piperacillin (1) oxacillin (1) temocillin (1) cefamandole (1) cefoperazone (1) cefotaxime (1) ceftriaxone (1) ceftazidime (6) cefepime (1) meropenem (6) imipenem/cilastatin (1)	Primarily GNB; HAP, VAP, CAP, bacteremia, sepsis, UTI, SSTI, cIAI, endocarditis, miscellaneous other infections; 18 studies of ICU patients	Significant reduction in mortality with CAI/PI (RR 0.66; 95% CI, 0.53–0.83) Significant improvement in clinical success with CAI/PI (RR 1.12; 95% CI, 1.03–1.21) Significantly reduced mortality with CAI/PI in non-randomized studies (RR 0.57; 95% CI, 0.43–0.76) but not in RCTs (RR 0.83; 95% CI, 0.57–1.21) No significant differences in clinical success in either non-randomized studies alone or RCTs alone (RR 1.34; 95% CI, 1.02–1.76; and RR 1.05; 95% CI, 0.99–1.12, respectively)

CAI = continuous antibiotic infusion; CAP = community-acquired pneumonia; CI = confidence interval; cIAI = complicated intra-abdominal infection; GNB = gram-negative bacilli; GPO = gram-positive organisms; HAP = hospital-acquired pneumonia; OR = odds ratio; PI = prolonged infusion; RCT = randomized controlled trial; RR = risk ratio; SSTI = skin and soft tissue infection; UTI = urinary tract infection; VAP = ventilator-associated pneumonia.

Several studies have examined the potential pharmacoeconomic benefits of continuous or prolonged β-lactam infusions, but the results of these studies are somewhat inconsistent and are highly dependent on study methodologies and the actual total daily dose of drug administered.[176,193-198] Although most studies have determined that alternative dosing strategies result in substantial cost savings relative to intermittent administration, particularly related to labor and supply costs, other studies have not shown such savings.[196] Although the potential for significant cost savings is somewhat institution-dependent and will vary with specific drugs and doses used, there is no question that β-lactam administration by constant and prolonged infusion regimens are associated with other potential advantages. Chief among these are the more reliable achievement of $fT>MIC$ targets and potential for improved clinical outcomes in high-risk patients who will likely derive the greatest benefit from optimization of PK/PD parameters.

Continuous Infusions of Vancomycin

It has been proposed that vancomycin, another time-dependent antibiotic, also benefits from administration by continuous infusion for reasons similar to those discussed for the β-lactam drugs. Increasing vancomycin MICs for methicillin-resistant *S. aureus* have been noted in recent years and are a great concern for the continued successful clinical use of vancomycin.[199] Higher MICs will reduce the AUC_{0-24}/MIC ratio achieved with any given dose, and desired AUC_{0-24}/MIC targets are unlikely to be achieved with standard vancomycin doses (i.e., 1 g every 12 hours) once the MIC increases to 1 mg/L and beyond.[200] In addition, vancomycin has been noted to have highly variable PK disposition in critically ill patients and to achieve subtherapeutic concentrations in a high proportion of patients after standard intermittent dosing.[201] Finally, the use of higher vancomycin doses in an effort to overcome the effects of increased MICs and still achieve desired AUC_{0-24}/MIC targets has been associated with higher rates of nephrotoxicity.[202] Continuous infusions of vancomycin have thus been advocated as a means of optimizing the PD of the drug while minimizing nephrotoxicity. Several studies report that continuous vancomycin infusions provide improved penetration and increased drug concentrations in cerebrospinal fluid and respiratory tissues.[203-206] Several studies, both retrospective and prospective, have also evaluated PK and clinical outcomes in patients receiving continuous infusions of vancomycin compared with standard intermittent dosing.[206-212] Studies have consistently shown that continuous infusion regimens more consistently achieve desired plasma concentrations of 20–25 mg/L (i.e., trough concentration with intermittent dosing, average concentration with continuous infusion) and in many cases are also able to achieve target concentrations significantly more rapidly after initiating therapy.[209,211] One study found that although there was no significant difference in AUC_{0-24}/MIC ratios between the two groups, patients receiving continuous infusions were markedly more likely to achieve and maintain desired plasma concentrations.[209] Other studies have also suggested that continuous vancomycin infusions either reduce the overall incidence of nephrotoxicity or substantially delay the onset.[210,211,213] However, what is significantly lacking in these studies are definitive data analyses showing improved response to vancomycin therapy and reductions in patient mortality. Individual studies have generally shown comparable efficacy between standard and continuous regimens. A meta-analysis evaluating continuous versus intermittent infusions of vancomycin for the treatment of gram-positive infections found no statistically significant difference in mortality rates in patients receiving the two regimens, although this analysis did find a significant reduction in nephrotoxicity in patients receiving continuous infusions (relative risk 0.63; 95% confidence interval, 0.43–0.94).[212] In summary, available data analyses suggest that continuous vancomycin infusions are a promising method of drug administration in patients with serious gram-positive infections. The ability to reach target drug concentrations more rapidly while having less PK/PD variability is potentially beneficial in the treatment of severe infections in high-risk patients, as is the possible reduction in nephrotoxicity. However, until more definitive data can provide evidence of clear benefits related to improved clinical outcomes, current guidelines recommend against the routine use of continuous infusions of vancomycin.[140,214] As with β-lactam drugs, if continuous vancomycin infusions are to be used, it is important that therapy be initiated with a loading dose of vancomycin before initiating the drug infusion.

Continuous Infusions of Linezolid

According to the previous discussions of continuous infusions of β-lactams and vancomycin, it is perhaps not surprising that continuous infusions of linezolid have also been explored. Linezolid, also a time-dependent drug, potentially has the same PK/PD limitations as the β-lactams and vancomycin, and it could perhaps benefit from continuous administration with respect to overcoming PK variability, improving tissue penetration of the drug, and maximizing achievement of PD targets. One study compared the PK/PD profile of standard intermittent infusions with continuous infusions of linezolid in critically ill patients with sepsis.[142] Continuous infusion was superior to intermittent infusions in achieving and maintaining PD targets. Of interest, a study of an animal model not only showed that continuous infusions of linezolid are more effective than intermittent infusions, but also that the drug behaved as a bactericidal rather than a bacteriostatic agent.[215] Clinical studies are needed to define whether continuous linezolid infusions are associated with improved patient outcomes and cannot be recommended at this time.

Extended-Interval Dosing of Aminoglycosides

Extended-interval dosing (or once-daily dosing) of aminoglycosides is perhaps the best-known example of direct application of PK/PD principles in the clinical care of patients. Being a concentration-dependent drug, aminoglycosides have been shown to eradicate organisms most effectively when peak plasma concentrations that are 10 times or greater above their MIC (i.e., Cmax/MIC of 10 or greater) are achieved. The concept behind extended-interval dosing is that by administering large doses at infrequent intervals (rather than smaller doses at frequent intervals), achievement of favorable Cmax/MIC ratios can be more reliably accomplished. If Cmax/MIC ratios were optimized early in therapy, it was expected that bacterial eradication would be increased and risk of resistance reduced, that the required therapy duration could be shortened, and that aminoglycoside exposure and toxicity would thereby be minimized because the ototoxicity and nephrotoxicity of aminoglycosides is best correlated with tissue accumulation rather than peak concentrations in serum.[216] The concept of extended-interval dosing of aminoglycosides was first widely advocated for in the early 1990s[217]; by 2000, about 75% of acute care hospitals were routinely using extended-interval regimens and had formal policies for their use.[218] Several clinical studies and many meta-analyses have firmly established the role of extended-interval aminoglycoside regimens, confirming that these regimens are at least as effective as traditional divided-dose regimens with respect to clinical response and bacteriological eradication, with the potential for reduced toxicities.[217,219-227] Further advantages of once-daily aminoglycoside dosing include reduction in supply and labor costs and the emergence of bacterial resistance.[228]

A common method for administration of extended-interval aminoglycoside regimens has been the use of dosing nomograms, among them the well-known Hartford nomogram in which a 7-mg/kg dose is administered at an interval determined by the calculated creatinine clearance.[229] The 7-mg/kg dose specified by the Hartford nomogram was designed to achieve peak plasma concentrations of 20 mg/L in order to provide favorable Cmax/MIC ratios against *P. aeruginosa*; many other nomograms have also been proposed.[230,231] These extended-interval regimens continue to be preferred dosing methods for aminoglycosides. However, several points need to kept in mind when using extended-interval regimens or dosing nomograms in critically ill patients. Although nomograms assume that adequate peak concentrations are achieved after administration of doses typically ranging from 5 to 7 mg/kg, many critically ill patients have a significantly increased Vss, which may lead to important reductions in peak plasma concentrations achieved after dosing. In addition, as previously discussed in this chapter, critically ill patients may have either increased or decreased clearance of renally cleared antibiotics, and estimates of renal function in ICU patients are often inaccurate. Because of these potential PK alterations, it cannot be assumed either that extended-interval regimens will produce desired Cmax/MIC ratios or that the aminoglycosides will be cleared from critically ill patients as expected. It is also important to remember that many patients with expected significant PK alterations have not been well represented in clinical studies of extended-interval dosing and/or were excluded from nomogram validation studies. Such patients include those with morbid obesity, pregnant females, patients with ascites or requiring renal replacement therapies, and patients with large total body surface area burns.[222,226,229-231] The other important issue related to use of extended-interval dosing in critically ill patients is that the bacterial pathogens often present in ICU patients have become less susceptible; as bacterial MICs rise, the probability of achieving optimal Cmax/MIC ratios becomes ever more problematic.[232-234] The combination of increased PK Vss values and increased pathogen MIC values means that substantially higher doses of aminoglycosides (e.g., tobramycin 10–12 mg/kg or more) will potentially be needed to achieve adequate Cmax/MIC ratios; such doses may also potentially increase toxicity risks and may not be acceptable for routine use despite PK/PD considerations regarding appropriate targets.[232-234] Whether the AUC_{0-24}/MIC ratio may be a better parameter for aminoglycosides in this setting is currently unknown. Careful monitoring of critically ill patients for lack of appropriate response to therapy and evidence of drug toxicities is obviously mandatory during aminoglycoside therapy, regardless of whether extended-interval regimens are used.

The question of whether extended-interval dosing is appropriate for patients receiving renal replacement therapy has been evaluated in several recent studies.[235-239] The FDA-approved regimen for adults undergoing hemodialysis consists of the administration of gentamicin 1–1.7 mg/kg at the end of each dialysis period. However, administration of relatively low doses does not optimize either Cmax/MIC or AUC_{0-24}/MIC ratios and may not be the most appropriate dosing strategy. Results of in vitro and clinical studies of patients requiring hemodialysis suggest that the administration of high, extended interval–like doses (6 mg/kg) of gentamicin to critically ill patients just before hemodialysis sessions allows for achievement of high peak concentrations and maximizes bacterial killing, whereas the subsequently rapid removal by hemodialysis minimizes total drug exposure and risk of toxicity. Administration of aminoglycosides to critically patients by this method has been shown to provide more optimal dosing and achievement of desired PK/PD targets.[239] Additional study is needed to document the clinical efficacy and safety of high-dose aminoglycosides in this setting, but this does appear to be a viable strategy from a PK/PD perspective.

High-Dose Fluoroquinolones

Certain principles of fluoroquinolone PD can readily be applied to the appropriate treatment of infections in critically ill patients. Because fluoroquinolones are concentration-dependent killers with Cmax/MIC or AUC_{0-24}/MIC ratios as the key PD parameters, optimizing the PD of the drug by administering higher doses should allow for more rapid and complete bacterial eradication. Fluoroquinolone PK are somewhat variable in the critically ill, and the drugs are often being used as empirical therapy for infections potentially caused by organisms with reduced fluoroquinolone susceptibility (i.e., higher MICs). Use of high doses (i.e., levofloxacin 750 mg rather than the lower 500-mg dose, ciprofloxacin 400 mg every 8 hours rather than 400 mg every 12 hours) may therefore help minimize the impact of variability in both PK and pathogen susceptibilities and optimize the concentration-dependent PD properties of the drugs in patients with severe infections. Although fluoroquinolones have concentration-dependent killing, excessively high serum concentrations of these agents can be associated with an increased risk of adverse reactions.[174,240] When a Cmax/MIC of 10 or greater cannot be reached without the use of very high doses because of high pathogen MICs, bacterial eradication becomes a function of concentration and time of exposure on the basis of the AUC_{0-24}/MIC ratio.[174] Fluoroquinolone AUC_{0-24}/MIC ratios are often adequate for clinical treatment of infections in ICU patients, even though adequate Cmax/MIC ratios cannot be achieved[145,152,153]; this is particularly true when critically ill patients have some degree of organ dysfunction because of the potentially decreased drug elimination and increased AUC that may result.

Use of higher fluoroquinolone doses can be particularly beneficial in the treatment of severe infections suspected or documented to be caused by pathogens with intrinsically higher MICs to the drugs (e.g., *P. aeruginosa* and *Acinetobacter* spp.). The fluoroquinolones readily penetrate most tissues and fluids of the body, but the use of high doses in the treatment of serious infections should also maximize tissue penetration and more reliably achieve adequate drug concentrations at the infection site. According to the PD properties of the fluoroquinolones, the intensity of dosing and ability to achieve favorable Cmax/MIC or AUC_{0-24}/MIC ratios should also minimize the development of resistance. However, of note, many pathogens found in critically ill patients (e.g., most of the enteric gram-negative bacilli, streptococci) are quite susceptible to the fluoroquinolones, and the use of high doses is not necessary to achieve concentrations adequate for the treatment of most infections. Moreover, note that the foregoing discussion primarily applies to levofloxacin and ciprofloxacin; moxifloxacin doses in excess of 400 mg/day are generally not recommended because of concerns regarding concentration-related prolongation of the electrocardiographic corrected QT (QTc) interval.[240]

Dosing of Antifungals

Fluconazole PK have been reported to be substantially altered in critically ill medical and surgical patients with varying levels of disease severity and normal renal function.[134,135,241,242] The Vss of fluconazole is predictably increased by about 50%–100% compared with that in normal volunteers; these changes are consistent with those expected of a highly hydrophilic drug in critically ill patients.[241,242] The fluconazole half-life is also generally increased by 50%–100% together with the changes in Vss. In contrast, fluconazole clearance appears to be somewhat variable and may be either increased or decreased; this is also consistent with the PK alterations expected in a critically ill population.[242,243]

According to currently available information from small studies involving heterogeneous patient populations, no definitive general conclusions can be made regarding fluconazole dosing in critically ill patients. Given the concentration-dependent properties of fluconazole and the consistently observed alterations in Vss that have been observed, care must be taken not to underdose fluconazole by administering too small a dose, which will result in low serum concentrations. However, once sufficiently high concentrations are reached, the increased half-life should allow maintenance of high AUCs and adequate drug exposures. This simplistic approach to optimizing fluconazole use in the ICU fails to account for the substantial variability that is typical of hydrophilic, renally cleared drugs in this setting. As discussed earlier in this chapter, allowing for PK variability while maintaining adequate drug exposures can be accomplished by administering aggressive doses. That fluconazole has few important toxicities makes this aggressive approach more acceptable from a patient safety perspective. Because of the potential for significantly increased half-life, it would also be reasonable to initiate fluconazole therapy with a loading dose, although this approach has not been widely recommended. Future studies focusing specifically on ICU populations are needed to establish definitive recommendations for fluconazole optimization.

According to CLSI susceptibility breakpoints and available clinical data, voriconazole plasma concentrations should be maintained above 2 mg/L over the entire dosing interval because this concentration is also correlated with a favorable $fAUC_{0-24}$/MIC for this concentration-dependent drug.[125,135,169,170,172] However, doses of 3–4 mg/kg every 12 hours in critically ill patients with or without renal impairment may be insufficient to reliably achieve trough concentrations above 2 mg/L for the entire dosing interval.[244,245] Considering the observed large interpatient variability in healthy volunteers and non-ICU patients[125] and the possibility of considerable PK variations in the critically ill, it is tempting to consider administering higher-than-normal doses in order to maximize the PD properties of this drug. Given the potential for serious concentration-related toxicities of voriconazole and the potential for many drug-drug interactions, use of higher doses is not recommended until additional clinical studies are available to support this strategy in critically ill patients.[124-126,133-135,163,164]

Similar to fluconazole and voriconazole, the $fAUC_{0-24}$/MIC is the PD parameter most associated with the activity of itraconazole. In a retrospective PK/PD analysis, a total AUC_{0-24} greater than 30 mg·hour/L was associated with optimal antifungal efficacy.[246] However, typical dosing regimens of 200 mg intravenously twice daily for four doses followed by 200 mg intravenously daily may not achieve the targeted $fAUC_{0-24}$/MIC greater than 25 in 20% of ICU patients or more.[246] Higher doses may be required for critically ill patients to achieve better clinical outcomes through dose-optimized administration, but again, specific data related to the use of high-dose itraconazole therapy in this population are lacking.

Echinocandins are concentration-dependent drugs for which $fCmax$/MIC and $fAUC_{0-24}$/MIC have been correlated with efficacy. These properties, together with the relatively long half-lives of these agents, support a dosing strategy in which large doses are administered infrequently.[133,163,172] As with the azoles, use of higher-than-normal doses would seem to be a reasonable option in patients who are not responding favorably to echinocandin therapy. Again, lack of specific data related to the effectiveness of increased doses of echinocandins in severely ill patients is a hindrance to optimizing therapy with these drugs in ICU patients. Lack of a complete understanding of the disposition of echinocandins (and other antifungal agents) in infected tissue sites also contributes to uncertainty regarding whether increased antifungal doses would actually improve clinical efficacy. Currently, use of echinocandin doses higher than those currently indicated in the product labeling is not routinely recommended.

With the increasing prevalence of invasive fungal infections in critically ill populations, optimization of antifungal therapy is critical to achieve favorable clinical outcomes and reduce the risk of toxicity. Some of the more commonly used antifungals, as noted earlier, have been shown to have large intra- and interpatient variations in serum concentrations. Together with the highly dynamic character of critically ill patients, these variations may be more significant and can potentially lead to treatment failure or toxicity. Therapeutic drug monitoring is a useful tool to optimize treatment with the various antifungals, and the role of TDM in antifungal therapy has been reviewed in detail elsewhere.[124,247,248] Despite the ability to perform TDM in many institutions and increased knowledge of antifungal PK/PD characteristics, optimal use of antifungals remains a challenge to ICU clinicians because of lack of key data in this population.

LIMITATIONS OF CLINICAL PK/PD APPLICATIONS IN CRITICALLY ILL

The severity of infections encountered in the ICU population and the need for adequate Cmax/MIC and AUC_{0-24}/MIC ratios are important considerations in severely ill patients. However, there is still much to learn regarding the direct application of PD principles to the routine care of critically ill patients. Although it is assumed that the serum concentrations of most drugs are related to their concentrations in various tissues, the use of serum Cmax/MIC and AUC_{0-24}/MIC ratios does not always accurately predict tissue concentrations of drugs. A particularly important limitation of PD principles in the routine care of ICU patients is that they have not been thoroughly clinically validated in critically ill populations. Several studies have shown that the PK of antimicrobials are often significantly altered in critical illness and that there is a high degree of interpatient (and even intrapatient) variability in this population.[13-20] Distribution of antimicrobials to infected tissues may also be affected by hemodynamic instability and regional or local changes in perfusion of various organs and tissues. The difficult combination of severe illness, PK variability, and life-threatening infections involving potentially drug-resistant pathogens makes the ICU population a difficult one in which to optimize drug therapy through appropriate application of PD principles. However, only through using these principles is optimization of antimicrobial therapy likely to be achieved in any consistent manner.

A basic limitation inherent in the clinical application of PK/PD principles is that the data necessary to make informed decisions for individual patients are simply not available. Optimization of antimicrobial therapy in individual patients (i.e., estimating patient-specific values for AUC_{0-24}/MIC, Cmax/MIC, and/or $fT>MIC$) requires that patient-specific PK and MIC data are able to be used. However, a large proportion of infections in critically ill patients are empirically treated for the duration of therapy; no specific pathogen is ever isolated and therefore the MIC of the pathogen causing the infection in an individual patient is never known. In addition, TDM is not available for most antimicrobials being used in clinical practice, and drug concentrations are rarely actually known. In actual practice, therefore, both PK parameters and MIC values must be estimated from other sources. This automatically imposes an inherent handicap on any attempts at individualization of antimicrobial therapy.

Using mathematical modeling, it is possible to apply PK-PD concepts to clinical practice in an effort to overcome some of these practical limitations. Monte Carlo simulation is used to integrate PK, PD, and MIC data to design rational antimicrobial drug regimens with a high probability of achieving favorable PD targets against organisms that are likely to be encountered in practice.[249] Monte Carlo simulation accounts for the variability in PK values within patient populations as well as the MIC distribution among the pathogens of interest in order to predict antibiotic exposure in entire populations of patients (i.e., MCS modeling simulates the variability in PK parameters that would be seen in a large population of individuals after administration of a specific drug dose or regimen). According to this PK variability, the probability of subsequently achieving specific PK/PD targets can then be determined. In summary, using this program, the probability of obtaining a target exposure that drives a microbiological effect for a given range of MIC values can be calculated.[249] Monte Carlo simulation has become an extremely common method of evaluating the adequacy of existing regimens and designing new regimens that optimize PK/PD exposure in various patient populations. Although MCS is a very valuable tool when applied correctly, many limitations exist. A major consideration for MCS is the PK model used to estimate variability in PK parameters (Vss, clearance, etc.) likely to be encountered in practice. Pharmacokinetic studies of healthy volunteers may be used in MCS, especially when PK data from specific populations such as the critically ill are lacking. However, there is a concern that PK parameters from healthy volunteer studies may not accurately reflect the magnitude or variability in PK alterations within severely ill populations and may overestimate the probabilities of achieving desired PD targets. Another major consideration of PK/PD modeling and MCS is ensuring that appropriate MIC data are used. As much as possible, microbiological data used for MCS must accurately reflect the range and frequency of MICs actually encountered in critically ill patients or, even more ideally, within a specific institution. The role of tissue penetration of antimicrobial and the most appropriate way to include tissue concentrations into MCS modeling are also somewhat controversial and not truly known.[250]

Although useful as a quantitative measure of drug activity or potency, the MIC itself is also not without several limitations.[174] The MIC does not mirror true physiological conditions; instead, it is a static measure that does not reflect fluctuating drug concentrations typically observed during the administering of many doses of a drug regimen. Because the MIC measures only inhibition of growth, it does not reflect the rate at which bacteria are actually killed by bactericidal agents. Furthermore, the MIC only quantifies net growth over an 18- to 24-hour observation period. Killing and regrowth may well occur during this period as long as the net growth is zero. Finally, the MIC does not account for the post-antibiotic effects of antibiotics.[174]

As previously discussed in this chapter, estimates of organ function are imprecise and pose another limitation to applying PK/PD principles in the clinical setting.

Assessments of renal and hepatic function and their effects on drug clearance within individual patients are potentially quite inaccurate. Related alterations in other PK parameters such as Vss, protein binding, and half-life are also difficult to estimate, and it can be quite difficult to individualize drug dosing with any precision.

Although the science and practice of PD has made significant progress during the past 30 years and clinical outcomes have undoubtedly been improved through rational application of PK/PD principles, the current state of the art is still actually quite crude. It is currently not possible to fully account for factors such as age, comorbidities, immune function, severity of illness, changes in pathophysiology, and affected PK parameters over time during therapy, yet these and other factors are known to influence patient outcomes in the treatment of infections. Characterization and application of PD parameters that primarily consider only PK and MIC variables obviously lacks a degree of sophistication and highlights how much there is yet to learn regarding how to "optimize" antimicrobial therapy in order to achieve the best possible patient outcomes. Indeed, it has been shown that predicting patient outcomes on the basis of population-based PK/PD parameters is difficult at best and does not accurately predict clinical outcomes in individual patients.[251]

Finally, it is important to recognize that most of what is known and recommended regarding antimicrobial PD targets has been derived from in vitro models, in vivo animal models, simulation modeling using techniques such as MCS, and retrospective data from humans. There are still relatively few prospective studies that were specifically conducted to validate PK/PD targets and to test whether the application of PD principles actually results in the desired outcomes, and until recently, well-designed prospective, randomized, controlled trials of the validity of PD principles were (and still are) almost nonexistent. There is clearly a need for additional prospective studies designed to specifically validate the PK/PD principles that are currently being applied to individual patients.

SUMMARY

Antimicrobial treatment of critically ill patients remains a significant challenge to clinicians. Many factors, over which clinicians may have little control, may influence the response of an individual patient to antimicrobial therapy; however, optimization of antimicrobial therapy through appropriate drug selection and dosing is one area in which clinicians can make an important difference. Optimization of antimicrobial therapy remains a high priority in the treatment of critically ill patients and requires that drugs be dosed in a manner that maximizes their pharmacologic activity while minimizing the risk of adverse effects and toxicities.

A wide variety of physiological alterations may occur in critically ill patients, many of which have the ability to significantly affect the PK/PD properties of drugs used in this patient population. Clinicians working with patients in the ICU must have a good working knowledge of many issues related to antimicrobial therapy: spectrum of activity of antimicrobials, potential PK alterations present in critically ill patients, how these alterations are likely to affect various types of antimicrobials, the PD properties of the drugs and how these are also likely to be affected in these patients, and how to appropriately apply knowledge of specific PK/PD targets to choose appropriate drugs and regimens that will provide favorable clinical outcomes. Understanding the rationale and limitations related to current clinical applications of antimicrobial PK/PD properties is also important with respect to the ability of clinicians to optimize antimicrobial use in ICU patients. Although appropriate application of these concepts will likely always remain a significant challenge, PK/PD principles also provide valuable tools by which clinicians can make significant improvements in the care and therapeutic outcomes of the patients they serve.

REFERENCES

1. Hidron AI, Edwards JR, Patel J, et al. NHSN annual update: antimicrobial-resistant pathogens associated with healthcare-associated infections: annual summary of data reported to the National Healthcare Safety Network at the Centers for Disease Control and Prevention, 2006-2007. Infect Control Hosp Epidemiol 2008;29:996-1011.

2. Boucher HW, Talbot GH, Bradley JS, et al. Bad bugs, no drugs: no ESKAPE! An update from the Infectious Diseases Society of America. Clin Infect Dis 2009;48:1-12.

3. Kallan AJ, Hidron AI, Patel J, et al. Multidrug resistance among gram-negative pathogens that caused healthcare-associated infections reported to the National Healthcare Safety Network, 2006-2008. Infect Control Hosp Epidemiol 2010;31:528-31.

4. Rice TW, Bernard GR. Therapeutic intervention and targets for sepsis. Annu Rev Med 2005;56:225-48.

5. Craig WA. Pharmacokinetic/pharmacodynamic parameters: rationale for antibacterial dosing of mice and men. Clin Infect Dis 1998;26:1-12.

6. Thomas JK, Forrest A, Bhavnani SM, et al. Pharmacodynamic evaluation of factors associated with the development of bacterial resistance in acutely ill patients during therapy. Antimicrob Agents Chemother 1998;42:521-527.

7. DeRyke CA, Lee SY, Kuti JL, et al. Optimising dosing strategies of antibacterials utilising pharmacodynamic principles: impact on the development of resistance. Drugs 2006;66:1-14.

8. Rybak MJ. Pharmacodynamics: relation to antimicrobial resistance. Am J Infect Control 2006;34:S38-45.

9. Roberts JA, Kruger P, Paterson DL, et al. Antibiotic resistance – what's dosing got to do with it? Crit Care Med 2008;36:2433-40.

10. Santos Filho L, Eagye KJ, Kuti JL, et al. Addressing resistance evolution in *Pseudomonas aeruginosa* using pharmacodynamic

11. Ambrose PG, Bhavnani SM, Rubina CM, et al. Pharmacokinetics-pharmacodynamics of antimicrobial therapy: it's not just for mice anymore. Clin Infect Dis 2007;44:79-86.

12. Roberts JA, Lipman J. Antibacterial dosing in intensive care. Pharmacokinetics, degree of disease and pharmacodynamics of sepsis. Clin Pharmacokinet 2006;45:755-73.

13. Pea F, Viale P, Furlanut M. Antimicrobial therapy in critically ill patients: a review of pathophysiological conditions responsible for altered disposition and pharmacokinetic variability. Clin Pharmacokinet 2005;44:1009-34.

14. Boucher BA, Wood GC, Swanson JM. Pharmacokinetic changes in critical illness. Crit Care Clin 2006;22:255-71.

15. Roberts JA, Lipman J. Pharmacokinetic issues for antibiotics in the critically ill patient. Crit Care Med 2009;37:840-51.

16. Goncalves-Pereira J, Povoa P. Antibiotics in critically ill patients: a systematic review of the pharmacokinetics of ß-lactams. Crit Care 2011;15:R206.

17. Macedo RS, Onita JH, Wille MP, et al. Pharmacokinetics and pharmacodynamics of antimicrobial drugs in intensive care unit patients. Shock 2013;39:24-8.

18. Carlier M, Carrette S, Stove V, et al. Does consistent piperacillin dosing result in inconsistent therapeutic concentrations in critically ill patients? A longitudinal study over an entire antibiotic course. Int J Antimicrob Agents 2014;43:470-3.

19. Udy AA, Roberts JA, Lipman J. Clinical implications of antibiotic pharmacokinetic principles in the critically ill. Intensive Care Med 2013;39:2070-82.

20. Felton TW, Hope WW, Roberts JA. How severe is antibiotic pharmacokinetic variability in critically ill patients and what can be done about it? Diagn Microbiol Infect Dis 2014;79:441-7.

21. Beale RJ, Hollenberg SM, Vincent JL, et al. Vasopressor and inotropic support in septic shock: an evidence-based review. Crit Care Med 2004;32(suppl):S455-65.

22. Johnston JD, Harvey CJ, Menzies IS, et al. Gastrointestinal permeability and absorptive capacity in sepsis. Crit Care Med 1996;24:1144-9.

23. Hassoun HT, Kone BC, Mercer DW, et al. Post-injury multiple organ failure: the role of the gut. Shock 2001;15:1-10.

24. Jacobi J, Fraser GL, Coursin DB, et al. Clinical practice guidelines for the sustained use of sedatives and analgesics in the critically ill adult. Crit Care Med 2002;30:119-41.

25. Hughes CA, Dowling RH. Speed of onset of adaptive mucosal hypoplasia and hypofunction in the intestine of parenterally fed rats. Clin Sci 1980;59:317-27.

26. Hernandez G, Velasco N, Wainstein C, et al. Gut mucosal atrophy after a short enteral fasting period in critically ill patients. J Crit Care 1999;14:73-7.

27. Glauser MP, Zanetti G, Baumgartner JD, et al. Septic shock: pathogenesis. Lancet 1991;338:732-6.

28. Suzuki A, Ishihara H, Hashiba E, et al. Detection of histamine-induced capillary protein leakage and hypovolaemia by determination of indocyanine green and glucose dilution method in dogs. Intensive Care Med 1999;25:304-10.

29. van der Poll T. Immunotherapy of sepsis. Lancet Infect Dis 2001;1:165-74.

30. Nuytinck HK, Offermans XJ, Kubat K, et al. Whole-body inflammation in trauma patients. An autopsy study. Arch Surg 1988;123:1519-24.

31. Gosling P, Sanghera K, Dickson G. Generalized vascular permeability and pulmonary function in patients following serious trauma. J Trauma 1994;36:477-81.

32. Etzel JV, Nafziger AN, Bertino JS Jr. Variation in the pharmacokinetics of gentamicin and tobramycin in patients with pleural effusions and hypoalbuminemia. Antimicrob Agents Chemother 1992;36:679-81.

33. Balogh Z, McKinley BA, Cocanour CS, et al. Supranormal trauma resuscitation causes more cases of abdominal compartment syndrome. Arch Surg 2003;138:637-42.

34. Conil JM, Georges B, Lavit M, et al. A population pharmacokinetic approach to ceftazidime use in burn patients: influence of glomerular filtration, gender and mechanical ventilation. Br J Clin Pharmacol 2007;64:27-35.

35. Beckhouse MJ, Whyte IM, Byth PL, et al. Altered aminoglycoside pharmacokinetics in the critically ill. Anaesth Intensive Care 1988;16:418-22.

36. Dasta JF, Armstrong DK. Variability in aminoglycoside pharmacokinetics in critically ill surgical patients. Crit Care Med 1988;16:327-30.

37. Botha FJ, van der Bijl P, Seifart HI, et al. Fluctuation of the volume of distribution of amikacin and its effect on once-daily dosage and clearance in a seriously ill patient. Intensive Care Med 1996;22:443-6.

38. Goonetilleke AK, Dev D, Aziz I, et al. A comparative analysis of pharmacokinetics of ceftriaxone in serum and pleural fluid in humans: a study of once daily administration by intramuscular and intravenous routes. J Antimicrob Chemother 1996;38:969-76.

39. Lugo G, Castaneda-Hernandez G. Amikacin Bayesian forecasting in critically ill patients with sepsis and cirrhosis. Ther Drug Monit 1997;19:271-6.

40. Teixeira LR, Sasse SA, Villarino MA, et al. Antibiotic levels in empyemic pleural fluid. Chest 2000;117:1734-9.

41. Lipman J, Wallis SC, Rickard CM, et al. Low cefpirome levels during twice daily dosing in critically ill septic patients: pharmacokinetic modelling calls for more frequent dosing. Intensive Care Med 2001;27:363-70.

42. Joukhadar C, Klein N, Mayer BX, et al. Plasma and tissue pharmacokinetics of cefpirome in patients with sepsis. Crit Care Med 2002;30:1478-82.

43. Makino J, Yoshiyama Y, Kanke M, et al. Pharmacokinetic study of penetration of meropenem into pleural effusion in patients with pleurisy. Jpn J Antibiot 2002;55:77-88.

44. Henriksen JH, Kiszka-Kanowitz M, Bendtsen F. Review article: volume expansion in patients with cirrhosis. Aliment Pharmacol Ther 2002;16(suppl 5):12-23.

45. Rea RS, Capitano B. Optimizing use of aminoglycosides in the critically ill. Semin Respir Crit Care Med 2007;28:596-603.

46. Rea RS, Capitano B, Bies R, et al. Suboptimal aminoglycoside dosing in critically ill patients. Ther Drug Monit 2008;30:674-81.

47. Boyer A, Gruson D, Bouchet S, et al. Aminoglycosides in septic shock. Drug Saf 2013;36:217-30.

48. McNamara PJ, Gibaldi M, Stoeckel K. Volume of distribution terms for a drug (ceftriaxone) exhibiting concentration-dependent protein binding. II. Physiological significance. Eur J Clin Pharmacol 1983;25:407-12.

49. Joynt GM, Lipman J, Gomersall CD, et al. The pharmacokinetics of once-daily dosing of ceftriaxone in critically ill patients. J Antimicrob Chemother 2001;47:421-9.

50. Toma O, Suntrup P, Stefanescu A, et al. Pharmacokinetics and tissue penetration of cefoxitin in obesity: implications for risk of surgical site infection. Anesth Analg 2011;113:730-7.

51. Muzevich KM, Lee KB. Subtherapeutic linezolid concentrations in a patient with morbid obesity and methicillin-resistant *Staphylococcus aureus* pneumonia: case report and review of the literature. Ann Pharmacother 2013;47:e25.

52. Longo C, Bartlett G, Macgibbon B, et al. The effect of obesity on antibiotic treatment failure: a historical cohort study. Pharmacoepidemiol Drug Saf 2013;22:970-6.

53. Hanley MJ, Abernethy DR, Greenblatt DJ. Effect of obesity on the pharmacokinetics of drugs in humans. Clin Pharmacokinet 2010;49:71-87.

54. Morrish GA, Pai MP, Green B. The effects of obesity on drug pharmacokinetics in humans. Exp Opin Drug Metab Toxicol 2011;7:697-706.

55. Pai MP, Bearden DT. Antimicrobial dosing considerations in obese adult patients. Pharmacotherapy 2007;27:1081-91.

56. Janson B, Thursky K. Dosing of antibiotics in obesity. Curr Opin Infect Dis 2012;25:634-9.

57. Polso AK, Lassiter JL, Nagel JL. Impact of hospital guideline for weight-based antimicrobial dosing in morbidly obese adult and comprehensive literature review. J Clin Pharm Ther 2014;39:584-608.

58. McKindley DS, Hanes SD, Boucher BA. Hepatic drug metabolism in critical illness. Pharmacotherapy 1998;18:759-78.

59. Tortorici MA, Kochanek PM, Poloyac SM. Effects of hypothermia on drug disposition, metabolism, and response: a focus of hypothermia-mediated alterations on the cytochrome 450 enzyme system. Crit Care Med 2007;35:2196-204.

60. Perkins MW, Dasta JF, DeHaven B. Physiologic implications of mechanical ventilation on pharmacokinetics. Drug Intell Clin Pharm 1989;23:316-23.

61. Meier-Hellmann A, Reinhart K, Bredle DL, et al. Epinephrine impairs splanchnic perfusion in septic shock. Crit Care Med 1997;25:399-404.

62. Obritsch MD, Bestul DJ, Jung R, et al. The role of vasopressin in vasodilatory septic shock. Pharmacotherapy 2004;24:1050-63.

63. Lugo G, Castaneda-Hernandez G. Relationship between hemodynamic and vital support measures and pharmacokinetic variability of amikacin in critically ill patients with sepsis. Crit Care Med 1997;25:806-11.

64. Mann HJ, Townsend RJ, Fuhs DW, et al. Decreased hepatic clearance of clindamycin in critically ill patients with sepsis. Clin Pharm 1987;6:154-9.

65. Boucher BA, Hanes SD. Pharmacokinetic alterations after severe head injury. Clinical relevance. Clin Pharmacokinet 1998;35:209-21.

66. Walter-Sack I, Klotz U. Influence of diet and nutritional status on drug metabolism. Clin Pharmacokinet 1996;31:47-64.

67. Benet LZ, Hoener BA. Changes in plasma protein binding have little clinical relevance. Clin Pharmacol Ther 2002;71:115-21.

68. Cockcroft DW, Gault MH. Prediction of creatinine clearance from serum creatinine. Nephron 1976;16:31-41.

69. Levey AS, Bosch JP, Lewis JB, et al. A more accurate method to estimate glomerular filtration rate from serum creatinine: a new prediction equation. Modification of Diet in Renal Disease Study Group. Ann Intern Med 1999;130:461-70.

70. Hoste EA, Damen J, Vanholder RC, et al. Assessment of renal function in recently admitted critically ill patients with normal serum creatinine. Nephrol Dial Transplant 2005;20:747-53.

71. Grootaert V, Williams L, Debaveye Y, et al. Augmented renal clearance in the critically ill: how to assess kidney function. Ann Pharmacother 2012;46:952-9.

72. Pickering JW, Frampton CM, Walker RJ, et al. Four hour creatinine clearance is better than plasma creatinine for monitoring renal function in critically ill patients. Crit Care 2012;16:R107-10.

73. Bragadottir G, Redfors B, Ricksten SE. Assessing glomerular filtration rate (GFR) in critically ill patients with acute kidney injury—true GFR versus urinary creatinine clearance and estimating equations. Crit Care 2013;17:R108-14.

74. Blasco V, Antonini F, Zieleskiewicz L, et al. Comparative study of three methods of estimation of creatinine clearance in critically ill patients. Ann Franc Anesth Reanimat 2014;33:e85-8.

75. Baptista JP, Neves M, Rodrigues L, et al. Accuracy of the estimation of glomerular filtration rate within a population of critically ill patients. J Nephrol 2014;27:403-10.

76. Casu GS, Hites M, Jacobs F, et al. Can changes in renal function predict variations in ß-lactam concentrations in septic patients? Int J Antimicrob Agents 2013;42:422-8.

77. Di Giantomasso D, May CN, Bellomo R. Norepinephrine and vital organ blood flow. Intensive Care Med 2002;28:1804-9.

78. Di Giantomasso D, May CN, Bellomo R. Norepinephrine and vital organ blood flow during experimental hyperdynamic sepsis. Intensive Care Med 2003;29:1774-81.

79. Di Giantomasso D, Bellomo R, May CN. The haemodynamic and metabolic effects of epinephrine in experimental hyperdynamic septic shock. Intensive Care Med 2005;31:454-62.

80. Udy AA, Putt MT, Shanmugathasan S, et al. Augmented renal clearance in the intensive care unit: an illustrative case series. Int J Antimicrob Agents 2010;35:606-8.

81. Udy AA, Roberts J, Boots RJ, et al. Augmented renal clearance: implications for antibacterial dosing in the critically ill. Clin Pharmacokinet 2010;49:1-16.

82. Udy AA, Roberts JA, Lipman J. Implications of augmented renal clearance in critically ill patients. Nat Rev Nephrol 2011;7:539-43.

83. Udy AA, Roberts J, De Waele J, et al. What's behind the failure of emerging antibiotics in the critically ill? Understanding the impact of altered pharmacokinetics and augmented renal clearance. Int J Antimicrob Agents 2012;39:455-7.

84. Udy AA, Roberts JA, Shorr AF, et al. Augmented renal clearance in septic and traumatized patients with normal plasma creatinine concentrations: identifying at-risk patients. Crit Care 2013;17:R35-43.

85. Udy AA, Baptista JP, Lim NL, et al. Augmented renal clearance in the ICU: results of a multicenter observational study of renal function in critically ill patients with normal plasma creatinine concentrations. Crit Care Med 2014;42:520-7.

86. Baptista JP, Sousa E, Martins PJ, et al. Augmented renal clearance in septic patients and implications for vancomycin monitoring. Int J Antimicrob Agents 2012;39:420-3.

87. Udy AA, Varghese JM, Altukroni M, et al. Subtherapeutic initial β-lactam concentrations in select critically ill patients. Association between augmented renal clearance and low trough drug concentrations. Chest 2012;142:30-9.

88. Claus BOM, Hoste EA, Colpaert K, et al. Augmented renal clearance is a common finding with worse clinical outcome in critically ill patients receiving antimicrobial therapy. J Crit Care 2013;28:695-700.

89. Troeger U, Drust A, Martens-Lobenhoffer J, et al. Decreased meropenem levels in intensive care unit patients with augmented renal clearance: benefit of therapeutic drug monitoring. Int J Antimicrob Agents 2012;40:370-2.

90. Carlier M, Carrette S, Roberts JA, et al. Meropenem and piperacillin/tazobactam prescribing in critically ill patients: does augmented renal clearance affect pharmacokinetic/pharmacodynamic target attainment when extended infusions are used? Crit Care 2013;17:R84.

91. Rybak MJ, Albrecht LM, Berman JR, et al. Vancomycin pharmacokinetics in burn patients and intravenous drug abusers. Antimicrob Agents Chemother 1990;34:792-5.

92. Boucher BA, Kuhl DA, Hickerson WL. Pharmacokinetics of systemically administered antibiotics in patients with thermal injury. Clin Infect Dis 1992;14:458-63.

93. Garrelts JC, Jost G, Kowalsky SF, et al. Ciprofloxacin pharmacokinetics in burn patients. Antimicrob Agents Chemother 1996;40:1153-6.

94. Boucher BA, King SR, Wandschneider HL, et al. Fluconazole pharmacokinetics in burn patients. Antimicrob Agents Chemother 1998;42:930-3.

95. Dailly E, Kergueris MF, Pannier M, et al. Population pharmacokinetics of imipenem in burn patients. Fundam Clin Pharmacol 2003;17:645-50.

96. Kiser TH, Hoody DW, Obritsch MD, et al. Levofloxacin pharmacokinetics and pharmacodynamics in patients with severe burn injury. Antimicrob Agents Chemother 2006;50:1937-45.

97. Barbot A, Venisse N, Rayeh F, et al. Pharmacokinetics and pharmacodynamics of sequential intravenous and subcutaneous teicoplanin in critically ill patients without vasopressors. Intensive Care Med 2003;29:1528-34.

98. Roberts JA, Pea F, Lipman J. The clinical relevance of plasma protein binding changes. Clin Pharmacokinet 2013;52:1-8.

99. Wise R, Gillett AP, Cadge B, et al. The influence of protein binding upon tissue fluid levels of six beta-lactam antibiotics. J Infect Dis 1980;142:77-82.

100. Gerding DN, Van Etta LL, Peterson LR. Role of serum protein binding and multiple antibiotic doses in the extravascular distribution of ceftizoxime and cefotaxime. Antimicrob Agents Chemother 1982;22:844-7.

101. Merrikin DJ, Briant J, Rolinson GN. Effect of protein binding on antibiotic activity in vivo. J Antimicrob Chemother 1983;11:233-8.

102. Joukhadar C, Frossard M, Mayer BX, et al. Impaired target site penetration of beta-lactams may account for therapeutic failure in patients with septic shock. Crit Care Med 2001;29:385-91.

103. Sauermann R, Delle-Karth G, Marsik C, et al. Pharmacokinetics and pharmacodynamics of cefpirome in subcutaneous adipose tissue of septic patients. Antimicrob Agents Chemother 2005;49:650-5.

104. Dahyot C, Marchand S, Bodin M, et al. Application of basic pharmacokinetic concepts to analysis of microdialysis data: illustration with imipenem muscle distribution. Clin Pharmacokinet 2008;47:181-9.

105. Roberts JA, Roberts MS, Robertson TA, et al. Piperacillin penetration into tissue of critically ill patients with sepsis—bolus vs continuous administration? Crit Care Med 2009;37:926-33.

106. Roberts JA, Kirkpatrick CMJ, Roberts MS, et al. Meropenem dosing in critically ill patients with sepsis and without renal dysfunction: intermittent bolus versus continuous administration? Monte Carlo dosing simulations and subcutaneous tissue distribution. J Antimicrob Chemother 2009;64:142-50.

107. DeFife R, Scheetz MH, Feinglass JM, et al. Effect of differences in MIC values on clinical outcomes in patients with bloodstream infections caused by gram-negative organisms treated with levofloxacin. Antimicrob Agents Chemother 2009;53:1074-9.

108. Doyle JS, Buising KL, Thursky KA, et al. Epidemiology of infections acquired in intensive care units. Semin Respir Crit Care Med 2011;32:115-38.

109. Sandiumenge A, Rello J. Ventilator-associated pneumonia caused by ESKAPE organisms: cause, clinical features, and management. Curr Opin Pulm Med 2012;18:187-93.

110. Laupland KB, Church DL. Population-based epidemiology and microbiology of community-onset bloodstream infections. Clin Microbiol Rev 2014;27:647-64.

111. Landelle, CA, Marimuthu KAB, Harbarth SA. Infection control measures to decrease the burden of antimicrobial resistance in the critical care setting. Curr Opin Crit Care 2014;20:499-506.

112. Tangden T, Giske CG. Global dissemination of extensively drug-resistant carbapenemase-producing Enterobacteriaceae: clinical perspectives on detection, treatment and infection control. J Int Med 2015;277:501-12.

113. Goncalves-Pereira J, Paiva JA. Dose modulation: a new concept of antibiotic therapy in the critically ill patient? J Crit Care 2013;28:341-6.

114. Roberts JA, Lipman J. Optimal doripenem dosing simulations in critically ill nosocomial pneumonia patients with obesity, augmented renal clearance, and decreased bacterial susceptibility. Crit Care Med 2013;41:489-95.

115. Cheatham SC, Fleming MR, Healy DP, et al. Steady-state pharmacokinetics and pharmacodynamics of piperacillin and tazobactam administered by prolonged infusion in obese patients. Int J Antimicrob Agents 2013;41:52-6.

116. Blot S, Lipman J, Roberts DM, et al. The influence of acute kidney injury on antimicrobial dosing in critically ill patients: are dose reductions always necessary? Diagn Microbiol Infect Dis 2014;79:77-84.

117. Roberts JA, Abdul-Aziz MH, Lipman J, et al. Individualised antibiotic dosing for patients who are critically ill: challenges and potential solutions. Lancet Infect Dis 2014;14:498-509.

118. Wells M, Lipman J. Measurements of glomerular filtration in the intensive care unit are only a rough guide to renal function. S Afr J Surg 1997;35:20-3.
119. Herrera-Gutierrez ME, Seller-Perez G, Banderas-Bravo E, et al. Replacement of 24-h creatinine clearance by 2-h creatinine clearance in intensive care unit patients: a single-center study. Intensive Care Med 2007;33:1900-6.
120. Udy A, Roberts JA, Boots RJ, et al. You only find what you look for: the importance of high creatinine clearance in the critically ill. Anaesth Intensive Care 2009;37:11-3.
121. Hayashi Y, Lipman J, Udy AA, et al. ß-Lactam therapeutic drug monitoring in the critically ill: optimising drug exposure in patients with fluctuating renal function and hypoalbuminaemia. Int J Antimicrob Agents 2013;41:162-6.
122. Roberts JA, Paul SK, Akova M, et al. DALI: defining antibiotic levels in intensive care unit patients: are current ß-lactam antibiotic doses sufficient for critically ill patients? Clin Infect Dis 2014;58:1072-83.
123. Wong G, Brinkman A, Benefield RJ, et al. An international, multicentre survey of ß-lactam antibiotic therapeutic drug monitoring practice in intensive care units. J Antimicrob Chemother 2014;69:1416-23.
124. Smith J, Andes D. Therapeutic drug monitoring of antifungals: pharmacokinetic and pharmacodynamic considerations. Ther Drug Monit 2008;30:167-72.
125. Hope WW, Billaud EM, Lestner J, et al. Therapeutic drug monitoring for triazoles. Curr Opin Infect Dis 2008;21:580-6.
126. Lewis RE. Current concepts in antifungal pharmacology. Mayo Clin Proc 2011;86:805-17.
127. Amsden JR. Fungla biomarkers, antifungal susceptibility testing, and therapeutic drug monitoring—practical applications for the clinician in a tertiary care center. Curr Fungal Infect Rep 2015;9:111-21.
128. Winterboer TM, Lecci KA, Olsen KM. Alternative approaches to optimizing antimicrobial pharmacodynamics in critically ill patients. J Pharm Pract 2010;23:6-18.
129. Lodise TP, Drusano GL. Pharmacokinetics and pharmacodynamics: optimal antimicrobial therapy in the intensive care unit. Crit Care Clin 2011;1-18.
130. Alvarez-Lerma F, Grau S. Management of antimicrobial use in the intensive care unit. Drugs 2012;72:447-70.
131. Rayner CR, Forrest A, Meagher AK, et al. Clinical pharmacodynamics of linezolid in seriously ill patients treated in a compassionate use programme. Clin Pharmacokinet 2003;42:1411-23.
132. Craig WA. Basic pharmacodynamics of antibacterials with clinical applications to the use of beta-lactams, glycopeptides, and linezolid. Infect Dis Clin North Am 2003;17:479-501.
133. Lewis RE. Pharmacodynamic implications for use of antifungal agents. Curr Opin Pharmacol 2007;7:491-7.
134. Lepak AJ, Andes DR. Antifungal PK/PD considerations in fungal pulmonary infections. Semin Respir Crit Care Med 2011;32:783-94.
135. Sinnollareddy M, Peake SL, Roberts MS, et al. Using pharmacokinetics and pharmacodynamics to optimise dosing of antifungal agents in critically ill patients: a systematic review. Int J Antimicrob Agents 2012;39:1-10.
136. Moise-Broder PA, Forrest A, Birmingham MC, et al. Pharmacodynamics of vancomycin and other antimicrobials in patients with *Staphylococcus aureus* lower respiratory tract infections. Clin Pharmacokinet 2004;43:925-42.
137. Jeffres MN, Isakow W, Doherty JA, et al. Predictors of mortality for methicillin-resistant *Staphylococcus aureus* health-care-associated pneumonia: specific evaluation of vancomycin pharmacokinetic indices. Chest 2006;130:947-55.
138. Del Mar Fernández de Gatta Garcia M, Revilla N, Calvo MV, et al. Pharmacokinetic/pharmacodynamic analysis of vancomycin in ICU patients. Intensive Care Med 2007;33:279-85.
139. Mohr JF, Murray BE. Point: vancomycin is not obsolete for the treatment of infection caused by methicillin-resistant *Staphylococcus aureus*. Clin Infect Dis 2007;44:1536-42.
140. Rybak MJ, Lomaestro B, Rotschafer JC, et al. Vancomycin therapeutic guidelines: a summary of consensus recommendations of Infectious Diseases Society of America, the American Society of Health-System Pharmacists, and the Society of Infectious Diseases Pharmacists. Clin Infect Dis 2009;49:325-7.
141. Zelenitsky S, Rubinstein E, Ariano R, et al.; the Cooperative Antimicrobial Therapy of Septic Shock-CATSS Database Research Group. Vancomycin pharmacodynamics and survival in patients with methicillin-resistant *Staphylococcus aureus*-associated septic shock. Int J Antimicrob Agents 2013;41:255-60.
142. Adembri C, Fallani S, Cassetta MI, et al. Linezolid pharmacokinetic/pharmacodynamic profile in critically ill septic patients: intermittent versus continuous infusion. Int J Antimicrob Agents 2008;31:122-9.
143. Moore RD, Lietman PS, Smith CR. Clinical response to aminoglycoside therapy: importance of the ratio of peak concentration to minimal inhibitory concentration. J Infect Dis 1987;155:93-9.
144. Highet VS, Forrest A, Ballow CH, et al. Antibiotic dosing issues in lower respiratory tract infection: population-derived area under inhibitory curve is predicative of efficacy. J Antimicrob Chem 1999;43(suppl A):55-63.
145. Zelenitsky SA, Harding GK, Sun S, et al. Treatment and outcome of *Pseudomonas aeruginosa* bacteraemia: an antibiotic pharmacodynamic analysis. J Antimicrob Chemother 2003;52:668-74.
146. Drusano GL, Ambrose PG, Bhavnani SM, et al. Back to the future: using aminoglycosides again and how to dose them optimally. Clin Infect Dis. 2007;45:753-60.
147. Schentag JJ, Nix DE, Adelman MH. Mathematical examination of dual individualization principles (I): relationships between AUC above MIC and area under the inhibitory curve for cefmenoxime, ciprofloxacin, and tobramycin. Drug Intell Clin Pharm 1991;25:1050-7.
148. Lacy MK, Nicolau DP, Nightingale CH, et al. The pharmacodynamics of aminoglycosides. Clin Infect Dis. 1998;27:23-7.
149. Preston SL, Drusano GL, Berman AL, et al. Pharmacodynamics of levofloxacin: a new paradigm for early clinical trials. JAMA 1998;279:125-9.
150. Lacy MK, Lu W, Xu X, et al. Pharmacodynamic comparisons of levofloxacin and ciprofloxacin against *Streptococcus pneumoniae* in an in vitro model of infection. Antimicrob Agents Chemother 1999;43:79-86.

151. Ambrose PG, Grasela DM, Grasela TH, et al. Pharmacodynamics of fluoroquinolones against *Streptococcus pneumoniae* in patients with community-acquired respiratory tract infections. Antimicrob Agents Chemother 2001;45:2793-7.

152. Drusano GL, Preston SL, Fowler C, et al. Relationship between fluoroquinolone area under the curve: minimum inhibitory concentration ratio and the probability of eradication of the infecting pathogen, in patients with nosocomial pneumonia. J Infect Dis 2004;189:1590-7.

153. Zelenitsky SA, Ariano RE. Support for higher ciprofloxacin AUC_{24}/MIC targets in treating Enterobacteriaceae bloodstream infection. J Antimicrob Chemother 2010;65:1725-32.

154. Dandekar PK, Tessier PR, Williams P, et al. Pharmacodynamic profile of daptomycin against *Enterococcus* species and methicillin-resistant *Staphylococcus aureus* in a murine thigh infection model. J Antimicrob Chemother 2003;52:405-11.

155. Safdar N, Andes D, Craig WA. In vivo pharmacodynamic activity of daptomycin. Antimicrob Agents Chemother 2004;48:63-8.

156. Firsov AA, Smirnova MV, Lubenko IY, et al. Testing the mutant selection window hypothesis with Staphylococcus aureus exposed to daptomycin and vancomycin in an in vitro dynamic model. J Antimicrob Chemother 2006;58:1185-92.

157. Cubicin® (daptomycin for injection) [package insert]. Lexington, MA: Cubist Pharmaceuticals U.S., July 2015.

158. Benvenuto M, Benziger DP, Yankelev S, et al. Pharmacokinetics and tolerability of daptomycin at doses up to 12 milligrams per kilogram of body weight once daily in healthy volunteers. Antimicrob Agents Chemother 2006;50:3245-9.

159. Falcone M, Russo A, Venditti M, et al. Considerations for higher doses of daptomycin in critically ill patients with methicillin-resistant Staphylococcus aureus bacteremia. Clin Infect Dis 2013;57:1568-76.

160. Zilberberg MD, Kollef MH, Arnold H, et al. Inappropriate empiric antifungal therapy for candidemia in the ICU and hospital resource utilization: a retrospective cohort study. BMC Infect Dis 2010;10:150-8.

161. Labelle AJ, Micek ST, Roubinian N, et al. Treatment-related risk factors for hospital mortality in *Candida* bloodstream infections. Crit Care Med 2008;36:2967-72.

162. Smith JA, Kauffman CA. Recognition and prevention of nosocomial invasive fungal infections in the intensive care unit. Crit Care Med 2010;38(suppl):S380-7.

163. Dodds Ashley ES, Lewis R, Lewis JS, et al. Pharmacology of systemic antifungal agents. Clin Infect Dis 2006;43(suppl 1):S28-39.

164. Wiederhold NP. Using antifungal pharmacodynamics to improve patient outcomes. Curr Fungal Infect Rep 2010;4:70-7.

165. Pfaller MA, Diekema DJ, Rex JH, et al. Correlation of MIC with outcome for *Candida* species tested against voriconazole: analysis and proposal for interpretive breakpoints for gram-negative aerobic bacteria based. J Clin Microbiol 2006;44:819-26.

166. Rodriguez-Tudela JL, Almirante B, Rodriguez-Pardo D, et al. Correlation of the MIC and dose/MIC ratio of fluconazole to the therapeutic response of patients with mucosal candidiasis and candidemia. Antimicrob Agents Chemother 2007;51:3599-604.

167. Pai MP, Turpin RS, Garey KW. Association of fluconazole area under the concentration-time curve/MIC and dose/MIC ratios with mortality in nonneutropenic patients with candidemia. Antimicrob Agents Chemother 2007;51:35-9.

168. Baddley JW, Patel M, Bhavnani SM, et al. Association of fluconazole pharmacodynamics with mortality in patients with candidemia. Antimicrob Agents Chemother 2008;52:3022-8.

169. Smith J, Safdar N, Knasinski V, et al. Voriconazole therapeutic drug monitoring. Antimicrob Agents Chemother 2006;50:1570-2.

170. Pascual A, Calandra T, Bolay S, et al. Voriconazole therapeutic drug monitoring in patients with invasive mycoses improves efficacy and safety outcomes. Clin Infect Dis 2008;46:201-11.

171. Hong Y, Shaw PJ, Nath CE, et al. Population pharmacokinetics of liposomal amphotericin B in pediatric patients with malignant diseases. Antimicrob Agents Chemother 2006;50:935-42.

172. Gumbo T. Impact of pharmacodynamics and pharmacokinetics on echinocandin dosing strategies. Curr Opin Infect Dis 2007;20:587-91.

173. Wiederhold NP, Kontoyiannis DP, Chi J, et al. Pharmacodynamics of caspofungin in a murine model of invasive pulmonary aspergillosis: evidence of concentration-dependent activity. J Infect Dis 2004;190:1464-71.

174. Quintiliani R Sr, Quintiliani R Jr. Pharmacokinetics/pharmacodynamics for critical care clinicians. Clin Care Clin 2008;24:335-48.

175. Frei CV, Burgess DS. Continuous infusion ß-lactams for intensive care unit pulmonary infections. Clin Microbiol Infect 2005;11:418-21.

176. Buck C, Bertram N, Ackermann T, et al. Pharmacokinetics of piperacillin-tazobactam: intermittent dosing versus continuous infusion. Int J Antimicrob Agents 2005;25:62-7.

177. Krueger WA, Bulitta J, Kinzig-Schippers M, et al. Evaluation by Monte Carlo simulation of the pharmacokinetics of two doses of meropenem administered intermittently or as a continuous infusion in healthy volunteers. Antimicrob Agents Chemother 2005;49:1881-9.

178. Lodise TP, Lomaestro BM, Drusano GL. Application of antimicrobial pharmacodynamic concepts into clinical practice: focus on ß-lactam antibiotics. Pharmacotherapy 2006;26:1320-32.

179. Nicolau DP. Pharmacokinetic and pharmacodynamic properties of meropenem. Clin Infect Dis 2008;47:S32-40.

180. Abdul-Aziz MH, Staatz CE, Kirkpatrick CMJ, et al. Continuous infusion vs. bolus dosing: implications for beta-lactam antibiotics. Minerva Anestesiol 2012;78:94-104.

181. Psathas PA, Kuzmission A, Ikeda K, et al. Stability of doripenem in vitro in representative infusion solutions and infusion bags. Clin Ther 2008;30:2075-87.

182. Kuti JI, Nightingale CH, Knault RF, et al. Pharmacokinetic properties of and stability of continuous-infusion meropenem in adults with cystic fibrosis. Clin Ther 2004;26:493-501.

183. Trissel LA. Handbook of Injectable Drugs, 18th ed. Bethesda, MD: American Society of Health-System Pharmacists, 2014.

184. Lomaestro BM, Drusano GL. Pharmacodynamic evaluation of extending the administration time of meropenem using a Monte Carlo simulation. Antimicrob Agents Chemother 2005;49:461-3.

185. Kim A, Sutherland CA, Kuti JL, et al. Optimal dosing of piperacillin-tazobactam for the treatment of *Pseudomonas*

186. MacVane SH, Kuti JL, Nicolau DP. Prolonging ß-lactam infusion: a review of the rationale and evidence, and guidance for implementation. Int J Antimicrob Agents 2014;43:105-13.

187. Lodise TP Jr, Lomaestro B, Drusano GL. Piperacillin-tazobactam for *Pseudomonas aeruginosa* infection: clinical implications of an extended-infusion dosing strategy. Clin Infect Dis 2007;44:357-63.

188. Kasiakou SK, Sermaides GJ, Michalopoulos A, et al. Continuous versus intermittent intravenous administration of antibiotics: a meta-analysis of randomised controlled trials. Lancet Infect Dis 2005;5:581-9.

189. Roberts JA, Webb S, Paterson D, et al. A systematic review on clinical benefits of continuous administration of ß-lactam antibiotics. Crit Care Med 2009;37:2071-8.

190. Falagas ME, Tansarli GS, Ikawa K, et al. Clinical outcomes with extended or continuous versus short-term intravenous infusion of carbapenems and piperacillin-tazobactam: a systematic review and meta-analysis. Clin Infect Dis 2013;56:272-82.

191. Teo J, Liew Y, Lee W, et al. Prolonged infusion versus intermittent boluses of ß-lactam antibiotics for treatment of acute infections: a meta-analysis. Int J Antimicrob Agents 2014;43:403-11.

192. Dulhunty JM, Roberts JA, Davis JS, et al. Continuous infusion of ß-lactam antibiotics in severe sepsis: a multicenter double-blind, randomized controlled trial. Clin Infect Dis 2013;56:236-47.

193. Nicolau DP, McNabb JC, Lacy MK, et al. Pharmacokinetic and pharmacodynamics of continuous and intermittent ceftazidime during the treatment of nosocomial pneumonia. Clin Drug Investig 1999;2:133-9.

194. Kuti JL, Maglio D, Nightingale CH, et al. Economic benefit of a meropenem dosage strategy based on pharmacodynamic concepts. Am J Health Syst Pharm 2003;60:565-8.

195. Florea NR, Kotapati S, Kuti JL, et al. Cost analysis of continuous versus intermittent infusion of piperacillin-tazobactam: a time-motion study. Am J Health Syst Pharm 2003;60:2321-7.

196. DeRyke CA, Kuti JL, Mansfield D, et al. Pharmacoeconomics of continuous versus intermittent infusion of piperacillin-tazobactam for the treatment of complicated intraabdominal infection. Am J Health Syst Pharm 2006;63:750-5.

197. Nicasio AM, Eagye KJ, Kuti EL, et al. Length of stay and hospital costs associated with a pharmacodynamic-based clinical pathway for empiric antibiotic choice for ventilator-associated pneumonia. Pharmacotherapy 2010;30:453-62.

198. Xamplas RC, Itokazu GS, Glowacki RC, et al. Implementation of an extended-infusion piperacillin-tazobactam program at an urban teaching hospital. Am J Health Syst Pharm 2010;67:622-8.

199. Sader HS, Fey PD, Fish DN, et al. Evaluation of vancomycin and daptomycin potency trends ("MIC creep") against methicillin-resistant *Staphylococcus aureus* collected in nine United States medical centers over five years (2002-2006). Antimicrob Agents Chemother 2009;53:4127-32.

200. Patel N, Pai MP, Rodvold KA, et al. Vancomycin: we can't get there from here. Clin Infect Dis 2011;52:969-74.

201. Blot S, Koulenti D, Akova M, et al. Does contemporary vancomycin dosing achieve therapeutic targets in a heterogeneous clinical cohort of critically ill patients? Data from the multinational DALI study. Crit Care 2014;18:R99.

202. Lodise TP, Lomaestro B, Graves J, et al. Larger vancomycin doses (at least four grams per day) are associated with an increased incidence of nephrotoxicity. Antimicrob Agents Chemother 2008;52:1330-6.

203. Brinquin L, Rousseau JM, Boulesteix G, et al. Continuous infusion of vancomycin in post-neurosurgical staphylococcal meningitis in adults. Presse Med 1993;22:1815-7.

204. Conil JM, Favarel H, Laguerre J, et al. Continuous administration of vancomycin in patients with severe burns. Presse Med 1994;23:1554-8.

205. Cruciani M, Gatti G, Lazzarini L, et al. Penetration of vancomycin into human lung tissue. J Antimicrob Chemother 1996;38:865-9.

206. Byl B, Jacobs F, Wallemacq P, et al. Vancomycin penetration of uninfected pleural fluid exudate after continuous or intermittent infusion. Antimicrob Agents Chemother 2003;47:2015-7.

207. Di Filippo A, De Gaudio AR, Novelli A, et al. Continuous infusion of vancomycin in methicillin-resistant staphylococcus infection. Chemotherapy 1998;44:63-8.

208. Albanese J, Leone M, Bruguerolle B, et al. Cerebrospinal fluid penetration and pharmacokinetics of vancomycin administered by continuous infusion to mechanically ventilated patients in an intensive care unit. Antimicrob Agents Chemother 2000;44:1356-8.

209. Wysocki M, Delatour F, Faurisson F, et al. Continuous versus intermittent infusion of vancomycin in severe staphylococcal infections: prospective multicenter randomized study. Antimicrob Agents Chemother 2001;45:2460-7.

210. Ingram PR, Lye DC, Fisher DA, et al. Nephrotoxicity of continuous versus intermittent infusion of vancomycin in outpatient parenteral antimicrobial therapy. Int J Antimicrob Agents 2009;34:570-4.

211. Vuagnat A, Stern R, Lotthe A, et al. High dose vancomycin for osteomyelitis: continuous vs intermittent infusion. J Clin Pharm Ther 2004;29:351-7.

212. Cataldo MA, Tacconelli E, Grilli E, et al. Continuous versus intermittent infusion of vancomycin for the treatment of gram-positive infections: systematic review and meta-analysis. J Antimicrob Chemother 2011;67:17-24.

213. Hutschala D, Kinster C, Skhirdladze MD, et al. Influence of vancomycin on renal function in critically ill patients after cardiac surgery. Anesthesiology 2009;111:356-65.

214. Liu C, Bayer A, Cosgrove SE, et al. Clinical practice guidelines by the Infectious Diseases Society of America for the treatment of methicillin-resistant *Staphylococcus aureus* infections in adults and children. Clin Infect Dis 2011;52:1-38.

215. Jacqueline C, Batard E, Perez L, et al. In vivo efficacy of continuous infusion versus intermittent dosing of linezolid compared to vancomycin in a methicillin-resistant *Staphylococcus aureus* rabbit endocarditis model. Antimicrob Agents Chemother 2002;46:3706-11.

216. Bennett WM, Plamp CE, Gilbert DN, et al. The influence of dosage regimen on experimental nephrotoxicity: dissociation of peak serum levels from renal failure. J Infect Dis 1979;140:576-80.

217. Galloe AM, Graudal N, Christensen HR, et al. Aminoglycosides: single or multiple daily dosing? Eur J Clin Pharmacol 1995;48:39-43.

218. Chuck SK, Raber SR, Rodvold KA, et al. National survey of extended-interval aminoglycoside dosing. Clin Infect Dis 2000;30:433-9.

219. Barza M, Ioannidis JP, Cappelleri JC, et al. Single or multiple daily doses of aminoglycosides: a meta-analysis. BMJ 1996;312:338-45.

220. Munckhof WJ, Grayson ML, Turnidge JD. A meta-analysis of studies on the safety and efficacy of aminoglycosides given either once daily or as divided doses. J Antimicrob Chemother 1996;37:645-63.

221. Ferriol-Lisart R, Alós-Almiñana M. Effectiveness and safety of once-daily cimonglycosides: a meta-analysis. Am J Health Syst Pharm 1996;53:1141-50.

222. Freeman CD, Strayer AH. Mega-analysis of meta-analysis: an examination of meta-analysis with an emphasis on once-daily aminoglycoside comparative trials. Pharmacotherapy 1996;16:1093-102.

223. Hatala R, Dinh TT, Cook DJ. Once-daily aminoglycoside dosing in immunocompetent adults: a meta-analysis. Ann Intern Med 1996;124:717-25.

224. Ali MZ, Goetz MB. A meta-analysis of the relative efficacy and toxicity of single daily dosing versus multiple daily dosing of aminoglycosides. Clin Infect Dis 1997;24:796-809.

225. Bailey TC, Little JR, Littenberg B, et al. A meta-analysis of extended-interval dosing versus multiple daily dosing of aminoglycosides. Clin Infect Dis 1997;24:786-95.

226. Hatala R, Dinh TT, Cook DJ. Single daily dosing of aminoglycosides in immunocompromised adults: a systemic review. Clin Infect Dis 1997;24:810-5.

227. Rybak MJ, Abate BJ, Kang SL, et al. Prospective evaluation of the effect of an aminoglycoside dosing regimen on rates of observed nephrotoxicity and ototoxicity. Antimicrob Agents Chemother 1999;43:1549-55.

228. Hitt CM, Klepser ME, Nightingale CH, et al. Pharmacoeconomic impact of once-daily aminoglycoside administration. Pharmacotherapy 1997;17:810-4.

229. Nicolau DP, Freeman CD, Belliveau PP, et al. Experience with a once-daily aminoglycoside program administered to 2:184 adult patients. Antimicrob Agents Chemother 1995;39:650-5.

230. Wallace AW, Jones M, Bertino JS Jr. Evaluation of four once-daily aminoglycoside dosing nomograms. Pharmacotherapy 2002;22:1077-83.

231. Stankowicz MS, Ibrahim J, Brown DL. Once-daily aminoglycoside dosing: an update on current literature. Am J Health Syst Pharm 2015;72:1357-64.

232. Rea RS, Capitano B. Optimizing use of aminoglycosides in the critically ill. Semin Respir Crit Care Med 2007;28:596-603.

233. Conil JM, Georges B, Ruiz S, et al. Tobramycin disposition in ICU patients receiving a once daily regimen: population approach and dosage simulations. Br J Clin Pharmacol 2010;71:61-71.

234. Zazo H, Martin-Suarez A, Lanao JM. Evaluating amikacin dosage regimens in intensive care unit patients: a pharmacokinetic/pharmacodynamic analysis using Monte Carlo simulation. Int J Antimicrob Agents 2013;42:155-60.

235. Matsuo H, Hayashi J, Ono K, et al. Administration of aminoglycosides to hemodialysis patients immediately before dialysis: a new dosing modality. Antimicrob Agents Chemother 1997;41:2597-601.

236. Teigen MM, Duffull S, Dang L, et al. Dosing of gentamicin in patients with end-stage renal disease receiving hemodialysis. J Clin Pharmacol 2006;46:1259-67.

237. Sowinski KM, Magner SJ, Lucksiri A, et al. Influence of hemodialysis on gentamicin pharmacokinetics, removal during hemodialysis, and recommended dosing. Clin J Am Soc Nephrol 2008;3:355-61.

238. O'Shea S, Duffull S, Johnson DW. Aminoglycosides in hemodialysis patients: is the current practice of post dialysis dosing appropriate? Semin Dial 2009;22:225-30.

239. Veinstein A, Venisse N, Badin J, et al. Gentamicin in hemodialyzed critical care patients: early dialysis after administration of a high dose should be considered. Antimicrob Agents Chemother 2013;57:977-82.

240. Fish DN. Fluoroquinolone adverse effects and drug interactions. Pharmacotherapy 2001;21(suppl):253S-72S.

241. Rosemurgy AS, Markowsky S, Goode SE, et al. Bioavailability of fluconazole in surgical intensive care unit patients: a study comparing routes of administration. J Trauma 1995;39:445-7.

242. Buijk SLCE, Gyssens IC, Mouton JW, et al. Pharmacokinetics of sequential intravenous and enteral fluconazole in critically ill surgical patients with invasive mycoses and compromised gastrointestinal function. Intensive Care Med 2001;27:115-21.

243. Zhou W, Nightingale CH, Davis GA, et al. Absolute bioavailability of fluconazole suspension in intensive care unit patients. J Infect Dis Pharmacother 2001;5:27-35.

244. Mohammedi I, Piens MA, Padoin C, et al. Plasma levels of voriconazole administered via a nasogastric tube to critically ill patients. Eur J Clin Microbiol Infect Dis 2005;24:358-60.

245. Myrianthefs P, Markantonis SL, Evaggelopoulou P, et al. Monitoring plasma voriconazole levels following intravenous administration in critically ill patients: an observational study. Int J Antimicrob Agents 2010;35:468-72.

246. Hagihara M, Kasai H, Umemura T, et al. Pharmacokinetic-pharmacodynamic study of itraconazole in patients with fungal infections in intensive care units. J Infect Chemother 2011;17:224-30.

247. Andes D, Pascua A, Marchetti O. Antifungal therapeutic drug monitoring: established and emerging indications. Antimicrob Agents Chemother 2009;53:24-34.

248. Goodwin ML, Drew RH. Antifungal serum concentration monitoring: an update. J Antimicrob Chemother 2008;61:17-25.

249. Roberts JA, Kirkpatrick CMJ, Lipman J. Monte Carlo simulations: maximizing antibiotic pharmacokinetic data to optimize clinical practice for critically ill patients. J Antimicrob Chemother 2011;66:227-31.

250. Theuretzbacher U. Tissue penetration of antibacterial agents: how should this be incorporated into pharmacodynamic analyses? Curr Opin Pharmacol 2007;7:498-504.

251. Fish DN, Kiser TH. Correlation of pharmacokinetic/pharmacodynamic-derived predictions of antibiotic efficacy with clinical outcomes in severely ill patients with *Pseudomonas aeruginosa* pneumonia. Pharmacotherapy 2013;33:1022-34.

Chapter 13

Laboratory Testing Considerations

Kali Martin, Pharm.D.; Shanna Cole, Pharm.D.; and Michael Klepser, Pharm.D.

LEARNING OBJECTIVES

1. Compare and contrast various platforms used to provide data regarding the identity and susceptibility of infecting pathogens.
2. Evaluate the benefits and limitations of rapid diagnostic tests used for infectious diseases.
3. Outline how rapids diagnostic tests should be used to optimize patient outcomes and return on investment.

ABBREVIATIONS IN THIS CHAPTER

MALDI-TOF MS	Matrix-assisted laser desorption ionization time-of-flight mass spectrometry	PNA FISH	Peptide nucleic acid fluorescence in situ hybridization
PCR	Polymerase chain reaction		

INTRODUCTION

An ever-important area of infectious diseases in the critical care setting remains identifying infecting microorganisms and determining antimicrobial susceptibility profiles in order to swiftly initiate appropriate antimicrobial therapy. However, the timely selection of an appropriate antibiotic continues to be a challenge for clinicians, especially for patients in the intensive care setting, where a delay of minutes can profoundly affect outcomes. Various studies have shown the significance of promptly administering appropriate antibiotics on survival in patients with high acuity.[1-3] Methods for culture and susceptibility testing remain suboptimal with respect to the timeliness of data availability. This delay leaves the clinician without critical information and places the patient at risk of suboptimal antimicrobial therapy. Conversely, de-escalation of antibiotics may be needlessly postponed without timely knowledge of the pathogen's identity and susceptibility, leading to overuse of broad-spectrum agents. Fortunately, advances in technology have presented substantial advances in rapid microbiological diagnostic testing. Various tests have been approved that can now provide vital data within hours rather than days and hold the promise of the decreasing mortality, length of hospital stay, and hospital costs that are associated with managing infectious processes.[4]

DIAGNOSTIC TESTS AVAILABLE FOR USE IN INFECTIOUS DISEASES

Cultures/Gram Stain

Culture and in vitro susceptibility testing remain the gold standard for identifying the causative pathogen and characterizing antimicrobial activity. Theoretically, these techniques allow for the detection of as few as 1 CFU of bacteria or fungi per unit of blood. Although culture-based methods for biochemical species identification and susceptibility determination have been used for decades, these techniques are far from ideal. Growing cultures is time- and resource-consuming. It can take more than 18 hours to get adequate bacterial growth from a specimen to use in subsequent biochemical tests. The time to detection of a microbe is considerably longer for some slow-growing bacteria and fungi.[5] Furthermore, the time required to detect the presence of a pathogen in a specimen can be prolonged when the amount of microbe in the collected specimen is low or if the patient has previously been exposed to antimicrobials. Another limitation of culture-based detection methods is that they can only detect viable organisms. Unfortunately, culture-based methods cannot identify cellular components such as antigens or genetic fragments that are released after cell lysis. In addition, even though blood is the most common specimen used for culture, circulation of viable organisms in the blood often does not consistently occur, which limits the sensitivity of these tests. In total, all of these limitations can result in delays in detecting and identifying a pathogen and adversely affect decisions regarding antimicrobial use.[5]

Despite their drawbacks, culture and susceptibility testing continue to serve as first line for identifying and characterizing infectious etiologies owing to the familiarity with the techniques and the relatively low cost associated with these tests.[6-9] As such, culture-based methods continue to be the standard against which new rapid detection tests are compared. A primary value of cultures is that they provide the microbial growth that is used in determining in vitro susceptibilities and nucleic acid testing. Although in vitro susceptibility testing has its own problems, these data continue to be used to direct patient care, construct antibiograms, and guide antibiotic selection and dosing decisions on the basis of optimizing pharmacodynamic parameters.

Nucleic Acid Testing

Decreasing the time in identifying an organism significantly decreases mortality and improves patient outcomes. As mentioned, culture and susceptibility, although widely used, are less than optimal, especially in critically ill patients because of the delayed time to obtaining results. For the past several years, the availability of rapid tests for organism detection has increased.[9] Examples of tests include those that are based on pathogen lysis, nucleic acid extraction and purification, nucleic acid amplification, and identification. Various methods to accomplish these tasks have been evaluated, including pathogen-specific assays for targeting species-specific genes, broad-range assays that target genomic sequences, and multiplex polymerase chain reaction (PCR) that focuses on species-specific targets of different organisms. Some of these tests are even intended to detect genes associated with antimicrobial resistance such as *mecA* in staphylococci or *vanA* and *vanB* in enterococci. Currently, many of these tests are used only as a complement to cultures, especially in serious clinical situations. The drawback of this approach is that the tests fail to overcome the technical and sensitivity issues of cultures.[10] Some nucleic acid tests, however, are considered first line for the diagnosis of pathogens such as hepatitis C virus, enteroviruses, *Bordetella pertussis*, herpes simplex virus (in the setting of herpes encephalitis), and *Chlamydia trachomatis*.

Historically, use of nucleic acid testing has been limited owing to cost, technical complexity, limited applicability, and the need to determine antimicrobial susceptibility after pathogen identification.[11] However, as test robustness continues to improve and isothermal methods are developed, these technologies may eventually supplant culture as the gold standard for pathogen identification.[12]

The primary limitations associated with the current generation of nucleic acid tests predominantly include the inability to assess antimicrobial susceptibility, complexity, and ability to differentiate between viable and non-viable organisms. Although tests capable of detecting broad arrays of pathogens may be of clinical value, their use may be limited because of the higher risk of contamination owing to the many steps involved in processing specimens. Furthermore, although many of these tests have quick turnaround times, actual timing may be longer because of issues such as transportation of specimens and availability of staff.[4]

One improvement already developed and implemented in nucleic acid testing is the use of nanoparticle probe technology. This technology improves specificity for both nucleic acid and protein detection. Nanosphere has developed the Verigene system. This system is a novel, multiplex platform that allows for the screening of a sample directly from positive culture medium. Following automated nucleic acid extraction and PCR amplification, the test uses nanoparticle probe technology resulting in target hybridization. The total run time post-inoculation is about 2.5 hours.[13-15] The gram-positive blood culture (BC-GP) nucleic acid test targets 12 genus- or species-specific targets and *mecA* and *vanA/B* genes (Table 13.1). The sensitivity and specificity for the various targets are

Table 13.1 Targets Identified by the Verigene Gram-Positive Blood Culture Test (BC-GP)

Species	
	Staphylococcus aureus
	Staphylococcus epidermidis
	Staphylococcus lugdunensis
	Streptococcus anginosus group
	Streptococcus agalactiae
	Streptococcus pneumoniae
	Streptococcus pyogenes
	Enterococcus faecalis
	Enterococcus faecium
Genus	
	Staphylococcus spp.
	Streptococcus spp.
	Listeria spp.
Resistance	
	mecA (methicillin)
	vanA (vancomycin)
	vanB (vancomycin)

92.6%–100% and 95.4%–100%, respectively.[16] The gram-negative blood culture (BC-GN) test is approved for eight genus- or species-specific targets and six resistance genes, including the extended-spectrum β-lactamase CTX-M and the carbapenemases IMP, KPC, NDM, OXA, and VIM (www.nanosphere.us/products/gram-negative-blood-culture-test). The percent agreement with this assay and routine methods for identifying and detecting resistance markers was 97.4% and 92.3%, respectively.[13] Although the tests perform well in monomicrobial cultures, test performance declines in the presence of polymicrobial cultures. Another limitation of the assay is its inability to associate a resistance determinate with a particular organism in a polymicrobial culture.

Several studies have assessed the impact of receipt of data from the Verigene test system compared with routine methods. On average, identification results are available 30–40 hours earlier with the Verigene system and susceptibility information 40–50 hours earlier.[15] When acted on in a timely manner, these data can significantly and positively affect treatment decisions. In one study, when results from the Verigene system were acted on by a critical care/infectious diseases pharmacist, the time to receipt of appropriate antibiotic therapy was decreased by 23.4 hours, length of hospitalization was 21.7 days shorter, and hospital costs were $60,729 lower.[17]

Polymerase Chain Reaction

Polymerase chain reaction allows for the amplification of a single copy of DNA or DNA fragment. The process involves repeated cycles of heating and cooling in the presence of primers and DNA polymerase, resulting in the amplification of the targeted sequence. Traditionally, results are determined when the presence or absence of the genetic fragment is noted on gel electrophoresis. Polymerase chain reaction can be a highly sensitive method for microbial detection; however, sensitivity is affected by primer and amplicon selection and contamination.[10] Some examples of U.S. Food and Drug Administration (FDA)-cleared PCR-based test systems include the Roche Molecular Systems LightCycler SeptiFast MecA, the BD GeneOhm Cdiff assay, the Cepheid Xpert C. difficile assay, and the Gen-Probe Prodesse ProGastro Cd.

Real-time PCR allows for monitoring of DNA amplification while the assay is in progress rather than at the end of the run. Real-time PCR assays can be used for analysis of genetic polymorphisms, gene expression, and species identification. The GeneXpert system uses real-time PCR with preparation and detection in a closed compartment to detect methicillin resistance or susceptibility. Depending on the cartridges selected, this system can be used to detect an array of pathogens/resistance determinants, including methicillin-resistant *Staphylococcus aureus* (MRSA), *Clostridium difficile*, *vanA* in enterococci, influenza virus, Norovirus, and resistance in *Mycobacterium tuberculosis*. For staphylococci, the system can detect *mecA* and *SCCmec* genes with a sensitivity of 100% and specificity of 98.6% for methicillin-susceptible *S. aureus* and a 98.3% sensitivity and 99.4% specificity for MRSA.[4,18] Results are available within 1 hour.

Broad-range or multiplex PCR provides the ability to rapidly and efficiently amplify different DNA sequences simultaneously using several sets of primers and DNA polymerases. Tests initially use PCR amplification, followed by downstream approaches for identification such as hybridization and sequencing. Examples of multiplex PCR tests currently available include the BD GeneOhm StaphSR assay, the Cepheid Xpert MRSA/SA BC and *C. difficile*/Epi assays, the Mobidiag Prove-it Sepsis, and the BioFire Diagnostics FilmArray blood culture identification (BCID). The value of these platforms is the rapid, simultaneous screenings of clinical samples for several pathogens. For example, the Prove-it Sepsis can screen for more than 60 bacteria and 13 fungi that produce more than 90% of sepsis-causing pathogens. In addition, resistance markers for genes such as *mecA* and *vanA* and *vanB* can be identified. Results are available in as few as 3 hours with a sensitivity of 95% and specificity of 99%.[19]

Real-time PCR tests are available to detect the genes encoding for *C. difficile* toxin B (*tcdB*) or the toxin regulatory gene (*tcdC*). Although these tests have sensitivities of 90% and specificities of 96%, their clinical value has been questioned. The positive predictive value (PPV) of these tests varies with the prevalence of disease.[20] When the prevalence of disease is low (less than 10%), the PPV for an accurate diagnosis is low. Conversely, when the prevalence of disease is high (greater than 20%), the PPV is higher, and the value of the test for making a diagnosis increases. The negative predictive value of the tests does not change with disease prevalence. Therefore, these tests may be of limited diagnostic value under endemic rates of disease but may be useful in ruling out infection. That the PCR tests detect genes rather than the gene product is another drawback. As a result, individuals colonized with non–toxin-producing strains of *C. difficile* may be inappropriately identified as being infected. Because it is possible to obtain false-positive results with PCR, clinicians must either use PCR in combination with initial screening using enzyme immunoassays for *C. difficile* glutamate dehydrogenase or toxins A and B or use PCR in select patients with a high probability of having *C. difficile* infection. Failure to use the tests judiciously can result in overtreatment of patients and excess cost and can foster antimicrobial resistance in collateral bacterial flora.

Real-time PCR systems greatly reduce the time that meaningful information regarding the causative pathogen and/or expression of resistance is available to clinicians. When appropriately disseminated and interpreted, these data and the ability to rapidly access them can affect antimicrobial use and patient outcome. A study by Carver and colleagues showed that when specimens from patients thought to have *S. aureus* infections underwent rapid screening with PCR for the *mecA* gene and data were acted on by an infectious diseases clinical pharmacist, the time to initiating appropriate antibiotic therapy was reduced by 25.4 hours.[21] Shortening the time to administering appropriate antibiotics may be associated with decreased mortality among patients with sepsis. Additional studies have shown that use of these tests is associated with decreased costs and length of stay owing to a reduction in the use of inappropriate antibiotics and decreased time to appropriate therapy.[22-24] However, if use of these tests is not coupled with an effective implementation strategy, their value for affecting antibiotic use may be limited.[25]

Peptide Nucleic Acid with Fluorescence In Situ Hybridization

Peptide nucleic acid fluorescence in situ hybridization (PNA FISH), a platform developed by AdvanDx (Woburn, MA), uses fluorescently labeled probes with neutral charges that penetrate the cell membrane and cell wall of intact organisms. Peptide nucleic acid probes are DNA mimics that rapidly hybridize to species-specific ribosomal RNA (rRNA) sequences. Bacteria and fungi produce an abundance of highly conserved, species-specific rRNA sequences; therefore, these represent good targets for molecular probes. In addition, because rRNA is naturally amplified in viable cells, targeting rRNA may be accomplished without additional amplification procedures, thus allowing for organism identification without cell rupture and with minimal risk of sample contamination.

A probe is a synthetic oligomer mimicking a DNA or an RNA sequence, and the target is the nucleic acid being detected. Probe detection is accomplished using a fluorescent microscope after hybridization. Results for first-generation tests took about 3 hours to obtain after a positive Gram stain. Newer QuickFISH tests have reduced this time to less than 30 minutes with high sensitivity and specificity. The PNA FISH and QuickFISH systems are available for detecting and differentiating *S. aureus* and coagulase-negative staphylococci, *Enterococcus faecalis* and *Enterococcus faecium*, gram-negative pathogens (i.e., *Escherichia coli*, *Klebsiella pneumoniae*, and *Pseudomonas aeruginosa*), and *Candida* spp. (i.e., *Candida albicans*, *Candida glabrata*, and *Candida parapsilosis*). In addition, newer XpressFISH assays can identify phenotypic resistance markers such as *mecA*. The diagnostic accuracy of this platform has been excellent. Rates of agreement between PNA FISH and other diagnostic methods have generally exceeded 95%.[26,27]

Several studies have determined that PNA FISH testing can help lead to decreased hospital costs, length of stay, and mortality for infections caused by a variety of pathogens, including various gram-positive, gram-negative, and *Candida* pathogens.[11,28-31] In one study, use of PNA FISH aided in detecting coagulase-negative *Staphylococcus* spp., resulting in decreased hospital length of stay from 6 to 4 days ($p<0.05$) and decreased hospital costs of about $4,000 per patient.[29] Similarly, in a study of 224 patients with hospital-acquired enterococcal bacteremia, the impact of PNA FISH with subsequent action by an antimicrobial team was examined. *E. faecalis* was identified 3 days earlier than with conventional culture, and *E. faecium* was identified 2.3 days earlier. This information resulted in decreased time to initiating appropriate antibiotics (1.3 vs. 3.1 days; $p<0.001$) and reduction in 30-day mortality (26% vs. 46%; $p=0.04$).[32] Similar benefits have been reported for PNA FISH for *Candida* and gram-negative pathogens.[26,30,31,33] Of note, reductions in cost and mortality are only observed when programs are implemented that allow for rapid alteration of antimicrobial therapy based on test results. A delay in response to the resultant information can negate any benefits gained from rapidly acquiring pathogen-identifying data.

Matrix-Assisted Laser Desorption Ionization Time-of-Flight

Matrix-assisted laser desorption ionization time-of-flight mass spectrometry (MALDI-TOF MS) can be used for determining the presence of various pathogens and resistance markers from a variety of sources (e.g., blood, urine, wound). To run, a sample colony is transferred from media to the target slide and covered with a chemical matrix. The target slide is placed in the analyzer and pulsed with a laser, resulting in ionic gas molecules that are accelerated through an electric field and into the time-of-flight analyzer. The rate at which particles travel through the tube and reach the particle detector depends on size. Measurements of particle flight times are converted into mass/velocity values, plotted on a mass spectrogram, and compared with a validated microbe library of results. Matrix-assisted laser desorption ionization time-of-flight mass spectrometry is an extremely versatile system that can be used to aid in detecting a variety of bacterial and fungal species. Run time is quick, with results available within in 1–2 hours. Sensitivities and specificities of up to 98% and greater than 96%, respectively, have been reported with MALDI-TOF MS. The two currently available MALDI-TOF MS systems are the MALDI Biotyper and the Vitek MS system.[4,6,18]

Historically, MALDI-TOF MS was performed on single-colony growth from a subculture of culture bottles. This process meant that results would be delayed until the subculture yielded growth. In an effort to decrease the time to obtain results from MALDI-TOF MS, protocols were developed that screened samples directly from positive culture vials. Although these protocols provided results much faster, several potential pitfalls were associated with this approach. It was noted that material in the blood culture vial such as human proteins, charcoal used to bind antibiotics, and components of the culture broth could produce a background signal that could affect the detection of pathogens.[34-36] Furthermore, the type of culture system used (i.e., BACTEC, VersaTREK, or BacT/ALERT) could affect identification rates.[34-36] Although problematic, background interference can be minimized by incorporating system-specific processing steps and performing internal validation to develop appropriate interpretative cutoff values.[37] Another complication that has been encountered with MALDI-TOF when direct identification from culture vials is used is difficulty identifying pathogens from polymicrobial samples. In this scenario, the proteins from the different pathogens affect the analyzer at overlapping time, thus making differentiation of species-specific peaks difficult.

The cost of acquiring a MALDI-TOF system ranges from about $160,000 to $250,000 and carries a significant annual maintenance cost.[38] However, per-test reagent costs can be 200 times less than conventional identification methods. From a clinical standpoint, use of MALDI-TOF can significantly affect the initiation of appropriate antimicrobials.[39] In one study where MALDI-TOF was used sequentially after Gram staining for gram-negative bacteremia, data from MALDI-TOF affected the empiric antimicrobial regimen selected in 35.1% of cases.[40] Shortening the time to starting appropriate antibiotic therapy has been associated with decreased lengths of stay and decreased hospital costs.[41-43] As with other tests that provide rapid identification of pathogens, benefit is only realized when results are acted on in a timely manner.

ANTIMICROBIAL STEWARDSHIP PROGRAM IMPLICATIONS

Rapid nucleic acid testing allows antimicrobial stewardship programs to improve patient outcomes and decrease antibiotic use. It is imperative that stewardship teams be thoroughly involved in using these tests and act as educators of the results of each test. The rapid results of the tests are of little value if not acted on in a timely manner. Stewardship teams can help outline which tests should be conducted depending on the prevalence of specific organisms in the hospital, sensitivity and specificity of each test, and price of the test supplies. It is beneficial if hospitals start with a short implementation period to compare factors such as costs of therapy, time to efficient therapy, readmission rate, and mortality. By determining the economic and clinical outcomes of each test, clinicians can appropriately reveal the benefit to patient care.

Regardless of the method used, it is important that the FDA guidelines be followed (GLP [Good Laboratory Practices]) in all steps of infectious disease testing. Standardization of the tests allows for quality assurance in order to increase accuracy.[39] Although many of the newer diagnostic tests are initially more expensive than the traditional cultures, they ultimately may save money and decrease the time to de-escalation from broad-spectrum antibiotics. Each institution should decide whether a particular test would be beneficial in its setting.

REFERENCES

1. Kumar A, Roberts D, Wood KE, et al. Duration of hypotension before initiation of effective antimicrobial therapy is the critical determinant of survival in human septic shock. Crit Care Med 2006;34:1589-96.
2. Kumar A, Ellis P, Arabi Y, et al.; Cooperative Antimicrobial Therapy of Septic Shock Database Research Group. Initiation of inappropriate antimicrobial therapy results in a fivefold reduction of survival in human septic shock. Chest 2009;136:1237-48.
3. Vallés J, Rello J, Ochagavía A, et al. Community-acquired bloodstream infection in critically ill adult patients: impact of shock and inappropriate antibiotic therapy on survival. Chest 2003;123:1615-24.
4. Afshari A, Schrenzel J, Ieven M, et al. Bench-to-bedside review: rapid molecular diagnostics for bloodstream infection—a new frontier? Crit Care 2012;16:222.
5. Fernandez J, Erstad BL, Petty W, et al. Time to positive culture and identification for *Candida* blood stream infections. Diagn Microbiol Infect Dis 2009;64:402-7.
6. Burillo A, Bouza E. Use of rapid diagnostic techniques in ICU patients with infections. BMC Infect Dis 2014;14:593.
7. Peralta G, Rodríguez-Lera MJ, Garrido JC, et al. Time to positivity in blood cultures of adults with *Streptococcus pneumoniae* bacteremia. BMC Infect Dis 2006;6:79.
8. Shah SS, Downes KJ, Elliott MR, et al. How long does it take to "rule out" bacteremia in children with central venous catheters? Pediatrics 2008;121:135-41.
9. Wolk DM, Dunne MD. New technologies in clinical microbiology. J Clin Microbiol 2011;49:S62-S67.
10. Okeke IN, Peeling RW, Goossens H, et al. Diagnostics as essential tools for containing antibacterial resistance. Drug Resist Updat 2011;14:95-106.
11. Olano JP, Walker DH. Diagnosing emerging and reemerging infectious diseases: the pivotal role of the pathologist. Arch Pathol Lab Med 2011;135:83-91.
12. Leggieri N, Rida A, François P, et al. Molecular diagnosis of bloodstream infections: planning to (physically) reach the bedside. Curr Opin Infect Dis 2010;23:311-9.
13. Dodemont M, De Mendonca R, Nonhoff C, et al. Performance of the Verigene gram-negative blood culture assay for rapid detection of bacteria and resistance determinants. J Clin Microbiol 2014;52:3085-7.
14. Beal SG, Ciurca J, Smith G, et al. Evaluation of the Nanosphere Verigene gram-positive blood culture assay with the VersaTREK blood culture system and assessment of possible impact on selected patients. J Clin Microbiol 2013;51:3988-92.
15. Wojewoda CM, Sercia L, Navas M, et al. Evaluation of the Verigene gram-positive blood culture nucleic acid test for rapid detection of bacteria and resistance determinants. J Clin Microbiol 2013;51:2072-6.

16. Buchan BW, Ginocchio CC, Manii R, et al. Multiplex identification of gram-positive bacteria and resistance determinants directly from positive blood culture broths: evaluation of an automated microarray-based nucleic acid test. PLoS Med 2013;10:e1001478.

17. Sango A, McCarter YS, Johnson D, et al. Stewardship approach for optimizing antimicrobial therapy through use of a rapid microarray assay on blood cultures positive for *Enterococcus* species. J Clin Microbiol 2013;51:4008-11.

18. Bauer KA, Perez KK, Forrest GN, et al. Review of rapid diagnostic tests used by antimicrobial stewardship programs. Clin Infect Dis 2014;59(suppl 3):S134-45.

19. Tissari P, Zumla A, Tarkka E, et al. Accurate and rapid identification of bacterial species from positive blood cultures with a DNA-based microarray platform: an observational study. Lancet 2010;375:224-30.

20. Deshpande A, Pasupleti V, Rolston DD, et al. Diagnostic accuracy of real-time polymerase chain reaction in detection of *Clostridium difficile* in the stool samples of patients with suspected *Clostridium difficile* infection: a meta-analysis. Clin Infect Dis 2011;53:e81-90.

21. Carver PL, Lin SW, DePestel DD, et al. Impact of *mecA* gene testing and intervention by infectious disease clinical pharmacists on time to optimal antimicrobial therapy for *Staphylococcus aureus* bacteremia at a university hospital. J Clin Microbiol 2008;46:2381-3.

22. Parta M, Goebel M, Thomas J, et al. Impact of an assay that enables rapid determination of *Staphylococcus* species and their drug susceptibility on the treatment of patients with positive blood culture results. Infect Control Hosp Epidemiol 2010;31:1043-8.

23. Bauer KA, West JE, Balada-Llasat JM, et al. An antimicrobial stewardship program's impact with rapid polymerase chain reaction methicillin-resistant *Staphylococcus aureus/S. aureus* blood culture test in patients with *S. aureus* bacteremia. Clin Infect Dis 2010;51:1074-80.

24. Wong JR, Bauer KA, Mangino JE, et al. Antimicrobial stewardship pharmacist interventions for coagulase-negative staphylococci positive blood cultures using rapid polymerase chain reaction. Ann Pharmacother 2012;46:1484-90.

25. Terp S, Krishnadasan A, Bowen W, et al. Introduction of rapid methicillin-resistant *Staphylococcus aureus* polymerase chain reaction testing and antibiotic selection among hospitalized patients with purulent skin infections. Clin Infect Dis 2014;58:e129-32.

26. Harris DM, Hata DJ. Rapid identification of bacteria and *Candida* using PNA-FISH from blood and peritoneal fluid cultures: a retrospective clinical study. Ann Clin Microbiol Antimicrob 2013;12:2.

27. Forrest GN, Mehta S, Weekes E, et al. Impact of rapid in situ hybridization testing on coagulase-negative staphylococci positive blood cultures. J Antimicrob Chemother 2006;58:154-8.

28. Ly T, Gulia J, Pyrgos V, et al. Impact upon clinical outcomes of translation of PNA FISH-generated laboratory data from the clinical microbiology bench to bedside in real time. Ther Clin Risk Manag 2008;4:637-40.

29. Forrest GN, Mehta S, Weekes E, et al. Impact of rapid in situ hybridization testing on coagulase-negative staphylococci positive blood cultures. J Antimicrob Chemother 2006;58:154-8.

30. Forrest GN, Mankes K, Jabra-Rizk MA, et al. Peptide nucleic acid fluorescence in situ hybridization-based identification of *Candida albicans* and its impact on mortality and antifungal therapy costs. J Clin Microbiol 2006;44:3381-3.

31. Parcell BJ, Orange GV. PNA-FISH assays for early targeted bacteraemia treatment. J Microbiol Methods 2013;95:253-5.

32. Forrest GN, Roghmann MC, Toombs LS, et al. Peptide nucleic acid fluorescent in situ hybridization for hospital-acquired enterococcal bacteremia: delivering earlier effective antimicrobial therapy. Antimicrob Agents Chemother 2008;52:3558-63.

33. Heil EL, Daniels LM, Long DM, et al. Impact of a rapid peptide nucleic acid fluorescence in situ hybridization assay on treatment of *Candida* infections. Am J Health Syst Pharm 2012;69:1910-4.

34. Romero-Gomez MP, Mingorance J. The effect of the blood culture bottle type in the rate of direct identification from positive cultures by matrix-assisted laser desorption/ionisation time-of-flight (MALDI-TOF) mass spectrometry. J Infect 2011;62:251-3.

35. Szabados F, Michels M, Kaase M, et al. The sensitivity of direct identification from positive BacT/ALERT (bioMérieux) blood culture bottles by matrix-assisted laser desorption ionization time-of-flight mass spectrometry is low. Clin Microbiol Infect 2011;17:192-5.

36. Schmidt V, Jarosch A, Marz P, et al. Rapid identification of bacteria in positive blood culture by matrix-assisted laser desorption ionization time-of-flight mass spectrometry. Eur J Clin Microbiol Infect Dis 2012;31:311-7.

37. Wuppenhorst N, Consoir C, Lorch D, et al. Direct identification of bacteria from charcoal-containing blood culture bottles using matrix-assisted laser desorption/ionisation time-of-flight mass spectrometry. Eur J Clin Microbiol Infect Dis 2012;31:2843-50.

38. Caliendo AM, Gilbert DN, Ginocchio CC, et al.; Infectious Diseases Society of America (IDSA). Better tests, better care: improved diagnostics for infectious diseases. Clin Infect Dis 2013;57(suppl 3):S139-S170.

39. Leli C, Cenci E, Cardaccia A, et al. Rapid identification of bacterial and fungal pathogens from positive blood cultures by MALDI-TOF MS. Int J Med Microbiol 2013;303:205-9.

40. Clerc O, Prod'hom G, Vogne C, et al. Impact of matrix-assisted laser desorption ionization time-of-flight mass spectrometry on the clinical management of patients with gram-negative bacteremia: a prospective observational study. Clin Infect Dis 2013;56:1101-7.

41. Perez KK, Olsen RJ, Musick WL, et al. Integrating rapid pathogen identification and antimicrobial stewardship significantly decreases hospital costs. Arch Pathol Lab Med 2013;137:1247-54.

42. Huang AM, Newton D, Kunapuli A, et al. Impact of rapid organism identification via matrix-assisted laser desorption/ionization time-of-flight combined with antimicrobial stewardship team intervention in adult patients with bacteremia and candidemia. Clin Infect Dis 2013;57:1237-45.

43. Tamma PD, Tan K, Nussenblatt VR, et al. Can matrix-assisted laser desorption ionization time-of-flight mass spectrometry (MALDI-TOF) enhance antimicrobial stewardship efforts in the acute care setting? Infect Control Hosp Epidemiol 2013;34:990-5.

Chapter 14: Antimicrobial Resistance in the Critical Care Environment

Andrew M. Roecker, Pharm.D.; and Steven J. Martin, Pharm.D.

LEARNING OBJECTIVES

1. Summarize the epidemiologic concerns associated with antimicrobial resistance, and describe the morbidity and mortality that results from organism resistance.
2. Differentiate the various mechanisms of resistance that occur in gram-positive and gram-negative bacteria.
3. Distinguish the relevant clinical manifestations of individual resistance phenotypes.
4. Explain urgent resistance concerns that are specific to the critical care setting.
5. Design individual patient- and population-based strategies to prevent or minimize resistance.

ABBREVIATIONS IN THIS CHAPTER

CDC	Centers for Disease Control and Prevention	ICU	Intensive care unit
CRE	Carbapenem-resistant Enterobacteriaceae	MDR	Multidrug resistant/resistance
ESBL	Extended-spectrum β-lactamase	MRSA	Methicillin-resistant *Staphylococcus aureus*
HAI	Health care–associated infection	PBP	Penicillin-binding protein
HAP	Hospital-acquired pneumonia	VAP	Ventilator-associated pneumonia
		VRE	Vancomycin-resistant *Enterococcus*

INTRODUCTION

Antimicrobial resistance has escalated in recent years. In intensive care units (ICUs) today, patients become infected with organisms for which no antibiotic treatment is effective. This post-antibiotic era in critical illness threatens to reverse significant improvements in survival and outcomes made possible through advanced technology, improved information systems, and novel treatment strategies. Antimicrobial resistance in critically ill patients increases morbidity, mortality, length of hospital stay, and health care costs. Unquestionably, the proliferation and overuse of antimicrobials is the driving factor behind resistance and the resulting adverse outcomes. This chapter will review current issues in antimicrobial resistance associated with critical illness and outline several strategies to reduce the expansion of resistance in individuals and populations.

The prevalence of antimicrobial resistance is increasing throughout the world, especially multidrug-resistant (MDR) bacteria, and this has become a significant threat today to patients in ICUs.[1] Multidrug-resistance is defined as when at least three different classes of antimicrobials no longer can eradicate the organism. Patients may acquire these bacteria during their stay in the ICU, but many patients have preexisting infection or colonization with resistant or MDR organisms before their entrance in the ICU.[2,3] Antimicrobial resistance is a barrier to the selection of appropriate antimicrobial therapy for serious infection, such as sepsis, pneumonia, or bloodstream infection.[4,5] Antimicrobial resistance and the resulting inappropriate initial antimicrobial treatment are important risk factors for mortality, increased duration of mechanical ventilation and ICU stay, higher rates of recurrence of infection, and higher costs.[6-9]

The annual yearly cost to the U.S. health system alone from antimicrobial resistance has been estimated at $21–$34 billion dollars and may account for more than 8 million additional hospital days.[10] In the United States, more than 23 million people each year develop infection with organisms that demonstrate antimicrobial resistance, accounting for 23,000 deaths annually.[11] The cost of care for patients with antimicrobial-resistant organisms is higher than for those with antimicrobial-susceptible organisms by $6,000–$30,000.[12]

The increased length of hospital stay and increased mortality, together with the excess costs associated with infection by resistant organisms, may be because of a variety of factors that include the patient, organisms, and treatment. The severity of the underlying disease in the patient may be synergistic with infection by resistant organisms, leading to poor outcomes.[12] For patients infected with resistant organisms, inappropriate treatment, ineffective dosage selection, delayed appropriate therapy, and treatment toxicity may lead to poor outcomes or higher costs.[12] Box 14.1 highlights important global concerns regarding antimicrobial resistance.

Inappropriate therapy because of antimicrobial resistance causes higher mortality rates in patients with ventilator-associated pneumonia (VAP).[5] The same poor outcomes have also been observed in patients with bacteremia from methicillin-resistant *Staphylococcus aureus* (MRSA) and vancomycin-resistant *Enterococcus* (VRE) bacteremia.[14,15] Increased mortality has been associated with infections from extended-spectrum β lactamase (ESBL)–producing *Klebsiella pneumoniae*.[16] In a recent study of 2,594 patients with sepsis or septic shock who had positive blood cultures, 788 did not survive, and resistance to cefepime or meropenem, the presence of MDR bacteria, non-abdominal surgery, and prior antibiotic use were identified through logistic regression as being independently associated with the administration of inappropriate antimicrobial treatment leading to death.[17] Box 14.2 lists antimicrobial resistance threats that may affect patients in the ICU.

Antibiotic exposure to bacteria in sublethal concentrations can promote subsequent resistance. Free radical production in the bacteria stimulated by the presence of antibiotic produces DNA mutations that can lead to protection from the antibiotic to which it was exposed, and often to other antibiotic classes.[18] Genetic mutations producing antimicrobial resistance are often stable and retained in bacteria even in the absence of ongoing exposure to the antibiotic.[19]

Bacteria are adaptable to their environment and quickly become tolerant of toxins in order to survive and reproduce. Low levels of genetic resistance may be common in most bacteria for protection against exposure of naturally occurring antibiotics produced by other microorganisms in the environment.[20] The exchange of genetic material by bacteria leads to the extension of resistant genes from organism to organism. Antibiotic resistance coded for on bacterial chromosomal DNA may also be exchanged among bacteria through mobile genetic elements such as plasmids. Plasmid-acquired resistance is largely driven by antimicrobial exposure.[18]

> **Box 14.1. Global Antimicrobial Resistance Concerns**[13]
>
> - 20% of people are persistent carriers of *S. aureus*;
> - $3 billion is the annual health care cost associated with MRSA in the United States;
> - 19,000 deaths each year are caused by MRSA in the United States;
> - 61% of *E. faecium* is resistant to vancomycin in the United States;
> - 40% of *S. pneumoniae* strains are resistant to penicillin;
> - 50% chance of contracting *C. difficile* after more than a 4-week hospital stay;
> - 30% increase in carbapenem-resistant *A. baumannii* strains from 1995 to 2004
> - 30% resistance to fluoroquinolones in *Enterobacter* spp.

The proliferation of various resistance genes has been promoted by widespread use of synthetic antimicrobial agents. Further regional or local concentrated drug use, such as through formulary or antimicrobial restriction, further exacerbates resistance through chromosomally mediated mechanisms.[21] The pressure of antimicrobial use can lead to mechanisms of resistance that often convey MDR. Efflux pumps are an example of a resistance mechanism that can often be non-specific conferring resistance to many types of drugs.[13,22] Horizontal gene transfer, which can spread resistance to several antibiotics in a single step, may also give rise to MDR.[22]

Specific patient risk factors for antimicrobial resistance include prior exposure to antibiotics, prior physical exposure to the health care environment (hospitals, nursing homes, etc.), comorbid conditions such as diabetes mellitus, advancing age, renal insufficiency and uremia, use of corticosteroids and other immunosuppressive medications, and radiation therapy.[23,24]

Antimicrobial exposure does not occur only during times of infection or suspected infection. Humans use antibiotics extensively at home and in hospitals, in such products as hand sanitizers and household cleaners. Antibiotics are used extensively in animals and agriculture. In the United States, antibiotics are still being given to animals to promote growth. Antibiotics are also sprayed on trees and other vegetation. Thus, resistance concerns in the ICU have their origin well outside the critical care and hospital setting.

GENERAL ANTIMICROBIAL RESISTANCE MECHANISMS

Antimicrobial resistance occurs by several different and disparate mechanisms. There is intrinsic or innate resistance in which an antimicrobial agent has no inherent activity against a specific pathogen. An example is vancomycin, which has no activity against gram-negative bacteria. Resistance of this type is a class phenomenon, is commonly understood by clinicians, and is not routinely confirmed by clinical laboratory susceptibility testing.[25] Most acquired resistance mechanisms can be categorized in general classes, with notable variety and degrees of mutation.

One general resistance class includes genetic mutations encoding for production or overproduction of medication-lysing enzymes. An example of this is production of β-lactamase that will enzymatically metabolize various β-lactam medications before their ability to bind to penicillin-binding proteins (PBPs) and damage the bacteria.[25] The PBP is important for the production of peptidoglycan, a key component of the cell wall. Normally, β-lactam antibiotics bind to the PBPs, disabling their ability to form a functional cell wall; the modifications prevent this from occurring. The extent of specificity for β-lactams by β-lactamases has waned over time, such that more problematic β-lactamases like ESBLs and metallo-β-lactamases have become more prevalent and render many more antimicrobials ineffective than earlier enzymes, which inhibited only penicillin or first-generation cephalosporins.[26]

Another general resistance class includes genetic mutations that either decrease binding to a specific mechanistic target or altogether change the target-binding site. These result in either suboptimal activity from an antimicrobial that previously inhibited the organism or complete resistance and antimicrobial failure. An example of this would include the *mecA* gene that codes for a change in PBP from PBP2 to PBP2a, resulting in resistance to medications that bind to that target, such as penicillins and cephalosporins.[25] Another example occurs in enterococci causing vancomycin resistance by alterations in the binding target from D-alanine-D-alanine by substituting a D-lactate instead of one of the D-alanines. This alters the binding site and results in drug resistance; it is often coded for by *vanA*, *vanB*, or *vanD* resistance genes.[27] There also may be mutations to intracellular binding sites, including mutations to DNA gyrase, topoisomerase IV, or genes that methylate ribosomal RNA.[28]

A third general resistance class is generation of efflux pumps that expel the antimicrobial agent before it reaches its binding site. This mechanism affects medications acting intracellularly.[25] Macrolides and tetracyclines are examples of agents that are affected by microbial efflux pumps because of their intracellular ribosomal binding targets. *S. aureus* may also produce efflux pumps effective against fluoroquinolones, which helps to explain their lack of activity in treating staphylococcal infections.[29]

The aforementioned three general resistance mechanisms occur as a result of an acquired genetic mutation. In contrast, microorganisms may pass genetic material through conjugation, transduction, or transformation. This often occurs through plasmid transference from one organism to another. If the genetic material on the plasmid contains resistance information, this mechanism explains the spread of antimicrobial class resistance between different genus and species of organism. The plasmid-transported *qnr* gene has been identified as a proliferation mechanism for fluoroquinolone resistance between bacterial pathogens.[25,29]

MAJOR RESISTANCE MECHANISMS IN CRITICAL CARE AREAS

All of the general resistance mechanisms described earlier occur in critical care patients, and the underlying comorbidities and severity of illness in these patients coupled with antimicrobial resistance often results in poor patient outcomes. Recognition of possible resistance is key to minimizing inappropriate antimicrobial therapy and poor treatment outcomes. Institution- and unit-specific antibiograms may identify local resistance patterns and help direct empiric drug selection. These data may also reduce overuse of broad-spectrum antimicrobial agents, reducing drug exposure and focusing activity on likely pathogens. Furthermore, some newer methods of rapidly diagnosing infections, as well as resistance, in critical care patients could greatly assist in timely and accurate use of antimicrobials. Urine antigen testing for *Streptococcus pneumoniae* and *Legionella pneumophila* has held utility for patients with diagnoses of community-acquired pneumonia. However, new technology using PCR (polymerase chain reaction), ELISA (enzyme-linked immunoassay)-based and "in situ" hybridization, and direct E-test may supplant traditional culture and susceptibility results for empiric antimicrobial therapy. Currently, some of these modalities are available to assist with catheter-related bloodstream infections, VAP, urinary tract infections, and skin and skin structure infections. Rapid diagnostic tests are useful as adjuncts to culture and susceptibility testing until specificity and sensitivity of the newer tests are better addressed. Ancillary measures of inflammation including C-reactive protein and procalcitonin can also aid in determining infectious versus non-infectious causes.[30]

CLINICAL RELEVANCE OF RESISTANCE

Reducing antimicrobial resistance requires minimizing the use of antimicrobials. During the past decade, advances in technical aspects of patient care and an emphasis on avoidance of nosocomial infection have led to notable decreases in many health care–associated infections (HAIs). The Centers for Disease Control and Prevention's (CDC's) HAI Progress Report notes reductions in central line–associated bloodstream infections (46% decrease) and surgical site infections (19% decrease) from 2008 to 2013.[31] Also reported were decreases in hospital-onset MRSA bacteremia (8% decrease) and hospital-onset *Clostridium difficile* infections (10% decrease) from 2011 to

2013.[31] Nonetheless, infection is still common in critical illness, and several antibiotic resistance issues are a concern in ICUs. The CDC published *Antibiotic Resistance Threats in the United States*, many of which will have direct application in the critical care environment (Box 14.2).[11]

Urgent Threats with Concern in Critical Care

Carbapenem-Resistant Enterobacteriaceae

Enterobacteriaceae are gram-negative bacilli typically found in the gastrointestinal (GI) tract. The most commonly reported Enterobacteriaceae associated with infection are *Escherichia coli*, *K. pneumoniae*, and *Enterobacter* spp.[32] Enterobacteriaceae cause an estimated 140,000 HAIs each year, with many in critically ill patients.[11] The increasing prevalence of ESBL infections has forced the expanded use of carbapenems, driving carbapenem-resistant Enterobacteriaceae (CRE).[32] The percentage of total Enterobacteriaceae that were carbapenem resistant has increased to 4.2% in 2012 from 1.2% in 2001.[32]

Hydrolyzing carbapenemases are responsible for CRE resistance. *K. pneumoniae* carbapenemase and VIM (Verona integrin-encoded metallo-β-lactamase) are the primary enzymes involved.[33] *K. pneumoniae* carbapenemase produces resistance to all cephalosporins, aztreonam, and currently available β-lactamase inhibitors (avibactam, clavulanate, and tazobactam).[33] *K. pneumoniae* carbapenemase is spread horizontally through plasmids and has also been identified in *E. coli*, *Klebsiella oxytoca*, *Enterobacter*, and *Serratia*.[34]

Infection with CRE has been associated with mortality rates of more than 40%, with most being from carbapenem-resistant *K. pneumoniae* (85.2%).[35]

Carbapenem-resistant Enterobacteriaceae bacteremia is associated with a 50% mortality rate.[11] Polymyxins such as colistin as well as tigecycline and aminoglycosides may retain activity against *K. pneumoniae* carbapenemase–producing organisms. Recent studies suggest that combinations of colistin-polymyxin B or tigecycline with a carbapenem lead to less mortality than monotherapy of colistin-polymyxin B or tigecycline for the treatment of *K. pneumoniae* carbapenemase–producing *K. pneumoniae* bacteremia.[36-39]

Serious Threats with Concern in Critical Care

Acinetobacter spp.

Multidrug-resistant *Acinetobacter* infections are classified as a serious threat by the CDC and are associated with bacteremia, pneumonia, urinary tract infection, and surgical site infections among critically ill populations.[11,40] Multidrug-resistant *Acinetobacter baumannii* may be defined as resistant to three or more classes of antibiotics. *Acinetobacter* is responsible for an estimated 12,000 infections yearly in the United States, with 61% (7,300) of those being classified as MDR.[11] Multidrug-resistant *Acinetobacter* infections result in 500 deaths annually.[11] *Acinetobacter* causes about 2% of all HAIs reported to the CDC but 7% of the infections reported in critically ill patients on mechanical ventilation.[11]

Resistance is usually acquired by *A. baumannii* through plasmids. Multidrug-resistant mechanisms include target site modification, enzymatic drug inactivation, efflux pumps, and porin channel modification. Multidrug-resistant *A. baumannii* can be difficult to treat because it is often resistant to many or, in some cases, all commercially available classes of antibiotics, including carbapenems, thereby leading to the need for more unconventional treatment combinations and more research into therapeutic options for those infections.[41] Colistin or other polymyxins in combination with other agents such as ampicillin/sulbactam, aminoglycosides, carbapenems, and rifampin has been used with mixed success to treat infections from MDR organisms. More recent data may also suggest that use of intravenous minocycline provides utility in treating resistant *A. baumannii* and other MDR organisms.[42]

Candida spp.

About 46,000 health care–associated *Candida* infections occur annually in hospitalized patients in the United States.[11] Fluconazole-resistant *Candida* infections result in 3,400 infections and 220 deaths and are considered a serious threat by the CDC.[11] Drug-resistant *Candida* bloodstream infections lead to about 30% mortality during hospitalization.[11] *Candida albicans* remains the most common fungal pathogen, but resistance is common in other *Candida* spp.[43] *Candida* are increasingly resistant to first- and second-line therapies such as azoles (fluconazole) and echinocandins (caspofungin, micafungin,

---

Box 14.2. Antimicrobial Resistance Threats in the Critical Care Setting[11]

Urgent Threats
- Carbapenem-resistant Enterobacteriaceae (CRE)

Serious Threats
- Multidrug-resistant *Acinetobacter*
- Fluconazole-resistant *Candida*
- Extended-spectrum β lactamase (ESBL)-producing Enterobacteriaceae
- Vancomycin-resistant *Enterococcus* (VRE)
- Multidrug-resistant *P. aeruginosa*
- Methicillin-resistant *S. aureus* (MRSA)
- Drug-resistant *S. pneumoniae*

Threats of Concern
- Vancomycin-resistant *S. aureus* (VRSA)

anidulafungin).[43] Systemic candidiasis may increase hospital length of stay by 3–13 days and add $6,000–$29,000 in direct costs.[11] Critical illness is a risk factor for systemic fungal infection, and drug-resistant candidemia leads to about a 30% mortality rate.[11]

Clinical laboratory susceptibility testing of fungi is still uncommon in the United States. The clinician must recognize potential inherent resistance issues among non-*albicans* Candida, as well as local resistance concerns among *C. albicans*. Although *C. albicans* drug resistance remains low, *C. glabrata* and *C. krusei* may produce drug-resistant candidemia.[44] Induction of efflux pumps is the most common acquired azole resistance mechanism for Candida spp.[44] Echinocandins retain excellent activity against most Candida spp. and should be considered first-line therapy for the treatment of candidemia.[44] *Candida parapsilosis* and *Candida guilliermondii* are inherently resistant to echinocandins, and *C. albicans*, *C. tropicalis*, *C. krusei*, *C. glabrata*, and *C. lusitaniae* may acquire echinocandin resistance through genetic mutation.[44] Critically ill patients whose echinocandin therapy for candidemia fails should undergo susceptibility testing to determine optimal drug treatment.

ESBL-Producing Enterobacteriaceae

Extended-spectrum β lactamase–producing Enterobacteriaceae infections constitute 19% (26,000) of all infections caused by Enterobacteriaceae, and *K. pneumoniae* and *E. coli* are the most common pathogens (17,000 and 9,000 cases, respectively).[11] Cephalosporin overuse is commonly cited as the primary cause of the proliferation of ESBLs. Extended-spectrum β lactamase–producing Enterobacteriaceae cause 1,700 deaths each year.[11] Bacteremia from an ESBL-producing pathogen produces a 57% higher mortality rate than non-ESBL pathogens.[11] The cost of infection with an ESBL-producing Enterobacteriaceae pathogen is more than $40,000.[11] Extended-spectrum β lactamase–producing Enterobacteriaceae are resistant to most extended-spectrum penicillins and cephalosporins, but they remain susceptible to carbapenems.[38]

The prevalence of ESBL-producing Enterobacteriaceae is less than 10% across all infection types, with more isolates identified in intra-abdominal and urinary tract infections than pneumonia or bacteremia. Critically ill patients are at high risk of ESBL-producing organisms because they commonly have invasive indwelling devices such as central venous catheters, urinary catheters, and endotracheal tubes. Prior exposure to the health care or hospital setting and prior antibiotic therapy increase the risk of ESBL production.

Almost all β-lactams are hydrolyzed by ESBLs, leaving carbapenems as the most active agents of the class against these organisms. Piperacillin/tazobactam may also remain active in infections with lower organism burden when the minimum inhibitory concentration (MIC) is 16 mcg/mL or less.

Cefepime in standard doses may be effective for ESBL-producing Enterobacteriaceae when the MIC for the organism is 2 mcg/mL or less, although most clinical laboratories routinely list it as resistant when an ESBL is suspected.[45] Higher cefepime doses may be considered for MICs in the 4- to 8-mcg/mL range.[45]

Ceftolozane/tazobactam, one of the first cephalosporin β-lactamase inhibitor combinations available, could provide some additional activity against ESBL-producing pathogens. The combination maintains activity against some ESBL-producing *E. coli*, but it may have no activity in ESBL-producing *Klebsiella* spp. where carbapenemases may be present. Its specific place in therapy is still to be determined, but it is an option for consideration when MDR occurs, particularly within the critical care areas.[46]

Enterococcus spp.

Enterococci are gram-positive cocci common to the GI tract. In the critically ill population, enterococci are common pathogens in mixed bacteria-intra-abdominal infections, urinary tract infections, surgical site and wound infections, and less commonly bloodstream infections. Vancomycin-resistant *Enterococcus* is responsible for about 20,000 infections and 1,300 deaths per year.[11] Almost one-third of bloodstream, urinary tract, and surgical site enterococcal infections are VRE.[11] The most common resistant species of VRE is *Enterococcus faecium*, which accounts for half of the cases and deaths associated with vancomycin resistance.[11] The rate of vancomycin-resistant *E. faecium* is much higher than that of vancomycin-resistant *Enterococcus faecalis*.[47]

Resistance to vancomycin in enterococci is mediated by binding site modifications in the terminal D-alanine that results in decreased vancomycin binding. The most common phenotypes of VRE are *vanA* and *vanB*. *vanA* produces broad resistance in vancomycin and teicoplanin, whereas *vanB* produces resistance to vancomycin but not teicoplanin.[48] These resistance genes are carried on plasmids and can be shared to other gram-positive bacteria including *S. aureus*.

Therapeutic options for VRE infection are oxazolidinone (linezolid or tedizolid), with other lipoglycopeptides such as daptomycin, telavancin, dalbavancin, or oritavancin possibly retaining activity.[49] Fosfomycin and nitrofurantoin may be effective in treating urinary tract infection, but they are only available for oral administration in the United States.

Pseudomonas aeruginosa

P. aeruginosa is a nonfermenting, aerobic gram-negative bacilli that is responsible for pneumonia, bloodstream infections, urinary tract infections, and surgical site infections in critical illness.[28] Multidrug resistance occurs in 13% of pseudomonal HAIs.[11] Multidrug resistance in *P. aeruginosa* is defined as resistant to three or more drug classes. Surveillance data analyses from the European Antimicrobial Resistance Surveillance Network reported that resistance rates for aminoglycosides, carbapenems, quinolones, and ceftazidime were 0%–51.9%, 9%–50.5%, 7.2%–51.9%, and 4%–48.5%, respectively.[50] Overall, 18% of isolates were recorded as being MDR.[50] Multidrug-resistant organisms are more prevalent in critically ill populations than in populations in other hospital wards.

Many resistance mechanisms are responsible for MDR *P. aeruginosa*. The organism produces chromosomally mediated AmpC β-lactamase and can obtain ESBLs and carbapenemases, such as metallo-β-lactamases.[51] Fluoroquinolone resistance is chromosomally mediated through DNA gyrase mutations. *P. aeruginosa* may also produce aminoglycoside-modifying enzymes and can modify porins and express efflux pumps to reduce drug entry into the cell.[51]

Combination therapy is recommended for empiric treatment to improve the likelihood of appropriate initial therapy. Although described in vitro, synergy between different classes of antibiotics against MDR *P. aeruginosa* is not considered an in vivo phenomenon. Combinations could include carbapenems or antipseudomonal β-lactams with aminoglycosides or colistin-polymyxin. Once susceptibility data are available, streamlining therapy with one effective agent is appropriate, although monotherapy with aminoglycosides may lead to drug resistance.

S. aureus

S. aureus is a gram-positive cocci that is a common pathogen in HAI. The organisms are commensal on skin and are introduced into sterile spaces through breaks in the dermal layer, such as with indwelling vascular catheters, or surgical incision. Methicillin resistance in *S. aureus* occurs through the chromosomally mediated production of the transpeptidase PBP2a. The PBP2a transpeptidase is encoded by the gene *mecA*, which is located on the staphylococcal cassette chromosome. The PBP2a transpeptidase has an altered binding affinity for β-lactams such that almost all β-lactams are rendered ineffective against MRSA.[52] Although methicillin is no longer used, MRSA is also resistant to all other semisynthetic penicillins, including oxacillin, nafcillin, and dicloxacillin.

Despite declining rates in recent years, invasive MRSA infections number 80,461 per year in the United States, resulting in 11,285 deaths.[11] Methicillin-resistant *S. aureus* became a clinical concern in the 1980s and 1990s, and the prevalence of MRSA among *S. aureus* in the United States today is about 24%.[11] Risk factors for MRSA include recent prior hospitalization or interaction with the health care setting, residence in a nursing home or long-term care facility, intravenous drug use, and hemodialysis.[52]

Community-acquired MRSA became a health concern in the 1990s and is defined as occurring in individuals who did not have the risk factors described earlier. It commonly produces skin and skin-structure infections. The terms *health care–associated MRSA* and *community-associated MRSA* became common to describe these two uniquely different infections. Community-associated MRSA is often susceptible to clindamycin, tetracycline, aminoglycosides, and fluoroquinolones, whereas health care–associated MRSA is typically resistant to those agents.[52,53]

Vancomycin remains the drug of choice for empiric treatment, but MICs to vancomycin have been increasing during the past decade. Recent data suggest that MRSA with a vancomycin MIC of 2 mcg/mL occurs in 5.1% of patients and is an independent predictor of mortality.[54] The MIC susceptibility breakpoint to determine vancomycin susceptibility for *S. aureus* was 4 mcg/mL, but in recent years, it has been lowered to 2 mcg/mL because of the clinical failures in patients with isolates with vancomycin MICs greater than 1 mcg/mL.[52]

Vancomycin-resistant *S. aureus* has been identified in the United States, but it remains uncommon. *vanA* transfer from VRE is responsible for vancomycin-resistant *S. aureus*. Vancomycin-intermediate *S. aureus* are organisms with a vancomycin MIC of 4 or 8 mcg/mL. Vancomycin-intermediate *S. aureus* may be constitutive (heterogeneous). When selective pressure occurs in the clinical setting, the organism induces modifications to the bacterial cell wall that reduce the ability of vancomycin to diffuse into the cell wall. Vancomycin susceptibility can return to the organism once the selective pressure is removed. Many antibiotics retain activity against vancomycin-intermediate *S. aureus*, including linezolid and tedizolid, tigecycline, minocycline, telavancin, oritavancin, and dalbavancin.[52] Heterogeneous vancomycin-intermediate *S. aureus* has created a potential clinical concern with microbiologic susceptibility testing. The organism may be interpreted as susceptible to vancomycin when tested in vitro, but the portion of the inoculum that is not inhibited by vancomycin could selectively grow and lead to vancomycin treatment failure.

Use of vancomycin to maintain serum trough concentrations at 15–20 mcg/mL has been recommended for MRSA infection, but the data are mixed on the success of this strategy and the potential for nephrotoxicity from exposure to high vancomycin concentrations.[52] Alternatives to vancomycin include linezolid, tedizolid, daptomycin, telavancin, oritavancin, dalbavancin, tigecycline, and ceftaroline. Linezolid may be an effective alternative to vancomycin for MRSA infections when the vancomycin MIC is greater than 1 mcg/mL, especially when the infection is in the lung, meninges, or other compartments into which vancomycin poorly diffuses.[52]

GENERAL STRATEGIES TO MINIMIZE ANTIBIOTIC RESISTANCE

Minimizing antimicrobial resistance is possible using multifaceted strategies that are directed at population-based and individual patient-based interventions. The Infectious Diseases Society of America/Society for Healthcare Epidemiology of America guidelines to minimize resistance recommend that all hospitals form antimicrobial stewardship teams.[40] Antimicrobial stewardship programs improve patient care and reduce costs.

Appropriate culture techniques leading to high-quality laboratory data allow for streamlining of antimicrobial therapy to a narrower-spectrum agent or discontinuation of antimicrobials in patients without infection. Hospital-acquired pneumonia (HAP) and VAP are examples of the need for high-quality culture techniques. Hospital-acquired pneumonia/VAP accounts for around 50% of antibiotic use in the hospital, yet clinical signs and symptoms are poor markers of disease.[55] The American Thoracic Society guidelines recommend using quantitative cultures from deep in the respiratory tract because a minority of patients (about 40%) who present with signs and symptoms of VAP actually have pneumonia when this technique is used.[56] Rapid diagnostic measures either addressing general inflammatory measures (C-reactive protein or procalcitonin) or pathogen- and resistance-specific testing could lead to more timely initiation or discontinuation of antimicrobial agents for HAP/VAP.

Antibiotics should be discontinued if cultures are negative and infection is unlikely. There are an increasing number of studies suggesting that antibiotics initiated empirically for suspected infection, such as HAP/VAP, can be safely discontinued in patients with negative cultures and resolving clinical signs.[57-62] For patients in whom microbiologic cultures have identified an organism, streamlining antibiotics to narrower-spectrum agents is recommended to reduce unnecessary exposure of antimicrobial agents.[63-65]

The optimal direction of therapy for most infections in the critically ill population has not been determined. Increasingly, data suggest shorter treatment duration is associated with infection resolution, minimizing unnecessary antibiotic exposure. For HAP/VAP, short-duration therapy (3–7 days) has been shown to be as effective as long-duration therapy (14–15 days) in recent trials, with the exception of infections caused by *P. aeruginosa*.[57-59] Shorter-duration therapy has also been associated with fewer relapses with resistant organisms.[66,67] Seven days of therapy may be adequate for bloodstream infections caused by selected pathogens, but organisms such as *S. aureus* do not respond well to short-duration therapy.[62,68]

Inappropriate antimicrobial dosing in critically ill patients may lead to suboptimal drug concentrations for organism eradication. Infections in spaces that have poor drug penetration, such as meninges or lung, as well as pharmacokinetic changes that occur in critical illness, such as increased distribution volume, may lead to ineffective therapy. Drug doses should be adjusted on the basis of individual pharmacodynamic targets for drug and organism and pharmacokinetic parameters to meet those targets at the infection site.

Use of local antibiograms is recommended for empiric antibiotic selection to allow the use of narrower-spectrum agents in patients who are not at high risk of infection with pathogens such as *P. aeruginosa* and MRSA and should be based on local organism patterns.[55,65] Antibiograms should routinely be updated, at a minimum, twice annually. Box 14.3 summarizes efforts to reduce antimicrobial resistance in critical care environments.

CONCLUSION

Other strategies to minimize resistance, such as antibiotic cycling and formulary restrictions, remain largely unproven. The focus of antimicrobial stewardship programs should be to reduce overall antibiotic use through the strategies outlined earlier.

Antimicrobial resistance remains a problem in managing infection in the critically ill population and leads to excessive morbidity and mortality. Despite continuing advances in drug design, microorganisms have evolved genetically to demonstrate a dynamic arsenal of mechanisms to reduce or eliminate the effectiveness of antimicrobial agents. Clinicians must identify risk factors for resistance in patients and engage in broad, population-based strategies to reduce the likelihood of resistance generation or spread of resistance in local ICUs. Early identification of pathogens and their resistance patterns will help target appropriate and effective therapy, resulting in improved outcomes.

Box 14.3. Methods to Minimize Resistance in Critical Care Environments[31,55,63-65]

- Use high-quality culture techniques for blood, sputum, urine, and wound cultures
- Use rapid diagnostics for isolate identification and resistance
- De-escalate or discontinue broad-spectrum antimicrobials when information is available to do so
- Use therapy durations appropriate for specific infection and causative pathogen, minimizing lengthy durations where data suggest them unnecessary
- Use appropriate patient-specific parameters to avoid under- and overdosing of antimicrobials
- Use updated local antibiogram information for empiric antimicrobial dosing and protocol development

REFERENCES

1. Arias CA, Murray BE. Antibiotic-resistant bugs in the 21st century—a clinical super-challenge. N Engl J Med 2009;360:439-43.
2. Kollef MH, Shorr A, Tabak YP, et al. Epidemiology and outcomes of health-care-associated pneumonia: results from a large US database of culture-positive pneumonia. Chest 2005;128:3854-62.
3. Shorr AF, Tabak YP, Killian AD, et al. Healthcare-associated bloodstream infection: a distinct entity? Insights from a large US database. Crit Care Med 2006;34:2588-95.
4. Nseir S, Di Pompeo C, Cavestri B, et al. Multiple-drug-resistant bacteria in patients with severe acute exacerbation of chronic obstructive pulmonary disease: prevalence, risk factors, and outcome. Crit Care Med 2006;34:2959-66.
5. Niederman MS. Use of broad-spectrum antimicrobials for the treatment of pneumonia in seriously ill patients: maximizing clinical outcomes and minimizing selection of resistant organisms. Clin Infect Dis 2006;42(suppl 2):S72-S81.
6. Mueller EW, Hanes SD, Croce MA, et al. Effect from multiple episodes of inadequate empiric antibiotic therapy for ventilator-associated pneumonia on morbidity and mortality among critically ill trauma patients. J Trauma 2005;58:94-101.
7. Nseir S, Deplanque X, Di Pompeo C, et al. Risk factors for relapse of ventilator-associated pneumonia related to nonfermenting gram-negative bacilli: a case-control study. J Infect 2008;56:319-25.
8. Ibrahim EH, Sherman G, Ward S, et al. The influence of inadequate antimicrobial treatment of bloodstream infections on patient outcomes in the ICU setting. Chest 2000;118:146-55.
9. Teixeira PJ, Seligman R, Hertz FT, et al. Inadequate treatment of ventilator- associated pneumonia: risk factors and impact on outcomes. J Hosp Infect 2007;65:361-7.
10. World Health Organization. Antimicrobial Resistance Global Report on Surveillance 2014. Available at apps.who.int/iris/bitstream/10665/112642/1/9789241564748_eng.pdf. Accessed March 1, 2015.
11. Centers for Disease Control and Prevention. Antibiotic Resistance Threats in the United States, 2013. Available at www.cdc.gov/drugresistance/pdf/ar-threats-2013-508.pdf. Accessed February 26, 2015.
12. Cosgrove SE. The relationship between antimicrobial resistance and patient outcomes: mortality, length of hospital stay, and health care costs. Clin Infect Dis 2006;42:S82-9.
13. Lodise TP, McKinnon PS, Swiderski L, et al. Outcomes analysis of delayed antibiotic treatment for hospital-acquired *Staphylococcus aureus* bacteremia. Clin Infect Dis 2003;36:1418-23.
14. Lodise TP, McKinnon PS, Tam VH, et al. Clinical outcomes for patients with bacteremia caused by vancomycin-resistant enterococcus in a level 1 trauma center. Clin Infect Dis 2002;34:922-9.
15. Lautenbach E, Patel JB, Bilker WB, et al. Extended-spectrum b-lactamase-producing *Escherichia coli* and *Klebsiella pneumoniae*: risk factors for infection and impact of resistance on outcomes. Clin Infect Dis 2001;32:1162-71.
16. Vazquez-Guillamet C, Scolari M, Zilberberg MD, et al. Using the number needed to treat to assess appropriate antimicrobial therapy as a determinant of outcome in severe sepsis and septic shock. Crit Care Med 2014;42:2342-9.
17. Kohanski MA, DePristo MA, Collins JJ. Sublethal antibiotic treatment leads to multidrug resistance via radical-induced mutagenesis. Mol Cell 2010;37:311-20.
18. Aiello AE, Larson EL, Levy SB. Consumer antibacterial soaps: effective or just risky? Clin Infect Dis 2007;45(suppl 2):S137-S147.
19. Khardori N. Antibiotics—past, present, and future. Med Clin North Am 2006;90:1049-76.
20. Neu HS. Current mechanisms of resistance to antimicrobial agents in microorganisms causing infection in the patient at risk for infection. Am J Med 1984;15:11-27.
21. Chang HH, Cohen T, Grad YH, et al. Origin and proliferation of multiple-drug resistance in bacterial pathogens. Microbiol Mol Biol Rev 2015;79:101-16.
22. Fair RJ, Tor Y. Antibiotics and bacterial resistance in the 21st century. Perspect Med Chem 2014;6 25-64.
23. Meier S, Weber R, Zbinden R, et al. Extended-spectrum β-lactamase-producing gram-negative pathogens in community-acquired urinary tract infections: an increasing challenge for antimicrobial therapy. Infection 2011;39:333-40.
24. Lee HY, Chen CL, Wu SR, et al. Risk factors and outcome analysis of *Acinetobacter baumannii* complex bacteremia in critical patients. Crit Care Med 2014;42:1081-8.
25. Tenover FC. Mechanisms of antimicrobial resistance in bacteria. Am J Med 2006;119:S3-S10.
26. Nordmann P, Cuzon G, Naas T. The real threat of *Klebsiella pneumoniae* carbapenemase producing bacteria. Lancet Infect Dis 2009;9:228-36.
27. Tacconelli E, Cataldo MA. Vancomycin-resistant enterococci (VRE): transmission and control. Int J Antimicrob Agents 2008;31:99-106.
28. Strahilevitz J, Jacoby GA, Hooper DC, et al. Plasmid-mediated quinolone resistance: a multifaceted threat. Clin Microbiol Rev 2009;22:664-89.
29. Rybak MJ. Resistance to antimicrobial agents: an update. Pharmacotherapy 2004;24(12 pt 2):203S-215S.
30. Burillo A, Bouza E. Use of rapid diagnostic techniques in ICU patients with infections. BMC Infect Dis 2014;14:1-12.
31. Centers for Disease Control and Prevention. Healthcare-Associated Infections (HAI) Progress Report, 2015. Available at www.cdc.gov/hai/progress-report/index.html. Accessed February 23, 2015.
32. Centers for Disease Control and Prevention (CDC). Vital signs: carbapenem-resistant Enterobacteriaceae. MMWR Morb Mortal Wkly Rep 2013;62:165-70.
33. Schwaber MJ, Carmeli Y. Carbapenem-resistant Enterobacteriaceae: a potential threat. JAMA 2008;300:98-705.
34. Nordmann P, Cuzon G. Naas T. The real threat of *Klebsiella pneumonia* carbapenemase-producing bacteria. Lancet Infect Dis 2009;9:228-36.
35. Patel G, Huprikar S, Factor SH, et al. Outcomes of carbapenem-resistant *Klebsiella pneumoniae* infection and the impact of antimicrobial and adjunctive therapies. Infect Control Hosp Epidemiol 2008;29:1099-106.

36. Qureshi ZA, Paterson DL, Potoski BA, et al. Treatment outcome of bacteremia due to KPC-producing *Klebsiella pneumoniae*: superiority of combination antimicrobial regimens. Antimicrob Agents Chemother 2012;56:2108-13.

37. Tumbarello M, Viale P, Viscoli C, et al. Predictors of mortality in bloodstream infections caused by *Klebsiella pneumoniae* carbapenemase-producing *K. pneumoniae*: importance of combination therapy. Clin Infect Dis 2012;55:943-50.

38. Hirsch EB, Tam VH. Detection and treatment options for *Klebsiella pneumoniae* carbapenemases (KPCs): an emerging cause of multi-drug resistant infection. J Antimicrob Chemother 2010;65:1119-25.

39. Cassir N, Rolain JM, Brouqui P. A new strategy to fight antimicrobial resistance: the revival of old antibiotics. Front Microbiol 2014;5:551.

40. Murray CK, Hospenthal DR. Acinetobacter infection in the ICU. Crit Care Clin 2008;24:237-48.

41. Kim BN, Peleg AY, Lodise TP, et al. Management of meningitis due to antibiotic-resistant *Acinetobacter* species. Lancet Infect Dis 2009;9:245-55.

42. Goff DA, Bauer KA, Mangino JE. Bad bugs need old drugs: a stewardship program's evaluation of minocycline for multidrug-resistant *Acinetobacter baumannii* infections. Clin Infect Dis 2014;59(S6):S381-7.

43. Pappas PG, Kauffman CA, Andes D, et al. Clinical practice guidelines for the management of candidiasis: 2009 update by the Infectious Diseases Society of America. Clin Infect Dis 2009;48:508-39.

44. Cleveland AA, Farley MM, Harrison LH, et al. Changes in incidence and antifungal drug resistance in candidemia: results from population-based laboratory surveillance in Atlanta and Baltimore 2008-2011. Clin Infect Dis 2012;55:1352-61.

45. Nguyen HM, Shier KL, Graber CJ. Determining a clinical framework for use of cefepime and β-lactam/β-lactamase inhibitors in the treatment of infections caused by extended-spectrum-β-lactamase-producing Enterobacteriaceae. J Antimicrob Chemother 2014;69:871-80.

46. Cho JC, Fiorenza MA, Estrada SJ. Ceftolozane/tazobactam: a novel cephalosporin/β-lactamase inhibitor combination. Pharmacotherapy 2015;35:701-15.

47. Sader HS, Moet GJ, Farrell DJ, et al. Antimicrobial susceptibility of daptomycin and comparator agents tested against methicillin-resistant Staphylococcus aureus and vancomycin-resistant enterococci: trend analysis of a 6-year period in US medical centers (2005-2010). Diagn Microbiol Infect Dis 2011;70:412-6.

48. Rivera AM, Boucher HW. Current concepts in antimicrobial therapy against select gram-positive organisms: methicillin-resistant *Staphylococcus aureus*, penicillin-resistant pneumococci, and vancomycin-resistant enterococci. Mayo Clin Proc 2011;86:1230-43.

49. Eliopoulos GM. Microbiology of drugs for treating multiple drug-resistant gram-positive bacteria. J Infect 2009;59(suppl 1):S17-S24.

50. Souli M, Galani I, Giamarellou H. Emergence of extensively drug-resistant and pandrug-resistant gram-negative bacilli in Europe. Eurosurveillance 2008;13:1-11.

51. Lister, PD, Wolter DJ, Hanson ND. Antibacterial-resistant *Pseudomonas aeruginosa*: clinical impact and complex regulation of chromosomally encoded resistance mechanisms. Clin Microbiol Rev 2009;22:582-610.

52. Liu C, Bayer A, Cosgrove CE, et al. Clinical practice guidelines by the Infectious Diseases Society of America for the treatment of methicillin-resistant *Staphylococcus aureus* infections in adults and children. Clin Infect Dis 2011;52:1-38.

53. Boucher HW, Corey GR. Epidemiology of methicillin-resistant *Staphylococcus aureus*. Clin Infect Dis 2008;46(suppl 5):S344-49.

54. Woods CJ, Chowdhury A, Patel VM, et al. Impact of vancomycin minimum inhibitory concentration on mortality among critically ill patients with methicillin-resistant *Staphylococcus aureus* bacteremia. Infect Control Hosp Epidemiol 2012;33:1246-9.

55. American Thoracic Society and the Infectious Diseases Society of America: guidelines for the management of adults with hospital-acquired, ventilator-associated, and healthcare-associated pneumonia. Am J Respir Crit Care Med 2005;171:388-416.

56. Chastre J, Fagon JY. Ventilator-associated pneumonia. Am J Respir Crit Care Med 2002;165:867-903.

57. Swanson JM, Wood GC, Croce MA, et al: Utility of preliminary bronchoalveolar lavage results in suspected ventilator-associated pneumonia. J Trauma 2008;65:1271-7.

58. Kollef MH, Kollef KE. Antibiotic utilization and outcomes for patients with clinically suspected ventilator-associated pneumonia and negative quantitative BAL culture results. Chest 2005;128:2706-13.

59. Micek ST, Ward S, Fraser VJ, et al. A randomized controlled trial of an antibiotic discontinuation policy for clinically suspected ventilator-associated pneumonia. Chest 2004;125:1791-9.

60. Croce MA, Fabian TC, Mueller EW, et al. The appropriate diagnostic threshold for ventilator-associated pneumonia using quantitative cultures. J Trauma 2004;56:931-6.

61. Miller PR, Meredith JW, Change MC. Optimal threshold for diagnosis of ventilator-associated pneumonia using bronchoalveolar lavage. J Trauma 2003;55:263-8.

62. Mermel LA, Allon M, Bouza E, et al. Clinical practice guidelines for the diagnosis and management of intravascular catheter-related infection: 2009 update by the Infectious Diseases Society of America. Clin Infect Dis 2009;49:1-45.

63. Dellit TH, Owens RC, McGowan JE, et al. Infectious Diseases Society of America and the Society for Healthcare Epidemiology of America guidelines for developing an institutional program to enhance antimicrobial stewardship. Clin Infect Dis 2007;44:159-77.

64. Centers for Disease Control and Prevention. Get Smart for Healthcare. May 2014. Available at www.cdc.gov/getsmart/healthcare. Accessed February 27, 2015.

65. Dellinger RP, Levy MM, Carlet JM, et al: Surviving Sepsis Campaign: international guidelines for management of severe sepsis and septic shock: 2008. Crit Care Med 2008;36:296-327.

66. Ibrahim EH, Ward S, Sherman G, et al. Experience with a clinical guideline for the treatment of ventilator-associated pneumonia. Crit Care Med 2001;29:1109-15.

67. Chastre J, Wolff M, Fagon JY, et al. Comparison of 8 vs. 15 days of antibiotic therapy for ventilator-associated pneumonia in adults: a randomized trial. JAMA 2003;290:2588-98.

68. Jensen AG, Wachmann CH, Espersen F, et al. Treatment and outcome of *Staphylococcus aureus* bacteremia: a prospective study of 278 cases. Arch Intern Med 2002;162:25-32.

Chapter 15: Severe Sepsis and Septic Shock

Seth R. Bauer, Pharm.D., FCCM, BCPS; Simon W. Lam, Pharm.D., FCCM, BCPS; and Lance J. Oyen, Pharm.D., FCCM, FCCP, BCPS

LEARNING OBJECTIVES

1. Construct an initial resuscitation pathway that includes quantitative resuscitation for patients with severe sepsis or septic shock.
2. Design an appropriate antimicrobial treatment strategy for adult patients with severe sepsis or septic shock that combines initial broad-spectrum therapies and subsequent de-escalation of therapy.
3. Evaluate the risks and benefits of volume resuscitation with crystalloids and colloids for patients with hemodynamic instability as the result of severe sepsis or septic shock.
4. Devise a treatment strategy for the hemodynamic management and monitoring of patients with severe sepsis or septic shock.
5. Distinguish scenarios in which the use of corticosteroids as an adjunct for septic shock is supported by the 2012 Surviving Sepsis Campaign (SSC) guidelines.
6. Develop a treatment pathway for the care of patients with severe sepsis or septic shock that incorporates the 2012 SSC guideline care bundles, new data since publication of the last guidelines, and National Quality Forum recommendations.

ABBREVIATIONS IN THIS CHAPTER

CVP	Central venous pressure	PCT	Procalcitonin
HES	Hydroxyethyl starch	SBP	Systolic blood pressure
ICU	Intensive care unit	$Scvo_2$	Central venous oxygen saturation
MAP	Mean arterial pressure	SSC	Surviving Sepsis Campaign

INTRODUCTION

Severe sepsis and septic shock are extreme conditions on the systemic infection disease continuum. In sepsis, an infecting pathogen elicits a systemic inflammatory response, which may be complicated by end-organ dysfunction (severe sepsis). Septic shock is characterized by acute circulatory failure leading to ineffective tissue perfusion and cellular hypoxia and is typically defined as arterial hypotension unresponsive to fluid administration.[1]

Overall, the in-hospital mortality associated with severe sepsis and septic shock is around 25%,[2] and mortality at 2 years is around 45%.[3] Classification of sepsis stage is important because mortality ranges from 15% with sepsis to as high as 70% with septic shock and multiorgan failure.[4] Prompt initiation of therapies is of utmost importance because patients may quickly progress through the stages of sepsis from systemic inflammatory response syndrome to septic shock. Further complicating matters is the fact that sepsis is common (annual U.S. incidence greater than 890,000), increasing in incidence (by about 13% per year), and costly, with annual costs in the United States exceeding $24 billion.[2] Septic shock is the most commonly encountered shock type, accounting for 62% of all cases of shock requiring vasopressors.[5] Fortunately, data evaluations suggest that outcomes in patients with severe sepsis and septic shock are improved through therapeutic intervention.[6] This should serve as a call to action for intensive care unit (ICU) practitioners.

The Surviving Sepsis Campaign (SSC), a joint collaboration between the Society of Critical Care Medicine and the European Society of Intensive Care Medicine, has published three iterations of international guidelines for the treatment of patients with severe sepsis and septic shock. The 2012 SSC guidelines, published in early 2013, were sponsored or endorsed by 30 international organizations[7]; a portion of the pharmacologic-related SSC recommendations is summarized in Box 15.1. Important differences between the 2008 and the 2012 SSC guideline recommendations can be found in Table 15.1. Translating the literature and treatment principles described in these guidelines to bedside care while incorporating an assessment of patient-specific data is necessary to design a comprehensive pharmacotherapeutic care plan for the patient with severe sepsis or septic shock.

PATHOPHYSIOLOGY

Severe sepsis and septic shock involve complex interactions between an infecting pathogen and the host inflammatory, immune, and coagulation response (Figure 15.1). The pattern recognition (e.g., toll-like) receptors on innate immune system cells recognize specific molecules present in microorganisms and signal the release of nuclear factor kappa B (NF-κB), which leads to the transcription of both proinflammatory cytokines (e.g., interleukin [IL]-1β, IL-6, tumor necrosis factor α) and anti-inflammatory cytokines (e.g., IL-10). The proinflammatory cytokines activate neutrophils and endothelial cells, leading to an increased expression of inducible nitric oxide synthase. Concomitantly, the coagulation cascade is activated by tissue factor presented by monocytes, and anticoagulant pathways are depressed; this leads to microvascular thrombosis and impaired tissue perfusion (Figure 15.2).[8] Although target-specific therapies are not currently in clinical use for sepsis, knowledge of these factors may lead to new therapeutic modalities.

Hypotension develops through inappropriate activation of vasodilatory mechanisms (increased nitric oxide synthesis) and failure of vasoconstrictive pathways (activation of ATP-dependent potassium channels in vascular smooth muscle cells and vasopressin deficiency), resulting in a vasodilatory shock. In addition, blood flow is inappropriately dispersed at the organ level or in the microcirculation (shunting), leading to distributive shock.[9] Vascular endothelial cell injury leads to shedding of the endothelial glycocalyx and loss of tight junctions between endothelial cells, resulting in capillary fluid leak and a decrease in cardiac preload. Venous dilation further exacerbates the decrease in cardiac preload and worsens hypotension. Tissue oxygen delivery may be further impaired through a decrease in cardiac output from myocardial stunting, inadequate arterial oxygen content (low hemoglobin concentration or saturation), or impaired oxygen unloading from hemoglobin. These multifactorial hemodynamic abnormalities lead to ineffective tissue perfusion, in which oxygen demand exceeds oxygen delivery, which results in cellular injury. This in turn further compounds the proinflammatory and procoagulant state, precipitating multiorgan dysfunction and possibly death.

DIAGNOSIS

There is no specific diagnostic test for severe sepsis or septic shock. Although bacteremia has been suggested as a fundamental, pathophysiological determinant of sepsis, positive blood cultures are infrequently established during sepsis.[10] This may be because of delays in obtaining blood cultures, prior antibiotic treatment, or inadequate culturing techniques. Because microbiological cultures are not always positive, the diagnosis of sepsis has traditionally required a known or suspected source of infection, together with two or more criteria of the systemic inflammatory response syndrome (i.e., fever/hypothermia, tachycardia, tachypnea, or leukocytosis/leukopenia).[1] Although using the systemic inflammatory response syndrome criteria is in accord with consensus guidelines, their diagnostic performance for patients with infection is suboptimal, with a high sensitivity and low specificity.[11] However, this finding is expected because of the design of the criteria, and these criteria are best used for ruling out, not ruling in, sepsis. Updated consensus criteria for the diagnosis of sepsis are currently being developed.

Early treatment is of paramount importance for severe sepsis and septic shock; hence, all diagnostic approaches should be performed simultaneously with the early administration of life-saving therapies. After a thorough history and physical examination, radiologic imaging should be done in an attempt to confirm a potential source of infection.[7] Recognizing that the lung (in about 45% of cases), abdomen (about 30%), and urinary tract (about 11%) account for most infectious sites,[12] microbial cultures should be sent from all suspected infectious sites and the blood as soon as possible. Cultures should be obtained before initiating antimicrobial therapy unless doing so would result in a significant (more than 45 minutes) delay in therapy.[7] Only 70% of patients with septic shock have positive microbial cultures (and only 30% have positive blood cultures), which creates therapeutic challenges for clinicians. Rapid, nonculture methods of microbial detection using molecular techniques are currently being studied to aid in faster pathogen identification and recognition of antimicrobial resistance mechanisms. In addition, biomarkers (e.g., procalcitonin [PCT]) may play a role in sepsis diagnosis or in guiding antibiotic decisions.

Box 15.1. Surviving Sepsis Campaign Pharmacologic-Related Recommendations for Patients with Severe Sepsis and Septic Shock[a]

Fluid Therapy

1. Crystalloids as the initial fluid of choice in the resuscitation of severe sepsis and septic shock (grade 1B)
2. Avoid the use of HES for fluid resuscitation of severe sepsis and septic shock (grade 1B).
3. Albumin in the fluid resuscitation of severe sepsis and septic shock when patients require a substantial amount of crystalloids (grade 2C)

Vasopressors and Inotropes

1. Vasopressor therapy initially to target a MAP of 65 mm Hg (grade 1C)
2. Norepinephrine as the first-choice vasopressor (grade 1B)
3. Epinephrine when an additional agent is needed to maintain adequate pressure (grade 2B)
4. Vasopressin (AVP) 0.03 unit/minute can be added to NE with the intent of either raising MAP or decreasing NE dosage (UG). AVP doses higher than 0.03–0.04 unit/minute should be reserved for salvage therapy (failure to achieve adequate MAP with other vasopressor agents) (UG)
5. Dopamine as an alternative vasopressor agent to NE only in highly selected patients (i.e., patients with low risk of tachyarrhythmias and absolute or relative bradycardia) (grade 2C)
6. Phenylephrine is not recommended in the treatment of septic shock except when (1) NE is associated with serious arrhythmias, (2) cardiac output is known to be high and blood pressure persistently low, or (3) used as salvage therapy when combined inotrope/vasopressor drugs and low-dose AVP have failed to achieve MAP targets (grade 1C)
7. A trial of dobutamine infusion (up to 20 mcg/kg/minute) may be administered or added to vasopressor (if in use) in the presence of (1) myocardial dysfunction as suggested by elevated cardiac filling pressures and low cardiac output or (2) ongoing signs of hypoperfusion, despite achieving adequate intravascular volume and adequate MAP (grade 1C)

Antimicrobial Therapy

1. Administration of effective intravenous antimicrobials within the first hour of recognition of septic shock (grade 1B) and severe sepsis without septic shock (grade 1C) should be the goal of therapy
2a. Initial empiric anti-infective therapy should include one or more drugs that have activity against all likely pathogens (bacterial, fungal, or both or viral) and that penetrate in adequate concentrations into the tissues presumed to be the source of sepsis (grade 1B)
2b. The antimicrobial regimen should be reassessed daily for potential de-escalation (grade 1B)
3. Low procalcitonin concentrations or similar biomarkers should be used to assist the clinician in discontinuing empiric antibiotics in patients who appear to have sepsis but have no subsequent evidence of infection (grade 2C)
4a. Combination empiric therapy for neutropenic patients with severe sepsis (grade 2B) and for patients with difficult-to-treat, multidrug-resistant bacterial pathogens such as *Acinetobacter* and *Pseudomonas* spp. (grade 2B)
4b. Combination therapy, when used empirically in patients with severe sepsis, should not be administered for longer than 3–5 days. De-escalation to the most appropriate single-agent therapy should be done as soon as the susceptibility profile of the pathogen(s) is known (grade 2B)
5. Therapy duration should typically be 7–10 days if clinically indicated. Longer courses may be appropriate in patients who have a slow clinical response, undrainable foci of infection, bacteremia with *Staphylococcus aureus*, some fungal and viral infections, or immunologic deficiencies, including neutropenia (grade 2C)
6. Antiviral therapy should be initiated as early as possible in patients with severe sepsis and septic shock of viral origin (grade 2C)
7. Antimicrobial agents should not be used in patients with severe inflammatory states determined to be of noninfectious cause (UG)

Corticosteroids

1. Not using intravenous hydrocortisone to treat adult patients with septic shock if adequate fluid resuscitation and vasopressor therapy can restore hemodynamic stability. If this is not achievable, intravenous hydrocortisone alone at a dose of 200 mg/day may be added (grade 2C)
2. Not using the ACTH stimulation test to identify those who should receive hydrocortisone (grade 2B)

[a]Strength and evidence level of recommendations listed in parentheses are according to the Grading of Recommendations Assessment, Development and Evaluation system. The system classifies strength of recommendations as strong (1) or weak (2), and quality of evidence as high (A), moderate (B), low (C), or very low (D). Recommendations not conducive for the grading process were regarded as ungraded (UG).

ACTH = adrenocorticotropic hormone; AVP = arginine vasopressin; HES = hydroxyethyl starch; MAP = mean arterial blood pressure; NE = norepinephrine.

Information from: Dellinger RP, Levy MM, Rhodes A, et al. Surviving Sepsis Campaign: international guidelines for management of severe sepsis and septic shock: 2012. Crit Care Med 2013;41:580-637.

Procalcitonin is a precursor of calcitonin that is up-regulated by bacterial toxins and certain bacterial proinflammatory mediators such as IL-1b, IL-6, and tumor necrosis factor α, but it is neutral to cytokines that are normally released for viral infections such as interferon-γ. As such, PCT has been studied as a diagnostic tool, a predictor of progression in sepsis stage, or a guidance tool for influencing antimicrobial decision-making.[13] Procalcitonin concentrations rise in response to severe bacterial infections; they also correlate with sepsis-related organ failure scores and outcomes. Thus, serum PCT concentrations may help assess the severity of sepsis when combined with clinical and laboratory variables. However, although PCT may perform well in less-severe infections, it may not reliably differentiate sepsis from other noninfectious causes of systemic inflammation (pooled sensitivity 0.77, pooled specificity 0.79, area under the receiver operating characteristic curve 0.85).[14] Thus, PCT requires further study before it can be recommended for widespread use as a diagnostic tool in sepsis. Using PCT to guide antibiotic decisions is addressed later in this chapter; other biomarkers and rapid diagnostics are discussed in detail in Chapter 13, "Laboratory Testing Considerations."

Recognizing patients who have signs of sepsis-induced end-organ hypoperfusion (progressing to severe sepsis and septic shock) is of paramount importance. Typically, hypoperfusion is secondary to low systemic blood pressure (i.e., systolic blood pressure [SBP] less than 90 mm Hg, mean arterial pressure [MAP] less than 70 mm Hg, or an SBP decrease of more than 40 mm Hg from baseline). However, signs of organ dysfunction such as altered mental status or decreased urine output may occur in the absence of hypotension.

Serum lactate concentrations may also be used to assess for tissue hypoperfusion. In sepsis, elevations in serum lactate concentrations (greater than 4 mmol/L) are generally a result of global hypoperfusion, but other causes (e.g., impaired lactate clearance, sepsis-induced mitochondrial dysfunction, reduced pyruvate dehydrogenase activity, increased aerobic glycolysis secondary to catecholamines) must be considered and ruled out. Chapter 10, "Shock Syndromes," contains an extensive discussion of hemodynamic values, monitoring devices, and methods to differentiate shock states. In patients with signs of sepsis-induced hypoperfusion (i.e., severe sepsis and septic shock), therapies to improve perfusion should be initiated promptly.

INITIAL AND SUBSEQUENT RESUSCITATION

The initial goals of therapy are to restore effective tissue perfusion (by administering intravenous fluids and vasoactive medications) while treating the underlying cause through antimicrobial administration and infectious source control, as applicable. Chapter 10 includes an extensive discussion of resuscitation end points and generalized treatment for shock.

Table 15.1 Key Updates in the 2012 Surviving Sepsis Campaign Guidelines

Category	2008 Recommendation	2012 Recommendation
Fluid type	Natural/artificial colloids or crystalloids	Crystalloids primarily, albumin use if high crystalloid volumes, do not use HES
Initial fluid challenge dose	≥ 1000 mL of crystalloids or 300–500 mL of colloids	≥ 30 mL/kg of crystalloids
Initial vasopressor	NE or dopamine	NE
Phenylephrine use	Not recommended as initial vasopressor (no discussion regarding other uses)	Not recommended except in certain circumstances (see Box 15.1)
Vasopressin use	May be added to NE with anticipation of an effect equivalent to that of NE alone	Added to NE with intent of either raising MAP or decreasing NE dosage
Hydrocortisone dose	≤ 300 mg/day	200 mg/day
Procalcitonin use	No recommendation made	Low concentrations should be used to discontinue empiric antibiotics in patients without evidence of infection
Drotrecogin use	Recommended in patients at high risk of death	No recommendation made (drug withdrawn from market)

HES = hydroxyethyl starch; MAP = mean arterial blood pressure; NE = norepinephrine.

Information from: Dellinger RP, Levy MM, Carlet JM, et al. Surviving Sepsis Campaign: international guidelines for management of severe sepsis and septic shock: 2008. Crit Care Med 2008;36:296-327; and Dellinger RP, Levy MM, Rhodes A, et al. Surviving Sepsis Campaign: international guidelines for management of severe sepsis and septic shock: 2012. Crit Care Med 2013;41:580-637. Adapted with permission from: Bauer SR, Lam SW. Severe sepsis and septic shock. In: Murphy JE, Lee MW, eds. Pharmacotherapy Self-Assessment Program, 2014 Book 1. Critical and Urgent Care. Lenexa, KS: American College of Clinical Pharmacy, 2014:219-35.

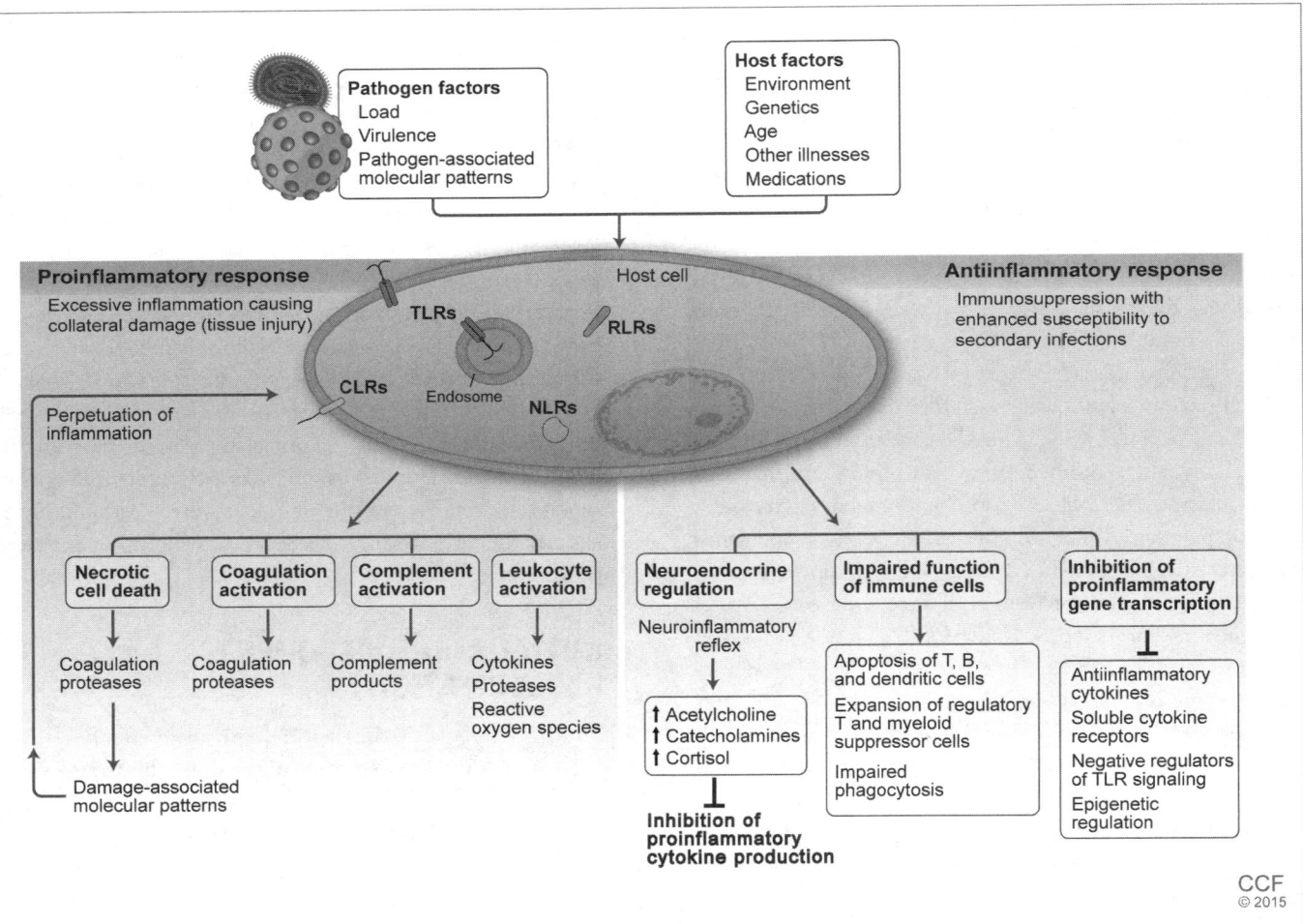

Figure 15.1 Host response in severe sepsis and septic shock.

In severe sepsis and septic shock, the host response includes both proinflammatory responses (left panel) and anti-inflammatory responses (right panel). Both pathogen and host factors contribute to the host response and contribute to the balance between pro- and anti-inflammatory response factors. The inflammatory response is commenced through detection of pathogen-associated molecular patterns (cell wall molecules expressed by pathogens) by pattern recognition receptors on the host immune cell surface (C-type lectin receptors [CLRs] and toll-like receptors [TLRs]), in the cytoplasm (nucleotide-binding oligomerization domain–like receptors [NLRs] and retinoic acid inducible gene 1–like receptors [RLRs]), or in the endosome (TLRs). Binding to these receptors leads to the activation of NF-B, which increases the transcription of both pro- and anti-inflammatory cytokines. An amplified proinflammatory response leads to tissue injury and necrotic cell death, which results in the release of damage-associated molecular patterns that perpetuate inflammation (possibly with the same pattern recognition receptors noted earlier). Concomitantly, the anti-inflammatory response can lead to immunosuppression and enhanced susceptibility to secondary infections. Reprinted with permission from the Cleveland Clinic.

Patients with severe sepsis and septic shock should first be administered a fluid challenge of crystalloid solution as quickly as possible. Typically, the fluid challenge target is 30 mL/kg or more of crystalloid solution.[7] Although recent randomized controlled trials simplified this requirement to the administration of 1 L of fluid challenge over 30–60 minutes for study inclusion, the patients who were included had on average about 30 mL/kg of intravenous fluids administered before randomization.[15,16] If blood pressure does not improve after the fluid challenge, or if the initial serum lactate concentration is greater than 4 mmol/L, quantitative resuscitation should be initiated. This strategy includes using intensive diagnostics and monitoring (e.g., echocardiography, placing a central venous [superior vena cava] catheter, or other mechanisms for monitoring fluid responsiveness), setting goals for hemodynamic support, and using therapies to achieve these goals (e.g., use and optimization of fluids, vasopressors, and oxygen delivery methods). Priority should be placed on early, aggressive fluid administration to optimize cardiac preload and improvement/preservation of organ perfusion pressure.

Early Quantitative Resuscitation

Quantitative resuscitation originated from the landmark study of early goal-directed therapy by Rivers and colleagues.[17] This study evaluated patients with severe sepsis and septic shock who were treated in the emergency department for the first 6 hours after presentation. Both study arms required insertion of central venous and arterial catheters and had treatment goals of central venous pressure (CVP) greater than 8 mm Hg, MAP greater than 65 mm Hg, and urine output greater than 0.5 mL/kg/hour. Patients in the standard therapy group were treated at the clinician's discretion, whereas patients in the intervention arm were uniformly treated with a protocol to achieve the resuscitation parameters, with the additional goal of central venous oxygen saturation ($Scvo_2$) of 70% or greater. Interventions used to increase $Scvo_2$ (if it was less than 70%) were packed red blood cell transfusion if the hematocrit value was 30% or below or dobutamine infusion if the hematocrit value was greater than 30%. Early, aggressive, goal-directed resuscitation was associated with a 16% absolute risk reduction in hospital mortality compared with standard therapy (30.5% vs. 46.5%, p<0.009). Several additional observational studies that included patients with early goal-directed therapy compared with historical controls have shown reduced mortality with bundle-based care.[10]

Despite these favorable results and support from all three iterations of the SSC guidelines, early goal-directed therapy was not universally adopted in emergency departments because of several factors. Given the design of the Rivers et al. study, it is unclear whether the use of a goal-directed protocol or the use of $Scvo_2$ as a treatment goal (or both) led to the study's positive findings. In addition, the study by Rivers and colleagues received several critiques, including a higher-than-expected mortality rate in the standard therapy arm, a high absolute risk reduction in mortality (16%), the incorporation of CVP as a resuscitation goal, the non-protocolized use of antimicrobials, and its single-center nature. Furthermore, many centers faced logistical and financial barriers to implementing the

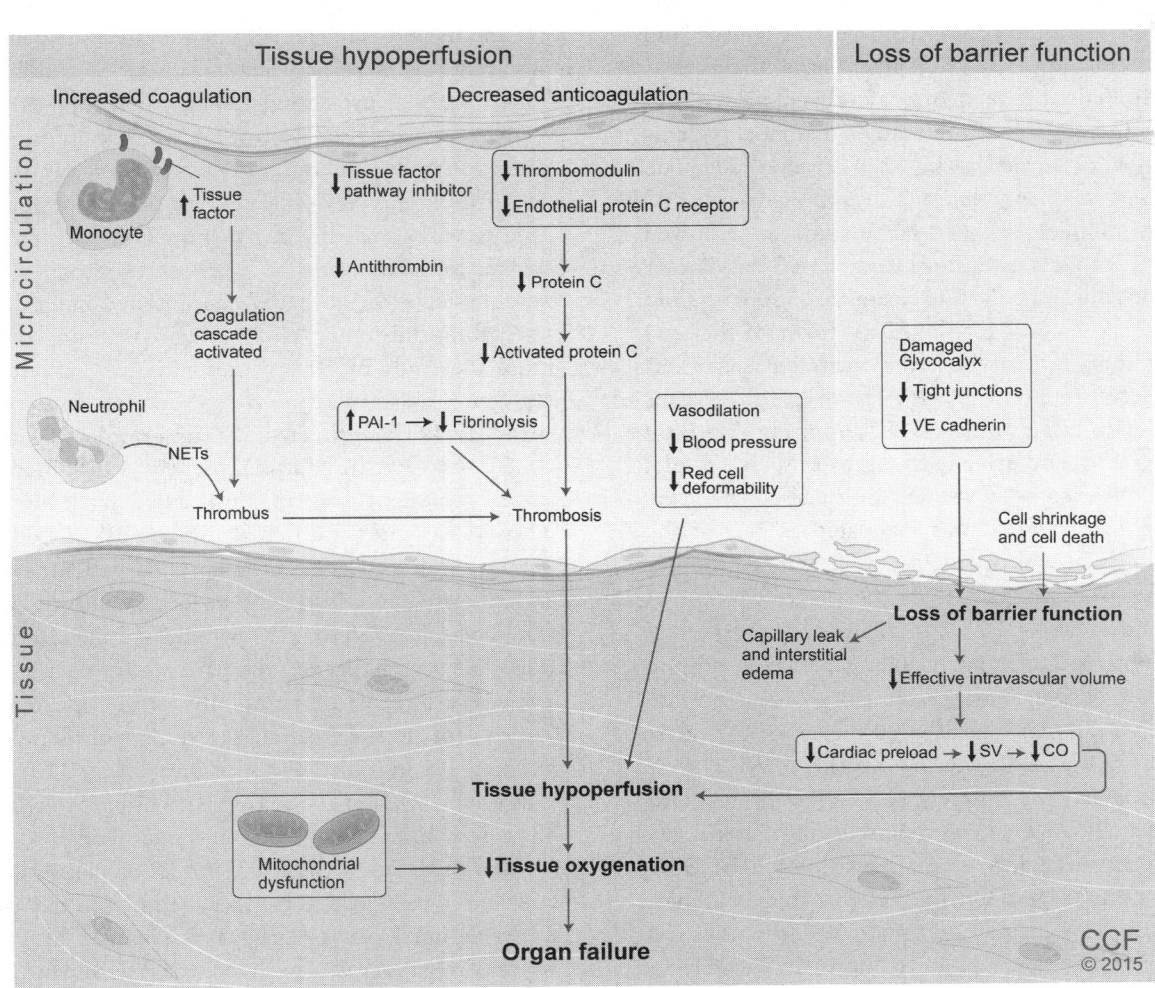

Figure 15.2 Mechanism of impaired tissue perfusion in severe sepsis and septic shock.

The coagulation cascade is activated in sepsis by expression of tissue factor on the vascular endothelium and on monocytes. Concomitantly, the endogenous anticoagulant pathway (tissue factor pathway inhibitor, activated protein C, and antithrombin) is impaired, and fibrinolysis is impaired (through release of plasminogen activator inhibitor type 1 [PAI-1]). As a result of an imbalance between pathways, microvascular thrombi form. Neutrophil extracellular traps (NETs) released from neutrophils further enhance thrombus generation. Microvascular thrombi and concomitant vasodilation, hypotension, and decreased red blood cell deformability further reduce tissue perfusion. Concurrently, damage to the endothelial glycocalyx layer, loss of endothelial cellular tight junctions, and impaired vascular endothelial (VE) cadherin lead to a loss of barrier function. The resultant capillary leak and interstitial edema contribute to ineffective intravascular volume, which impairs cardiac preload, stroke volume (SV), and cardiac output (CO), leading to further tissue hypoperfusion. Reprinted with permission from the Cleveland Clinic.

protocols. As such, alternative approaches to quantitative resuscitation were developed and studied.

A large, multicenter, noninferiority study was designed to evaluate whether incorporating $Scvo_2$ as a treatment goal is a necessary component of a quantitative resuscitation protocol.[18] This study randomized patients to a quantitative resuscitation protocol that incorporated $Scvo_2$ as a treatment goal or to a quantitative resuscitation protocol that was similar in all components except that it incorporated a lactate clearance of 10% or greater, instead of $Scvo_2$, as a treatment goal. The lactate clearance strategy was determined to be noninferior to the $Scvo_2$ strategy (in-hospital mortality 17% vs. 23%, respectively; 95% confidence interval [CI] for mortality difference -3% to 15% [greater than the -10% predefined noninferiority threshold]). Of note, only 10% of the patients in each arm received a therapy specifically directed to improve either lactate clearance or $Scvo_2$, which could have biased the study toward finding no difference between treatment arms (and incorrect rejection of a true null hypothesis of the existence of a difference between groups in this noninferiority study; a type I error). Equally relevant is that most patients in this study with septic shock (90%) achieved adequate oxygen delivery with only fluids and vasopressors.

Another multicenter, open-label study randomized ICU patients with a lactate concentration of 3 mmol/L or greater to the addition of lactate clearance of 20% or more (evaluated every 2 hours for the first 8 hours of therapy) or standard therapy (in which the treatment team was blinded for lactate concentrations).[19] Both treatment arms had resuscitation targets of CVP 8–12 mm Hg, MAP 60 mm Hg or greater, and urine output greater than 0.5 mL/kg/hour. Monitoring of $Scvo_2$ was optional in the standard therapy group, but it was mandated as part of the lactate clearance group. In the lactate clearance group, if the $Scvo_2$ was 70% or greater but the lactate concentrations did not decrease by 20%, vasodilators (e.g., nitroglycerin) were initiated to improve microvascular perfusion. Adding lactate clearance as a treatment goal was not associated with a difference in hospital mortality on bivariate analysis (33.9% vs. 43.5%, p=0.067). However, after adjustment for baseline differences between groups with multivariate analysis, there was a significant difference favoring the lactate clearance group (hazard ratio 0.61; 95% CI, 0.43–0.87; p=0.006). On the basis of these findings, in a low-level recommendation (grade 2C), the SSC has suggested targeting resuscitation to normalize lactate in patients with elevated lactate concentrations.[7]

Three recently published multicenter studies further evaluated the utility of quantitative resuscitation protocols. The first study published, the Protocolized Care for Early Septic Shock (ProCESS) study, was conducted in academic medical centers in the United States. The study aimed to evaluate (1) if a quantitative resuscitation protocol was associated with improved patient outcomes compared with usual care and (2) if a quantitative resuscitation protocol was superior to usual care whether the specific protocol used by Rivers and colleagues was superior to an alternative protocol.[16] The study randomized patients in the emergency department to one of three treatment arms: (1) early goal-directed therapy according to the protocol of Rivers and colleagues; (2) protocol-based standard care that did not require the use of a central venous catheter but that used clinician judgment for fluid administration and hypoperfusion, together with a shock index (heart rate/SBP) less than 0.8 and an SBP greater than 100 mm Hg as resuscitation targets; or (3) usual care (treatment according to the bedside physician). There was no difference in 60-day mortality between the treatment arms (early goal-directed therapy 21.0% vs. protocol-based standard care 18.2% vs. usual care 18.9%, p=0.83 for a comparison of the two protocol-based groups combined and the usual care group, p=0.55, for the three-group comparison).

The second published evaluation, the Australasian Resuscitation in Sepsis Evaluation (ARISE) study, also enrolled patients presenting to the emergency department with severe sepsis or septic shock.[15] The study was conducted in both academic and nonacademic centers mainly in Australia and New Zealand, and patients were randomized to early goal-directed therapy (with a protocol very similar to the one used by Rivers and colleagues) or usual care. Patients had to have been initiated on antimicrobials before study entry (eliminating a potential confounder from the study by Rivers and colleagues). There was no difference in 90-day mortality between the treatment arms (early goal-directed therapy 18.6% vs. usual care 18.8%, p=0.90). In addition, there was no difference between treatment arms in prespecified subgroup analyses or mortality rates at different time points (including hospital mortality). Because the enrolled patients had lower severity-of-illness scores and lower mortality at 90 days, it could be suggested that the patients enrolled in this study were less acutely ill than the patients enrolled in the U.S. early goal-directed therapy study. However, about 70% of the patients in the Australasian study had septic shock at randomization (only 54% of patients in the U.S. trial met this criterion), suggesting that the patients were critically ill and the intended population was studied.

The third study, the ProMISe (Protocolised Management in Sepsis) trial, was conducted by the UK Intensive Care National Audit & Research Centre and used a research design identical to that of the ARISE study to evaluate the utility of goal-directed resuscitation.[20] The study enrolled 1,260 patients randomized equally to either early goal-directed therapy or usual care. Similar to the previous studies, no difference in 90-day mortality was seen between those treated with early goal-directed therapy and those treated with usual care (29.5% vs. 29.2%, p=0.90). The mortality rate in this study was in range with the mortality rates from the ARISE and ProCESS studies, all of which were notably lower than in the initial study by Rivers and colleagues. These consistent findings of lower mortality rates in the contemporary studies suggests that care of patients with septic shock has evolved since the Rivers et al. study and that, with ubiquitous early recognition and aggressive resuscitation, protocolized care may no longer be mandatory. Indeed, the progression of care and resultant improvement in outcomes for patients with severe sepsis and septic shock during the past 10–15 years has been remarkable.[21]

The recently published quantitative resuscitation studies highlight the benefits of timely administration of antibiotics and intravenous fluids, which should be a focus of the early care of patients with severe sepsis and septic shock. Quantitative resuscitation efforts and use of monitoring devices should be individualized for patients on the basis of assessments of blood pressure, adequate end-organ perfusion, lack of fluid responsiveness, and adequate oxygen delivery; these components are reviewed in detail in the Shock Syndromes chapter. After an initial fluid challenge, fluid therapy should be continued as long as the patient continues to be fluid responsive. Vasopressors should be applied to initially target a MAP of 65–70 mm Hg, but the MAP goal may subsequently be adjusted if adequate organ perfusion is not attained (particularly in patients with chronic hypertension). Adequate tissue oxygen delivery should be ensured, likely through a combination of lactate clearance and an $Scvo_2$ of 70% or greater as treatment goals.

Other Resuscitation Goals

As discussed in Chapter 10, MAP is the true driving pressure for peripheral blood flow (and end-organ perfusion) and is preferred to SBP as a therapeutic target. A multicenter open-label study randomized patients with septic shock to resuscitation with a MAP goal of either 65–70 mm Hg (low-target group) or 80–85 mm Hg (high-target group).[22] The higher MAP target was achieved through vasopressor administration; patients in the high-target group had a significantly higher infusion rate and longer duration of vasopressors than did patients in the low-target group, but there was no difference between groups in total volume of fluid administration. Nor was there any difference between treatment arms in 28-day mortality (34.0% in the low-target group vs. 36.6% in the high-target group, p=0.57). However, the incidence of atrial fibrillation was significantly higher in the high-target group (6.7% vs. 2.8%, p=0.02). In an a priori–defined subgroup analysis of patients with chronic hypertension (with randomization stratified according to this covariate), those randomized to the high-target group had a lower incidence of a doubling of the serum creatinine concentration (38.9% vs. 52.0%, p=0.02, stratum interaction p=0.009) and less need for renal replacement therapy (31.7% vs. 42.2%, p=0.046, stratum interaction p=0.04). Analyses of these data suggest that an initial MAP goal of 65–70 mm Hg (as suggested in the SSC guidelines) should be used, but the MAP goal may need to be adjusted if the patient has persistent signs of hypoperfusion.

Transfusions of packed red blood cells are often given to patients with shock and evidence of hypoperfusion to increase oxygen delivery. This practice was incorporated into the early goal-directed therapy algorithm from Rivers and colleagues noted earlier (if the hematocrit value was less than 30%) and was previously endorsed by the SSC guidelines. A multicenter study compared two different transfusion thresholds in patients with septic shock.[23] The study enrolled patients with septic shock and a hemoglobin concentration below 9 g/dL to receive a packed red blood cell transfusion if their hemoglobin concentration was 7 g/dL or less (lower threshold) or 9 g/dL or less during their ICU stay. As expected, patients allocated to the lower-threshold group less commonly received a packed red blood cell transfusion and had lower hemoglobin concentrations. There was no difference between treatment arms in 90-day mortality (43.0% in the lower-threshold group vs. 36.6% in the higher-threshold group, p=0.44). Patients in the lower-threshold group did not have a higher incidence of ischemic events in the ICU (7.2% vs. 8.0%, p=0.64), and there was no difference in outcomes between groups in the subgroup of patients with chronic cardiovascular disease (relative risk [RR] 1.08 [95% CI, 0.75–1.40], p=0.25 for heterogeneity of treatment effect by subgroup; only 14% of the overall population had chronic cardiovascular disease). Although the study did not specifically evaluate the practice of transfusing blood in patients with evidence of hypoperfusion (low $Scvo_2$ or elevated lactate concentrations) associated with a low hemoglobin concentration, the median $Scvo_2$ at baseline was less than 70%, and lactate concentrations were greater than 2 mmol/L in both groups, suggesting that most patients had evidence of hypoperfusion. Evaluations of these data suggest that using a hemoglobin transfusion threshold of 7 g/dL or lower is safe for most patients, including those with severe sepsis and septic shock.[24]

Resuscitation targeted to improving microcirculatory perfusion is a potential new therapeutic frontier. Studies have shown the following: microcirculation is often altered in patients with sepsis, persistent microvascular alterations are associated with multisystem organ failure and death, alterations are more severe in non-survivors than in survivors, and improvements in microcirculatory blood flow correspond with improved patient outcomes.[25] Impaired microcirculatory perfusion may at least partly explain why patients have elevated lactate concentrations despite achieving (macrovascular) hemodynamic goals.

Several strategies to improve microcirculatory perfusion have been investigated with mixed results. In a nonrandomized trial, fluid resuscitation improved microvascular perfusion in early, but not late, sepsis.[26] Another study found that microcirculatory perfusion improved with passive leg raising or fluid administration in patients who were fluid responsive.[27] Using vasopressors to increase MAP and tissue perfusion is theoretically attractive, but using norepinephrine to increase MAP to greater than 65 mm Hg has not been associated with correction of impaired microcirculatory perfusion.[28-30] Likewise, vasodilators may induce capillary vasodilation and improve blood flow, but in a randomized trial of patients who underwent quantitative resuscitation, adding nitroglycerin was not associated with improved microcirculatory blood flow. In-hospital mortality was numerically higher in patients allocated to nitroglycerin than in placebo, but this difference was not statistically significant (34.3% vs. 14.2%, p=0.09).[31] In addition, initiating inhaled nitric oxide after quantitative resuscitation did not improve microcirculatory flow or lactate clearance.[32] As such, neither vasopressors nor vasodilators can currently be recommended solely for improving microcirculatory blood flow. Finally, the effects of inodilators (e.g., dobutamine) and a pure inotrope (levosimendan) on microcirculatory blood flow have been studied. A prospective open-label study evaluated the effects of dobutamine 5 mcg/kg/minute initiated after quantitative resuscitation (but within the first 48 hours of presentation). Dobutamine significantly improved microcirculatory perfusion compared with baseline.[33] In a small study, levosimendan improved microcirculatory blood flow more effectively than did dobutamine,[34] but levosimendan is not available for use in the United States. Of interest, the beneficial effects of dobutamine and levosimendan in these studies were unrelated to changes in cardiac index or blood pressure, suggesting a mechanism of benefit separate from (or in addition to) the inotropic effects of the agents. In summary, fluid resuscitation and the initiation of dobutamine appear to improve microcirculatory perfusion, but widespread use of these agents solely to improve microcirculatory blood flow cannot be recommended at this time.[25] Currently, it is still unknown whether using these therapies to improve microcirculatory perfusion can improve patient outcomes such as mortality.

Severe Sepsis and Septic Shock Management Bundle

The SSC guidelines include a core set of initial process steps and treatment goals grouped into a care bundle for the treatment of patients with severe sepsis and septic shock. These bundles were developed as a quality improvement program, in conjunction with the Institute for Healthcare Improvement, with a goal of reducing patient mortality by integrating the recommendations from the SSC guidelines into bedside care. Previous versions of the SSC guidelines included both a resuscitation bundle and a management bundle to be completed within the first 6 hours and 24 hours of presentation, respectively.

As part of a performance improvement initiative (SSC phase III), hospitals were invited to contribute data regarding bundle compliance and patient outcomes in exchange for educational materials and feedback regarding performance. An analysis of more than 15,000 patients from 165 hospitals in Europe, South America, and the United States showed that compliance with both the resuscitation bundle and the management bundle increased linearly each quarter during a 2-year period.[6] Although compliance improved over time, fulfillment of every bundle element at the end of the 2-year observation period was relatively low (31.3% for the resuscitation bundle and 36.1% for the management bundle). During the same observation period, unadjusted hospital mortality decreased from 37% to 30.8% (p=0.001). On multivariate analysis, each quarter that a site participated in the initiative was independently associated with a 3% decrease in hospital mortality (odds ratio [OR] 0.97; 95% CI, 0.96–0.99; p=0.0006). Although a cause-and-effect relationship cannot be established from these data, the association between bundle implementation and decreased mortality suggests that using a care bundle is an effective way to improve the care of patients.

After further analysis of data from SSC phase III, the management bundle was removed, and the resuscitation bundle was broken into two parts (items to be completed within 3 and 6 hours) as a care bundle in the 2012 SSC guidelines. In 2015, in response to the new evidence from the three previously noted quantitative resuscitation studies, the SSC Executive Committee released an update to the SSC bundles.[35] The update acknowledges the findings of the three studies and amends the bundles to use techniques in addition to CVP and $Scvo_2$ to reassess fluid responsiveness and tissue perfusion. These techniques include either use of a repeat focused examination by a licensed practitioner to evaluate for vital signs, cardiopulmonary findings, capillary refill, heart rate, and skin findings or use of at least two of the following: CVP, $Scvo_2$, bedside ultrasonography, or dynamic markers of fluid responsiveness.

A severe sepsis and septic shock care bundle was adopted by the National Quality Forum (NQF)[36] with a goal of improving early recognition and treatment of patients with severe sepsis and septic shock. Of note, the care bundle from the NQF differs from that published in the 2012 SSC guidelines[7] but is very similar to the updated SSC bundle (Box 15.2).[35] The care bundle from the NQF has been adopted by the Centers for Medicare & Medicaid Services as a chart-abstracted quality measure, with reimbursement to be influenced beginning in 2017.[37]

The adjustment of the SSC bundle and the implementation of sepsis as a quality measure will likely lead to a shift in resuscitation approaches for many clinicians. To prepare for and implement this new quality measure, practitioners should systematically evaluate their institutional compliance and implement broad process steps to ensure compliance. These steps may include, but are not limited to, patient identification by clinical decision support tools in the electronic medical record and implementation of care paths and order sets for treatment. The SSC has distributed a guidance document for implementing the 2012 SSC guidelines, which may serve as a valuable resource for initiating and optimizing quality initiatives related to the new quality measure.[38]

Continued Care Beyond Initial Resuscitation

Uncertainty persists regarding resuscitation end points and hemodynamic targets after the first 6 hours of patient presentation. Therapy should be directed toward maintaining adequate end-organ perfusion and normalization of lactate concentrations, but the specific methods to achieve these goals should be patient-specific. A strategy of systematically increasing cardiac output to predefined "supranormal" levels was not associated with a mortality benefit; hence, it is not recommended.[39]

The liberal use of fluid boluses during the early stages of resuscitation should be undertaken with caution beyond the initial hours to avoid giving excessive fluids. In a retrospective analysis of data from a randomized controlled trial of patients with septic shock, patients in the highest quartile of fluid balance had a significantly higher mortality rate than did patients in the lowest two quartiles. This association was present when fluid balance was evaluated at both 12 hours and 4 days after study enrollment. In the same analysis, a CVP greater than 12 mm Hg conferred a higher risk of mortality than did a lower CVP.[40] Fluid administration can be limited by only giving fluid in patients who are proved or predicted to respond to fluid. This is best accomplished using dynamic markers of fluid responsiveness, as discussed in Chapter 10.

ANTIMICROBIALS

Because infection is the underlying cause of septic shock, antimicrobial therapy should be initiated at the same time as initial resuscitation efforts. The SSC guidelines recommend that adequate empiric antibiotics be initiated within 1 hour after recognition of severe sepsis or septic shock.[7] This recommendation is informed by a multicenter, retrospective study of patients with septic shock, which found that within the first 6 hours from the onset of hypotension, each hour of delay in the administration of appropriate antibiotics was associated with a 7.6% decrease in hospital survival.[41] Other studies have further shown the importance of empiric antimicrobials used in conjunction with a quantitative resuscitation protocol, associating the administration of antimicrobials either before shock or within the initial hour of shock with improved survival.[42,43] Source control measures (e.g., drainage of an abscess, debridement of infected necrotic tissue, or removal of a potentially infected device [including intravascular access devices]), as applicable, should also be undertaken as soon as possible (within 12 hours after the diagnosis is made).

Initial empiric therapy should include one or more drugs with activity against all likely pathogens. The most commonly isolated pathogens in critically ill patients are

---

Box 15.2. Severe Sepsis and Septic Shock Management Bundle[a]

Accomplished within 3 hours of presentation[b]
A. Measure lactate concentration
B. Obtain blood cultures before administering antibiotics
C. Administer broad-spectrum antibiotics

If septic shock is present,[c] additional measures to be accomplished within 6 hours of presentation[b]
D. Administer crystalloid 30 mL/kg for hypotension or lactate ≥ 4 mmol/L[d]
E. Apply vasopressors (for hypotension that does not respond to initial fluid resuscitation to maintain a mean arterial blood pressure ≥ 65 mm Hg)
F. If persistent arterial hypotension after initial fluid administration (mean arterial blood pressure < 65 mm Hg) or if initial was lactate ≥ 4 mmol/L, reassess volume status and tissue perfusion, and document findings[e]
G. Remeasure lactate if the initial lactate concentration was elevated[f]

---

[a]Applies to all patients presenting with severe sepsis and septic shock. Patients are excluded from the measure if they have advanced directives for comfort care, if they have clinical conditions that preclude total measure completion (i.e., mortality within the first 6 hours of presentation), if a central line is clinically contraindicated, if a central line was tried but could not be successfully inserted, if a patient or surrogate decision-maker declined or is unwilling to consent to such therapies or central line placement, or if a patient was transferred to an acute care facility from another acute care facility.

[b]Time of presentation is defined as the time of triage in the emergency department or, if the patient is located in another care venue, from the earliest chart annotation consistent with all elements of severe sepsis or septic shock ascertained through chart review.

[c]Septic shock defined as either hypotension (to systolic blood pressure [SBP] less than 90 mm Hg, mean arterial blood pressure less than 70 mm Hg, or an SBP decrease greater than 40 mm Hg for known baseline) or a lactate concentration of 4 mmol/L or greater.

[d]In the Centers for Medicare & Medicaid Services quality measure, crystalloid 30 mL/kg must be administered within 3 hours of presentation if septic shock is present.

[e]To meet the requirements, one of the following must be documented: (1) a focused examination by a licensed independent practitioner, including vital signs, cardiopulmonary, capillary refill, heart rate, and skin findings, or (2) any two of the following: measure central venous pressure, measure central venous oxygen saturation, perform bedside cardiovascular ultrasonography, or perform dynamic assessment of fluid responsiveness with passive leg raise or fluid challenge.

[f]In the Centers for Medicare & Medicaid Services quality measure, this is defined as a lactate concentration ≥ 2 mmol/L.

Information from: Surviving Sepsis Campaign. Updated Bundles in Response to New Evidence [homepage on the Internet]. Available at www.survivingsepsis.org/SiteCollectionDocuments/SSC_Bundle.pdf. Accessed July 23, 2015.

gram-negative bacteria (62%), gram-positive bacteria (47%), and fungi (19%)⁴⁴; a careful analysis of an individual patient's risk factors for each pathogen should be undertaken, with the appropriate therapy administered. In an observational study of more than 5,700 patients with septic shock, patients who received initial appropriate antimicrobials had a significantly higher hospital survival rate than did those who received initial inappropriate antimicrobials (52.0% vs. 10.3%, p<0.0001).[45]

Using combination antibacterial therapy (at least two different classes of antibiotics) increases the likelihood that at least one drug will be effective against the pathogen, particularly in the setting of known or suspected multidrug-resistant organisms such as *Pseudomonas aeruginosa*. Combination therapy is likely indicated for patients who are severely ill with a high baseline chance of mortality, perhaps restricted to those with septic shock. A randomized controlled trial of patients with severe sepsis that allocated patients to meropenem monotherapy or combination therapy with meropenem and moxifloxacin did not detect a difference between groups in mean Sequential Organ Failure Assessment scores over 14 days (7.9 points vs. 8.3 points, p=0.36) or in mortality rates at 28 days or 90 days.[46] Important caveats to this study are that the patient population studied was at a low risk of resistant pathogens (half of the patients had community-acquired infection) and that moxifloxacin does not adequately cover pathogens with a high likelihood for multidrug resistance (e.g., *P. aeruginosa* and *Acinetobacter* spp.). A meta-analysis that included 50 studies and more than 8,500 patients with sepsis did not detect an overall mortality benefit of combination antibacterial therapy compared with monotherapy (pooled OR of death 0.86; 95% CI, 0.71–1.03, p=0.09); however, a stratified analysis showed significantly lower mortality with combination therapy in more severely ill patients (monotherapy risk of death greater than 25%, pooled OR of death with combination therapy 0.54; 95% CI, 0.45–0.66, p<0.001). The benefit of combination therapy was confined to patients with septic shock (with no benefit of combination therapy in patients without shock). In addition, a meta-regression analysis, which tried to elucidate the differences in the benefit seen with combination therapy on the basis of baseline mortality risk, showed a significant benefit of combination therapy with a mortality risk greater than 25%.[47] Analyses of these data suggest that severely ill patients will likely benefit from combination antibacterial therapy. Empiric combination therapy is recommended for a maximum of 3–5 days[7]; the use of combination therapy for definitive treatment is beyond the scope of this chapter.

As noted in Chapter 12, severe sepsis and septic shock can significantly affect the probability of attaining the antimicrobial PK/PD target. Most notably, the volume of distribution of hydrophilic antibiotics (e.g., β-lactams, aminoglycosides, and vancomycin) will be increased. Clearance may either be increased (in the setting of augmented renal clearance) or decreased (in the presence of end-organ dysfunction).[48] A PK/PD study of the first dose of β-lactams in patients with severe sepsis and septic shock suggested that the PK/PD target was attained in less than 50% of the patients given ceftazidime 2 g (28% target attainment), cefepime 2 g (16%), and piperacillin/tazobactam 4 g/0.5 g (44%). The PK/PD target was attained in 75% of patients receiving meropenem 1 g. For each antibiotic, the volume of distribution was higher and the clearance was lower than in healthy volunteers.[49] Similarly, a multicenter cross-sectional study of β-lactam concentrations in critically ill patients found that the minimum PK/PD target of at least 50% of free drug time above the minimum inhibitory concentration (MIC) (50% $fT>MIC$) was not achieved in 16% of patients with an infection. Of importance, achievement of 50% $fT>MIC$ or 100% $fT>MIC$ was independently associated with a higher likelihood of a positive outcome on multivariable analysis (OR 1.02; 95% CI, 1.01–1.04 and OR 1.56; 95% CI, 1.15–2.13, respectively).[50] Analyses of these data suggest that a loading dose approach for these antibiotics in patients with severe sepsis and septic shock is likely necessary. In addition, the impact of methods to improve the $fT>MIC$ should be studied further.

Antimicrobial therapy should be evaluated on a daily basis to determine whether opportunities for de-escalation or discontinuation exist. Continued use of broad-spectrum antimicrobial therapy may cause untoward adverse effects and promote the development of resistant pathogens. Whether to use de-escalation may be a clear-cut decision in infections in which a contributive pathogen has been identified; in such cases, antimicrobial therapy should be reduced to the narrowest-spectrum agent with adequate activity. However, de-escalation may be more challenging in patients with culture-negative sepsis, where clinical judgment, baseline suggestion of infection, local pathogen epidemiology, and likely source will dictate further changes in antimicrobials. For patients with proven or high suggestion of infection, antimicrobials are typically continued for 7–10 days,[7] although longer courses may be indicated in patients with a poor clinical response, those with bacteremia, and those who are immunocompromised.

Procalcitonin has been studied as a tool to assist with clinical decisions regarding antibiotic use and duration, and its use was endorsed as a low-level (grade 2C) recommendation by the 2012 SSC guidelines.[7] The assay and corresponding algorithms have been evaluated for antibiotic initiation, antibiotic cessation, and the combination of both strategies. These strategies assume PCT availability from an institutional laboratory. If the PCT turnaround time is more than 24 hours, the effects of minimizing antimicrobial treatment days may be limited. According to current evidence, PCT should not routinely be measured in patients without signs and symptoms of infection. The decision to initiate patients on antibiotics without signs and symptoms of infection using PCT alone would probably lead to antimicrobial overuse and possible adverse effects associated with antimicrobial therapy. In the largest PCT study of critically ill patients to date, 1,200 patients were randomized to either a PCT alert strategy or standard of care. For those randomized to intervention, a PCT concentration greater than 1.0 mcg/L generated an alert that mandated clinical intervention, which included use of microbiological cultures, additional radiologic assessment, and initiation or expansion of antimicrobial coverage. Overall, this strategy did not lead to an improvement in mortality or time to appropriate antibiotics. However, patients had a greater need for mechanical ventilation, a prolonged ICU length of stay, and prolonged antibiotic use.[51]

In critically ill patients with signs and symptoms of infection, including those with severe sepsis and septic shock, a baseline PCT (at the time of the symptoms) should not be used to determine whether antibiotics should be initiated. Withholding antimicrobials in patients with severe sepsis and septic shock and a low PCT concentration may have severe negative consequences. In addition, the compliance rate for withholding antibiotics for a low PCT in this scenario has consistently been low in randomized studies. The compliance rate in clinical practice is likely even lower than that in clinical studies; however, this has not been evaluated. If a baseline PCT is obtained, it should only be used to trend the PCT concentration for possible early discontinuation of antibiotics. In a study of patients with signs and symptoms of infections to determine whether a PCT-guided strategy would limit the initiation of antibiotics, no difference in antibiotic use was seen.[52] However, this finding was likely confounded by a 36% clinician compliance rate with the recommendation to withhold antimicrobials when the PCT was low. This is in sharp contrast to the 86% compliance rate with the recommendation to initiate antibiotics when the PCT was high.

It may be helpful to obtain a baseline PCT for trending purposes in critically ill patients with signs and symptoms of infection. A low PCT (or a substantial decrease from baseline) during antibiotic treatment should be used to shorten the duration of antimicrobial therapy.[7] This can be accomplished by either eliminating unnecessary antibiotics in patients without signs and symptoms of infection or shortening the course of therapy for patients with an infection. Several studies have evaluated the utility of a PCT-guided strategy for determining the appropriate time to discontinue or de-escalate antibiotics.[53-60] These studies consistently show that PCT guidance for discontinuing antimicrobial therapy led to decreases in antibiotic use without an untoward outcome effect.[61] This has also been shown in various ICU patient populations with differing severity of illness, including patients with severe sepsis and septic shock. Ideally, if a PCT algorithm is implemented, it should be combined with formalized antimicrobial stewardship efforts. In fact, when a PCT algorithm was combined with twice-weekly infectious stewardship rounds in a randomized trial aimed at limiting the duration of antibiotics, compliance with PCT algorithm recommendations was greater than 97%.[58] Many different PCT guidance algorithms exist; Figure 15.3 represents a reasonable approach to using PCT for antibiotic cessation.

AGENTS USED TO TREAT SHOCK

Fluid Therapy

Crystalloids

Resuscitation fluids are commonly given for patients in the ICU, with 37% of patients receiving this therapy in a 24-hour period in a cross-sectional study.[62] Crystalloids (i.e., 0.9% sodium chloride or lactated Ringer solution) are the initial fluid type of choice,[7] particularly for an initial fluid challenge. The Saline versus Albumin Fluid Evaluation (SAFE) study compared 0.9% sodium chloride with 4% albumin in a heterogeneous ICU population of almost 7,000 patients. Overall, the study did not detect a difference in 28-day mortality between groups (20.9% vs. 21.1%, p=0.87).[63] Of note, however, this was not a study of strictly initial fluid resuscitation because the allocated study fluid was used for all fluid resuscitation in the ICU until death, discharge, or 28 days after randomization. Despite some limitations, evaluations of these data have informed the SSC recommendation of crystalloids as the initial fluid type, particularly given their low cost.

Crystalloid solutions with relatively low chloride content ("chloride-poor" or "balanced salt" solutions) are an attractive alternative to 0.9% sodium chloride (see Chapter 10 for further discussion). Administration of chloride-rich fluids may lead to afferent renal arteriole vasoconstriction (leading to a decrease in renal perfusion and kidney injury) and may cause a metabolic acidosis by lowering the strong ion difference. As such, crystalloids that better approximate the electrolyte composition of plasma (e.g., lactated Ringer solution) have been evaluated. A propensity-matched retrospective cohort study of medical ICU patients with sepsis found that receipt of a balanced solution compared with 0.9% sodium chloride was associated with a lower incidence of in-hospital mortality (19.6% vs. 22.8%, p=0.001). Unlike in analyses of general critical care patients, this study did not detect a difference in the incidence of acute renal failure between groups, which leads to questions regarding the mechanism of the detected mortality difference between groups.[64] In addition, a recently published systematic review and network meta-analysis of patients with sepsis suggested a lower mortality rate in patients resuscitated with balanced solutions than in patients resuscitated with 0.9% sodium chloride (OR 0.78, credibility interval 0.58–1.05; low confidence in estimate of effect).[65] Balanced salt solutions are not without adverse effects; they may lead to hyponatremia and hypotonicity (with lactated Ringer solution) or cardiotoxicity (with acetate-containing solutions) when administered

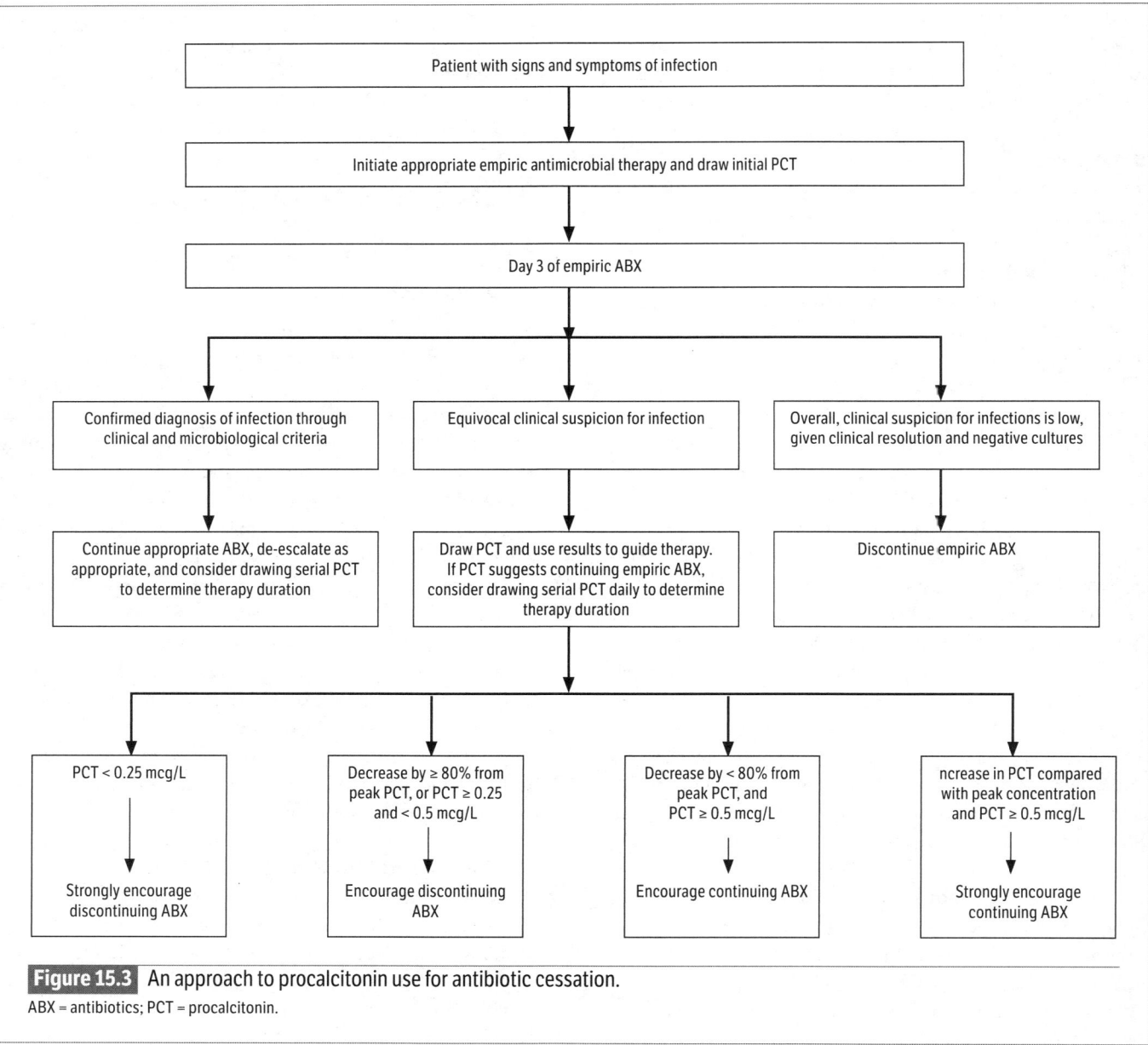

Figure 15.3 An approach to procalcitonin use for antibiotic cessation.
ABX = antibiotics; PCT = procalcitonin.

in large volumes. Although intriguing, analyses of these data do not definitively support the benefit of balanced salt solutions, and a large randomized trial comparing these crystalloid solutions is eagerly awaited.

Colloids

Albumin for Resuscitation

Iso-oncotic (4%–5%) albumin may be used as a component of the fluid resuscitation strategy. Despite decades of research, though, the choice between crystalloids and albumin for fluid resuscitation in patients with severe sepsis and septic shock remains controversial. A prospectively defined subgroup analysis of the SAFE study evaluated the effect of albumin 4% compared with that of 0.9% sodium chloride in patients with severe sepsis and septic shock. The unadjusted RR of death with albumin was 0.87 (95% CI, 0.74–1.02) in patients with severe sepsis and 1.05 (95% CI, 0.94–1.17) in patients without severe sepsis (p=0.06 for heterogeneity of treatment effect by subgroup). In a multivariate analysis that accounted for baseline factors, albumin was associated with a lower mortality risk (OR 0.71; 95% CI, 0.52–0.97; p=0.03).[66] A systematic review and fixed-effect meta-analysis of albumin compared with alternative fluids for resuscitation in patients with sepsis found an association between albumin use and lower mortality (OR 0.82; 95% CI, 0.67–1.0; p=0.047). The benefit of albumin was retained when the analysis was restricted to crystalloids as the comparator (OR 0.78; 95% CI, 0.62–0.99; p=0.04). These data should be interpreted with caution, however, because many of the included studies had poor methodological quality, and when a random-effects model was used, the results for the overall analysis were not statistically significant (OR 0.84; 95% CI, 0.69–1.02, p=0.08).

These data have renewed interest in 4%–5% albumin as a resuscitation fluid for patients with severe sepsis and septic shock. Indeed, the 2012 SSC guidelines suggest albumin as a component of the fluid resuscitation regimen when patients require a substantial amount of crystalloids.[7]

Many clinicians find this recommendation from the SSC challenging to implement into practice because there is no clear definition of a "substantial amount" of crystalloids, and the recommendation is weak with low-quality evidence (grade 2C). Proponents of crystalloids note the predominant use of crystalloids in quantitative resuscitation studies, the patient enrollment after initial resuscitation in most studies in the previously noted meta-analysis, the lack of a prospective study favoring albumin that enrolled only patients with severe sepsis, and the high cost of albumin. Advocates for albumin note its more efficacious plasma volume expansion, its non-fluid (e.g., ligand binding and antioxidant) properties, and the subgroup and meta-analysis findings noted earlier. Until further data are available, it seems reasonable to use crystalloids preferentially to iso-oncotic albumin for initial fluid resuscitation, particularly for the initial fluid challenge.

If a component of a patient's fluid resuscitation strategy includes colloids, it may be challenging to calculate the total amount of "crystalloid-equivalent" fluid a patient has received. This is particularly important when colloids are used as a component of initial resuscitation and at least 30 mL/kg of crystalloid must be administered. Approximate intravenous fluid equivalencies for crystalloids and colloids are included in Table 15.2 to assist with this calculation.[67]

Hydroxyethyl Starch for Resuscitation

Synthetic colloids such as hydroxyethyl starch (HES) have been suggested as an alternative therapy for fluid resuscitation. Two large studies comparing resuscitation with HES to resuscitation with crystalloids in patients having severe sepsis and septic shock have been completed with similar findings (studies evaluating HES in nonselected critically ill patients are discussed in Chapter 10). In the first study, patients with severe sepsis who were allocated to pentastarch (a HES formulation) had a significantly higher incidence of acute renal failure (34.9% vs. 22.8%, p=0.002) and a greater need for renal replacement therapy (31.0% vs. 18.8%, p=0.001) than did patients with severe sepsis allocated to lactated Ringer solution, with no difference in 28-day mortality (26.7% vs. 24.1%, p=0.48).[68] In a more recent study, patients with severe sepsis randomized to receive HES had a significantly higher 90-day mortality (51% vs. 43%, p=0.03) and need for renal replacement therapy (22% vs. 16%, p=0.04) than did patients with severe sepsis randomized to receive Ringer acetate solution.[69] The findings in this study did not appear to depend on the time duration between ICU admission and study enrollment, surgery, type of fluid given before randomization, or markers of shock severity in a post hoc subgroup analysis.[70] A systematic review and meta-analysis of tetrastarch (a HES formulation) in patients with severe sepsis found an association between HES use and 90-day mortality (RR 1.13; 95% CI, 1.02–1.25; p=0.02), renal replacement therapy (RR 1.42; 95% CI, 1.09–1.85; p=0.01), and blood product transfusion (RR 1.21; 95% CI, 1.08–1.36; p=0.001).[71] The increased mortality and increased need for renal replacement therapy led to a strong recommendation against the use of HES for fluid resuscitation in patients with severe sepsis and septic shock in the 2012 SSC guidelines.[7]

Albumin Replacement

Hyperoncotic (20%–25%) albumin replacement may be beneficial in patients with septic shock. An open-label study compared albumin replacement (with 20% albumin) with a goal serum albumin concentration of 3 g/dL plus crystalloid solution administration with crystalloid solution administration alone in patients with severe sepsis or septic shock. There was no difference between the albumin and crystalloid groups in the incidence of 28-day mortality (31.8% vs. 32.0%, p=0.94), but patients allocated

Table 15.2 Crystalloid and Colloid Equivalency Chart

Fluid	Equivalent Dose[a]
0.9% sodium chloride	20 mL/kg
Lactated Ringer solution	20 mL/kg
Albumin	0.24 g/kg
4%–5% albumin	5.2 mL/kg
20%–25% albumin	1.1 mL/kg
Hetastarch	0.29 g/kg
3% hetastarch	9.7 mL/kg
6% hetastarch	4.8 mL/kg
10% hetastarch	2.9 mL/kg
10% pentastarch	0.30 g/kg (3 mL/kg)
10% dextran-40	0.30 g/kg (3 mL/kg)
3% dextran-60, 6% dextran-70	0.19 g/kg
3% dextran-60	6.3 mL/kg
6% dextran-70	3.1 mL/kg
Gelatins (succinylated and crosslinked 2.5, 3.0, 4.0%; urea linked 3.5%)	0.23 g/kg

[a]For percentage solutions, listed milligrams per kilogram were calculated from the grams per kilogram data.

Information from: American Thoracic Society. Evidence-based colloid use in the critically ill: American Thoracic Society consensus statement. Am J Respir Crit Care Med 2004;170:1247-59.

to albumin had a shorter time to cessation of vasoactive agents (median 3 days vs. 4 days, p=0.007). A post hoc subgroup analysis of patients with septic shock at enrollment showed that those randomized to albumin had a lower 90-day mortality rate (RR 0.87; 95% CI, 0.77–0.99); there was no difference in 90-day mortality in patients without septic shock (RR 1.13; 95% CI, 0.92–1.39; p=0.03 for heterogeneity).[72] Of note, in multivariable analysis, depending on which variables were entered into the model, the significant difference in 90-day mortality was no longer seen. Analyses of these data suggest that albumin replacement does not improve outcomes in patients with severe sepsis but that albumin replacement may have hemodynamic (and potentially mortality) advantages in patients with septic shock. Hence, the role of albumin replacement in patients with septic shock warrants further study.

Vasoactive Agents and Inotropes

Catecholamine Vasopressors

Vasoactive agents should be initiated in patients who have signs of end-organ hypoperfusion despite fluid resuscitation, with the goal of attaining an initial MAP of 65 mm Hg. Selecting the most appropriate drug depends on the goal of therapy: either to increase systemic vascular resistance (for which vasopressors are used) or to improve cardiac output (for which inotropes are used). Norepinephrine and dopamine have traditionally been the go-to vasopressors for patients with septic shock, although no strong data existed to guide selection between the two. However, a large, randomized trial compared blinded norepinephrine and dopamine administration in patients with shock (62% had septic shock). Overall, there was no significant difference in 28-day mortality between the norepinephrine and dopamine groups (48.5% vs. 52.5%, p=0.10). Of importance, however, patients randomized to norepinephrine had significantly fewer days on vasopressors and a lower incidence of arrhythmias (12.4% vs. 24.1%, p<0.001).[5] In addition, a meta-analysis of randomized trials that compared norepinephrine with dopamine for the treatment of patients with septic shock found a higher risk of short-term mortality (RR 1.12; 95% CI, 1.01–1.20; p=0.035) and arrhythmias (RR 2.34; 95% CI, 1.46–3.77; p=0.001) in patients allocated to dopamine.[73] In light of these data, the SSC strongly recommends norepinephrine as the first-choice vasopressor in patients with septic shock.

The optimal approach to using vasoactive agents and inotropes beyond the choice of initial vasopressor is unclear, but the choice should be based on patient-specific clinical factors. Potential interventions could include the use of norepinephrine monotherapy (with appropriate dose escalation) or the initiation of an additional therapy (i.e., a second catecholamine vasopressor, arginine vasopressin, corticosteroids, an inotrope, or a combination of these therapies). The optimal time or norepinephrine dose at which to consider additional therapies is unknown. Moreover, a dose that constitutes the failure of norepinephrine is not well defined in the literature, and the maximal doses used by clinicians (or institutions) are variable and often subjective.

The SSC guidelines recommend epinephrine (added to or potentially substituted for norepinephrine) when a vasoactive agent is needed in addition to norepinephrine. Although epinephrine is not commonly used in the United States, its use in Europe and other parts of the world is more common because of its relatively low cost. Two large studies have compared the effects of epinephrine with those of norepinephrine in patients with shock. In the first study, patients with septic shock were randomized to norepinephrine with or without dobutamine or epinephrine. There was no difference between groups in 28-day mortality (40% vs. 34%, p=0.31), but patients allocated to epinephrine had significantly higher lactate concentrations on day 1 (p=0.003) and lower arterial pH values on each of the first 4 study days.[74] Caution should be used in concluding that a difference in mortality between epinephrine and norepinephrine does not exist because the study was powered to detect a 20% absolute difference in mortality rates, and a smaller difference between agents cannot be ruled out. In a second study of patients with mixed shock types (55% had septic shock) randomized to norepinephrine or epinephrine, there was no difference between agents in the time to achievement of a goal MAP (median 40 hours vs. 35.1 hours, p=0.26) or in the median number of vasopressor-free days at day 28 (25.4 days vs. 26.0 days, p=0.31). Patients allocated to epinephrine, though, had higher heart rates and lactic acid concentrations on the first study day (but not on subsequent days) and were more often withdrawn from the study by the treating clinician (12.9% vs. 2.8%, p=0.002).[75] Analyses of these data suggest that epinephrine offers no efficacy benefits over norepinephrine and that epinephrine is associated with an increased incidence of adverse effects (at least initially).

The benefit of adding epinephrine to norepinephrine (whether this approach has a norepinephrine-sparing effect or whether it is best used in norepinephrine failure) is unclear. Although norepinephrine may cause tachycardia or tachyarrhythmias (often the impetus to limit doses), adding catecholamine vasopressors with β_1-adrenergic properties such as epinephrine to augment MAP in patients receiving norepinephrine is unlikely to prevent these tachyarrhythmias. In addition, epinephrine may preclude the use of lactate clearance as an initial resuscitation goal because epinephrine increases lactate concentrations through increased production by aerobic glycolysis (by stimulating skeletal muscle β_2-adrenergic receptors), an effect that likely wanes with continued epinephrine administration. It seems most prudent to use epinephrine in patients receiving norepinephrine with a low MAP and requiring cardiac output augmentation. Dobutamine may be an acceptable option in this scenario as well.

Phenylephrine, essentially a sole α_1-adrenergic receptor augmenter, is an attractive alternative for patients who develop tachyarrhythmias on norepinephrine. Because of its profound afterload augmentation effects (without β_1-adrenergic properties), phenylephrine may theoretically decrease stroke volume and cardiac output. As such, it is not recommended as a first-line vasopressor in patients with septic shock who have decreased cardiac output because of inadequate preload. A small study (n=32) that randomized patients with septic shock to phenylephrine or norepinephrine as first-line therapy found no difference in hemodynamic measures (including cardiac output) between agents in the first 12 hours of therapy.[76] Evaluations of these data contrast the theoretical concerns with phenylephrine, which warrants further study in larger trials. The SSC guidelines recommend that phenylephrine be reserved for the patients with the following: (1) a tachyarrhythmia on norepinephrine, (2) a confirmed high cardiac output with a blood pressure that is still low despite use of norepinephrine, or (3) an unachieved goal MAP with other vasoactive agents, including low-dose arginine vasopressin.

Dopamine is best used in a select patient population, including patients with a low risk of tachyarrhythmias (which is difficult to predict) and those with bradycardia-induced hypotension. Low-dose ("renal dose" 2 mcg/kg/minute) dopamine should not be used to improve renal blood flow and urine output (renal protection).[77]

Vasopressin

Arginine vasopressin offers an alternative mechanism of vasoconstriction to the α_1-adrenergic receptor augmenting actions of catecholamines. Vasopressin constricts vascular smooth muscle directly (through actions on the V_1 receptor) and indirectly (by decreased nitric oxide–mediated vasodilation). In patients with septic shock, a relative vasopressin deficiency may exist, and patients are sensitive to the vasoconstrictive effects of arginine vasopressin. In light of these effects, arginine vasopressin has been used in patients with septic shock as both an endocrine replacement therapy (with a fixed-dose infusion) and a vasopressor (titrated to MAP). A randomized trial compared the effects of adding arginine vasopressin (0.01–0.03 unit/minute) to norepinephrine with the effects of norepinephrine monotherapy. Overall, the study found no difference in 28-day mortality between treatment arms (35.4% vs. 39.3%, p=0.26), but norepinephrine requirements were significantly lower during the first 4 study days in the patients allocated to receive arginine vasopressin (p<0.001). There was no difference in adverse effects between groups. In an a priori–defined subgroup analysis of patients based on shock severity (less-severe shock defined as a baseline norepinephrine dose of 5–14 mcg/minute), with randomization stratified according to this covariate, 28-day mortality in the less-severe shock stratum was lower in patients randomized to arginine vasopressin plus norepinephrine (26.5% vs. 35.7%, p=0.05) and no different between groups in the more-severe shock stratum (44.0% vs. 42.5%, p=0.76, stratum interaction p=0.10).

To further investigate the effects of high-dose arginine vasopressin, a study of patients with vasodilatory shock (about half with septic shock) requiring high-dose norepinephrine (greater than 0.6 mcg/kg/minute) randomized patients to arginine vasopressin 0.033 unit/minute versus arginine vasopressin 0.067 unit/minute. The study was designed to evaluate hemodynamic changes, not mortality. Patients randomized to the higher arginine vasopressin dose had a more pronounced reduction in norepinephrine requirements than did those allocated to the lower arginine vasopressin dose (p=0.006).[78] High-dose arginine vasopressin did not lead to a significantly lower cardiac index than did low-dose arginine vasopressin (as might be anticipated), but this finding is difficult to interpret because most patients in the study were receiving concomitant inotropes, and the study was likely underpowered to assess this outcome. Of note, however, large studies evaluating the efficacy and safety of high-dose arginine vasopressin have not been conducted, and this dosing strategy should be reserved for salvage therapy. In the setting of salvage therapy, each additional therapy (e.g., phenylephrine, epinephrine, high-dose arginine vasopressin) has the potential for negative consequences, which the clinician should carefully consider during the therapeutic decision-making process.

Conflicting findings regarding the effects of arginine vasopressin (and its analogs) on mortality have been seen in meta-analyses. One meta-analysis found a decreased mortality risk in patients with septic shock allocated to arginine vasopressin (RR 0.87; 95% CI, 0.75–1.0; p=0.05),[79] whereas another found no significant benefit with arginine vasopressin (RR 0.91; 95% CI, 0.79–1.05; p=0.21).[80] Both meta-analyses found a significant benefit of arginine vasopressin in decreasing norepinephrine doses. Despite the unclear benefits of arginine vasopressin on mortality, this agent offers an alternative mechanism to catecholamines for vasoconstriction, and low-dose arginine vasopressin is commonly used in practice (often as the second vasoactive medication).[81] In an ungraded recommendation, the 2012 SSC guidelines recommend adding arginine vasopressin (up to 0.03 unit/minute) to norepinephrine, with the intent of raising the MAP to goal or sparing norepinephrine.

Prospective randomized studies have shown no significant difference in the rate of adverse effects when catecholamine monotherapy was compared with the addition of arginine vasopressin to catecholamines. Similar to phenylephrine, arginine vasopressin is a pure vasoconstrictor and may decrease stroke volume and cardiac output. Thus, the previously mentioned randomized trial excluded patients with acute coronary syndrome or underlying chronic heart failure (New York Heart Association class III or IV). Vasopressin should be used with caution in patients with these disorders or with low cardiac output from other causes. Concerns for severe adverse effects (mainly cardiac arrest) from arginine vasopressin doses above 0.03–0.04 unit/minute have largely been based on retrospective, noncomparative reports when causality could not be established.[82]

Inotropes

A low cardiac output is common in early septic shock, but this is often corrected with fluid resuscitation alone. However, myocardial dysfunction may persist despite fluid resuscitation, with 39% of patients having left ventricular hypokinesia on ICU admission, despite fluid resuscitation, and an additional 21% with hypokinesia developing 24–48 hours after ICU admission (potentially attributable to norepinephrine) in one series.[83] Patients with signs of hypoperfusion despite adequate cardiac filling pressures, MAP, and hemoglobin concentration should have an assessment of cardiac output (i.e., echocardiography, arterial pressure waveform analysis, or pulmonary artery catheterization). If myocardial dysfunction leads to significant impairment in oxygen delivery, an inotrope such as dobutamine may be indicated to improve cardiac output. Variable effects on systemic hemodynamics have been seen in studies of dobutamine administration in unselected patients with septic shock.[84,85] Indeed, the SSC guidelines recommend that a trial of dobutamine infusion (up to 20 mcg/kg/minute) be administered or added to the vasopressor (if in use) only in patients with the presence of (1) myocardial dysfunction, as suggested by elevated cardiac filling pressures and low cardiac output; or (2) ongoing signs of hypoperfusion, despite adequate intravascular volume and adequate MAP. However, this recommendation is based on low-quality evidence. Dobutamine has commonly been used as a component of quantitative resuscitation to increase $Scvo_2$; this approach must be individualized, and the decision to initiate dobutamine should include evidence of end-organ perfusion (e.g., elevated lactate concentrations and low urine output) as noted earlier.

Corticosteroids

For patients with septic shock, corticosteroids are an attractive treatment option because of their anti-inflammatory effects (through inhibition of NF-κB) and their ability to improve blood pressure response to catecholamines (through up-regulation of adrenergic receptors and potentiation of vasoconstrictor actions). However, using corticosteroids for patients with septic shock has been a source of controversy for many years. In studies of short courses of high-dose corticosteroids in patients with severe sepsis and septic shock, corticosteroids did not lead to improved patient outcomes and may have increased mortality.[86] Two large studies have evaluated the effects of longer courses of low-dose corticosteroids. In the first study, a French trial of patients with septic shock and vasopressor-unresponsive shock (i.e., inability to increase SBP greater than 90 mm Hg for 1 hour despite fluids and vasopressors), those randomized to low-dose hydrocortisone and fludrocortisone had improved survival in a time-to-event analysis (hazard ratio 0.71; 95% CI, 0.53–0.97) and time-to-shock reversal.[87] The mortality benefit with corticosteroids was limited to patients unable to increase their cortisol concentration by more than 9 mcg/dL in response to adrenocorticotropic hormone administration (nonresponders). In the second study—the larger, multicenter Corticosteroid Therapy for Septic Shock (CORTICUS) study, which had less-stringent inclusion criteria—hydrocortisone administration was not associated with improved survival in adrenocorticotropic hormone nonresponders (28-day mortality 39.2% vs. 36.1%, p=0.69).[88] However, patient inclusion in the two trials was quite different, as shown by a placebo-arm 28-day mortality rate of 61% in the French study[87] and a corresponding mortality rate of 31% in the CORTICUS study.[88] These differences in patient characteristics suggest that severity of illness affects the benefit (or lack thereof) of corticosteroids in altering mortality in patients with septic shock.

In a meta-analysis of only high-quality trials, corticosteroid administration was not associated with improved survival in the overall analysis. When patients were analyzed according to severity of illness, a systematic review of three randomized controlled trials did not detect a mortality benefit with corticosteroid use in patients at a low risk of death (placebo mortality rate less than 50%). In those with a high risk of death (placebo mortality rate greater than 60%), there was a numerical, although not statistically significant, mortality benefit with corticosteroid use (RR 0.77; 95% CI, 0.56–1.05).[7] Another meta-analysis also found a significant relationship between severity of illness and patient outcomes with corticosteroids; low-dose corticosteroids were harmful in less severely ill patients and beneficial in more severely ill patients.[86] In meta-analyses, corticosteroid administration has consistently been associated with improvements in shock reversal, but, as noted previously, this has not led to a consistent benefit on patient mortality. These findings have further fueled the controversy regarding the role of corticosteroids in patients with septic shock. The SSC guidelines recommend that corticosteroids be used only in patients with septic shock who do not achieve resuscitation goals despite fluid resuscitation and vasopressors, but these guidelines do not explicitly define poor response to initial therapy. If a clinician were considering adding corticosteroids to decrease a patient's mortality risk, it would seem prudent to initiate corticosteroids in severely ill patients. One approach to operationalize the SSC guideline recommendation is to reserve corticosteroids only for patients receiving norepinephrine doses greater than 40 mcg/minute (the mean maximal norepinephrine dose in the CORTICUS study was about this dose).

When corticosteroid use is deemed appropriate, hydrocortisone (without fludrocortisone) should be initiated immediately. Because of immunoassay imprecision and the inconsistent benefit of identifying patient response, the adrenocorticotropic hormone test should not be used to identify patients for corticosteroid administration.[7] Unfortunately, the optimal dose, administration method, and therapy duration of hydrocortisone have not been fully elucidated. Although different hydrocortisone doses have not directly been compared in studies, 200 mg/day is now the dosage recommended by the SSC guidelines. Emerging data suggest that even this lower dose is too aggressive because of impaired hydrocortisone clearance in critically ill patients.[89]

In low-level (grade 2D) recommendations, the SSC guidelines suggest that hydrocortisone be administered as a continuous infusion (rather than as a bolus injection) to avoid glucose fluctuations; the guidelines also suggest that hydrocortisone be tapered, to avoid rebound hypotension or inflammation, when patients no longer require vasopressors. Clinicians must balance the potential benefit of decreased glucose variability with the need for dedicated intravenous access and drug y-site incompatibility with a hydrocortisone infusion. In addition, tapered doses will likely lead to longer treatment courses, and thus, adverse effects may occur more often with prolonged corticosteroid administration.

SUPPORTIVE THERAPIES

Drotrecogin alfa (activated), or recombinant human activated protein C, was used for more than a decade as the only therapy with a U.S. Food and Drug Administration–approved labeling for use in severe sepsis. However, clinical controversy regarding the risk-benefit ratio surrounded the agent, leading to the completion of another placebo-controlled phase III trial. Patients with septic shock and clinical evidence of hypoperfusion were randomized to receive a drotrecogin alfa or placebo infusion for 96 hours. There was no difference in 28-day mortality between the drotrecogin alfa and placebo groups (26.4% vs. 24.2%, p=0.31). Nonserious bleeding events were higher in patients allocated to drotrecogin alfa (8.6% vs. 4.2%, p=0.002); there was no difference between groups in the rate of serious bleeding.[12] In light of these findings, the manufacturer of drotrecogin alfa voluntarily withdrew the agent from the market in October 2011.

Infusion of intravenous immunoglobulins in patients with severe sepsis and septic shock has the potential to neutralize bacterial antigens (e.g., endotoxin from gram-negative bacteria) and modulate the inflammatory response. However, randomized controlled trials and meta-analyses have yielded conflicting results regarding the effect of intravenous immunoglobulins on patient outcomes. Indeed, the largest randomized study of adult patients with severe sepsis did not detect a difference in 28-day mortality between patients allocated to intravenous immunoglobulin G or placebo (39.3% vs. 37.3%, p=0.67).[90] However, a meta-analysis that analyzed the effect of immunoglobulin infusion in adults, children, and neonates found an association between immunoglobulin infusion and lower mortality (RR 0.79; 95% CI, 0.69–0.90; p≤0.0003).[91] This meta-analysis did not use strict criteria to identify sources of bias and did not explicitly state the criteria used for assessing trial quality. In another meta-analysis, when only high-quality studies were considered, there was no association between immunoglobulin infusion and mortality (RR 0.96; 95% CI, 0.71–1.30; p=0.78).[92] However, there seems to be a difference in patient response between intravenous immunoglobulin preparations, with products containing immunoglobulins G, M, and A having superior benefits to those containing only immunoglobulin G.[93] Of note, the intravenous immunoglobulin products available in the United States do not have immunoglobulin M, and they contain low levels of immunoglobulin A. In light of the conflicting data, the SSC guidelines suggest not using intravenous immunoglobulins for the treatment of patients with severe sepsis and septic shock.[7]

TREATMENT PATHWAYS AND ORDER SETS

The SSC guidelines provide no explicit instructions for the timing and addition of particular pharmacotherapeutic agents for every patient. Instead, the approach should be individualized while incorporating the recommendations from guidelines and the data from the primary literature. A treatment pathway should provide the flexibility to initiate appropriate agents according to an assessment of altered hemodynamic parameters. Using an order set is one way to increase compliance with treatment pathways and guideline recommendations. Grouping of specific orders into an order set can help users operationalize the approach outlined in a treatment pathway.

Implementing order sets for the treatment of severe sepsis and septic shock can improve treatment processes and patient outcomes. In fact, several studies have noted increased volume of fluid administered within the first 6 hours of patient presentation, decreased time to antibiotic initiation, and even decreased mortality after order set implementation.[94,95] Educating all patient caregivers regarding the components of the order set is essential to the success of the endeavor.

CONCLUSION

Severe sepsis and septic shock are associated with high patient mortality and morbidity. Optimal treatment of these patients is complex and requires frequent patient reassessment. Treatment of patients with severe sepsis and septic shock requires timely application of evidence-based therapies, as outlined in the SSC guidelines. Translating the literature and treatment principles described in these guidelines to bedside care while incorporating an assessment of patient-specific data is necessary to design a comprehensive pharmacotherapeutic care plan for the patient with severe sepsis or septic shock.

REFERENCES

1. Levy MM, Fink MP, Marshall JC, et al. 2001 SCCM/ESICM/ACCP/ATS/SIS international sepsis definitions conference. Crit Care Med 2003;31:1250-6.
2. Gaieski DF, Edwards JM, Kallan MJ, et al. Benchmarking the incidence and mortality of severe sepsis in the United States. Crit Care Med 2013;41:1167-74.
3. Karlsson S, Ruokonen E, Varpula T, et al. Long-term outcome and quality-adjusted life years after severe sepsis. Crit Care Med 2009;37:1268-74.
4. Martin GS, Mannino DM, Eaton S, et al. The epidemiology of sepsis in the United States from 1979 through 2000. N Engl J Med 2003;348:1546-54.
5. De Backer D, Biston P, Devriendt J, et al. Comparison of dopamine and norepinephrine in the treatment of shock. N Engl J Med 2010;362:779-89.
6. Levy MM, Dellinger RP, Townsend SR, et al. The Surviving Sepsis Campaign: results of an international guideline-based performance improvement program targeting severe sepsis. Crit Care Med 2010;38:367-74.
7. Dellinger RP, Levy MM, Rhodes A, et al. Surviving Sepsis Campaign: international guidelines for management of severe sepsis and septic shock: 2012. Crit Care Med 2013;41:580-637.
8. Angus DC, van der Poll T. Severe sepsis and septic shock. N Engl J Med 2013;369:840-51.
9. Landry DW, Oliver JA. The pathogenesis of vasodilatory shock. N Engl J Med 2001;345:588-95.
10. Cunha BA. Sepsis and septic shock: selection of empiric antimicrobial therapy. Crit Care Clin 2008;24:313-34, ix.
11. Zhao H, Heard SO, Mullen MT, et al. An evaluation of the diagnostic accuracy of the 1991 American College of Chest Physicians/Society of Critical Care Medicine and the 2001 Society of Critical Care Medicine/European Society of Intensive Care Medicine/American College of Chest Physicians/American Thoracic Society/Surgical Infection Society sepsis definition. Crit Care Med 2012;40:1700-6.
12. Ranieri VM, Thompson BT, Barie PS, et al. Drotrecogin alfa (activated) in adults with septic shock. N Engl J Med 2012;366:2055-64.
13. Kopterides P, Siempos II, Tsangaris I, et al. Procalcitonin-guided algorithms of antibiotic therapy in the intensive care unit: a systematic review and meta-analysis of randomized controlled trials. Crit Care Med 2010;38:2229-41.
14. Wacker C, Prkno A, Brunkhorst FM, et al. Procalcitonin as a diagnostic marker for sepsis: a systematic review and meta-analysis. Lancet Infect Dis 2013;13:426-35.
15. Peake SL, Delaney A, Bailey M, et al. Goal-directed resuscitation for patients with early septic shock. N Engl J Med 2014;371:1496-506.
16. Yealy DM, Kellum JA, Huang DT, et al. A randomized trial of protocol-based care for early septic shock. N Engl J Med 2014;370:1683-93.
17. Rivers E, Nguyen B, Havstad S, et al. Early goal-directed therapy in the treatment of severe sepsis and septic shock. N Engl J Med 2001;345:1368-77.
18. Jones AE, Shapiro NI, Trzeciak S, et al. Lactate clearance vs central venous oxygen saturation as goals of early sepsis therapy: a randomized clinical trial. JAMA 2010;303:739-46.
19. Jansen TC, van Bommel J, Schoonderbeek FJ, et al. Early lactate-guided therapy in intensive care unit patients: a multicenter, open-label, randomized controlled trial. Am J Respir Crit Care Med 2010;182:752-61.
20. Mouncey PR, Osborn TM, Power GS, et al. Trial of early, goal-directed resuscitation for septic shock. N Engl J Med 2015;372:1301-11.
21. Kaukonen KM, Bailey M, Suzuki S, et al. Mortality related to severe sepsis and septic shock among critically ill patients in australia and new zealand, 2000-2012. JAMA 2014;311:1308-16.
22. Asfar P, Meziani F, Hamel JF, et al. High versus low blood-pressure target in patients with septic shock. N Engl J Med 2014;370:1583-93.
23. Holst LB, Haase N, Wetterslev J, et al. Lower versus higher hemoglobin threshold for transfusion in septic shock. N Engl J Med 2014;371:1381-91.
24. Hebert PC, Carson JL. Transfusion threshold of 7 g per deciliter—the new normal. N Engl J Med 2014;371:1459-61.
25. De Backer D, Orbegozo Cortes D, Donadello K, et al. Pathophysiology of microcirculatory dysfunction and the pathogenesis of septic shock. Virulence 2014;5:73-9.
26. Ospina-Tascon G, Neves AP, Occhipinti G, et al. Effects of fluids on microvascular perfusion in patients with severe sepsis. Intensive Care Med 2010;36:949-55.
27. Pottecher J, Deruddre S, Teboul JL, et al. Both passive leg raising and intravascular volume expansion improve sublingual microcirculatory perfusion in severe sepsis and septic shock patients. Intensive Care Med 2010;36:1867-74.
28. Boerma EC, Ince C. The role of vasoactive agents in the resuscitation of microvascular perfusion and tissue oxygenation in critically ill patients. Intensive Care Med 2010;36:2004-18.
29. Dubin A, Pozo MO, Casabella CA, et al. Increasing arterial blood pressure with norepinephrine does not improve microcirculatory blood flow: a prospective study. Crit Care 2009;13:R92.
30. Jhanji S, Stirling S, Patel N, et al. The effect of increasing doses of norepinephrine on tissue oxygenation and microvascular flow in patients with septic shock. Crit Care Med 2009;37:1961-6.
31. Boerma EC, Koopmans M, Konijn A, et al. Effects of nitroglycerin on sublingual microcirculatory blood flow in patients with severe sepsis/septic shock after a strict resuscitation protocol: a double-blind randomized placebo controlled trial. Crit Care Med 2010;38:93-100.
32. Trzeciak S, Glaspey LJ, Dellinger RP, et al. Randomized controlled trial of inhaled nitric oxide for the treatment of

32. microcirculatory dysfunction in patients with sepsis. Crit Care Med 2014;42:2482-92.

33. De Backer D, Creteur J, Dubois MJ, et al. The effects of dobutamine on microcirculatory alterations in patients with septic shock are independent of its systemic effects. Crit Care Med 2006;34:403-8.

34. Morelli A, Donati A, Ertmer C, et al. Levosimendan for resuscitating the microcirculation in patients with septic shock: a randomized controlled study. Crit Care 2010;14:R232.

35. Surviving Sepsis Campaign. Updated bundles in response to new evidence. 2015. Available at www.survivingsepsis.org/SiteCollectionDocuments/SSC_Bundle.pdf. Accessed August 11, 2015

36. National Quality Forum. Severe Sepsis and Septic Shock: Management Bundle. 2013. Available at www.qualityforum.org/QPS/0500. Accessed August 11, 2015.

37. Centers for Medicare & Medicaid Services. Fact Sheets: CMS to Improve Quality of Care During Hospital Inpatient Stays. 2014. Available at https://www.cms.gov/Newsroom/MediaReleaseDatabase/Fact-sheets/2014-Fact-sheets-items/2014-08-04-2.html. Accessed August 11, 2015.

38. Surviving Sepsis Campaign. Implementation and Improvement Guide. 2013. Available at www.survivingsepsis.org/SiteCollectionDocuments/SSC-Implementation-Guide.pdf. Accessed August 11, 2015.

39. Gattinoni L, Brazzi L, Pelosi P, et al. A trial of goal-oriented hemodynamic therapy in critically ill patients. Svo2 Collaborative Group. N Engl J Med 1995;333:1025-32.

40. Boyd JH, Forbes J, Nakada TA, et al. Fluid resuscitation in septic shock: a positive fluid balance and elevated central venous pressure are associated with increased mortality. Crit Care Med 2011;39:259-65.

41. Kumar A, Roberts D, Wood KE, et al. Duration of hypotension before initiation of effective antimicrobial therapy is the critical determinant of survival in human septic shock. Crit Care Med 2006;34:1589-96.

42. Gaieski DF, Mikkelsen ME, Band RA, et al. Impact of time to antibiotics on survival in patients with severe sepsis or septic shock in whom early goal-directed therapy was initiated in the emergency department. Crit Care Med 2010;38:1045-53.

43. Puskarich MA, Trzeciak S, Shapiro NI, et al. Association between timing of antibiotic administration and mortality from septic shock in patients treated with a quantitative resuscitation protocol. Crit Care Med 2009;39:2066-71.

44. Vincent JL, Rello J, Marshall J, et al. International study of the prevalence and outcomes of infection in intensive care units. JAMA 2009;302:2323-9.

45. Kumar A, Ellis P, Arabi Y, et al. Initiation of inappropriate antimicrobial therapy results in a fivefold reduction of survival in human septic shock. Chest 2009;136:1237-48.

46. Brunkhorst FM, Oppert M, Marx G, et al. Effect of empirical treatment with moxifloxacin and meropenem vs meropenem on sepsis-related organ dysfunction in patients with severe sepsis: a randomized trial. JAMA 2012;307:2390-9.

47. Kumar A, Safdar N, Kethireddy S, et al. A survival benefit of combination antibiotic therapy for serious infections associated with sepsis and septic shock is contingent only on the risk of death: a meta-analytic/meta-regression study. Crit Care Med 2010;38:1651-64.

48. Roberts JA, Lipman J. Pharmacokinetic issues for antibiotics in the critically ill patient. Crit Care Med 2009;37:840-51; quiz 859.

49. Taccone FS, Laterre PF, Dugernier T, et al. Insufficient beta-lactam concentrations in the early phase of severe sepsis and septic shock. Crit Care 2010;14:R126.

50. Roberts JA, Paul SK, Akova M, et al. Dali: defining antibiotic levels in intensive care unit patients: are current beta-lactam antibiotic doses sufficient for critically ill patients? Clin Infect Dis 2014;58:1072-83.

51. Jensen JU, Hein L, Lundgren B, et al. Procalcitonin-guided interventions against infections to increase early appropriate antibiotics and improve survival in the intensive care unit: a randomized trial. Crit Care Med 2011;39:2048-58.

52. Layios N, Lambermont B, Canivet JL, et al. Procalcitonin usefulness for the initiation of antibiotic treatment in intensive care unit patients. Crit Care Med 2012;40:2304-9.

53. Deliberato RO, Marra AR, Sanches PR, et al. Clinical and economic impact of procalcitonin to shorten antimicrobial therapy in septic patients with proven bacterial infection in an intensive care setting. Diagn Microbiol Infect Dis 2013;76:266-71.

54. Hochreiter M, Kohler T, Schweiger AM, et al. Procalcitonin to guide duration of antibiotic therapy in intensive care patients: a randomized prospective controlled trial. Crit Care 2009;13:R83.

55. Nobre V, Harbarth S, Graf JD, et al. Use of procalcitonin to shorten antibiotic treatment duration in septic patients: a randomized trial. Am J Respir Crit Care Med 2008;177:498-505.

56. Schroeder S, Hochreiter M, Koehler T, et al. Procalcitonin (PCT)-guided algorithm reduces length of antibiotic treatment in surgical intensive care patients with severe sepsis: results of a prospective randomized study. Langenbecks Arch Surg 2009;394:221-6.

57. Stolz D, Smyrnios N, Eggimann P, et al. Procalcitonin for reduced antibiotic exposure in ventilator-associated pneumonia: a randomised study. Eur Respir J 2009;34:1364-75.

58. Shehabi Y, Sterba M, Garrett PM, et al. Procalcitonin algorithm in critically ill adults with undifferentiated infection or suspected sepsis. A randomized controlled trial. Am J Respir Crit Care Med 2014;190:1102-10.

59. Annane D, Maxime V, Faller JP, et al. Procalcitonin levels to guide antibiotic therapy in adults with non-microbiologically proven apparent severe sepsis: a randomised controlled trial. BMJ Open 2013;3.

60. Bouadma L, Luyt CE, Tubach F, et al. Use of procalcitonin to reduce patients' exposure to antibiotics in intensive care units (prorata trial): a multicentre randomised controlled trial. Lancet 2009;375:463-74.

61. Matthaiou DK, Ntani G, Kontogiorgi M, et al. An esicm systematic review and meta-analysis of procalcitonin-guided antibiotic therapy algorithms in adult critically ill patients. Intensive Care Med 2012;38:940-9.

62. Finfer S, Liu B, Taylor C, et al. Resuscitation fluid use in critically ill adults: an international cross-sectional study in 391 intensive care units. Crit Care 2010;14:R185.

63. Finfer S, Bellomo R, Boyce N, et al. A comparison of albumin and saline for fluid resuscitation in the intensive care unit. N Engl J Med 2004;350:2247-56.

64. Raghunathan K, Shaw A, Nathanson B, et al. Association between the choice of iv crystalloid and in-hospital mortality among critically ill adults with sepsis. Crit Care Med 2014;42:1585-91.

65. Rochwerg B, Alhazzani W, Sindi A, et al. Fluid resuscitation in sepsis: a systematic review and network meta-analysis. Ann Intern Med 2014;161:347-55.

66. Finfer S, McEvoy S, Bellomo R, et al. Impact of albumin compared to saline on organ function and mortality of patients with severe sepsis. Intensive Care Med 2011;37:86-96.

67. American Thoracic Society. Evidence-based colloid use in the critically ill: American Thoracic Society consensus statement. Am J Respir Crit Care Med 2004;170:1247-59.

68. Brunkhorst FM, Engel C, Bloos F, et al. Intensive insulin therapy and pentastarch resuscitation in severe sepsis. N Engl J Med 2008;358:125-39.

69. Perner A, Haase N, Guttormsen AB, et al. Hydroxyethyl starch 130/0.42 versus Ringer's acetate in severe sepsis. N Engl J Med 2012;367:124-34.

70. Muller RG, Haase N, Wetterslev J, et al. Effects of hydroxyethyl starch in subgroups of patients with severe sepsis: exploratory post hoc analyses of a randomised trial. Intensive Care Med 2013;39:1963-71.

71. Patel A, Waheed U, Brett SJ. Randomised trials of 6% tetrastarch (hydroxyethyl starch 130/0.4 or 0.42) for severe sepsis reporting mortality: systematic review and meta-analysis. Intensive Care Med 2013;39:811-22.

72. Caironi P, Tognoni G, Masson S, et al. Albumin replacement in patients with severe sepsis or septic shock. N Engl J Med 2014;370:1412-21.

73. De Backer D, Aldecoa C, Njimi H, et al. Dopamine versus norepinephrine in the treatment of septic shock: a meta-analysis. Crit Care Med 2012;40:725-30.

74. Annane D, Vignon P, Renault A, et al. Norepinephrine plus dobutamine versus epinephrine alone for management of septic shock: a randomised trial. Lancet 2007;370:676-84.

75. Myburgh JA, Higgins A, Jovanovska A, et al. A comparison of epinephrine and norepinephrine in critically ill patients. Intensive Care Med 2008;34:2226-34.

76. Morelli A, Ertmer C, Rehberg S, et al. Phenylephrine versus norepinephrine for initial hemodynamic support of patients with septic shock: a randomized, controlled trial. Crit Care 2008;12:R143.

77. Bellomo R, Chapman M, Finfer S, et al. Low-dose dopamine in patients with early renal dysfunction: a placebo-controlled randomised trial. Australian and New Zealand Intensive Care Society (ANZICS) Clinical Trials Group. Lancet 2000;356:2139-43.

78. Torgersen C, Dunser MW, Wenzel V, et al. Comparing two different arginine vasopressin doses in advanced vasodilatory shock: a randomized, controlled, open-label trial. Intensive Care Med 2010;36:57-65.

79. Serpa Neto A, Nassar APJ, Cardoso SO, et al. Vasopressin and terlipressin in adult vasodilatory shock: a systematic review and meta-analysis of nine randomized controlled trials. Crit Care 2012;16:R154.

80. Polito A, Parisini E, Ricci Z, et al. Vasopressin for treatment of vasodilatory shock: an esicm systematic review and meta-analysis. Intensive Care Med 2012;38:9-19.

81. Hsu JL, Liu V, Patterson AJ, et al. Potential for overuse of corticosteroids and vasopressin in septic shock. Crit Care 2012;16:447.

82. Bauer SR, Lam SW. Arginine vasopressin for the treatment of septic shock in adults. Pharmacotherapy 2010;30:1057-71.

83. Vieillard-Baron A, Caille V, Charron C, et al. Actual incidence of global left ventricular hypokinesia in adult septic shock. Crit Care Med 2008;36:1701-6.

84. Enrico C, Kanoore Edul VS, Vazquez AR, et al. Systemic and microcirculatory effects of dobutamine in patients with septic shock. J Crit Care 2012;27:630-8.

85. Jellema WT, Groeneveld AB, Wesseling KH, et al. Heterogeneity and prediction of hemodynamic responses to dobutamine in patients with septic shock. Crit Care Med 2006;34:2392-8.

86. Minneci PC, Deans KJ, Eichacker PQ, et al. The effects of steroids during sepsis depend on dose and severity of illness: an updated meta-analysis. Clin Microbiol Infect 2009;15:308-18.

87. Annane D, Sebille V, Charpentier C, et al. Effect of treatment with low doses of hydrocortisone and fludrocortisone on mortality in patients with septic shock. JAMA 2002;288:862-71.

88. Sprung CL, Annane D, Keh D, et al. Hydrocortisone therapy for patients with septic shock. N Engl J Med 2008;358:111-24.

89. Boonen E, Vervenne H, Meersseman P, et al. Reduced cortisol metabolism during critical illness. N Engl J Med 2013;368:1477-88.

90. Werdan K, Pilz G, Bujdoso O, et al. Score-based immunoglobulin G therapy of patients with sepsis: the SBITS study. Crit Care Med 2007;35:2693-701.

91. Kreymann KG, de Heer G, Nierhaus A, et al. Use of polyclonal immunoglobulins as adjunctive therapy for sepsis or septic shock. Crit Care Med 2007;35:2677-85.

92. Laupland KB, Kirkpatrick AW, Delaney A. Polyclonal intravenous immunoglobulin for the treatment of severe sepsis and septic shock in critically ill adults: a systematic review and meta-analysis. Crit Care Med 2007;35:2686-92.

93. Werdan K. Mirror, mirror on the wall, which is the fairest meta-analysis of all? Crit Care Med 2007;35:2852-4.

94. Barochia AV, Cui X, Vitberg D, et al. Bundled care for septic shock: an analysis of clinical trials. Crit Care Med 2010;38:668-78.

95. Micek ST, Roubinian N, Heuring T, et al. Before-after study of a standardized hospital order set for the management of septic shock. Crit Care Med 2006;34:2707-13.

Chapter 16: Invasive Fungal Infections

Kathryn R. Matthias, Pharm.D., BCPS-AQ ID

LEARNING OBJECTIVES

1. Classify intrinsic and acquired antifungal therapy resistance patterns for fungi.
2. Distinguish between antifungal interpretive breakpoints for *Candida* spp.
3. Develop an algorithm for selecting an appropriate antifungal therapy regimen based on current resistance patterns and risk factors for patients in a critical care setting.

ABBREVIATIONS IN THIS CHAPTER

ICU	Intensive care unit	MIC	Minimum inhibitory concentration
IFI	Invasive fungal infection		

INTRODUCTION

Invasive fungal infections (IFIs) from organisms including *Candida* spp., *Aspergillus* spp., and *Rhizopus* spp. represent a major burden of mortality and morbidity for patients in critical care settings.[1-3] Although new antifungal therapy options and rapid diagnostic testing capabilities for yeasts and molds have expanded treatment and prophylaxis options, knowledge of known risk factors for treatment efficacy based on fungi genus and species together with drug characteristics has become paramount to individualize antifungal therapy for patients admitted to intensive care units (ICUs).[4,5] Although several species of fungal organisms can be isolated from human culture samples, this chapter will focus on the common yeasts and molds that are known to cause IFIs in critically ill patients.

Antifungal Therapy

A variety of antifungal therapy options are available for the treatment of IFIs, but most are within three drug classes, as shown in Table 16.1, Table 16.2, and Table 16.3.[6-17] Although many of the pharmacologic, pharmacokinetic, and pharmacodynamic properties within each of these drug classes are similar, several of the differences between the triazole agents may affect the selection of a drug for a critically ill patient with an IFI. Approved triazole agents with indications for fungal infections in the United States are fluconazole, itraconazole, isavuconazole (formulated as prodrug isavuconazonium sulfate), posaconazole, and voriconazole. Although these agents have a similar mechanism of action by inhibiting the cytochrome P450 (CYP)-dependent enzyme lanosterol 14-α-demethylase, there is significant variability in the spectrum of activity, drug characteristics, and appropriateness of use in patients who are critically ill, as shown in Table 16.2. All of these triazole agents are available in an intravenous formulation except for itraconazole in the United States. In patients with critical illness but adequate gastrointestinal (GI) function, each of these agents is available in oral formulations, although the delayed-release tablet posaconazole formulation should not be crushed and administered through feeding tubes. Conversely, the oral suspension posaconazole formulation that can be administered through a feeding tube can have significantly lower and unpredictable absorption compared with the delayed-release tablet formulation.[18]

Antifungal Therapy Resistance Patterns

The in vitro interpretive criteria result for drug susceptibility testing should correlate with clinical outcomes and be associated with drug resistance mechanisms. Certain antifungal interpretive criteria were recently revised by the Clinical and Laboratory Standards Institute committee, as shown in Table 16.4.[19,20] The revised susceptibility minimum inhibitory concentration (MIC) breakpoints for several *Candida* spp. were lowered because of recent studies evaluating the association of resistance mechanism, clinical outcomes, and reported MIC values. Interpretive criteria have not been established for antifungal agents for certain yeasts and molds because testing results have not clearly predicted clinical success and failure rates.[20] A more detailed discussion of resistance mechanisms and antifungal therapy options for certain groups of yeasts and molds that are known to cause IFIs appears in the text that follows.

YEASTS

The two main types of yeasts that cause IFI in critically ill patients are *Candida* and *Cryptococcus* spp.

Candidiasis

Candida spp. are normal GI and oropharyngeal flora, but isolation from deeper sites and blood in a patient should not be ignored or considered a contaminant. *Candida* spp. isolated from blood requires appropriate antifungal treatment regardless of whether a visceral source is known.[21] Conversely, 30%–50% of invasive *Candida* infections have negative blood cultures because of low sensitivity of traditional blood culture methods, so no growth from blood cultures does not exclude the diagnosis of a deep-seated *Candida* infection. *Candida* spp. endophthalmitis can occur from hematogenous seeding. An ophthalmologist examination is recommended for all patients with candidemia, and the presence of *Candida* endophthalmitis can increase the recommended antifungal therapy duration.[21] If a patient is given a diagnosis of *Candida* endocarditis, combined surgical and medical interventions should be considered. Conversely, pneumonia caused by *Candida* spp. is considered rare. *Candida* spp. isolated through respiratory samples such as sputum, tracheal, or bronchial lavage are normally considered a contaminant from normal oropharyngeal flora.[21]

More than 200 *Candida* spp. have been known to cause medically significant disease.[21] Although many *Candida* spp. have predictable susceptibility patterns, recent increased rates of acquired resistance to fluconazole and echinocandin agents for certain species may change treatment recommendations for IFIs, as shown in Table 16.5 and Table 16.6.[4,22-31] *Candida albicans* isolates continue to have low antifungal therapy resistance rates and remain the most commonly isolated species even in ICU settings, but

Table 16.1 Properties of Amphotericin B Agents to Consider in Critically Ill Patients[6,7]

	Amphotericin B Deoxycholate (conventional)	Amphotericin B (lipid complex)	Amphotericin B (liposomal)
Weight-based dosing for treatment (adult)	Yes		
Dosage weight in patients with obesity	Lean body weight		
Urine concentrations	High	Low	
Potential infusion-related reactions	Yes, associated with TNFα, IL-1, IL-6, and prostaglandins		
	Rare are IgG-mediated allergic reactions		
Potential for hepatotoxicity	Yes, liver function testing monitoring recommended		
Potential for anemia	Yes, normochromic and normocytic		
Potential for nephrotoxicity	Yes, serum creatinine, potassium, and magnesium concentration monitoring recommended. Avoid other nephrotoxic agents, if possible		
Concurrent non-antifungal agents or fluids	Adequate fluid hydration recommended (incompatible with 0.9% NaCl; use D_5W^a flush)		
	Severity of infusion-related reactions may be decreased with agents including acetaminophen, antiemetic, diphenhydramine, meperidine, hydrocortisone (selection of drugs dependent on individual patient characteristics)		
Combination therapy with other antifungals	Based on disease state, published data, and patient characteristics		
	Potential synergy or antagonism[b]		
Mechanisms of resistance	*ERG2, ERG3, ERG5, ERG6, ERG11* gene mutations (membrane sterol composition)		

[a] Flush venous access catheter with D_5W before and after each dose of amphotericin B if normal saline or other incompatible agent used for hydration through that catheter.

[b] Antagonism between antifungal agents may occur (i.e., triazole agents decrease ergosterol synthesis by inhibiting sterol 14α-demethylase, and amphotericin B binds to ergosterol in the cytoplasmic membrane). Clinical benefits and use of combination antifungal therapy (amphotericin B, echinocandins, triazole, and other antifungal agents including terbinafine and flucytosine) controversial for many invasive fungal infections.

D_5W = dextrose 5%; IgG = immunoglobulin G; IL = interleukin; TNF = tumor necrosis factor.

Table 16.2 Properties of Triazole Agents to Consider in Critically Ill Patients[6-16]

	Fluconazole	Itraconazole	Voriconazole	Posaconazole	Isavuconazole
Weight-based dosing for treatment (adult)	Yes	No	Yes	No	
Dosage weight in patients with obesity	Total body weight	—	Lean body weight	—	
Loading dose recommended for treatment	Yes	No	Yes		
Intravenous formulation	Yes	Not in the United States	Yes		
Oral solution or suspension (feeding tubes)	Yes				No
Oral tablet or capsule formulation	Yes				
Absorption altered by food	No	Variable	Variable	Variable	No
Absorption altered by changes in gastric pH	No	Variable	No	Variable	No
Volume of distribution (L/kg)	Low	Very high	High		
Cerebrospinal fluid concentrations	High	Low	High	Low	Low
Urine concentrations	High	Low			
Elimination (major)	Renal	Hepatic	Hepatic	Fecal	Hepatic
Clearance by dialysis	Yes	No	No	Variable	No
Sulfobutyl ether β-cyclodextrin vehicle	No	No, polyethylene glycol (oral solution)	Yes (intravenous)	Yes (intravenous)	No
CYP metabolism 2C9 inhibitor	Strong	—	Moderate	—	Mild
CYP metabolism 2C19 inhibitor	Strong	—	Moderate	—	Mild
CYP metabolism 3A4 inhibitor	Moderate	Strong			
P-glycoprotein efflux transporters	—	Yes	Yes	Substrate	Yes
Target serum concentrations for efficacy (mcg/mL)	Not routinely performed[a]	>1[b]	>1–2	>0.7–1.25[c]	Not established[d]
Target serum concentrations for toxicity (mcg/mL)	Not routinely performed	<5	<5.5	Not established	Not established
Potential for QT-wave prolongation	Yes	Yes, potential to worsen congestive heart failure	Yes	Yes	No, shorten
Potential for hepatotoxicity	Yes, potential ALT/AST increases (usually transient) and rare hepatitis				
Mechanisms of resistance	Various mechanisms depending on organism and agent including drug efflux [ATP-binding cassette or major facilitator superfamily], ERG3 mutations, overproduction of enzyme Erg11p, CYP51A gene, and lanosterol 14-α-demethylase mutation				

[a]One study recommends a goal of 24-hour area under the curve (AUC24)/MIC of more than 400, which was associated with higher 30-day survival for patients with *C. albicans* but not non-*albicans Candida* bloodstream infections.

[b]Depending on assay method. Separate measurement of active metabolite (hydroxyitraconazole) concentration can be considered if high-performance liquid chromatography (HPLC) is used instead of a bioassay.

[c]Goal posaconazole serum concentrations have not been clearly established for the treatment of invasive fungal infections with delayed-release tablet and intravenous formulations.

[d]Mean isavuconazole trough concentration was 3 mcg/mL after 25 days of therapy

proportional rates of *Candida* spp. including *C. glabrata*, *C. parapsilosis*, *C. tropicalis*, and *C. krusei* with decreased susceptibility to fluconazole are changing.[32,33] One of the associated risk factors for non-*albicans* candidemia in the ICUs (medical and surgical) at two U.S. tertiary care medical centers was previous fluconazole exposure (odds ratio [OR] 11.6; 95% confidence interval [CI], 2.3–58.9).[34]

In addition to reduced susceptibility to fluconazole, the other main resistance concern for *Candida* spp. is reduced susceptibility to echinocandin agents from *FKS* gene mutations, which can decrease the amount of glucan synthesis available in the cell wall that is the binding site for echinocandin agents.[35,36] *FKS* gene mutations are found in *C. krusei* and *C. parapsilosis* together with other *Candida* spp., but the prevalence of *C. glabrata* isolates with *FKS1* or *FKS2* gene mutation appears to be increasing, at least in certain geographic locations in the United States. Unlike with *C. parapsillosis*, the presence of *FKS1* mutation in *C. glabrata* is associated with echinocandin treatment failures.[37,38] In a single-center study at a U.S. tertiary care hospital, 18% of the *C. glabrata* bloodstream isolates from 2009 through 2012 had an *FKS* mutation.[39] Echinocandin treatment failure occurred in 60% of patients with *C. glabrata* isolates with an *FKS* mutation compared with 23% of patients without an *FKS* mutation, and *FKS* mutations were associated with prior echinocandin exposure (OR 8.3; 95% CI, 1.7–40.4).[39] In a prospective multicenter study in France, increased prevalence of non-*albicans Candida* spp. such as *C. glabrata* and *C. krusei* was associated with previous recent exposure to fluconazole (OR 2.17; 95% CI, 1.51–3.13), and *Candida* spp. with decreased susceptibility to caspofungin were associated with previous recent exposure to caspofungin (OR 4.79; 95% CI, 2.47–9.28).[40]

Because there are known differences in susceptibility to antifungal agents for certain *Candida* spp., decreasing the time to species identification may decrease the time to appropriate antifungal therapy. As shown in Table 16.7, certain rapid diagnostic testing methods for specific yeasts are now being evaluated and approved for use in the United States by the U.S. Food and Drug Administration (FDA).[5,41-50] Instead of waiting several days for species identification, some of these testing methods allow for direct testing of blood samples so that *Candida* spp. identification can be reported on the day the blood sample was obtained.[51] If a specific *Candida* spp. is isolated from blood or a deep site, susceptibility testing should be considered if few published data are found regarding susceptibility patterns or if there is significant risk of reduced susceptibility. To improve time to appropriate therapy, especially for *Candida* spp. with known acquired or intrinsic resistance to commonly used empiric antifungal therapy, a practitioner with knowledge of these patterns and the associated risk factors can use these testing methods to de-escalate or escalate antifungal therapy.

Candidiasis Treatment

The 2009 Infectious Diseases Society of America guidelines recommend echinocandins or fluconazole as an alternative regimen for empiric therapy in patients who are critically ill with suspected candidemia, depending on absolute neutrophil count.[21] When this guideline statement was published, *C. glabrata* isolates were known to have clinically significant rates of reduced susceptibility and resistance to fluconazole. Since then, increasing rates of *C. glabrata* echinocandin resistance with and without coresistance to fluconazole have been reported in the United States. Other antifungal therapy options may be considered if a patient has recent fluconazole and echinocandin exposure before isolation of *C. glabrata* because of concern for reduced susceptibility to these agents.

For *Candida* spp., cross-resistance for triazole agents may be best associated with fluconazole resistance.[52] For *Candida* spp. with a fluconazole MIC of 64 mcg/mL or higher, there are increased rates of reduced susceptibility for itraconazole, isavuconazole, posaconazole, and voriconazole. For *C. glabrata*, fluconazole resistance is associated with reduced

Table 16.3 Properties of Echinocandin Agents to Consider in Critically Ill Patients[7,17]

	Caspofungin	Micafungin	Anidulafungin
Loading dose recommended for treatment	Yes	No	Yes
Urine concentrations	Low		
Potential infusion-related reactions	Yes, histamine-mediated reaction (improved with slower infusion)		
Potential for hepatotoxicity	Yes, liver function test monitoring recommended		
Potential paradoxical effect[a]	Yes		
Mechanisms of resistance	*FKS* genes (glucan synthase) by *Candida* spp.		

[a]Paradoxical effect of resistance to killing may occur when higher-than-approved dosage is used that causes relatively high concentrations of echinocandin.

activity of posaconazole and voriconazole. In contrast, *C. krusei* is often susceptible to voriconazole despite being considered intrinsically resistant to fluconazole.

Multi-antifungal (fluconazole, echinocandin, and amphotericin B agents) resistance for *Candida* spp. has been reported in a few case reports and case series, but most of these cases involved patients who had prolonged periods of severe immunosuppression.[53] Resistance to fluconazole and echinocandin agents is more common without resistance to amphotericin B agents.[54] Therapy selection in these cases depends on susceptibility results, infection site, and each patient's response to therapy.

Cryptococcosis

Cryptococcus neoformans is an encapsulated yeast that can cause IFIs in patients with significant immunosuppression (especially T lymphocytes) such as organ transplant recipients or patients with a diagnosis of AIDS, leukemia, or lymphomas.[55] Patients often present to an acute care setting with symptoms consistent with chronic meningitis.

Cryptococcosis Treatment

In critically ill patients without a diagnosis of AIDS or history of an organ transplant with central nervous system (CNS) or severe pulmonary cryptococcosis, amphotericin B deoxycholate with or without flucytosine is recommended

Table 16.4 Revised In Vitro Interpretive Criteria for *Candida* spp.[19,20]

		Susceptible MIC (mcg/mL)	Susceptible-Dose Dependent MIC (mcg/mL)	Intermediate MIC (mcg/mL)	Resistant MIC
Polyenes (amphotericin B)					
Candida spp.[a]	All products	Not available[b]			
Echinocandins (caspofungin, micafungin, anidulafungin)					
C. guilliermondii *C. parapsilosis*	All products	≤ 2	Not available	4	≥ 8
C. albicans *C. krusei*	All products	≤ 0.25		0.5	≥ 1
C. glabrata	Caspofungin Andulafungin	≤ 0.12		0.25	≥ 0.5
	Micafungin	≤ 0.06		0.12	≥ 0.25
Triazoles					
C. glabrata	Fluconazole[c]	Not available	≤ 32	Not available	≥ 64
C. albicans *C. guilliermondii* *C. parapsillosis* *C. tropicalis*		≤ 2	4	Not available	≥ 8
Candida spp.[a]	Isavuconazole	Not available			
C. albicans	Itraconazole	≤ 0.12	0.25–0.5	Not available	≥ 1
Candida spp.[a]	Posaconazole	Not available			
C. krusei	Voriconazole[d]	≤ 0.5	Not available	1	≥ 2
C. albicans *C. parapsillosis* *C. tropicalis*		≤ 0.12	Not available	0.25–0.5	≥ 1

[a]*Candida* spp. including *C. albicans, C. glabrata, C. guilliermondii, C. krusei, C. parapsillosis,* and *C. tropicalis.*
[b]MIC of 2 mcg/mL or higher is often associated with suboptimal efficacy.
[c]No breakpoints are available for *C. krusei* with fluconazole from the Clinical and Laboratory Standards Institute (CLSI). All isolates are considered resistant.
[d]No breakpoints are available for *C. glabrata* with voriconazole from CLSI.
MIC values for *Candia* spp. originally published in: *Clinical and Laboratory Standards Institute (CLSI). Reference Method for Broth Dilution Antifungal Susceptibility Testing of Yeasts, 4th Informational Supplement. CLSI Document M27-54.* Wayre, PA: CLSI, 2012.

for induction therapy that can be changed to fluconazole monotherapy for maintenance therapy.[55] If the patient has a history of organ transplantation, the use of amphotericin B liposomal with fluconazole is recommended for induction therapy, followed by fluconazole maintenance therapy. For a patient with a diagnosis of AIDS and CNS cryptococcosis, amphotericin B deoxycholate with flucytosine or fluconazole is recommended. Maintenance therapy with fluconazole, itraconazole, or amphotericin B deoxycholate is recommended until the patient is asymptomatic and evidence of active disease has resolved.

MOLDS

Although not as common a cause of IFIs as *Candida* spp., several molds have been reported to cause IFIs with high morbidity rates and mortality.[2,3,56,57] For certain mold species, antifungal therapy options are limited.

Aspergillosis

Although *Candida* spp. are the most common cause of IFIs in ICUs, invasive *Aspergillosis* spp. infection rates have surpassed *Candida* spp. infection rates in patients with hematologic malignancy in the United States.[2,58]

Table 16.5 Resistance Patterns for *Candida* spp. with Triazole Agents[4,22-29]

	Significant Acquired or Inducible Resistance Rates				
Candida spp.	Fluconazole	Itraconazole	Voriconazole	Posaconazole	Isavuconazole
C. albicans					
C. glabrata	X	X	X		X[a]
C. krusei	Intrinsic				
C. lusitaniae					
C. parapsilosis	X	X			
C. tropicalis		X			
Other species	Variable[b,c]	Variable[d]	Variable[e]		

[a]Decreased susceptibility to isavuconazole has been associated with *C. glabrata* isolates that have decreased susceptibility to fluconazole and/or voriconazole.
[b]Cases of fluconazole-resistant isolates have been reported for *Candida* spp. including *C. dubliniensis*, *C. famata* (> 50% isolates), *C. guilliermondii*, *C. haemulonii* (> 90% isolates), *C. inconspieua*, *C. kefyr*, *C. norvegensis* (> 70% isolates), *C. pelliculosa*, *C. rugosa*, and *C. valida* (> 70% isolates).
[c]Inducible fluconazole resistance has been reported for *C. utilis*.
[d]Cases of itraconazole-resistant isolates have been reported for *Candida* spp. including *C. guilliermondii*, *C. haemulonii* (> 90% isolates), *C. pelliculosa* (> 70% isolates), *C. rugosa*, and *C. utilis* (> 50% isolates).
[e]Cases of voriconazole-resistant isolates have been reported for *Candida* spp. including *C. dubliniensis*, *C. famata*, *C. guilliermondii*, *C. haemulonii*, and *C. valida*.

Table 16.6 Resistance Patterns for *Candida* spp. with Polyene, Echinocandin, and Miscellaneous Antifungal Agents[29-31]

	Significant Acquired or Inducible Resistance Rates					
Candida spp.	Amphotericin B	Caspofungin	Micafungin	Anidulafungin	Terbinafine	Flucytosine
• C. albicans						
• C. glabrata		X	X	X	No activity	
• C. krusei					No activity	
• C. lusitaniae	Inducible					
• C. parapsilosis						
• C. tropicalis					No activity	
• Other species	Variable[a]					Variable[b]

[a]Cases of amphotericin B–resistant isolates have been reported for *Candida* spp. including *C. haemulonii* (> 70%) and *C. krusei*.
[b]Cases of flucytosine-resistant isolates have been reported for *Candida* spp. including *C. haemulonii*, *C. krusei* (> 70%), *C. pelliculosa*, and *C. utilis* (> 50%).

Most *Aspergillus* spp. are reported to have low MIC values for commonly used therapy such as voriconazole and amphotericin B agents, but recent increases in resistance have been reported for specific species. *A. terreus* isolates tend to have high amphotericin B MIC values, whereas *A. calidostus* and *A. lentulus* isolates have reduced susceptibility to a variety of antifungal agents. Certain isolates of *A. fumigatus* have been reported to be resistant to voriconazole ($TR_{46}/Y121F/T289A$ mutation), itraconazole, and/or posaconazole, and higher mortality rates have been reported in patients infected with these isolates.[59]

Posaconazole, itraconazole, and isavuconazole all have potential efficacy for the treatment of invasive aspergillosis. In a noninferiority trial that compared isavuconazole with voriconazole, all-cause mortality rates through day 42 were 18.6% and 20.2%, respectively.[60] Combination salvage therapy with an echinocandin and voriconazole or amphotericin B has been reported. The mortality rates of 47 patients with invasive aspergillosis were significantly lower in patients who received voriconazole plus caspofungin than in those who received voriconazole monotherapy (OR 0.28; 95% CI, 0.28–0.92).[61]

Aspergillosis Treatment

Voriconazole is recommended as monotherapy as first line because of a multicenter, randomized unblinded, clinical trial that compared the use of voriconazole with that of amphotericin B deoxycholate in patients with invasive aspergillosis.[2] The voriconazole and amphotericin B group survival rates at 12 weeks were 70.8% and 57.9%, respectively (hazard ratio 0.59; 95% CI, 0.4–0.88).[62] In critically ill patients with suspected invasive aspergillosis, initial use of an amphotericin B agent has been recommended to cover for both mucormycosis and aspergillosis until *Aspergillus* spp. infection has been confirmed, especially if the patient had recently received voriconazole.[2,3]

Mucormycosis

The rapidly growing organisms that cause mucormycosis (previously known as zygomycosis) include *Absidia*, *Apophysomyces*, *Cunninghamella*, *Mucor*, *Rhizomucor*, *Rhizopus*, and *Saksenaea* spp.[3] The most common infection sites are rhino-orbital-cerebral or pulmonary in patients who are immunocompromised, received a diagnosis of diabetes, are intravenous drug users, or are receiving deferoxamine therapy for iron overload (enhanced growth of organisms). Although invasive *Candida* infection rates have decreased in patients with hematologic malignancies, rates of mucormycosis have increased. The use of voriconazole in this patient population has been associated as being an independent risk factor for disease (OR 10.4; 95% CI, 2.1–39).[63]

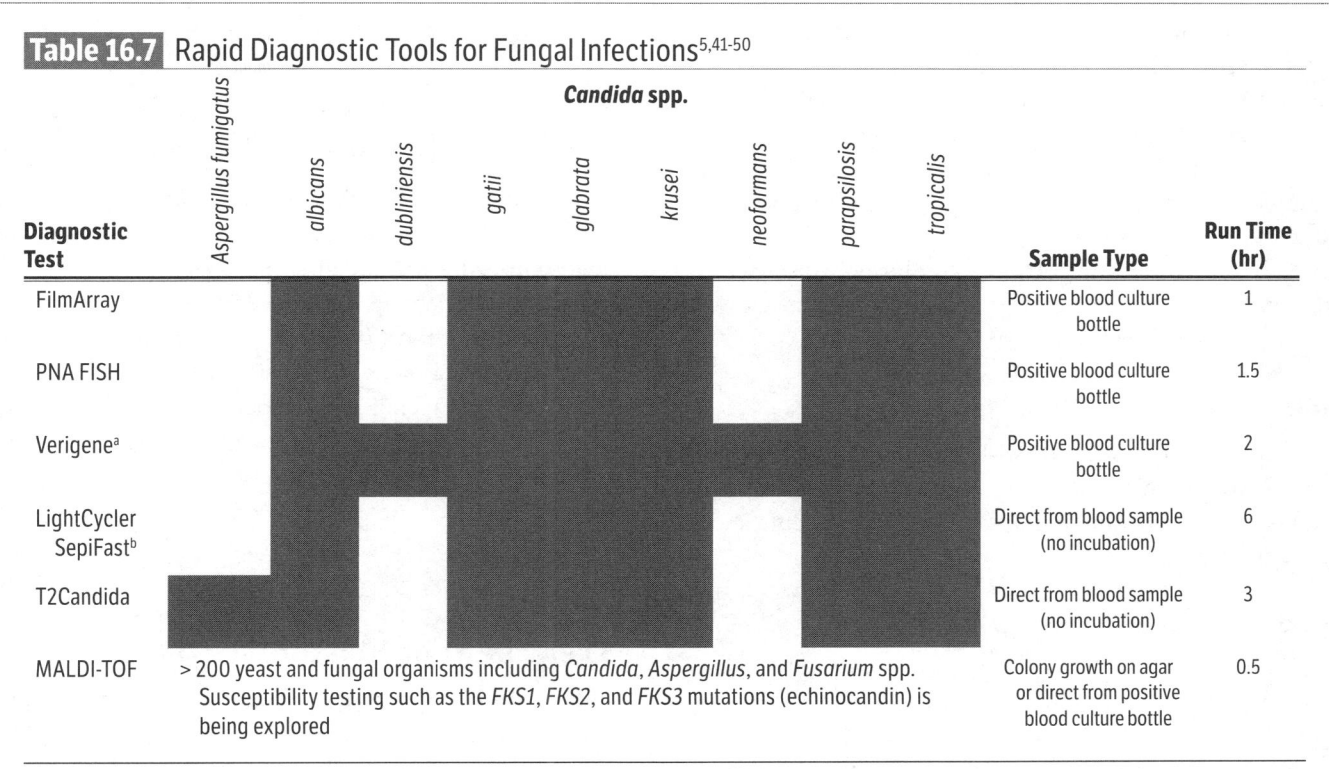

Table 16.7 Rapid Diagnostic Tools for Fungal Infections[5,41-50]

Diagnostic Test	*Aspergillus fumigatus*	*Candida* spp. albicans	dubliniensis	gatii	glabrata	krusei	neoformans	parapsilosis	tropicalis	Sample Type	Run Time (hr)
FilmArray		■	■		■	■		■	■	Positive blood culture bottle	1
PNA FISH		■			■	■		■	■	Positive blood culture bottle	1.5
Verigene[a]		■			■	■		■	■	Positive blood culture bottle	2
LightCycler SepiFast[b]		■			■	■		■	■	Direct from blood sample (no incubation)	6
T2Candida		■			■	■		■	■	Direct from blood sample (no incubation)	3
MALDI-TOF	> 200 yeast and fungal organisms including *Candida*, *Aspergillus*, and *Fusarium* spp. Susceptibility testing such as the *FKS1*, *FKS2*, and *FKS3* mutations (echinocandin) is being explored									Colony growth on agar or direct from positive blood culture bottle	0.5

[a]Research use only.
[b]LightCycler SeptiFast test not available in the United States.
MALDI-TOF = matrix-assisted laser desorption/ionization time-of-flight (mass spectrometry); PNA FISH = peptide nucleic acid fluorescence in situ hybridization.

Mucormycosis Treatment

Primary treatment of mucormycosis is surgical intervention with early antifungal therapy together with decreasing immunosuppression or other risk factors, if possible.[3] Appropriate early antifungal therapy within 6 days of diagnosis for mucormycosis is associated with decreased mortality rates (49% vs. 83%).[64] Lipid formulations of amphotericin B are used for initial therapy. Double coverage with posaconazole or isavuconazole is controversial because of the high mortality rate for patients with mucormycosis who receive amphotericin B monotherapy and the potential antagonism with triazole therapy. Before FDA approval of the labeled uses of the delayed-release tablet and intravenous formulations of posaconazole together with the oral and intravenous formulation of isavuconazole, the oral suspension formulation of posaconazole was used for the treatment of mucormycosis.

According to posaconazole 24-hour area under the curve comparison, the bioavailability of the delayed-release formulation of posaconazole is higher than that of the oral suspension, so the tablet formulation may be preferred for mucormycosis treatment.[18] Isavuconazole has an FDA-approved indication for the treatment of invasive mucormycosis. In an open-label study of isavuconazole for patients with probable or proven mucormycosis, the all-cause mortality rate was 47% at day 180.[65]

Echinocandin agents in combination with amphotericin B products have been reported.[66] Echinocandin agents have no in vitro activity against the organisms that cause mucormycosis. One retrospective study evaluated 41 patients with rhino-orbital or rhino-orbital-cerebral mucormycosis. Six of the 41 patients received a combination of caspofungin and amphotericin B agents, whereas the remaining patients received monotherapy with amphotericin B.[66] Using multivariate logistic regression analysis with an end point of success at 30 days after hospital discharge, the combination therapy patient group had higher success rates (OR 10.9; 95% CI, 1.3–∞).

Scedosporiosis

Scedosporiosis is associated with high mortality rates in immunocompromised patients, and infection outcomes are associated with the immune function of patients and surgical interventions.[56]

Scedosporiosis Treatment

Antifungal susceptibility testing is recommended because of variable reported resistance to *Scedosporium* spp.[55] Voriconazole is often used as the primary antifungal agent for infections caused by *S. apiospermum* (asexual form of *Pseudallescheria boydii*). Therapy options are limited for *S. prolificans* because high antifungal MIC (amphotericin B, flucytosine, triazole agents) and minimum effective concentration (echinocandin) values have been reported for most isolates. Combination therapy of voriconazole with micafungin, miltefosine, or terbinafine based on in vitro synergy testing has been reported.

Fusariosis

Certain *Fusarium* spp. have been reported to cause IFIs with high mortality rates in immunocompromised patients, especially those with a T-cell immunodeficiency or severe neutropenia.[57] Treatment successes are associated with improved outcomes with immune reconstitution. Agents such as interferon-γ and granulocyte colony-stimulating factor have been prescribed to patients with invasive fusariosis, but efficacy rates with these types of agents are not fully understood.

Fusariosis Treatment

High MIC values have been reported for a variety of antifungal agents including echinocandin and amphotericin B agents with *Fusarium* spp. and triazole agents, specifically with *F. solani* and *F. verticillioides*.[57] Despite in vitro results, lipid formulations of amphotericin B and/or voriconazole have been used to treat invasion fusariosis, with 90-day survival rates reported as 28%–53% with amphotericin B agents and 60% with voriconazole.[57] Posaconazole has been used as salvage therapy, whereas combinations of amphotericin B agents with caspofungin, terbinafine, or voriconazole have been reported.

DIMORPHIC FUNGI—OPPORTUNISTIC ENDEMIC FUNGAL INFECTIONS

Some fungi are dimorphic because these organisms can grow as either a mold or a yeast, depending on growth conditions. Many of the dimorphic fungi that cause IFIs in critically ill patients are considered endemic to certain geographic locations. *Blastomyces dermatitidis*, *Coccidioides* spp., and *Histoplasma capsulatum* may be causative organisms of IFIs, depending on a patient's exposure history in the United States.[67-69] Treatment of endemic IFIs depends on the site and severity of disease together with patient characteristics. Amphotericin B or triazole (including fluconazole or itraconazole) is commonly used as first-line therapy.

Treatment of Blastomycosis

Pulmonary blastomycosis is commonly treated with itraconazole or amphotericin B, as recommended by the 2008 Infectious Diseases Society of America guideline statement.[67] Therapy recommendations start with amphotericin B agents rather than itraconazole for severe disseminated blastomycosis.

Treatment of Coccidioidomycosis

Endemic to the U.S. Southwest, *Coccidioides* spp. infections often need no treatment.[68] Most patients will be asymptomatic after initial exposure. Pulmonary or disseminated disease can develop in some infected patients. Amphotericin B agents are often used first line for symptomatic critically ill patients, with fluconazole or other triazole agents used as stepdown therapy or as initial therapy for less severe disease. If a patient is given a diagnosis of meningitis, fluconazole or alternative triazole therapy is normally recommended to be continued for the duration of the patient's life because of high relapse rates if triazole therapy is discontinued. For refractory cases, other triazole agents have been prescribed, but comparison data are limited. Interferon-γ has been used in salvage therapy in combination with antifungal therapy for patients with interferon-γ receptor 1 deficiency.[70]

Treatment of Histoplasmosis

Infection with *H. capsulatum* is often asymptomatic, but certain critically ill patients, especially if immunocompromised, may require antifungal therapy.[69] As discussed in the 2007 Infectious Diseases Society of America guideline statement, amphotericin B is often used as first-line therapy for moderate to severe pulmonary histoplasmosis, and methylprednisolone can be prescribed in combination if the patient develops acute respiratory distress syndrome. Itraconazole can be used as outpatient therapy.

PROPHYLAXIS FOR IFIs

As shown in Table 16.8, patients in a critical care setting can have a variety of risk factors that have been associated with the increased invasive *Candida* infection rates, including degree of immunosuppression, exposure to broad-spectrum antibiotics, parenteral nutrition, and use of devices including dialysis and extracorporeal life support.[21,33,71-74] The use of antifungal prophylaxis and screening tests such as (1,3)-beta-D-glucan or galactomannan antigen detection assays has been evaluated for patients with certain risk factors for the prevention and detection of IFIs.[75-78] Please see chapter 13, "Laboratory Testing Considerations"; chapter 18, "Antimicrobial Prophylaxis"; and chapter 50, "Care of Immunocompromised Patient," for specific information regarding fungi screening assays and antifungal prophylaxis in critically ill patients.

CONCLUSION

Specialists with a knowledge of antifungal therapy pharmacology and pharmacokinetics together with interpretive susceptibility breakpoints can influence the appropriate use of these agents in patients with IFIs in critical care settings. As yeast and mold rapid diagnostic detection advances, practitioners' ability to develop antifungal therapy algorithms and protocols for drug selection and monitoring on the basis of therapy outcomes, patient characteristics, and known resistance patterns will become important to decrease the time to appropriate antifungal therapy.

REFERENCES

1. Pappas PG, Kauffman CA, Andes D, et al. Clinical practice guidelines for the management of candidiasis: 2009 update by the Infectious Diseases Society of America. Clin Infect Dis 2009;48:503-35.

Table 16.8 Risk Factors for Invasive *Candida* Infections[21,33,71-73]

Infection Site	Associated Risk Factors Include
General risk factors for invasive infection	Immunocompromised state (hematologic malignancies, HSCT, solid organ transplantation, corticosteroids), central venous catheters, parenteral nutrition, exposure to broad-spectrum antibiotics, renal dysfunction (acute), diabetes, surgical procedures
	Specific risk factors based on diagnosis:
Bloodstream infection (candidemia)	• ICU admission
Empyema	• Candidemia
Endocarditis	• Prosthetic heart values, intravenous drug use, central venous catheters, prolonged candidemia
Meningitis	• Candidemia
Pericarditis	• Candidemia, thoracic surgery
Peritonitis	• Peritoneal dialysis, GI perforation, anastomotic leaks, acute necrotizing pancreatitis

HSCT = hematopoietic stem cell transplantation; ICU = intensive care unit.

2. Walsh TJ, Anaissie EJ, Denning DW, et al. Treatment of aspergillosis: clinical practice guidelines of the Infectious Diseases Society of America. Clin Infect Dis 2008;46:327-60.

3. Cornely OA, Arikan-Akdagli S, Dannaoui E, et al. ESCMID and ECMM joint clinical guidelines for the diagnosis and management of mucormycosis 2013. Clin Microbiol Infect 2014;20:5-26.

4. Pfaller MA, Rhomberg PR, Messer SA, et al. Isavuconazole, micafungin, and 8 comparator antifungal agents' susceptibility profiles for common and uncommon opportunistic fungi collected in 2013: temporal analysis of antifungal drug resistance using CLSI species-specific clinical breakpoints and proposed epidemiological cutoff values. Diagn Microbiol Infect Dis 2015;82:303-13.

5. Kothari A, Morgan M, Haake DA. Emerging technologies for rapid identification of bloodstream pathogens. Clin Infect Dis 2014;59:272-8.

6. Amsden JR, Slain D. Antifungal dosing in obesity: a review of the literature. Curr Fungal Infect Rep 2011;5:83-91.

7. Maubon D, Garnaud C, Calandra T, et al. Resistance of *Candida* spp. to antifungal drugs in the ICU: where are we now? Intensive Care Med 2014;40:1241-55.

8. Goodwin ML, Drew RH. Antifungal serum concentration monitoring: an update. J Antimicrob Chemother 2008;61:17-25.

9. Schmitt-Hoffmann A, Roos B, Maares J, et al. Multiple-dose pharmacokinetics and safety of the new antifungal triazole BAL4815 after intravenous infusion and oral administration of its prodrug, BAL8557, in healthy volunteers. Antimicrob Agents Chemother 2006;50:286-93.

10. Falci DR, Pasqualotto AC. Profile of isavuconazole and its potential in the treatment of severe invasive fungal infections. Infect Drug Resist 2013;6:163-74.

11. Sinnollareddy M, Peake SL, Roberts MS, et al. Pharmacokinetic evaluation of fluconazole in critically ill patients. Expert Opin Drug Metab Toxicol 2011;7:1431-40.

12. Brosh-Nissimov T, Ben-Ami R. Differential association of fluconazole dose and dose/MIC ratio with mortality in patients with *Candida albicans* and non-*albicans* bloodstream infection. Clin Microbiol Infect. 2015;21:1011-7.

13. Ray J, Campbell L, Rudham S, et al. Posaconazole plasma concentrations in critically ill patients. Ther Drug Monit 2011;33:387-92.

14. Pascual A, Calandra T, Bolay S, et al. Voriconazole therapeutic drug monitoring in patients with invasive mycoses improves efficacy and safety outcomes. Clin Infect Dis 2008;46:201-11.

15. Koselke E, Kraft S, Smith J, et al. Evaluation of the effect of obesity on voriconazole serum concentrations. J Antimicrob Chemother 2012;67:2957-62.

16. Fish DN. Antifungal dosing in dialysis and continuous renal replacement therapy. Curr Fungal Infect Rep 2011;5:75-82.

17. Muilwijk EW, Schouten JA, van Leeuwen HJ, et al. Pharmacokinetics of caspofungin in ICU patients. J Antimicrob Chemother 2014;69:3294-9.

18. Krishna G, Ma L, Martinho M, et al. Single-dose phase I study to evaluate the pharmacokinetics of posaconazole in new tablet and capsule formulations relative to oral suspension. Antimicrob Agents Chemother 2012;56:4196-201.

19. Clinical and Laboratory Standards Institute (CLSI). Reference Method for Broth Dilution Antifungal Susceptibility Testing of Yeasts; 4th Informational Supplement. CLSI Document M27-S4. Wayne, PA: CLSI, 2012.

20. Pfaller MA, Diekema DJ, Andes D, et al. Clinical breakpoints for the echinocandins and *Candida* revisited: integration of molecular, clinical, and microbiological data to arrive at species-specific interpretive criteria. Drug Resist Updat 2011;14:164-76.

21. Pappas PG, Kauffman CA, Andes D, et al. Clinical practice guidelines for the management of candidiasis: 2009 update by the Infectious Diseases Society of America. Clin Infect Dis 2009;48:503-35.

22. Eschenauer GA, Nguyen MH, Shoham S, et al. Real-world experience with echinocandin MICs against *Candida* species in a multicenter study of hospitals that routinely perform susceptibility testing of bloodstream isolates. Antimicrob Agents Chemother 2014;58:1897-906.

23. Oberoi JK, Wattal C, Goel N, et al. Non-*albicans Candida* species in blood stream infections in a tertiary care hospital at New Delhi, India. Indian J Med Res 2012;136:997-1003.

24. Howard SJ, Lass-Flörl C, Cuenca-Estrella M, et al. Determination of isavuconazole susceptibility of *Aspergillus* and *Candida* species by the EUCAST method. Antimicrob Agents Chemother 2013;57:5426-31.

25. Grossman NT, Pham CD, Cleveland AA, et al. Molecular mechanisms of fluconazole resistance in *Candida parapsilosis* isolates from a U.S. surveillance system. Antimicrob Agents Chemother 2015;59:1030-7.

26. Pfaller MA, Messer SA, Rhomberg PR, et al. In vitro activities of isavuconazole and comparator antifungal agents tested against a global collection of opportunistic yeasts and molds. J Clin Microbiol 2013;51:2608-16.

27. Pfaller MA, Castanheira M, Lockhart SR, et al. Frequency of decreased susceptibility and resistance to echinocandins among fluconazole-resistant bloodstream isolates of *Candida glabrata*. J Clin Microbiol 2012;50:1199-203.

28. Jensen RH, Astvad KM, Silva LV, et al. Stepwise emergence of azole, echinocandin and amphotericin B multidrug resistance in vivo in *Candida albicans* orchestrated by multiple genetic alterations. J Antimicrob Chemother 2015;70:2551-5.

29. Pfaller MA, Messer SA, Moet GJ, et al. *Candida* bloodstream infections: comparison of species distribution and resistance to echinocandin and azole antifungal agents in intensive care unit (ICU) and non-ICU settings in the SENTRY Antimicrobial Surveillance Program (2008-2009). Int J Antimicrob Agents 2011;38:65-9.

30. Ryder NS, Wagner S, Leitner I. In vitro activities of terbinafine against cutaneous isolates of *Candida albicans* and other pathogenic yeasts. Antimicrob Agents Chemother 1998;42:1057-61.

31. Bourgeois N, Laurens C, Bertout S, et al. Assessment of caspofungin susceptibility of *Candida glabrata* by the Etest®, CLSI, and EUCAST methods, and detection of FKS1 and FKS2 mutations. Eur J Clin Microbiol Infect Dis 2014;33:1247-52.

32. Pfaller MA, Jones RN, Castanheira M. Regional data analysis of *Candida* non-*albicans* strains collected in United States medical sites over a 6-year period, 2006-2011. Mycoses 2014;57:602-11.

33. Fernández-Ruiz M, Puig-Asensio M, Guinea J, et al. *Candida tropicalis* bloodstream infection: incidence, risk factors

34. Chow JK, Golan Y, Ruthazer R, et al. Factors associated with candidemia caused by non-*albicans Candida* species versus *Candida albicans* in the intensive care unit. Clin Infect Dis 2008;46:1206-13.

35. Martí-Carrizosa M, Sánchez-Reus F, March F, et al. Implication of *Candida parapsilosis* FKS1 and FKS2 mutations in reduced echinocandin susceptibility. Antimicrob Agents Chemother 2015;59:3570-7.

36. Beyda ND, Liao G, Endres BT, et al. Innate inflammatory response and immunopharmacologic activity of micafungin, caspofungin, and voriconazole against wild-type and FKS mutant *Candida glabrata* isolates. Antimicrob Agents Chemother 2015;59:5405-12.

37. Fernández-Ruiz M, Aguado JM, Almirante B, et al. Initial use of echinocandins does not negatively influence outcome in *Candida parapsilosis* bloodstream infection: a propensity score analysis. Clin Infect Dis 2014;58:1413-21.

38. Pfaller MA, Moet GJ, Messer SA, et al. Geographic variations in species distribution and echinocandin and azole antifungal resistance rates among *Candida* bloodstream infection isolates: report from the SENTRY Antimicrobial Surveillance Program (2008 to 2009). J Clin Microbiol 2011;49:396-9.

39. Beyda ND, John J, Kilic A, et al. FKS mutant *Candida glabrata*: risk factors and outcomes in patients with candidemia. Clin Infect Dis 2014;59:819-25.

40. Lortholary O, Desnos-Ollivier M, Sitbon K, et al. Recent exposure to caspofungin or fluconazole influences the epidemiology of candidemia: a prospective multicenter study involving 2,441 patients. Antimicrob Agents Chemother 2011;55:532-8.

41. Chalupová J, Raus M, Sedlářová M, et al. Identification of fungal microorganisms by MALDI-TOF mass xpectrometry. Biotechnol Adv 2014;32:230-41.

42. De Carolis E, Vella A, Florio AR, et al. Use of matrix-assisted laser desorption ionization–time of flight mass spectrometry for caspofungin susceptibility testing of *Candida* and *Aspergillus* species. J Clin Microbiol 2012;50:2479-83.

43. Abdelhamed AM, Zhang SX, Watkins T, et al. Multicenter evaluation of Candida QuickFISH BC for identification of *Candida* species directly from blood culture bottles. J Clin Microbiol 2015;53:1672-6.

44. Beyda ND, Alam MJ, Garey KW. Comparison of the T2Dx instrument with T2Candida assay and automated blood culture in the detection of *Candida* species using seeded blood samples. Diagn Microbiol Infect Dis 2013;77:324-6.

45. Mylonakis E, Clancy CJ, Ostrosky-Zeichner L, et al. T2 magnetic resonance assay for the rapid diagnosis of candidemia in whole blood: a clinical trial. Clin Infect Dis 2015;60:892-9.

46. Stone NR, Gorton RL, Barker K, et al. Evaluation of PNA-FISH yeast traffic light for rapid identification of yeast directly from positive blood cultures and assessment of clinical impact. J Clin Microbiol 2013;51:1301-2.

47. Altun O, Almuhayawi M, Ullberg M, et al. Clinical evaluation of the FilmArray blood culture identification panel in identification of bacteria and yeasts from positive blood culture bottles. J Clin Microbiol 2013;51:4130-6.

48. Martinez RM, Bauerle ER, Fang FC, et al. Evaluation of three rapid diagnostic methods for direct identification of microorganisms in positive blood cultures. J Clin Microbiol 2014;52:2521-9.

49. Garnaud C, Botterel F, Sertour N, et al. Next-generation sequencing offers new insights into the resistance of *Candida* spp. to echinocandins and azoles. J Antimicrob Chemother 2015;70:2556-65.

50. Dudiuk C, Gamarra S, Jimenez-Ortigosa C, et al. Quick detection of FKS1 mutations responsible for clinical echinocandin resistance in *Candida albicans*. J Clin Microbiol 2015;53:2037-41.

51. Fernandez J, Erstad BL, Petty W, et al. Time to positive culture and identification for *Candida* blood stream infections. Diagn Microbiol Infect Dis 2009;64:402-7.

52. Castanheira M, Messer SA, Rhomberg PR, et al. Isavuconazole and nine comparator antifungal susceptibility profiles for common and uncommon *Candida* species collected in 2012: application of new CLSI clinical breakpoints and epidemiological cutoff values. Mycopathologia 2014;178:1-9.

53. Cho EJ, Shin JH, Kim SH, et al. Emergence of multiple resistance profiles involving azoles, echinocandins and amphotericin B in *Candida glabrata* isolates from a neutropenia patient with prolonged fungaemia. J Antimicrob Chemother 2015;70:1268-70.

54. Tavernier E, Desnos-Ollivier M, Honeyman F, et al. Development of echinocandin resistance in *Candida krusei* isolates after exposure to micafungin and caspofungin in a BM transplant unit. Bone Marrow Transplant 2015;50:158-60.

55. Perfect JR, Dismukes WE, Dromer F, et al. Clinical practice guidelines for the management of cryptococcal disease: 2010 update by the Infectious Diseases Society of America. Clin Infect Dis 2010;50:291-322.

56. Troke P, Aguirrebengoa K, Arteaga C, et al. Treatment of scedosporiosis with voriconazole: clinical experience with 107 patients. Antimicrob Agents Chemother 2008;52:1743-50.

57. Nucci M, Marr KA, Vehreschild MJ, et al. Improvement in the outcome of invasive fusariosis in the last decade. Clin Microbiol Infect 2014;20:580-5.

58. Sipsas NV, Kontoyiannis DP. Invasive fungal infections in patients with cancer in the Intensive Care Unit. Int J Antimicrob Agents 2012;39:464-71.

59. Gregson L, Goodwin J, Johnson A, et al. In vitro susceptibility of *Aspergillus fumigatus* to isavuconazole: correlation with itraconazole, voriconazole, and posaconazole. Antimicrob Agents Chemother 2013;57:5778-80.

60. Kontoyiannis D, Giladi M, Lee M, et al. A Phase 3, Randomized, Double-blind, Non-inferiority Trial to Evaluate Efficacy and Safety of Isavuconazole versus Voriconazole in Patients with Invasive Mold Disease (SECURE): Outcomes in Invasive Aspergillosis Patients. Available at idsa.confex.com/idsa/2014/webprogram/Paper46236.html. Accessed July 6, 2015.

61. Marr KA, Boeckh M, Carter RA, et al. Combination antifungal therapy for invasive aspergillosis. Clin Infect Dis 2004;39:797-802.

62. Herbrecht R, Denning DW, Patterson TF, et al. Voriconazole versus amphotericin B for primary therapy of invasive aspergillosis. N Engl J Med 2002;347:408-15.

63. Kontoyiannis DP, Lionakis MS, Lewis RE, et al. Zygomycosis in a tertiary-care cancer center in the era of Aspergillus-active antifungal therapy: a case-control observational study of 27 recent cases. J Infect Dis 2005;191:1350-60.

64. Chamilos G, Lewis RE, Kontoyiannis DP. Delaying amphotericin B-based frontline therapy significantly increases mortality among patients with hematologic malignancy who have zygomycosis. Clin Infect Dis 2008;47:503-9.

65. Marty FM, Perfect JR, Cornely OA, et al. An Open-label Phase 3 Study of Isavuconazole (VITAL): Focus on Mucormycosis. Available at idsa.confex.com/idsa/2014/webprogram/Paper45645.html. Accessed July 6, 2015.

66. Reed C, Bryant R, Ibrahim AS, et al. Combination polyene-caspofungin treatment of rhino-orbital-cerebral mucormycosis. Clin Infect Dis 2008;47:364-71.

67. Chapman SW, Dismukes WE, Proia LA, et al. Clinical practice guidelines for the management of blastomycosis: 2008 update by the Infectious Diseases Society of America. Clin Infect Dis 2008;46:1801-12.

68. Galgiani JN, Ampel NM, Blair JE, et al. Coccidioidomycosis. Clin Infect Dis 2005;41:1217-23.

69. Wheat LJ, Freifeld AG, Kleiman MB, et al. Clinical practice guidelines for the management of patients with histoplasmosis: 2007 update by the Infectious Diseases Society of America. Clin Infect Dis 2007;45:807-25.

70. Vinh DC, Masannat F, Dzioba RB, et al. Refractory disseminated coccidioidomycosis and mycobacteriosis in interferon-γ receptor 1 deficiency. Clin Infect Dis 2009;49:e62-5.

71. Serefhanoglu K, Timurkaynak F, Can F, et al. Risk factors for candidemia with non-*albicans Candida* spp. in intensive care unit patients with end-stage renal disease on chronic hemodialysis. J Formos Med Assoc 2012;111:325-32.

72. Montagna MT, Caggiano G, Lovero G, et al. Epidemiology of invasive fungal infections in the intensive care unit: results of a multicenter Italian survey (AURORA Project). Infection 2013;41:645-53.

73. Wisplinghoff H, Ebbers J, Geurtz L, et al. Nosocomial bloodstream infections due to *Candida* spp. in the USA: species distribution, clinical features and antifungal susceptibilities. Int J Antimicrob Agents 2014;43:78-81.

74. Gardner AH, Prodhan P, Stovall SH, et al. Fungal infections and antifungal prophylaxis in pediatric cardiac extracorporeal life support. J Thorac Cardiovasc Surg 2012;143:689-95.

75. Timsit JF, Azoulay E, Cornet M, et al. EMPIRICUS micafungin versus placebo during nosocomial sepsis in *Candida* multi-colonized ICU patients with multiple organ failures: study protocol for a randomized controlled trial. Trials 2013;14:399-408.

76. Prattes J, Hoenigl M, Rabensteiner J, et al. Serum 1,3-beta-d-glucan for antifungal treatment stratification at the intensive care unit and the influence of surgery. Mycoses 2014;57:679-86.

77. Fontana C, Gaziano R, Favaro M, et al. (1-3)-β-D-glucan vs galactomannan antigen in diagnosing invasive fungal infections (IFIs). Open Microbiol J 2012;6:70-3.

78. Krause R, Zollner-Schwetz I, Salzer HJ, et al. Elevated levels of interleukin 17A and kynurenine in candidemic patients, compared with levels in noncandidemic patients in the intensive care unit and those in healthy controls. J Infect Dis 2015;211:445-51.

Chapter 17: Invasive Viral Infections in the Intensive Care Unit

P. Brandon Bookstaver, Pharm.D., FCCP, BCPS-AQ ID, AAHIVP;
and Caroline B. Derrick, Pharm.D., BCPS

LEARNING OBJECTIVES

1. Describe and familiarize the reader with viral infections that may be present in the intensive care unit (ICU).
2. Discuss typical patient presentations of these viral infections.
3. List standard diagnostic tools used to differentiate typical viral infections in ICU patients.
4. Recommend appropriate pharmacologic therapy for common viral infections in the ICU.

ABBREVIATIONS IN THIS CHAPTER

CDC	Centers for Disease Control and Prevention	IRIS	Immune reconstitution inflammatory syndrome
CMV	Cytomegalovirus	IVIG	Intravenous immunoglobulin
CoV	Coronavirus	MERS	Middle East respiratory syndrome
CSF	Cerebrospinal fluid	PCR	Polymerase chain reaction
EBV	Epstein-Barr virus	RSV	Respiratory syncytial virus
HAART	Highly active antiretroviral therapy	SARS	Severe acute respiratory syndrome
HSV	Herpes simplex virus	VHF	Viral hemorrhagic fever
ICU	Intensive care unit	VZV	Varicella zoster virus
		WNV	West Nile virus

INTRODUCTION

Viruses play a predominant role in many infectious-related hospital admissions ranging from mild gastroenteritis to life-threatening meningoencephalitis. Intensive care unit (ICU) admissions are also commonplace both in acute viral infections (e.g., respiratory, encephalitis) and among those with chronic infections including HIV and hepatitis. The emergence of viral hemorrhagic fevers (VHFs) and vaccine-preventable diseases such as measles is becoming more prevalent in recent times, requiring new therapeutic advances and renewal of once-forgotten therapies. Many patients admitted to the ICU with viral infections will require mechanical ventilation, vasopressor support, and further invasive management.[1] Although viral pathogens are probably community acquired, there are several reports of hospital acquisition of enteric pathogens such as rotavirus and norovirus, influenza, and cytomegalovirus (CMV).[2,3] Many hospital-acquired infections can be limited through proper education combined with continued hand hygiene, appropriate employee vaccination, and early recognition of a potential outbreak.[3-5]

Although significant, morbidity and mortality vary depending on the viral pathogen and the underlying immune status of the host. The increasing burden of viral disease in hospitalized patients, especially among immunocompromised hosts, has concurrently increased the need for and value of early diagnosis.[6,7] Molecular-based rapid diagnostics such as nucleic acid amplification tests, which are becoming more readily available, allow for early identification of viral pathogens.[8,9] Although causality cannot always be established because of the limitations of such tests, they can help direct targeted pharmacotherapy and promote antimicrobial stewardship in combination with additional laboratory assessment and clinical correlation. Pharmacologic therapy includes not only direct antiviral therapy, but also supportive care measures including hemodynamic management, corticosteroids, and management of common sequelae such as seizures, acute kidney injury, and post-viral bacterial infections. Despite their effectiveness, many antivirals are associated with significant adverse drug events and require careful monitoring. Continuing of home medications for chronic viral infections, specifically HIV, is essential to avoid the development of resistance and an iatrogenic nonadherence.[10] In addition, challenges in drug administration and dosing are created with ICU patients, with frequent interruptions in oral access, intravenous compatibility issues, dynamic renal function, and altered pharmacokinetics.[10] This chapter discusses the clinical presentation, diagnoses, and management of both the common and emerging viral infections seen in the ICU.

HUMAN HERPES VIRUS

The *Herpesviridae* is a family of double-stranded DNA viruses with eight distinct varieties identified as human pathogens. Exposure to these endemic viruses is common, and transmission is often through sexual contact such as with herpes simplex virus (HSV) or casual contact with Epstein-Barr virus (EBV).[11] Although infections in immunocompetent hosts are common, underlying immunocompromise from malignancy, solid-organ or blood and marrow transplantation, or HIV places patients at a heightened risk of invasive herpes infections.[12] In addition to HSV-1 and HSV-2 infections, other important invasive human herpes viruses in hospitalized patients include CMV and varicella zoster virus (VZV).

Herpes Simplex Virus Types 1 and 2

Herpes simplex virus exposure in the general population occurs commonly at an early age with an 80%–90% seropositivity rate.[13] Herpes simplex virus type 1 preferentially establishes latency in the trigeminal ganglion near the ear, typically causing oral lesions, whereas HSV-2 primarily establishes latency in the sacral ganglion at the base of the spine, leading to genital infections. Transmission is through direct contact, by the oral or genital route.[14] Although many infections secondary to HSV are often superficial, HSV is responsible for invasive diseases including meningoencephalitis and, less commonly, pneumonia. Herpes simplex virus is the most prevalent pathogen in encephalitis, identified in 40%–50% of encephalitis cases with a known cause and in about 20% overall.[1,15,16] Table 17.1 provides an overview

Table 17.1 Viral Etiologies of Encephalitis with Diagnostic Testing[a]

Viral Pathogen	Proportion of Total Cases	Diagnostic Endocrine and Metabolic Disorders Testing Method
Herpes simplex virus (HSV-1)	11%–22%	PCR (CSF)
Varicella zoster virus (VZV)	4%–14%	PCR (CSF)
Enterovirus	1%–4%	PCR (CSF)
Arboviruses	Varies by location and season	PCR (CSF)
(Japanese encephalitis virus; West Nile virus [WNV]; tickborne encephalitis virus [TBEV]; Murray Valley encephalitis virus; St. Louis encephalitis virus; La Crosse encephalitis virus [LCEV])	North America: WNV and LCEV Europe: TBEV, WNV	Serology (blood and CSF)
Other herpes viruses (EBV, HHV-6, CMV)	Rare, except in immunocompromised hosts	PCR (CSF) Serology
JC virus (PML)	Only in immunocompromised	PCR (CSF) Serology
Respiratory viruses (influenza, adenovirus)	Rare, except during outbreaks	PCR (respiratory samples, CSF)
Rabies	Rare	PCR saliva, CSF; serology Brain biopsy
Mumps, measles	Rare	Serology (blood)

[a]Unknown cause in 37%–70% of cases.

CMV = cytomegalovirus; EBV = Epstein-Barr virus; HHV = human herpes virus; PML = progressive multifocal leukoencephalopathy.

of viral causes of encephalitis. Although HSV-2 may cause aseptic meningitis, HSV-1 is the predominant type in encephalitis cases. The incidence does not appear to change significantly on the basis of age or sex.[1,13]

Universally, patients with viral encephalitis present with altered mental status, although coma is less common, occuring in about 25% of patients with HSV. For coma to occur, there must be significant cerebral edema raising intracranial pressure or disruption of the ascending reticular activating system (RAS), a neuronal network responsible for wakefulness.[17] Disruption of the RAS is especially common with the temporal lobe involvement seen with HSV encephalitis. Fever occurs in more than 75% of patients. Overt seizures have been reported in up to 65% of patients; however, encephalitis in general is among the most common cause of nonconvulsive status epilepticus, which can only be reliably diagnosed with electroencephalogram (EEG). Seizures are an independent predictor of worse outcomes, and chronic epilepsy is common after treatment.[18,19] Diagnosis is achieved through radiology, cerebrospinal fluid (CSF) examination after lumbar puncture, and CSF polymerase chain reaction (PCR) for HSV. Magnetic resonance imaging (MRI) is abnormal in 90% of cases, whereas computed tomography (CT) scans are abnormal more than 50% of the time. On CSF examination, patients typically have a predominance (80%) of lymphocytes with elevated protein. The presence of red blood cells or xanthochromia may be caused by hemorrhagic inflammation secondary to HSV. Serologic testing is unhelpful, and the test of choice is PCR on the CSF. The sensitivity, which is about 100%, may decrease slightly over time if obtaining CSF is delayed for several days. Viral culture has a low sensitivity and is not commonly performed in standard laboratories.[20,21]

According to several randomized controlled trials (RCTs), antiviral therapy with intravenous acyclovir should be initiated empirically if HSV is in the diagnostic differential (Table 17.2).[22,23] Acyclovir is activated by the viral enzyme thymidine kinase, present in essentially all strains of HSV. Therapy delays beyond 2 days have been associated with poorer outcomes, and initiation within the first 48 hours of suspicion has resulted in reduced mortality rates below 10%.[24] Acyclovir is typically dosed on ideal body weight, although this recommendation is based on very limited data.[25] Associated toxicities commonly include nephrotoxicity and, less commonly, headache, gastrointestinal (GI) effects, altered mental status, and bone marrow suppression. The mechanism of nephrotoxicity is thought to be obstructive secondary to the crystallization of acyclovir in the renal tubules exceeding maximum solubility. Intravenous hydration is an important mechanism of prevention and should be initiated in critically ill patients. Rapid administration may also contribute to the development of acute kidney injury.[10] Therapy duration is typically 14–21 days, despite the original RCTs targeting 10 days of therapy,[24] because of the long-term neuropyschological effects commonly seen among survivors. A recent trial of extended 3-month therapy with oral valacyclovir showed no improved outcomes compared with placebo; however, the rate of neuropyschological decline in this population was less than 15%, lower than in previous reports.[26] Oral valacyclovir, a prodrug of acyclovir, has excellent bioavailability and, at doses of 1,000 mg every 8 hours, has shown sustained CSF concentrations above target during a 20-day treatment period.[27,28] Although treatment data are limited, this may be a potential option when intravenous access or intravenous acyclovir is unavailable. Rarely, HSV has tolerance or resistance to acyclovir, primarily because of deficiency or mutations in thymidine kinase. In these cases, alternative antiviral therapies, including foscarnet or less commonly cidofovir, should be considered. Ganciclovir, a thymidine kinase–dependent antiviral, should not be used routinely in suspected acyclovir resistance or clinical failures.[11] Foscarnet and cidofovir dosing is available in Table 17.2 and discussed in more detail in the Cytomegalovirus section.

Comprehensive symptomatic care is also important for these patients to prevent secondary brain injury, including management of hypotension, hypoxemia, intracranial hypertension, hyperthermia, hypo- and hyperglycemia, anemia, and seizures.[1] Adjunctive use of corticosteroids, specifically dexamethasone, was studied in a limited fashion in a single study of 45 patients with HSV encephalitis.[29] Although corticosteroids were a predictor of improved outcomes in combination with acyclovir, they are not routinely recommended at this time. Management of status epilepticus in accordance with current national guidelines is initially with intravenous lorazepam and establishment of a second agent to prevent recurrence, which may include one of several intravenous options including phenytoin, fosphenytoin, valproate, levetiracetam, and lacosamide.[30]

Cytomegalovirus

Cytomegalovirus is a large double-stranded type 5 β-herpesvirus most closely related to human herpesviruses 6 and 7.[6] Viral replication takes place in human fibroblasts and can be found in an array of cell types including hematopoietic cells, epithelial cells, endothelial cells, fibroblasts, and smooth muscle cells.[31] Similar to other herpesviruses, CMV remains latent in the human body after primary infection and may reactivate throughout a host's life span, causing severe disease in immunocompromised individuals. Asymptomatic viral shedding (urine, saliva, semen, breast milk, and cervical secretions) continues after primary infection; the virus is passed from the infected host through direct contact with body fluids, including sexual contact, blood transfusions, and transplanted organs, with oral and respiratory secretions being the primary route of transmission.[32,33]

Table 17.2 Antiviral Properties and Dosing

Antiviral	Mechanism of Action	Typical Dosing for Invasive Disease	Adverse Events	Antiviral Activity/ Common Use[a]
Acyclovir	DNA polymerase inhibitor; thymidine kinase direct dependent activity	IV: 10 mg/kg every 8 hr according to IBW; renal dose adjustment required for CrCl < 50 mL/min/1.73 m²	Nephrotoxicity, HA, AMS, GI, BMS	HSV; VZV
Valacyclovir	Acyclovir prodrug; DNA polymerase inhibitor; thymidine kinase-dependent activity	PO: 1,000 mg every 8 hr; renal dose adjustment required for CrCl < 50 mL/min/1.73 m²	HA, BMS, transaminitis	HSV; VZV
Ganciclovir	DNA polymerase inhibitor; viral kinase–dependent activity	IV: 5 mg/kg every 12 hr (induction); renal dose adjustment required for CrCl < 70 mL/min/1.73 m²	BMS, GI, nephrotoxicity	CMV; HSV
Valganciclovir	Ganciclovir prodrug; DNA polymerase inhibitor; viral kinase–dependent activity	PO: 900 mg twice daily (induction); 900 mg once daily (maintenance/prophylaxis); renal dose adjustment required for CrCl < 60 mL/min/1.73 m²	GI, BMS, edema	CMV; HSV
Foscarnet	DNA polymerase inhibitor	IV: 90 mg/kg every 12 hr or 60 mg/kg every 8 hr (induction); renal dose adjustment required for CrCl < 1.4 mL/min//1.73 m²/kg[a]	Nephrotoxicity, electrolyte abnormalities, anemia, genital ulceration	CMV; Acyclovir-resistant HSV, VZV
Cidofovir	DNA polymerase inhibitor	IV: 5 mg/kg once weekly x 2 wk (induction); then once every 2 wk (maintenance); each dose must be given with probenecid. Probenecid 2 g 3 hr before infusion; 1 g 2 and 8 hr after completion of cidofovir infusion (4 g total per dose). Renal dose adjustment required for SCr increases of 0.3–0.4 mg/dL above baseline	Nephrotoxicity, proteinuria, neutropenia	CMV; poxvirus; adenovirus; BK polyomavirus; HPV. Can be used in acyclovir-resistant HSV, VZV
Oseltamivir	Neuraminidase inhibitor	PO: 75 mg twice daily; increases to 150 mg twice daily may be indicated. Renal dose adjustment required with CrCl < 60 mL/min/1.73 m²	Neurotoxicity, GI	Influenza B; H1N1; H3N2; resistance emerged to H7N9
Peramivir	Neuraminidase inhibitor	IV: 600 mg daily dose for at least 5 days. Renal dose adjustment required with CrCl < 50 mL/min/1.73 m²	GI, neurotoxicity	Influenza types A and B
Ribavirin	RNA polymerase inhibitor preventing viral protein synthesis	PO: 15–20 mg/kg/day divided and give three times daily (round to available tablet size); renal dose adjustment should be considered < 50 mL/min	Anemia, nephrotoxicity, rash	HCV; RSV; viral hemorrhagic fevers

Table 17.2 Antiviral Properties and Dosing (continued)

Antiviral	Mechanism of Action	Typical Dosing for Invasive Disease	Adverse Events	Antiviral Activity/ Common Use[a]
IVIG	Polyvalent IgG antibodies conferring passive immunity	IV: 400–500 mg/kg daily or every other day	Infusion reaction, aseptic meningitis, hyponatremia, or pseudohyponatremia	Variable use
Palivizumab	Recombinant humanized monoclonal antibody providing passive immunity	IM: 15 mg/kg monthly	Acute hypersensitivity reactions including anaphylaxis	RSV

AMS = altered mental status; BMS = bone marrow suppression; CrCl = creatinine clearance; HA = headache; HCV = hepatitis C virus; HPV = human papillomavirus; HSV = herpes simplex virus (types 1 and 2); IBW = ideal body weight; IM = intramuscular; IV = intravenous; IVIG = intravenous immunoglobulin; PO = by mouth; RSV = respiratory syncytial virus; VZV = varicella zoster virus.

Cytomegalovirus causes complications in the fetus, neonate, and immunocompromised host but rarely in the healthy adult.[34,35] The Centers for Disease Control and Prevention (CDC) reports that 50%–80% of all adults within the United States are infected with CMV by age 40.[33] About 1% of infants are congenitally infected in the United States.[33] Cannon and colleagues found a higher seroprevalence of 45%–100% among women of reproductive ability. Seronegativity within this population places patients at risk of primary infection while pregnant. Variation exists in seropositive percentages across the United States.[34]

In the immunocompetent host, children and adults may be asymptomatic. However, CMV often presents similar to a mononucleosis-like syndrome, comparable with that caused by EBV.[12] Cytomegalovirus causes host-dependent diseases, resulting in immunocompromised hosts developing invasive disease.[6] Specifically in the immunocompromised host, CMV often presents with end-organ damage (e.g., colitis, esophagitis, and neurologic diseases). Solid-organ transplant recipients may have CMV-associated leukopenia, and bone marrow recipients often present with interstitial pneumonitis or pneumonia. In severely immunocompromised patients with AIDS, disease manifestations include gastroenteritis and chorioretinitis leading to potential blindness.[12] Cytomegalovirus retinitis is the most common HIV-associated CMV infection and usually presents at CD4 counts below 100 cells/mm^3. Acute flares may be associated with initiating highly active antiretroviral therapy (HAART) against HIV correlating with an immune reconstitution syndrome.

Cytomegalovirus viremia is detected primarily by PCR, although antigen assays and culture are also available. End-organ disease should not be diagnosed by CMV antigen because of the potential for false-negative tests.[7] Antibody presence in breast milk does not confer protective immunity but may defend against serious disease in the newborn. Antibody titers during acute and chronic illness are usually performed with enzyme immunoassays and indirect and anticomplement immunofluorescence assays. The CMV-immunoglobulin (Ig)M test is highly sensitive but is restricted because of the cross-reaction of acute EBV and the presence of rheumatoid factors.[9] A 4-fold increase in serologies is used to assist in diagnosing infection; however, false positives may occur, and serology testing should not be used alone. Cytomegalovirus may be detected in a blood, urine, throat, and lung culture (from bronchoalveolar lavage or washing) as well as in a lung biopsy. The tissue culture method (shell vial assay) involves centrifugation and an immunocytochemical detection, which uses monoclonal antibodies directed at early CMV antigen.[36]

In the solid-organ transplant recipient, CMV is one of the most important pathogens causing significant morbidity and mortality posttransplantation. More than 50% of solid-organ transplant recipients show evidence of CMV infection. The serostatus of the recipient and donor determines the response after transplantation. The patient with the strongest risk of infection and invasive disease is a serologically negative recipient receiving an organ from a serologically positive donor. However, CMV infection in hematopoietic stem cell transplant recipients is primarily through reactivation of a latent virus of a seropositive recipient.[12,35] Infection can occur if the recipient or donor is serologically positive; however, the disease severity is lessened. The T cell–mediated immune response primarily controls CMV replication, placing immunodeficient hosts at higher infection rates. Cytomegalovirus pneumonitis is rare together with pneumonia, but it represents the most troublesome infection in this patient population, which presents with fever, cough, and infiltrates on chest radiography. Clinicians prefer to see diagnostic "owl's-eye" inclusion bodies on lung biopsy for confirmation.[7,35]

The widespread use of HAART in the United States against HIV has led to a decreased prevalence of CMV retinitis within this population. Retinitis is still the most common CMV-associated end-organ disease and often presents unilaterally. Bilateral progression occurs without appropriate therapy or recovery of the immune system.[7] Cytomegalovirus retinitis affects populations discordantly; men who have sex with men have a higher rate of latent infection, with estimates as high as above 90%.[37]

Therapy for CMV-associated infections should be individualized.[38] Location and severity of infection should be considered before initiating therapy. Primary treatment with ganciclovir (or valganciclovir) is indicated in patients with confirmed, invasive disease. Foscarnet and cidofovir are alternative therapeutic regimens. Patients with HIV infection remain on secondary prophylaxis until CD4 counts recover to greater than 100 cells/mm^3 for 3–6 months.[7,38] Patients receiving solid-organ or bone marrow transplants usually receive prophylaxis for about 3 months.

Ganciclovir requires triphosphorylation to a substrate that competitively inhibits viral DNA synthesis by inhibiting the binding of deoxyguanosine triphosphate to DNA polymerase. The first phosphorylation is known as the rate-limiting step and is induced by enzymes produced by CMV. This unique mechanism renders acyclovir inactive against CMV. The oral prodrug of ganciclovir, valganciclovir, is commonly used in CMV infections. Valganciclovir is rapidly converted to ganciclovir and has about 60% bioavailability. Both agents are renally dose adjusted and require close monitoring.[7,39,40] The predominant adverse effects are moderate to severe neutropenia followed by thrombocytopenia and central nervous system (CNS) events such as confusion and dizziness. Fever and GI adverse events are also documented. Valganciclovir adverse drug events include hypertension, headache, insomnia, and tremor, which are more associated with the use of valganciclovir than with ganciclovir. Cerebrospinal fluid concentrations of ganciclovir are about 50% of serum concentrations. This agent should be continued and monitored closely as maintenance therapy after induction is complete, given the high relapse rates if prematurely discontinued. Ganciclovir may also be administered intraocularly every 5–8 months for CMV retinitis.[7,39,40]

Foscarnet is a pyrophosphate analog that acts as a noncompetitive inhibitor of many viral RNA and DNA polymerases as well as HIV reverse transcriptase. Foscarnet is a highly toxic agent causing considerable nephrotoxicity and electrolyte disturbances (hypomagnesemia, hypokalemia, hypocalcemia). Aggressive hydration is used to decrease renal toxicity, and appropriate dose adjustments must be made in patients with preexisting renal dysfunction. An infusion pump, at a rate not to exceed 1 mg/kg/minute, is necessary for administration. Other documented adverse events are genital ulcers, dysuria, nausea, and paresthesia. This agent does not require phosphorylation to be active; therefore, it can be used to treat ganciclovir-resistant isolates.[7,41]

Cidofovir acts through inhibition of viral DNA synthesis by incorporating cidofovir into replicating viral DNA. Infusion must take place over 1 hour with 1 L of 0.9% normal saline administered intravenously before cidofovir infusion. A second liter may be administered over 1–3 hours immediately after infusion, if tolerated. Serum creatinine (SCr) must be monitored for dose adjustments, and contraindications to cidofovir include SCr values greater than 1.5 mg/dL, creatinine clearance greater than 55 mL/minute/1.73 m^2, history of clinically severe hypersensitivity to probenecid or other sulfa-containing medications, and use of nephrotoxic agents within 7 days. Although renal toxicity is the primary adverse effect of cidofovir administration, GI, hematologic (black box warning for neutropenia), and CNS effects have been reported.[42,43]

Varicella Zoster Virus

Varicella zoster virus is a human neurotropic DNA virus. Primary varicella infection or chickenpox was once commonplace in children in the United States until the vaccine was licensed in 1995. The causative agent, VZV, remains latent in the cranial nerve, dorsal root, and autonomic ganglia along the entire neuroaxis. More than 90% of adults are latently infected with VZV.[44] With the decline in VZV cell-mediated immunity, reactivation occurs in older adults, especially those older than 85 years, and in those with severe immunocompromise, including organ transplantation, malignancy, and HIV.[1,44] Reactivation may occur at any point during the immunocompromised state, although it has been the presenting condition before an HIV diagnosis. On reactivation, herpes zoster presents classically as a vesicular rash after dermatomes with sharp, radiating pain exacerbated by touch. Varicella zoster virus is also the most common cause of viral encephalitis in immunocompromised hosts. Other systemic manifestations include cerebellitis, meningoencephalitis, myelopathy, and ocular disease. Ocular involvement usually manifests as acute retinal necrosis or progressive outer retinal necrosis, of which VZV is the most common cause. This typically occurs in patients with HIV and a CD4 count less than 10 cells/mm^3. Varicella zoster virus infection in the cerebral arteries often leads to ischemic or hemorrhagic stroke.[45-47] Postherpetic neuralgia is also extremely common.

Vasculopathy is a common theme in patients with systemic varicella CNS disease, and some investigators have argued that most VZV CNS infections represent vasculopathy as opposed to encephalitis. Patients may have both small and large vessel involvement. Although most patients will develop CNS involvement after zoster, up to 33% of patients will develop encephalitis in the absence of rash.[45,46,48] In addition, MRI scans are abnormal in most cases; however, some changes on CT and MRI can be seen in patients with rash in the absence of neurological changes. Patients who present with transient ischemic attack or ischemic stroke, chronic headaches, or severe altered mental status with a history of zoster should be evaluated for VZV CNS disease. In addition, those with severe immunocompromise with or without preceding zoster should be evaluated for VZV disease when other common causes of altered mental status have been ruled out. Compared with HSV encephalitis, however, milder CNS-specific symptoms and fever should be expected.[1,44]

Together with imaging findings, patients with confirmed disease will have a CSF pleocytosis in approximately 66% of cases. Angiography has revealed abnormal findings in 70% of patients. With a high specificity, VZV PCR on CSF may be the initial diagnostic test, but with a low sensitivity, a negative PCR can be seen in up to 70% of patients.[1,44] Anti-VZV IgG in the CSF is present in more than 90% of patients with active CNS infection and should be considered the optimal diagnostic test. Patients in the ICU are less likely to have VZV optic disease because of the protracted disease course; however, it may occur concomitantly with CNS disease.[48]

Recommended management of invasive VZV disease is intravenous acyclovir 10–15 mg/kg every 8 hours.[1,24,49] Compared with HSV, higher doses of acyclovir may be required because targeted concentrations against VZV are relatively higher in some strains. Controlled trials supporting this recommendation are limited; however, reduction in disease severity and recovery time has been shown. Therapy should not be delayed because of lack of confirmed diagnostics from CSF if suspicion of VZV is high. Many patients will have concomitant immunocompromising states (e.g., malignancy and HIV) that require management of these conditions. Toxicities associated with acyclovir, which are often dose-dependent, remain significant and may be exacerbated in immunocompromised patients with underlying renal dysfunction. Therapy duration should be 14 days; however, 21 days should be strongly considered in patients with underlying immunocompromise.[1,24,48] Use of oral agents such as valacyclovir has not been studied and cannot be recommended at this time. Because of the accompanying vasculitis, adjunct corticosteroids are recommended by many experts. A prednisone equivalent dose of 1 mg/kg/day should be considered. Limited use in varicella pneumonia has had some beneficial effects.[2] No definite duration for prednisone has been established, although some have recommended 3–5 days of therapy.[1,50,51] Short-course therapy may still be associated with significant adverse drug events and should be evaluated and managed as required. In patients with VZV optic disease—specifically, progressive outer retinal necrosis—acyclovir monotherapy has produced suboptimal results. Ganciclovir or foscarnet, or in combination, should be considered first-line therapy. Dosage is consistent with that of other invasive viral diseases (Table 17.2).

Because of the immunocompromised state of many of these patients, specialist management, including infectious diseases consultation, is recommended. Although many patients recover from the VZV infection itself, full recovery is highly dependent on disease manifestations (e.g., stroke) and the patient's immune status.[44]

Epstein-Barr Virus

Epstein-Barr virus is commonly known as the causative pathogen of infectious mononucleosis. Although it can rarely be responsible for other invasive viral syndromes in immunocompetent hosts, including encephalitis, most patients at risk of EBV disease are severely immunocompromised. Epstein-Barr virus is primarily transmitted through saliva.[52] In immunocompetent hosts, EBV preferentially infects circulating B lymphocytes and the epithelium in the oropharynx and of the cervix. These infected B lymphocytes lead to infiltration of other organs. The lymphocytosis seen with EBV infection is primarily that of T lymphocytes, indicative of the extreme immune response mounted against infected B cells.[52,53] In immunocompromised hosts, especially those with HIV/AIDS and those after solid-organ or blood and marrow stem cell transplantation, EBV is responsible for many infections including hairy leukoplakia (HLP), lymphoproliferative syndromes, and several associated malignancies. In HLP, EBV replicates at high numbers in associated lesions; however, EBV remains in a latent state in other associated syndromes and malignancies.[53]

Treatment of these patients is targeted at restoring T-cell (and B-cell) immune function and supportive care. Antiviral therapy, including acyclovir, has activity in vitro; however, clinical trials have failed to show morbidity or mortality benefit.[54,55] This may be because of a lack of phosphorylation, and thus activation, of the antivirals by viral enzymes. In addition, failure to concentrate in circulating infected B lymphocytes and inability to target the virus in the latent state may be contributing factors. Corticosteroids are used in the acute phase of these infections by some experts, although clinical data to support outcomes are lacking.[1,55]

HUMAN IMMUNODEFICIENCY VIRUS

Establishment of HIV infection depletes the T lymphocytes and therefore promotes an immunosuppressive state. About 3–6 weeks after an initial HIV infection, more than half of infected individuals experience an acute HIV infection syndrome.[56] The term *acute* refers to the time during which the virus is detectable within the blood and serum but antibodies have not yet formed.[57] Symptoms vary in severity but resemble an acute infectious mononucleosis. The decrease in CD4 T lymphocytes and the perpetual increase in viral load lead to the acute HIV response. After this response, described in further detail in the following text, an immune response will mount from the host in an attempt to fight the infection. The immunity formed from the host does not completely hinder viral replication, and the decrease in viremia does not persist.[58,59] Immunity is decreased by the infected CD4 T lymphocytes, and opportunistic infections are most common at CD4 T-cell counts less than 200/mm^3. To prevent this progressive decrease in immune function, the mainstay of treatment is initiating antiretroviral therapy.[60]

During initial HIV infection, patients often present with fever, pharyngitis, lymphadenopathy, headache, muscle pain, fatigue, weight loss, and GI symptoms (nausea, vomiting, and diarrhea). Patients may also have a maculopapular rash on the trunk and extremities and/or genital ulcers. Presentation with sexually transmitted infections (HSV, gonorrhea, syphilis, hepatitis viruses) is common, and coinfection rates are high. This nonspecific syndrome leads to a diagnostic challenge for clinicians. Antibody formation is undetectable on initial infection and may not be present during the acute infectious stage. Acute HIV is therefore often undiagnosed, leading to negative patient outcomes and necessitating high clinical suspicion.[58,59]

On entry into the health care system, it is recommended that all patients be tested for HIV with an opt-out setting. Initial HIV infection presents with a high viral load, and patients may not know they are infected. Rosenberg and colleagues found that early treatment with antiretrovirals increased HIV-1–specific CD4 and CD8 T-cell responses, boosting host immunity.[60]

Initiating HAART may precipitate an immune reconstitution inflammatory syndrome (IRIS), often called immune reconstitution disease if not stemming from an autoimmune process.[56] Variations in epidemiologic statistics exist, but early retrospective data showed that about 30% of patients who are at risk of IRIS develop the clinical syndrome. More recent data support a lower incidence overall, about 15%, with higher percentages of almost 38% for patients with CMV retinitis specifically.[61] Opportunistic infections that have not been treated may reactivate, causing an exacerbation of clinical symptoms. Cytomegalovirus retinitis, tuberculosis, *Mycobacterium avium* complex, *Pneumocystis jiroveci* pneumonia, cryptococcosis, progressive multifocal leukoencephalopathy, and herpes zoster infection represent most of the causative opportunistic infections outlined by Walker and colleagues detailing HIV-associated IRIS specifically. Previously undiagnosed infection is termed *unmasking*, and exacerbation or recurrence of symptoms is termed *paradoxical worsening*.[62]

Risk factors for IRIS consist of a lower CD4 count (less than 100 cells/mm^3), high viral load, and suboptimal treatment of opportunistic infections before initiating HAART.[63] Immune reconstitution, which may occur days to months after HAART, is accompanied by an increase in CD4 cells. The pathophysiology of the response is not clearly defined and cannot completely be explained by this increase. Cytokines as well as innate and adaptive immune responses, together with the host immune functional capacity, have been proposed as important factors. Patients may have symptoms of inflammation—specifically, fever, malaise, and lymphadenitis. If an opportunistic infection was not previously treated, the symptoms specific to this infection may present.[64] Shelbourne et al. performed a retrospective chart review of patients with HIV infection with *Mycobacterium tuberculosis*, *M. avium* complex, or *Cryptococcus neoformans* and evaluated risk factors for IRIS.[65] When the opportunistic infection was diagnosed, affected patients were more likely to have started HAART close to diagnosis, to have been antiretroviral naive, and to have had a more rapid initial fall in HIV-1 RNA levels in response to HAART. Cytomegalovirus retinitis–associated IRIS has sight-threatening implications; therefore, patients with HIV infection having a history of CMV retinitis should have a dilated ophthalmologic examination every 3 months for the first year after initiation of ARV therapy or if visual acuity changes or floaters develop. Wiselz and colleagues detail three case reports of acute respiratory failure after introducing HAART to patients with severe *P. jiroveci* pneumonia. In the ICU, this clinical picture may present as a therapeutic challenge. Reintroducing steroids or suspending HAART was necessary for these patients to recover.[65]

In all cases, appropriate diagnostics must be performed to identify whether an opportunistic infection has activated. If identified, the opportunistic infection must be treated appropriately. Overall, symptomatic treatment is the mainstay of therapy. If the IRIS is severe, steroids may be administered for 1–2 weeks and tapered to discontinuation. Doses have not been standardized; however, some experts recommend 1–2 mg/kg of prednisone daily. For mild IRIS, nonsteroidal anti-inflammatory agents can be used for fever and inflammation; if pulmonary inflammation presents, inhaled steroids are therapeutic options. In general, a delay in, or holding of, antiretroviral therapy is not currently recommended because of the life-saving nature of the therapy.[66] However, if life-threatening symptoms occur or if permanent sequelae may result, HAART should be deferred. Dheda and colleagues evaluated patients coinfected with tuberculosis and HIV and concluded that initiating HAART reduced immediate and long-term risk of death and AIDS-defining illnesses.[67] In addition, patients with a CD4$^+$ cell count less than 100 cells/mm^3 are at higher risk of death or new AIDS-defining illnesses during the early phase of tuberculosis treatment and more prone to immune reconstitution. Treating opportunistic infections before HAART will assist in preventing IRIS and decreasing bacterial burden.[7,30,67]

Patients with long-standing HIV infection are often admitted to the ICU for noninfectious causes.[45] It is imperative to consider reinitiating antiretroviral therapy as soon as clinically feasible. Failure to reinitiate antiretroviral therapy may lead to an iatrogenic nonadherence. Antiretroviral errors are very common in the hospitalized setting and may occur in up to 70% of inpatients.[68] In the ICU specifically, high rates of acute kidney injury and use of acid-suppressing agents may lead to dosing errors and drug-drug interactions, respectively. In addition, knowledge of crushable administration is important in the ICU, and maintaining available formulations of solutions and suspensions will help ensure the continuity of antiretroviral therapy.[69]

RESPIRATORY VIRUSES

Viral infections may play a prominent role in respiratory disease in the ICU, both community acquired and less commonly through nosocomial acquisition.[2,70] Community-acquired viruses such as influenza, specifically H1N1, have resulted in significant acute respiratory diseases prompting ICU admission (Table 17.3).[7] This is more likely to occur in the older adult or immunocompromised population and is often associated with community outbreaks. Reactivation of endogenous viruses including HSV and CMV can also occur in immunocompromised patients. Histologic assessment and open lung biopsy of previously healthy intubated patients with suspected ventilator-associated pneumonia have revealed that almost 30% had findings compatible with CMV lung disease, whereas only 3% had HSV.[71] Patients with documented CMV infections have had increased duration of mechanical ventilation and longer ICU and overall hospital length of stay; these infections were inconsistently associated with increased mortality.[71,72] In addition, these patients had higher rates of bacterial and fungal superinfections, which may also be reflected in the immunocompromised state of most of these patients. Herpes simplex virus appears less likely to be associated with a true pneumonia or bronchopneumonitis, as opposed to a tracheobronchitis.[2,73] Patients with HSV often have outcomes similar to those with nonviral infections. If active CMV infection is suspected, management with ganciclovir is appropriate; however, consultation with infectious diseases specialists is recommended.[74] Preemptive or prophylactic management of viral infections in acute respiratory distress syndrome is limited to a single prospective study of intravenous acyclovir showing no clinical benefit in ventilated patients. Despite the unknown contribution of CMV and HSV as viral pathogens in respiratory disease in the ICU, these patients are susceptible to nosocomial outbreaks of viruses including influenza.[75] Both patients and health care workers may serve as potential vectors. Procalcitonin has been investigated specifically in patients with concurrent influenza to determine the presence or absence of bacterial infection. The available data suggest that in patients with concurrent respiratory viral disease, procalcitonin is helpful to determine the need for antibiotics; however, it should not be used as a stand-alone test.[76,77] The availability of rapid diagnostics outside conventional antigen testing with influenza and respiratory synctial virus (RSV) using nucleic acid amplification tests and PCR technologies is becoming more prevalent.[9] Commericially available multiplex testing allows for simultaneous investigation of not only several viruses but also atypical bacteria. Use of multiplex PCR for viral pathogens specifically offers several potential advantages in the ICU population: optimizing treatment with both antibacterials and antivirals, limiting the overuse of antibiotics and the subsequent development of resistance, reducing the need for superfluous diagnostic testing, and allowing for proper isolation. Installing multiplex PCR has shown a reduction in the use of antibiotics, primarily in a hematology-oncology population.[9,32,49] Data for use in a medical or surgical ICU are limited to date; however, this is a quickly evolving area of study and development. Several other viral pathogens including RSV, adenovirus, parainfluenza, metapneumovirus, and rhinovirus have been implicated in causing primarily respiratory disease. Although most of these pathogens are typically associated with self-limiting infections, serious, life-threatening disease is not uncommon, especially in children younger 1 year and older adults, often with accompanying immunocompromise. Management of these viruses is primarily symptomatic care, and identification by PCR, including commercially available multiplex PCR, is increasingly common for high-volume institutions. The clinical relevance of identifying these pathogens in the presence of respiratory disease remains debatable, although a growing body of evidence supports their causality of lower respiratory tract infections in immunocompromised adults. Viruses, including virulent strains of coronavirus (CoV) and enterovirus, although naturally common, have been associated with severe outbreaks globally and in the United States, respectively.

Influenza

Influenza types A and B are known to cause serious infection in humans and are typically associated with seasonal outbreaks, typically peaking in the winter months. Unlike influenza B, influenza A can be further subtyped by the surface proteins hemagglutinin and neuraminadase. There are 18 different hemagglutinin (H1–H18) and 11 different neuraminidase (N1–N11) subtypes.[78] Viruses are named

Table 17.3 Causes of Viral Respiratory Disease in the Intensive Care Unit

Virus	Endogenous	Exogenous
Community	HSV, CMV	Influenza, parainfluenza, adenovirus, rhinovirus, CoV, metapneumovirus, enterovirus
Nosocomial	HSV, CMV	Mimivirus, CMV (transfusion), influenza (H1N1), CoV

CoV = coronavirus.

in accordance with the internationally accepted World Health Organization (WHO) nomenclature originally published in 1980.[79] Each year, 5%–20% of the U.S. population will be infected with influenza, resulting in more than 200,000 hospitalizations.[78] Most of these hospitalizations do not result in critical illness except in patients of extreme age or with immunocompromise. However, since 2009, with the emergence of the endemic H1N1 (an influenza type A) strain, young and middle-aged adults have more commonly been admitted to the ICU with severe acute respiratory distress syndrome.[80] This may be because of the relatively lower immunization rate in this population (less than 50% nationally) and the prior immunity acquired in older patients from exposure to antigenic similar strains.[54,80] This 2009 strain has now replaced the previously circulating H1N1 virus in humans. The annual deaths associated with influenza range from 3,000 to up to 35,000 annually, and most recently, most are associated with the H1N1 strain.[78] Patients with obesity (body mass index greater than 30 kg/m²) and pregnant women are among the higher-risk populations for critical illness with influenza infection. Proinflammatory cytokines occur at a high rate in the lungs of influenza-positive patients and are responsible for much of the significant morbidity associated with the disease.[7,81]

Rapid diagnosis is important because many patients will deteriorate 4–5 days after onset of illness, which is associated with typical flu-like symptoms including fever, fatigue, cough, rhinorrhea, and myalgias.[8] Although the historic gold standard for influenza diagnosis is viral cell culture, delays in diagnosis and required laboratory resources make this impractical for routine patient diagnosis, especially during influenza season.[82] The use of rapid diagnostics, specifically molecular-based PCR testing, is recommended for hospitalized patients. Reverse-transcriptase PCR testing is available in both single and multiplex design. Table 17.4 lists commonly available testing methods. The sensitivity of rapid diagnostic tests is typically 50%–70% but ranges from 10% to 80%, depending on the viral replication and specimen collection, storage, and transport.[82,83] Testing within 3–4 days of onset of influenza infection is more likely to yield positive test results. Specificity is quite high (more than 95%), and false positives are unlikely.[83,84] A false positive may be achieved if a patient has received the live attenuated virus vaccine within 7 days and an upper respiratory tract sample is used. In addition, if a patient tests positive to both influenza A and influenza B, the unlikely result of having both viruses simultaneously should prompt additional testing at a reference laboratory. False negatives are more common during peak season, and of importance, a negative test should not preclude targeted antiviral therapy during peak season and in the setting of high pretest probability. In an outbreak, testing several patients will significantly increase the sensitivity.[83]

On deterioration, patients will develop hypoxemia, shock, and multiorgan dysfunction. Careful monitoring of hemodynamics is required for prompt and timely

Table 17.4 Commonly Available Influenza Diagnostic Testing Methods[83]

Testing Method	Influenza Types Detected	Acceptable Specimens	Time to Results
Viral tissue cell culture	A and B	NP or throat swab; NP or bronchial wash; nasal or ET aspirate; sputum	3–10 days
Rapid cell culture	A and B	NP or throat swab; NP or bronchial wash; ET or nasal aspirate; sputum	1–3 days
Immunofluorescence, direct or indirect fluorescent antibody testing	A and B	NP swab; NP or bronchial wash; ET or nasal aspirate	1–4 hr
Reverse-transcriptase PCR testing (single or multiplex)	A and B	NP or throat swab; NP or bronchial wash; ET or nasal aspirate; sputum	Variable; typically 1–8 hr
Rapid molecular assay	A and B	NP swab; nasal aspirate, wash, or swab	< 30 min
Rapid influenza diagnostic tests	A and B	NP and throat swab; nasal wash, aspirate	< 30 min

ET = endotracheal; NP = nasopharyngeal.

Adapted from: Centers for Disease Control and Prevention (CDC). Guidance for Clinicians on the Use of Rapid Influenza Diagnostic Tests. Available at www.cdc.gov/flu/professionals/diagnosis/clinician_guidance_ridt.htm. Accessed October 9, 2015.

intubation. Patients may also present with concomitant bacterial pneumonia, especially *Staphylococcus aureus*, including methicillin-resistant *S. aureus*, *Streptococcus pneumoniae*, or *Streptococcus pyogenes*.[85] The acute respiratory distress syndrome associated with influenza requires low-tidal volume lung-protective ventilation and an open-lung approach with increased positive end-expiratory pressure. Appropriate fluid management is also essential to recovery. Many patients may not respond to conventional management and may require advanced care to include extracorporeal membrane oxygenation, neuromuscular blockade, nitric oxide, and lung recruitment maneuvers.[7] Outcomes with these interventions are inconsistent and should be considered on a patient-specific basis.

Antiviral therapy is recommended for all hospitalized patients with influenza.[78] Neuramindase inhibitors, including oseltamivir, zanamavir, and most recently peramivir, are recommended for both influenza A and influenza B.[78,86,87] Oral oseltamivir is recommended by the CDC as first-line therapy for hospitalized, critically ill patients. Zanamavir is available as inhaled version and may be difficult to administer in critically ill patients, especially if intubated. Zanamavir is also contraindicated in patients with underlying respiratory disease such as asthma or chronic obstructive pulmonary disease.[86,88] Intravenous zanamavir is currently under investigation and available on limited access.[78] Oseltamivir is orally adminsterd as a prodrug that is rapidly converted to the active form. Oral bioavailability is high and reaches peak concentrations within 1 hour of administration. Standard dosing (75 mg twice daily) for a minimum of 5 days is recommended (Table 17.2), although longer durations should be considered in critically ill patients, depending on clinical response.[78,86,88] Higher doses of 150 mg twice daily have also been suggested in critically ill patients, although limited data suggest that serum concentrations are adequate with conventional dosing.[89] Limited pharmacokinetic studies in morbid obesity and pregnancy also suggest that standard doses provide adequate concentrations, despite some clinician practices to increase the dosing to 150 mg.[90] In critically ill patients, oseltamivir administered by oro- or nasogastric tube was well absorbed, including in those on continuous renal replacement therapy and extracorporeal membrane oxygenation.[90-92] If absorption is questioned or oral access is not established, intravenous peramivir is recommended.[78,87] Although intravenous peramivir compared with standard of care had no clinical benefit in hospitalized patients during clinical trials, it was well tolerated.[87] Treatment should be 600 mg daily for at least 5 days.[78] A small subset of patients with influenza A may have resistance to oseltamivir. Zanamavir often maintains activity against oseltamivir-resistant strains, and its use should be strongly considered.[54,88]

Despite the recommendations and widespread use of the neuraminidase inhibitors for influenza, there are questions regarding their effectiveness. In a 2014 Cochrane review, data from 46 clinical trials showed a modest 14.4- to 16.8-hour reduction in time to first symptom alleviation for oseltamivir and zanamivir.[93] However, complications of influenza were not carefully examined in most studies, and lack of consistent definitions did not allow for full assessment if a reduction occurred in these influenza-related complications including pneumonia. Prophylactic oseltamivir appeared to reduce symptomatic influenza but did not reduce hospitalizations.[93] Despite the relative lack of effectiveness shown and general lack of good outcomes data in hospitalized patients, our treatments are limited to aggressive antiviral therapies and supportive care. Ultimate recovery is variable and dependent on the total care of the patient beyond antiviral therapies. Prevention is likely to be the best mode of treatment for most patients. Patients with influenza are more susceptible to bacterial pathogens, as mentioned previously. Postinfluenza *S. aureus*, including methicillin-resistant *S. aureus* (MRSA), pneumonia is often common.[94] In patients with a recent history of influenza infection or severe viral pneumonia, MRSA pneumonia should be considered in the differential and may direct empiric therapy, even in community-acquired infections.

Prevention through vaccination is primarily the responsibility of health care workers, including pharmacists. Many hospitals have introduced mandated vaccine protocols for workers with direct patient care responsibilities.[95] Despite the limitations in viral coverage associated with the recent available vaccine therapy, use has been shown to reduce influenza infections and prevent health care worker-to-patient transfer and thus the potential for associated outbreaks.

Respiratory Syncytial Virus

Respiratory syncytial virus is an RNA virus in the *Pneumovirus* genus that is responsible for more than 50,000 hospitalizations each year in children younger than 5 years.[96] An additional 175,000 hospitalizations with almost 15,000 deaths in adults older than 65 years are reported in the United States.[97] Infants younger than 1 year are at highest risk. By age 3, virtually all children have been infected. Respiratory syncytial virus is a seasonal virus peaking between October and May in the United States.[97] Respiratory syncytial virus may be responsible for up to 2% of nursing home deaths in older adults. The disease manifestations range from common cold symptoms to severe lower respiratory tract disease.[98] The air trapping that results leads to a rapid respiratory rate, a palpable spleen and liver, and typical radiographic findings of hyperinflation and diffuse atelectasis. Bronchiolitis may lead to respiratory failure requiring mechanical ventilation. Around 1%–2% of patients will require admission to the ICU.[96,98]

Treatment of these patients is primarily supportive care, although many treatments have been studied. Most clinical data remain in pediatric patients.[96] Bronchodilators and corticosteroids have not been shown to improve clinical outcomes and are not currently recommended. Bronchodilators may be used on a trial basis and continued if there is objective improvement.[96,99,100] Ribavirin is U.S. Food and Drug Administration (FDA) approved for the management of RSV, despite large controlled studies showing a lack of benefit in clinical end points. The aerosolized form has been used anecdotally with some success and is recommended in pediatric patients with severe, clinical disease and potentially underlying immunocompromise. Administration is continuous or intermittent for 8–24 hours daily for 3–5 days and requires a special device for aerosol delivery (Table 17.2).[52] Ribavirin is also considered a hazardous agent according to the National Institute for Occupational Safety and Health. Precautions during preparation and administration are required.[101] Ribavirin is category X and is contraindicated in pregnancy.[28] Exposure to ribavirin has been seen by health care workers administering the drug, with minor adverse effects including headaches and nausea. Although improvements in delivery continue, pregnant health care workers should be cautioned in delivering the aerosolized drug. On rare occasions, it can worsen bronchospasms for the patient.[28] Palivizumab, a humanized monoclonal antibody derived from murine samples, and polyclonal immunoglobulins have been used in adults and children with mixed results in a treatment modality.[102]

Palivizumab is FDA approved for the prophylaxis of RSV in high-risk pediatric patients. The American Academy of Pediatrics updates recommendations on the basis of additional evidence.[102] The most recent update in the summer of 2014 included premature infants (younger than 29 weeks) who are younger than 12 months at the start of the RSV season, especially those with congenital heart or lung disease.

Coronavirus

Coronavirus infections are caused by one of six serotypes, four of which are extremely common, and most adults have been infected with one or more during their lifetime.[103,104] Typically, these are responsible for mild, self-limiting upper respiratory tract diseases. Two strains in particular, SARS-CoV and MERS-CoV, are responsible for global outbreaks of severe acute respiratory syndrome (SARS) and Middle East respiratory syndrome (MERS), respectively.[94] In 2002, an outbreak of SARS, which began in China, was responsible for almost 8,100 infections and more than 750 deaths. Since 2004, however, there have been no documented cases of SARS worldwide.[94,105] The SARS-CoV strain disproportionally infects adults and carries a case fatality rate of almost 10%.[5] Most patients present with 5–7 days of fever, dyspnea, cough, malaise, and other generalized respiratory symptoms. About 25% will have diarrhea, and of concern, 20% will develop severe respiratory distress requiring mechanical ventilation. Transmission occurs from human-to-human contact and peaks during the second week of illness (day 10) concurrently with peaks in viral load. Management is primarily symptomatic care, although several agents have been studied in humans.[5,106] Ribavirin, interferon, and lopinavir/ritonavir have all shown antiviral activity in vitro.[103,107] Clinical studies, however, do not support the routine use of these agents. Corticosteroids and intravenous immunoglobulin (IVIG) also failed to show improved outcomes.[5,103] Patients who received ribavirin or corticosteroids also had higher rates of significant adverse drug events, and those who received pulse-dose methylprednisolone specifically had higher rates of 30-day mortality, which should be considered before administration.[5] Proper isolation and infection control measures are essential to prevent patient-to-health care worker or patient-to-patient transmission in an institutional setting.

The MERS-CoV strain was responsible for a recent outbreak, which began in 2012 in Jordan. Since then, as of June 2015, about 1,200 cases have been reported to WHO.[107] Outside the Middle East, where most cases have been reported, South Korea has also had a significant outbreak of almost 200 cases. Only two cases have been reported in the United States, both from international travelers from the Middle East.[108] Like with SARS-CoV, bats are thought to be the primary vector of infection.[109] However, unlike with SARS-CoV, human-to-human transmission, although possible and documented, appears to be somewhat less of a concern. Adults are primarily affected (in more than 90% of cases), and the median age is around 50.[94,109] Most patients with MERS-CoV infection, about 75%, have had associated comorbidities, and more than 75% of patients have required hospitalization. Respiratory failure is common, requiring mechanical ventilation. Patients often have laboratory abnormalities including leukopenia, lymphopenia, thrombocytopenia, and elevated lactate dehydrogenase. The case fatality rate appears to be 35%–45%.[94,108,109] Table 17.5 offers a detailed comparison of SARS-CoV and MERS-CoV. Early recognition and diagnosis remains difficult in patients with MERS infection. The primary method of diagnosis is MERS-CoV PCR testing and is available on respiratory, blood, and stool samples. There are reports of false negatives, especially on inadequate upper respiratory tract samples early in the disease process. Retesting of patients with high pretest probability may be required at this time.[109] Most state reference laboratories in the United States are equipped to handle specimen testing; however, contact with the CDC for suspected cases is required. Treatment of these patients is primarily symptomatic care, recognizing the aggressive and virulent nature of this virus. Interferon, ribavirin, cyclosporine A, and mycophenolic acid have shown effects in vitro; however, none has shown positive clinical outcomes to date.[106,109] Limited knowledge of the viral kinetics currently limits targeted therapies. Convalescent serum from survivors may be considered in the absence of other proven therapies.[106,107]

Table 17.5 Comparison of Common Characteristics Between SARS and MERS[94]

Characteristic	MERS-CoV	SARS-CoV
First reported case	April 2012 – Jordan	November 2002 – China
Incubation period	5.2 days (2–13 days)	4.6 days (2–14 days)
Age group affected	Adults > 90%	Adults > 90%
Mortality	~35%	~10%
Sex	Male: ~65%	Male: ~43%
Symptoms		
Fever	98%	99%–100%
Chills/rigors	87%	15%–73%
Cough	83%	62%–100%
Hemoptysis	17%	0%–1%
Myalgia	32%	45%–61%
Shortness of breath	72%	40%–42%
Laboratory results		
Chest radiograph abnormalities	100%	94%–100%
Leukopenia	14%	25%–35%
Lymphopenia	32%	68%–85%
Thrombocytopenia	36%	40%–45%
Elevated LDH	48%	50%–71%
Elevated ALT/AST	11%–14%	20%–30%
Ventilatory support required	80%	14%–20%

LDH = lactate dehydrogenase; MERS = Middle East respiratory syndrome; SARS = systemic acute respiratory syndrome.

Adapted from: Hui DS, Memish ZA, Zumla A. Severe acute respiratory syndrome vs. the Middle East respiratory syndrome. Curr Opin Pulm Med 2014;20:233-41.

Enterovirus

In 2014, a nationwide outbreak of enterovirus infection occurred in the United States, infecting almost 1,200 people, primarily infants and young children.[110,111] This population is primarily affected because of the lack of natural immunity acquired from exposure to related viruses. The virus strain in this particular outbreak of severe disease, enterovirus D68 (EV-D68), is only one of almost 100 identified non-polio enteroviruses. Patients present with severe hypoxemia, wheezing, and difficulty breathing. Many of these patients have underlying asthma (75%). Very few (about 25%) patients have fever on initial presentation.[110] Consideration of enterovirus diagnosis is important to prevent human-to-human transmission, which may occur through droplets. Management of underlying lung disease and acute respiratory decline is essential, which may often include corticosteroids.[110,112] There is no conclusive evidence of the effectiveness of pharmacologic interventions, aside from symptomatic care of acute respiratory syndrome. The death rate appears to be about 1%. During the 2014 outbreak, about 100 patients were also given a diagnosis of an acute flaccid myelitis, first reported in Colorado.[112] Although it has not been conclusively proven, evidence suggests and experts agree that this is a unique presentation of EV-D68. Many of these patients have remained symptomatic, and only a small percentage of patients have fully recovered. Therapeutic interventions including corticosteroids, IVIG, and convalescent serum have been tried, but no evidence supports their benefit at this time.[110,112]

VIRAL HEMORRHAGIC FEVERS

Viral hemorrhagic fevers represent a group of viruses from four distinct families: arenaviruses, filoviruses, bunyaviruses, and flaviviruses. All are RNA viruses enveloped in a lipid bilayer that require an animal or insect as the vector. Outbreaks of these infections are primarily relegated to the geographic areas where the natural hosts live.[22] However, in the example of Marburg virus, the first reported cases in 1978 were in Marburg and Frankfurt, Germany, and Yugoslavia secondary to exposure to infected monkeys from the host region.[113] Transmission may occur from human-to-human contact for some VHFs, including Ebola, Marburg, and Lassa. Recent outbreaks of Ebola virus disease in 2014 that affected the United States and other Western countries have increased the sensitivity and need for preparedness for VHFs.[22,61] Global transportation has brought the world much closer, shrinking once-distinct geographic regions for disease.

Patients often present with typical, generalized viral illness symptoms including fatigue, fever, weakness, and muscle aches. Severe disease is associated with bleeding, although this is not necessarily present in most patients, and patients often die secondary to severe hypovolemia and multiorgan failure. Treatment is primarily symptomatic care, although emerging antiviral and convalescent serum therapies are under development or have some limited experimental data. Ribavirin has been used effectively in patients with Lassa fever and hemorrhagic fever renal syndrome.[114] The CDC has developed practical, institutional guidelines for managing and preventing VHFs.[61] Guidelines are often updated on the emergence of new outbreaks and availability of new data. Understanding and management of these infections is limited in part because of the relative youth in discovery of many of these VHFs as well as because much of the burden of disease has been isolated to the developing world in Sub-Saharan Africa. Ebola virus disease, highlighted in detail in the following text, can serve as an example in management and prevention for other VHFs.

Ebola virus, a member of the flavivirus family, was first identified in 1976 near the Ebola River in the present-day Democratic Republic of the Congo. Although a vector has not been fully confirmed, many experts agree that the fruit bat is the most likely host. The virus affects both humans and primates. Several outbreaks have been reported historically, localized primarily to Central Africa and the eastern coastline. The most recent outbreak, which began in March 2014 in Guinea, has resulted in almost 28,000 infected individuals and more than 11,000 deaths.[115] In June 2015, at least several small pockets of disease remain in Sierra Leone. The incubation period can be as short as 2 days and as long as 3 weeks; however, the average onset of symptoms is typically 8–10 days from infection.[115] Transmission can be directly from the infected primate or the vector or between humans through contact with infected body fluids including blood, sweat, urine, and saliva. Viral RNA typically peaks 3–5 days after infection and is higher among fatal cases than among survivors.

Like with many other VHFs, patients often present with generalized symptoms including fever, fatigue, malaise, generalized weakness, hiccups, and muscle aches.[22,116,117] Gastrointestinal symptoms typically appear in the first 5 days and are common. Diarrhea is very severe, with volumetric losses mimicking those of severe cholera. Severe hypovolemia preempting additional sequelae (e.g., acute kidney injury) is often the primary reason for ICU admission. Despite volume losses of up to 10 L/day, patients have increased body weights of 15–20 kg because of extreme third spacing. Electrolyte abnormalities including hyponatremia, hypokalemia, and hypocalcemia are severe and require prompt attention. In severe cases, patients have multiorgan failure and other effects including seizures and arrhythmias.[22,116,118]

Prompt diagnosis, followed by isolation, is the first and most important intervention to prevent further exposure and limit spread of disease. Diagnosis is based initially on appropriate travel history and corresponding symptoms. Ebola PCR testing is available but, because it is not routinely available in institutions, requires a delay for send-out testing at a reference laboratory.[22,61,119] Rapid diagnostic testing is not currently commercially available but is under investigation. To prevent transmission, a level 4 biocontainment facility setup is required. In general, the patient requires 24 hours/day, 7 days/week one-to-one or two-to-one nursing care using strict isolation and appropriate personal protection equipment (PPE).[22,61] Staff must be specially trained on the donning and doffing of PPE. Laboratory specimens for testing require point-of-care testing or designated equipment in a centralized laboratory. Although medication transfer and administration are managed by the nurse, medication safety checks and balances such as bar scanning should be maintained, whenever possible. The CDC outlines the appropriate development of a biocontainment team and isolation ward.[61]

Treatment of these patients is primarily symptomatic care because no antiviral agents have shown effectiveness on a large scale. Some experts recommend the use of lactated Ringer solution (20 mL/kg) boluses with aggressive intravenous electrolyte replacement.[22,118] Sequelae such as disseminated intravascular coagulation, hypotension, arrhythmias, and/or seizures should be managed like in other critically ill patients. Antibiotics are not indicated unless a secondary bacterial infection develops.[22,118] Experimental antivirals have been used with success, and several are currently under development. Without controlled trials, little is currently known about the safety and effectiveness of these antivirals in humans. Convalescent serum from survivors has also been used with success.[120] Antibodies that develop to Ebola virus disease are thought to remain for about 10 years.[62] At least one reinfection case has been documented.[115]

ARBOVIRUSES

Arboviruses represent a broad group of viruses with arthropod vectors, most commonly mosquitoes and ticks. The most common arboviruses and their characteristics are listed in Table 17.6.[1,121,122] Knowledge and discovery of these viruses varies significantly because the first reports of Dengue fever date to AD 992 in the *Encyclopedia of Chinese Medicine*.[123] West Nile virus (WNV) was first identified in 1937, since being recognized in the United States at the turn of the 20th century.[124] Throughout history, these viruses have caused sporadic epidemics globally, but rarely have they caused a significant burden of disease in the United States. Globalization with enhanced international travel during the past 3–4 decades has increased the spread of the disease and emergence in new parts of the world. The incubation period ranges from 2 days to 2 weeks in most patients.[124] Many infected patients have self-limiting disease; however, severe infections requiring hospitalization result in a subset of patients. Symptoms range from general "flu-like" illness to severe respiratory distress, multiorgan failure, and shock. Symptomatic care is the hallmark of treatment with no active antiviral therapies available. In some instances, IVIG has been used on a limited basis with mixed results. In a pediatric population in Nepal with Japanese encephalitis, IVIG at 400 mg/kg/day for 5 days resulted in higher antibodies and interleukin (IL)-4 and IL-6 levels in treated patients than in those receiving standard of care.[125] Clinical outcomes, however, remained the same in both groups. Sporadic case reports show mixed results on the effectiveness in WNV encephalitis.[1] Immunoglobulin lots obtained from endemic areas are likely to have higher viral titers specific to many of these viral infections and potentially enhanced effects. In viral encephalitis, some

Table 17.6 List of Common Arboviruses and Corresponding Properties

Arbovirus	Typical Incubation	Symptoms	Complications/ Case Fatality Rate	Vector	Geographic Distribution
Chikungunya	3–7 days (range 1–12 days)	Most patients have self-limiting disease; fever and polyarthralgia; HA, muscle pain, joint swelling, or rash	Persistent joint pain; rarely myelitis, meningoencephalitis 1/1,000 case fatality	Mosquito	Africa, Asia, Indian, and Pacific oceans. Caribbean islands
Dengue fever	5–7 days (range 3–10 days)	80% of patients are asymptomatic; fever (high temperature), HA, N/V, pain behind eyes, mild bleeding, leukopenia, thrombocytopenia	24–48 hr after resolution of fever, an increase in capillary permeability leads to shock and multiorgan failure 1%–10% case fatality rate	Mosquito	Tropics including Asia, South America, and Central America
Japanese encephalitis virus	5–10 days	Fever, HA, vomiting; mental status changes, movement disorders and seizures (especially in children)	Encephalitis case fatality rate is 20%–30% 30%–50% of survivors have cognitive, neurologic, or psychiatric symptoms	Mosquito	East Asia, Indian Ocean
Tickborne encephalitis virus	8 days (range 4–28 days)	33% of patients have a nonspecific febrile illness, HA, myalgia, fatigue; 33% of these patients progress to second phase with CNS involvement	CNS involvement occurs in 10% of patients; case fatality rate of 2% in the European subtype, 20%–40% in Far Eastern subtype, and 2%–3% in Siberian subtype	Tick (*Ixodes* spp.)	Europe, Far East Asia, Siberia
West Nile virus	5–15 days	20% of patients develop West Nile fever; HA, weakness, body aches, rash on trunk, lymphadenopathy	1 in 150 individuals develop neuroinvasive disease 5% case fatality rate	Mosquito	Africa, Europe, the Middle East, North America, and West Asia
Yellow fever virus	3–6 days	Initial phase of disease fever, chills, HA, generalized weakness; after a remission, about 15% progress to severe form of disease	Severe disease characterized by high temperature, jaundice, bleeding, shock, and multiorgan failure 20%–50% case fatality rate in severe disease	Mosquito	Africa, South America

N/V = nausea and vomiting.

experts suggest using intrathecal or intraventricular administration to enhance antibody exposure across the blood-CSF barrier. Although IVIG may be considered in many of the flavivirus infections with progression despite aggressive symptomatic care, caution should be used with untoward effects. The optimal dosing and route of administration for a suspected CNS infection are unknown.[1,124]

Dengue Fever

Dengue fever is the most common arbovirus infection, only behind malaria for infection-related sequelae in the tropics. The mosquito in the genus *Aedes* is the primary vector, and human-to-human transfer of disease is not confirmed. Infection occurs with one of four serotypes, DEN 1–4, and infection with one serotype does not offer protection against the others.[123] Subsequent infections, in fact, with different serotypes may increase the severity of disease and the likelihood of associated hemorrhagic fever or shock. The infection rate worldwide has increased 30-fold in the past 50 years.[123] Dengue fever worldwide is primarily a disease of infants and children, although disease in a returning traveler from an area where Dengue fever is endemic may occur in adults as well. Diagnosis is based on travel history, together with fever and two of the following criteria: nausea/vomiting, rash, aches and pains, positive tourniquet test, leukopenia, or one of the warning signs for severe disease. Viral serologies are also available for Dengue, which are often used for confirmation. The hemagglutination inhibition assay and the IgG and IgM enzyme immunoassays are available, with the IgM enzyme immunoassay test being the most commonly used. Rapid PCR testing is also available that can diagnose the disease early in the infection window (less than 48 hours), but it requires a reference laboratory for most institutions.[124,126] Dengue infection occurs in three distinct phases over an average 10-day period: febrile, critical, and recovery.[123,126] The hallmark of the clinical course is an increase in capillary permeability and a resultant plasma leakage and increase in hematocrit. Plasma leakage peaks over a 24- to 48-hour period during the critical phase. This is accompanied by a significant decrease in white blood cell and platelet counts. The severity of the plasma leakage may lead to other sequelae including shock and multiorgan failure, although this is rare. Other laboratory abnormalities seen in the critical phase include hypoalbuminemia, elevated liver enzymes, thrombocytopenia and leukopenia, and abnormal coagulation profile.[1,126]

Management of severe Dengue fever is primarily symptomatic care and focused on appropriate fluid balance. Repeated boluses may be needed in severe plasma leak; however, maintenance fluids should be carefully balanced and adjusted according to patient requirement.[126] Further management of resultant hypotension beyond intravenous fluids may be required in rare situations. Electrolyte shifts are also common. Antibiotics are not indicated unless a secondary bacterial infection occurs. The mortality rate is less than 1%, and many patients can be treated as outpatients, with proper education and knowledge of immune status. Prevention is a primary focus with the lack of antiviral therapies. Avoiding mosquito acquisition is the best current strategy. Vaccine development is under investigation, although no timeline is available.[1,123]

Other Zoonotic Infections

The rabies virus is an RNA virus transmitted through the saliva of an infected animal vector. In the United States, bats, raccoons, skunks, and foxes are the primary sources of infection, depending on the geographic region. Each year in the United States, about 6,000 animals, 92% of which are nondomestic, and two or three humans are infected with rabies. Worldwide, however, almost 75,000 cases occur annually.[127] The case fatality rate is 100%, and only three survivors who have not received postexposure prophylaxis with immunoglobulin or the rabies vaccine have been reported.[128] After exposure to an infected animal, the average incubation period is 20–90 days, although time to presentation is quite variable.[41,129] Patients often have localized symptoms after the initial bite has healed, including localized pain, numbness, tingling, and paresthesias together with generalized viral syndrome of fatigue, malaise, and fever. The two distinct forms of rabies are encephalitic in 80% of patients and paralytic in 20% of patients. It is not clearly understood why and how each may manifest. The encephalitic form has a greater burden of disease involving the spinal cord and peripheral nerves. Patients have episodes of hyperexcitability separated by lucid periods. Autonomic dysfunction is common. The hallmark feature is hydrophobia, which involves diaphragmatic spasms lasting 5–15 seconds on attempts to swallow. This can also be triggered by the sight of liquids and draft of air. Patients quickly progress to coma and multiorgan failure. Paralytic rabies typically begins at the bite location with spread to quadriparesis and bilateral facial weakness. Hydrophobia does not typically occur in this form of rabies, although progression to coma and organ failure is imminent but often delayed compared with progression with the encephalitic form.[41,130]

Early presentation after a bite but before the onset of symptoms will trigger a proactive response to determine the necessary prophylaxis. Animal testing can be done quickly using direct fluorescent antibody testing on the brain tissue. If it is determined that a high-risk exposure has occurred, the previously unvaccinated patient will receive a single dose of human rabies immunoglobulin (HRIG) infiltrated into the wound and surrounding areas.[128,129] Patients will also receive a four-dose series of rabies vaccine, with the first dose beginning the same day and subsequent doses given on days 3, 7, and 14. The vaccine should be administered intramuscularly in the deltoid area at a site distant from the HRIG. If the entire volume of the HRIG cannot be administered local to the bite, the remaining volume can be administered intramuscularly at a site distant from the vaccine. This is to reduce the potential inactivation of the rabies vaccine. Patients who were previously vaccinated should receive two doses of the vaccine, but HRIG is not indicated.[128]

Among the three survivors known to date who did not receive postexposure prophylaxis, a 15-year-old girl who survived was placed in a therapeutic coma with intravenous midazolam and supplemental phenobarbital for a burst-suppression pattern on EEG. In addition, she was maintained on continuous infusion ketamine and provided antiviral therapy with ribavirin and amantadine. This protocol, based on very limited evidence, has been labeled the "Milwaukee protocol."[128,131] Despite success in this patient, at least 20 failures have been documented using a similar approach since its publication.[132] Although these agents are under investigation, no evidence currently suggests that this pharmacologic approach promotes clearance of rabies or resolution of symptoms.

SUMMARY

Pharmacists contribute daily to improving patient care in the ICU through improving medication safety, promoting evidence-based practice, optimizing medication delivery, and reducing unnecessary costs. For many critical care pharmacists, managing infectious diseases is a primary function of day-to-day patient care activities.[10] Viral infections play a critical role in the burden of infectious diseases in the ICU. Although many of these are acquired in the community, the risk of nosocomial viral infections is increasingly prevalent. Pharmacists should always practice and promote appropriate infection control measures, abiding by institutional guidelines. Good hand hygiene is a simple but proven effective measure for reducing the transmission of nosocomial pathogens from health care workers to patients or between patients.[4] The continued development of rapid diagnostics and the availability of new testing platforms for viral pathogens such as multiplex PCR provide an additional, integral role for pharmacists. Knowledge and interpretation of such tests are important for properly managing unnecessary antibiotics, discussing the potential need for targeted antiviral therapy, or communicating the need for infection control measures. Supportive care is the cornerstone of management for many invasive viral infections; however, some of the more prevalent viral infections in the ICU have proven, available, evidence-based, antiviral therapies. For antivirals, which are usually much less commonly used than antibacterials, knowledge of appropriate dosing, administration, and adverse effects is limited to a select few members of the treatment team. Many of these patients will also have accompanying immunocompromised states, requiring a working knowledge of immunomodulators and immunodeficiencies. Research is significantly lacking in the management of many invasive viral infections, priming pharmacists for an opportunity to help lead efforts to enhance the clinical investigation of these patients.

REFERENCES

1. Kramer AH. Viral encephalitis in the ICU. Crit Care Clin 2013;29:621-49.
2. Chiche L, Forel JM, Papazian L. The role of viruses in nosocomial pneumonia. Curr Opin Infect Dis 2011;24:152-6.
3. Bobo LD, Dubberke ER. Recognition and prevention of hospital-associated enteric infections in the intensive care unit. Crit Care Med 2010;38:S324-34.
4. Tschudin-Sutter S, Pargger H, Widmer AF. Hand hygiene in the intensive care unit. Crit Care Med 2010;38:S299-305.
5. Stockman LJ, Bellamy R, Garner P. SARS: systematic review of treatment effects. PLoS Med 2006;3:e343.
6. Ljungman P, Hakki M, Boeckh M. Cytomegalovirus in hematopoietic stem cell transplant recipients. Hematol Oncol Clin North Am 2011;25:151-69.
7. Mauskopf J, Klesse M, Lee S, et al. The burden of influenza complications in different high-risk groups: a targeted literature review. J Med Econ 2013;16:264-77.
8. Peaper DR, Landry ML. Rapid diagnosis of influenza: state of the art. Clin Lab Med 2014;34:365-85.
9. Caliendo AM. Multiplex PCR and emerging technologies for the detection of respiratory pathogens. Clin Infect Dis 2011;52(suppl 4):S326-30.
10. Hernandez JO, Norstrom J, Wysock G. Acyclovir-induced renal failure in an obese patient. Am J Health Syst Pharm 2009;66:1288-91.
11. James SH, Prichard MN. Current and future therapies for herpes simplex virus infections: mechanism of action and drug resistance. Curr Opin Virol 2014;8:54-61.
12. El Amari EB, Combescure C, Yerly S, et al. Clinical relevance of cytomegalovirus viraemia. HIV Med 2011;12:394-402.
13. Steiner I, Kennedy PGE, Pachner AR. The neurotropic herpes viruses: herpes simplex and varicella-zoster. Lancet Neurol 2007;6:1015-28.
14. Engelberg R, Carrell D, Krantz E, et al. Natural history of genital herpes simplex virus type 1 infection. Sex Transm Dis 2003;30:174-7.
15. Gable MS, Sheriff H, Dalmau J, et al. The frequency of autoimmune N-methyl-D-aspartate receptor encephalitis surpasses that of individual viral etiologies in young individuals enrolled in the California Encephalitis Project. Clin Infect Dis 2012;54:899-904.
16. Granerod J, Ambrose HE, Davies NWS, et al. Causes of encephalitis and differences in their clinical presentations in England: a multicentre, population-based prospective study. Lancet Infect Dis 2010;10:835-44.
17. Almond MH, McAuley DF, Wise MP, et al. Influenza-related pneumonia. Clin Med 2012;12:67-70.

18. Steiner I, Budka H, Chaudhuri A, et al. Viral meningoencephalitis: a review of diagnostic methods and guidelines for management. Eur J Neurol 2010;17:999-e57.
19. Misra UK, Tan CT, Kalita J. Viral encephalitis and epilepsy. Epilepsia 2008;49(suppl 6):13-8.
20. Tindall B, Cooper DA. Primary HIV infection: host responses and intervention strategies. AIDS 1991;5:1-14.
21. Shelbourne SA, Darcourt J, White AC Jr, et al. The role of immune reconstitution inflammatory syndrome in AIDS-realted Cryptococcus neoformans disease in the era of highly active antiretroviral therapy. Clin Infect Dis 2005;40:1049-52.
22. Toner E, Adalja A, Inglesby T. A primer on Ebola for clinicians. Disaster Med Public Health Prep 2015;9:33-7.
23. Volling C, Hassan K, Mazzulli T, et al. Respiratory syncytial virus infection-associated hospitalization in adulats: a retrospective cohort study. BMC Infect Dis 2014;14:665.
24. Tunkel AR, Glaser CA, Bloch KC, et al. The management of encephalitis: clinical practice guidelines by the Infectious Diseases Society of America. Clin Infect Dis 2008;47:303-27.
25. Davis RL, Quenzer RW, Weller S, et al. Acyclovir Pharmacokinetics in Morbid Obesity. Presented at: Interscience Conference on Antimicrobial Agents and Chemotherapy; 1991; Washington, DC. Abstract 765.
26. Gnann JW Jr, Skoldenberg B, Hart J, et al. Herpes simplex encephalitis: lack of clinical benefit of long-term valacyclovir therapy. Clin Infect Dis 2015.
27. Pouplin T, Pouplin JN, Van Toi P, et al. Valacyclovir for herpes simplex encephalitis. Antimicrob Agents Chemother 2011;55:3624-6.
28. Lycke J, Malmestrom C, Stahle L. Acyclovir levels in serum and cerebrospinal fluid after oral administration of valacyclovir. Antimicrob Agents Chemother 2003;47:2438-41.
29. Kamei S, Sekizawa T, Shiota H, et al. Evaluation of combination therapy using aciclovir and corticosteroid in adult patients with herpes simplex virus encephalitis. J Neurol Neurosurg Psychiatry 2005;76:1544-9.
30. Brophy GM, Bell R, Claassen J, et al. Guidelines for the evaluation and management of status epilepticus. Neurocrit Care 2012;17:3-23.
31. Sinzger C, Digel M, Jahn G. Cytomegalovirus cell tropism. Curr Top Microbiol Immunol 2008;325:63-83.
32. Kurath S, Halwachs-Baumann G, Muller W, et al. Transmission of cytomegalovirus via breast milk to the prematurely born infant: a systematic review. Clin Microbiol Infect 2010;16:1172-8.
33. Centers for Disease Control and Prevention (CDC). Cytomegalovirus (CMV) and Congenital CMV Infection. Available at www.cdc.gov/cmv/index.html. Accessed July 29, 2015.
34. Cannon MJ, Schmid DS, Hyde TB. Review of cytomegalovirus seroprevalence and demographic characteristics associated with infection. Rev Med Virol 2010;20:202-13.
35. Crough T, Khanna R. Immunobiology of human cytomegalovirus: from bench to bedside. Clin Microbiol Rev 2009;22:76-98, Table of Contents.
36. Hirsch HH, Lautenschlager I, Pinsky BA, et al. An international multicenter performance analysis of cytomegalovirus load tests. Clin Infect Dis 2013;56:367-73.
37. Jabs DA, Ahuja A, Van Natta M, et al. Course of cytomegalovirus retinitis in the era of highly active antiretroviral therapy: five-year outcomes. Ophthalmology 2010;117:2152-61 e1-2.
38. Jabs DA, Ahuja A, Van Natta M, et al.; Studies of the Ocular Complications of ARG. Comparison of treatment regimens for cytomegalovirus retinitis in patients with AIDS in the era of highly active antiretroviral therapy. Ophthalmology 2013;120:1262-70.
39. Cytovene [package insert]. South San Francisco, CA: Genentech USA.
40. Valcyte [package insert]. South San Francisco, CA: Genentech USA.
41. Foscavir [package insert]. North Ryde NSW: AstraZeneca.
42. Lea AP, Bryson HM. Cidofovir. Drugs 1996;52:225-30.
43. Vistide [package insert]. Foster City, CA: Gilead Sciences, September 2010.
44. Nagel MA, Gilden D. Neurological complications of varicella zoster virus reactivation. Curr Opin Neurol 2014;27:356-60.
45. Palacios R, Hidalgo A, Reina C, et al. Effect of antiretroviral therapy on admission of HIV-infected patients to an intensive care unit. HIV Med 2006;7:193-6.
46. Kalpoe JS, van Dehn CE, Bollemeijer JG, et al. Varicella zoster virus (VZV)-related progressive outer retinal necrosis (PORN) after allogeneic stem cell transplantation. Bone Marrow Transplant 2005;36:467-9.
47. Gilden D. Varicella zoster virus and central nervous system syndromes. Herpes 2004;11(suppl 2):89A-94A.
48. Hagiya H, Kimura M, Miyamoto T, et al. Systemic varicella-zoster virus infection in two critically ill patients in an intensive care unit. Virol J 2013;10:225.
49. Zumla A, Al-Tawfiq JA, Enne VI, et al. Rapid point of care diagnostic tests for viral and bacterial respiratory tract infections—needs, advances, and future prospects. Lancet Infect Dis 2014;14:1123-35.
50. Wood AJ, Johnson RW, McKendrick MW, et al. A randomized trial of acyclovir for 7 days or 21 days with and without prednisolone for treatment of acute herpes zoster. N Engl J Med 1994;330:896-900.
51. Whitley RJ, Weiss H, Gnann JW Jr, et al. Acyclovir with and without prednisone for the treatment of herpes zoster. Ann Intern Med 1996;125:376-83.
52. Young LS, Rickinson AB. Epstein-Barr virus: 40 years on. Nat Rev Cancer 2004;4:757-68.
53. Young LS, Murray PG. Epstein-Barr virus and oncogenesis: from latent genes to tumours. Oncogene 2003;22:5108-21.
54. Rafailidis PI, Mavros MN, Kapaskelis A, et al. Antiviral treatment for severe EBV infections in apparently immunocompetent patients. J Clin Virol 2010;49:151-7.
55. Gershburg E, Pagano JS. Epstein-Barr virus infections: prospects for treatment. J Antimicrob Chemother 2005;56:277-81.
56. Chun TW, Fauci AS. HIV reservoirs: pathogenesis and obstacles to viral eradication and cure. AIDS 2012;26:1261-8.
57. Pilcher CD, Eron JJ, Galvin S, et al. Acute HIV revisited: new opportunities for treatment and prevention. J Clin Invest 2004;113:937-45.
58. Cohen MS, Shaw GM, McMichael AJ, Haynes BF. Acute HIV-1 infection. N Eng J Med 2011;364:1943-54.

59. Panel on Antiretroviral Guidelines for Adults and Adolescents. Guidelines for the use of antiretroviral agents in HIV-1 infected adults and adolescents. Department of Health and Human Services. Available at http://www.aidsinfo.nih.gov/ContentFiles/AdultandAdolescentGL.pdf.
60. Rosenberg RS, Altfeld M, Poon SH, et al. Immune control of HIV-1 after early treatment of acute infection. Nature 2000;407:523-6.
61. Müller M, Wandel S, Colebunders R, et al. Immune reconstitution inflammatory syndrome in patients starting antiretroviral therapy for HIV infection: a systematic review and meta-analysis. Lancet Infect Dis 2010;10:251-61.
62. Walker NF, Scriven J, Meintjes G, et al. Immune reconstitution inflammatory syndrome in HIV-infected patients. HIV AIDS (Auckl) 2015;7:49-64.
63. Grant PM, Komarow L, Andersen J, et al. Risk factor analyses for immune reconstitution inflammatory syndrome in a randomized study of early vs. deferred ART during an opportunistic infection. PLoS One 2010;5:e11416.
64. Phillips P. How infrequent are opportunistic diseases and immune reconstitution syndromes among HIV-infected individuals who have favorable CD4+ cell count responses to antiretroviral therapay? Clin Infect Dis 40:1379-80.
65. Wislez M, Bergot E, Antoine M, et al. Acute respiratory failure following HAART introduction in patients treated for *Pneumocystis carinii* pneumonia. Am J Respir Crit Care Med 2001;164:847-51.
66. Carr A, Zolopa AR, Andersen J, et al. Early antiretroviral therapy reduces AIDS progression/death in individuals with acute opportunistic infections: a multicenter randomized strategy trial. PLoS One 2009;4:e5575.
67. Dheda K, Lampe FC, Johnson MA, Lipman MC. Outcome of HIV-associated tuberculosis in the era of highly active antiretroviral therapy. J Infect Dis 2004; 190:1670-101.
68. Kelly LS, Caulder CR, Bookstaver PB. Timely formulary management for preventing errors related to antiretroviral drugs. Am J Health Syst Pharm 2013;70:1014-5.
69. Duggan JM, Akpanudo B, Shukla V, et al. Alternative antiretroviral therapy formulations for patients unable to swallow solid oral dosage forms. Am J Health Syst Pharm 2015;72:1555-65.
70. Limaye AP, Boeckh M. CMV in critically ill patients: pathogen or bystander? Rev Med Virol 2010;20:372-9.
71. Chiche L, Forel JM, Roch A, et al. Active cytomegalovirus infection is common in mechanically ventilated medical intensive care unit patients. Crit Care Med 2009;37:1850-7.
72. Mosca F, Pugni L. Cytomegalovirus infection: the state of the art. J Chemother 2007;19 Suppl 2:46-8.
73. Luyt CE, Combes A, Deback C, et al. Herpes simplex virus lung infection in patients undergoing prolonged mechanical ventilation. Am J Respir Crit Care Med 2007;175:935-42.
74. Osawa R, Singh N. Cytomegalovirus infection in critically ill patients: a systematic review. Crit Care 2009;13:R68.
75. Cameron RJ, de Wit D, Welsh TN, et al. Virus infection in exacerbations of chronic obstructive pulmonary disease requiring ventilation. Intensive Care Med 2006;32:1022-9.
76. Wu MH, Lin CC, Huang SL, et al. Can procalcitonin tests aid in identifying bacterial infections associated with influenza pneumonia? A systematic review and meta-analysis. Influenza Other Respir Viruses 2013;7:349-55.
77. Wacker C, Prnko A, Brunkhorst FM, Schlattmann P. Procalcitonin as a diagnostic marker for sepsis: a systematic review and meta-analysis. Lancet Infect Dis 2013 May;13(5):426-35.
78. Centers for Disease Control and Prevention (CDC). Influenza (Flu). Available at www.cdc.gov/flu/. Accessed August 19, 2015.
79. World Health Organization (WHO). A revision of the system of nomenclature for influenza viruses: a WHO memorandum. Bull World Health Organ 1980;58:585-91.
80. Lee EH, Wu C, Lee EU, et al. Fatalities associated with the 2009 H1N1 influenza A virus in New York City. Clin Infect Dis 2010;50:1498-504.
81. Fezeu L, Julia C, Henegar A, et al. Obesity is associated with higher risk of intensive care unit admission and death in influenza A (H1N1) patients: a systematic review and meta-analysis. Obes Rev 2011;12:653-9.
82. Kumar S, Henrickson KJ. Update on influenza diagnostics: lessons from the novel H1N1 influenza A pandemic. Clin Microbiol Rev 2012;25:344-61.
83. Centers for Disease Control and Prevention (CDC). Guidance for Clinicians on the Use of Rapid Influenza Diagnostic Tests. Available at www.cdc.gov/flu/professionals/diagnosis/clinician_guidance_ridt.htm. Accessed October 9, 2015.
84. Leland DS, Ginocchio CC. Role of cell culture for virus detection in the age of technology. Clin Microbiol Rev 2007;20:49-78.
85. Corneli HM, Zorc JJ, Mahajan P, et al. A multicenter, randomized, controlled trial of dexamethasone for bronchiolitis. N Engl J Med 2007;357:331-9.
86. Louie JK, Yang S, Acosta M, et al. Treatment with neuraminidase inhibitors for critically ill patients with influenza A (H1N1) pdm09. Clin Infect Dis 2012;55:1198-204.
87. de Jong MD, Ison MG, Monto AS, et al. Evaluation of intravenous peramivir for treatment of influenza in hospitalized patients. Clin Infect Dis 2014;59:e172-85.
88. Razonable RR. Antiviral drugs for viruses other than human immunodeficiency virus. Mayo Clin Proc 2011;86:1009-26.
89. Lee N, Hui DS, Zuo Z, et al. A prospective intervention study on higher-dose oseltamivir treatment in adults hospitalized with influenza A and B infections. Clin Infect Dis 2013;57:1511-9.
90. Pai MP, Lodise TP Jr. Oseltamivir and oseltamivir carboxylate pharmacokinetics in obese adults: dose modification for weight is not necessary. Antimicrob Agents Chemother 2011;55:5640-5.
91. Kromdijk W, Sikma MA, van den Broek MP, et al. Pharmacokinetics of oseltamivir carboxylate in critically ill patients: each patient is unique. Intensive Care Med 2013;39:977-8.
92. Ariano RE, Sitar DS, Zelenitsky SA, et al. Enteric absorption and pharmacokinetics of oseltamivir in critically ill patients with pandemic (H1N1) influenza. CMAJ 2010;182:357-63.
93. Jefferson T, Jones MA, Doshi P, et al. Neuraminidase inhibitors for preventing and treating influenza in adults and children. Cochrane Database Syst Rev 2014;4:CD008965.
94. Hui DS, Memish ZA, Zumla A. Severe acute respiratory syndrome vs. the Middle East respiratory syndrome. Curr Opin Pulm Med 2014;20:233-41.

95. Drees M, Wroten K, Smedley M, et al. Carrots and sticks: achieving high healthcare personnel influenza vaccination rates without a mandate. Infect Control Hosp Epidemiol 2015;36:717-24.
96. Turner TL, Kopp BT, Paul G, et al. Respiratory syncytial virus: current and emerging treatment options. Clinicoecon Outcomes Res 2014;6:217-25.
97. Centers for Disease Control and Prevention (CDC). Respiratory Syncytial Virus Infection (RSV). Available at www.cdc.gov/rsv/. Accessed August 20, 2015.
98. Vincent B, Timsit JF, Auburtin M, et al. Characteristics and outcomes of HIV-infected patients in the ICU: impact of the highly active antiretroviral treatment era. Intensive Care Med 2004;30:859-66.
99. Lado M, Walker NF, Baker P, et al. Clinical features of patients isolated for suspected Ebola virus disease at Connaught Hospital, Freetown, Sierra Leone: a retrospective cohort study. Lancet Infect Dis 2015;15:1024-33.
100. Jones SM, Feldmann H, Stroher U, et al. Live attenuated recombinant vaccine protects nonhuman primates against Ebola and Marburg viruses. Nat Med 2005;11:786-90.
101. Department of Health and Human Services. NIOSH List of Antineoplastic and Other Hazardous Drugs in Healthcare Settings 2012. Updated June 2012. Available at www.cdc.gov/niosh/eNews.
102. Horwitz CA, Henle W, Henle G, et al. Clinical and laboratory evaluation of cytomegalovirus-induced mononucleosis in previously healthy individuals. Report of 82 cases. Medicine (Baltimore) 1986;65:124-34.
103. Wong SS, Yuen KY. The management of coronavirus infections with particular reference to SARS. J Antimicrob Chemother 2008;62:437-41.
104. Centers for Disease Control and Prevention (CDC). Middle East Respiratory Syndrome (MERS). Available at www.cdc.gov/coronavirus/mers/. Accessed September 1, 2015.
105. Centers for Disease Control and Prevention (CDC). Severe Acute Respiratory Syndrome (SARS). Available at www.cdc.gov/sars/. Accessed September 9, 2015.
106. Adedeji AO, Sarafianos SG. Antiviral drugs specific for coronaviruses in preclinical development. Curr Opin Virol 2014;8:45-53.
107. Chu CM. Role of lopinavir/ritonavir in the treatment of SARS: initial virological and clinical findings. Thorax 2004;59:252-6.
108. World Health Organization (WHO). Middle East Respiratory Syndrome Coronavirus (MERS-CoV): Summary of Current Situation, Literature Update and Risk Assessment. July 7, 2015. Available at http://apps.who.int/iris/bitstream/10665/179184/2/WHO_MERS_RA_15.1_eng.pdf. Accessed November 25, 2015.
109. Sharif-Yakan A, Kanj SS. Emergence of MERS-CoV in the Middle East: origins, transmission, treatment, and perspectives. PLoS Pathog 2014;10:e1004457.
110. Khan F. Enterovirus D68. Emerg Med Clin North Am 2015;33:e19-e32.
111. Centers for Disease Control and Prevention (CDC). Non-polio Enterovirus. Available at www.cdc.gov/non-polio-enterovirus/. Accessed September 7, 2015.
112. Greninger AL, Naccache SN, Messacar K, et al. A novel outbreak enterovirus D68 strain associated with acute flaccid myelitis cases in the USA (2012–14): a retrospective cohort study. Lancet Infect Dis 2015;15:671-82.
113. Centers for Disease Control and Prevention (CDC). Marburg Hemorrhagic Fever (Marburg HF). Available at www.cdc.gov/vhf/marburg/. Accessed September 7, 2015.
114. Centers for Disease Control and Prevention (CDC). Lassa Fever. Available at www.cdc.gov/vhf/lassa/. Accessed September 7, 2015.
115. World Health Organization (WHO). Ebola Virus Disease. Available at www.who.int/mediacentre/factsheets/fs103/en/. Accessed September 7, 2015.
116. Lado M, Walker NF, Baker P, et al. Clinical features of patients isolated for suspected Ebola virus disease at Connaught Hospital, Freetown, Sierra Leone: a retrospective cohort study. Lancet Infect Dis 2015;9:1024-33.
117. Peacock G, Uyeki TM, Rasmussen SA. Ebola virus disease and children: what pediatric health care professionals need to know. JAMA Pediatr 2014;168:1087-8.
118. Fowler RA, Fletcher T, Fischer WA II, et al. Caring for critically ill patients with ebola virus disease. Perspectives from West Africa. Am J Respir Crit Care Med 2014;190:733-7.
119. Hill CE, Burd EM, Kraft CS, et al. Laboratory test support for ebola patients within a high-containment facility. Lab Med 2014;45:e109-11.
120. World Health Organization (WHO). Use of Convalescent Whole Blood or Plasma Collected from Patients Recovered from Ebola Virus Disease for Transfusion as an Empirical Treatment During Outbreaks. Version 1.0, September 2014. Available at http://www.searo.who.int/entity/emerging_diseases/ebola/who_his_sds_2014.8_eng.pdf. Accessed November 25, 2015.
121. Go YY, Balasuriya UB, Lee CK. Zoonotic encephalitides caused by arboviruses: transmission and epidemiology of alphaviruses and flaviviruses. Clin Exp Vaccine Res 2014;3:58-77.
122. Weaver SC, Forrester NL. Chikungunya: evolutionary history and recent epidemic spread. Antiviral Res 2015;120:32-9.
123. Halstead SB, Cohen SN. Dengue hemorrhagic fever at 60 years: early evolution of concepts of causation and treatment. Microbiol Mol Biol Rev 2015;79:281-91.
124. Weaver SC, Reisen WK. Present and future arboviral threats. Antiviral Res 2010;85:328-45.
125. Rayamajhi A, Nightingale S, Bhatta NK, et al. A preliminary randomized double blind placebo-controlled trial of intravenous immunoglobulin for Japanese encephalitis in Nepal. PLoS One 2015;10:e0122608.
126. Ranjit S, Kissoon N. Dengue hemorrhagic fever and shock syndromes. Pediatr Crit Care Med 2011;12:90-100.
127. Centers for Disease Control and Prevention (CDC). Rabies. Available at www.cdc.gov/rabies/. Accessed September 7, 2015.
128. Jackson AC. Current and future approaches to the therapy of human rabies. Antiviral Res 2013;99 61-7.
129. Jackson AC. Rabies. Neurol Clin 2008;26:717-26.
130. Fu ZF, Jackson AC. Neuronal dysfunction and death in rabies virus infection. J Neurovirol 2005;11:101-6.
131. Zimmerman RF, Belanger ES, Pfeiffer CD. Skin infections in returned travelers: an update. Curr Infect Dis Rep 2015;17:467.
132. Caicedo Y, Paez A, Kuzmin I, et al. Virology, immunology and pathology of human rabies during treatment. Pediatr Infect Dis J 2015;34:520-8.

Chapter 18: Antimicrobial Prophylaxis

Keith M. Olsen, Pharm.D., FCCP, FCCM; and Gregory Peitz, Pharm.D., BCPS

LEARNING OBJECTIVES

1. Determine the correct use of antibiotics during surgical prophylaxis pertaining to indication, dose, duration, and timing.
2. Identify risk factors for surgical site infections (SSIs) and the unique risks faced by critically ill patients.
3. Identify differences in the causative pathogens for SSIs among intensive care unit (ICU) patients.
4. Synthesize an antibiotic prophylactic approach for the ICU patient receiving antibiotics for a concomitant infection.
5. Describe which procedures performed at the ICU bedside warrant antibiotic prophylaxis and the preferred regimen.

ABBREVIATIONS IN THIS CHAPTER

AASLD	American Association for the Study of Liver Diseases	ISHLT	International Society for Heart & Lung Transplantation
ANC	Absolute neutrophil count	LVAD	Left ventricular assist device
BMI	Body mass index	MRSA	Methicillin-resistant *Staphylococcus aureus*
CIED	Cardiovascular implantable electronic device	PPDs	Permanent pacemaker devices
		PQRS	Project and Physician Quality Reporting System
CMS	Centers for Medicare & Medicaid Services	SBP	Spontaneous bacterial peritonitis
CSF	Cerebrospinal fluid	SSI	Surgical site infection
ECMO	Extracorporeal membrane oxygenation	TAH	Total artificial heart
HCT	Hematopoietic stem cell transplantation	VAD	Ventricular assist device
ICU	Intensive care unit	VAP	Ventilator-associated pneumonia

INTRODUCTION: BASICS OF SURGICAL PROPHYLAXIS

Surgical site infections (SSIs) precipitate a cascade of events that often result in significant morbidity, increased mortality, and substantial costs to health care systems and patients. Prevention of these SSIs is fundamental to clinical practice whether the patient originates in the intensive care unit (ICU), hospital ward, skilled nursing facility, or is admitted from home. Antimicrobial prophylaxis plays an important role in the prevention of infections, but their administration is only one step in a comprehensive infection prevention program. Basic infection control practices are the core of preventing SSIs and should include controllable factors such as targeted temperature control, blood glucose control, hair clipping versus shaving, venous thromboembolism prophylaxis, and perioperative β-blocker administration. Equally important are controllable factors of antimicrobial administration that include which surgical cases may benefit antibiotic selection, antibiotic dosing, timely administration before surgical incision, and duration of postoperative prophylaxis. Pharmacists have been involved in collaborative improvement efforts on the national, state, local, and institutional level to improve antimicrobial use during the perioperative period. Major national initiatives developed by the Centers for Medicare & Medicaid Services (CMS), including the Surgical Care Improvement Project and Physician Quality Reporting System (PQRS), have resulted in dramatic improvements in standardizing antimicrobial administration and infectious control practices centered on the surgical procedure. For example, CMS requires collection and reporting of administration of antibiotic prophylaxis through the PQRS, which is shown electronically on public access websites to allow the consumer to compare performance among hospitals on specific surgical procedures.

Many questions remain unanswered with perioperative antimicrobial prophylaxis. An area that is largely absent in recommendations from CMS and SSI prevention guidelines is the decision-making process for patients receiving antibiotics for other infections, including patients residing in the ICU. The pharmacist and surgeon are often left without guidance regarding the correct approach to antimicrobial prophylaxis among these patients. Very few answers to these questions are found in the literature; however, a basic understanding of antimicrobial prophylaxis and the targeted organisms that cause these infections provides evidence for best practices. These are important considerations for patient safety, potential antimicrobial resistance, burden of antimicrobial use, and ties to CMS reimbursement policies. This chapter will examine the fundamentals of antimicrobial surgical prophylaxis, review surgical procedures in the ICU and surgical suite, and address antibiotic administration in patients receiving active treatment for infection.

Principles of Prophylaxis

Surgical Site Infections

The National Healthcare Safety Network has defined the criteria for determining an SSI. Infections can be classified in three categories: superficial incisional site SSI, deep incisional SSI, and organ space SSI.[1,2] Superficial infections usually occur within 30 days of the operative procedure and involve the skin and/or surrounding subcutaneous tissue of the incision site plus the clinical findings of purulent wound drainage, aseptically isolated organisms from the wound, and at least one sign of infection: pain or tenderness, or localized swelling, redness, or heat. Additionally, any culture positive or noncultured superficial incision that is deliberately opened by or determined by a surgeon or another clinician as an incisional SSI, is classified as a superficial infection. Deep incisional infections also occur within 30 days, or if an implant is left in place, the period is extended to 1 year, and the SSI appears related to the procedure. Deep tissue infections involve the fascial and muscle layer and/or deep soft tissue. An SSI is confirmed if the surgical site has purulent drainage or the incision spontaneously dehisces or is opened by the surgeon and is culture positive. If not cultured, the patient must have other signs of infection that include fever (temperature greater than 38°C), localized pain or tenderness, abscess, or other evidence of infection found on examination or during reoperation, histopathologic or radiologic evidence, or visual diagnosis by the clinician. Organ space SSIs may occur in a part of the body excluding infections isolated to superficial or deep tissues (e.g., those of the skin incision, fascia, or layers of muscle) and is more likely to result in systemic culture of infecting pathogens. Organ space infections follow the same 30-day and 1-year criteria of deep incisional SSIs and meet the criteria of purulent drainage from a drain placed through the wound, organism isolated aseptically, abscess or radiologic or histopathologic evidence, or direct examination with evidence of infection. Complete descriptions of these criteria are found elsewhere.[3]

Surgical Site Pathogens

Common pathogens associated with SSIs are usually associated with skin flora that include *Staphylococcus aureus* and coagulase-negative organisms such as *Staphylococcus epidermidis*. In procedures that penetrate areas harboring other pathogens (e.g., intra-abdominal, colon), the pathogens associated with SSI also include *Enterococcus* sp., enteric gram-negative rods (e.g., *Escherichia coli*, *Proteus* sp.), and anaerobes (e.g., *Bacteroides* sp.). There is an increasing understanding of pathogen access to the surgical wound by hematogenous spread, through drains, or through slow-healing wounds.[4] In addition to preoperative risk factors, postoperative factors that have been associated with SSIs may include prolonged hospital stay or ICU admission, admission from a long-term care facility, poor wound healing, anticoagulation, respiratory insufficiency, and prolonged antimicrobial administration beyond the first postoperative 24 hours.

Antimicrobial Resistance

Antibiotic resistance is an increasing cause of SSIs that has led to increased morbidity and mortality and associated costs of care for these complicated infections.[5] The incidence of methicillin-resistant *S. aureus* (MRSA) and *S. epidermidis* has gradually risen and is now a major cause of SSIs in some health centers. Awad and colleagues showed a greater than 45% rise in MRSA isolates from 288 surgical cases requiring surgical debridement.[6] A comparison of SSIs caused by methicillin-sensitive *S. aureus* (MSSA) and MRSA showed a 90-day postoperative mortality rate of 6.7% versus 20.7% (p<0.001) and a longer length of hospital stay in the MRSA group than in the MSSA group.[7] This study showed that the longer a patient remains in the ICU, the more likely the causative pathogen for the SSI will be multidrug resistant and include not only MRSA but also gram-negative Enterobacteriaceae and vancomycin-resistant *Enterococcus* sp.

Antibiotic Selection

In general, antibiotic prophylaxis immediately before surgical incision reduces the overall incidence of SSIs. The choice of antibiotics should target the most common pathogens associated with a specific surgical procedure. *S.*

aureus and *S. epidermidis* are the most common causes of SSI; therefore, a regimen that includes coverage of these pathogens is warranted. Cefazolin, based on its wide availability, low cost, and activity against these common pathogens, is included in most single-agent or multidrug regimens. Surgical procedures and recommended antibiotics are listed in Table 18.1. Because of the changing sensitivity patterns of pathogens, vancomycin has been added to some regimens. The routine use of vancomycin is discouraged because of the risk of indiscriminate use and development of resistance.[3] Each institution must carefully look at its MRSA rates in SSIs and decide the proper use of vancomycin. It has been argued that health care centers with a high incidence of MRSA should routinely use vancomycin, although the definition of "high incidence" has yet to be determined. Because vancomycin has a long half-life, a single dose before surgery is adequate in most patients. In patients allergic to β-lactam antibiotics, either clindamycin or vancomycin is a reasonable alternative guided by the institution resistance patterns.[8] In some surgical procedures (i.e., intra-abdominal), aerobic and anaerobic gram-negative bacteria cause more SSIs, and in these cases, prophylactic coverage should be expanded to antibiotics with activity against these pathogens, such as cefoxitin, cefotetan, or ertapenem. Extended-spectrum agents are generally not recommended for routine antimicrobial prophylaxis because of broad exposure to bacterial flora and the potential for developing resistance.

Antibiotic Delivery

Perhaps the most important factor in preventing SSI after selecting the correct antibiotic is the timing of administration in relation to the initial incision. Many would say that the pre-incision timing of the antimicrobial is as important as, if not more important than, the agent selection because a common error in prescribing presurgical antimicrobials is coverage that is too wide. If the dose is given too late, infection can occur. In a 1961 study, Burke showed that, in an animal model, administration of antibiotics before the incision was more efficacious than administration after incision.[9] These data were confirmed by a landmark prospective human study by Classen and colleagues, which showed that, in 2,847 patients undergoing elective clean or "clean-contaminated" surgical procedures, administration of antibiotics within 2 hours of the initial incision was associated with a significantly lower rate of SSI.[10] Administration before the 2-hour window or after the incision was similar to placebo administration in the incidence of SSIs. More recent data analyses from a hospital largely noncompliant with this recommendation showed a reduction in SSIs from 21.6% to 4% when administered within 30 minutes of the incision.[11] Since the Classen et al. study, investigators have tried to find the optimal delivery time for the antibiotic before incision. Currently, 60 minutes or less is recommended, but this broad recommendation is being questioned. A multicenter study of prophylactic antibiotic administration in 1,922 patients undergoing total hip arthroplasty showed the lowest infection rate among patients receiving antibiotics within 30 minutes of the incision versus 31–60 minutes.[12] Substantially higher infection rates occurred if the prophylactic antibiotic was administered 61–90 or 91–200 minutes before surgery and 0–30 minutes or greater than 30 minutes post-incision. Examination of more than 32,000 cases in a retrospective cohort study of antibiotic surgical prophylaxis showed a small increase in the incidence of SSI if the antibiotics were administered within 15 minutes of the incision.[13] Vancomycin, which requires a minimum 1-g/hour infusion rate, was studied in more than 2,000 patients undergoing coronary artery bypass grafting or valve replacement surgery. The incidence of SSIs coinciding with initiating the vancomycin infusion before the incision was 3.4% (16–60 minutes), 26.7% (0–15 minutes), 7.7% (61–120 minutes), and 6.9% (121–180 minutes).[14] Other studies have found similar results.[15] Thus, the optimal antibiotic administration appears to be 15–60 minutes before the incision, but confirmatory randomized controlled trials are needed to confirm this as the optimal interval.

Duration of Prophylaxis

The number of doses, or the duration of antibiotic delivery post-surgery, has remained controversial. Although several studies have compared short- and long-term administration with the same antibiotic, the shorter duration has not been universally accepted. National data analyses show that postoperative durations are now in compliance with national guidelines for less than 24 hours or less than 48 hours for cardiovascular surgical procedures. National quality measures have forced compliance with these guidelines. The main duration controversies are in patients with indwelling drains, or in patients on antibiotics for a primary infection before the procedure. McDonald conducted a 1998 systematic review of single- versus multidose antimicrobial prophylaxis for major surgery.[16] Twenty-eight studies were identified that compared the same antibiotic administered as a single dose or as multiple doses. The results showed no difference in SSIs of single versus multiple doses or the length of the dose (greater than 24 hours vs. 24 hours or less) or by the type of surgery. The results showed no clear benefit for prolonged antimicrobial prophylaxis to prevent SSIs. Some surgical procedures may be at greater risk of SSI and require several doses of antibiotics postoperatively. Cefmetazole was compared as a single dose versus three doses (over 24 hours) in colorectal surgery with a resulting SSI rate of 14.2% and 4.3%, respectively.[17] This is the only study to show that multiple doses are better than a single dose. A Cochrane review of antimicrobial prophylaxis for colorectal surgery suggested a slightly higher, but not statistically significant increase in SSI with single dose versus multiple dose over 24 hours.[18]

Table 18.1 Prophylactic Antibiotic Choices for Select Surgical Procedures[a,b]

Surgical Procedure	Preferred Antibiotics	Comments
Cardiovascular		
Coronary artery bypass	Cefazolin; cefuroxime	There is no clearance guidance on the duration. Prophylaxis should be limited to ≤ 48 hr
Cardiac device	Cefazolin; cefuroxime	
Ventricular assist device	Cefazolin; cefuroxime	
Cardiothoracic		
Thoracic	Cefazolin; ampicillin/sulbactam	
Noninvasive procedures	Cefazolin; ampicillin/sulbactam	
GI		
Intra-abdominal (bariatric, pancreas)	Cefazolin	A single dose is recommended
Noninvasive to GI tract		
Biliary		
Open		
Laparoscopic	Cefazolin, cefoxitin, ceftriaxone, ampicillin/sulbactam	For low-risk elective procedures, no prophylaxis is required
Appendectomy, uncomplicated	Cefoxitin, cefotetan, cefazolin + metronidazole	Both anaerobic and aerobic gram-negative enteric pathogens
Small bowel		
Non-obstructed	Cefazolin	
Obstructed	Cefazolin + metronidazole; cefoxitin, cefotetan	Single dose if no obstruction; broad gram-negative in obstruction
Hernia	Cefazolin	Single dose recommended
Colorectal	Cefazolin + metronidazole; cefoxitin, cefotetan, ampicillin/sulbactam, ceftriaxone + metronidazole; ertapenem	Both anaerobic and aerobic gram-negative enteric pathogens; antimicrobial coverage should be limited to 24 hr
Head and neck		
Clean with prosthesis placement	Cefazolin	SSIs are primarily associated with gram-positive pathogens; *S. aureus* and *S. epidermidis*
Clean-contaminated, including cancer	Cefazolin + metronidazole, cefuroxime + metronidazole, ampicillin/sulbactam	
Neurosurgery		
Craniotomy	Cefazolin	SSIs are primarily associated with gram-positive organisms
CSF shunt	Cefazolin	
Intrathecal pump implant	Cefazolin	
Hysterectomy		
Vaginal or abdominal	Cefazolin, cefotetan, cefoxitin, ampicillin/sulbactam	Trials with placebo resulted in > 14% SSIs

Table 18.1 Prophylactic Antibiotic Choices for Select Surgical Procedures[a,b] (continued)

Surgical Procedure	Preferred Antibiotics	Comments
Orthopedic		
Clean; no implants	None	No differences between antibiotics including cephalosporin generations
Spinal	Cefazolin	
Hip fracture	Cefazolin	
Total joint replacement	Cefazolin	
Transplantation		
Heart	Cefazolin	Cefazolin; same as cardiovascular procedures
Lung and heart-lung	Cefazolin	First-generation cephalosporin if negative donor cultures
Liver	Piperacillin/tazobactam or cefotaxime + ampicillin	Modify regimen on the basis of isolated pathogens from donor; gram-negative aerobes, staphylococci, enterococci most common
Pancreas and pancreas-kidney	Cefazolin ± fluconazole	A wide range of pathogens including gram-negative may necessitate broader coverage
Kidney	Cefazolin or ceftriaxone	Two separate studies with single-dose cefazolin or ceftriaxone resulted in 0% SSI
Plastic		
Clean or clean contaminated	Cefazolin or ampicillin/sulbactam	Clean procedures without risk factors do not require prophylaxis

[a]Clindamycin or vancomycin may be administered in β-lactam allergy for gram-positive coverage.
[b]Aztreonam, aminoglycoside, and, occasionally, a fluoroquinolone may be added for additional gram-negative coverage or gram-negative coverage with β-lactam allergy.
SSI = surgical site infection.
Adapted from: Bratzler DW, Dellinger EP, Olsen KM, et al. Clinical practice guidelines for antimicrobial prophylaxis in surgery. Am J Health Syst Pharm 2013;70:195-283.

The authors did not mention whether a second dose of antibiotic was administered intraoperatively in prolonged surgical procedures. However, they did conclude that high-quality evidence showed that antibiotics targeting both aerobic and anaerobic pathogens were more effective. Ertapenem is the only U.S. Food and Drug Administration label-approved antibiotic for single-dose prophylaxis in colorectal surgical procedures. Few studies have compared a short duration of prophylaxis in cardiovascular surgical procedures. A study of more than 2,800 patients undergoing prolonged cardiovascular surgical procedures compared the SSI rate of 48 hours or less with more than 48 hours of antimicrobial prophylaxis. The results showed no difference in the SSI rate between the two durations; however, with the longer duration, when an infection did occur, it was more likely (odds ratio 1.6% [95% confidence interval, 1.1–2.6]) caused by an antimicrobial-resistant pathogen.[17]

Repeat Dosing

Antibiotics with short half-lives require repeated dosing in prolonged surgical procedures to ensure adequate tissue concentrations at the surgical site. If the surgery exceeds 2 half-lives of the antibiotic, repeat dosing is necessary.[3] For example, cefazolin with a half-life of 2 hours should be redosed if the time from the start of antibiotic administration and the surgical procedure exceeds 4 hours. Antibiotics with a longer half-life (e.g., ceftriaxone with an 8-hour half-life) generally do not require repeat dosing. With repeated dosing guidance now available, institutions should consider developing additional guidelines for the frequency of intraoperative dosing to avoid excessive under- and overdosing of antimicrobials.

Dose

To achieve adequate tissue concentration preoperatively, the antimicrobial dose should be chosen on the basis of the type of surgery, antibiotic pharmacokinetics, and individual characteristics of the patient. Early studies of antimicrobial prophylaxis used fixed dosing; however, weight-based dosing is increasingly recognized as ensuring adequate drug concentration at the incision site. Standardized fixed doses do have merit because they avoid the common pitfalls of calculations that lead to dosing errors and compromise patient safety.[3] Obesity rates have been rising in the United States, with estimates of more than 66% of adult Americans classified as overweight or obese, which may affect tissue concentrations of antibiotics at the point of incision.[19]

The most recent guidelines for surgical prophylaxis recommend intravenous cefazolin 2 g for patients weighing more than 80 kg and 3 g for those weighing more than 120 kg.[3] However, only a few studies have addressed dosing in the patient with obesity, most of which have been directed toward the patient with morbid obesity undergoing bariatric surgery. Nonetheless, the clinician should be aware of the potential impact of obesity on antimicrobial penetration into fat tissue and to the surgical incision site. The pharmacokinetics of a single dose of cefazolin were examined in 25 patients (body mass index [BMI] range 43.7–55.7 kg/m^2) undergoing elective surgical procedures. Patients were divided into four groups according to their BMI and then assigned to receive cefazolin 2 g intravenous push, 2 g by 30-minute infusion (two different groups), and 3 g by 30-minute infusion. Serum cefazolin concentrations were determined in sequential format before surgery through 360 minutes after initiating the infusion. At all BMIs and doses, the cefazolin pharmacokinetics exhibited similar mean concentrations at 30 minutes after the dose and displayed concentrations of 67.1–84.8 mcg/mL and 22.9–40.8 mcg/mL at 120 and 360 minutes post-dose, respectively. The authors concluded that a single 2-g cefazolin dose provided adequate serum concentrations regardless of BMI for surgical procedures of less than 5 hours.[20] In contrast, 38 patients undergoing Roux-en-Y gastric bypass for morbid obesity were given cefazolin 2 g intravenously followed by a second dose 3 hours later. Patients were assigned to one of three groups according to their BMI (40–49, 50–59, 60 kg/m^2 or greater). Serum cefazolin concentrations were inadequate in 52%, 68%, and 73%, with therapeutic tissue concentrations achieved in only 48.1%, 28.6%, and 10.2%, respectively.[21] Pharmacists responsible for dosing antibiotics in surgical prophylaxis should be knowledgeable of pharmacokinetics and pharmacodynamics in applying weight-based dosing, and weight-based dosing, versus standard dosing, should be the new standard of practice. Aminoglycosides and vancomycin are examples of antibiotics used in surgical prophylaxis with the dose based on weight. Traditionally, a 1-g dose of vancomycin has been administered for surgical prophylaxis. In a study of 216 patients who screened positive for MRSA before elective total joint or spine surgical procedures, a vancomycin 1-g dose was compared with a weight-based dose of 15 mg/kg. A total of 149 patients (69%) were determined to be underdosed, and an additional 22 patients (10%) were overdosed. The predicted vancomycin value was less than 15 mg/L in 60% of patients receiving the 1-g dose.[22]

Antibiotic dosing should be appropriately adjusted for renal dysfunction. In single-dose administration, the dose usually needs no adjustment for renal impairment; however, multidose regimens may need the dose reduced or the interval extended, depending on the estimated glomerular filtration rate and antibiotic renal clearance.

ICU Patients

Many ICU patients receive antibiotics for other infections before their surgical procedure. This scenario often raises the question of whether additional antibiotics are required before the procedure. Unfortunately, there are no randomized trials to guide the clinician in this decision. Rather, the decision must be made considering the antibiotics being used to treat the infection, their antimicrobial coverage, the length of hospital stay, and the most recent dose in proximity to the surgical procedure. If the antibiotics used for the infection are substantially different in coverage from what would be used for surgical prophylaxis, the recommended dose of the antibiotic commonly used in the procedure should be administered at the appropriate time and duration. However, if the antibiotics being used for the existing infection consistently cover the potential pathogens associated with the procedure, a prudent approach would be to adjust the time of administration to coincide with the usual administration of prophylaxis, or if the times are considerably different from what would be required for the procedure, an additional dose may be given within 1 hour before the incision.

ICU Specifics and Risks of SSIs

Many factors, including several comorbidities, depressed host defenses, the presence of invasive devices, prolonged antibiotic courses, immunosuppressive therapy, and exposure to resistant bacteria, make infectious complications in the critically ill population of concern. Specifically, infectious insults in the ICU environment are more common than infectious complications in non-ICU patients, with at least twice the risk of mortality as in patients who are not affected by an infection.[23,24] These increases in prevalence and suboptimal outcomes are a result of several variables encountered by critically ill patients.[23,25]

Many patients admitted to the ICU have comorbidities or acute syndromes that precipitate an immunocompromised state. This transient state of depressed immune function predisposes critically ill patients to infection. Even previous immunocompetent hosts who are exposed to surgical or traumatic procedures are particularly susceptible to a bacterial insult because of an excessive inflammatory response affecting cell-mediated immunity.[26] In addition to acute changes in immune status, other challenges faced by the critically ill population include perioperative glucose management. Hyperglycemia (blood glucose greater than 150 mg/dL), which can impair macrophage chemotaxis and function, has been shown to occur in patients in the perioperative setting and to increase the likelihood of postoperative infections.[27]

Colonization with virulent pathogens also carries an increased risk of infectious complications in the ICU. Nasal colonization of MRSA in medically ICU patients has been shown to have a significant increase in subsequent MRSA infections over that in patients not colonized with the bacteria.[28,29]

Many critically ill patients also receive foreign devices such as central venous catheters, ventricular assist devices (VADs), cardiovascular implantable electronic devices (CIEDs), and neurosurgical devices,[30,31] which may be prone to the formation of biofilm. Although data are sparse regarding the ability of perioperative prophylaxis to affect biofilm development in all device implantation, using effective preoperative antibiotics may be important to minimize the risk of any inoculum propagating biofilm after surgery.[31,32]

Although critically ill patients are perhaps at a greater risk of infection related to surgical procedures, this population is also susceptible to other infectious complications because of patients' various risk factors. Prophylactic antibiotic regimens in this population have been shown to reduce infectious complications. This review is intended to focus on specific ICU indications for antimicrobial prophylaxis and, in addition to ICU procedures, the need for antimicrobial prophylaxis that has not been fully elucidated in previous literature or guidelines. It is not intended to be fully comprehensive in addressing all potential ICU infections.

ANTIBIOTIC PROPHYLAXIS IN ICU PATIENT POPULATIONS

Prophylaxis in Nonsurgical ICU Patients

Spontaneous Bacterial Peritonitis Prophylaxis

Spontaneous bacterial peritonitis (SBP) is a common complication of cirrhotic ascites that causes inflammation and infection of the abdominal cavity membrane. It affects more than 10% of patients admitted with cirrhotic ascites[33-35] and has an attributable mortality rate of up to 50%,[36] with a higher risk of death if the infection occurs within 48 hours of a variceal bleeding event.[34] Patients with cirrhosis who present with suspected SBP are recommended to be promptly initiated on appropriate antibiotic therapy, but the outcomes associated with empiric antibiotic initiation have been more compelling in the resolution of infection than in having an impact on mortality.[35] Empiric antibiotic therapy for SBP is warranted if at least one risk factor is present, including (1) temperature greater than 37.8°C, (2) abdominal pain or tenderness, (3) acute mental status changes, or (4) polymorphonuclear leukocytes greater than 250 cells/mm^3 in the ascitic fluid.[35,37]

Patients with cirrhosis having no outward indication for empiric SBP treatment should be evaluated for the inclusion of SBP prophylaxis. Spontaneous bacterial peritonitis prophylaxis has not only been shown to reduce the risk of infections by 30%,[38] but has also delayed the development of hepatorenal syndrome,[39] reduced variceal rebleeding,[40] and improved patients' hemodynamics[41] and has shown a mortality benefit.[38,39,42]

Because of concerns that the widespread use of antibiotics in all patients with cirrhosis may lead to subsequent colonization with multidrug-resistant organisms, the AASLD (American Association for the Study of Liver Diseases) guidelines have provided specific indications for the provision of SBP prophylaxis. Their recommendations and level of support can be seen in Table 18.2.[35]

The most common isolated organisms during cirrhotic bleeding events are aerobic gram-negative bacilli of enteric origin including *E. coli* and *Klebsiella* sp., but gram-positive organisms have also been isolated.[39,43] Few studies have evaluated various antibiotics and regimens regarding prophylaxis against SBP. Norfloxacin was once the preferred agent for SBP prophylaxis,[44] but ceftriaxone (1 g daily) has been proven superior in the setting of cirrhosis complicated by gastrointestinal (GI) bleeding[39] and is recommended as initial intravenous prophylaxis.[35] Prophylaxis for SBP should continue for 7 days in patients who present with an acute GI bleed, but once the patient can take oral medications, transitioning to an oral twice-daily norfloxacin regimen would be appropriate. Norfloxacin is not available in the United States; thus, ciprofloxacin 500 mg daily orally can be used. In summary, ceftriaxone 1 g daily or ciprofloxacin 500 mg daily for 7 days is recommended for SBP prophylaxis.

Fungal Prophylaxis

Although a relatively rare occurrence, the development of an invasive fungal infection in the ICU portends high mortality, particularly with delays in effective treatment.[45,46] Overall mortality may reach 60%, with outcomes worse in medical patients than in surgical patients.[45,47,48] Preexisting diabetes mellitus, concurrent immunosuppression, mechanical ventilation, and temperatures greater than 38.2°C are associated with increased mortality.[49] In ICU patients without neutropenia, the incidence of fungemia is less than 0.5%, with most cases attributable to *Candida* spp.[48,49] Because of the considerably poor outcomes

Table 18.2 Indications for Spontaneous Bacterial Peritonitis Prophylaxis in Patients with Cirrhosis	
Recommendation	Level of Evidence
Patients with concurrent GI bleeding	Class I, Level A
Patients having ≥ 1 episode of SBP	Class I, Level A
Patients with concurrent ascites AND aseitic fluid protein > 1.5 g/dL with concurrent renal dysfunction (creatinine > 1.2 mg/dL; BUN > 25 mg/dL or serum sodium < 130 mEq/L) or liver failure (Child-Pugh score > 9 and bilirubin > 3 mg/dL)	Class I, Level A

Adapted from: Runyon BA, AASLD. Introduction to the revised American Association for the Study of Liver Diseases practice guideline management of adult patients with ascites due to cirrhosis 2012. Hepatology 2013;57:1651-3.

observed in these infectious insults, initiating early appropriate antifungal therapy is of paramount importance for success. To aid in identifying patients at risk of fungal infections, research efforts have investigated the use of clinical prediction tools to identify patients who may empirically benefit from antifungal prophylaxis.[50-54] These clinical prediction tools have collated various risk factors for invasive candidiasis found in ICU patients without neutropenia. Common risk factors identified by these studies include colonization with *Candida* spp.,[53,55] concurrent antibiotic use,[52,55] surgical procedures,[53] the presence of a foreign device,[55] acute kidney injury or dialysis,[52,55] prolonged intubation,[50] and increased severity of illness,[56] among others. Each prediction tool is different because each incorporates different variables into its risk assessment; thus, each tool has variations in both sensitivity and specificity to predict the critically ill patients who would benefit from antifungal prophylaxis.[50-54,56] Several of these prediction tools have not been validated in prospective multicenter trials. In addition, several have failed to consistently predict infection, and their potential role as standard surveillance for the general critically ill population remains undetermined.

Eight major prospective studies have evaluated fungal prophylaxis in the critically ill population. Although specific trials and subsequent meta-analyses have shown a reduction in the incidence of *Candida* infections after fungal prophylaxis in the ICU,[57-61] survival benefits have been equivocal and have mainly been shown in surgical/trauma ICU patients.[59] High-risk surgical patients, particularly those with intestinal perforations or anastomotic leaks, have benefited from empiric prophylactic antifungal therapy.[57] A small study evaluated 49 patients with recurrent GI perforations or anastomotic leakage treated with intravenous fluconazole 400 mg/day or placebo.[62] The investigators showed a significant decrease in *Candida* peritonitis (4% vs. 35%) and *Candida* infections (9% vs. 35%) in the fluconazole arm of the study.[62] In addition to these high-risk surgical patients, routine prophylaxis is beneficial in these patients after solid organ transplantation, or in patients with neutropenia.[63,64] Otherwise, routine prophylaxis in the ICU is only recommended if a patient's risk is presumed to be greater than 10%.[65] Fluconazole dosed at 400 mg daily is the preferred prophylactic agent of choice as described by the 2009 Infectious Diseases Society of America (IDSA) guidelines, but there is evidence that fluconazole resistance may be emerging (these guidelines are currently under revision).[66] In an effort to curb *Candida* resistance to azole therapy and optimize the benefits of fungal prophylaxis, there may be utility in analyzing institution-specific risk factors for invasive fungal infections and applying necessary prophylactic antifungals according to local culture data including albicans and non-albicans *Candida* spp. A study of prophylaxis showed a favorable outcome with oral fluconazole versus placebo in 260 critically ill surgery patients with greater than a 3-day expected length of stay. The patients who received fluconazole had a statistically lower rate of *Candida* infections; however, this did not occur until day 14, when only 20 patients remained in the study.[61] A more recent study examined the impact of caspofungin prophylaxis versus placebo followed by preemptive therapy for invasive candidiasis in high-risk adults in the ICU. A total of 222 patients who were in the ICU for at least 3 days; who were mechanically ventilated; who received antibiotics, with central line present; and who had at least one other risk factor were included in the study. The primary end point was proven or probable invasive candidiasis. The caspofungin arm of the study had lower or proven invasive candidiasis, but this was not statistically significant, nor was the overall mortality of 16.7% and 14.3% in the two study arms.[67] At this time, prophylactic, presumptive, or even empiric therapy cannot be routinely recommended in the ICU patient. For patients with GI leakage into the abdominal cavity or those with an overall calculated fungemia risk of 10% or higher, fluconazole 400 mg intravenously daily can be recommended for prophylaxis.

Hematopoietic Cell Transplantation

Hematopoietic cell transplantation (HCT) is a therapeutic option for many bloodborne syndromes including lymphoma, leukemia, myelodysplastic syndrome, myeloproliferative disorders, and autoimmune conditions, among others.[68]

Transplanted hematopoietic stem cells can be obtained from the recipient patient (autologous HCT) or from another donor (allogenic HCT). Hematopoietic cell transplantation is often preceded by either a myeloablative or a nonmyeloablative conditioning regimen that is facilitated to eradicate malignant cells of the offending disease process and prevent rejection of an allogenic stem cell transplant. Myeloablative and nonmyeloablative therapies differ in their chemotherapeutic intensity depending on the specific type of conditioning regimen and respective malignant disorder. Consequently, these regimens vary in their degree of cytotoxicity and bone marrow suppression. Substantial pancytopenia is commonly precipitated by these conditioning regimens, placing patients at an increased risk of infection. In addition to neutropenia, these immunosuppressive regimens can cause damage to normal mucosal barriers and further increase the infectious risks of HCT recipients.[69]

After a patient's initial conditioning therapy and subsequent HCT, the infectious pathogenic risks change as each patient's immune system recovers and specific immune-regulating cell lines are regenerated. Early after the conditioning phase, patients are at the highest risk of an infection caused by gram-negative bacteria or *Candida* spp. Compelling factors that may contribute to infectious threats include the type of transplant (autologous HCT vs. allogenic HCT), severity of the patient's underlying malignant disorder, degree of donor matching, and time from conditioning therapy to the patient's stem cell transplant. As patients recover from their neutropenia and progress further from transplantation, their infectious risk profile shifts from predominant bacterial causes to viral and invasive fungal pathogens as the cellular-mediated immunity remains deficient.[68] The long-term prophylactic regimens necessary for managing these risks will be discussed elsewhere in this book, and the prophylactic strategies described in this chapter will focus on the immediate posttransplant period.

Immediately after stem cell infusion, patients should receive an antibiotic with gram-negative coverage. Levofloxacin 500 mg orally daily is recommended and should continue until a patient's neutropenia has resolved.[68,70] Evidence does not support the inclusion of broad-spectrum gram-positive agents to the initial prophylactic regimen. The understanding and application of local bacterial resistance patterns should be used when deciding on a prophylactic strategy. If a patient has had recurrent MRSA infections, mupirocin has been used to reduce the MRSA burden by applying the ointment twice daily for 5 days directly to the nares or to any visible wounds for up to 2 weeks, but this strategy has insufficient evidence to recommend universally.[68]

Anti-infective Prophylaxis After Neutropenia

Neutropenia is defined as a reduction in the absolute neutrophil count (ANC) in a patient's peripheral blood. Although neutropenia can occur secondary to autoimmune disorders,[71,72] the focus of this section will be directed at neutropenia experienced in patients with cancer, which can be defined as an ANC less than 500 cells/m^3.[73] After a course of chemotherapy or a bone marrow transplant, patients are at an increased risk of life-threatening infectious complications, particularly when profound neutropenia (ANC less than 100 cells/m^3) exists. Bodey and colleagues showed that in patients with leukemia having an ANC less than 100 cells/m^3, there was an overall risk of 43 infectious episodes per 1,000 patient-days.[74]

During neutropenia, infectious insults are often recognized by observing a patient's temperature because fever continues to be detectable early in a neutropenic infection.[75] Fever, defined as a single temperature of 38.3°C or greater for 1 hour by the Infectious Diseases Society of America (IDSA)[73] and the National Comprehensive Cancer Network (NCCN) guidelines,[70] can be realized in up to 50% and greater than 80% of patients who receive chemotherapy for solid tumors and hematologic malignancies, respectively.[73]

Despite the high rates of febrile episodes, less than 30% of these patients will have a verified clinical infection during the period of febrile neutropenia.[73] Gram-positive organisms, particularly coagulase-negative staphylococci, have become the most common organisms isolated in bloodstream infections in patients with neutropenia.[76] Gram-negative pathogens including *E. coli*, *Klebsiella* sp., *Enterobacter* sp., and other Enterobacteriaceae are isolated less commonly but are associated with a higher mortality rate than are gram-positive bacterial infections in the neutropenic population.[73]

Although the definitive yield of infectious cause may be poor, prompt and appropriate treatment of patients who develop febrile neutropenia is imperative to improve outcomes, with improvements in mortality observed with early antibiotic initiation on detection of fever in the patient with neutropenia.[77]

Although early initiation of antibiotics is critical in a patient with neutropenia and fever, preventing infection during the neutropenic phase after chemotherapy is also important. Antibiotic prophylaxis in the patient with neutropenia is recommended by the NCCN and IDSA guidelines with considerations given to low- and high-risk populations for infection. Antibiotic prophylaxis is recommended by both organizations, specifically in high-risk populations. High-risk patients are identified as those with an ANC less than 100 cells/m^3 or an anticipated duration of neutropenia of greater than 7 days. The NCCN guidelines[70] also encourage prophylactic antibiotics for patients being treated for multiple myeloma or chronic lymphocytic leukemia and in those who are receiving a purine analog as their chemotherapeutic agent.[70]

Fluoroquinolones are the preferred antibacterial prophylactic agents for these patients during their high-risk period of neutropenia. Levofloxacin 500 mg daily orally has shown a reduced rate of infection and hospitalization in two randomized prospective clinical trials, but it had no mortality benefits.[78,79] Adding gram-positive prophylaxis is not recommended in the initial regimen for patients with neutropenia.

Fungal prophylaxis with fluconazole 400 mg daily either intravenously or orally is warranted as well in high-risk patients with neutropenia, particularly in those who are receiving allogeneic HCT or being treated with intense chemotherapy for remission or salvage therapy in acute leukemia.[73] Prophylaxis should continue throughout neutropenia.

Prophylaxis with the antiviral agent acyclovir is recommended for patients who test positive for herpes simplex virus and have undergone induction therapy for allogenic HCT or leukemia.

Viral prophylaxis after HCT is dependent on the presence of specific viral findings in pretransplant serum testing. Prophylaxis for cytomegalovirus (CMV) infection after HCT is determined by the patient's and donor's serum CMV status in allogeneic HCT. For any patients who require CMV prophylaxis (CMV-seropositive HCT recipients or CMV-seropositive donors), available prophylactic options include high-dose acyclovir therapy (500 mg/m^2 intravenously three times daily or 800 mg orally four times daily), valacyclovir (2 g three or four times daily), or intravenous ganciclovir. For patients who receive ganciclovir therapy, it is recommended to include induction therapy of 5 mg/kg twice daily for 5–7 days; this should be initiated when HCT occurs and then continued daily for 100 days post-HCT.[68]

To prevent reactivation of herpes simplex virus, prophylactic acyclovir is recommended for all individuals who test seropositive before transplantation. Acyclovir 400–800 mg orally twice daily or 250 mg/m^2 per dose every 12 hours intravenously should commence during the initial conditioning phase and be continued until the patient has appropriate engraftment or resolution of mucositis.[68]

Fluconazole 400 mg orally or intravenously daily is recommended as prophylaxis for all patients receiving allogeneic HCT and for those with autologous HCT who have had intense conditioning regimens or who are experiencing mucositis. Fungal prophylaxis should ensue until at least 7 days after the ANC is greater than 1,000 cells/mm^3.

Prophylaxis in Cardiac Critical Care Procedures

Ventricular Assist Devices

The rate and precision of VAD implantation has dramatically increased since the first report of an artificial ventricle in 1963. As the placement of these devices has become more common, efforts have continued to improve their longevity in addition to minimizing the associated complications. One specific improvement of note is the increasing prevalence of the implantation of continuous-flow devices such as the HeartMate II, which have shown more favorable outcomes, including infectious complications, than pulsatile-flow left ventricular assist devices (LVADs).[80] Although data from the 2014 Interagency Registry for Mechanically Assisted Circulatory Support report indicate that infection rates for VADs have decreased, infection remains a common complication associated with VAD placement.[81] Despite this information, there is a lack of consensus on the management of these patients' infectious prophylaxis, particularly in the perioperative setting.

The main infectious risks immediately after VAD implementation are driveline infections, pump pocket infections, bacteremia, and endocarditis.[82] The pathogenic insults to these patients may include gram-positive organisms, gram-negative bacilli, and fungi.[83,84] The principal source of inoculum comes from the skin surface, which is a primary source of staphylococcal species. These isolates have a high capacity to adhere to foreign device material and form biofilm and evade the immunological system, thereby becoming very difficult to eradicate,[32,85,86] making antistaphylococcal prophylaxis of paramount importance in the perioperative period. Although staphylococcal coverage is deemed of utmost importance for VAD perioperative prophylaxis, coverage for other pathogens remains common in most VAD centers. In addition to driveline infections, surgical pocket infection is common. Because of a high mortality rate associated with fungemia, fungal prophylaxis often joins the perioperative antibiotic prophylactic regimen. In addition, coverage of gram-negative pathogens is often added.

Several studies have evaluated various perioperative antibiotic regimens in the setting of VAD placement, but inconsistent choice, timing, and duration of prophylactic antimicrobial therapy and differing definitions of LVAD infection make a direct comparison of stated infection rates difficult.[87] Unfortunately, large prospective trials are lacking regarding the appropriateness of perioperative antibiotic management in VAD transplantation, and recommendations in the International Society for Heart & Lung Transplantation (ISHLT) guidelines are largely based on expert opinion. The 2013 update on perioperative management recommends broad-spectrum gram-positive and gram-negative coverage within 60 minutes of the first incision before implantation. Because of the high rate of staphylococcal driveline infections, the opinion expressed in the document calls for patients to undergo nasal swab screening for MRSA preoperatively with the desire for topical treatment with mupirocin to be incorporated if positive. Gram-negative and fungal coverage inclusion should be tailored according to institution-specific epidemiologic data, colonization rates, and other high-risk patient-specific data. Fungal coverage may be warranted in regions known to have higher risks of virulent fungal pathogens. There are no specific recommendations on which antibiotics to choose or address toward antifungal coverage, but there is evidence that advocates against using prolonged vancomycin in high-risk general cardiac surgery patients.[18,88] The recommended therapy duration is 24–48 hours, but the evidence with the longer duration is scarce.[83] The optimal regimen for antibiotic prophylaxis in patients undergoing LVAD placement is not known. Guidelines indicate that a single dose of cefazolin or cefuroxime can be used before LVAD transplantation,[3] but the 2013 ISHLT guidelines[83] advocate for MRSA coverage with 24–48 hours of antimicrobial coverage.

Many centers use a combination of vancomycin (15 mg/kg intravenously 1 hour before surgery; then every 12 hours), rifampin (600 mg orally 1–2 hours before surgery; then every 24 hours), levofloxacin (500 mg intravenously 1 hour before surgery; then every 24 hours), and fluconazole (200 mg intravenously 1 hour before surgery; then every 24 hours) for a total of 48 hours postoperatively as recommended in the Randomized Evaluation of Mechanical Assistance for the Treatment of Congestive Heart Failure (REMATCH) trial.[89,90] Data analyses on the use of alternative MRSA prophylactic strategies other than vancomycin are scarce in LVAD transplantation, but if a contraindication to vancomycin exists, daptomycin may be an alternative prophylactic strategy.

Artificial Heart Implantation

The availability of total artificial heart (TAH) implantation has improved short-term survival rates in patients who do not meet the criteria for VAD placement or who do not have an opportunity for an immediate heart transplant.[91] Postoperative complications, including infections, are major deterrents to the success after TAH placement. Infectious complications can occur in more than 80% of TAH recipients, potentially delaying the patient's ability to receive a heart transplant.[91,92] At least half of all infections occur within the first 30 days post-implantation,[93] but most documented infectious complications originate from pulmonary or urinary sources.[92,93] In addition to these infectious insults, patients with TAH are predisposed to bacteremia, driveline infections, and superficial sternal infections, potentially because of exposure to organisms during the perioperative period. These infectious risks are notably higher than in other patients, potentially because of the nature of the mechanical device itself. A TAH system is composed of metals and polymers that are in contact with tissues and hemodynamic surfaces. These surfaces pose a medium susceptible to biofilm development that is believed to promote bacterial colonization and predicate biomaterial-centered infections.[85]

Unfortunately, prophylactic antibiotic regimens are poorly described in the literature, and there are no specific recommendations for the choice of antimicrobial agent or duration of prophylaxis in the perioperative management of TAH. Because of the nature of the surgical procedure necessary for a TAH placement, antibiotic administration with agents similar to those used in other cardiac surgical procedures such as intravenous cefazolin of cefuroxime for 24 hours would be advocated. Patients with penicillin allergies should receive vancomycin or clindamycin as surgical prophylaxis.

Extracorporeal Membrane Oxygenation Cannulation

The prevalence of extracorporeal membrane oxygenation (ECMO) initiation has continually increased during the past 2 decades in both the neonatal and the adult critical care populations. As more adult patients have acute needs for ECMO initiation, it is evident that coinciding management strategies will have to continue evolving to improve delivery and minimize complications. Currently, infectious complications during ECMO management are the second most frequent setback after hemorrhagic issues.[94] Potential issues that pose infection risks to patients initiated on ECMO therapy are the presence of several large-bore catheters that are exposed to the environment after surgical placement. In addition, depending on the selection of site of the ECMO cannulation that is chosen, infectious risks differ. Venovenous ECMO therapy typically uses a femoral access site that may carry an additional infectious risk because of higher contamination rates similar to the placement of femoral central lines.[95]

Several studies have investigated potential infections related to ECMO initiation. In a study by Aubron et al., the investigators found that 14.4% of 146 patients had a bloodstream infection related to ECMO cannulation within 8 days of the procedure.[95] Although they showed that the only independent risk of perioperative infection was related to the patient's present severity of illness, this is not in accordance with all studies as a risk factor. The independent relationship between patient severity before ECMO initiation and bloodstream infection occurrence is controversial, possibly because of the variations in design between studies, including differences in periods and methods used for assessing severity and patient populations. Similar to TAH, there are no published standardized prophylactic antibiotic strategies or associated infectious outcomes with their use during the initiation of ECMO therapy, but using cefazolin or cefuroxime (or vancomycin or clindamycin in penicillin-allergic patients) would be appropriate, especially in the setting of central cannulation.

Cardiac Implantable Electronic Devices

Cardiovascular implantable devices, including both PPDs (permanent pacemaker devices) and ICDs (implantable cardioverter-defibrillators), have increased in prevalence by at least 19% and 60%, respectively, since 1999,[96] with more procedures being done in older patients with more comorbidities.[96,97] As the overall patient age and acuity of these device recipients continues to increase, there is an increasing probability that critical care practitioners will provide care to this population after a new cardiac event while these patients are in the ICU.

Two primary categories of infections are seen after CIED implantation: pocket infection and deeper infections. Pocket infection is a particular risk during CIED implantation and is most consistent with gram-positive bacteria, specifically *S. aureus*.[98] Overall, infectious complications after CIEDs are relatively low in the perioperative window, but infections after the implantation of these devices portend high morbidity, costs, and mortality up to 18% at 6 months.[98] Like other cardiovascular devices, CIEDs have the risk of biofilm development, which can contribute antibiotic resistance.[98] These devices can also become infected secondary to bacteremia or intraoperative contamination.

To minimize the risk of perioperative infection with CIED placement, it is recommended to administer a parenteral antibiotic within 1 hour of the procedure. This is supported by findings from a double-blind randomized trial in which preoperative cefazolin had a postoperative infection rate of 0.63% compared with 3.28% without prophylaxis.[99] Additional support for preoperative antibiotics can be seen in two multivariate analyses,[100,101] both of which have shown preoperative antibiotics to have a protective effect against infections after CIED. A one-time dose of cefazolin or cefuroxime (vancomycin or clindamycin for β-lactam allergy) given within 1 hour of the procedure is sufficient prophylaxis before CIED placement.

Prophylaxis in Neurocritical Care Procedures

Neurosurgical procedures are stratified into one of five categories according to a neurosurgical classification score investigated by Narotam and colleagues (Table 18.3).[102] The classification system delineates variation in infectious risks according to the type of neurosurgical procedure. Clean neurosurgical procedures carry the lowest infection risk (1.9%–5.8%)[102-104] if perioperative antimicrobial prophylaxis is used. The absence of antibiotic prophylaxis has been shown to increase the risk of postoperative infections by up to 10% in this patient population.[103,104]

Specific risk factors can compound the likelihood of postoperative infections in neurosurgical patients. Diabetes mellitus, emergency surgery, prolonged procedural times, cerebrospinal fluid (CSF) leaks, or the surgical placement of a foreign body increases the infection risk. Neurosurgical infectious complications are typically attributed to either superficial SSIs or the development of deeper central nervous system (CNS) infectious such as meningitis, epidural abscesses, or subdural empyemas.[105,106] Antimicrobial prophylaxis has resulted in lower postoperative infections when perioperative antibiotics are included in low-risk neurosurgical procedures. The American Society of Health-System Pharmacists and Society for Healthcare Epidemiology of America (SHEA) guidelines for surgical guidelines for antibiotic prophylaxis recommend a single dose of antibiotic within 60 minutes before the incision.[3] There is no overall consensus on the choice of antibiotics in the neurosurgical population.[107] Perioperative antibiotics should be directed at gram-positive organisms such as *S. aureus* and coagulase-negative staphylococcus, which account for most infectious insults.[108,109] Gram-negative organisms are less commonly reported but are indicated in up to 20% of cases. *Pseudomonas aeruginosa* and other resistant gram-negative organisms' prevalence is indicated in less than 5% of cases.[104] Antibiotic selection should

Table 18.3 Narotam Classification of Neurosurgical Procedures

Clean	Elective procedure under ideal operative conditions
Clean with foreign body implantation	All other criteria for a clean procedure with the placement of permanent or temporary foreign material, including shunt, intracranial monitory, reservoirs, or ventricular draining device
Clean-contaminated	Procedure with entry into the paranasal sinuses, cranial base fracture, surgery for greater than 2 hr, or breach in standard procedures
Contaminated	Contamination of operative site, compound skull fractures, open lacerations for greater than 4 hr, CSF leakage, or operation within the same incision site within the previous 4 wk
Dirty	Procedure occurring during sepsis at the time of operation; confounding infection including abscess, subdural empyema, ventriculitis, osteitis, or skin infection

Adapted from: Narotam PK, van Dellen JR, du Trevou MD, et al. Operative sepsis in neurosurgery: a method of classifying surgical cases. Neurosurgery 1994;34:409-15; discussion 415-6.

include an agent active against gram-positive organisms and ideally tailored to local resistant and susceptibility patterns. A common antimicrobial used for prophylaxis in neurosurgical procedures includes cefazolin, or vancomycin if severe allergy or if MRSA resistance rates are high at the individual institution.

In addition to clean neurosurgical procedures, surgical procedures that involve the placement of foreign devices for intracranial monitoring or CSF shunting are common in the critically ill population.[110] These devices have been indicated as specific risks of postoperative infection in the neurosurgical population.[109,111,112]

Intracranial Pressure (ICP) Monitoring and CSF Shunting Devices

External ventricular drains are commonly used for CSF diversion from the cranial space as well as for intracranial pressure (ICP) monitoring in the setting of traumatic brain injury, intracranial hemorrhage, or hydrocephalus. Although these devices are used for monitoring and management, they portend infectious complications cumulating around 10%,[113] with the incidence of infection increasing with prolonged ventricular catheterization.[112,113] Similar to the microbiologic sources seen in the clean procedural infections, most pathogenic organisms are gram-positive cocci.[113] Studies supporting the routine use of prophylactic antibiotics in these populations are equivocal. Retrospective analyses have shown no benefit with prophylactic antibiotics over no prophylaxis after ICP placement in infectious outcomes.[112,114] The provision of broad-spectrum perioperative antibiotics (ceftriaxone or ciprofloxacin) has also not been advantageous versus narrow-spectrum antibiotics (cefazolin or vancomycin) after ICP placement.[115] In addition, it has been shown that either broad-spectrum antibiotics or prolonged use of antibiotics may expose patients to resistant gram-negative organisms in future infections.[114,115] To contrast these findings, however, two meta-analyses have shown a reduction in infection rates using antibiotic prophylaxis in CSF shunting procedures.[116,117] Antibiotic-impregnated shunts are available for use, but further data may be needed before universal use.[3] Because of the high risk of complications associated with a CSF-related infection and available data, the SHEA surgical antibiotic guidelines committee gave a level A recommendation for a one-time preoperative dose of cefazolin before shunting procedures.[3] Clindamycin and vancomycin are recommended for patients allergic to penicillin.

Subdural Grids

Subdural grid placement may occur in a select set of patients with a history of intractable antiepileptic medication-resistant epilepsy,[118] which often requires close observation, possibly in a neuro-ICU. Placement of a subdural grid with depth electrodes for seizure foci identification is done by craniectomy. By definition, this is a clean procedure with a foreign body implantation and carries more than a minimal risk of perioperative infection as classified by Narotam et al.[102] There currently are no guidelines or specific recommendations for antibiotic coverage during the placement and period of subdural grid. A meta-analysis involving 21 studies (20 retrospective) indicated that although the overall prevalence of neurologic infections is relatively low, they are the most commonly identified complication in these cases. Particular infectious insults were described as superficial surgical infections (3%), pyogenic neurologic infections (2.3%), and CSF bacterial colonization (7.1%). Thirteen of the 21 studies indicated that systemic antibiotics were administered, but the choice of antibiotics and duration of use were variable, with cephalosporins being the most likely used antibiotic class. Prophylaxis is extended for the duration of the subdural grid placement in most cases. Because of the paucity of randomized trials of antibiotic prophylaxis, a standard recommendation cannot be made at this time, but antibiotics with adequate CNS penetration that target superficial gram-positive flora such as cefazolin or cefotaxime would be reasonable while the subdural grid is in place.

Prophylaxis in Unique ICU Procedures

Antibiotics at Intubation

Patients who are intubated during their ICU stay have an increased risk of developing pneumonia. Ventilator-associated pneumonia (VAP) may occur in up to 15% of ventilated patients and portends worse outcomes such as longer length of stay, increased costs, and higher mortality rates.[119] The estimated mortality associated with VAP may be as high as 10%.[120]

Identified risk factors for VAP include concurrent organ failure, age older than 60, prior antibiotic exposure, and failure to elevate the head of the bed after intubation.[121] Although the inoculum responsible for VAP commonly comes from pathogens that are colonized in the oropharynx and upper GI tract, targeted bacteria should be based on a patient's medical history, prior antibiotic exposure, and institutional microbial patterns.[122]

Specifically recommended prophylactic measures for VAP include the coordination of daily interruption of sedation and spontaneous breathing trials, incorporation of early mobility measures, use of noninvasive mechanically ventilation when possible, and changing of the ventilator circuit only when necessary.[123] Although there is moderate evidence for using both prophylactic probiotics and chlorhexidine-based oral care in mechanically ventilated patients, evidence remains sparse describing the utility of prophylactic antibiotics during intubation or mechanical ventilation.

Some trials have investigated the benefit of prophylactic antibiotics post-intubation. Cefuroxime given as prophylaxis for two doses after intubation had a protective effect against early-onset VAP in patients with head injury.[124] Another prospective trial that studied the impact of a single dose of ceftriaxone, ertapenem, or levofloxacin given before intubation showed a reduction in the incidence of early-onset VAP. However, it showed no benefit regarding late-onset VAP, tracheobronchitis, or mortality.[125] Neither of these single-center trials assessed the impact on developing resistant pathogens, possibly overlooking any ramification on antimicrobial stewardship efforts. The SHEA guidelines do not address the utility of prophylactic antibiotics in VAP.[123] Because of the absence of larger multicenter randomized trials, the delivery of prophylactic antibiotics at intubation cannot be recommended.

Nasal Packing

Although epistaxis is a relatively normal occurrence at some point in a patient's lifetime, only 6% of these events result in the need for medical attention,[126] and many bleeding events occurring in the anterior septum are self-limiting. For the patients who have bleeding events that require nasal packing, however, there may be a need for more aggressive management and closer observation, occasionally in the ICU. Complications that can ensue after nasal packing include aspiration, angina, myocardial infarction, respiratory distress, and hypoxia.[126-128] Patients with nasal packing are also at an increased risk of toxic shock syndrome (TSS), an insult that is rapidly precipitated after toxin production by colonized *S. aureus* in the nasal membranes. Although the rate of TSS is reportedly low in postoperative nasal packing (16 per 100,000 packings), antibiotics are routinely prescribed to these patients.[129] However, there has been no clear evidence that using antibiotics reduces the rate of *S. aureus* infection, rates of nasal colonization, or episodes of TSS.[130-132] Antimicrobial prophylaxis may not be necessary for TSS prophylaxis in the setting of nasal packing, but if used, agents that have antistaphylococcal activity such as amoxicillin/clavulanate 500 mg orally three times daily or cephalexin 500 mg orally twice daily could be considered for the duration of the nasal packing.

SUMMARY

Because of the increased risk of adverse events attributed to SSIs, adherence to antimicrobial prophylactic strategies in the critically ill population is of paramount importance and should be directed by best practices. Pharmacists practicing in an ICU environment should be aware of the surgical risks and necessary precautions to minimize poor outcomes in many unique surgical and non-surgical scenarios. Various recommendations have been provided throughout this chapter according to the available evidence and guidelines, but the chapter does not provide insight into all potential ICU procedures or infectious events. However, this chapter can serve as a guide to the ICU clinician when fully elucidated recommendations may not be available in other available guidelines.

REFERENCES

1. Mangram AJ, Horan TC, Pearson ML, et al. Guideline for prevention of surgical site infection, 1999. Hospital infection control practices advisory committee. Infect Control Hosp Epidemiol 1999;20:250-78; quiz 279-80.
2. Horan TC, Andrus M, Dudeck MA. CDC/NHSN surveillance definition of health care-associated infection and criteria for specific types of infections in the acute care setting. Am J Infect Control 2008;36:309-32.
3. Bratzler DW, Dellinger EP, Olsen KM, et al. Clinical practice guidelines for antimicrobial prophylaxis in surgery. Am J Health Syst Pharm 2013;70:195-283.
4. Manian FA. The role of postoperative factors in surgical site infections: time to take notice. Clin Infect Dis 2014;59:1272-6.
5. Centers for Disease Control and Prevention (CDC). Antibiotic Resistance Threats in the United States. 2013. Available at www.cdc.gov/antibioticresistancethreats.pdf. Accessed July 22, 2015.
6. Awad SS, Elhabash SI, Lee L, et al. Increasing incidence of methicillin-resistant *Staphylococcus aureus* skin and soft-tissue infections: reconsideration of empiric antimicrobial therapy. Am J Surg 2007;194:606-10.
7. Engemann JJ, Carmeli Y, Cosgrove SE, et al. Adverse clinical and economic outcomes attributable to methicillin resistance among patients with *Staphylococcus aureus* surgical site infection. Clin Infect Dis 2003;36:592-8.
8. Engelman R, Shahian D, Shemin R, et al. The Society of Thoracic Surgeons practice guideline series: antibiotic prophylaxis in cardiac surgery, part II: antibiotic choice. Ann Thorac Surg 2007;83:1569-76.
9. Burke JF. The effective period of preventative antibiotic action in experimental incisions and dermal lesions. Surgery 1961;50:161-8.
10. Classen DC, Evans RS, Pestotnik SL, et al. The timing of prophylactic administration of antibiotics and the risk of surgical-wound infection. N Engl J Med 1992;326:281-6.
11. Saxer F, Widmer A, Fehr J, et al. Benefit of a single preoperative dose of antibiotics in a Sub-Saharan district hospital: minimal input, massive impact. Ann Surg 2009;249:322-6.
12. van Kasteren ME, Mannien J, Ott A, et al. Antibiotic prophylaxis and the risk of surgical site infections following total hip arthroplasty: timely administration is the most important factor. Clin Infect Dis 2007;44:921-7.
13. Hawn MT, Richman JS, Vick CC, et al. Timing of surgical antibiotic prophylaxis and the risk of surgical site infection. JAMA Surg 2013;148:649-57.
14. Garey KW, Rege M, Pai MP, et al. Time to initiation of fluconazole therapy impacts mortality in patients with candidemia: a multi-institutional study. Clin Infect Dis 2006;43:25-31.
15. Weber WP, Marti WR, Zwahlen M, et al. The timing of surgical antimicrobial prophylaxis. Ann Surg 2008;247:918-26.

16. McDonald M, Grabsch E, Marshall C, et al. Single- versus multiple-dose antimicrobial prophylaxis for major surgery: a systematic review. Aust N Z J Surg 1998;68:388-96.

17. Harbarth S, Samore MH, Lichtenberg D, et al. Prolonged antibiotic prophylaxis after cardiovascular surgery and its effect on surgical site infections and antimicrobial resistance. Circulation 2000;101:2916-21.

18. Nelson RL, Gladman E, Barbateskovic M. Antimicrobial prophylaxis for colorectal surgery. Cochrane Database Syst Rev 2014;5:CD001181.

19. Wang Y, Beydoun MA. The obesity epidemic in the United States—gender, age, socioeconomic, racial/ethnic, and geographic characteristics: a systematic review and meta-regression analysis. Epidemiol Rev 2007;29:6-28.

20. Ho VP, Nicolau DP, Dakin GF, et al. Cefazolin dosing for surgical prophylaxis in morbidly obese patients. Surg Infect (Larchmt) 2012;13:33-7.

21. Edmiston CE, Krepel C, Kelly H, et al. Perioperative antibiotic prophylaxis in the gastric bypass patient: do we achieve therapeutic levels? Surgery 2004;136:738-47.

22. Catanzano A, Phillips M, Dubrovskaya Y, et al. The standard one gram dose of vancomycin is not adequate prophylaxis for MRSA. Iowa Orthop J 2014;34:111-7.

23. Vincent JL, Rello J, Marshall J, et al. International study of the prevalence and outcomes of infection in intensive care units. JAMA 2009;302:2323-9.

24. Suljagic V, Cobeljic M, Jankovic S, et al. Nosocomial bloodstream infections in ICU and non-ICU patients. Am J Infect Control 2005;33:333-40.

25. Colpan A, Akinci E, Erbay A, et al. Evaluation of risk factors for mortality in intensive care units: a prospective study from a referral hospital in turkey. Am J Infect Control 2005;33:42-7.

26. Kimura F, Shimizu H, Yoshidome H, et al. Immunosuppression following surgical and traumatic injury. Surg Today 2010;40:793-808.

27. van den Berghe G, Wouters P, Weekers F, et al. Intensive insulin therapy in critically ill patients. N Engl J Med 2001;345:1359-67.

28. Keene A, Lemos-Filho L, Levi M, et al. The use of a critical care consult team to identify risk for methicillin-resistant Staphylococcus aureus infection and the potential for early intervention: a pilot study. Crit Care Med 2010;38:109-13.

29. Corbella X, Dominguez MA, Pujol M, et al. Staphylococcus aureus nasal carriage as a marker for subsequent staphylococcal infections in intensive care unit patients. Eur J Clin Microbiol Infect Dis 1997;16:351-7.

30. Padera RF. Infection in ventricular assist devices: the role of biofilm. Cardiovasc Pathol 2006;15:264-70.

31. Braxton EE Jr, Ehrlich GD, Hall-Stoodley L, et al. Role of biofilms in neurosurgical device-related infections. Neurosurg Rev 2005;28:249-55.

32. Padera RF. Infection in ventricular assist devices: the role of biofilm. Cardiovasc Pathol 2006;15:264-70.

33. Caly WR, Strauss E. A prospective study of bacterial infections in patients with cirrhosis. J Hepatol 1993;18:353-8.

34. Bleichner G, Boulanger R, Squara P, et al. Frequency of infections in cirrhotic patients presenting with acute gastrointestinal haemorrhage. Br J Surg 1986;73:724-6.

35. Runyon BA, AASLD. Introduction to the revised American Association for the Study of Liver Diseases practice guideline management of adult patients with ascites due to cirrhosis 2012. Hepatology 2013;57:1651-3.

36. Runyon BA. Spontaneous bacterial peritonitis: an explosion of information. Hepatology 1988;8:171-5.

37. Such J, Runyon BA. Spontaneous bacterial peritonitis. Clin Infect Dis 1998;27:669-74; quiz 675-6.

38. Bernard B, Grange JD, Khac EN, et al. Antibiotic prophylaxis for the prevention of bacterial infections in cirrhotic patients with gastrointestinal bleeding: a meta-analysis. Hepatology 1999;29:1655-61.

39. Fernandez J, Ruiz del Arbol L, Gomez C, et al. Norfloxacin vs ceftriaxone in the prophylaxis of infections in patients with advanced cirrhosis and hemorrhage. Gastroenterology 2006;131:1049-56; quiz 1285.

40. Hou MC, Lin HC, Liu TT, et al. Antibiotic prophylaxis after endoscopic therapy prevents rebleeding in acute variceal hemorrhage: a randomized trial. Hepatology 2004;39:746-53.

41. Rasaratnam B, Kaye D, Jennings G, et al. The effect of selective intestinal decontamination on the hyperdynamic circulatory state in cirrhosis: A randomized trial. Ann Intern Med. 2003;139:186-93.

42. Soares-Weiser K, Brezis M, Tur-Kaspa R, et al. Antibiotic prophylaxis of bacterial infections in cirrhotic inpatients: a meta-analysis of randomized controlled trials. Scand J Gastroenterol 2003;38:193-200.

43. Fernandez J, Acevedo J, Castro M, et al. Prevalence and risk factors of infections by multiresistant bacteria in cirrhosis: a prospective study. Hepatology 2012;55:1551-61.

44. Rimola A, Garcia-Tsao G, Navasa M, et al. Diagnosis, treatment and prophylaxis of spontaneous bacterial peritonitis: a consensus document. International Ascites Club. J Hepatol 2000;32:142-53.

45. Fraser VJ, Jones M, Dunkel J, et al. Candidemia in a tertiary care hospital: epidemiology, risk factors, and predictors of mortality. Clin Infect Dis 1992;15:414-21.

46. Garey KW, Rege M, Pai MP, et al. Time to initiation of fluconazole therapy impacts mortality in patients with candidemia: a multi-institutional study. Clin Infect Dis 2006;43:25-31.

47. Charles PE, Doise JM, Quenot JP, et al. Candidemia in critically ill patients: difference of outcome between medical and surgical patients. Intensive Care Med 2003;29:2162-9.

48. Nolla-Salas J, Sitges-Serra A, Leon-Gil C, et al. Candidemia in non-neutropenic critically ill patients: analysis of prognostic factors and assessment of systemic antifungal therapy. study group of fungal infection in the ICU. Intensive Care Med 1997;23:23-30.

49. Leroy O, Gangneux JP, Montravers P, et al. Epidemiology, management, and risk factors for death of invasive Candida infections in critical care: a multicenter, prospective, observational study in France (2005-2006). Crit Care Med 2009;37:1612-8.

50. Michalopoulos AS, Geroulanos S, Mentzelopoulos SD. Determinants of candidemia and candidemia-related death in cardiothoracic ICU patients. Chest 2003;124:2244-55.

51. Dupont H, Bourichon A, Paugam-Burtz C, et al. Can yeast isolation in peritoneal fluid be predicted in intensive care unit patients with peritonitis? Crit Care Med 2003;31:752-7.
52. Paphitou NI, Ostrosky-Zeichner L, Rex JH. Rules for identifying patients at increased risk for candidal infections in the surgical intensive care unit: approach to developing practical criteria for systematic use in antifungal prophylaxis trials. Med Mycol 2005;43:235-43.
53. Leon C, Ruiz-Santana S, Saavedra P, et al. Usefulness of the "candida score" for discriminating between Candida colonization and invasive candidiasis in non-neutropenic critically ill patients: a prospective multicenter study. Crit Care Med 2009;37:1624-33.
54. Ostrosky-Zeichner L, Sable C, Sobel J, et al. Multicenter retrospective development and validation of a clinical prediction rule for nosocomial invasive candidiasis in the intensive care setting. Eur J Clin Microbiol Infect Dis 2007;26:271-6.
55. Wey SB, Mori M, Pfaller MA, et al. Risk factors for hospital-acquired candidemia. A matched case-control study. Arch Intern Med 1989;149:2349-53.
56. Pittet D, Monod M, Suter PM, et al. Candida colonization and subsequent infections in critically ill surgical patients. Ann Surg 1994;220:751-8.
57. Eggimann P, Francioli P, Bille J, et al. Fluconazole prophylaxis prevents intra-abdominal candidiasis in high-risk surgical patients. Crit Care Med 1999;27:1066-72.
58. Playford EG, Webster AC, Sorrell TC, et al. Antifungal agents for preventing fungal infections in non-neutropenic critically ill and surgical patients: systematic review and meta-analysis of randomized clinical trials. J Antimicrob Chemother 2006;57:628-38.
59. Cruciani M, de Lalla F, Mengoli C. Prophylaxis of Candida infections in adult trauma and surgical intensive care patients: a systematic review and meta-analysis. Intensive Care Med 2005;31:1479-87.
60. Shorr AF, Chung K, Jackson WL, et al. Fluconazole prophylaxis in critically ill surgical patients: a meta-analysis. Crit Care Med 2005;33:1928-35; quiz 1936.
61. Pelz RK, Hendrix CW, Swoboda SM, et al. Double-blind placebo-controlled trial of fluconazole to prevent candidal infections in critically ill surgical patients. Ann Surg 2001;233:542-8.
62. Eggimann P, Francioli P, Bille J, et al. Fluconazole prophylaxis prevents intra-abdominal candidiasis in high-risk surgical patients. Crit Care Med 1999;27:1066-72.
63. Bow EJ, Evans G, Fuller J, et al. Canadian clinical practice guidelines for invasive candidiasis in adults. Can J Infect Dis Med Microbiol 2010;21:e122-50.
64. Pappas PG, Kauffman CA, Andes D, et al. Clinical practice guidelines for the management of candidiasis: 2009 update by the Infectious Diseases Society of America. Clin Infect Dis 2009;48:503-35.
65. Pappas PG, Kauffman CA, Andes D, et al. Clinical practice guidelines for the management of candidiasis: 2009 update by the Infectious Diseases Society of America. Clin Infect Dis 2009;48:503-35.
66. Kanafani ZA, Perfect JR. Antimicrobial resistance: resistance to antifungal agents: mechanisms and clinical impact. Clin Infect Dis 2008;46:120-8.
67. Ostrosky-Zeichner L, Shoham S, Vazquez J, et al. MSG-01: a randomized, double-blind, placebo-controlled trial of caspofungin prophylaxis followed by preemptive therapy for invasive candidiasis in high-risk adults in the critical care setting. Clin Infect Dis 2014;58:1219-26.
68. Tomblyn M, Chiller T, Einsele H, et al. Guidelines for preventing infectious complications among hematopoietic cell transplantation recipients: a global perspective. Biol Blood Marrow Transplant 2009;15:1143-238.
69. Metzger KE, Rucker Y, Callaghan M, et al. The burden of mucosal barrier injury laboratory-confirmed bloodstream infection among hematology, oncology, and stem cell transplant patients. Infect Control Hosp Epidemiol 2015;36:119-24.
70. National Comprehensive Cancer Network (NCCN). NCCN clinical practice guidelines in oncology: prevention and treatment of cancer-related infection. Updated 2015. Available at http://www.nccn.org/professionals/physician_gls/pdf/infections.pdf. Accessed October 22, 2015.
71. Akhtari M, Curtis B, Waller EK. Autoimmune neutropenia in adults. Autoimmun Rev 2009;9:62-6.
72. Nossent JC, Swaak AJ. Prevalence and significance of haematological abnormalities in patients with systemic lupus erythematosus. Q J Med 1991;80:605-12.
73. Freifeld AG, Bow EJ, Sepkowitz KA, et al. Clinical practice guideline for the use of antimicrobial agents in neutropenic patients with cancer: 2010 update by the Infectious Diseases Society of America. Clin Infect Dis 2011;52:e56-93.
74. Bodey GP, Buckley M, Sathe YS, et al. Quantitative relationships between circulating leukocytes and infection in patients with acute leukemia. Ann Intern Med 1966;64:328-40.
75. Pizzo PA. Management of fever in patients with cancer and treatment-induced neutropenia. N Engl J Med 1993;328:1323-32.
76. Wisplinghoff H, Seifert H, Wenzel RP, et al. Current trends in the epidemiology of nosocomial bloodstream infections in patients with hematological malignancies and solid neoplasms in hospitals in the United States. Clin Infect Dis 2003;36:1103-10.
77. Zuckermann J, Moreira LB, Stoll P, et al. Compliance with a critical pathway for the management of febrile neutropenia and impact on clinical outcomes. Ann Hematol 2008;87:139-45.
78. Bucaneve G, Micozzi A, Menichetti F, et al. Levofloxacin to prevent bacterial infection in patients with cancer and neutropenia. N Engl J Med 2005;353:977-87.
79. Cullen M, Steven N, Billingham L, et al. Antibacterial prophylaxis after chemotherapy for solid tumors and lymphomas. N Engl J Med 2005;353:988-98.
80. Slaughter MS, Rogers JG, Milano CA, et al. Advanced heart failure treated with continuous-flow left ventricular assist device. N Engl J Med 2009;361:2241-51.
81. Kirklin JK, Naftel DC, Pagani FD, et al. Sixth INTERMACS annual report: a 10,000-patient database. J Heart Lung Transplant 2014;33:555-64.
82. Gordon RJ, Quagliarello B, Lowy FD. Ventricular assist device-related infections. Lancet Infect Dis 2006;6:426-37.
83. Feldman D, Pamboukian SV, Teuteberg JJ, et al. The 2013 International Society for Heart and Lung Transplantation guidelines for mechanical circulatory support: executive summary. J Heart Lung Transplant 2013;32:157-87.

84. Gordon SM, Schmitt SK, Jacobs M, et al. Nosocomial bloodstream infections in patients with implantable left ventricular assist devices. Ann Thorac Surg 2001;72:725-30.

85. Gristina AG, Dobbins JJ, Giammara B, et al. Biomaterial-centered sepsis and the total artificial heart. Microbial adhesion vs tissue integration. JAMA 1988;259:870-4.

86. Shoham S, Miller LW. Cardiac assist device infections. Curr Infect Dis Rep 2009;11:268-73.

87. Acharya MN, Som R, Tsui S. What is the optimum antibiotic prophylaxis in patients undergoing implantation of a left ventricular assist device? Interact Cardiovasc Thorac Surg 2012;14:209-14.

88. Eyler RF, Butler SO, Walker PC, et al. Vancomycin use during left ventricular assist device support. Infect Control Hosp Epidemiol 2009;30:484-6.

89. Rose EA, Gelijns AC, Moskowitz AJ, et al. Long-term use of a left ventricular assist device for end-stage heart failure. N Engl J Med 2001;345:1435-443.

90. Holman WL, Park SJ, Long JW, et al. Infection in permanent circulatory support: experience from the REMATCH trial. J Heart Lung Transplant 2004;23:1359-65.

91. Copeland JG, Smith RG, Arabia FA, et al. Cardiac replacement with a total artificial heart as a bridge to transplantation. N Engl J Med 2004;351:859-67.

92. Roussel JC, Senage T, Baron O, et al. CardioWest (jarvik) total artificial heart: a single-center experience with 42 patients. Ann Thorac Surg 2009;87:124-9; discussion 130.

93. Copeland JG, Copeland H, Gustafson M, et al. Experience with more than 100 total artificial heart implants. J Thorac Cardiovasc Surg 2012;143:727-34.

94. Aubron C, Cheng AC, Pilcher D, et al. Factors associated with outcomes of patients on extracorporeal membrane oxygenation support: a 5-year cohort study. Crit Care 2013;17:R73.

95. Aubron C, Cheng AC, Pilcher D, et al. Infections acquired by adults who receive extracorporeal membrane oxygenation: risk factors and outcome. Infect Control Hosp Epidemiol 2013;34:24-30.

96. Zhan C, Baine WB, Sedrakyan A, et al. Cardiac device implantation in the united states from 1997 through 2004: a population-based analysis. J Gen Intern Med 2008;23(suppl 1):13-9.

97. Uslan DZ, Tleyjeh IM, Baddour LM, et al. Temporal trends in permanent pacemaker implantation: a population-based study. Am Heart J 2008;155:896-903.

98. Baddour LM, Epstein AE, Erickson CC, et al. Update on cardiovascular implantable electronic device infections and their management: a scientific statement from the American Heart Association. Circulation 2010;121:458-77.

99. de Oliveira JC, Martinelli M, Nishioka SA, et al. Efficacy of antibiotic prophylaxis before the implantation of pacemakers and cardioverter-defibrillators: results of a large, prospective, randomized, double-blinded, placebo-controlled trial. Circ Arrhythm Electrophysiol 2009;2:29-34.

100. Klug D, Balde M, Pavin D, et al. Risk factors related to infections of implanted pacemakers and cardioverter-defibrillators: results of a large prospective study. Circulation 2007;116:1349-55.

101. Sohail MR, Uslan DZ, Khan AH, et al. Risk factor analysis of permanent pacemaker infection. Clin Infect Dis 2007;45:166-73.

102. Narotam PK, van Dellen JR, du Trevou MD, et al. Operative sepsis in neurosurgery: a method of classifying surgical cases. Neurosurgery 1994;34:409-15; discussion 415-6.

103. Barker FG II. Efficacy of prophylactic antibiotics against meningitis after craniotomy: a meta-analysis. Neurosurgery 2007;60:887-94; discussion 887-94.

104. Korinek AM, Golmard JL, Elcheick A, et al. Risk factors for neurosurgical site infections after craniotomy: a critical reappraisal of antibiotic prophylaxis on 4,578 patients. Br J Neurosurg 2005;19:155-62.

105. Borges LF. Infections in neurologic surgery. host defenses. Neurosurg Clin North Am 1992;3:275-8.

106. McClelland S III, Hall WA. Postoperative central nervous system infection: incidence and associated factors in 2111 neurosurgical procedures. Clin Infect Dis 2007;45:55-9.

107. Hosein IK, Hill DW, Hatfield RH. Controversies in the prevention of neurosurgical infection. J Hosp Infect 1999;43:5-11.

108. Korinek AM, Baugnon T, Golmard JL, et al. Risk factors for adult nosocomial meningitis after craniotomy: role of antibiotic prophylaxis. Neurosurgery 2006;59:126-33; discussion 126-33.

109. Lietard C, Thebaud V, Besson G, et al. Risk factors for neurosurgical site infections: an 18-month prospective survey. J Neurosurg 2008;109:729-34.

110. Curry WT Jr, Butler WE, Barker FG II. Rapidly rising incidence of cerebrospinal fluid shunting procedures for idiopathic intracranial hypertension in the United States, 1988-2002. Neurosurgery 2005;57:97-108; discussion 97-108.

111. Korinek AM, Baugnon T, Golmard JL, et al. Risk factors for adult nosocomial meningitis after craniotomy: role of antibiotic prophylaxis. Neurosurgery 2008;62(suppl 2):532-9.

112. Rebuck JA, Murry KR, Rhoney DH, et al. Infection related to intracranial pressure monitors in adults: analysis of risk factors and antibiotic prophylaxis. J Neurol Neurosurg Psychiatry 2000;69:381-4.

113. Lozier AP, Sciacca RR, Romagnoli MF, et al. Ventriculostomy-related infections: a critical review of the literature. Neurosurgery 2008;62(suppl 2):688-700.

114. Alleyne CH Jr, Hassan M, Zabramski JM. The efficacy and cost of prophylactic and periprocedural antibiotics in patients with external ventricular drains. Neurosurgery 2000;47:1124-7; discussion 1127-9.

115. May AK, Fleming SB, Carpenter RO, et al. Influence of broad-spectrum antibiotic prophylaxis on intracranial pressure monitor infections and subsequent infectious complications in head-injured patients. Surg Infect (Larchmt) 2006;7:409-17.

116. Langley JM, LeBlanc JC, Drake J, et al. Efficacy of antimicrobial prophylaxis in placement of cerebrospinal fluid shunts: meta-analysis. Clin Infect Dis 1993;17:98-103.

117. Haines SJ, Walters BC. Antibiotic prophylaxis for cerebrospinal fluid shunts: a meta-analysis. Neurosurgery 1994;34:87-92.

118. Hedegard E, Bjellvi J, Edelvik A, et al. Complications to invasive epilepsy surgery workup with subdural and depth electrodes: a prospective population-based observational study. J Neurol Neurosurg Psychiatry 2014;85:716-20.

119. Klompas M, Branson R, Eichenwald EC, et al. Strategies to prevent ventilator-associated pneumonia in acute care hospitals: 2014 update. Infect Control Hosp Epidemiol 2014;35:915-36.

120. Melsen WG, Rovers MM, Koeman M, et al. Estimating the attributable mortality of ventilator-associated pneumonia from randomized prevention studies. Crit Care Med 2011;39:2736-42.

121. Kollef MH. Ventilator-associated pneumonia. A multivariate analysis. JAMA 1993;270:1965-70.

122. Park DR. The microbiology of ventilator-associated pneumonia. Respir Care 2005;50:742-63; discussion 763-5.

123. Klompas M, Branson R, Eichenwald EC, et al. Strategies to prevent ventilator-associated pneumonia in acute care hospitals: 2014 update. Infect Control Hosp Epidemiol 2014;35:915-36.

124. Sirvent JM, Torres A, El-Ebiary M, et al. Protective effect of intravenously administered cefuroxime against nosocomial pneumonia in patients with structural coma. Am J Respir Crit Care Med 1997;155:1729-34.

125. Valles J, Peredo R, Burgueno MJ, et al. Efficacy of single-dose antibiotic against early-onset pneumonia in comatose patients who are ventilated. Chest 2013;143:1219-25.

126. Schlosser RJ. Clinical practice. epistaxis. N Engl J Med 2009;360:784-9.

127. Corrales CE, Goode RL. Should patients with posterior nasal packing require ICU admission? Laryngoscope 2013;123:2928-9.

128. Pollice PA, Yoder MG. Epistaxis: a retrospective review of hospitalized patients. Otolaryngol Head Neck Surg 1997;117:49-53.

129. Jacobson JA, Kasworm EM. Toxic shock syndrome after nasal surgery: case reports and analysis of risk factors. Arch Otolaryngol Head Neck Surg 1986;112:329-32.

130. Biswas D, Mal RK. Are systemic prophylactic antibiotics indicated with anterior nasal packing for spontaneous epistaxis? Acta Otolaryngol 2009;129:179-81.

131. Pennekamp A, Tschirky P, Grossenbacher R. Significance of staphylococcus aureus in nose operations. risk of toxic shock syndrome? HNO 1995;43:664-8.

132. Jacobson JA, Stevens MH, Kasworm EM. Evaluation of single-dose cefazolin prophylaxis for toxic shock syndrome. Arch Otolaryngol Head Neck Surg 1988;114:326-7.

Section 3

Neurocritical Care

Chapter 19
Status Epilepticus and Acute Seizure Management

Eljim P. Tesoro, Pharm.D., BCPS; Karen Berger, Pharm.D., BCPS; and Gretchen M. Brophy, Pharm.D., FCCP, FCCM, FNCS, BCPS

LEARNING OBJECTIVES

1. Identify risk factors for seizures in critically ill patients.
2. Recommend appropriate dosing and monitoring of urgent and emergent therapy.
3. Compare and contrast antiepileptic agents used in the management of status epilepticus (SE).
4. Customize drug therapy management in special populations with altered pharmacokinetic parameters.
5. Develop a patient-specific treatment algorithm for the management of refractory SE in intubated and non-intubated patients.

ABBREVIATIONS IN THIS CHAPTER

cEEG	Continuous electroencephalogram	NMDA	*N*-methyl-D-aspartate
EEG	Electroencephalogram	RSE	Refractory status epilepticus
GABA	γ-Aminobutyric acid	SE	Status epilepticus
ICU	Intensive care unit	TH	Therapeutic hypothermia
NCSE	Non-convulsive status epilepticus		

INTRODUCTION

Seizures are a serious medical complication of the central nervous system (CNS) that can lead to considerable morbidity and mortality. They can occur along a spectrum of syndromes, from the focal seizure to status epilepticus (SE), which in turn can evolve into refractory status epilepticus (RSE) and super-refractory status epilepticus. Most isolated seizures are self-resolving, but any seizure that persists beyond 5 minutes or a series of seizures between which a patient does not regain consciousness should be considered SE.[1] In intensive care units (ICUs), this diagnosis may be difficult to make because of severe underlying neurological disease or drugs that may mask outward signs of seizures. Although outcomes are improved with faster identification and timely pharmacologic treatment, clinicians are still challenged by the hemodynamic instability, numerous drug interactions, and end-organ dysfunction often seen in critically ill patients. Several guidelines have been published to help promote evidence-based practice,[2,3] but the ICU remains a challenging area. Use of published algorithms and pathways and development of institutional protocols can expedite treatment to terminate SE.

This chapter will focus on the treatment of SE in critically ill patients with a brief discussion of the role of seizure prophylaxis. The goals of therapy for SE are to (1) rapidly terminate seizure activity, both physiologic and electrographic; (2) identify and treat the cause, if possible; and (3) prevent future seizures, if needed, with the appropriate use of anticonvulsants.

EPIDEMIOLOGY

A recent study described the epidemiology of SE in the United States over 12 years.[4] Although an increase in incidence was seen (3.5–12.5 per 100,000), there was no change for in-hospital mortality. This increased incidence may have occurred partly because of the change in definition of SE as well as increased use of electroencephalogram (EEG) monitoring and, therefore, SE diagnosis during the past decade.[5] A higher incidence of SE was seen at each end of the age spectrum (younger than 10 years and older than 50 years), but in-hospital mortality was much higher for older adults than for children (20.2% vs. 2.6%). Men have higher incidence and mortality rates than do women; men also have SE at a younger age. Racial disparities are seen in SE, with a higher incidence among blacks (13.7 per 100,000) than among whites (6.9 per 100,000), although in-hospital mortality rates are higher for whites (10%; 95% CI, 9.8–10) than for blacks (7.4%; 95% CI, 7.3–7.6). The number of patients discharged to home declined over time, whereas discharge to long-term care facilities almost doubled.

Most seizures occurring in ICU patients are convulsive in nature—around 90% in a recent series of medical and surgical patients,[6] although 50% of these patients had a history of epilepsy. Hospital mortality was reported to be 21% and was highly predicted by age, lower Glasgow Coma Scale score at baseline, and severity of SE. Treatment of SE in a neuro-ICU versus a medical ICU did not result in decreased mortality or morbidity or a shorter length of stay,[7] although the use of continuous electroencephalogram (cEEG) monitoring was greater in the neuro-ICU.

Mortality for SE has been reported to be around 4% for inpatients with generalized tonic-clonic SE.[8] Additional mortality risk factors include mechanical ventilation, female sex, comorbidity index, and anoxic brain injury. Other cohort studies report higher case fatality rates of around 22%, but they include all types of SE. Increasing age and anoxic brain injury continue to be driving contributors for death after SE and are commonly seen in ICU patients. Status epilepticus after CNS infection also confers a poor prognosis. Patients without epilepsy who develop SE tend to have worse outcomes.[9]

ETIOLOGY

Seizures in the ICU can arise from existing neurological conditions or as a complication of systemic illness (see Table 19.1). Neurotrauma, stroke, CNS infections or tumors, and epilepsy are common neurological etiologies of SE. Hypoxia, substance abuse/toxicity, drug-drug interactions, renal or

Table 19.1 Etiology and Selected Prevalence and Mortality in Status Epilepticus

Etiology	Prevalence (%)[a]	Mortality (%)[a]	Prophylaxis Recommended?[b]
Ischemic stroke	6.0	20.5	No
Metabolic abnormalities	5.7	12.5	No
• Hypoglycemia			
• Hyper/hypoglycemia			
• Hypocalcemia			
• Hypomagnesemia			
• Uremia/hyperosmolality			
• Anoxia	3.5	42.4	
Infection			No
• CNS (e.g., meningitis)	2.3	24.2	
• Systemic (e.g., sepsis)			
Traumatic brain injury	1.1	15.6	Yes (7-day course of phenytoin; levetiracetam may be reasonable option)
Subarachnoid hemorrhage			Yes (3-day course of AED may be sufficient)
Intracerebral hemorrhage			No
Drugs			No
• Subtherapeutic anticonvulsant concentration			
• Alcohol withdrawal			
• Toxicity/overdose	2.2	5.9	
• Toxins			
Tumors	1.8	23.6	No
Congenital	5.9	1.1	Unknown

[a]Data from: Dham BS, Hunter K, Rincon F. The epidemiology of status epilepticus in the United States. Neurocrit Care 2014;20:476-83.
[b]Data from: Rowe AS, Goodwin H, Brophy GM, et al. Seizure prophylaxis in neurocritical care: a review of evidence-based support. Pharmacotherapy 2014;34:396-409.
AED = antiepileptic drug.

hepatic dysfunction, and acute metabolic disturbances may also lead to the development of SE in the critically ill patient. Electrolyte imbalances are common in ICU patients, and acute fluctuations in sodium, calcium, and magnesium can lead to seizure activity.[10] Drugs may also be implicated in acute seizures. Bupropion, diphenhydramine, tricyclic antidepressants, tramadol, amphetamines, isoniazid, and venlafaxine have all been implicated in seizures or SE in overdose cases.[11] A clinical tool was recently developed to aid clinicians in evaluating potential etiologies in patients with SE,[12] which may result in more timely treatment and resolution. The most common determinants for SE included subtherapeutic anticonvulsant concentrations, brain tumors, acute intracerebral hemorrhage, history of epilepsy, infection (both CNS and systemic), traumatic brain injury, alcohol withdrawal/intoxication, and benzodiazepine withdrawal.

PATHOPHYSIOLOGY

Traditionally, the cause of SE has been described as an imbalance of excitatory and inhibitory neurotransmitter activity in the CNS. It may be a condition of excess excitation, insufficient inhibition, or a combination of both. Clinically, it is difficult to differentiate, but current treatments focus on increasing overall inhibitory activity. Glutamate, substance P, and neurokinin B are the more common excitatory neurotransmitters, whereas γ-aminobutyric acid (GABA) and neuropeptide Y moderate neuronal inhibition. Most isolated seizures occur when inhibitory mechanisms are transiently overwhelmed.

Glutamate normally produces depolarization of neurons through its effects on postsynaptic N-methyl-D-aspartate (NMDA) and α-amino-3-hydroxy-5-methyl-isoxazole-4-propionate (AMPA) receptors. γ-aminobutyric acid mediates postsynaptic hyperpolarization through the opening of chloride channels. More recent literature has shed light on additional mechanisms and potential treatment strategies.[13]

An alteration in GABA activity over time may explain the refractoriness of GABA-ergic drugs as SE progresses.[14,15] Internalization of synaptic $GABA_A$ receptors has been reported to increase with ongoing seizure activity, resulting in the decreased efficacy of benzodiazepines as well as other GABA-ergic drugs.[16] Clinically, this pharmacoresistance begins soon after seizures begin, persists beyond 30 minutes, and may contribute to increased morbidity in these patients because of delayed diagnosis and proper intervention. Use of benzodiazepines early on in SE may be successful, but response quickly declines as time progresses between onset and treatment.[17] This highlights the importance of rapidly identifying seizure activity with immediate administration of benzodiazepines to optimize control, followed by urgent and refractory treatments as necessary.

Distinct physiological phases are seen with classic generalized tonic-clonic SE. Within 10 minutes of seizure activity (early or phase I), increases in serum concentrations of norepinephrine and epinephrine as well cortisol can be seen, leading to cardiovascular hyperactivity (e.g., hypertension, tachycardia, and arrhythmias), fever, and hyperglycemia.[18] Prolonged muscle contraction from uncontrolled tonic-clonic convulsions results in lactic acid production, and subsequent acidosis can be severe. Normally, this resolves once convulsions stop, but in critically ill patients with an underlying acidosis from other conditions or compromised tissue perfusion, it may persist and warrant further therapy.

After 30 minutes of continuous seizing (late or phase II), systems begin to fail as compensatory mechanisms are overwhelmed. Hypotension, bradycardia, and hypoglycemia can be seen; cerebral perfusion pressure is compromised as mean arterial pressure falls, whereas cerebral demand remains high because of unrelenting electrical activity. In critically ill patients with poor reserve or unrecognized SE, this phase may occur earlier and require emergent treatment. Unrelenting tonic-clonic activity can lead to rhabdomyolysis and subsequent renal failure.[19]

DIAGNOSIS

Timely clinical identification of SE is important because of the time-sensitive response of treatment strategies. Most generalized seizures in the ICU are well recognized,[20] but it can be difficult to detect subtle seizure types such as non-convulsive status epilepticus (NCSE) where the traditional tonic-clonic movements of the extremities are not visibly apparent (Table 19.2). A cEEG is a useful tool in these cases to help identify such patients and direct therapy. Any unexplained acute changes in mental status should be investigated with EEG for evidence of seizure

Table 19.2 Clinical Features of Seizures

Seizure Type	Physical Findings	Sensorium
Focal motor	Focal facial or limb twitching	No alteration
Complex partial	Automatisms/involuntary activity	Disturbed
Generalized tonic-clonic	Generalized convulsions	Loss of consciousness
Non-convulsive status epilepticus	No twitching/convulsions	Altered sensorium or loss of consciousness

activity. Patients who lack response to drug therapy will also benefit from EEG monitoring. Figure 19.1 and Figure 19.2 represent EEG findings in patients with convulsive and non-convulsive seizures, respectively.

PROPHYLAXIS

For patients with known risk factors for seizures, prophylactic therapy can reduce the risk of SE. In patients with provoked SE, it is essential to treat both the seizure and the underlying cause. For some ICU patients, it may be difficult to assess the cause of the SE because of several risk factors and difficulty in identifying the exact onset of the seizure activity. Some etiologies such as anoxic brain injury, most commonly seen after cardiac arrest, are more difficult to treat and tend to have poorer outcomes.[20]

Certain ICU patients at high risk of seizures should receive short-term prophylaxis (e.g., traumatic brain injury and aneurysmal subarachnoid hemorrhage; see Table 19.1). Guidelines have been published to identify high-risk populations, describe the risk of seizures after brain injury, and recommend suitable timing of therapy.[21] Seizures, and potentially SE, may occur in these patients if dosing is not optimized, prophylaxis is not initiated in a timely manner, or therapy is interrupted or inadvertently altered (e.g., drug interactions). Prophylaxis should only be provided during the high-risk period and discontinued afterward unless actual seizures occur because these agents are not without considerable adverse effects. ICU patients who are pharmacologically sedated and paralyzed should remain on seizure prophylaxis until these agents are cleared systemically because of the possible masking of any physiologic signs of seizures unless cEEG monitoring can confirm the absence of seizure activity.

TREATMENT

The treatment of SE is complex, often requiring the use of multiple agents, drugs with narrow therapeutic indexes, aggressive dosing targeting higher serum concentrations, and frequent titrations to a goal of seizure cessation. Although a variety of treatment options are available, evidence is lacking to support one treatment strategy over another. Many of the current treatment data are from non-randomized, retrospective studies that have small sample sizes and lack standardized dosing strategies and treatment durations. Newer anticonvulsants have easier, non–weight-based dosing, fewer drug interactions, and better adverse event profiles. Although they may be more desirable, the data surrounding their use, particularly as first-line agents, are less robust than for historical agents. These agents were also excluded from many of the earlier comparator trials.[22] Regardless of which drugs are selected, the primary treatment goal remains the same: cessation of seizures, including clinical and subclinical (electrographic) seizures. Management of airway, breathing, and circulation should occur simultaneously with targeted treatment for SE. Other goals include achievement of therapeutic drug concentrations, liberation from mechanical ventilation (particularly if the initial treatment required respiratory support), identification and treatment of the underlying cause, and selection of regimens that produce acceptable

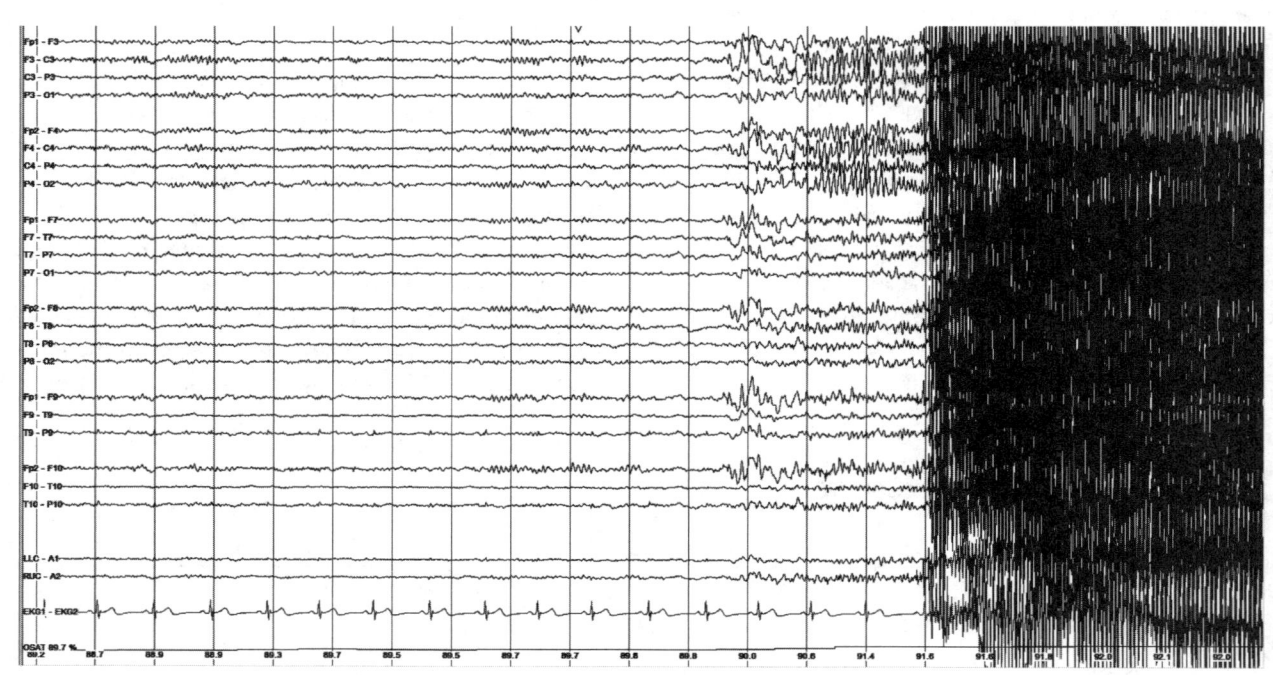

Figure 19.1 EEG of patient with tonic-clonic seizures. Normal brain waves are seen initially followed by evidence of seizure activity.

adverse effect profiles. Emergent therapy should be initiated within the first 5 minutes of seizure onset and urgent control treatment, immediately after or within the first 10 minutes of seizure onset.[3]

It is important to be familiar with all available agents so that an individualized, stepwise approach to the treatment of SE can be selected. Pharmacologic options may be classified as emergent, urgent, and refractory and are generally initiated in this order, although sometimes, the addition of a drug or the titration of a continuous infusion occurs simultaneously. Table 19.3 describes the most commonly used drugs for SE.

Emergent Initial Treatment: Benzodiazepines

Benzodiazepines, GABA receptor agonists, are considered first-line agents in the treatment of SE. Lorazepam, midazolam, and diazepam are the most commonly used benzodiazepines, and all are available intravenously. When used emergently for SE, intravenous benzodiazepine administration is preferred; however, nasal, buccal, or rectal routes are acceptable alternative routes of administration.[3] Historically, drugs such as midazolam and diazepam were preferred for their ability to quickly cross the blood-brain barrier; however, they carry a risk of rebound seizures because of their rapid redistribution out of the brain and into adipose tissue.[23] Intravenous lorazepam, a less lipophilic benzodiazepine than diazepam, is the preferred first-line treatment for SE.[3,22,24] A randomized trial comparing lorazepam (2–4 mg), diazepam (5–10 mg), and placebo for out-of-hospital SE found an SE termination rate of 59%, 43%, and 21%, respectively.

Although the only statistically significant difference was between both benzodiazepines and the placebo group, there was a trend toward faster termination and better control of SE in the lorazepam group.[25] Another study found numerically better success rates with lorazepam 2 mg over diazepam 5 mg (78% vs. 58% seizure termination after one dose), but the results were not statistically significant. Similar results were seen after two doses of each drug; a total of 4 mg of lorazepam and 10 mg of diazepam terminated seizures in 89% and 76%, respectively.[26] The VA Cooperative Trial compared four different treatment regimens (lorazepam, phenobarbital, diazepam plus phenytoin, and phenytoin) and found that lorazepam was more successful than phenytoin in overt status cases (64.9% vs. 43.6%; p=0.002). Because of the formulation of lorazepam and diazepam with propylene glycol, midazolam is the preferred agent when given intramuscularly. In a randomized controlled trial, midazolam 10 mg intramuscularly was found as effective as lorazepam 4 mg intravenously for prehospital seizure control.[27] Diazepam is preferred for rectal administration, although this route should only be used when intravenous and intramuscular options are unavailable or contraindicated.[3] Although respiratory depression is a concern with benzodiazepine administration, studies have shown no difference in respiratory depression compared with placebo and non-benzodiazepines when administered for SE.[22,25]

Urgent Control Treatment

Urgent treatment uses non-benzodiazepine anticonvulsants. Drugs are initiated in a stepwise fashion and quickly titrated to therapeutic doses. No prospective, comparative data past

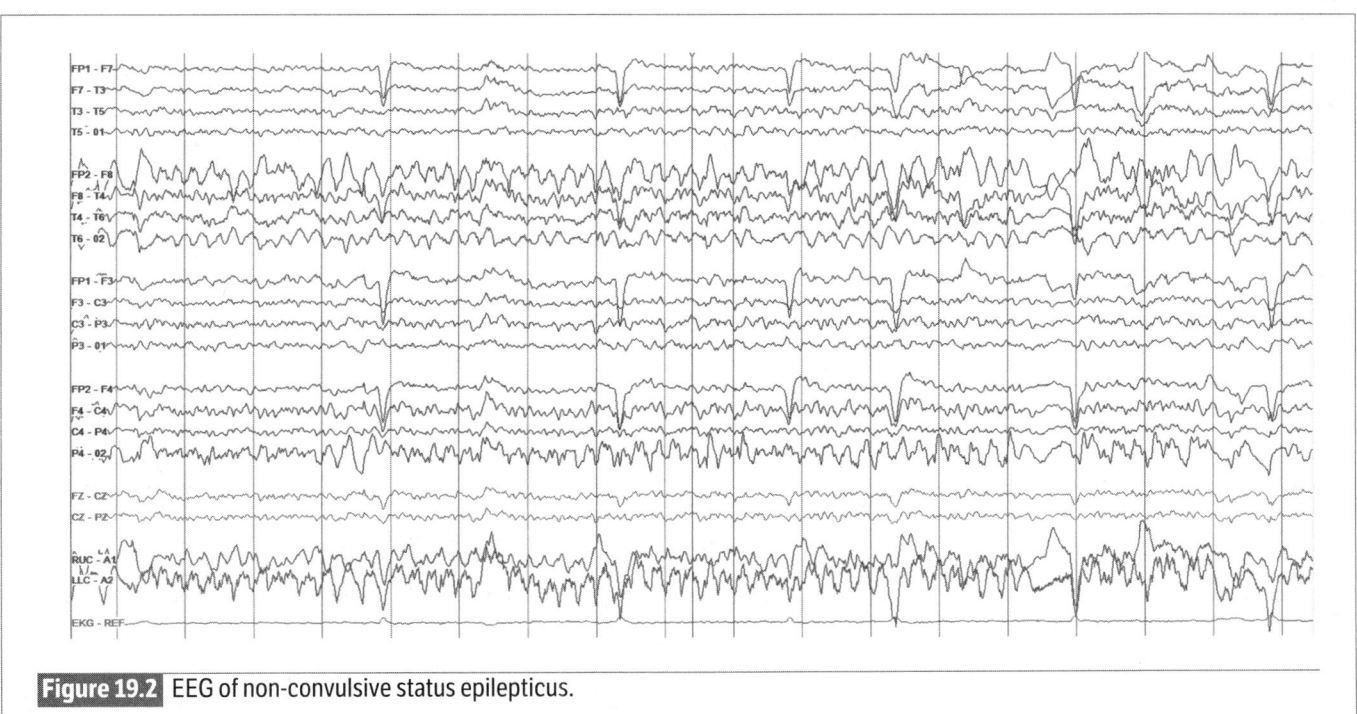

Figure 19.2 EEG of non-convulsive status epilepticus.

Table 19.3 Treatment Summary Chart

	Mechanism of Action	Bolus Dose	Dose Range	Metabolism/ Renal Elimination	Half-life (hr)	Drug Interactions	Significant Adverse Effects	Comments
Emergent Initial Treatment: Benzodiazepines								
Diazepam	GABA agonist	0.15 mg/kg IV up to 10 mg/dose *May repeat in 5 min *0.2 mg/kg rectally	10–20 mg	Hepatic, active metabolite	33–45	CYP 2C19 and 3A4 substrate	Hypotension	IV contains propylene glycol; Respiratory depression; Up to 5 mg/min IV; May be administered rectally
Lorazepam	GABA agonist	0.1 mg/kg IV up to 4 mg/dose *May repeat in 5–10 min	4–10 mg	Hepatic	14	Non-significant	Hypotension; Respiratory depression	IV contains propylene glycol; Up to 2 mg/min IV
Midazolam	GABA agonist	0.2 mg/kg IM up to 10 mg/dose	10–20 mg	Hepatic, active metabolite renally eliminated	2–7	CYP3A4 substrate	Hypotension; Respiratory depression	Accumulates in fat tissue; May be administered IM, buccally
Urgent Control Treatment: Anticonvulsants								
Phenytoin	Sodium channel blocker	20 mg/kg IV *May give additional 5–10 mg/kg	5–7 mg/kg per day in two or three divided doses	Hepatic	7–42	CYP 2B, 2C and 3A4 inducer PgP	Hypotension; Arrhythmias; Purple glove syndrome	Maximum infusion rate 50 mg/min; Only stable in NS; Highly protein bound; TDC: 10–25 mcg/mL (free 1–2.5 mcg/mL)
Fosphenytoin	Sodium channel blocker	20 mg PE/kg IV *May give additional 5–10 mg PE/kg	5–7 mg PE/kg per day in two or three divided doses	Hepatic	7–42	CYP 2B, 2C, and 3A4 inducer PgP	Hypotension; Arrhythmias	Maximum infusion rate 150 mg PE/min; Prodrug of phenytoin (15 min conversion rate to active drug); Highly protein bound; May be administered IM; TDC: 10–25 mcg/mL (free 1–2.5 mcg/mL)
Valproic acid	Enhances GABA	20–40 mg/kg IV *May give additional 20 mg/kg	500–1,000 mg q6–8hr	Hepatic	9–19	CYP2C9 inhibitor; weak CYP2A6 inducer	Thrombocytopenia; Hepatotoxicity; Hyperammonemia; Pancreatitis; Tremor	Can be rapidly administered (up to 6 mg/kg/min); Highly protein bound; TDC: 50–140 mcg/mL (free 4–11 mcg/mL)
Phenobarbital	Barbiturate; GABA agonist	20 mg/kg IV *May give additional 5–10 mg/kg	1–3 mg/kg per day in two or three divided doses	Hepatic	53–140	CYP 2C9 and 3A4 inducer	Hypotension; Respiratory depression	TDC: 20–50 mcg/mL
Levetiracetam	Enhances GABA, calcium channel blocker	1–3 g IV	1.5–3 g per day in two to four divided doses	Renal	6–8	Nonsignificant	Agitation; Anxiety; Lethargy; Aggression	Renal dose adjustment; TDC: N/A (12–45 mcg/mL has been suggested)
Lacosamide	Sodium channel slow inactivation	200–400 mg IV	100–200 mg q12hr	Renal and hepatic	13	Nonsignificant	PR prolongation	Renal dose adjustment

Table 19.3 Treatment Summary Chart (continued)

	Mechanism of Action	Bolus Dose	Dose Range	Metabolism/ Renal Elimination	Half-life (hr)	Drug Interactions	Significant Adverse Effects	Comments
Refractory Treatment: Anticonvulsants and Continuous Infusions								
Ketamine	NMDA antagonist	1.5 mg/kg *May repeat q3–5min	5–167 mcg/kg/min (0.3–7.7 mg/kg/hr) CI	Hepatic	2.5	CYP2B6, 2C9 and 3A4 substrate	Hypertension ICP elevations Hallucinations Confusion	No respiratory depression
Topiramate	Sodium channel blocker, enhances GABA, glutamate antagonist	200–400 mg PO	300–1,600 mg/day (divided two to four times daily)	Renal and hepatic	21	CYP3A4 inducer; 2C19 inhibitor	Metabolic acidosis Lethargy	No IV available
Propofol	Anesthetic; GABA agonist, NMDA antagonist	1–2 mg/kg *May repeat q3–5min	200 mcg/kg/min CI *May increase infusion rate by 5–10 mcg/kg/min q5min	Hepatic	0.5–7	Non-significant	PRIS Hypotension Respiratory depression Hypertriglyceridemia	Consider 1 mg/kg bolus with increases in CI Accumulates in fat tissue
Pentobarbital	Barbiturate; GABA agonist	5–15 mg/kg IV *May give additional 5–10 mg/kg	0.5–5 mg/hr CI *May increase infusion rate by 0.5–1 mg/kg/hr q12hr	Hepatic	15–50	CYP2A6 inducer; 3AY inducer	Hypotension Bradycardia Respiratory depression	Consider 5 mg/kg bolus with increases in CI Accumulates after prolonged use TDC: 10–50 mcg/ml
Midazolam infusion	GABA agonist	0.2 mg/kg IV	0.05–2 mg/kg/hr CI *May increase infusion rate by 0.05–0.1 mg/kg/hr q3–4hr	Hepatic, active metabolite renally eliminated	2–7	CYP3A4 substrate	Hypotension Respiratory depression	Consider 0.1- to 0.2-mg/kg bolus with increases in CI. Accumulates in fat tissue Active metabolite accumulates in renal insufficiency or after prolonged use

CI = continuous infusion; ICP = intracranial pressure; IM = intramuscular(ly); IV = intravenous(ly); NS = normal saline; PgP = p-glycoprotein; PO = oral(ly); PRIS = propofol-related infusion syndrome; q = every; TDC = target drug concentration.

Adapted from: Brophy GM, Bell R, Claassen J, et al. Guidelines for the evaluation and management of status epilepticus. Neurocrit Care 2012;17:3-23; Tanaka E. Clinically significant pharmacokinetic drug interactions with benzodiazepines. J Clin Pharm Ther 1999;24:347-55. Tanaka E. Clinically significant pharmacokinetic drug interactions between antiepileptic drugs. J Clin Pharm Ther 1999;24:87-92; Limdi NA, Shimpi AV. Faught E. et al. Efficacy of rapid IV administration of valproic acid for status. Neurology 2005;64:353-5.

the first benzodiazepine and non-benzodiazepine drug combination suggest the superiority of any third-line agent. Because of the suboptimal success rate with second and third anticonvulsants, some prescribers opt to skip urgent control treatment and move directly to continuous infusions, whereas others may initiate anticonvulsants concurrently with continuous infusions. Regardless, most prescribers will at least administer one anticonvulsant after the initial benzodiazepine before ordering a continuous infusion.[28] This option is especially desirable in non-intubated patients who may benefit from a trial of anticonvulsants in order to avoid the intubation required for most anesthetic infusions. Urgent therapy with anticonvulsants often requires bolus dosing, rapid and aggressive titration, and, at times, addition of several drugs concomitantly or in rapid succession. Dose adjustments for renal or hepatic dysfunction are not required for loading doses. Because treatment delays of greater than 30 minutes are associated with a delayed response, the initiation and titration of urgent therapy should occur rapidly.[29] Commonly used agents are detailed in the following sections and are listed in descending order according to the amount of data surrounding their use.

Phenytoin/Fosphenytoin

Phenytoin is one of the most commonly studied drugs in the treatment of SE. Phenytoin is a substrate of cytochrome

P450 (CYP) 2C19 (major), 2C9 (minor), and 3A4 (minor) as well as a potent CYP3A4, CYP2C19, and CYP2C9 PgP inducer. Because of its interference with major metabolic enzymes, phenytoin is associated with several drug interactions and can decrease concentrations of drugs that are commonly coadministered in the ICU such as quetiapine, midazolam, methadone, nimodipine, and atorvastatin. Additional interactions occur with other highly protein-bound agents. Coadministration with warfarin may result in increased serum concentration of each drug. Because of its effects on sodium channels, phenytoin is considered a class 1B antiarrhythmic, and it can lead to arrhythmias and hemodynamic instability. It is formulated with propylene glycol, which further potentiates its risk of hypotension, especially with faster administration rates. Thus, the rate of administration is limited to 50 mg/minute or less.

Fosphenytoin, a prodrug of phenytoin, is often preferred to phenytoin because it is not stabilized with propylene glycol and can be administered at a faster maximum rate of 150 mg/minute. The less basic pH of the formulation decreases the risk of purple glove syndrome and phlebitis compared with phenytoin and allows for intramuscular administration. Whereas phenytoin is only compatible with normal saline, fosphenytoin is compatible with many diluents, including 5% dextrose. Phenytoin and fosphenytoin both carry other significant adverse effects including thrombocytopenia, leukopenia, and hepatotoxicity.

Phenytoin follows Michaelis-Menten kinetics, which requires thoughtful dose titration because small increases in dose may result in large, nonlinear increases in serum concentrations. For example, a simple doubling of the dose may lead to an exponentially higher-than-expected drug concentration, increasing the risk of toxicity. In addition, high serum concentrations may take days or weeks to return to the therapeutic or desired range because of phenytoin's long half-life, which is concentration-dependent. Phenytoin is highly protein bound, and free serum concentrations may be needed to properly assess phenytoin concentrations in patients who are critically ill or otherwise hypoalbuminemic. Although correction equations exist to adjust for low albumin, studies have found conflicting results regarding their accuracy in estimating true free concentrations.[30,31]

Valproic Acid

Although less commonly used than phenytoin, valproic acid is another commonly studied second-line anticonvulsant. Valproic acid has shown efficacy comparable with phenytoin in SE.[32,33] A meta-analysis of benzodiazepine-resistant SE assessed the relative efficacy of anticonvulsants in patients who did not respond to benzodiazepines and found the mean efficacy of valproate to be 75.5% compared with phenytoin (50.2%), levetiracetam (68.5%), and phenobarbital (73.6%).[34]

Valproic acid has many adverse effects, including hepatotoxicity, pancreatitis, hyperammonemia, and thrombocytopenia, but it lacks the cardiac toxicity associated with phenytoin. It affects the metabolism of other CYP substrates through its inhibition of CYP2C9, resulting in increased concentrations of CYP2C9 substrates. Valproic acid can displace phenytoin from protein binding sites as well as inhibit its hepatic metabolism,[35] warranting a close follow-up with free serum concentrations of both drugs to optimize efficacy. Several drugs may also affect valproate acid concentrations through interactions not directly related to the CYP hepatic enzymes. Of note, carbapenems can significantly decrease valproic acid concentrations, often making it challenging to reach therapeutic targets. This combination should be avoided whenever possible when treating SE. Valproic acid concentrations should be monitored routinely, particularly at initiation of therapy, with dosage changes, and when interacting drugs are concomitantly used. Free concentrations of phenytoin are more readily available than for valproic acid, which is also known to be highly protein bound. In these cases, it is helpful to assess the serum albumin concentration as well as the free phenytoin to total phenytoin fraction (for patients receiving both agents) to help interpret total valproic acid concentrations. For instance, a patient with low albumin, a subtherapeutic total phenytoin concentration, and a therapeutic free phenytoin concentration may be expected to have a higher free valproic acid concentration (active drug) than generally observed. This may help prevent unnecessary rebolusing and dose escalations for patients with resolving SE in whom dose de-escalation is warranted.

Phenobarbital

Phenobarbital is a barbiturate that exerts an effect by its actions on GABA receptors, but at a different subunit from where benzodiazepines act. In the VA Cooperative Trial, its efficacy was similar to that of lorazepam; however, it is rarely administered as a first-line agent.[22] Its long half-life, drug interactions, and adverse effect profile (i.e., sedation) make it less desirable than the alternatives for urgent control treatment. Accumulation of phenobarbital can occur after repeated doses, making it difficult to assess a patient's neurological examination, even after doses have been tapered or weaned off completely. Phenobarbital is a reasonable option for patients who require third-line therapy but are not yet eligible for a continuous infusion, such as patients without ventilator support or those who are outside an ICU setting.

Levetiracetam

The use of levetiracetam for SE has grown in recent years because of the availability of an intravenous formulation. It offers advantages over historical agents in being easy to dose (non–weight-based dosing) and free of significant drug interactions. It does not require therapeutic drug concentration monitoring, has very low protein binding, and does not cause respiratory depression. Some laboratories will report drug concentrations for levetiracetam; although a therapeutic range has been recommended, it has not been correlated with therapeutic outcomes in SE.[36] Thus, the role of levetiracetam monitoring is unclear in the general population; however, it may be considered in patients with pharmacokinetic alterations such as obesity and continuous renal replacement therapy. In addition, levetiracetam concentrations may be helpful in assessing adherence in patients who were prescribed levetiracetam and present with breakthrough seizures. Levetiracetam can be titrated quickly, and doses higher than those used in chronic epilepsy have been safely used in SE. For these reasons, it has become a staple of urgent control treatment regimens.[3] One study randomized 44 patients with SE to phenytoin intravenously (20 mg/kg) or levetiracetam intravenously (20 mg/kg) after administration of lorazepam 0.1 mg/kg intravenously. In patients receiving phenytoin versus levetiracetam, there was no difference in clinical termination of seizure activity within 30 minutes (68.2% vs. 59.1%), seizure recurrence within 24 hours (72.7% vs. 59.1%), adverse effects (9.1% vs. 0%), need for mechanical ventilation (27.3% vs. 18.2%), or mortality (9.1% vs. 9.1%).[37] Another study retrospectively compared phenytoin, valproic acid, and levetiracetam as second-line agents for SE. In 167 patients, 198 seizure episodes were identified, and treatment failures were reported in 25%, 41%, and 48% of valproic acid, phenytoin, and levetiracetam patients, respectively (p=0.032 with valproic acid as the comparator). After adjusting for SE severity and etiology, levetiracetam was associated with a higher risk of treatment failure than was valproic acid (OR 2.7; 95% CI, 1.2–6.1), but not phenytoin, and there was no difference in mortality between the three groups.[38] Levetiracetam is not as well studied as phenytoin, valproic acid, and phenobarbital; however, its pharmacokinetic profile makes it an attractive adjunctive agent in the treatment of SE.

Lacosamide

Like with levetiracetam, lacosamide's intravenous availability, ease of dosing, lack of major drug interactions, and well-tolerated adverse effect profile have led to its off-label use in SE. Lacosamide can cause changes on electrocardiogram (ECG) (i.e., PR prolongation), which may warrant ECG monitoring when used at the higher doses for SE, especially in patients with underlying cardiac abnormalities. One analysis of 19 RSE studies of patients treated with lacosamide reported an overall success rate of 56% in 136 cases. Lacosamide was generally well tolerated (dose range 50–600 mg), with sedation being the most common adverse effect (25%) and one patient who developed third-degree atrioventricular block.[39] One study compared two loading-dose regimens of lacosamide in 25 patients with RSE. The overall response rate was 36% for both groups, with a numerically higher overall response in the 400-mg group versus the 200-mg group (50% vs. 18%, p=0.2). The maintenance dose of 200 mg every 12 hours was the same in both groups.[40] The use of lacosamide as an adjunctive treatment for status has also increased during the past few years; however, more data are needed to confirm its place in SE algorithms.

RSE Treatment

Status epilepticus that is unresponsive to first-line (emergent) or second-line (urgent) therapies is considered RSE. Treatment of RSE uses anesthetics and continuous intravenous infusions. The results of studies evaluating these treatment modalities are difficult to interpret, partly because of the heterogeneous patient populations, non-standardized treatment regimens, and variable dosing strategies. Given the lack of superiority data establishing a standard of care, patient-specific characteristics, such as hemodynamic stability as well as physician preference and institutional algorithms, generally guide agent selection. Continuous infusions may be implemented as refractory treatment, after failure of initial anticonvulsants, or earlier to allow the traditional anticonvulsants enough time to be initiated and to reach therapeutic concentrations. When continuous infusions are titrated, they should be rebolused with every increase in the continuous infusion rate. Commonly, 24–48 hours of seizure control is recommended before continuous infusions and drugs are tapered; however, practices varies widely among clinicians, particularly in super-refractory status epilepticus treatment.[3] Several anticonvulsants may be used adjunctively, particularly when trying to wean off the anesthetic infusions.

Propofol

Propofol is a very short-acting anesthetic that acts on GABA receptors and may have an effect on NMDA receptors. It causes significant hypotension at treatment doses for SE, which are often higher than that required for continuous sedation, necessitating the use of vasopressors. The risk of propofol-related infusion syndrome (PRIS) associated with higher doses and long durations of propofol makes it less ideal for treatment of RSE, where high doses are often needed for extended periods. Triglycerides (TG) should be evaluated every 48–72 hours in patients receiving propofol, with TG concentrations greater than 400 mg/dL necessitating a potential dose reduction, discontinuation, or change to alternative therapy. One prospective, randomized study of 23 patients with RSE randomized patients to barbiturates (pentobarbital 5-mg/kg bolus and thiopental 2-mg/kg bolus) or propofol (2 mg/kg bolus) titrated to burst suppression. The median doses for each agent were propofol 5.5 mg/kg/hour (range 2–10.9), thiopental 7 mg/kg/hour (range 4–20), and pentobarbital 2.5 mg/kg/hour (range 2–3). Investigators of this study found no difference in mortality between propofol and barbiturates, but they did find a longer duration of mechanical ventilation with barbiturates and a nonsignificant increase in RSE control with propofol (43% vs. 22%). One patient in the propofol group was determined to have PRIS.[41]

Midazolam Continuous Infusion

Continuous infusion midazolam is the benzodiazepine of choice for RSE treatment because of its lack of propylene glycol diluent, which allows it to be administered at high doses for long durations without risk of toxicity and metabolic acidosis. Midazolam is a CYP3A4 substrate and is affected by CYP3A4 inducers and inhibitors (including other concomitantly used anticonvulsants). Although the parent drug undergoes hepatic metabolism, it has an active metabolite that is renally eliminated; thus, its half-life is prolonged in older adult patients or those with renal failure. After prolonged infusions, midazolam distributes into adipose tissues and can prolong sedative effects. Midazolam causes respiratory depression requiring intubation, and high doses often cause hypotension requiring vasopressors, although generally less so than propofol. A retrospective study of 20 patients found no difference in clinical seizure suppression (64% vs. 67%) or electrographic seizure suppression (78 vs. 67%) between propofol and midazolam, respectively, as well as no difference in infection, duration of mechanical ventilation, or hemodynamic compromise. Mortality was nonsignificantly higher in the propofol group (57% vs. 17%), although patients receiving propofol had a longer duration of SE before treatment. Propofol was administered as a bolus (1–3 mg/kg) in some, but not all, patients, followed by a continuous infusion range of 1–10 mg/kg/hour. Midazolam was administered as a bolus (2–12 mg) and continuous infusion of 0.05–0.8 mg/kg/hour.[42] Another study identified 33 patients with continuous EEG monitoring who received midazolam (0.1- to 0.2-mg/kg bolus, followed by an infusion at 0.05–0.4 mg/kg/hour) for RSE. Seizure termination was seen within the first hour in 82% of patients, and breakthrough seizures were seen in 56% of patients who were treated for more than 6 hours. Midazolam did not control RSE in 18% of cases and required switching to an alternative continuous infusion anesthetic.[43]

Pentobarbital

Pentobarbital is a long-acting barbiturate that can be used in place of propofol or midazolam for RSE. Pentobarbital is known to cause significant cardiovascular depression and hypotension, leading to cardiovascular collapse and the requirement of vasopressors in order to maintain therapeutic infusion rates. Mechanical ventilation is required before initiation due to respiratory depression. Pentobarbital has a half-life of 15–48 hours, but it may take days to weeks for complete elimination. Its long half-life complicates neurological examinations and prognostication. For patients evaluated for brain death, pentobarbital may confound the examination, and serum concentrations typically come back elevated for significant periods after the drug has been discontinued. In addition, adverse effects are noted even after the infusion has been discontinued, leading to possible prolonged mechanical ventilation and hypotension, higher risk of infections, and reduced gastrointestinal motility. One systematic review that assessed pentobarbital, propofol, and midazolam for the treatment of RSE in 193 patients and 28 studies found no difference in mortality between the three treatments. Pentobarbital was associated with less short-term treatment failure and fewer breakthrough seizures than the other agents; however, fewer patients received cEEG monitoring than in the propofol and midazolam groups, making it possible to have missed some breakthrough seizures. Pentobarbital was more frequently titrated to burst suppression rather than seizure termination, and titration to EEG suppression was associated with fewer breakthrough seizures (4 vs. 53%, p<0.001) regardless of treatment arm. However, most of the patients treated to a goal of EEG burst suppression were in the pentobarbital group, making it difficult to draw conclusions on efficacy from these results. Moreover, the maximum infusion rate of midazolam (0.23 mg/kg/hour) was much lower than that recommended in the current guidelines.[3] Pentobarbital was associated with more hypotension requiring vasopressors than were propofol and midazolam (77% vs. 42% and 30%, p<0.001).[44] Another review of 31 patients treated with pentobarbital (10–15 mg/kg loading dose and continuous infusion of 0.5–4 mg/kg/hour) for RSE found a 90% control rate but a 48% recurrence rate while weaning the continuous infusion, even in patients who had achieved burst suppression. Complications surrounding pentobarbital exposure included pneumonia (32%), hypotension requiring vasopressors (32%), urinary tract infections (13%), deep venous thromboses (10%), and ileus (10%).[45]

Ketamine

Ketamine is a NMDA receptor antagonist that may be beneficial in RSE when changes in GABA receptor affinity and regulation may be altered. Although all the other continuous infusions used for RSE cause hypotension, ketamine has a stable hemodynamic profile, sometimes even resulting in elevated blood pressure, which may be desirable when used with other agents that may cause hypotension. Because ketamine may increase intracranial pressure, it should be used cautiously when intracranial hypertension is present or suspected. In one retrospective review of 11 patients with RSE, ketamine was added to a continuous infusion anesthetic.[46] Patients received boluses of 1–2 mg/kg and were initiated on weight-based infusions of 0.45–2.1 mg/kg/hour (7.5–35 mcg/kg/minute). All patients had resolution of RSE, and 73% of patients were able to have the concomitant anesthetic infusion weaned off within 72 hours. Six of seven patients (85%) who required hemodynamic support were able to be weaned off vasopressors after ketamine initiation. In another study, 60 patients with RSE received ketamine as add-on therapy, administered as a bolus dose (median 1.5 mg/kg, maximum 5 mg/kg) and continuous infusion (median 2.75 mg/kg/hour [46 mcg/kg/minute], maximum 10 mg/kg/hour [167 mcg/kg/minute]).[47] Fifty-seven percent of patients achieved permanent RSE control. Ketamine is an attractive treatment option in RSE; however, current data support its use when initiated as an adjunctive continuous infusion, followed by slow titration of other continuous infusions.

Topiramate

Topiramate is an oral agent used in the management of chronic epilepsy. It is a sodium channel blocker, but it also causes enhanced effects of GABA and glutamate inhibition at AMPA/kainate receptors. Because topiramate's effects on GABA are independent of the GABAa receptor, it may theoretically help when benzodiazepine resistance is suspected in later stages of SE. Its inhibitory effects on glutamate transmission also provide an added mechanism of action in SE treatment and make it a useful adjunctive agent. In one case series, six patients who received topiramate (300–1600 mg) in addition to their treatment regimens for RSE had resolution of seizure activity and were discharged from the hospital.[48] The main disadvantage of topiramate is its lack of an intravenous formulation. For this reason, it is generally reserved as adjunctive therapy after more rapid intravenous therapies have been initiated. It is also a weak carbonic anhydrase inhibitor and can cause metabolic acidosis when used at high doses. Topiramate may be useful when patients are weaned off interacting drugs or when the adverse effect profile is unacceptable (e.g., increasing liver function tests). When used in SE, the dose should be rapidly titrated to a maximum of 1600 mg/day in divided doses.[3]

Inhaled Anesthetics

Efficacy with the inhaled anesthetics isoflurane and desflurane for the treatment of RSE has been reported in case reports or case series as an adjunct to conventional SE treatment (a combination of benzodiazepines, barbiturates, and anticonvulsants). Their use may be associated with cognitive changes, sedation, and hypotension; however, their rapid onset and elimination allow for easy titration if the adverse effects become unmanageable. Administration of inhaled anesthetics may be technically difficult because of unfamiliarity with the dosing and administration outside the operating room setting. In addition, monitoring of these agents without appropriately trained providers may be logistically challenging and require institution-specific protocols to do so safely within the ICU. Availability of an end-tidal anesthetic monitor may delay the initiation of inhaled anesthetics and offset the benefits of their rapid onset of activity.[49-51]

Nonpharmacologic Treatment

In addition to the available treatment options, nonpharmacologic strategies including the ketogenic diet, vagal nerve stimulation, electroconvulsant therapy, induced hypothermia, and surgical management have been evaluated; however, there is insufficient evidence to support their routine use. These strategies are best used as an adjunct to drug therapy, if at all. Correction and identification of an underlying cause such as hypoglycemia and alcohol withdrawal seizures is critical and may lead to different treatment algorithms. Induced hypothermia is the most common nonpharmacologic treatment management used in the ICU setting, although robust studies are lacking. In one case series of four patients with RSE, the addition of therapeutic hypothermia (TH) (31°C–35°C) resulted in seizure cessation in all four patients and burst suppression in three.[52]

Special consideration should be given to drug dosing in patients undergoing TH because of alterations seen in metabolism and volume of distribution of agents used in SE. The metabolism of propofol decreases in TH, increasing the risk of toxicity with normally used doses.[53] Clinicians should consider close titration of propofol using EEG monitoring for patients undergoing TH. Midazolam does not seem to be affected by TH.[54] Phenytoin metabolism is decreased in TH by about 70% in mild TH,[55] but specific dosing guidelines have not been published. It is probably most prudent to dose by free serum concentrations in this situation.

Treatment Considerations

Given the lack of randomized controlled trials comparing various treatment options, the treatment of SE has become prescriber-, institution-, and patient-specific. Potential considerations when selecting pharmacotherapy treatments include cost, availability of an intravenous formulation, adverse effect profile, hospital formulary options, and drug shortages. Additional unanswered questions surrounding continuous infusions include the timing of titrations, most appropriate titration dosing strategy, and duration of continuous infusions. Once the decision has been made to transition from a continuous infusion to intermittent therapy, clinicians should determine which anticonvulsants to continue, discontinue, or dose adjust. Often, many anticonvulsants are added almost simultaneously, but the continuation of five or six agents after seizure termination is unnecessary and may contribute to added adverse effects and potential drug interactions. Continuous infusions may be necessary in the treatment of RSE, but the preferred agents and duration of treatment are unknown. Several studies have shown that outcome is not influenced by the choice of continuous infusion.[41,42,56] A worse outcome, including increased mortality, infections, and length of stay, has also been documented in patients managed with therapeutic coma; however, these are all retrospective in nature and subject to possible selection bias of sicker patients.[56-58] Once continuous infusions have been weaned off (or, in many cases, while they are still being administered), de-escalation of therapy and transition from intravenous to oral therapy can occur during cEEG monitoring. Commonly, 24–48 hours of seizure control is recommended before tapering of continuous infusions and drugs.[3] There are no established guidelines on weaning off continuous infusions; however, considerations include duration the patient was on the infusion, half-life of the infused drug, and the patient's renal and hepatic function. For example, an older adult patient with compromised renal function who has received continuous infusion midazolam for several days can be weaned faster than can a younger patient with good renal function receiving only 1 day of therapy because the active metabolite has not had the opportunity to accumulate. There is also no consensus regarding the optimal treatment duration, the precise tapering mechanism, or the total number of maintenance anticonvulsants for patients whose seizures resolve. These decisions, as well as when to consider alternative or salvage therapy, are often left to the discretion of the treating physician or neuro-ICU team. Algorithms are provided for initial SE treatment (Figure 19.3) and RSE treatment (Figure 19.4) that include many of the previously mentioned therapeutic considerations as well as expert opinion and clinical experience.

MONITORING

Electroencephalography

Continuous EEG monitoring is recommended for all patients with active SE and should be reviewed often throughout the day.[3,23] Because NCSE may be intermittent, spot (e.g., 6 hours) EEG monitoring is often inadequate and may miss more than 50% of the seizure episodes that are subsequently captured in cEEG.[59] The target goal for dose titrations with EEG monitoring remains controversial, with some clinicians treating toward cEEG burst suppression patterns and others treating toward seizure termination.[3,23,28,60] One systematic review showed fewer breakthrough seizures (53% vs. 4%, p<0.001) and more hypotension (76% vs. 29%, p<0.001), but no difference in treatment failure or withdrawal seizures, with a goal of EEG burst suppression compared with seizure suppression.[44] Data regarding the duration of cEEG are lacking. After termination of seizures, the decision of when to discontinue continuous monitoring and use spot EEGs is left to the discretion of the clinician, often dependent on concomitant therapy and duration of SE.[3,60,61] Surveys of neurologists, neurophysiologists, and neurointensivists reported that 47%–50% would continue cEEG for 24 hours after non-convulsive seizure termination.[60,62] Current guidelines recommend cEEG for 24 hours after seizure termination on EEG or during anticonvulsant weaning trials and 48 hours for comatose patients.[3] In general, more stable patients who have been weaned off continuous infusions are considered for discontinuations of cEEG.[23]

Laboratory

Several anticonvulsants that can be measured in the serum have known target drug concentration ranges that correlate with efficacy. These drugs include phenytoin and fosphenytoin (phenytoin concentrations assessed), valproic acid,

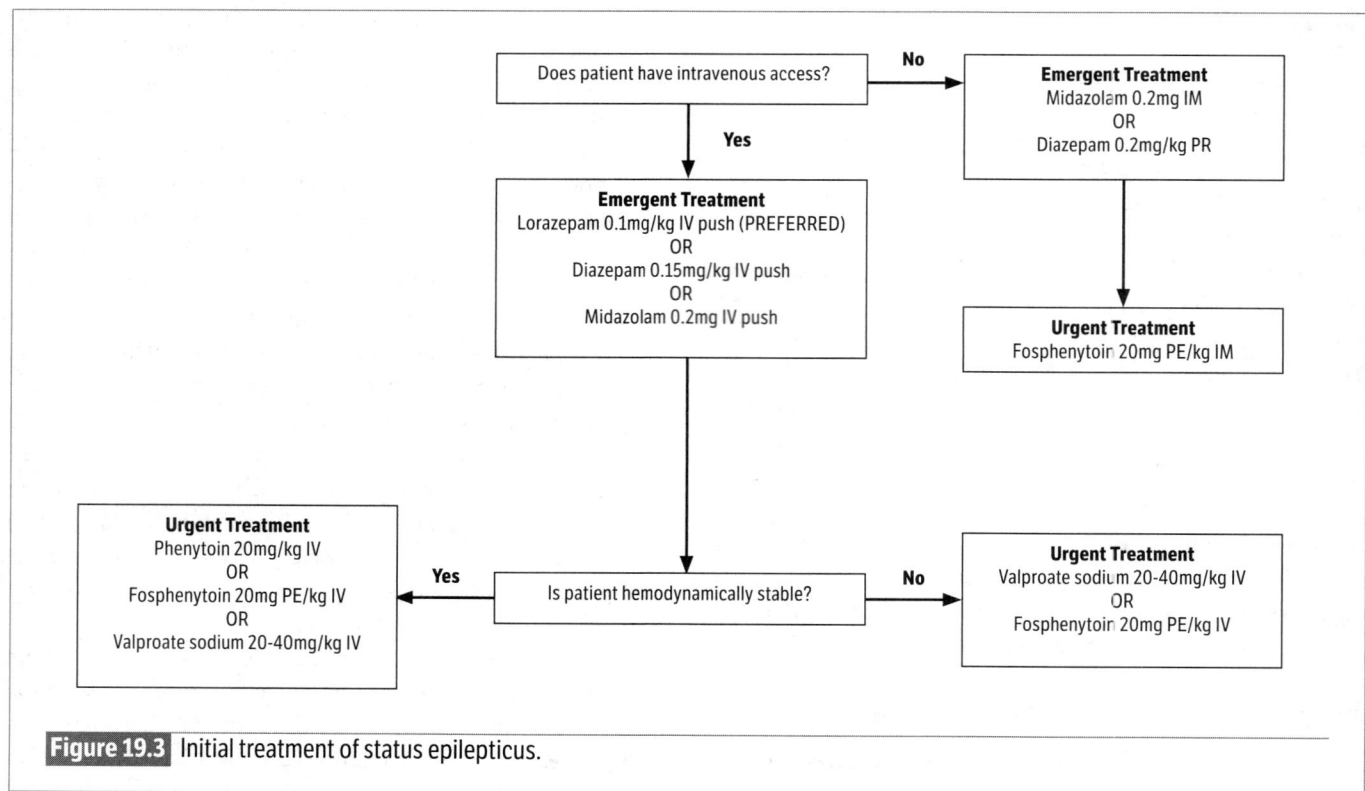

Figure 19.3 Initial treatment of status epilepticus.

phenobarbital, and carbamazepine. Weight-based loading doses should achieve target concentrations in most patients; however, in patients where pharmacokinetic variables are assumed to be altered (e.g., traumatic brain injury patients), post-load concentrations (2 hours after a dose) can be obtained to ensure adequate therapeutic concentrations for individual patients. Monitoring trough anticonvulsant concentrations about 24 hours after the loading dose and then 48 hours later may be reasonable to ensure continued therapeutic targets. Although therapeutic ranges exist for chronic treatment of epilepsy, clinicians often target the higher end of these ranges during the treatment of SE and sometimes concentrations above the therapeutic range. In these cases, the benefit of more aggressive seizure management is deemed to outweigh the low risk of acute drug toxicities.[23] Free trough concentrations should be checked whenever possible; however, proper knowledge of institutional protocols and turnaround time is important because in-house assays for free concentrations are not always available and may take longer to obtain results. Where drug concentration monitoring is not available, especially for many of the newer anticonvulsants, monitoring renal function may help guide dosing adjustments in renally eliminated drugs, and monitoring for toxicity will help determine dose reductions or the need to switch to an alternative drug. Baseline laboratory values including a basic metabolic panel, toxicology screen, and blood gas are also helpful and should be ordered according to the individual patient and clinical scenario. Liver function tests should be ordered at baseline and about every 72 hours in patients receiving phenytoin, fosphenytoin, or valproic acid or more often for patients having liver function test elevations or receiving other hepatotoxic drugs.

SPECIAL POPULATIONS

Children

The approach to the treatment of SE in critically ill children is similar to that in adults, and various guidelines have been published for pediatric SE.[63] Special consideration must be made for increased hepatic metabolism seen in pediatric patients[64] as well as for difficulties in obtaining intravenous access. The use of buccal,[65] nasal,[66] rectal,[67] intramuscular,[68] and intraosseous routes has been published in children.

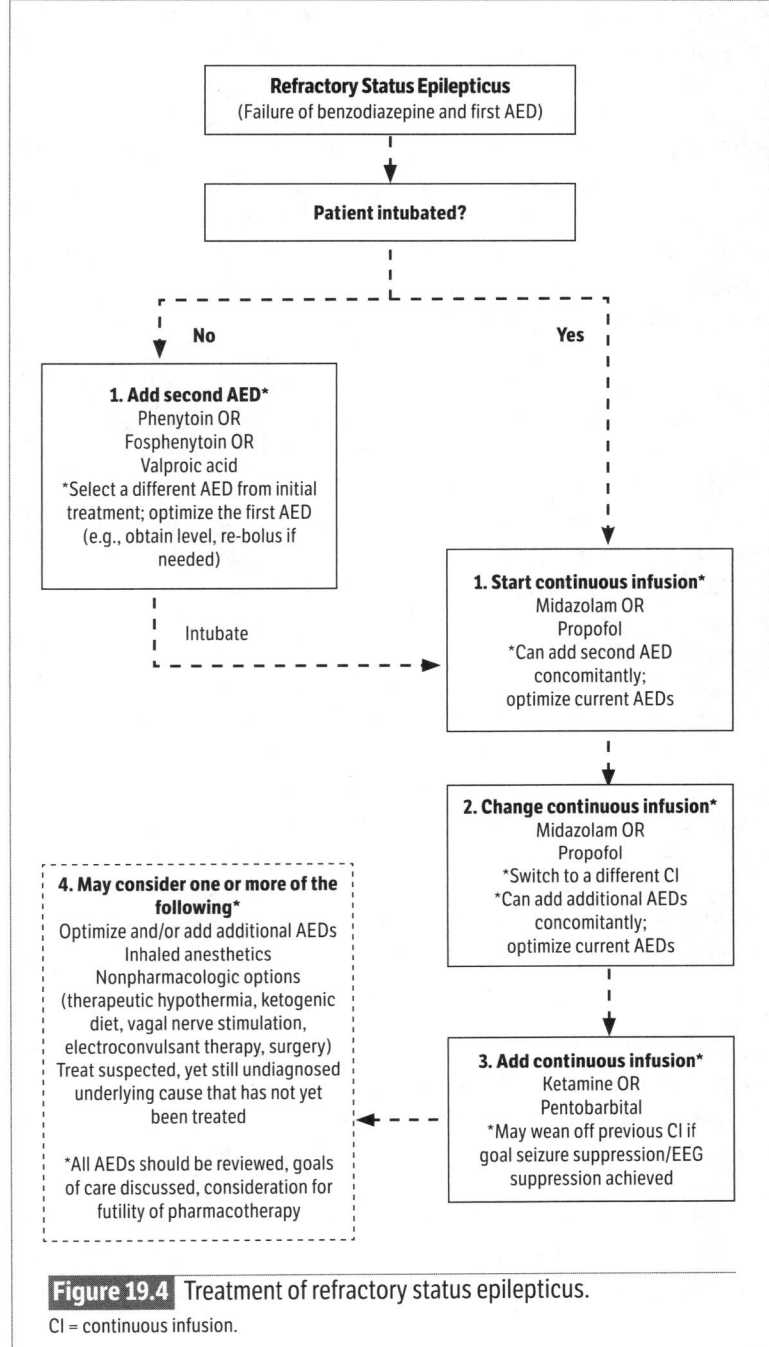

Figure 19.4 Treatment of refractory status epilepticus.
CI = continuous infusion.

Older Adults

The proportion of older adult patients admitted to the ICU has increased during the past several years and, unfortunately, so has the mortality in this patient population, even after controlling for underlying comorbidities.[69] Older adult patients have a higher incidence of SE and a higher mortality rate than do younger patients.[70] Mortality rates approach 50% in patients older than 80 years who have generalized convulsive SE; lower rates of 30% were reported for patients with partial SE. Stroke is a major cause of SE in older adults and is associated with 60% of cases; other common causes include trauma, anoxia, metabolic disturbances, and subtherapeutic anticonvulsant concentrations. Anoxic brain injury incurs the poorest prognosis, with almost complete fatality (70%–100%).[70] Because signs and symptoms in the older adult critically ill patient may be difficult to observe,[71] cEEG is recommended for timely diagnosis and treatment,[70] especially when NCSE is suspected. Partial SE is more common in the older adult than are generalized tonic-clonic types, and signs may be as subtle as confusion, atypical behavior, or depressed consciousness. In one study, it was reported that about 16% of patients with unprovoked confusion were actually in NCSE.[72] Another study examining older adult patients with delirium had EEG findings consistent with NCSE in about 28% of patients.[73] Sedation and narcotic use, which are common treatments in the ICU, may mask these signs and potentially delay treatment.

Treatment of SE in the older adult generally follows contemporary management, despite the lack of representation in the few randomized clinical trials in SE to date. This patient population requires special attention to drug dosing because of decreased volume of distribution, decreased protein binding, decreased renal and hepatic function, and potential for drug interactions because of polypharmacy. To minimize adverse effects in the older adult, accurate weights should be used to calculate doses, and doses should be individualized. Electrocardiogram and blood pressure should be monitored closely, especially with parenteral agents containing propylene glycol because hypotension and arrhythmias are common. Infusion rates should be decreased when necessary, especially in patients with tenuous or unstable cardiac conditions. Older adult patients are particularly sensitive to the respiratory depressant effects of barbiturates, so consideration for intubation should be made before intravenous administration. Valproic acid is an attractive agent to use in the older adult because of its low risk of hypotension, respiratory depression, and sedation compared with other agents. Levetiracetam is also attractive for the same reasons but has the additional benefit of minimal drug interactions. No published studies show the superiority of one agent over another. Therapeutic drug monitoring, when appropriate, is essential to minimize toxicity, especially when concomitant renal and hepatic dysfunction exists.

Pregnancy

Very little has been published regarding SE in pregnancy, especially in patients being treated in an ICU. In a prospective registry of pregnant women with epilepsy, SE was reported in 0.6% of all pregnancies (0.3% were categorized as convulsive).[74] No maternal or fetal deaths were attributed to SE in this series. Uncontrolled seizures could theoretically compromise fetal blood pressure, heart rate, and oxygenation and be associated with poor postnatal cognitive development.[75] No data are available regarding the mortality of SE in pregnancy. Seizure control in women with epilepsy requires adherence to anticonvulsant therapy because withdrawal can lead to SE and subsequent complications.[76] Consideration must be given to addressing the changes in pharmacokinetics seen during pregnancy and making appropriate adjustments in therapy.

The acute treatment of SE in pregnancy follows general guidelines because the priority is control of both physiological and electrical manifestations in order to minimize adverse effects on the mother and fetus. Although many of the anticonvulsants used in SE have associated teratogenicity, there is no evidence to suggest that limited, acute treatment leads to any fetal complications. If the source of the provoked seizures can be identified and treated, there may be no need to initiate anticonvulsant therapy. Input from neurology and obstetrical services is important in the intensive care management of these patients (enrollment in an antiepileptic drug pregnancy registry may be recommended). Drug dosing can be challenging in this population because various pharmacokinetic parameters change during pregnancy: the volume of distribution increases and protein binding decreases because of increases in weight and a decline in albumin production, respectively.[77] In addition to SE, any underlying critical illness must be addressed and treated.

Obesity

Drug dosing can be challenging in critically ill patients with obesity, and there are limited recommendations for drugs used in SE. Changes in volume of distribution typically affect loading doses of drugs while having minimal impact on maintenance regimens. Of the anticonvulsants, only phenytoin/fosphenytoin and phenobarbital have specific dosing recommendations in obesity.[78,79] A dosing weight (DW) for phenytoin can be calculated from ideal body weight (IBW) and actual body weight (ABW) using the following calculation: $DW = IBW + 1.33(ABW - IBW)$. This dosing weight can then be used to calculate a volume of distribution (Vd): $Vd = 0.7$ L/kg. Finally, a loading dose (LD) can be estimated: $LD = C_{target} \times Vd$, where C_{target} is the goal serum concentration (typically 15–20 mg/L). Intravenous doses of phenobarbital can be dosed using total body weight.[79] Some institutions may cap loading doses for patients with obesity as a safety precaution; extremely large loading doses may be divided into smaller doses given sequentially, using post-load concentration monitoring, clinical response, or both as a guide.

Renal/Hepatic Failure

Renal and hepatic dysfunction are common conditions encountered in ICU patients. Most cases of SE in renal failure stem from drug toxicity caused by impaired clearance. Particularly notable are antibiotics,[80] especially penicillins and β-lactams.[81,82] Fluoroquinolones are also implicated in drug-induced seizures and SE.[83-85] These patients typically respond to benzodiazepines and anticonvulsants, although once the suspected offending agent is discontinued or dose adjusted, long-term prophylactic therapy is probably unwarranted.

Patients with renal failure who are receiving continuous renal replacement therapy deserve special consideration. For some anticonvulsants, drug clearance may increase above normal ranges during some modes of continuous renal replacement therapy such as continuous venovenous hemofiltration, requiring more frequent dosing than expected.[86,87] Because of the changes in protein binding and volume of distribution seen in patients with renal failure, the free fraction of highly bound drugs may be altered, and free serum concentrations of anticonvulsants should be measured to ensure appropriate clinical response.[88]

Liver dysfunction can be prevalent in the ICU and can complicate drug selection in SE. Drugs that are not hepatically metabolized to active metabolites or hepatotoxic moieties are preferred agents to use in SE.[89] Lorazepam, levetiracetam, and lacosamide are attractive agents from this standpoint. Hepatic encephalopathy can confound the presence of SE in patients with cirrhosis,[90] and lactulose has been reported to be effective in rare cases.[91] Patients with encephalopathy may need continuous EEG monitoring to help identify the onset or presence of seizures.

Genetics

Very little has been reported on genetic considerations in SE or treatment of SE. Although there appear to be differences among ethnicities with respect to incidence of SE and mortality, there is no genetic test to predict the risk of SE in the general population. Genomic testing is available for certain anticonvulsants, but only to decrease the risk of serious and potentially fatal dermatologic adverse effects. Patients with the *HLA-B*1502* allele may be predisposed to the development of Stevens-Johnson syndrome or toxic epidermal necrolysis when administered phenytoin or lamotrigine.[92] The use of genetic screening in the setting of a patient with SE is unclear. Critically ill patients with a history of the *HLA-B*1502* allele should not be given phenytoin or fosphenytoin in the setting of SE.

CONCLUSIONS AND FUTURE AREAS OF DEVELOPMENT

Many options are available in the treatment armamentarium for SE; however, robust comparison data are lacking. Specifically, no prospective, randomized trials directly compare second- and third-line agents added to a standardized treatment regimen. There are also a paucity of randomized controlled trials assessing the role of newer agents in the treatment of SE. Finally, there is little guidance on the role of continuous infusions early on in status management compared with the addition or dose escalation of more anticonvulsants. This leaves agent selection to a combination of institution-specific treatment algorithms and clinician experience and preference. Future studies should use standardized protocols to evaluate the addition of second-, third-, and fourth-line treatment strategies against a consistent background of therapy. Doses as well as drug concentrations at the time of seizure cessation should be reported. Reasons for drug discontinuation should be clearly described. Goals for weaning of continuous infusions should be provided, as well as the specific weaning strategy, parameters for tapering the continuous infusion, and cEEG titration goals (burst suppression vs. seizure termination). Pharmacoeconomic studies should evaluate different treatment strategies, considering overall patient outcomes as well as cost of newer drugs, need for drug concentration monitoring, and duration of mechanical ventilation with continuous infusions. Studies should also clearly define their patient populations and aim to identify subgroups of patients or specific characteristics that may predict better response. Added resources such as faster cEEG interpretation, improved turnaround time on drug concentration assays, and earlier identification of patients in SE may shorten the time to treatment initiation and escalation.[3]

REFERENCES

1. Lowenstein DH, Bleck T, Macdonald RL. It's time to revise the definition of status epilepticus. Epilepsia 1999;40:120-2.
2. Tesoro EP, Brophy GM. Pharmacological management of seizures and status epilepticus in critically ill patients. J Pharm Pract 2010;23:441-54.
3. Brophy GM, Bell R, Claassen J, et al. Guidelines for the evaluation and management of status epilepticus. Neurocrit Care 2012;17:3-23.
4. Dham BS, Hunter K, Rincon F. The epidemiology of status epilepticus in the United States. Neurocrit Care 2014;20:476-83.
5. Betjemann JP, Josephson SA, Lowenstein DH, et al. Trends in status epilepticus-related hospitalizations and mortality: redefined in US practice over time. JAMA Neurol 2015;72:650-5.
6. Legriel S, Mourvillier B, Bele N, et al. Outcomes in 140 critically ill patients with status epilepticus. Intensive Care Med 2008;34:476-80.
7. Varelas PN, Corry J, Rehman M, et al. Management of status epilepticus in neurological versus medical intensive care unit: does it matter? Neurocrit Care 2013;19:4-9.
8. Koubeissi M, Alshekhlee A. In-hospital mortality of generalized convulsive status epilepticus: a large US sample. Neurology 2007;69:886-93.
9. Cook AM, Castle A, Green A, et al. Practice variations in the management of status epilepticus. Neurocrit Care 2012;17:24-30.
10. Castilla-Guerra L, del Carmen Fernandez-Moreno M, Lopez-Chozas JM, et al. Electrolytes disturbances and seizures. Epilepsia 2006;47:1990-8.
11. Thundiyil JG, Kearney TE, Olson KR. Evolving epidemiology of drug-induced seizures reported to a Poison Control Center System. J Med Toxicol 2007;3:15-9.
12. Alvarez V, Westover MB, Drislane FW, et al. Evaluation of a clinical tool for early etiology identification in status epilepticus. Epilepsia 2014;55:2059-68.

13. Rajasekaran K, Zanelli SA, Goodkin HP. Lessons from the laboratory: the pathophysiology, and consequences of status epilepticus. Semin Pediatr Neurol 2010;17:136-43.

14. Scharfman HE, Brooks-Kayal AR. Is plasticity of GABAergic mechanisms relevant to epileptogenesis? Adv Exp Med Biol 2014;813:133-50.

15. Kapur J, Lothman EW, DeLorenzo RJ. Loss of GABAA receptors during partial status epilepticus. Neurology 1994;44:2407-8.

16. Goodkin HP, Yeh JL, Kapur J. Status epilepticus increases the intracellular accumulation of GABAA receptors. J Neurosci 2005;25:5511-20.

17. Goodkin HP, Kapur J. Responsiveness of status epilepticus to treatment with diazepan decreases rapidly as seizure duration increases. Epilepsy Curr 2003;3:11-2.

18. Simon RP. Physiologic consequences of status epilepticus. Epilepsia 1985;26(suppl 1):S58-66.

19. Guven M, Oymak O, Utas C, et al. Rhabdomyolysis and acute renal failure due to status epilepticus. Clin Nephrol 1998;50:204.

20. Mirski MA, Varelas PN. Seizures and status epilepticus in the critically ill. Crit Care Clin 2008;24:115-47, ix.

21. Rowe AS, Goodwin H, Brophy GM, et al. Seizure prophylaxis in neurocritical care: a review of evidence-based support. Pharmacotherapy 2014;34:396-409.

22. Treiman DM, Meyers PD, Walton NY, et al. A comparison of four treatments for generalized convulsive status epilepticus. Veterans Affairs Status Epilepticus Cooperative Study Group. N Engl J Med 1998;339:792-8.

23. Costello DJ, Cole AJ. Treatment of acute seizures and status epilepticus. J Intensive Care Med 2007;22:319-47.

24. Prasad M, Krishnan PR, Sequeira R, et al. Anticonvulsant therapy for status epilepticus. Cochrane Database Syst Rev 2014;9:CD003723.

25. Alldredge BK, Gelb AM, Isaacs SM, et al. A comparison of lorazepam, diazepam, and placebo for the treatment of out-of-hospital status epilepticus. N Engl J Med 2001;345:631-7.

26. Leppik IE, Derivan AT, Homan RW, et al. Double-blind study of lorazepam and diazepam in status epilepticus. JAMA 1983;249:1452-4.

27. Silbergleit R, Durkalski V, Lowenstein D, et al. Intramuscular versus intravenous therapy for prehospital status epilepticus. N Engl J Med 2012;366:591-600.

28. Claassen J, Hirsch LJ, Mayer SA. Treatment of status epilepticus: a survey of neurologists. J Neurol Sci 2003;211:37-41.

29. Eriksson K, Metsaranta P, Huhtala H, et al. Treatment delay and the risk of prolonged status epilepticus. Neurology 2005;65:1316-8.

30. Kane SP, Bress AP, Tesoro EP. Characterization of unbound phenytoin concentrations in neurointensive care unit patients using a revised Winter-Tozer equation. Ann Pharmacother 2013;47:628-36.

31. Mlynarek ME, Peterson EL, Zarowitz BJ. Predicting unbound phenytoin concentrations in the critically ill neurosurgical patient. Ann Pharmacother 1996;30:219-23.

32. Agarwal P, Kumar N, Chandra R, et al. Randomized study of intravenous valproate and phenytoin in status epilepticus. Seizure 2007;16:527-32.

33. Misra UK, Kalita J, Patel R. Sodium valproate vs phenytoin in status epilepticus: a pilot study. Neurology 2006;67:340-2.

34. Yasiry Z, Shorvon SD. The relative effectiveness of five antiepileptic drugs in treatment of benzodiazepine-resistant convulsive status epilepticus: a meta-analysis of published studies. Seizure 2014;23:167-74.

35. Bruni J, Gallo JM, Lee CS, et al. Interactions of valproic acid with phenytoin. Neurology 1980;30:1233-6.

36. Naik GS, Kodagali R, Mathew BS, et al. Therapeutic drug monitoring of levetiracetam and lamotrigine: is there a need? Ther Drug Monit 2015;37:437-44.

37. Chakravarthi S, Goyal MK, Modi M, et al. Levetiracetam versus phenytoin in management of status epilepticus. J Clin Neurosci 2015;22:959-63.

38. Alvarez V, Januel JM, Burnand B, et al. Second-line status epilepticus treatment: comparison of phenytoin, valproate, and levetiracetam. Epilepsia 2011;52:1292-6.

39. Hofler J, Trinka E. Lacosamide as a new treatment option in status epilepticus. Epilepsia 2013;54:393-404.

40. Legros B, Depondt C, Levy-Nogueira M, et al. Intravenous lacosamide in refractory seizure clusters and status epilepticus: comparison of 200 and 400 mg loading doses. Neurocrit Care 2014;20:484-8.

41. Rossetti AO, Milligan TA, Vulliemoz S, et al. A randomized trial for the treatment of refractory status epilepticus. Neurocrit Care 2011;14:4-10.

42. Prasad A, Worrall BB, Bertram EH, et al. Propofol and midazolam in the treatment of refractory status epilepticus. Epilepsia 2001;42:380-6.

43. Claassen J, Hirsch LJ, Emerson RG, et al. Continuous EEG monitoring and midazolam infusion for refractory nonconvulsive status epilepticus. Neurology 2001;57:1036-42.

44. Claassen J, Hirsch LJ, Emerson RG, et al. Treatment of refractory status epilepticus with pentobarbital, propofol, or midazolam: a systematic review. Epilepsia 2002;43:146-53.

45. Pugin D, Foreman B, De Marchis GM, et al. Is pentobarbital safe and efficacious in the treatment of super-refractory status epilepticus: a cohort study. Crit Care 2014;18:R103.

46. Synowiec AS, Singh DS, Yenugadhati V, et al. Ketamine use in the treatment of refractory status epilepticus. Epilepsy Res 2013;105:183-8.

47. Gaspard N, Foreman B, Judd LM, et al. Intravenous ketamine for the treatment of refractory status epilepticus: a retrospective multicenter study. Epilepsia 2013;54:1498-503.

48. Towne AR, Garnett LK, Waterhouse EJ, et al. The use of topiramate in refractory status epilepticus. Neurology 2003;60:332-4.

49. Kofke WA, Young RS, Davis P, et al. Isoflurane for refractory status epilepticus: a clinical series. Anesthesiology 1989;71:653-9.

50. Kofke WA, Bloom MJ, Van Cott A, et al. Electrographic tachyphylaxis to etomidate and ketamine used for refractory status epilepticus controlled with isoflurane. J Neurosurg Anesthesiol 1997;9:269-72.

51. Mirsattari SM, Sharpe MD, Young GB. Treatment of refractory status epilepticus with inhalational anesthetic agents isoflurane and desflurane. Arch Neurol 2004;61:1254-9.

52. Corry JJ, Dhar R, Murphy T, et al. Hypothermia for refractory status epilepticus. Neurocrit Care 2008;9:189-97.

53. Bjelland TW, Klepstad P, Haugen BO, et al. Effects of hypothermia on the disposition of morphine, midazolam,

54. Bastiaans DE, Swart EL, van Akkeren JP, et al. Pharmacokinetics of midazolam in resuscitated patients treated with moderate hypothermia. Int J Clin Pharm 2013;35:210-6.

55. Iida Y, Nishi S, Asada A. Effect of mild therapeutic hypothermia on phenytoin pharmacokinetics. Ther Drug Monit 2001;23:192-7.

56. Hocker SE, Britton JW, Mandrekar JN, et al. Predictors of outcome in refractory status epilepticus. JAMA Neurol 2013;70:72-7.

57. Kowalski RG, Ziai WC, Rees RN, et al. Third-line antiepileptic therapy and outcome in status epilepticus: the impact of vasopressor use and prolonged mechanical ventilation. Crit Care Med 2012;40:2677-84.

58. Marchi NA, Novy J, Faouzi M, et al. Status epilepticus: impact of therapeutic coma on outcome. Crit Care Med 2015;43:1003-9.

59. Pandian JD, Cascino GD, So EL, et al. Digital video-electroencephalographic monitoring in the neurological-neurosurgical intensive care unit: clinical features and outcome. Arch Neurol 2004;61:1090-4.

60. Abend NS, Dlugos DJ, Hahn CD, et al. Use of EEG monitoring and management of non-convulsive seizures in critically ill patients: a survey of neurologists. Neurocrit Care 2010;12:382-9.

61. Wasim M, Husain AM. Nonconvulsive seizure control in the intensive care unit. Curr Treat Options Neurol 2015;17:340.

62. Gavvala J, Abend N, LaRoche S, et al. Continuous EEG monitoring: a survey of neurophysiologists and neurointensivists. Epilepsia 2014;55:1864-71.

63. Mishra D, Sharma S, Sankhyan N, et al. Consensus guidelines on management of childhood convulsive status epilepticus. Indian Pediatr 2014;51:975-90.

64. Dodson WE. Special pharmacokinetic considerations in children. Epilepsia 1987;28(suppl 1):S56-70.

65. Kutlu NO, Dogrul M, Yakinci C, et al. Buccal midazolam for treatment of prolonged seizures in children. Brain Dev 2003;25:275-8.

66. Wolfe TR, Macfarlane TC. Intranasal midazolam therapy for pediatric status epilepticus. Am J Emerg Med 2006;24:343-6.

67. Brigo F, Nardone R, Tezzon F, et al. Nonintravenous midazolam versus intravenous or rectal diazepam for the treatment of early status epilepticus: a systematic review with meta-analysis. Epilepsy Behav 2015;49:325-36.

68. Momen AA, Azizi Malamiri R, Nikkhah A, et al. Efficacy and safety of intramuscular midazolam versus rectal diazepam in controlling status epilepticus in children. Eur J Paediatr Neurol 2015;19:149-54.

69. Nielsson MS, Christiansen CF, Johansen MB, et al. Mortality in elderly ICU patients: a cohort study. Acta Anaesthesiol Scand 2014;58:19-26.

70. Towne AR. Epidemiology and outcomes of status epilepticus in the elderly. Int Rev Neurobiol 2007;81:111-27.

71. de Assis TM, Costa G, Bacellar A, et al. Status epilepticus in the elderly: epidemiology, clinical aspects and treatment. Neurol Int 2012;4:e17.

72. Cheng S. Non-convulsive status epilepticus in the elderly. Epileptic Disord 2014;16:385-94.

73. Naeije G, Depondt C, Meeus C, et al. EEG patterns compatible with nonconvulsive status epilepticus are common in elderly patients with delirium: a prospective study with continuous EEG monitoring. Epilepsy Behav 2014;36:18-21.

74. Battino D, Tomson T, Bonizzoni E, et al. Seizure control and treatment changes in pregnancy: observations from the EURAP epilepsy pregnancy registry. Epilepsia 2013;54:1621-7.

75. Sveberg L, Svalheim S, Tauboll E. The impact of seizures on pregnancy and delivery. Seizure 2015;28:35-8.

76. Putta S, Pennell PB. Management of epilepsy during pregnancy: evidence-based strategies. Future Neurol 2015;10:161-76.

77. Anderson GD. Pregnancy-induced changes in pharmacokinetics: a mechanistic-based approach. Clin Pharmacokinet 2005;44:989-1008.

78. Abernethy DR, Greenblatt DJ. Phenytoin disposition in obesity. Determination of loading dose. Arch Neurol 1985;42:468-71.

79. Wilkes L, Danziger LH, Rodvold KA. Phenobarbital pharmacokinetics in obesity. A case report. Clin Pharmacokinet 1992;22:481-4.

80. Misra UK, Kalita J, Chandra S, et al. Association of antibiotics with status epilepticus. Neurol Sci 2013;34:327-31.

81. Martinez-Rodriguez JE, Barriga FJ, Santamaria J, et al. Nonconvulsive status epilepticus associated with cephalosporins in patients with renal failure. Am J Med 2001;111:115-9.

82. Shaheen T, Volles D, Calland F, et al. Cefepime-associated status epilepticus in an ICU patient with renal failure. J Chemother 2009;21:452-4.

83. Isaacson SH, Carr J, Rowan AJ. Ciprofloxacin-induced complex partial status epilepticus manifesting as an acute confusional state. Neurology 1993;43:1619-21.

84. Koussa SF, Chahine SL, Samaha EI, et al. Generalized status epilepticus possibly induced by gatifloxacin. Eur J Neurol 2006;13:671-2.

85. Mazzei D, Accardo J, Ferrari A, et al. Levofloxacin neurotoxicity and non-convulsive status epilepticus (NCSE): a case report. Clin Neurol Neurosurg 2012;114:1371-3.

86. Oltrogge KM, Peppard WJ, Saleh M, et al. Phenytoin removal by continuous venovenous hemofiltration. Ann Pharmacother 2013;47:1218-22.

87. Rosenborg S, Saraste L, Wide K. High phenobarbital clearance during continuous renal replacement therapy: a case report and pharmacokinetic analysis. Medicine 2014;93:e46.

88. de Maat MM, van Leeuwen HJ, Edelbroek PM. High unbound fraction of valproic acid in a hypoalbuminemic critically ill patient on renal replacement therapy. Ann Pharmacother 2011;45:e18.

89. Shepard PW, St Louis EK. Seizure treatment in transplant patients. Curr Treat Options in Neurol 2012;14:332-47.

90. Jhun P, Kim H. Nonconvulsive status epilepticus in hepatic encephalopathy. West J Emerg Med 2011;12:372-4.

91. Eleftheriadis N, Fourla E, Eleftheriadis D, et al. Status epilepticus as a manifestation of hepatic encephalopathy. Acta Neurol Scand 2003;107:142-4.

92. Li X, Yu K, Mei S, et al. HLA-B*1502 increases the risk of phenytoin or lamotrigine induced Stevens-Johnson syndrome/toxic epidermal necrolysis: evidence from a meta-analysis of nine case-control studies. Drug Res 2015;65:107-11.

Chapter 20
Traumatic Brain Injury and Acute Spinal Cord Injury

A. Shaun Rowe, Pharm.D., BCPS; and Bradley A. Boucher, Pharm.D., BCPS

LEARNING OBJECTIVES

1. Discuss the epidemiology and pathophysiology of traumatic brain injury (TBI) and acute spinal cord injury (SCI).
2. Compare various treatment options for elevated intracranial pressure.
3. Choose the most appropriate pharmacotherapy for TBI and acute SCI.
4. Describe current investigational pharmacotherapies for TBI and acute SCI.

ABBREVIATIONS IN THIS CHAPTER

AANS	American Association of Neurological Surgeons	ICP	Intracranial pressure
		LMWH	Low-molecular-weight heparin
ASIA	American Spinal Injury Association	NMB	Neuromuscular blockade
BTF	Brain Trauma Foundation	SCI	Spinal cord injury
CNS	Congress of Neurological Surgeons	TBI	Traumatic brain injury
FOUR score	Full Outline of Unresponsiveness (score)	VTE	Venous thromboembolism
GCS	Glasgow Coma Scale		

TRAUMATIC BRAIN INJURY

Epidemiology and Pathophysiology

Traumatic brain injury (TBI) is a medical condition that can have devastating effects on patients and families. Traditionally, the severity of TBI has been classified using the Glasgow Coma Scale (GCS). However, sedatives, neuromuscular blocking agents, and intubation can potentially decrease the GCS thereby, increasing the severity classification of TBI.[1] This limitation has led to the development of other coma scales such as the Full Outline of Unresponsiveness (FOUR) score.[2] Unlike the GCS, the FOUR score allows for assessment of brain stem function and responsiveness in patients unable to speak (Table 20.1). When used to classify the severity of TBI, the goal of these coma scales is to correlate a potentially poor outcome (e.g., death, disability) with the scale score. Patients who have the highest potential for a poor outcome and require critical care can be classified as having severe TBI (GCS 3–8). Although the mortality associated with severe TBI has declined, a recent report suggested a mortality of 14.1% in patients who sustained a severe TBI while involved in a motor vehicle collision.[3,4] Mortality that is associated with severe TBI is multifactorial. Compared with those who lived in high-income countries, patients with severe TBI who live in low- and middle-income countries had a higher chance of death.[5] In addition, patients with a systolic blood pressure higher or lower than 120–140 mm Hg on admission may have a higher probability of death.[6] Increasing age, prehospital hypoxemia (Spo$_2$ [peripheral capillary oxygen saturation] less than 90%), and prehospital hypothermia (temperature less than 35°C) may be risk factors for increased mortality as well.[7]

The pathophysiology of severe TBI can be broadly categorized as primary and secondary injury. Primary injury occurs during the initial trauma as energy is transferred to the brain and surrounding central nervous system tissues. The initial impact can cause shearing of axons, contusions, swelling, and dysregulation of blood flow leading to ischemia.[8,9] Secondary brain injury is a complex disease state that can begin minutes to hours to days after the initial injury. Soon after the initial injury, the brain is inundated with high levels of excitatory neurotransmitters. The primary excitatory neurotransmitter in this setting, glutamate, binds to NMDA (*N*-methyl-D-aspartate) receptors and AMPA (α-amino-3-hydroxy-5-methyl;-4-isoxazolepropionic acid) receptors, causing an influx of calcium into the cells. Ultimately, this excess of excitatory neurotransmitters leads to cell damage, necrosis, and apoptosis. In addition, the blood-brain barrier is disrupted during the primary injury, allowing an influx of peripheral immune cells and cytokines into the brain parenchyma. Neutrophils from the peripheral blood driven by increases in local iNOS (inducible nitric oxide synthase), COX-2 (cyclooxygenase-2), NADPH (nicotinamide adenine dinucleotide phosphate), and other cytokines increase oxidative activity. This further damages the brain parenchyma and degrades the blood-brain barrier. Activation of the brain microglia and astrocytes by cellular debris and cytokines increases the production of many proinflammatory markers (interleukin [IL]-1β, IL-6, tumor necrosis factor

Table 20.1 Glasgow Coma Scale Score and FOUR Score Comparison

	Score	Glasgow Coma Scale	FOUR Score
Best eye opening response	0	N/A	Eyelids remain closed with pain
	1	No response	Eyelids closed but open to pain
	2	To pain	Eyelids closed but open to loud voice
	3	To speech	Eyelids open but not tracking
	4	Spontaneously	Eyelids open or opened, tracking, or blinking on command
Best motor response	0	N/A	No response to pain or generalized myoclonus status
	1	No response	Extension response to pain
	2	Abnormal extension	Flexion response to pain
	3	Abnormal flexion	Localizing to pain
	4	Withdraws to pain	Thumbs-up, fist, or peace sign
	5	Localizes to pain	N/A
	6	Obeys verbal commands	N/A
Best verbal response	1	No response	N/A
	2	Incomprehensible sounds	N/A
	3	Inappropriate words	N/A
	4	Confused	N/A
	5	Oriented	N/A
Brain stem reflexes	0	N/A	Absent pupil, corneal, and cough reflex
	1	N/A	Pupil and corneal reflexes absent
	2	N/A	Pupil or corneal reflexes absent
	3	N/A	One pupil wide and fixed
	4	N/A	Pupil and corneal reflexes present
Respiration	0	N/A	Breathes at ventilator rate or apnea
	1	N/A	Breathes above ventilator rate
	2	N/A	Not intubated, irregular breathing
	3	N/A	Not intubated, Cheyne-Stokes breathing pattern
	4	N/A	Not intubated, regular breathing pattern

N/A = not applicable.

alpha) and anti-inflammatory markers (IL-10, transforming growth factor beta).[8,10] These pro- and anti-inflammatory markers have a very complex role in the pathophysiology of severe TBI. Studies have not consistently found a correlation of increased pro- and anti-inflammatory markers with poor outcomes. In part, this contradiction in patient outcome and inflammatory markers may be the result of differences in sampling time and fluid type sampled (i.e., cerebrospinal fluid vs. peripheral blood vs. extracellular fluid).[11] Edema secondary to the primary injury and increased inflammatory markers increases the intracranial pressure (ICP). This further decreases cerebral blood flow, which in turn leads to further cerebral ischemia and cell death.

The mechanisms of secondary injury after severe TBI offer many potential therapeutic targets for improving the clinical outcomes of patients who have experienced severe TBI. In 2007, the Brain Trauma Foundation (BTF) revised its treatment guidelines for the management of severe TBI. These are the most authoritative recommendations for the treatment of these patients. Where appropriate, levels of evidence from the BTF severe TBI guidelines will be cited. Treatment algorithms for TBI can be found in Figures 20.1 and 20.2.

ICP Control

Hyperventilation

Hyperventilation and the induction of hypocapnia ($Paco_2$ less than 35 mm Hg) results in cerebral vasoconstriction and decreased blood flow to the brain. At the price of reduced cerebral blood flow, decreased oxygen delivery to the brain, and ischemia, ICP is quickly reduced.[12] Prolonged use of this therapy is related to worse outcomes at 3 and 6 months after injury[13] and may be associated with increased mortality and when overused before hospital arrival. Dumont et al. retrospectively evaluated patients with TBI and grouped them according to their presenting $Paco_2$. The authors found that compared with normocapnic patients, those with a $Paco_2$ less than 35 mm Hg had increased mortality (77% vs. 15%).[14] The BTF guidelines give level II evidence that recommends against the use of prophylactic hyperventilation and level III recommendations that hyperventilation should only be used as a "temporizing measure for the reduction of

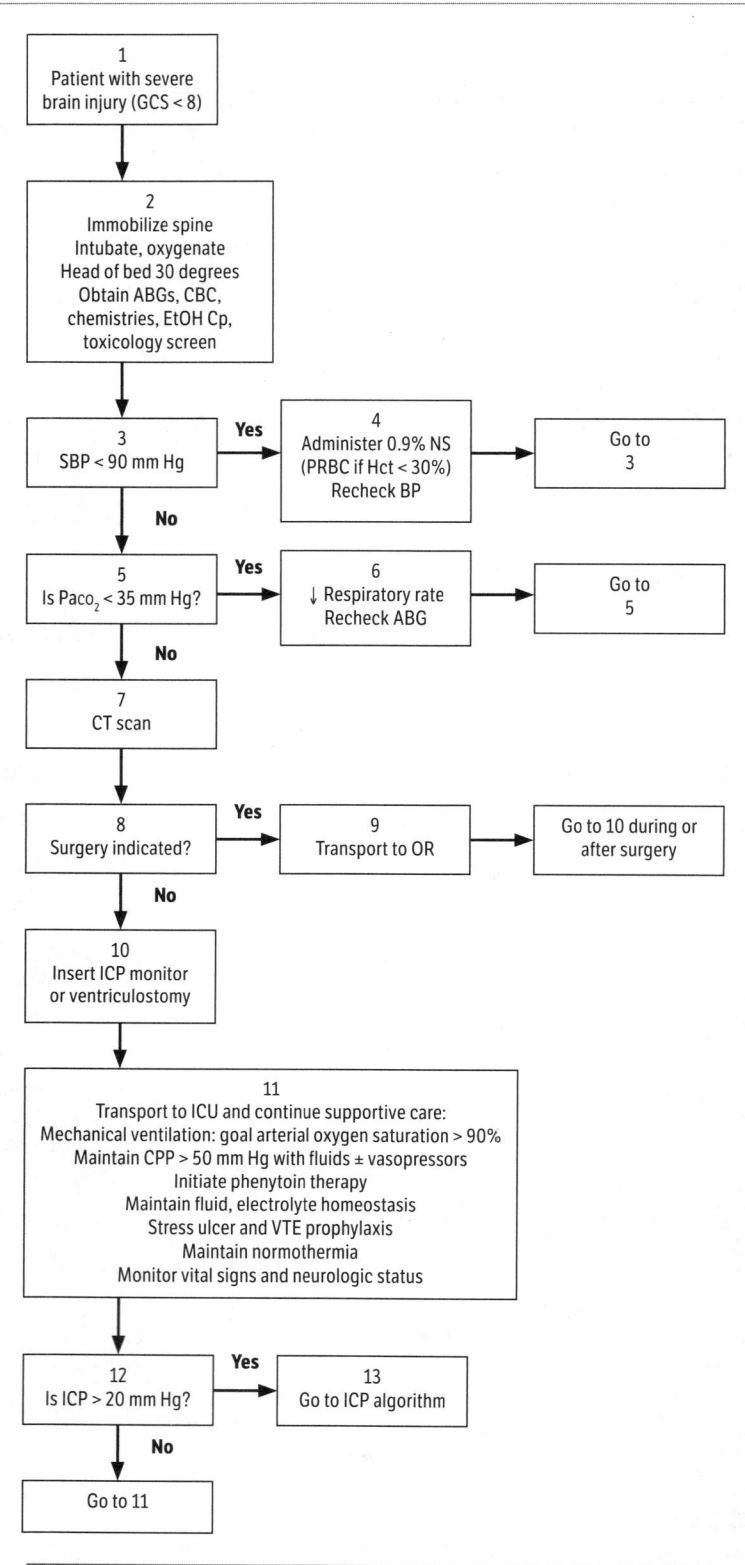

Figure 20.1 Algorithm for the acute management of traumatic brain injury.

ABG = arterial blood gas; CBC = complete blood cell count; Cp = plasma concentration; CPP = cerebral perfusion pressure; GCS = Glasgow Coma Scale; ICP = intracranial pressure; NS = normal saline; OR = operating room; PRBC = packed red blood cell; SBP = systolic blood pressure; VTE = venous thromboembolism.

Adapted from: Boucher BA. Neurotrauma. Pharmacotherapy Self-Assessment Program, 3rd ed. Module 2: Critical Care, Lenexa, KS: American College of Clinical Pharmacy, 1995:215-38.

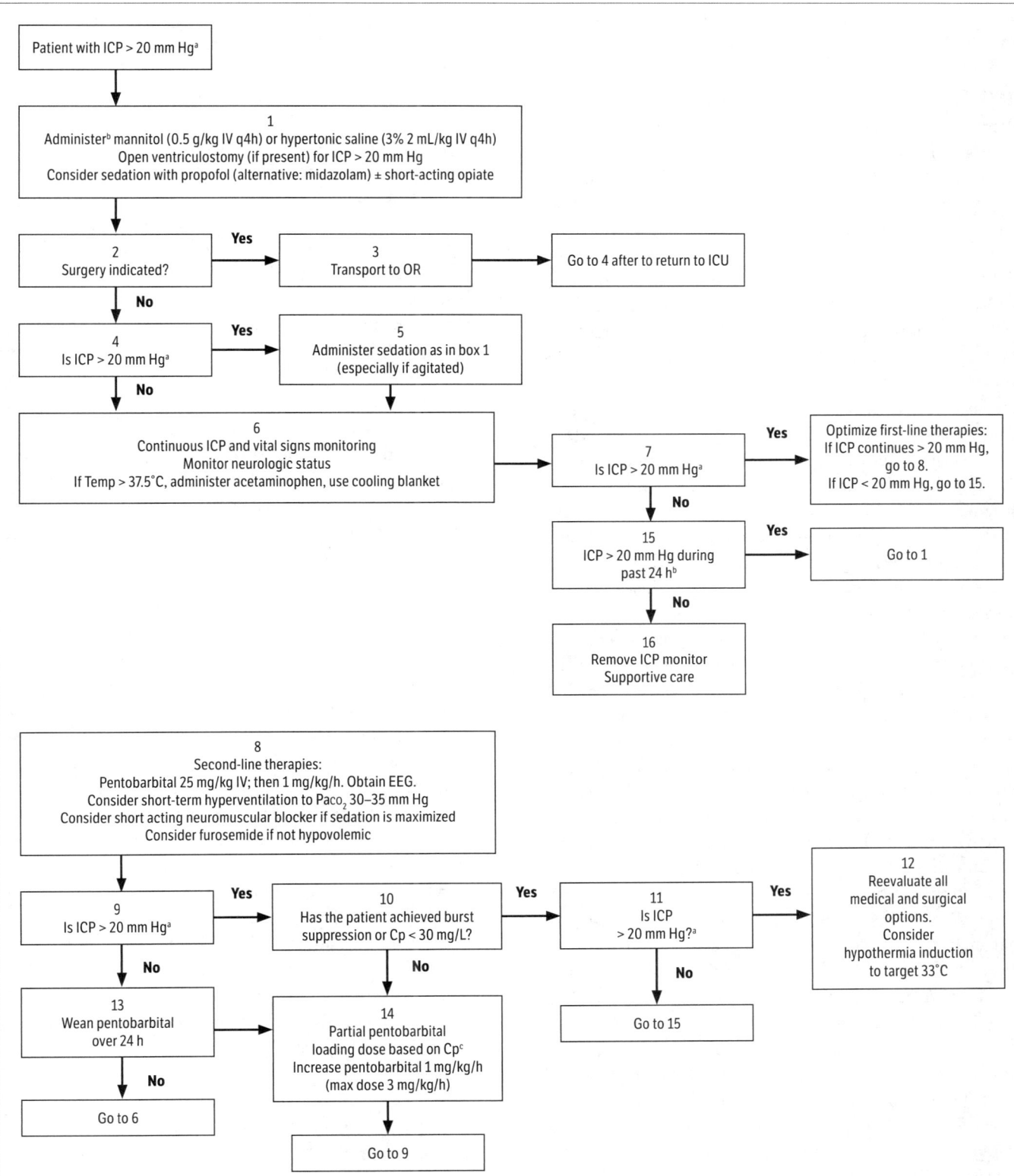

Figure 20.2 Algorithm for the management of ICP.

[a]Treatment thresholds: ICP 20–29 mm Hg for > 15 min, ICP 30–39 mm Hg for > 2 min, ICP > 40 mm Hg for > 1 min. Note: Transient increases may occur after respiratory procedures (e.g., suctioning, chest physiotherapy, bronchoscopy, intubation).

[b]Hold if serum osmolality > 320 mOsm/kg or mOsm gap > 20.

[c]Partial pentobarbital loading dose (mg) = (30 mg/L − measured Cp) (1 L/kg × wt(kg))

EEG = electroencephalogram; IV = intravenously; q = every.

Adapted from: Boucher BA. Neurotrauma. Pharmacotherapy Self-Assessment Program, 3rd ed. Module 2: Critical Care, Lenexa, KS: American College of Clinical Pharmacy, 1995:215-38.

elevated intracranial pressure" and that "hyperventilation should be avoided during the first 24 hours after injury."[15]

Hyperosmolar Therapy

The two primary agents used for hyperosmotic therapy to control ICP are mannitol and hypertonic saline. Mannitol is a sugar alcohol that is usually prepared for intravenous administration as a 20%–25% solution. Mannitol can be administered by a central venous catheter or a peripheral venous catheter. Mannitol affects the cerebral blood flow and ICP though two primary mechanisms of action. Immediately after infusion of mannitol, blood viscosity is decreased, thus increasing cerebral blood flow throughout the brain. When autoregulation is intact, this increase in cerebral blood flow causes a compensatory vasoconstriction and rapid reduction in ICP. The osmotic effect of mannitol occurs about 15 minutes after infusion. Mannitol causes a dehydration of brain tissue and hyperosmolarity through diuresis. This in turn decreases ICP.[16-18] Because mannitol is a strong osmotic diuretic, significant hypotension and significant fluid shifts can occur after administration. These rapid fluid shifts may be detrimental to patients with significant comorbidities (e.g., heart failure). Although the mechanism is not fully elucidated, mannitol can cause renal insufficiency in the setting of extreme hyperosmolarity. The dogmatic approach has been to discontinue or limit mannitol once the serum osmolarity reaches 320 mOsm; however, in clinical practice, this value is routinely exceeded. Acute renal insufficiency associated with mannitol may be related to accumulating mannitol plasma concentrations and cumulative mannitol dose.[19] The serum osmole gap, calculated as (measured osmolarity – calculated osmolarity), correlates with accumulating plasma concentrations better than serum osmolarity.[20] Compared with serum osmolarity, the serum osmole gap may be a better monitor for mannitol toxicity. Literature suggests that maintaining a serum osmole gap of less than 55 reduces the risk of renal insufficiency[21,22]; however, many practitioners conservatively target an osmolar gap of less than 18–20. In addition, mannitol is renally eliminated. Thus, in patients with significant renal insufficiency, mannitol may accumulate, necessitating a change in treatment agent. Hypertonic saline, usually prepared in concentrations of 1.5%–23.4%, must be administered by a central venous catheter when concentrations are greater than 3%. It decreases ICP by directly causing hyperosmolarity. This effectively dehydrates brain tissue, thus decreasing ICP. Hypertonic saline has been administered as a bolus or continuous infusion. The bolus dose varies depending on the concentration of sodium chloride; however, the osmolarity of the dose administered should be comparable with that of a therapeutic mannitol dose.[23] Table 20.2 contains equimolar doses of mannitol and hypertonic saline. Unlike mannitol, hypertonic saline does not cause diuresis and will expand the intravascular volume. Consequently, care should be taken when using hypertonic saline in patients when expanded intravascular volume would be deleterious (e.g., patients with heart failure). In addition, there is concern for osmotic demyelinating syndrome when using hypertonic saline in patients with chronic hyponatremia. Therefore, in patients with chronic hyponatremia, hypertonic saline therapy for increased ICP should be avoided.[24]

The BTF guidelines only give recommendations for the use of mannitol to control intracranial hypertension. They state that "mannitol is effective for control of raised ICP at doses of 0.25 gm/kg to 1 g/kg body weight. Arterial hypotension (systolic blood pressure less than 90 mm Hg) should be avoided (level II evidence)."[24] Since those guidelines were published in 2007, a significant amount of data comparing hypertonic saline and mannitol for the control of ICP have been published. A 2011 meta-analysis by Kamel et al. evaluated five trials that compared equimolar doses of mannitol and hypertonic saline. The authors found that patients treated with hypertonic saline had a better risk of achieving ICP control (relative risk [RR] 1.16; 95% confidence interval [CI], 1.00–1.13).[25] A second meta-analysis from 2012 found 12 studies that compared hypertonic saline with mannitol. Of those, nine found hypertonic saline superior to mannitol for reduction of ICP. Eight studies compared hypertonic saline and mannitol with respect to treatment failure or insufficient ICP reduction. Compared with patients treated with mannitol, significantly fewer patients had treatment failure or insufficiency when treated with hypertonic saline (odds ratio 0.36; 95% CI, 0.19–0.68).[23] This meta-analysis compared non-equimolar doses of agents; thus, it may overestimate the treatment effect of hypertonic saline. However, because the results are similar to those of previous meta-analyses, the trend of less treatment failure with hypertonic saline remains.

Choice of the most appropriate hyperosmolar therapy to decrease ICP must be linked not only to efficacy but also to speed of agent availability, access for administration (i.e., central vs. peripheral catheter), and patient-specific considerations (e.g., volume status, presence of hyponatremia, renal dysfunction). Therefore, a single approach

Table 20.2 Equivalent Doses of Hyperosmolar Agents Based on Osmolality

Therapeutic Agent	Dose	
Mannitol	1 g/kg	≅5.5 mOsm/kg
1.5% NaCl	10.8 mL/kg	
3% NaCl	5.4 mL/kg	
5% NaCl	3.2 mL/kg	
23.4% NaCl	0.69 mL/kg	

cannot be taken with these agents. Although data suggest that hypertonic saline is more effective at reducing ICP, mannitol remains a useful agent.

Barbiturate Therapy

Compared with hyperosmotic therapy, barbiturates are not as effective at reducing ICP.[26-30] However, barbiturates may have a role in control of refractory ICP. The BTF guidelines give level II evidence for the use of barbiturates "to control elevated ICP refractory to maximum standard medical and surgical treatment."[31] Many barbiturate regimens have been used, but most commonly, medications are titrated to induce and maintain electroencephalographic burst suppression.[27,28,32-35] There is little correlation between barbiturate plasma concentrations and achievement of electroencephalographic burst suppression; thus, barbiturate plasma concentrations should not be used to monitor the efficacy of a treatment regimen. Table 20.3 lists the most commonly used barbiturate regimens. A 2012 meta-analysis evaluated the effect of barbiturate coma and found no effect on outcome. In addition, the investigators found a significant risk of hypotension associated with the use of barbiturate coma, which may decrease this treatment's clinical significance.[30] A prospective cohort of five European countries was used to evaluate the use of barbiturates in patients with TBI. Compared with the time before barbiturate administration, patients who received high-dose barbiturates had a significant reduction in time with ICP greater than 25 mm Hg (6.4 hours ± 7.05 hours vs. 4.2 hours ± 5.9 hours; $p<0.05$), but they also had more time with a mean arterial pressure less than 70 mm Hg (6.2 hours ± 6.1 hours vs. 9.4 hours ± 8.2 hours; $p<0.05$). When survival was adjusted for age, GCS score, and injury severity score, no mortality benefit was associated with high-dose barbiturates.

Although barbiturate coma may play a role in management of refractory ICP management, data are sparse suggesting this therapy will benefit long-term clinical outcomes. Currently, these agents should be considered only if all other efforts to control ICP have been exhausted.

Close monitoring for, and management of, hypotension should be employed when using these agents for the treatment of elevated ICP.

Neuromuscular Blockade

The role of neuromuscular blockade (NMB) is not clearly defined in patients with severe TBI. However, it is often considered for control of ICP. The potential advantages of NMB include prevention of ventilator dyssynchrony, prevention of coughing during stimulating procedures (e.g., endotracheal suctioning), prevention of shivering during targeted temperature management, and decreased metabolic demand. All of these potential advantages decrease the ICP or decrease metabolic demand.

The literature surrounding these advantages is less clear. A 2015 systematic review identified 32 articles related to this topic. The data were too diverse to perform a meta-analysis, and there was no consistent theme of benefit or harm.[36] The authors concluded that if NMB was considered in the treatment of severe TBI, a nondepolarizing NMB agent would be the most appropriate choice. This was based primarily on the safety profile and, with respect to ICP reduction, less variability across the literature.

Neuromuscular blocking agents should only be used in patients who have received adequate analgesia and sedation. In addition, NMB has potential adverse effects that should be considered. With prolonged use of NMB, there is potential for critical care polyneuropathy and myopathy. In addition, the use of NMB may prolong ventilator and intensive care unit (ICU) duration. However, given that many patients with severe TBI will have prolonged ventilator courses, the association between NMB and prolonged ventilator use has not been adequately studied in severe TBI.

Targeted Temperature Management

The maintenance of normothermia or induction of hypothermia is a debated topic in the care of patients with severe TBI. The BTF guidelines do not recommend or

Table 20.3	Commonly Used Barbiturate Regimens	
	Bolus	**Infusion**
Eisenberg 1988[28]	Pentobarbital – 10 mg/kg followed by 5 mg/kg × 3 doses hourly	1 mg/kg/h
Perez-Barcena 2008[33]		
Levy 1995[32]	Pentobarbital – 2.5 mg/kg every 15 minutes for 1 h. 10 mg/kg × 4 doses hourly	1.5 mg/kg/h
Perez-Barcena 2008[33]	Thiopental – 2 mg/kg with second bolus of 3 mg/kg if no response	3 mg/kg/h
Saul 1982[34]	Pentobarbital – 10 mg/kg/h × 4 h	1.6 mg/kg/h
Schwartz 1984[35]	Pentobarbital – 10 mg/kg	0.5–3 mg/kg/h
Ward 1985[27]	Pentobarbital – 5–10 mg/kg	1–3 mg/kg/h

dissuade practitioners from using prophylactic hypothermia, but they do mention that level III evidence suggests use of hypothermia is associated with better clinical outcomes.[37] Since 2007, some key articles have been published on this management strategy. The NABIS: H II (National Acute Brain Injury Study: Hypothermia II) trial evaluated the early use of hypothermia in patients with nonpenetrating head injuries. Patients were rapidly cooled to 33°C and maintained at that temperature for 48 hours. Overall, the trial failed to show that the use of hypothermia was beneficial in this population.[38] A meta-analysis in 2008 evaluated the use of normothermia and hypothermia in patients with neurologic injury. Although the investigators did not find an association with improved outcomes with lowering of body temperature, they consistently found that fever and higher body temperature were associated with worse clinical outcomes (e.g., Glasgow Outcome Scale, Barthel Index, Modified Rankin Scale).[39] A more recent meta-analysis also evaluated the use of hypothermia in patients with neurologic injury but did not find a statistically significant difference in clinical outcome.[40] Because of these results and the recommendations by the BTF, it is conservative to say that hyperthermia is inappropriate in this patient population; however, with respect to improved clinical outcomes, the data surrounding the use of hypothermia versus the maintenance of normothermia are more equivocal.

If practitioners choose to use hypothermia or actively maintain normothermia, consideration should be given to changes in the pharmacokinetic profile of commonly used medications. In the setting of hypothermia, many medications have been shown to have prolonged elimination times, thus increasing the potential for toxicity in these patients.[41,42]

Steroids

Progesterone

Animal studies and small human trials evaluating the use of progesterone early after TBI showed promising results. In fact, in the phase II Progesterone for the Treatment of Traumatic Brain Injury trial (ProTECT), patients who received progesterone had significantly less mortality at 30 days compared with placebo (RR 0.43; 95% CI, 0.18–0.99).[43] In a separate study, patients with diffuse axonal injury who received progesterone had improved clinical outcomes.[44] These results were very encouraging to practitioners caring for patients with severe TBI.

Unfortunately, when progesterone was evaluated in a large-scale phase III trial, PROTECT III, the results were not as robust as in earlier trials. The trial included a much larger sample of 1,140 patients (100 patients in ProTECT II) and did not show an improvement in favorable outcomes (RR 0.95; 95% CI, 0.85–1.06; p=0.35).[45] In a second large study, the SYNAPSE (Study of the Neuroprotective Activity of Progesterone in Severe Traumatic Brain Injuries) trial, progesterone did not show a significant difference in mortality or clinical outcome.[46] The results of these trials were based on the evaluation of the Glasgow Outcome Scale - Extended (GOSE). The GOSE may not be precise enough to find a difference in this patient population. Therefore, the results currently suggest that in patients with severe TBI, progesterone does not improve clinical outcomes. Reevaluation of this treatment modality may be warranted if more precise outcome tools are developed.

Corticosteroids

Corticosteroids should not be used in patients with TBI. The BTF guidelines give level I evidence against the use of corticosteroids for improving outcomes or reducing ICP.[47] These recommendations were based on a wide range of evidence but primarily on the results of the Corticosteroid Randomisation After Significant Head Injury (CRASH) trial. This trial evaluated the use of high-dose methylprednisolone (2-g intravenous load followed by 0.4 g/hour) in patients with TBI having a GCS of less than 14. The trial planned to enroll 20,000 people but was terminated early after the corticosteroid group was shown to have a higher mortality rate.[48]

Supportive Care

Seizure Prophylaxis

Posttraumatic seizures are relatively common in patients with severe TBI. The BTF guidelines give level II evidence to support the use of anticonvulsants up to 7 days for the prevention of early posttraumatic seizures. However, the use of anticonvulsants is not associated with decreased rates of late seizure activity (i.e., seizures after 7 days post ictus).[49] This is primarily based on the work of N.R. Temkin and others, who evaluated the use of phenytoin and other anticonvulsants for the prevention of seizures after TBI.[50-54] It is not usually recommended to use valproate because of the potential risk of increased mortality.

The use of anticonvulsants with fewer adverse events compared with phenytoin has been of interest to practitioners.[55] The data suggest that levetiracetam is as effective as phenytoin at preventing seizures, but with fewer adverse events.[56-58] In one study by Jones et al., patients who received levetiracetam 500 mg intravenously every 12 hours for 7 days were compared with a historical control of patients who received phenytoin for 7 days. Although there was no difference in the number of seizures, patients who received levetiracetam had a higher incidence of abnormal electroencephalography readings.[59] However, compared with other trials, the dose used by Jones et al. may have been too low. In an evaluation of levetiracetam pharmacokinetics in neurocritical care patients, patients receiving 500 mg intravenously every 12 hours had a low probability of achieving a trough concentration of 6–20 mcg/mL. Doses of up to 1,500–2,000 mg every 12 hours were needed to have the best probability of achieving an appropriate serum concentration of levetiracetam.[60] Given this and levitiracetam's pharmacokinetic properties, some practitioners have considered a loading dose of 15–20 mg/kg followed by a maintenance dose of 1000–1500 mg every 12 hours. However, data are sparse to suggest the most appropriate dose of levetiracetam for seizure prophylaxis in patients with TBI. In addition, some data suggest that levetiracetam has neuroprotective activity. A trial by Szaflarski et al. found that, compared with patients treated with phenytoin, patients treated with levetiracetam had a lower 3-month disability rating scale.[61] Although not particularly robust, the results do suggest that patients treated with levetiracetam had a better clinical outcome but no difference in mortality. Thus, the use of levetiracetam may be considered a viable alternative to phenytoin for the prevention of early seizures after TBI.

Venous Thromboembolism Prophylaxis

Patients who experience a severe TBI should be considered at high risk of developing a venous thromboembolism (VTE). The benefit of using chemical VTE prophylaxis in this patient population must be balanced against the risk of increasing intracranial hemorrhage. The BTF guidelines quote level III evidence to recommend the use of "low-molecular-heparin or low-dose unfractionated heparin in combination with mechanical prophylaxis." They note that this recommendation comes with the risk of worsened intracranial hemorrhage.[62] Recent data from a retrospective study suggest that the use of chemical VTE prophylaxis did not increase intracranial hemorrhage volume.[63] However, because of the low observed rate of increased intracranial hemorrhage, these results may be the product of a type II statistical error.

A small study addressed the question of when VTE prophylaxis should be implemented in these patients. The study evaluated the use of enoxaparin or placebo in 62 patients with unchanged cranial computed tomography (CT) scans at 24 hours after injury. The study found that, with respect to hematoma expansion, there was no difference between the two groups. However, this study included only patients with mild to moderate TBI and those with small radiographic findings. These results may not be applicable to patients with larger radiographic findings or patients with severe TBI.[64] In a retrospective study by the Western Trauma Association, patients who received low-molecular-weight heparin (LMWH) were compared with those who did not receive systemic anticoagulation. These patients had moderate to severe TBI, and patients in the LMWH group appeared to have worse injuries. Although the patients who received LMWH had a higher percentage of hemorrhage progression compared with those who did not receive LMWH, the timing of when the LMWH was initiated did not affect hemorrhage progression rates.[65] Thus, the worse injuries in the LMWH group could have confounded the outcome on hemorrhage progression but should not have influenced the results associated with the timing of administration.

According to the observed data and the BTF guidelines, the use of chemical VTE prophylaxis in addition to mechanical VTE prophylaxis is warranted. In addition, the conservative approach to the addition of LMWH or low-dose unfractionated heparin would be to start within 24–48 hours of the last stable cranial CT scan.

Tranexamic Acid

The CRASH-2 trial has shown a potential mortality benefit for using tranexamic acid in bleeding trauma patients. A subanalysis of that trial showed that patients who received tranexamic acid had smaller hematoma expansions than did patients not receiving tranexamic acid. However, this result did not reach statistical significance.[66] This has led to the development of CRASH-3, which will be a large study evaluating mortality in patients with severe TBI who receive tranexamic acid.[67] Until the results of this trial are released— and given the significant risk of thrombosis associated with tranexamic acid—the use of tranexamic acid in patients with severe TBI is undefined.

Investigational Therapies

Most pharmacotherapeutic modalities for severe TBI are aimed at the prevention or modulation of secondary injury. The mechanisms for secondary injury are diverse and largely ill defined. Thus, many potential therapies are being investigated. Many of these such as statin use,[68,69] growth hormone replacement,[70] prostacyclin supplementation,[71,72] and bradykinin B_2 receptor antagonists[73] are aimed at reducing the inflammatory process. However, these potential treatment strategies are early in development.

ACUTE SPINAL CORD INJURY

Epidemiology and Pathophysiology

Acute spinal cord injury (SCI) is a physically and emotionally devastating traumatic event warranting ICU care to minimize morbidity and mortality in patients surviving the initial event. Acute mortality ranges from 48% to 79%, and another 4.4%–16% of patients will die before hospital discharge.[74] Perhaps even more tragic is that more than half of the cases are individuals between age 16 and 30, with just less than 80% being males according to the National Spinal Cord Injury Statistical Center.[75] The average age for patients with SCI is 29 years. The prevalence of acute SCI is estimated at 17,000 new cases (54 cases per 1 million) annually in the United States according to 2012 data.[76] This is a modest increase from 1993.[76] This does not include those who die at the scene of the accident. About 31% of SCI cases are a result of motor vehicle collisions.[76]

The next most common etiology is falls (40.4%), followed by firearm injuries (5.4%).[76] The incidence of falls has increased significantly during the past 2 decades, largely in older adult patients.[76] Median hospital length of stay for SCI is 11 days since 2010, resulting in average first-year expenses of $342,111–$1.05 million, depending on injury severity. Less than 1% of patients with SCI have complete neurologic recovery by the time of hospital discharge.

It is recommended that evaluations of acute SCI use the American Spinal Injury Association (ASIA) International Standards for Neurological Classification of Spinal Cord Injury recommendations (level II).[77] The ASIA examination worksheet can be downloaded free of charge at the ASIA website. Motor and sensory assessments are done with these instruments, resulting in the classification of patients according to the injury spine level (e.g., cervical spine 5 [C5], thoracic spine 6 [T6]). Patients are also classified as having complete or incomplete injuries. The latter reflects sensory and/or motor function preserved below the specified level. Three ASIA incomplete injury subcategories are available to further delineate patients for assessment and prognosis (see Box 20.1). *Central cord syndrome* is yet another classification for patients with acute SCI.[78] This term is used for patients with the atypical presentation of relative preservation of lower extremity function compared with the upper extremities. Patients with tetraplegia have sustained injuries to one of the eight cervical segments of the spinal cord, whereas patients with paraplegia have had cord injuries in the thoracic, lumbar, or sacral regions.[75] Incomplete tetraplegia (40.6%) followed by incomplete paraplegia (18.7%) are the most common neurologic categories among patients with SCI. Complete tetraplegia injuries occur in about 12% of patients with SCI.

Similar to acute TBI, the pathophysiology of acute SCI involves both primary and secondary injuries.[79] Primary injury results from a mechanical insult to the spinal cord from compression, contusion, laceration, flexion, extension, rotation, or shearing forces.[74] Ischemia caused by damage to the adjacent vasculature, systemic hypotension, and hypoxemia is also integral to the pathophysiology of acute SCI in addition to direct damage to the spinal cord.[80] The concept of secondary injury encompasses many processes ranging from edema and inflammation to apoptosis and necrosis. No therapy to date has been shown to attenuate these processes resulting in improved outcomes after acute SCI. Nevertheless, there are data that treating patients with acute SCI within an ICU setting is beneficial in minimizing morbidity and mortality as well as reducing the economic burden for patients after this catastrophic injury.[81] This occurs through prompt and aggressive hemodynamic and respiratory stabilization and subsequent prevention of associated complications. Unstable spine fractures and/or dislocation must be recognized and surgically managed in a timely manner as well.[79]

The Joint Section on Disorders of the Spine and Peripheral Nerves of the American Association of Neurological Surgeons (AANS) and the Congress of Neurological Surgeons (CNS) has published comprehensive and evidence-based guidelines for the management of acute cervical spine and SCIs.[82] The AANS/CNS guidelines, first published in 2002 and revised in 2013, provide the most authoritative recommendations for the treatment of these patients. The evidence levels from the AANS/CNS guidelines are listed where applicable. A treatment algorithm for SCI can be found in Figure 20.3.

Acute Cardiopulmonary Management

Ventilation

Concurrent with spine stabilization to prevent further injury, the initial priority in patients with acute SCI is cardiopulmonary management.[81] Acute SCI can have profound effects on the mechanics of ventilation because of the loss of diaphragmatic function above C5 and loss of accessory muscles with damage in the C4–C8 regions of the spinal

---

Box 20.1. ASIA Impairment Scale (AIS)

A = Complete. No sensory or motor function is preserved in the sacral segments S4–5.

B = Sensory Incomplete. Sensory but not motor function is preserved below the neurologic level and includes the sacral segments S4–5 (light touch or pinprick at S4–5 or deep anal pressure) AND no motor function is preserved more than three levels below the motor level on either side of the body.

C = Motor Incomplete. Motor function is preserved at the most caudal sacral segments for voluntary anal contraction (VAC) OR the patient meets the criteria for sensory incomplete status (sensory function preserved at the most caudal sacral segments (S4–5) by LT, PP, or DAP) and has some sparing of motor function more than three levels below the ipsilateral motor level on either side of the body.

(This includes key or non-key muscle functions to determine motor incomplete status.) For AIS C – less than half of key muscle functions below the single NLI have a muscle grade ≥ 3.

D = Motor Incomplete. Motor incomplete status as defined above, with at least half (half or more) of key muscle functions below the single NLI having a muscle grade ≥ 3.

E = Normal. If sensation and motor function as tested with the ISNCSCI are graded as normal in all segments, and the patient had prior deficits, the AIS grade is E. Someone without an initial SCI does not receive an AIS grade.

Using ND: To document the sensory, motor, and NLI levels; the ASIA Impairment Scale grade; and/or the zone of partial preservation (ZPP) when they are unable to be determined according to the examination results.

S = sacral; L = lumbar; LT = light touch; PP = pinprick, DNP = deep anal pressure; NLI = neurologic level of injury.

Adapted from: American Spinal Injury Association (ASIA) International Standards for Neurological Classification of Spinal Cord Injury (ISNCSCI). Available at www.asia-spinalinjury.org/elearning/ASIA_ISCOS_high.pdf.

cord. Relative hypoxemia and exacerbated spinal cord hypoxemia can also occur because of diaphragmatic function. Thus, patients with acute SCI often require intubation and mechanical ventilation. The duration of mechanical ventilation typically depends on injury level and complete versus incomplete injury. A tracheostomy is warranted in some patients requiring long-term mechanical ventilation (greater than 2 weeks).[74] Although mechanical ventilation is lifesaving for many patients with SCI, pneumonia is an inevitable risk because of this supportive care.[83] As such, prevention of pneumonia through reducing oropharyngeal secretion aspiration and possible alteration of digestive flora should be a priority in patients with SCI to minimize morbidity and mortality.[84]

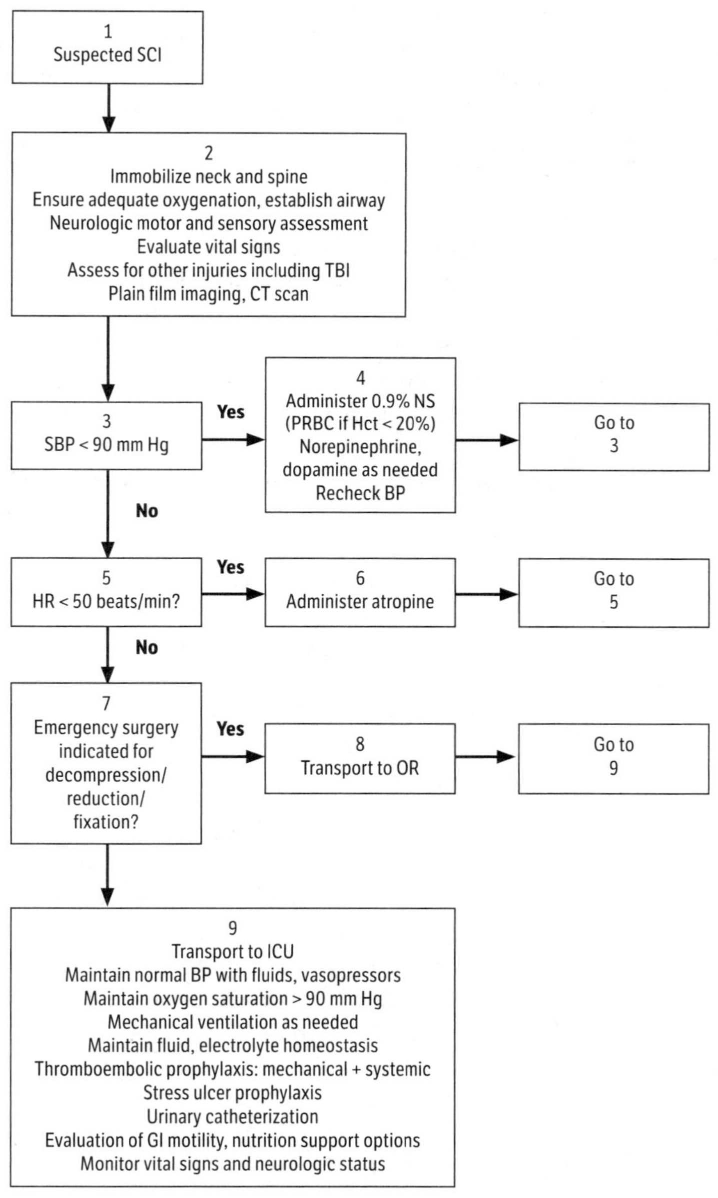

Not unlike any other critically ill patients with ventilator-associated pneumonia, patients with SCI developing pneumonia should promptly begin broad-spectrum antimicrobial therapy.

Blood Pressure Stabilization

Reversal of hypotension (systolic blood pressure less than 90 mm Hg) is recommended as soon as possible (level III) with a goal mean arterial pressure of 85–90 mm Hg for the first 7 days (level II).[81] Augmentation of blood pressure reduces morbidity and mortality and reduces the length of stay. Because of trauma-related hypovolemia from concurrent injuries or neurogenic shock, hypotension may be present. Neurogenic shock is a form of distributive shock that occurs secondary to loss of sympathetic innervation to blood vessels and the heart as well as unopposed parasympathetic tone in patients with injuries above T6.[74] The incidence of neurogenic shock is about 19% in patients with cervical cord injuries and 7% in patients with thoracic injury.[85] This complication manifests as vasodilation, decreased heart rate, and decreased cardiac output. Aggressive fluid resuscitation with crystalloids or red blood cell transfusion if the patient is anemic is often required for restoration of blood pressure together with adrenergic agents such as dopamine and norepinephrine. Although albumin therapy may be considered an alternative to crystalloid fluid resuscitation after acute SCI, a retrospective analysis of 460 patients with TBI showed an increase in mortality (33.2%) compared with patients receiving 0.9% normal saline, indirectly bringing this practice into question.[86] Atropine is often used in patients with neurogenic shock having bradycardia.[74] Phenylephrine should be avoided in patients with hypotension and bradycardia because it is essentially devoid of beta activity. Invasive monitoring is usually needed in patients requiring vasopressor support. Orthostatic hypotension in the subacute period may be seen. Pharmacologic therapy for this complication includes fludrocortisone, midodrine, and pseudoephedrine.[74,87]

Thermoregulation

Temperature dysregulation with resultant hypothermia and hyperthermia also commonly occurs after SCI.[80] Furthermore, patients with acute SCI may have sweating disturbances (i.e., hyperhidrosis and anhidrosis).[80] These can occur secondary to damage to autonomic

Figure 20.3 Algorithm for the acute management of the patient with SCI.
BP = blood pressure; HR = heart rate; SCI = spinal cord injury; TBI = traumatic brain injury.

1. Suspected SCI

2. Immobilize neck and spine
Ensure adequate oxygenation, establish airway
Neurologic motor and sensory assessment
Evaluate vital signs
Assess for other injuries including TBI
Plain film imaging, CT scan

3. SBP < 90 mm Hg — Yes → 4. Administer 0.9% NS (PRBC if Hct < 20%) Norepinephrine, dopamine as needed Recheck BP → Go to 3

5. HR < 50 beats/min? — Yes → 6. Administer atropine → Go to 5

7. Emergency surgery indicated for decompression/reduction/fixation? — Yes → 8. Transport to OR → Go to 9

9. Transport to ICU
Maintain normal BP with fluids, vasopressors
Maintain oxygen saturation > 90 mm Hg
Mechanical ventilation as needed
Maintain fluid, electrolyte homeostasis
Thromboembolic prophylaxis: mechanical + systemic
Stress ulcer prophylaxis
Urinary catheterization
Evaluation of GI motility, nutrition support options
Monitor vital signs and neurologic status

pathways to the skin. As such, close attention to body temperature in patients after acute SCI is warranted. Hypothermia may require warming techniques, whereas hyperthermia may necessitate cooling of the patient.

Prevention and Management of Acute Complications

Prevention of a VTE after acute SCI is another priority for patients with SCI after cardiopulmonary stabilization. The greatest risk of a VTE is 72 hours to 2 weeks post-injury, with an incidence that may exceed 80%.[74] As such, both the American College of Chest Physicians Antithrombotic Therapy and Prevention of Thrombosis guidelines and the AANS/CNS guidelines recommend early prophylaxis to prevent VTE formation and associated morbidity in patients with acute SCI (level I).[88,89] Neither sequential compression devices nor low-dose unfractionated heparin alone is deemed adequate.[88] Alternatively, combination therapy with mechanical devices and prophylactic dosing of an LMWH or unfractionated heparin is recommended (level I).[88] Consideration of placement of a vena cava filter in patients with therapeutic failure is noted but not recommended as a routine prophylactic measure (level III).[88] Physical examination monitoring for deep venous thrombosis is especially important in patients with SCI because the symptom of pain that usually accompanies this complication may be absent.

Musculoskeletal, visceral, and neuropathic pain at or below the injury level are common after SCI. This complication can have a major effect on the quality of life and psychological well-being of the patient, often leading to anxiety and depression. The International SCI Pain Basic Data Set is recommended as the preferred means to assess pain in patients with SCI (level I).[77] This tool, which is available on the NINDS (National Institute of Neurological Disorders and Stroke) website, evaluates pain severity, physical functioning, and emotional functioning. Depression after acute SCI is common and can occur independently of the pain often associated secondarily with other psychiatric illnesses.[90,91] Psychotherapy and/or pharmacologic treatment may be needed for both pain and psychological management, acutely and chronically.[80] However, no specific recommendations are available for patients with acute SCI having these conditions. As such, therapy should be individualized to the greatest extent possible, including if and when pharmacologic therapy should be initiated. Relative to neuropathic pain, anticonvulsants are commonly used in the management of this condition in patients with acute SCI, not unlike other patient populations.[92]

Nutrition support should begin as soon as feasible (less than 72 hours) after SCI (level III).[93] The rationale for this supportive care in patients with SCI is the hypermetabolism, inherent immobility, and muscle atrophy typically present after injury. Although nutrition support is safe, no effect on neurologic outcome has been shown (e.g., decreased infection, ventilator hours, length of stay).[94] Noteworthy is that impaired peristalsis, a gastrointestinal (GI) complication of acute SCI, may initially compromise the use of enteral feedings in patients with SCI. Close monitoring of bowel sounds, gastric residual volumes, and bowel movements is needed to facilitate nutrition support of patients with SCI having no complications (e.g., aspiration). Use of stool softeners and laxatives is also commonly needed as adjunctive therapy to facilitate stool evacuation in patients with SCI. Prophylaxis therapy for stress-related mucosal disease (e.g., histamine-2 receptor antagonists, proton pump inhibitors) should usually be administered acutely in patients with SCI, especially those requiring intubation and/or with evidence of relative hypotension. After the risk of stress-related mucosal disease diminishes (e.g., cardiopulmonary stabilization, extubation), discontinuation of these agents is advocated.

Pneumonia is not the only acute infectious complication experienced after SCI. Urinary tract infections are also very common in patients with SCI because of impaired bladder emptying associated with a neurogenic bladder and the inherent need for urinary catheters continuously or intermittently. Evaluating patients with SCI for evidence of a urinary tract infection, including urinary cultures, is warranted in any patient with fever, leukocytosis, and other generalized systemic signs of infection. Patients with acute and chronic SCI should also receive meticulous skin care because they are at risk of developing pressure ulcers that can become secondarily infected. Log-rolling patients and using rotokinetic beds are strategies for avoiding this challenging complication.

Neuroprotective Therapy

Corticosteroids

Interest in using glucocorticoids as a pharmacologic strategy for improving neurologic outcomes in SCI has existed for decades.[74,95] Postulated mechanisms for the beneficial effects of corticosteroids in SCI include increasing cell membrane integrity, decreasing inflammation and free radical production, and limiting vasogenic edema through stabilization of the blood–spinal cord barrier. Three major clinical trials investigating the efficacy of methylprednisolone have been conducted since the 1980s. These trials are usually called the National Acute Spinal Cord Injury Study (NASCIS) I–III. The first of these studies (NASCIS I) compared motor and sensory scores in individuals with SCI after administration of either a 100- or 1000-mg bolus dose of methylprednisolone followed by a daily dose for 10 days without a placebo control.[96] No differences in outcomes were seen between the two groups. In NASCIS II, the dose of methylprednisolone was increased, and individuals with SCI were randomized to three different treatments: (1) methylprednisolone (30-mg/kg bolus followed by 5.4 mg/kg/hour for 23 hours), (2) the opioid antagonist naloxone (5.4-mg/kg bolus followed by 4.0 mg/kg/hour for 23 hours), and (3) placebo.[97] In a post hoc analysis, the investigators reported improved motor and sensory scores at 6 months if methylprednisolone was administered within 8 hours of injury. This finding was immediately embraced as the standard of care for acute SCI. A third trial (NASCIS III) randomized patients to receive methylprednisolone for 24 or 48 hours or the antioxidant tirilazad mesylate for 48 hours after a bolus of methylprednisolone.[98] Neurologic outcomes were similar for all treatment groups if initiated within 3 hours of injury. When comparing individuals treated between 3 and 8 hours after injury, motor scores and functional measures were improved at 6 weeks and 6 months in participants treated with methylprednisolone for 48 hours. The findings from this study became the new standard of care for 15 years thereafter.

Despite having many advocates, the NASCIS trials were always deemed questionable by many clinicians and scientists. One major reservation was the association of methylprednisolone administration with an increased incidence of pulmonary embolism, pneumonia, wound infection, sepsis, and GI complications in NASCIS II and III.[74,95] Other methodological flaws have also been identified, including a post hoc versus prospectively defined administration time window (i.e., 8 hours), inclusion of patients with minimal deficits and lesions below T12, lack of functional measures, and no standardization with respect to surgical or medical treatment. On review of these data, the AANS/CNS guidelines recommend against using methylprednisolone in the management of SCI (level I), reversing the standard of care for more than 2 decades.[95]

Gangliosides

In addition to corticosteroids, an agent known as GM1 ganglioside was one of the most widely studied pharmacologic agents in acute SCI in the past.[95] This was based on animal studies showing increased neural plasticity, decreased excitotoxicity, and apoptosis in SCI models. Unfortunately, a large prospective, multicenter, randomized trial of low-dose GM1 ganglioside, high-dose GM1 ganglioside, and placebo in 797 patients with acute SCI was unable to show any difference in neurologic outcome between the treatment groups.[99] Noteworthy and potentially confounding the study results, all patients enrolled in this trial received methylprednisolone as described in the NASCIS II study.

Other Therapies

In light of no single pharmacologic agent being available to heal the injured spinal cord and restore function, other investigational strategies have been evaluated. These other approaches have usually paralleled clinical studies of patients with TBI. One example is progesterone that has been investigated as a neuroprotective agent in animal models of acute SCI.[100] Interest in local or systemic therapeutic hypothermia has existed for years, based on preclinical studies.[79,101] The rationale of therapeutic hypothermia is to attenuate the secondary inflammatory processes after acute SCI.[79] However, there are a paucity of controlled comparative clinical data relative to the beneficial effects of this treatment strategy after acute SCI. As such, the AANS/CNS issued a level IV recommendation stating that evidence is insufficient for or against this practice.[102] One unique therapy is antihuman Nogo-A antibody administered intrathecally.[79] Nogo-A is an inhibitory molecule that limits regenerative sprouting of injured axons. A prospective, multicenter trial of this agent is currently under way in patients with complete and incomplete SCI.[103] In addition, other targeted anti-inflammatory agents offer promise in modulating the inflammatory response after acute SCI.[79] Finally, using mesenchymal stem cell transplantation as a regeneration strategy for restoring the injured spinal cord is being investigated.[79] However, many challenges await clinical application of this treatment approach.[104]

REFERENCES

1. Stocchetti N, Pagan F, Calappi E, et al. Inaccurate early assessment of neurological severity in head injury. J Neurotrauma 2004;9:1131-40.

2. Kornbluth J, Bhardwaj A. Evaluation of coma: a critical appraisal of popular scoring systems. Neurocrit Care 2011;1:134-43.

3. Brain Trauma Foundation, American Association of Neurological Surgeons, Congress of Neurological Surgeons, et al. Guidelines for the management of severe traumatic brain injury. Introduction. J Neurotrauma 2007;24:S1-2.

4. Leijdesdorff HA, van Dijck JT, Krijnen P, et al.; Regional Trauma Center West-Netherlands' Research G. Injury pattern, hospital triage, and mortality of 1250 patients with severe traumatic brain injury caused by road traffic accidents. J Neurotrauma 2014;5:459-65.

5. De Silva MJ, Roberts I, Perel P, et al. Patient outcome after traumatic brain injury in high-, middle- and low-income countries: analysis of data on 8927 patients in 46 countries. Int J Epidemiol 2009;2:452-8.

6. Fuller G, Hasler RM, Mealing N, et al. The association between admission systolic blood pressure and mortality in significant traumatic brain injury: a multi-centre cohort study. Injury 2014;3:612-7.

7. Tohme S, Delhumeau C, Zuercher M, et al. Prehospital risk factors of mortality and impaired consciousness after severe traumatic brain injury: an epidemiological study. Scand J Trauma Resusc Emerg Med 2014;22:1.

8. Algattas H, Huang JH. Traumatic brain injury pathophysiology and treatments: early, intermediate, and late phases post-injury. Int J Mol Sci 2014;1:309-41.

9. Maas AI, Stocchetti N, Bullock R. Moderate and severe traumatic brain injury in adults. Lancet Neurol 2008;8:728-41.

10. Andriessen TM, Jacobs B, Vos PE. Clinical characteristics and pathophysiological mechanisms of focal and diffuse traumatic brain injury. J Cell Mol Med 2010;10:2381-92.

11. Hinson HE, Rowell S, Schreiber M. Clinical evidence of inflammation driving secondary brain injury: a systematic review. J Trauma Acute Care Surg 2015;1:184-91.

12. Yundt KD, Diringer MN. The use of hyperventilation and its impact on cerebral ischemia in the treatment of traumatic brain injury. Crit Care Clin 1997;1:163-84.

13. Muizelaar JP, Marmarou A, Ward JD, et al. Adverse effects of prolonged hyperventilation in patients with severe head injury: a randomized clinical trial. J Neurosurg 1991;5:731-9.

14. Dumont TM, Visioni AJ, Rughani AI, et al. Inappropriate prehospital ventilation in severe traumatic brain injury increases in-hospital mortality. J Neurotrauma 2010;7:1233-41.

15. Bratton SL, Chestnut RM, Ghajar J, et al. Guidelines for the management of severe traumatic brain injury. XIV. Hyperventilation. J Neurotrauma 2007;24:S87-90.

16. Mendelow AD, Teasdale GM, Russell T, et al. Effect of mannitol on cerebral blood flow and cerebral perfusion pressure in human head injury. J Neurosurg 1985;1:43-8.

17. Muizelaar JP, Lutz HA III, Becker DP. Effect of mannitol on ICP and CBF and correlation with pressure autoregulation in severely head-injured patients. J Neurosurg 1984;4:700-6.

18. Diringer MN, Scalfani MT, Zazulia AR, et al. Effect of mannitol on cerebral blood volume in patients with head injury. Neurosurgery 2012;5:1215-8; discussion 19.

19. Kim MY, Park JH, Kang NR, et al. Increased risk of acute kidney injury associated with higher infusion rate of mannitol in patients with intracranial hemorrhage. J Neurosurg 2014;6:1340-8.

20. García-Morales EJ, Cariappa R, Parvin CA, et al. Osmole gap in neurologic-neurosurgical intensive care unit: its normal value, calculation, and relationship with mannitol serum concentrations. Crit Care Med 2004;4:986-91.

21. Visweswaran P, Massin EK, Dubose TD Jr. Mannitol-induced acute renal failure. J Am Soc Nephrol 1997;6:1028-33.

22. Rabetoy GM, Fredericks MR, Hostettler CF. Where the kidney is concerned, how much mannitol is too much? Ann Pharmacother 1993;1:25-8.

23. Mortazavi MM, Romeo AK, Deep A, et al. Hypertonic saline for treating raised intracranial pressure: literature review with meta-analysis. J Neurosurg 2012;1:210-21.

24. Bratton SL, Chestnut RM, Ghajar J, et al. Guidelines for the management of severe traumatic brain injury. II. Hyperosmolar therapy. J Neurotrauma 2007;24:S14-20.

25. Kamel H, Navi BB, Nakagawa K, et al. Hypertonic saline versus mannitol for the treatment of elevated intracranial pressure: a meta-analysis of randomized clinical trials. Crit Care Med 2011;3:554-9.

26. Levin AB, Duff TA, Javid MJ. Treatment of increased intracranial pressure: a comparison of different hyperosmotic agents and the use of thiopental. Neurosurgery 1979;5:570-5.

27. Ward JD, Becker DP, Miller JD, et al. Failure of prophylactic barbiturate coma in the treatment of severe head injury. J Neurosurg 1985;3:383-8.

28. Eisenberg HM, Frankowski RF, Contant CF, et al. High-dose barbiturate control of elevated intracranial pressure in patients with severe head injury. J Neurosurg 1988;1:15-23.

29. Cordato DJ, Herkes GK, Mather LE, et al. Barbiturates for acute neurological and neurosurgical emergencies—do they still have a role? J Clin Neurosci 2003;3:283-8.

30. Roberts I, Sydenham E. Barbiturates for acute traumatic brain injury. Cochrane Database Syst Rev 2012;12:CD000033.

31. Brain Trauma Foundation, American Association of Neurological Surgeons, Congress of Neurological Surgeons, et al. Guidelines for the management of severe traumatic brain injury. XI. Anesthetics, analgesics, and sedatives. J Neurotrauma 2007;24(suppl 1):S71-6.

32. Levy ML, Aranda M, Zelman V, et al. Propylene glycol toxicity following continuous etomidate infusion for the control of refractory cerebral edema. Neurosurgery 1995;2:363-9; discussion 69-71.

33. Perez-Barcena J, Llompart-Pou JA, Homar J, et al. Pentobarbital versus thiopental in the treatment of refractory intracranial hypertension in patients with traumatic brain injury: a randomized controlled trial. Crit Care 2008;4:R112.

34. Saul TG, Ducker TB. Effect of intracranial pressure monitoring and aggressive treatment on mortality in severe head injury. J Neurosurg 1982;4:498-503.

35. Schwartz ML, Tator CH, Rowed DW, et al. The University of Toronto head injury treatment study: a prospective, randomized comparison of pentobarbital and mannitol. Can J Neurol Sci 1984;4:434-40.

36. Sanfilippo F, Santonocito C, Veenith T, et al. The role of neuromuscular blockade in patients with traumatic brain injury: a systematic review. Neurocrit Care 2015;22:325-34.

37. Brain Trauma Foundation, American Association of Neurological Surgeons, Congress of Neurological Surgeons, et al. Guidelines for the management of severe traumatic brain injury. III. Prophylactic hypothermia. J Neurotrauma 2007;24:S21-5.

38. Clifton GL, Valadka A, Zygun D, et al. Very early hypothermia induction in patients with severe brain injury (the National Acute Brain Injury Study: Hypothermia II): a randomised trial. Lancet Neurol 2011;2:131-9.

39. Greer DM, Funk SE, Reaven NL, et al. Impact of fever on outcome in patients with stroke and neurologic injury: a comprehensive meta-analysis. Stroke 2008;11:3029-35.

40. Li P, Yang C. Moderate hypothermia treatment in adult patients with severe traumatic brain injury: a meta-analysis. Brain Inj 2014;8:1036-41.

41. Empey PE, de Mendizabal NV, Bell MJ, et al. Therapeutic hypothermia decreases phenytoin elimination in children with traumatic brain injury. Crit Care Med 2013;10:2379-87.

42. Morbitzer KA, Jordan JD, Rhoney DH. Vancomycin pharmacokinetic parameters in patients with acute brain injury undergoing controlled normothermia, therapeutic hypothermia, or pentobarbital infusion. Neurocrit Care 2015;22:258-64.

43. Wright DW, Kellermann AL, Hertzberg VS, et al. ProTECT: a randomized clinical trial of progesterone for acute traumatic brain injury. Ann Emerg Med 2007;4:391-402, 402 e1-2.

44. Shakeri M, Boustani MR, Pak N, et al. Effect of progesterone administration on prognosis of patients with diffuse axonal

injury due to severe head trauma. Clin Neurol Neurosurg 2013;10:2019-22.

45. Wright DW, Yeatts SD, Silbergleit R, et al. Very early administration of progesterone for acute traumatic brain injury. N Engl J Med 2014;26:2457-66.

46. Skolnick BE, Maas AI, Narayan RK, et al. A clinical trial of progesterone for severe traumatic brain injury. N Engl J Med 2014;26:2467-76.

47. Brain Trauma Foundation, American Association of Neurological Surgeons, Congress of Neurological Surgeons, et al. Guidelines for the management of severe traumatic brain injury. XV. Steroids. J Neurotrauma 2007;24:S91-5.

48. Wasserberg J. The MRC CRASH trial—a large, simple randomised trial of steroids in head injury. Acta Neurochir Suppl 2004;89:109-12.

49. Brain Trauma Foundation, American Association of Neurological Surgeons, Congress of Neurological Surgeons, et al. Guidelines for the management of severe traumatic brain injury. XIII. Antiseizure prophylaxis. J Neurotrauma 2007;24:S83-6.

50. Temkin NR, Dikmen SS, Anderson GD, et al. Valproate therapy for prevention of posttraumatic seizures: a randomized trial. J Neurosurg 1999;4:593-600.

51. Angeleri F, Majkowski J, Cacchio G, et al. Posttraumatic epilepsy risk factors: one-year prospective study after head injury. Epilepsia 1999;9:1222-30.

52. Temkin NR, Dikmen SS, Wilensky AJ, et al. A randomized, double-blind study of phenytoin for the prevention of post-traumatic seizures. N Engl J Med 1990;8:497-502.

53. Young B, Rapp RP, Norton JA, et al. Failure of prophylactically administered phenytoin to prevent late posttraumatic seizures. J Neurosurg 1983;2:236-41.

54. McQueen JK, Blackwood DH, Harris P, et al. Low risk of late post-traumatic seizures following severe head injury: implications for clinical trials of prophylaxis. J Neurol Neurosurg Psychiatry 1983;10:899-904.

55. Kruer RM, Harris LH, Goodwin H, et al. Changing trends in the use of seizure prophylaxis after traumatic brain injury: a shift from phenytoin to levetiracetam. J Crit Care 2013;5:883 e9-13.

56. Rowe AS, Goodwin H, Brophy GM, et al. Seizure prophylaxis in neurocritical care: a review of evidence-based support. Pharmacotherapy 2014;4:396-409.

57. Gabriel WM, Rowe AS. Long-term comparison of GOS-E scores in patients treated with phenytoin or levetiracetam for posttraumatic seizure prophylaxis after traumatic brain injury. Ann Pharmacother 2014;11:1440-4.

58. Cook AM, Goodwin HE, Brophy GM, et al. Antiepileptics for seizure prophylaxis after traumatic brain injury. Am J Health Syst Pharm 2013;23:2062, 2064.

59. Jones KE, Puccio AM, Harshman KJ, et al. Levetiracetam versus phenytoin for seizure prophylaxis in severe traumatic brain injury. Neurosurg Focus 2008;4:E3.

60. Spencer DD, Jacobi J, Juenke JM, et al. Steady-state pharmacokinetics of intravenous levetiracetam in neurocritical care patients. Pharmacotherapy 2011;10:934-41.

61. Szaflarski JP, Sangha KS, Lindsell CJ, et al. Prospective, randomized, single-blinded comparative trial of intravenous levetiracetam versus phenytoin for seizure prophylaxis. Neurocrit Care 2010;2:165-72.

62. Brain Trauma Foundation, American Association of Neurological Surgeons, Congress of Neurological Surgeons, et al. Guidelines for the management of severe traumatic brain injury. V. Deep vein thrombosis prophylaxis. J Neurotrauma 2007;24:S32-6.

63. Farooqui A, Hiser B, Barnes SL, et al. Safety and efficacy of early thromboembolism chemoprophylaxis after intracranial hemorrhage from traumatic brain injury. J Neurosurg 2013;6:1576-82.

64. Phelan HA, Wolf SE, Norwood SH, et al. A randomized, double-blinded, placebo-controlled pilot trial of anticoagulation in low-risk traumatic brain injury: the Delayed Versus Early Enoxaparin Prophylaxis I (DEEP I) study. J Trauma Acute Care Surg 2012;6:1434-41.

65. Kwiatt ME, Patel MS, Ross SE, et al. Is low-molecular-weight heparin safe for venous thromboembolism prophylaxis in patients with traumatic brain injury? A Western Trauma Association multicenter study. J Trauma Acute Care Surg 2012;3:625-8.

66. Effect of tranexamic acid in traumatic brain injury: a nested randomised, placebo controlled trial (CRASH-2 Intracranial Bleeding Study). BMJ 2011;343:d3795.

67. Dewan Y, Komolafe EO, Mejia-Mantilla JH, et al. CRASH-3 – tranexamic acid for the treatment of significant traumatic brain injury: study protocol for an international randomized, double-blind, placebo-controlled trial. Trials 2012;13:87.

68. Sanchez-Aguilar M, Tapia-Perez JH, Sanchez-Rodriguez JJ, et al. Effect of rosuvastatin on cytokines after traumatic head injury. J Neurosurg 2013;3:669-75.

69. Tapia-Perez J, Sanchez-Aguilar M, Torres-Corzo JG, et al. Effect of rosuvastatin on amnesia and disorientation after traumatic brain injury (NCT003229758). J Neurotrauma 2008;8:1011-7.

70. Moreau OK, Cortet-Rudelli C, Yollin E, et al. Growth hormone replacement therapy in patients with traumatic brain injury. J Neurotrauma 2013;11:998-1006.

71. Olivecrona M, Rodling-Wahlstrom M, Naredi S, et al. Prostacyclin treatment and clinical outcome in severe traumatic brain injury patients managed with an ICP-targeted therapy: a prospective study. Brain Inj 2012;1:67-75.

72. Grande PO, Moller AD, Nordstrom CH, et al. Low-dose prostacyclin in treatment of severe brain trauma evaluated with microdialysis and jugular bulb oxygen measurements. Acta Anaesthesiol Scand 2000;7:886-94.

73. Shakur H, Andrews P, Asser T, et al. The BRAIN TRIAL: a randomised, placebo controlled trial of a bradykinin B2 receptor antagonist (Anatibant) in patients with traumatic brain injury. Trials 2009;10:109.

74. Evans LT, Lollis SS, Ball PA. Management of acute spinal cord injury in the neurocritical care unit. Neurosurg Clin North Am 2013;3:339-47.

75. National Spinal Cord Injury Statistical Center (NSCISC). Spinal Cord Injury Facts and Figures at a Glance, February 2013. Available at www.uab.edu/nscisc. Accessed December 12, 2014.

76. Jain NB, Ayers GD, Peterson EN, et al. Traumatic spinal cord injury in the United States, 1993-2012. JAMA 2015;313:2236-43.

77. Hadley MN, Walters BC, Aarabi B, et al. Clinical assessment following acute cervical spinal cord injury. Neurosurgery 2013;72(suppl 2):40-53.

78. Aarabi B, Hadley MN, Dhall SS, et al. Management of acute traumatic central cord syndrome (ATCCS). Neurosurgery 2013;72:195-204.

79. Stahel PF, VanderHeiden T, Finn MA. Management strategies for acute spinal cord injury: current options and future perspectives. Curr Opin Crit Care 2012;6:651-60.

80. Hagen EM. Acute complications of spinal cord injuries. World J Orthop 2015;1:17-23.

81. Ryken TC, Hurlbert RJ, Hadley MN, et al. The acute cardiopulmonary management of patients with cervical spinal cord injuries. Neurosurgery 2013;72:84-92.

82. Hadley MN, Walters BC. Introduction to the Guidelines for the Management of Acute Cervical Spine and Spinal Cord Injuries. Neurosurgery 2013;72:5-16.

83. Roquilly A, Seguin P, Mimoz O, et al. Risk factors for prolonged duration of mechanical ventilation in acute traumatic tetraplegic patients—a retrospective cohort study. J Crit Care 2014;2:313 e7-13.

84. Roquilly A, Marret E, Abraham E, et al. Pneumonia prevention to decrease mortality in intensive care unit: a systematic review and meta-analysis. Clin Infect Dis 2015;1:64-75.

85. Guly HR, Bouamra O, Lecky FE, et al. The incidence of neurogenic shock in patients with isolated spinal cord injury in the emergency department. Resuscitation 2008;1:57-62.

86. Cooper DJ, Myburgh J, Heritier S, et al. Albumin resuscitation for traumatic brain injury: is intracranial hypertension the cause of increased mortality? J Neurotrauma 2013;7:512-8.

87. Wood GC, Boucher AB, Johnson JL, et al. Effectiveness of pseudoephedrine as adjunctive therapy for neurogenic shock after acute spinal cord injury: a case series. Pharmacotherapy 2014;1:89-93.

88. Dhall SS, Hadley MN, Aarabi B, et al. Deep venous thrombosis and thromboembolism in patients with cervical spinal cord injuries. Neurosurgery 2013;72:244-54.

89. Guyatt GH, Akl EA, Crowther M, et al., American College of Chest Physicians Antithrombotic T, et al. Executive summary: Antithrombotic Therapy and Prevention of Thrombosis, 9th ed: American College of Chest Physicians Evidence-Based Clinical Practice Guidelines. Chest 2012;2(suppl):7S-47S.

90. Ullrich PM, Smith BM, Blow FC, et al. Depression, healthcare utilization, and comorbid psychiatric disorders after spinal cord injury. J Spinal Cord Med 2014;1:40-5.

91. Williams R, Murray A. Prevalence of depression after spinal cord injury: a meta-analysis. Arch Phys Med Rehabil 2015;1:133-40.

92. Guy S, Mehta S, Leff L, et al. Anticonvulsant medication use for the management of pain following spinal cord injury: systematic review and effectiveness analysis. Spinal Cord 2014;2:89-96.

93. Dhall SS, Hadley MN, Aarabi B, et al. Nutritional support after spinal cord injury. Neurosurgery 2013;72:255-9.

94. Dvorak MF, Noonan VK, Belanger L, et al. Early versus late enteral feeding in patients with acute cervical spinal cord injury: a pilot study. Spine (Phila Pa 1976) 2004;9:E175-80.

95. Hurlbert RJ, Hadley MN, Walters BC, et al. Pharmacological therapy for acute spinal cord injury. Neurosurgery 2013;72:93-105.

96. Bracken MB, Collins WF, Freeman DF, et al. Efficacy of methylprednisolone in acute spinal cord injury. JAMA 1984;1:45-52.

97. Bracken MB, Shepard MJ, Collins WF, et al. A randomized, controlled trial of methylprednisolone or naloxone in the treatment of acute spinal-cord injury. Results of the Second National Acute Spinal Cord Injury Study. N Engl J Med 1990;20:1405-11.

98. Bracken MB, Shepard MJ, Holford TR, et al. Administration of methylprednisolone for 24 or 48 hours or tirilazad mesylate for 48 hours in the treatment of acute spinal cord injury. Results of the Third National Acute Spinal Cord Injury Randomized Controlled Trial. National Acute Spinal Cord Injury Study. JAMA 1997;20:1597-604.

99. Geisler FH, Coleman WP, Grieco G, et al.; Sygen Study G. The Sygen multicenter acute spinal cord injury study. Spine (Phila Pa 1976) 2001;24(suppl):S87-98.

100. Deutsch ER, Espinoza TR, Atif F, et al. Progesterone's role in neuroprotection, a review of the evidence. Brain Res 2013;1530:82-105.

101. Ahmad FU, Wang MY, Levi AD. Hypothermia for acute spinal cord injury—a review. World Neurosurg 2014;1-2:207-14.

102. O'Toole JE, Wang MC, Kaiser MG. Hypothermia and Human Spinal Cord Injury: Updated Position Statement and Evidence Based Recommendations from the AANS/CNS Joint Sections on Disorders of the Spine & Peripheral Nerves and Neurotrauma & Critical Care. Available at www.spinesection.org/files/pdfs/Hypothermia%20Position%20Statement%20Mar%202014.pdf. Accessed February 4, 2015.

103. Zorner B, Schwab ME. Anti-Nogo on the go: from animal models to a clinical trial. Ann N Y Acad Sci 2010;1198:E22-34.

104. Volarevic V, Erceg S, Bhattacharya SS, et al. Stem cell-based therapy for spinal cord injury. Cell Transplant 2013;8:1309-23.

Chapter 21: Acute Management of Stroke

Martina Holder, Pharm.D., BCPS; and Stacy Voils, Pharm.D., M.Sc., BCPS

LEARNING OBJECTIVES

1. Recognize the risk factors, signs, and symptoms of acute ischemic stroke (AIS).
2. Determine eligibility for thrombolytic medications using patient-specific factors.
3. Manage and monitor blood pressure in patients with AIS.
4. Define the role of endovascular treatment for AIS including the role of intra-arterial tissue plasminogen activator.
5. Prevent hospital complications by providing supportive care to patients with AIS.
6. Discuss the etiology, risk factors, and clinical presentation of hemorrhagic stroke.
7. Using patient-specific factors, recommend an optimal medication regimen for blood pressure management in the setting of hemorrhagic stroke.
8. Provide recommendations for reversal of anticoagulation in patients receiving warfarin and the non-vitamin K antagonist oral anticoagulants.
9. Prevent complications associated with hemorrhagic stroke.
10. Understand the role of dedicated stroke units in the care of patients with stroke.

ABBREVIATIONS IN THIS CHAPTER

AIS	Acute ischemic stroke	PCC	Prothrombin complex concentrate
FFP	Fresh frozen plasma	PT	Prothrombin time
ICH	Intracerebral hemorrhage	TIA	Transient ischemic attack
MCA	Middle cerebral artery	TPA	Tissue plasminogen activator
NINDS	National Institute of Neurological Disorders and Stroke	VKA	Vitamin K antagonist
		VTE	Venous thromboembolism
NOAC	Non-vitamin K antagonist oral anticoagulant		

INTRODUCTION: ACUTE ISCHEMIC STROKE

Ischemic stroke, or brain attack, is a debilitating condition that often leads to disability, family hardship, increase in direct and indirect health care costs, and death. Transient ischemic attack (TIA), termed *mini-stroke*, precedes stroke in 60% of patients and should be viewed as a warning sign for impending stroke. Symptoms of TIA are similar to those of stroke but resolve in less than 24 hours. However, this definition is problematic because up to one-third of patients with symptoms for less than 24 hours have evidence of infarction. This has led to a new "tissue-based" definition for TIA as a transient episode of stroke symptoms without radiologic evidence of infarction.[1]

EPIDEMIOLOGY

Each year, around 800,000 people in the United States have a stroke, with about 90% of those related to ischemia. Ischemic strokes are further classified as atherosclerotic, cardioembolic (e.g., atrial fibrillation, valvular disease), lacunar, atypical (e.g., dissection, drug abuse), and cryptogenic in up to one-third of cases. Prevalence of ischemic stroke is highest in African Americans and American Indians or Alaskan natives.[2] Strokes are more common in the southeastern United States than in other areas. These are the so-called "stroke belt" states.

PATHOPHYSIOLOGY

Whether because of atherosclerosis or embolism, the initiating event in patients with acute ischemic stroke (AIS) is cerebral arterial occlusion. Depending on the severity and duration of the occlusion, ischemic brain injury may occur as a result of several pathobiologic processes. The ischemic penumbra is an area thought to surround the core ischemic area and may represent salvageable neurons. Blood flow to this area is below normal but may be augmented by the presence of collateral flow from surrounding blood vessels. Under normal conditions, cerebral blood vessels dilate in an attempt to maintain consistent blood flow, which is termed *autoregulation* (Figure 21.1). For instance, normotensive patients "autoregulate" within a mean arterial pressure (MAP) zone of about 50–150 mm Hg, whereas hypertensive patients have a shift of the autoregulation curve to the right and autoregulate at higher MAP ranges.[3] However, autoregulation is impaired in the penumbra (area of ischemic but viable brain tissue), and a decrease in blood pressure can lead to a decrease in cerebral blood flow. Pharmacologic interventions may be most effective in preventing ischemic injury within the penumbra. Without emergency restoration of perfusion to the penumbra, propagation of neuronal cell death occurs.

CLINICAL PRESENTATION

Symptoms of AIS commonly include sudden onset of numbness or weakness in the face or extremities, especially on one side of the body. Visual and speech impairment are also common, as are dizziness, loss of balance, and headache. Depending on the location of the stroke, very distinct patterns of impairment may manifest. Strokes occurring in the upper lobes of the brain (cerebrum) may cause hemiparesis (weakness) or hemiplegia (paralysis) on the contralateral side. In addition, other common deficits include visual, memory, speech, and cognition. Cerebellar strokes may cause headache, nausea, vomiting, and problems with coordination and balance (ataxia). Finally, brain stem strokes may lead to loss of respiratory stimulation, heart function, temperature regulation, and ability to chew or swallow.

DISEASE CLASSIFICATION, RISK FACTORS, AND DIAGNOSIS

Eighty-seven percent of all strokes are ischemic and can further be classified as atherosclerotic, penetrating artery disease, cardiogenic (e.g., atrial fibrillation, myocardial infarction), and cryptogenic. Nonmodifiable risk factors for AIS include age older than 55 years, male sex, family history, prior stroke or TIA, and African American race. Modifiable risk factors include hypertension (most important), atrial fibrillation, diabetes mellitus, hyperlipidemia, drug use (smoking, alcohol abuse, cocaine), physical inactivity/obesity, carotid stenosis, and oral contraceptive use. Although increasing age is an important risk factor for stroke, the average age of stroke onset has been declining, and in 2009, about one-third of patients hospitalized with stroke were younger than 65 years.[4] In addition to an increase in prevalence of traditional risk factors, stroke in younger adults has been associated with migraines, drug use (e.g., cocaine and cannabis), patent foramen ovale, pregnancy, and oral contraceptive use.[5]

Emergency medical service personnel can identify patients with stroke before arrival to the hospital using assessment tools such as the Cincinnati Prehospital Stroke Scale or the Los Angeles Prehospital Stroke Screen (Table 21.1).

TREATMENT

On arrival to the hospital, the American Heart Association has published detailed guidelines regarding the management of stroke in the emergency department (ED).[6] These guidelines include several interventions that should be performed in a timely manner according to recommendations from the National Institute of Neurological Disorders and Stroke (NINDS) (Figure 21.2). One of the most important steps

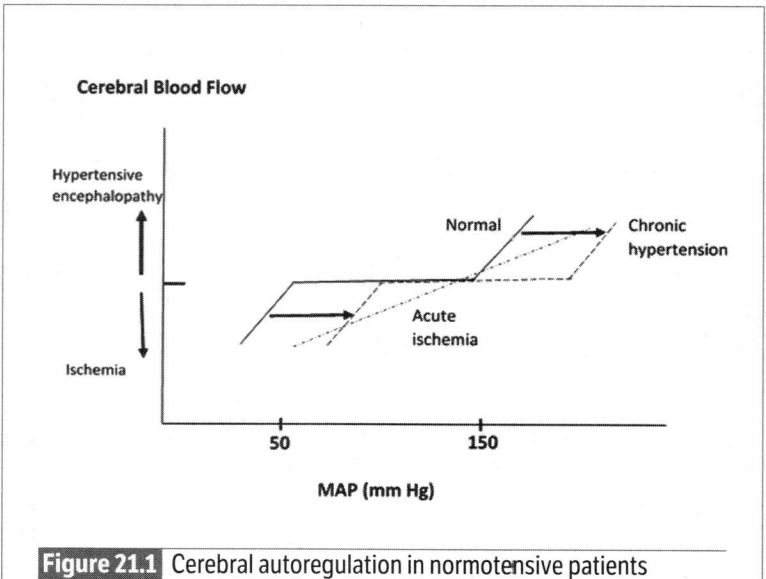

Figure 21.1 Cerebral autoregulation in normotensive patients (solid line, sideways "Z"), hypertensive patients (dotted line, sideways "Z"), and those with acute ischemia (straight, dashed line).

is performing a detailed patient history and clearly identifying the time of symptom onset. Neurologic assessment should be done within 25 minutes of ED arrival, usually incorporating the National Institutes of Health Stroke Scale (NIHSS). Computed tomography (CT) scanning of the head should be done and evaluated within 45 minutes of ED arrival to exclude hemorrhagic stroke. Intravenous tissue plasminogen activator (TPA) should be administered to eligible patients within 60 minutes of arrival to the hospital. Of note, these time goals are "worst-case scenario" because AIS is a medical emergency requiring interventions as soon as possible ("time is brain tissue"). Clinical scenarios that may mimic stroke signs need to be ruled out before a diagnosis of stroke and include hypoglycemia, encephalopathies, postictal state, mass lesions (e.g., brain tumor, brain abscess, head injury), conversion disorder, drug toxicities, and complicated migraine.

Criteria for Intravenous TPA Administration

Intravenous TPA is the only medication shown to improve outcome in AIS and should be administered as soon as possible to all eligible patients. Criteria for administration of intravenous TPA within 3 hours of symptom onset are directed by the NINDS protocol, whereas additional exclusion criteria for administration 3–4.5 hours from symptom onset are guided by the European Cooperative Acute Stroke Study (ECASS) III protocol (Box 21.1).[7,8]

Although several laboratory and diagnostic studies are recommended in the evaluation of a patient with AIS, the only laboratory result required before intravenous TPA administration is blood glucose concentration (because this is a stroke mimic). However, if a bleeding abnormality is expected or the patient has a known or uncertain anticoagulation status, it is reasonable to await the results of coagulation studies before intravenous TPA administration. In patients receiving direct oral anticoagulants (e.g., factor Xa inhibitors or direct thrombin inhibitors) with an unclear history regarding the last dose taken,

Table 21.1 Assessment Tools for Identifying Potential Stroke

Cincinnati Prehospital Stroke Scale

Facial droop (have patient smile)
- Normal: both sides of face move equally
- Abnormal: one side of face does not move as well as the other

Arm drift (have patient close eyes and hold both arms out straight for 10 seconds)
- Normal: arms stay parallel or move in conjunction
- Abnormal: arms not parallel or one arm "drifts"

Abnormal speech
- Normal: no slurring and uses correct words
- Abnormal: slurs speech, uses incorrect words, or is unable to speak

Interpretation: Any abnormal findings, probability of stroke is 72%.

Los Angeles Prehospital Stroke Screen (LAPSS)

Criteria	Yes	No	Unknown
1. Age > 45 years			
2. Absent history of seizures			
3. Symptom duration < 24 hours			
4. Not wheelchair bound/bedridden			
5. Blood glucose 60–400 mg/dL			
6. Obvious unilateral asymmetry in:			
a. Facial smile/grimace			
b. Grip			
c. Arm strength			

Interpretation: All items checked "yes" or "unknown," 97% will have stroke.

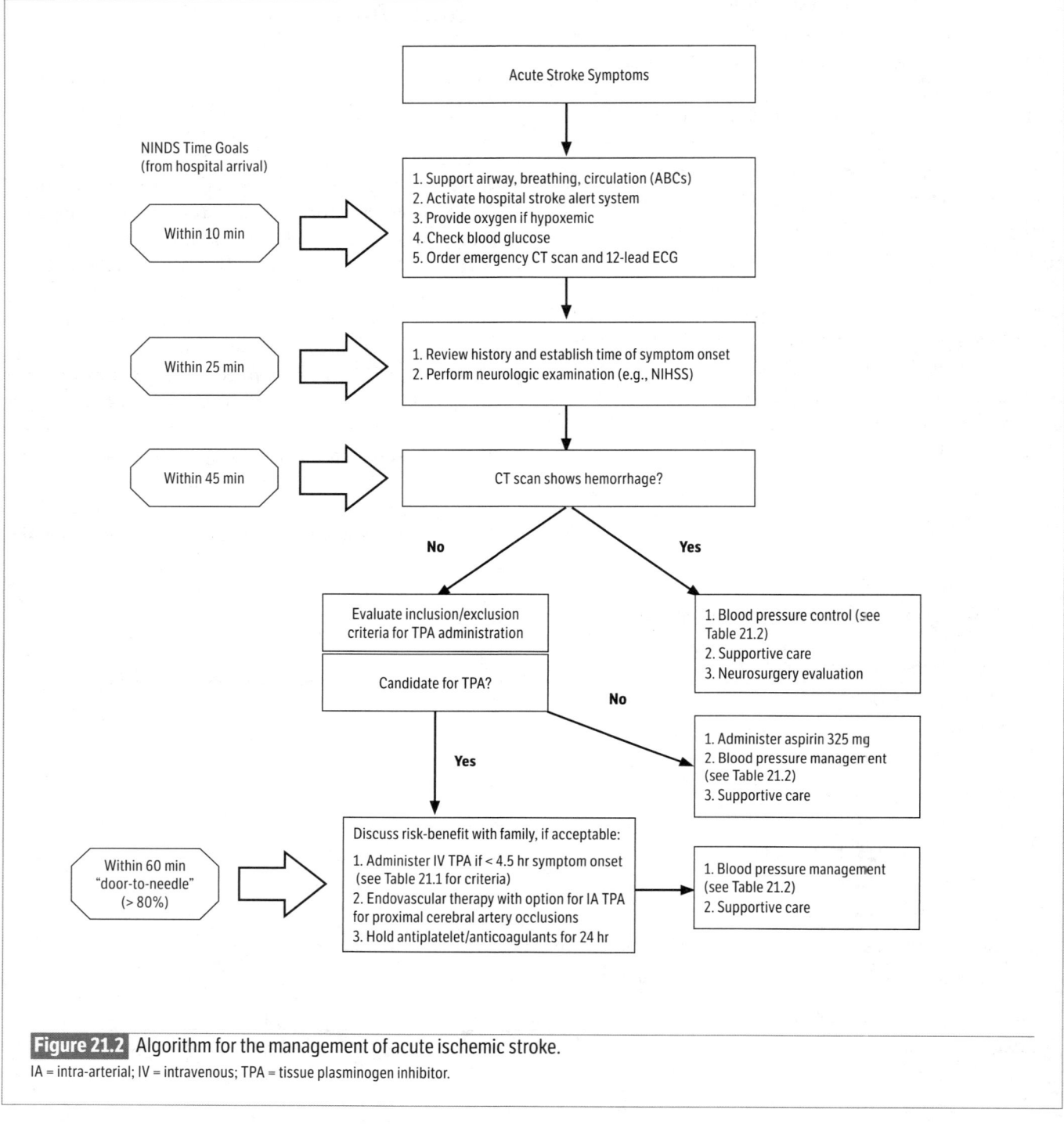

Figure 21.2 Algorithm for the management of acute ischemic stroke.
IA = intra-arterial; IV = intravenous; TPA = tissue plasminogen inhibitor.

laboratory assessment may be helpful to assess the risk-benefit of intravenous TPA administration. For direct thrombin inhibitors, a normal TT (thrombin time) and aPTT (activated partial thromboplastin time) suggest that the concentration of dabigatran is very low. Anti-factor Xa assays are preferred to confirm the concentration of factor Xa inhibitors but may not be available at many institutions. In this instance, prothrombin time (PT) may be used instead, but PT may be normal with "on-therapy" rivaroxaban concentrations because the effect on PT is highly dependent on the reagent used in the PT test.[9]

Monitoring and Adverse Effects of Intravenous TPA

Bleeding is the most worrisome adverse effect associated with intravenous TPA administration, with intracerebral hemorrhage (ICH) the most serious (termed *hemorrhagic conversion*). The rate of symptomatic ICH was 6.4% in the NINDS trial and 7.9% in ECASS III when using the same definition as in NINDS.[8,10] Because of the importance of strict adherence to administration criteria for intravenous TPA, a 15.7% rate of symptomatic ICH was reported in a cohort of patients who often received the drug outside the therapeutic window or had protocol violations.[11] Other factors that increase the risk of ICH after intravenous TPA administration include increasing age and stroke severity, hyperglycemia, presence of edema/mass effect on the initial head CT, and hypertension. Recommendations and treatment options for blood pressure monitoring are summarized in Table 21.2.

Neurological monitoring should be performed often during and for the initial 24 hours after intravenous TPA administration. Patients who develop severe headache, acute hypertension, nausea, vomiting, or seizure or who have a worsening neurological examination should have intravenous TPA discontinued and an emergency head CT performed.

Angioedema is another potentially serious adverse effect of intravenous TPA, occurring in 1.3%–5.1% of patients. The proposed mechanism is an increase in the vasodilator bradykinin caused by cleavage with TPA-generated plasmin of high-molecular-weight kininogen.[12] Risk factors include African American race, use of angiotensin-converting enzyme inhibitor medications, and strokes involving the insular and frontal cortex. Monitoring should include visual inspection of the tongue, lips, and oropharynx. Symptoms may be asymmetric and appear on the side contralateral to the ischemic infarct.[13] Mechanical ventilation may be necessary if edema involves the larynx, hypopharynx, oropharynx, or palate as opposed to edema isolated to the lips or anterior tongue. Medical treatments described in case reports have been variable, but a short course of corticosteroids and antihistamines is probably warranted in patients requiring mechanical ventilation.[12]

Other Fibrinolytic Agents

Although intravenous TPA is the only U.S. Food and Drug Administration (FDA)-approved fibrinolytic for AIS in the United States, tenecteplase, bioengineered from 3 amino acid substitutions on human tissue plasminogen activator (alteplase), has increased fibrin specificity, has a longer half-life (22 minutes vs. 3.5 minutes), and is less susceptible to PAI-1 (plasminogen activator inhibitor-1) compared to alteplase.[14] In a randomized controlled phase IIb trial of patients with AIS presenting within 6 hours of symptoms, patients who received tenecteplase had significantly improved reperfusion, NIHSS scores, and excellent or good recovery at 90 days compared with alteplase, with a nonsignificant decrease in intracerebral bleeding.[15] Tenecteplase also has a practical advantage over alteplase because it may be administered as a rapid intravenous bolus compared with a 1-hour infusion for alteplase. A large Norwegian phase III randomized trial is ongoing (NOR-TEST) to compare 3-month clinical outcomes in alteplase- versus tenecteplase-treated patients presenting within 4.5 hours of AIS symptom onset.[16] Derived from bat saliva, desmoteplase has a very high fibrin selectivity compared with intravenous TPA, but a recent study (DIAS-3) reported no improvement in functional outcome in patients who received desmoteplase compared with placebo when administered between 3 and 9 hours of symptom onset in AIS.[17] As such, this drug is no longer in development for the indication of AIS.

Endovascular Interventions

Treatment of AIS has evolved beyond intravenous administration of TPA to include endovascular interventions such as

---

Box 21.1. Criteria for Administration of Intravenous TPA

Within 3 hours of symptom onset

Inclusion criteria

1. Age ≥ 18 years
2. Clinical diagnosis of AIS with a *measurable* neurologic deficit
3. Clearly established time of symptom onset < 3 hours

Exclusion criteria

1. Evidence of intracranial hemorrhage on CT scan
2. Multilobar infarction (hypodensity > 1/3 cerebral hemisphere)
3. History of intracranial hemorrhage
4. Blood pressure remaining > 185/110 mm Hg at time of intravenous TPA administration despite treatment
5. Arteriovenous malformation, neoplasm, or aneurysm
6. Witnessed seizure at stroke onset
7. Active internal bleeding or acute trauma (fracture)
8. Platelet count < 100,000/mm³
9. Heparin administration within 48 hours resulting in aPTT > upper limit of normal
10. Anticoagulant use with INR > 1.7 or PT > 15 seconds
11. Intracranial or intraspinal surgery, serious head trauma, or previous stroke within 3 months
12. Arterial puncture at noncompressible site within 7 days

Relative contraindications

1. Minor or rapidly improving stroke symptoms
2. Major surgery/trauma within 14 days
3. GI or urinary tract hemorrhage within 21 days
4. Myocardial infarction within 3 months
5. Post-myocardial infarction pericarditis
6. Blood glucose concentration < 50 or > 400 mg/dL
7. Additional criteria 3–4.5 hours from symptom onset

Exclusion criteria

1. Age > 80 years
2. Severe stroke defined as NIHSS > 25
3. Taking oral anticoagulant regardless of INR
4. History of both diabetes and previous AIS

AIS = acute ischemic stroke; TPA = tissue plasminogen activator.

Table 21.2 Management of Hypertension in Patients with Acute Ischemic Stroke

Patient Characteristic	Goal Blood Pressure, mm Hg	Pharmacotherapy	Monitoring
Eligible for IV TPA	< 185/110 before administration	Labetalol 10–20 mg IV over 1–2 min; may repeat × 1 or Nicardipine 5 mg/hr; titrate by 2.5 mg/hr every 5 min up to 15 mg/hr	If blood pressure does not decline and remains > 185/110 mm Hg, do not administer IV TPA
During and after IV TPA administration	< 180/105 for 24 hr after administration	Systolic 180–230 or diastolic 105–120: Labetalol 10–20 mg IV over 1–2 min; may repeat every 10–20 min or Labetalol 10 mg IV × 1; then 2–8 mg/min infusion Systolic > 230 or diastolic 121–140: Labetalol 10–20 mg IV over 1–2 min; may repeat every 10–20 min or Labetalol 10 mg IV × 1; then 2–8 mg/min infusion or Nicardipine 5 mg/hr; titrate by 2.5 mg/hr every 5 min up to 15 mg/hr Uncontrolled by above measures: Nitroprusside 0.5 mcg/kg/min	Monitor blood pressure every 15 min during IV TPA treatment and then every 15 min for the next 2 hr; then every 30 min for 6 hr; then every 1 hr for 16 hr (first 24 hr after IV TPA)
Not eligible for IV TPA	< 220/120	Systolic > 220 or diastolic 121–140: Labetalol 10–20 mg IV over 1–2 min; may repeat every 10–20 min or Nicardipine 5 mg/hr; titrate by 2.5 mg/hr every 5 min up to 15 mg/hr Diastolic > 140: Nitroprusside 0.5 mcg/kg/min	Frequent monitoring of blood pressure with goal reduction of 10%–15% diastolic in first 24 hr

IV = intravenous(ly).

intraarterial TPA, mechanical clot aspiration (e.g., Penumbra device) or retrieval (e.g., Merci catheter, Trevo retriever, Solitaire stent retriever), and angioplasty and stenting. These interventions are often used in combination, and in addition to intravenous TPA. For instance, patients eligible for intravenous TPA may receive this intervention followed by endovascular treatment with intra-arterial TPA and clot retrieval. Although intravenous TPA is considered the "gold standard" for AIS, it may be less effective for certain types of strokes such as large middle cerebral artery (MCA) occlusions. Of note, the same "time is brain" principle also applies to any endovascular intervention.

Intra-arterial TPA

Patients with AIS may have a contraindication to intravenous TPA therapy, commonly presentation outside the time window for intravenous TPA window. Although intra-arterial TPA is not FDA approved for this indication, two clinical trials that used other fibrinolytic agents provide most of the (extrapolated) evidence for intra-arterial TPA. In the Prolyse in Acute Cerebral Thromboembolism II (PROACT II) study, patients who received recombinant pro-urokinase within 6 hours of symptom onset for MCA occlusions had improved modified Rankin scores at 90 days and better recanalization than control. Symptomatic ICH was numerically higher in the treatment group (10%) than in control (2%), but this was not statistically significant.[18] In the MELT (middle cerebral artery embolism local fibrinolytic intervention trial) study, patients who received urokinase within 6 hours of AIS were more likely to have modified Rankin scores of 0–1 (no significant disability) than was control. Symptomatic ICH occurred in 9% of patients, similar to that seen in PROACT II.[19] Current guidelines recommend intra-arterial fibrinolysis within 6 hours of symptom onset in patients with large MCA strokes who are ineligible for intravenous TPA (class I recommendation) and those with other types of stroke who have a contraindication to intravenous TPA (class IIa recommendation).[7]

Combination Intravenous Fibrinolysis and Endovascular Interventions

Patients with proximal cerebral artery occlusions (e.g., MCA) often have large clot burdens, greater neurologic deficits, and subsequently increased likelihood of intravenous TPA failure. In this setting, eligible patients receive intravenous TPA and then endovascular administration of intra-arterial TPA if necessary ("salvage" or "rescue" therapy). In the Interventional Management of Stroke (IMS)-1 and IMS-2 trials, patients presenting within 3 hours of symptom onset received a reduced dose of intravenous TPA 0.6 mg/kg (max of 60 mg), followed by intra-arterial TPA up to 22 mg administered by a standard microcatheter or the EKOS microinfusion catheter. Good clinical outcome was reported in both studies (modified Rankin score 0–2) as well as better outcomes than the placebo group from NINDS.[20,21] Rescue intra-arterial fibrinolysis is currently considered a reasonable approach in patients with large artery occlusion.[7]

As discussed previously, endovascular interventions are often used in combination. A recent multicenter randomized open-label Dutch study (MR CLEAN) compared endovascular therapy (intra-arterial fibrinolysis, mechanical treatment, or both) plus usual care (mostly intravenous TPA) with usual care alone.[22] Patients were required to receive intra-arterial treatment within 6 hours of symptom onset and have an occlusion of the distal intracranial carotid artery, MCA, or anterior cerebral artery. Intra-arterial fibrinolysis consisted of either alteplase or urokinase with maximum doses of 30 mg and 400,000 international units if intravenous TPA was given (87% of the intervention group). Most patients in the intervention group received mechanical intra-arterial therapy, although the proportion of patients who received intra-arterial fibrinolysis is unclear. At 90 days, 32.6% of patients were functionally independent (as defined by a modified Rankin score of 0–2) compared with only 19.1% in the usual care group. Symptomatic ICH was reported in 7.7% of patients in the intervention group compared with 6.4% of patients in the usual care group, which was not statistically significant and was similar to bleeding rates from studies of patients who received intravenous TPA only. Of note, 82% of patients in the intervention group from this study received treatment with "modern" retrievable stents, which are more effective than first-generation devices. Success of combination therapy has been confirmed in the ESCAPE (Endovascular treatment for Small Core and Anterior circulation Proximal occlusion with Emphasis on minimizing CT to recanalization times) and EXTEND-IA (Extending the Time for Thrombolysis in Emergency Neurological Deficits–Intra-arterial) studies because endovascular treatment (with primarily the Solitaire stent retrieval device) was superior to intravenous TPA alone.[23,24]

Early Antiplatelet Administration

The CAST (Chinese Acute Stroke Trial) and IST (International Stroke Trial) trials both reported a small benefit from aspirin 160–300 mg/day administered early during hospitalization for AIS.[25,26] Current recommendations are to administer aspirin 325 mg/day orally beginning within 48 hours of stroke onset.[7] In patients who receive fibrinolysis, an antithrombotic should not be initiated until 24 hours afterward, but may be initiated on hospital day 1 in patients who do not receive fibrinolysis. Patients who fail swallowing studies and have no enteral access may receive aspirin rectally. In patients with aspirin allergy, there is little evidence regarding alternative antiplatelet medications, but it is reasonable to administer clopidogrel with the understanding that a loading dose is necessary to rapidly achieve inhibition of platelet aggregation. Administration of antithrombotic medications by the end of hospital day 2 is a performance measure of the Joint Commission Stroke National Hospital Inpatient Quality Measures for certified stroke centers.

SUPPORTIVE CARE

Temperature Control

Fever is common in patients with AIS and has been associated with poor neurological outcomes. However, hypothermia may be neuroprotective by decreasing metabolic demand, acidosis, calcium influx, free radical production, and production of inflammatory cytokines and excitatory amino acids. Current recommendations are to lower body temperature in patients with a temperature greater than 38°C using antipyretic medications.[7] Surface cooling devices (e.g., Arctic Sun) may also be used in patients with fever who do not respond appropriately to medications. Induced hypothermia for the purpose of neuroprotection is not recommended because of a lack of robust clinical evidence.

Glucose Control

Hyperglycemia on admission and while in hospital has been associated with poor outcomes in AIS and may increase the risk of hemorrhagic conversion. Hypoglycemia may mimic stroke but, when prolonged, can also lead to ischemia and should be urgently treated in patients with AIS. The target blood glucose concentration is unclear, but current recommendations suggest a goal of 140–180 mg/dL.[7]

Intravenous Fluids

Most patients with AIS are either euvolemic or hypovolemic, the latter often requiring administration of intravenous fluids in the acute setting because of impaired swallowing or altered mental status. Hypovolemia may decrease cerebral perfusion and worsen ischemic injury, whereas hypervolemia may exacerbate ischemic brain edema and increase stress on the heart; therefore, euvolemia is recommended in patients with AIS. Intravenous solutions containing substantial amounts of free water (e.g., dextrose 5%, 0.45% sodium chloride) should be avoided because of the potential to increase brain swelling.[7]

Prophylaxis

Venous Thromboembolism

Deep venous thrombosis and pulmonary embolism are potential complications in patients with AIS, likely because of the combination of immobility and the presence of other risk factors for venous thromboembolism (VTE). Mechanical prophylaxis should be used in all patients with immobility and combined with pharmacologic prophylaxis, with the caveat that all anticoagulant medications should be held for 24 hours after fibrinolytic administration. One clinical trial found enoxaparin 40 mg daily to be superior to unfractionated heparin 5,000 units twice daily for the prevention of VTE in patients with AIS, but this trial has been criticized because of the small dose of heparin used.[27] In the absence of conclusive studies, either low-molecular-weight heparin or unfractionated heparin (5,000 units three times daily for most patients) is a reasonable option for VTE prophylaxis in patients with AIS.

Seizure

Seizures after AIS are less common than in patients with ICH, but the incidence may be increased in patients who have hemorrhagic transformation. It is currently not recommended to administer medications for seizure prophylaxis in patients with AIS.[7] Clinical seizures should be treated, and the risk of non-convulsive seizures should be appreciated in patients with neurological injuries.

INTRODUCTION: HEMORRHAGIC STROKE

Stroke consistently ranks as the second leading cause of death around the world, claiming 6.7 million lives in 2012.[28] Although hemorrhagic stroke accounts for 10%–20% of strokes, it appears to carry with it a higher mortality rate. One study in Denmark showed a 49.2% mortality in the hemorrhagic subcategory, whereas ischemic stroke had a mortality of 25.9%.[29] The National Stroke Association estimates that although hemorrhagic strokes account for only about 15% of strokes, more than 30% of stroke deaths can be attributed to hemorrhages.[30] A hemorrhagic stroke is defined by a cerebral blood vessel leaking blood into the brain and can be divided further into two categories: ICH and aneurysmal subarachnoid hemorrhage (aSAH). Intracerebral hemorrhage describes a vessel rupture in the brain parenchyma resulting in the formation of a hematoma.[31] In contrast, aSAH represents the subcategory of stroke that occurs when blood enters the subarachnoid space.[32] The focus of this chapter will be ICH.

Epidemiology, Incidence, and Risk

The incidence of ICH is about 24.6 per 100,000 person-years, making it the most common subtype of hemorrhagic stroke.[31] The yearly incidence in the United States is about 795,000 people per year, with most being new strokes.[33] Intracranial hemorrhage appears to be less common in women and has a strong association with age. Those 85 years and older appear to have an almost 10-fold higher yearly risk compared with those 45–54 years. Modifiable risk factors include hypertension (most important), smoking, alcohol use, diabetes mellitus, and anticoagulant/antiplatelet use. Of interest, lower cholesterol and triglyceride concentrations are associated with a higher risk. Other, non-modifiable risk factors include genetic predisposition, cerebral amyloid angiopathy, and Asian ethnicity.[31] The incidence of ICH secondary to hypertension has decreased over time because of better treatment, yet the overall incidence of ICH has remained steady throughout the years. This has been explained by the increasing incidence of ICH caused by anticoagulant use.[34]

Pathophysiology

Although the pathophysiology of hemorrhagic stroke is not quite as well defined as that of ischemic stroke, it is known that the damage is both mechanical and chemical. The mechanical damage is secondary to mass effect. A hemorrhage with a volume greater than 30 mL is associated with a significant increase in morbidity and mortality. Mass effect can lead to increased intracranial pressure (ICP), herniation, and death,[32,33] although the chemical changes occur secondary to the blood components and products of degradation.

Intracerebral hemorrhage occurs after a rupture of a cerebral artery leading to blood entering the parenchymal space. This can be secondary to a complication from a preexisting lesion (e.g., vascular malformation or tumor) and is called secondary ICH. A primary ICH is the result of a hemorrhage in the absence of a clear underlying lesion. Primary is the most common ICH subcategory.[31] As the hematoma starts to expand, there is an increase in ICP, causing a disruption in local tissue integrity and the blood-brain barrier. The hematoma also leads to an obstruction in venous outflow, thereby causing the release of tissue thromboplastin, leading to local coagulopathy. Cerebral edema then begins to form around the hematoma and can continue to develop over days after the initial insult. In up to 40% of cases, the hemorrhage extends into the cerebral ventricles, leading to another condition known as intraventricular hemorrhage, which is associated with a significantly worse prognosis. The onset of edema can cause mass effect in addition to the hematoma formation, leading to compression of local tissue and neurological dysfunction.[33]

Clinical Presentation, Diagnosis, and Severity

The patient with classic ICH presents with focal neurological deficits progressing over minutes to hours, rather than the typically more abrupt progression seen in AIS. The patient with ICH often has accompanying headache, nausea, vomiting, increased blood pressure, and decreased level of consciousness. The symptoms are typically because of an increase in ICP and evidenced from the Cushing triad (hypertension, bradycardia, irregular respiration). Often, dysautonomia accounting for hyperventilation, tachypnea, bradycardia, fever, hypertension (systolic blood pressure greater than 220 mm Hg), and hyperglycemia is also present.[33] Because the symptoms are relatively indistinct, neuroimaging is imperative to diagnosis. Computed tomography is considered the gold standard for identification and is very sensitive for acute hemorrhage identification. Although magnetic resonance imaging (MRI) can be as sensitive for acute identification, it is more sensitive for prior hemorrhage than is CT. However, time, cost, and patient tolerance are some of the considerations that can inhibit emergency MRI. Intracerebral hemorrhage is a medical emergency, and rapid deterioration is not uncommon within the hours after onset. It has been shown that more than 15% of patients have a GCS (Glasgow Coma Scale) score decrease of 2 points or more within the first hour of hospital presentation.[35,36]

Although there is no widely used standard of grading for the severity of ICH, the most widely validated scoring tool is the ICH score (Table 21.3). It represents a 6-point scale that stratifies the severity according to the five risk factors that were deemed independent 30-day mortality indicators. Table 21.4 represents the 30-day mortality associated with the scoring in the original trial.[37] Of note, no scoring system for ICH should be used as a solitary prognostic indicator.

Treatment

Anticoagulant Reversal

As mentioned before, although the incidence of stroke secondary to hypertension is decreasing because of better medical management, those presenting with hemorrhagic stroke secondary to oral anticoagulant use are now estimated to represent 12%–14% of patients with ICH. Therefore, identifying an underlying coagulopathy as a cause and risk of expansion should be at the forefront of the clinician's mind.

Vitamin K Antagonists

If the ICH is related to a vitamin K antagonist (VKA), vitamin K 5-10 mg intravenously should still be given for international normalized ratio (INR) reversal; however, the onset of even intravenous vitamin K typically begins at around 2 hours and therefore should not be used as the sole reversal agent, but should be part of the reversal algorithm for all VKA-related bleeds. Fresh frozen plasma (FFP), dosed at 10–15 mL/kg, was historically the adjunctive agent used with vitamin K in reversal of VKA, but its use is limited secondary to processing and thawing time, volume to be delivered, and immunologic reactions. The goal of INR reversal varies within the literature but ranges from less than 1.3 to less than 1.5.[35,38] In more recent years, especially with the addition of the non-vitamin K antagonist oral anticoagulants (NOACs), direct thrombin inhibitors and factor Xa inhibitors to the market, factor products have gained much attention in the treatment of these bleeds. Prothrombin complex concentrates (PCCs) are plasma-derived concentrates that were developed to treat hemophilia. Three-factor PCCs contain

Table 21.3 ICH Score

Component	Value Associated
GCS	
3–4	2
5–12	1
13–15	0
Volume, cm^3	
≥ 30	1
< 30	0
IVH	
Yes	1
No	0
Infratentorial origin	
Yes	1
No	0
Age, years	
≥ 80	1
< 80	0

GCS = Glasgow Coma Scale (score); IVH = intraventricular hemorrhage.

Table 21.4 30-Day Mortality Association with the ICH Score

Score	30-Day Mortality (%)	N
0	0	26
1	13	32
2	26	27
3	72	32
4	97	29
5	100	6
6	Unknown	0

factors II, IX, and X, whereas four-factor PCCs also contain factor VII. These products can rapidly be prepared for administration, do not require prolonged administration times, and do not have to be cross-matched, making them operationally advantageous to FFP. A study published in 2013 compared four-factor PCCs with FFP for emergency warfarin reversal with acute bleed (24 were patients with ICH) and found that the rate of achieving an INR less than 1.3 within 30 minutes was 62.2% and 9.6% for four-factor PCC and FFP, respectively.[39] The study also showed similar between-group thromboembolic event rates (7.8% PCC and 6.4% FFP) but described fluid overload more commonly in the FFP group (12.8% vs. 4.9%). However, the literature comparing three- and four-factor PCC is not abundant. A study published in 2015 comparing the effectiveness of three- and four-factor PCC showed that patients who received four-factor PCC and patients who had an INR reversal to 1.5 or less regardless of product were more likely to survive.[40] In the United States, four-factor PCC is labeled for use in emergency reversal of warfarin, and dosing can be found in Table 21.5.[41] However, of note, the four-factor product used in the United States does contain heparin and would be contraindicated in a patient with a history of heparin-induced thrombocytopenia; therefore, a three-factor PCC product (Profilnine) could be considered as an alternative because the three-factor product Bebulin also contains heparin. Recombinant activated factor VII (rFVIIa) would not be expected to restore the thrombin generation inhibited by a VKA as well as PCC because it does not contain all the inhibited factors and is therefore not recommended for routine use in warfarin reversal.[42,43] In addition, rFVIIa has been shown to have an increased risk of thromboembolic event,[44] and adding rFVIIa to a three-factor PCC product would not be recommended. A higher risk of thromboembolic events would also be expected when using activated PCCs (factor eight inhibitor bypassing activity [FEIBA]) because of their activated prothrombotic components.

Non-vitamin K Antagonist/NOACs

Although the literature describing the reversal of VKA provides needed guidance, the data describing the reversal of the NOACs is much less dense. Although PCC has been evaluated for use, the data are inconsistent. Increasing the levels of circulating factors is the rationale for using PCCs for VKA; however, in NOACs, the purpose of these products and of factor replacement, in general, is more an attempt to overcome the inhibition by creating a supranormal factor level.[45] One study that evaluated the use of four-factor PCC (50 units of factor IX per kilogram) did show a correction of the prolonged PT and abnormal endogenous thrombin potential in healthy subjects taking rivaroxaban.[46] However, the data regarding reversal of direct thrombin inhibitors (e.g., dabigatran) are not as convincing.[47] Activated PCCs (FEIBA) have also been studied for use in NOAC reversal and showed the ability to normalize abnormal thrombin generation times as well as reducing clot initiation time in patients receiving dabigatran. Therefore, it has been suggested that PCC has more of a role in reversal of factor Xa inhibitors, whereas patients with bleeds secondary to direct thrombin inhibitors may benefit from FEIBA (80 international units/kg).[47] These suggested antidotes for NOACs do not actually affect the ongoing inhibition of the drugs on factors IIa and Xa, and although they may limit the extent of bleeding, the actual outcome in relation to morbidity or mortality is likely minimal.[48] It is also prudent to note that if doses were recently ingested, charcoal may be an option, and dabigatran is not highly protein bound; therefore, circulating levels can be successfully removed by dialysis. In general, PCC and FEIBA are both reasonable options for the reversal of NOACs in the setting of life-threatening ICH. The results are preliminary, but FEIBA may be a better option in the setting of bleeding secondary to a direct thrombin inhibitor, whereas four-factor PCC may be a more appropriate first-line option for factor Xa inhibitors. Of note, use of these products for this indication is off-label, and consultation with a hematology service is recommended, if available, and reasonable in the setting of the emergency. Although the current options and data for NOAC reversal are not well researched, new targeted antidotes are on the horizon, with idarucizumab for dabigatran reversal gaining significant attention, having just gained accelerated approval by the FDA on October 16, 2015.[49]

Antiplatelet Reversal

Although anticoagulants have been reliably linked to ICH, the data are more conflicting on the effects of prior antiplatelet treatment. It has been shown that platelet transfusion within 12 hours of symptom onset is associated with smaller final hemorrhage and even level of independence at 3 months.[50] There are currently ongoing studies evaluating platelet transfusion in patients with ICH on prior antiplatelet therapy, which will hopefully elucidate the topic.

Table 21.5 Four-Factor PCC Dosing for Emergency VKA Reversal

INR before treatment	2 to ≤ 4	4–6	> 6
Dose (units of factor IX)/kg, maximum weight 100 kg	25	35	50

PCC = prothrombin complex concentrate; VKA = vitamin K antagonist.

Blood Pressure Management

It is unsurprising that elevated blood pressure is a common presentation in patients with ICH. This presentation can be related to persistent and pre-ICH elevations, as well as stress, pain, and increased ICP. Nonetheless, it is well documented that elevated systolic blood pressure is associated with hematoma expansion, neurological deterioration, and death or dependency after an event.[51-53] Although the safety and efficacy of systolic blood pressure lowering to 140 mm Hg or less has been well established in the literature,[54-57] there is only a paucity of data relating to the safety and efficacy of this goal for those presenting with a systolic blood pressure greater than 220 mm Hg. Nonetheless, it may still be reasonable to explore aggressive blood pressure lowering in those patients.[35] Reasonable options for initial blood pressure lowering include bolus doses of labetalol or hydralazine or more aggressive management by a nicardipine or esmolol infusion.[36]

Surgical Intervention

In addition to the medical interventions that can be made, surgical intervention is an option. Surgical interventions typically include clot removal or craniotomy. These procedures are typically reserved for rapidly deteriorating patients and are generally not recommended in early aggressive treatment of the non-rapidly deteriorating patient.[35]

Supportive Care

Location of Initial Care

It is recommended that the initial care of the patient with ICH occur in a dedicated stroke unit or an ICU. In fact, care in a dedicated unit has been shown to improve mortality.[58] Patients require close monitoring, and it is ideal to have staff trained specifically in the care of neurological injury.

Temperature Control

One parameter that should be monitored is temperature. A temperature fluctuation in the patient with ICH is a predictor of outcome, and fever is a common occurrence in these patients and may be an indicator of hematoma expansion or increased ICP.[59] Therefore, treatment of fever in patients with ICH is a reasonable clinical decision.[55] Although there is a paucity of data to suggest that cooling reduces edema, the treatment is still considered experimental at this time.[35]

VTE Prophylaxis

Patients presenting with an ICH are also at an increased risk of thromboembolic events, with women and African Americans being at the highest risk; therefore, consideration must be given to prevention of such complications during the patient's admission. It is generally accepted that these patients should use an intermittent pneumatic compression device in addition to compression stockings for prevention.[60-62] Although it may seem counterintuitive, these patients may also benefit from prophylaxis with low-molecular-weight or unfractionated heparin. A meta-analysis published in 2011 showed that early use of chemical thromboprophylaxis was associated with a reduction in pulmonary embolism. There was no difference in hematoma enlargement between groups.[35,63] The ideal timing of initiation of pharmacologic prophylaxis is unclear.

Glucose Management

Glucose monitoring is an important component of post-ICH management. Although clearly defined goals have not so far been established, both hyperglycemia and hypoglycemia are associated with worse outcomes. Therefore, therapy should be initiated to prevent hyperglycemia and hypoglycemia.[64,65]

Seizure Prophylaxis

Secondary to the neurologic nature of ICH injury, patients are at risk of seizures, and ICH has an early seizure (within 1 week) frequency of about 16%. Although antiepileptic drugs reduce the number of clinical seizures, this has yet to be associated with improved neurologic outcome or mortality. However, data suggest that prophylaxis with these medications (especially phenytoin) is associated with increased mortality and disability. Therefore, routine use of seizure prophylaxis is not currently recommended and should be used when patient examination indicates a suspicion of seizure.[35]

REFERENCES

1. Furie KL, Kasner SE, Adams RJ, et al. Guidelines for the prevention of stroke in patients with stroke or transient ischemic attack: a guideline for healthcare professionals from the American Heart Association/American Stroke Association. Stroke 2011;42:227-76.

2. Go AS, Mozaffarian D, Roger VL, et al. Heart disease and stroke statistics—2014 update: a report from the American Heart Association. Circulation 2014;129:e28-e292.

3. Varon J, Marik PE. The diagnosis and management of hypertensive crises. Chest 2000;118:214-27.

4. Hall MJ, Levant S, DeFrances CJ. Hospitalization for stroke in U.S. hospitals, 1989-2009. NCHS Data Brief 2012;95:1-8.

5. Maaijwee NA, Rutten-Jacobs LC, Schaapsmeerders P, et al. Ischaemic stroke in young adults: risk factors and long-term consequences. Nat Rev Neurol 2014;10:315-25.

6. Jauch EC, Cucchiara B, Adeoye O, et al. Part 11: adult stroke: 2010 American Heart Association guidelines for cardiopulmonary resuscitation and emergency cardiovascular care. Circulation 2010;122(18 suppl 3):S818-28.

7. Jauch EC, Saver JL, Adams HP Jr, et al. Guidelines for the early management of patients with acute ischemic stroke: a guideline for healthcare professionals from the American

Heart Association/American Stroke Association. Stroke 2013;44:870-947.

8. Hacke W, Kaste M, Bluhmki E, et al. Thrombolysis with alteplase 3 to 4.5 hours after acute ischemic stroke. N Engl J Med 2008;359:1317-29.

9. Francart SJ, Hawes EM, Deal AM, et al. Performance of coagulation tests in patients on therapeutic doses of rivaroxaban. A cross-sectional pharmacodynamic study based on peak and trough plasma levels. Thromb Haemost 2014;111:1133-40.

10. Tissue plasminogen activator for acute ischemic stroke. The National Institute of Neurological Disorders and Stroke rt-PA Stroke Study Group. N Engl J Med 1995;333:1581-7.

11. Katzan IL, Furlan AJ, Lloyd LE, et al. Use of tissue-type plasminogen activator for acute ischemic stroke: the Cleveland area experience. JAMA 2000;283:1151-8.

12. Fugate JE, Kalimullah EA, Wijdicks EF. Angioedema after tPA: what neurointensivists should know. Neurocrit Care 2012;16:440-3.

13. Maertins M, Wold R, Swider M. Angioedema after administration of tPA for ischemic stroke: case report. Air Med J 2011;30:276-8.

14. Tanswell P, Modi N, Combs D, et al. Pharmacokinetics and pharmacodynamics of tenecteplase in fibrinolytic therapy of acute myocardial infarction. Clin Pharmacokinet 2002;41:1229-45.

15. Parsons M, Spratt N, Bivard A, et al. A randomized trial of tenecteplase versus alteplase for acute ischemic stroke. N Engl J Med 2012;366:1099-107.

16. Logallo N, Kvistad CE, Nacu A, et al. The Norwegian tenecteplase stroke trial (NOR-TEST): randomised controlled trial of tenecteplase vs. alteplase in acute ischaemic stroke. BMC Neurol 2014;14:106-2377-14-106.

17. Albers GW, von Kummer R, Truelsen T, et al. Safety and efficacy of desmoteplase given 3-9 h after ischaemic stroke in patients with occlusion or high-grade stenosis in major cerebral arteries (DIAS-3): a double-blind, randomised, placebo-controlled phase 3 trial. Lancet Neurol 2015;14:575-84.

18. Furlan A, Higashida R, Wechsler L, et al. Intra-arterial prourokinase for acute ischemic stroke. the PROACT II study: a randomized controlled trial. prolyse in acute cerebral thromboembolism. JAMA 1999;282:2003-11.

19. Ogawa A, Mori E, Minematsu K, et al. Randomized trial of intraarterial infusion of urokinase within 6 hours of middle cerebral artery stroke: the middle cerebral artery embolism local fibrinolytic intervention trial (MELT) Japan. Stroke 2007;38:2633-9.

20. IMS Study Investigators. Combined intravenous and intra-arterial recanalization for acute ischemic stroke: the interventional management of stroke study. Stroke 2004;35:904-11.

21. IMS II Trial Investigators. The interventional management of stroke (IMS) II study. Stroke 2007;38:2127-35.

22. Berkhemer OA, Fransen PS, Beumer D, et al. A randomized trial of intraarterial treatment for acute ischemic stroke. N Engl J Med 2015;372:11-20.

23. Campbell BC, Mitchell PJ, Kleinig TJ, et al. Endovascular therapy for ischemic stroke with perfusion-imaging selection. N Engl J Med 2015;372:1009-18.

24. Goyal M, Demchuk AM, Menon BK, et al. Randomized assessment of rapid endovascular treatment of ischemic stroke. N Engl J Med 2015;372:1019-30.

25. CAST: randomised placebo-controlled trial of early aspirin use in 20,000 patients with acute ischaemic stroke. CAST (Chinese Acute Stroke Trial) collaborative group. Lancet 1997;349:1641-9.

26. The International Stroke Trial (IST): a randomised trial of aspirin, subcutaneous heparin, both, or neither among 19435 patients with acute ischaemic stroke. International Stroke Trial Collaborative Group. Lancet 1997;349:1569-81.

27. Sherman DG, Albers GW, Bladin C, et al. The efficacy and safety of enoxaparin versus unfractionated heparin for the prevention of venous thromboembolism after acute ischaemic stroke (PREVAIL study): an open-label randomised comparison. Lancet 2007;369:1347-55.

28. World Health Organization. The Top 10 Causes of Death 2014. Available at www.who.int/mediacentre/factsheets/fs310/en/index4.html. Accessed October 14, 2015.

29. Andersen KK, Olsen TS, Dehlendorff C, et al. Hemorrhagic and ischemic strokes compared: stroke severity, mortality, and risk factors. Stroke 2009;40:2068-72.

30. National Stroke Association. Hemorrhagic Stroke Fact Sheet. 2009. Available at www.stroke.org/stroke-resources/library/hemorrhagic-stroke. Accessed October 14, 2015.

31. Ikram MA, Wieberdink RG, Koudstaal PJ. International epidemiology of intracerebral hemorrhage. Curr Atheroscler Rep 2012;14:300-6.

32. Fagan SC, Hess DC. Stroke. In: DiPiro JT, Talbert RL, Yee GC, et al., eds. Pharmacotherapy: A Pathophysiologic Approach. New York: McGraw-Hill, 2008:373-81.

33. Magistris F, Bazak S, Martin J. Intracerebral hemorrhage: pathophysiology, diagnosis and management. MUMJ 2013;10:15-22.

34. Lovelock CE, Molyneux AJ, Rothwell PM. Change in incidence and aetiology of intracerebral haemorrhage in Oxfordshire, UK, between 1981 and 2006: a population-based study. Lancet Neurol 2007;6:487-93.

35. Hemphill JC III, Greenberg SM, Anderson CS, et al. Guidelines for the management of spontaneous intracerebral hemorrhage: a guideline for healthcare professionals from the American Heart Association/American Stroke Association. Stroke 2015;46:2032-60.

36. Morgenstern LB, Hemphill JC III, Anderson C, et al. Guidelines for the management of spontaneous intracerebral hemorrhage: a guideline for healthcare professionals from the American Heart Association/American Stroke Association. Stroke 2010;41:2108-29.

37. Hemphill JC III, Bonovich DC, Besmertis L, et al. The ICH score: a simple, reliable grading scale for intracerebral hemorrhage. Stroke 2001;32:891-7.

38. Connolly ES Jr, Rabinstein AA, Carhuapoma JR, et al. Guidelines for the management of aneurysmal subarachnoid hemorrhage: a guideline for healthcare professionals from the American Heart Association/American Stroke Association. Stroke 2012;43:1711-37.

39. Sarode R, Milling TJ Jr, Refaai MA, et al. Efficacy and safety of a 4-factor prothrombin complex concentrate in patients on vitamin K antagonists presenting with major bleeding: a

40. Voils SA, Holder MC, Premraj S, et al. Comparative effectiveness of 3- versus 4-factor prothrombin complex concentrate for emergent warfarin reversal. Thromb Res 2015;136:595-8.

41. Behring C. Frequently Asked Questions 2014. Available at www.kcentra.com/professional/resources/frequently-asked-questions.aspx?role=pharmacist.

42. Rosovsky RP, Crowther MA. What is the evidence for the off-label use of recombinant factor VIIa (rFVIIa) in the acute reversal of warfarin? ASH evidence-based review 2008. Hematology Am Soc Hematol Educ Program 2008:36-8.

43. Tanaka KA, Szlam F, Dickneite G, Levy JH. Effects of prothrombin complex concentrate and recombinant activated factor VII on vitamin K antagonist induced anticoagulation. Thromb Res 2008;122:117-23.

44. Mayer SA, Brun NC, Begtrup K, et al. Recombinant activated factor VII for acute intracerebral hemorrhage. N Engl J Med 2005;352:777-85.

45. Dickneite G, Hoffman M. Reversing the new oral anticoagulants with prothrombin complex concentrates (PCCs): what is the evidence? Thromb Haemost 2014;111:189-98.

46. Eerenberg ES, Kamphuisen PW, Sijpkens MK, et al. Reversal of rivaroxaban and dabigatran by prothrombin complex concentrate: a randomized, placebo-controlled, crossover study in healthy subjects. Circulation 2011;124:1573-9.

47. Siegal DM, Cuker A. Reversal of novel oral anticoagulants in patients with major bleeding. J Thromb Thrombolysis 2013;35:391-8.

48. Lazo-Langner A, Lang ES, Douketis J. Clinical review: clinical management of new oral anticoagulants: a structured review with emphasis on the reversal of bleeding complications. Crit Care 2013;17:230.

49. Pollack CV Jr, Reilly PA, Eikelboom J, et al. Idarucizumab for dabigatran reversal. N Engl J Med 2015;373:511-20.

50. Naidech AM, Liebling SM, Rosenberg NF, et al. Early platelet transfusion improves platelet activity and may improve outcomes after intracerebral hemorrhage. Neurocrit Care 2012;16:82-7.

51. Rodriguez-Luna D, Pineiro S, Rubiera M, et al. Impact of blood pressure changes and course on hematoma growth in acute intracerebral hemorrhage. Eur J Neurol 2013;20:1277-83.

52. Sakamoto Y, Koga M, Yamagami H, et al. Systolic blood pressure after intravenous antihypertensive treatment and clinical outcomes in hyperacute intracerebral hemorrhage: the stroke acute management with urgent risk-factor assessment and improvement-intracerebral hemorrhage study. Stroke 2013;44:1846-51.

53. Zhang Y, Reilly KH, Tong W, et al. Blood pressure and clinical outcome among patients with acute stroke in Inner Mongolia, China. J Hypertens 2008;26:1446-52.

54. Anderson CS, Heeley E, Huang Y, et al. Rapid blood-pressure lowering in patients with acute intracerebral hemorrhage. N Engl J Med 2013;368:2355-65.

55. Anderson CS, Huang Y, Wang JG, et al. Intensive blood pressure reduction in acute cerebral haemorrhage trial (INTERACT): a randomised pilot trial. Lancet Neurol 2008;7:391-9.

56. Arima H, Huang Y, Wang JG, et al. Earlier blood pressure-lowering and greater attenuation of hematoma growth in acute intracerebral hemorrhage: INTERACT pilot phase. Stroke 2012;43:2236-8.

57. Qureshi AI, Palesch YY, Martin R, et al. Effect of systolic blood pressure reduction on hematoma expansion, perihematomal edema, and 3-month outcome among patients with intracerebral hemorrhage: results from the antihypertensive treatment of acute cerebral hemorrhage study. Arch Neurol 2010;67:570-6.

58. Diringer MN, Edwards DF. Admission to a neurologic/neurosurgical intensive care unit is associated with reduced mortality rate after intracerebral hemorrhage. Crit Care Med 2001;29:635-40.

59. Schwarz S, Hafner K, Aschoff A, et al. Incidence and prognostic significance of fever following intracerebral hemorrhage. Neurology 2000;54:354-61.

60. Dennis M, Sandercock P, Reid J, et al. Effectiveness of intermittent pneumatic compression in reduction of risk of deep vein thrombosis in patients who have had a stroke (CLOTS 3): a multicentre randomised controlled trial. Lancet 2013;382:516-24.

61. Dennis M, Sandercock P, Reid J, et al. The effect of graduated compression stockings on long-term outcomes after stroke: the CLOTS trials 1 and 2. Stroke 2013;44:1075-9.

62. Dennis M, Sandercock PA, Reid J, et al. Effectiveness of thigh-length graduated compression stockings to reduce the risk of deep vein thrombosis after stroke (CLOTS trial 1): a multicentre, randomised controlled trial. Lancet 2009;373:1958-65.

63. Paciaroni M, Agnelli G, Venti M, et al. Efficacy and safety of anticoagulants in the prevention of venous thromboembolism in patients with acute cerebral hemorrhage: a meta-analysis of controlled studies. J Thromb Haemost 2011;9:893-8.

64. Oddo M, Schmidt JM, Carrera E, et al. Impact of tight glycemic control on cerebral glucose metabolism after severe brain injury: a microdialysis study. Crit Care Med 2008;36:3233-8.

65. Fogelholm R, Murros K, Rissanen A, et al. Admission blood glucose and short term survival in primary intracerebral haemorrhage: a population-based study. J Neurol Neurosurg Psychiatry 2005;76:349-53.

Chapter 22
Critical Care Management of Aneurysmal Subarachnoid Hemorrhage

Denise H. Rhoney, Pharm.D., FCCP, FCCM, FNCS; Kathryn Morbitzer, Pharm.D.; and J. Dedrick Jordan, M.D., Ph.D.

LEARNING OBJECTIVES

1. Describe the epidemiology and risk factors of aneurysmal subarachnoid hemorrhage (aSAH).
2. Explain the complex pathophysiological mechanisms of early brain injury and delayed cerebral ischemia.
3. Discuss the clinical presentation of patients with aSAH and clinical severity scores.
4. Outline the predictors of outcome after aSAH.
5. Recognize the common neurological and medical complications associated with aSAH.
6. Develop an evidence-based treatment plan for preventing and treating each neurological and medical complication.

ABBREVIATIONS IN THIS CHAPTER

aSAH	Aneurysmal subarachnoid hemorrhage	GCS	Glasgow Coma Scale
CPP	Cerebral perfusion pressure	ICP	Intracranial pressure
CSF	Cerebrospinal fluid	ICU	Intensive care unit
DCI	Delayed cerebral ischemia	TCD	Transcranial Doppler
DVT	Deep venous thrombosis		

INTRODUCTION

Subarachnoid hemorrhage refers to bleeding that occurs in the subarachnoid space, between the pia and the arachnoid membranes, and can be spontaneous or secondary to trauma. The focus of this chapter will be spontaneous subarachnoid hemorrhage, which is caused by the rupture of a saccular aneurysm in 80% of cases. Aneurysmal subarachnoid hemorrhage (aSAH) accounts for about 7% of all strokes and is associated with high morbidity and mortality.[1] The disease course can be prolonged and can be associated with serious neurological and medical complications that compromise patient outcomes. The clinical effects of aSAH are biphasic, consisting of early brain injury as a result of the initial impact of the hemorrhage, followed by several secondary pathophysiological events. As a result, patients are routinely admitted to an intensive care unit (ICU) and are ideally cared for by a multidisciplinary care team.

Epidemiology

The annual incidence of aSAH varies widely in different regions of the world, from 2 to 20 cases per 100,000.[2] Studies from the World Health Organization report an age-adjusted annual incidence of 2 cases per 100,000 population in China to 22.5 cases per 100,000 in Finland.[1] Overall, the incidence is higher in Finland and Japan and lower in South and Central America. In the United States, the incidence is estimated at 14.5 cases per 100,000 annually.[3] This may be an underestimate, however, because up to 15% of patients die before receiving medical care.[2]

The incidence of aSAH is reported to be 1.24 times (95% confidence interval [CI], 1.09–1.42) higher in women than in men and increases with age, with the typical age of onset at 50 years or older.[1,3,4] Race and ethnicity also affect aSAH incidence, with African Americans and Hispanics having a higher incidence than white Americans.[5]

Risk Factors

Independent modifiable risk factors include hypertension, smoking, alcohol use, and use of sympathomimetic drugs, whereas nonmodifiable risk factors include sex, age, size of aneurysm, and family history.[6,7] When assessing risk factors, it is important to consider the risk factors for aneurysm formation and growth together with aSAH.

Cigarette smoking has been identified as an important risk factor for aneurysm formation, growth, and rupture.[6,8-10] Hypertension can be considered a significant risk factor for aSAH but may be less of a risk than in other types of stroke. Data on the role of hypertension on aneurysm formation and growth are inconsistent; however, hypertension should be treated for many other reasons, and in doing so, the risk of aSAH may be reduced. If the systolic blood pressure exceeds 130 mm Hg, the risk is twice as high, and if the systolic blood pressure is above 170 mm Hg, the risk is 3 times as high.[6,10,11] The role of alcohol use is a less-established risk factor than cigarette smoking, with several studies showing that excessive alcohol consumption (greater than 150 g/week) increases the risk of aSAH.[9,10] More traditional cardiovascular risk factors like diabetes and hypercholesterolemia have a less-defined relationship for aSAH or aneurysm formation and growth.

A family history of intracranial aneurysms suggests a genetic component to this disease. Siblings of patients with aSAH have a 6-fold increased risk of developing aSAH, and there is a 3–7 times higher risk in first-degree relatives of patients with aSAH than in the general population.[12] Familial aneurysms are usually larger at the time of rupture and are more likely located in the middle cerebral artery; also, the age at presentation is typically younger.[12] Other risk factors for forming intracranial aneurysms include sickle cell disease, α_2-antitrypsin deficiency, polycystic kidney disease, and inheritable connective tissue disorders (e.g., fibromuscular dysplasia).

Outcomes

Although mortality rates have declined throughout the past 3 decades, aSAH remains a devastating neurological disease. Estimations of current mortality rates show that 10%–15% of patients die before reaching the hospital, whereas 40% die within the first week and 50% die within the first 6 months. Rebleeding also carries a high mortality rate of 51%–80%.[13] Of those who survive, up to 50% have some degree of cognitive dysfunction long term.[14] Survivors commonly have deficits in memory, executive function, and language that significantly affect their day-to-day function. These deficits in cognition are further compounded by anxiety, depression, fatigue, and sleep disturbances.[15] The most important predictive factors for an acute prognosis after aSAH include the following[16-19]:

- Level of consciousness and neurological grade on admission
- Patient age (younger patients do better)
- Amount of blood on the initial head computed tomography (CT) scan and location of blood (presence of intraventricular hemorrhage carries a worse prognosis)
- Presence of comorbid conditions and the hospital course (e.g., infections, myocardial ischemia, anemia)
- Location of aneurysm (anterior circulation aneurysms carry a more favorable prognosis)
- Aneurysm rebleeding
- Global cerebral edema
- Hyperglycemia

The rebleeding rate is 2%–4% within the first 24 hours and 15%–20% within the first 2 weeks if the aneurysm is not secured and is a significant cause of poor outcomes early on. Factors associated with poor outcomes that develop later include cerebral infarction, delayed cerebral ischemia (DCI), fever, and use of anticonvulsant agents, particularly phenytoin.[16]

PATHOPHYSIOLOGY

Aneurysm Formation

The pathogenesis of intracranial aneurysms is complex. Historically, congenital causes were thought to play a major role in aneurysm development; however, only 10% of cases appear to be attributable to genetic/familial causes. The current theory is that aneurysms develop gradually throughout an individual's lifetime because of acquired changes in the intracranial arterial wall. In patients without the previously discussed risk factors, the prevalence of aneurysms is only 2.3%.[20] Inflammation may also play a role in aneurysm formation, with several inflammatory cytokines being implicated in endothelial injury and remodeling.[21] Inflammation is becoming an attractive therapeutic target because aspirin may reduce the rate of aneurysm rupture, given its anti-inflammatory properties; however, more definitive studies are required.[22]

Saccular or berry aneurysms account for 80% of aSAH cases and are specific to intracranial arteries because their walls lack an external elastic lamina and contain a very thin adventitia. Rupture of arteriovenous malformations is the second most identifiable cause of aSAH, accounting for 10% of cases. The remaining cases can result from rupture of these pathologic entities: mycotic aneurysm, angioma, neoplasm, or cortical thrombosis.

The circle of Willis is the most common area in the cerebral circulation for the development of cerebral aneurysms (see Figure 22.1). The bifurcations of these major vessels are particularly vulnerable to aneurysm formation because of hemodynamic factors such as wall sheer stress and mechanical stretch.[23] Most ruptured aneurysms (89%) arise from the anterior circulation.[24] In 25% of cases, aneurysms are present.

Most aneurysms do not rupture according to radiographic and autopsy studies, which report a higher incidence of intracranial saccular aneurysms than of aSAH.[25] The probability of rupture is related to the tension on the artery wall and is directly related to the aneurysm size. Aneurysms with a diameter of 5 mm or less have a 2.5% risk of rupture, whereas 41% of those with a diameter of 6–10 mm have already ruptured on diagnosis. Aneurysms larger than 10 mm in diameter are 5 times more likely to rupture than small aneurysms. The annual risk of rupture for aneurysms less than 10 mm is 0.7%. The exact mechanism for aneurysm rupture is not fully understood, but it may be precipitated in activities that result in a sudden increase in arterial blood pressure (e.g., sneezing, exercise, sexual intercourse) in less than one-third of cases.[26]

Early Brain Injury

Early brain injury has been used to describe the mechanisms of acute (first 72 hours) neurological deterioration after aSAH and is the result of physiological derangements such as increased intracranial pressure (ICP), decreased cerebral blood flow, and global cerebral ischemia. These physiologic derangements result in blood-brain barrier dysfunction, inflammation, and oxidative cascades that lead to neuronal cell death. The consequences can result in death or severe neurological deficits. Although vasospasm is thought to be the main cause of clinical deterioration after aSAH, more recent thinking has focused on the fact that vasospasm is not the only pathophysiological factor contributing to poor patient outcomes.[27] Recently, a study showed an increase in the neuroinflammatory response after aSAH at days 2–3 with no evidence angiographically of vasospasm, and this response was associated with a poor outcome at 3 months.[28] Evidence also suggests that the cascade of events set in motion in early brain injury contributes to the delayed neurological deterioration traditionally attributed to vasospasm.[27] Figure 22.2 describes the complex pathophysiological events after aSAH that lead to early brain injury and DCI.

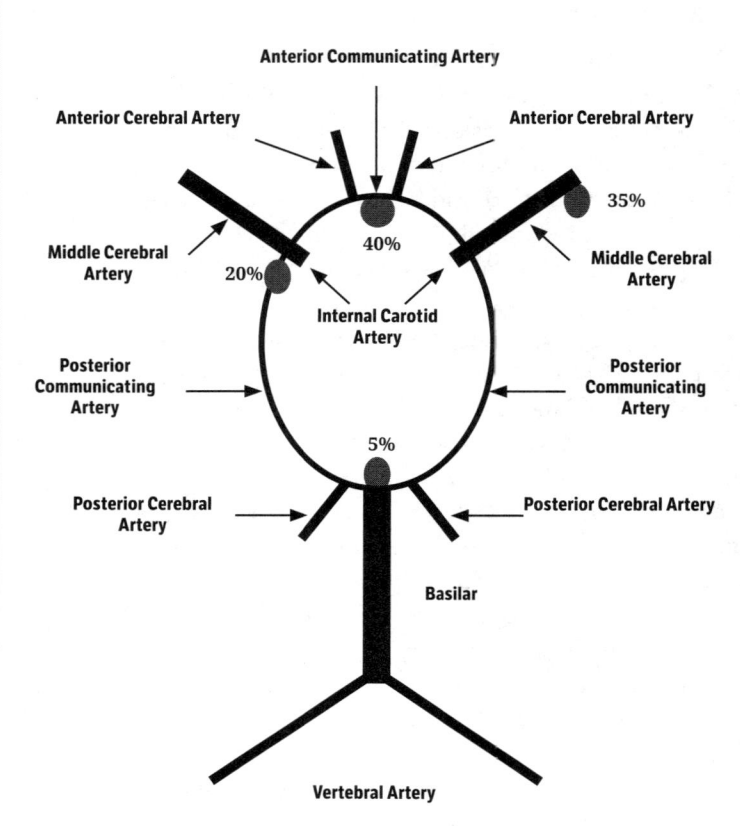

Figure 22.1 Location of aneurysm responsible for subarachnoid hemorrhage in the "circle of Willis." Most (85%) saccular aneurysms arise in the vessels that constitute the circle of Willis at the base of the brain. The anterior circulation comprises the anterior cerebral arteries that are joined by a single anterior communicating artery that is paired with the internal carotid arteries. Most aneurysms are within the anterior circulation. The posterior circulation is composed of the posterior communicating arteries that are paired with the posterior cerebral arteries that originate at the bifurcation of the basilar terminus of the basilar artery.

Early brain injury starts with the initial response of increased ICP because of the blood in the subarachnoid space and sometimes the cerebral ventricle and brain parenchyma. The quantity of the initial bleed drives the degree of ICP elevation the patient experiences. With this increase in ICP, the cerebral perfusion pressure (CPP) decreases, causing cerebral ischemia through a reduction in cerebral blood flow because cerebral autoregulation may be disturbed. The presence of blood and its degraded products in the cerebral ventricles produces obstructive hydrocephalus, which also results in an increase in ICP. As a result, global ischemia may occur, which produces oxidative damage to neural tissue and then neuronal death. Oxidative mediators can also disrupt the blood-brain barrier and lead to the production of cytotoxic cerebral edema, which results in more ischemia.[27] The global ischemia experienced varies in severity, with about 30% of patients having necrosis throughout the brain and the remainder, a degree of ischemia not as severe but in which both apoptosis and necrosis may be present. Overall, brain injury occurs from transient global ischemia and from the direct effects of the intracranial blood.

The ischemic insults to the brain after aSAH stimulate several complex pathways that can lead to stimulation of apoptotic mechanisms in the hippocampus, blood-brain barrier, and vasculature, resulting in early brain injury. Some of the proposed different mechanisms for early brain injury include nitric oxide dysregulation, oxidative injury, generation of matrix metalloproteinase-9, modulation of nuclear factor erythroid-2 related factor 2 and antioxidant-response element pathway, interleukin-1 beta activation, vascular endothelial growth factor, activation of c-Jun N-terminal kinase pathway, mitogen-activation protein kinase, and iron overload.[29-33] Currently, interventions targeting early brain injury are mainly experimental, but they deserve further investigation because the cerebral infarction that occurs in aSAH not only occurs after vasospasm but also as a result of the physiologic changes that occur with the initial bleed.

Delayed Neurological Deterioration

Neurological worsening that occurs days after aSAH can be ascribed to DCI (see Figure 22.2). Throughout the literature, various terms are used that may be confused as being interchangeable: symptomatic vasospasm, DCI, and angiographic vasospasm. Delayed cerebral ischemia is a clinical syndrome that encompasses symptomatic deterioration in the neurological examination together with radiographic evidence of ischemia or infarction.[34] Not all patients with DCI have angiographic vasospasm, and not all patients with angiographic spasm have DCI. Delayed cerebral ischemia occurs in about 30% of patients 3–14 days after the initial hemorrhage and is the most important cause of mortality and morbidity in the patients who survive the initial bleed.[35]

Angiographic vasospasm occurs within 3–14 days after aneurysm rupture in almost 70% of patients, 30% of whom develop significant global or focal neurological deficits.[36] The severity and duration of vasospasm are related to the thickness, density, location, and persistence of the subarachnoid blood.[37] The most likely mechanism for development is an inflammatory reaction in the blood vessel wall. Extravasated blood and its by-products in the cerebrospinal fluid (CSF) are thought to be responsible for this complication. Many spasmogens such as oxyhemoglobin, histamine, eicosanoids, endothelin, nitrous

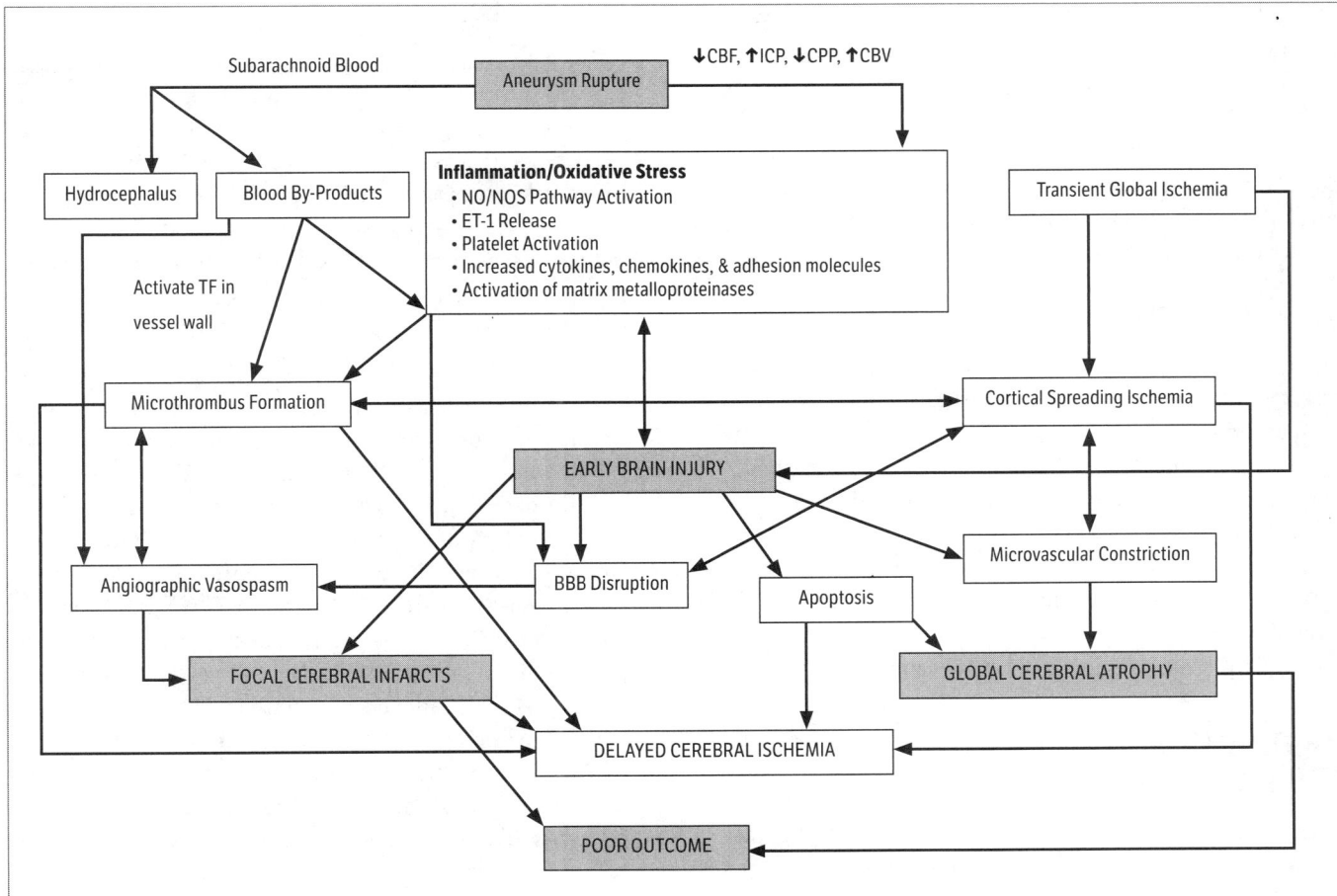

Figure 22.2 Pathophysiology of early brain injury and delayed cerebral ischemia after aSAH. The etiology starts with early brain injury as a result of the initial bleeding event, leading to transient global cerebral ischemia. This process starts a complex cascade of pathophysiological changes leading to secondary brain injury.

aSAH = aneurysmal subarachnoid hemorrhage; BBB = blood-brain barrier; CBF = cerebral blood flow; CBV = cerebral blood volume; CPP = cerebral perfusion pressure; ET-1 = endothelin-A; ICP = intracranial pressure; NO = nitric oxide; NOS = nitric oxide synthase; TF = tissue factor.

oxide, and 2-hydrosy-3-methylglutarylcoenayme have been implicated in the development of vasospasm. These spasmogenic substances cause endothelial damage and smooth muscle contraction and can result in cerebral hypoperfusion, DCI, and infarction.[38] The true connection between vasospasm and DCI is under question because interventions have shown that significant reductions in angiographic vasospasm do not improve outcome.[39] Clinical and physiological factors that influence whether angiographic vasospasm causes cerebral infarction include genetic variations (*APOE* [apolipoprotein E] alleles, polymorphisms of *eNOS* [endothelial nitric oxide synthase] and plasminogen activator inhibitor-1), epigenetic variations, DNA polymorphisms, cerebral metabolic demand, autoregulation, variations in collateral and anastomotic blood flow, cardiac output, and ICP.[27]

Angiographic vasospasm may be associated with DCI, but other pathophysiological factors may also play a role in DCI development such as microthrombosis, cortical spreading ischemia, microcirculatory constriction, and apoptosis.[27] Nimodipine is currently the only pharmacologic agent that has shown an improvement in outcome after aSAH, and it is indicated for use by the U.S. Food and Drug Administration (FDA). In clinical trials, nimodipine did not show a significant improvement in angiographic vasospasm, which led to other theories surrounding the benefit of this agent. It is proposed that nimodipine slightly attenuates vasospasm but also inhibits cortical spreading ischemia and reduces microthrombi through its fibrinolytic activity.[27]

Systemic Effects

The extent of injury after aSAH also affects other organ systems like the heart and lung. There is an increase in sympathetic nervous system activity that can contribute to the development of acute lung injury, pulmonary edema, and cardiac dysfunction (takotsubo cardiomyopathy, stunned myocardium, ECG changes).[40] The most prevalent systemic response that occurs in up to 60% of patients with aSAH is a systemic inflammatory response characterized by increased or decreased body temperature, tachypnea, tachycardia, and leukocytosis or leukopenia.[41]

CARE SETTINGS AND MULTIDISCIPLINARY TEAM

Aneurysmal subarachnoid hemorrhage is a complex disease with a prolonged course that requires expertise from a multidisciplinary team. Ideally, the management of patients with aSAH should take place in a neuro-ICU or an ICU similarly equipped that treats a high volume of patients with aSAH. The available data analyses show that high-volume centers (defined as greater than 60 cases per year) had the best outcomes and that low-volume centers with less than 20 cases per year had the worst outcomes.[42,43] The most recent guidelines by both the Neurocritical Care Society (NCS) Multidisciplinary Consensus Conference and the American Heart Association/American Stroke Association (AHA/ASA) recommend that patients with aSAH be treated at high-volume centers and that low-volume hospitals consider early transfer of these patients to high-volume centers.[44,45] A multidisciplinary neurocritical care team in a specialized neuro-ICU is independently associated with improved hospital discharge disposition for patients with aSAH.[46] This improved outcome may not be a result of the single addition of any type of personnel; rather, it may be the overall impact of a consistent and organized approach to patient management that contributes to improved outcomes.

INITIAL STABILIZATION IN EMERGENCY DEPARTMENT

Clinical Features

The clinical presentation of aSAH can vary dramatically from what is described as "the worst headache of my life" to coma or death. Often, patients have nausea, vomiting, neck stiffness, and photophobia in addition to the sudden-onset severe headache. With more severe presentations, patients may have an altered level of consciousness with states of confusion, lethargy, or coma. Furthermore, focal neurological deficits such as motor weakness, aphasia, special neglect, or cranial nerve palsies may be present. Commonly, patients may have had a severe headache similar in nature several days before presentation, which has been termed a *sentinel bleed*.

Diagnostic Approaches to aSAH

The diagnosis of aSAH must be considered when patients present with the classic symptoms; however, because many of the symptoms are nonspecific, the diagnosis is commonly missed on initial presentation to a medical provider.[47] Because patients who are initially misdiagnosed have a higher rate of complications, an accurate and sensitive workup must be initiated at presentation.[48]

The sensitivity for noncontrast head CT has been validated and is 98%–100% within 12 hours from onset and 93% at 24 hours.[49,50] After 3 days, however, the sensitivity decreases to 73% and after 7 days, to 50%, which results in a high likelihood of a false-negative study.[49,50] If the clinical suspicion is high, a lumbar puncture to evaluate for xanthochromia is warranted. This should be done at least 12 hours after the onset of headache for a negative study to be valid because it takes this amount of time for xanthochromia to develop from red blood cell breakdown.[47] Magnetic resonance imaging (MRI) is up to 100% sensitive in the detection of aSAH and can be considered as an alternative to lumbar puncture; however, it is not available at many hospitals and is not cost-effective.[51] For patients in whom the diagnosis of aSAH has not been effectively ruled out, a further imaging study is required. Computed tomography angiography, a high-resolution CT scan of the cerebral arteries that is obtained after intravenous contrast injection, is comparable with the gold standard procedure, digital subtraction angiography of the cerebral blood vessels.[52] When an aneurysm is not identified in this circumstance, repeat imaging in a delayed fashion after 1–2 weeks is supported, given that an undetected untreated aneurysm has high morbidity and mortality.[53]

Clinical Severity Scores

Many scoring algorithms have been developed with the aim of predicting the outcome and risk of neurological complications after aSAH (Table 22.1). The most widely used clinical scoring systems to predict outcome include the Hunt and Hess score and the World Federation of Neurological Surgeons score. With both scales, the higher the score, the higher the likelihood of a poor outcome.[54,55] The Hunt and Hess score is an ordinal scale from 1 to 5 that is based on the level of consciousness as well as focal neurological deficits. Patients who score a 1 are asymptomatic or have a mild headache, whereas those who score a 5 are comatose with reflexive motor response only. The World Federation of Neurological Surgeons score is based on two components: the overall neurological status according to the Glasgow Coma Scale (GCS), range 3–15, and the absence or presence of motor deficits. Patients with a normal GCS of 15 and no neurological deficits are given a score of I, whereas those with a GCS score of 3–6 with or without motor deficits are given a V.

The Fisher grade was developed to predict the risk of cerebral vasospasm after aSAH according to the amount of blood revealed on head CT at presentation.[37] Patients with no hemorrhage or with a hemorrhage of minimal thickness have a very low rate of vasospasm, whereas those with a hemorrhage greater than 1 mm in thickness have a high rate of developing clinical vasospasm and a worse outcome.[37,56]

MANAGEMENT AND PREVENTION OF NEUROLOGICAL COMPLICATIONS

The primary strategies used in the management of aSAH are to provide initial supportive therapy and to prevent both neurological and medical complications (see Table 22.2 and Table 22.3).

Rebleeding

Recurrent bleeding of an aneurysm after the initial hemorrhage is often fatal, and early measures should be in place to reduce this risk.[57] The highest risk is within the

continued on page 425

Table 22.1 Aneurysmal Subarachnoid Hemorrhage Grading Scales

	Grade	Description	
Hunt and Hess score[55]	I	Asymptomatic, or minimal headache and slight nuchal rigidity	
	II	Moderate to severe headache, nuchal rigidity, no neurological deficits other than cranial nerve palsy	
	III	Drowsiness, confusion, or mild focal deficit	
	IV	Stupor, moderate to severe hemiparesis	
	V	Deep coma, decerebrate posturing	
WFNS score[54]		GCS Score	Motor Deficit
	I	15	Absent
	II	13–14	Absent
	III	13–14	Present
	IV	7–12	Absent or present
	V	3–6	Absent or present
Fisher grade[37]	1	No hemorrhage	
	2	Subarachnoid hemorrhage < 1 mm thickness	
	3	Subarachnoid hemorrhage > 1 mm thickness	
	4	Presence of intraventricular or intraparenchymal hemorrhage	

GCS = Glasgow Coma Scale; WFNS = World Federation of Neurological Surgeons

Table 22.2 General Overview of Patient Management for Aneurysmal Subarachnoid Hemorrhage

	Pre-securing Aneurysm (day 0)	Post-securing Aneurysm (days 1–3)	Symptomatic Vasospasm Period (days 3–14)
Monitoring	• Frequent neurological examinations q1–2hr • BP • Fluid status • ICP/CPP • Temp • ECG • SaO_2	• Frequent neurological examinations q1–2hr • BP • Fluid status • ICP/CPP • Temp • Serum chemistry/CBC	• Frequent neurological examinations q1–2hr • BP • Fluid status • ICP/CPP • Temp • TCD • Serum chemistry/CBC
Goals	• SBP < 160 mm Hg • Euvolemia • Temp ≤ 37°C • ICP < 20 mm Hg • CPP > 60 mm Hg • GEDI: Avoid < 680 mL/m² • ELWI < 10 mL/kg • Hgb > 8 mg/dL • SaO_2 > 93%	• SBP 100–180 mm Hg • Euvolemia • Temp ≤ 37°C • ICP < 20 mm Hg • CPP > 60 mm Hg • GEDI: Avoid < 680 mL/m² • ELWI < 10 mL/kg • Hgb > 8 mg/dL • Blood glucose ≤ 200 mg/dL (avoid hypoglycemia) • Serum magnesium > 2 mg/dL • Serum sodium > 135 mEq/L	• SBP 140–220 mm Hg • Euvolemia • Temp ≤ 37°C • ICP < 20 mm Hg • CPP > 60 mm Hg • GEDI: Avoid < 680 mL/m² • ELWI < 10 mL/kg • Hgb > 8 mg/dL • Blood glucose ≤ 200 mg/dL (avoid hypoglycemia) • Serum magnesium > 2 mg/dL • Serum sodium > 135 mEq/L • Mean cerebral blood flow velocity < 120 cm/s
Intervention(s)	• Early aneurysm repair • Oral/enteral nimodipine 60 mg PO q4hr x 21 days • Control agitation/maintain adequate analgesia/sedation (if intubated) • Nausea/vomiting treatment • Bowel regimen • Continuous infusion BP-lowering agent (nicardipine/clevidipine) • 0.9% NaCl 1–1.5 mL/kg/hr • Consider anticonvulsant agent for 3–7 days • Maintain head of bead elevation 20°–30° • Graduated compression devices • Swallow assessment before oral intake	• Oral/enteral nimodipine 60 mg PO q4hr x 21 days • Control agitation/maintain adequate analgesia/sedation (if intubated) • Treat ICP using stepwise approach as indicated • Consider anticonvulsant agent for 3–7 days • 0.9% NaCl 1–1.5 mL/kg/hr • VTE prophylaxis (heparin 5000 units SC q8–12hr or LMWH 40 mg q24hr) + graduated compression devices • Maintain head of bed elevation 20°–30° • Consider hypertonic saline if hyponatremic	• Oral/enteral nimodipine 60 mg PO q4hr x 21 days • Control agitation/maintain adequate analgesia/sedation (if intubated) • Treat ICP using stepwise approach as indicated • Induced hypertension with vasopressors (phenylephrine or norepinephrine) and/or hemodynamic augmentation with inotropes (dobutamine or milrinone) for symptomatic vasospasm • 0.9% NaCl 1–1.5 mL/kg/hr • DVT prophylaxis (heparin 5000 units SC q8–12hr or LMWH 40 mg q24hr) • Maintain head of bed elevation 20°–30° • Consider hypertonic saline if hyponatremic • Consider anticonvulsant agent for 3–7 days • Bowel regimen

BP = blood pressure; CPP = cerebral perfusion pressure; ELWI = extravascular lung water index; GEDI = global end-diastolic volume index; ICP = intracranial pressure; LMWH = low-molecular-weight heparin; NaCl = sodium chloride; PO = orally; q = every; SaO_2 = arterial oxygen saturation; SBP = systolic blood pressure; SC = subcutaneously; TCD = transcranial Doppler; VTE = venous thromboembolism.

Table 22.3 Pharmacotherapy Recommendations from Clinical Guidelines

Recommendation	AHA/ASA Guideline[44]		NCS Consensus Statements[45]	
	Class of Evidence	Level of Evidence	Quality of Evidence	Recommendation
Prevention of Rebleeding:				
Between the time of aSAH symptom onset and aneurysm obliteration, BP should be controlled with titratable agent	I	B	—	—
Magnitude of BP control has not been established, but a decease to < 160 mm Hg is reasonable	IIa	C	—	—
For patients with an unavoidable delay in obliteration of aneurysm, a significant risk of rebleeding, and no compelling medication contraindications, short-term (< 72 hr) therapy with tranexamic acid or aminocaproic acid is reasonable to reduce the risk of early aneurysm rebleeding	IIa	B	Low	Weak
Antifibrinolytic therapy is relatively contraindicated in patients with risk factors for thromboembolic complications	—	—	Moderate	Strong
Antifibrinolytic therapy should be discontinued 2 hr before planned endovascular aneurysm ablation	—	—	Very low	Weak
Treatment/Prevention of DCI:				
Oral nimodipine (60 mg q4hr x 21 days) is indicated to reduce poor outcome related to aSAH	I	A	High	Strong
If nimodipine administration results in hypotension, dosing intervals should be changed to more frequent lower doses. If hypotension continues to occur, nimodipine may be discontinued	—	—	Low	Strong
Patients clinically suspected of having DCI should undergo a trial of induced hypertension; choice of vasopressor should be based on the other pharmacologic properties of the agents (e.g., inotropy, tachycardia)	—	—	Moderate	Strong
BP augmentation should progress in a stepwise fashion with assessment of neurologic function at each MAP level to determine whether a higher BP target is appropriate	—	—	Poor	Strong
Induction of hypertension is recommended for patients with DCI unless BP is elevated at baseline or cardiac status precludes it	I	B	—	—
Maintenance of euvolemia and normal circulating blood volume is recommended to prevent DCI	I	B	Moderate	Strong
Prophylactic hypervolemia or balloon angioplasty before the development of angiographic spasm is not recommended	III	B	High	Strong
In patients with a persistent negative fluid balance, use of fludrocortisone or hydrocortisone may be considered	—	—	Moderate	Weak
Consider a saline bolus to increase CSF in areas of ischemia as a prelude to other interventions	—	—	Moderate	Weak
Isotonic crystalloid is the preferred agent for volume replacement	—	—	Moderate	Weak
If patients with DCI do not improve with BP augmentation, a trial of inotropic therapy may be considered	—	—	Low	Strong
Inotropes with prominent β_2-agonist properties (e.g., dobutamine) may lower MAP and require increase in vasopressor dosage	—	—	High	Strong
Hemodilution in an attempt to improve rheology should not be undertaken except in cases of erythrocythemia	—	—	Moderate	Strong
Patients should receive packed RBC transfusions to maintain hemoglobin concentration above 8–10 g/dL	—	—	Moderate	Strong

Table 22.3 Pharmacotherapy Recommendations from Clinical Guidelines (continued)

Recommendation	AHA/ASA Guideline[44] Class of Evidence	AHA/ASA Guideline[44] Level of Evidence	NCS Consensus Statements[45] Quality of Evidence	NCS Consensus Statements[45] Recommendation
Higher hemoglobin concentrations may be appropriate for patients at risk of DCI, but whether transfusion is useful cannot be determined from the available data	—	—	No	Strong
Endovascular treatment using intra-arterial vasodilators and/or angioplasty may be considered for vasospasm-related DCI	IIa	B	Moderate	Strong
The timing and triggers of endovascular treatment of vasospasm remain unclear, but generally, rescue therapy should be considered for ischemic symptoms that remain refractory to medical treatment	—	—	Moderate	Strong
Seizure Prophylaxis:				
Routine use of anticonvulsant prophylaxis with phenytoin is not recommended after aSAH	—	—	Low	Strong
Routine use of other anticonvulsants for prophylaxis may be considered	—	—	Very low	Weak
If anticonvulsant prophylaxis is used, a short course (3–7 days) is recommended	—	—	Low	Weak
In patients who have a seizure after presentation, anticonvulsants should be continued for a duration defined by local practice	—	—	Low	Weak
The use of prophylactic anticonvulsants may be considered in the immediate posthemorrhagic period	IIa	B	—	—
The routine long-term use of anticonvulsants is not recommended	III	B	—	—
May consider use of long-term anticonvulsants in patients considered at risk of delayed seizures such as prior seizure, intracerebral hematoma, intractable hypertension, infarction, or aneurysm at the middle cerebral artery	IIb	B	—	—
General Critical Care Management:				
Hypoglycemia (serum glucose < 80 mg/dL) should be avoided	—	—	High	Strong
Serum glucose should be maintained at < 200 mg/dL	—	—	Moderate	Strong
Careful glucose management with strict avoidance of hypoglycemia may be considered as part of the general critical care management of patients with aSAH	IIb	B	—	—
Unfractionated heparin for prophylaxis could be initiated 24 hr after undergoing surgery	—	—	Moderate	Strong
Unfractionated heparin and LMWH should be withheld 24 hr before and after intracranial procedures	—	—	Moderate	Strong
LMWH or unfractionated heparin for prophylaxis should be withheld in patients with unprotected aneurysms who are expected to undergo surgery	—	—	Low	Strong
The duration of DVT prophylaxis is presently uncertain, but may be based on patient mobility	—	—	Low	Weak
Sequential compression devices should be routinely used in all patients	—	—	High	Strong
Heparin-induced thrombocytopenia and DVT are relatively common complications after aSAH. Early identification and targeted treatment are recommended, but further research is needed to identify the idea screening paradigms	I	B	—	—

Table 22.3 Pharmacotherapy Recommendations from Clinical Guidelines (continued)

Recommendation	AHA/ASA Guideline[44]		NCS Consensus Statements[45]	
	Class of Evidence	Level of Evidence	Quality of Evidence	Recommendation
Aggressive control of fever to target normothermia using standard or advanced temperature-modulating systems is reasonable in the acute phase of aSAH	IIa	B	—	—
Antipyretic agents (acetaminophen, ibuprofen) should be used as first-line therapy, even though efficacy is low	—	—	Moderate	Strong
Surface cooling or intravascular devices should be used when antipyretics fail if fever control is highly desirable	—	—	High	Strong
During the period of risk for DCI, control of fever is desirable; intensity should reflect the individual patient's relative risk of ischemia	—	—	Low	Strong
Hypomagnesemia should be avoided	—	—	Moderate	Strong
The use of fludrocortisone acetate and hypertonic saline solution is reasonable for preventing and correcting hyponatremia	IIa	B	Moderate	Weak
Do not treat hyponatremia with fluid restriction	—	—	Weak	Strong
Early treatment with hydrocortisone or fludrocortisone may be used to limit natriuresis and hyponatremia	—	—	Moderate	Weak
Mild hypertonic saline solutions can be used to correct hyponatremia	—	—	Very low	Strong
Extreme caution to avoid hypovolemia is needed if vasopressin-receptor antagonists are used for treatment of hyponatremia	—	—	Weak	Strong
Free water intake by intravenous and enteral routes should be limited	—	—	Very low	Strong
Hormonal replacement with stress-dose corticosteroids for patients with vasospasm and unresponsiveness to induced hypertension may be considered	—	—	Weak	Weak
High-dose corticosteroids are not recommended	—	—	High	Weak
Consider hypothalamic dysfunction in patients unresponsive to vasopressors	—	—	Moderate	Weak
Patients taking statins before presenting with aSAH should have their medication continued in the acute phase	—	—	Low	Strong

SAH = aneurysmal subarachnoid hemorrhage; DCI = delayed cerebral ischemia.

continued from page 421

first 24 hours; therefore, treatment of the underlying aneurysm should be completed on an emergency basis.[44,45] Furthermore, medical management should include therapies aimed at risk reduction, including strict blood pressure control and the consideration of antifibrinolytics. Other important supportive interventions include the use of bed rest, stool softeners to prevent straining, and pain management because pain is associated with a transient elevation in blood pressure, which can increase the risk of rebleeding.

Strict blood pressure control in the acute phase until the aneurysm is secured is reasonable to reduce the risk of rebleeding. Although no prospective studies show a reduction in rebleeding with aggressive blood pressure control, the consensus guidelines recommend a treatment systolic blood pressure threshold of 160 mm Hg.[44,45] If antihypertensive therapy is indicated, an intravenous agent that is easily titratable to goal blood pressure and that has minimal negative effects on cerebral hemodynamics should be used.[58] The use of intermittent bolus doses of antihypertensives such as labetalol may be effective; however, intermittent bolus dosing may lead to significant blood pressure variability. A continuous intravenous infusion such as nicardipine or clevidipine can be titrated more effectively to maintain the blood pressure goal.[59] Please see Table 22.4 for a comparison of the acute blood pressure–lowering agents that can be used to manage blood pressure before securing the aneurysm.

The use of antifibrinolytics (tranexamic acid or aminocaproic acid) in the immediate period after hemorrhage and before treatment of the aneurysm is reasonable; antifibrinolytics should be considered primarily in patients who cannot have the aneurysm secured in a timely manner. Data have been conflicting regarding the effectiveness and safety of these agents; however, much of the debate surrounds the timing and duration of treatment. Patients treated with antifibrinolytic therapy for a prolonged period appear to have an increased risk of DCI.[60] A recent Cochrane analysis does not support the use of antifibrinolytics to reduce the risk of rebleeding; however, this analysis included only one study that limited the use to 72 hours.[61] More recent studies limiting the use of therapy to 72 hours have shown a benefit in reducing the risk of rebleeding from about 10% to 3%.[62-64] Short-term treatment with antifibrinolytics can be considered, especially for patients who cannot be treated immediately.[44,45] The definitive prevention for rebleeding is aneurysmal coiling or clipping, and any benefit from antifibrinolytics in SAH is likely to be a temporary measure until the offending aneurysm is secured. Delayed (greater than 48 hours from ictus) or prolonged (greater than 3 days) use of antifibrinolytic agents exposes patients to adverse effects such as cerebral infarction during the time for which the risk of rebleeding is reduced and vasospasm is increased and thus should be avoided.[45]

The key treatment in aSAH is stabilizing the aneurysm to prevent rebleeding. Two approaches can be taken: surgical clipping and endovascular coiling. In endovascular coiling, a catheter is placed in the artery to gain access to the aneurysm, after which platinum coils are placed inside the aneurysm to embolize the aneurysm. Clipping is an invasive surgical intervention whereby a surgical clip is placed over the aneurysm, obliterating it and blocking blood flow into the aneurysm. Long-term controversy exists on which intervention is preferred because both interventions are effective. To date, the International Subarachnoid Aneurysm Trial (ISAT) has been the largest study (more than 2,100 patients) to compare coiling and clipping.[65,66] The results showed that endovascular coiling was associated with a lower 1-year mortality rate compared with surgical clipping (absolute risk reduction 7.4%; relative risk reduction 23.9%). However, long-term follow-up showed that rebleeding rates and the need for additional coiling were more frequent in patients treated with intravascular coiling. The risk of death at 5 years was significantly lower in the coiling group.[67] Attempts have been made to identify subgroups of patients for which one approach may be preferred to the other. Most clinicians agree that clipping may be preferred in patients presenting with large (greater than 50 mL) intraparenchymal hematomas and middle cerebral artery aneurysms, whereas endovascular coiling may be considered in older adults (older than 70 years), those presenting with poor-grade aSAH (World Federation of Neurological Surgeons classification IV/V), and those with aneurysms of the basilar tip.[44] Overall, the current guidelines recommend that surgical clipping or coiling be done as early as feasible in most patients to reduce the rate of rebleeding (class I; level of evidence B), and the determination of treatment should be a multidisciplinary decision based on characteristics of the patient and the aneurysm (class I; level of evidence C).[44]

Seizures

Seizures after aSAH are of concern because of their association with early complications, such as rebleeding and poor outcomes.[68,69] The reported incidence of seizures remains highest at the time of aneurysm rupture, with a rate varying from 4% to 26%. This discrepancy in reported events is partly because of the occurrence of both seizures and seizure-like phenomena, which may be difficult to distinguish, at the time of aneurysm rupture.[69-73]

After aneurysm treatment, the incidence of seizures appears low and may be related to the method in which the aneurysm was secured, thickness of the subarachnoid clot, aneurysm location, presence of subdural hematoma, and secondary cerebral infarction.[72] The ISAT study reported that the frequency of seizures was 0.65% after hospitalization but before treatment and 2.3% between treatment and discharge. The frequency of seizures after treatment and before discharge was doubled in patients treated with surgical clipping (3.1%) compared with patients undergoing endovascular treatment (1.5%).[66] In a 14-year follow-up, 10.9% of patients enrolled in ISAT had a seizure. During this period, there was a higher incidence of posttreatment seizures in patients who underwent surgical clipping compared with endovascular coiling (13.6% vs. 8.3%, p=0.014).[74]

Appropriate management of seizures related to aSAH remains an area of debate. Although the use of prophylactic antiepileptic drugs in the setting of aSAH is common, there is a paucity of evidence showing the safety and efficacy of this practice. This has led to highly variable practice between institutions and physicians.[69] Most literature evaluating the use of prophylactic antiepileptic drugs in the setting of aSAH is observational and focuses mainly on phenytoin. One of the first studies published evaluating this area described the early use of a short perioperative course of phenytoin for seizure prophylaxis in low-risk patients. Patients without a history of seizure disorder, cerebral ischemia, parenchymal clot, postoperative hematoma, or concomitant arteriovenous malformation received a phenytoin 900- to 1100-mg load, followed by 300 mg/day for an average of 5.3 days. The overall seizure rate was 5.4% with an average follow-up of 2.4 years, leading the authors to advocate for no more than 7 days of phenytoin for seizure prophylaxis in most patients with aSAH.[75] A retrospective review of 453 patients built on these data by comparing phenytoin prophylaxis (1000-mg loading dose, followed by 300 mg/day) through hospital discharge (average 14 days) to 3 days. This review found a similar incidence of seizures between the two groups during hospitalization (discharge 1.3% vs. 3 days 1.9%, p=0.6) and at follow-up (5.7% vs. 4.6%, p=0.6; follow-up ranged from 3 to 12 months).[76] Of note, few of these studies included a high percentage of patients who were treated with coiling of the aneurysm, so most of the data are from aneurysm clipping.

The use of phenytoin is not without risk because several studies have shown phenytoin to have a negative impact on neurological outcomes.[77,78] In addition, phenytoin is a significant inhibitor and inducer of many hepatic enzymes, leading to potential drug-drug interactions.[72]

Literature regarding the use of alternative antiepileptic drugs for seizure prophylaxis in the setting of aSAH is scarce, with the most support currently for levetiracetam. One retrospective study (n=442) compared short-course levetiracetam (500 mg twice daily; median therapy duration 3.6 days) with extended-duration phenytoin (15- to 20-mg/kg loading dose, followed by maintenance dose; median therapy duration 13.7 days) for seizure prophylaxis after aSAH. The levetiracetam group had a higher incidence of in-hospital seizures (8.3% vs. 3.4%, p=0.03); however, this was driven by the increased incidence of late seizures in the levetiracetam group, which suggests a longer duration of prophylaxis is needed.[79] Levetiracetam was also compared with phenytoin for seizure prophylaxis in a prospective, single-center, randomized trial of patients with severe traumatic brain injury or subarachnoid hemorrhage (n=52; 89% of patients included in the trial had a primary diagnosis of severe traumatic brain injury). Patients received either phenytoin (20 mg/kg load, followed by 5 mg/kg/day) or levetiracetam (20 mg/kg load, followed by 1000 mg twice daily) for 7 days. No difference was observed in seizure occurrence (phenytoin group: 16.7% vs. levetiracetam group 14.7%, p=1.0), and patients in the levetiracetam group had better outcomes in Disability Rating Scale scores and higher Glasgow Outcomes Scale-Extended scores at 3 and 6 months.[80]

The lack of high-quality literature available regarding seizure prophylaxis in this population is reflected in the current guidelines (see Table 22.3). The NCS guidelines recommend against the use of phenytoin for seizure prophylaxis, although they state that the role of other antiepileptic drugs is unclear. Both guidelines state that the use of prophylactic antiepileptic drugs may be considered in the immediate posthemorrhagic period for a short duration (NCS guidelines 3–7 days). A longer duration may be considered for patients with risk factors for a delayed seizure disorder such as a prior seizure or in those who have a seizure after presentation.[44,45]

Hydrocephalus

Hydrocephalus is a common acute complication of aSAH occurring in about 15%–20% of patients.[81,82] This complication occurs because of either the obstructed circulation of CSF or the impairment in absorption of CSF that occurs by the arachnoid granulations.[83] When symptomatic hydrocephalus occurs, the standard treatment is CSF diversion through an external ventricular drain. Placement of this type of drain allows for both the drainage of CSF and the measurement of ICP. When significant intraventricular blood is present, aggressive treatment with CSF diversion and drainage of the ventricular clot may reduce the risk of cerebral vasospasm.[84] The alteration in CSF flow dynamics or reabsorption can be transient, during which the drain can be removed; however, it can also be permanent, necessitating the placement of a permanent shunt.

In patients with an altered level of consciousness, the evaluation for hydrocephalus can be more difficult. An alteration in the level of consciousness is the most common symptom of hydrocephalus; therefore, a combination of clinical judgment and imaging are required to determine whether CSF diversion and ICP monitoring is indicated. Commonly, a GCS score of 8 or lower is used to determine when a patient requires ICP monitoring, which can be done through an external ventricular drain or an intraparenchymal ICP monitor. In those with hydrocephalus on head CT and a clinical picture consistent with symptomatic hydrocephalus, CSF diversion is warranted regardless of the GCS score.

When ICP monitoring is used, the goal is to maintain the ICP within a normal range and to ensure adequate cerebral perfusion. The CPP is calculated by subtracting the ICP from the mean arterial pressure (MAP). The pressure differential, which is what drives perfusion of the brain, is termed the *CPP*. The goals are to maintain the ICP less than 20 mm Hg and the CPP greater than 60 mm Hg. Often, vasopressors (phenylephrine or norepinephrine) are required to increase the MAP or hyperosmolar therapy (mannitol or hypertonic saline) is used to decrease the ICP, both of which lead to an increase in the CPP. Intracranial hypertension is defined as a sustained (more than 5 minutes) elevation of ICP greater than 20 mm Hg. Please see the article titled "Emergency Neurological Life Support: Intracranial Hypertension and Herniation" for a tiered treatment protocol.[85]

DELAYED CEREBRAL ISCHEMIA

Cerebral vasospasm has traditionally been regarded as the cause of DCI, which occurs after aSAH and leads to cerebral infarction and poor neurological outcomes. However, data from more recent studies argue against a pure focus on vasospasm as the sole cause of DCI. Research is now intensifying on methods for intervention in the early brain injury pathophysiological process, which also contributes to DCI. Narrowing of the cerebral arteries through vasospasm resulting in a reduction in cerebral blood flow may lead to ischemia and infarction.[86] About two-thirds of patients may develop angiographic evidence of vasospasm, although only 20%–30% have clinical symptoms.[35] In up to 25% of patients, the delayed infarcts revealed on CT scans are not located in the vascular territory of the spastic artery, or they occur in patients who develop vasospasm.[87,88] The predictive value of radiographic vasospasm for DCI is only about 67%.[89] More recent studies using perfusion imaging methods now suggest that only severe vasospasm with at least a 50% luminal narrowing produces sufficient reductions in cerebral blood flow to cause symptomatic ischemia.[90] Studies have tried to predict the patients more likely to develop vasospasm after aSAH.[91] The strongest risk factor appears to be the volume of subarachnoid clot present, with patients having larger clot volumes being at highest risk.[92] Several other risk factors have also been shown to be predictive of vasospasm, including clinical grade on admission, history of cigarette smoking, history of hypertension, and cocaine use.[93,94]

Nomenclature

Many terms are used somewhat interchangeably in the literature when describing delayed neurological deficits. As previously discussed, many investigators use the terms *vasospasm* and *DCI* interchangeably, making it difficult to evaluate treatments and associated outcomes from research studies. Cerebral vasospasm can be defined as the delayed narrowing of the large arteries within the basal cisterns, which may be associated with clinical or radiographic signs of ischemia in the areas of the brain supplied by the spastic artery. Delayed cerebral ischemia is an umbrella term in the literature that encompasses several clinical entities, including symptomatic vasospasm, delayed ischemic neurological deficit, and asymptomatic delayed cerebral infarction. Not all patients who develop vasospasm develop DCI. *Delayed ischemic neurological deficit* is a much broader term that includes delayed neurological deficits that occur with or without angiographic vasospasm. Ultimately, DCI is a clinical diagnosis of exclusion that may be difficult to recognize in patients with poor clinical grade aSAH. In 2010, a consensus statement by a multidisciplinary panel proposed new definitions for clinical deterioration caused by DCI and cerebral infarction after aSAH that were further supported by the 2011 NCS consensus guidelines.[45,95] Overall both consensus groups advocated for a separation of DCI from vasospasm after aSAH.

- DCI = the occurrence of focal neurological impairment (e.g., hemiparesis, aphasia, apraxia, neglect) or a decrease of at least two points on the GCS (either the total scale or one component of the scale). This should last for at least 1 hour, not be apparent immediately after the aneurysm occlusion, and not be attributed to other causes.
- Cerebral infarction = the presence of cerebral infarction by CT or MRI within 6 weeks after aSAH, not present between 24 and 48 hours after early occlusions, and not attributable to other causes such as surgical clipping or endovascular treatment.

Measuring and Monitoring Cerebral Vasospasm

The easiest form of vasospasm monitoring involves a vigilant clinical examination. Frequent neurological examinations should be done to establish each patient's baseline neurologic status and to detect any changes. Newly identified deficits should be worked up immediately to rule out other causes such as hydrocephalus, seizures, and metabolic abnormalities. Although clinical examination can detect subtle changes in patients with low-grade aSAH, these same changes may not be apparent in a patient who is comatose; therefore, clinical examination alone cannot be used to screen for vasospasm.

Transcranial Doppler (TCD) monitoring was introduced in the 1980s as a less-invasive approach for monitoring cerebral vasospasm and has become a mainstay of vasospasm monitoring in the ICU at many centers. This provides an indirect measure of the vessel diameter by measuring cerebral blood flow velocity. When the proximal cerebral arteries narrow, the velocity of blood flow in those arteries increases and can be detectable by TCD. Absolute velocity of blood flow in the middle cerebral artery shows a strong correlation with the lack or presence of vasospasm when it is low (less than 120 cm/second is low risk for vasospasm) or very high (greater than 200 cm/second is high risk for vasospasm) but does not correlate well in the intermediate range.[44] The Lindegaard ratio is also predictive of vasospasm and is the middle cerebral artery velocity compared with the velocity in the proximal extracranial internal carotid artery (V_{MCA}/V_{ICA}). A value greater than 3 is consistent with vasospasm.[96] The disadvantage of this approach is the high interrater variability that is dependent on the operator. In addition, many patients may have dense temporal bone windows that prohibit an accurate measurement, and it is inadequate to identify spasm of more distal arteries. Even with these limitations, however, this tool can be used in the ICU to evaluate trends and complement the clinical examination.

Imaging with perfusion methods such as CT, MRI, and/or positron emission tomography is being used to screen and confirm vasospasm and DCI. These perfusion studies can be combined with noninvasive arteriography to acquire more complete information. Computed tomography angiography is correlated with conventional angiography for large artery narrowing and can be used as a screening tool.[45] Computed tomography perfusion imaging provides a measure of tissue perfusion. Severe vasospasm is associated with absolute cerebral blood flows of less than 25 mL/100 g/minute and mean transit times greater than 6.4 seconds or 20% higher than average.[97] The current consensus recommendations suggest that a mean transient time greater than 6.4 seconds on perfusion imaging is additive to CT angiography for predicting DCI. Serial use of these techniques can be limited by cumulative radiation exposure, higher cost, lower availability, and the need for patients to be admitted or transported to centers with this imaging capability.

The gold standard diagnostic method for identifying vasospasm is digital subtraction angiography, which is invasive and expensive and carries the risk of other complications.[45] The serious complication rate is 1%–2% and includes risk of the anesthetic regimen, puncture site complications, contrast nephropathy, allergic reactions, embolic or thrombotic strokes, perforation of the cerebral artery, and intracranial hemorrhage.[98] The advantage of angiography is that is provides the opportunity to treat vasospasm by endovascular approaches; however, using this invasive approach is not appropriate for surveillance monitoring of vasospasm.

Other tools can be used in the ICU to evaluate the physiologic impact of vasospasm, including electroencephalogram, brain tissue oxygen monitoring, and cerebral microdialysis.[45] Electroencephalography has been used to detect reversible cerebral ischemia since the 1970s, and specific patterns have now been correlated with vasospasm.[99,100] Continuous quantitative electroencephalogram monitoring that focuses on the ratio of fast alpha activity and slow delta activity, alpha variability, and the alpha/delta ratio may precede clinical signs of cerebral ischemia. Relative decreased alpha variability precedes clinical diagnosis of vasospasm by 3 days.[101] Microdialysis may provide a modality for assessing bedside comparisons of neurochemical changes with the patient's neurological examination. Lactate and glutamate are sensitive markers of impending cerebral ischemia.[102] Brain tissue oxygenation, thermal diffusion cerebral blood flow, and near-infrared spectroscopy have also been used to monitor patients with aSAH with some success, although the value of these approaches is currently unknown. The NCS published consensus statements on multimodality monitoring that provide a more comprehensive review of these monitoring approaches.[103]

Prevention Strategies

Calcium Channel Blockers

The only pharmacologic intervention that improves outcome after aSAH is the calcium channel antagonist, nimodipine.[104] Nimodipine is a dihydropyridine calcium channel blocker that shows cerebral vascular selectivity by preferentially dilating cerebral blood vessels to a greater degree than the peripheral and coronary vasculature.[105] Nimodipine has become the standard of care in the United States, according to a clinical trial published in 1983 in which 13% of patients who were randomized to the placebo group had severe neurologic deficits compared with 1.7% of patients randomized to nimodipine.[106] A larger trial showed reductions of 34% in ischemic stroke and 40% in poor outcome at 3 months in patients treated with nimodipine compared with placebo.[107] A subsequent meta-analysis that evaluated nine prospective randomized trials including 1,514 patients showed a significantly reduced incidence of delayed neurological deficits by 38% (odds ratio [OR] 0.62; 95% CI, 0.5–0.78) and cerebral infarcts by 48% (OR 0.52; 95% CI, 0.41–0.66).[108]

Originally, it was hypothesized that the benefit from nimodipine was related to a reduction in vasospasm; however, clinical trials did not show a reduction in vasospasm, even while showing an overall improvement in outcome. Clinical trials that have shown the benefit of enteral nimodipine in patients with aSAH used a dose of 60 mg every 4 hours for 21 days. The most common adverse effect is hypotension, which is reported to occur in about 7.7% of patients. This can be a serious concern because hemodynamic lability is independently associated with death or severe disability after aSAH.[100] Avoiding blood pressure fluctuations is key in the management of these patients, so alterations in the dosing strategy of nimodipine (30 mg every 2 hours) have been suggested in patients who have hypotension, but this has not been evaluated in clinical trials. Nimodipine has also been shown to be cost-effective, given that it increased patient life-years at a very low incremental cost.[109] The two guidelines recommend that oral nimodipine (60 mg every 4 hours) be given for 21 days after aSAH.[44,45] Common practice in patients with a good Hunt and Hess grade aSAH is to discontinue nimodipine as patients are discharged from the hospital, provided there have been no complications from the aSAH or intervention. This practice is not based on evidence, but only on the clinical knowledge that patients with good Hunt and Hess grades are less likely to develop DCI beyond post-aSAH day 10. Similarly, if hypotension is too pervasive, nimodipine may have to be held in an effort to support cerebral perfusion, but this is not based on evidence.

Some serious drug errors have been reported when oral nimodipine is administered intravenously instead of through a nasogastric tube when patients are unable to swallow the capsule. The drug comes with instructions for making a hole in both ends of the capsule with a standard 18-gauge needle for removing the contents with a syringe and then administering through the nasogastric tube. Because these needles do not fit on an oral syringe, an intravenous syringe is used, which has resulted in intravenous administration. Intravenous administration can result in cardiac arrest, dramatic drops in blood pressure, or other cardiovascular adverse events. The FDA issued a drug safety communication in 2010, for which it reported 25 intravenous nimodipine-prescribing or administration errors, where four of the patients died and five had near-death events.[110] In 2013, the FDA approved a new oral nimodipine solution in an effort to reduce drug errors because this dosage form eliminated the need for needle extraction of nimodipine from the capsules.[111] There are also potentials for drug interactions between nimodipine and strong inhibitors and inducers of cytochrome P450 (CYP) 3A4. The clinical significance of these drug interactions is the possibility of significant hypotension when administered with CYP3A4 inhibitors and lack of effectiveness when coadministered with CYP3A4 inducers.

The future direction for non-enteral delivery of nimodipine compared with enteral nimodipine is currently being investigated in clinical trials. EG-1962 is a novel polymeric nimodipine microparticle that is administered directly into the cerebral ventricles and provides sustained drug exposure throughout 21 days. EG-1962 uses a programmable, biodegradable polymer-based development platform known as Precisa. This delivery system allows for targeted drug delivery to the site of injury to provide sustained drug exposure while avoiding systemic toxicities. This site-specific delivery of nimodipine microparticles reduces angiographic vasospasm after aSAH in dogs.[112] EG-1962 is currently being evaluated in a phase I/II study, NEWTON (Nimodipine Microparticles to Enhance Recovery While Reducing Toxicity After Subarachnoid Hemorrhage), for safety, tolerability and pharmacokinetic properties.[113,114]

Nicardipine is another calcium channel blocker that has been evaluated for prophylactic use after aSAH. Intravenous nicardipine (0.15 mg/kg/hour for up to 14 days) was compared with placebo. In contrast to the results reported for nimodipine, nicardipine was associated with lower symptomatic vasospasm but was not associated with improvement in neurological outcome at 3 months. Hypotension, the main concern with the use of intravenous nicardipine, occurred in 34.5% of nicardipine-treated patients compared with 17.5% of placebo-treated patients. The potential positive effect on outcome may have been negated by the 3% incidence of life-threatening hypotension that developed.[115,116]

Statins

Statins have generated much interest for the prevention of vasospasm after aSAH because of their pleiotropic effects, which include anti-inflammatory properties, up-regulation of endothelial nitric oxide synthase, anti-adhesive effects on endothelium, amelioration of glutamate-mediated excitotoxicity, and inhibition of platelet aggregation.[117,118] Because of strong experimental evidence, several studies examined the clinical effect of simvastatin and pravastatin for prevention of vasospasm and DCI. The primary difference between these statins is that simvastatin has a higher affinity for hydroxymethylglutaryl coenzyme A reductase and is more lipophilic than pravastatin, so it has higher blood-brain barrier penetration.[119] The results of these studies were critically appraised in two meta-analyses that included four published randomized trials with a total of 190 patients.[95,120] Simvastatin 80 mg was used in three of the four studies, and pravastatin 40 mg was used in the other study. There was no statistical difference in TCD-detected vasospasm, incidence of DCI, or neurologic outcomes between statin treatment and placebo. The other meta-analysis included these four trials together with two unpublished randomized trials and five observational studies.[120] Similar to the previous meta-analysis, there was no significant difference in the incidence of DCI. The results of these meta-analyses should be viewed cautiously because the definitions of DCI were inconsistent. Atorvastatin 40 mg/day for 21 days was studied in 142 patients to evaluate whether this statin could reduce vasospasm-induced ischemia by measuring serum S100B (biomarker for cerebral ischemia) and ischemic lesion volume by CT. Atorvastatin reduced the incidence of cerebral vasospasm, severity of vasospasm, volume of ischemia, and serum S100B concentrations, but there were no differences in clinical outcomes at 1 year.[121]

The STASH study (Simvastatin in Aneurysmal Subarachnoid Hemorrhage), a phase III randomized trial of 803 patients that compared simvastatin 40 mg with placebo for up to 21 days, was recently published.[122] Despite showing no safety concerns, this trial failed to show any short- or long-term benefit in outcome, and the investigators concluded that simvastatin should not be routinely used during the acute stages. Several experimental and clinical studies suggest that sudden withdrawal of statins can suppress endothelial nitric oxide production, leading to a higher risk of hemorrhage and vasospasm.[123,124] The current guidelines state that statins may be initiated in statin-naive patients for reducing DCI after aSAH, but these were published before the STASH results; therefore, statins should not be used in statin-naive patients. However, the guidelines do mention continuing patients on statins if they were receiving statins before presenting with aSAH.[44,45]

Magnesium

Magnesium is a noncompetitive calcium antagonist and is thought to result in smooth muscle relaxation and vessel dilation. Magnesium may also have neuroprotective properties because it decreases glutamate release and reduces calcium entry into cells.[125,126] Hypomagnesemia occurs in more than 50% of patients with aSAH and is associated with poor outcome and a predictor of DCI.[127] Several clinical trials have investigated the effects of magnesium after aSAH.[128-136] The first phase III randomized controlled trial enrolled 327 patients within 48 hours of aSAH to either magnesium 20 mmol (5 g) over 30 minutes, followed by an infusion of 80 mmol (20 g)/day for up to 14 days posthemorrhage, or placebo (0.9% sodium chloride). The magnesium infusion was adjusted to achieve a magnesium concentration twice the patient's baseline up to a maximum of 2.5 mmol/L. There were no significant differences in 6-month outcomes or in the percentage of patients with clinical vasospasm.[135] The MASH-2 (Magnesium for Aneurysmal Subarachnoid Hemorrhage) study is another phase III randomized placebo-controlled trial of 1,204 patients that did not find significant benefit of intravenous magnesium infusion on favorable outcome.[136] The investigators of this trial also completed a meta-analysis and confirmed the lack of benefit of magnesium after aSAH.[136]

Magnesium was administered intravenously in these clinical trials; however, this route of administration does not result in a significant increase in CSF magnesium values, even if the serum magnesium level is increased by 50% or more.[137] Direct administration of magnesium into the basal cisterns may be a more effective approach, although there are currently no ongoing clinical trials investigating magnesium after aSAH.[138,139] Intravenous administration of magnesium is not currently recommended. However, hypomagnesemia should be avoided.[44,45]

Clearance of Subarachnoid Spaces

Because the breakdown by-product of the subarachnoid clot is believed to play a key role in the development of vasospasm and DCI, removal of the hemorrhage would appear to be a rational preventive strategy. Some evidence suggests that subarachnoid clot removal achieved by way of intracisternal injections of recombinant tissue plasminogen activator reduces the risk of vasospasm.[140] The recombinant tissue plasminogen activator is usually administered at the time of aneurysm clipping, and because endovascular approaches to aneurysm stabilization are increasingly being used, this approach is not practical for all patients. In addition, the results appear to be inconclusive, and this approach can increase the risk of intracerebral hemorrhage. Currently, the use of intracisternal thrombolytics cannot be recommended.

Intraventricular administration of thrombolytic agents has been investigated as a method for preventing the development of vasospasm. A meta-analysis of five trials that included 465 patients showed significant reductions in the development of vasospasm and DCI.[141] The results of this meta-analysis should be viewed cautiously, given that there were considerable differences in the study methodology of the trials included in the meta-analysis; as such, routine use cannot be currently recommended.

The use of lumbar drains is another approach for clearing subarachnoid blood. A current clinical trial is investigating the benefit of this approach (EARLYDRAIN).[142]

Endothelin-1 Antagonist

Endothelin-1 is a 21-amino acid peptide and one of the most potent vasoconstrictors produced in endothelial cells on stimulation by ischemia. It has been suggested that endothelin-1 contributes to an imbalance in vasoconstriction and vasodilation during aSAH. Endothelin-1 can be found in high concentrations in the CSF on day 5 post-ictus, and it corresponds with increased cerebral blood flow velocity.[143] Clazosentan is a selective endothelin-A receptor antagonist that decreases and reverses cerebral vasospasm in experimental aSAH. The CONSCIOUS-1 (Clazosentan to Overcome Neurological Ischemia and Infarct Occurring After Subarachnoid Hemorrhage) trial showed significant dose-dependent effects on the angiographic incidence of vasospasm with a 65% reduction at the highest dose.[144] The phase III trial, CONSCIOUS-2, was designed to target patients at highest risk of vasospasm and DCI, such as those with substantial blood clot thickness who had undergone surgical clipping. The results of the CONSCIOUS-2 trial showed that clazosentan at 5 mg/hour had no significant effect on mortality, vasospasm-related morbidity, or functional outcome. Pulmonary complications, anemia, and hypotension were more common in the patients who received clazosentan.[145] A similar study of patients who were treated with coiling (CONSCIOUS-3) was stopped early after 577 of the 1,500 patients were enrolled.[146] The results of CONSCIOUS-3 showed findings similar to CONSCIOUS-2 for the 5-mg/hour dose; however, the 15-mg/hour doses significantly reduced vasospasm-related morbidity and all-cause mortality but did not lead to improved outcomes at week 12. The CONSCIOUS-2 and CONSCIOUS-3 trials have raised questions regarding the efficacy of endothelin-1 antagonists in preventing vasospasm; however, the possibility remains that these agents have clinical utility as part of a complex treatment regimen for aSAH.

Treatment Strategies

Hemodynamic and Fluid Goals

Hemodynamic therapy known as triple-H therapy has been a popular approach to managing symptomatic vasospasm in patients who have secured aneurysms, despite the moderate quality of evidence supporting this intervention. Triple-H refers to hypervolemia (central venous pressures 10–12 mm Hg), hypertension (systolic blood pressure 180–220 mm Hg), and hemodilution (hematocrit 30%–35%).[147] The rationale for this therapy is for maintaining high circulating blood volume, increased CPPs, and decreased blood viscosity that will enhance cerebral blood flow in the face of vasoconstriction. There is currently no supportive evidence from randomized controlled trials that triple-H therapy or its separate components improve cerebral blood flow or clinical outcome in patients with aSAH.[148,149] The role of triple-H therapy has also been investigated as a prophylactic approach to prevent DCI, with the data showing no benefit and a higher risk of serious adverse effects and death; thus, this approach should be reserved for managing patients with symptomatic vasospasm.[150,151]

Hemodilution is the most controversial component of triple-H therapy. Although cerebral blood flow increases with a decreasing hematocrit, this approach is also associated with decreased oxygen-carrying capacity and increased volume of ischemic areas of the brain.[152] Higher hemoglobin values are associated with decreased rates of cerebral infarction, poor outcome, and death after aSAH.[152] However, blood transfusions are associated with increased rates of angiographic vasospasm, cerebral ischemia, and worse functional outcomes.[153] There are no convincing data to support an ideal hematocrit; thus, induced hemodilution to achieve a lower hemoglobin or hematocrit to improve blood rheology should be avoided. The current guidelines recommend maintaining hemoglobin concentrations of greater than 8–10 g/dL with packed red cells, although higher thresholds may be appropriate in patients at high risk of DCI.[44,45] Transfusion with packed red blood cells, however, is not without risk, and a recent retrospective cohort study reported that transfusion with red cells was independently associated with increased mortality in patients with aSAH.[154]

Hypovolemia, which can commonly occur after aSAH, should be avoided because it is associated with worse clinical outcomes. Hypovolemia appears to be a cumulative process and is more prevalent 6–72 hours after aSAH for patients who undergo surgical intervention.[155] Prophylactic hypervolemia does not improve cerebral blood flow or prevent symptomatic vasospasm or DCI and is associated with increased risk of cardiopulmonary complications because of the fluid overload.[151] A recent survey showed that medical centers without a dedicated neuro-ICU are more likely to use prophylactic hypervolemia.[156] The approach to intravascular volume management should target euvolemia with isotonic crystalloids rather than prophylactic hypervolemia.[44,45]

The choice of fluid for use in aSAH is typically isotonic crystalloids, which is specifically mentioned in the guidelines. However, other fluid choices have been assessed in patients with aSAH. Hypertonic saline has not been part of the traditional regimen for triple-H therapy, although this fluid can be commonly used for the reduction of ICP and may have clinical benefits in patients with poor-grade aSAH. A prospective study administered a 2-mL/kg infusion of 23.4% sodium chloride over 10–30 minutes to 44 patients with poor-grade aSAH and showed that hypertonic saline increased systemic blood pressure, reduced ICP, and improved cerebral blood flow, cerebral oxygenation, and brain tissue pH. The effects lasted 2–4 hours after administration. Although these data evaluations are limited, hypertonic saline may be an alternative fluid for use in patients with poor-grade aSAH.[157]

Albumin is another fluid currently being investigated because it is believed to possess neuroprotective properties through several mechanisms, including increasing serum oncotic pressure, improving microcirculatory blood flow, decreasing the inflammatory response, and free radical scavenging properties.[158] Many of the triple-H regimens evaluated in the literature included albumin as part of their regimen, but there is no good study comparing albumin with crystalloids. A retrospective evaluation of high doses of 25% human albumin used to increase the central venous pressure above 8 mm Hg reported an association with improved outcomes and reduced costs in patients with aSAH.[159] A phase I dose-escalation study evaluated the safety and efficacy of 25% albumin in doses of 0.625, 1.25, 1.875, and 2.5 g/kg/day for up to 7 days.[160] Doses up to 1.25 g/kg/day were well tolerated, but the study was terminated early once the dose reached 1.875 g/kg/day because of the development of pulmonary edema. Albumin in Subarachnoid Hemorrhage (ALISAH) II, a phase III randomized placebo-controlled trial powered to test the efficacy of albumin, is planned. Until the results of this study are complete, it is not recommended to routinely use albumin in the management of these patients because patients with traumatic brain injury have shown increased mortality with the administration of albumin.[161] However, a recent survey reported that almost one-half (45.9%) of the respondents commonly administer albumin to their patients with aSAH, but they also acknowledged the need for a randomized clinical trial.[162]

Although prophylactic hypervolemia is no longer recommended, this approach is still commonly used for the treatment of cerebral vasospasm, though even in this setting, the safety and efficacy of hypervolemia are being reconsidered. In a study of 16 patients with severe vasospasm documented with angiography, the impact of hypervolemia (1,000 mL/day colloid plus 3,740 mL/day crystalloid; mean central venous pressure increase from 5.4 cm H_2O to 7.4 cm H_2O), induced hypertension with phenylephrine (MAP increase from 102 mm Hg to 132 mm Hg), or enhanced cardiac output with dobutamine (mean cardiac index increased from 4.1 L/minute/m^2 to 5 L/minute/m^2) was compared using cerebral blood flow as the outcome measurement. Improvements in cerebral blood flow were only observed in patients who received phenylephrine or dobutamine.[163] Similar results were reported in an observational study of 45 patients wherein induced hypertension increased brain tissue oxygenation in 90% of patients with an 8% complication rate, whereas hypervolemia was only effective in 12% of patients but had a 53% complication rate.[164] The role of hypervolemia as a single component of triple-H therapy does not appear to be supported by these small studies. The NCS consensus recommendations suggest considering a saline bolus to increase cerebral blood flow in areas of ischemia as a prelude to other interventions, like induced hypertension.[45]

Case series have linked induced hypertension with improved neurological improvement and increased cerebral blood flow, especially in patients with angiographic vasospasm or in brain regions that are hypoperfused.[165-168] Administering vasoactive agents produces a sustained increase in systemic blood pressure that results in improved CPP, cerebral blood flow, and cerebral tissue oxygenation. In clinical studies, induced hypertension was more effective at improving cerebral oxygenation than aggressive hypervolemia.[164,169] Induced hypertension improves regional cerebral blood flow and brain tissue oxygenation, but these benefits disappear after induction of hypervolemia.[169] A computational model approach evaluated the effect of hypertension and hemodilution in managing vasospasm.[170]

This study found that in cases of severe vasospasm, the systemic blood pressure should be increased in order to reverse vasospasm. Any decreases in hematocrit had minimal impact on cerebral blood flow in a constricted vessel. Two systematic reviews have been published assessing the different components of triple-H therapy.[148,149] The large heterogeneity in interventions and populations studied prohibited conducting a meta-analysis. Hypervolemia did not appear to be superior to normovolemia, but hypervolemia was associated with more adverse effects.[149] Hemodilution was not associated with a change in cerebral blood flow, and hypertension was associated with higher cerebral blood flow, regardless of the volume status.[148,149]

Several vasopressors can be used to induce hypertension, including phenylephrine, norepinephrine, and dopamine. In a prospective case series, the use of high-dose phenylephrine had an acceptable safety profile.[171] There are no studies comparing the effect of different agents on cerebral blood flow. Both phenylephrine and norepinephrine are equally used to induce hypertension.[156] Vasopressin is an effective vasopressor agent but is not routinely used in patients with aSAH because of its potential to exacerbate the hyponatremia that can occur in these patients. When vasopressin (0.01–0.04 unit/minute) was added to maximal phenylephrine therapy (4–5 mcg/kg/minute) in patients with clinically symptomatic vasospasm, vasopressin was effective in reducing the phenylephrine dosage without reducing serum sodium concentrations or causing detrimental effects on cerebral perfusion or worsening vasospasm.[172] Different approaches with respect to defining the blood pressure targets are used in clinical practice. Some clinicians target a percent increase from baseline blood pressure, whereas others target an arbitrary number. Pressure should be increased in a stepwise fashion, as guided by an assessment of the neurological examination, neuromonitoring, or radiological evidence of improved perfusion.[45]

Cardiac output augmentation is an alternative method for increasing cerebral blood flow.[163] In addition to treatment of vasospasm, patients with aSAH may have reduced cardiac output because of "stunned myocardium." An alternative to induced hypertension is the use of inotropic agents like milrinone or dobutamine to induce a hyperdynamic state. One concern with routine use of these agents is the potential to lower blood pressure. Milrinone may be more potent than dobutamine in increasing cardiac output and is more effective in patients with normal vascular resistance and normal blood pressure yet reduced systolic function.[173] Dobutamine may be a preferred option when vascular resistance or blood pressure is reduced.[173] Inotropic agents may be useful in patients who lack response to induced hypertension or have poor cardiac function, but these agents cannot be recommended for prophylactic administration.

Volume status should be routinely monitored in these patients. Although a target central venous pressure of 8 mm Hg or greater has been recommended, it is important to understand the lack of reliability of central venous pressure in estimating intravascular volume; therefore, the approach must be individualized. Goal-directed hemodynamic management using PiCCO has been successfully used in patients with aSAH.[174,175] The specific targets that have been suggested include the following:

- Cardiac index greater than 3.0 L/minute/m^2
- Global end-diastolic volume index equal to 700–900 mL/m^2
- Extravascular lung water index less than 14 mL/kg

Larger randomized controlled trials are needed to validate the usefulness of goal-directed hemodynamic monitoring in patients with aSAH.

The current clinical guidelines recommend maintaining euvolemia and inducing hypertension in patients with DCI, except in those who have elevated blood pressure at baseline or have comorbid cardiac disease, which precludes its use.[44] In patients with preexisting cardiac disease and older adults, the risk of complications with hypervolemic/hypertensive therapy is increased; risks include cardiac failure, pulmonary edema, cerebral edema, and elevated ICP.[171]

Locally Administered Pharmacologic Agents

Targeted delivery of pharmacologic agents through intra-arterial, intraventricular, or intrathecal administration is a method for treating cerebral vasospasm. It is important to evaluate the products directly administered into the central nervous system (CNS) and assess the potential risk of the diluent and other excipients that are contained in the product.[176] Papaverine is a vasodilator agent that preferentially vasodilates cerebral and coronary vascular smooth muscle. Intra-arterial administration of papaverine (150–600 mg) has shown success in treating cerebral vasospasm in published reports of clinical experience.[177-183] The limitation with the use of papaverine is the potential for the development of neurotoxicity because of altered mitochondrial cellular respiration with high exposure.[184] Other adverse events include increased ICP, hemiplegia, seizures, agitation, altered mental status, and hypotension.[185] Because of these significant safety concerns, papaverine is no longer recommended.

Nicardipine has shown promise when administered by intra-arterial, intrathecal, or intraventricular routes of administration for treating cerebral vasospasm.[186-190] Intra-arterial administration involves diluting intravenous nicardipine with 0.9% sodium chloride to a concentration of 0.1 mg/mL and administering in 1-mL aliquots through the microcatheter to a maximum of 5 mg per vessel. Nicardipine is effective at inducing vasodilation and reducing mean peak systolic velocities on TCD from pretreatment for 4 days after the infusion. Overall, neurologic improvement was reported in 42% of patients.[186] Intraventricular administration of nicardipine is an attractive treatment option because it can be administered in the ICU and avoids transport of the patient to the angiography suite. The evidence for this treatment approach is limited to a small case series of eight patients in which nicardipine 4 mg every 12 hours for 5–17 days was administered through the intraventricular catheter. The drug was well tolerated, and seven of the eight patients had good functional outcomes.[188] There are several other more recent studies, two of which report a significant and sustained reduction in mean cerebral blood flow velocity after intraventricular nicardipine; however, neither study was powered for clinical outcomes.[191,192]

Verapamil is another calcium channel antagonist that has been used by way of intra-arterial administration for treating cerebral vasospasm. The published data are from retrospective evaluations in which verapamil was administered at dosages of 25–369 mg per vessel by continuous infusion.[193-196] Verapamil was effective in reversing vasospasm, but close hemodynamic monitoring is advised because the most common complications include hypotension and bradycardia.

Sodium nitroprusside is another vasodilating agent that has been administered by the intraventricular route. In a prospective study of 25 patients with aSAH, nitroprusside 4 mg/mL was given in escalating doses (8–30 mg) and frequency according to mean blood flow velocity on TCD. An improvement in blood flow velocity was reported, together with hypotension and vomiting.[197]

Intra-arterial milrinone has also been used to treat cerebral vasospasm.[198-200] Milrinone is a bipyridine inotropic vasodilator that inhibits peak III cyclic adenosine monophosphate phosphodiesterase isozyme. Combining intra-arterial milrinone (8 mg over 30 minutes repeated up to a maximum of 24 mg) with intravenous milrinone 0.5–1.5 mcg/kg/minute until day 14 after the initial bleed was safe and effective for reversing cerebral vasospasm and was usually well tolerated.[199]

Local administration of all the agents discussed provides a more targeted approach for treating cerebral vasospasm. To date, most of the data for this approach are limited to small case series or case reports, making it difficult to provide definitive recommendations, which in turn leads to significant practice variation across centers treating these patients.

Transluminal Balloon Angioplasty

For significant symptomatic vasospasm in the proximal cerebral arteries, transluminal balloon angioplasty is an effective approach to immediately produce dilation of the involved artery and increase distal cerebral blood flow.[201] Transluminal balloon angioplasty has two limitations: suitability limited to vessels with a diameter of 2 mm or greater and the variability in effectiveness that is based on the operator's expertise. This intervention also has the potential for serious complication rates of about 5%, including vessel rupture, thromboembolic complications, and delayed stenosis.[202] The results of this intervention tend to be more durable compared with those of pharmacologic intervention. No current randomized trials confirm the clinical efficacy, although the current clinical guidelines state that angioplasty is reasonable in symptomatic patients who do not respond to medical therapies, including induced hypertension.[44]

MANAGEMENT AND PREVENTION OF MEDICAL COMPLICATIONS

Renal Complications

Intravascular Volume

As discussed previously, hypovolemia is a common complication after aSAH, and it should be avoided because it is associated with worse clinical outcomes.[155,203] Intravascular volume management should target euvolemia, with isotonic crystalloid the preferred agent for volume replacement. Assessment of intravascular volume in patients after aSAH is essential to daily management. In many institutions, fluid management is guided by calculations of the daily fluid balance of the patient. However, several studies have determined that fluid balance may not accurately reflect intravascular volume status after aSAH.[203-205]

Accurate monitoring of volume status may be accomplished using minimally invasive techniques. One such method is using transpulmonary hemodynamic monitoring (PiCCO). Transpulmonary thermodilution measurements that are obtained using the PiCCO system correlate well with pulmonary artery catheter measurements and provide an effective tool for the fluid management of patients.[175,206] The PiCCO system for monitoring has fewer cardiac complications as well as fewer episodes of symptomatic vasospasm (p<0.05) compared with standard therapy.[207]

Although recognizing that fluid balance may not accurately reflect intravascular volume, the NCS guidelines recommend that the primary assessment of intravascular volume status be close monitoring of fluid balance and clinical assessment. These guidelines continue to state that other invasive and noninvasive modalities may be used to provide supplemental information but that they should not be used in isolation. They also recommend against the routine use of pulmonary artery catheters and dependence on central venous pressure targets. As described in an earlier section, prophylactic hypervolemia therapy is not recommended.[45]

Hyponatremia

Hyponatremia (sodium less than 135 mEq/L) is the most common electrolyte abnormality in patients with aSAH, with a reported incidence as high as 50%.[45,208] Although it is difficult to determine the contribution of hyponatremia to poor patient outcomes, the most feared complication of hypotonic hyponatremia is worsening of cerebral edema.[209] Cerebral salt wasting and syndrome of inappropriate antidiuretic hormone secretion are the two most common causes of this abnormality after aSAH.[147] Both cerebral salt wasting and syndrome of inappropriate antidiuretic hormone secretion are associated with hypotonic hyponatremia, with high urinary sodium content; however, the pathogenesis of the condition is different. Cerebral salt wasting is thought to be caused by an increased secretion of natriuretic peptides, mediated by activation of the sympathetic nervous system, leading to excessive excretion of sodium in the urine. The high intratubular sodium content then creates an osmotic gradient that results in increased water elimination. Therefore, cerebral salt wasting is associated with intravascular volume contraction.[208,209] The syndrome of inappropriate antidiuretic hormone secretion is caused by excessive release of antidiuretic hormone, resulting in retention of free water. Consequently, the syndrome of inappropriate antidiuretic hormone secretion results in normal or slightly expanded intravascular volume.[208,209] Although often thought to be mutually exclusive conditions, cerebral salt wasting and syndrome of inappropriate antidiuretic hormone secretion may also coexist in the same patient.[209]

It is important to determine the cause of hyponatremia because the management for the different causes is vastly different. The focus of management for cerebral salt wasting is replacing the salt and water losses with the use of intravenous sodium solutions with or without mineralocorticoids. Treatment of syndrome of inappropriate antidiuretic hormone secretion is focused on treating the underlying cause or, if that is not possible, using agents that target the excessive antidiuretic hormone secretion.

Most studies in this area have evaluated preventive strategies, aiming to maintain normal serum sodium concentrations (135–145 mEq/L). Several studies have evaluated the use of mineralocorticoids, such as fludrocortisone and hydrocortisone, to prevent hyponatremia and have found them to be effective when initiated early after aSAH.[210,211] The exact approach for use in treating hyponatremia should be directed toward the severity of symptoms and hyponatremia, together with the duration of hyponatremia. Acute cases (less than 48 hours) with severe symptoms should be treated with hypertonic saline (3%), for which a rate of 1 mL/kg/hour increases serum sodium by about 1 mEq/L/hour, and correction should be no more than 12 mEq/L in 24 hours to minimize the risk of overcorrection and osmotic demyelination syndrome. After acute correction, continuing sodium replacement should be no faster than 0.5 mEq/hour.[212] In euvolemic or hypervolemic conditions, vasopressin-receptor antagonists such as conivaptan and tolvaptan are effective in the treatment of hyponatremia. Use of these agents in patients with aSAH may lead to hypovolemia with an increased risk of worse outcomes; hence, careful monitoring has to be enacted if used in this population.[209,213,214]

The NCS guidelines state that current practice varies, with free water restriction, hypertonic saline, and fludrocortisone administration being the most common methods used to manage hyponatremia in the aSAH population. Although acknowledging the weak and low quality of evidence currently available, the NCS guidelines recommend that fluid restriction not be used to treat hyponatremia because of the potential increased risk of cerebral ischemia with hypovolemia. Both the NCS guidelines and the AHA/ASA guidelines state that early treatment with hydrocortisone or fludrocortisone may be used to limit natriuresis and hyponatremia. In addition, they both recommend limiting free water intake. The NCS guidelines further state that mild hypertonic solutions can be used to correct hyponatremia and that extreme caution to avoid hypovolemia is needed if vasopressin-receptor antagonists are administered.[44,45]

Endocrine: Glucose Management

Depending on the definition, hyperglycemia can occur in 30%–100% of patients with aSAH. Several studies have shown associations between admission hyperglycemia or sustained hyperglycemia and worse outcomes.[215-218] Although there are currently no studies that have randomized patients with aSAH to either liberal or tight glucose management, several observational studies exist that have described patients with aSAH who were managed clinically according to various target glucose regimens.[218-220] Risks found associated with hyperglycemia include increased infection and occurrence of vasospasm, whereas targeting tight glucose control (80–110 mg/dL) increased the risk of hypoglycemic events.[221,222] However, limited evidence exists showing a specific target serum glucose range after aSAH. The NCS guidelines recommend avoiding hypoglycemia (serum glucose less than 80 mg/dL) while maintaining serum glucose below 200 mg/dL.[45]

Hematologic

Venous Thromboembolism

Aneurysmal SAH is thought to induce a prothrombotic state, potentially leading to the development of deep venous thrombosis (DVT) and/or pulmonary embolism. The incidence of DVT has ranged from 1.5% to 18%, whereas the incidence of symptomatic pulmonary embolism has been reported to be 3%.[223-225] The wide range reported for DVT is a result of how DVT screening was done, with the higher incidence shown using venous ultrasonography screening. Nonpharmacologic prophylaxis using sequential compression devices is recommended on admission.[45] The risk associated with the use of pharmacologic prophylaxis is hemorrhagic complications; however, literature is lacking to direct the optimal timing for initiating venous thromboembolism prophylaxis as well as the best pharmacologic agent. The current recommendation to withhold pharmacologic DVT prophylaxis until 24 hours after undergoing surgery or an intracranial procedure is extrapolated from the literature evaluating patients with traumatic brain injury and the general neurosurgical population.[45,226,227] No distinction has been made between the use of unfractionated heparin and low-molecular-weight heparin as the agent of choice for venous thromboembolism prophylaxis.

Anemia

Anemia after aSAH is common, with more than 80% of patients reportedly having hemoglobin concentrations less than 11 g/dL. Anemia typically develops 3–4 days after hemorrhage with an average hemoglobin concentration drop of 3 g/dL.[228-230] Factors contributing to anemia after aSAH include an aSAH-related reduction in red blood cell mass, combined with blood losses because of phlebotomy and invasive procedures, as well as hemodilution from fluid administration.[208]

A primary concern in patients who develop anemia after aSAH is that anemia may exacerbate the reduction in oxygen delivery that underlies DCI. Several observational trials have linked anemia or a larger hemoglobin reduction in aSAH with unfavorable outcomes, such as infarction, dependency, and mortality.[228,229,231,232] The optimal hemoglobin threshold for patients with aSAH remains unclear. Limited evidence is currently available suggesting that hemoglobin less than 10 g/dL is associated with brain hypoxia and cerebral tissue injury, although one study showed that a hemoglobin greater than 11 g/dL was associated with less cerebral infarction and improved outcomes after aSAH.[152,233,234]

It also remains unknown whether red blood cell transfusion is the appropriate management strategy to increase the hemoglobin concentration. Red blood cell transfusion is associated with medical complications such as immunosuppression and infections in both general critical care patients and patients with aSAH.[228,235] Although higher hemoglobin targets may be desirable in patients with aSAH, risks associated with red blood cell transfusion need to be considered. The AHA/ASA guidelines state that the use of red blood cell transfusion may be reasonable in patients with aSAH who are at risk of cerebral ischemia, although they state that the optimal hemoglobin goals are still to be determined. Similarly, the NCS guidelines state that patients should receive red blood cell transfusions to maintain hemoglobin concentrations above 8–10 mg/dL and that higher hemoglobin concentrations may be appropriate for patients at risk of DCI, but the use of transfusion is unknown.[44,45]

Cardiac and Pulmonary

Observational studies have reported a high frequency of myocardial injury after aSAH, which is likely related to sympathetic stimulation and catecholamine discharge. The incidence of elevations of troponin I values, arrhythmias, and wall motion abnormalities on echocardiography is about 35%, 35%, and 25%, respectively.[17,236-238] Neurogenic stunned myocardium, thought to be the most severe form of cardiac injury after aSAH, manifests as chest pain, dyspnea, hypoxemia, and cardiogenic shock with pulmonary edema and elevated cardiac markers within hours after aSAH. A wide spectrum of severity exists, including sudden death reported in about 12% of patients. Normal myocardial function commonly returns after 1–3 days; however, evidence of regional wall motion abnormalities has been shown to persist through day 9 after aSAH.[208]

The most important risk factors for cardiac abnormalities appear to be poor clinical grade and DCI. Patients who have cardiac complications are more likely to have a poor outcome because left ventricular dysfunction and low cardiac output are independent risk factors for symptomatic vasospasm.[239,240] Minor cardiac enzyme elevations commonly occur after aSAH, but their significance remains unknown.[45,208] Monitoring of cardiac function may be beneficial in the setting of hemodynamic dysfunction, but it is unclear whether this improves outcomes. The NCS guidelines recommend using best medical practices in the management of cardiac complications.[45]

Symptomatic pulmonary complications such as pulmonary edema, acute lung injury, or acute respiratory distress syndrome are reported to occur in more than 20% of patients with aSAH, with evidence of impaired oxygenation occurring in up to 80% of patients.[241-243] Similar to cardiac complications, the mechanism of pulmonary dysfunction is believed to be related to sympathetic hyperactivity. For the management of pulmonary complications, the NCS guidelines again state to follow the general principles of pulmonary management, including avoiding excessive fluid intake and using diuretics to target euvolemia.[45]

Temperature Modulation

Fever (body temperature of 38.3°C or greater) is a common complication in patients with aSAH (41%–72%) and is associated with worse outcome and increased length of stay, with detrimental effects independent of vasospasm.[244] In addition, in a study using microdialysis measurements, fever induced cerebral metabolic distress, which was reduced with fever control.[245] Although infection as the cause of fever should always be considered, noninfectious fever is common in patients with aSAH, typically starting within the first 3 days after injury. The strongest predictors of fever are a poor Hunt and Hess grade and the presence of intraventricular blood.[246,247]

Several different pharmacologic and nonpharmacologic methods have been evaluated to treat fever. Antipyretics are traditionally used first line to control fever. However, agents such as acetaminophen and ibuprofen are not effective in most patients with aSAH, perhaps because of the impaired thermoregulatory mechanisms seen in brain-damaged patients.[244,248,249] Using continuous infusions of NSAIDs may be more effective in normalizing temperature in patients with aSAH.[250] External nonpharmacologic cooling methods, such as the use of fanning, evaporative cooling, cool cloths, sponging, ice packs, and cooling, are largely ineffective in aSAH. Hydrogel-coated water-circulating energy transfer pads applied externally have efficacy in reducing the fever burden. However, the time to induction of normothermia is usually slow, and problematic shivering may occur.[244,251,252] A new approach to temperature control uses intravascular systems, which are more effective than external cooling devices.[253,254] An important consideration when treating fever is the potential for shivering. Shivering has been reported to occur in up to 40% of patients undergoing therapeutic normothermia with nonpharmacologic strategies. The metabolic consequences of shivering include an increase in resting energy expenditure, carbon dioxide production, and systemic oxygen consumption and a decrease in brain tissue oxygen tension. Interventions such as surface counter-warming and pharmacologic agents such as buspirone, meperidine, propofol, and other sedatives reduce shivering, but the relative efficacy of these strategies remains unknown.[208,244]

Infectious Disease

Nosocomial infections are common in critically ill patients, with serious implications on functional outcome, mortality, and cost of care. In general, neurological and neurosurgical patients may be at an increased risk of nosocomial infections because of the increased incidence of abnormal mental status, coma, aspiration, and concomitant trauma.[255] The overall frequency of nosocomial infections in neuro-ICUs ranges from 14 to 36 per 100 patients.[256,257] In a study looking specifically at patients with aSAH, the most prevalent nosocomial infections were pneumonia (20%), urinary tract infection (13%), bloodstream infection (8%), and meningitis/ventriculitis (5%). Pneumonia and bloodstream infection independently predicted death or disability at 3 months, whereas prolonged length of stay was significantly associated with all infection types. Hunt and Hess scores of 3 or greater, DCI, ICU length of stay, and intubation/mechanical ventilation were all risk factors associated with many infection types.[255]

As stated previously, it is important to rule out infection as the cause of fever in febrile patients. Other infection control measures, such as hand hygiene, elevation of head of bed to prevent aspiration, ventilator weaning trials, management of blood glucose, and early extubation when possible have been adopted in many institutions to prevent nosocomial infections.[45,255]

Pain and Sedation

Headache is the most common complaint of patients after aSAH. Untreated pain can increase sympathetic activity, leading to systemic hypertension, increased cerebral blood flow, oxygen consumption, and elevated ICP. Because of the variety of complications that can occur, adequate assessment and management of headache is important in patients with aSAH.[258,259] A recent retrospective study evaluated the nature, severity, and treatment of headache caused by aSAH. The study showed that headache pain after aSAH is significant and can persist through 7 days after ictus. Patients who developed cerebral vasospasm early after aSAH had a significantly higher pain score than did patients without vasospasm. Furthermore, patients who reported a pain score of 8/10 or higher usually developed vasospasm earlier than patients who reported a pain score less than 4/10.[259]

In patients with aSAH, treatment strategies should be aimed at providing adequate analgesia without confounding the neurologic examination or contributing to morbidity. Monitoring of pain management in critically ill patients is often difficult because of patients' inability to provide a subjective assessment of their pain level. Pain assessment tools such as the Behavioral Pain Scale and the Critical-Care Pain Observation Tool have been validated in ICU patients.[260] These scales use indicators such as facial expression, body movements, and compliance with the ventilator to provide a pain score. In patients who are awake and interactive, pain scales such as the numerical rating scale and/or the visual analog scale can be used.[261,262]

Patients with cognitive dysfunction are also prone to increased fear, restlessness, and agitation from the inability to understand their predicament, thus requiring sedation agents. The Society of Critical Care Medicine has recommended a bundled approach to pain/sedation, promoting a pain-first approach (analagosedation).[260] If a patient's pain is adequately managed and sedation is still required, several agents are often used (see Chapter 6). Short-acting agents are typically preferred in the neurocritically ill population because of the frequency of neurological examinations.

No recommendations are currently available regarding the optimal pain/sedation assessment and management strategy in patients with aSAH. Ultimately, an individualized approach should be used, with specific aspects of drug selection requiring consideration, such as drug-drug interactions, drug-disease interactions, and cost-effectiveness.[261] For more information on pain and sedation in critically ill patients, please see the Society of Critical Care Medicine clinical practice guidelines for the management of pain, agitation, and delirium in adult patients in the ICU.[260]

Paroxysmal Sympathetic Hyperactivity

Acute aSAH can be accompanied by an excess of sympathoadrenal activity that can be termed *paroxysmal sympathetic hyperactivity*, *CNS storming*, *autonomic storming*, and *dysautonomic hyperactivity*. Clinically, this is characterized as sudden onset with hypertension, sinus tachycardia, hyperventilation, facial flushing, hyperemia, diaphoresis, hypertonia, hyperreflexia, and fever.[263] Although this may occur in any patient with an acute brain injury, patients with aSAH who develop this may have prolonged ICU and hospital lengths of stay, increased medical complications, and poor long-term functional outcomes. Several pharmacologic agents have been used to treat paroxysmal sympathetic hyperactivity, including benzodiazepines, bromocriptine, opioids, β-blockers, baclofen, α_2-agonists, and antiepileptic drugs.[263]

SUMMARY AND KEY LEARNING POINTS

Aneurysmal subarachnoid hemorrhage is a devastating disease and is associated with poor outcome and high mortality in a large proportion of patients. The management of patients with aSAH demands expertise to anticipate, recognize, and treat many of the neurological and systemic complications that may occur. Despite the progress made throughout the past decades, there is still a paucity of high-quality evidence to guide the management of these patients. Treatment is focused on three main areas: supportive measures, prevention of complications, and treatment of complications as they arise.

- Many mechanisms are involved in the pathogenesis of the delayed insult after aSAH.
- Managing patients with aSAH is challenging, requires a multidisciplinary team approach, and is best done at high-volume centers.
- Rebleeding is associated with a worse outcome and an increased risk of death; therefore, emergency treatment of a ruptured aneurysm is warranted.
- Medical therapies, including aggressive blood pressure control and the consideration of antifibrinolytic therapy, are recommended until the ruptured aneurysm is treated.
- The use of antiepileptic drugs for seizure prophylaxis remains controversial; it appears reasonable to limit the use of phenytoin in this role; a duration beyond 7 days for seizure prophylaxis does not seem warranted unless risk factors exist for a delayed seizure disorder.
- Nimodipine is the only pharmacologic agent that has shown beneficial effects on patient outcomes; it should be routinely used for all patients with aSAH.
- Hypertension is the best component of triple-H therapy for improving cerebral perfusion and oxygenation, with clinical practice guidelines recommending a euvolemic-induced hypertension approach to managing clinical vasospasm.
- DCI can be treated with combinations of blood pressure or cardiac output augmentation, angioplasty of proximal vasospastic vessels, and local administration of vasodilators.
- Hypovolemia is a common complication after aSAH, and intravascular volume status should be closely monitored.
- Hyponatremia is the most common electrolyte abnormality after aSAH and can be caused by cerebral salt wasting or syndrome of inappropriate antidiuretic hormone secretion; it is important to differentiate the cause because this can dictate management.
- It is recommended to avoid hypoglycemia (serum glucose less than 80 mg/dL) while maintaining serum glucose below 200 mg/dL.
- Venous thromboembolism prophylaxis is recommended using both nonpharmacologic and pharmacologic agents; the optimal time of initiation, agent, and dose remains unknown.
- More than 80% of patients with aSAH have hemoglobin concentrations less than 11 g/dL; although higher hemoglobin concentration goals in patients with aSAH compared with general critically ill patients may be beneficial, the adverse effects associated with red blood cell transfusions need to be considered.
- It is recommended to follow current best medical practices in managing cardiac and pulmonary complications.
- Fever is a common occurrence after aSAH; although fever can result from a noninfectious origin, infection as the cause should always be considered; nonpharmacologic mechanisms such as hydrogel-coated water-circulating energy transfer pads and intravascular cooling devices are effective in temperature control.
- The most prevalent nosocomial infections in patients with aSAH are pneumonia, urinary tract infections, bloodstream infections, and meningitis/ventriculitis; it is recommended that infection control measures be instituted.
- Headache is the most common complaint of patients after aSAH; treatment strategies should be aimed at providing adequate analgesia without confounding the neurologic examination or contributing to other morbidity.

REFERENCES

1. Ingall T, Asplund K, Mahonen M, et al. A multinational comparison of subarachnoid hemorrhage epidemiology in the WHO MONICA stroke study. Stroke 2000;31:1054-61.
2. Feigin VL, Lawes CM, Bennett DA, et al. Worldwide stroke incidence and early case fatality reported in 56 population-based studies: a systematic review. Lancet Neurol 2009;8:355-69.
3. Shea AM, Reed SD, Curtis LH, et al. Characteristics of nontraumatic subarachnoid hemorrhage in the United States in 2003. Neurosurgery 2007;61:1131-7, discussion 7-8.
4. de Rooij NK, Linn FH, van der Plas JA, et al. Incidence of subarachnoid haemorrhage: a systematic review with emphasis on region, age, gender and time trends. J Neurol Neurosurg Psychiatry 2007;78:1365-72.

5. Labovitz DL, Halim AX, Brent B, et al. Subarachnoid hemorrhage incidence among Whites, Blacks and Caribbean Hispanics: the Northern Manhattan Study. Neuroepidemiology 2006;26:147-50.

6. Feigin VL, Rinkel GJ, Lawes CM, et al. Risk factors for subarachnoid hemorrhage: an updated systematic review of epidemiological studies. Stroke 2005;36:2773-80.

7. Kernan WN, Viscoli CM, Brass LM, et al. Phenylpropanolamine and the risk of hemorrhagic stroke. N Engl J Med 2000;343:1826-32.

8. Juvela S, Poussa K, Porras M. Factors affecting formation and growth of intracranial aneurysms: a long-term follow-up study. Stroke 2001;32:485-91.

9. Juvela S, Hillbom M, Numminen H, et al. Cigarette smoking and alcohol consumption as risk factors for aneurysmal subarachnoid hemorrhage. Stroke 1993;24:639-46.

10. Qureshi AI, Suri MF, Yahia AM, et al. Risk factors for subarachnoid hemorrhage. Neurosurgery 2001;49:607-12; discussion 12-3.

11. Sandvei MS, Romundstad PR, Muller TB, et al. Risk factors for aneurysmal subarachnoid hemorrhage in a prospective population study: the HUNT study in Norway. Stroke 2009;40:1958-62.

12. Krischek B, Inoue I. The genetics of intracranial aneurysms. J Hum Genet 2006;51:587-94.

13. Naval NS, Chang T, Caserta F, et al. Impact of pattern of admission on outcomes after aneurysmal subarachnoid hemorrhage. J Crit Care 2012;27:532 e1-7.

14. Kreiter KT, Copeland D, Bernardini GL, et al. Predictors of cognitive dysfunction after subarachnoid hemorrhage. Stroke 2002;33:200-8.

15. Al-Khindi T, Macdonald RL, Schweizer TA. Cognitive and functional outcome after aneurysmal subarachnoid hemorrhage. Stroke 2010;41:e519-36.

16. Rosengart AJ, Schultheiss KE, Tolentino J, et al. Prognostic factors for outcome in patients with aneurysmal subarachnoid hemorrhage. Stroke 2007;38:2315-21.

17. Wartenberg KE, Mayer SA. Medical complications after subarachnoid hemorrhage: new strategies for prevention and management. Curr Opin Crit Care 2006;12:78-84.

18. Dorhout Mees SM, van Dijk GW, Algra A, et al. Glucose levels and outcome after subarachnoid hemorrhage. Neurology 2003;61:1132-3.

19. Frontera JA, Fernandez A, Claassen J, et al. Hyperglycemia after SAH: predictors, associated complications, and impact on outcome. Stroke 2006;37:199-203.

20. Rinkel GJ, Djibuti M, Algra A, et al. Prevalence and risk of rupture of intracranial aneurysms: a systematic review. Stroke 1998;29:251-6.

21. Aoki T, Nishimura M. Targeting chronic inflammation in cerebral aneurysms: focusing on NF-kappaB as a putative target of medical therapy. Expert Opin Ther Targets 2010;14:265-73.

22. Hasan DM, Mahaney KB, Brown RD Jr, et al. Aspirin as a promising agent for decreasing incidence of cerebral aneurysm rupture. Stroke 2011;42:3156-62.

23. Penn DL, Komotar RJ, Sander Connolly E. Hemodynamic mechanisms underlying cerebral aneurysm pathogenesis. J Clin Neurosci 2011;18:1435-8.

24. Brisman JL, Song JK, Newell DW. Cerebral aneurysms. N Engl J Med 2006;355:928-39.

25. Stehbens WE. Aneurysms and anatomical variation of cerebral arteries. Arch Pathol 1963;75:45-64.

26. Anderson C, Ni Mhurchu C, Scott D, et al. Triggers of subarachnoid hemorrhage: role of physical exertion, smoking, and alcohol in the Australasian Cooperative Research on Subarachnoid Hemorrhage Study (ACROSS). Stroke 2003;34:1771-6.

27. Macdonald RL. Delayed neurological deterioration after subarachnoid haemorrhage. Nat Rev Neurol 2014;10:44-58.

28. Chou SH, Feske SK, Atherton J, et al. Early elevation of serum tumor necrosis factor-alpha is associated with poor outcome in subarachnoid hemorrhage. J Investig Med 2012;60:1054-8.

29. Lee JY, Keep RF, He Y, et al. Hemoglobin and iron handling in brain after subarachnoid hemorrhage and the effect of deferoxamine on early brain injury. J Cereb Blood Flow Metab 2010;30:1793-803.

30. Sozen T, Tsuchiyama R, Hasegawa Y, et al. Role of interleukin-1beta in early brain injury after subarachnoid hemorrhage in mice. Stroke 2009;40:2519-25.

31. Yatsushige H, Ostrowski RP, Tsubokawa T, et al. Role of c-Jun N-terminal kinase in early brain injury after subarachnoid hemorrhage. J Neurosci Res 2007;85:1436-48.

32. Sabri M, Ai J, Macdonald RL. Nitric oxide related pathophysiological changes following subarachnoid haemorrhage. Acta Neurochir Suppl 2011;110(pt 1):105-9.

33. Guo Z, Sun X, He Z, et al. Matrix metalloproteinase-9 potentiates early brain injury after subarachnoid hemorrhage. Neurol Res 2010;32:715-20.

34. Frontera JA, Fernandez A, Schmidt JM, et al. Defining vasospasm after subarachnoid hemorrhage: what is the most clinically relevant definition? Stroke 2009;40:1963-8.

35. Dorsch N. A clinical review of cerebral vasospasm and delayed ischaemia following aneurysm rupture. Acta Neurochir Suppl 2011;110(pt 1):5-6.

36. Kassell NF, Sasaki T, Colohan AR, et al. Cerebral vasospasm following aneurysmal subarachnoid hemorrhage. Stroke 1985;16:562-72.

37. Fisher CM, Kistler JP, Davis JM. Relation of cerebral vasospasm to subarachnoid hemorrhage visualized by computerized tomographic scanning. Neurosurgery 1980;6:1-9.

38. Dhar R, Scalfani MT, Blackburn S, et al. Relationship between angiographic vasospasm and regional hypoperfusion in aneurysmal subarachnoid hemorrhage. Stroke 2012;43:1788-94.

39. Etminan N, Vergouwen MD, Ilodigwe D, et al. Effect of pharmaceutical treatment on vasospasm, delayed cerebral ischemia, and clinical outcome in patients with aneurysmal subarachnoid hemorrhage: a systematic review and meta-analysis. J Cereb Blood Flow Metab 2011;31:1443-51.

40. Hinson HE, Sheth KN. Manifestations of the hyperadrenergic state after acute brain injury. Curr Opin Crit Care 2012;18:139-45.

41. Tam AK, Ilodigwe D, Mocco J, et al. Impact of systemic inflammatory response syndrome on vasospasm, cerebral infarction, and outcome after subarachnoid hemorrhage: exploratory analysis of CONSCIOUS-1 database. Neurocrit Care 2010;13:182-9.

42. Berman MF, Solomon RA, Mayer SA, et al. Impact of hospital-related factors on outcome after treatment of cerebral aneurysms. Stroke 2003;34:2200-7.

43. Cross DT III, Tirschwell DL, Clark MA, et al. Mortality rates after subarachnoid hemorrhage: variations according to hospital case volume in 18 states. J Neurosurg 2003;99:810-7.

44. Connolly ES Jr, Rabinstein AA, Carhuapoma JR, et al. Guidelines for the management of aneurysmal subarachnoid hemorrhage: a guideline for healthcare professionals from the American Heart Association/American Stroke Association. Stroke 2012;43:1711-37.

45. Diringer MN, Bleck TP, Claude Hemphill J III, et al. Critical care management of patients following aneurysmal subarachnoid hemorrhage: recommendations from the Neurocritical Care Society's Multidisciplinary Consensus Conference. Neurocrit Care 2011;15:211-40.

46. Samuels O, Webb A, Culler S, et al. Impact of a dedicated neurocritical care team in treating patients with aneurysmal subarachnoid hemorrhage. Neurocrit Care 2011;14:334-40.

47. Edlow JA, Caplan LR. Avoiding pitfalls in the diagnosis of subarachnoid hemorrhage. N Engl J Med 2000;342:29-36.

48. Kowalski RG, Claassen J, Kreiter KT, et al. Initial misdiagnosis and outcome after subarachnoid hemorrhage. JAMA 2004;291:866-9.

49. Sames TA, Storrow AB, Finkelstein JA, et al. Sensitivity of new-generation computed tomography in subarachnoid hemorrhage. Acad Emerg Med 1996;3:16-20.

50. van der Wee N, Rinkel GJ, Hasan D, et al. Detection of subarachnoid haemorrhage on early CT: is lumbar puncture still needed after a negative scan? J Neurol Neurosurg Psychiatry 1995;58:357-9.

51. Mitchell P, Wilkinson ID, Hoggard N, et al. Detection of subarachnoid haemorrhage with magnetic resonance imaging. J Neurol Neurosurg Psychiatry 2001;70:205-11.

52. Jayaraman MV, Mayo-Smith WW, Tung GA, et al. Detection of intracranial aneurysms: multi-detector row CT angiography compared with DSA. Radiology 2004;230:510-8.

53. Bakker NA, Groen RJ, Foumani M, et al. Repeat digital subtraction angiography after a negative baseline assessment in nonperimesencephalic subarachnoid hemorrhage: a pooled data meta-analysis. J Neurosurg 2014;120:99-103.

54. Report of World Federation of Neurological Surgeons Committee on a Universal Subarachnoid Hemorrhage Grading Scale. J Neurosurg 1988;68:985-6.

55. Hunt WE, Hess RM. Surgical risk as related to time of intervention in the repair of intracranial aneurysms. J Neurosurg 1968;28:14-20.

56. Claassen J, Bernardini GL, Kreiter K, et al. Effect of cisternal and ventricular blood on risk of delayed cerebral ischemia after subarachnoid hemorrhage: the Fisher scale revisited. Stroke 2001;32:2012-20.

57. Fujii Y, Takeuchi S, Sasaki O, et al. Ultra-early rebleeding in spontaneous subarachnoid hemorrhage. J Neurosurg 1996;84:35-42.

58. Rhoney DH, Liu-DeRyke X. Effect of vasoactive therapy on cerebral circulation. Crit Care Clin 2006;22:221-43.

59. Liu-Deryke X, Janisse J, Coplin WM, et al. A comparison of nicardipine and labetalol for acute hypertension management following stroke. Neurocrit Care 2008;9:167-76.

60. Roos YB, Rinkel GJE, Vermeulen M, et al. Antifibrinolytic therapy for aneurysmal subarachnoid haemorrhage. Cochrane Database Sys Rev 2003;2:CD001245.

61. Baharoglu MI, Germans MR, Rinkel GJ, et al. Antifibrinolytic therapy for aneurysmal subarachnoid haemorrhage. Cochrane Database Syst Rev 2013;8:CD001245.

62. Harrigan MR, Rajneesh KF, Ardelt AA, et al. Short-term antifibrinolytic therapy before early aneurysm treatment in subarachnoid hemorrhage: effects on rehemorrhage, cerebral ischemia, and hydrocephalus. Neurosurgery 2010;67:935-9; discussion 9-40.

63. Hillman J, Fridriksson S, Nilsson O, et al. Immediate administration of tranexamic acid and reduced incidence of early rebleeding after aneurysmal subarachnoid hemorrhage: a prospective randomized study. J Neurosurg 2002;97:771-8.

64. Starke RM, Kim GH, Fernandez A, et al. Impact of a protocol for acute antifibrinolytic therapy on aneurysm rebleeding after subarachnoid hemorrhage. Stroke 2008;39:2617-21.

65. Molyneux A, Kerr R, Stratton I, et al. International Subarachnoid Aneurysm Trial (ISAT) of neurosurgical clipping versus endovascular coiling in 2143 patients with ruptured intracranial aneurysms: a randomised trial. Lancet 2002;360:1267-74.

66. Molyneux AJ, Kerr RSC, Yu LM, et al. International subarachnoid aneurysm trial (ISAT) of neurosurgical clipping versus endovascular coiling in 2143 patients with ruptured intracranial aneurysms: a randomised comparison of effects on survival, dependency, seizures, rebleeding, subgroups, and aneurysm occlusion. Lancet 2005;366:809-17.

67. Molyneux AJ, Kerr RS, Birks J, et al. Risk of recurrent subarachnoid haemorrhage, death, or dependence and standardised mortality ratios after clipping or coiling of an intracranial aneurysm in the International Subarachnoid Aneurysm Trial (ISAT): long-term follow-up. Lancet Neurol 2009;8:427-33.

68. Butzkueven H, Evans AH, Pitman A, et al. Onset seizures independently predict poor outcome after subarachnoid hemorrhage. Neurology 2000;55:1315-20.

69. Lanzino G, D'Urso PI, Suarez J; Participants in the International Multi-disciplinary Consensus Conference on the Critical Care Management of Subarachnoid H. Seizures and anticonvulsants after aneurysmal subarachnoid hemorrhage. Neurocrit Care 2011;15:247-56.

70. Pinto AN, Canhao P, Ferro JM. Seizures at the onset of subarachnoid haemorrhage. J Neurol 1996;243:161-4.

71. Rhoney DH, Tipps LB, Murry KR, et al. Anticonvulsant prophylaxis and timing of seizures after aneurysmal subarachnoid hemorrhage. Neurology 2000;55:258-65.

72. Rowe AS, Goodwin H, Brophy GM, et al. Seizure prophylaxis in neurocritical care: a review of evidence-based support. Pharmacotherapy 2014;34:396-409.

73. Ibrahim GM, Fallah A, Macdonald RL. Clinical, laboratory, and radiographic predictors of the occurrence of seizures following aneurysmal subarachnoid hemorrhage. J Neurosurg 2013;119:347-52.

74. Hart Y, Sneade M, Birks J, et al. Epilepsy after subarachnoid hemorrhage: the frequency of seizures after clip occlusion or coil embolization of a ruptured cerebral aneurysm: results from

74. the International Subarachnoid Aneurysm Trial. J Neurosurg 2011;115:1159-68.
75. Baker CJ, Prestigiacomo CJ, Solomon RA. Short-term perioperative anticonvulsant prophylaxis for the surgical treatment of low-risk patients with intracranial aneurysms. Neurosurgery 1995;37:863-70; discussion 70-1.
76. Chumnanvej S, Dunn IF, Kim DH. Three-day phenytoin prophylaxis is adequate after subarachnoid hemorrhage. Neurosurgery 2007;60:99-102; discussion 102-3.
77. Rosengart AJ, Huo JD, Tolentino J, et al. Outcome in patients with subarachnoid hemorrhage treated with antiepileptic drugs. J Neurosurg 2007;107:253-60.
78. Naidech AM, Kreiter KT, Janjua N, et al. Phenytoin exposure is associated with functional and cognitive disability after subarachnoid hemorrhage. Stroke 2005;36:583-7.
79. Murphy-Human T, Welch E, Zipfel G, et al. Comparison of short-duration levetiracetam with extended-course phenytoin for seizure prophylaxis after subarachnoid hemorrhage. World Neurosurg 2011;75:269-74.
80. Szaflarski JP, Sangha KS, Lindsell CJ, et al. Prospective, randomized, single-blinded comparative trial of intravenous levetiracetam versus phenytoin for seizure prophylaxis. Neurocrit Care 2010;12:165-72.
81. Graff-Radford NR, Torner J, Adams HP Jr, et al. Factors associated with hydrocephalus after subarachnoid hemorrhage. A report of the Cooperative Aneurysm Study. Arch Neurol 1989;46:744-52.
82. van Gijn J, Hijdra A, Wijdicks EF, et al. Acute hydrocephalus after aneurysmal subarachnoid hemorrhage. J Neurosurg 1985;63:355-62.
83. Doczi T, Nemessanyi Z, Szegvary Z, et al. Disturbances of cerebrospinal fluid circulation during the acute stage of subarachnoid hemorrhage. Neurosurgery 1983;12:435-8.
84. Findlay JM, Kassell NF, Weir BK, et al. A randomized trial of intraoperative, intracisternal tissue plasminogen activator for the prevention of vasospasm. Neurosurgery 1995;37:168-76; discussion 77-8.
85. Stevens RD, Huff JS, Duckworth J, et al. Emergency neurological life support: intracranial hypertension and herniation. Neurocrit Care 2012;17(suppl 1):S60-5.
86. Dankbaar JW, Rijsdijk M, van der Schaaf IC, et al. Relationship between vasospasm, cerebral perfusion, and delayed cerebral ischemia after aneurysmal subarachnoid hemorrhage. Neuroradiology 2009;51:813-9.
87. Rabinstein AA, Weigand S, Atkinson JL, et al. Patterns of cerebral infarction in aneurysmal subarachnoid hemorrhage. Stroke 2005;36:992-7.
88. Brown RJ, Kumar A, Dhar R, et al. The relationship between delayed infarcts and angiographic vasospasm after aneurysmal subarachnoid hemorrhage. Neurosurgery 2013;72:702-7; discussion 7-8.
89. Rabinstein AA, Friedman JA, Weigand SD, et al. Predictors of cerebral infarction in aneurysmal subarachnoid hemorrhage. Stroke 2004;35:1862-6.
90. Mir DI, Gupta A, Dunning A, et al. CT perfusion for detection of delayed cerebral ischemia in aneurysmal subarachnoid hemorrhage: a systematic review and meta-analysis. AJNR Am J Neuroradiol 2014;35:866-71.
91. Gonzalez NR, Boscardin WJ, Glenn T, et al. Vasospasm probability index: a combination of transcranial doppler velocities, cerebral blood flow, and clinical risk factors to predict cerebral vasospasm after aneurysmal subarachnoid hemorrhage. J Neurosurg 2007;107:1101-12.
92. Reilly C, Amidei C, Tolentino J, et al. Clot volume and clearance rate as independent predictors of vasospasm after aneurysmal subarachnoid hemorrhage. J Neurosurg 2004;101:255-61.
93. Conway JE, Tamargo RJ. Cocaine use is an independent risk factor for cerebral vasospasm after aneurysmal subarachnoid hemorrhage. Stroke 2001;32:2338-43.
94. Harrod CG, Bendok BR, Batjer HH. Prediction of cerebral vasospasm in patients presenting with aneurysmal subarachnoid hemorrhage: a review. Neurosurgery 2005;56:633-54; discussion 633-54.
95. Vergouwen MD, Vermeulen M, van Gijn J, et al. Definition of delayed cerebral ischemia after aneurysmal subarachnoid hemorrhage as an outcome event in clinical trials and observational studies: proposal of a multidisciplinary research group. Stroke 2010;41:2391-5.
96. Lindegaard KF, Nornes H, Bakke SJ, et al. Cerebral vasospasm diagnosis by means of angiography and blood velocity measurements. Acta Neurochir (Wien) 1989;100:12-24.
97. Rabinstein AA, Lanzino G, Wijdicks EF. Multidisciplinary management and emerging therapeutic strategies in aneurysmal subarachnoid haemorrhage. Lancet Neurol 2010;9:504-19.
98. Cloft HJ, Joseph GJ, Dion JE. Risk of cerebral angiography in patients with subarachnoid hemorrhage, cerebral aneurysm, and arteriovenous malformation: a meta-analysis. Stroke 1999;30:317-20.
99. Claassen J, Hirsch LJ, Kreiter KT, et al. Quantitative continuous EEG for detecting delayed cerebral ischemia in patients with poor-grade subarachnoid hemorrhage. Clin Neurophysiol 2004;115:2699-710.
100. Claassen J, Vu A, Kreiter KT, et al. Effect of acute physiologic derangements on outcome after subarachnoid hemorrhage. Crit Care Med 2004;32:832-8.
101. Vespa PM, Nuwer MR, Juhasz C, et al. Early detection of vasospasm after acute subarachnoid hemorrhage using continuous EEG ICU monitoring. Electroencephalogr Clin Neurophysiol 1997;103:607-15.
102. Nilsson OG, Brandt L, Ungerstedt U, et al. Bedside detection of brain ischemia using intracerebral microdialysis: subarachnoid hemorrhage and delayed ischemic deterioration. Neurosurgery 1999;45:1176-84; discussion 84-5.
103. Le Roux P, Menon DK, Citerio G, et al. Consensus summary statement of the International Multidisciplinary Consensus Conference on Multimodality Monitoring in Neurocritical Care: a statement for healthcare professionals from the Neurocritical Care Society and the European Society of Intensive Care Medicine. Intensive Care Med 2014;40:1189-209.
104. Dorhout Mees SM, Rinkel GJ, Feigin VL, et al. Calcium antagonists for aneurysmal subarachnoid haemorrhage. Cochrane Database Syst Rev 2007;3:CD000277.
105. Liu-Deryke X, Rhoney DH. Cerebral vasospasm after aneurysmal subarachnoid hemorrhage: an overview of pharmacologic management. Pharmacotherapy 2006;26:182-203.

106. Allen GS, Ahn HS, Preziosi TJ, et al. Cerebral arterial spasm--a controlled trial of nimodipine in patients with subarachnoid hemorrhage. N Engl J Med 1983;308:619-24.

107. Pickard JD, Murray GD, Illingworth R, et al. Effect of oral nimodipine on cerebral infarction and outcome after subarachnoid haemorrhage: British aneurysm nimodipine trial. BMJ 1989;298:636-42.

108. Liu GJ, Luo J, Zhang LP, et al. Meta-analysis of the effectiveness and safety of prophylactic use of nimodipine in patients with an aneurysmal subarachnoid haemorrhage. CNS Neurol Disord Drug Targets 2011;10:834-44.

109. Karinen P, Koivukangas P, Ohinmaa A, et al. Cost-effectiveness analysis of nimodipine treatment after aneurysmal subarachnoid hemorrhage and surgery. Neurosurgery 1999;45:780-4; discussion 4-5.

110. FDA Drug Safety Communication. 2010. Serious Medication Errors from Intravenous Administration of Nimodipine Oral Capsules. Available at www.fda.gov/Drugs/DrugSafety/PostmarketDrugSafetyInformationforPatientsandProviders/ucm220386.htm. Accessed February 28, 2015.

111. FDA Approves Nymalize—First Nimodipine Oral Solution for Use in Certain Brain Hemorrhage Patients. 2013. Available at www.fda.gov/NewsEvents/Newsroom/PressAnnouncements/ucm352280.htm. Accessed February 28, 2015.

112. Cook DJ, Kan S, Ai J, et al. Cisternal sustained release dihydropyridines for subarachnoid hemorrhage. Curr Neurovasc Res 2012;9:139-48.

113. Etminan N, Macdonald RL, Davis C, et al. Intrathecal application of the nimodipine slow-release microparticle system eg-1962 for prevention of delayed cerebral ischemia and improvement of outcome after aneurysmal subarachnoid hemorrhage. Acta Neurochir Suppl 2015;120:281-6.

114. Hanggi D, Etminan N, Macdonald RL, et al. NEWTON: Nimodipine Microparticles to Enhance Recovery While Reducing Toxicity After Subarachnoid Hemorrhage. Neurocrit Care. 2015 Feb 13. [Epub ahead of print]

115. Haley EC Jr, Kassell NF, Torner JC. A randomized trial of nicardipine in subarachnoid hemorrhage: angiographic and transcranial Doppler ultrasound results. A report of the Cooperative Aneurysm Study. J Neurosurg 1993;78:548-53.

116. Haley EC Jr, Kassell NF, Torner JC. A randomized controlled trial of high-dose intravenous nicardipine in aneurysmal subarachnoid hemorrhage. A report of the Cooperative Aneurysm Study. J Neurosurg 1993;78:537-47.

117. McGirt MJ, Lynch JR, Parra A, et al. Simvastatin increases endothelial nitric oxide synthase and ameliorates cerebral vasospasm resulting from subarachnoid hemorrhage. Stroke 2002;33:2950-6.

118. O'Driscoll G, Green D, Taylor RR. Simvastatin, an HMG-coenzyme A reductase inhibitor, improves endothelial function within 1 month. Circulation 1997;95:1126-31.

119. Thelen KM, Rentsch KM, Gutteck U, et al. Brain cholesterol synthesis in mice is affected by high dose of simvastatin but not of pravastatin. J Pharmacol Exp Ther 2006;316:1146-52.

120. Kramer AH, Fletcher JJ. Statins in the management of patients with aneurysmal subarachnoid hemorrhage: a systematic review and meta-analysis. Neurocrit Care 2010;12:285-96.

121. Sanchez-Pena P, Nouet A, Clarencon F, et al. Atorvastatin decreases computed tomography and S100-assessed brain ischemia after subarachnoid aneurysmal hemorrhage: a comparative study. Crit Care Med 2012;40:594-602.

122. Kirkpatrick PJ, Turner CL, Smith C, et al. Simvastatin in aneurysmal subarachnoid haemorrhage (STASH): a multicentre randomised phase 3 trial. Lancet Neurol 2014;13:666-75.

123. Moskowitz SI, Ahrens C, Provencio JJ, et al. Prehemorrhage statin use and the risk of vasospasm after aneurysmal subarachnoid hemorrhage. Surg Neurol 2009;71:311-7; discussion 7-8.

124. Risselada R, Straatman H, van Kooten F, et al. Withdrawal of statins and risk of subarachnoid hemorrhage. Stroke 2009;40:2887-92.

125. Macdonald RL, Curry DJ, Aihara Y, et al. Magnesium and experimental vasospasm. J Neurosurg 2004;100:106-10.

126. Pyne GJ, Cadoux-Hudson TA, Clark JF. Magnesium protection against in vitro cerebral vasospasm after subarachnoid haemorrhage. Br J Neurosurg 2001;15:409-15.

127. van den Bergh WM, Algra A, van der Sprenkel JW, et al. Hypomagnesemia after aneurysmal subarachnoid hemorrhage. Neurosurgery 2003;52:276-81; discussion 81-2.

128. Bradford CM, Finfer S, O'Connor A, et al. A randomised controlled trial of induced hypermagnesaemia following aneurysmal subarachnoid haemorrhage. Crit Care Resusc 2013;15:119-25.

129. Muroi C, Terzic A, Fortunati M, et al. Magnesium sulfate in the management of patients with aneurysmal subarachnoid hemorrhage: a randomized, placebo-controlled, dose-adapted trial. Surg Neurol 2008;69:33-9; discussion 9.

130. van den Bergh WM, Albrecht KW, Berkelbach van der Sprenkel JW, et al. Magnesium therapy after aneurysmal subarachnoid haemorrhage a dose-finding study for long term treatment. Acta Neurochir (Wien) 2003;145:195-9; discussion 9.

131. van den Bergh WM, Algra A, van Kooten F, et al. Magnesium sulfate in aneurysmal subarachnoid hemorrhage: a randomized controlled trial. Stroke 2005;36:1011-5.

132. Veyna RS, Seyfried D, Burke DG, et al. Magnesium sulfate therapy after aneurysmal subarachnoid hemorrhage. J Neurosurg 2002;96:510-4.

133. Westermaier T, Stetter C, Vince GH, et al. Prophylactic intravenous magnesium sulfate for treatment of aneurysmal subarachnoid hemorrhage: a randomized, placebo-controlled, clinical study. Crit Care Med 2010;38:1284-90.

134. Wong GK, Boet R, Poon WS, et al. Intravenous magnesium sulphate for aneurysmal subarachnoid hemorrhage: an updated systemic review and meta-analysis. Crit Care 2011;15:R52.

135. Wong GK, Poon WS, Chan MT, et al. Intravenous magnesium sulphate for aneurysmal subarachnoid hemorrhage (IMASH): a randomized, double-blinded, placebo-controlled, multicenter phase III trial. Stroke 2010;41:921-6.

136. Dorhout Mees SM, Algra A, Vandertop WP, et al. Magnesium for aneurysmal subarachnoid haemorrhage (MASH-2): a randomised placebo-controlled trial. Lancet 2012;380:44-9.

137. Brewer RP, Parra A, Borel CO, et al. Intravenous magnesium sulfate does not increase ventricular CSF ionized magnesium concentration of patients with intracranial hypertension. Clin Neuropharmacol 2001;24:341-5.

138. Mori K, Miyazaki M, Hara Y, et al. Novel vasodilatory effect of intracisternal injection of magnesium sulfate solution on spastic cerebral arteries in the canine two-hemorrhage model of subarachnoid hemorrhage. J Neurosurg 2009;110:73-8.

139. Mori K, Yamamoto T, Nakao Y, et al. Initial clinical experience of vasodilatory effect of intra-cisternal infusion of magnesium sulfate for the treatment of cerebral vasospasm after aneurysmal subarachnoid hemorrhage. Neurol Med Chir (Tokyo) 2009;49:139-44; discussion 44-5.

140. Amin-Hanjani S, Ogilvy CS, Barker FG III. Does intracisternal thrombolysis prevent vasospasm after aneurysmal subarachnoid hemorrhage? A meta-analysis. Neurosurgery 2004;54:326-34; discussion 34-5.

141. Kramer AH, Fletcher JJ. Locally administered intrathecal thrombolytics following aneurysmal subarachnoid hemorrhage: a systematic review and meta-analysis. Neurocrit Care 2011;14:489-99.

142. Bardutzky J, Witsch J, Juttler E, et al. EARLYDRAIN – outcome after early lumbar CSF-drainage in aneurysmal subarachnoid hemorrhage: study protocol for a randomized controlled trial. Trials 2011;12:203.

143. Kastner S, Oertel MF, Scharbrodt W, et al. Endothelin-1 in plasma, cisternal CSF and microdialysate following aneurysmal SAH. Acta Neurochir (Wien) 2005;147:1271-9; discussion 9.

144. Macdonald RL, Kassell NF, Mayer S, et al. Clazosentan to overcome neurological ischemia and infarction occurring after subarachnoid hemorrhage (CONSCIOUS-1): randomized, double-blind, placebo-controlled phase 2 dose-finding trial. Stroke 2008;39:3015-21.

145. Macdonald RL, Higashida RT, Keller E, et al. Clazosentan, an endothelin receptor antagonist, in patients with aneurysmal subarachnoid haemorrhage undergoing surgical clipping: a randomised, double-blind, placebo-controlled phase 3 trial (CONSCIOUS-2). Lancet Neurol 2011;10:618-25.

146. Macdonald RL, Higashida RT, Keller E, et al. Randomized trial of clazosentan in patients with aneurysmal subarachnoid hemorrhage undergoing endovascular coiling. Stroke 2012;43:1463-9.

147. Rhoney DH, McAllen K, Liu-DeRyke X. Current and future treatment considerations in the management of aneurysmal subarachnoid hemorrhage. J Pharm Pract 2010;23:408-24.

148. Dankbaar JW, Slooter AJ, Rinkel GJ, et al. Effect of different components of triple-H therapy on cerebral perfusion in patients with aneurysmal subarachnoid haemorrhage: a systematic review. Crit Care 2010;14:R23.

149. Treggiari MM, Deem S. Which H is the most important in triple-H therapy for cerebral vasospasm? Curr Opin Crit Care 2009;15:83-6.

150. Egge A, Waterloo K, Sjoholm H, et al. Prophylactic hyperdynamic postoperative fluid therapy after aneurysmal subarachnoid hemorrhage: a clinical, prospective, randomized, controlled study. Neurosurgery 2001;49:593-605; discussion 605-6.

151. Lennihan L, Mayer SA, Fink ME, et al. Effect of hypervolemic therapy on cerebral blood flow after subarachnoid hemorrhage: a randomized controlled trial. Stroke 2000;31:383-91.

152. Naidech AM, Jovanovic B, Wartenberg KE, et al. Higher hemoglobin is associated with improved outcome after subarachnoid hemorrhage. Crit Care Med 2007;35:2383-9.

153. Smith MJ, Le Roux PD, Elliott JP, et al. Blood transfusion and increased risk for vasospasm and poor outcome after subarachnoid hemorrhage. J Neurosurg 2004;101:1-7.

154. Festic E, Rabinstein AA, Freeman WD, et al. Blood transfusion is an important predictor of hospital mortality among patients with aneurysmal subarachnoid hemorrhage. Neurocrit Care 2013;18:209-15.

155. Nakagawa A, Su CC, Sato K, et al. Evaluation of changes in circulating blood volume during acute and very acute stages of subarachnoid hemorrhage: implications for the management of hypovolemia. J Neurosurg 2002;97:268-71.

156. Meyer R, Deem S, Yanez ND, et al. Current practices of triple-H prophylaxis and therapy in patients with subarachnoid hemorrhage. Neurocrit Care 2011;14:24-36.

157. Al-Rawi PG, Tseng MY, Richards HK, et al. Hypertonic saline in patients with poor-grade subarachnoid hemorrhage improves cerebral blood flow, brain tissue oxygen, and pH. Stroke 2010;41:122-8.

158. Horstick G, Lauterbach M, Kempf T, et al. Early albumin infusion improves global and local hemodynamics and reduces inflammatory response in hemorrhagic shock. Crit Care Med 2002;30:851-5.

159. Suarez JI, Shannon L, Zaidat OO, et al. Effect of human albumin administration on clinical outcome and hospital cost in patients with subarachnoid hemorrhage. J Neurosurg 2004;100:585-90.

160. Suarez JI, Martin RH, Calvillo E, et al. The Albumin in Subarachnoid Hemorrhage (ALISAH) multicenter pilot clinical trial: safety and neurologic outcomes. Stroke 2012;43:683-90.

161. Investigators SS, Australian, New Zealand Intensive Care Society Clinical Trials G, Australian Red Cross Blood S, George Institute for International H, Myburgh J, et al. Saline or albumin for fluid resuscitation in patients with traumatic brain injury. N Engl J Med 2007;357:874-84.

162. Suarez JI, Martin RH, Calvillo E, et al. Human albumin administration in subarachnoid hemorrhage: results of an international survey. Neurocrit Care 2014;20:277-86.

163. Joseph M, Ziadi S, Nates J, et al. Increases in cardiac output can reverse flow deficits from vasospasm independent of blood pressure: a study using xenon computed tomographic measurement of cerebral blood flow. Neurosurgery 2003;53:1044-51; discussion 51-2.

164. Raabe A, Beck J, Keller M, et al. Relative importance of hypertension compared with hypervolemia for increasing cerebral oxygenation in patients with cerebral vasospasm after subarachnoid hemorrhage. J Neurosurg 2005;103:974-81.

165. Kassell NF, Peerless SJ, Durward QJ, et al. Treatment of ischemic deficits from vasospasm with intravascular volume expansion and induced arterial hypertension. Neurosurgery 1982;11:337-43.

166. Muizelaar JP, Becker DP. Induced hypertension for the treatment of cerebral ischemia after subarachnoid hemorrhage. Direct effect on cerebral blood flow. Surg Neurol 1986;25:317-25.

167. Otsubo H, Takemae T, Inoue T, et al. Normovolaemic induced hypertension therapy for cerebral vasospasm after subarachnoid haemorrhage. Acta Neurochir (Wien) 1990;103:18-26.

168. Touho H, Karasawa J, Ohnishi H, et al. Evaluation of therapeutically induced hypertension in patients with delayed cerebral vasospasm by xenon-enhanced computed tomography. Neurol Med Chir (Tokyo) 1992;32:671-8.

169. Muench E, Horn P, Bauhuf C, et al. Effects of hypervolemia and hypertension on regional cerebral blood flow, intracranial pressure, and brain tissue oxygenation after subarachnoid hemorrhage. Crit Care Med 2007;35:1844-51; quiz 52.

170. Robinson JS, Walid MS, Hyun S, et al. Computational modeling of HHH therapy and impact of blood pressure and hematocrit. World Neurosurg 2010;74:294-6.

171. Miller JA, Dacey RG Jr, Diringer MN. Safety of hypertensive hypervolemic therapy with phenylephrine in the treatment of delayed ischemic deficits after subarachnoid hemorrhage. Stroke 1995;26:2260-6.

172. Muehlschlegel S, Dunser MW, Gabrielli A, et al. Arginine vasopressin as a supplementary vasopressor in refractory hypertensive, hypervolemic, hemodilutional therapy in subarachnoid hemorrhage. Neurocrit Care 2007;6:3-10.

173. Naidech A, Du Y, Kreiter KT, et al. Dobutamine versus milrinone after subarachnoid hemorrhage. Neurosurgery 2005;56:21-61; discussion 6-7.

174. LeTourneau JL, Pinney J, Phillips CR. Extravascular lung water predicts progression to acute lung injury in patients with increased risk. Crit Care Med 2012;40:847-54.

175. Mutoh T, Kazumata K, Ajiki M, et al. Goal-directed fluid management by bedside transpulmonary hemodynamic monitoring after subarachnoid hemorrhage. Stroke 2007;38:3218-24.

176. Cook AM, Mieure KD, Owen RD, et al. Intracerebroventricular administration of drugs. Pharmacotherapy 2009;29:832-45.

177. Clouston JE, Numaguchi Y, Zoarski GH, et al. Intraarterial papaverine infusion for cerebral vasospasm after subarachnoid hemorrhage. AJNR Am J Neuroradiol 1995;16:27-38.

178. Firlik KS, Kaufmann AM, Firlik AD, et al. Intra-arterial papaverine for the treatment of cerebral vasospasm following aneurysmal subarachnoid hemorrhage. Surg Neurol 1999;51:66-74.

179. Kassell NF, Helm G, Simmons N, et al. Treatment of cerebral vasospasm with intra-arterial papaverine. J Neurosurg 1992;77:848-52.

180. Little N, Morgan MK, Grinnell V, et al. Intra-arterial papaverine in the management of cerebral vasospasm following subarachnoid haemorrhage. J Clin Neurosci 1994;1:42-6.

181. Liu JK, Tenner MS, Gottfried ON, et al. Efficacy of multiple intraarterial papaverine infusions for improvement in cerebral circulation time in patients with recurrent cerebral vasospasm. J Neurosurg 2004;100:414-21.

182. Numaguchi Y, Zoarski GH. Intra-arterial papaverine treatment for cerebral vasospasm: our experience and review of the literature. Neurol Med Chir (Tokyo) 1998;38:189-95.

183. Polin RS, Hansen CA, German P, et al. Intra-arterially administered papaverine for the treatment of symptomatic cerebral vasospasm. Neurosurgery 1998;42:1256-64; discussion 64-7.

184. Smith WS, Dowd CF, Johnston SC, et al. Neurotoxicity of intra-arterial papaverine preserved with chlorobutanol used for the treatment of cerebral vasospasm after aneurysmal subarachnoid hemorrhage. Stroke 2004;35:2518-22.

185. Carhuapoma JR, Qureshi AI, Tamargo RJ, et al. Intra-arterial papaverine-induced seizures: case report and review of the literature. Surg Neurol 2001;56:159-63.

186. Badjatia N, Topcuoglu MA, Pryor JC, et al. Preliminary experience with intra-arterial nicardipine as a treatment for cerebral vasospasm. AJNR Am J Neuroradiol 2004;25:819-26.

187. Ehtisham A, Taylor S, Bayless L, et al. Use of intrathecal nicardipine for aneurysmal subarachnoid hemorrhage-induced cerebral vasospasm. South Med J 2009;102:150-3.

188. Goodson K, Lapointe M, Monroe T, et al. Intraventricular nicardipine for refractory cerebral vasospasm after subarachnoid hemorrhage. Neurocrit Care 2008;8:247-52.

189. Linfante I, Delgado-Mederos R, Andreone V, et al. Angiographic and hemodynamic effect of high concentration of intra-arterial nicardipine in cerebral vasospasm. Neurosurgery 2008;63:1080-6; discussion 6-7.

190. Tejada JG, Taylor RA, Ugurel MS, et al. Safety and feasibility of intra-arterial nicardipine for the treatment of subarachnoid hemorrhage-associated vasospasm: initial clinical experience with high-dose infusions. AJNR Am J Neuroradiol 2007;28:844-8.

191. Lu N, Jackson D, Luke S, et al. Intraventricular nicardipine for aneurysmal subarachnoid hemorrhage related vasospasm: assessment of 90 days outcome. Neurocrit Care 2012;16:368-75.

192. Webb A, Kolenda J, Martin K, et al. The effect of intraventricular administration of nicardipine on mean cerebral blood flow velocity measured by transcranial Doppler in the treatment of vasospasm following aneurysmal subarachnoid hemorrhage. Neurocrit Care 2010;12:159-64.

193. Albanese E, Russo A, Quiroga M, et al. Ultrahigh-dose intraarterial infusion of verapamil through an indwelling microcatheter for medically refractory severe vasospasm: initial experience. J Neurosurg 2010;113:913-22.

194. Feng L, Fitzsimmons BF, Young WL, et al. Intraarterially administered verapamil as adjunct therapy for cerebral vasospasm: safety and 2-year experience. AJNR Am J Neuroradiol 2002;23:1284-90.

195. Flexman AM, Ryerson CJ, Talke PO. Hemodynamic stability after intraarterial injection of verapamil for cerebral vasospasm. Anesth Analg 2012;114:1292-6.

196. Keuskamp J, Murali R, Chao KH. High-dose intraarterial verapamil in the treatment of cerebral vasospasm after aneurysmal subarachnoid hemorrhage. J Neurosurg 2008;108:458-63.

197. Agrawal A, Patir R, Kato Y, et al. Role of intraventricular sodium nitroprusside in vasospasm secondary to aneurysmal subarachnoid haemorrhage: a 5-year prospective study with review of the literature. Minim Invasive Neurosurg 2009;52:5-8.

198. Arakawa Y, Kikuta K, Hojo M, et al. Milrinone for the treatment of cerebral vasospasm after subarachnoid hemorrhage: report of seven cases. Neurosurgery 2001;48:723-8; discussion 8-30.

199. Fraticelli AT, Cholley BP, Losser MR, et al. Milrinone for the treatment of cerebral vasospasm after aneurysmal subarachnoid hemorrhage. Stroke 2008;39:893-8.

200. Schmidt U, Bittner E, Pivi S, et al. Hemodynamic management and outcome of patients treated for cerebral vasospasm with

intraarterial nicardipine and/or milrinone. Anesth Analg 2010;110:895-902.

201. Firlik AD, Kaufmann AM, Jungreis CA, et al. Effect of transluminal angioplasty on cerebral blood flow in the management of symptomatic vasospasm following aneurysmal subarachnoid hemorrhage. J Neurosurg 1997;86:830-9.

202. Pierot L, Aggour M, Moret J. Vasospasm after aneurysmal subarachnoid hemorrhage: recent advances in endovascular management. Curr Opin Crit Care 2010;16:110-6.

203. Hoff RG, van Dijk GW, Algra A, et al. Fluid balance and blood volume measurement after aneurysmal subarachnoid hemorrhage. Neurocrit Care 2008;8:391-7.

204. Hoff RG, Rinkel GJ, Verweij BH, et al. Nurses' prediction of volume status after aneurysmal subarachnoid haemorrhage: a prospective cohort study. Crit Care 2008;12:R153.

205. Hoff R, Rinkel G, Verweij B, et al. Blood volume measurement to guide fluid therapy after aneurysmal subarachnoid hemorrhage: a prospective controlled study. Stroke 2009;40:2575-7.

206. Mutoh T, Ishikawa T, Nishino K, et al. Evaluation of the FloTrac uncalibrated continuous cardiac output system for perioperative hemodynamic monitoring after subarachnoid hemorrhage. J Neurosurg Anesthesiol 2009;21:218-25.

207. Mutoh T, Kazumata K, Ishikawa T, et al. Performance of bedside transpulmonary thermodilution monitoring for goal-directed hemodynamic management after subarachnoid hemorrhage. Stroke 2009;40:2368-74.

208. Wartenberg KE, Mayer SA. Medical complications after subarachnoid hemorrhage. Neurosurg Clin N Am 2010;21:325-38.

209. Rabinstein AA, Bruder N. Management of hyponatremia and volume contraction. Neurocrit Care 2011;15:354-60.

210. Katayama Y, Haraoka J, Hirabayashi H, et al. A randomized controlled trial of hydrocortisone against hyponatremia in patients with aneurysmal subarachnoid hemorrhage. Stroke 2007;38:2373-5.

211. Moro N, Katayama Y, Kojima J, et al. Prophylactic management of excessive natriuresis with hydrocortisone for efficient hypervolemic therapy after subarachnoid hemorrhage. Stroke 2003;34:2807-11.

212. Rahman M, Friedman WA. Hyponatremia in neurosurgical patients: clinical guidelines development. Neurosurgery 2009;65:925-35; discussion 35-6.

213. Murphy T, Dhar R, Diringer M. Conivaptan bolus dosing for the correction of hyponatremia in the neurointensive care unit. Neurocrit Care 2009;11:14-9.

214. Rabinstein AA. Vasopressin antagonism: potential impact on neurologic disease. Clin Neuropharmacol 2006;29:87-93.

215. Lanzino G, Kassell NF, Germanson T, et al. Plasma glucose levels and outcome after aneurysmal subarachnoid hemorrhage. J Neurosurg 1993;79:885-91.

216. Kruyt ND, Biessels GJ, de Haan RJ, et al. Hyperglycemia and clinical outcome in aneurysmal subarachnoid hemorrhage: a meta-analysis. Stroke 2009;40:e424-30.

217. Lee SH, Lim JS, Kim N, Yoon BW. Effects of admission glucose level on mortality after subarachnoid hemorrhage: a comparison between short-term and long-term mortality. J Neurol Sci 2008;275:18-21.

218. Schlenk F, Vajkoczy P, Sarrafzadeh A. Inpatient hyperglycemia following aneurysmal subarachnoid hemorrhage: relation to cerebral metabolism and outcome. Neurocrit Care 2009;11:56-63.

219. Bilotta F, Spinelli A, Giovannini F, et al. The effect of intensive insulin therapy on infection rate, vasospasm, neurologic outcome, and mortality in neurointensive care unit after intracranial aneurysm clipping in patients with acute subarachnoid hemorrhage: a randomized prospective pilot trial. J Neurosurg Anesthesiol 2007;19:156-60.

220. Bell DA, Strong AJ. Glucose/insulin infusions in the treatment of subarachnoid haemorrhage: a feasibility study. Br J Neurosurg 2005;19:21-4.

221. Badjatia N, Topcuoglu MA, Buonanno FS, et al. Relationship between hyperglycemia and symptomatic vasospasm after subarachnoid hemorrhage. Crit Care Med 2005;33:1603-9.

222. Naidech AM, Levasseur K, Liebling S, et al. Moderate hypoglycemia is associated with vasospasm, cerebral infarction, and 3-month disability after subarachnoid hemorrhage. Neurocrit Care 2010;12:181-7.

223. Mack WJ, Ducruet AF, Hickman ZL, et al. Doppler ultrasonography screening of poor-grade subarachnoid hemorrhage patients increases the diagnosis of deep venous thrombosis. Neurol Res 2008;30:889-92.

224. Kim KS, Brophy GM. Symptomatic venous thromboembolism: incidence and risk factors in patients with spontaneous or traumatic intracranial hemorrhage. Neurocrit Care 2009;11:28-33.

225. Ray WZ, Strom RG, Blackburn SL, et al. Incidence of deep venous thrombosis after subarachnoid hemorrhage. J Neurosurg 2009;110:1010-4.

226. Norwood SH, McAuley CE, Berne JD, et al. Prospective evaluation of the safety of enoxaparin prophylaxis for venous thromboembolism in patients with intracranial hemorrhagic injuries. Arch Surg 2002;137:696-701; discussion-2.

227. Collen JF, Jackson JL, Shorr AF, et al. Prevention of venous thromboembolism in neurosurgery: a meta-analysis. Chest 2008;134:237-49.

228. Kramer AH, Gurka MJ, Nathan B, et al. Complications associated with anemia and blood transfusion in patients with aneurysmal subarachnoid hemorrhage. Crit Care Med 2008;36:2070-5.

229. Kramer AH, Zygun DA, Bleck TP, et al. Relationship between hemoglobin concentrations and outcomes across subgroups of patients with aneurysmal subarachnoid hemorrhage. Neurocrit Care 2009;10:157-65.

230. Sampson TR, Dhar R, Diringer MN. Factors associated with the development of anemia after subarachnoid hemorrhage. Neurocrit Care 2010;12:4-9.

231. Le Roux PD; Participants in the International Multi-disciplinary Consensus Conference on the Critical Care Management of Subarachnoid H. Anemia and transfusion after subarachnoid hemorrhage. Neurocrit Care 2011;15:342-53.

232. Wartenberg KE, Schmidt JM, Claassen J, et al. Impact of medical complications on outcome after subarachnoid hemorrhage. Crit Care Med 2006;34:617-23; quiz 24.

233. Kurtz P, Schmidt JM, Claassen J, et al. Anemia is associated with metabolic distress and brain tissue hypoxia after subarachnoid hemorrhage. Neurocrit Care 2010;13:10-6.

234. Oddo M, Milby A, Chen I, et al. Hemoglobin concentration and cerebral metabolism in patients with aneurysmal subarachnoid hemorrhage. Stroke 2009;40:1275-81.

235. Levine J, Kofke A, Cen L, et al. Red blood cell transfusion is associated with infection and extracerebral complications after subarachnoid hemorrhage. Neurosurgery 2010;66:312-8; discussion 8.

236. Banki N, Kopelnik A, Tung P, et al. Prospective analysis of prevalence, distribution, and rate of recovery of left ventricular systolic dysfunction in patients with subarachnoid hemorrhage. J Neurosurg 2006;105:15-20.

237. Deibert E, Barzilai B, Braverman AC, et al. Clinical significance of elevated troponin I levels in patients with nontraumatic subarachnoid hemorrhage. J Neurosurg 2003;98:741-6.

238. Hravnak M, Frangiskakis JM, Crago EA, et al. Elevated cardiac troponin I and relationship to persistence of electrocardiographic and echocardiographic abnormalities after aneurysmal subarachnoid hemorrhage. Stroke 2009;40:3478-84.

239. Crago EA, Kerr ME, Kong Y, et al. The impact of cardiac complications on outcome in the SAH population. Acta Neurol Scand 2004;110:248-53.

240. Okabe T, Kanzaria M, Rincon F, et al. Cardiovascular protection to improve clinical outcomes after subarachnoid hemorrhage: is there a proven role? Neurocrit Care 2013;18:271-84.

241. Friedman JA, Pichelmann MA, Piepgras DG, et al. Pulmonary complications of aneurysmal subarachnoid hemorrhage. Neurosurgery 2003;52:1025-31; discussion 31-2.

242. Solenski NJ, Haley EC Jr, Kassell NF, et al. Medical complications of aneurysmal subarachnoid hemorrhage: a report of the multicenter, cooperative aneurysm study. Participants of the Multicenter Cooperative Aneurysm Study. Crit Care Med 1995;23:1007-17.

243. Vespa PM, Bleck TP. Neurogenic pulmonary edema and other mechanisms of impaired oxygenation after aneurysmal subarachnoid hemorrhage. Neurocrit Care 2004;1:157-70.

244. Scaravilli V, Tinchero G, Citerio G; Participants in the International Multi-disciplinary Consensus Conference on the Critical Care Management of Subarachnoid H. Fever management in SAH. Neurocrit Care 2011;15:287-94.

245. Oddo M, Frangos S, Milby A, et al. Induced normothermia attenuates cerebral metabolic distress in patients with aneurysmal subarachnoid hemorrhage and refractory Fever. Stroke 2009;40:1913-6.

246. Commichau C, Scarmeas N, Mayer SA. Risk factors for fever in the neurologic intensive care unit. Neurology 2003;60:837-41.

247. Rabinstein AA, Sandhu K. Non-infectious fever in the neurological intensive care unit: incidence, causes and predictors. J Neurol Neurosurg Psychiatry 2007;78:1278-80.

248. Dippel DW, van Breda EJ, van Gemert HM, et al. Effect of paracetamol (acetaminophen) on body temperature in acute ischemic stroke: a double-blind, randomized phase II clinical trial. Stroke 2001;32:1607-12.

249. Mayer S, Commichau C, Scarmeas N, et al. Clinical trial of an air-circulating cooling blanket for fever control in critically ill neurologic patients. Neurology 2001;56:292-8.

250. Cormio M, Citerio G. Continuous low dose diclofenac sodium infusion to control fever in neurosurgical critical care. Neurocrit Care 2007;6:82-9.

251. Mayer SA, Kowalski RG, Presciutti M, et al. Clinical trial of a novel surface cooling system for fever control in neurocritical care patients. Crit Care Med 2004;32:2508-15.

252. Price T, McGloin S, Izzard J, et al. Cooling strategies for patients with severe cerebral insult in ICU (Part 2). Nurs Crit Care 2003;8:37-45.

253. Diringer MN; Neurocritical Care Fever Reduction Trial G. Treatment of fever in the neurologic intensive care unit with a catheter-based heat exchange system. Crit Care Med 2004;32:559-64.

254. Hoedemaekers CW, Ezzahti M, Gerritsen A, et al. Comparison of cooling methods to induce and maintain normo- and hypothermia in intensive care unit patients: a prospective intervention study. Crit Care 2007;11:R91.

255. Frontera JA, Fernandez A, Schmidt M, et al. Impact of nosocomial infectious complications after subarachnoid hemorrhage. Neurosurgery 2008;62:80-7; discussion 7.

256. Daschner FD, Frey P, Wolff G, et al. Nosocomial infections in intensive care wards: a multicenter prospective study. Intensive Care Med 1982;8:5-9.

257. Dettenkofer M, Ebner W, Els T, et al. Surveillance of nosocomial infections in a neurology intensive care unit. J Neurol 2001;248:959-64.

258. Diringer MN. Management of aneurysmal subarachnoid hemorrhage. Crit Care Med 2009;37:432-40.

259. Swope R, Glover K, Gokun Y, et al. Evaluation of headache severity after aneurysmal subarachnoid hemorrhage. Interdisciplinary Neurosurgery 2014;1:119-22.

260. Barr J, Fraser GL, Puntillo K, et al. Clinical practice guidelines for the management of pain, agitation, and delirium in adult patients in the intensive care unit. Crit Care Med 2013;41:263-306.

261. Makii JM, Mirski MA, Lewin JJ III. Sedation and analgesia in critically ill neurologic patients. J Pharm Pract 2010;23:455-69.

262. Mirski MA, Hemstreet MK. Critical care sedation for neuroscience patients. J Neurol Sci 2007;261:16-34.

263. Perkes I, Baguley IJ, Nott MT, et al. A review of paroxysmal sympathetic hyperactivity after acquired brain injury. Ann Neurol 2010;68:126-35.

Section 4

Hematology

Chapter 23: Prevention and Treatment of Venous Thromboembolism

William E. Dager, Pharm.D., FCCP, FCCM, FCSHP, FASHP, MCCM, BCPS; and A. Josh Roberts, Pharm.D., BCPS

LEARNING OBJECTIVES

1. Understand the risks involved with the occurrence and management of a venous thrombotic (VTE) event.
2. Describe common risk factors for a VTE present in the critically ill patient.
3. Describe the various approaches to VTE prophylaxis in the intensive care unit.
4. Implement an anticoagulation regimen in the setting of a new VTE event.
5. Discuss approaches to monitor a patient receiving prophylaxis or treatment of a VTE.
6. Describe the reversal of an antithrombotic agent.

ABBREVIATIONS IN THIS CHAPTER

ACS	Acute coronary syndromes	ICU	Intensive care unit
aPCC	Activated prothrombin complex concentrate	LMWH	Low-molecular-weight heparin
		PCC	Prothrombin complex concentrate
aPTT	Activated partial thromboplastin time	PE	Pulmonary embolism
AT	Antithrombin	rFVIIa	Recombinant activated factor II
DTI	Direct thrombin inhibitor	TE	Thromboembolism
DVT	Deep venous thrombosis	UFH	Unfractionated heparin
HIT	Heparin-induced thrombocytopenia	VTE	Venous thromboembolism

INTRODUCTION

Although not a common reason for being in the intensive care unit (ICU), thromboembolism (TE) either in the cardiac chamber or on the venous and arterial vessels, together with the challenges in providing the necessary management, can affect outcomes. The occurrence of venous thromboembolism (VTE) can be high and potentially devastating in the ICU, with risks of developing it related to the presence of comorbid conditions including venous stasis, hypercoagulable conditions, and endothelial damage, which are the main components of Virchow triad.[1] The number of risk factors present, together with the magnitude of their expression, can determine the related risk and incidence of VTE. The incidence of deep venous thrombus (DVT) has been reported as high as 28%–32% in the medical ICU population and up to 60%–70% with trauma or ischemic stroke.[2] For DVT, the most common locations include the lower extremity, but it can also occur in the upper extremity, especially in regions where venous access lines or catheters existed.[3] Although most TEs may be asymptomatic and undetected, symptomatic VTE including pulmonary embolism (PE) can potentially be devastating. Consequences include chronic thromboembolic pulmonary hypertension, post-thrombotic syndrome, and venous stasis ulcers. Massive PE can lead to pulseless electrical activity–related cardiac arrest and sudden death.

Management of anticoagulation carries an increased risk of bleeding complications. As such, in the presence of anticoagulation, procedures may be avoided or done differently, blood product transfusions or corrective procedures for bleeding may occur, and duration of ICU stay may be prolonged, creating additional risks for the patient. Because of this, acutely ill patients, including those in the ICU, may receive mechanical or pharmacologic VTE prophylaxis as a preventive measure. Guidelines have been developed to address the prevention or treatment of various forms of VTE, but these may be limited in the critical care setting because of bleeding, invasive procedures, loss of sites to administer injections, or just being overlooked. Given the notable challenges because of the countless variables and heterogeneity that exist and exclusion factors in clinical trials, well-controlled studies in the ICU setting are limited. Many of our current management approaches for VTE in the ICU continue to be based on clinical experiences or on limited, smaller studies. Suggestions regarding anticoagulant agent selection and the dosing regimen may not have considered challenges that may exist in the critically ill patient such as planned invasive procedures, extent of endothelial damage, transient imbalance between drivers for thrombosis and hemostasis, excessive fluid, impact of vasoactive agents on subcutaneous delivery, multisystem organ failure, low platelet counts, liver disease–related coagulopathy, or presence of mechanical circulatory devices, to just name a few. Because of the devastating consequences of VTE and related anticoagulation management, various agencies have developed and implemented regulations or outcomes measures to encourage best practices. Examples include protocols on the initiation and maintenance of anticoagulation therapy, education, and follow-up monitoring (www.jointcommission.org/standards_information/npsgs.aspx).

PREVENTION OF VTE

Current guidelines have explored various forms of VTE prevention in the ICU setting. Key concepts include avoiding delays in implementing prophylaxis, understanding limitations with the use of pharmacologic agents when the risk of bleeding is high, providing agent selection dose, and understanding potential need for modifications in selected ICU populations (e.g., renal insufficiency).[4] The ICU patient may be unable to ambulate or may have to be kept in a position that promotes venous stasis. If ambulation is at all possible, it should be encouraged. As mentioned, several risk factors for VTE can occur in the ICU, with some being transient and others long term. The presence of endothelial damage from invasive procedures, including use of catheters or related trauma of the venous vascular bed, also increases VTE risks. Other causes of venous stasis include heart failure, sepsis (which can be a multiple trigger), and the result of major surgery. Hypercoagulable conditions occurring in the ICU, although too many to explore in detail, should always be considered. Some may be hereditary and may not lead to a VTE event until combined with additional risk factors. Long-term risk factors can include cancer, obesity, long-term effects of trauma, or history of VTE. Transient hypercoagulable conditions may be the result of exposure to drivers for thrombosis. Examples include surgery, immobility, the use of concentrated clotting factors, immune-mediated heparin-induced thrombocytopenia (HIT), impairment of natural factors protecting against thrombosis such as loss of antithrombin (AT), acute blood loss, excessive hemoglobin from erythropoiesis-stimulating agents, cardiopulmonary failure, use of vasopressors, presence of mechanical devices within the cardiovascular system (e.g., extracorporeal life support), pregnancy, drugs such as steroids, and oral contraceptives.

Management decisions should balance the risk of VTE and bleeding when implementing or holding anticoagulation therapy and may occur on a moment-by-moment basis in more unstable situations. This may especially be true when invasive procedures are necessary or when other drivers for bleeding must be balanced with the concurrent risks of thrombosis. Common risks of bleeding include a history of bleeding complications (e.g., gastrointestinal bleeding); consequences of invasive procedures including neuraxial anesthesia; trauma; deficiency in the hemostatic process, such as loss of clotting factors; continued presence of an anticoagulant or antiplatelet agent; kidney or liver failure; and the inability to transfuse, if necessary. Bleeding at any surgical site is a concern, especially if it is closed and an accumulation of blood increases the risk of complications. The presence of a drain and the ability to transfuse may at times ease this concern. The potential volume of blood and the regions in which it occurs may also factor in. Small amounts of blood in critical surgical sites such as the central nervous system (CNS), selected ocular regions, or cardiac regions may be of especial concern. Because the risk of VTE can be high after surgical procedures, prophylaxis is encouraged as soon as possible unless bleeding-related risks exceed the risk of a VTE. In the United States, guidelines and benchmarkers encourage the initiation of prophylaxis within 24 hours of the procedure.[5] Clinicians should be aware of and avoid any barriers for initiating prophylaxis. One example is standard dosing times and the ordering of prophylaxis postoperatively to avoid the initial dose being administered more than 24 hours after surgery. Order sets during admission and transfer in or out of the ICU should include assessment for VTE and initiation of any necessary management approaches to avoid being missed. Informatic systems should be developed to assist clinical staff in optimizing the recognition, prevention, and treatment of a VTE.

Risk assessment tools for bleeding and thrombosis have been explored but have not been validated in the ICU population. Because of the many factors mentioned, such tools may need to be combined with an individual assessment of the patient's risk of bleeding or thrombosis. This can be especially challenging in the postprocedure period when the risk of both bleeding and thrombosis may be high. Although VTE may not be on the problem list, all patients in the ICU should be evaluated for VTE and implementation of prophylaxis unless it is contraindicated or unless the patient is sufficiently mobile and at very low risk. Mechanical prophylaxis, although common and unrelated to the risks with pharmacologic prophylaxis, may be the only approach present in high bleeding risk situations. Support stockings may include TED support hose, which is a stocking without a compression gradient, and graduated compression stockings that provide a gradual decline in pressure from the distal to the proximal end. Intermittent pneumatic compression devices involve pressurized air into segmental diaphragms that are secured around the leg for a fixed period, which are then relaxed. These devices reduce the incidence of DVT compared with graduated compression stockings in high-risk patients with or without pharmacologic prophylaxis.[6] This provides a wavelike effect to move flow through the veins and prevent the pooling of blood. When pharmacologic prophylaxis is not an option, it is important to assess whether mechanical approaches have been considered or whether they are present and are actually being done. Stockings can be uncomfortable, and at times, they are found in the room but not on the patient. As such, the use of stockings on the patients should be assessed each day. Weight loss or changes in swelling may alter the effectiveness of the stockings, and cornstarch or talcum may be applied at times to assist patients with moist skin in pulling them up. For effective DVT prophylaxis, compression gradients of 20–40 mm Hg may be targeted. If the compression devices are only in the foot region, compression pressures on the higher end may be considered.

In some situations, an inferior vena cava (IVC) filter (which may be temporary or permanent) may be placed. However, thrombus formation within the filter creates challenges in removal and, in some cases, can lead to a need for systemic anticoagulation. In rare cases, the device could migrate, so for a combative patient, use of restraints should not run over the abdominal region, where any abrupt motion and resulting pressure in the region of the filter can dislodge the IVC. In general, the use of IVC filters has been discouraged unless the risk of VTE is high and other means of prophylaxis are not feasible.[4,7] In addition, continuous assessment to determine when pharmacologic prophylaxis can be added should be a component of the ICU stay. Routine use of ultrasonography to detect VTE should be avoided, in general, because it is unclear whether this changes the incidence of symptomatic events, and a positive finding could be noted as an event irrespective of being treated. The various pharmacologic agents used for VTE treatment and prophylaxis are listed in Table 23.1. Considerations and doses for these agents in VTE prophylaxis are listed in Table 23.2.

TREATMENT OF VTE

The occurrence of a DVT, either preexisting and still under anticoagulation therapy or occurring during admission, creates a more compelling situation. In acute VTE, higher levels of anticoagulation may initially be considered, creating a

Table 23.1 Properties of Commonly Used Anticoagulants in the Critically Ill Patient[8]

Agent	Mechanism of Action	Half-life[a]	Half-life in Renal Dysfunction	Elimination Site (approximated %)	Removed by Hemodialysis	Comments
UFH	Indirect IIa, Xa inhibitor	1–2 hr	1–2 hr	Hepatic	No	Low conc of AT may affect anticoagulant activity
Enoxaparin	Indirect Xa inhibitor	5–7 hr	6–9 hr	Renal (40%)	No	Low conc of AT may affect anticoagulant activity
Dalteparin	Indirect Xa inhibitor	2–5 hr	4–8 hr	Renal	No	Low conc of AT may affect anticoagulant activity
Fondaparinux	Indirect Xa inhibitor	17–21 hr	> 21 hr	Renal (70%)	No	Low conc of AT may affect anticoagulant activity
Warfarin	Inhibitors II, VII, IX, X	25 min	3.5 hr	Hepatic	No	
Dabigatran	Direct IIa inhibitor	39–51 min	0.5–1 hr	Renal (80%)	Yes	Do not open capsule
Rivaroxaban	Direct Xa inhibitor	1 wk	1 wk	Renal (36%)	No (minimal)	
Apixaban	Direct Xa inhibitor	12–17 hr	28 hr	Renal (25%)	No (minimal)	
Edoxaban	Direct Xa inhibitor	5–9 hr	10 hr	Renal (50%)	No (minimal)	

[a]Half-life listed was determined in normal healthy individuals, and not in the critically ill for which it can be considerably longer.
AT = antithrombin; UFH = unfractionated heparin; Hr = hours; Conc = plasma concentration; wk = week; min = minutes.

higher risk of bleeding. Decisions to treat or continue treatment may depend on the location and timing of the VTE. In general, VTEs occurring above the knee may be treated for at least 3 months for a first occurrence, and potentially for life if sustained risk factors are present or recurrent.[10] Venous thromboembolism may also be defined as provoked, meaning that it occurred in relation to a specific event (e.g., elective knee surgery) and carries a lower concern for extended therapy. Non-provoked VTE occurs when the VTE was not related to an identified high-risk situation, occurring more spontaneously. It may be a more difficult decision to hold anticoagulation therapy with non-provoked VTE, especially in the ICU setting when risk factors for thrombosis are present.

Initial therapy for an acute VTE may depend on the location of the thrombosis, its size, and any additional symptoms. Pulmonary embolisms may be classified as massive when congestion in the pulmonary circulation leads to expanded volume in the right ventricle upstream where the cardiac wall presses against the left ventricle, reducing stroke volume and leading to hemodynamic insufficiency. In this situation, initial therapy may include thrombolytic agents followed by a heparin infusion and eventually a long-term oral anticoagulant. For a submassive PE, the decision to use thrombolytic therapy may be weighed against the risks involved and the potential benefits. Most of the symptomatic PEs in the ICU are initially treated with a parenteral anticoagulant, followed by a long-term anticoagulant for at least 3 months, if possible (Table 23.3).

Table 23.2 Considerations with Anticoagulants for VTE Prophylaxis[8,9]

Agent	Common VTE Prophylactic Dose	Dose Adjustment in Renal Insufficiency	Dialysis Dose Adjustment
UFH	IV Anti-Xa 0.2–0.3 units/mL SC 5,000 units SC q8/q12hr 7,500 units q12hr	No adjustment	No adjustment
Enoxaparin	30 mg SC q12hr 40 mg SC q24hr	CrCl 15–30 mL/min/1.73 m^2: 30 mg q24hr Dialysis: 30 mg q24hr	30 mg SC q24hr
Dalteparin	5,000 units SC q24hr	CrCl > 20 mL/min – no adjustment; 5,000 units q24hr	—
Fondaparinux	2.5 mg SC q24hr	CrCl < 30 mL/min/1.73 m^2: 2.5 mg SC q48hr	—
Bivalirudin	0.12–0.15 mg/kg/hr	CrCl 30-60 mL/min/1.73 m^2: 0.08–0.1 mg/kg/hr CrCl 15–30 mL/min/1.73 m^2: 0.03–0.5 mg/kg/hr	IHD: 0.5 mg/kg/min CRRT: 0.7 mg/kg/min SLEDD: 0.7 mg/kg/min
Argatroban	0.2 mcg/kg/min	Decrease 0.1–0.6 mcg/kg/min for each 30-mL/min drop in CrCl has been suggested	No dose adjustment
Warfarin	Varies (INR 2–3)	No adjustment	Smaller-than-average doses may be warranted
Dabigatran	—	—	Contraindicated
Rivaroxaban	10 mg PO q24hr[a]	VTE prophylaxis post-elective orthopedic surgery. Avoid use if CrCl < 30 mL/min/1.73 m^2	No recommendation available
Apixaban	2.5 mg PO q12hr[a]	VTE prophylaxis post-elective orthopedic surgery. Patients with CrCl < 30 mL/min/1.73 m^2 were excluded in the prophylaxis trials	No recommendation available
Edoxaban	—	—	No recommendation available

[a]Orthopedic hip/knee prophylaxis.

CrCl = creatinine clearance; CRRT = continuous renal replacement; IHD = intermittent hemodialysis; INR = international normalized ratio; IV = intravenous(ly); kg = kilogram; PO = oral(ly); q = every; SC = subcutaneous(ly); SLEDD = slow duration dialysis; VTE = venous thromboembolism.

Often, patients admitted to the ICU with pulmonary symptoms may have PE included in the potential problem list. The diagnosis of the PE may be assessed by a chest computed tomography (CT) or a ventilation/perfusion scan. Because the consequences of a VTE, and especially a PE, can include sudden death or long-term pulmonary insufficiency (pulmonary hypertension), therapy should not be delayed for the results of diagnostic test results, but instead, instituted promptly and continued until a VTE or PE is ruled in or out. Additional approaches to therapy can include surgical removal or catheter-directed thrombolysis (Table 23.4).

In the ICU, parenteral anticoagulation for at least 5 days is desired, and include transitioning (bridging) to long-term anticoagulation; typically, warfarin is used if there is no need to discontinue anticoagulation. This in part may be attributed to its ability to be rapidly reverse heparin and warfarin if necessary. Anticoagulation plans using longer-acting agents should address any planned procedures with risks of bleeding and be held until resolved. When transitioning to warfarin, the parenteral agent should be continued until the international normalized ratio (INR) is above 2. Guidelines suggest that INR greater than 2 plus 1 additional day; however, specific benefits of this particular timing has not been tested in clinical trials.[10] Newer options include the direct-acting oral anticoagulants; however, most of these have been explored outside the critical care setting. Several limitations may exist, including the potential need to adjust dosing in organ failure, ability to measure the degree of effect or loss of effect for invasive procedures, and ability to reverse their effects. It is unclear whether they may be beneficial for other indications such as mechanical devices or in concurrent acute coronary syndromes (ACS) when other, more established agents have been used. Other options include 3 weeks of rivaroxaban 15 mg orally twice daily, followed by a dose deescalation to 20 mg daily, or apixaban 10 mg orally twice weekly for 7 days, followed by 5 mg twice daily. Dabigatran and edoxaban have been explored in VTE treatment but initiated after an initial period of parenteral anticoagulant therapy. With the use of the newer agents, there is no need to overlap with another anticoagulant. If the ICU stay is short and the patient can be discharged home, transitioning to long-term oral anticoagulation can be completed on an outpatient basis if the therapy can safely be implemented and the follow-up management arranged.

Other modalities for VTE management may include invasive procedures such as thrombolysis by intravenous infusion, which is considered for a massive PE and hemodynamic instability as the result of congestion in the right ventricle compressing against the left ventricle and reducing cardiac output. This strategy may also be considered in selected submassive PEs as well on a case-by-case basis. Catheter-directed thrombolysis incorporating thrombolytic therapy (e.g., EKOS catheters) or surgical thrombectomy can be used to remove the clot. For very high bleeding concerns outweighing those of the thrombosis when anticoagulation therapy is held, or if a lower intensity of anticoagulation is necessary, monitoring of a DVT can include repeat ultrasonography to determine whether the thrombosis is extending.

ANTICOAGULATION AGENTS

Unfractionated Heparin

Unfractionated heparin (UFH) is administered parenterally either by bolus or continuous intravenous infusion or subcutaneously for many indications in the critically ill patient. Heparin administered intravenously is completely bioavailable, but it is reduced to about 30% when administered subcutaneously, depending on the site of injection or the presence of vasopressors, which can decrease absorption.[17] Heparin can be used to coat catheters to prevent thrombosis on their surface as well as prophylactically to prevent VTE, or it can be used in the acute management of VTE as well as several other situations. The advantage of heparin is its rapid onset of effect, its rapid removal out of the system, and the ability to reverse its effects rapidly with protamine. Heparin is available in many concentrations, and it is important to use standard concentrations for the various uses to minimize potential errors. For the treatment of VTE, premixed solutions of heparin are available, and it is best to choose one standard concentration and incorporate that into VTE management guidelines, order sets, and products that are dispensed from the pharmacy. Because heparin is removed by the liver, the dose need not be adjusted for renal insufficiency. It can be reconstituted in either dextrose or saline, providing options in selected situations when another option may be preferred.

For VTE prophylaxis, UFH may be administered subcutaneously or by continuous intravenous infusion. In the International Medical Prevention Registry on Venous Thromboembolism (IMPROVE), a multicenter registry involving 15,156 acutely ill hospitalized medical patients of whom 5% were in the ICU, a marked variation in practices was seen in dosing frequency of low-dose UFH used to prevent VTE.[18] Combined with other comparisons and the low quality of evidence, including the lack of head-to-head comparative trials exploring twice- versus three-times-daily dosing, no compelling evidence exists to support a benefit of three-times-daily low-dose UFH compared with twice-daily dosing for reduction in VTE or increase in bleeding.[19] What is unclear is identifying the optimal approach in special populations that were not the focus of clinical trials such as surgical versus medical critically ill populations, populations with obesity, or populations with the presence of a hypercoagulable or bleeding state. This is evidenced by the fact that 7.7% of 3,746 medical-surgical ICU patients developed a DVT despite adequate thromboprophylaxis with either low-dose UFH

Table 23.3 Considerations with Anticoagulants for Treatment of VTE[a,b,9,11-13,21]

Agent	Common Treatment Dose	Dose Adjustment in Renal Insufficiency	Dialysis Dose Adjustment[a]
UFH	IV aPTT[b] Anti-Xa 0.3–0.7 units/mL (or aPTT calibrated to anti-Xa target range) SC 1.2 × total 24-hr dose divided BID/TID	No adjustment	No adjustment
Enoxaparin	1 mg/kg SC q12hr (acute) 1.5 mg/kg SC q24hr (history of)	CrCl 30–60 mL/min/1.73 m^2: Can lower 25% or to the next lower syringe size CrCl 15–30 mL/min/1.73 m^2: 1 mg/kg SC q24hr	IHD: 0.6–0.7 mg/kg SC q24hr
Dalteparin	200 units/kg SC q24hr (acute) 150 units/kg SC q24hr (> 30 days since acute event)	CrCl > 20 mL/min/1.73 m^2 – no adjustment; no recommendations < 20 mL/min/1.73 m^2	Not explored in VTE treatment
Fondaparinux	Weight < 50 kg: 5 mg SC daily Weight 50–100 kg: 7.5 mg SC daily Weight > 100 kg: 10 mg SC daily	CrCl < 30 mL/min/1.73 m^2: 2.5 mg SC q48hr	0.03–0.05 mg/kg SC q48hr –TIW or 2.5 mg SC q48hr has been explored in IHD
Bivalirudin	0.12–0.15 mg/kg/hr	CrCl 30-60 mL/min/1.73 m^2: 0.08–0.1 mg/kg/hr CrCl 15–30 mL/min/1.73 m^2: 0.03–0.5 mg/kg/hr	IHD: 0.5 mg/kg/min CRRT: 0.7 mg/kg/min SLEDD: 0.7 mg/kg/min
Argatroban	0.2 mcg/kg/min	Decrease 0.1–0.6 mcg/kg/min for each 30-mL/min drop in CrCl has been suggested	No dose adjustment specifically during dialysis. Reduce dose 75% in severe hepatic impairment
Warfarin	Varies (INR 2–3)	No adjustment – doses are generally 20%–25% lower as renal function declines	Smaller-than-average doses may be warranted
Dabigatran	150 mg PO BID after initial parenteral therapy	No recommendations in VTE	Contraindicated
Rivaroxaban	20 mg PO q24hr	CrCl ≥ 30 mL/min: no adjustment	No recommendation available for CrCl < 30 mL/min/1.73 m^2
Apixaban	5 mg PO q12hr. After 6 months, the dose can be reduced to 2.5 mg twice daily if continued	CrCl > 25 mL/min/1.73 m^2 or SCr > 2.5 mg/dL: no adjustment	No recommendation available because these patients were excluded. Dialysis dosing exists for atrial fibrillation according to a small pharmacokinetic study, but not in VTE treatment
Edoxaban	60 mg PO daily after initial parenteral therapy	CrCl 15–50 mL/min/1.73 m^2 (or weight ≤ 60 kg): 30 mg daily	No recommendation available with CrCl < 15 mL/min/1.73 m^2 or in dialysis

[a]Dosing in hemodialysis describes the approach the dose that was explored and may not apply to other forms of dialysis.

[b]Values for the aPTT depend on the reagent lot and range that fits within the 0.3–0.7 anti-Xa unit samples (typically, 30 heparin patient samples are used for the calibration). In the treatment of acute VTE, values in the upper range (e.g., 0.5–0.7 anti-Xa units) may be considered unless bleeding risks are high.

BID = twice daily; TID = three times daily; TIW = three times weekly.

or low-molecular-weight heparin (LMWH). A multivariate regression analysis suggests that patients with a personal or family history of TE, those with an elevated body mass index (BMI), and those receiving vasopressors appear more likely to have had failed standard thromboprophylaxis strategies.[20] Although patients may prefer fewer daily injections, the lower dose can be presumed to lower the level of anticoagulation and increase the risk of thrombosis, but as mentioned previously, this has not been shown in clinical trials. Empirically, patients at an advanced age (e.g., older than 80 years) with a low body weight (e.g., less than 50 kg) may have a more pronounced effect from heparin. In such cases, 5,000 units twice daily may be considered, or a trough activated partial thromboplastin time (aPTT) can be measured to assess whether a higher-than-desired anticoagulation effect is present. Although there is no supporting evidence on using continuous infusions for prophylaxis, it is another consideration when target goals are a small 10-second rise in aPTT over baseline or when measuring an anti-factor Xa (anti-Xa) activity concentration of 0.2–0.3 unit/mL. When using heparin for prophylaxis in the absence of an acute clot, a bolus dose may be unnecessary.

In the treatment of acute VTE, heparin is commonly used in the ICU and initiated as an intravenous bolus followed by a continuous infusion, with a desire to achieve and sustain target goals as soon as possible. The approach to dosing may depend on additional factors such as the concurrent use of a thrombolytic agent or concurrent bleeding issues. For example, a patient with an acute major bleeding episode who subsequently develops a VTE may be dosed on the basis of a risk assessment of the VTE (including location and severity) versus the risk of additional bleeding. The initial bolus may vary, if done at all, and may empirically be based on a set number of units (e.g., 2,500–5,000 units) or loading doses individualized using the patient's weight (e.g., 80 units/kg initially and potentially a lower amount when subsequent aPTT or anti-Xa activity concentrations are below target). If the bleeding concerns are very high, a lower bolus, if any at all, and a lower infusion rate may be considered.

Currently, no standard proven approach to the optimal infusion rate of target therapy goals has been established. A variety of approaches to continuous dosing exist, with dosing at 18 units/kg/hour being the most commonly used starting rate for an acute VTE.[21] The aPTT or anti-Xa activity can be measured 4–8 hours after initiating the infusion and the dose subsequently adjusted. The duration of effect by the bolus on the measured activity may be longer with higher doses. If no bolus is used, activity assessment can be done at 4 hours. A delay of 6–8 hours may

Table 23.4 Thrombolytic Therapy for Acute VTE[14-16]

Agent	Dose	Monitoring	Comments
Alteplase	PE: - 100 mg IV over 2 hr	Fibrinogen, Hgb/Hct	- Massive PE: patients < 65 kg: consider 50 mg IV over 2 hr: significantly fewer bleeding events than with 100-mg dose.
	Catheter directed ≤ 0.01 mg/kg/hr		- Bolus regimens may incur more bleeding without significant improvement in massive PE
	Pharmacomechanical and percutaneous mechanical: - Dosing strategies may vary depending on the device		- Surgical and older adult populations may benefit from smaller doses infused over longer periods (> 2 hr)
Tenecteplase	PE: < 60 kg = 30 mg 60–69 kg = 35 mg 70–79 kg = 40 mg 80–89 kg = 45 mg ≥ 90 kg = 50 mg	Hgb/Hct	Full-dose LMWH administered before tenecteplase administration Enoxaparin 1 mg/kg q12hr Dalteparin 200 units/kg daily
Reteplase	PE: 10 mg IV, with 10 mg IV 30 min after first dose	Hgb/Hct	

Hct = hematocrit; Hgb = hemoglobin; hr = hours; IV = intravenous; kg = kilogram; LMWH = low-molecular-weight heparin; mg = milligram; PE = pulmonary embolism.

be required, however, if a bolus is given to avoid elevated values driven in part by the bolus and resulting in infusion rates that may be below target.[22] Monitoring patients on anticoagulation with a VTE includes assessing the VTE and, if it is continuing to expand, the bleeding or potential complications such as HIT. Typically, a complete blood cell count and aPTT or anti-Xa activity is checked before initiating the infusion and then periodically as needed to assess the impact of the therapy.

In rare cases, such as in the loss of intravenous access or if long-term heparin is needed, a subcutaneous route may be considered. To determine a subcutaneous dose from a currently administered intravenous infusion, the following equation may be used:

$$\text{dose SC administered every 12 hours} = (\text{last IV infusion rate/hr} \times 24) \times (1.2)/2$$

where IV is intravenous, SC is subcutaneously, and "1.2" reflects the 20% or so loss of bioavailability with the subcutaneous route.

The common 250 unit/kg every 12 doses for VTE treatment is based on the concept of 20% over the common 18-unit/kg/hr intravenous infusion rate used in VTE.

There are several approaches to measuring the intensity of heparin therapy. Target ranges have in general been determined from experiences using the aPTT; however, discordance between the aPTT and the other assay approaches exist.[23-28] Previously, a target aPTT prolonged to 1.5–2.5 times the patient's normal baseline value was used.[29-31] However, it was recently observed that different assay reagent sensitivities exist, leading to subtherapeutic or excessive doses of heparin. Several factors can drive the variability in reported laboratory results with either the aPTT or the anti-Xa activity value. These include the reagent used and its sensitivity to heparin, presence of other factors influencing the result such as prolongation of the aPTT that is seen with lupus anticoagulant antibodies, certain congenital factor deficiencies, excessive factor VIII, fibrinogen or warfarin in the case of the aPTT, and AT deficiency for the anti-Xa activity assay.

The current recommendations of the American College of Chest Physicians and the College of American Pathologists indicate that patients should be treated with intravenous UFH to prolong the aPTT to a range that corresponds with a whole-blood heparin concentration of 0.3–0.7 unit/mL by the anti-Xa heparin assay or 0.2–0.4 unit/mL by protamine titration.[32,33] In recent years, some institutions have shifted from measuring the aPTT to using anti-Xa activity. Institutions that have made the change have noted fewer dosing titrations and earlier achievement of target goals.[34] However, hard outcomes such as any differences in the resulting heparin dose, incidence of thrombosis, or incidence of bleeding have not been determined. Given the high variability in reagents and the reported results between laboratories for both the aPTT and the anti-Xa assays, it is important to know the specifics of the assay used to adjust heparin (or LMWH) therapy.[35,36]

Several challenges can occur with the management of heparin infusions. A diurnal pharmacokinetic elimination pattern has been shown with heparin infusions where higher aPTT or anti-Xa values can occur during sleeping times and then lower values during awake cycles.[37] Because sleep cycles are often inconsistent in the ICU, it is difficult to coordinate them with measuring the level of anticoagulation. Another challenge is the observation of "heparin resistance," in which the aPTT or anti-Xa concentration does not increase despite titration to higher heparin infusion rates (e.g., above 25 units/kg/hour and values are still at baseline). Causes include elevated fibrinogen or factor VIII concentrations, which may limit the aPTT response, and depression in AT, which may blunt the action of heparin and potentially be missed if an anti-Xa assay is used that incorporates supplemented AT within the assay. To determine whether resistance is present, an AT, aPTT, anti-Xa assay, fibrinogen, and factor VIII concentration, if available, may be considered. Another means of determining potential resistance to heparin is to measure either the aPTT or the anti-Xa assay shortly after a bolus dose. If there is no response with either test, consider other approaches to anticoagulation management. Alternative tests such as activated clotting time (ACT) may be another consideration to assess whether an anticoagulation response is present. For VTE management, the low-range ACT is suggested because it may be better at detecting heparin concentrations in the target range.[35]

Low-Molecular-Weight Heparin

Another option in patients at lower concern for bleeding and with no perceived need to immediately reverse anticoagulation includes use of an LMWH or one of the newer oral anticoagulants. This may also be a consideration when intravenous access is limited or there is inability to measure laboratory values to adjust therapy. The LMWHs are now commonly used for the prevention and treatment of VTE and may be seen in the ICU if emergency reversal is not a concern. The low-molecular-weight tinzaparin (no longer available in the United States), dalteparin, and enoxaparin have been determined to be safe and effective in the prevention and treatment of VTE; however, most of the studies with them involved patients outside the ICU.

Low-molecular-weight heparins administered subcutaneously are about 87%–92% bioavailable (F = 0.87–0.92), which is considerably greater than that with subcutaneous doses of UFH (30%; F = 0.3).[38] The degree of bioavailability may be lower in the critically ill surgical or medical patient.[39-41] An impaired response to standard dosing as measured by anti-Xa, possibly leading to a greater incidence of VTE, has been seen.[42,43] Site of administration may be a factor. In one analysis of enoxaparin, the measured anti-Xa activity was significantly lower in patients with obesity when administered in the thigh than when administered in the abdomen.[44]

Compared with UFH, the LMWHs have a longer half-life and a more predictable anticoagulant response to weight-adjusted doses, allowing for either once- or twice-daily administration. The actual body weight should be considered for dosing, and it is suggested to avoid capping the dose at a certain weight (Table 23.2 and Table 23.3).[45]

When switching from UFH to an LMWH, the LMWH can generally be given when discontinuing the UFH infusion to simplify the process. Acute thrombus or bleeding is unlikely to occur when a slight difference in the time between discontinuing the UFH and initiating the LMWH occurs. For transitioning from an LMWH to a UFH infusion, consider initiating the UFH infusion when the next LMWH dose would be administered. A bolus dose of UFH is probably unnecessary.

The management end point for anticoagulation therapy should focus on potential bleeding and thrombosis or other related undesirable events. Studies comparing various agents in general have shown no significant differences in lowering either thrombosis or bleeding.[46,47] Clinicians should be cautious with measuring anti-Xa activity and applying the results to a dosing modification, especially when doses are outside those studied in clinical trials as supporting literature with hard outcomes is very limited. This would also hold true with special populations, including those with obesity and renal failure. It can be problematic to have a level drive a dosing modification in a direction that is very uncomfortable given the current clinical situation.

Fondaparinux

Fondaparinux is a synthetic pentasaccharide that mimics the 5-sugar moiety binding sequence that gives heparin the ability to activate AT. Fondaparinux is highly selective for factor Xa inhibition with no appreciable inhibition of factor IIa (thrombin). Fondaparinux rapidly binds to AT, causing an irreversible conformational change. It is subsequently released, allowing binding to other AT molecules. The ability of fondaparinux to trigger an immune-mediated HIT response is potentially less likely given its small molecular size and the absence of the additional side chains. Although HIT cases attributed to fondaparinux have been reported, fondaparinux is now an optional alternative anticoagulant in the management of HIT, or for VTE prophylaxis when there is a history of HIT.[48]

Fondaparinux is available in several different strengths (2.5, 5, 7.5, and 10 mg) for once-daily subcutaneous injection. Evaluated in several phase II trials, fondaparinux is approved for VTE prophylaxis in hip and knee replacement, treatment of acute DVT and PE, and treatment of ACS. Fondaparinux dosing in the treatment of a VTE is based on weight: 5 mg (weight less than 50 kg), 7.5 mg (weight 50–99 kg), and 10 mg (100 kg or greater). However, the dose for ACS or VTE prophylaxis post-hip or knee is a fixed 2.5 mg regardless of patient weight. In one phase II dose-response trial, there were no observed differences in recurrent VTE rates or bleeding events between patients weighing 50–100 kg receiving fondaparinux 5, 7.5, or 10 mg subcutaneously daily.[49] In a larger randomized phase III trial, weight-adjusted fondaparinux was as effective as continuous infusion UFH and weight-adjusted enoxaparin in the treatment of VTE, with a slight decrease in thrombotic events countered by a small increase in bleeding events.[50,51] Another phase II trial of ACS evaluating doses of 2.5, 4, 8, and 12 mg showed no difference in the primary end point of myocardial infarction, recurrent ischemia, death, or bleeding. Overall, fondaparinux is effective in the prophylaxis against and treatment of VTE and may be more potent than originally perceived.

Fondaparinux is almost entirely renally eliminated and has a long half-life; thus, its use in patients with moderate to severe renal impairment is discouraged. To date, fondaparinux doses of 1.5 mg daily and 2.5 mg every other day in severe renal impairment have been described only in case reports and case series and a single cohort analysis.[52,53] Fondaparinux use in hemodialysis seems to provide an adequate level of anticoagulation when properly dose adjusted. Dosing in dialysis appears to require a further dose reduction to either 0.05 mg/kg or 2.5 mg before the dialytic session.[54] Providers should consider residual renal function because anuric patients are potentially more likely to accumulate fondaparinux at a faster rate, thus increasing the risk of a potential bleeding event compared with oliguric patients.

Much of the data regarding the use of fondaparinux for VTE prophylaxis and treatment in obesity are confined to observational studies and subgroup analyses of larger randomized controlled trials. Fondaparinux is given as a single 10-mg subcutaneous, once-daily injection for patients weighing more than 100 kg. In one subgroup analysis, fondaparinux 10 mg subcutaneously daily was evaluated in patients weighing as much as 166 kg with a BMI of 46 kg/m^2. Fondaparinux appeared to be as effective as therapeutic twice-daily enoxaparin and intravenous UFH in the initial treatment of VTE. Fondaparinux had numerically fewer recurrent VTE and major bleeding events than did enoxaparin and UFH.[55] Use of fondaparinux in the obese population provides the opportunity for improved compliance compared with a twice-daily therapy, using multiple syringes, together with the convenience of a single once-daily injection.

Dosing fondaparinux for VTE prophylaxis is even less clear. The current U.S. Food and Drug Administration (FDA)-approved dose of 2.5 mg subcutaneously daily has been debated regarding whether the dose should be increased for those with morbid obesity or at a certain weight cutoff. Some authors have suggested a dose increase to 5 mg subcutaneously daily in weights greater than 120 kg because of a lack of data for the approved prophylactic dose in this population.[56] Anti-Xa activity within range greater than half of the time in the patient with morbid obesity (BMI less than 50 kg/m^2; weight less than 150 kg) with fondaparinux 2.5 mg subcutaneously daily has also been seen.[57]

Reversing Heparin and LMWH Effect

The effects of UFH and, to a lesser degree, LMWH can be neutralized using protamine sulfate. In general, each milligram of protamine sulfate neutralizes around 100 units of heparin calcium, with a maximum of 50 mg as a single dose suggested.[21] Excessive dosing of protamine should be avoided because it can independently promote bleeding. Protamine should be administered slowly over at least 10 minutes to reduce the possibility of hypotension and anaphylaxis.

When dosing protamine, the clinician should consider how long heparin has been held. Because UFH administered intravenously has an elimination half-life of 60–90 minutes, only heparin given during the preceding several hours needs to be considered when calculating the dose of protamine sulfate. For example, a heparin infusion at 1,250 units/hour requires about 30 mg of protamine sulfate for neutralization. Neutralization of UFH administered by subcutaneous injection may require a prolonged infusion or repeat doses of protamine sulfate because of continued absorption from the site of administration. The effectiveness of the neutralization can be assessed by measuring either the aPTT or the anti-Xa activity.[33] For the LMWHs, protamine only partly neutralizes their effects, with a potentially greater response to higher sulfated compounds (tinzaparin > dalteparin > enoxaparin); however, the clinical significance of this is unclear.[58] A 1-mg dose of protamine for every 100 anti-Xa international units of dalteparin or 1 mg of enoxaparin has been recommended for reversal if less than 8 hours has elapsed since the dose of LMWH.

Fondaparinux is currently without a specific antidote. Protamine is ineffective in neutralizing the anticoagulant effect of fondaparinux because of the lack of sulfations in the synthetic pentasaccharide. Doses of recombinant activated factor II (rFVIIa) up to 90 mcg/kg have shown only partial correction in the thrombin-generating capacity of an ex vivo analysis, whereas a low dose (20 units/kg) of the activated prothrombin complex concentrate (aPCC) factor eight inhibitor bypassing activity (FEIBA) showed a complete correction in the assay.[59]

Direct Thrombin Inhibitors

The parenteral direct thrombin inhibitors (DTIs), typically administered by continuous infusion, provide an alternative option when commonly used therapies such as UFH or LMWH cannot be used (Table 23.5). This may occur in patients who have heparin allergies, concerns for HIT, or AT deficiency. The two currently available parenteral DTIs are argatroban and bivalirudin. Most of the experiences with these agents in the management of VTE arise in the setting of acute HIT-with or without associated thrombosis, HIT post-initial therapy for VTE, or history of HIT requiring VTE prophylaxis. Fondaparinux may be

Table 23.5 DTIs in the Management of VTE[22]

	Argatroban	Bivalirudin
FDA-approved indication	HIT, PCI	PCI
Route of elimination	Hepatic	Renal (20%); proteolytic cleavage
Elimination half-life	39–51 min	25 min
Common dose	1.6 mcg/kg/min	0.12–0.15 mg/kg/hr
aPTT target	1.5–3 × baseline; not to exceed 100 seconds	1.5–2.5 baseline
Assay approach	aPTT,[a] TT, dTT,[a] ECT[a]	
Dose in critically ill	0.5–1.2 mcg/kg/min	0.08–0.17 mg/kg/hr
Dose in renal failure	Decrease 0.1–0.6 mcg/mL/min for each 30-mL/min decrease in CrCl	CrCl 30–60 mL/min: 0.08–0.1 mg/kg/hr CrCl < 30 mL/min: 0.03–0.05 mg/kg/hr
Dose in hepatic failure	≤ 0.5 mcg/kg/min	No adjustment

[a]No nationally standardized test; thus, test results and sensitivity may vary between institutions.

aPTT = activated partial thromboplastin time; dTT = diluted thrombin time; ECT = ecarin clotting time; HIT = heparin-induced thrombocytopenia; min = minute; TT = thrombin time; PCI = percutaneous coronary intervention.

an option in some cases where use of a DTI infusion is not desired and a long acting agent is permissible. The elimination half-lives for argatroban and bivalirudin are relatively short, according to an analysis of healthy individuals. In the critically ill patient, especially in the presence of heart, kidney, or liver dysfunction, elimination rates can be considerably longer, thus taking longer to reach steady state and longer for the effects to leave after discontinuing the infusion. In addition, the amount of drug needed to achieve treatment targets may be lower. The infusion rate is typically adjusted on the basis of observed aPTT or dilute thrombin time values.[22,60] The aPTT target concentrations are based on achieving ratios of 1.5–2.5 for bivalirudin and 1.5–3.0 for argatroban from the patient's baseline value. The upper end of the range is commonly targeted in patients at higher thrombosis concerns such as for acute thrombosis, and the lower end for thromboprophylaxis. Although the aPTT is also used for heparin, the target value during DTI therapy may be different.

Argatroban is primarily eliminated in the liver, but it also requires dosing reductions in renal insufficiency.[61,62] The aPTT target is 1.5–3 times control according to the range set in the ARG 911 trial. Although the prescribing information notes starting at 2 mcg/kg/minute, the mean dose in the ARG 911 and the subsequent postmarketing ARG 915 trial was lower at 1.5–1.6 mcg/kg/minute. Experiences with the use of argatroban in the critically ill patient suggest even lower doses less than 1 mcg/kg/minute.[63] For liver failure with a Child-Pugh score greater than 6 or a total bilirubin greater than 1.5 mg/dL, the dose should be reduced to 25% of normal, or 0.5 mcg/kg/minute; however, lower doses may occur.[22] For renal insufficiency, the observations have suggested a dose reduction of 0.1–0.6 mcg/kg/minute for every 30-mL/minute decrease in CrCl.[11] There is no known reversal agent for argatroban, and it is not removed by hemodialysis.

Bivalirudin is another DTI primarily developed for use in ACS; however, there are several postmarket, single-center experiences describing its use in the management of HIT at much lower doses. The commonly targeted aPTT value is 1.5–2.5 times control, and it is eliminated primarily by enzymatic degradation by thrombin; however, the dose may need to be reduced as renal function declines. The common dose is 1.5 mg/kg/hour; however, lower doses are commonly seen in the critically ill patient as well. Unlike argatroban, bivalirudin may be removed by hemodialysis, and enzymatic elimination may be impaired in hypothermia.[9,64] The aPTT should not be measured during, or for several hours after, intermittent hemodialysis. In the setting of continuous renal replacement therapy, a higher dose may be necessary to account for removal by hemofiltration.[9] Although package labeling suggests that steady state may occur within hours, it may take considerably longer in the critically ill patient. One strategy is to assess an aPTT within a few hours of initiating the infusion, and if the value is in the upper part of the target range or above (and before reaching steady state), an excessive level of anticoagulation could shortly occur. As such, the infusion rate may tapered down earlier as a precaution.[65] In a bleeding patient with acute thrombosis concerns, the infusion can be initiated at a lower rate and titrated to effect using more frequent aPTT assessments.[65]

Management of bleeding during parenteral DTI therapy includes targeting lower aPTT values, giving blood transfusions as needed, and providing hemofiltration, if necessary, for bivalirudin. Concentrated clotting factors, fresh frozen plasma, and vitamin K do not expedite removal; however, in theory and according to very limited case experiences, it is possible that the thrombin burst with rFVIIa can accelerate the enzymatic removal of bivalirudin.[64]

Of additional note, heparin and the parenteral DTIs can independently cause an increase in measured INR values. These are not thought to reflect independent pharmacologic activity, but they are the result of influencing the INR assay.[35,66] The higher the drug concentration, the greater the impact on the observed INR value, which may vary between laboratories and the assay used. Some laboratories perform an additional step and neutralize the heparin before measuring the INR, eliminating the influence. It is important to know whether your laboratory does this neutralization step because many clinicians may otherwise target an INR of 2.5 or higher with warfarin before discontinuing heparin to account for the assay differences. In the absence of warfarin, an INR value at or above target ranges does not indicate a need to discontinue the infusion, but it could be an indication of excessive anticoagulation effect from the DTI, again depending on the sensitivity of the INR assay to the DTI.

For the DTIs, the INR assay is more sensitive to argatroban followed by bivalirudin.[66] This can be an advantage in patients for whom the aPTT response is not very robust. In some patients, the aPTT response curve may flatten and may not increase despite significant increases in the infusion rate. In such situations, a thrombin time can be measured, and if a very high result is noted, excessive anticoagulation can be present despite a low aPTT. In such situations, the dose can empirically be capped and the patient monitored for thrombosis and bleeding. The effect on the aPTT could be transient, so it should continue to be measured, and if excessive values subsequently occur, the infusion rate might need to be reassessed.

ORAL AGENTS

Vitamin K Antagonists

For longer-term anticoagulation, the vitamin K antagonists have been the preferred agent for treatment of a VTE after initial management with a parenteral anticoagulant, or prevention of VTE. This class of agents, for which warfarin is the most common agent used in North America, decreases the production of the vitamin K–dependent clotting factors (II, VII, IX, and X) in the liver to lower concentrations, blunting the drive for thrombosis. The INR is the common means for measuring the intensity of anticoagulation with vitamin K antagonists, where target values of 2–3 are typically used in the management of VTE. Many factors can influence the dose response to warfarin; these are described in detail elsewhere.[67] Many can be present in the critically ill patient, typically leading to lower doses. Examples include renal, liver, and heart failure; concurrent drug interactions; inflammatory responses; infections, and low vitamin K stores. Some such as rifampin or continuous tube feeds, or improvement in organ function and resolution of an infection, may lead to a dosing increase.

For an acute VTE, warfarin can be initiated once anticoagulation with a parenteral agent has been established. This would be 4 hours after an LMWH dose or when a therapeutic aPTT value on UFH occurs. When initiating therapy, the clotting factor with the shortest life span, factor VII, is eliminated faster than is factor II. Because factor II remains longer and is the primary driver for thrombosis, rapidly rising INR values may underpredict the level of anticoagulation.[68] Before initiating warfarin, a baseline INR should be determined and then measured daily, if possible, at least 8–10 hours post-dose (longer may be preferred, if feasible) to assess any early potential dose response. Because warfarin is eliminated through the liver, lower doses may be common in liver disease. However, renal failure may also block the elimination of selected cytochrome enzymes (in the case of warfarin 2C19), resulting in lower warfarin dosing.[69] If the INR is not a feasible test because of other influencing factors (e.g., lupus anticoagulant), clotting factors such as factor II or X can be directly measured. For acute VTE, the parenteral bridge therapy may be discontinued once the INR is greater than 2 and determined to be believable. Unexpected INR values may be repeated to determine if the result is believable or not before a dosing decision.

Warfarin can be crushed, and the effects of a particular dose may not reach maximal influence for several days; however, in some patients, a marked response may be seen after 8–12 hours. Thus, an INR may be measured at some point after the first dose to determine whether the patient is very sensitive to it.

Directing Acting Oral Anticoagulants

Until recently, warfarin was the mainstay of prolonged VTE therapy; however, dosing can be difficult because of the many influencing factors. Several new agents recently became available and have been approved for VTE management. Dabigatran is a DTI, and rivaroxaban, apixaban, and edoxaban are factor Xa antagonists. Patients enrolled in the clinical trials exploring the use of these agents for VTE were probably not critically ill, limiting any clear insights of any advantages over warfarin. The designs of the VTE trials were also very different. Although most patients received heparin or an LMWH initially while being randomized, initial therapy for edoxaban and dabigatran included a parenteral agent for 1 week or so, which was then switched to oral therapy. For rivaroxaban, a higher dose of 15 mg twice daily was administered for 3 weeks, followed by a lower 20-mg once-daily dose. For apixaban, the initial dose was 10 mg orally twice daily for 7 days, followed by 5 mg twice daily in VTE treatment. Rivaroxaban and apixaban can be crushed and mixed for nasogastric administration; however, the dabigatran capsule should not be opened; rather, it should be given as manufactured because any alterations can substantially increase the bioavailability 8- to 10-fold.[70-72]

Critically ill patients such as those with severe liver failure or high risk of bleeding were pre-determined exclusions in the clinical trials. Unlike warfarin, which requires invasive INR tests for adjusting dosing, the newer agents do not require or have commonly available measures of anticoagulation intensity and subsequent dosing adjustments. However, drug interactions do exist with the newer agents, and the presence of organ failure can result in higher levels of anticoagulation that may be difficult to recognize. Assays to directly measure the intensity of anticoagulation with the newer agents have been developed or are under development; however, they are not commonly available.

The thrombin time is very sensitive to the presence of dabigatran and can be used to detect its presence; however, it can exceed maximum values when normal serum concentrations are present.[73] For the INR, prothrombin time, and aPTT, the various assay regents available can respond differently to the presence of the newer agents, depending on their sensitivity. Elevated values beyond what may be expected for a selected assay may be a signal for excessive anticoagulation, especially if a clinical condition (e.g., overdose, organ failure, or a drug interaction) is present. Anti-Xa activity can be increased depending on the assay and the calibrator used, creating notable variability in results and limiting its usefulness.[74,75] Several agents that can directly reverse the DOACs (direct oral anticoagulants) are currently under development. Idarucizumab is a monoclonal antibody fragment (Fab) currently in phase III trials but recently approved by the FDA specifically binds to dabigatran and rapidly neutralizes its anticoagulant effect in minutes.[76,77] It has no activity against other anticoagulants. In the REVERSE-AD phase III trial, the median time for hemostasis took 11 hours.[77] As such, it is unclear in situations with massive hemorrhage whether concurrent use of a concentrated clotting factor or tranexamic acid is necessary if rapid hemostasis is critical. Andexanet alfa is a modified recombinant version of factor Xa that works as a decoy to block any anticoagulant with anti-Xa activity.[78] Both agents are initiated with a bolus dose;

however, andexanet may require continued therapy with a continuous infusion.

During anticoagulation therapy, situations may arise in which the concerns for bleeding outweigh those for thrombosis, either for high bleeding risk situations, including necessary invasive procedures, or active bleeding. Approaches can include reducing the level of anticoagulation, holding anticoagulation, expediting removal, or independently promoting hemostasis. Agent-specific reversal strategies are listed in Table 23.6. For a bleeding event, if a patient has a history of VTE, the reversal approach may consider the brevity of the situation. If severe morbidity or mortality is perceived and no emergency reversal occurs, more aggressive management may be considered. If time permits or a desire not to fully reverse effects is present, more conservative reversal regimens can be considered and titrated to the desired effect.

In the critical bleeding situation, administration of reversal approaches should be accomplished without delay. For heparin or LMWH, protamine can be administered. For warfarin, a prothrombin complex concentrate (PCC) together with parenteral vitamin K can be given. Three-factor PCCs (which have a lower amount of factor VII compared with factors II, IX, and X); four-factor PCCs, which have all four factors; and, to a limited extent, aPCCs, which have all four factors with factor VII in a activated form, have been explored.[79] In addition, recombinant activated factor VIIa (rVIIa) has been explored for reversing anticoagulants. The dosing of PCCs to reverse warfarin may depend on the observed INR; however, waiting for a value to return before dosing may delay therapy. If the INR is not yet available, therapy can be initiated with the initial three or four factor PCC dose of 25 units/kg using a weight up to 100 kg, and if the INR suggests a higher dose, an additional agent can be given. To avoid delays in the admixture of several vials, therapy with a single 1,000-IU vial can be reconstituted and given while the remaining dose is determined and prepared. One of the challenges with using PCCs is their association with increased risk of thrombosis. Combined with a history of VTE, the concern for an additional VTE can be even greater.

In the setting of warfarin, vitamin K can be given orally or parenterally. Parenteral vitamin K has a more rapid onset in INR reduction; however, little difference is seen between the two routes after 24 hours. Recent experiences have suggested that doses greater than 2 mg intravenously provide no additional reduction in the INR after 24 hours, but more prolonged reversal.[80] If the goal is a partial reversal of the INR, low doses of vitamin K (e.g., 0.25–0.5 mg intravenously) can be considered. If anticoagulation is reinitiated shortly, higher doses of vitamin K may lead to prolonged bridge therapy before a response to warfarin occurs. If there is no plan to reinitiate therapy, a vitamin K dose of 10 mg is feasible.

For the newer oral anticoagulants, approaches to reverse their effects have not been established. Dabigatran can be removed by hemodialysis, and given the potential for tissue rebound, prolonged dialysis may be necessary.[81] However, recent availability of an antibody to dabigatran, idarucizumab, may limit the need for hemodialysis. Case reports have suggested that an aPCC can establish hemostasis; however, the optimal dose has not been established.[81-84] The effectiveness of non-activated PCC is less clear. For rivaroxaban, edoxaban, and apixaban, any difference between aPCC and non-activated PCC is unclear. Ideally, the lowest effective dose necessary to establish hemostasis may be preferred. If time permits, a lower dose can be used and titrated to effect depending on hemoglobin values and symptoms of bleeding.

Once the bleeding issue resolves, reinitiating anticoagulation may be a consideration. For a previous VTE, obtaining the history of the previous VTE event, including whether it was provoked or non-provoked, the previous number of events, and the duration elapsed, can assist in determining the subsequent management plan. If it has been more than 3 months after a provoked VTE, continued anticoagulation may be unnecessary. In contrast, if there is a history of several non-provoked VTE events, continued therapy may be strongly encouraged.

CONSIDERATIONS IN SPECIAL POPULATIONS

Because the critically ill patient is at high risk of VTE, prevention and management decisions continually require assessment each day instead of just during times of admission or transferring between services. Mechanical methods, unless there is a specific reason not to use them, should be used and will be effective as long as they are in use. If anticoagulation therapy is not an option in the presence of a VTE, clinicians may consider temporary placement of an inferior vena cava (IVC) filter. These filters may prevent subsequent PEs, but they have also been associated with a higher rate of VTE; thus, it is preferred that they be removed once it is safe to do so.[85] Decisions to initiate systemic anticoagulation in the presence of an IVC filter should include the plan for filter removal.

The dynamics of a critically ill patient can also continuously be changing between degrees of instability and more stable conditions. The dynamics of other patients, although requiring ICU-level care, can be for the most part very stable, and response to therapy may be consistent with the post-ICU setting. In the unstable patient, decisions on pharmacologic therapy should include the current risk of bleeding and thrombosis as well as any trends or future events that may alter them. In addition, decisions should include timely assessment of the patient's clinical presentation such as improving or declining trends, together with trends in organ function. Assessing such trends in

Table 23.6 Reversal Approaches to Anticoagulation

Anticoagulant	Examples of Laboratory Assays to Consider	Pharmacologic Reversal Agents	Comment
UFH	aPTT or anti-Xa	Protamine	For urgent situations. Effects of heparin dissipate several hours after holding. Post-cardiopulmonary bypass, an aPTT rebound may be detected after up to 6 hours requiring an additional dose of protamine (~25 mg)
LMWH	Anti-Xa drawn 4 hr post-dose in selected situations	Protamine	Partial reversal of effects with protamine. Degree of reversal and ability to reduce bleeding is unclear
Fondaparinux	Anti-Xa has been proposed, but no known effect on outcomes. Not recommended at this time	Unclear	One assessment showed a greater impact with an aPCC of 25 units/kg than with rFVIIa
Argatroban	aPTT ACT in selected cardiac procedures		Effective means to reverse argatroban has not been established
Bivalirudin	aPTT ACT in selected cardiac procedures	Hemofiltration	Limited evidence suggests that rFVIIa (e.g., 1–2 mg) reverses effects
Warfarin	INR	Vitamin K, PCC (three or four factor), FFP	Vitamin K doses (0.25–10 mg IV) take 12–48 hours for full effect PCC4 (Kcentra) dosing: Max dosing weight 100 kg INR 2–4: 25 units/kg (actual body weight) INR 4.1–6: 35 units/kg (actual body weight) INR > 6: 50 units/kg (actual body weight) If INR > 1.5 and severe bleeding, can consider a PCC Some experience with low-dose aPCC (500–1,000 units ×1) Option: Administer 1,000 units PCC4 up front, and balance when INR is back. Some products have heparin and are not recommended in HIT. Repeat INR 10–15 min post-dose
Dabigatran	TT, aPTT, INR, and if available – ECT- or dTT-derived dabigatran conc INR may be elevated at high concentrations	Idarucizumab aPCC or PCC Hemodialysis	Idarucizumab 5 gm can be rapidly administered as a bolus or infusion to neutralize the anticoagulation effects of Dabigatran. Another option is hemodialysis to remove dabigatran, depending on the amount present in the plasma. Drug concentrations have been shown to rebound on cessation of hemodialysis from tissue rebound; therefore, prolonged dialysis may be warranted in selected situations (can consider lowering the blood flow rate). For minor bleeding, monitor and recheck laboratory values Major bleeding: Consider tranexamic acid or PCC for more rapid hemostasis. Some limited data analyses have shown positive effects with an aPCC (FEIBA) 8–50 units/kg have been explored. PCC dose is 25–50 units/kg may be another consideration. Can consider starting at low doses and titrating to effect. Can administer just before catheter placement for hemodialysis

Table 23.6 Reversal Approaches to Anticoagulation *(continued)*

Anticoagulant	Examples of Laboratory Assays to Consider	Pharmacologic Reversal Agents	Comment
Rivaroxaban, apixaban, edoxaban	aPTT, chromogenic anti-Xa (consider calibrating to agent involved). UHF and LMWH calibrators can be used, but results may vary	PCC or aPCC	Data on the agent and dose to reverse the effects of rivaroxaban has not been established. Not dialyzable
			Minor bleeding, monitor and recheck laboratory values
			Major bleeding: PCC or aPCC
			Some limited data analyses have observed positive effects with an aPCC (FEIBA) of 8–50 units/kg. PCC dose is 25–50 units/kg
			Can consider initiating at low doses and titrating to effect

ACT = activated clotting time; aPCC = activated prothrombin complex concentrate (FEIBA or factor eight inhibitor bypassing activity is a aPCC); aPTT = activated partial thromboplastin time; dTT = diluted thrombin time; ECT = ecarin clotting time; FPP = fresh frozen plasma; HIT = heparin-induced thrombocytopenia; LMWH = low-molecular-weight heparin; UFH = unfractionated heparin; PCC = prothrombin complex concentrate (PCC4 = four factor PCC); rFVIIa = recombinant activated factor VII; TT = thrombin time.

today's management decisions will help clinicians achieve goals in subsequent days.

For acute decompensated heart failure or notable hypotension, poor perfusion to the kidney or liver may lead to reduced drug clearance and increased levels of anticoagulation and lower dosing requirements. Reductions in the liver's capacity to produce clotting factors may also occur. Acute and transient changes in response to warfarin may be seen with an infection or new interacting drug added. As the transient influencing factors such as heart function recover or the infection diminishes, drug elimination will recover, and dosing may need to be increased. For such situations with warfarin, for example, and with a desire to sustain its effects, the INR may be notably elevated and dosing held or reduced. As the INR begins to drop, the dosing should be reinstituted or increased before the INR drops to the target range. Holding warfarin until reaching target range after several days of low or no doses may result in a continued drop below target range and require bridge therapy, especially if there was a recent VTE event. Bedside observations and timely assessment of the patient's clinical presentation, including shifts in factors influencing decisions for management trends in advance, may allow earlier adjustments and minimize time outside the treatment goals.

Acute changes in renal function can alter the dynamics of anticoagulation therapy as well as the balance between bleeding and thrombosis for many factors. Unfortunately, patients with severe forms of renal failure or the requirements for renal replacement therapy have been poorly studied and excluded from large clinical trials. Dosing of renally influenced agents as noted earlier can also be difficult to manage when kidney function is unstable. Having the ability to measure the level of anticoagulation, if available, may assist in assessing the regimen. In this setting, heparin therapy may be considered because the kidney does not alter its elimination. However, at times, it may not be feasible to use heparin if there is no intravenous access or ability to measure. One option recently explored and included for acutely ill patients requiring hemodialysis was enoxaparin dosed at about 0.6–0.7 mg/kg daily.[12] Anti-Xa activity was not measured in this analysis because it may not accurately describe the balance between thrombosis and hemostasis effects of enoxaparin in this setting as other drivers notable in renal failure may influence outcomes.[53] Anticoagulation in acute liver injury and/or failure, including chronic conditions, can be difficult to manage, not only because of altered effects of the drugs and some assays but also between the balance of thrombosis and the bleeding potential. Although indicators such as the INR may suggest poor clotting factor production and a hypocoagulable state, other factors such as the natural anticoagulants may also be impaired.[86,87] Management decisions must carefully weigh this. In some cases, acute reductions in liver function could also be caused by portal thrombosis, which would require a separate management approach. When initiating warfarin in the setting of an elevated INR, it has not been established what the subsequent target range should be, and this is typically determined on a case-by-case basis. Use of newer anticoagulants in severe liver impairment is unclear because this population was excluded.

When initiating warfarin in an unstable setting such as liver disease or other factors that may suggest an increased response to a dose, consider allowing as much time as possible between the dose and the subsequent INR to unmask the sensitivity. Remember that when the INR is abruptly rising, it is mainly being driven by a fall in factor VII instead of factor II. As such, the INR may suggest a higher level of anticoagulation than truly exists.

Anticoagulation management decisions relative to invasive procedures should consider the risk of thrombosis and bleeding before, during, and after surgery. In the preoperative setting, a bridge to a shorter-acting agent may be considered if the VTE risk is high. Heparin can typically be turned off several hours before the procedure. For LMWH, the last dose may be 24–48 hours prior, and for warfarin, the INR may be allowed to drop to a predetermined level on the basis of bleeding assessments. For other anticoagulants, holds may depend on the perceived time for effects to diminish. If neuroaxial anesthesia is being considered, a longer hold of the anticoagulant to allow the complete absence of anticoagulation may be preferred. This may be used for up 5 days for some agents if their effects cannot immediately be reversed.[88]

Postprocedure management decisions should consider outcomes of the procedure and potential complications or requirements for additional procedures. Anticoagulation may be initiated slowly after procedures with higher risks for bleeding, especially if the CNS or other critical areas are involved when there is no drain in place or ability to transfuse. In some situations, such as in the eye, heart, or spine, a small amount of blood can be devastating. Once bleeding risks subside, either prophylaxis or full anticoagulation therapy can be initiated. With the exception of reinitiating warfarin, bridging between agents is unnecessary.

In some situations, other indications for anticoagulation may be present. In these settings, target ranges or doses may be considered, typically using the higher of the two variables unless there is a bleeding-related issue suggesting the lower intensity. For some of the agents approved for use in VTE, the anticoagulant may need to be switched to an agent that has been determined to be effective in both settings.

HEPARIN-INDUCED THROMBOCYTOPENIA

Immune-mediated HIT is a rare complication associated with exposure to heparin or LMWH that can lead to venous and arterial thrombosis or death. Heparin-induced thrombocytopenia can occur in three time settings: immediate exposure (within minutes with recent previous exposure to heparin), typical exposure (5–10 days after exposure to heparin), and delayed exposure (up to 40 days after heparin exposure). Because of delayed-onset HIT, patients presenting with acute thrombosis and recent heparin exposure should have their platelet count checked before initiating heparin or LMWH. The presence of antibodies related to immune HIT can be determined using selected assays as a means of separating this from other causes of thrombocytopenia. Common assays include the enzyme-linked immunosorbent assay and the serotonin release assay, which is more specific but may take longer for results to be reported. The process of ordering a test for HIT and for knowing when alternative therapy should be initiated creates notable decisions on how to proceed with anticoagulation management. When making decisions to test for HIT, consider the impact of results because there is the potential for false-positive observations. Because thrombocytopenia for many reasons can occur in the critically ill patient, clinicians should carefully think about adding in HIT testing as part of a global approach to determining the cause for the low platelet count unless clinical suspicion is sufficient. Commonly used HIT predictive tools such as the 4T score include the magnitude of the platelet count drop, timing in relation to heparin exposure, presence of new thrombosis after initiating heparin, and absence of other causes of thrombocytopenia.[48] Platelet counts can commonly drop post-cardiopulmonary bypass surgery, and here, the pattern for HIT is the presence of platelet count recovery, followed by a second drop in platelet count. Other common devices in the ICU such as aortic balloon pumps can commonly cause thrombocytopenia and are not suggestive of HIT.

For HIT, alternative anticoagulation with a DTI or fondaparinux is suggested. Holding heparin or LMWH alone is not recommended. Once platelet counts are sufficiently recovering or have recovered, warfarin can be considered for prolonged anticoagulation. The parenteral anticoagulant should be continued until the INR adjusted for any assay influenced by the DTI is greater than 2.0. At times in the ICU, other causes of thrombocytopenia may be present, and platelet counts may not recover, resulting in a prolonged course of parenteral anticoagulation.

Alternative anticoagulation in the setting of isolated HIT should be continued until the platelet count has recovered and the risk of thrombosis is resolved. For thrombosis, either as the reason for initial anticoagulation or for thrombosis attributed to HIT (heparin-induced thrombocytopenia thrombosis or HITTS), anticoagulation should be continued for at least 3 months. Given that the antibody response driving HIT is transient, lasting for around 3 months, alternative anticoagulants such as fondaparinux or a DTI may be considered.[48] Such decisions should weigh the risks involved. If transitioning the patient to warfarin, current observations encourage continuing the initial parenteral therapy until the INR is in a target range adapted to the false elevation caused by the DTI. This can be determined by looking at the INR on the DTI before initiating warfarin and adding the elevation to the INR target. For example, if the INR on argatroban is 2.0 before initiating warfarin, an INR above 3.0 should be observed before discontinuing the DTI. Minimal change in the DTI dose between the two INR determinations would be preferred to limit changes in the DTI effect in the INR.

Caution should be exercised against dosing that leads to having excessive effects from warfarin during initiation of therapy because it may pose a risk of venous limb gangrene. In addition, guidelines suggest waiting for the platelet count to recover to more than 150,000/mm^3.[48] However, in the critically ill patient especially, platelet counts may not recover, resulting in prolonged DTI therapy. One recent observation noted no difference between the strategies of waiting for platelet count recovery compared with initiating warfarin in conservative dosing once two consecutive rising platelet counts had occurred.[89]

REFERENCES

1. Mammen EF. Pathogenesis of venous thrombosis. Chest 1992;102(6 suppl):640S-4S.
2. Chan CM, Shorr AF. Venous thromboembolic disease in the intensive care unit. Semin Respir Crit Care Med 2010;31:39-46.
3. Kearon C, Akl EA, Comerota AJ, et al. Antithrombotic therapy for VTE disease: Antithrombotic Therapy and Prevention of Thrombosis, 9th ed: American College of Chest Physicians Evidence-Based Clinical Practice Guidelines. Chest 2012;141:e419S-e494S
4. Geerts WH, Bergqvist D, Pineo GF, et al. Prevention of venous thromboembolism: American College of Chest Physicians Evidence-Based Clinical Practice Guidelines, 8th ed. Chest 2008;133:381S-453S.
5. Centers for Medicare & Medicaid Services and The Joint Commission. Specifications Manual for National Hospital Inpatient Quality Measures. Version 4.4a. Available at http://manual.jointcommission.org. Accessed October 5, 2015.
6. MacLellan DG, Fletcher JP. Mechanical compression in the prophylaxis of venous thromboembolism. ANZ J Surg 2007;77:418-23.
7. Dobesh P, Stacy Z. Venous thromboembolism prevention. In: Dager WE, Gulseth MP, Nutescu EA, eds. Anticoagulation Therapy: A Point-of-Care Guide. Bethesda, MD: American Society of Health-System Pharmacists, 2011:201-29.
8. Dager WE, Tsu LV, Pon TK. Considerations for systemic anticoagulation in ESRD. Semin Dial 2015;28:354-62.
9. Tsu LV, Dager WE. Bivalirudin dosing adjustments for reduced renal function with or without hemodialysis in the management of heparin-induced thrombocytopenia. Ann Pharmacother 2011;45:1185-92.
10. Kearon C, Akl EA, Comerota AJ, et al. Antithrombotic therapy for VTE disease: Antithrombotic Therapy and Prevention of Thrombosis, 9th ed: American College of Chest Physicians Evidence-Based Clinical Practice Guidelines. Chest 2012;141:e419S-e494S.
11. Hursting MJ, Murray PT. Argatroban anticoagulation in renal dysfunction: a literature analysis. Nephron Clin Pract 2008;109:c80-94.
12. Pon TK, Dager WE, Roberts AJ, et al. Subcutaneous enoxaparin for therapeutic anticoagulation in hemodialysis patients. Thromb Res 2014;133:1023-8.
13. Mahieu E, Claes K, Jacquemin M, et al. Anticoagulation with fondaparinux for hemodiafiltration in patients with heparin-induced thrombocytopenia: dose-finding study and safety evaluation. Artif Organs 2013;37:482-7.
14. Brandt K, McGinn K, Quedado J. Low-dose systemic alteplase (tPA) for the treatment of pulmonary embolism. Ann Pharmacother 2015;49:818-24.
15. Jaff MR, McMurtry MS, Archer SL, et al. Management of massive and submassive pulmonary embolism, iliofemoral deep vein thrombosis, and chronic thromboembolic pulmonary hypertension: a scientific statement from the American Heart Association. Circulation 2011;123:1788-830.
16. Kline JA, Nordenholz KE, Courtney DM, et al. Treatment of submassive pulmonary embolism with tenecteplase or placebo: cardiopulmonary outcomes at 3 months: multicenter double-blind, placebo-controlled randomized trial. J Thromb Haemost 2014;12:459-68.
17. Bara L, Billaud E, Gramond G, et al. Comparative pharmacokinetics of a low molecular weight heparin (PK 10 169) and unfractionated heparin after intravenous and subcutaneous administration. Thromb Res 1985;39:631-6.
18. Spyropoulos AC, Anderson FA Jr, Fitzgerald G, et al. Predictive and associative models to identify hospitalized medical patients at risk for VTE. Chest 2011;140:706-14.
19. Kahn SR, Lim W, Dunn AS, et al. Prevention of VTE in nonsurgical patients: Antithrombotic Therapy and Prevention of Thrombosis, 9th ed: American College of Chest Physicians Evidence-Based Clinical Practice Guidelines. Chest 2012;141:e195S-226S.
20. Lim W, Meade M, Lauzier F, et al. Failure of anticoagulant thromboprophylaxis: risk factors in medical-surgical critically ill patients. Crit Care Med 2015;43:401-10.
21. Garcia DA, Baglin TP, Weitz JI, et al. Parenteral anticoagulants: Antithrombotic Therapy and Prevention of Thrombosis, 9th ed: American College of Chest Physicians Evidence-Based Clinical Practice Guidelines. Chest 2012;141:e24S-e43S.
22. Dager WE. Parenteral direct thrombin inhibitors. In: Dager WE, Gulseth MP, Nutescu EA, eds. Anticoagulation Therapy: A Point-of-Care Guide. Bethesda, MD: American Society of Health-System Pharmacists, 2011:77-99.
23. Basu D, Gallus A, Hirsh J, et al. A prospective study of the value of monitoring heparin treatment with the activated partial thromboplastin time. N Engl J Med 1972;287:324-7.
24. Frugé KS, Lee YR. Comparison of unfractionated heparin protocols using antifactor Xa monitoring or activated partial thrombin time monitoring. Am J Health Syst Pharm 2015;72(17 suppl 2):S90-7.
25. van Roessel S, Middeldorp S, Cheung YW, et al. Accuracy of aPTT monitoring in critically ill patients treated with unfractionated heparin. Neth J Med 2014;72:305-10.
26. Fuentes A, Gordon-Burroughs S, Hall JB, et al. Comparison of anti-Xa and activated partial thromboplastin time monitoring for heparin dosing in patients with cirrhosis. Ther Drug Monit 2015;37:40-4.
27. Aarab R, van Es J, de Pont AC, et al. Monitoring of unfractionated heparin in critically ill patients. Neth J Med 2013;71:466-71.
28. Takemoto CM, Streiff MB, Shermock KM, et al. Activated partial thromboplastin time and anti-Xa measurements in heparin monitoring. Am J Clin Pathol 2013;139:450-6.
29. Kearon C, Kahn SR, Agnelli G, et al. Antithrombotic therapy for venous thromboembolic disease: American College of Chest Physicians Evidence-Based Clinical Practice Guidelines, 8th ed. Chest 2008;133:454S-545S.
30. Cipolle RJ, Rodvold KA. Heparin. In: Evans WE, Schentag JJ, Jusko WJ, eds. Applied Pharmacokinetics: Principles of Therapeutic Drug Monitoring, 2nd ed. Spokane, WA: Applied Therapeutics, 1986:908-43.

31. McDonald MM, Jacobson LJ, Hay WW Jr, et al. Heparin clearance in the newborn. Pediatr Res 1981;15:1015-8.

32. Harrington RA, Becker RC, Cannon CP, et al. Antithrombotic therapy for non–ST-segment elevation acute coronary syndromes: American College of Chest Physicians Evidence-Based Clinical Practice Guidelines. Chest 2008;133:670S-707S.

33. Hirsh J, Bauer KA, Donati MB, et al. Parenteral anticoagulants: American College of Chest Physicians Evidence-Based Clinical Practice Guidelines. Chest 2008;133:141S-159S.

34. Groce JB III, Gal P, Douglas JB, et al. Heparin dosage adjustment in patients with deep-vein thrombosis using heparin concentrations rather than activated partial thromboplastin time. Clin Pharm 1987;6:216-22.

35. Gosselin RC, Smythe MA. Coagulation laboratory considerations. In: Dager WE, Gulseth MP, Nutescu EA, eds. Anticoagulation Therapy: A Point-of-Care Guide. Bethesda, MD: American Society of Health-System Pharmacists, 2011:391-425.

36. Dager WE. Unfractionated heparin. In: Dager WE, Gulseth MP, Nutescu EA, eds. Anticoagulation Therapy: A Point-of-Care Guide. Bethesda, MD: American Society of Health-System Pharmacists, 2011:33-59.

37. Decousus HA, Croze M, Levi FA, et al. Circadian changes in anticoagulant effect of heparin infused at a constant rate. Br Med J (Clin Res Ed) 1985;290:341-4.

38. Dager WE, Roberts AJ. Unfractionated heparin, low molecular weight heparin, and fondaparinux. In: Murphy JE, ed. Clinical Pharmacokinetics, 5th ed. Bethesda, MD: American Society of Health-System Pharmacists, 2012:203-27.

39. Mayr AJ, Dünser M, Jochberger S, et al. Antifactor Xa activity in intensive care patients receiving thromboembolic prophylaxis with standard doses of enoxaparin. Thromb Res 2002;105:201-4.

40. Dörffler-Melly J, de Jonge E, Pont AC, et al. Bioavailability of subcutaneous low-molecular-weight heparin to patients on vasopressors. Lancet 2002;359:849-50.

41. Priglinger U, Delle Karth G, Geppert A, et al. Prophylactic anticoagulation with enoxaparin: is the subcutaneous route appropriate in the critically ill? Crit Care Med 2003;31:1405-9.

42. Malinoski D, Jafari F, Ewing T, et al. Standard prophylactic enoxaparin dosing leads to inadequate anti-Xa levels and increased deep venous thrombosis rates in critically ill trauma and surgical patients. J Trauma 2010;68:874-80.

43. Robinson S, Zincuk A, Larsen UL, et al. A comparative study of varying doses of enoxaparin for thromboprophylaxis in critically ill patients: a double-blinded, randomised controlled trial. Crit Care 2013;17:R75.

44. Hacquard M, Mainard D, de Maistre E, et al. Influence of injection site on prophylactic dose enoxaparin bioavailability in obese patients. J Thromb Haemost 2007;5(suppl 2):P-M-669.

45. Nutescu EA, Spinler SA, Wittkowsky A, et al. Low-molecular-weight heparins in renal impairment and obesity: available evidence and clinical practice recommendations across medical and surgical settings. Ann Pharmacother 2009;43:1064-83.

46. Levine M, Gent M, Hirsh J, et al. A comparison of low-molecular-weight heparin administered primarily at home with unfractionated heparin administered in the hospital for proximal deep-vein thrombosis. N Engl J Med 1996;334:677-81.

47. Koopman MM, Prandoni P, Piovella F, et al. Treatment of venous thrombosis with intravenous unfractionated heparin administered in the hospital as compared with subcutaneous low-molecular-weight heparin administered at home. The Tasman study group. N Engl J Med 1996;334:682-7.

48. Linkins LA, Dans AL, Moores LK, et al. Treatment and prevention of heparin-induced thrombocytopenia: Antithrombotic Therapy and Prevention of Thrombosis, 9th ed: American College of Chest Physicians Evidence-Based Clinical Practice Guidelines. Chest 2012;141:e495S-530S.

49. The Rembrandt Investigators. Treatment of proximal deep vein thrombosis with a novel synthetic compound (SR90107A/ORG31540) with pure anti-factor Xa activity: a phase II evaluation. Circulation 2000;102:2726-31.

50. Büller HR, Davidson BL, Decousus H, et al. Subcutaneous fondaparinux versus intravenous unfractionated heparin in the initial treatment of pulmonary embolism. N Engl J Med 2003;349:1695-702.

51. Büller HR, Davidson BL, Decousus H, et al. Fondaparinux or enoxaparin for the initial treatment of symptomatic deep venous thrombosis: a randomized trial. Ann Intern Med 2004;140:867-73.

52. Ageno W, Riva N, Noris P, et al. Safety and efficacy of low-dose fondaparinux (1.5 mg) for the prevention of venous thromboembolism in acutely ill medical patients with renal impairment: the FONDAIR study. J Thromb Haemost 2012;10:2291-7.

53. Dager WE, Kiser TH. Systemic anticoagulation considerations in chronic kidney disease. Adv Chronic Kidney Dis 2010;17:420-7.

54. Speeckaert MM, Devreese KM, Vanholder RC, et al. Fondaparinux as an alternative to vitamin K antagonists in haemodialysis patients. Nephrol Dial Transplant 2013;28:3090-5.

55. Davidson BL, Büller HR, Decousus H, et al. Effect of obesity on outcomes after fondaparinux, enoxaparin, or heparin treatment for acute venous thromboembolism in the Matisse trials. J Thromb Haemost 2007;5:1191-4.

56. Nagler M, Haslauer M, Wuillemin WA. Fondaparinux – data on efficacy and safety in special situations. Thromb Res 2012;129:407-17.

57. Martinez L, Burnett A, Borrego M, et al. Effect of fondaparinux prophylaxis on anti-factor Xa concentrations in patients with morbid obesity. Am J Health Syst Pharm 2011;68:1716-22.

58. Crowther MA, Berry LR, Monagle PT, et al. Mechanisms responsible for the failure of protamine to inactivate low-molecular-weight heparin. Br J Haematol 2002;116:178-86.

59. Desmurs-Clavel H, Huchon C, Chatard B, et al. Reversal of the inhibitory effect of fondaparinux on thrombin generation by rFVIIa, aPCC and PCC. Thromb Res 2009;123:796-8.

60. Love JE, Ferrell C, Chandler WL. Monitoring direct thrombin inhibitors with a plasma diluted thrombin time. Thromb Haemost 2007;98:234-42.

61. Reddy BV, Grossman EJ, Trevino SA, et al. Argatroban therapy in patients with heparin-induced thrombocytopenia requiring renal replacement therapy. Ann Pharmacother 2005;39:1601-5.

62. Arpino PA, Hallisey RK. Effect of renal function on the pharmacodynamics of argatroban. Ann Pharmacother 2004;38:25-9.

63. Smythe MA, Koerber JM, Forsyth LL, et al. Argatroban dosage requirements and outcomes in intensive care versus non-intensive care patients. Pharmacotherapy 2009;29:1073-81.

64. Nagle EL, Tsu LV, Dager WE. Bivalirudin for anticoagulation during hypothermic cardiopulmonary bypass and recombinant factor VIIa for iatrogenic coagulopathy. Ann Pharmacother 2011;45:e47.

65. Dager WE. Considerations for drug dosing post coronary artery bypass graft surgery. Ann Pharmacother 2008;42:421-4.

66. Gosselin RC, Dager WE, King JH, et al. Effect of direct thrombin inhibitors, bivalirudin, lepirudin, and argatroban, on prothrombin time and INR values. Am J Clin Pathol 2004;121:593-9.

67. Dager WE. Initiating warfarin therapy. Ann Pharmacother 2003;37:905-8.

68. Ageno W, Gallus AS, Wittkowsky A, et al. Oral anticoagulant therapy: Antithrombotic Therapy and Prevention of Thrombosis, 9th ed: American College of Chest Physicians Evidence-Based Clinical Practice Guidelines. Chest 2012;141:e44S-88S.

69. Wittkowsky A. Warfarin. In: Dager WE, Gulseth MP, Nutescu EA, eds. Anticoagulation Therapy: A Point-of-Care Guide. Bethesda, MD: American Society of Health-System Pharmacists, 2011:11-31.

70. Xarelto [package insert]. Titusville, NJ: Janssen, 2011. Revised 2015.

71. Eliquis [package insert]. New York: Pfizer, 2015.

72. Pradaxa [package insert]. Ridgefield, CT: Boehringer Ingelheim, 2015.

73. Dager WE, Gosselin RC, Kitchen S, et al. Dabigatran effects on the international normalized ratio, activated partial thromboplastin time, thrombin time, and fibrinogen: a multicenter, in vitro study. Ann Pharmacother 2012;46:1627-36.

74. Gosselin RC, Francart SJ, Hawes EM, et al. Heparin-calibrated chromogenic anti-Xa activity measurements in patients receiving rivaroxaban: can this test be used to quantify drug level? Ann Pharmacother 2015;49:777-83.

75. Dale BJ, Ginsberg JS, Johnston M, et al. Comparison of the effects of apixaban and rivaroxaban on prothrombin and activated partial thromboplastin times using various reagents. J Thromb Haemost 2014;12:1810-5.

76. Schiele F, van Ryn J, Canada K, et al. A specific antidote for dabigatran: functional and structural characterization. Blood 2013;121:3554-62.

77. Pollack CV Jr, Reilly PA, Eikelboom J, et al. Idarucizumab for dabigatran reversal. N Engl J Med 2015;373:511-20.

78. Lu G, DeGuzman FR, Hollenbach SJ, et al. A specific antidote for reversal of anticoagulation by direct and indirect inhibitors of coagulation factor Xa. Nat Med 2013;19:446-51.

79. Kalus JS. Pharmacologic interventions for reversing the effects of oral anticoagulants. Am J Health Syst Pharm 2013;70:S12-S21.

80. Tsu LV, Dienes JE, Dager WE. Vitamin K dosing to reverse warfarin based on INR, route of administration, and home warfarin dose in the acute/critical care setting. Ann Pharmacother 2012;46:1617-26.

81. Chang DN, Dager WE, Chin AI. Removal of dabigatran by hemodialysis. Am J Kidney Dis 2013;61:487-9.

82. Dager WE, Gosselin RC, Roberts AJ. Reversing dabigatran in life-threatening bleeding occurring during cardiac ablation with factor eight inhibitor bypassing activity. Crit Care Med 2013;41:e42-6.

83. Dager W, Roberts AJ, Gosselin R, et al. Low dose FEIBA and hemodialysis for managing major bleeding on dabigatran. J Thromb Haemost 2015;13:S881.

84. Dager W, Roberts AJ, Gosselin R, et al. Effective use of low dose activated prothrombin complex concentrates in managing major GI bleeding on rivaroxaban. J Thromb Haemost 2015;13:S883.

85. Huang W, Goldberg R, Anderson F, et al. Risk-assessment model of recurrence within 3 months after a first episode of acute venous thromboembolism: Worcester venous thromboembolism study. J Thromb Haemost 2015;13:S716.

86. Mannucci PM, Tripodi A. Hemostatic defects in liver and renal dysfunction. Hematology Am Soc Hematol Educ Program 2012;2012:168-73.

87. Tripodi A, Mannucci PM. The coagulopathy of chronic liver disease. N Engl J Med 2011;365:147-56.

88. Horlocker TT, Wedel DJ, Rowlingson JC, et al. Regional anesthesia in the patient receiving antithrombotic or thrombolytic therapy: American Society of Regional Anesthesia and Pain Medicine Evidence-Based Guidelines (3rd ed). Reg Anesth Pain Med 2010;35:64-101.

89. Chen LD, Dager WE, Roberts AJ. Safety and efficacy of starting warfarin after two consecutive platelet rises in patients with heparin-induced thrombocytopenia. J Thromb Haemost 2015;13:S866.

Chapter 24: Hemostatic Agents for the Prevention and Management of Hemorrhage in the ICU

Robert MacLaren, Pharm.D., MPH, FCCP, FCCM; Bradley A. Boucher, Pharm.D., FCCP, FCCM; and Laura Baumgartner, Pharm.D.

LEARNING OBJECTIVES

1. Describe the physiologic integration of coagulation, fibrinolysis, platelets, and the vessel wall to achieve optimal hemostasis.
2. Delineate the extrinsic and intrinsic coagulation pathways, and compare the common laboratory values used to measure their activities.
3. Define coagulopathy and thrombocytopenia, and outline common etiologies of both in critically ill patients.
4. Explain the pathophysiologic mechanisms contributing to coagulopathy for hypothermia, acidosis, dilutional, inflammation (disseminated intravascular coagulopathy), hepatic dysfunction, renal dysfunction, inherited abnormalities, and medications.
5. Formulate a treatment plan and goals of therapy for fluid resuscitation during hemorrhage.
6. Compare and contrast the blood products (red blood cells, platelets, fresh frozen plasma, prothrombin complex concentrates, and cryoprecipitate) with respect to indications, goals of therapy, and adverse events.
7. Compare and contrast the pharmacologic agents (local hemostatics, vitamin K, recombinant activated factor VII, desmopressin, conjugated estrogen, and fibrinogen concentrate) with respect to indications, goals of therapy, and adverse events.
8. Develop a plan for the prevention and management of hemorrhage associated with surgery, trauma, hepatic dysfunction, obstetric, and anticoagulants.

ABBREVIATIONS IN THIS CHAPTER

ADP	Adenosine diphosphate	PPH	Postpartum hemorrhage
aPTT	Activated partial thromboplastin time	PRBC	Packed red blood cell
ATP	Adenosine triphosphate	RBC	Red blood cell
DIC	Disseminated intravascular coagulation	rFVIIa	Recombinant activated factor VII
DTI	Direct thrombin inhibitor	ROTEG	Rotational thromboelastography
FFP	Fresh frozen plasma	TACO	Transfusion-associated cardiac overload
GP	Glycoprotein	TEG	Thromboelastography
ICU	Intensive care unit	TRALI	Transfusion-related acute lung injury
INR	International normalized ratio	TRIM	Transfusion-related immunomodulation
MTP	Massive transfusion protocol	vWF	von Willebrand factor
PCC	Prothrombin complex concentrate		

INTRODUCTION

Hemostatic pathways act to promote and maintain blood flow. Coagulation is an orchestration of interactions between blood vessels, procoagulant mediators, anticoagulant mediators, and platelets. Several etiologies may disrupt these homeostatic processes, leading to hemorrhage. The clinician must understand these pathologic causes in order to facilitate appropriate management and monitoring. Therapies may include blood products, pharmacologic agents, and nonpharmacologic interventions, each with their own considerations that must be understood to optimize treatment and prevent further hemorrhage. This chapter will review the common causes of disruption to the hemostatic pathways; delineate the properties of blood products, pharmacologic agents, and nonpharmacologic interventions that clinicians need to consider when applying them in a clinical scenario; and discuss appropriate management for common types of hemorrhage.

AN OVERVIEW OF HEMOSTASIS

Hemostasis is a complex homeostatic system that integrates coagulation, fibrinolysis, platelets, and the vessel wall to limit hemorrhage and prevent thrombus propagation. Under normal conditions, the endothelial cells have antithrombotic properties such as heparin-like glycosaminoglycans, platelet inhibitors, coagulation inhibitors, and activators of fibrinolysis. In contrast, the subendothelium is highly thrombotic with mediators that include collagen, von Willebrand factor (vWF), and platelet adhesion molecules. This hemostatic balance, however, may be disrupted by pathological conditions such as trauma/surgery, blood abnormalities, or inflammation.[1,2]

Any vascular insult results in arteriolar vasospasm, mediated by reflex neurogenic mechanisms and the release of local mediators like endothelin and platelet-derived thromboxane A_2. Platelets are disc shaped and normally do not adhere to intact vascular endothelium. Vessel injury releases vWF, a glycoprotein (GP) always present to some degree in plasma, to cause platelets to undergo a morphological change that increases their surface area. von Willebrand factor also promotes platelet adhesion by acting as a bridge between endothelial collagen and platelet surface receptors GPIb. After adhesion, platelets are activated and undergo degranulation that causes the release of P-selectin; factors I (also called fibrinogen), V, and VIII; platelet factor IV; platelet-derived growth factor; tumor growth factor α; adenosine triphosphate (ATP); adenosine diphosphate (ADP); calcium; serotonin; histamine; and epinephrine. Hypoxia from blood loss or other causes up-regulates P selectin and can initiate coagulation through the recruitment of factor III (also called tissue factor) containing monocytes. Calcium binds to phospholipids to provide a surface for the assembly of various coagulation factors. Thromboxane A_2 and ADP stimulate further platelet aggregation leading to the formation of a platelet plug, which temporarily seals the vascular injury. Adenosine diphosphate binding also causes a conformational change in GPIIb/IIIa receptors on the platelet surface leading to the deposition of fibrinogen and platelet clumping. Thrombin generation catalyzes the conversion of fibrinogen to fibrin, which stabilizes the platelet plug by forming a matrix for additional adhesion.[1,2]

Comprehending the tissue factor pathway (extrinsic pathway) and the contact activation pathway (intrinsic pathway) is necessary to understand the coagulation cascade, the possible disorders associated with major hemorrhage, and the laboratory values that describe coagulation and define coagulopathy (Figure 24.1).[1,2] Most clotting factors are precursors of proteolytic enzymes and circulate in an inactive form. With the exception of tissue factor and factors IV and VIII, clotting factors are produced in the liver. Factors II (also called prothrombin), VII, IX, and X undergo post-translational modification by vitamin K–dependent carboxylation of the glutamic acid residues. Naturally occurring anticoagulants include antithrombin (which inactivates thrombin and factors IXa, Xa, XIa, and XIIa), tissue factor plasminogen inhibitor, proteins C and S, thrombomodulin, and protein Z.

The extrinsic pathway is plasma-mediated hemostasis. It is activated by tissue factor that is expressed in the subendothelial tissue and exposed during direct vascular injury, functional injury (activation of circulating tissue factor), hypoxia, malignancy, or inflammation. Tissue factor binds to calcium to activate factor VII (now called factor VIIa), which further activates factors X, V, and II. The intrinsic pathway is a parallel pathway to the extrinsic system. It is initiated by collagen exposure, which activates factor XII, which in turn activates factors XI, IX, and VIII to form tenase complex on a phospholipid surface. The propagation requires calcium, high-molecular-weight kininogen, and prekallikrein. The extrinsic and intrinsic pathways merge at the common pathway where activated factor X, cofactor V, tissue and platelet phospholipids, and calcium form a prothrombinase complex. This complex converts prothrombin to thrombin to cleave fibrinogen to fibrin and activates factor XIII. This leads to the formation of covalent crosslinks of fibrin (polymers) that are incorporated in the platelet plug.[1,2] The intrinsic pathway also augments thrombin generation primarily initiated by the extrinsic pathway.

Coagulation can be described as four steps: initiation, amplification, propagation, and stabilization. During the initiation phase, the expression of tissue factor from the inured vessel complexes with factor VIIa, which activates factor IX. The tissue factor-VIIa complex represents a bridge between the two pathways as factor Xa activates thrombin. The generation of thrombin is not robust and can be terminated by tissue factor pathway inhibitor. This thrombin is often called "priming thrombin" because it

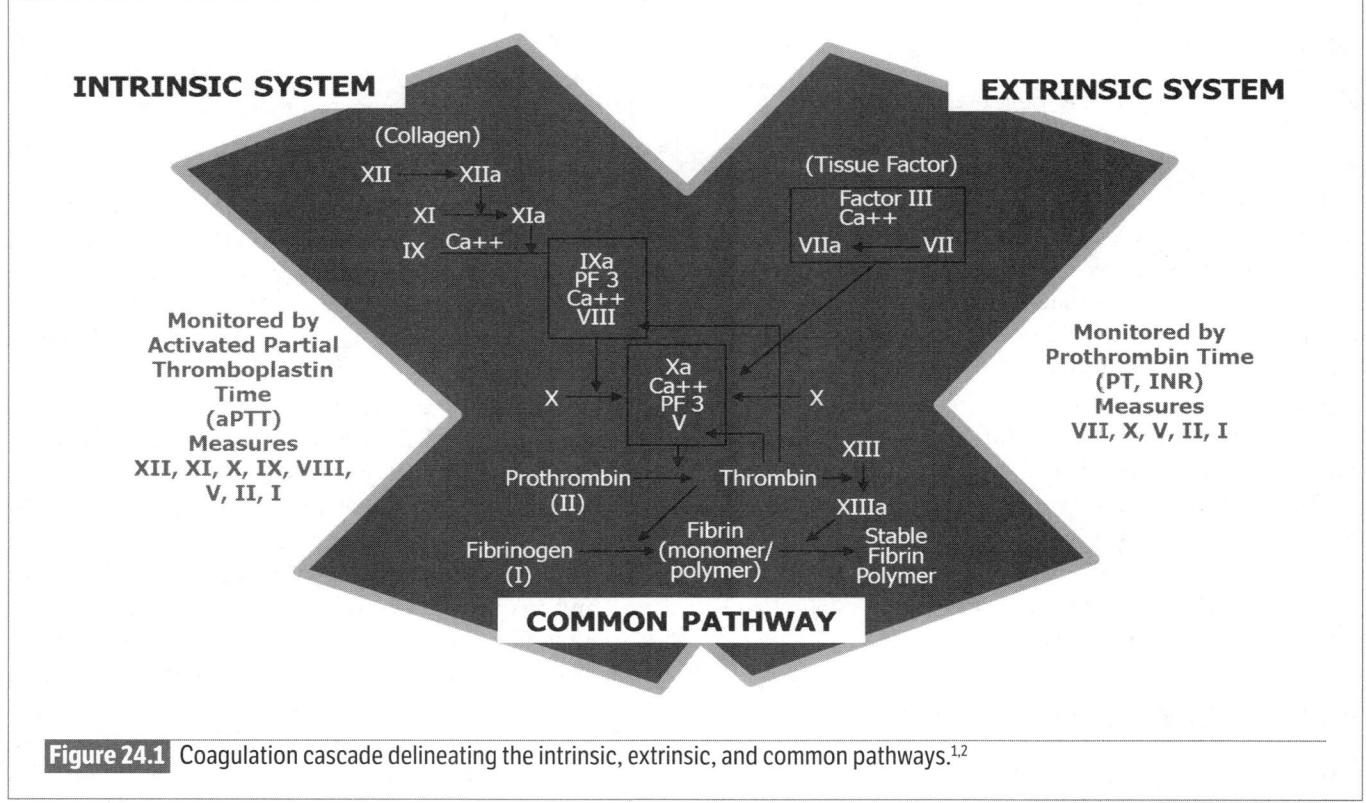

Figure 24.1 Coagulation cascade delineating the intrinsic, extrinsic, and common pathways.[1,2]

binds to platelets to activate them and factors V and VIII, the latter of which serves as a cofactor in the prothrombinase complex and accelerates the formation factor Xa. This process represents amplification. Propagation occurs when the accumulated enzyme complexes (tenase and prothrombinase) on the platelet surface produce robust thrombin, often called a thrombin burst, which further activates platelets creating a positive loop. This ensures continuous thrombin generation and fibrin production in sufficient amounts to form a stable clot. Stabilization is the factor XIIIa process of forming covalently linked fibrin polymers that provide strength to the platelet plug. Thrombin also activates thrombin activatable fibrinolysis inhibitor, which protects the clot from degradation.[1,2]

Measuring Hemostasis

To fully comprehend the limitations of treatments used to promote hemostasis, it is necessary to understand the assays used to measure coagulation (Figure 24.1).[2] The prothrombin time (PT) and the international normalized ratio (INR) monitor the extrinsic pathway (tissue factor pathway) and common portions of the clotting cascade.[3,4] Platelets are removed from citrate anticoagulated plasma by centrifugation to isolate the role of the soluble clotting factors to which tissue factor and calcium are added to initiate clotting. This process preferentially activates factor VII, which in turn activates factors X, V, and II to ultimately convert fibrinogen to fibrin; this last step is captured optically or electrically and measured in seconds.[3,4] Because factor VII circulates in the highest abundance of any factor, the PT is relatively resistant to change and requires single factor levels to decline to less than 10% of normal before becoming prolonged.[3,4] The only factor unique to this pathway is factor VII, so the only manner in which PT can be prolonged without affecting PTT is a selective factor VII deficiency.[3,4] The PT is commonly referenced to an international standard (INR) because the sensitivities of the reagents measuring PT vary. The INR is calibrated to assess anticoagulation in patients receiving stable warfarin therapies. Its applicability to other causes of an elevated PT is uncertain, although commonly done. In hepatic dysfunction, the extent of coagulopathy as measured by the PT or INR is not predictive of bleeding complications.[3,4] Normal values for PT and INR are 12–13 seconds and 0.8–1.2, respectively.

The activated partial thromboplastin time (aPTT) measures the intrinsic pathway and is more complex than the PT. A particulate contact activator (hence the name "activated") like ellagic acid, kaolin, celite, or silica is added to platelet-poor citrate anticoagulated plasma to which a "partial thromboplastin" (lacking tissue factor) is added and the citrate reversed with calcium.[3,4] The particulate activates factor XII, which in turn activates factors XI, IX, and VIII and the common sequence of factor X through fibrin formation. Like PT, aPTT is measured in seconds with normal reference values of 25–35 seconds, but unlike PT, single factors unique to the aPTT must decline to only 15%–30% of normal values for the aPTT to be prolonged.[3,4] This may reflect the lengthier clotting sequence contributing to the aPTT and/or the fact that these clotting factors are already lower in concentration than factor VII. Milder deficiencies of many factors can prolong the aPTT, so it may be more sensitive than PT for assessing factor changes, especially factors VIII and IX.[3,4] Prekallikrein, high-molecular-weight kininogen, antiphospholipid antibodies, and factor XII deficiencies prolong aPTT, but none increases the risk of hemorrhage.

Other tests used to measure coagulation include anti-Xa activity, activated clotting time, and assessments of fibrinolysis. Anti-Xa activity is often used to assess anticoagulation in patients receiving low-molecular-weight heparins, especially in patients at the extremes of weight or those with reduced or increased kidney function.[3,4] Activated clotting time nonspecifically measures the time for an activating agent to produce clot in whole blood and is often used to monitor unfractionated heparin or direct thrombin inhibitors (DTIs) during surgery. Fibrinolysis is the process of dispersing and dissolving clot. This process may be described by the term *fibrin degradation product* or D-dimer. The fibrin degradation product assay refers to the breakdown products of fibrin and fibrinogen produced by plasmin.[3,4] The nonspecific fibrin degradation product or fibrin split product assay may be present in the absence of clot. In contrast, the D-dimer is only formed from the degradation of fibrin from an intact clot. Both assays lack specificity and are commonly positive in critically ill patients regardless of the presence of thromboembolic disease or coagulopathy.[3,4] In addition, fibrin degradation product and D-dimer are hepatically eliminated, so liver function may influence their specificities. Moreover, various commercially available assay methods differ significantly (e.g., latex or red blood cell [RBC] agglutination, enzyme-linked immunoassays) resulting in varying sensitivities. Normal values for D-dimer are below 500 ng/mL.

Measuring Platelet Function

Platelet function may be assessed for a variety of reasons including identifying bleeding disorders, monitoring response to antiplatelet therapies, evaluating perioperative hemostasis, and guiding platelet transfusion therapy.[5,6] Several tests are available to assess platelet function and include light transmission platelet aggregation, impedance aggregometry on whole blood, lumi-aggregometry, platelet activation by flow cytometry, and shear stress platelet activation.[5,6] Light transmission platelet aggregation is considered the gold standard test and incorporates in vitro platelet-to-platelet clump formation in a GPIIb/IIIa-dependent manner. The assay measures the light transmission after platelet-rich plasma is activated with various platelet agonists (e.g., collagen, ADP, thrombin, epinephrine, arachidonic acid). Light transmission increases as platelets aggregate. Although this method can assess different platelet aggregation pathways and is sensitive to antiplatelet therapy, it is time-consuming and not reflective of whole blood activity because it uses platelet-rich plasma. It also requires relatively large volumes of blood to generate platelet-rich plasma. Impedance aggregometry, which uses smaller volumes of citrated whole blood, is based on the principle that activated platelets stick by their surface receptors to artificial surfaces of electrodes within the sample. Electrical impedance is generated by aggregated platelets, which is measured by diminishing current between electrodes. This method is available as point-of-care testing and is sensitive to antiplatelet therapy. Lumi-aggregometry measures the ATP released from platelets that are activated in vitro by various agonists. The ATP reacts with a luciferin-luciferase reagent, and the intensity of light emitted is proportional to the ATP concentration. This method may be used to assess several platelet aggregation pathways and is particularly useful for assessing platelet function when thrombocytopenia is present. Flow cytometry, which uses citrate anticoagulated whole blood, is based on the optical and fluorescence evaluation of the physical and antigenic properties of platelets. Therefore, it assesses the internal complexity and conformational changes of platelets in response to in vitro platelet activation. Antibodies that bind to specific proteins on the platelet surface or inside the platelet are conjugated to fluorescence dyes so that light is emitted on platelet activation. The results are expressed as a histogram with fluorescence intensity plotted against platelet number. This method is sensitive to antiplatelet therapy and may be used when thrombocytopenia is present. Shear stress platelet activation applies physical stress to citrate anticoagulated whole blood and measures either the time taken for platelets to occlude a collagen-coated orifice or the percentage of a polystyrene plate covered by platelet aggregates. This method is available as point-of-care testing and is sensitive to antiplatelet therapy.

COAGULOPATHY AND THROMBOCYTOPENIA IN CRITICALLY ILL PATIENTS

Hemostatic abnormalities are common in critically ill patients, ranging from an isolated laboratory abnormality to complex derangements. By far the most common causes of abnormal clotting assays and low platelet counts are errors incurred during sample collection or laboratory analyses, so laboratory aberrations should always be confirmed, especially in the absence of clinical manifestations. As discussed in the previous section, coagulation and hemostasis require complex interactions between the vessel wall, platelets, and soluble coagulation factors. Hemostatic abnormalities can result when any one of these three systems is defective. However, several causes may contribute to the mechanisms of abnormal hemostasis, making it difficult to diagnose and manage hemostatic derangements in critically ill patients.[7-10]

Coagulopathy

Alterations in coagulation factors, including decreased levels of coagulation factors, reduced levels of endogenous anticoagulants, and enhanced fibrinolysis, all contribute to hemostatic abnormalities in critically ill patients.[7-10] Despite their poor reflection of in vivo hemostasis, laboratory values such as aPTT, PT or INR and platelet counts are often used to assess the degree of coagulopathy (Table 24.1).[3,4,7-11] Up to one-third of patients in the intensive care unit (ICU) have coagulopathy, as defined by an INR of 1.5 or greater or an aPTT of 1.5-fold or greater than the upper limit of normal.[10] The presence of coagulopathy increases the likelihood of hemorrhage by 4- to 5-fold and is an independent risk factor for mortality (odds ratio [OR] 1.5–4.3).[12] Causes of coagulopathy are generally categorized by the extent that either or both the PT/INR and the aPTT are prolonged (Table 24.1).[3,4,7-11] Mechanisms contributing to coagulopathy include hypothermia, acidosis, dilution from administration of fluids and blood products, disseminated intravascular coagulation (DIC), liver dysfunction, renal dysfunction, inherited disorders, and medications.[4,7-11]

Hypothermia

Hypothermia may be the result of several causes, including iatrogenic etiologies such as therapeutic hypothermia, surgery, or invasive interventions (e.g., dialysis, extracorporeal membrane oxygenation, plasmapheresis) or non-iatrogenic etiologies such as prolonged exposure to cold ambient temperatures, impaired thermoregulation (e.g., injuries to the central nervous system, hypothyroidism), or excessive heat loss (e.g., thermal injuries, drug intoxication).[12] The mechanisms of hypothermia-induced coagulopathy vary with the magnitude of hypothermia, and the extent of coagulopathy grows exponentially as the core body temperature decreases.[13] Although temperatures of 35°C and greater have very little effect on coagulation, temperatures of 32°C–34°C alter platelet number and function by reducing platelet adhesion and aggregation.[14,15] Temperatures of 33°C or less decrease the synthesis and kinetics of coagulation factors.

Therapeutic hypothermia to temperatures of 32°C–34°C for up to 24 hours may improve neurologic recovery in comatose patients with the return of spontaneous circulation after cardiac arrest.[16] The occurrence of bleeding requiring transfusions in the setting of therapeutically-induced hypothermia is 6%.[17] The risk of hemorrhage should not be viewed as a reason to withhold therapeutic hypothermia treatment in patients who are not actively bleeding. In patients who are at high bleeding risk or are actively bleeding, the hemorrhage risk should be considered in the context of possible neurologic benefit.[17] Hypothermia should be reversed and core body temperatures maintained at 35°C or greater when hypothermia is the result of other iatrogenic or non-iatrogenic etiologies.

Table 24.1 Causes of Coagulopathies as Defined by Laboratory Values[3,4,7-11]

Prothrombin Time	Activated Partial Thromboplastin Time	Coagulation Pathway Abnormality	Likely Causes
Prolonged	Normal	Extrinsic pathway	Factor VII deficiency
			Mild vitamin K deficiency
			Vitamin K antagonist administration
			Mild hepatic dysfunction
Normal	Prolonged	Intrinsic pathway	Factor VIII, IX, XI, XII deficiency
			Antiphospholipid syndrome
			Heparin administration
			DTI administration
Prolonged	Prolonged	Common pathway	Factor X, V, II, or fibrinogen deficiency
			Severe vitamin K deficiency
			Vitamin K antagonist administration
			Factor Xa inhibitor administration
			Global clotting factor deficiency
			• DIC
			• Hepatic dysfunction
			• Massive blood loss

DIC = disseminated intravascular coagulopathy; DTI = direct thrombin inhibitor.

Acidosis

Acidosis is a common clinical problem in critically ill patients and is a known predictor of coagulopathy in the ICU. Acidosis can present as a result of both respiratory and metabolic disturbances; however, coagulopathy is often caused by a hypoperfused state resulting in increased lactate generation. Coagulopathy is heightened when hypothermia is also present as acidosis and hypothermia synergistically impair coagulation.[18,19] The clinical effects include both prolonged clotting times and increased bleeding times, with a direct correlation between the extent of acidosis and coagulation impairment.[19]

The mechanisms of acidosis-induced coagulopathy primarily involve severe inhibition of the propagation phase of thrombin generation and increased fibrinogen degradation.[20] However, clotting factor function is also significantly impaired because acidotic environments hinder protease activity and limit anion exposure of phospholipids. When pH drops below 7.2, the functional activities of factor VIIa, tissue factor-factor VIIa complex, and the factor Xa/Va complex are diminished. As a result, clotting time is prolonged, and overall clot strength is weakened.[18-20] Although few studies have reported on outcome assessments looking strictly at acidosis-induced coagulopathy, it is usually regarded as a poor prognostic sign.[18] It is common practice before giving procoagulants to ensure that pH values are 7.2 or greater by temporarily inducing hyperventilation or administering intravenous bicarbonate.

Dilutional

Critically ill patients often require rapid resuscitation with large volumes of crystalloids, colloids, or RBCs if critical bleeding is present. As a result, these patients often have dilutional coagulopathy, a combination of decreased plasma concentrations of coagulation factors and platelets.[10-12,21] The degree of coagulopathy is directly related to the total volume transfused, in addition to preexisting hemostatic abnormalities, and the effects are synergistic with coagulopathy from hypothermia and acidosis.[22]

Dilutional coagulopathy is the result of an uncompensated loss of platelets and coagulation factors. This occurs most commonly during situations involving major blood loss or large-volume resuscitation, but it can also occur in critically ill patients with increased consumption or sequestration of platelets.[10,21,22] Red blood cell concentrates contain negligible amounts of platelets and coagulation factors, so they can further exacerbate a patient's risk of developing dilutional coagulopathy when transfused in large quantities. A platelet count of less than $50 \times 10^9/L$ is expected when two blood volumes have been replaced by fluid and RBC concentrates.[22] Similarly, coagulation factor deficiencies occur after blood volume losses exceed 150% because fibrinogen concentrations fall first, followed by other labile coagulation factors such as prothrombin and factors V and VII.[22] Hospital-specific "massive transfusion protocols" (MTPs) help reduce the incidence of dilutional coagulopathy by augmenting RBC supplementation with platelets, fresh frozen plasma (FFP), cryoprecipitate, and pharmacologic agents.[10,11,21,22]

Disseminated Intravascular Coagulopathy

Disseminated intravascular coagulopathy is an acquired syndrome characterized by systemic intravascular activation of coagulation that can occur in up to 25% of critically ill patients.[7,23] It originates secondary to fibrin deposition and intravascular microthrombi and may lead to significant complications including major bleeding and multiorgan dysfunction.[10,24] Critically ill patients with DIC often have rapidly decreasing platelet counts, low plasma concentrations of coagulation factors, prolonged coagulation tests, increased markers of fibrinogen formation, and hyperfibrinolysis. These abnormalities often lead to bleeding as the first sign of DIC, with only 5%–10% of cases presenting with microthrombi alone.[7] A DIC scoring tool developed by the International Society on Thrombosis and Haemostasis assigns points according to the extent of thrombocytopenia (platelet counts of $50-100 \times 10^9/L$ = 1 point, platelet counts less than $50 \times 10^9/L$ = 2 points), fibrin concentrations (moderate rise = 2 points, strong rise = 3 points), PT prolongation (3–6 seconds = 1 point, greater than 6 seconds = 2 points), and fibrinogen concentrations (less than 100 mg/dL = 1 point).[5] A score of at least 5 points in the presence of an underlying disorder associated with DIC is indicative of DIC.[5,23,24]

There are several etiologies of DIC among critically ill patients, with the most common cause being sepsis, followed by systemic infection, trauma, surgery, malignancy, thermal injury, and pancreatitis.[9,24] Less common etiologies include immunologic reactions (e.g., transplant rejection, host vs. graft disease, transfusion reactions, venomous bites or stings), vascular abnormalities, and cardiopulmonary bypass.[9,11,24,25] The mechanism of DIC is multifactorial but is commonly mediated by pathogen-associated molecular patterns and the generation of an overwhelming inflammatory response. Proinflammatory cytokines activate mononuclear cells and endothelial cells, which in turn express tissue factor, the main initiator of the extrinsic pathway of coagulation.[9,11,24,25] The physiological anticoagulation mechanism and endogenous fibrinolysis are stimulated but are inadequate to counterbalance the thrombin generation and intravascular fibrin formation. This, in combination with continuous consumption of platelets and clotting factors, leads to multiorgan failure and severe bleeding complications. Treatment with anticoagulants (e.g., heparin, DTIs) may be attempted, but this often hastens the development of hemorrhage. Instead, therapies usually focus on preventing hemorrhage and reversing the underlying disorder causing the proinflammatory state.[7,9,11]

Hepatic Dysfunction

Hepatic insufficiency is the most common cause of acquired coagulation abnormalities.[1,7] Thrombopoietin and most hemostatic proteins are synthesized in the liver; thus, reduced hepatic function often results in prolonged coagulation tests.[7] Splenic sequestration of platelets can also occur, further contributing to thrombocytopenia. Recent data suggest that patients with hepatic insufficiency are not naturally "auto-anticoagulated," as once believed.[26-28] Therefore, these patients may be at increased risk of both hemorrhage and thrombosis.[26-28]

The coagulopathy abnormalities seen in patients with hepatic insufficiency are complex. Anticoagulation occurs because hepatic synthesis of coagulation factors II, V, VII, IX, and X is reduced, the metabolism of tissue plasminogen activator is impaired, and fibrinogen production is lessened.[7,9,11] In addition, moderate to severe vitamin K deficiencies can occur in hepatic insufficiency. In contrast, levels of factor VIII and vWF, potent drivers of thrombin generation, are increased to enhance coagulation. In addition, there is a concomitant reduction in endogenous anticoagulants (proteins C, S, and Z; antithrombin; and Z-dependent protease inhibitor) and fibrinolytic mediators (thrombin activatable fibrinolysis inhibitor) that enhance coagulation and clot stability.[7,9,11] Thus, patients with hepatic insufficiency and prolonged coagulation tests may not be at increased bleeding risk.[3,12,26,27] Because discerning the likelihood of hemorrhage is clinically impossible, most clinicians try to minimize the extent of the coagulopathy before invasive procedures or during a bleeding event. It is plausible that bleeding in patients with hepatic insufficiency is the result of other etiologies of coagulopathy acquired from the acute situation (e.g., a systemic infection causing DIC).

Renal Dysfunction

Kidney failure produces uremia-induced qualitative defects in platelets that arise from insufficient vWF, decreased production of thromboxane A_2, increased cyclic adenosine monophosphate and cyclic guanosine monophosphate, and anemia.[7,27] In addition, the quantity of GPIIb receptors on platelet surfaces is diminished. Platelet function is improved with dialysis.[27,29] The anemia that commonly accompanies renal disease reduces ADP production and diminishes laminar flow in the vasculature, which hampers platelet and clotting factor migration, ultimately leading to prolonged clotting times and coagulopathy. Treatment of the anemia with erythropoiesis-stimulating agents or the administration of RBC transfusions helps reverse the coagulopathy.[27,29] Renal dysfunction also leads to impaired fibrinolysis and reduced generation of factor VIII–related antigen, impairing both clot breakdown and formation, respectively.[27,29]

Inherited Abnormalities

Consideration should be given to an inherited bleeding disorder if unexplained coagulation abnormalities are present in a critically ill patient.[1,7] Although uncommon, hemophilia and von Willebrand disease can pose significant bleeding complications among critically ill patients.[11] Hemophilia A is characterized by deficiencies in factor VIII, whereas hemophilia B is characterized by deficiencies in factor IX. Both disorders are inherited X-chromosome–linked conditions that range in severity from mild surgery or trauma-related bleeding to severe spontaneous bleeding into muscles and joints.[1,7] Acquired hemophilia is a rare but potentially life-threatening bleeding disorder caused by the development of autoantibodies (inhibitors) directed against plasma coagulation factors, most commonly factor VIII. In general, spontaneous bleeding occurs only in cases with less than 2% of coagulation factors.[27] However, patients with greater than 10% of coagulation factors may be at risk of excessive hemorrhage after trauma, surgery, or other invasive procedures.[27] von Willebrand disease is characterized by a deficiency in vWF, which plays an essential role in both platelet adhesion and binding to factor VIII to prevent rapid degradation of factor VIII.[1,11] Other rare congenital disorders that lead to coagulation abnormalities include factor V Leiden deficiency, factor XI deficiency (also known as Rosenthal syndrome or hemophilia C), factor VII deficiency, prothrombin deficiency, fibrinogen disorders, and plasminogen activator inhibitor deficiency.[1,9]

Medications

Coagulation abnormalities can also occur in critically ill patients taking or receiving medications that alter the coagulation cascade or interfere with platelet function. Therapeutic anticoagulation with agents such as unfractionated heparin, low-molecular-weight heparins, warfarin, anti-Xa inhibitors, and/or DTIs inhibits coagulation and increases a patient's risk of bleeding.[7,30,31] In addition, fibrinolytic medications or medications that interfere with platelet aggregation can alter a patient's ability to maintain hemostasis (Table 24.2).[7,11,12,30-33] Anticoagulants, platelet inhibitors, and fibrinolytic agents are commonly administered to patients for therapeutic reasons or to prevent clot formation during surgical procedures (e.g., cardiopulmonary procedures) or when invasive devices (e.g., dialysis, extracorporeal membrane oxygenation) are used.[30-33]

Thrombocytopenia

Thrombocytopenia in the ICU ranges from 15% to 60%, depending on the definition used and the population evaluated, with trauma/surgery patients having a higher prevalence than medical patients.[7,34] Thrombocytopenia is typically defined as a platelet count less than 150×10^9/L or a decrement of 50% or greater from a recent previous

Table 24.2 Drug-Induced Therapeutic Coagulopathies and Reversal Options[7,11,12,30-33]

Agent(s)	Mechanism of Action	Half-Life and Duration of Action	Reversal Options
Aspirin	Antiplatelet by irreversible inhibition of cyclooxygenase-1 and cyclooxygenase-2	$t_{1/2}$ = 20 min but effect can last 5–7 days	Platelet transfusion ± desmopressin
Dipyridamole	Antiplatelet by increasing adenosine and cyclic adenosine monophosphate and inhibiting thromboxane A_2	$t_{1/2}$ = 6–15 hr but effect can last 5–7 days Hold 5–7 days before procedure	Platelet transfusion ± desmopressin
Clopidogrel, prasugrel, ticagrelor	Antiplatelet by antagonizing $P2Y_{12}$ ADP receptor	$t_{1/2}$ = 6–15 hr but effect can last 5–7 days Hold 5–7 days before procedure	Platelet transfusion
Abciximab, eptifibatide, tirofiban	Antiplatelet by antagonizing binding of fibrinogen to GPIIb/IIIa receptors (eptifibatide and tirofiban are reversible inhibitors; abciximab is an irreversible inhibitor)	Abciximab $t_{1/2}$ = 0.5–4 hr Eptifibatide = 2.5 hr Tirofiban = 2 hr	No specific antidote
Unfractionated heparin	Potentiates the action of antithrombin to inactivate thrombin	$t_{1/2}$ = 30–90 min Hold 2–12 hr before procedure	Protamine
Enoxaparin, dalteparin	Similar to unfractionated heparin but with greater inhibition of factor Xa	$t_{1/2}$ = 4–7 hr; prolonged in renal impairment Hold 12–24 hr before procedure	Protamine (partial reversal) + FFP or PCCs
Fondaparinux	Antithrombin-mediated inhibition of factor Xa	$t_{1/2}$ = 17–20 hr; prolonged in renal impairment Hold 48 hr before procedure	aPCC ± rFVIIa
Bivalirudin	Reversible DTI	$t_{1/2}$ = 25 min; prolonged in renal impairment Hold 1–2 hr before procedure	aPCC ± rFVIIa + hemodialysis or plasmapheresis
Argatroban	Direct inhibition of free and fibrin-bound thrombin	$t_{1/2}$ = 39–51 min; prolonged in hepatic impairment Hold 1–2 hr before procedure	PCCs or aPCC ± rFVIIa
Warfarin	Inhibition of vitamin K–dependent clotting factors (II, VII, IX, and X) and proteins C and S	$t_{1/2}$ = 20–60 hr; highly variable among patients (effects can last up to 5 days)	Vitamin K (IV 5–10 mg) + FFP or PCCs ± rFVIIa
Dabigatran	Direct inhibition of both free and fibrin-bound thrombin	$t_{1/2}$ = 11–17 hr; prolonged in renal impairment Hold 2–5 days before procedure	aPCC ± rFVIIa + hemodialysis (idarucizumab when available)
Rivaroxaban, apixaban	Direct inhibition of factor Xa	Apixaban $t_{1/2}$ = 9–14 hr Rivaroxaban $t_{1/2}$ = 5–13 hr Hold 18–48 hr before procedure	Four-factor PCCs ± rFVIIa
Alteplase, tenecteplase	Fibrinolytic; converts plasminogen to plasmin	Alteplase $t_{1/2}$ = 5–10 min (effects may last for up to 1 hr) Tenecteplase $t_{1/2}$ = 20–120 min	Antifibrinolytic + cryoprecipitate

aPCC = activated prothrombin complex concentrate; FFP = fresh frozen plasma; IV = intravenous; PCC = prothrombin complex concentrate; rFVIIa = recombinant activated factor VII.

measurement.[35-37] The presence of platelet counts less than 50×10^9/L increases the likelihood of hemorrhage by 4- to 5-fold and is an independent risk factor for mortality (OR 1.9–4.2).[34-37] The incidence of spontaneous hemorrhage, however, is low for patients with a platelet count exceeding 10×10^9/L.[35] Although fewer than 5% of ICU patients develop platelet counts of 20×10^9/L or less, this value is often used as a threshold to maintain in an effort to prevent hemorrhage.[34,35] Values of $30–50 \times 10^9$/L are targeted when hemorrhage is present.[34-37]

Platelets participate in hemostasis through several mechanisms, including the release of vasoactive substances (e.g., thromboxane A_2 and serotonin), activation of the coagulation cascade by releasing attractants for additional platelets (e.g., thromboxane A_2 and ADP), provision of a phospholipid scaffold formed when activated platelets bind to circulating fibrinogen, and adherence and aggregation at the site of injury to form a platelet plug.[1,35] Causes of thrombocytopenia are generally categorized according to decreased platelet production in the bone marrow, sequestration of platelets in the spleen, or enhanced platelet destruction (immunological or non-immunological, mechanical) (Table 24.3).[7,8,34-37] Rare inherited platelet disorders include Glanzmann disease and Bernard-Soulier disease.

Screening tests to investigate the source of thrombocytopenia should include a confirmatory platelet count, full blood count with peripheral blood film, coagulation tests, platelet function tests, fibrinogen, B_{12}, folate, renal function tests, liver function tests, HIV, hepatitis C, and imaging to examine for the presence of portal hypertension or splenomegaly.[5,6,8,34-37] Up to 25% of critically ill patients develop drug-induced thrombocytopenia (Table 24.4).[7,34,35] With the exception of heparin-induced thrombocytopenia, drug-induced causes are etiologies of exclusion that often necessitate careful examination of the daily platelet count profile and the medication administration record.[7,34,35]

HEMORRHAGE PREVENTION, RESUSCITATION, AND MANAGEMENT

The prevention of hemorrhage is targeted at avoiding excessive coagulopathy and thrombocytopenia. Although few data exist, the goals of therapy are to lower the INR less than 1.5 and the aPTT less than 1.5-fold the upper limit of normal and maintain platelet counts of $20 \times 10^9/L$ or greater.[1,2,7,8,35-38] Several etiologies exist for coagulopathy and thrombocytopenia, and providing procoagulant therapies may be relatively or absolutely contraindicated in some circumstances (e.g., DIC, cases of immune-mediated thrombocytopenia like heparin-induced thrombocytopenia). In practice, the reversal of coagulopathy and thrombocytopenia to prevent bleeding is similar to the correction of these during hemorrhage, except that time is of less concern during prevention so that the causative etiology may be investigated and possibly therapeutically targeted, whereas early support of coagulation is required during hemorrhagic resuscitation. Agents used to reverse coagulopathy include vitamin K, FFP, prothrombin complex concentrates (PCCs), and recombinant activated factor VII (rFVIIa).[1-4] Platelet administration is used to correct thrombocytopenia.[35-38]

The basic goals of therapy in the management of hemorrhage are achieving fluid resuscitation and bleeding cessation by correcting anemia, reversing coagulopathy, optimizing platelet activity, and inhibiting fibrinolysis, all while minimizing adverse events and bleeding sequelae.[13,39-41] Early resuscitation is often characterized by uncertainty regarding the exact source of the bleeding, quantity of blood loss, and anticipated duration of hemorrhage. The manifestations of hemorrhage, however, may be used as a crude estimate of blood loss. Tachycardia and lightheadedness are often evident after 15%–30% blood volume depletion, hypotension develops after 30% or greater depletion, and severely altered sensorium usually requires 40% or greater depletion. Initial resuscitation is targeted at rapidly repleting intravascular volume and is commonly performed with the administration of a warmed isotonic crystalloid solution.[39,40] The initial response to 1–2 L of normal saline indicates the extent of hemorrhage and may help predict the need for additional therapies.[39,40] The return of normal vital signs suggests the hemorrhage was mild-moderate (estimated blood loss less than 2 L) and likely ceased, so the need for additional resuscitation is unlikely. A transient improvement in vital signs suggests the hemorrhage was moderate (estimated blood loss of 2–3 L) and likely ongoing, so the need for additional resuscitation and blood product administration is probable. Little to no change in vital signs suggests the hemorrhage was severe (estimated blood loss of greater than 3 L) with ongoing active bleeding, so the need for additional resuscitation and blood product administration is immediate. The patients with little to no change in vital signs require emergency medical therapy to treat the etiology of the hemorrhage, necessitating the planning process for many possible interventions by several services (e.g., interventional radiology, general or specialized surgery services, trauma, gastroenterology, critical care, nursing, pharmacy). In all cases, rapidly controlling the source of hemorrhage must be a priority, and delaying an intervention while obtaining a laboratory or radiological study, placing an invasive monitor, or awaiting other therapies increases the likelihood of exsanguination.

Fluid Resuscitation

Initial resuscitation should be administered through a large-bore intravenous catheter using either normal saline or lactated Ringer solutions.[13,42,43] Specialty infusion systems provide real-time warming and have high-flow capacities with built-in filters so that resuscitation fluids and blood products can be administered rapidly in emergency situations. Saline solutions may induce hyperchloremic acidosis, whereas lactated Ringer solutions may worsen lactic acidosis or induce hyperkalemia if hepatic impairment or renal dysfunction is present, respectively.[13,42,43] Racemic lactated Ringer solutions may be proinflammatory and induce apoptosis. Other resuscitation fluids include hypertonic saline solutions and colloid fluids. Hypertonic saline solutions increase transmembrane sodium gradients, may produce more rapid hemodynamic improvement with less cumulative fluid volume than isotonic solutions, and have been shown in rodent models to ameliorate immunodepression.[13,42,43] Colloid fluids are usually reserved for patients with moderate hypovolemia without adequate response to crystalloid or showing manifestations of pulmonary or cerebral edema or cardiac overload.[13,42,43] Although the Committee on Trauma of the American College of Surgeons recommends lactated Ringer solutions, the choice of fluid will ultimately be guided by local practice patterns, prescriber preferences, and perhaps cost.[12,42]

The goals of resuscitation should focus on restoring tissue perfusion and hemodynamic status.[13] Although adequate resuscitation should optimize oxygen delivery and stabilize hemodynamic deviations, systolic blood pressures of 80–90 mm Hg should be the goal of resuscitation because the bleeding rate and cumulative blood loss are lessened with permissive or deliberate hypotension.[1,41] Overly aggressive fluid resuscitation shifts the Frank-Starling curve to increase cardiac output, which causes a reflex vasodilation, both of which increase blood flow to the injured vasculature to possibly enhance the rate of blood loss. Increased blood pressure may also wash away early clot formation, and the resuscitation fluid will decrease the blood viscosity and dilute clotting factors, RBCs, and platelets at the site of injury.[11] These reasons may explain the results of a recent systematic review that found liberal fluid resuscitation strategies were associated with higher mortality than restrictive strategies (risk ratio [RR] 1.25; 95% confidence interval [CI], 1.01–1.55) across three randomized trials of trauma patients.[44] As a result, clinical goals have shifted from the traditional approach of rapid bolus fluid administration to a systematic approach that includes supporting coagulation while providing the least amount of fluid to reverse hemodynamic compromise without overly increasing cardiac output.[13] Therefore, early resuscitation requires substantial clinical judgment and experience, so management recommendations are guidelines and not standards of care.

Global tissue perfusion may be assessed by blood lactate concentrations with restored perfusion indicated by declining lactate values over minutes to hours because lactate production is a function of anaerobic metabolism in the presence of tissue hypoxia.[13,42,43] The adequacy of regional perfusion can be assessed by

Table 24.3 Causes of Thrombocytopenia[7,8,34-37]

Differential Diagnosis	Mechanism of Thrombocytopenia
Cancers • Acute leukemia • Metastatic bone marrow infiltration • Myelodysplasia	• Decreased production
Congestive cardiac failure	• Sequestration
Disseminated intravascular coagulation	• Increased destruction/consumption
Drug induced (see Table 24.4 for further information)	• Decreased production • Increased destruction/consumption
HELLP syndrome	• Increased destruction/consumption
Hepatic insufficiency/cirrhosis	• Sequestration
Irradiation	• Decreased production
Immune mediated • Antiphospholipid syndrome • ITP • Post-infusion purpura • Systemic lupus erythematosus	• Increased destruction/consumption
Infections • Chronic (hepatitis B, HIV, malaria) • Transient (mumps, rubella, varicella, EBV, CMV)	• Decreased production • Increased destruction
Intravascular devices • Extracorporeal membrane oxygenation • Intraaortic balloon pump • Post-cardiopulmonary bypass • Renal dialysis	• Increased destruction/consumption
Massive blood loss	• Hemodilutional
Malnutrition • B_{12} or folate deficiency	• Decreased production
Sepsis	• Decreased production • Increased destruction/consumption • Sequestration
Thrombotic microangiographies • Clot formation • Hemolytic-uremic syndrome • TTP	• Increased destruction/consumption

CMV = cytomegalovirus; EBV = Epstein-Barr virus; HELLP = hemolysis, elevated liver enzymes, and low platelet count associated with pregnancy; ITP = immune thrombocytopenic purpura; TTP = thrombotic thrombocytopenic purpura.

Table 24.4 Examples of Drugs Commonly Associated with Thrombocytopenia in the Intensive Care Unit[a,7,34,35]

Medication	Mechanism	Resulting Effect	Time to Mean Platelet Nadir	Time to Platelet Recovery
Antiarrhythmics (amiodarone, procainamide)	Bone marrow suppression and immune mediated	Decreased production and increased destruction/consumption	9–71 days after initiation	5–11 days after discontinuation
β-Lactam antibiotics	Immune mediated – hapten-dependent antibody	Increased destruction/consumption	Dose/drug-dependent	Dose/drug-dependent
Fluoroquinolones	Immune mediated	Increased destruction/consumption	10 days after initiation	8 days after discontinuation
GPIIb/IIIa inhibitors	Immune mediated; binds to platelet – GPIIb/IIIa complex and induces neoepitope formation	Increased destruction/consumption	Abrupt reduction (within 2 hr after initiation); may be prolonged with abciximab therapy	Eptifibatide, tirofiban = immediately after discontinuation; Abciximab = 2–5 days after discontinuation
Heparin	Nonimmune mediated (type I) or immune mediated (type II) – formation of immunoglobulin G antibodies that cause platelet activation by binding to platelet-heparin-factor-4 complexes	Increased destruction/consumption	Type I = 1–4 days after initiation; Type II = 5–14 days after initiation	Type I = 2–4 days after discontinuation; Type II = 2–14 days after discontinuation
Histamine-2 receptor antagonists	Bone marrow suppression and immune mediated	Decreased production and increased destruction/consumption	14 days after initiation	7 days after discontinuation
Linezolid	Bone marrow suppression and immune mediated	Decreased production and increased destruction/consumption	14–40 days after initiation	4–13 days after discontinuation
Phenytoin	Immune mediated	Increased destruction/consumption	Variable	Variable
Rifampin	Immune mediated	Increased destruction/consumption	Unknown	Unknown
Trimethoprim/sulfamethoxazole	Immune mediated	Increased destruction/consumption	9 days after initiation	7 days after discontinuation
Vancomycin	Immune mediated	Increased destruction/consumption	~8 days after initiation	~8 days after discontinuation

[a]Recent exposure to chemotherapeutic agents or transplant anti-rejection (immunosuppressive) medications can cause thrombocytopenia.

indices of specific organ perfusion. These measurements may include the following[13,39-41]:

- normalization of coagulation abnormalities,
- improvement in renal dysfunction as indicated by adequate urine production (greater than 0.5 mL/kg/hour) and/or decreasing serum concentrations of blood urea nitrogen and creatinine,
- improvement in hepatic parenchymal dysfunction as indicated by normalizing serum concentrations of transaminases and bilirubin,

- change in extremities from cool and mottled to warm with rapid capillary refill and normalizing temperature gradient between the toe and core body,
- normalization of elevated troponin concentrations from cardiac ischemia,
- reversal of altered sensorium.

Correction of Anemia

Red blood cell administration is used clinically to increase hemoglobin with the intent of enhancing oxygen-carrying capacity and tissue perfusion. About 2 units of packed RBCs (PRBCs) are procured from each whole blood donation.[2,38] Packed RBCs are stored at 1°C–6°C in a solution containing citrate, phosphate, dextrose, adenine, and nutrients. Each unit has a shelf-life of 42 days.[2,38]

Major or massive blood loss is defined as a loss of 100% of the circulating blood volume within 24 hours, at least 50% within 3 hours, the transfusion of 6 units of PRBCs in a 12-hour period, or a bleeding rate of 1.5 mL/kg/hour or greater.[13] Clinical practice guidelines recommend maintaining hemoglobin values of 7 g/dL, primarily on the basis of studies of non-bleeding critically ill patients and patients with upper gastrointestinal (GI) hemorrhage. The combined results of these studies found lower mortality rates, fewer cardiopulmonary adverse events, and reduced ongoing hemorrhage in patients allocated to restrictive transfusion strategies aimed at a hemoglobin value of 7 g/dL.[39,40,45-47] Retrospective data from hemorrhaging Jehovah's Witness patients support limited detrimental outcomes of permissive anemia.[46-49] The transfusion threshold may be increased to 8 g/dL in patients with preexisting cardiovascular disease or active cardiac ischemia.

The decision to transfuse PRBCs must consider intravascular volume status, the presence of shock, the duration and extent of anemia and coagulopathy, cardiopulmonary parameters, and the extent of lactic acidosis. Packed RBCs are usually required only when the estimated blood loss exceeds 1.5–2 L.[40,42,47] In general, hemorrhaging patients should receive a single unit of PRBC at a time with response assessed thereafter; however, the patient with massive hemorrhage or in hypovolemic shock may need several units rapidly transfused simultaneously.[3,13,27,47] In the stable patient of average size, 1 unit of PRBC will elevate hemoglobin by about 1 g/dL or the hematocrit by 3%.[47] Increases less than these thresholds may be the result of dilution from the concomitant administration of crystalloid solutions, or it may indicate ongoing hemorrhage, which warrants further investigation. The process of compatibility testing takes 45 minutes to complete and includes ABO and Rhesus blood typing and antibody screening.[27,38] In emergency situations, O/Rh-negative blood is used without antibody screening.

Several concerns surround PRBC administration. First, many evaluations have failed to show meaningful increases in end-organ oxygen delivery and use despite increases in hemoglobin.[38] This is contradictory to the common goal of using allogenic administration of PRBCs to enhance tissue perfusion. This contradiction may be explained by the timing of the intervention relative to the onset of hemorrhage. Alternatively, storage of the RBCs may induce biochemical changes in rheology to enhance microcirculatory occlusion and increase hemoglobin's affinity for oxygen (rapid decline in S-nitrosohemoglobin, 2,3-diphosphoglycerate, and ATP) to reduce oxygen disassociation and promote tissue ischemia.[38,48]

Allogenic RBC administration may contribute to coagulopathy because RBCs contain citrate, which binds calcium, a cofactor for many clotting factors, and are stored at pH values of 6.5–7 (lactate concentrations increase 15-fold, and pH declines to 6.7 after 3 weeks of storage).[38] Many transfusion protocols recommend monitoring systemic ionized calcium values and preemptively administering intravenous calcium when 4 units of PRBCs have been given.[38] Each PRBC unit also provides about 7–10 mEq of potassium because potassium leaks from RBCs during storage.[38] Allogeneic PRBCs may also promote coagulation by activating host platelets through thromboxane generated by the stored RBC and by producing thrombin in the host in response to phospholipid exposure caused by membrane vesiculation of the stored RBC. A recent study of "fresh" (average storage time of 6.1 ± 4.9 days) versus "old" (average storage time of 22 ± 8.4 days) PRBC transfusions in critically ill patients without hemorrhage showed similar outcomes of mortality, length of stay, transfusion reactions, and duration of organ-specific support.[49]

Another concern of allogenic RBC transfusions, and other allogeneic blood products, is the profound effects they have on the recipient's immune function, which contributes to transfusion-related acute lung injury (TRALI) and transfusion-related immunomodulation (TRIM).[38,50-52] Transfusion-related acute lung injury is defined as new-onset acute lung injury occurring within 6 hours after completing the transfusion of a plasma-containing blood product. The pathogenesis of TRALI relates to blood products that contain antibodies to the recipient's human leukocyte antigen or human neutrophil antigen.[50] Allorecognition leads to the activation of neutrophils that are marginated in the lung to cause inflammation and disruption of the lung-alveolar-capillary permeability barrier. Monocytes and activated platelets also contribute. Experimental models have also implicated cell membrane phospholipids, specifically lysophosphatidylcholine, which are generated during storage of cellular blood products and can prime neutrophils. The incidence of TRALI is 1 in 12,000 PRBC transfusions, and the mortality rate is 6%, substantially lower than the estimate for other forms of acute lung injury.[38,50,51] Excluding females with a pregnancy history as blood donors lowers the TRALI rate by 10- to 20-fold because these females are more likely to have anti–human leukocyte antigen or anti–human neutrophil antigen antibodies given their exposure to fetal blood.[38,50,51] The process of leukoreduction by specialized filtration or irradiation of donated blood also reduces the likelihood of TRALI. Irradiated blood products are indicated in severely immunocompromised patients or transplant populations where leukocytes are speculated to contribute to graft-vs.-host disease; however, the process reduces RBC viability and increases the release of intracellular potassium. Leukocyte-reduced blood components contain less than 5×10^6/L of leukocytes. Around 70% of transfused PRBCs are leukoreduced in the United States.[50,51]

Transfusion-related immunomodulation refers to a state of proinflammation and immunosuppression associated with transfusions of allogeneic blood products. The pathogenic mechanism is still speculative, but the process is likely mediated by allogeneic mononuclear cells, white blood cell–derived soluble mediators, and soluble human leukocyte antigen peptides circulating in allogeneic plasma.[38,50-52] During RBC storage, cytokines and inflammatory mediators such as interleukin (IL)-1, IL-6, and tumor necrosis factor also accumulate and may contribute to the pathogenesis of TRIM. Transfusion-related immunomodulation likely contributes to the association of the administration of blood products with acquired infections and organ failures.[52] Leukoreduction of donated blood decreases the likelihood of TRIM.

Transfusion-associated cardiac overload (TACO) is acute pulmonary edema secondary to congestive heart failure precipitated by the volume of fluid in transfusions that overwhelm the recipient's circulatory system.[38,50,51] Risk factors for TACO include both the total volume and the transfusion administration rate, number of blood products administered, preexisting fluid balance, renal dysfunction, preexisting cardiac dysfunction, and extremes of age.[38,50,51] Transfusion-associated cardiac overload is not as prevalent as TRALI but is associated with higher morbidity and mortality. Other concerns of PRBCs include hemolytic reactions from the transfusion of mismatched blood products caused by the recipient's complement antibodies attaching to donor RBC antigens, fevers and rigors associated with nonhemolytic immunological responses, other allergic reactions like urticaria and anaphylaxis, and the transmission of infectious diseases (HIV risk is 1 in 2 million units; hepatitis B, C, and A risks are each 1 in 250–500,000 units).[38,50-53] Costs of PRBCs vary depending on what expenses are included, but estimates per unit range from $250 as a rudimentary approximation to $750 when all costs associated with donation and procurement, processing, storage, matching, preparation, and administration are included.[54,55]

Reversal or Prevention of Coagulopathy

The presence of coagulopathy is an independent risk factor for mortality during hemorrhage, and many factors may contribute to its development.[10] The general goals for reversing coagulopathy are an INR less than 1.5, an aPTT less than 1.5-fold the upper limit of normal, platelet count of $30–50 \times 10^9$/L or greater (or 20×10^9/L or greater to prevent hemorrhage), optimizing platelet function, fibrinogen of 100 mg/dL or greater, arterial pH of 7.20 or greater, core body temperature of 35°C or greater, and normal blood values of ionized calcium.[1,2,7,8,35-38] Several agents are available that may be tried to reverse prolonged clotting times (Table 24.5 and Table 24.6).[2,3,7,35-38,56-66] These include vitamin K, FFP, PCC products, and rFVIIa.

Vitamin K

Vitamin K_1, also known as phytonadione or phylloquinone, is a fat-soluble compound that aids in the carboxylation of glutamate residues of certain proteins to form γ-carboxyglutamate residues, which can then bind calcium to activate these proteins. Within the realm of coagulation, vitamin K_1 activates factors II, VII, IX, and X and proteins C, S, and Z by oxidative carboxylation in the liver.[2,57,67] Activation of these coagulation factors is essential for hemostasis and normal functioning of the coagulation cascade. Variables contributing to the development of vitamin K_1 deficiency include inadequate diet; malabsorption; hepatic dysfunction, antibiotic therapy, which alters the GI flora; lack of vitamin K_1 supplementation; major surgery; and the use of warfarin.[67] Critically ill patients, who may have many of these variables,[67] are at high risk of developing coagulopathy associated with vitamin K_1 deficiency.[2] Reports indicate that as many as 51% of hospitalized patients have vitamin K_1 deficiency,[10,11] with 34% resulting in hemorrhage and 24% associated with mortality.[67]

Vitamin K_1 is commonly administered to patients with coagulopathies thought to be from vitamin K_1 deficiency and/or hepatic dysfunction.[2,57] It may be administered enterally, subcutaneously, or intravenously. Although either the enteral or the intravenous route of administration is recommended for urgent coagulopathy reversal, a recent study found that intravenous administration lowers INR quicker.[2] If given intravenously, the rate of administration should not exceed 1 mg/minute to avoid immunoglobulin E–mediated anaphylactoid reactions that are associated with the solubilizing vehicle. For patients with an elevated INR because of warfarin, the American College of Chest Physicians recommends oral vitamin K for an INR greater than 10 and no signs of bleeding and intravenous vitamin K 5–10 mg for all major hemorrhage regardless of the INR.[68] Cumulative intravenous doses of 20–30 mg are required to lower the INR from other causes of vitamin K deficiency; however, the efficacy of vitamin K is unpredictable,

Table 24.5 Procoagulant Blood Products[2,3,7,35-38,56-66]

Product	Contents	Indications and Usual Dosage Regimen	Considerations
Platelets	Thrombocytes in plasma	-Platelet < 30–50 × 10⁹/L (bleeding) -Platelet < 20 × 10⁹/L (prevention)	-Stored at ~24°C -Bacterial contamination ~1/2000–1/3000 units -Requires ABO/Rh typing and antibody screening -Contributes to TRALI, TRIM, and TACO -Worsens immune reactions -Likely contributes to thrombosis -Variable costs
FFP	Coagulation factors and fibrinogen in variable amounts	-Use early in massive bleeding -Prevention of bleeding if INR ≥ 1.5 -15 mL/kg ~30% factor replacement	-Stored at -18°C and requires thawing -Requires ABO/Rh typing and antibody screening -Limited effectiveness at reducing INR < 1.5 -Hypervolemia -TRALI (1/5–10,000) -Contributes to TRIM -TACO (6%) -Likely contributes to thrombosis -Variable costs
Prothrombin complex concentrates	Factors II, VII, IX, X and prothrombin, proteins C, S, Z in variable amounts	-Use early in massive bleeding -Prevention of bleeding if INR ≥ 1.5 -25–50 IU/kg (based on factor IX)	-Faster onset than FFP -Variable amounts of factors and limited factor VII in some products -May contain heparin -Several donors -Thrombosis (0.9%–2.3%) -No TRALI or TRIM -Substantially less fluid than FFP -Costly
Cryoprecipitate	Factors VIII, XIII, vWF, fibrinogen, fibronectin	-Fibrinogen < 100 mg/dL -1 unit will ↑ fibrinogen ~5–10 mg/dL -vWF deficiency	-Stored at -18°C and requires thawing -Requires ABO typing -Contributes to TRALI and TRIM -Contributes to thrombosis -Costly

TACO = transfusion-associated cardiac overload; TRALI = transfusion-related acute lung injury; TRIM = transfusion-related immunomodulation; vWF = von Willebrand factor.

especially in the more severely ill and those with hepatic dysfunction.[67] The half-life of vitamin K is 1.5–3 hours, and its full effect is achieved only after 6–12 hours.[2] Therefore, vitamin K's activity is slow, but the duration of action may last several days, irrespective of the route of administration. It is inexpensive and readily available.

Fresh Frozen Plasma

Fresh frozen plasma is derived from donated blood that has been centrifuged and separated from the cellular components.[2,56,57] Each 250- to 300-mL unit contains soluble clotting factors and inhibitors, 1–2.5 mg/mL of fibrinogen, complement, albumin, and proteins C and S. Once

Table 24.6 Procoagulant Pharmacologic Products[2,3,7,35-38,56-66]

Product	Contents	Indications and Usual Dosage Regimens	Considerations
Local hemostatics	Cellulose based		May not adhere, swelling-induced stenosis
	Fibrin (human or bovine) ± fibrinolytic inhibitor ± thrombin		Immune reaction, infection transmission, may contain aprotinin, costly
	Thrombin (human or bovine)		Immune reaction
	Zeolite that causes exothermic reaction		Heat-induced tissue damage
	Chitosan (chitin) that activates platelets and electrophysiologic endothelial attraction of RBCs		May not adhere
Vitamin K	Cofactor for activation of factors II, VII, IX, K	-INR ≥ 1.5 -0.5–20 mg	-Very slow onset but long duration -Variable SC absorption -Limited effectiveness for reversing INR for causes other than warfarin -IV requires administration > 1 mg/min to avoid anaphylactic reactions
Recombinant factor VIIa	Activates platelets to augment thrombin burst	-Refractory hemorrhage related to surgery or trauma -10–90 mcg/kg IV	-Rapid onset but short acting -Thrombosis (~10%) -Costly -No human elements -No TRALI, TRIM, TACO -No compatibility testing
Desmopressin	Selective V_2 agonist to release factor VIII, vWF, and PA	-Platelet dysfunction -0.3 mcg/kg IV	-Short-acting -Tachyphylaxis and ↑ bleeding risk with repeated doses
Conjugated estrogen	↓ Antithrombin and protein S while ↑ factors VII, VIII, IX, X, prothrombin	-Platelet dysfunction -25–50 mg IV	-Slow acting -Slow offset
Fibrinogen concentrate	Fibrinogen	-Fibrinogen < 100 mg/dL -Dose in mg/kg = (desired fibrinogen concentration − measured fibrinogen concentration)/1.7 or 70 mg/kg if measured concentration unknown	-Rapid onset -Contributes to thrombosis -Costly -No TRALI or TRIM -No compatibility testing
Antifibrinolytics (EACA, TA)	Inhibit plasminogen proteases and some anti-inflammation	-Prevention of surgical/trauma blood loss -Major hemorrhage related to surgery or trauma ± indications of clot dissolution -EACA: 150 mg/kg (10,000 mg); then 15 mg/kg/hr (2000 mg/hr) -TA: 10–30 mg/kg; then 1–16 mg/kg/hr (< 400 mg/hr)	-Thrombosis -Hypotension (TA)

EACA = ε-aminocaproic acid; INR = international normalized ratio; IV = intravenous(ly); SC = subcutaneous; TA = tranexamic acid; TACO = transfusion-associated cardiac overload.

frozen, plasma is kept at -18°C and can be stored for 12 months.[2,56,57] After thawing, it must be kept at 1°C–6°C, labeled as "thawed plasma," and transfused within 4 days. The process of freezing and thawing may affect the temperature labile clotting factors. The low and varying amounts of fibrinogen in FFP means that large volumes are often required to reverse coagulopathy; a dose of 15 mL/kg restores clotting factor levels to 30% of normal, and doses exceeding 30 mL/kg are required to increase fibrinogen concentrations.[10,57] A target INR of less than 1.5 may never be reached by solely administering FFP because the fibrinogen concentration of FFP is below the target fibrinogen concentration required to fully reverse the coagulopathy.[10,57] Normalization of the INR occurs in only 0.8% of patients, and a dose-response effect is inconsistent. The need for large doses, however, heightens the risk of fluid overload that may contribute to ongoing hemorrhage, cerebral edema, portal hypertension in the presence of liver dysfunction, and TACO, which occurs in 6% of patients receiving FFP.[10,51,57] Hypervolemia leading to edema is of particular concern in patients with preexisting renal, cardiac, and pulmonary disorders.[51] Plasma is also associated with TRALI at estimated rates of 1 in 5–10,000 units, a risk exceeding that of PRBC transfusions.[10,51,57] Transfusion-related immunomodulation is also associated with FFP at occurrence rates exceeding RBC transfusions. Another concern is that extensive preparation time is required before FFP is ready to administer. After determining appropriate compatibility with the recipient, FFP must be thawed, which can take 30–60 minutes to process. Clinically, it is often difficult to estimate the number of FFP units that should be thawed for a given situation. Some centers ensure they have a constant supply of thawed or never-frozen plasma that is universally compatible; however, this can lead to units being wasted and may not be cytomegalovirus safe.[57] Like other procoagulants, FFP is associated with thromboembolic adverse effects. The cost per unit of FFP is $70–$350.[54,55]

Despite the aforementioned concerns, the use of FFP increased 23% between 2005 and 2012.[2] Clinically applicable indications for FFP include replacement of an inherited single coagulation factor for which a virus-safe fractionated product does not exist, replacement of a specific protein deficiency such as C-1 esterase inhibitor, replacement of many coagulation factor deficiencies (DIC, hemorrhage), replacement of removed plasma during plasmapheresis in cases of thrombotic thrombocytic purpura, reversal of warfarin-associated hemorrhage, prevention of dilutional coagulopathy during hemorrhage, and prevention of bleeding in patients with advanced hepatic dysfunction and coagulopathy awaiting an invasive procedure or surgery.[2,38,57] The most common reason to administer FFP in the United States is to prevent hemorrhage in patients with prolonged coagulation tests awaiting an invasive procedure. Limited data support this indication because a prophylactic dose of 12 mL/kg lowered the INR to less than 1.5 in only 54% of patients and did not lower the rate of bleeding after various invasive procedures compared with placebo.[8] Moreover, clinically relevant bleeding problems in patients with hepatic dysfunction may be precipitated by increased venous pressures that may be associated with the large volume of fluid that accompanies FFP administration. Rather than trying to shorten clotting times, a conservative approach to plasma therapy in these patients using clinical judgment may prove beneficial. Fresh frozen plasma's duration of action is typically 6–12 hours.[2,57]

Prothrombin Complex Concentrates

Prothrombin complex concentrates are an inactive concentrate of variable, yet balanced, amounts of the vitamin K–dependent clotting factors. The concentration of vitamin K–dependent clotting factors in PCCs is about 25-fold higher than in plasma, and usual doses are equivalent to about 2 L of FFP.[2] Prothrombin complex concentrates are purified from pooled human plasma and lyophilized, which allows them to be reconstituted, as opposed to frozen and thawed.[57,58] This provides significant advantages over FFP, including rapid administration, avoidance of compatibility testing, and the absence of risk of TRALI and TRIM.[57,58] Like allogenic blood products, however, PCCs carry the potential risk of transmitting infectious microbes. Prothrombin complex concentrates contain factors II, IX, and X and are available with low amounts of factor VII (three-factor PCCs) and higher concentrations of factor VII (four-factor PCCs). Unlike three-factor PCCs, four-factor PCCs also contains albumin, proteins C and S, antithrombin, and heparin. Although the inclusion of anticoagulants theoretically reduces the occurrence of thromboembolic events that are associated with rapid induction of coagulation, they need to be considered in patients with known sensitivities to them (e.g., heparin-induced thrombocytopenia).[2,57,58] The weighted mean average of thrombotic events with PCCs through 2008 was 2.3%, with higher rates associated with larger and repeated doses.[57] A lower rate of 0.9% was identified in a review of eight clinical trials, although all of these studies included patients requiring warfarin reversal.[57] Because of their rapid effect at reversing coagulopathy, PCCs may slightly increase the risk of thromboembolic events compared with FFP.[57,58] Prothrombin complex concentrates are derived from human plasma, so patients declining blood products should be consulted before PCCs are administered. Dosage regimens of PCCs typically involve the administration of 50–200 mL of total fluid, so TACO and other manifestations of fluid overload are unlikely to occur. The acquisition costs of PCCs vary but are about $1.30 per unit with typical doses exceeding 2,000 units, and it is common practice to round to the nearest vial size.[57,58] Prothrombin complex concentrates are available as a kit that contains the lyophilized powder and a provided diluent that is commonly mixed at the bedside but must be administered within 4 hours of reconstitution. Institutional procurement, storage, and distribution may originate from the blood bank rather than the pharmacy department.

In the United States, three-factor PCCs are only indicated for the prevention and control of bleeding in patients with factor IX deficiency caused by hemophilia B.[57,58] In contrast, four-factor PCCs are labeled for rapid reversal of acquired coagulation deficiency induced by warfarin in adult patients with acute major bleeding or the need for urgent surgery or an invasive procedure.[57,58] The general consensus of several guidelines that have been published regarding the use of PCCs to reverse anticoagulation indicates that four-factor PCCs are the preferred therapy, FFP may be needed if three-factor PCCs are used, and FFP is likely not needed if four-factor PCCs are used.[57] One guideline suggests that rFVIIa can be considered in addition to three-factor PCCs when emergency reversal is required.[57] The results of studies comparing four-factor PCCs with FFP in patients receiving anticoagulation with vitamin K antagonists show that four-factor PCCs reverse INR more rapidly with less fluid administration and achieve greater rates of effective hemostasis.[69,70] The dosage regimens are based on units of factor IX, but an adjustment for four-factor PCCs includes the INR (INR of 2–4 = 25 units/kg, INR of 4–6 = 35 units/kg, INR of greater than 6 = 50 units/kg). This latter adjustment for the INR is often applied to dosage regimens of all products when they are used in clinical scenarios of prolonged clotting in the absence of anticoagulation. In a retrospective assessment of patients with coagulopathy caused by trauma, adding PCCs to FFP accelerated INR reversal, reduced the number of units of PRBCs and FFP administered, lessened the total costs associated with procoagulant administration, and lowered mortality.[71] Although not systematically studied for the prevention of bleeding in patients with coagulopathies owing to causes other than anticoagulation and awaiting surgery or an invasive procedure, PCCs likely reverse INR more rapidly than does FFP with substantially less fluid and may expedite the time to the intervention. The duration of action depends on the dose of PCC administered but is typically 12–24 hours.[57,58]

Activated PCC or factor VIII inhibitor bypassing complex (FEIBA; Baxter Healthcare, Westlake Village, CA) is an anti-inhibitor coagulation complex used in the management of hemorrhage in patients with hemophilia and acquired factor VIII inhibitors.[61] It is composed of factors II, IX, and X; small amounts of activated factor VII; and factor VIII antigen. It acts by facilitating thrombin generation on the surface of activated platelets and activating factor X. It is not commonly used to manage or prevent hemorrhage in patients without factor VIII inhibitors, but case reports show it may successfully reverse new oral anticoagulant agents.[61] It is associated with thrombosis and the propagation of DIC, and it may pose a risk of transmitting infectious microbes because it is manufactured from human blood pools.

Recombinant Activated Factor VII

Recombinant activated factor VII is indicated for the treatment and prevention of bleeding in patients with hemophilia with inhibitors, cases of factor VII deficiency, and individuals with Glanzmann thrombasthenia with little to no response to platelets.[57] Recombinant activated factor VII stimulates the extrinsic pathway by interacting with exposed endothelial tissue factor to activate factors IX and X. At pharmacologic doses, rFVIIa bypasses the need for tissue factor by generating thrombin on the surface of activated platelets that are localized to the site of injury.[67] Both mechanisms ultimately produce activated factor X, which drives thrombin burst to cleave fibrinogen to fibrin. Factor VII levels are often extremely low in patients with major hemorrhage. To optimize the activity of rFVIIa, patients should be normothermic with an arterial pH greater than 7.20.[67,72] Results from studies using dosage regimens of 10–90 mcg/kg are mixed with respect to reducing hemorrhage expansion and limiting the administration of other procoagulant products and/or PRBCs in bleeding cases associated with vitamin K antagonists, liver disease, liver transplant, trauma- and surgery-associated coagulopathy, cardiothoracic surgery, and spontaneous intracranial hemorrhage.[57,72] None of these studies, however, has shown clinical benefits of morbidity or mortality.[57] Recombinant activated factor VII reduces prolonged clotting times within 15–30 minutes of administration and typically lasts 2–6 hours. Reversal time is faster than that of PCCs and FFP, but duration may be shorter. Several studies comparing rFVIIa with FFP show that rFVIIa may expedite invasive procedures or surgery in patients with coagulopathies from causes other than anticoagulants. These nonproprietary indications represent more than 95% of rFVIIa use in the United States.[57,72] Some have recommended against the use of rFVIIa in favor of PCCs for INR reversal, regardless of the etiology of prolonged clotting, because rFVIIa may not adequately restore thrombin generation over time to the same extent as other products, resulting in a duration of action that is substantially shorter.[2,57] The rate of thromboembolic events associated with rFVIIa administration is 11.1% across studies, but only the rate of arterial events exceeds that of placebo (5.5% vs. 3.2%, $p<0.003$).[72-74] The occurrence of thromboembolic events increases with patient age and rFVIIa dose. Recombinant activated factor VII contains no human elements and may be administered to patients not accepting products derived from human sources. The cost of rFVIIa is around $1,800 per milligram, and it is common practice to round to the nearest milligram.[57] Institutional procurement, storage, and distribution may originate from the blood bank rather than the pharmacy department. As with PCCs, rFVIIa is available as a lyophilized powder in a kit with a syringe that contains a histidine diluent, and it must be administered within 3 hours of reconstitution.

Platelet Optimization

The activity of platelets may be improved by increasing the platelet count through administering platelets or enhancing their functionality using desmopressin or estrogen.

Platelets

Platelets are essential for primary hemostasis because they form a plug at the site of endothelial injury. Circulating platelets are activated by exposed collagen when the integrity of the endothelial lining is compromised. Signaling molecules (vWF, fibrinogen, platelet-derived growth factor, ADP, serotonin) lead to conformational changes in platelets, specifically of the GPIIb/IIIa receptors on the surface.[1] Endothelial release of vWF also decelerates platelets at sites of high shear stress (rapid blood flow though narrow blood vessels) and enhances platelet adhesiveness.[35] Further platelet recruitment occurs as activated platelets secrete thromboxane A_2 and ADP, and the platelet phospholipid surfaces and calcium potentiate factors V, VIII, IX, and X. Activated platelets also bind to circulating fibrinogen, which forms and stabilizes local platelet aggregates to form plugs.

Bleeding risk is minimal when platelet counts exceed 50×10^9/L but increases dramatically when counts drop below 10×10^9/L.[38] These data, however, are derived mostly from patients with bone marrow failure and compromised thrombopoiesis, so application to critically ill patients is indeterminate. A consensus regarding the optimal platelet count to prevent bleeding or maintain during hemorrhage has not been well established. In general, platelet counts of 20×10^9/L or greater is used as a minimum threshold to prevent bleeding and $30-50 \times 10^9$/L or greater is targeted during hemorrhage, respectively.[34,35] Higher thresholds of 100×10^9/L may be warranted in some patient-specific scenarios such as neurosurgery or orthopedic surgery. In addition, platelet dysfunction may occur because of issues other than low platelet counts (e.g., low vWF, IIb/IIIa inhibition).

Platelets are separated from RBCs and concentrated by repeated centrifugation. Platelets are stored at 22°C for up to 8 days but require constant agitation. Bacterial contamination increases and the efficacy of transfusion decreases after 5 days of storage.[35] Compatibility testing is performed before platelets are administered. Each platelet transfusion is dosed in "six-packs," with each containing 6 units of platelets from several donors or a single apheresis unit. A 6-unit transfusion should raise the platelet count by $25-50 \times 10^9$/L and last up to 72 hours.[35] Refractoriness, defined by a platelet rise less than 5×10^9/L within 1 hour of transfusion, indicates the presence of alloimmunization or platelet antibodies (e.g., heparin-induced thrombocytopenia, idiopathic thrombocytopenic purpura), and additional administration of platelets may heighten the immune response and further aggregate platelet destruction.[37] The rate of alloimmunization is less than 1%, but as many as 70% of patients receiving several RBC or platelet transfusions may temporarily develop alloantibodies.[37] The use of leukoreduced blood products delays or prevents this phenomenon.

As with PRBCs and FFP, platelets are high-volume products and share many of the same risks, including TRALI, TRIM, TACO, acute hemolysis, and anaphylaxis. A concern unique to platelets is transfusion-related sepsis with bacterial contamination of stored platelets at room temperature.[35] Platelet administration is also associated with thrombotic complications. Each 6-unit transfusion is estimated to cost $350–$500.[57,58]

Enhancing Platelet Function

Desmopressin is a synthetic analog of endogenous human antidiuretic hormone.[2] Traditionally, it was used to treat inherited bleeding disorders such as vWF deficiency and mild forms of factor VIII deficiency hemophilia A. Desmopressin causes the release of vWF, factor VIII, and tissue plasminogen activator from the endothelium, increasing their plasma concentrations by 2- to 20-fold within 30 minutes of an intravenous dose of 0.3 mcg/kg.[2] von Willebrand factor acts as a carrier protein binding to factor VIII and promotes platelet adhesion at sites of endothelial injury.[2] The duration of action is about 4 hours.[2] Desmopressin may be particularly useful if platelet dysfunction is caused by aspirin or dipyridamole. It has been shown to shorten bleeding time in patients with uremia and reduce blood loss during hemorrhage.[2] Repeated doses for short periods should be avoided because this may facilitate fibrinolysis by stimulating the release of plasminogen activator from the endothelium.[2]

High doses of intravenous estrogen also enhance platelet function by increasing factors VII, VIII, IX, X, and prothrombin.[2] It also reduces antithrombin and protein S. The slow onset of action limits the practicality of estrogen for promoting hemostasis, but it may be tried in refractory cases of presumed platelet dysfunction.

Inhibiting Fibrinolysis

Fibrinogen is a required protein for hemostasis. Produced in the liver, it circulates at the highest concentration of all clotting proteins. It is the physiologic substrate of thrombin, activated factor VIII, and plasmin. Activated thrombin cleaves fibrinogen and catalyzes fibrin polymerization to form a structural network that is the basis of each clot.[63] Cross-linking of fibrin polymers is induced by factor VIIIa and increases the elasticity of clots to enhance resistance to fibrinolysis. Fibrinogen also serves as a ligand for GPIIb/IIIa receptors on platelets to enhance platelet adhesion.

Fibrinogen

Although the half-life of fibrinogen is about 3.8 days, fibrinogen catabolism exceeds synthesis during major hemorrhage, especially in cases of liver dysfunction.[63] Ongoing hemorrhage and dilutional coagulopathy can cause fibrinogen concentrations to decline, and it is often the first factor to be relatively depleted during uncontrolled bleeding. Low concentrations are an independent risk factor for bleeding during surgery.[62] Despite little supporting evidence, several guidelines recommend maintaining fibrinogen concentrations of 80–100 mg/dL.[62] Higher target thresholds may be required to optimize hemostasis because clot strength increases linearly with fibrinogen concentration, even up to 1,000 mg/dL.[62] Hypofibrinogenemia will prolong clotting assays.

Fibrinogen is available from three sources: FFP, cryoprecipitate, and factor concentrate.[62] The amount of fibrinogen in FFP is minimal, and the dosing requirements to achieve adequate fibrinogen concentrations are usually limited by the fluid volume of FFP. Each unit of cryoprecipitate is prepared from the centrifugation of 1 unit of FFP using a method that precipitates high-molecular-weight proteins such as factor VIII, vWF, and fibrinogen.[62] The insoluble precipitate is reconstituted in 20–40 mL of plasma as cryoprecipitate and stored at -18°C for up to 12 months.[62] The amount of fibrinogen in cryoprecipitate varies substantially but is about 1,500 mg/dL. Each unit should increase fibrinogen concentrations by 5–10 mg/dL.[62] It also contains factor VIII (80 IU or greater), factor XIII VIII (30% of original plasma content), vWF (about 50% of original plasma content), and fibronectin.[62] It is considered to be leukoreduced without additional filtration and does not require antibody screening. Like other blood products, cryoprecipitate requires ABO compatibility testing, and it is associated with TRALI, TRIM, and thrombosis but is less likely to cause TACO or hypervolemia.[62] Fibrinogen concentrate is manufactured from plasma and commercially available as a pasteurized lyophilized powder that is virus free. Currently, only one product (RiaSTAP; CSL Behring, King of Prussia, PA) is available in the United States, and it is indicated for the treatment of acute bleeding episodes in patients with conditions of hypofibrinogenemia.[62] It is reconstituted in sterile water to a final vial concentration of 20 g/L and contains 900–1300 mg of fibrinogen per vial.[62] It also contains human albumin. Although not recommended by the manufacturer, it may be infused over seconds to minutes to rapidly replete fibrinogen. Unlike cryoprecipitate, it does not require ABO compatibility testing and is not associated with TRALI or TRIM, but unfounded concerns exist that the concentrate may increase thrombotic events. The costs of each product must consider that the procurement of cryoprecipitate also produces PRBCs and cryosupernatant, but the concentrate does not require thawing and compatibility testing and is not associated with TRALI and TRIM.

Antifibrinolysis

The blood products and pharmacologic agents discussed to this point enhance coagulation and/or improve clot stability. Antifibrinolytic agents inhibit the enzymatic degradation of clot. Antifibrinolytic agents currently in use are the synthetic lysine analogs ε-aminocaproic acid and tranexamic acid.[2] These agents reversibly bind to the lysine-binding site of the fibrin clot to competitively inhibit the binding of plasminogen to fibrin at the same lysine-binding site. This prevents the conversion of plasminogen to plasmin and subsequent plasmin-mediated fibrinolysis. The antifibrinolytic activity of tranexamic acid in vitro is about 10-fold higher than that of ε-aminocaproic acid.[2] Most centers use tranexamic acid because it is slightly less expensive with acquisition costs of $50–$70 per 1,000-mg vial or $250–$500 for most therapeutic dosage regimens. Both agents are associated with thrombosis, and rapid administration of tranexamic acid may cause hypotension.

SPECIFIC PATIENT POPULATIONS

Hemostatic management varies by the etiology causing coagulopathy or thrombocytopenia. This section will review preventive strategies and management options of hemorrhage in specific patient populations.

Perioperative/Surgical Bleeding

Historically, management of perioperative bleeding was reactive and focused on restitution of intravascular volume with blood products at the time of hemorrhage. Today, greater attention is given to preventing blood loss from the outset because few data show a favorable benefit-risk ratio related to blood product administration.[21,38,41] Bleeding and transfusions independently increase morbidity and mortality as well as increase costs. These latter economic consequences relate to prolonged hospital length of stay and operating room time, greater laboratory testing, and the costs associated with blood products. Blood management programs aimed at minimizing the use of blood products in surgical patients improve patient outcomes and resource use. Some centers offer "blood-free" operating rooms as a result of practice initiatives that minimize bleeding risks preoperatively and limit blood loss intraoperatively.

The process of minimizing allogeneic blood products begins with preoperative identification of surgical patients at high risk of bleeding through completion of a structured history.[39,41,75] This history should include clinical conditions (e.g., renal disease, liver disease) associated with bleeding as well as family bleeding history (e.g., hemophilia, factor deficiencies). Advanced age increases the risk of hemorrhage. In addition, liver, spine, craniofacial, cardiopulmonary, and major urological surgical procedures are prone to bleeding. Two modifiable factors that may be targeted in these patients are managing preoperative anemia and reversing preexisting coagulopathy.[39,41,75] Strategies used to increase RBC mass in elective surgery patients include iron replacement therapy when iron-deficient anemia is present, the administration of erythropoiesis-stimulating agents (epoetin alfa or darbepoetin alfa) when iron deficiency has been ruled out, and autologous blood donation.[39,41,75] All three strategies require planning weeks before surgery and implementation at least several days before the procedure. Managing preexisting coagulopathy includes the discontinuation and/or reversal of systemic anticoagulants preoperatively. This includes heparin, low-molecular-weight heparins, antiplatelet agents, and oral anticoagulants such as warfarin or the new agents. These latter agents are particularly challenging in emergency surgery cases because pharmacologic reversal agents are unpredictable or not yet available. Selected herbal agents with anticoagulant activity should also be discontinued preoperatively (e.g., garlic, ginseng, saw palmetto), as should any other pharmacologic agents that may increase bleeding (e.g., valproic acid, selective serotonin reuptake inhibitors). The timing of discontinuing these agents will depend on their pharmacologic half-lives and the potential lack of reversibility.[75] Point-of-care testing for platelet function should aid in determining the appropriate time to discontinue antiplatelet therapies.

Intraoperative strategies aimed at reducing blood loss include patient positioning, operative technique and environment, regional anesthesia, ventilation, controlled hypotension, acute normovolemic hemodilution, RBC salvage or recovery, and the use of topical hemostats.[64-66] (Table 24.7).[39,41,75] Ideally, patients are positioned during surgery to reduce arterial pressure and maximize venous drainage away from the wound. Operative techniques vary, but blood loss is minimized using tourniquets, infiltrating the surgical site with local vasoconstrictors, and using advanced surgical techniques (e.g., laparoscopic, endoscopic, robotic, transcatheter). Regional anesthesia using central neuraxial blocks such as spinal/epidural anesthesia reduces blood loss by 25%–30% by inducing sympathetic blockade to minimize perfusion of the surgical site and decreasing venous tone to enhance drainage. Ventilator settings that minimize positive end expiratory pressure and use low tidal volumes under general anesthesia decrease mean intrathoracic pressure to increase venous return and reduce blood loss. The environment refers to ensuring that laboratory values are normalized (e.g., pH, ionized calcium, fibrinogen) and that core body temperature is 35°C or greater. Controlled hypotension reduces arterial blood flow to the surgical site to minimize blood loss. During acute normovolemic hemodilution, several units of blood are collected from the patient preoperatively and replaced with crystalloid or colloid solutions so that blood loss during the procedure contains fewer RBCs. Collected blood is stored at the patient's bedside during the surgery to minimize the administrative costs and is given back to the patient at a predefined transfusion trigger or the conclusion of surgery. Autologous blood cell salvage is the process of recovering the patient's blood from the surgical field, washing and filtering, and reinfusing to the patient. Cell recovery is cost-effective when blood loss is expected to be high. In all cases, surgical procedures should use a restrictive hemoglobin transfusion trigger of 6–7 g/dL, which will also reduce blood transfusions. In addition, using extracorporeal systems with mini-circuits, minimizing phlebotomy, collecting samples in small-volume (pediatric) collection tubes, or using alternative sampling methods when possible (e.g., pulse oximetry rather than blood gas analyses) during and after surgery reduces blood loss. In general, phlebotomy should be minimized across all patients. Although surgical drains reduce hematoma expansion and compression of vital structures, they are associated with increased blood loss and enhanced transfusion rates of up to 40%. Reinfusion of the blood from wound drains is safe if the volume is less than 1 L and the process is completed within 6 hours.

Topical hemostats, surgical sealants, and adhesives are adjunctive approaches to control bleeding together with blood products, systemic agents, and direct approaches (e.g., pressure at bleeding site, suture ligation, hemoclips, electrocautery).[64-66] They may also be used when the latter approaches are not feasible (e.g., surgical fields with diffuse oozing). These agents are most commonly used in the operating room, although they can be used in other settings to augment hemostasis (e.g., uncontrollable epistaxis,

Table 24.7 Perioperative Blood Conservation Strategies[39,41,75]

Options	Units of Blood Conserved
Preoperative techniques:	
Increase preoperative RBC mass	2
Preoperative autologous donation	1–2
Intraoperative techniques:	
Meticulous hemostasis and operative technique	1–2
	≥1
Regional anesthesia	0.5–1
Ventilator techniques	1–2
Controlled hypotension	1–2
Acute normovolemic hemodilution	≥1
Blood salvage	≥1
Tolerance of anemia (reduced transfusion trigger)	
Postoperative techniques	
Restricted phlebotomy	1
Drain removal or reinfusion of blood from drain	≥1

dermal bleeds, or oral-pharyngeal hemorrhage). The ideal topical hemostat is one that is safe, provides prompt and reliable hemostasis, is easy to use, is simple to store and prepare, and is affordable. Although an ever-expanding number of these agents are commercially available, no agent meets all of these criteria. Inadvertent intravascular administration of these products is also a risk. Because many of the topical hemostats are considered devices rather than drugs, institutional procurement and distribution often originates from materials management rather than the pharmacy department.[65]

Topical hemostats are generally categorized into mechanical agents, biologically active agents, flowables, and fibrin sealants (Table 24.6).[2,3,7,35-38,56-66] Mechanical hemostats provide a matrix on which blood clotting can occur as well as a bleeding barrier. The source materials for these physical matrices are gelatin, collagen, cellulose, and polysaccharide starches. These materials are supplied in a wide variety of forms including sponges, foams, sheets, and spheres. Biologically active hemostats all contain thrombin that has an integral enzymatic role in clot formation by stimulating the formation of fibrin from its precursor, fibrinogen. Three thrombin products are available in the United States and vary in their origin: bovine derived, human plasma derived, and recombinant human derived.[65] The potential safety issue distinguishing these three products is the development of antibodies, depending on the thrombin source. Flowable hemostats are characterized by their consistency and gel-like properties rather than their mechanical counterparts. Limited clinical data suggest the superiority of at least one flowable agent to mechanical hemostats relative to the rates of hemostasis and shorter time to hemostasis in cardiothoracic surgery patients.[66] As with the mechanical hemostats, flowable agents can be combined with thrombin to provide physical and active hemostasis. Fibrin sealants are unique because they combine human thrombin with human fibrinogen to promote clot formation. Unlike the active hemostats, they do not require patient-supplied fibrinogen at the active bleeding site to promote hemostasis. Surgical sealants and synthetic adhesives are used for hemostasis but have broader indications as well. Examples for surgical sealants include vascular reconstruction procedures, dural repairs during cranial surgery, and pleural repairs. In contrast, synthetic adhesives can be used to seal adjacent skin surfaces together and closure of skin incisions or lacerations. Sutures, however, are significantly better for minimizing surgical wound dehiscence.

As mentioned, several types of surgery are associated with major bleeding complications. Cardiac surgery, which has the most data for managing hemorrhage, will be discussed in detail. Of note, most surgeons are willing to accept a state of relative hypocoagulation, assuming the hemorrhage is not life threatening. Around 20% of patients undergoing cardiac surgery have perioperative hemostatic abnormalities, and 15% of all blood products in the United States are used in cases of cardiac surgery.[39] In the 2%–6% of cardiac cases requiring surgical revision, coagulopathy is present in 53%, and an identifiable source of bleeding is found in only 67%.[67] Reexploration is associated with a 3- to 4-fold increase in mortality.[67] Acutely, hemorrhage may lead to shock, cardiac tamponade, and cardiac decompensation, and hemorrhage increases the likelihood of infection, arrhythmias, pulmonary complications, and other organ dysfunctions. These surgical patients often develop coagulopathies from many etiologies including iatrogenic anticoagulation to prevent catastrophic clot formation during extracorporeal circulation, DIC, dilutional, hypothermia, acidosis, and the use of anticoagulant or antiplatelet agents before surgery.[76] In extracorporal circulation, blood contact with artificial surfaces and air bubbles simultaneously activates coagulation factors, especially factor VII, to further stimulate thrombin generation while enhancing fibrinolysis.[76] Heparin is the primary anticoagulant used during extracorporeal circulation and is easily reversed with protamine; however, protamine can inhibit coagulation, paradoxically increasing the risk of hemorrhage.[76]

Treatment goals for these patients are aimed at maximizing clot formation and stabilization by enhancing coagulation and reducing fibrinolysis, rapidly controlling hemorrhage, and reducing the likelihood of reexploration.[39] These goals are applicable to hemorrhage associated with other types of surgery and trauma. An added level of complexity is hemorrhage associated with surgery that involves grafting such as coronary artery bypass grafting or solid organ transplant because graft patency is vital and may limit administration of procoagulant and antifibrinolytic agents.[76] Conventional therapies used to reverse coagulopathy and/or minimize the severity of hemorrhage during surgery include PRBCs, FFP, PCCs, platelets, cryoprecipitate, antifibrinolytics, desmopressin, and topical hemostatic agents (Table 24.6 and Table 24.8).[2,3,7,35-40,56-66] In general, these agents are used to achieve or maintain the aforementioned laboratory goals for INR, platelet count, and fibrinogen concentrations and/or normal point-of-care viscoelastic hemostatic parameters (Table 24.9; Figure 24.2)[67,77,78] (see Traumatic Injury section for more detail). A meta-analysis of tranexamic acid use in surgery across 104 trials and 8,030 subjects found that it reduced blood loss by 34% (OR 0.66; 95% CI, 0.65–0.67; p<0.001) consistently across all types of surgery (cardiac, orthopedic, head and neck, obstetrical and gynecologic, urological, and hepatic), irrespective of whether it was administered pre- or post-incision, and without increasing thromboembolic events.[79,80] Recombinant activated factor VII is a controversial therapy because results of studies of surgical patients are mixed with respect to the amount of blood loss, transfusion requirements, or hemorrhage control.[57] No study has shown improved morbidity or

Table 24.8 Guidelines for the Use of Procoagulants During Cardiothoracic Surgery and Trauma[39,40]

Recommendation	Cardiothoracic Surgery	Trauma
PCCs for urgent warfarin reversal	2A	—
Use of topical agents to control bleeding	2B	1B
Early FFP in massive bleed (15 mL/kg)	2B	1B
Platelets to achieve ≥ 100 × 10^9/L with ongoing bleed or ≥ 50 × 10^9/L if discontinued	2A	2C/1C
Cryoprecipitate to achieve fibrinogen > 100–200 mg/dL in massive hemorrhage	—	1C
Use of rFVIIa if major bleeding persists despite standard therapies	2B	2C (blunt trauma only)
Use of antifibrinolytics to control bleeding/blood conservation	3A/1A	1B[a]
Use of desmopressin if refractory bleeding and received platelet inhibitor or uremic	2B	2C

1 = recommend; 2 = suggest; 3 = consider.

[a]Recommendation provided administration is within 3 hr of injury.

PCC = prothrombin complex concentrate.

Table 24.9 Interpretation of TEG Parameters[67,77,78]

Parameter (normal values)	Interpretation	Therapy
r (15–23 min)	-Latency time from placement of blood specimen to TEG tracing amplitude of 2 mm -Reflects quantity or action of clotting factors	FFP or PCCs
K (5–10 min)	-Latency time for TEG tracing amplitude to increase from 2 mm to 20 mm -Reflects rate of clot formation and fibrinogen amount	Fibrinogen (cryoprecipitate) ± rFVIIa
α (22°–38°)	-Angle of the slope of the line connecting r and K times -Reflects rate of clot formation and fibrinogen amount	Fibrinogen (cryoprecipitate) ± rFVIIa
MA (47–58 mm)	-The greatest vertical amplitude of the TEG tracing -Reflects strength of clot and platelet activation	Platelets ± desmopressin
A$_{60}$ (usually > 90%)	-The amplitude 60 min after MA as a percentage of MA -Reflects fibrinolysis	Antifibrinolytics
LY$_{30}$ (< 7.5%)	-The rate of amplitude reduction 30 min after MA -Reflects fibrinolysis	Antifibrinolytics

LY = lysed; MA = maximum amplitude; TEG = thromboelastogram.

mortality with rFVIIa when applied to surgical patients.[57] None of the aforementioned therapies, however, should supplant rapid surgical intervention.

Traumatic Injury

Hemorrhagic shock is most commonly seen after acute injury. However, non-trauma cases of massive hemorrhage include patients with GI bleeding, obstetrical patients, and surgical procedures with the potential for massive bleeding complications. The overarching goal in hemorrhagic shock is improving patient outcomes through source control, restoration of adequate end-organ perfusion, increased oxygen-carrying capacity of the circulating blood, and reversal of the hypocoagulable state often accompanying massive blood loss. As with surgery, coagulopathy from trauma is the consequence of many factors including hypothermia, acidosis, DIC, and dilution.[75,81] About 9% of patients with trauma present with hypothermia, and about 65% of hypothermia can be attributed to radiant heat loss from removal of clothing, muscle relaxation, frequent removal of blankets for examinations, or resuscitation with cold intravenous fluids.[12,40] Unlike elective surgery where normovolemic hemodilution conserves blood, excessive resuscitation during trauma with crystalloid fluids dilutes clotting factors, increases hydrostatic pressure, and reduces quality clot formation.

Acute coagulopathy of trauma is recognized as a distinct entity as patients progress from an early hypocoagulable/profibrinolytic phase to a prothrombotic phase.[12,81,82] The defining etiology is traumatic shock leading to systemic hypoperfusion, which slows the clearance of thrombin.[81,82] Enhanced binding of thrombin to endothelial thrombomodulin activates protein C, inactivates factors Va and VIIIa, and abrogates plasminogen activator inhibitor and thrombin activatable plasminogen inhibitor to produce greater fibrinolysis. Tissue hypoperfusion generates new expression of thrombomodulin, furthering the hypocoagulable state. In contrast, massive tissue destruction also releases damage-associated molecular pattern molecules such as histones and mitochondrial DNA, which lead to microvascular thrombosis by inducing platelet activation, promoting thrombin generation, and impairing protein C activation. Tissue injury also releases the proinflammatory cytokines, IL-1β and tumor necrosis factor α, which elicit tissue factor expression on the surface of monocytes and endothelium to propagate thrombosis and possibly incite DIC. Traumatic brain injury also causes the release of tissue factor from injured neurons.[81,82]

The reversal of coagulopathy with blood products and pharmacologic agents is critical because coagulopathy is an independent risk factor for morbidity and mortality in trauma patients with hemorrhagic shock (Table 24.8).[39,40] Massive transfusion protocols were developed in an effort to minimize RBC transfusions and crystalloids in trauma patients with hemorrhagic shock (Figure 24.3).[12,38,40] Increasing the speed and efficiency of transfusions are other potential benefits of MTPs. Massive transfusion protocols are processes for administering RBCs, plasma, and platelets in a set ratio, as well as hemostatic agents in a standardized manner versus guiding blood product administration on the basis of laboratory data.[83-87] These protocols are often initiated by an order set or telephone call to the blood bank, and the blood products

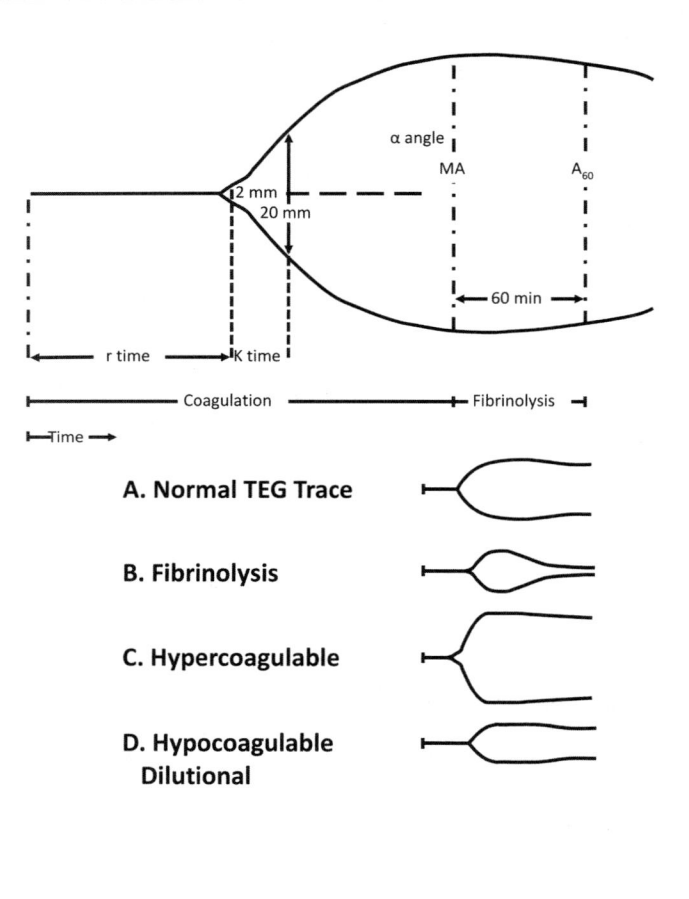

Figure 24.2 Schematic diagram of thromboelastogram showing reaction time (r), clot formation time (K), alpha (α) angle, maximum amplitude (MA), and maximum amplitude (A_{60}).

Compared with a normal trace (A), fibrinolysis (B) is associated with prolonged r and K times, reduced MA and A_{60}, greater LY_{30}, and possibly obtuse α angle; hypercoagulation (C) is associated with shorter r and K times, heightened MA and A_{60}, relatively normal LY_{30}, and acute α angle; hypocoagulation (D) is associated with lengthened r and K times, reduced MA and A_{60}, relatively normal LY_{30}, and obtuse α angle.[67,77,78]

are delivered to the bedside ready to use. The first MTP used a ratio of 1:1:1 (PRBC/plasma/platelets) for civilian trauma patients and was based on military data.[12,38] Massive transfusion protocols are physiologically rational because whole blood has an RBC/plasma ratio of 1:1.[12,38] Although studies are almost uniformly positive, most were observational and usually based on before-after methodology at single centers.[12,38] The Prospective, Observational, Multicenter, Major Trauma Transfusion (PROMMTT) study was conducted across 10 U.S. level 1 trauma centers and evaluated 1,245 patients who received at least 1 PRBC unit within 6 hours of admission.[88] Findings from the PROMMTT study indicate that ratios of RBC to FFP of 1:1 or less and ratios of RBC to platelets less than 1:2 within 6 hours of admission were independently associated with decreased 30-day mortality rates. A follow-up study examining the optimal PRBC/FFP/platelet ratios, known as the Pragmatic Randomized Optimal Platelet and Plasma Ratios (PROPPR) study, randomized 680 hemorrhaging patients to PRBC/plasma/platelets in ratios of 1:1:1 to 2:1:1.[89] The results showed similar mortality rates between groups at 24 hours and 30 days despite fewer deaths from exsanguination within 24 hours (9.2% vs. 14.6%, p=0.03) and greater achievement of hemostasis in the 1:1:1 group (86% vs. 78%, p=0.006). Most trauma centers have an MTP in place, but significant variability exists relative to the fixed ratio of blood products within the protocol. An average of 10 MTP studies of more than 4,000 trauma patients showed a mean RBC/plasma ratio of less than 3:2 and an RBC/platelet ratio less than 2:1.[86,87]

A significant limitation of studies examining MTPs is survival bias. Plasma must be thawed before administration, so patients bleeding profusely may die after receiving PRBCs but before receiving FFP.[12] In addition, administering platelet transfusions in trauma patients without thrombocytopenia is questionable, and the "shotgun" approach may result in over-replacement of products with limited supply and contribute to adverse events and/or the propagation of DIC.[12] In many cases, systemic pharmacologic agents or factor-specific products are included in these MTPs.[86,87] Consideration of other blood products for inclusion in MTPs such as PCCs, cryoprecipitate, and fibrinogen concentrates

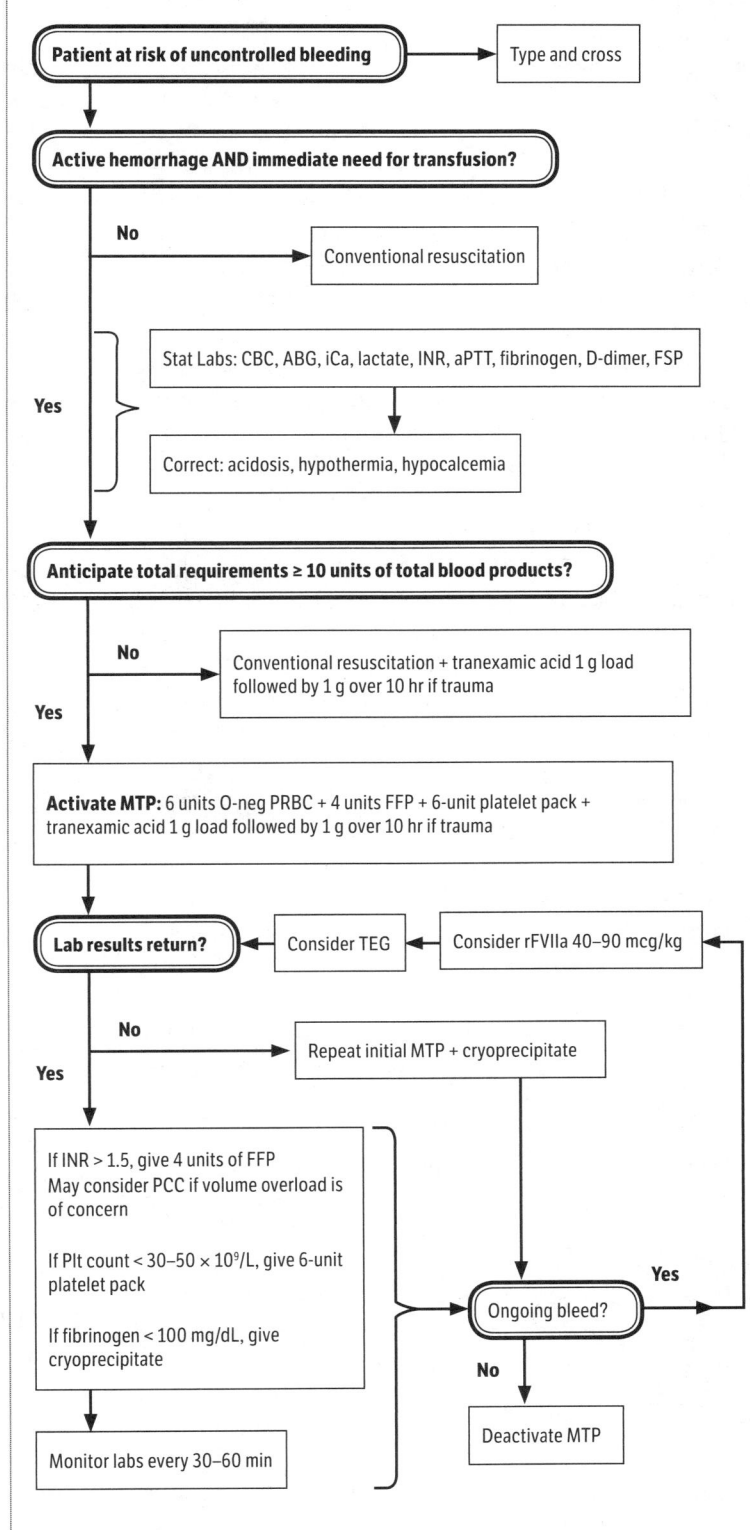

Figure 24.3 Example of a massive transfusion protocol showing the considerations and incorporation of blood product ratios, pharmacologic agents, laboratory parameters, and thromboelastogram.[12,38,40]

ABG = arterial blood gas; aPTT = activated partial thromboplastin time; CBC = complete blood count; FSP = fibrin split product; iCa = ionized calcium; INR = international normalized ratio; MTP = massive transfusion protocol; Plt = platelet; rFVIIa = recombinant activated factor VII; TEG = thromboelastogram.

may also be directed by this strategy.[86,87] Massive transfusion protocols are often applied to etiologies of hemorrhage other than trauma.[87]

There is a trend toward using a hybrid, more individualized approach to treating patients, which combines viscoelastic testing data and a structured MTP. Thromboelastography (TEG) or rotational TEG (ROTEG) is an integral element of this point-of-care management approach.[77,78] The primary advantage of these tests over other conventional tests used during surgery and trauma is that they offer delineated assessments of coagulation, clot stability, and fibrinolysis (Table 24.9; Figure 24.2).[67,77,78] Disadvantages of the TEG or ROTEG include cost, differences in results, and time to obtain results on the basis of technique and device.[67] Several reports suggest that viscoelastic testing used during surgery or trauma to specifically direct the appropriate use of therapies improves coagulation, minimizes fibrinolysis, and limits patient exposure to unnecessary blood products.[77,78] Used in this way, these tests can facilitate the efficient use of blood products and hemostatic agents while reducing blood loss and potentially improving clinical outcomes.[77,78] Of note, these viscoelastic hemostatic assays are commonly used during non-trauma surgical procedures to monitor coagulation and guide therapies and are becoming more commonly applied across ICUs in nonsurgical types of hemorrhage.[77,78]

Tranexamic acid and rFVIIa are two pharmacologic products that have been systematically studied in trauma patients at high risk of hemorrhage. The Clinical Randomisation of an Antifibrinolytic in Significant Haemorrhage (CRASH)-2 trial was a multicenter study of 274 hospitals in 40 countries that randomized 20,211 adult trauma patients actively hemorrhaging or at high risk of hemorrhage and within 8 hours of injury to tranexamic acid (loading dose 1 g over 10 minutes; then infusion of 1 g over 8 hours) or matching placebo.[90] All-cause 28-day hospital mortality, the primary outcome, was lower with tranexamic acid (14.5% vs. 16%; RR 0.91; 95% CI, 0.85–0.97, p=0.0035). The risk of death caused by bleeding was also lower (4.9% vs. 5.7%; RR 0.85; 95% CI, 0.76–0.96, p=0.0077). The greatest survival benefit was most evident for the day of injury and when treatment was initiated within 3 hours of injury.[91,92] Exploratory analyses of the CRASH-2 trial found that treatment given after 3 hours increased the risk of death caused by bleeding (4.4% vs. 3.1%; RR 1.44; 95% CI, 1.12–1.84, p=0.004).[92-94] The contrasting survival benefit, given the timing of administration, may pertain to the pathophysiology of coagulopathy from acute trauma because early administration may help control the hypocoagulable/profibrinolytic phase seen shortly after trauma.[92,93] Vascular occlusive events (1.7% vs. 2%; RR 0.84; 95% CI, 0.68–1.02, p=0.084) and the use of blood products were similar between groups.[91-93] Cost-effectiveness analyses show that the incremental cost of using tranexamic acid per life-year gained is less than $100, especially when administered within 3 hours of injury.[94,95] Because of these results, most trauma centers administer tranexamic acid when patients present within 3 hours of injury. Considerable controversy exists about the administration beyond 3 hours.

Before tranexamic acid was studied, rFVIIa was evaluated in 301 bleeding patients with blunt or penetrating trauma across 32 hospitals.[96] Patients requiring 6 units of PRBCs within 4 hours of injury were randomized to receive rFVIIa 200 mcg/kg, followed by two doses of 100 mcg/kg 1 and 3 hours after the first dose or placebo. In blunt trauma, rFVIIa reduced RBC transfusions within 48 hours (2.6 units, p=0.02), the primary outcome, and the need for massive transfusion, as defined by greater than 20 PRBC units (14% vs. 33%, p=0.03).[96] The rate of acute respiratory distress syndrome was also decreased (29% vs. 42%, p=0.03). These results were not statistically different for the penetrating trauma group. Mortality and thromboembolic rates were similar between groups. A subgroup analysis showed that the greatest benefit occurred when coagulopathy was present.[97] A phase III study of patients who bled 4–8 RBC units within 12 hours of injury and were still bleeding despite resuscitation and operative management using a similar dosing scheme was terminated early after 573 patients (481 with blunt trauma) of 1,502 planned subjects because mortality rates (11% vs. 10.7%, respectively) were lower than anticipated, resulting in futility concerns.[98,99] Similar to the previous study, blunt trauma patients randomized to rFVIIa received fewer PRBC units (7.8 ± 10.6 vs. 9.1 ± 11.3, p=0.04) and total units of allogenic blood products (19 ± 27.1 vs. 23.5 ± 28, p=0.04). Thromboembolic rates were similar between groups. Because of the cost of rFVIIa and the newer data with tranexamic acid, most trauma centers reserve rFVIIa use for patients with refractory hemorrhage and often use dosage regimens of 40–90 mcg/kg rather than the cumulative dose of 400 mcg/kg that was studied.

Management and Prevention of Bleeding in Patients with Cirrhosis

The complex nature of the coagulation system in patients with hepatic insufficiency makes management difficult and often controversial. Traditionally, clinicians associated hepatic insufficiency with an anticoagulated state and increased bleeding tendency, so management was targeted at reversing coagulation tests such as PT/INR.[26-28] However, recent literature suggests that patients with hepatic insufficiency have a balanced coagulation system and that prolonged coagulation tests do not correlate with bleeding risk.[26-28] The focused use of blood products in clinical scenarios is currently the mainstay of therapy for these patients, in addition to the potential use of vitamin K, rFVIIa, and PCCs.[7,27,28] Concomitant renal dysfunction is common in patients with hepatic insufficiency and hemorrhage, so desmopressin may be administered if uremia is present in an effort to improve platelet function.[7,28]

Despite the lack of literature proving their efficacy, blood products (FFP, platelets, and cryoprecipitate) are commonly administered in patients with hepatic insufficiency to control active bleeding or reverse PT/INR before invasive procedures. Fresh frozen plasma may partly reverse prolonged values of PT/INR; however, achievement of an INR less than 1.5 occurs in fewer than 10% of cases.[8] Similarly, correlation between a corrected PT/INR and clinically significant bleeding cessation or occurrence in the case of prophylactic administration has not been established in this patient population.[4,26] The amount of plasma needed to consistently reduce the PT/INR is often 10–15 mL/kg, which exposes these patients to increased volume expansion and subsequent risks of TACO, TRALI, and cerebral edema and worsening portal pressure to promote ongoing hemorrhage.[10,57] In addition, the effects of FFP are short lived, which is consistent with the short half-life of factor VII. The lack of clinical evidence and the risks associated with the administration of FFP in this patient population argue against its routine use; however, many clinicians are compelled to try to reverse the coagulopathy in cases of hemorrhage and to prevent bleeding.

Administration of cryoprecipitate may aid in restoring "normal" concentrations of fibrinogen in patients with hepatic insufficiency who may have lower concentrations of fibrinogen and impaired aggregation of fibrin monomers.[28,62] The exact target concentration of fibrinogen has not been established, and systemic fibrinogen concentrations may not give an accurate assessment of bleeding risk, given the uncertainty regarding the degree of dysfibrinogenemia found in patients with hepatic insufficiency. However, in clinical practice, doses of cryoprecipitate are typically titrated to achieve a fibrinogen concentration of 100–120 mg/dL in the setting of bleeding, and they typically range from 1 to 2 units/kg of body weight.[28,62] Caution should be taken during administration because cryoprecipitate lacks certain clotting factors and can worsen the already imbalanced coagulation system seen in patients with hepatic insufficiency.

The quantity and quality of platelets is also important to achieve primary hemostasis, and patients with hepatic insufficiency often have abnormalities in their platelet production and function.[4,26] Transfusions of platelets typically result in an immediate rise in platelet counts; however, the target platelet concentration in this patient population remains poorly defined. In-vitro studies have shown that platelet counts of 50×10^9/L or greater enable adequate thrombin generation, whereas concentrations of 100×10^9/L or greater may enable optimal thrombin generation. In clinical practice, it is reasonable to aim for platelet counts of 50×10^9/L or greater in the setting of active bleeding or of 20×10^9/L or greater to prevent hemorrhage in high-risk procedures.[26,28,34,35]

Vitamin K deficiency is a common complication of hepatic insufficiency and may occur because of malnutrition and malabsorption. In addition, vitamin K–dependent clotting factors (II, VII, IX, and X) are synthesized in the liver and are often deficient in patients with hepatic insufficiency.[11,37] Prothrombin time and INR tests are nonspecific for vitamin K–dependent clotting factors and are often insensitive in patients with hepatic insufficiency because these patients may have an elevated PT/INR despite having normal concentrations of vitamin K.[7,9,11,67] Despite the lack of literature proving its efficacy, vitamin K is commonly administered to patients with hepatic insufficiency to help correct their coagulopathy. Given the high safety profile and nominal cost of vitamin K, the risk-benefit profile of vitamin K will often favor its administration. There is no standardized dosing regimen; however, intravenous doses of 10 mg daily for 48–72 hours adequately replace vitamin K deficiency.[2,28,67]

Replacing factor VII in hepatic insufficiency with rFVIIa is physiologically reasonable because these patients often have low levels of factor VII, and the small volume needed to administer rFVIIa may improve safety compared with FFP.[28] Although several studies show that rFVIIa effectively normalizes prolonged values of PT/INR in patients with cirrhosis, the efficacy of rFVIIa for reducing clinically significant bleeding remains unclear. Bosch et al. conducted a double-blind study that randomized 245 patients with cirrhosis with upper GI bleeding to receive either eight doses of rFVIIa 100 mcg/kg or placebo, in addition to pharmacologic and endoscopic treatment.[100] No significant differences were seen regarding the primary composite end point (failure to control upper GI bleeding within 24 hours after the first dose, or failure to prevent rebleeding at 24 hours and day 5, or death within 5 days). However, subgroup analysis showed that administering rFVIIa in patients with Child-Pugh class B and C cirrhosis was more effective than placebo at improving the primary composite end point, whereas administration of rFVIIa in Child-Pugh A patients had no benefit. As a result of this subgroup analysis, the same investigators carried out a second randomized clinical trial that examined the same primary composite end point, but solely in patients with Child-Pugh class B and C cirrhosis.[101] Results showed no significant differences between rFVIIa and placebo in these patients. As a result of these studies and the cost of rFVIIa, it is rarely administered to manage hemorrhage in patients with hepatic insufficiency.

The role of rFVIIa in the management of bleeding secondary to major surgical operations such as liver transplantation, resections, and/or liver biopsies also remains unclear.[74] A multicenter, randomized, double-blind study examining the efficacy and safety of repeated perioperative doses of rFVIIa in liver transplantation secondary to cirrhosis failed to show any significant differences between placebo and rFVIIa with respect to perioperative PRBC transfusion requirements.[102] Furthermore, there were no differences in requirements of FFP, platelets, and fibrinogen, and overall blood loss and length of hospital stay were similar. Other trials examining the use of rFVIIa in this patient population provide inconclusive evidence, and use has not been widely accepted during major surgical procedures secondary to hepatic insufficiency.[74]

Finally, the prophylactic use of rFVIIa for invasive procedures in patients with acute liver failure is still highly debated. Limited data have shown that rFVIIa at a dose of 40 mcg/kg may be useful during invasive procedures, particularly the placement of intracranial pressure monitors.[74,103] Compared with FFP alone, rFVIIa rapidly normalized PT/INR values, allowing for a higher number of successful intracranial pressure monitor placements. Despite the small amount of literature available, the role of rFVIIa as a prophylactic agent for invasive procedures remains uncertain, particularly because the normalization of coagulation tests in these patients has not been associated with clinically significant cessation of bleeding.[103]

Similar to rFVIIa, the role of PCCs for the management or prevention of bleeding associated with hepatic insufficiency is currently undefined, with much less data to support its use.[2,57,58] Like rFVIIa, PCCs provide much smaller volumes of administration than FFP. Although data from large, randomized trials are lacking, several smaller studies have examined the safety and efficacy of PCC use in bleeding patients with hepatic insufficiency. In general, four-factor PCCs reverse prolonged PT/INR values in these patients, whereas three-factor PCCs require the addition of rFVIIa to be effective. Thromboelastography- or ROTEG-guided use of PCCs in bleeding associated with liver transplantation further reduces the need for RBCs, FFP, and platelets with no change in thromboembolic or ischemic events. Most data analyses currently available for the use of PCCs for bleeding associated with hepatic insufficiency were done using PT/INR as a surrogate marker of efficacy, yet these parameters do not predict bleeding risk in these patients.[2,57,58] Prothrombin complex concentrates are often substituted for FFP to reverse PT/INR in patients with cirrhosis about to undergo invasive procedures because PCCs act more predictably and rapidly and require less volume administration. Further studies are ongoing and will help guide the clinical use of PCCs for bleeding associated with hepatic insufficiency. Continued caution is warranted when using PCCs because it is unknown whether a disruption of the coagulation system in these patients could place them at an increased risk of thrombosis.

Major Obstetric Hemorrhage

Pregnancy is associated with a hypercoagulable state because levels of factors V, VII, VIII, IX, X, and XII; vWF; and fibrinogen are increased with concomitant decreases in the anticoagulants protein C and S and heparin cofactor II and depressed antifibrinolytic activity.[104,105] The transfusion rate in obstetrics in the United States is relatively low, from 0.9% to 2.3%. The incidence of postpartum hemorrhage (PPH), however, is increasingly driven by the greater prevalence of uterine atony caused by higher rates of cesarian deliveries and the older average age of women at childbirth. Postpartum hemorrhage is defined as persistent bleeding of greater than 500–1,000 mL within 24 hours of birth that continues despite the use of initial measures.[104,105] Fortunately, massive transfusion of 10 units or greater of blood products occurs in only 6 of every 10,000 deliveries. Although uterine atony represents about 80% of the causes of PPH, placental problems account for 27% of all cases of massive transfusion.[104,105] Other etiologies of PPH include genital tract trauma and systemic medical disorders. Obstetrical DIC can occur secondary to placental abruption, amniotic fluid embolism, dead fetus syndrome, or massive hemorrhage.

First-line treatment of PPH consists of identifying and correcting the cause (e.g., removal of a retained placenta), using uterotonic agents (e.g., oxytocin, carboprost, or misoprostol) that improve uterine tone and cause local vasoconstriction to reduce blood flow to the uterus, and using mechanical manipulations (e.g., massage, uterine tamponade, packing).[104,105] Persistent hemorrhage should mandate the activation of the MTP (Figure 24.3)[12,38,40] with therapies directed to achieve or maintain the aforementioned laboratory goals for INR, platelet count, and fibrinogen concentrations (Table 24.6 and Table 24.8)[2,3,7,35-40,56-66] or normal viscoelastic hemostatic parameters (Table 24.9; Figure 24.2)[67,77,78] (see Traumatic Injury section for more detail). In some cases, topical hemostats may be applied. The results of a randomized, double-blind study of 144 women with PPH (greater than 800 mL of estimated blood loss after vaginal delivery) found that tranexamic acid (4 g loading dose, followed by 1 g/hour for 6 hours) significantly reduced blood loss, RBC transfusion requirement, bleeding duration, and progression to severe PPH.[106] Although guidelines suggest the use of tranexamic acid in persistent PPH, a large, multicenter study is ongoing that will investigate the impact of tranexamic acid on the rates of hysterectomy and mortality. Recombinant activated factor VII may also cease or slow PPH, but it has only been assessed in retrospective cohort studies, most commonly at doses of 90 mcg/kg.[104,105] Recombinant activated factor VII may be a plausible option before the definitive treatment of a hysterectomy is performed.

Managing Hemorrhage Associated with Anticoagulants

About 1%–10% of patients receiving anticoagulation therapies will have a hemorrhagic complication.[67] In all cases of hemorrhage, the benefit of reversing the anticoagulant in an effort to stop the bleed must be considered against the risk of thrombosis for which the anticoagulant is being used. In general, life-threatening bleeding events or those with long-term severe morbidities such as intracranial hemorrhage, retroperitoneal hemorrhage, GI hemorrhage, or intraocular hemorrhage mandate the temporary discontinuation and reversal of the anticoagulant. The extent of anticoagulation, if assessable, must be considered. In addition, the projected duration of effective anticoagulation after discontinuing the anticoagulant must be considered because reversal agents may have shorter half-lives than the anticoagulant, especially when organ dysfunction is present. For some bleeding sources, invasive or surgical procedures may be warranted.

Until recently, vitamin K antagonists such as warfarin were the only oral anticoagulants available for the prevention of thrombosis. In intracranial hemorrhage, the mortality rate doubles when it is associated with warfarin.[1,2] Early hematoma expansion is associated with neurological deterioration and poor clinical outcomes.[7,8] In severe or life-threatening intracranial hemorrhage, rapid reversal of anticoagulation is associated with clinical improvements, likely because hematoma expansion is minimized.[9,10] Conventional therapies used to reverse the anticoagulant effects of warfarin include vitamin K, FFP, and PCCs (Table 24.5 and Table 24.6).[2,3,7,35-38,56-66] Early administration of these agents is associated with greater reversal of INR, so these and other therapies should not be delayed for the results of coagulation tests.[9,10] Intravenous vitamin K 5–10 mg should be administered in cases of major hemorrhage. Four-factor PCCs reduce INR more rapidly than FFP and have become the primary reversal option for warfarin-associated hemorrhage. Recombinant activated factor VII is the most effective agent at reversing INR, but its use is controversial because it is costly and short acting relative to the duration of action of warfarin, and few studies have evaluated it for warfarin reversal. Studies evaluating rFVIIa for warfarin reversal are poor quality, and the results of studies of patients with spontaneous intracranial hemorrhage are mixed with respect to neurological improvement, although rFVIIa consistently reduces hematoma expansion at the risk of increasing thromboembolic events.

Target-specific oral anticoagulants include dabigatran (DTI) and the factor Xa inhibitors (rivaroxaban, apixaban, and edoxaban). These newer agents have rapid onset of action and predictable pharmacokinetics, allowing for fixed dosing and mitigation of laboratory monitoring. Unlike warfarin, however, they do not currently have a known antidote. Several reversal agents are in development or at various stages of testing. The furthest along is idarucizumab, a monoclonal antibody that binds to free and thrombin-bound dabigatran and was recently shown to normalize clotting times in patients (79% at 24 hours) requiring urgent or emergency reversal of dabigatran.[107] However, most data to treat hemorrhage associated with these agents are derived from animal models, in vitro studies of plasma from patients, or healthy volunteer studies that used outcomes of coagulation parameters or surrogate markers of clot formation such as thrombin generation (Table 24.2).[7,11,12,30-33] Although dabigatran may be removed through dialysis, the factor Xa inhibitors cannot. Four-factor PCCs inconsistently reverse the effects of dabigatran, whereas they appear effective at promoting coagulation when anticoagulation is from factor Xa inhibitors. Both aPCCs and rFVIIa improve thrombin generation when anticoagulation is with dabigatran.

Other anticoagulants include heparin (stimulate antithrombin), low-molecular-weight heparins (stimulate antithrombin and anti-Xa activity), fondaparinux (indirect anti-Xa activity), other DTIs, and fibrinolytic agents (Table 24.2).[7,11,12,30-33] The effects of heparin are reversed with protamine (1.0–1.5 mg protamine sulfate for every 100 U of heparin, not to exceed 50 mg). Reversal of the anti-Xa activity of low-molecular-weight heparins can be 60% achieved with protamine, so FFP or PCCs are commonly administered as adjunctive therapy to replace additional factors. Anticoagulation associated with fondaparinux or the DTIs may partly be reversed by PCCs, aPCCs, or rFVIIa. Bleeding associated with fibrinolytic agents may be treated with antifibrinolytics and fibrinogen replacement with cryoprecipitate. Platelets and desmopressin are often administered to reverse the effects of antiplatelet agents (Table 24.2).[7,11,12,30-33]

CONCLUSION

This chapter reviewed the common causes of disruption to the hemostatic pathways; delineated the properties of blood products, pharmacologic agents, and nonpharmacologic interventions; and discussed the appropriate management for common types of hemorrhage. Many questions remain regarding the pathophysiology of coagulopathy and hemorrhage and the appropriate use of procoagulant strategies.

REFERENCES

1. Palta S, Saroa R, Palta A. Overview of the coagulation system. Indian J Anaesth 2014;58:515-23.
2. Paterson TA, Stein DM. Hemorrhage and coagulopathy in the critically ill. Emerg Med Clin North Am 2014;32:797-810.
3. Hunt BJ. Bleeding and coagulopathies in critical care. N Engl J Med 2014;370:847-59.
4. Retter A, Barrett NA. The management of abnormal haemostasis in the ICU. Anaesthesia 2015;70(suppl 1):121-7.
5. Paniccia R, Piora R, Liotta AA, et al. Platelet function tests: a comparative review. Vasc Health Risk Manag 2015;11:133-48.

6. Han JH, Li S, Choi JL. Platelet function tests: a review of progresses in clinical application. Biomed Res Int 2014;2014:456569.
7. Marks PW. Coagulation disorders in the ICU. Clin Chest Med 2009;30:123-9.
8. Levi M, Opal SM. Coagulation abnormalities in critically ill patients. Crit Care 2006;10:222.
9. Zimmerman LH. Causes and consequences of critical bleeding and mechanisms of blood coagulation. Pharmacotherapy 2007;27(9 pt 2):S45-56.
10. Wheeler AP, Rice TW. Coagulopathy in critically ill patients. Part 2 – soluble clotting factors and hemostatic testing. Chest 2010;137:185-94.
11. Dutton RP. Haemostatic resuscitation. Br J Anaesth 2012;109(suppl 1):i39-i46.
12. Ruzicka J, Stengl M, Bolek L, et al. Hypothermic anticoagulation: testing individual responses to graded severe hypothermia with thromboelastography. Blood Coagul Fibrinolysis 2012;23:285-9.
13. Rohrer MJ, Natale AM. Effect of hypothermia on the coagulation cascade. Crit Care Med 1992;20:1402-5.
14. Wolberg AS, Meng ZH, Monroe DM, et al. A systemic evaluation of the effect of temperature on coagulation enzyme activity and platelet function. J Trauma 2004;56:1221-8.
15. Hazinski MF, Nolan JP, Billi JE, et al. Executive summary: 2010 international consensus on cardiopulmonary resuscitation and emergency cardiovascular care science with treatment recommendations. Circulation 2010;122:250-75.
16. Polderman KH. Mechanisms of action, physiological effects, and complications of hypothermia. Crit Care Med 2009;37:186-202.
17. Dirkmann D, Hanke AA, Gorlinger K, et al. Hypothermia and acidosis synergistically impair coagulation in human whole blood. Anesth Analg 2008;106:1627-32.
18. Thorsen K, Ringdal KG, Strand K, et al. Clinical and cellular effects of hypothermia, acidosis, and coagulopathy in major injury. Br J Surg 2011;98:894-907.
19. Martini WZ. Coagulopathy by hypothermia and acidosis: mechanisms of thrombin generation and fibrinogen availability. J Trauma 2009;67:202-8.
20. D'Angelo MR, Dutton RP. Management of trauma-induced coagulopathy: trends and practices. AANA J 2010;78:35-40.
21. Sihler KC, Napolitano LM. Complications of massive transfusion. Chest 2010;137:209-20.
22. Gando S, Saitoh D, Ogura H, et al. Natural history of disseminated intravascular coagulation diagnosed based on the newly established diagnostic criteria for critically ill patients: results of a multi-center, prospective study. Crit Care Med 2008;36:145-50.
23. Levi M, Toh CH, Thachil J, et al. Guidelines for the diagnosis and management of disseminated intravascular coagulation. British Committee for Standards in Haematology. Br J Haematol 2009;145:24-33.
24. Levi M, van der Poll T. Coagulation in patients with severe sepsis. Semin Thromb Hemost 2015;41:9-15.
25. Schaden E, Saner FH, Goerlinger K. Coagulation pattern in critical liver dysfunction. Curr Opin Crit Care 2013;19:142-8.
26. Gopinath R, Sreekanth Y, Yadav M. Approach to bleeding patient. Indian J Anaesth 2014;58:595-602.
27. Dasher K, Trotter JF. Intensive care unit management of liver-related coagulation disorders. Crit Care Clin 2012;28:389-98.
28. Levy JH, Szlam F, Wolberg AS, et al. Clinical use of the activated partial thromboplastin time and prothrombin time for screening: a review of the literature and current guidelines for testing. Clin Lab Med 2014;34:453-77.
29. Oudemans-van Straaten H. Hemostasis and thrombosis in continuous renal replacement treatment. Semin Thromb Hemost 2015;41:91-8.
30. Miller MP, Trujillo TC, Nordenholz KE. Practical considerations in emergency management of bleeding in the setting of target-specific oral anticoagulants. Am J Emerg Med 2014;32:375-82.
31. Kalus JS. Pharmacologic interventions for reversing the effects of oral anticoagulants. Am J Health Syst Pharm 2013;70(suppl 1):S12-21.
32. Nutescu EA, Dager WE, Kalus JS, et al. Management of bleeding and reversal strategies for oral anticoagulants: clinical practice considerations. Am J Health Syst Pharm 2013;70:1914-29.
33. Yorkgitis BK, Ruggia-Check C, Dujon JE. Antiplatelet and anticoagulation medications and the surgical patient. 2014;207:95-101.
34. Parker RI. Etiology and significance of thrombocytopenia in critically ill patients. Crit Care Clin 2012;28:399-411.
35. Wang HL, Aguilera C, Knopf KB, et al. Thrombocytopenia in the intensive care unit. 2013;28:268-80.
36. Rice TW, Wheeler AP. Coagulopathy in critically ill patients. Part 1: platelet disorders. Chest 2009;136:1622-30.
37. Thiele T, Selleng K, Selleng S, et al. Thrombocytopenia in the intensive care unit-diagnostic approach and management. Semin Hematol 2013;50:239-50.
38. Kor DJ, Gajic O. Blood product transfusion in the critical care setting. Curr Opin Crit Care 2010;16:309-16.
39. Ferraris VA, Brown JR, Despotis GJ, et al. 2011 update to the Society of Thoracic Surgeons and the Society of Cardiovascular Anesthesiologists blood conservation clinical practice guidelines. Ann Thorac Surg 2011;91:944-82.
40. Spahn DR, Bouillon B, Cerny V, et al. Management of bleeding and coagulopathy following major trauma: an updated European guideline. Crit Care 2013;17:R76.
41. Kozek-Langenecker SA. Coagulation and transfusion in the postoperative bleeding patients. Curr Opin Crit Care 2014;20:460-6.
42. Gill R. Practical management of major blood loss. Anaesthesia 2015;70(suppl 1):54-7.
43. Dutton RP. Management of traumatic haemorrhage – the US perspective. Anaesthesia 2015;70(suppl 1):108-27.
44. Wang CH, Hsieh WH, Chou HC, et al. Liberal versus restricted fluid resuscitation strategies in trauma patients: a systematic review and meta-analysis of randomized controlled trials and observational studies. Crit Care Med 2014;42:954-61.
45. Carson JL, Grossman BJ, Kleinman S, et al. Red blood cell transfusion: a clinical practice guideline from the AABB. Ann Intern Med 2012;157:49-58.

46. Carson JL, Carless PA, Hebert PC. Transfusion thresholds and other strategies for guiding allogeneic red blood cell transfusion. Cochrane Database Syst Rev 2012;4:CD002042.

47. Retter A, Wyncoll D, Pearse R, et al. Guidelines on the management of anaemia and red cell transfusion in adult critically ill patients. Br J Haematol 2013;160:445-64.

48. Hess JR. Measures of stored red blood cell quality. Vox Sang 2014;107:1-9.

49. Lacroix J, Hébert PC, Fergusson DA, et al. Age of transfused blood in critically ill adults. N Engl J Med 2015;372:1410-8.

50. Sayah DM, Looney MR, Toy P. Transfusion reactions: newer concepts on the pathophysiology, incidence, treatment, and prevention of transfusion-related acute lung injury. Crit Care Clin 2012;28:363-72.

51. Osterman JL, Arora S. Blood product transfusions and reactions. Emerg Med Clin North Am 2014;32:727-38.

52. Hart S, Cserti-Gazdewich CN, McCluskey SA. Red cell transfusion and the immune system. Anaesthesia 2015;70(suppl 1):38-45.

53. Rohde JM, Dimcheff DE, Blumberg N, et al. Health care-associated infection after red blood cell transfusion: a systematic review and meta-analysis. JAMA 2014;311:1317-26.

54. Toner RW, Pizzi L, Leas B, et al. Costs to hospitals of acquiring and processing blood in the US: a survey of hospital-based blood banks and transfusion services. Appl Health Econ Health Policy 2011;9:29-37.

55. Shander A, Hofmann A, Ozawa S, et al. Activity-based costs of blood transfusions in surgical patients at four hospitals. Transfusion 2010;50:753-65.

56. Grotke O. Coagulation management. Curr Opin Crit Care 2012;18:641-6.

57. Goodnough LT. A reappraisal of plasma, prothrombin complex concentrates, and recombinant factor VIIa in patient blood management. Crit Care Clin 2012;28:413-26.

58. Ferreira J, DeLosSantos M. The clinical use of prothrombin complex concentrate. J Emerg Med 2013;44:1201-10.

59. Spahn DR, Goodnough LT. Blood transfusion 2. Alternatives to blood transfusion. Lancet 2013;381:1855-65.

60. McQuilten ZK, Crighton G, Engelbrecht S, et al. Transfusion interventions in critical bleeding requiring massive transfusion: a systematic review. Transfus Med Rev 2015;29:127-37.

61. Cromwell C, Aledort LM. FEIBA: a prohemostatic agent. Semin Thromb Hemost 2012;38:265-7.

62. Nascimento B, Goodnough LT, Levy JH. Cryoprecipitate therapy. Br J Anaesth 2014;113:922-34.

63. Levy JH, Welsby I, Goodnough LT. Fibrinogen as a therapeutic target for bleeding: a review of critical levels and replacement therapy. Transfusion 2014;54:1389-405.

64. Gabay M, Boucher BA. An essential primer for understanding the role fo topical hemostats, sugical sealants, and adhesives for maintaining hemostasis. Pharmacotherapy 2013;33:935-55.

65. Spotnitz WD, Burks S. Hemostats, sealants, and adhesives III: a new update as well as cost and regulatory considerations for components of the surgical toolbox. Transfusion 2012;52:2243-55.

66. Achneck HE, Sileshi B, Jamiolkowski RM, et al. A comprehensive review of topical hemostatic agents: efficacy and recommendations for use. Ann Surg 2010;251:217-28.

67. MacLaren R. Key concepts in the management of difficult hemorrhagic cases. Pharmacotherapy 2007;27(9 pt 2):S93S-102.

68. Guyatt GH, Akl EA, Crowther M, et al. Introduction to the ninth edition: Antithrombotic Therapy and Prevention of Thrombosis, 9th ed: American College of Chest Physicians Evidence-Based Clinical Practice Guidelines. Chest 2012;141(suppl 2):S48-52.

69. Goldstein JN, Refaai MA, Milling TJ Jr, et al. Four-factor prothrombin complex concentrate versus plasma for rapid vitamin K antagonist reversal in patients needing urgent surgical or invasive interventions: a phase 3b, open-label, non-inferiority, randomised trial. Lancet 2015;385:2077-87.

70. Khorsand N, Kooistra HA, van Hest RM, et al. A systematic review of prothrombin complex concentrate dosing strategies to reverse vitamin K antagonist therapy. Thromb Res 2015;135:9-19.

71. Joseph B, Aziz H, Pandit V, et al. Prothrombin complex concentrate versus fresh-frozen plasma for reversal of coagulopathy of trauma: is there a difference? World J Surg 2014;38:1875-81.

72. Levi M, Peters M, Buller HR. Efficacy and safety of recombinant factor VIIa for treatment of severe bleeding: a systemic review. Crit Care Med 2005;33:883-90.

73. Yank V, Tuohy CV, Logan AC, et al. Systematic review: benefit and harms of in-hospital use of recombinant factor VIIa for off-label indications. Ann Intern Med 2011;154:529-40.

74. Levi M, Levy JH, Andersen HF, et al. Safety of recombinant activated factor VII in randomized clinical trials. N Engl J Med 2011;363:1791-800.

75. Manjuladevi M, Vasudeva Upadhyaya KS. Perioperative blood management. Indian J Anaesth 2014;58:573-80.

76. Ranucci M. Hemostatic and thrombotic issues in cardiac surgery. Semin Thromb Hemost 2015;41:84-90.

77. da Luz TL, Nascimento B, Rizoli S. Thromboelastography (TEG®): practical consideration on its clinical use in trauma resuscitation. Scand J Trauma Resusc Emerg Med 2013;21:29.

78. Hunt H, Stanworth S, Curry N, et al. Thromboelastography (TEG) and rotational thromboelastometry (ROTEM) for trauma induced coagulopathy in adult trauma patients with bleeding. Cochrane Database Syst Rev 2015;2:CD010438.

79. Ker K, Prieto-Merino D, Roberts I. Systemic review, meta-analysis and meta-regression of the effect of tranexamic acid on surgical blood loss. Br J Surg 2013;100:1271-9.

80. Ker K, Edwards P, Perel P, et al. Effect of tranexamic acid on surgical bleeding: systematic review and cumulative meta-analysis. BMJ 2012;344:e3054.

81. Gando S. Hemostasis and thrombosis in trauma patients. Semin Thromb Hemost 2015;41:26-34.

82. Ward KR. The microcirculation: linking trauma and coagulopathy. Transfusion 2013;53:S38-47.

83. Godier A, Samama CM, Susen S. Plasma/platelets/red blood cell ratio in the management of the bleeding traumatized patient: does it matter? Curr Opin Anaesthesiol 2012;25:242-7.

84. Kutcher ME, Kornblith LZ, Narayan R, et al. A paradigm shift in trauma resuscitation: evaluation of evolving massive transfusion practices. JAMA Surg 2013;148:834-40.

85. Malone DL, Hess JR, Fingerhut A. Massive transfusion practices around the globe and a suggestion for a common massive transfusion protocol. J Trauma 2006;60:S91-96.

86. Lal, DS, Shaz BH. Massive transfusion: blood component ratios. Curr Opin Hematol 2013;20:521-5.

87. McDaniel LM, Etchill EW, Raval JS, et al. State of the art: massive transfusion. Transfusion Med 2014;24:138-44.

88. Holcomb JB, Del Junco DJ, Fox EE, et al. The prospective, observational multicenter, major trauma transfusion (PROMMTT) study: comparative effectiveness of a time varying treatment with competing risks. JAMA Surg 2013;148:127-36.

89. Holcomb JB, Tilley BC, Baraniuk S, et al. Transfusion of plasma, platelets, and red blood cells in a 1:1:1 vs a 1:1:2 ratio and mortality in patients with severe trauma: the PROPPR randomized clinical trial. JAMA 2015;313:471-82.

90. Shakur H, Roberts I, Bautista R, et al. Effects of tranexamic acid on death, vascular occlusive events, and blood transfusion in trauma patients with significant haemorrhage (CRASH-2): a randomised, placebo-controlled trial. Lancet 2010;376:23-32.

91. Roberts I, Prieto-Merino D, Manno D. Mechanism of action of tranexamic acid in bleeding trauma patients: an exploratory analysis of data from the CRASH-2 trial. Crit Care 2014;18:685.

92. Roberts I, Shakur H, Afolabi A, et al. The importance of early treatment with tranexamic acid in bleeding trauma patients: an exploratory analysis of the CRASH-2 randomised controlled trial. Lancet 2011;377:1096-101.

93. Roberts I, Prieto-Merino D. Applying results from clinical trials: tranexamic acid in trauma patients. J Intensive Care 2014;2:56.

94. Roberts I, Shakur H, Coats T, et al. Effect of tranexamic acid on mortality in patients with traumatic bleeding: prespecified analysis of data from randomised controlled trial. BMJ 2012;345:e5839.

95. Roberts I, Shakur H, Coats T, et al. The CRASH-2 trial: a randomised controlled trial and economic evaluation of the effects of tranexamic acid on death, vascular occlusive events and transfusion requirement in bleeding trauma patients. Health Technol Assess 2013;17:1-79.

96. Boffard KD, Riou B, Warren B, et al. Recombinant factor VIIa as adjunctive therapy for bleeding control in severely injured trauma patients: two parallel randomized, placebo-controlled, double-blind clinical trials. J Trauma 2005;59:8-15.

97. Rizoli SB, Boffard KD, Riou B, et al. Recombinant activated factor VII as an adjunctive therapy for bleeding control in severe trauma patients with coagulopathy: subgroup analysis from two randomized trials. Crit Care 2006;10:R178.

98. Hauser CJ, Boffard K, Dutton R, et al. Results of the CONTROL trial: efficacy and safety of recombinant activated factor VII in the management of refractory traumatic hemorrhage. J Trauma 2010;69:489-500.

99. Dutton RP, Parr M, Tortella BJ, et al. Recombinant activated factor VII safety in trauma patients: results from the CONTROL trial. J Trauma 2011;71:12-9.

100. Bosch J, Thabut D, Bendtsen F. Recombinant factor VIIa for upper gastrointestinal bleeding in patients with cirrhosis: a randomized, double-blind trial. Gastroenterology 2004;127:1123-30.

101. Bosch J, Thabut D, Albillos A, et al. Recombinant factor VIIa for variceal bleeding in patients with advanced cirrhosis: a randomized controlled trial. Hepatology 2008;47:1604-14.

102. Planinsic RM, van der Meer J, Testa G, et al. Safety and efficacy of a single bolus administration of recombinant factor VIIa in liver transplantation due to chronic liver disease. Liver Transpl 2005;11:895-900.

103. Caldwell SH, Chang C, Macik BG. Recombinant factor VII (rVIIa) as a hemostatic agent in liver disease: a break from convention in need of controlled trials. Hepatology 2004;39:592-8.

104. Abdul-Kadir R, McLintock C, Ducloy AS, et al. Evaluation and management of postpartum hemorrhage: consensus from an international expert panel. Transfusion 2014;54:1756-68.

105. Butwick AJ, Goodnough LT. Transfusion and coagulation management in major obstetric hemorrhage. Curr Opin Anaesthesiol 2015;28:275-84.

106. Ducloy-Bouthors AS, Jude B, Duhamel A, et al. High-dose tranexamic acid reduces blood loss in postpartum haemorrhage. Crit Care 2011;15:R117.

107. Pollack CV Jr, Reilly PA, Eikelboom J, et al. Idarucizumab for dabigatran reversal. N Engl J Med 2015;373:511-20.

Chapter 25

Laboratory Testing with Anticoagulation

Tyree H. Kiser, Pharm.D., FCCP, FCCM, BCPS

LEARNING OBJECTIVES

1. Describe the most common laboratory methods for evaluating anticoagulation in critically ill patients.
2. Discuss the potential limitations of laboratory tests used to evaluate anticoagulation in critically ill patients.
3. Identify patient characteristics common to critically ill patients that should be considered when interpreting laboratory tests used for monitoring anticoagulation.
4. Compare and contrast different laboratory methods used to evaluate commonly prescribed anticoagulants.

ABBREVIATIONS IN THIS CHAPTER

ACT	Activated clotting time	MA	Maximum amplitude
aPTT	Activated partial thromboplastin time	PT	Prothrombin time
DOAC	Direct-acting oral anticoagulant	ROTEM	Rotational thromboelastography
DTI	Direct thrombin inhibitor	TEG	Thromboelastography
dTT	Dilute thrombin time or plasma diluted thrombin time	TT	Thrombin time
		UFH	Unfractionated heparin
ICU	Intensive care unit	VTE	Venous thromboembolism
LMWH	Low-molecular-weight heparin		

INTRODUCTION

Coagulation tests are often used within critical care medicine. Accurate measurement of the coagulation status can be crucial for the correct treatment of an intensive care unit (ICU) patient. Coagulation tests may be used to evaluate patients for coagulation abnormalities or comorbidities, for diagnostic purposes, or to monitor antithrombotic medications.[1] Many variables, including critical illness, must be considered when interpreting coagulation tests in the ICU because they may affect the accuracy of test results.[2] This chapter will review most of the coagulation tests available for critical care clinicians. When interpreting information provided within this chapter, it is important to understand that different instruments and testing approaches are used depending on the health care institution. Therefore, tests may be used differently, and variability in reported values should be expected when comparing information provided within this chapter, data from available clinical studies, and laboratory results in your clinical setting. Of note, laboratory tests used for monitoring anticoagulants are by definition a surrogate marker for anticoagulation outcomes. In many situations, laboratory tests and therapeutic ranges have been developed according to in vitro mechanisms and have not been formally evaluated in clinical trials to determine their correlation with definitive outcomes such as thromboembolism or bleeding. It is critical that interpretation of the results from the coagulation tests used be confirmed with the clinical scenario observed at the bedside.

METHODS OF COAGULATION TESTING

Coagulation testing can be conducted by different methodologies, with most tests being either functional or antigenic (Box 25.1). Clot-based assays typically use citrated platelet-poor plasma. The testing is performed with the use of reagents at normal body temperature (37°C). Some tests (e.g., activated partial thromboplastin time [aPTT]) require a short incubation period to allow activator and phospholipids

Box 25.1. Coagulation Test Methodology[3]

Functional tests:
Clotting end point – Adding patient plasma to reagent(s) and then determining the amount of clot formation. Examples: PT (prothrombin time), aPTT (activated partial thromboplastin time), ACT (activated clotting time), TT (thrombin time), fibrinogen, factor activity

Chromogenic testing – Adding patient plasma to reagent(s) and then determining the amount of color formation. Examples: Factor activity, anti-Xa, antithrombin activity

Aggregation – Adding patient plasma (platelet poor or containing platelets) to platelets and/or agonist(s) and measuring light scattering (agglutination) or platelet clumping (aggregation). Examples: Heparin-induced thrombocytopenia, platelet function

Antigenic tests:
Immunologic – Adding patient plasma or serum to beads or microwells containing target antigen or antibody and then assessing color changes, changes in agglutination, hemagglutination, etc. Examples: Fibrinogen, factor activity, D-dimer, heparin-induced thrombocytopenia, antithrombin

to interact with plasma factors. The clotting end point is determined by changes in light scattering because of turbidity induced by fibrin formation.[3] Chromogenic versions of assays use a color formed after the addition of reagent to determine the anticoagulant activity present (Figure 25.1). Antibody-related assays incorporate an antigen/antibody complex to measure a specific antigen or antibody present within the patient sample. Some assays must be performed by a laboratory, whereas others can be conducted at or near the bedside (commonly called point-of-care testing). Point-of-care testing, which has increased in availability and popularity, is often used in operating rooms and in some critical care specialty units. As a rule, point-of-care testing results should be evaluated in comparison with central laboratory results. Bias in results should be expected, especially at the low and high ends of the testing range for many tests.[3]

Most screening coagulation assays (e.g., prothrombin time [PT] or aPTT) are based on how rapidly fibrin clots form in patient samples. The type of activator used will trigger different coagulation pathways. For example, thromboplastin is used to trigger the extrinsic pathway, kaolin is used to trigger the intrinsic pathway, and viper venoms are used to trigger the common pathway. There are different methods of detecting the formation of fibrin in these assays, including visual, mechanical, photo-optical, and viscoelastographic techniques (Figure 25.2).

REGULATORY REQUIREMENTS FOR CLINICAL USE OF LABORATORY TESTS

Clinical Laboratory Improvement Amendments (CLIA) regulations govern the use of laboratory tests in patients. The U.S. Food and Drug Administration (FDA)-approved commercially available tests must comply with these regulations. However, in many coagulation tests, institutions must individually determine the accuracy, precision, and reportable ranges. Any modifications to an FDA-approved test, the use of a "for research purposes only test," or the use of a homegrown test requires that the laboratory evaluate the performance of the assay according to the CLIA regulations, with additional testing for sensitivity and specificity.

OBTAINING A RELIABLE SAMPLE FOR TESTING

Acquiring and appropriately delivering a patient sample to the laboratory for analysis is a critical step in evaluating anticoagulant intensity. The sample should be free of tissue and intravenous solutions delivered through indwelling lines. Obtaining a proper sample is most problematic in patients with a central venous catheter, particularly those being used for extracorporeal circuits or that have large volumes of medication infusions running through them. If syringes are used for collecting the sample, immediate (within 1 minute) transfer to the collection tube will minimize alterations in coagulation test results. Adequate techniques should be used to avoid dilution of the sample or contamination with infusing medications during the collection process. Samples should not be placed on ice because this can affect factor and platelet function. Withdrawal and waste of 5–10 mL of volume may be necessary before a proper blood draw can be obtained. Once the sample is obtained, it should be sent to the laboratory quickly and preferably tested within 2 hours. Prolonged

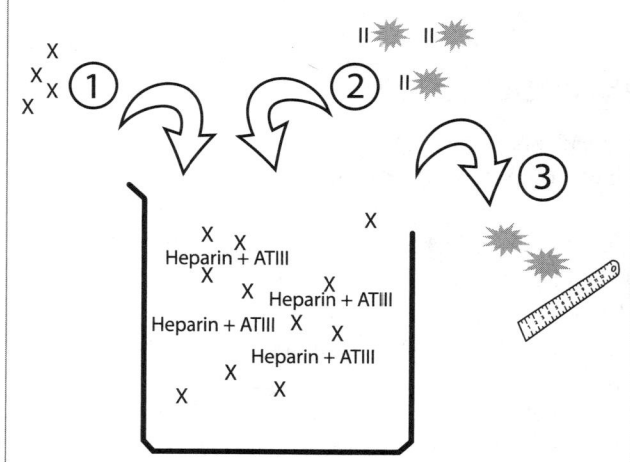

Figure 25.1 Chromogenic anti-Xa test.

Figure 25.1 depicts how the chromogenic anti-Xa assay is performed. Blood activates the patient's antithrombin III, and they both act to deactivate the factor X. As heparin level in the blood increases, more factor X is deactivated, and the less active Xa is left in the test tube. Factor II (marked with a yellow marker) is added into the test tube. The active Xa remaining interacts with the factor II, and the yellow marker is released. This is then measured. The amount of heparin is deduced from the amount of color change.

incubation at room temperature for greater than 24 hours can result in significantly altered activity of clotting factors.[4] The appropriateness of a blood draw should be considered any time a result is discordant with what is being observed clinically in a patient. If the test is believed to be misrepresenting the clinical scenario, repeating a test may be necessary before making clinical decisions.

BASELINE LABORATORY STUDIES FOR PATIENTS INITIATED ON ANTICOAGULATION

All critically ill patients should have certain laboratory tests measured before initiation of anticoagulation therapy. At a minimum, a baseline complete blood cell count to evaluate platelets, hemoglobin, and hematocrit and an assessment of renal function and hepatic function tests should be considered. Platelet monitoring should continue during therapy for patients taking heparin products (see Chapter 23, "Prevention and Treatment of Venous Thromboembolism"). Laboratory tests to evaluate for thrombophilias such as lupus anticoagulant (e.g., dilute Russell viper venom time and lupus-sensitive PTT) should be considered in patients with an unexplained thrombosis in a vein or artery, recurrent miscarriages, or an unexplained prolonged PTT test.

For many anticoagulant tests, it is important to determine whether the patient's baseline values are within normal limits so that clinicians can determine whether alterations in the target therapeutic range or additional testing is needed. These include the PT/international normalized ratio (INR) (if initiating Coumadin) and the aPTT (if initiating UFH or a direct thrombin inhibitor [DTI]). The patient's weight and creatinine clearance should be measured for any weight-based medications that are renally eliminated. The decision to monitor these laboratory values and the frequency of monitoring throughout anticoagulation therapy should be considered depending on the anticoagulant chosen, laboratory test, and clinical situation. Physical examination findings, ultrasonography, Doppler, computed tomography, or other imaging studies may be useful for evaluating the presence or extension of thromboembolism and should be evaluated as appropriate in addition to coagulation tests to assist with anticoagulant choice, dosing, and monitoring strategies.

ALTERATIONS IN COAGULATION TESTING

When interpreting the results of a coagulation test, it is critically important to determine whether the test is providing an accurate assessment of the patient's coagulation status. To do this, everything from the time of the blood draw until the result is reported from the laboratory must be evaluated. Most blood samples collected for coagulation

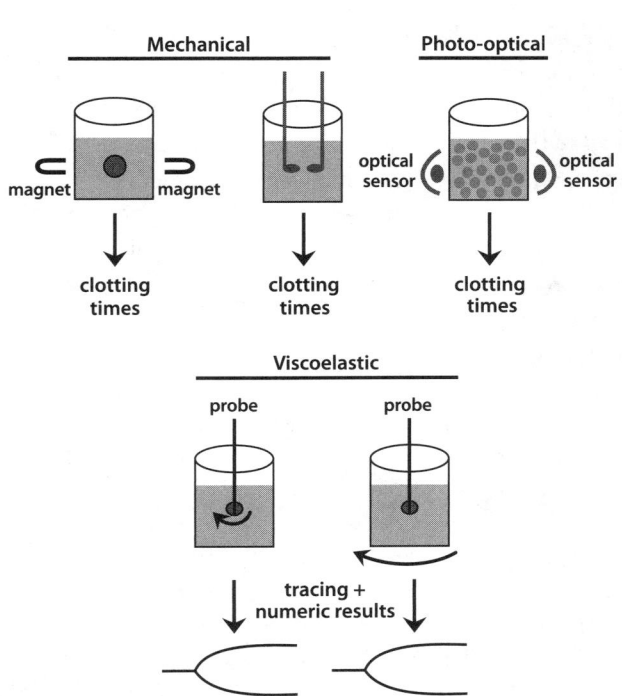

Figure 25.2 Methods of clot detection.

Mechanical: There are different mechanical methods, but these are either based on the movement of a metal ball between two magnets or based on the movement of two probes inserted within the patient sample. Fibrin formation restricts movement of the magnetic ball or movement of the probe in relation to each other, resulting in a finite end point, which is recorded as the clotting time.

Photo-optical: With this technique, fibrin formation is detected by the change in optical density or turbidity of the sample. The results are usually recorded as the time to clot; however, some analyzers also provide a curve of clot formation.

Viscoelastic: With this technique, a probe is inserted into a cup containing the patient sample. Then, either the probe is rotated within the cup or the cup is rotated around a fixed probe. Changes in the movement of the cup in relation to the probe result in a tracing that reflects the kinetics of fibrin formation and fibrinolysis, with numerical measurements pertaining to these kinetics and the strength of the resulting fibrin clot.

testing will be placed in a tube containing citrate, which inhibits coagulation by binding to calcium. As mentioned previously, it is preferred to use systems that allow for direct transfer from a vascular device to the collection tube. In addition to alterations in results because of improper acquisition or handling of the sample, patient factors or conditions can affect laboratory tests. Common conditions affecting PT and aPTT are listed in Table 25.1. In certain situations listed in Table 25.1, the CLSI (Clinical & Laboratory Standards Institute) guidelines require special processing of specimens. For example, in specimens from patients with polycythemia or hematocrit values greater than 55%, a spurious prolongation of coagulation studies may occur because of a relative excess of citrate anticoagulant in relation to plasma volume. If the citrate concentration is not adjusted in this situation, citrate may bind to calcium added to initiate the clotting process and slow its initiation, leading to prolonged PT and aPTT.[5]

The complex interplay of patient, sample, and laboratory environment factors makes communication with the laboratory an important part of patient care. Alerting laboratory staff to the anticoagulant being monitored and the condition of the patient may provide them with enough information to allow for sample alteration (e.g., dilution of sample), additional testing, or correction of values. They can also provide clinicians with specific information regarding the reagents being used and their sensitivity to outside influences commonly occurring in critically ill patients.

PT AND INR

The PT is a measure of the extrinsic and final common pathway of clotting. This consists of tissue factor, fibrinogen (I), and coagulation factors II, V, VII, and X (Figure 25.3). In hospitalized patients, the PT is done on a venipuncture-acquired sample and analyzed using a laboratory-based coagulation analyzer. In the test, clotting is initiated by recalcifying citrated patient plasma in the presence of thromboplastin. The PT measures the time it takes plasma to form a fibrin clot after the addition of calcium and thromboplastin. The clot can be detected by visual, optical, or electromechanical means. The PT result is expressed in seconds. Variations in PT occur because of the source of thromboplastin and the type of instrument used for clot detection. Therefore, thromboplastin reagent sensitivity is expressed using the term *international sensitivity index* (*ISI*). The INR was created as a mechanism to adjust for variation in PTs because of thromboplastin reagent sensitivity.

The equation for the INR is as follows:

$$INR = [\text{patient PT/laboratory's geometric mean for normal patients}]^{ISI}$$

The PT/INR is sensitive to the vitamin K–dependent clotting factors (e.g., factors II, VII, and X); therefore, it is commonly used to evaluate the anticoagulant effects of vitamin K antagonists. Of note, the INR describes only the activity of factors II, VII, and X, and not factor IX or protein C and S. Most PT reagents also contain heparin-binding chemicals to block the effect of unfractionated heparin (UFH), low-molecular-weight heparin (LMWH), and fondaparinux.

Table 25.1 Common Diseases or Conditions Affecting the Accuracy of PT or aPTT Results

Increased PT and/or aPTT	Decreased PT and/or aPTT
Low-volume sample (increased citrate/plasma ratio)	Decreased hematocrit (< 25%)
Elevated hematocrit (> 55%)	Elevated calcium concentrations
Prolonged time between draw and analysis	Administration of plasma products (e.g., FFP, cryoprecipitate, prothrombin complex concentrates)
Hemodilution	
Contamination with infusing medication (e.g., heparin, citrate)	
Hypothermia	
Deficiency in factor II, V, VII, VIII, IX, X, XI, or XII	
Hereditary factor deficiencies	
Antiphospholipid antibodies	
Hepatic disease	
Consumptive coagulopathy	
Disseminated intravascular coagulation	
Excess PRBC transfusion	
Citrate administration	
Volume expansion (e.g., starches)	
Medications:	
Daptomycin	
Activated protein C	
Direct thrombin inhibitors	
Heparin or LMWH	
Thrombolytics	

aPTT = activated partial thromboplastin time; PRBC = packed red blood cell; PT = prothrombin time.

However, at high heparin levels, the heparin binders may become saturated, and the PT may be prolonged.

For most patients taking warfarin, the goal steady-state INR for most indications is 2–3. The full anticoagulant effect of warfarin is delayed until the normal clotting factors are eliminated from the circulation. The INR is less accurate during the initial few days of warfarin therapy because the INR is most reflective of reductions in factor VII, which has a much shorter half-life than factor II. This may lead a clinician to assume that a greater degree of anticoagulation is present in the patient than actually exists. In contrast, as warfarin is held or removed, an increase in factor VII activity may have a reduction in INR that underestimates the degree of anticoagulation present. Inaccuracies can also occur because of errors in ISI reporting or use and differences in laboratory instrumentation. Co-morbidities such as hepatic disease and the presence of lupus anticoagulant can prolong the INR. The use of anticoagulants such as DTIs can prolong the PT/INR in a dose-dependent fashion. The DTIs interact with the coagulation test, and of note, a prolonged PT/INR is not indicative of their anticoagulant effect. The elevation in INR can be significant, particularly with the parenteral anticoagulants, with argatroban causing greater increases than bivalirudin, lepirudin, and desirudin. The effects of dabigatran on the INR are less pronounced.

CHROMOGENIC FACTOR X ACTIVITY

The chromogenic factor X assay is an alternative to the INR for monitoring patients taking warfarin. The chromogenic factor X assay is a phospholipid-independent test, which prevents it from being altered by coagulation abnormalities such as lupus anticoagulant. In this case, the chromogenic factor X activity can be measured at same interval as the INR would typically be completed. Chromogenic factor X results are reported as a percentage of normal activity and are inversely related to INR values. A chromogenic factor X level of 20%–25% approximates an INR of 3, and a level of 40%–45% approximates an INR of 2. The main drawbacks of the test include its expense and availability. Results may take 24–72 hours depending on the availability of the laboratory within the institution.

In addition to using it in patients with altered INR values at baseline, the chromogenic factor X activity assay may be useful for monitoring warfarin in critically ill patients who are taking DTIs and transitioning to warfarin therapy. Interpretation of the INR can be difficult in these patients because DTIs inhibit thrombin and prevent fibrin clot formation. This results in a falsely elevated PT and INR in a concentration-dependent manner. Because DTIs do not affect factor X, a potential option to evaluate the effects of warfarin without having to hold DTI therapy is to use the chromogenic factor X assay. The chromogenic factor X assay is capable of evaluating the effects of warfarin while excluding the anticoagulant effects of DTIs. Similar to patients on warfarin monotherapy, a chromogenic factor X level of less than 45% predicts an INR of 2 or greater with around 80% specificity and 60%–90% sensitivity.[6,7] Once this level is achieved, a therapeutic INR for warfarin should be verified by discontinuing the DTI and measuring a PT/INR after the DTI has been appropriately cleared (typically 4 hours or more after discontinuing the DTI) from the systemic circulation. Although this approach is likely to be reasonable for most critically ill patients, the reliability of the chromogenic factor X assay is diminished in patients with hepatic dysfunction or vitamin K deficiency.

ACTIVATED PARTIAL THROMBOPLASTIN TIME

The aPTT is a global assay of coagulation. The aPTT can be used to screen for inhibitors and deficiencies of the intrinsic pathway (prekallikrein, high-molecular-weight kininogen, factors XII, XI, IX, and VIII) and the final common pathway (factors II, X, V, prothrombin) and fibrinogen (Figure 25.3). The aPTT is performed by recalcifying citrated plasma in the presence of a thromboplastic material that does not have tissue factor activity and

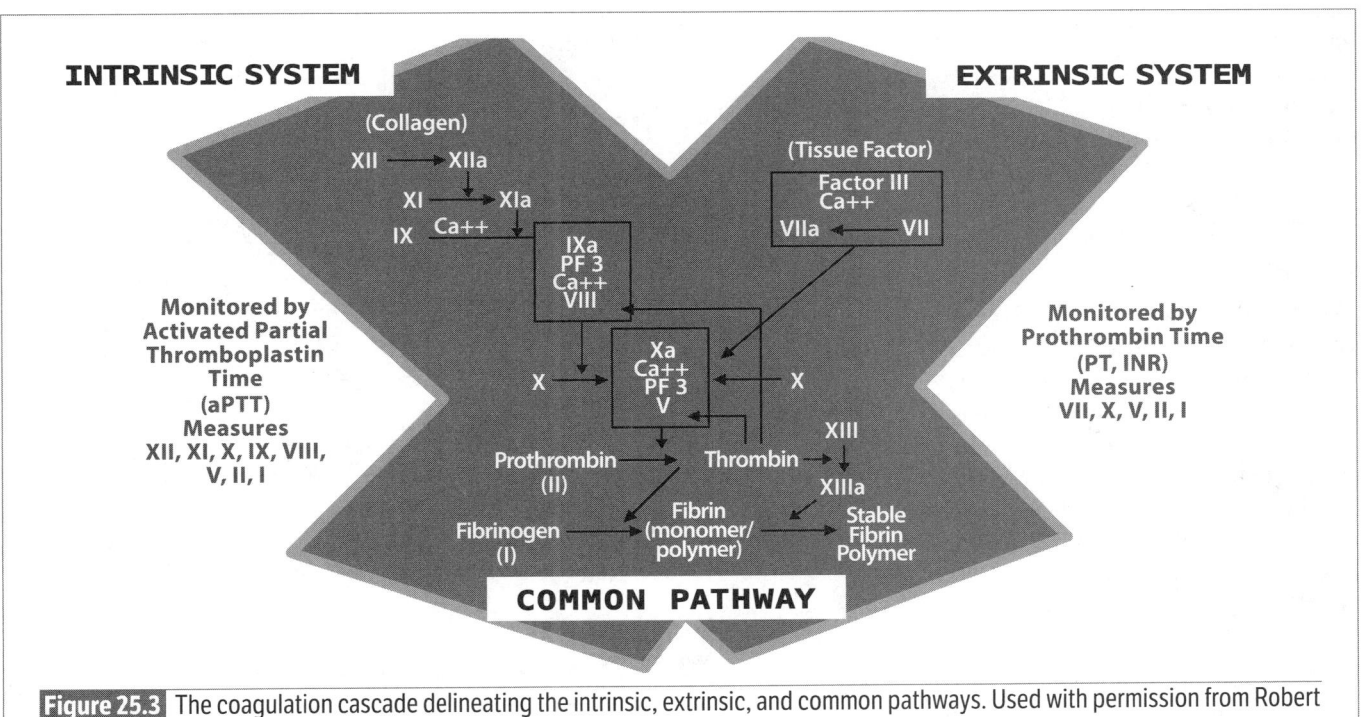

Figure 25.3 The coagulation cascade delineating the intrinsic, extrinsic, and common pathways. Used with permission from Robert MacLaren, Chapter 24, page 470.

a negatively charged substance (e.g., kaolin), which results in contact factor activation, thereby initiating coagulation by the intrinsic pathway. Several variables can affect the aPTT including sample timing, site of sample, citrate concentration, and sample handling and processing time (Table 25.1). The reagents used for the aPTT vary in type of contact activator, phospholipid composition, and concentration. Deficiency in all clotting factors except factor VII can cause prolongation of the aPTT. The relationship between the factor activity in the blood and the aPTT result is logarithmic. For elevated baseline aPTTs, a lower level of change is needed for additional prolongation.

The aPTT is the most common test used for monitoring UFH therapy, although the evidence for adjusting the UFH dose to maintain a therapeutic aPTT range is based on a post hoc analysis of a prospective descriptive study.[8,9] Most patients evaluated (n=162) were receiving heparin therapy for venous thromboembolism (VTE). Heparin was titrated to an aPTT between 1.5 and 2.5 times control values, and the analysis showed that an aPTT greater than 1.5 times control was associated with reduced recurrent VTE.[9] Therefore, this goal aPTT range became widely accepted in clinical practice. Unfortunately, this therapeutic range has not been confirmed by a randomized clinical trial, and it does not account for significant variability in the aPTT test observed both within and between institutions. Because of this, the goal therapeutic aPTT range varies, depending on the aPTT reagent, the instrument, and the reagent's responsiveness to each lot of UFH. Therefore, the traditional reported therapeutic range of 60–80 seconds (e.g., about 1.5–2.5 times control) cannot accurately be used within hospital settings without evaluation of a specific aPTT reagent's sensitivity to heparin. The therapeutic range is calculated using a regression analysis evaluating values obtained from samples containing known levels of heparin and samples from patients on UFH therapy by aPTT versus the anti-factor Xa (anti-Xa) activity (e.g., heparin levels). In the original study described previously, the investigators established that an aPTT ratio of 1.5–2.5 corresponded to a heparin level of 0.2–0.4 international units/mL by protamine titration and a heparin level of 0.3–0.7 international units/mL measured by anti-Xa assay.[9] Therefore, most institutions set their aPTT goal range for VTE at 0.3–0.7 international units/mL of anti-Xa activity (Figure 25.4).[8] The goal therapeutic aPTT range for other UFH indications is less clear, which commonly results in a variety of goal ranges depending on the type of critically ill patient and the therapeutic end points. The sensitivity of a reagent will determine the aPTT response, with more sensitive reagents resulting in steeper regression slopes and higher aPTT goal ranges. It is important for institutions to use plasma samples from patients on heparin treatment rather than simply using spiked heparin samples because using spiked samples often results in therapeutic ranges higher than those calibrated from actual patient samples. The heparin therapeutic range needs to be reevaluated with each new lot number of reagent or change in reagent manufacturer. If there is a clinically significant change in the therapeutic range (e.g., greater than 5–10 seconds), adjustment of the therapeutic range reported by the laboratory is needed. In addition, protocols used throughout the health system should be adjusted as appropriate (Figure 25.5).

Monitoring anticoagulants by the aPTT can be problematic for many reasons and may be reflective of factors independent of the anticoagulant being used. As mentioned previously, results vary depending on the aPTT reagent and lot number. The aPTT can be shortened or prolonged because of deficiency or excess of coagulation factors. In addition, the phospholipids within the assay make it vulnerable to interference from lupus inhibitors. Discordance between anti-Xa activity and aPTT results can occur in a significant number of hospitalized patients on UFH. As seen in Figure 25.6, patients with a goal aPTT measurement may actually have a sub- or supratherapeutic anti-Xa level. Conversely, patients with an aPTT outside the goal range may actually have a therapeutic anti-Xa level. For this reason, many institutions have changed to monitoring UFH according to anti-Xa results; however, consideration of the concordance or discordance with aPTT values in critically ill patients may provide a clearer picture of global coagulation and correlate better with clinical outcomes. In a recent study of 2,321 paired values from 539 patients, 42% of data pairs had

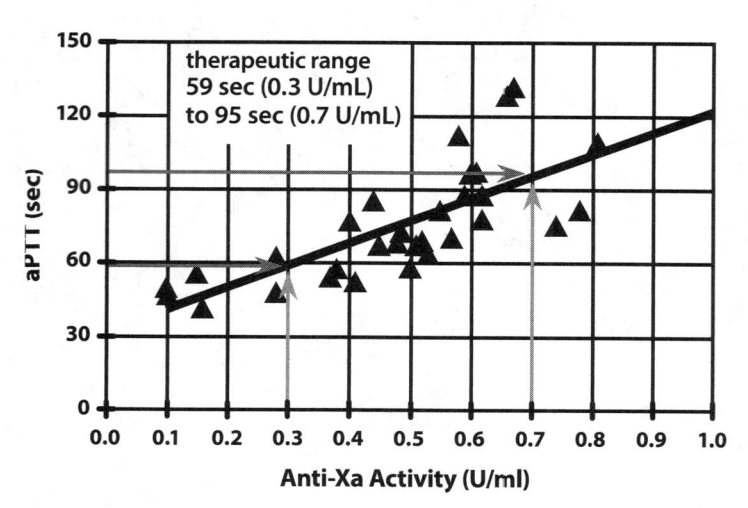

Figure 25.4 Calibrating the goal activated partial thromboplastin time range that corresponds to an anti-Xa activity of 0.3–0.7 for unfractionated heparin.

Standard-Dose Heparin Therapy (DVT/PE Treatment) Goal aPTT range is equivalent to heparin level of 0.3–0.7 units/mL			Lower-Dose Heparin Therapy (ACS/MI, Stroke, AF, Other) Goal aPTT Range is equivalent to 1.5–2.5 times baseline aPTT		
aPTT(s)	aPTT(s)	Dose Adjustment	aPTT(s)	aPTT(s)	Dose Adjustment
< 40	< ___	Bolus 40 units/kg, Increase infusion by 3 units/kg/hr	< 30	< ___	Increase infusion by 3 units/kg/hr
40–53	___ - ___	Bolus 20 units/kg, Increase infusion by 2 units/kg/hr	30–39	___ - ___	Increase infusion by 2 units/kg/hr
54–67	___ - ___	Increase infusion by 1 unit/kg/hr	40–49	___ - ___	Increase infusion by 1 unit/kg/hr
68–90	___ - ___	Goal Range. No Change	50–80	___ - ___	Goal Range. No Change
91–104	___ - ___	Decrease infusion by 1 unit/kg/hr	81–90	___ - ___	Decrease infusion by 1 unit/kg/hr
105–118	___ - ___	Hold infusion for 0.5 hour, decrease infu-sion by 2 units/kg/hr	91–100	___ - ___	Hold infusion for 0.5 hour, decrease in-fusion by 2 units/kg/hr
119–200	___ - ___	Hold infusion for 1 hour, decrease infusion by 3 units/kg/hr	101–200	___ - ___	Hold infusion for 1 hour, decrease infu-sion by 3 units/ kg/hr
> 200	> ___	Send **stat** aPTT, contact physician, HOLD infusion until aPTT < 200 (check q6hr), then decrease infusion by 4 units/kg/hr	> 200	> ___	Send stat aPTT, contact physician, HOLD infusion until aPTT < 200 (check q6hr); then decrease infusion by 4 units/kg/hr

ACS = acute coronary syndromes; AF = atrial fibrillation; DVT = deep venous thrombosis; MI = myocardial infarction; PE = pulmonary embolism; q = every.

Figure 25.5 Creation of goal aPTT targets and titration algorithms according to the correlation between anti-Xa and activated partial thromboplastin time results.

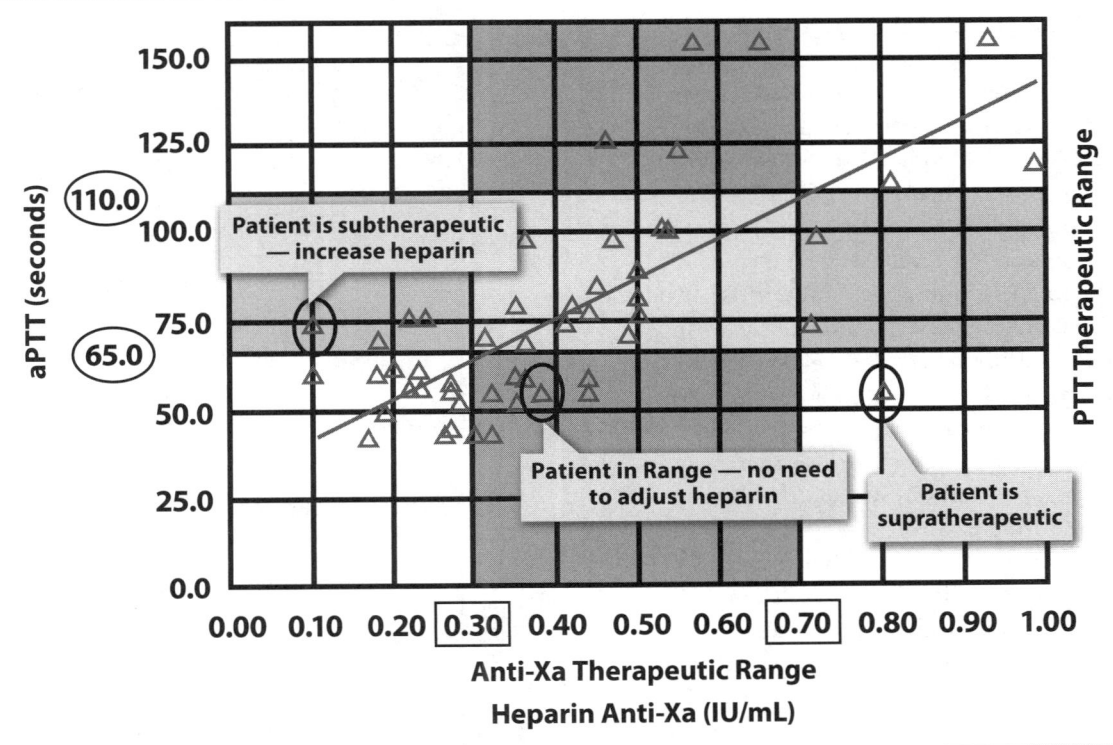

Figure 25.6 Discordance between activated partial thromboplastin time and anti-Xa measurement.

a high aPTT value relative to the anti-Xa value. Patients with elevated baseline PT/INR or aPTT often had disproportionate relative prolongation of the aPTT. Patients with at least two consecutive high aPTT to anti-Xa values had increased 21-day major bleeding (9% vs. 3%; p=0.0316) and 30-day mortality (14% dead vs. 5% dead at 30 days; p=0.0202) compared with patients with consistently concordant values.[10] The results of this study call for the potential need to evaluate both tests at least initially to identify patients with significantly discordant aPTT and anti-Xa findings to proactively determine whether they may be at risk of bleeding or thrombosis.

Unfractionated heparin resistance can also be identified by failure to obtain a therapeutic aPTT despite escalating doses of UFH (e.g., greater than 25 units/kg/hour). If this occurs, evaluation of antithrombin III activity may need to be considered. However, the low response to heparin may be because of increased clearance, increased binding to heparin-binding proteins, or increases in acute-phase reactants such as factor VIII or fibrinogen.[8]

The aPTT is the most common test used for monitoring parenteral DTI therapy (e.g., argatroban or bivalirudin). Although the aPTT is used to monitor DTIs, the dose-response is not linear, and the aPTT reaches a ceiling threshold with high concentrations of the drug in plasma. The goal therapeutic aPTT range for parenteral DTIs is not the same as the heparin-calibrated curve by the anti-Xa regression analysis. Many centers simply use the DTI package insert–recommended aPTT goals and create an individualized goal aPTT range on the basis of the patient's baseline aPTT (goal aPTT 1.5–3 times baseline aPTT for argatroban or 1.5–2.5 times baseline aPTT for bivalirudin). Alternative options are to create a titration algorithm that is based on the mean of the normal aPTT range (or, in some cases, the upper end of the normal range) to create a standard aPTT goal for all patients (Figure 25.7).[11,12] Given that many critically ill patients do not have a normal aPTT at baseline, this approach may be limited. Laboratories can also create a therapeutic range that is based on spiked normal plasma with known concentrations of each DTI. This may allow for detecting different reagent lot sensitivities to the DTIs. However, the concentration versus aPTT regression line is curvilinear, and little evidence is currently available linking a goal range of DTI plasma concentrations to therapeutic and safety outcomes. Other options include the development of aPTT range using ecarin chromogenic or dilute thrombin time or plasma diluted thrombin time (dTT) assays, but these require a clinical laboratory to perform significant validation steps throughout the process and are more cumbersome than the methods mentioned earlier.

The timing of aPTT monitoring varies between institution, DTI, and organ function and expected time to steady state (extended time to steady state would be expected for argatroban in patients with hepatic impairment and bivalirudin in patients with renal impairment). When developing an aPTT monitoring plan for parenteral DTIs, an aPTT should be monitored within 2–4 hours of initiation or after any dosing change. After this, the aPTT can be monitored every 4–6 hours until at least two consecutive aPTTs are within the goal range. Once this occurs, the frequency can be extended to once daily.[8,11,12]

ANTI-Xa MONITORING

The anti-Xa can be measured using a functional assay to determine anticoagulation intensity for anticoagulants that directly or indirectly affect factor Xa. The test is performed by adding patient plasma to a reagent factor Xa and measuring factor Xa activity using a substrate that releases a color compound when cleaved. The premise of the assay depends on the fact that the factor Xa activity is proportional to the amount of anticoagulant in the plasma. The most common

---

MONITORING

Nursing to titrate argatroban or bivalirudin infusion according to aPTT result using orders and the table below:

- ✓ Check aPTT at baseline, 2 hours after initiation, every 4 hours after any dosing change, and then every morning after two consecutive aPTTs in goal.
- ✓ Goal aPTT for argatroban and bivalirudin is 50–80 seconds (about 1.5–2.5 times the baseline aPTT). Standard aPTT goal and dosage adjustment will be used unless prescriber fills out "patient-specific aPTT goal" ranges in the table below

☐ Standard aPTT Goal	☐ Patient-Specific aPTT Goal	Dose Adjustment
Less than 35	Less than ____	Increase dose by 50%
35–44	____ – ____	Increase dose by 25%
45–49	____ – ____	Increase dose by 10%
50–80	____ – ____	**Goal Range. No Change**
81–90	____ – ____	Decrease dose by 10%
91–100	____ – ____	Hold infusion × 1 hour, decrease dose by 25%
Greater than 100	Greater than ____	Hold infusion × 2 hours, decrease dose by 50%

If aPTT greater than 200 seconds at any time point: hold infusion, send stat aPTT, and contact house officer.

If aPTT goal not achieved within 24 hours of initiation, contact house officer.

Figure 25.7 Example of a monitoring and titration algorithm for direct thrombin inhibitor therapy.

anti-Xa activity assays currently used are chromogenic because clot-based assays may underestimate activity.

Institutions may use a single hybrid anti-Xa curve for UFH and LMWH, or create separate titration curves. Anti-Xa assays are typically calibrated using UFH. It is important to verify that the correct calibrated anti-Xa curve is being used for the anticoagulant being tested. Of note, use of the UFH-derived curve to evaluate LMWH can underestimate the LMWH effect, whereas use of the LMWH curve for measuring UFH can overestimate the UFH effect. Because of these differences in calibration, target anti-Xa levels may vary between laboratories. In addition, the activity of fondaparinux and the direct-acting oral anticoagulants (DOACs) requires a separate anti-Xa calibration before the results can accurately be interpreted.

The anti-Xa goal range was originally established using protamine sulfate titration. Variability in assay performance can occur because of different lots of heparin, the addition of exogenous antithrombin, or variations in the process of creating the standard curve. Antithrombin supplementation or the administration of antithrombin either directly or indirectly (e.g., through the administration of fresh frozen plasma) may result in altered anti-Xa results. Other outside influences listed as having a potential to interfere with the reagent include plasma concentrations greater than 1.5 g/L hemoglobin (0.15 g% or greater plasma free hemoglobin), greater than 288 mg/L conjugated bilirubin (28.8 mg% or greater direct bilirubin), greater than 138 mg/L unconjugated bilirubin (13.8 g% or greater indirect bilirubin), and greater than 6.9 g/L triglycerides (690 mg% or greater triglycerides).

Despite the potential effects of outside influences, the anti-Xa provides a potentially more accurate measurement of UFH therapy. For this reason, many institutions have moved to monitoring UFH by anti-Xa rather than aPTT. The anti-Xa may be preferred to the aPTT for monitoring UFH in patients with suspected heparin resistance, lupus anticoagulant, or antiphospholipid antibodies or when the aPTT results do not appear to correlate with UFH dosing adjustments. In general, anti-Xa monitoring of UFH results in fewer variations in results, reduced testing, fewer dose changes, and more time within the therapeutic range. However, limited data are available regarding the use of anti-Xa–based titration and clinical outcomes, and as mentioned in the aPTT section within this chapter, discordance between the anti-Xa result and aPTT may be a predictor for risk of bleeding or thrombosis.[10] Monitoring of both the anti-Xa activity and the aPTT may be prudent in certain critically ill patients, such as those with hepatic disease, prolonged baseline clotting time, and significant thrombosis or risk of bleeding and those with factor inhibitors. However, there is little guidance on what clinicians should do if the aPTT and anti-Xa results are discordant. Ultimately, a decision on which assay to use will have to be made according to which laboratory test appears to be correlating best with the patient's clinical scenario.

The anti-Xa assay can be used similarly to the aPTT when dose adjusting heparin. The anti-Xa activity (heparin level) should be drawn at intervals similar to those recommended for the aPTT (e.g., every 6 hours initially and then at least daily after two consecutive levels in goal are achieved). Heparin nomograms can be used for titrating heparin in a fashion similar to those derived from the aPTT (Figure 25.8).

The anti-Xa assay is the preferred measurement for LMWH; however, monitoring is typically needed only in special populations. Such critical care populations include those with extremes of body weight (e.g., less than 50 kg or more than 150 kg), those with reduced creatinine clearance (e.g., less than 30 mL/minute), pediatric patients, trauma patients, patients with a potential for altered subcutaneous absorption (e.g., significant edema), pregnant patients with mechanical valves, or those with unexpected bleeding or thrombosis during therapy. Unlike UFH, where an anti-Xa level can be monitored anytime during the infusion, timing is important when monitoring LMWHs. A peak concentration should be drawn 4 hours after the subcutaneous dose of the LMWH. The goal anti-Xa varies depending on whether once- or twice-daily dosing is used, which LMWH is being administered, treatment versus prophylactic dosing, and the calibration of the assay by the laboratory. For example, the goal concentration for 1 mg/kg of twice-daily enoxaparin may be 0.6–1 IU/mL, and the goal concentration for 200 units/kg of once-daily dalteparin may be 1–2 IU/mL.[8] A peak concentration of 0.2–0.4 IU/mL or a trough concentration greater than 0.1 IU/mL has been suggested as a target for prophylactic dosing strategies.[13-15] Of note, a specifically calibrated assay must be used for monitoring fondaparinux. Goal concentrations for fondaparinux are not well established, but anti-Xa peak levels are about 0.39–0.5 mg/L for 2.5-mg/day doses and about 1.2 mg/L for 7.5-mg/day dosing. Clinicians should consult with their laboratory to determine the therapeutic ranges for the LMWH and dosing strategy used in their patient.

The heparin-calibrated chromogenic anti-Xa assay can also be used to quantitate the newer DOACs.[16] Currently, calibration kits for rivaroxaban and apixaban are available for research use only. However, hospitals may choose to calibrate their standard anti-Xa assay to measure these DOACs. Of note, the returned values for the DOAC will be significantly higher than those reported for UFH, and dilution of the sample may be required to fit the results within the laboratory's testing range. Although the PT may provide a quick qualitative assessment of the presence of a DOAC in the patient, the correlation with drug concentration is much higher with the anti-Xa assay than with the PT.[16] See Figure 25.9 through Figure 25.14.

HEPARIN TITRATION BY ANTI-Xa

Titrate heparin infusion according to heparin levels (if baseline aPTT value abnormal, consider consulting hematology):

- ✓ Check aPTT at baseline
- ✓ Check heparin level 6 hours after heparin initiation, 6 hours after any dosing change, and then every morning if two or more consecutive therapeutic heparin levels.
- ✓ Adjust heparin dosage using titration algorithm chosen below. Use standard heparin level titration ranges unless prescriber fills out individualized heparin level column in the table below.

(Choose high- or low-dose heparin therapy depending on treatment indication; round all doses to nearest 50 units/hour.)

☐ Lower-Dose Heparin Therapy (ACS, MI, Stroke, Other)			☐ High-Dose Heparin Therapy (DVT/PE Treatment)		
Heparin Level (units/mL)	Heparin Level (units/mL)	Adjustment	Heparin Level (units/mL)	Heparin Level (units/mL)	Adjustment
< 0.2	< ____	Increase infusion by 3 units/kg/hr	< 0.2	< ____	Bolus 40 units/kg, increase infusion by 3 units/kg/hr
0.2–0.25	____ - ____	Increase infusion by 2 units/kg/hr	0.2–0.25	____ - ____	Bolus 20 units/kg, increase infusion by 2 units/kg/hr
0.26–0.29	____ - ____	Increase infusion by 1 unit/kg/hr	0.26–0.29	____ - ____	Increase infusion by 1 unit/kg/hr
0.3–0.6	____ - ____	**No Change**	**0.3–0.7**	____ - ____	**No Change**
0.61–0.8	____ - ____	Decrease infusion by 1 unit/kg/hr	0.71–0.9	____ - ____	Decrease infusion by 1 unit/kg/hr
0.81–0.9	____ - ____	Hold infusion for 0.5 hour, decrease infusion by 2 units/kg/hr	0.91–1	____ - ____	Hold infusion by 0.5 hour, decrease infusion by 2 units/kg/hr
> 0.9	____ - ____	Hold infusion for 1 hour, decrease infusion by 3 units/kg/hr	> 1	____ - ____	Hold infusion for 1 hour, decrease infusion by 3 units/kg/hr

If heparin level > 1.5 units/mL at any time point: hold heparin infusion, send stat heparin level and aPTT, and contact house officer.

Figure 25.8 Example of an anti-Xa monitoring and titration algorithm for unfractionated heparin therapy.

HEPTEST AND HEPTEST-STAT

The Heptest and Heptest-Stat are clot-based assays that measure heparin or LMWHs and fondaparinux in human plasma, respectively. The assay consists of incubating plasma samples with an equal volume of factor Xa. This mixture is then recalcified by adding a reagent containing optimal concentrations of calcium chloride and brain cephalin in a bovine plasma fraction rich in factor V and fibrinogen. The amount of anticoagulant present in the sample is interpolated from a standard curve of clotting times versus known heparin levels.

The Heptest has a high correlation with the anti-Xa chromogenic assay for heparin and LMWH and may more accurately measure the anticoagulant effects of heparins than the aPTT because it is less influenced by high factor VIII levels and lupus anticoagulant.[17] The Heptest-Stat is most likely to be useful for low-dose heparin monitoring, including dialysis and pediatric patients. The Heptest-Stat has been used for monitoring VTE prophylaxis in pregnant women with and without prosthetic valves because it is unaffected by the hormonal changes common in these patients.[18]

ACTIVATED CLOTTING TIME

The activated clotting time (ACT) is one of the few point-of-care methods used for monitoring anticoagulant therapy in critically ill patients. The ACT is performed by adding an activating agent (e.g., kaolin) to a sample of freshly drawn whole blood and measuring the time to clot formation. The results for time to clot are presented in seconds. The ACT devices use a low- and high-range cassette, which provide different responses depending on the heparin level present. Because the aPTT becomes infinitely prolonged when heparin levels exceed 1 unit/mL, the ACT is typically used to monitor high-dose UFH or DTI therapy during cardiopulmonary bypass or other invasive intravascular procedures such as cardiac angiography and intervention, extracorporeal membrane oxygenation, vascular surgery, or carotid endarterectomy. The ACT is capable of showing a graded response to heparin levels at 1–5 units/mL. Low- and high-dose cartridges are available depending on the dose of anticoagulation and type of procedure being performed.

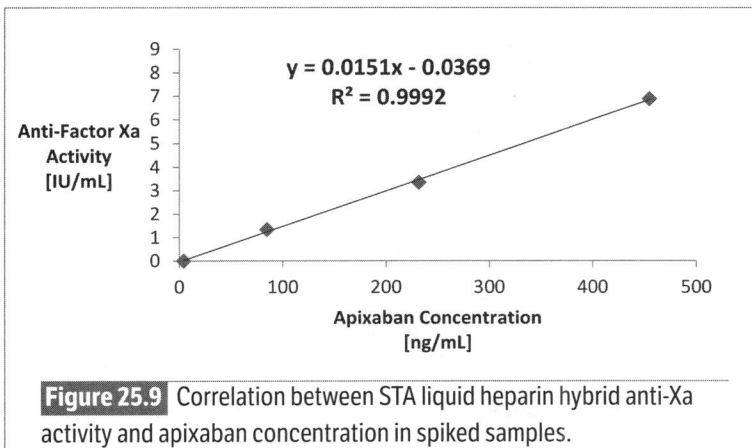

Figure 25.9 Correlation between STA liquid heparin hybrid anti-Xa activity and apixaban concentration in spiked samples.

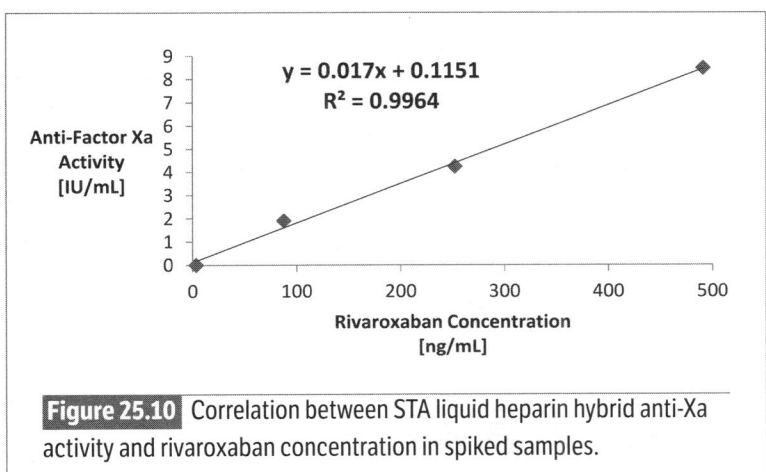

Figure 25.10 Correlation between STA liquid heparin hybrid anti-Xa activity and rivaroxaban concentration in spiked samples.

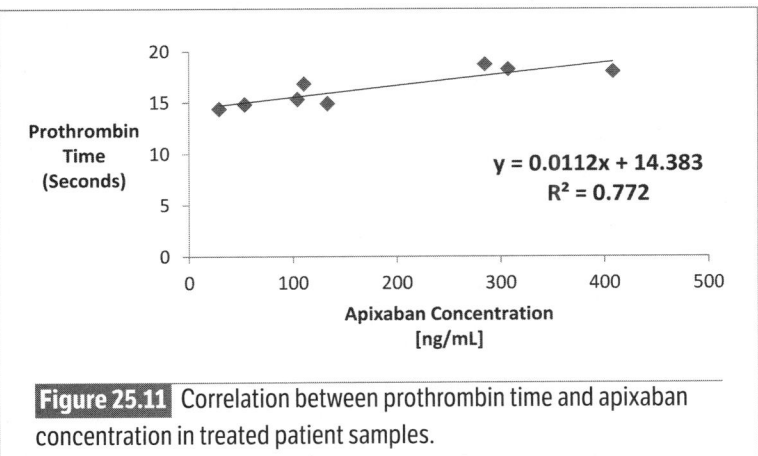

Figure 25.11 Correlation between prothrombin time and apixaban concentration in treated patient samples.

The ACT results can be affected by many factors including platelet count, platelet function, lupus anticoagulants, factor deficiencies, blood volume, temperature, and hemodilution (Figure 25.15). The presence of other anticoagulants (e.g., warfarin) or antiplatelet agents (e.g., glycoprotein IIb/IIIa inhibitors) can also increase the ACT.

The optimal goal range for the ACT is not well established, which therefore leads to variability in goals among various procedures and settings. A linear relationship between ACT and thrombosis and bleeding outcomes in percutaneous coronary intervention has not been established; however, increased rates of death, myocardial infarction, and target vessel revascularization have been observed in patients with ACTs of 300 seconds or less.[19] In patients undergoing cardiopulmonary bypass, a minimal ACT goal may range from greater than 350 to greater than 500 seconds; however, many institutions target a value between 400 and 480 seconds.[20] The ACT correlates well with heparin level only after the initial bolus of UFH in patients undergoing cardiopulmonary bypass. This correlation decreases significantly during cardiopulmonary bypass, potentially because of hemodilution, hypothermia, and platelet dysfunction (Figure 25.15).[21] Adding normal plasma to the patient sample may improve the correlation.[22] Reduced heparin sensitivity (e.g., heparin resistance) can also be picked up on if the ACT does not increase as expected with a given UFH dose (Figure 25.16). An arbitrary cutpoint of failure to achieve an ACT of greater than 480 seconds despite 500 units/kg of UFH has been a common definition of heparin insensitivity.[23,24] The clinical importance of identifying heparin resistance is unknown, and considerable debate exists about whether patients should simply be given higher doses of UFH or whether exogenous antithrombin III should be administered.

ECARIN CLOTTING TIME OR ECARIN CHROMOGENIC ASSAY

The ecarin clotting time test uses a known quantity of ecarin (thrombin activatable snake venom) and adds this to the plasma of a patient treated with a DTI. Ecarin activates prothrombin through a specific proteolytic cleavage, which produces meizothrombin, a prothrombin-thrombin intermediate that retains the full molecular weight of prothrombin but possesses a low level of procoagulant enzymatic activity. This activity is inhibited by DTIs, but not by heparin. The ecarin clotting time is also unaffected by prior treatment with warfarin or the presence of phospholipid-dependent anticoagulants, such as lupus anticoagulant. Thus, the ecarin clotting time is prolonged in a specific and linear fashion with increasing concentrations of DTIs.

An enhancement of the ecarin clotting time is the ecarin chromogenic assay in which diluted sample is mixed with an excess of purified prothrombin, and the generated meizothrombin is measured with a specific chromogenic substrate. This assay shows no interference from prothrombin or fibrinogen in the sample and is suitable for measuring all DTIs.[25,26] Unfortunately, this test is not yet FDA approved for use in the United States. Even if the test becomes available, many questions remain regarding the optimal drug concentration and correlation of the ecarin chromogenic assay to patient outcomes.

THROMBIN TIME AND DTT

The thrombin time (TT) measures the conversion of fibrinogen to fibrin, the final step in the clotting pathway. The test measures the time it takes for a clot to form in the plasma of a blood sample containing anticoagulant after an excess of thrombin has been added. It is typically used to diagnose blood coagulation disorders and to assess the effectiveness of fibrinolytic therapy. The TT compares the rate of clot formation with that of a sample of normal pooled plasma. Thrombin is added to the samples of plasma. If the time it takes for the plasma to clot is prolonged, a quantitative (fibrinogen deficiency) or qualitative (dysfunctional fibrinogen) defect is present. Thrombin time can be prolonged by anticoagulants (e.g., heparin or DTIs), fibrin degradation products, and fibrinogen deficiency or abnormality. The assay can be affected by fibrinogen concentrations, with fibrinogen concentrations greater than 600 mg/dL causing as much as a 5%–20% decrease in expected dTT compared with samples with normal fibrinogen values.[27]

The TT has a high sensitivity to anticoagulants, particularly DTIs.[27] For example, if used to monitor DTIs, this unmodified TT will provide results above the threshold for the assay (e.g., greater than 200 seconds). Therefore, the assay is typically diluted with pooled normal patient plasma by a 1:4 ratio yielding a dTT. The dTT may provide an alternative to the aPTT for monitoring UFH or DTIs, but because of the availability of other laboratory options for UFH, its use is more common with DTIs.[28] Potential advantages of the assay compared with the aPTT are avoidance of interference by lupus inhibitors, deficiency in vitamin K–dependent factor levels, or elevated D-dimer concentrations. Although the dTT can be run by automated machines, additional work must be done at individual institutions to dilute the patient samples and calibrate the assay according to

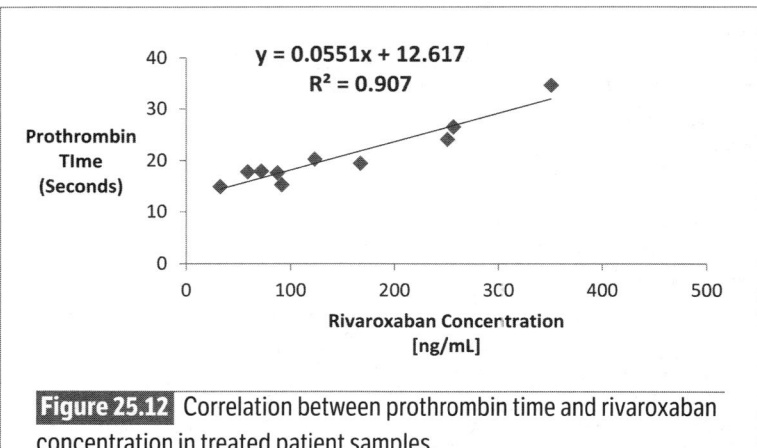

Figure 25.12 Correlation between prothrombin time and rivaroxaban concentration in treated patient samples.

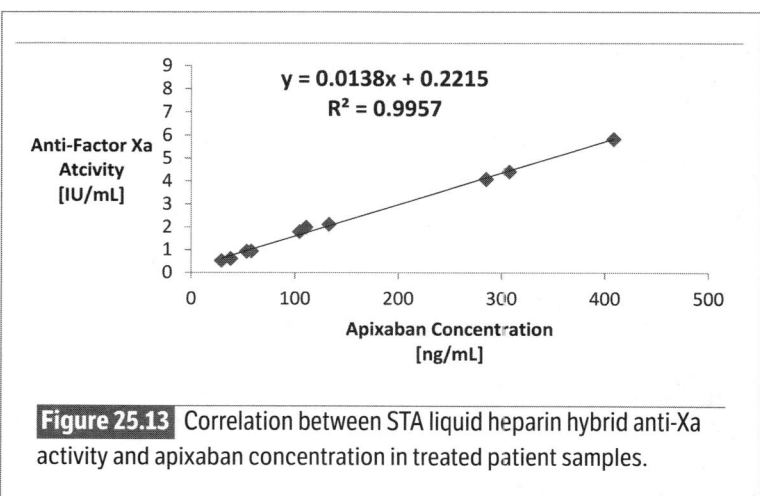

Figure 25.13 Correlation between STA liquid heparin hybrid anti-Xa activity and apixaban concentration in treated patient samples.

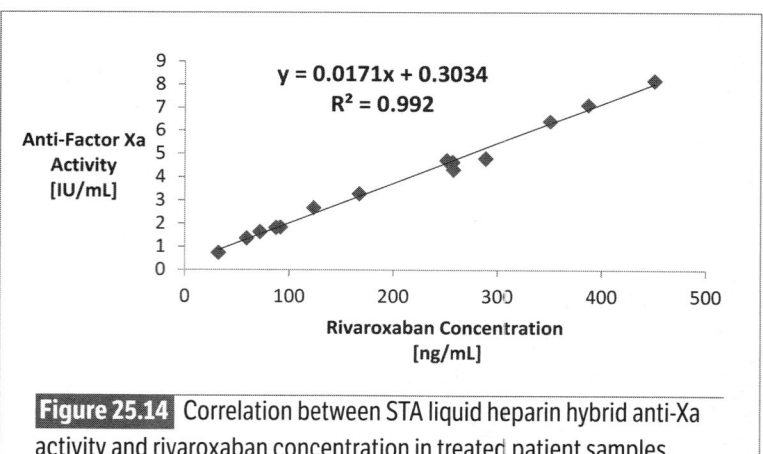

Figure 25.14 Correlation between STA liquid heparin hybrid anti-Xa activity and rivaroxaban concentration in treated patient samples.

DTI plasma concentrations (Figure 25.17). Additional considerations are the appropriateness of choosing the target therapeutic range for the dTT test because the goal therapeutic concentrations for DTIs vary depending on the source. For example, published argatroban goal concentrations equivalent to an aPTT of about 1.5–3 times baseline aPTT have been reported as 0.5–1.5 mcg/mL, 1–2 mcg/mL, and 0.4–1.1 mcg/mL.[29-31] The predominance of pharmacokinetic information with bivalirudin is

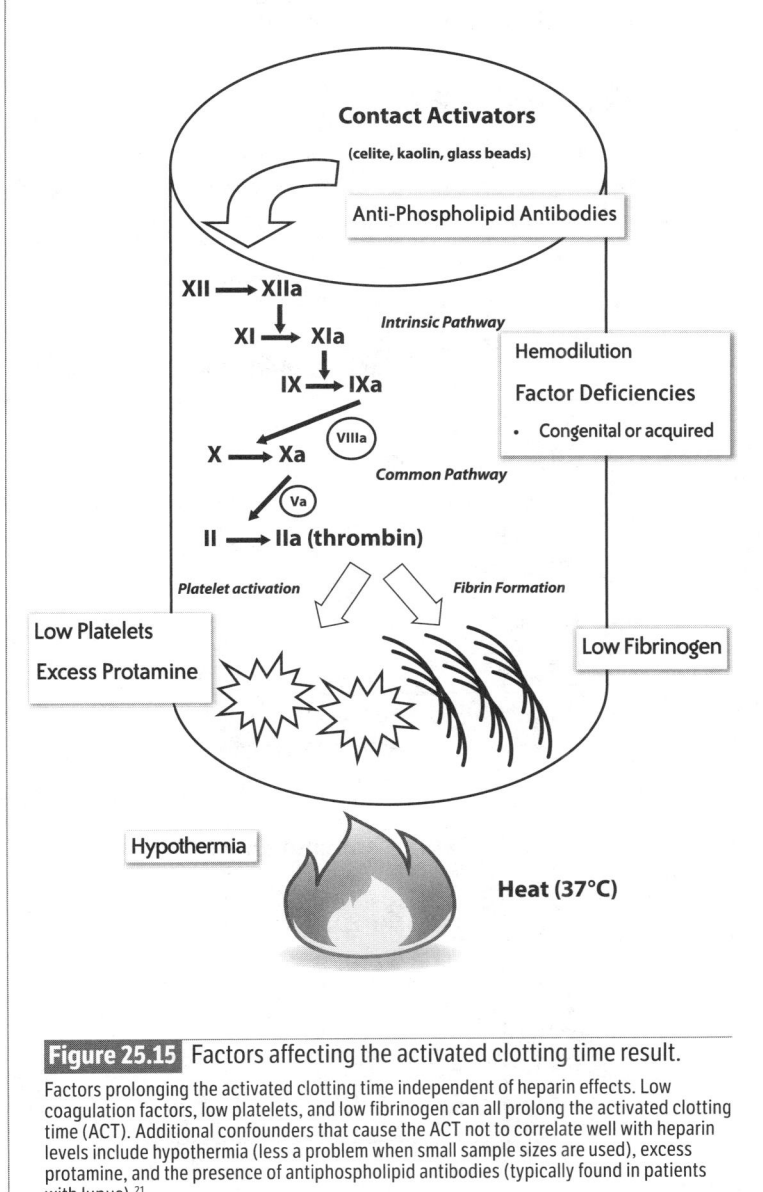

Figure 25.15 Factors affecting the activated clotting time result.

Factors prolonging the activated clotting time independent of heparin effects. Low coagulation factors, low platelets, and low fibrinogen can all prolong the activated clotting time (ACT). Additional confounders that cause the ACT not to correlate well with heparin levels include hypothermia (less a problem when small sample sizes are used), excess protamine, and the presence of antiphospholipid antibodies (typically found in patients with lupus).[21]

in patients undergoing percutaneous coronary intervention or coronary artery bypass grafting, which uses significantly higher doses and yields concentrations of 1–15 mcg/mL.[32] This range is even less well defined for bivalirudin in patients with heparin-induced thrombocytopenia and is approximated to be anywhere from 0.25 to 1.5 mcg/mL.[27] To account for this, some institutions have decided to truncate the goal range to a mean of the concentrations reported in the literature (e.g., 0.8–1.2 mcg/mL). However, more data are needed linking therapeutic concentrations to clinical outcomes before a specific goal can be recommended. Furthermore, individual ICU patient considerations, treatment goals, and risk-benefit of thrombosis and bleeding should be considered when designing a patient's therapeutic goal. Use of the test for DTIs should likely be reserved for patients with altered baseline aPTT values (e.g., patients with lupus anticoagulant) or those with an unexpected aPTT response in concordance with usual DTI dosing strategies.

PROTHROMBINASE-INDUCED CLOTTING TIME ASSAY

The prothrombinase-induced clotting time (PiCT) assay is a clotting assay that is sensitive to factor Xa and IIa. The assay adds factor Xa and Russell viper venom to platelet-poor plasma. After incubation, the plasma is recalcified, and the clotting time is determined. The PiCT is a relatively new test that has mainly been studied ex vivo. A mostly linear dose response is observed when evaluating UFH, LMWHs, argatroban, and fondaparinux.[33] A study comparing the PiCT assay with the ecarin chromogenic and dTT tests for monitoring argatroban, bivalirudin, and dabigatran showed greater variations in results with the PiCT test.[11] More studies are needed of critically ill patients before recommendations can be made to use the PiCT test in clinical practice.

HEMOCLOT THROMBIN INHIBITOR ASSAY

The Hemoclot thrombin inhibitor assay is a chronometric assay used for the quantitative measurement of both parenteral (argatroban) and oral (dabigatran) DTIs. During the Hemoclot thrombin inhibitor test, the patient's plasma is first diluted with normal pooled human plasma. Clotting is then initiated by adding a constant amount of highly purified human thrombin. The clotting time measured is directly related to the concentration of the DTI in plasma. Preliminary studies have shown a higher correlation between the Hemoclot thrombin inhibitor test and DTI concentrations in plasma than in the aPTT; however, little is known about the use of this test in clinical practice.[34,35] The test is relatively new in the United States and currently has no calibrators for bivalirudin.

THROMBIN GENERATION TEST

Thrombin generation assays measure the ability of a plasma sample to generate thrombin after activation of coagulation with tissue factor or another trigger. Thrombin generation assays also probe the propagation and termination phases. The thrombin generation curve shows and integrates all procoagulant and anticoagulant reactions that regulate the formation and inhibition of thrombin. Currently, there is poor standardization for the assay among institutions, which significantly limits its application in clinical practice.[36]

REPTILASE TIME

Reptilase is an enzyme similar to thrombin. It is different from thrombin because it resists inhibition by heparin through antithrombin. In addition, it is unaffected by DTIs. Reptilase time is useful for detecting abnormalities in fibrinogen and in detecting whether heparin or DTIs are causing a prolongation of the TT.

THROMBOELASTOGRAPHY

Thrombelastography (TEG) is a common method of performing point-of-care monitoring of coagulation. It provides clinicians with real-time results of whole blood coagulation status and is applicable at the bedside. More specifically, the TEG device provides graphic representation of the rate of fibrin polymerization, platelet function, and clot strength and stability through in vivo interactions of the coagulation system with platelets and red blood cells at the patient's actual temperature.

TERMINOLOGY

Thromboelastography was first described in 1948 as a research device to assess global viscoelastic changes in coagulation of a single blood sample.[37] In 1996, thromboelastograph

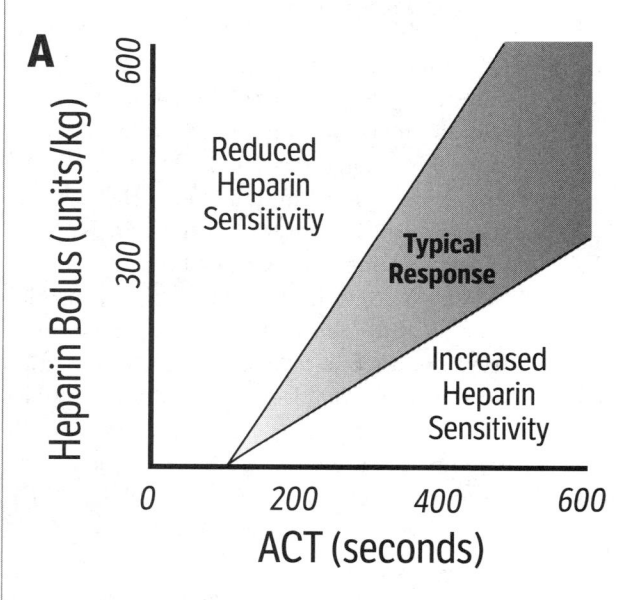

Figure 25.16 Dose-response graph for initial heparin bolus as measured by the activated clotting time.

Dose-response graph for initial heparin bolus as measured by the activated clotting time. (A) Before commencing cardiopulmonary bypass (CPB), the relationship of an intravenous heparin bolus and the resulting ACT is relatively linear. This relationship does not continue during CPB. (B) The heparin sensitivity index (HSI) is the dose-response slope. It is calculated by subtracting the baseline ACT measurement from the ACT obtained after the loading dose (both measured in seconds) and dividing that by the loading dose of heparin given (in units per kilogram).[21]

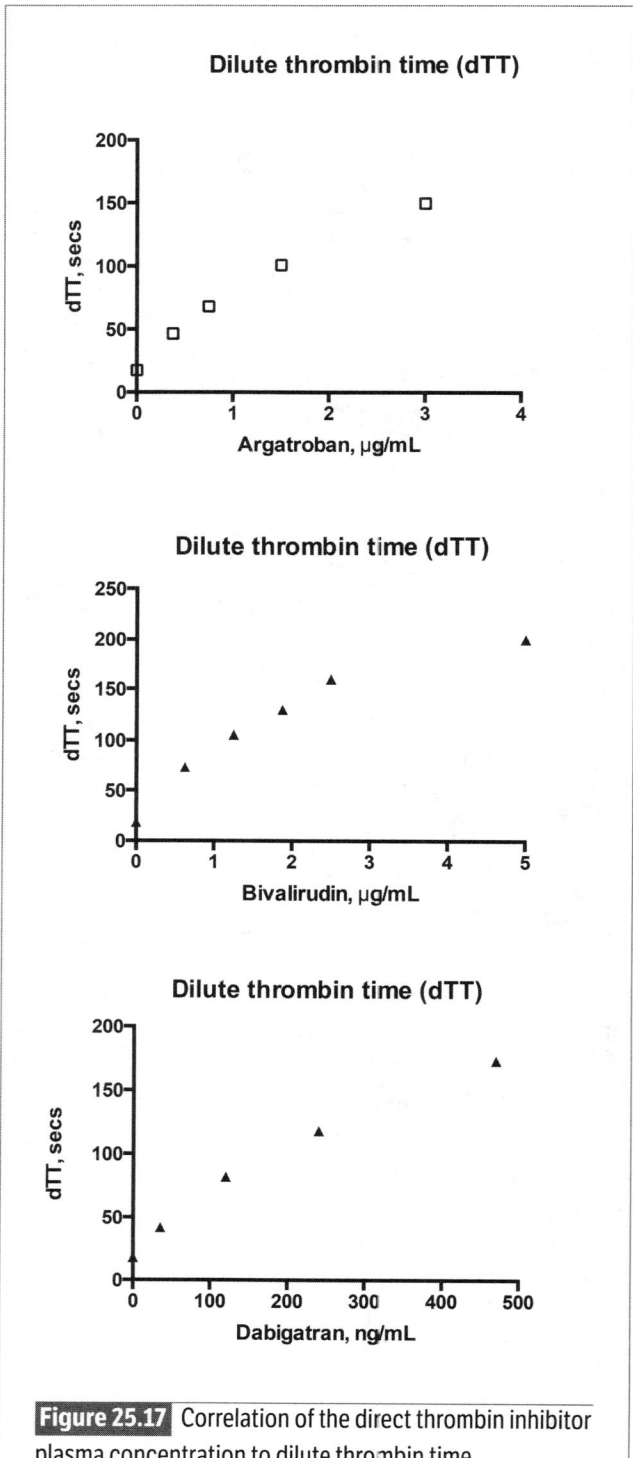

Figure 25.17 Correlation of the direct thrombin inhibitor plasma concentration to dilute thrombin time.

and TEG became registered trademarks of the Haemoscope Corporation (Niles, IL) and now describe the assay performed using Haemoscope instrumentation only. Rotational thromboelastography (ROTEM) also measures the viscoelastic properties of coagulation and differs from TEG in proprietary components and coagulation activators but has similar graphic results.

PRINCIPLES OF THROMBELASTOGRAPHY

The TEG/ROTEM devices both assess the viscoelastic physical properties of clotting whole blood, but they do so in a blood sample cup; this negates the high shear forces otherwise found in the vessels of the circulatory system. Because the TEG measures coagulation status under a no-flow (static) state in a blood sample cup (in vitro), it is important to emphasize that the results should be interpreted in context of the clinical scenario.[38] The TEG device uses a stationary cylindrical blood sample cup and oscillates through an angle of 4° 45' with each rotation lasting 10 seconds.[6] An immersed pin is suspended in the blood by a torsion wire and is monitored for motion. Torque is generated between the oscillation of the blood sample cup and the pin only after fibrin-platelet bonding has linked the cup and pin together. The graphic output of the rotational movement is related to the magnitude of strength of these fibrin-platelet bonds for the immersed pin. The TEG device may graphically represent robust or weak fibrin-platelet bond interactions depending on the level of coagulation and fibrinolysis the sampled blood is experiencing.[38] The ROTEM device uses modified technology compared with the TEG device using an optical detector rather than a torsion wire, and the mechanical oscillation originates from the pin, not the blood sample cup. Furthermore, the ROTEM instrument uses different plastic for the pin and cup that enhances contact activation with the sample; it also is equipped with an automatic pipette device and has proprietary formulas for coagulation activators different from those of the TEG system.[37,38]

Table 25.2 describes the TEG/ROTEM viscoelastic measurements and the variable nomenclature that represent the different stages of developing and resolving clot. The time until initial fibrin formation is the reaction (R) time (TEG) or clotting time (CT) (ROTEM); the kinetics of fibrin formation and clot development is the kinetic (K) or alpha angle (α) (TEG) or the clot formation time or alpha angle (α) (ROTEM); the strength and stability of the fibrin clot is the maximum amplitude (MA) (TEG) or maximum clot firmness (MCF) (ROTEM) and clot lysis (CL) (TEG) or clot lysis (LY) (ROTEM).

USE OF TEG FOR MONITORING ANTICOAGULANT THERAPY

Thromboelastography produces a tracing that depicts parameters measured throughout the life span of a clot

Table 25.2 Nomenclature and Reference Values of Thromboelastography and Thromboelastometry[6]

	TEG	ROTEM
Clotting time (period to 2 mm amplitude)	R (reaction time)	CT (clotting time)
	N (WB) 4–8 min	N (Cit, in-TEM) 137–246 s
	N (Cit, kaolin) 3–8 min	N (Cit, ex-TEM) 42–74 s
Clot kinetics (period from 2 to 20 mm amplitude)	K (kinetic time)	CFT (clot formation time)
	N (WB) 1–4 min	N (Cit, in-TEM) 40–100 s
	N (Cit, kaolin) 1–3 min	N (Cit, ex-TEM) 46–148 s
Clot strengthening (α angle)	α (slope between r and k)	α (slope of tangent at 2 mm amplitude)
	N (WB) 47°–74°	N (Cit, in-TEM) 71°–82°
		N (Cit, ex-TEM) 63°–81°
Amplitude (at set time)	A	A
Maximum strength	MA (maximum amplitude)	MCF (maximum clot firmness)
	N (WB) 55–73 mm	N (Cit, in-TEM) 52–72 mm
	N (Cit, kaolin) 51–69 mm	N (Cit, ex-TEM) 49–71 mm
		N (Cit, fib-TEM) 9–25 mm
Lysis (at fixed time)	CL30, CL60	LY30, LY60

TEG (thromboelastography): N = normal values for kaolin activated TEG in native whole blood (WB) or citrated and recalcified blood samples (Cit) (Haemoscope Corp.) or ROTEM using contact (partial thromboplastin phospholipids, in-TEM), tissue factor (ex-TEM), and tissue factor plus platelet inhibitor cytochalasin D (fib-TEM) activated citrated and recalcified blood samples. Reference value depends on reference population, blood sampling technique, and other re-analytic factors and coagulation activator.

(Figure 25.18). Alterations because of anticoagulation therapy or coagulopathies result in alteration of the tracing. Interpretation of the tracing (Figure 25.19) or output results (Table 25.3) can provide insight into the contributions of anticoagulant therapy versus those of other contributors to alterations in the clotting cascade that may be present in critically ill patients on anticoagulation.

Thromboelastography can be used to evaluate the effect of heparin, either exogenous or endogenous, by placing the sample into cups coated with heparinase. This enzyme, unlike protamine, will antagonize the effects of heparin without affecting TEG/ROTEM variables. The heparinase-coated cup samples can be analyzed in parallel with non-coated cup samples to determine whether heparin is still present (e.g., in the case of protamine reversal)[39] or to monitor coagulation in the presence of full-dose heparin therapy. The difference in R time between the simultaneously performed TEG with and without heparinase provides a linear relationship between heparin level and R time and allows for the determination of heparin dosing in patients.[40] The test times of TEG and ROTEM are typically 20 minutes or less, which offers a convenient point-of-care option if the machine is located near the patient. The downside to the TEG for monitoring heparin is the lack of clinical outcomes associated with the results provided. This makes it difficult to establish the goal R time and an appropriate recommendation for dosage adjustment that is based on the result. Although the use of the TEG for monitoring heparin therapy is a plausible option, it still becomes a distant alternative to the aPTT and anti-Xa assay for routine monitoring of heparin therapy.

In addition to monitoring UFH, TEG can detect the anticoagulant effects of LMWHs. Thromboelastography has been compared with anti-Xa activity using a variety of end points including R time, α angle, and maximum amplitude. Most, but not all, studies have shown a good correlation between the anti-Xa results and TEG R time or change in R time.[41-43] The goal R time or change in R time is unknown, but a study of coronary care unit patients showed that every 10% increase in milligram per kilogram dose of enoxaparin resulted in an increase in R time of 2.7 (95% confidence interval, 0.6–4.7).[41] Almost all patients

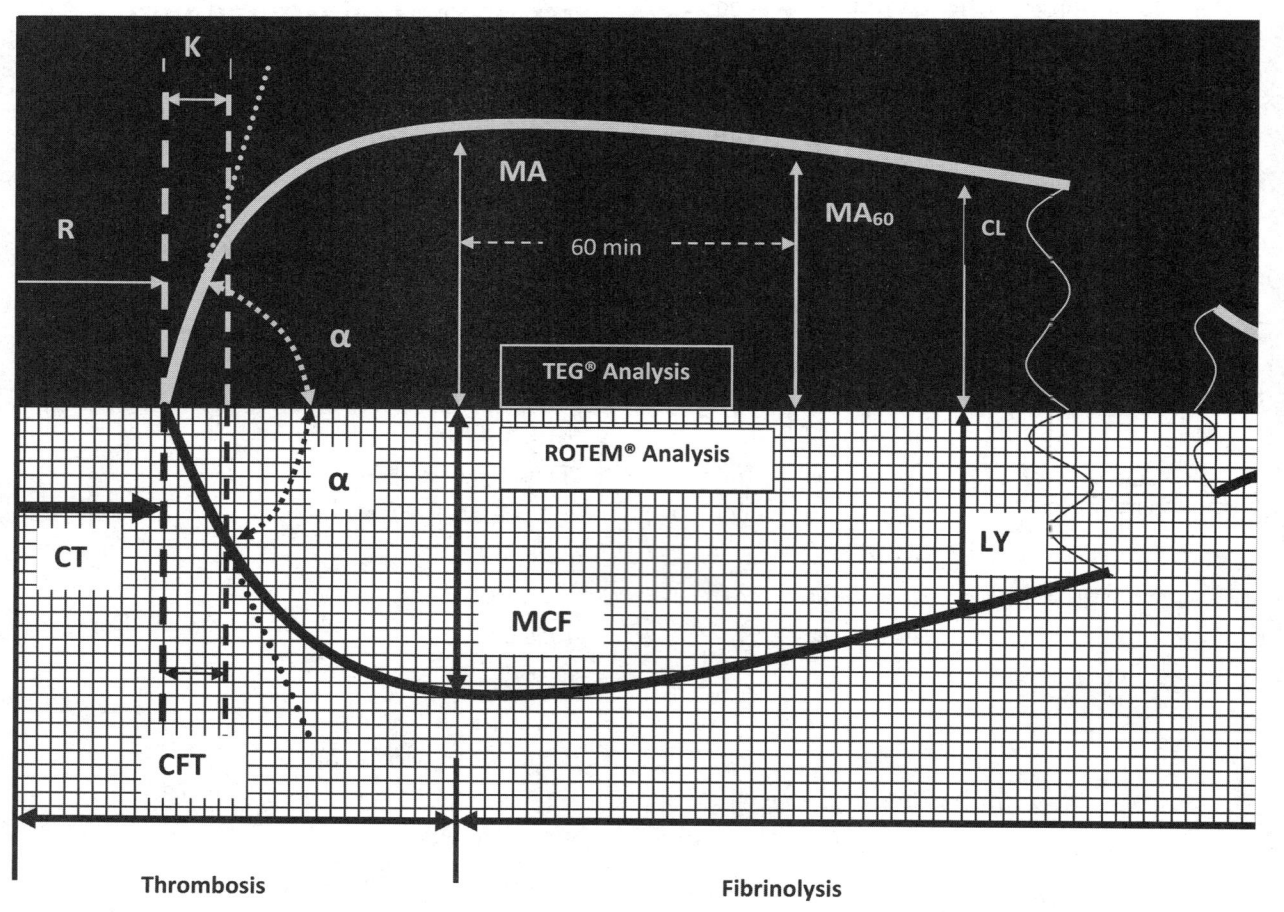

Figure 25.18 Thromboelastography tracing and measured parameters.

Normal viscoelastic tracing of TEG/ROTEM. Upper side: Thromboelastography (TEG) tracing: α = slope between R and K; CL = clot lysis; K time = kinetic time; MA = maximum amplitude; MA_{60} = maximum amplitude 60 min after initial maximum amplitude; R = reaction time. Lower side: Rotation thromboelastography (ROTEM) tracing: α = slope of tangent at 2 mm amplitude; CFT = clot formation time; CT = clotting time; LY = lysis; MCF = maximum clot formation firmness.

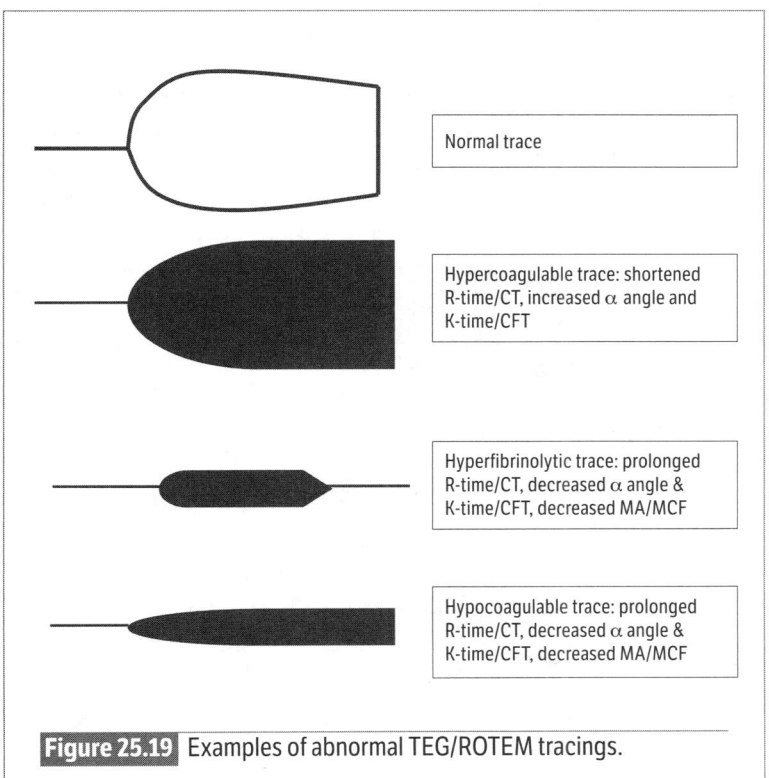

Figure 25.19 Examples of abnormal TEG/ROTEM tracings.

had an R time of more than 8 minutes when peak levels were drawn 4 hours after a 1-mg/kg subcutaneous enoxaparin dose. Most studies to date are too small to correlate TEG results to clinical outcomes in patients on LMWH. A study of 87 trauma and general surgery patients used TEG-guided enoxaparin dosing to increase the R time by 1–2 minutes. They compared this TEG-adjusted regimen with a standard 30-mg twice-daily regimen. Thromboelastography-guided therapy resulted in increased LMWH dosing and anti-Xa levels, but no decrease in VTE.[44] Therefore, at this time, TEG may be considered an additional tool for monitoring LMWH when the anti-Xa assay is not readily available or there is a question about the accuracy of the reported results.

Thromboelastography assays using ecarin can be used as an alternative method to monitor DTIs.[45-47] Adding ecarin to the TEG initiates coagulation, and the effect of bivalirudin is measured by the change in R time. Compared with the ACT, correlation of the ecarin TEG with bivalirudin concentration was significantly higher with the TEG (r^2 = 0.75) versus the ACT (r^2 = 0.31) [$p<0.001$].[46] For a range of bivalirudin concentrations from 2 to 11 mcg/mL, the R time increased from 144 ± 109 seconds to 557 ± 105 seconds in a linear fashion. The TEG may provide an alternative option to the aPTT and dTT, but routine use cannot be recommended at this time.

Thromboelastography can also be used for detecting the newer DOACs.[48] In patients taking dabigatran, apixaban, rivaroxaban, or edoxaban, the kaolin test reaction time (R time) and the time to maximum rate of thrombus generation are elevated in a dose proportional response relationship. The RapidTEG reagent also appears effective at detecting the DOACs. This allows laboratories to create a dose-response curve to determine the amount of drug in the system. The clinical utility of TEG for monitoring DOACs requires further elucidation, but it may be useful in patients undergoing emergency procedures or those requiring anticoagulation reversal while taking a DOAC.

Thromboelastography platelet mapping can be used to quantify the response to antiplatelet therapy including both $P2Y_{12}$ inhibitors and IIB/IIIA inhibitors.[49-52] The effects of platelet inhibitors can be observed in the parameters measured by TEG with the standard kaolin activator, with the MA being the predominant component to evaluate.[49] Modification of the TEG assay using reptilase and factor XIIIa is used to generate a whole blood crosslinked clot in the absence of thrombin generation or platelet activation. This increases the sensitivity of the TEG for measuring platelet contribution to shear elasticity of the clot and allows for measurement of a larger range of antiplatelet activity. This modification also permits convenient monitoring of patients receiving antiplatelet therapy during interventional procedures. Further studies are needed to establish the goal target MA range and the ability of the TEG to predict patient outcomes.

Overall, the TEG or ROTEM tests have the potential to monitor all current anticoagulant and antiplatelet therapies. This, plus the ability to differentiate the contribution of anticoagulants and/or antiplatelet agents versus endogenous factors affecting the coagulation pathway, makes it a very intriguing option to use in critically ill patients. Despite our increasing familiarity and potential applications of the TEG/ROTEM, the paucity of clinical data and the lack of routine availability of the test in many hospitals currently limit its use.

D-DIMER

Plasmin cleaves fibrin-releasing fibrin degradation products. D-dimer is one of the main fibrin degradation products, which consists of two D domains from adjacent fibrin monomers that have been crosslinked by activated factor XIII. An elevated plasma D-dimer indicates recent or ongoing intravascular blood coagulation. A D-dimer will be detectable at concentrations greater than 500 ng/mL in almost all patients with VTE. Therefore, a D-dimer is often used to rule out thrombosis and has a greater than 96% negative predictive value.[53-57] However, how to evaluate elevated D-dimer concentrations is more controversial. Critically ill patients may have many reasons to have an elevated D-dimer

(Table 25.4); therefore, it is unlikely that a single D-dimer would be helpful in monitoring anticoagulation therapy. It is conceivable that following trends in D-dimer could provide evidence of the effectiveness of the anticoagulant to prevent clot formation. In patients on extracorporeal membrane oxygenation therapy, an increasing D-dimer may be a marker for early diagnosis of thrombus formation and dysfunction of heparin-coated membrane oxygenators.[58,59] It is possible that monitoring D-dimer changes on a daily basis will provide insight into the effectiveness of anticoagulation for other indications, but more research is needed before this can routinely be recommended.

PLATELET REACTIVITY TESTS

Platelet function testing can now be conducted and applied at the bedside to help determine the degree of platelet reactivity and identify whether an adjustment to therapy is warranted to reduce the risks of both ischemic and bleeding complications. Specific tests are available for $P2Y_{12}$ inhibitors (e.g., VerifyNow PRU test), aspirin (e.g., VerifyNow aspirin test), and IIb/IIIa inhibitors (e.g., VerifyNow IIb/IIIa test). Each test is based on the ability of activated platelets to bind fibrinogen. Fibrinogen-coated microparticles aggregate in whole blood in proportion to the number of expressed platelet GP IIB/IIa receptors. Light transmittance increases as activated platelets bind and aggregate fibrinogen-coated beads. The instrument measures this change in optical signal caused by aggregation and reports results in platelet aggregation units (platelet activity units, IIb/IIIa test), $P2Y_{12}$ reaction units (platelet reactivity units, $P2Y_{12}$ inhibitors), or aspirin reactivity units. Most tests take about 10 minutes to produce results.

The need for platelet monitoring is based on the premise that it will improve patient outcomes. However, data analyses to date are mixed regarding any clinical outcome

Table 25.3 Interpretation of Thromboelastography Parameters

Parameter (normal values)	Interpretation
r (15–23 minutes)	-Latency time from placement of blood specimen to TEG tracing amplitude of 2 mm
	-Reflects quantity or action of clotting factors
K (5–10 minutes)	-Latency time for TEG tracing amplitude to increase from 2 to 20 mm
	-Reflects rate of clot formation and fibrinogen amount
α (22°–38°)	-Angle of the slope of the line connecting r and K times
	-Reflects rate of clot formation and fibrinogen amount
MA (47–58 mm)	-The greatest vertical amplitude of the TEG tracing
	-Reflects strength of clot and platelet activation
A_{60} (usually > 90%)	-The amplitude 60 minutes after MA as a percentage of MA
	-Reflects fibrinolysis
LY_{30} (< 7.5%)	-The rate of amplitude reduction 30 minutes after MA
	-Reflects fibrinolysis

FFP = fresh frozen plasma; LY = lysed; MA = maximum amplitude; PCC = prothrombin complex concentrate; rFVIIa = recombinant factor VIIa.

Table 25.4 Disorders Associated with Increased Plasma Concentrations of Fibrin D-dimer

Arterial thromboembolic disease
Myocardial infarction
Stroke
Acute limb ischemia
Atrial fibrillation
Intracardiac thrombus
Venous thromboembolic disease
Deep venous thrombosis
Pulmonary embolism
Disseminated intravascular coagulation
Preeclampsia and eclampsia
Abnormal fibrinolysis; use of thrombolytic agents
Cardiovascular disease, congestive failure
Severe infection/sepsis/inflammation
Surgery/trauma (e.g., tissue ischemia, necrosis)
Systemic inflammatory response syndrome
Vasoocclusive episode of sickle cell disease
Severe liver disease (decreased clearance)
Malignancy
Renal disease
Nephrotic syndrome (e.g., renal vein thrombosis)
Acute renal failure
Chronic renal failure and underlying cardiovascular disease
Normal pregnancy
Venous malformations

improvements.⁶⁰⁻⁶³ A recent randomized multicenter study of 2,440 patients scheduled for coronary stenting was unable to show any significant improvements in clinical outcomes with platelet function monitoring with dose adjustment compared with standard antiplatelet therapy without monitoring.[61] Given the lack of a clear benefit in most patients, point-of-care monitoring of platelet activity should likely be reserved for patients with significant drug interactions with their antiplatelet medications, those with concerns about oral antiplatelet absorption, and those with a significant risk of bleeding.

FUTURE DIRECTIONS IN LABORATORY ANTICOAGULATION TESTING

Despite the many tests available and the vast experience with antithrombotic agents, bleeding and thrombosis are still substantial contributors to morbidity and mortality in the ICU. The problem with many anticoagulant laboratory tests is their evaluation of only a portion of the coagulation process and their susceptibility to outside influences. Many tests may be a good surrogate for an anticoagulant's contribution to a specific portion of thrombus generation, but they may lead to a lack of understanding of the entire hemostatic process that places a patient at risk of unintended outcomes. Many believe that global assays of hemostasis (e.g., TEG) are more reflective of likely clinical outcomes such as VTE, bleeding, length of stay, and mortality. However, their lack of standardization and limited data showing their sensitivity and specificity for predicting clinically important outcomes preclude their use as a standard of care for most ICU patients. Novel global assays in development build on currently available tests and include thrombin and plasmin generation, thrombodynamics, and flow perfusion chambers.[64] Despite the potential advantages of these new options, most of these tests are in their infancy. Large patient cohorts will be necessary to determine whether they offer any clinically meaningful advantage over current laboratory options. Given that the data generated will have to show both a statistically and a clinically meaningful difference, clinicians are likely to have to choose a monitoring strategy from the currently available laboratory tests for the near future.

CONCLUSION

Routine anticoagulant laboratory tests, including the PT, aPTT, and anti-Xa, are commonly ordered to assess clotting function in critically ill patients. Many variables commonly present in critically ill patients must be considered when interpreting the results of coagulation laboratory tests. Newer laboratory tests are available that may be more specific for monitoring certain anticoagulants; however, data correlating results to clinical outcomes are limited. Many assays are performed on several platforms using different reagents between institutions, making standardization difficult to accomplish. Critical care clinicians should have a close working relationship with the anticoagulation laboratory and hematologists to ensure appropriate use of coagulation testing and interpretation.

REFERENCES

1. Bates SM, Weitz JI. Coagulation assays. Circulation 2005;112:e53-60.
2. Funk DM. Coagulation assays and anticoagulant monitoring. Hematology Am Soc Hematol Educ Program 2012;2012:460-5.
3. Dager WE, Gulseth MP, Nutescu EA, eds. Anticoagulation Therapy: A Point-of-Care Guide. Bethesda, MD: American Society of Health-Systems Pharmacists, 2011.
4. Zurcher M, Sulzer I, Barizzi G, et al. Stability of coagulation assays performed in plasma from citrated whole blood transported at ambient temperature. Thromb Haemost 2008;99:416-26.
5. Marlar RA, Potts RM, Marlar AA. Effect on routine and special coagulation testing values of citrate anticoagulant adjustment in patients with high hematocrit values. Am J Clin Pathol 2006;126:400-5.
6. Arpino PA, Demirjian Z, Van Cott EM. Use of the chromogenic factor X assay to predict the international normalized ratio in patients transitioning from argatroban to warfarin. Pharmacotherapy 2005;25:157-64.
7. Austin JH, Stearns CR, Winkler AM, et al. Use of the chromogenic factor X assay in patients transitioning from argatroban to warfarin therapy. Pharmacotherapy 2012;32:493-501.
8. Garcia DA, Baglin TP, Weitz JI, et al. Parenteral anticoagulants: Antithrombotic Therapy and Prevention of Thrombosis, 9th ed: American College of Chest Physicians Evidence-Based Clinical Practice Guidelines. Chest 2012;141:e24S-43S.
9. Basu D, Gallus A, Hirsh J, et al. A prospective study of the value of monitoring heparin treatment with the activated partial thromboplastin time. N Engl J Med 1972;287:324-7.
10. Price EA, Jin J, Nguyen HM, et al. Discordant aPTT and anti-Xa values and outcomes in hospitalized patients treated with intravenous unfractionated heparin. Ann Pharmacother 2013;47:151-8.
11. Kiser TH, Mann AM, Trujillo TC, et al. Evaluation of empiric versus nomogram-based direct thrombin inhibitor management in patients with suspected heparin-induced thrombocytopenia. Am J Hematol 2011;86:267-72.
12. Arpino PA, Goeller AJ, Fatalo A, et al. Evaluation of 2 nomogram-based strategies for dosing argatroban in patients with known or suspected heparin-induced thrombocytopenia. Clin Appl Thromb Hemost 2015;21:260-5.
13. Samama MM, Poller L. Contemporary laboratory monitoring of low molecular weight heparins. Clin Lab Med 1995;15:119-23.
14. Costantini TW, Min E, Box K, et al. Dose adjusting enoxaparin is necessary to achieve adequate venous thromboembolism prophylaxis in trauma patients. J Trauma Acute Care Surg 2013;74:128-33; discussion 34-5.
15. Malinoski D, Jafari F, Ewing T, et al. Standard prophylactic enoxaparin dosing leads to inadequate anti-Xa levels and

16. Gosselin RC, Francart SJ, Hawes EM, et al. Heparin-calibrated chromogenic anti-Xa activity measurements in patients receiving rivaroxaban: can this test be used to quantify drug level? Ann Pharmacother 2015;49:777-83.
17. Hellstern P, Bach J, Simon M, et al. Heparin monitoring during cardiopulmonary bypass surgery using the one-step point-of-care whole blood anti-factor-Xa clotting assay heptest-POC-Hi. J Extra Corpor Technol 2007;39:81-6.
18. Dempfle CE, Zharkowa U, Elmas E, et al. Heptest-STAT, a new assay for monitoring of low-molecular-weight heparins, is not influenced by pregnancy-related changes of blood plasma. Thromb Haemost 2009;102:1001-6.
19. Ducrocq G, Jolly S, Mehta SR, et al. Activated clotting time and outcomes during percutaneous coronary intervention for non-ST-segment-elevation myocardial infarction: insights from the FUTURA/OASIS-8 Trial. Circ Cardiovasc Interv 2015;8.
20. Lobato RL, Despotis GJ, Levy JH, et al. Anticoagulation management during cardiopulmonary bypass: a survey of 54 North American institutions. J Thorac Cardiovasc Surg 2010;139:1665-6.
21. Sniecinski RM, Levy JH. Anticoagulation management associated with extracorporeal circulation. Best Pract Res Clin Anaesthesiol 2015;29:189-202.
22. Koster A, Despotis G, Gruendel M, et al. The plasma supplemented modified activated clotting time for monitoring of heparinization during cardiopulmonary bypass: a pilot investigation. Anesth Analg 2002;95:26-30, table of contents.
23. Staples MH, Dunton RF, Karlson KJ, et al. Heparin resistance after preoperative heparin therapy or intraaortic balloon pumping. Ann Thorac Surg 1994;57:1211-6.
24. Williams MR, D'Ambra AB, Beck JR, et al. A randomized trial of antithrombin concentrate for treatment of heparin resistance. Ann Thorac Surg 2000;70:873-7.
25. Lange U, Nowak G, Bucha E. Ecarin chromogenic assay—a new method for quantitative determination of direct thrombin inhibitors like hirudin. Pathophysiol Haemost Thromb 2003;33:184-91.
26. Nowak G. The ecarin clotting time, a universal method to quantify direct thrombin inhibitors. Pathophysiol Haemost Thromb 2003;33:173-83.
27. Love JE, Ferrell C, Chandler WL. Monitoring direct thrombin inhibitors with a plasma diluted thrombin time. Thromb Haemost 2007;98:234-42.
28. Lind SE, Boyle ME, Fisher S, et al. Comparison of the aPTT with alternative tests for monitoring direct thrombin inhibitors in patient samples. Am J Clin Pathol 2014;141:665-74.
29. Ahmad S, Ahsan A, George M, et al. Simultaneous monitoring of argatroban and its major metabolite using an HPLC method: potential clinical applications. Clin Appl Thromb Hemost 1999;5:252-8.
30. Fenyvesi T, Jorg I, Harenberg J. Monitoring of anticoagulant effects of direct thrombin inhibitors. Semin Thromb Hemost 2002;28:361-8.
31. Harenberg J, Jorg I, Fenyvesi T, et al. Treatment of patients with a history of heparin-induced thrombocytopenia and anti-lepirudin antibodies with argatroban. J Thromb Thrombolysis 2005;19:65-9.
32. Koster A, Chew D, Grundel M, et al. Bivalirudin monitored with the ecarin clotting time for anticoagulation during cardiopulmonary bypass. Anesth Analg 2003;96:383-6, table of contents.
33. Calatzis A, Peetz D, Haas S, et al. Prothrombinase-induced clotting time assay for determination of the anticoagulant effects of unfractionated and low-molecular-weight heparins, fondaparinux, and thrombin inhibitors. Am J Clin Pathol 2008;130:446-54.
34. Samos M, Stanciakova L, Ivankova J, et al. Monitoring of dabigatran therapy using Hemoclot((R)) Thrombin Inhibitor assay in patients with atrial fibrillation. J Thromb Thrombolysis 2015;39:95-100.
35. Guy S, Kitchen S, Maclean R, et al. Limitation of the activated partial thromboplastin time as a monitoring method of the direct thrombin inhibitor argatroban. Int J Lab Hematol 2015.
36. Castoldi E, Rosing J. Thrombin generation tests. Thromb Res 2011;127(suppl 3):S21-5.
37. Luddington RJ. Thrombelastography/thromboelastometry. Clin Lab Haematol 2005;27:81-90.
38. Ganter MT, Hofer CK. Coagulation monitoring: current techniques and clinical use of viscoelastic point-of-care coagulation devices. Anesth Analg 2008;106:1366-75.
39. Levin AI, Heine AM, Coetzee JF, et al. Heparinase thromboelastography compared with activated coagulation time for protamine titration after cardiopulmonary bypass. J Cardiothorac Vasc Anesth 2014;28:224-9.
40. Schaden E, Jilch S, Hacker S, et al. Monitoring of unfractionated heparin with rotational thromboelastometry using the prothrombinase-induced clotting time reagent (PiCT(R)). Clin Chim Acta 2012;414:202-5.
41. White H, Sosnowski K, Bird R, et al. The utility of thromboelastography in monitoring low molecular weight heparin therapy in the coronary care unit. Blood Coagul Fibrinolysis 2012;23:304-10.
42. Klein SM, Slaughter TF, Vail PT, et al. Thromboelastography as a perioperative measure of anticoagulation resulting from low molecular weight heparin: a comparison with anti-Xa concentrations. Anesth Analg 2000;91:1091-5.
43. Carroll RC, Craft RM, Whitaker GL, et al. Thromboelastography monitoring of resistance to enoxaparin anticoagulation in thrombophilic pregnancy patients. Thromb Res 2007;120:367-70.
44. Louis SG, Van PY, Riha GM, et al. Thromboelastogram-guided enoxaparin dosing does not confer protection from deep venous thrombosis: a randomized controlled pilot trial. J Trauma Acute Care Surg 2014;76:937-42; discussion 42-3.
45. Solbeck S, Meyer MA, Johansson PI, et al. Monitoring of dabigatran anticoagulation and its reversal in vitro by thrombelastography. Int J Cardiol 2014;176:794-9.
46. Carroll RC, Chavez JJ, Simmons JW, et al. Measurement of patients' bivalirudin plasma levels by a thrombelastograph ecarin clotting time assay: a comparison to a standard activated clotting time. Anesth Analg 2006;102:1316-9.
47. Engstrom M, Rundgren M, Schott U. An evaluation of monitoring possibilities of argatroban using rotational thromboelastometry and activated partial thromboplastin time. Acta Anaesthesiol Scand 2010;54:86-91.

48. Dias JD, Norem K, Doorneweerd DD, et al. Use of thromboelastography (TEG) for detection of new oral anticoagulants. Arch Pathol Lab Med 2015;139:665-73.
49. Craft RM, Chavez JJ, Bresee SJ, et al. A novel modification of the Thrombelastograph assay, isolating platelet function, correlates with optical platelet aggregation. J Lab Clin Med 2004;143:301-9.
50. Katori N, Szlam F, Levy JH, et al. A novel method to assess platelet inhibition by eptifibatide with thrombelastograph. Anesth Analg 2004;99:1794-9, table of contents.
51. Kettner SC, Panzer OP, Kozek SA, et al. Use of abciximab-modified thrombelastography in patients undergoing cardiac surgery. Anesth Analg 1999;89:580-4.
52. Khurana S, Mattson JC, Westley S, et al. Monitoring platelet glycoprotein IIb/IIIa-fibrin interaction with tissue factor-activated thromboelastography. J Lab Clin Med 1997;130:401-11.
53. Aschwanden M, Labs KH, Jeanneret C, et al. The value of rapid D-dimer testing combined with structured clinical evaluation for the diagnosis of deep vein thrombosis. J Vasc Surg 1999;30:929-35.
54. Lennox AF, Delis KT, Serunkuma S, et al. Combination of a clinical risk assessment score and rapid whole blood D-dimer testing in the diagnosis of deep vein thrombosis in symptomatic patients. J Vasc Surg 1999;30:794-803.
55. Wells PS, Anderson DR, Bormanis J, et al. Application of a diagnostic clinical model for the management of hospitalized patients with suspected deep-vein thrombosis. Thromb Haemost 1999;81:493-7.
56. Le Gal G, Righini M, Roy PM, et al. Value of D-dimer testing for the exclusion of pulmonary embolism in patients with previous venous thromboembolism. Arch Intern Med 2006;166:176-80.
57. Righini M, Le Gal G, De Lucia S, et al. Clinical usefulness of D-dimer testing in cancer patients with suspected pulmonary embolism. Thromb Haemost 2006;95:715-9.
58. Dornia C, Philipp A, Bauer S, et al. D-dimers are a predictor of clot volume inside membrane oxygenators during extracorporeal membrane oxygenation. Artif Organs 2015.
59. Lubnow M, Philipp A, Dornia C, et al. D-dimers as an early marker for oxygenator exchange in extracorporeal membrane oxygenation. J Crit Care 2014;29:473 e1-5.
60. Steinhubl SR, Kottke-Marchant K, Moliterno DJ, et al. Attainment and maintenance of platelet inhibition through standard dosing of abciximab in diabetic and nondiabetic patients undergoing percutaneous coronary intervention. Circulation 1999;100:1977-82.
61. Collet JP, Cuisset T, Range G, et al. Bedside monitoring to adjust antiplatelet therapy for coronary stenting. N Engl J Med 2012;367:2100-9.
62. Steinhubl SR, Talley JD, Braden GA, et al. Point-of-care measured platelet inhibition correlates with a reduced risk of an adverse cardiac event after percutaneous coronary intervention: results of the GOLD (AU-Assessing Ultegra) multicenter study. Circulation 2001;103:2572-8.
63. Tamberella MR, Bhatt DL, Chew DP, et al. Relation of platelet inactivation with intravenous glycoprotein IIb/IIIa antagonists to major bleeding (from the GOLD study). Am J Cardiol 2002;89:1429-31.
64. Lipets EN, Ataullakhanov FI. Global assays of hemostasis in the diagnostics of hypercoagulation and evaluation of thrombosis risk. Thromb J 2015;13:4.

Section 5

Acute Kidney Injury

Chapter 26
Acute Kidney Injury—Prevention and Management

Curtis L. Smith, Pharm.D., BCPS; and Thomas C. Dowling, Pharm.D., Ph.D., FCCP, FCP

LEARNING OBJECTIVES

1. Describe the basic etiology, common causes, and prognosis of acute kidney injury (AKI).
2. Differentiate prerenal azotemia, intrinsic AKI, and postrenal causes of AKI.
3. Explain how laboratory tests are used to differentiate between various types of AKI.
4. Discuss approaches to prevent and treat AKI.
5. Explain measures the critical care pharmacist may use to predict, prevent, and manage drug-induced AKI.

ABBREVIATIONS IN THIS CHAPTER

ACEI	Angiotensin-converting enzyme inhibitor	ICU	Intensive care unit
AKI	Acute kidney injury	KDIGO	Kidney Disease Improving Global Outcomes
AKIN	Acute Kidney Injury Network		
ARB	Angiotensin receptor blocker	NSAID	Nonsteroidal anti-inflammatory drug
ATN	Acute tubular necrosis	RIFLE	Risk, injury, failure, loss of kidney function, end-stage kidney disease
BUN	Blood urea nitrogen		
FENa	Fractional excretion of sodium	RRT	Renal replacement therapy
GFR	Glomerular filtration rate		

INTRODUCTION

Monitoring kidney function and hemodynamics is a mainstay of intensive care medicine. Acute kidney injury (AKI), previously called acute renal failure, is characterized by a rapid decline in glomerular filtration rate (GFR) and excretory function in the kidneys. The traditional assumptions about acute changes in kidney function have been challenged within the past decade, with a renewed focus on earlier, mild injury associated with adverse clinical outcomes, particularly in the critically ill population. This chapter will review the most recent approaches to preventing, defining, staging, and managing AKI with an emphasis on patient care.

Incidence and Prognosis

Acute kidney injury reportedly affects almost 500 people per 1 million each year, including 5% of all hospitalized patients,[1] with around 40% of these requiring acute renal replacement therapy (RRT).[2] The timeline for developing AKI after an acute insult ranges from hours to days or weeks and has been reported to occur in up to 20% of hospital admissions.[3] The reported incidence of AKI in postsurgical populations ranges from 0.8% (minor surgery) to 36.7% (major surgery), with mortality (90 day and 5 year) increasing 2- to 3-fold in the presence of AKI.[4] The incidence of AKI in intensive care unit (ICU) patients is even higher, approaching 50% in patients with early AKI.[5]

The prognosis of patients with AKI is associated with the degree of reduced urine output and the duration and severity of AKI. For example, it is widely reported that a urine output of less than 0.5 mL/kg/hour for 6 hours is associated with increased mortality even in the absence of changes in serum creatinine.[6] However, lower thresholds for urine output have been associated with worse outcomes. In a critical care cohort study, Ralib et al. reported that a urine output below 0.3 mL/kg/hour for 6 hours was associated with a marked increase in mortality.[7] The length of time serum creatinine remains elevated, or the duration of AKI, has also been associated with worse outcomes. Long-term survival was associated with the duration of AKI in patients post-cardiac surgery[8] and in patients with diabetes non-cardiac surgery,[9] where the mortality for patients with 3–6 days of initial AKI was greater than 2 or fewer days of more advanced stages of AKI.

Etiology

Acute kidney injury is highly preventable and usually reversible, with recovery taking days to weeks. If prolonged, AKI can progress to end-stage kidney disease requiring chronic RRT. Thus, identifying risk factors for AKI (see Table 26.1) is critical to prevent it from developing.

According to NCEPOD (the UK National Confidential Enquiry into Patient Outcome and Death), around 20%–30% of all AKI events are predictable and avoidable. In reviewing more than 1,500 AKI-related deaths, this expert advisory group found that only 50% of patients receiving care for AKI met acceptable medical practice standards (defined as "good").[10] A likely contributor to inadequate care for patients with AKI is failure to recognize and manage the condition. For example, azotemia, defined as a nonspecific elevation in serum urea nitrogen concentration, is common in patients with gastrointestinal bleeding, severe catabolism, oliguria, intravascular volume depletion, and after administering drugs that alter renal hemodynamics. Other confounding factors include nonspecific elevations in serum creatinine, as noted in patients with increased muscle mass, associated with increased dietary protein intake, or after severe muscle injury or rhabdomyolysis. Thus, a complete clinical assessment is needed before an accurate diagnosis of AKI can be made. Regardless of the etiology of AKI, both ischemic injury and directly toxic injury to the kidney can ultimately lead to AKI, including acute tubular necrosis (ATN). Acute kidney injury in the ICU population is often complicated by several organ system failures occurring simultaneously. These critically ill patients may be receiving pharmacologic and life-support treatments, including RRT to maintain adequate homeostasis.

PATHOPHYSIOLOGY

The two fundamental mechanisms contributing to AKI are hypoxia and cellular injury. The kidneys receive almost 20% of cardiac output to meet the high tissue oxygen demands. The tubular regions in the loop of Henle have the highest oxygen extraction ratio (relative to O_2 delivery) of any cell in the human body, with almost 80% of delivered oxygen being used.[11] Most of the oxygen consumption is related to ATP-dependent sodium transporters that drive the major fluid homeostasis mechanism of the body. This activity is coupled with GFR, where increased ultrafiltrate delivery leads to higher sodium reabsorption and greater oxygen consumption. The three primary mechanisms of AKI are conventionally classified according to relative hemodynamics and vascular anatomy.

Prerenal Azotemia

Azotemia classified as "prerenal" indicates that an acute decrease in GFR has occurred in an otherwise normal kidney, in response to hypovolemia or hypoperfusion. As an initial response to hypoperfusion, blood flow is redistributed to the hypoxic regions of the kidney (medulla). Renal ischemia and tissue hypoperfusion, if present for a prolonged duration, can ultimately lead to loss of renal cellular integrity and tissue necrosis. In severe ischemia, tubular sodium reabsorption is compromised, leading to urinary sodium loss and activation of the renin-angiotensin-aldosterone system (RAAS). This leads to heightened afferent arteriolar tone and a decrease in GFR. Without this RAAS-mediated negative feedback mechanism, the GFR would remain unchanged, and severe dehydration and death would rapidly ensue. The reduced GFR and urine output (oliguria) in the face of AKI serves as a mechanism that sacrifices GFR to maintain life. This functional feedback loop is often called "acute renal success" as opposed to renal failure.

Table 26.1 Examples of Risk Factors Associated with AKI[35,125-127]		
Preexisting liver disease	Hypovolemic states (hemorrhage, volume depletion, burns, cardiovascular shock)	Obesity
Preexisting renal disease		Cardiovascular disease
Concomitant nephrotoxins (i.e., amphotericin B, aminoglycosides)	Low cardiac output (heart failure)	ACEIs/ARBs
	Anaphylaxis	Surgery or trauma
Advanced age	Severity of illness	Multiple comorbidities
Impaired renal vasoconstriction/vasodilation		Respiratory disease
		Vasopressors
		Diuretics

ACEI = angiotensin-converting enzyme inhibitor; AKI = acute kidney injury; ARB = angiotensin receptor blocker.

Intrarenal (Intrinsic) AKI

Intrinsic renal causes are important sources of AKI and are usually categorized by the mechanism of direct injury that typically occurs in each condition. The most common forms of intrinsic AKI likely to be seen in ICU settings include sepsis, ATN, ischemia/vascular, and endogenous nephrotoxins.

Sepsis

Sepsis is the most common form of AKI occurring in the ICU population (greater than 30%). The exact mechanism is not fully understood, but it likely involves a complex interplay between initial reduction in vascular resistance, hypoperfusion, ischemia/reperfusion, and apoptosis.[12,13]

Acute Tubular Necrosis

Acute tubular necrosis is the leading cause of non-sepsis AKI in the ICU. Because of the close association of ATN with prerenal azotemia, it is important to distinguish the two forms using clinical signs, medical history, and laboratory criteria (see Table 26.2). The time course of ATN is often described by a three-part series of events: initiation, maintenance, and recovery. The initiation phase is characterized by an acute decline in GFR, followed by a rapid rise in serum creatinine and blood urea nitrogen (BUN) concentrations. The maintenance phase is characterized by a sustained reduction in GFR, continuing for up to 2 weeks. Because GFR is severely compromised during this phase, serum creatinine and BUN continue to rise. During the recovery phase, tubular function is restored, leading to an increase in urine output and a return of the BUN and serum creatinine concentrations to their pre-injury levels. The extent of tubule cell damage and nephrotoxicity in ATN depends on the kidneys' capacity to recover from the initial insult, intrarenal vasoconstriction, and any intratubular obstruction.

Ischemia/Vascular

Ischemic ATN is often closely related to prerenal azotemia, given that both conditions are caused by similar insults. Ischemic ATN occurs after prolonged hypoperfusion, where the initial autoregulatory responses in the kidney are overwhelmed. Here, severe hypoperfusion leads to cell injury and cell death.

Endogenous Nephrotoxins

Conditions associated with traumatic injury or muscle toxicity can lead to rhabdomyolysis-induced AKI. Extensive hemolysis caused by severe blood transfusion reactions can lead to myoglobin-induced AKI. Acute crystal-induced nephropathy is another endogenous form of AKI, caused by myeloablative cancer treatments associated with high cell turnover (and release of uric acid crystals), but it may also be caused by acute ingestions of ethylene glycol or high-dose vitamin C.

Exogenous Nephrotoxins

Many nephrotoxic drugs that are associated with ATN are commonly used in the ICU. Individual nephrotoxic drugs are rarely the sole cause of AKI, unless given in high doses over a long period. Nephrotoxic drugs used in high-risk patients with preexisting conditions such as chronic kidney disease, sepsis, dehydration, or hypotension, or the use of vasopressors, can increase the likelihood of AKI in the ICU. Examples of drug-induced ATN include the following:

- Aminoglycoside-related toxicity occurs in 10%–30% of patients receiving aminoglycosides, even when serum drug concentrations are within the typical therapeutic range. This is the result of direct toxicity in proximal tubular cells, where uptake is mediated by megalin receptors.[14]

Table 26.2 Common Clinical Laboratory Evaluation of AKI

Test	Intrarenal AKI	Prerenal Azotemia	Postrenal AKI
BUN/SCr ratio	10–15:1	> 20:1	10–15:1
Urine osmolality (mOsm/kg)	< 450	> 500	< 450
Urine specific gravity	≤ 1.010	> 1.020	≤ 1.010
Urine sodium (mEq/L)	> 40	< 20	> 20
Urine/SCr ratio	< 20	> 40	< 20
FENa (%)	> 2	< 1	> 2
Urine examination	Tubular casts, leukocytes,[a] WBC casts,[a] epithelial cells, other debris	Normal or hyaline casts	Cellular debris

[a]Often seen in acute interstitial nephritis.

FENa = fractional excretion of sodium; SCr = serum creatinine.

- Amphotericin B nephrotoxicity is often dose-related, where risk is related to the maximum daily dose (greater than 3 g) and therapy duration. The mechanism is likely related to the combined effects of sterol binding in cell membranes and direct vasoconstriction. The increased membrane permeability can lead to the renal wasting of electrolytes, such as potassium and magnesium, as well as a back-leak of hydrogen ions in the collecting duct, causing distal renal tubular acidosis. Direct vasoconstriction at the afferent arteriole can further contribute to acute changes in GFR and alterations in the tubuloglomerular feedback mechanism.

- Radiographic contrast media can cause contrast-induced nephropathy or radiocontrast nephropathy. These agents cause renal medullary vasoconstriction, decreased renal blood flow, and direct tubular toxicity.[15] Radiocontrast nephropathy is associated with several risk factors, including preexisting chronic kidney disease, diabetic nephropathy, heart failure, volume depletion and drugs (i.e., diuretics, nonsteroidal anti-inflammatory drugs [NSAIDs], angiotensin-converting enzyme inhibitors [ACEIs], and angiotensin receptor blockers [ARBs]).

- Nonsteroidal anti-inflammatory drugs can have adverse renal effects that are explained by two distinct pathological processes. The first mechanism of AKI is the result of reduced renal plasma flow caused by a decrease in prostaglandin synthesis, which regulates vasodilation at the glomerular level. Nonsteroidal anti-inflammatory drugs block the compensatory vasodilation response of renal prostaglandins, leading to unopposed vasoconstriction. A second mechanism of AKI is an acute allergic reaction, also known as acute interstitial nephritis. This typically occurs after short-term exposure (less than 7 days) and is characterized by the presence of an inflammatory cell infiltrate in the interstitium of the kidney.

- Calcineurin inhibitors (such as cyclosporin and tacrolimus) often cause acutely severe afferent arteriolar vasoconstriction that impairs glomerular blood flow, leading to decreased GFR. Chronic exposure to these drugs can lead to tubulointerstitial fibrosis, further increasing the risk of AKI when combined with other risk factors, including vasopressors such as norepinephrine, which are commonly used in ICU settings.

Postrenal AKI

Postrenal AKI is often caused by an obstruction in the urinary tract downstream from the kidneys, disrupting normal urine outflow. It occurs less often than intrinsic AKI or ATN in ICU settings. Conditions that may lead to postrenal AKI include kidney stones, an enlarged prostate, and neurological conditions leading to incomplete bladder emptying. For example, urinary calculi can be caused by metabolic abnormalities induced by loop diuretics, carbonic anhydrase inhibitors, and laxatives or supersaturation/crystallization with ciprofloxacin, triamterene, and sulfonamide antibiotics. In most cases, normal kidney function is regained if the etiology is identified and corrected promptly.

DISEASE ASSESSMENT

History and Physical Examination

A detailed and accurate medical history is critical for understanding the cause(s) of AKI in a given patient. This information is needed to distinguish acute from chronic kidney disease, where symptoms of fatigue, weight loss, anorexia, and pruritus are more common. Findings in the medical history that may predispose an individual to AKI include significant fluid or blood loss (i.e., gastroenteritis, recent surgery), trauma, and exposure to nephrotoxic drugs or heavy metals (mercury, lead, cadmium) that are considered an occupational hazard for welders and miners. Certain preexisting conditions can place patients at an elevated risk of developing AKI, including hypertension, chronic heart failure, diabetes, and autoimmune disorders.

The physical examination may provide evidence of intravascular hypovolemia depending on cardiovascular signs (heart rate, blood pressure) and peripheral edema. The presence of skin lesions may indicate trauma or acute allergic/immune reactions. Abdominal examination may help identify bladder obstruction caused by cancer or an enlarged prostate.

Estimating urine output for the past 3–5 days together with recent hourly fluid intake and output can yield important information about the time of onset and severity of AKI. Oliguria, defined as a urine output less than 400 mL/day, commonly occurs in prerenal and intrinsic AKI, whereas abrupt anuria (less than 50 mL/day) suggests acute urinary obstruction. A slower rate of urine output decline may indicate urethral or bladder outlet obstruction related to prostate hypertrophy.

Serum and Urinary Measures

The criteria most widely used to define AKI are based on (1) rate of rise of serum creatinine and (2) urine output. Until recently, there were no clear guidelines, definitions, or terminology related to AKI, making it difficult to directly compare ICU populations and outcomes in clinical studies. In 2004, the RIFLE approach to categorizing and staging AKI according to risk, injury, failure, loss of kidney function, and end-stage kidney disease was introduced by the ADQI (Acute Dialysis Quality Initiative) to grade the severity of AKI in the ICU.[16] In 2007, a set of uniform standards for describing and classifying AKI was proposed by the Acute Kidney Injury Network (AKIN).[17] In 2012, a third set of criteria was introduced by the Kidney Disease Improving Global Outcomes (KDIGO) group that incorporates parts of both the RIFLE and the AKIN definitions.[18] A comparison of these approaches is shown in Table 26.3.

The AKIN criteria include a shorter time interval for the rise of serum creatinine (within 48 hours) and include an absolute increase in serum creatinine of 0.3 mg/dL or greater or 50% or greater from baseline. Both RIFLE and AKIN criteria include a reduction in urine output of less than 0.5 mL/kg per hour for more than 6 hours. The KDIGO group further simplified the approach to include a basic definition of AKI, together with severity criteria (similar to AKIN), to provide a single definition that could be applied to practice, research, and public health.

Cystatin C is another surrogate marker used to detect acute changes in kidney function. It has been suggested that the rise in serum cystatin C from baseline occurs earlier than for serum creatinine and is a better early indicator of AKI. Herget-Rosenthal et al. reported that an increase in cystatin C of 50% occurred almost 2 days earlier than a similar rise in serum creatinine.[19] Nejat et al. studied more than 400 ICU patients and reported that changes in urinary cystatin C were detected earlier than for creatinine in patients with AKI, and urinary cystatin C was independently associated with AKI, sepsis, and death within 30 days.[20]

In addition to measuring urine output and classifying/staging AKI according to the criteria given previously, measuring the fractional excretion of sodium (FENa) provides an index of the percentage of filtered sodium excreted in the urine that can be used to distinguish prerenal

Table 26.3 Common Criteria Used for AKI Severity Staging

Consensus Group	AKI Severity Classification	GFR Cutoff	Serum Creatinine Change	Urine Output
RIFLE (2004)	RIFLE – R (Risk)	Decrease > 25%	Increase ≥ 1.5 x from baseline[a,b]	< 0.5 mL/kg/hr for 6 hr
	RIFLE – I (Injury)	Decrease > 50%	Increase ≥ 2 x from baseline[a,b]	< 0.5 mL/kg/hr for 12 hr
	RIFLE – F (Failure)	Decrease > 75%	Increase ≥ 3 x from baseline OR increase ≥ 0.5 mg/dL if baseline ≥ 4.0 mg/dL[a,b]	< 0.3 mL/kg/hr for 24 hr OR Anuria for 12 hr
	RIFLE – L (Loss of Kidney Function)	No GFR > 3 wk	—	—
	RIFLE – E (End-Stage Kidney disease)	No GFR > 4 mo	—	—
AKIN (2007)	Stage 1	—	Increase ≥ 0.3 mg/dL OR Increase ≥ 1.5–2 x within 48 hr	< 0.5 mL/kg/hr for more than 6 hr
	Stage 2	—	Increase > 2–3 x within 48 hr	< 0.5 mL/kg/hr for more than 12 hr
	Stage 3	—	Increase > 3 x within 48 hr OR increase ≥ 0.4 mg/dL if baseline ≥ 4.0 mg/dL[c]	< 0.3 mL/kg/hr for 24 hr OR Anuria for 12 hr
KDIGO (2012)	Stage 1	—	(Same as AKIN stage 1)	< 0.5 mL/kg/hr for 6–12 hr
	Stage 2	—	(Same as AKIN stage 2)	< 0.5 mL/kg/hr for ≥ 12 hr
	Stage 3	—	(Same as AKIN stage 3)	< 0.3 mL/kg/hr for ≥ 24 hr OR Anuria for ≥ 12 hr

[a]Within the past 7 days.
[b]Recommended to use MDRD (Modification of Diet in Renal Disease) with estimated GFR of 75–100 mL/minute/1.73m^2 to estimate baseline creatinine when missing.
[c]Stage 3 also includes any patients with at least stage 1 AKI requiring RRT (renal replacement therapy).
AKIN = Acute Kidney Injury Network; KDIGO = Kidney Disease Improving Global Outcomes; RIFLE = risk, injury, failure, loss of kidney function, and end-stage kidney disease.

from intrarenal (ATN) causes of AKI (Table 26.1). This nonspecific index of tubular function should not be used alone to evaluate AKI because many other conditions can alter FENa values, including renal salt wasting and diuretic therapy. The FENa is included as part of the comprehensive evaluation of AKI, including medical history, clinical and laboratory evaluation, and urine microscopy.

Calculating FENa requires measuring the filtered sodium load, which is the product of the creatinine clearance [urine creatinine (UCr) × urine volume (V) divided by serum creatinine (SCr)] and the serum sodium concentration (SNa). The urinary sodium excretion is equal to the product of the urine sodium concentration (UNa) and the urine volume (V).

This results in the following equation:

$$\text{FENa (\%)} = \frac{(\text{UNa} \times \text{SCr} \times 100)}{(\text{SNa} \times \text{UCr})}$$

Although no definitive tests predict AKI, measuring urine output in response to a diuretic challenge has been proposed. For example, a furosemide stress test, consisting of a single dose of furosemide 1 mg/kg in naive patients or 1.5 mg/kg in previously exposed patients, in early AKI (defined as AKIN stage I or II) significantly predicts the patients who will progress to a higher AKI stage.[21] After receiving the furosemide dose, patients were significantly more likely to progress if their subsequent urine output in 2 hours was less than 200 mL (100 mL/hour). The sensitivity and specificity of this test are 87.1% and 84.1%, respectively. Adding other renal biomarkers did not improve the predictive quality of the test.

Urine Microscopy

Urine microscopy is readily available and inexpensive and is an important part of the differential diagnosis of AKI. Evaluating the urinary sediment is most useful to distinguish between ATN and prerenal AKI. Urinary microscopy in patients with ATN often reveals renal tubular epithelial cells, cellular casts, granular casts, and muddy brown or mixed cellular casts. In a study of 267 consecutive patients with AKI, a urinary sediment scoring system was a strong predictor of ATN.[22] In the absence of pyelonephritis, the presence of leukocytes, red blood cells (RBCs), and white blood cell (WBC) casts in the urine of patients with AKI can indicate drug-induced acute interstitial nephritis. In contrast, patients with prerenal AKI may have no abnormal findings on microscopy, or occasional hyaline casts.

Renal Imaging and Biopsy Studies

Renal ultrasonography is particularly important for identifying postrenal causes of AKI. For example, the presence of residual postvoiding urine volumes greater than 100 mL can indicate a urine outflow obstruction. Other extrarenal causes of obstruction, such as tumors, can be detected using computed tomography or magnetic resonance imaging. Kidney biopsies are usually reserved for when pre- and postrenal causes of AKI have been excluded and the cause of intrinsic renal injury is unclear. Renal biopsy can be used to confirm acute glomerular and interstitial nephritis (acute interstitial nephritis) that may be related to drug-induced AKI.

Novel Biomarkers

Many novel urinary protein biomarkers have been shown to predict the occurrence and severity of AKI in ICU settings. Haase et al. compiled the results of several studies and found that neutrophil gelatinase-associated lipocalin (NGAL), across different time points, predicted the need for dialysis and death.[23] Similarly, Koyner et al. reported that urine NGAL, measured post-cardiac surgery, was a strong predictor of stage 3 AKI and that preoperative urine KIM-1 (kidney injury molecule 1) levels were less predictive.[24] Parikh et al. reported that urine IL-18 (interleukin-18) was significantly associated with mortality in a subgroup of ICU patients within the ARDS (Acute Respiratory Distress Syndrome) Network trial.[25] More recent studies have evaluated novel combinations of biomarkers for their ability to predict AKI. Prowle et al. studied a group of 93 high-risk patients undergoing cardiopulmonary bypass together with combinations of biomarkers to predict RIFLE-R (see Table 26.3) within 5 days after surgery.[26] Of the 25 patients who developed AKI, the ratio of urinary NGAL to creatinine measurement postoperatively, followed by urinary hepcidin to creatinine at 24 hours, best identified the patients in the high-, intermediate-, and low-risk AKI groups. In 2013, a combination test was introduced that measures urinary tissue inhibitor of metalloproteinase 2 (TIMP-2) and urinary insulin-like growth factor binding protein 7 (IGFBP-7). The rationale for studying these two biomarkers is that they are both involved in the G1 cell cycle arrest of renal tubular cells during the early period of cell injury. Derivation and validation of the "TIMP-2 × IGFBP-7" biomarker algorithm in more than 500 patients accurately predicted AKI after cardiac surgery in high-risk patients,[27,28] resulting in the FDA approval of NephroCheck (Astute Medical, San Diego, CA) as a urinary diagnostic device for AKI in September 2014.[29]

PREVENTION AND TREATMENT

General Approaches

Because of limited treatment options, preventing AKI is essential. Patients at risk of AKI should be identified early, with steps taken to avoid potential renal insults (see Table 26.4). Patient characteristics associated with a greater risk of AKI are included in Table 26.1. Once high-risk patients are identified, instituting general measures lessens the occurrence of AKI. These measures include maintaining appropriate fluid status and, when possible, avoiding diuretics; maintaining adequate blood pressure; and minimizing the use of potential nephrotoxins, including drugs.

Loop diuretics are used in many patients with AKI to either treat or prevent renal failure.[30] Because data regarding the use of loop diuretics in AKI are usually from observational or small clinical trials, often with conflicting results, several meta-analyses have clarified their role.[31,32] These meta-analyses conclude that loop diuretics have little to no impact on the outcome of AKI. Whether loop diuretics were used to prevent renal deterioration or treat AKI, there was no effect on mortality or the requirement for RRT. The results were mixed regarding number of dialysis sessions and urine output, with one analysis concluding that loop diuretics shorten the duration of RRT and increase urine output, and the other showing no difference. One of the analyses showed a significantly greater incidence of ototoxicity in the loop diuretic group. Loop diuretics also have not proven beneficial in renal recovery after the completion of AKI-related RRT.[33] Overall, using loop diuretics in AKI remains controversial.

There are no definitive trials of critically ill patients, and at this time, the benefit or harm of loop diuretics in AKI is unsubstantiated. The soon-to-be-published SPARK (Furosemide in Early Acute Kidney Injury) study may provide more definitive guidance.[34]

Hypovolemia

Hypovolemia and volume depletion are significant risk factors for AKI.[35] Although no clinical trials substantiate the use of fluids in preventing and treating AKI, their importance in this setting is well accepted. In addition, no large randomized controlled trials analyze the amount of fluid that should be administered to prevent or treat AKI. In the large trials that have compared colloids (e.g., albumin, hetastarches) with crystalloids (e.g., 0.9% saline, lactated Ringer solution) and chloride-liberal with chloride-restricted fluids, the amount of fluid given was at the discretion of the treating clinician.

Many trials have compared colloids with crystalloids for volume depletion in ICU patients. The SAFE (Saline versus Albumin Fluid Evaluation) trial compared the administration of albumin with that of crystalloids (normal saline) in patients who required fluid administration to maintain intravascular volume.[36] Although the number of patients who subsequently developed AKI was not specifically delineated in the trial, there were no differences in the number of patients with new single or multiorgan failure. Another study that looked at adding albumin to crystalloid resuscitation in patients with septic shock found similar results.[37] Patients received albumin infusions on a daily basis for 28 days, and crystalloids were given according to sepsis guidelines and at the discretion of the clinician. No differences existed in the number of patients who developed AKI or required RRT at 28 days. The CRISTAL (Colloids versus Crystalloids for the Resuscitation of the Critically Ill) trial compared crystalloids with several different colloids (albumin, gelatins, dextrans, hydroxyethyl starches) in patients with hypovolemic shock.[38] Results showed no difference in the percentage of patients requiring RRT within 7 or 28 days. Of interest, using hydroxyethyl starches for resuscitation in this trial did not increase the requirement for RRT as it had in other trials.[39] In fact, a meta-analysis has shown that the use of hydroxyethyl starches for resuscitation increases the risk of AKI and the need for RRT.[40] These data suggest that other than hydroxyethyl starches, which may increase the risk of AKI, the choice of resuscitation fluid, colloid or crystalloid, does not affect the subsequent development of AKI.

Early goal-directed therapy in sepsis is designed to administer fluids to achieve a central venous pressure of 8–12 mm Hg; mean arterial pressure of 65 mm Hg or greater; urine output of 0.5 mL/kg/hour or greater; superior vena cava oxygenation saturation ($Scvo_2$) or mixed venous oxygen saturation (Svo_2) of 70% or 65%, respectively; and normalization of lactate concentrations.[41,42] The results of the

Table 26.4 General AKI Prevention/Treatment Strategies

General interventions	• Identify at-risk patients • Maintain appropriate fluid status • Avoid diuretics • Maintain adequate blood pressure • Minimize nephrotoxic medications • Use alternative, less nephrotoxic agents when possible • Discontinue the offending agent as soon as possible • Provide general supportive measures including fluids and RRT, if necessary
Loop diuretics	• Minimize use to prevent AKI • Little to no benefit in preventing or treating AKI
Crystalloids	• Equal in efficacy to colloids at preventing AKI in volume-depleted patients. • Recommended over colloids (KDIGO) • Use chloride-restricted fluids

RRT = renal replacement therapy.

original trial showing mortality benefits with goal-directed therapy did not specifically evaluate the benefits related to AKI.[41] However, several organ functioning scores were improved with the therapy. Subsequent trials evaluating the impact of early goal-directed therapy in sepsis did not find any benefit in the fluid strategy for either mortality or AKI.[43,44] The number of patients requiring RRT and the duration of RRT were not statistically different between groups. There is also concern that fluid accumulation, which may occur in early goal-directed therapy in patients who are volume depleted or hypotensive, may actually increase the risk of AKI.[45] In this trial, patients with fluid overload had greater mortality at 30 days and less recovery of renal function after AKI. In the FACTT study (Fluids and Catheters Treatment Trial), which evaluated conservative versus liberal fluid management of patients with acute lung injury, there was no difference in the incidence of AKI in the two fluid management groups.[46]

Another important factor related to fluid resuscitation is choosing between chloride-liberal and chloride-restricted fluids. Excess chloride is believed to have a negative impact on renal perfusion. Therefore, administering large volumes of chloride-rich fluids may increase the risk of AKI. Most patients who receive crystalloids for shock receive normal saline (0.9% sodium chloride), which contains 154 mEq of chloride per liter. Chloride-restricted fluids include Ringer lactate and PlasmaLyte (109 and 98 mEq of chloride per liter, respectively). In a large trial of almost 3,000 patients, the use of a chloride-restricted fluid resuscitation strategy resulted in fewer patients with moderate to severe AKI and a lower requirement for RRT.[47] The fluids used were either crystalloids or colloids, but the chloride-restricted fluids all had chloride concentrations less than 110 mEq/L. An even larger retrospective study of more than 7,000 patients matched patients receiving normal saline for resuscitation with patients receiving a chloride-restricted crystalloid approach (combination of Ringer lactate and normal saline).[48] Although in-hospital mortality was significantly lower in the balanced fluid group, there were no differences in the percentage of patients experiencing AKI with or without the need for dialysis. A meta-analysis of perioperative and critical care fluid resuscitation with chloride-liberal versus chloride-restricted fluids found no difference in mortality between the different crystalloids.[49] However, chloride-restricted resuscitation decreased the incidence of acute renal failure and hyperchloremic metabolic acidosis. In this analysis, the significant effect was mostly driven by the results of the Yunos et al. trial, which was the only trial in the analysis that included colloids.[47]

The KDIGO AKI guidelines recommend crystalloids for expanding intravascular volume over albumin or starches.[50] They do not address the issue of hyperchloremic crystalloids, but most of the literature in this area was published after publication of the KDIGO guidelines. The Kidney Disease Outcomes Quality Initiative (KDOQI) commentary related to the KDIGO AKI guidelines does address the issue of harm related to hyperchloremic fluids but suggests that better prospective data are still warranted before advocating the preferential use of these fluids.[18] Both KDIGO and KDOQI recommend that vasopressors be used with fluids to prevent AKI in patients with hypovolemic shock, with KDOQI commentators recommending cautious use of dopamine as a first-line vasopressor. Finally, the KDIGO guidelines recommend using a protocol to manage hemodynamic instability (e.g., early goal-directed therapy). However, because the original early goal-directed therapy trial in sepsis did not specifically assess the incidence of AKI and because more recent trials have not shown a benefit to early goal-directed therapy at preventing AKI, the KDOQI commentators do not endorse management by a protocol. It should be noted that the lack of benefit with early goal-directed therapy in more recent trials may be related to an overall improvement in the standard of care (the comparative arm in these trials) for the fluid management of sepsis. Given all of this, to prevent AKI in hypovolemic patients, it seems prudent to use chloride-restricted crystalloids with vasopressors when necessary, as part of a fluid management protocol.

Drug-Induced AKI

Specific recommendations for preventing or treating drug-induced AKI are limited (see Table 26.5). For most drugs, understanding the risk and using alternative, less nephrotoxic agents in patients at high risk of renal failure is the best preventive strategy. Treatment involves supportive care and discontinuing the offending agent as soon as possible. Fortunately, most drug-related causes of AKI are reversible if caught early, with subsequent discontinuation of the nephrotoxin. Medications most associated with renal failure include NSAIDs and selective cyclooxygenase 2 inhibitors; ACEIs and ARBs; vasopressors; β-lactam, sulfonamide, aminoglycoside, and glycopeptide antibiotics; amphotericin B; acyclovir and cisplatin; carboplatin and oxaliplatin; cyclosporine and tacrolimus; and radiocontrast agents. Drug classes with specific recommendations are listed in the paragraphs that follow with the data supporting prevention or treatment strategies.

ACEIs and ARBs

Although there are no specific prevention or treatment recommendations for ACEI- or ARB-induced AKI, two important points should be stressed. First, ACEI- or ARB-induced AKI is more likely to occur in patients receiving NSAIDs or diuretics, or in patients who are volume depleted.[51] These risk factors reduce renal perfusion pressure and exacerbate the ACEI or ARB effect on the kidneys. In patients with these risk factors, ACEIs and ARBs should be initiated at low doses and titrated slowly. Even when someone is stabilized on an ACEI/ARB, volume depletion or adding an NSAID or diuretic can increase the likelihood of decreasing GFR.[51]

Table 26.5	Drug-Induced AKI Prevention/Treatment Strategies
Medication	
ACEIs and ARBs	• Avoid concomitant use with NSAIDs and diuretics, if possible • Maintain adequate volume status • Start at low doses and titrate slowly
Aminoglycosides	• Avoid prolonged courses, elevated trough concentrations, hypovolemia, concurrent nephrotoxic agents, and over-diuresis • Use high-dose extended-interval dosing, if possible
Vancomycin	• Close monitoring when targeting higher trough concentrations • Close monitoring when used concomitantly with either aminoglycosides or piperacillin/tazobactam
Amphotericin B	• Use a lipid formulation • Liberalize sodium intake, including normal saline boluses before and after administration
Sulfonamides, acyclovir, methotrexate (crystalluria)	• Adequate fluid (e.g., normal saline) to achieve a urine output of 100–150 mL/hr • For sulfonamide or methotrexate crystalluria, alkalinize the urine
Cisplatin	• Adequate fluid (e.g., normal saline) to achieve a urine output of 100–150 mL/hr • Begin fluid administration 12 hr before infusion and continue for 24 hr • In ovarian cancer, may consider administering amifostine before each dose • Reduce the dose or use carboplatin instead
Calcineurin inhibitors (cyclosporine, tacrolimus)	• Monitor therapeutic drug concentrations closely • Avoid drug interactions that increase serum concentrations
Radiocontrast agents	• Use lower doses and minimize diagnostic tests requiring radiocontrast agents • Normal saline or sodium bicarbonate infusions up to 12 hr before and 12 hr after administration • Moderate- or high-dose statins (for cardiac procedures using contrast) • Ascorbic acid (for cardiac procedures using contrast)

NSAID = nonsteroidal anti-inflammatory drug.

Second, an increase in serum creatinine after administering ACEIs/ARBs is not a reason to discontinue therapy. An increase in creatinine of up to 30% is common in the first few weeks after initiating an ACEI/ARB.[51] This increase will remain but will stabilize in the first month of therapy. Only if a patient's creatinine increases greater than 30% over baseline when initiating an ACEI/ARB should the dose be reduced or the drug discontinued altogether.

Aminoglycosides

Nephrotoxicity is a well-known complication of aminoglycoside therapy. Fortunately, this adverse event is reversible after discontinuation because renal cells can regenerate.[52] Controversy exists regarding the risk factors associated with aminoglycoside nephrotoxicity. Various controlled studies relate certain factors to subsequent toxicity, including a prolonged course or recent course, persistently elevated trough concentrations, hypovolemia, advanced age, liver disease, concurrent nephrotoxic agents, and overdiuresis.[52,53]

No specific interventions consistently prevent aminoglycoside nephrotoxicity. General measures (e.g., hydrating the patient and avoiding concomitant nephrotoxins) are important. Maintaining appropriate serum concentrations is also recommended; however, no data correlate nephrotoxicity with specific serum concentrations or with therapeutic drug monitoring.[54] In an effort to decrease toxicity and improve efficacy, high-dose extended-interval ("once daily") aminoglycoside dosing is recommended. Many studies have evaluated the nephrotoxicity of once-daily dosing compared with traditional dosing, and many meta-analyses have subsequently tried to aggregate the results.[55-62] In two of eight of these meta-analyses, once-daily dosing was associated with less nephrotoxicity, a 26%–40% relative risk reduction. In the others, there was no difference between the two dosing strategies. Although controversial, it seems prudent to use once-daily dosing whenever possible and to institute other general preventive strategies, including therapeutic drug monitoring, when using aminoglycosides.

Vancomycin

The understanding of vancomycin nephrotoxicity has changed over the years. Early in its use, vancomycin contained many impurities that were believed to lead to nephrotoxicity. Once the clinical formulation was purified, the incidence of nephrotoxicity was 5%–17% in various clinical trials.[63–68] This rate increased to as high as 35% of patients when vancomycin was combined with aminoglycosides. In guidelines published in 2009, higher vancomycin trough values (10–20 mcg/mL) were recommended to decrease resistance, enhance tissue penetration, and improve clinical outcomes, especially in serious MRSA (methicillin-resistant *Staphylococcus aureus*) infections.[69] After these recommendations, several studies and a meta-analysis of a variety of hospitalized patients with gram-positive infections showed an increased nephrotoxicity of vancomycin to as high as 34% of patients.[70-73] A few other factors were related to this high level, including ICU residence and longer lengths of therapy, but higher trough concentrations had the biggest impact.

As with aminoglycosides, no specific interventions definitively prevent or treat vancomycin nephrotoxicity. Because recent studies suggest that higher vancomycin trough concentrations increase the risk of nephrotoxicity, closer monitoring is advised when targeting trough concentrations above 15 mcg/mL. Certain infections may require these higher concentrations because of the location or the MIC (minimum inhibitory concentration) of the causative organism. In these situations, using an alternative antibiotic may be the most appropriate method to prevent AKI. The incidence of nephrotoxicity is also significantly higher when vancomycin is combined with aminoglycosides[63,67] or piperacillin/tazobactam.[68,74,75] Because these are antibiotic combinations commonly used in the ICU patient, diligence is warranted in monitoring serum concentrations, maintaining adequate volume status, and avoiding any other nephrotoxins.

Amphotericin B

Amphotericin B nephrotoxicity occurs commonly, with the GFR falling within the first few weeks of initiating therapy.[76] Most patients stabilize at 20%–60% of normal renal function, but acute renal failure can occur.[77] The exact mechanism of nephrotoxicity is uncertain but is probably related to decreases in renal blood flow and amphotericin binding to cholesterol in the tubular epithelium, causing tubular necrosis. The decrease in function is also believed to be the result of a feedback mechanism in the kidney where the ion load created by amphotericin in the urine causes vasoconstriction of the afferent arteriole.[77] Newer lipid formulations of amphotericin significantly decrease the incidence of renal toxicity, with rates decreasing from 40%–50% to 8%–20%.[78–81] This lower incidence is believed to be because of a slower release of amphotericin B in the bloodstream and less of the drug available to interact directly with the renal tubules.

Because there is no specific treatment for amphotericin renal toxicity, prevention is key. Treatment usually consists of interrupting amphotericin therapy, which is problematic in patients with certain resistant fungal infections. Newer antifungals, such as the azoles and echinocandins, are not considered nephrotoxic and are appropriate alternatives for certain fungal infections (e.g., candidiasis and aspergillosis) in patients at risk of nephrotoxicity.[82] Lipid formulations of amphotericin should be used whenever possible to decrease the risk of nephrotoxicity. One of the best nephrotoxicity prevention strategies for either amphotericin deoxycholate or one of the lipid formulations is salt loading.[77,83] Because of the proposed renal feedback mechanism for nephrotoxicity, maintaining an adequate osmolality in the blood decreases the renal response to the high ionic load in the renal tubules. Liberalizing salt intake and using normal saline for maintenance fluid and intravenous medications is beneficial. In addition to increasing sodium intake, 500 mL of normal saline should be administered over the 30 minutes immediately before and immediately after the amphotericin infusion.[77] Ideally, the goal is to induce a urinary sodium excretion of 250–300 mmol per day. If not instituted preventively, sodium loading may be beneficial as a treatment to allow for continued amphotericin B administration. The only other method with data supporting its effectiveness in preventing nephrotoxicity is continuous infusion amphotericin.[84] Acetylcysteine and mannitol are not beneficial in preventing amphotericin toxicity.[85,86]

Sulfonamides, Acyclovir, and Methotrexate

Certain medications cause AKI by crystallizing in the urine and causing tubular obstruction. Examples of these drugs include sulfonamides, acyclovir, and methotrexate. This crystallization can be prevented by administering adequate fluids. Patients should receive fluid to maintain a urine output of 100–150 mL/hour while on these agents.[87] For crystallization secondary to sulfonamides and methotrexate, giving sodium bicarbonate to alkalinize the urine increases crystal solubility.

Cisplatin

Because of its efficacy as a cancer chemotherapeutic agent, cisplatin is still commonly used, even though it causes significant direct cellular toxicity in the proximal tubule. Many agents have been evaluated for their potential protection against this nephrotoxicity.[88] At this time, the best method appears to be administering fluid, starting at least 12 hours before cisplatin. This fluid volume should achieve a urine output of at least 100–125 mL/hour. In addition, cisplatin should be infused in normal saline. Fluid administration should then continue for 24 hours after cisplatin administration. Data on administering diuretics such as furosemide or mannitol do not consistently support their effectiveness over saline alone.[89] In ovarian cancer, administering amifostine before each cisplatin dose may be considered to prevent renal oxidative stress and subsequent cisplatin-related nephrotoxicity.[90] Amifostine cost and adverse events, especially hypotension, may limit its use. Finally, cisplatin dose reduction or use of the less nephrotoxic platinum drug carboplatin decreases the risk of nephrotoxicity.

Calcineurin Inhibitors

The calcineurin inhibitors, cyclosporine and tacrolimus, are both acutely and chronically nephrotoxic.[91] This can add to the complexity of their therapeutic use, especially when used to prevent renal transplant rejection. Acutely, these agents cause vasoconstriction of afferent arterioles, leading to nephrotoxicity that is reversed with dosage alterations. Chronically, they cause an irreversible tubular toxicity and progressive, ischemic glomerulosclerosis.[92] Patients receiving these agents should take the standard precautions for preventing toxicity (i.e., avoid other nephrotoxic agents, maintain appropriate fluid volume, etc.). Both medications should have drug concentrations monitored closely and doses adjusted accordingly. Concomitant medications should be used carefully to avoid drug interactions that may increase concentrations and associated nephrotoxicity.

Radiocontrast Agents

Whether radiocontrast agents are nephrotoxic is controversial. Studies with control groups are rare (all nonrandomized) and have found no difference in AKI between those that do and do not receive these agents.[93] The proposed mechanism of nephrotoxicity associated with radiocontrast agents is unknown but is believed to be the result of a combination of decreased renal blood flow and direct tubular toxicity. Many studies have evaluated strategies for preventing nephrotoxicity, primarily focusing on normal saline, sodium bicarbonate, acetylcysteine, and statins. Several meta-analyses and guidelines have been developed using these studies. As with amphotericin, an effective preventive strategy appears to be sodium loading.[94] Recommendations include using normal saline at a rate of 100 mL/hour 6–12 hours before and 4–12 hours after administering radiocontrast agents. Obviously, in emergency cases, the pre-administration salt loading may not be possible. Studies have also shown that sodium bicarbonate infusions are more effective than normal saline at preventing radiocontrast-induced AKI, and most subsequent meta-analyses have confirmed this superior benefit.[95-99] Acetylcysteine has been studied to prevent radiocontrast-induced AKI in several clinical trials with subsequent meta-analyses. These meta-analyses have generally not supported this intervention because of inconsistent results, but using higher doses may be beneficial.[100-103] Many studies have evaluated the use of statins in either moderate or high doses to prevent contrast-induced nephropathy after coronary angiography and percutaneous coronary intervention. Several meta-analyses of these trials have shown a consistent benefit of statins in preventing AKI.[104-107] Ascorbic acid is also effective at preventing AKI after contrast use for coronary angiography.[108] Theophylline has shown benefit in preventing contrast-induced nephrotoxicity, but primarily in patients with normal serum creatinine.[109] Other agents that have been tried without success in this setting are mannitol, furosemide, and fenoldopam.[110] Nonpharmacologic measures such as using lower doses of contrast, minimizing diagnostic tests with contrast, or spacing out these tests can also be used to prevent toxicity.

Ineffective Agents for Renal Protection

For years, low- or renal-dose dopamine was used to maintain renal perfusion and prevent AKI. At doses of 0.5–5 mcg/kg/minute, dopamine has preferential effects on the kidney, causing increased renal perfusion. Many meta-analyses and a large clinical trial have looked at several different outcomes when using low-dose dopamine, including mortality, increases in serum creatinine, development of acute renal failure, need for RRT, and hospital and ICU lengths of stay.[111-114] Urine output increases in the first 24 hours after adding low-dose dopamine, but that effect diminishes within 48 hours.[114] Low-dose dopamine is therefore no longer recommended for renal protection.[42]

Fenoldopam, a D_1-specific dopamine agonist, has also been suggested as an agent to prevent or treat AKI in critical care patients. A meta-analysis of studies in cardiac surgery patients found that the incidence of AKI was significantly decreased by fenoldopam.[115] Patients receiving fenoldopam had a higher incidence of hypotension and vasopressor use, and there was no d   tients undergoing noncardiac surgery.[124] Although the primary outcomes of POISE-2 were death or nonfatal MI, a substudy evaluated the impact of the two drugs on AKI. Neither drug decreased the risk of AKI perioperatively; however, there was an increased risk of major bleeding and hypotension as the result of aspirin and clonidine, respectively. Patients who had either a major bleed or hypotension had a higher risk of subsequent AKI.

CONCLUSION

In summary, AKI often occurs in ICU settings. It is rarely attributed to a single factor, and most critically ill patients who develop AKI do so as a result of several renal insults occurring simultaneously or in sequence (hemodynamic, septic, and nephrotoxic). The clinical picture is further complicated in patients with underlying kidney disease and in those receiving nephrotoxic medications. Because many forms of AKI are preventable, patients at risk should be identified early and steps taken to avoid potential renal insults. Treatment of established AKI involves fluids, drug dose adjustment or discontinuation, and supportive care.

REFERENCES

1. Waikar SS, Liu KD, Chertow GM. The incidence and prognostic significance of acute kidney injury. Curr Opin Nephrol Hypertens 2007;16:227-36.
2. Hilton R. Acute renal failure. BMJ 2006;333:786-90.
3. Kellum JA. Acute kidney injury. Crit Care Med 2008;36:S141-145.
4. Hansen MK, Gammelager H, Mikkelsen MM, et al. Post-operative acute kidney injury and five-year risk of death, myocardial infarction, and stroke among elective cardiac surgical patients: a cohort study. Crit Care 2013;17:R292.
5. Mandelbaum T, Scott DJ, Lee J, et al. Outcome of critically ill patients with acute kidney injury using the Acute Kidney Injury Network criteria. Crit Care Med 2011;39:2659-64.
6. Macedo E, Malhotra R, Bouchard J, et al. Oliguria is an early predictor of higher mortality in critically ill patients. Kidney Int 2011;80:760-7.
7. Ralib AM, Pickering JW, Shaw GM, et al. The urine output definition of acute kidney injury is too liberal. Crit Care 2013;17:R112.
8. Brown JR, Kramer RS, Coca SG, et al. Duration of acute kidney injury impacts long-term survival after cardiac surgery. Ann Thorac Surg 2010;90:1142-9.
9. Coca SG, King JT, Rosenthal RA, et al. The duration of postoperative acute kidney injury is an additional parameter predicting long-term survival in diabetic veterans. Kidney Int 2010;78:926-33.
10. Stewart J, Findlay G, Smith N, et al. Adding insult to injury: a review of the care of patients who died in hospital with a primary diagnosis of acute kidney injury (acute renal failure). A Report by the National Confidential Enquiry into Patient Outcome and Death (2009). Available at www.ncepod.org.uk/2009aki.htm. Accessed February 28, 2015.
11. Ricksten SE, Bragadottir G, Redfors B. Renal oxygenation in clinical acute kidney injury. Crit Care 2013;17:221.
12. Bagshaw SM, George C, Bellomo R. Early acute kidney injury and sepsis: a multicentre evaluation. Crit Care 2008;12:R47.
13. Bellomo R, Wan L, Langenberg C, et al. Septic acute kidney injury: the glomerular arterioles. Contrib Nephrol 2011;174:98-107.
14. Watanabe A, Nagai J, Adachi Y, et al. Targeted prevention of renal accumulation and toxicity of gentamicin by aminoglycoside binding receptor antagonists. J Control Release 2004;95:423-33.
15. Heyman SN, Rosen S, Rosenberger C. Renal parenchymal hypoxia, hypoxia adaptation, and the pathogenesis of radiocontrast nephropathy. Clin J Am Soc Nephrol 2008;3:288-96.
16. Bellomo R, Ronco C, Kellum JA, et al. Acute renal failure – definition, outcome measures, animal models, fluid therapy and information technology needs: the Second International Consensus Conference of the Acute Dialysis Quality Initiative (ADQI) Group. Crit Care 2004;8:R204-12.
17. Ronco C, Levin A, Warnock DG, et al. AKIN Working Group. Improving outcomes from acute kidney injury (AKI): report on an initiative. Int J Artif Organs 2007;30:373-6.
18. Palevsky PM, Liu KD, Brophy PD, et al. KDOQI US commentary on the 2012 KDIGO clinical practice guideline for acute kidney injury. Am J Kidney Dis 2013;61:649-72.
19. Herget-Rosenthal S, Marggraf G, Hüsing J, et al. Early detection of acute renal failure by serum cystatin C. Kidney Int 2004;66:1115-22.
20. Nejat M, Pickering JW, Walker RJ, et al. Rapid detection of acute kidney injury by plasma cystatin C in the intensive care unit. Nephrol Dial Transplant 2010;25:3283-9.
21. Chawla LS, Davison DL, Brasha-Mitchell E, et al. Development and standardization of a furosemide stress test to predict the severity of acute kidney injury. Crit Care 2013 Sep 20;17(5):R207.
22. Perazella MA, Coca SG, Kanbay M, et al. Diagnostic value of urine microscopy for differntial diagnosis of acute kidney injury in hospitalized patients. Clin J Am Soc Nephrol 2008;31615-9.
23. Haase M, Bellomo R, Devarajan P, et al. Accuracy of neutrophil gelatinase-associated lipocalin (NGAL) in diagnosis and prognosis in acute kidney injury: a systematic review and meta-analysis. Am J Kidney Dis 2009;54:1012-24.
24. Koyner JL, Vaidya VS, Bennett MR, et al. Urinary biomarkers in the clinical prognosis and early detection of acute kidney injury. Clin J Am Soc Nephrol 2010;5:2154-65.
25. Parikh CR, Abraham E, Ancukiewicz M, et al. Urine IL-18 is an early diagnostic marker for acute kidney injury and predicts mortality in the intensive care unit. J Am Soc Nephrol 2005;16:3046-52.
26. Prowle JR, Calzavacca P, Licari E, et al. Combination of biomarkers for diagnosis of acute kidney injury after cardiopulmonary bypass. Ren Fail 2015;14:1-9.
27. Wetz AJ, Richardt EM, Wand S, et al. Quantification of urinary TIMP-2 and IGFBP-7 – an adequate diagnostic test to predict acute kidney injury after cardiac surgery? Crit Care 2015;19:3.
28. Hoste EA, McCullough PA, Kashani K, et al. Derivation and validation of cutoffs for clinical use of cell cycle arrest biomarkers. Nephrol Dial Transplant 2014;29:2054-61.
29. U.S. Food and Drug Administration (FDA). FDA Allows Marketing of the First Test to Assess Risk of Developing Acute Kidney Injury. September 5, 2014. Available at www.fda.gov/NewsEvents/Newsroom/PressAnnouncements/ucm412910.htm. Accessed February 28, 2015.
30. Uchino S, Doig GS, Bellomo R, et al.; Beginning and Ending Supportive Therapy for the Kidney (B.E.S.T. Kidney) Investigators. Diuretics and mortality in acute renal failure. Crit Care Med 2004;32:1669-77.
31. Ho KM, Sheridan DJ. Meta-analysis of frusemide to prevent or treat acute renal failure. BMJ 2006;333:420.
32. Bagshaw SM, Delaney A, Haase M, et al. Loop diuretics in the management of acute renal failure: a systematic review and meta-analysis. Crit Care Resusc 2007;9:60-8.
33. van der Voort PH, Boerma EC, Koopmans M, et al. Furosemide does not improve renal recovery after hemofiltration for acute renal failure in critically ill patients: a double blind randomized controlled trial. Crit Care Med 2009;37:533-8.
34. Bagshaw SM, Gibney RT, McAlister FA, et al. The SPARK study: a phase II randomized blinded controlled trial of the effect of furosemide in critically ill patients with early acute kidney injury. Trials 2010;11:50.

35. Piccinni P, Cruz DN, Gramaticopolo S, et al.; NEFROINT Investigators. Prospective multicenter study on epidemiology of acute kidney injury in the ICU: a critical care nephrology Italian collaborative effort (NEFROINT). Minerva Anestesiol 2011;77:1072-83.

36. Finfer S, Bellomo R, Boyce N, et al.; SAFE Study Investigators. A comparison of albumin and saline for fluid resuscitation in the intensive care unit. N Engl J Med 2004;350:2247-56.

37. Caironi P, Tognoni G, Masson S, et al.; ALBIOS Study Investigators. Albumin replacement in patients with severe sepsis or septic shock. N Engl J Med 2014;370:1412-21.

38. Annane D, Siami S, Jaber S, et al.; CRISTAL Investigators. Effects of fluid resuscitation with colloids vs crystalloids on mortality in critically ill patients presenting with hypovolemic shock: the CRISTAL randomized trial. JAMA 2013;310:1809-17.

39. Myburgh JA, Finfer S, Bellomo R, et al.; CHEST Investigators; Australian and New Zealand Intensive Care Society Clinical Trials Group. Hydroxyethyl starch or saline for fluid resuscitation in intensive care. N Engl J Med 2012;367:1901-11.

40. Zarychanski R, Abou-Setta AM, Turgeon AF, et al. Association of hydroxyethyl starch administration with mortality and acute kidney injury in critically ill patients requiring volume resuscitation: a systematic review and meta-analysis. JAMA 2013;309:678-88. Erratum in: JAMA 2013;309:1229.

41. Rivers E, Nguyen B, Havstad S, et al.; Early Goal-Directed Therapy Collaborative Group. Early goal-directed therapy in the treatment of severe sepsis and septic shock. N Engl J Med 2001;345:1368-77.

42. Dellinger RP, Levy MM, Rhodes A, et al.; Surviving Sepsis Campaign Guidelines Committee including the Pediatric Subgroup. Surviving Sepsis Campaign: international guidelines for management of severe sepsis and septic shock: 2012. Crit Care Med 2013;41:580-637.

43. ARISE Investigators; ANZICS Clinical Trials Group, Peake SL, et al. Goal-directed resuscitation for patients with early septic shock. N Engl J Med 2014;371:1496-506.

44. ProCESS Investigators; Yealy DM, Kellum JA, et al. A randomized trial of protocol-based care for early septic shock. N Engl J Med 2014;370:1683-93.

45. Bouchard J, Soroko SB, Chertow GM, et al.; Program to Improve Care in Acute Renal Disease (PICARD) Study Group. Fluid accumulation, survival and recovery of kidney function in critically ill patients with acute kidney injury. Kidney Int 2009;76:422-7.

46. National Heart, Lung, and Blood Institute Acute Respiratory Distress Syndrome (ARDS) Clinical Trials Network; Wiedemann HP, Wheeler AP, et al. Comparison of two fluid-management strategies in acute lung injury. N Engl J Med 2006;354:2564-75.

47. Yunos NM, Bellomo R, Glassford N, et al. Chloride-liberal vs. chloride-restrictive intravenous fluid administration and acute kidney injury: an extended analysis. Intensive Care Med 2015;41:257-64.

48. Raghunathan K, Shaw A, Nathanson B, et al. Association between the choice of IV crystalloid and in-hospital mortality among critically ill adults with sepsis. Crit Care Med 2014;42:1585-91.

49. Krajewski ML, Raghunathan K, Paluszkiewicz SM, et al. Meta-analysis of high- versus low-chloride content in perioperative and critical care fluid resuscitation. Br J Surg 2015;102:24-36.

50. Kidney Disease: Improving Global Outcomes (KDIGO) Acute Kidney Injury Work Group. KDIGO Clinical Practice Guideline for Acute Kidney Injury. Kidney Int Suppl 2012;2:1-138.

51. Bakris GL, Weir MR. Angiotensin-converting enzyme inhibitor-associated elevations in serum creatinine: is this a cause for concern? Arch Intern Med 2000;160:685-93.

52. Lietman PS, Smith CR. Aminoglycoside nephrotoxicity in humans. Rev Infect Dis 1983;5(suppl 2):S284-S292.

53. Appel GB. Aminoglycoside nephrotoxicity. Am J Med 1990;88:16S-20S; discussion 38S-42S.

54. McCormack JP, Jewesson PJ. A critical reevaluation of the "therapeutic range" of aminoglycosides. Clin Infect Dis 1992;14:320-39.

55. Ali MZ, Goetz MB. A meta-analysis of the relative efficacy and toxicity of single daily dosing versus multiple daily dosing of aminoglycosides. Clin Infect Dis 1997;24:796-809.

56. Bailey TC, Little JR, Littenberg B, et al. A meta-analysis of extended-interval dosing versus multiple daily dosing of aminoglycosides. Clin Infect Dis 1997;24:786-95.

57. Ferriols-Lisart R, Alós-Almiñana M. Effectiveness and safety of once-daily aminoglycosides: a meta-analysis. Am J Health Syst Pharm 1996;53:1141-50.

58. Hatala R, Dinh T, Cook DJ. Once-daily aminoglycoside dosing in immunocompetent adults: a meta-analysis. Ann Intern Med 1996;124:717-25.

59. Munckhof WJ, Grayson ML, Turnidge JD. A meta-analysis of studies on the safety and efficacy of aminoglycosides given either once daily or as divided doses. J Antimicrob Chemother 1996;37:645-63.

60. Barza M, Ioannidis JP, Cappelleri JC, et al. Single or multiple daily doses of aminoglycosides: a meta-analysis. BMJ 1996;312:338-45.

61. Blaser J, König C. Once-daily dosing of aminoglycosides. Eur J Clin Microbiol Infect Dis 1995;14:1029-38.

62. Galløe AM, Graudal N, Christensen HR, et al. Aminoglycosides: single or multiple daily dosing? A meta-analysis on efficacy and safety. Eur J Clin Pharmacol 1995;48:39-43.

63. Farber BF, Moellering RC Jr. Retrospective study of the toxicity of preparations of vancomycin from 1974 to 1981. Antimicrob Agents Chemother 1983;23:138-41.

64. Mellor JA, Kingdom J, Cafferkey M, et al. Vancomycin toxicity: a prospective study. J Antimicrob Chemother 1985;15:773-80.

65. Sorrell TC, Collignon PJ. A prospective study of adverse reactions associated with vancomycin therapy. J Antimicrob Chemother 1985;16:235-41.

66. Cimino MA, Rotstein C, Slaughter RL, et al. Relationship of serum antibiotic concentrations to nephrotoxicity in cancer patients receiving concurrent aminoglycoside and vancomycin therapy. Am J Med 1987;83:1091-7.

67. Downs NJ, Neihart RE, Dolezal JM, et al. Mild nephrotoxicity associated with vancomycin use. Arch Intern Med 1989;149:1777-81.

68. Meaney CJ, Hynicka LM, Tsoukleris MG. Vancomycin-associated nephrotoxicity in adult medicine patients: incidence, outcomes, and risk factors. Pharmacotherapy 2014;34:653-61.

69. Rybak MJ, Lomaestro BM, Rotschafer JC, et al. Vancomycin therapeutic guidelines: a summary of consensus recommendations from the infectious diseases Society of America, the American Society of Health-System Pharmacists, and the Society of Infectious Diseases Pharmacists. Clin Infect Dis 2009;49:325-7. Erratum in: Clin Infect Dis 2009;49:1465.

70. Lodise TP, Patel N, Lomaestro BM, et al. Relationship between initial vancomycin concentration-time profile and nephrotoxicity among hospitalized patients. Clin Infect Dis 2009;49:507-14.

71. Bosso JA, Nappi J, Rudisill C, et al. Relationship between vancomycin trough concentrations and nephrotoxicity: a prospective multicenter trial. Antimicrob Agents Chemother 2011;55:5475-9.

72. van Hal SJ, Paterson DL, Lodise TP. Systematic review and meta-analysis of vancomycin-induced nephrotoxicity associated with dosing schedules that maintain troughs between 15 and 20 milligrams per liter. Antimicrob Agents Chemother 2013;57:734-44.

73. Carreno JJ, Jaworski A, Kenney RM, et al. Comparative incidence of nephrotoxicity by age group among adult patients receiving vancomycin. Infect Dis Ther 2013;2:201-8.

74. Burgess LD, Drew RH. Comparison of the incidence of vancomycin-induced nephrotoxicity in hospitalized patients with and without concomitant piperacillin-tazobactam. Pharmacotherapy 2014;34:670-6.

75. Gomes DM, Smotherman C, Birch A, et al. Comparison of acute kidney injury during treatment with vancomycin in combination with piperacillin-tazobactam or cefepime. Pharmacotherapy 2014;34:662-9.

76. Gallis HA, Drew RH, Pickard WW. Amphotericin B: 30 years of clinical experience. Rev Infect Dis 1990;12:308-29.

77. Branch RA. Prevention of amphotericin B-induced renal impairment. A review on the use of sodium supplementation. Arch Intern Med 1988;148:2389-94.

78. Falci DR, da Rosa FB, Pasqualotto AC. Comparison of nephrotoxicity associated to different lipid formulations of amphotericin B: a real-life study. Mycoses 2015;58:104-12.

79. Cannon JP, Garey KW, Danziger LH. A prospective and retrospective analysis of the nephrotoxicity and efficacy of lipid-based amphotericin B formulations. Pharmacotherapy 2001;21:1107-14.

80. Wade RL, Chaudhari P, Natoli JL, et al. Nephrotoxicity and other adverse events among inpatients receiving liposomal amphotericin B or amphotericin B lipid complex. Diagn Microbiol Infect Dis 2013;76:361-7.

81. Hamill RJ. Amphotericin B formulations: a comparative review of efficacy and toxicity. Drugs 2013;73:919-34.

82. Limper AH, Knox KS, Sarosi GA, et al.; American Thoracic Society Fungal Working Group. An official American Thoracic Society statement: treatment of fungal infections in adult pulmonary and critical care patients. Am J Respir Crit Care Med 2011;183:96-128.

83. Karimzadeh I, Farsaei S, Khalili H, et al. Are salt loading and prolonging infusion period effective in prevention of amphotericin B-induced nephrotoxicity? Expert Opin Drug Saf 2012;11:969-83.

84. Falagas ME, Karageorgopoulos DE, Tansarli GS. Continuous versus conventional infusion of amphotericin B deoxycholate: a meta-analysis. PLoS One 2013;8:e77075.

85. Karimzadeh I, Khalili H, Farsaei S, et al. Role of diuretics and lipid formulations in the prevention of amphotericin B-induced nephrotoxicity. Eur J Clin Pharmacol 2013;69:1351-68.

86. Karimzadeh I, Khalili H, Dashti-Khavidaki S, et al. N-acetyl cysteine in prevention of amphotericin-induced electrolytes imbalances: a randomized, double-blinded, placebo-controlled, clinical trial. Eur J Clin Pharmacol 2014;70:399-408.

87. Perazella MA. Crystal-induced acute renal failure. Am J Med 1999;106:459-65.

88. dos Santos NA, Carvalho Rodrigues MA, Martins NM, et al. Cisplatin-induced nephrotoxicity and targets of nephroprotection: an update. Arch Toxicol 2012;86:1233-50.

89. Santoso JT, Lucci JA III, Coleman RL, et al. Saline, mannitol, and furosemide hydration in acute cisplatin nephrotoxicity: a randomized trial. Cancer Chemother Pharmacol 2003;52:13-8.

90. Hensley ML, Hagerty KL, Kewalramani T, et al. American Society of Clinical Oncology 2008 clinical practice guideline update: use of chemotherapy and radiation therapy protectants. J Clin Oncol 2009;27:127-45.

91. Naesens M, Kuypers DR, Sarwal M. Calcineurin inhibitor nephrotoxicity. Clin J Am Soc Nephrol 2009;4:481-508.

92. Nankivell BJ, Borrows RJ, Fung CL, et al. The natural history of chronic allograft nephropathy. N Engl J Med 2003;349:2326-33.

93. McDonald JS, McDonald RJ, Comin J, et al. Frequency of acute kidney injury following intravenous contrast medium administration: a systematic review and meta-analysis. Radiology 2013;267:119-28.

94. Weisbord SD, Palevsky PM. Prevention of contrast-induced nephropathy with volume expansion. Clin J Am Soc Nephrol 2008;3:273-80.

95. Jang JS, Jin HY, Seo JS, et al. Sodium bicarbonate therapy for the prevention of contrast-induced acute kidney injury – a systematic review and meta-analysis. Circ J 2012;76:2255-65.

96. Trivedi H, Nadella R, Szabo A. Hydration with sodium bicarbonate for the prevention of contrast-induced nephropathy: a meta-analysis of randomized controlled trials. Clin Nephrol 2010;74:288-96.

97. Kunadian V, Zaman A, Spyridopoulos I, et al. Sodium bicarbonate for the prevention of contrast induced nephropathy: a meta-analysis of published clinical trials. Eur J Radiol 2011;79:48-55.

98. Zoungas S, Ninomiya T, Huxley R, et al. Systematic review: sodium bicarbonate treatment regimens for the prevention of contrast-induced nephropathy. Ann Intern Med 2009;151:631-8.

99. Navaneethan SD, Singh S, Appasamy S, et al. Sodium bicarbonate therapy for prevention of contrast-induced nephropathy: a systematic review and meta-analysis. Am J Kidney Dis 2009;53:617-27.

100. Sun Z, Fu Q, Cao L, et al. Intravenous N-acetylcysteine for prevention of contrast-induced nephropathy: a meta-analysis of randomized, controlled trials. PLoS One 2013;8:e55124.

101. Nallamothu BK, Shojania KG, Saint S, et al. Is acetylcysteine effective in preventing contrast-related nephropathy? A meta-analysis. Am J Med 2004;117:938-47.

102. Gonzales DA, Norsworthy KJ, Kern SJ, et al. A meta-analysis of N-acetylcysteine in contrast-induced nephrotoxicity: unsupervised clustering to resolve heterogeneity. BMC Med 2007;5:32.

103. Trivedi H, Daram S, Szabo A, et al. High-dose N-acetylcysteine for the prevention of contrast-induced nephropathy. Am J Med 2009;122:874.e9-15.

104. Zhang BC, Li WM, Xu YW. High-dose statin pretreatment for the prevention of contrast-induced nephropathy: a meta-analysis. Can J Cardiol 2011;27:851-8.

105. Ukaigwe A, Karmacharya P, Mahmood M, et al. Meta-analysis on efficacy of statins for prevention of contrast-induced acute kidney injury in patients undergoing coronary angiography. Am J Cardiol 2014;114:1295-302.

106. Giacoppo D, Capodanno D, Capranzano P, et al. Meta-analysis of randomized controlled trials of preprocedural statin administration for reducing contrast-induced acute kidney injury in patients undergoing coronary catheterization. Am J Cardiol 2014;114:541-8.

107. Gandhi S, Mosleh W, Abdel-Qadir H, et al. Statins and contrast-induced acute kidney injury with coronary angiography. Am J Med 2014;127:987-1000.

108. Sadat U, Usman A, Gillard JH, et al. Does ascorbic acid protect against contrast-induced acute kidney injury in patients undergoing coronary angiography: a systematic review with meta-analysis of randomized, controlled trials. J Am Coll Cardiol 2013;62:2167-75.

109. Dai B, Liu Y, Fu L, et al. Effect of theophylline on prevention of contrast-induced acute kidney injury: a meta-analysis of randomized controlled trials. Am J Kidney Dis 2012;60:360-70.

110. Kelly AM, Dwamena B, Cronin P, et al. Meta-analysis: effectiveness of drugs for preventing contrast-induced nephropathy. Ann Intern Med 2008;148:284-94.

111. Kellum JA, M Decker J. Use of dopamine in acute renal failure: a meta-analysis. Crit Care Med 2001;29:1526-31.

112. Marik PE. Low-dose dopamine: a systematic review. Intensive Care Med 2002;28:877-83.

113. Bellomo R, Chapman M, Finfer S, et al. Low-dose dopamine in patients with early renal dysfunction: a placebo-controlled randomised trial. Australian and New Zealand Intensive Care Society (ANZICS) Clinical Trials Group. Lancet 2000;356:2139-43.

114. Friedrich JO, Adhikari N, Herridge MS, et al. Meta-analysis: low-dose dopamine increases urine output but does not prevent renal dysfunction or death. Ann Intern Med 2005;142:510-24.

115. Zangrillo A, Biondi-Zoccai GG, et al. Fenoldopam and acute renal failure in cardiac surgery: a meta-analysis of randomized placebo-controlled trials. J Cardiothorac Vasc Anesth 2012;26:407-13.

116. Bove T, Zangrillo A, Guarracino F, et al. Effect of fenoldopam on use of renal replacement therapy among patients with acute kidney injury after cardiac surgery: a randomized clinical trial. JAMA 2014;312:2244-53.

117. Landoni G, Biondi-Zoccai GG, Tumlin JA, et al. Beneficial impact of fenoldopam in critically ill patients with or at risk for acute renal failure: a meta-analysis of randomized clinical trials. Am J Kidney Dis 2007;49:56-68.

118. Chen HH, Anstrom KJ, Givertz MM, et al.; NHLBI Heart Failure Clinical Research Network. Low-dose dopamine or low-dose nesiritide in acute heart failure with renal dysfunction: the ROSE acute heart failure randomized trial. JAMA 2013;310:2533-43.

119. Witteles RM, Kao D, Christopherson D, et al. Impact of nesiritide on renal function in patients with acute decompensated heart failure and pre-existing renal dysfunction a randomized, double-blind, placebo-controlled clinical trial. J Am Coll Cardiol 2007;50:1835-40.

120. Wang DJ, Dowling TC, Meadows D, et al. Nesiritide does not improve renal function in patients with chronic heart failure and worsening serum creatinine. Circulation 2004;110:1620-5.

121. Ejaz AA, Martin TD, Johnson RJ, et al. Prophylactic nesiritide does not prevent dialysis or all-cause mortality in patients undergoing high-risk cardiac surgery. J Thorac Cardiovasc Surg 2009;138:959-64.

122. Lingegowda V, Van QC, Shimada M, et al. Long-term outcome of patients treated with prophylactic nesiritide for the prevention of acute kidney injury following cardiovascular surgery. Clin Cardiol 2010;33:217-21.

123. Mentzer RM Jr, Oz MC, Sladen RN, et al.; NAPA Investigators. Effects of perioperative nesiritide in patients with left ventricular dysfunction undergoing cardiac surgery: the NAPA trial. J Am Coll Cardiol 2007;49:716-26.

124. Garg AX, Kurz A, Sessler DI, et al.; POISE-2 Investigators. Perioperative aspirin and clonidine and risk of acute kidney injury: a randomized clinical trial. JAMA 2014;312:2254-64.

125. Hoste EA, Clermont G, Kersten A, et al. RIFLE criteria for acute kidney injury are associated with hospital mortality in critically ill patients: a cohort analysis. Crit Care 2006;10:R73.

126. Bagshaw SM, George C, Dinu I, et al. A multi-centre evaluation of the RIFLE criteria for early acute kidney injury in critically ill patients. Nephrol Dial Transplant 2008;23:1203-10.

127. Taber SS, Mueller BA. Drug-associated renal dysfunction. Crit Care Clin 2006;22:357-74.

Chapter 27: Drug Dosing in Acute Kidney Injury and Extracorporeal Therapies

Melanie S. Joy, Pharm.D., Ph.D., FCCP, FASN; Michael L. Bentley, Pharm.D.; and Katja M. Gist, D.O., M.A., MSCS

LEARNING OBJECTIVES

1. Understand how solute transfer occurs between different modes of intermittent and continuous renal replacement.
2. Compare the advantages and disadvantages of intermittent hemodialysis and continuous renal replacement therapy.
3. List anticoagulation options used for extracorporeal dialytic therapies.
4. Understand how renal replacement therapy fluids affect the transfer of electrolytes during therapy.
5. List filter characteristics that affect solute movement during renal replacement therapies.
6. Identify pharmacokinetic alterations in patients with critical illness.
7. Understand the drug characteristics that promote clearance by continuous renal replacement therapies.
8. Appreciate the impact of diffusion versus convection on drug clearance.
9. Understand how to develop drug dosing regimens using pharmacokinetic data in patients receiving continuous renal replacement strategies.
10. Understand the drug characteristics that promote clearance by plasmapheresis.
11. Appreciate how different components and conditions of the plasmapheresis procedure can affect drug clearance.
12. Know when to dose drugs in patients receiving plasmapheresis.
13. Describe the components of the extracorporeal membrane oxygenation (ECMO) circuit.
14. Identify the factors responsible for alterations in drug pharmacokinetics in patients on ECMO.
15. Recognize the drugs known or predicted to be sequestered by the ECMO circuit.

ABBREVIATIONS IN THIS CHAPTER

AUC	Area under the plasma concentration time curve	ECMO	Extracorporeal membrane oxygenation
Cl	Total body clearance	EDD	Extended daily hemodialysis
Cp	Concentration in the plasma	IHD	Intermittent hemodialysis
Cp_{ss}	Concentration in the plasma at steady state	ICU	Intensive care unit
CVVH	Continuous venovenous hemofiltration	Q	Flow rate determining delivery of a drug to the extracting organ or device
CVVHD	Continuous venovenous hemodialysis	SCUF	Slow continuous ultrafiltration
CVVHDF	Continuous venovenous hemodiafiltration	SLED	Sustained low-efficiency hemodialysis
E	Extraction of a drug across an organ or device	Vd	Volume of distribution

INTRODUCTION

Renal replacement therapy comprises a group of techniques that provide dialytic and fluid removal support either alone or in combination. It is estimated that 6% of patients admitted to the intensive care unit (ICU) will receive renal replacement therapy during their hospitalization.[1] In addition to patients with a history of dialysis-dependent chronic kidney disease, patients in the ICU are at increased risk of requiring renal replacement therapy because of acute kidney injury induced by drugs, sepsis, exacerbation of autoimmune diseases, and so forth.[2] The primary goals of renal replacement therapy in ICU patients are to reduce kidney injury and complications related to decreased kidney function.[2]

Prescribed renal replacement therapies can be intermittent or continuous in duration. Intermittent therapies include conventional intermittent hemodialysis (IHD), sustained low-efficiency hemodialysis (SLED) or extended daily hemodialysis (EDD), and intermittent peritoneal dialysis. Continuous renal replacement therapies include two forms of peritoneal dialysis (CAPD [continuous ambulatory peritoneal dialysis] and CCPD [continuous cycler-assisted peritoneal dialysis]) and several forms of dialysis and ultrafiltration (slow continuous ultrafiltration [SCUF], continuous venovenous hemofiltration [CVVH], continuous venovenous hemodialysis [CVVHD], and continuous venovenous hemodiafiltration [CVVHDF]). A discussion of each technique will follow later in this chapter. An excellent review that discusses the various continuous renal replacement therapies has been published.[3]

In general, renal replacement therapy techniques are capable of removing water and metabolic waste products (often called solute) by transport across a semipermeable membrane. What differentiates each technique is the method in which water and solute are removed. Ultrafiltration is the process of water removal without the appreciable loss of solutes. Hypervolemic conditions (e.g., heart failure) are indications for isolated ultrafiltration or SCUF. When ultrafiltration flow rates are increased (usually greater than 1,000 mL per hour), solute is removed as water carries it across a semipermeable membrane in response to a transmembrane pressure gradient. The process of removing solute with water from blood is termed *hemofiltration*. When it is performed in a continuous mode (e.g., CVVH), replacement fluid is adjusted at either the prefilter or the postfilter location. Ultrafiltration through CVVH can remove larger molecular weight solutes than diffusion alone (e.g., CVVHD). Because CVVHD uses diffusion to remove solutes, a dialysate is needed to create a concentration gradient. To effectively remove both solute and fluid, several extracorporeal techniques, including IHD, SLED/EDD, and CVVHDF, can be used. Choosing a modality is controversial and is usually determined by the ICU physician and/or nephrologist depending on the clinical needs of the patient. However, continuous forms of renal replacement therapy are preferred over IHD in patients who are hemodynamically unstable or who have increased intracranial pressure or brain edema (e.g., acute brain injury).[2]

Outcomes with Renal Replacement Therapy

Patients developing acute kidney injury tend to have prolonged ICU and hospital stays and have in-hospital mortality rates of 50%–70%.[4-8] For survivors, health-related quality of life is reduced compared with the general population.[9] For ICU survivors with and without acute kidney injury, the health-related quality of life is similar at 6 months; however, it is still lower than in the general population.[10] There is considerable interest in determining the effect of different renal replacement therapies on long-term kidney function recovery. Studies evaluating short-term kidney function recovery have not found a difference between continuous renal replacement therapy and IHD.[11,12] For long-term recovery comparisons, observational and cohort studies have suggested that patients receiving continuous renal replacement therapy compared with intermittent therapies are less likely to progress to chronic kidney disease requiring maintenance hemodialysis.[13-15] Although a cause and effect has not been determined, it is believed that less hemodynamic instability occurs during continuous renal replacement therapy.[16,17] Many patients regaining kidney function after acute kidney injury will have advanced kidney disease compared with their baseline kidney function.[18,19]

RENAL REPLACEMENT THERAPY

Of the available forms of renal replacement therapy, IHD and continuous therapies are used most commonly in adult critically ill patients in developed countries. Peritoneal dialysis is infrequently used because of its inability to effectively and rapidly remove metabolic waste products in hypercatabolic critically ill patients. In addition, it has a relative contraindication in patients with recent intra-abdominal surgery and pathologies.[20] Pediatric and neonatal patients with acute kidney injury often receive peritoneal dialysis, but controversy remains regarding the most appropriate therapy.[21] In developing countries, peritoneal dialysis provides a means for renal replacement therapy when other, more technical procedures may not be feasible.[20]

COMPONENTS OF THERAPIES

Filters and Dialyzers

Technologies to improve the biocompatibility and permeability of filters used in IHD and continuous renal replacement therapies have evolved over several decades, from cellulosic membranes primary used in early IHD to synthetic polymers (e.g., polysulfone, polyamide, polymethylmethacrylate, polyacrylonitrile) used most often today. Other important features of newer filter membranes include a larger, more uniform pore size, increased hydrophobicity, and greater biocompatibility. Binding to these filters has been described for select drugs (e.g., aminoglycosides)[22] and cytokines.[23] Attempts at removing cytokines during continuous renal replacement therapies have been investigated using both hemodialysis and hemofiltration. Cytokine removal during CVVH would likely require a highly permeable membrane with production of a large amount of filtrate. Cytokines may also adsorb to these membranes. However, because the surface area of these filters quickly becomes saturated, frequent filter changes may be required. Cole et al. investigated the adsorption of several interleukins and tissue necrosis factor to a polyacrylonitrile membrane (AN69) using donated blood from six healthy volunteers in an ex vivo model of CVVHD and CVVH. Cytokine adsorption was only minor.[24] Several studies have failed to show a correlation between cytokine removal and improved outcomes.[25,26]

The permeability of a filter directly correlates with the ability of water to cross and is described as the ultrafiltration coefficient (Kuf). The Kuf is determined by the volume of fluid that crosses the membrane in milliliters per hour per millimeter of mercury. If the membrane Kuf is low, its permeability to water is also low, and a higher transmembrane pressure is required to generate an ultrafiltrate. Membranes with a higher Kuf produce a greater amount of ultrafiltrate at equivalent or lower transmembrane pressures. Small solutes (e.g., urea) are primarily removed by diffusion. In addition to size, the ability of solutes to cross a membrane is a function of the thickness and porosity and is expressed as the diffusion coefficient.

To remove larger solutes, convection is needed. The rate of convection is related to how fast water crosses the membrane, size of the solute, and pore size of the membrane. The ability of solutes to cross a membrane during convection is determined by the solute's sieving coefficient. A solute with a sieving coefficient of 1.0 crosses the membrane, whereas a solute with a value of zero is impermeable. For IHD, filters with a greater urea clearance are required because of the short therapy duration. For continuous renal replacement therapies, however, lower urea clearance is acceptable because of the continuous duration. For convection (CVVH), the Kuf must be greater than 6–8 mL/hour/mm Hg to produce an ultrafiltration rate of 15–20 mL/minute. For diffusive clearance (IHD, CVVHD, or CVVHDF), solutes must pass through the membrane quickly to prevent equilibration between the plasma and the dialysate.

Anticoagulation

Activation of the intrinsic and extrinsic coagulation pathway occurs, in addition to platelet activation, when blood contacts the surface of an extracorporeal circuit. Because of this blood-circuit interface, anticoagulation is needed for most patients. In patients who are critically ill, this may be problematic because many have an increased tendency for bleeding given concomitant hepatic impairment. The need for anticoagulation must be balanced with the increased risk of bleeding. One advantage of peritoneal dialysis over IHD and continuous renal replacement therapy is that no anticoagulation is required.

Anticoagulation during IHD usually consists of a heparin bolus given at the beginning of treatment with an additional bolus dose or infusion given during treatment. For patients at high risk of bleeding, a "no-heparin" or minimum-dose heparin option is usually chosen. Other anticoagulation options include trisodium citrate dialysate or regional anticoagulation with trisodium citrate or prostacyclin. In heparin-induced thrombocytopenia, a no-heparin approach is preferred with a direct thrombin inhibitor as the anticoagulant of choice. The choice of an anticoagulant and its dose should be patient-specific to reduce the likelihood of bleeding events.

Several agents have been used to anticoagulate the extracorporeal circuit in continuous renal replacement therapy including unfractionated heparin, low-molecular-weight heparin, trisodium citrate, direct thrombin inhibitors, and prostacyclin. Regional trisodium citrate is generally preferred in the absence of a contraindication (e.g., severe liver failure). Although trisodium citrate has the advantage of reduced bleeding, metabolic acidosis and hypocalcemia can occur in patients with reduced liver function. Other complications include alkalosis, hypernatremia, and hypercalcemia. The largest disadvantage of trisodium citrate is its complexity of administration and monitoring. However, with the use of a specific protocol, it can safely be used. Unfractionated heparin has several advantages over trisodium citrate including its wide availability, familiarity, and easy of monitoring. The disadvantages of unfractionated heparin include increased risk of bleeding, unpredictable kinetics, risk of heparin-induced thrombocytopenia, and heparin resistance.[2] Regardless of the anticoagulant selected for use, each institution should have a protocol in place to reduce the possibility of unwanted adverse effects.

Composition of Dialysate and Replacement Fluids

In general, dialysate fluids for IHD, peritoneal dialysis, and continuous renal replacement therapies mimic physiological consistency. However, they can be modified to enhance the elimination of electrolytes. For example, if hypercalcemia is present, the dialysate will contain a lower amount of calcium. Replacement fluids can also be tailored to ensure that blood solutes have a composition that is physiologic. Although there are several choices for commercial premade solutions, Table 27.1 gives examples of the different types of dialysate and replacement fluids used in IHD, peritoneal dialysis, CVVH, and CVVHD.

TYPES OF RENAL REPLACEMENT

Intermittent Techniques

Intermittent Hemodialysis

Solute removal during IHD and CVVHD occurs primarily by diffusion. The principal differences between CVVHD and IHD are the duration and frequency of treatment and the flow rates for blood and dialysate. Table 27.2 lists flow rate characteristics (blood, dialysate, and ultrafiltration), mechanisms for solute removal, and therapy durations for both continuous and intermittent renal replacement therapies. Several advantages and disadvantages are associated with each of these therapies (Table 27.3). An advantage of IHD is the rapid removal of solutes and water. This is most important in the setting of hyperkalemia, certain intoxications, and severe fluid overload. However, hypotension is a common cause for interrupting or stopping IHD and occurs during 20%–30% of treatments. Patients with acute kidney injury are often intolerant of IHD, and it is estimated that up to 10% of these patients cannot tolerate this form of therapy.[27]

Sustained Low-Efficiency Dialysis and Extended Daily Dialysis

Sustained low-efficiency dialysis and EDD are performed using conventional hemodialysis machines, but with modified blood and dialysate flow rates. A typical blood flow rate is 200 mL/minute during SLED/EDD versus up to about 450 mL/minute with conventional IHD. Dialysate flow rate is about 300 mL/minute during SLED/EDD versus up to 800 mL/minute with conventional IHD sessions. The therapy duration is longer during SLED/EDD (6–12 hours) than

Table 27.1 Composition of Dialysate and Replacement Fluids

	IHD	PD	CVVHD	CVVH
Sodium (mEq/L)	137	132	140	140
Chloride (mEq/L)	105	96	108	113
Potassium (mEq/L)	2.0	0	2.0	4.0
Calcium (mEq/L)	3.0	3.5	0	2.5
Magnesium (mEq/L)	0.75	0.5	1.0	1.5
Acetate/lactate (mEq/L)	4.0	40	3.0	3.0
Bicarbonate (mEq/L)	33		32	33
Dextrose (mg/dL)	200	1.5, 2.5, 4.25	110	100

CVVHD = continuous venovenous hemodialysis; CVVH = continuous venovenous hemofiltration; IHD = intermittent hemodialysis; PD = peritoneal dialysis.

Table 27.2 Typical Conditions During Renal Replacement Therapies[40,119]

Therapy	Typical Flow Rates[a]				
Intermittent Therapies	Blood Flow (mL/min)	Dialysate Flow (mL/min)	Ultrafiltration Flow (mL/hr)	Duration (hr)	Solute Removal
IHD	300–500	500–800	Not applicable	3–4	Diffusion
SLED/EDD	160–200	100–300	Not applicable	6–12	Diffusion
Continuous Therapies	Blood Flow (mL/min)	Dialysate Flow (mL/hr)	Ultrafiltration Flow (mL/hr)	Duration (hr)	Solute Removal
CVVH	50–300	Not applicable	500–4,000	24	Convection
CVVHD	50–300	500–4,000	0–350[b]	24	Diffusion
CVVHDF	50–300	500–4,000	500–4,000	24	Diffusion and convection

[a]Dialysate flow rates are in milliliters per minute for intermittent and milliliters per hour for continuous therapies.
[b]Because of the slow rate at which fluid is removed during CVVHD, ultrafiltration has no impact on solute removal.
CVVH = continuous venovenous hemofiltration; EDD = extended daily dialysis; SLED = sustained low-efficiency dialysis; IHD = intermittent hemodialysis; CVVHD = continuous venovenous hemodialysis; CVVHDF = continuous venovenous hemodiafiltration

during conventional IHD (4 hours), but it is shorter than during continuous renal replacement therapy. Longer treatment duration allows for better hemodynamic stability than with IHD. In addition, because of its intermittent nature, SLED/EDD enables time away from therapy to perform various tests and procedures without affecting solute clearance and fluid management treatment goals.

Peritoneal Dialysis (intermittent or continuous)

Peritoneal dialysis differs from intermittent or continuous renal replacement therapies because it uses the lining of the abdominal cavity to act as a dialysis membrane. However, dialysate is also needed for peritoneal dialysis in order to create a concentration gradient to enable solute and water removal. Several commercial dialysate solutions are available for peritoneal dialysis, and all contain a mixture of electrolytes, lactate, and glucose.

Continuous Renal Replacement Techniques

Slow Continuous Ultrafiltration

Ultrafiltration uses pressure to force plasma water across a semipermeable membrane. The driving force for flow is dependent on the difference between the positive pressure that is created on the blood side of the membrane and the negative pressure that is created on the opposite side of the membrane. Although the hydrostatic pressure has a large impact on removal of fluid, there is a minimal effect on solute removal. When isolated ultrafiltration is provided in a continuous mode, it is typically termed *SCUF*. Figure 27.1 represents a typical SCUF circuit.

Continuous Venovenous Hemodialysis

Diffusion occurs when a solute moves across a semipermeable membrane in response to a concentration gradient. The ability to transverse the membrane depends on membrane porosity and the molecular weight of the solute. The ability to diffuse is inversely proportional to the solute molecular weight. For diffusion, the greatest impact on solute clearance is for low-molecular-weight molecules (less than 500 g/mol). Other factors that influence solute clearance are membrane characteristics (e.g., surface area and thickness) and solution temperature.[28] For diffusion to occur, a concentration gradient must be maintained. Blood (containing a high-solute concentration) flows across the hollow fiber membranes, whereas dialysate (containing an absent or low-solute concentration) flows countercurrent on the other side of the dialyzer membrane. If the dialysate contains a higher concentration of solute than blood, diffusion will occur in the opposite direction (e.g., from dialysate to blood). In general, this "backward flow" is undesirable. One exception may be the backward flow of

Table 27.3 Advantages and Disadvantages of Renal Replacement Therapies

Therapy	Advantages and Disadvantages
IHD	**Advantages**
	• Less expensive than SLEDD and CRRT
	• Rapid control of hyperkalemia
	Disadvantages
	• Can cause hemodynamic compromise in critically ill patients
	• May require frequent treatments (e.g., daily for several days) early in therapy course
SLEDD	**Advantages**
	• Better hemodynamic stability than IHD
	• Less expensive than CRRT
	• Allows for out-of-unit test and procedures
	Disadvantages
	• Requires two nurses (ICU and dialysis) for the treatment duration at most institutions
	• Limited drug dosing recommendations
CRRT	**Advantages**
	• Can be used in most hemodynamically unstable critically ill patients
	• Several options to choose from (i.e., CVVH, CVVHD, CVVHDF)
	• Allows for full nutritional support
	• May be safer for patients with brain injuries
	• May have a beneficial effect in patients in septic shock
	• May increase the likelihood of renal recovery
	Disadvantages
	• Requires the purchase of specific devices
	• Higher cost for supplies
	• Requires a dedicated ICU nurse
	• Usually requires continuous anticoagulation
	• Can cause hypothermia
	• Can cause life-threating depletion of several electrolytes if not monitored closely and replaced

bicarbonate in metabolic acidosis. In 2004, an ISMP Canada Safety Bulletin reported the deaths of two patients who inadvertently received dialysate containing about 57 mEq per liter of potassium chloride.[29] Because dialysate fluid is not under a condition of recirculation, equilibrium is not obtained. Figure 27.2 shows the diffusion process as it occurs in IHD (and CVVHD). However, although conventional IHD usually occurs over 4 hours, CVVHD is a form of continuous renal replacement therapy. Figure 27.3 is a graphical depiction of CVVHD.

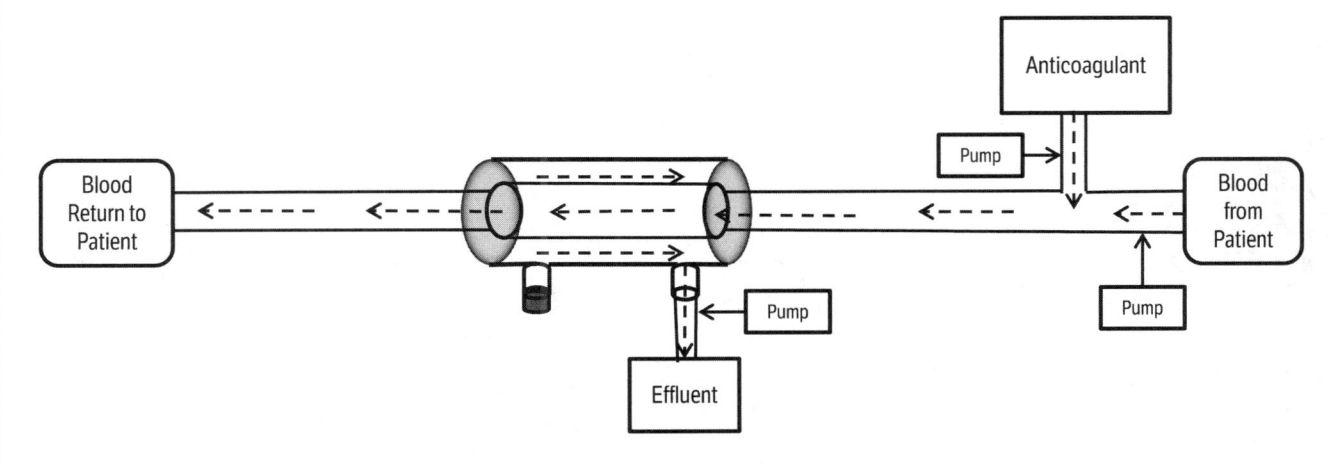

Figure 27.1 Slow continuous ultrafiltration (SCUF) circuit.
For slow continuous ultrafiltration (SCUF), blood is filtered through a semipermeable membrane under pressure, producing an ultrafiltrate. Because fluid removal is minimal, a replacement solution is not needed. The primary indication for SCUF is volume overload.

Continuous Venovenous Hemofiltration

The ability to remove medium- and high-molecular-weight solutes (up to 15,000 g/mol) using extracorporeal techniques requires convection. Convection occurs when solutes are transported across a semipermeable membrane with the flow of water under the influence of a pressure gradient. The hemofilter membranes have enhanced permeability to enable removal of higher molecular weight solutes.[30,31] Figure 27.4 shows the blood, water, and ultrafiltration components of convection. The clearance of solute shown during convection occurs though solvent drag.

Hemofiltration differs from ultrafiltration in that the flow across the filter is increased. To provide adequate hemofiltration, at least 1 L of water per hour should cross the membrane.[32] Figure 27.5 provides an example of a typical CVVH circuit showing both pre- and postfilter replacement fluid administration.

Continuous Venovenous Hemodiafiltration

Continuous venovenous hemodiafiltration uses both diffusion and convection to remove water and solute (Figure 27.6).

> **Box 27.1. Characteristics of Drugs That Enhance Dialytic Clearance**
>
> ↓ Molecular weight/size
> ↑ Hydrophilicity
> ↓ Protein binding
> ↓ Volume of distribution
> ↑ Percentage of clearance by kidneys
> ↑ Percentage of clearance by nonrenal routes significantly altered by critical illness

DRUG-RELATED CHARACTERISTICS AND CLEARANCE BY CONTINUOUS EXTRACORPOREAL DIALYTIC TECHNIQUES

The removal of drugs by continuous as well as intermittent dialytic techniques is dependent on the physicochemical characteristics of the drugs and the characteristics of the dialytic procedure. The primary physicochemical characteristics that predict whether a drug will be removed by a dialytic technique are its molecular weight, degree of hydrophilicity, protein binding, volume of distribution (Vd), and whether the kidneys represent the primary clearance pathway (Box 27.1).

Molecular Weight

A drug with a molecular weight of less than 500 g/mol is readily removed by extracorporeal clearance methods that use diffusion. The clearance of drugs with higher molecular weights is enhanced with techniques that use high-flux membranes.

Hydrophilicity vs. Lipophilicity

Drugs are classified by their lipophilic to hydrophilic status by log P values. The log P is a partition coefficient defined as the log of the ratio of the concentration of nonionized drug between oil (lipophilic) and aqueous (hydrophilic) phases. It is often necessary to adjust the pH of the aqueous phase to optimize for the presence of the nonionized form of the drug when determining partition coefficients. A lower log P value indicates that the drug is more hydrophilic, whereas higher log P values indicate improved lipophilicity. Drugs that are more hydrophobic have a greater ability to diffuse through lipid bilayers of cells. Hydrophilic drugs, because of their charges, require transporters to move across cellular membranes.

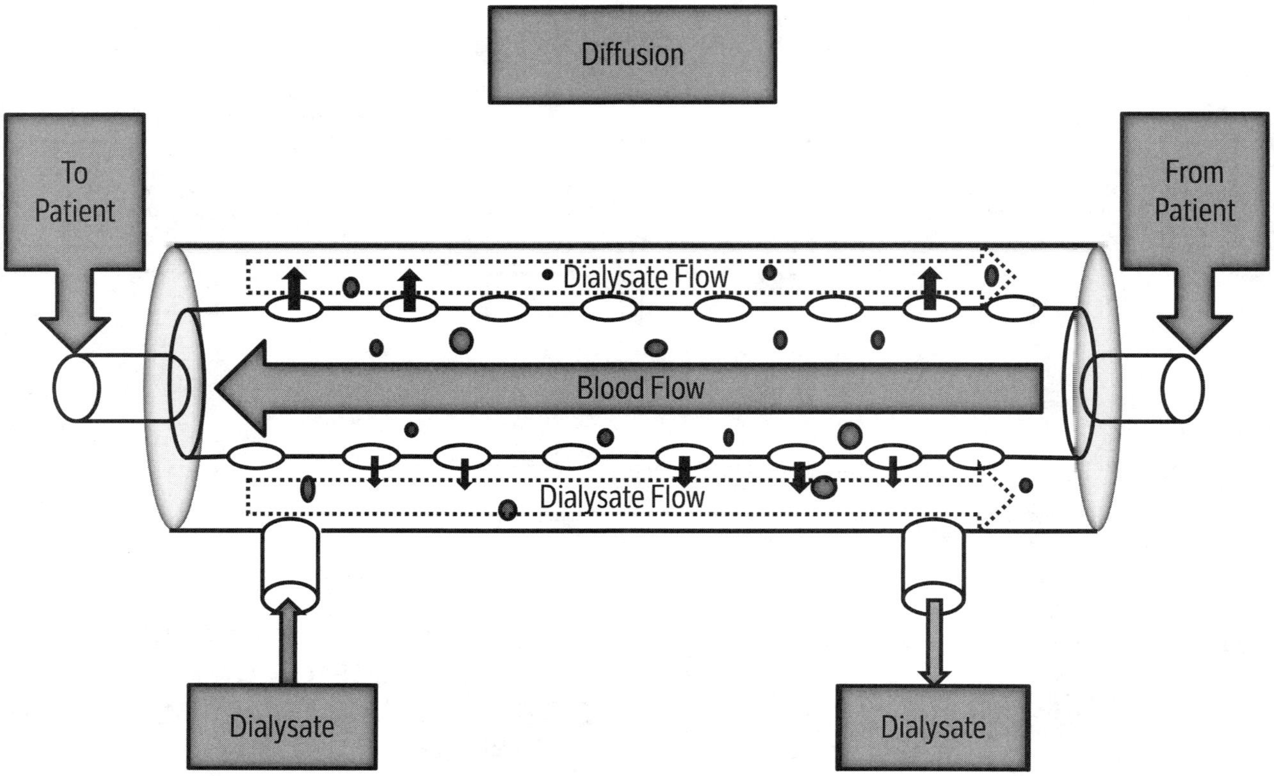

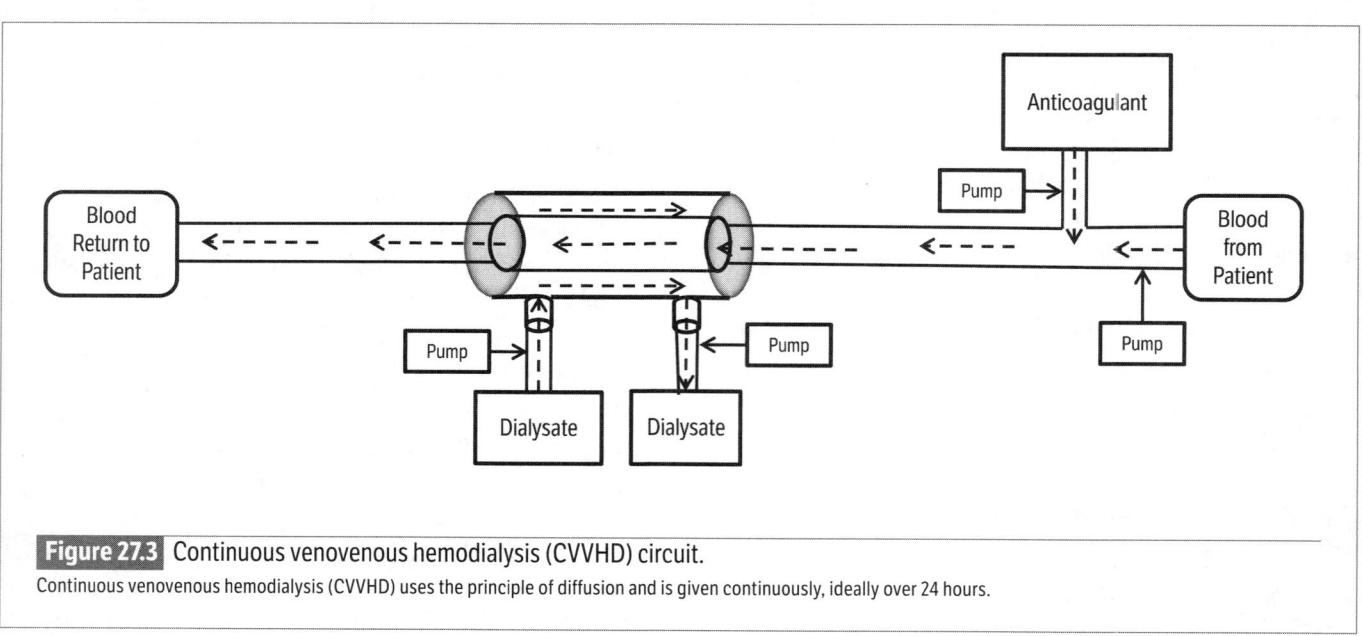

Figure 27.2 Intermittent hemodialysis circuit.
Diffusion occurs when solute moves from an area of higher concentration to an area of lower concentration. Renal replacement therapies that use diffusion do not allow for equilibrium. To prevent equilibrium, these therapies use a countercurrent dialysate solution (e.g., a dialysate). Diffusion is responsible for removing small molecular weight molecules.

Figure 27.3 Continuous venovenous hemodialysis (CVVHD) circuit.
Continuous venovenous hemodialysis (CVVHD) uses the principle of diffusion and is given continuously, ideally over 24 hours.

The hydrophilic/hydrophobic characteristics can influence the absorption, distribution, and excretion of drugs. Drugs and metabolites that are cleared by the kidney are typically hydrophilic. They are typically cleared by dialytic techniques because of their presence in the intravascular compartment (the eliminating compartment for dialytic techniques). For hydrophilic compounds, charges (positive or negative) can result in interactions with extracorporeal membranes that can lead to drug adsorption. Determination of adsorption requires the assessment of

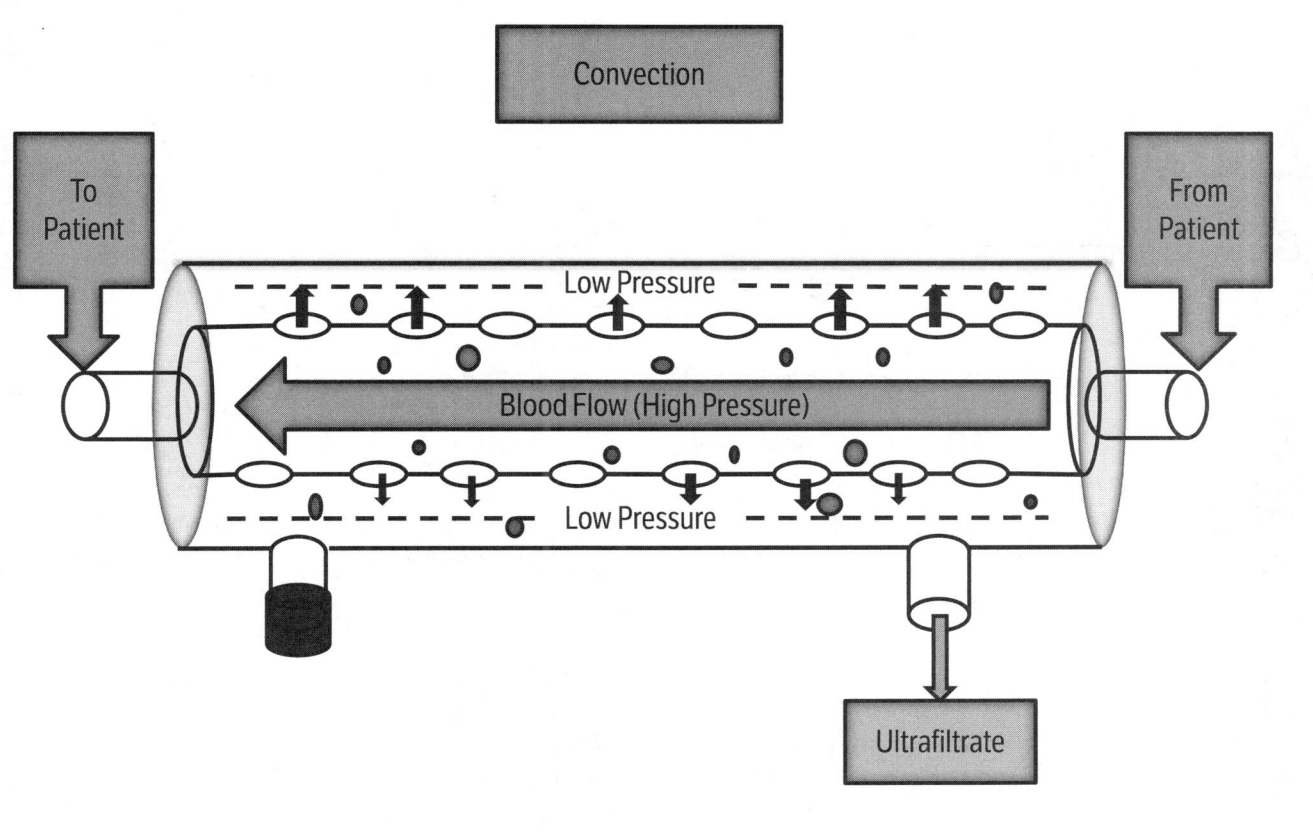

Figure 27.4 Continuous venovenous hemofiltration circuit demonstrating movement of blood flow and solutes.

Convection occurs when solutes are transported across a semipermeable membrane with the flow of water and under the influence of pressure. As flow increases, so does the movement of solutes. This movement is called "solute drag." Convection can remove middle to large molecular weight molecules.

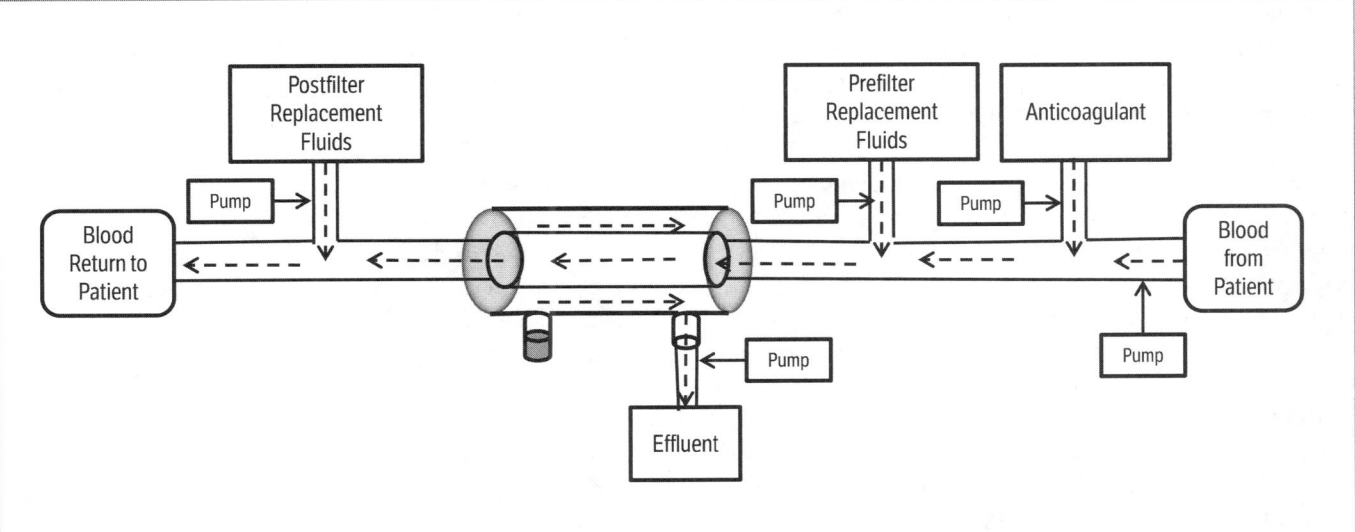

Figure 27.5 Continuous venovenous hemofiltration (CVVH) circuit incorporating pre- and post-filter replacement fluids.

Continuous venovenous hemofiltration (CVVH) uses the principle of convection. Because CVVH requires the production of a large ultrafiltrate, replacement fluids are added either prefilter (predilution) or postfilter (postdilution), or both. Convection removes middle to large molecular weight molecules.

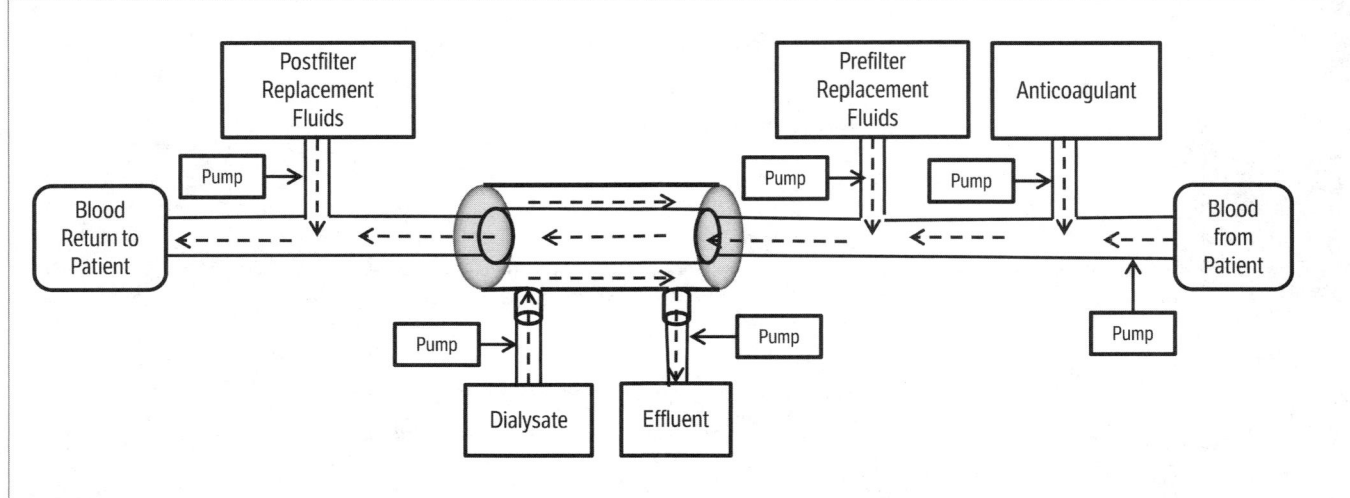

Figure 27.6 Circuitry of continuous venovenous hemodiafiltration (CVVHDF) with pre- and post-filter fluid replacement.
Circuitry of continuous venovenous hemodiafiltration with pre- and postfilter fluid replacement. Continuous venovenous hemodiafiltration (CVVHDF) uses both diffusive and convective clearance. Therefore, both dialysate and replacement fluids are required. CVVHDF removes both small and middle molecules.

drug concentrations in the effluent and not just arterial and venous port measurements. Gentamicin (log P -3.1) is an example of a drug that is documented to adsorb to the polyacrylonitrile extracorporeal filter membrane.[22,33] A recent publication showed adsorption of teicoplanin by polysulfone and polymethylmethacrylate membranes.[34]

Protein Binding

The extent of protein binding is important for determining the Vd and exposure of a drug to its tissue sites compared with the intravascular compartment. The clearance of drugs by dialytic methods, as with filtration clearance by the endogenous kidney, is dependent on the fraction of unbound drug. Drugs that are more highly protein bound (e.g., greater than 80% protein bound) are less likely to be removed by dialytic techniques. Bound drugs are complexed with high-molecular-weight proteins, with albumin (69,000 g/mol) being a common protein for binding acidic drugs. It is customary to consult common drug dosing references and product literature to ascertain the reported unbound fraction of a drug. However, the sieving coefficient can also be determined experimentally under conditions of isolated ultrafiltration[35] or referenced from the literature. The sieving coefficient is the ratio of drug concentration in the ultrafiltrate to the prefilter plasma concentration. Either the sieving coefficient or the unbound fraction is necessary for estimating drug clearance during continuous renal replacement therapy. Sieving coefficients typically, but not always, correspond to the unbound fraction.

The degree of protein binding can be decreased by competitive displacers in the plasma including other concomitant highly protein bound drugs and uremic toxins.[36,37] Decreased albumin concentrations in kidney and hepatic diseases can also reduce protein binding. Increased protein binding can result from increased α_1-acid glycoprotein concentrations found in acute care and inflamed patients.[38] Because α_1-acid glycoprotein binds basic drugs, increased binding will not be observed for acidic drugs. The systemic pH can also influence the protein binding of drugs in critical care patients.

Volume of Distribution

The Vd of a drug is defined as a theoretical volume that the total amount of administered drug would have to occupy, if uniformly distributed, to provide the same concentration as blood plasma. It is most influenced by protein binding and log P. Drugs that have high plasma protein binding have small Vd values. Drugs that have high tissue protein binding and low plasma protein binding typically have large Vd values. Factors described earlier (under Protein Binding) will also influence the Vd of drugs. Because extracorporeal techniques remove solutes from blood or plasma, drugs with smaller Vd values (e.g., less than 1 L/kg) are more likely to be removed by dialytic techniques. The duration of the dialytic technique will also affect the degree of influence of Vd on drug clearance. The likelihood of clearance for drugs with large Vd values increases as the duration of the dialytic procedure increases. The increased time allows drugs to transfer between tissue and vascular compartments. This is particularly important for drugs with larger Vd values. Moxifloxacin (Vd 1.7–2.7 L/kg) is an example whereby clearance is 95 mL/minute with conventional IHD and 33 mL/minute with extended daily dialysis.[39] However, the moxifloxacin half-life is shorter on extended dialysis (6 hours) than on IHD (12 hours).[39] Readers are referred to a recent review on antibiotic dosing during extended dialysis.[40]

Clearance Pathways

The clearance pathway for a drug is also important for determining the impact of dialytic clearance on total body clearance. In acute and chronic kidney diseases, dialytic modalities are important for enhancing the clearance of drugs that undergo a significant percentage of clearance by the renal route. As kidney function declines, the total body clearance of drugs that are excreted primarily by the renal route declines significantly. The contribution of clearance by extracorporeal techniques, renal pathways, and nonrenal pathways to total body clearance is determined by equation 27.1:

$$\text{clearance}_{total} = \text{clearance}_{nonrenal} + \text{clearance}_{residual\ renal} + \text{clearance}_{extracorporeal} \text{ (equation 27.1)}$$

The terms in this equation are total body clearance (clearance$_{total}$), nonrenal clearance (clearance$_{nonrenal}$), renal clearance (clearance$_{residual\ renal}$), and extracorporeal clearance (clearance$_{extracorporeal}$). The equation shows that clearance processes are additive.

Several clinical cases require particular attention with respect to clearance. Special consideration is required in drug conditions where nonrenal clearance can also decline as kidney function declines since the drug product literature values for unaltered nonrenal clearance may not be valid under this condition. As an example, cytochrome P450 (CYP) 3A expression and function is significantly reduced in chronic kidney disease.[41] Patients receiving drugs that undergo predominant nonrenal clearance through CYP3A will likely have reductions in this clearance pathway necessitating drug dosing adjustments. Another special consideration is the case of drug combinations. In this scenario, one compound may have a predominant renal clearance pathway, whereas the other compound is predominantly cleared through nonrenal routes. Another consideration is the contribution of residual renal function to total body clearance. It is often assumed that patients in the ICU who require dialytic techniques have a drug clearance$_{residual\ renal}$ of 0 mL/minute. However, some patients can have significant kidney function that can result in a drug clearance that is considerably higher than predicted. In these circumstances, it is important to remember to add the estimated residual renal clearance to the clearance by nonrenal and extracorporeal pathways to avoid drug underdosing.

CLEARANCE PROCESSES OF DRUGS DURING EXTRACORPOREAL TECHNIQUES

Diffusion

Drug clearance during continuous renal replacement therapies using a dialysis component occurs through diffusion. Several equations can be used to estimate this clearance. In the body or by extracorporeal devices, clearance is calculated as $Q \times E$, where Q is a flow rate, and E is the extraction of the drug across the organ or device. The extraction across the dialyzer is governed by the unbound fraction of the drug. Extraction can be measured by the difference between the prefilter (arterial) concentration and the postfilter (venous) concentration divided by the prefilter concentration: E = (arterial − venous)/arterial. The clearance can be estimated either by the unbound fraction or by E multiplied by the dialysate flow rate (equation 27.2). Dialytic clearance estimates by this approach are amenable for use in the clinical environment.

$$\text{clearance} = f_{ub} \text{ (or E)} \times Q_{dialysate} \text{ (equation 27.2)}$$

The dialytic clearance can also be measured during the continuous renal replacement procedure, but this requires more laborious methods that are usually reserved for research studies. These methods are analogous to the calculations used to measure drug clearance by the renal route. For these assessments, the dialysate effluent is collected at intervals, the volume is measured, and the concentration of drug is determined by an analytic method. After multiplying dialysate volumes by their respective concentrations, drug amount determinations are obtained. The amounts are then summed over the intervals and divided by the area under the plasma concentration time curve (AUC) that corresponds to this total time period; this is shown in equation 27.3. Determination of the AUC requires serial blood sampling over the collection period.

$$\text{clearance}_{dialysis} = [\Sigma \text{ (concentration}_{dialysate} \times \text{volume)}] / \text{AUC}_{over\ collection\ time} \text{ (equation 27.3)}$$

Convection/Ultrafiltration

Drug clearance during continuous renal replacement therapies using an ultrafiltration component occurs through convection. Several clearance equations can be used to estimate convection clearance. Clearance is calculated as $Q \times E$; where Q is the ultrafiltration flow rate, and E is the extraction of the drug across the filter. The extraction across the filter is governed by the available unbound fraction of the drug. Extraction is measured by the ratio of drug in the ultrafiltrate to the prefilter concentration: E = [ultrafiltrate]/[arterial]. This determination of E is also called the sieving coefficient. A value of 1 indicates free passage of the solute across the membrane under the condition of isolated ultrafiltration. The clearance can be estimated either by the unbound fraction or by E multiplied by the ultrafiltration flow rate (equation 27.4). Equation 27.4 is used when fluids are administered postdilution.

$$\text{clearance} = f_{ub} \text{ (or E)} \times Q_{ultrafiltration} \text{ (equation 27.4)}$$

If fluids are administered in the predilution mode, equation 27.5 should be used.

$$\text{clearance} = f_{ub} \text{ (or E)} \times Q_{ultrafiltration} \times [Q_{blood}/(Q_{blood} + Q_{replacement})] \text{ (equation 27.5)}$$

Clearance estimates by these approaches can be used in the clinical environment.

The ultrafiltration clearance, like the dialysate clearance, can also be measured during continuous renal replacement therapy. For these assessments, the ultrafiltration effluent is collected at intervals, the volume measured, and the concentration of drug determined by an analytic method. After multiplying ultrafiltrate volumes by their respective concentrations, drug amount results are obtained. These amounts are then summed over the intervals and divided by the AUC that corresponds to this total time period; this is shown in equation 27.6. Determination of the AUC requires serial blood sampling over the collection period.

$$\text{clearance}_{\text{ultrafiltration}} = [\Sigma (\text{concentration}_{\text{ultrafiltrate}} \times \text{volume})]/\text{AUC}_{\text{over collection time}} \quad (\text{equation } 27.6)$$

Combined Dialysis with Convection/Ultrafiltration

It is now common in the ICU to use a combination of dialysis and ultrafiltration during continuous renal replacement therapy. Therefore, the clinician needs to know how to account for clearance through this combination. The clearance by the combination of dialysis and ultrafiltration can be estimated by multiplying the unbound fraction by the total effluent rate, which is composed of the combination of dialysate flow rate and ultrafiltration flow rate (equation 27.7). Clearance estimates by this approach are used in the clinical environment.

$$\text{clearance} = \text{fub} \times (Q_{\text{dialysate}} + Q_{\text{ultrafiltration}}) \quad (\text{equation } 27.7)$$

For measuring clearance through the combination of dialysis and ultrafiltration, the total effluent is collected at intervals, the volume is measured, and the concentration of drug is determined through an analytic method. After multiplying effluent volumes by their respective concentrations, drug amounts result. These amounts are then summed over the intervals and divided by the AUC that corresponds to this total time; this is shown in equation 27.8.

$$\text{clearance}_{\text{effluent}} = [\Sigma (\text{concentration}_{\text{effluent}} \times \text{volume})]/\text{AUC}_{\text{over collection time}} \quad (\text{equation } 27.8)$$

As mentioned at the beginning of this section, to adequately determine drug clearance, an assessment of determinants of total clearance is required. Therefore, the nonrenal clearance and residual renal clearance of the drug must be added to the clearance estimated or measured from the continuous renal replacement therapy (equation 27.1). Box 27.2 summarizes the clearance equations discussed in this section. Table 27.4 provides the abstracted clearance data for drugs during various continuous renal replacement therapies.

ACUTE VS. CHRONIC KIDNEY DISEASE AND PHARMACOKINETIC ALTERATIONS

There is a considerable body of literature to show the influence of chronic kidney disease on the pharmacokinetics of drugs.[42-44] However, there is a paucity of comparable data in patients with acute kidney injury. According to the available data, it is reasonable to assume similar changes in acute and chronic kidney diseases. However, there are differences that require consideration (Table 27.5), which are discussed in the following sections. Patients with acute kidney disease typically receive continuous versus intermittent dialytic techniques. The longer treatment duration will affect drugs with a large Vd secondary to more time for net transfer from tissue to vascular compartments. The incorporation of convection with high-flux membranes in continuous renal replacement therapy will enhance the removal of drugs with high molecular weights. Drug pharmacokinetics can be altered in critical care patients secondary to the physiological changes induced by organ alterations such as acute kidney injury, hepatic disease, cardiac failure, or generalized inflammatory states, occurring alone or in combination. Changes to drug absorption, distribution, metabolism, and excretion processes are reported and are reviewed.

Absorption

Because many medications are administered by the intravenous route to patients in the ICU, changes to oral bioavailability secondary to alterations in absorption may be less problematic. However, medication administered by other extravascular routes, including subcutaneous and intramuscular, can result in alterations in absorption and for subsequent bioavailability. Several processes are responsible

continued on page 552

Box 27.2. Equations for Clearance Determination in Continuous Renal Replacement Therapies

Diffusion

Eq. 2: Clearance = fub (or E) × $Q_{\text{dialysate}}$

Eq. 3: Clearance$_{\text{dialysis}}$ = [Σ (concentration$_{\text{dialysate}}$ × volume)]/AUC$_{\text{over collection time}}$

Convection

Eq. 4: Clearance = fub (or E) × $Q_{\text{ultrafiltration}}$ (if using predilution fluids)

Eq. 5: Clearance = fub (or E) × $Q_{\text{ultrafiltration}}$ × [Q_{blood}/(Q_{blood} + $Q_{\text{Replacement}}$)] (if using postdilution fluids)

Eq. 6: Clearance$_{\text{ultrafiltration}}$ = [Σ (concentration$_{\text{ultrafiltrate}}$ × volume)]/AUC$_{\text{over collection time}}$

Diffusion + Convection

Eq. 7: Clearance = fub × ($Q_{\text{dialysate}}$ + $Q_{\text{ultrafiltration}}$)

Eq. 8: Clearance$_{\text{effluent}}$ = [Σ (concentration$_{\text{effluent}}$ × volume)]/AUC$_{\text{over collection time}}$

Table 27.4 Drug Clearance Data During Continuous Renal Replacement Therapies

Drugs	MW (g/mol)	Vd	Log P	PB (%)	Cl_{TB} (mL/min)	Cl_{RRT} (mL/min)	Filter	SA	DFR (mL/hr)	UFR (mL/hr)	REF	Effluent Rate (mL/hr)
Amikacin	585.6	24 L	-8.6	0%–11%	39 ± 4.6	16.4	PS	0.25, 0.6	0	1,152	120	1,152
					10.5	10.1	PS	0.25	0	600	121	600
Amrinone	187.2	1.2 L/kg	-0.57	10%–49%	41–46	2.4-14.4	PS	NR	0	533	122	533
Atracurium	929.1	0.116–0.390 L/kg	-0.96	82%	503 ± 135	8.25±4.5	PA	2	0	1,140	123	1,140
Cefepime	480.6	18.0 ± 2.0 L	-4.3	20%	114	23	AN69	0.9	167	1,580	124,125	1,747
					105	40	PS	1.4	1,000	1,500	124,125	2,500
					47 ± 0.12	26 ± 5	AN69	0.6	957	1,044	126	2,001
					36 ± 6	13 ± 4	AN69	0.6	0	948	126	948
Cefotiam	525.6	0.5 L/kg	-3.1	40%	10–35	8.5–32.5	PS	1.35	0	1,113	127	1,113
Ceftazidime	546.6	0.28–0.4 L/kg	-4.1	<10%	25 ± 1.8	13 ± 1.3	AN69	0.43	1,000	448	128	1,448
					25 ± 1.8	15 ± 1.3	AN69	0.43	2,000	448	128	2,448
					98.7 ±	32.1 ± 7.9	PS	0.7	0	2,820	129	2,820
					NR	22 ± 2.2	AN69	0.6	2,000	0	130	2,000
					NR	28 ± 3.7	PS	0.65	2,000	0	130	2,000
					NR	24 ± 5.2	PMMA	2.1	2,000	0	130	2,000
					62 ± 4.8	34 ± 4	AN69	0.6	1,000	1,500	131	2,500
					149	23	AN69	0.9	750	1,000	132	1,750
Ceftriaxone	554.6	5.78–13.5 L	-1.8	97%	NR	3.3±1.2	AN69	0.6	2,000	0	133	2,000
					NR	4.4±1.5	PS	0.65	2,000	0	133	2,000
					NR	6.1 ± 2.3	PMMA	2.1	2,000	0	133	2,000
Cefuroxime	424.4	NR	-0.9	50%	32 ± 7.5	11 ± 5.2	PS	0.6	0	850	134	850
					22 ± 7.9	14 ± 2.2	AN69	0.43	1,000	448	128	1,448
					22 ± 7.9	14±2.2	AN69	0.43	2,000	448	128	2,448
Cidofovir	279.2	0.5 L/kg	-3.4	<6%	3.7	3.5±0.5	PES	1.2	0	1,500	135	1,500
Cilastatin	358.5	NR	-1.3	NR	29 ± 29	4±2.3	PS	NR	0	450	136	450
					13	10 ± 3	AN69	0.6	1,000	500	137	1,500
					21	18 ± 4	AN69	0.6	3,000	500	137	3,500
Ciprofloxacin	331.3	1.2–2.7 L/kg	-0.81	20%–40%	264 ± 73	16 ± 2.5	AN69	0.43	1,000	434	138	1,434
					264 ± 73	20 ± 3.1	AN69	0.43	2,000	434	138	2,434
					203 ± 72	37 ± 7	AN69	0.6	1,000	2,000	139	3,000
Clavulanic acid	199.2	39–52 L	-1.5	22%–30%	129 ± 56	25 ± 6	PS	0.25	0	890	140	890
Colistin	1155.5	12.4 L	-8.1	NR	67	12.2	PS	0.71	NR	NR	141	2,050
Daptomycin	1620.7	0.1 L/kg	NR	90%–93%	11 ± 4.7	55 ± 26	PS	1.5	2,132	574	142	2,706

Table 27.4 Drug Clearance During Continuous Renal Replacement Therapies (continued)

Drugs	MW (g/mol)	Vd	Log P	PB (%)	Cl_{TB} (mL/min)	Cl_{RRT} (mL/min)	Filter	SA	DFR (mL/hr)	UFR (mL/hr)	REF	Effluent Rate (mL/hr)
Doripenem	420.6	16.8 L	-3.65	8%–10%	82 ± 35	22 ± 5	AN69	0.9	0	2,000	143	2,000
					82 ± 35	25 ± 5	AN69	0.9	2,000	0	143	2,000
Fluconazole	306.3	0.56–0.82 L/kg	0.56	11%–12%	22	25	AN69	0.43	1,000	0	144	1,000
					57	NR	CTA	1.5	75	135	145	210
					38	31	AN69	0.9	1,000	1,163	146	2,163
					25	18	AN69	0.9	0	1,163	146	1,163
Fosfomycin	138.1	2.4 L/kg	-0.74	0%–3%	107 ± 127	18 ± 3.3	PES	1.2	0	1,500	147	1,500
Ganciclovir	255.2	0.74 ± 0.15 L/kg	-2.2	1%–2%	32 ± 6.2	5.2 ± 1.8	AN69	0.43	1,000	0	148	1,000
Gentamicin	477.6	0.29–0.37 L/kg	-3.1	0%–30%	11.6 ± 6.4	3.5 ± 2.0	PS	0.25	0	267	149	267
					NR	1.5 ± 13	PS	0.6	0	322	150	322
					21 ± 6.9	5.2 ± 1.8	AN69	0.43	1,000	420	151	1,420
Imipenem	317.4	NR	-3.9	20%	108 ± 14	13	PS	0.25	0	1,000	152	1,000
					64 ± 11	13	PS	NR	0	1,000	152	1,000
					103 ± 34	6.6 ± 5.6	PS	NR	0	450	136	450
					134	16 ± 7	AN69	0.6	1,000	500	137	1,500
					134	16 ± 7	AN69	0.6	3,000	500	137	3,500
					145 ± 18	36 ± 13	AN69	0.6	0	1,140	153	1,140
					178 ± 18	57 ± 28	AN69	0.6	973	6,060	153	7,033
Linezolid	337.3	40–50 L	0.64	31%	85	37	PS	1.6	2,000	774	154	2,774
					155 ± 58	32 ± 13	PS	1.2	0	2,520	155	2,520
					155 ± 58	25	PS	0.9	0	2,340	155	2,340
					NR	20	AN69	1.65	0	2,240	156	2,240
					189	16	PAN	1	1,200	200	157	1,400
Lithium carbonate	73.9	0.7–1.4 L/kg	-0.809	0%	55	46	AN69	0.6, 0.9	3,200	2	158	3,202
					NR	54	CTA	1.9	0	5,000	159	5,000
Lomefloxacin	351.3	1.82–2.54 L/kg	-0.39	10%–21%	47	21	AN69	0.9	0	1,300	160	1,300
					54 ± 23	26 ± 4.7	AN69	0.9	1,000	100	161	1,100
					48 ± 20	16 ± 2.7	AN69	0.9	0	1,000	161	1,000
Meropenem	383.5	12–20 L	-4.4	2%	450 ± 265	25 ± 6.9	AN69, PS	0.9, 1.15	0	1,500	162	1,500
					76 ± 15	17 ± 7	PAN	0.6	0	1,600	163	1,600
					55 ± 38	NR	PS	0.7	0	400	164	400
					79 ± 45	NR	PS	0.7	1,000	400	164	1,400
					95 ± 60	NR	PS	0.7	2,000	400	164	2,400
					72	NR	PS	1.4	NR	1,900	165	1,900
					75	27	AN69	0.9	1,177	130	166	1,307

Table 27.4 Drug Clearance During Continuous Renal Replacement Therapies *(continued)*

Drugs	MW (g/mol)	Vd	Log P	PB (%)	Cl$_{TB}$ (mL/min)	Cl$_{RRT}$ (mL/min)	Filter	SA	DFR (mL/hr)	UFR (mL/hr)	REF	Effluent Rate (mL/hr)
					83 ± 22	24±8.0	AN69	0.9	0	1,600	167	1,600
Micafungin	1270.3	0.39 L/kg	-6.3	>99%	23 ± 12	NR	PMMA	1	750	1,050	168	1,800
Midazolam	325.8	1.0–2.5 L/kg	3.33	95%	484	2.8	AN69	NR	1,000	0	169	1,000
Moxifloxacin	401.4	1.7–2.7 L/kg	-0.5	30%–50%	318 ± 137	27±5.5	AN69	0.9	1,000	1,000	170	2,000
Mycophenolic acid	320.3	4 L/kg	3.53	97%		0.84	NR	NR	0	3,500	171	3,500
						1.5	NR	NR	1,250	750	171	2,000
Ofloxacin	361.4	2.4–3.5 L/kg	0.65	20%–32%	278 ± 28	90±4.5	PS	0.7	0	2,460	172	2,460
Phenytoin	252.3	0.5–1.0 L/kg	2.15	90%	NP	1	PS	NR	0	165	173	165
Piperacillin	517.6	0.18–0.3 L/kg	-0.26	16%	64.5 ± 59.7	27.6±15.2	AN69	06, 0.9	2,375	0	174	2,375
									1,663	1,663	174	3,326
					65 ± 20	NR	PS	0.7	0	800	175	800
					84 ± 28	NR	PS	0.7	1,000	800	175	1,800
					91 ± 35	NR	PS	0.7	2,000	800	175	2,800
					47	22	AN69	0.6	1,500	140	176	1,640
					66	38	AN69	1.5	1,000	1,000	177	2,000
Quinine	324.4	2.5–7.1 L/kg	2.51	70%	100 ± 12	1.33	PA	2	0	1,380	178	1,380
Tazobactam	300.3	14–16 L	-1.4	30%	40 ± 12	NR	PS	0.7	0	800	175	800
					52 ± 11	NR	PS	0.7	1,000	800	175	1,800
					65 ± 20	NR	PS	0.7	2,000	800	175	2,800
					30	17	AN69	0.6	1,500	140	176	1,640
Ticarcillin	384.4	12–16 L	0.6	45%	30 ± 18	12 ± 2.3	PS	0.25	0		140	0
Tobramycin	467.5	85.1 L	-6.5	0%	12 ± 6.4	3.5 ± 1.9	PS	0.25	0	267	149	267
					0.63	0.32–0.91	PS	0.25	0	25	179	25
Vancomycin	1449.3	0.864 L/kg	-4.4	55%	22	23	PA	2	0	1,000	180	1,000
					185	153 ± 22	PA	NR	0	12,312	181	12,312
					1.9	0.27–0.80	PS	0.25	0	25	179	25
					29	6.7–13	PS	0.25	0	13	48	13
					31 ± 13	12 ± 5.7	AN69	0.43	1,000	570	138	1,570
					31 ± 13	17 ± 5.7	AN69	0.43	2,000	570	138	2,570
					39 ± 4.3	4.2 ± 1.3	AN69	0.43	500	4,747	182	5,247
					17 ± 5.0	8.1 ± 3.2	AN69	0.43	1,000	162	183	1,162
					NR	13 ± 6.7	AN69	0.6	2,000	0	35	2,000
					NR	22 ± 9.3	PS	0.65	2,000	0	35	2,000
					NR	27 ± 5.6	PMMA	2.1	2,000	0	35	2,000

Table 27.4 Drug Clearance During Continuous Renal Replacement Therapies (continued)

Drugs	MW (g/mol)	Vd	Log P	PB (%)	Cl$_{TB}$ (mL/min)	Cl$_{RRT}$ (mL/min)	Filter	SA	DFR (mL/hr)	UFR (mL/hr)	REF	Effluent Rate (mL/hr)
					42 ± 12	30 ± 6.7	AN69	1.15	NR	NR	184	NR
Voriconazole	349.3	4.6 L/kg	1.82	58%	338	20	AN69	0.9	1,000	500	185	1,500
					90	23	PES	1.9	0	1,000	186	1,000
					215 ± 112	18 ± 5	AN69	0.9	1,000	1,000	187	2,000

Cl$_{TB}$ = total body clearance; Cl$_{RRT}$ = renal replacement therapy clearance; DFR = dialysate flow rate; MW = molecular weight; NR = not reported; PB = protein binding; REF = reference; SA = surface area; UFR = ultrafiltration flow rate; Vd = volume of distribution.

continued from page 548

changes to the systemic bioavailability of medications in the critical care population and are described.

Slowing of gastric emptying, or gastroparesis, is common in the ICU patient and can decrease the rate of drug absorption, resulting in a prolonged time (Tmax) to reach the maximum plasma concentration (Cmax). In addition, patients may have concomitant diseases such as diabetes mellitus or be prescribed medications (e.g., opiates, tricyclic antidepressants, phenothiazines, and calcium channel blockers) that can slow gastric emptying.

Metabolic acidosis is common in critical care patients and can change the fraction of drug in the ionized versus nonionized state, resulting in changes to bioavailability. In addition, critical care patients are often prescribed ulcer prophylaxis and/or treatment regimens that contain drugs that can increase gastric pH, resulting in changes to the systemic bioavailability of prescribed medications. Concomitant use of proton pump inhibitors will reduce the absorption of iron, calcium, magnesium, and vitamin B$_{12}$. The pH can also influence the availability of active pharmaceuticals from prodrug formulations. Binding of medications in the gut, such as the interaction between sucralfate and fluoroquinolones, can reduce oral bioavailability.

Reduction in first-pass metabolism can occur in critically ill patients secondary to decreases in the function of CYP metabolizing enzymes in the gut and liver. This can result in increases in the systemic bioavailability of CYP substrates. Other conditions such as edema of the gut and impaired small bowel function can also change the bioavailability of medications in the critical care population.

Distribution

Distribution volume is related to plasma protein binding and tissue binding. Two common plasma proteins are albumin (which binds acidic drugs) and α_1-acid glycoprotein (which binds basic drugs). Although chronic kidney disease is associated with reduced plasma protein concentrations, acute care patients can have increased protein binding of basic drugs secondary to increased α_1-acid glycoprotein concentrations.[38] This scenario would predict

Table 27.5 Differences Between Acute and Chronic Kidney Diseases That May Impact Drug Pharmacokinetics

Acute	Chronic
Use of continuous RRT	Use of intermittent RRT
Redistribution of plasma proteins	Decreased plasma proteins
↑ Vd for hydrophilic drugs	↓ Vd for hydrophilic drugs
↑ Residual renal clearance	↓ Residual renal clearance
Addition of ECMO	Metabolism and transport alterations

RRT = renal replacement therapy.

a potential increase in the removal of acid drugs and a decrease in the removal of basic drugs during continuous renal replacement therapies. Patients with acute illness can also have redistribution of albumin from the intravascular to the extravascular compartments secondary to capillary leak syndrome, resulting in significant changes to the Vd of hydrophilic drugs.[45] Common antibiotic examples include ceftriaxone, ertapenem, daptomycin, and aztreonam.[46] It is often recommended to consider using loading doses of hydrophilic drugs in critical care patients. Alterations in drug to albumin binding have recently been extensively reviewed.[46] Increases in body water that occur with volume overload in acute kidney disease can result in increases in the distribution volume of hydrophilic drugs (e.g., aminoglycoside antibiotics).

Metabolism

Cytochrome P450 enzymes can be decreased up to 35%, according to studies using experimental models of chronic kidney disease, and decreased up to 63%, according to clinical studies.[41-44] In addition, in patients with chronic kidney disease, the function of CYP3A4 can be improved immediately after hemodialysis.[41] The function of metabolic pathways in acute kidney injury and other representative diseases in critically ill patients is not well defined. Reductions in the nonrenal clearance of imipenem and vancomycin have been reported in patients with acute kidney injury.[47] The clearance reduction was reported to be less severe than in patients with chronic kidney disease requiring IHD: 90 mL/minute versus 50 mL/minute, respectively, for imipenem and 15 mL/minute versus 5 mL/minute, respectively, for vancomycin.[47] The duration of acute kidney injury can also influence the reduction in nonrenal clearance. Macias et al. reported that as the length of continuous renal replacement therapy increased, the nonrenal clearance was more significantly affected.[48]

Excretion

Drugs that undergo excretion primarily through the kidneys (aminoglycosides, penicillins) will have significant reductions in total body clearance through decreases in renal clearance. The Dettli method[49-51] is used to predict the fraction of clearance of a patient with chronic kidney disease relative to the expected clearance in a healthy individual (e.g., Q factor). It can be used to predict changes in the dose, interval, or combination of dose and interval in patients with chronic kidney disease. However, it has not been tested under acutely changing kidney function conditions.

Endogenous clearance (both renal and nonrenal) can be different in acute versus chronic kidney diseases. It is generally recognized that residual renal clearances will be higher in the setting of acute versus chronic kidney disease. In addition, clearance can be increased in critically ill patients secondary to concomitant drugs prescribed to maintain adequate perfusion pressure.[52] Mechanical ventilation can also contribute to increased clearance.[53] A recent review provides additional discussion of the potential for augmented renal clearance in critical care patients.[54] Several transport proteins (e.g., P-glycoprotein, organic anion and cation transporters) contribute to drug secretion in the kidney tubules and can be affected by chronic kidney disease. The effects of critical illness on transport processes have not been evaluated. In addition, the influence of metabolic by-products (e.g., uremic toxins) on transporters in acute kidney injury is currently unknown.[36,37,42,44]

DRUG DOSING STRATEGIES/ PHARMACOKINETICS

A previous section of this chapter reviewed the basic equations for estimating and measuring clearance during continuous renal replacement techniques. However, in addition to clearance determinations, clinicians must be able to recommend appropriate medication doses according to the clearance values, pharmacodynamic goals, and other individual concerns. This is important because the available drug dosing references are not written to be personalized for the patient in your care. Individual patients may have specific therapeutic goals or may be receiving different dialytic techniques or concomitant medications that could affect the plasma and tissue concentrations of drugs. The following sections will review drug dosing equations that use the clearance determinations from continuous renal replacement modalities (Table 27.6). These equations can also be used for dosing drugs in patients with chronic kidney disease. Additional information for drug clearance and dosing in chronic kidney disease can be found in several manuscripts and reviews.[49,51,55-58] The equations will empower the clinician to calculate the plasma concentrations likely to result under given administration scenarios. In addition, the equations can be rearranged to solve for dose to enable the dosing revisions required to reach targeted plasma concentrations. The equations described in the following sections are applicable to drugs that are described by a one-compartment model.

Intravenous Bolus

Intravenous bolus administration implies an instantaneous administration of drug into the central compartment of the body. Many drugs (e.g., morphine, diphenhydramine) are administered as a direct intravenous bolus in the critical care unit. In addition, intravenous bolus administration can be used to provide a loading dose of medications and will be followed by an intravenous infusion. The maximal plasma concentration (Cp) after intravenous bolus administration is described by the dose and Vd (equation 27.9).

$$Cp = dose/Vd \text{ (equation 27.9)}$$

Table 27.6 Equations for Drug Dosing[a]

IV Bolus	
Eq. 9	$Cp = dose/Vd$
IV Infusion	
Eq. 10 (during infusion):	$Cp = Ko/Cl \times [1 - e^{-ke \cdot t}]$
Eq. 11 (at steady state):	$Cp_{ss} = Ko/Cl$
Eq. 12 (at end of infusion):	$Cp = Ko/Cl \times [1 - e^{-ke \cdot T}]$
Eq. 13 (after end of infusion):	$Cp = Cp_{at\ time = T} \cdot e^{-ke \cdot [time - T]}$
Extravascular	
Eq. 14:	$Cp = [F \times dose \times Ka]/[Vd (Ka - Ke)] \times [e^{-ke \cdot t} - e^{-ka \cdot t}]$
Eq. 15:	$Dose = (Cpss \times Cl \times tau)/(S \times F)$

[a]The equations are representative of one-compartment models.
IV = intravenous.

As shown in the equation, a good estimation of the Vd for the drug in the critically ill patient will suffice for determining concentration without respect to clearance. If the concentration is less than expected, the Vd of the drug in the patient was higher than predicted by literature values. The equation can be rearranged to inform about the Vd in the particular patient. Subsequent intravenous bolus doses can be modified according to the actual Vd to achieve a targeted peak plasma concentration. The decline of the plasma concentration after intravenous bolus administration will suggest whether the drug follows a one-, two-, or three-compartment model.

Intravenous Infusion (during infusion)

Although an intravenous bolus is straightforward, infusions are more complicated. For intravenous infusions, it must be realized that clearance processes during the infusion will affect the obtained concentration in the plasma. The plasma concentration (Cp) can be computed at any time point (t) during the intravenous infusion according to equation 27.10, considering the rate of infusion (Ko), total body clearance (Cl), and amount remaining as defined by the term $1 - e^{-ke*t}$.

$$Cp = Ko/Cl \times [1 - e^{-ke*t}] \text{ (equation 27.10)}$$

As suggested earlier, the total body clearance should be the sum of the residual renal, nonrenal, and renal replacement therapy clearance. The duration of the renal replacement therapy will further affect the clearance. This condition (equation 27.10) does not represent steady state. Equation 27.10 will be helpful to use to determine where the plasma concentrations fall during an infusion and to calculate the infusion rates needed to achieve a targeted drug concentration.

Intravenous Infusion (at steady state)

The plasma concentration at steady state (Cp_{ss}) can be computed for drug therapy that requires an intravenous infusion according to equation 27.11, considering the rate of infusion (Ko) and total body clearance (Cl). Note that the amount remaining term is not included because, by definition, steady state would imply that the rate in equals the rate out.

$$Cp_{ss} = Ko/Cl \text{ (equation 27.11)}$$

This method can also be useful to determine rates of infusion needed given a known clearance and targeted Cp_{ss}.

Intravenous Infusion (at end of infusion)

The plasma concentration at the end of an infusion (time is T) can be computed according to equation 27.12, considering the rate of infusion (Ko), total body clearance (Cl), and amount remaining term $(1 - e^{-ke*T})$ that incorporates the end of infusion time term (T).

$$Cp = Ko/Cl \times [1 - e^{-ke*T}] \text{ (equation 27.12)}$$

This equation will be helpful to determine where the plasma concentrations fall at the end of one infusion rate in order to guide changes to infusion rates for subsequent doses to achieve a targeted drug concentration.

Intravenous Infusion (after end of infusion)

Finally, the plasma concentration at any time point after the end of an intravenous infusion (time) can be computed according to equation 27.13, considering the concentration at the end of the infusion (Cp at T) and the loss of drug between the end of the infusion and T ($e^{-ke*[time-T]}$).

$$Cp = Cp_{at\ time\ =\ T}\ e^{-ke*[time-T]}$$
$$\text{(equation 27.13)}$$

Extravascular Route

The calculation of the plasma concentration after administration of a drug by the extravascular route is more complicated (equation 27.14). It requires the bioavailability term (F), dose, Vd, and rate constants for elimination (Ke) and absorption (ka).

$$Cp = [F \times dose \times Ka]/[Vd (Ka - Ke)] \times [e^{-ke*t} - e^{-ka*t}]$$
$$\text{(equation 27.14)}$$

If the usual condition of the absorption rate being faster than the elimination rate is not met, the drug is said to have flip-flop pharmacokinetics. Given the potential absorption issues in critical care patients, clinical scenarios whereby flip-flop pharmacokinetics are shown are highly likely.

At steady state, an extravascular dose can be calculated as shown in equation 27.15.

$$Dose = (Cpss \times Cl \times Tau)/(S \times F)$$
$$\text{(equation 27.15)}$$

In equation 27.15, the numerator is the product of the concentration in plasma at steady state (Cpss), total body clearance (Cl), and dosing frequency (Tau), whereas the denominator is the product of the salt form of the drug (S) and bioavailability (F).

More advanced pharmacokinetic modeling and simulation using population approaches are warranted to fully understand the differences in pharmacokinetics in discrete populations within the ICU. In addition, population modeling techniques enable the determination of patient, clinical, and renal replacement therapy covariates that could affect pharmacokinetic parameters and interindividual variability.[59]

IMPLICATIONS OF DRUG DOSING ON PHARMACODYNAMIC EFFECTS

It has been suggested that despite attention to adjustments of drugs in patients receiving renal replacement therapies, patients with infections who are receiving antibiotics often have inadequate outcomes.[60,61] Because of variations in drug clearance by renal replacement therapies, it is highly recommended that clinicians treat infections aggressively, especially during the early phase of treatment, using loading doses to reach targeted plasma concentrations sooner. For antibiotics, the targeted plasma concentrations should consider the desired concentrations at the infection site. It is necessary for clinicians to consult their local laboratory to obtain susceptibility data (minimum inhibitory concentrations [MICs]) for antibiotics to ensure that targeted concentrations are adequate. Clinicians also need to identify whether the selected antibiotics have time- or concentration-dependent killing.[62] For drugs that have time-dependent killing, previous data analyses have suggested that maximal bactericidal effects occur when concentrations above the MIC are obtained for a defined percentage of the dosing interval: for cephalosporins, about 60%–70%; penicillins, 50%; and carbapenems, 40%.[63] These targeted times have been used as pharmacodynamic measures for therapy outcomes.[64] In the study by Seyler et al., 90% of patients receiving antibiotic therapy (meropenem, piperacillin/tazobactam, cefepime, or ceftazidime) had plasma concentrations deemed adequate for concentration breakpoints of Enterobacteriaceae, but inadequate for most other microorganisms.[64] According to Seyler et al., the dosing ranges suggested for the antibiotics mentioned previously in critical care patients receiving renal replacement therapies would have resulted in poor pharmacodynamic responses given the percentage of the antibiotic dosing interval in which drug concentrations are greater than the MIC.[64]

These data analyses suggest that clinicians should use the combined pharmacokinetic-pharmacodynamic simulation tools available in many commercial pharmacokinetics software packages to more accurately estimate how dosing recommendations may affect pharmacodynamic outcomes. Strategies proposed during continuous renal replacement therapies to optimize the attainment of adequate concentrations of antibiotics with time-dependent killing include continuous or prolonged infusions, shorter dosing intervals, supplemental dosing, and weight-based dosing.[65] For antibiotics that have concentration-dependent dosing (e.g., aminoglycosides, colistin, daptomycin, fluoroquinolones, linezolid, macrolides, metronidazole, vancomycin), strategies such as loading doses, extended dosing intervals, and weight-based dosing have been proposed to optimize pharmacodynamic outcomes.[65] A paucity of literature exists for other classes of drugs and pharmacodynamic outcomes in patients undergoing continuous renal replacement therapies.

CLINICIAN DOSING AND OUTCOMES

Despite clinicians providing dosing consultations for drugs in patients receiving renal replacement therapies, there are limited publications that show outcomes. One publication reported more than 180 recommendations for dosing adjustment of antimicrobials in critical care patients.[66] Changing continuous renal replacement therapy conditions was reportedly the most common reason for dosing errors, showing the need to adequately monitor for these changes and incorporate them into clearance and drug dosing equations. Of importance, clinician dosing recommendations had positive clinical outcomes, including reduced length of stay in the ICU by 3 days as compared with a control group not receiving targeted recommendations.[66] Another recent publication evaluated prescribing patterns of antimicrobials in patients receiving sustained low-efficiency dialysis.[67] Results indicated that antimicrobial under-dosing was a predominant problem, with failures to reach clinical cures. These data show the potential for the positive impacts clinicians can have on outcomes in patients receiving renal replacement therapies.

ONGOING CONSIDERATIONS FOR CONTINUOUS RENAL REPLACEMENT THERAPIES

According to the available published data for the pharmacokinetics of drugs during continuous renal replacement therapy, it is clear that most evaluated drugs have been antibiotics. Given the polypharmacy in the ICU population, future studies should assess pharmacokinetic alterations and dosing guidance for other classes of drugs. Most published research evaluating drug pharmacokinetics during renal replacement has focused on adults. However, given the increased frequency of these therapies in the pediatric population and the inherent pharmacokinetic differences between adult and pediatric patients, future research should include this patient subgroup as well.

Continuous renal replacement therapies have been in clinical use since the 1990s. However, the therapy conditions have evolved over time with new hemofilters composed of different materials and higher effluent rates. It is necessary to note the therapy conditions in published research in order to determine the relevance to individual patients today. It may be necessary to recalculate the expected clearance for a drug of interest according to the differences in effluent rates in the past versus the present. Pharmacokinetic-pharmacodynamic modeling and simulation can assist with achieving targeted concentrations and clinical outcomes.

Finally, given the widespread use of continuous renal replacement therapies, it is now necessary to provide education and experiential training to students and clinicians who train or practice in the critical care setting.

PLASMAPHERESIS

Plasmapheresis is a continuous flow procedure that involves the extracorporeal separation of plasma from other blood components through intravenous access. The plasma is discarded and exchanged with a physiological replacement fluid that varies depending on the clinical scenario and typically contains albumin or fresh frozen plasma. Replacement fluid is necessary to maintain oncotic pressure and intravascular blood volume in order to avoid hypovolemic shock. Replacement fluid in conjunction with the patient's blood and cellular components is returned to the patient through the intravenous access.

There are many clinical indications for the use of plasmapheresis. Disease indications include thrombotic thrombocytopenic purpura, myasthenia gravis, acute/chronic inflammatory demyelinating polyneuropathy, acute antibody-mediated rejection related to a variety of solid organ transplant types, and other autoimmune processes. In addition, plasmapheresis has been reported to be effective for the treatment of medication overdoses and venomous exposures.[68-70] Apart from the intended use of plasmapheresis for the treatment of medical conditions and toxicological problems, there is an unintended effect of plasmapheresis on the loss of prescribed medications. The impact of plasmapheresis on the pharmacokinetics of medications commonly prescribed in the ICU setting is not insignificant. There continues to be a paucity of evidence-based guidelines on the impact of plasmapheresis on drug clearance.

Limited studies in the literature report formal pharmacokinetic evaluations of drugs during plasmapheresis.[71] In 2007, Ibrahim et al. described the existing limitations of the available published literature on this topic including (1) heterogeneity of plasma exchange procedures with respect to the duration, volume, and type of replacement fluid used; (2) lack of uniformity in plasma sampling times for pharmacokinetic evaluation among studies, and the relationship of this sampling to initiation of plasmapheresis; (3) use of different analyses to ascertain removal such as declines in drug plasma concentration versus the total quantity of drug removed during plasmapheresis; (4) statistical flaws; and (5) inappropriate extrapolations between patient populations (e.g., adult data extrapolated to neonates).[71]

DRUG CHARACTERISTICS FOR CLEARANCE BY PLASMAPHERESIS

There are specific drug- and plasmapheresis-dependent factors that influence the likelihood of a drug being cleared by this extracorporeal technique[72] (Table 27.7). To provide a framework for the extent of solute removal during plasmapheresis, one study reported that a single exchange of 1 plasma volume (about 3 L in a 70-kg adult patient) removes around 63% of all solutes in the plasma, and an increase to a 1.5 exchange volume removes about 78% of solutes.[73] Solute elimination by plasma exchange is passive and described by linear kinetics.[73] The time between the drug administration and plasmapheresis initiation is considered to be the most important and critical factor affecting drug removal.[74] Several early studies evaluating the disposition and removal of ceftriaxone, ceftazidime, phenobarbital, vancomycin, gentamicin, thyroxine, and aspirin reported increased drug removal when plasmapheresis was initiated immediately or

Table 27.7 Important Determinants of the Effectiveness of Plasmapheresis in Removal of Drugs[72]

Drug-Dependent

Time between dose administration and plasmapheresis initiation
    The higher the drug plasma concentration at the time of plasmapheresis initiation, the more likely it will be removed (a function of the drug's distribution half-life)

Protein binding
    The lower a drug's protein binding, the less likely it will be removed

Volume of distribution
    The higher the drug's volume of distribution, the less likely it will be removed

Plasmapheresis-Dependent

Duration of plasmapheresis

Successive plasmapheresis sessions

Volume of plasma removed

Plasmapheresis replacement fluid (equivocal)

Reprinted with permission. Adapted from: Ibrahim RB, Balogun RA. Medications in patients treated with therapeutic plasma exchange: prescription dosage, timing and drug overdose. Semin Dial 2012;25:176-89.

shortly after drug administration. These data are consistent with more recent findings such as those described for cefepime removal by plasmapheresis.[74-81] Ibrahim et al. also reported data showing that 75% of mycophenolate mofetil was recovered in the volume of plasma removed when it was concurrently administered by intravenous infusion during the plasmapheresis procedure.[72]

Drugs with a higher degree of protein binding have enhanced removal during plasmapheresis. In general, a drug whose protein binding is greater than 80% will be removed by plasmapheresis.[71,72] It is suggested that for a drug bound to albumin, a linear relationship exists between the fraction eliminated during the plasmapheresis session and the fraction of the drug present in the extracellular fluid.[82] Plasma proteins and bound drugs are removed in tandem with fluid in plasmapheresis. Of importance, this scenario is contrary to what is known about drug protein binding and clearance during extracorporeal dialysis techniques. During dialysis procedures (intermittent or continuous), drugs with increased protein binding are not significantly removed. The unbound fraction of drugs is cleared through dialysis procedures (as described earlier in this chapter).

Drugs with a lower Vd (less than 0.2 L/kg) are more likely to be removed by plasmapheresis.[72] This is intuitive because drugs must be in the plasma compartment to be eliminated by plasmapheresis. A drug with increased Vd has reduced clearance by plasma exchange. Calculating patient-specific Vd values for medications will enable an estimate of total body drug stores. This method is the most stringent for determining the drug fraction eliminated during plasmapheresis.[83] Single-dose drug studies of plasmapheresis are limited because the Vd after a single dose may vary from the Vd at steady state and is one of the limitations of many of the published studies.[84] Hydrophilic drugs with small volumes of distribution and high protein binding would be predicted to be cleared, especially if administered around the time of the plasmapheresis procedure. However, lipophilic drugs have large Vd and would not be expected to have significant clearance by plasmapheresis.[72] For example, voriconazole, a lipophilic drug with a large Vd (4 L/kg) and moderate protein binding (58%), was not significantly removed by plasmapheresis.[85]

PLASMAPHERESIS CONDITIONS AND DRUG CLEARANCE

Several plasmapheresis-specific factors are implicated in drug clearance including the duration of the plasmapheresis procedure, need for successive plasmapheresis sessions, volume of plasma removed, and type of replacement fluid used (Table 27.8).[71,72]

Table 27.8 Drug Characteristics for Removal by Plasmapheresis[a]

Drug	Vd (in liters except where noted)	Plasma Protein Binding (%)	Drug Removal by Plasmapheresis	Other Properties/Need Dose Adjustment
Prednisone	0.6–0.7	90–95	No, 0.83% of total dose	No need to adjust dose
Cyclosporine	13	90–98	No, 1% fraction eliminated from whole blood and plasma	No need to adjust dose
Tacrolimus	0.85–1.4 L/kg	Unknown but low	No	No need to adjust dose
Rituximab	3.1	None	Yes, pre-plasmapheresis level was reduced by 65%	No, because no impact on immediate effect (t½ 1–3 days)
Amiodarone	5,000	> 98	No	No need to adjust dose
Digoxin	5–8	25	No	No need to adjust dose
Propranolol	4	90	Yes, mean elimination t½ decreased from 4.3 to 1.1 hr	Removal may not affect clinical/biological effect
Aspirin	0.1–0.2	80–90	Variable, 7%–32% was removed	Unpredictable, removed in some patients secondary to nonlinear kinetics
Heparin	0.04–0.07	Unknown	Yes	Increase dose or give after session
Tobramycin	0.25	10	Yes	Administer after plasmapheresis
Ampicillin	0.2–0.3	20	Yes, 35.2% drop in concentration	Administer after plasmapheresis

[a]This is not a comprehensive list of medications. A more comprehensive list can be found in Ibrahim RB, Balogun RA. Medications in patients treated with therapeutic plasma exchange: prescription dosage, timing and drug overdose. Semin Dial 2012;25:176-89.

t½ = half-life.

Most commonly, plasmapheresis sessions last 1–3 hours. The duration of the sessions can vary depending on the patient's hemodynamics during exchange of the desired plasma volume and the overall therapeutic goals. Although some drugs have a large Vd and will not be removed by plasmapheresis, others that are highly protein bound will have increased removal, as previously discussed. An extended duration of each session may result in increased drug removal. It is, however, important to realize that although some drugs such as β-blockers are heavily removed by plasmapheresis, blood concentrations do not correlate with their biologic effect. As such, removal by plasmapheresis may not always predict changes in pharmacodynamics. However, out of an abundance of caution, it is recommended that drugs with a small Vd and high degree of protein binding be administered after the plasmapheresis session.

In some clinical scenarios, several plasmapheresis sessions may be required, often on a daily basis, depending on the intended outcome. As discussed previously, waiting to dose drugs with small distribution volumes and increased protein binding until after the plasmapheresis session is complete may allow for enhanced benefits from the therapies.

Because dilution of plasma occurs secondary to the administration of replacement fluid, the targeted substances of interest cannot completely be removed from the circulation. For example, for each 1–1.5 plasma volume exchanged, about 60%–70% of the substances present in the plasma at the start of that plasma volume will be removed. As additional plasma volumes are exchanged, the absolute amount removed becomes lower, although the removal of a fixed 60%–70% still occurs. For this reason, routine practice is to exchange only 1–1.5 plasma volumes during a single plasmapheresis session. Plasmapheresis volumes beyond 1.5 plasma volumes remove smaller, less clinically important amounts of pathologic substances present in the plasma while prolonging the procedure and exposing patients to more replacement fluid with an increasing risk of complications.[86] Similar to the removal of pathologic substances, plasma volume can also affect the removal of drug solutes.

The composition of the replacement fluid influences the effects of plasmapheresis on the patient. It is known that about one-third of the replacement fluid administered at the beginning of a session will be present by the end, with the other two-thirds removed. Administering plasma as a replacement fluid at the beginning of a session exposes the patient to blood products without additional clinical benefit. The most commonly used replacement fluid is 5% albumin in physiological saline. This fluid mixture has several advantages because it decreases the risk of disease transmission from the use of blood products and transfusion-related reactions such as acute lung injury. This specific replacement fluid has a higher oncotic pressure than plasma and thus may result in expansion of the intravascular volume. The albumin concentrations in the replacement fluids may affect drug clearance through protein binding.

DRUG PHARMACODYNAMICS WITH PLASMAPHERESIS

As mentioned previously, plasma concentrations of drugs and therapeutic proteins do not always correlate with clinical effects. Therefore, plasmapheresis may not alter the biologic effect of a drug despite reducing the plasma concentration. This scenario has been shown for rituximab, a monoclonal antibody used for the treatment of a variety of conditions. Rituximab has a moderate Vd (3.1 L), no protein binding, and a half-life of 9–70 days. Despite these pharmacokinetic parameters, significant removal of rituximab is seen when it is dosed within 24 hours of a plasmapheresis session. The main mechanism for rituximab removal by plasmapheresis is unknown but is thought to be related to the removal of the therapeutic antibody or antibody complexes and resulting inflammatory cytokines, or the transient depletion of complement.[68] However, an assessment of pharmacodynamic markers (peripheral CD19 B cells and ADAMST12 immunoglobulin G, and increased ADAMST13 activity) has suggested that the drug response was unaltered.[87] Given this example, it can be concluded that the removal of therapeutic proteins by plasmapheresis does not necessarily translate to a loss of pharmacologic effects. The optimal timing between drug administration and plasmapheresis initiation for different drugs remains ill defined, and the correlation between drug pharmacokinetics and clinical outcomes requires further study.

Plasmapheresis may have effects on drugs because of the clearance of other circulating components necessary for drug effectiveness. Plasmapheresis is known to reduce levels of antithrombin III,[71] and can therefore have an effect on achieving therapeutic anticoagulation. A study evaluating anti-factor 10a activity during plasmapheresis found decreased anti-factor 10a and a 40% loss in a patient receiving low-molecular-weight heparin. This is thought to be related to the extraction of antithrombin III alone or the complex of heparin and antithrombin III.[88] Patients on plasmapheresis who require simultaneous anticoagulation with heparin may require higher doses to achieve therapeutic effects.

Patients receiving plasmapheresis often have other comorbidities that can influence the pharmacokinetics of drugs. For example, acute renal or hepatic failure can alter pharmacokinetics, independent of plasmapheresis. Clinicians should review the characteristics of prescribed drugs (protein binding, Vd) before plasmapheresis initiation so that they can be aware of the medications that should be closely monitored for decreased efficacy secondary to increased clearance.[89] Ibrahim et al. have published two excellent reviews from the literature (case reports and randomized studies) on the impact of plasmapheresis on drug removal.[71,72] Table 27.8 is a summary of drug clearance by plasmapheresis. Finally, if the pharmacokinetic and pharmacodynamic effects of plasmapheresis on the drug are not well described, administration of drugs after a plasmapheresis session remains a viable and conservative approach. Therapeutic drug monitoring should also be considered when available.

EXTRACORPOREAL MEMBRANE OXYGENATION

Extracorporeal membrane oxygenation (ECMO) is a type of extracorporeal life support and, depending on its configuration, can be used to provide oxygenation, carbon dioxide removal, and/or perfusion to vital organs for days to weeks in critically ill patients with lung and/or cardiac dysfunction. Its use spans a wide variety of populations, including neonates, children, adolescents, and adults. The first successful use of ECMO was in 1972, but initial enthusiasm was dampened when a randomized controlled trial of ECMO for adult acute respiratory distress syndrome (ARDS) was terminated because of futility.[90] Although there have been some advances in technology, enthusiasm for this technique in adults has been renewed because of recent randomized and cohort studies of patients with severe ARDS, and in particular H1N1-related ARDS where reductions in mortality were reported.[91,92]

The two separate modes of ECMO are venovenous and venoarterial. Venovenous ECMO is used for isolated respiratory failure, and its use increased dramatically in adults during the H1N1 influenza outbreak.[91] In this mode, systemic blood flow and pressure are the result of native cardiac function unrelated to extracorporeal flow. Venoarterial ECMO is used for isolated cardiac failure or combined cardiopulmonary failure. Systemic flow is a combination of that established by the extracorporeal circuit plus the amount of blood passing through the native heart and lungs. Systemic oxygen and carbon dioxide concentrations are determined by a mix of blood passing through the lungs and heart and oxygenated blood that is reinfused from the circuit into the arterial circulation.

ECMO Components

Several circuit components are known to affect drug pharmacokinetics. A clear understanding of each of the circuit components, including the tubing, oxygenator, type of circuit (roller vs. centrifugal pump), and venous reservoir, is necessary to understand how they may affect drug pharmacokinetics. Several excellent reviews have been published that describe these components and their function.[93-96] Figure 27.7 depicts the standard ECMO circuit setup.[94]

The purpose of the pump is to push blood through the oxygenator and back to the patient. Flow in the centrifugal pump is dependent on the blood volume from the patient, systemic vascular resistance, size of the cannula, and pump speed. The main advantage of the centrifugal pump is that it creates less negative pressure on the blood, and therefore less hemolysis. Flow in the roller pump depends on the size of the tubing in the raceway, occlusion pressures of the rollers, pump speed, and blood volume. One of the major disadvantages of the roller pump is increased hemolysis and continued rotation of the pump independent of blood volume or air entrapment.[93,97]

The two main devices used for gas exchange in the ECMO circuit are the silicone membrane oxygenator and the hollow fiber oxygenator. The hollow fiber oxygenator has major advantages, including priming that is easy and fast, presence of a coating that reduces the risk of clot formation, smaller surface area to reduce platelet activation and inflammation, and lower pressure gradient across the membrane to reduce shear stress on the red blood cells and subsequent hemolysis.

Different types of ECMO tubing exist, each with different components, and are beyond the scope of this chapter. However, remember that each of these tubing types can influence drug pharmacokinetics in patients on ECMO.

An ECMO circuit may also include a venous reservoir or bladder located on the venous line before the pump and serves as an air bubble trap and volume buffer as it sits at the lowest point on the ECMO circuit. Clot formation in the reservoir poses a significant risk. Pooling of medications may occur in the venous reservoir, especially if the specific gravity of the medication is less than that of blood. For this reason, it is recommended that medications be administered in the circuit at a location after the reservoir.[98] Many centers no longer use a venous reservoir as part of the ECMO circuit.

Factors Responsible for Alterations in Drug Pharmacokinetics in ECMO

Extracorporeal membrane oxygenation can alter the pharmacokinetics and pharmacodynamics of medications for a variety of reasons in a population (e.g., critically ill patients) already known to have altered drug pharmacokinetics. The addition of ECMO increases the degree of systemic inflammation because of the interaction between the patient's blood and the artificial membranes, hemodilution, transfusions, organ dysfunction, and renal replacement therapy.[99,100] Extracorporeal membrane oxygenation treatment can lead to drug sequestration and changes to Vd and clearance. The addition of continuous renal replacement therapy to the ECMO circuit (Figure 27.7) can result in further changes to drug pharmacokinetics (as described earlier in this chapter). Although the body of literature on the effects of ECMO on drug clearance is growing, data

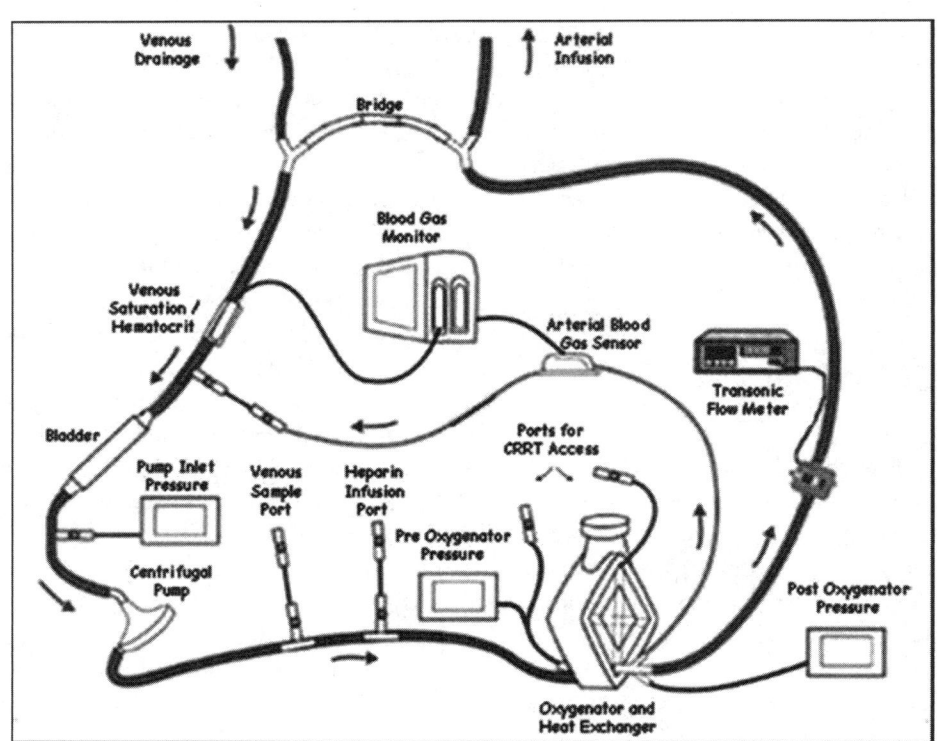

Figure 27.7 Standard extracorporeal membrane oxygenation (ECMO) circuit.

Venous blood drains from the patient and passes through a venous saturation sensor and a bladder before being pumped to the oxygenator/heat-exchanger device. The oxygenated warmed blood passes the ECMO circuit bridge before infusing back into the patient into the arterial (venoarterial) or venous (venovenous) system. There are many infusion and access ports, as well as pressure and flow monitors, along the way.

CRRT = continuous renal replacement therapy.

Reprinted with permission from: Lequier L, Horton SB, McMullan DM, et al. Extracorporeal membrane oxygenation circuitry. Pediatr Crit Care Med 2013;14:S7-12.

are currently insufficient to make meaningful recommendations for drug dosing adjustments.[101] Ongoing studies continue to investigate altered pharmacokinetics and related outcomes for a variety of drugs commonly administered to patients requiring ECMO.[102,103] These studies fall into three general categories: in vitro studies related to the physiochemical properties of drugs (e.g., drug binding to ECMO circuitry), classical pharmacokinetic studies, and clinical trials evaluating outcomes.[89]

Drug Sequestration and Influence of ECMO Circuit Components and Drug Characteristics

Drug sequestration on ECMO is well known but poorly characterized. It is influenced by specific drug properties, including molecular size, degree of ionization, lipophilicity, and plasma protein binding.[104] Sequestration is a function of binding to a biosynthetic surface. The most common biosynthetic surface is the standard polyvinyl chloride tubing. In addition, there are a variety of other coated tubing types, including Maquet Safeline (synthetic immobilized albumin), Maquet Softline (heparin-free biopassive polymer), Maquet Bioline (recombinant human albumin plus heparin) by Maquet Cardiopulmonary AG (Hirrlingen, Germany), Terumo X Coating (poly2methoxylacrylate) by Terumo Cardiovascular Systems Corporation (Ann Arbor, MI), and Medtronic Carmeda (covalently bonded heparin) and Medtronic Trillium (covalently bonded heparin) by Medtronic (Minneapolis, MN). Sequestration can vary depending on the circuit components (pump, oxygenator, tubing, venous reservoir), circuit priming, and age of the circuit.[105,106] Most of the available data on drug disposition have been derived from neonatal studies using older-generation ECMO circuits.[107] In these studies, significant sequestration by the ECMO circuit was observed and was dependent on the physiochemical properties of drugs and the type and age of the circuits used.[104,107,108]

In an adult ex vivo model of ECMO using contemporary circuitry, Shekar et al. hypothesized that lipophilic and protein bound drugs have enhanced sequestration in ECMO circuits.[109] The authors used four identical ECMO circuits comprising centrifugal pumps and polymethylpentene oxygenators to investigate the influence of plasma protein binding on drug disposition. Drug recovery was defined as the amount of drug recovered from the ex vivo circuit at the end of the study and after accounting for sequestration. Ceftriaxone, ciprofloxacin, linezolid, fluconazole, caspofungin, and thiopentone were selected for evaluation on the basis of lipophilicity and protein binding values. Lipophilicity (log P) and protein binding values for these drugs appear in Table 27.9. The circuit conditions (oxygen tension, temperature, activated clotting times, pH) were kept stable in order to discern differences in sequestration related to drug characteristics. Study drugs were injected post-oxygenator as a single bolus dose, with doses selected on the basis of producing concentrations that were similar to expected clinical concentrations. Larger doses were chosen for drugs having high protein binding in order to achieve concentrations that were similar to clinical concentrations. Equivalent doses of drugs were injected into four polypropylene jars containing fresh human whole blood in order to serve as study controls and for stability testing. Serial blood samples were collected from the ECMO circuits and control reservoirs over 24 hours. Drugs with a significant decrease in plasma concentration at 24 hours had a high degree of protein binding (greater than 80%), were highly lipophilic (log P greater than 2.3), or both, with a recovery of less than 20%.[109] However, meropenem, a drug with a low degree of protein binding (2%) and hydrophilic (log P -0.6), had a very low plasma concentration remaining at 24 hours, which was attributed to its instability at physiological temperature. This situation highlights the need to study and identify the impact of ECMO on the sequestration of thermolabile medications.[108,110,111] Despite this robust study, it remains unclear whether protein binding and lipophilicity definitively have an additive effect on drug sequestration in the circuit. In addition, drugs with a similar lipophilicity but different protein binding can have variable recovery from the circuit, suggesting that protein binding determines circuit drug sequestration.[109]

A significant loss of ampicillin, a hydrophilic drug (log P -2.0) with low protein binding (15%–25%), was reported in ex vivo blood primed circuits compared with crystalloid primed circuits.[111] This suggests that ECMO circuits can bind blood proteins and drugs, and it is unclear whether there is a competitive binding between them, and if so, whether this phenomenon is concentration-dependent.

The mechanisms that lead to circuit sequestration of highly protein bound drugs are unclear. In ex vivo neonatal circuits, 80% of fentanyl (85% protein bound, log P 3.9) was sequestered in the absence of an oxygenator, and an additional 6% sequestration occurred when the oxygenator was added.[112] It has been postulated that circuit sites that bind albumin and other proteins on priming or after the passage of blood lead to binding of administered drugs that have high protein binding. In a recent study evaluating different circuit types, there were significant differences in drug recovery rates between roller and centrifugal pumps, respectively, for fentanyl (0.4% vs. 34%) and midazolam (0.6% vs. 63%).[108,113] Similar to fentanyl, midazolam is 92% protein bound and has a log P value of 3.9. Age of the ECMO circuit can also influence drug sequestration. Midazolam sequestration in the first 10 minutes in a used ECMO circuit was lower than in a new ECMO circuit (4.1% vs. 26.1%, p=0.0004), but this difference disappeared after 180 minutes.[106] For both midazolam and fentanyl, there was a failure to reach steady state, and ongoing drug losses suggest the presence of a greater amount of binding sites within the ECMO circuit for these drugs than for other evaluated compounds. This study, however, did not identify where the loss of drugs occurred.[106] Although all drugs are clinically administered before the oxygenator in the circuit to decrease the risk of air embolus, given the results, it can be hypothesized that fentanyl and perhaps other highly lipophilic drugs have less therapeutic effectiveness when administered pre-oxygenator in the ECMO circuit. Hence, these drugs should be administered directly to the patient to minimize sequestration.[106]

It is known that drug adsorption by polymers (silicone and rubber) is related to lipophilicity.[113] As the total adsorptive capacity is linked to total surface area, ECMO circuits with larger membrane oxygenators and longer tubing may result in more adsorption. It has been reported that polyvinyl chloride tubing with newer surface coatings such as the Maquet tubing (including Bioline) led to a decrease in morphine concentration in the circuit to 51% of baseline compared with 35% of baseline in other types of tubing, suggesting that adsorption by certain tubing types is significantly reduced.[113]

Several unanswered questions remain regarding sequestration of drugs during ECMO. Controversy currently exists

Table 27.9	Lipophilicity (log P) and Percent (%) Protein Binding of Drugs Prone to Sequestration in ECMO	
Drug	Lipophilicity (log P)	Protein Binding (%)
Ciprofloxacin	2.3	20–40
Fluconazole	0.4	12
Linezolid	0.9	31
Ceftriaxone	-1.7	95
Caspofungin	0.1	80
Fentanyl	3.9	85
Midazolam	3.9	92
Meropenem	-0.6	2
Vancomycin	-3.1	55
Morphine	0.8	30
Thiopentone	2.3	80

over whether new or old circuits have more drug sequestration, with studies showing significant variability.[106,108,114] It remains unclear how fast saturation occurs for the protein and drug-binding sites in the ECMO circuit. The impact of competitive binding to blood proteins and circuit components from administration of concomitant drugs also remains unknown. When dye was administered to the venous limb of the circuit, it pooled at the loop of the reservoir.[98] Newer types of reservoirs such as the collapsible Better Bladder (Circulatory Technology, Oyster Bay, NY), which is vertically oriented, may decrease this pooling by regulating forward flow through the ECMO pump.

In summary, the circuit loss of a drug through sequestration may represent a balance between the binding to the circuit components and the extent of drug protein binding. In addition, critically ill patients can have reductions in serum proteins that can influence protein binding of drugs in addition to the effects of binding to the circuit. Sequestration of drugs in the circuit may have implications in both choice and dosing of particular drugs during ECMO. The circuit may also release the sequestered molecules once a drug infusion is ceased. This situation is unpredictable and may prolong the pharmacologic effect in an undesirable manner. Interpatient variability inherent to critically ill children and adult patients contributes to altered pharmacokinetics observed on ECMO. Therefore, therapeutic drug monitoring is highly recommended, when available. It is also recommended to refer to routine drug dosing handbooks and recent ECMO literature for information pertaining to drug protein binding and Vd information and factors responsible for ECMO clearance.[103,109,115]

VOLUME OF DISTRIBUTION

Volume of distribution is the theoretical volume of fluid into which the total drug administered will have to be diluted to produce a concentration equal to that observed in plasma. It has been suggested that ECMO represents another pharmacokinetic compartment, similar to extracorporeal dialysis techniques. Extracorporeal membrane oxygenation can lead to a SIRS (systemic inflammatory response syndrome) that increases the Vd, resulting in low serum concentrations and therapeutic failure (Figure 27.8).[101] The inflammatory response can down-regulate CYP enzymes in the liver and increase the Vd within the extracellular fluid.

Extracorporeal membrane oxygenation alters the Vd of medications (Table 27.10).[101] The circuit may lead to a doubling in the patient's extracellular fluid volume. This

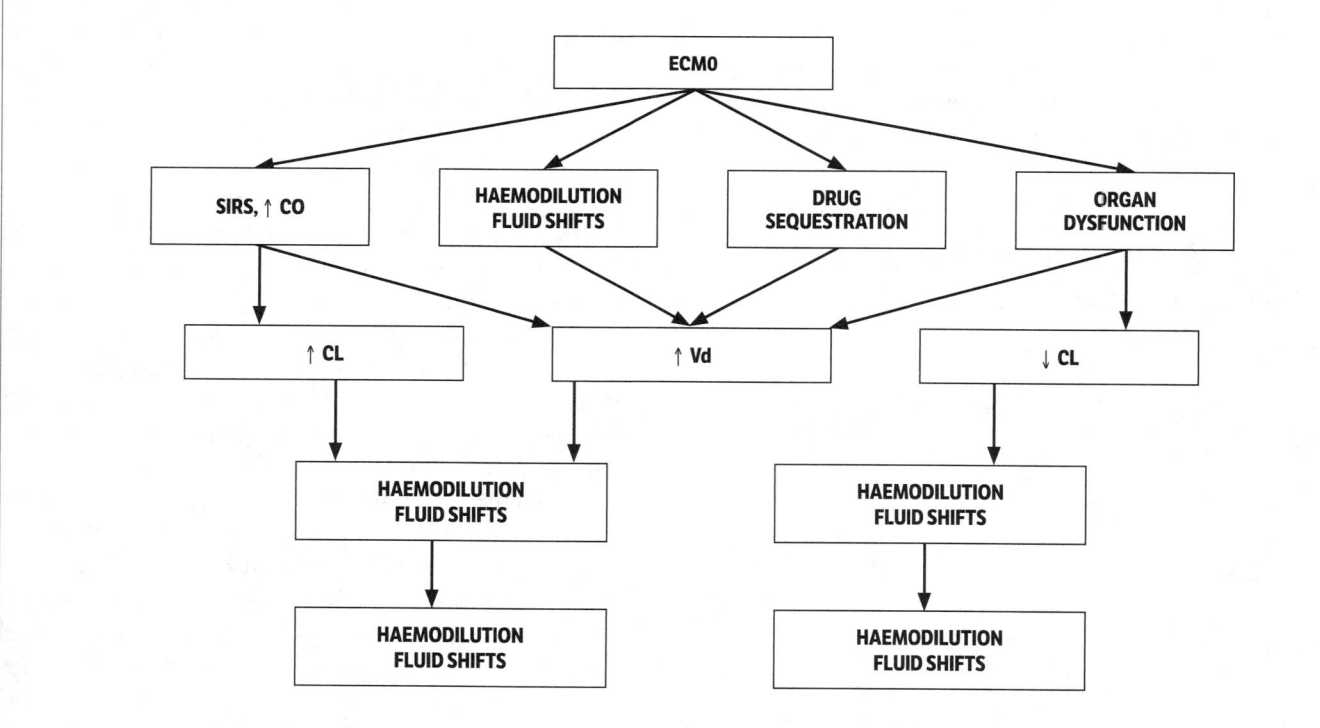

Figure 27.8 Impact of critical illness, inflammation and ECMO on drug pharmacokinetics.

Impact of critical illness, inflammation, and extracorporeal membrane oxygenation on drug pharmacokinetics.
CO = cardiac output; ECMO = extracorporeal membrane oxygenation; SIRS = systemic inflammatory response syndrome.
Reprinted with permission from: Shekar K, Fraser JF, Smith MT, et al. Pharmacokinetic changes in patients receiving extracorporeal membrane oxygenation. J Crit Care 2012;27:741 e9-18.

Table 27.10 Impact of Pharmacokinetic (PK) Changes During ECMO and Clinical Implications

	Changes in PK	Therapeutic implication	Drugs affected
Priming/transfusion			
Hemodilution	↑ Vd ↓ Cmax	↑ Loading dose	Hydrophilic drugs, eg, β-lactams and aminoglycosides
	↑ Free drug concentrations	↑ Loading dose ↑ Frequency	Highly protein-bound drugs, eg, teicoplanin and ceftriaxone
Circuit-related factors			
Drug sequestration	↑ Vd ↓ Cmax	↑ Loading dose	Lipophilic drugs, eg, fluoroquinolones fentanyl, and midazolam
Drug inactivation	↑ CL ↓ Bioavailability	↑ Frequency regarding dose with circuit changes	
Patient factors			
Systemic inflammation/sepsis	↑ Vd ↓ Cmax ↑ CL	↑ Loading dose	Hydrophilic drugs, eg, β-lactams and glycopeptides
Organ failures	↓ CL ↑ Vd	↓ Frequency	Renally or hepatically excreted drugs
Drug factors			
Hydrophilicity	↑ Vd ↓ Cmax ↑↓ CL (dependent on renal function)	↑ Loading dose ↑↓ Frequency	For example, β-lactams aminoglycosides
Lipophilicity	Vd largely unchanged ↑ Circuit sequestration ↓↑ CL (dependent on hepatic function)	↑ Loading dose ↑ Frequency	For example, fluoroquinolones, macrolides, and propofol

Cmax indicates peak concentrations.

Reprinted with permission from: Shekar K, Fraser JF, Smith MT, et al. Pharmacokinetic changes in patients receiving extracorporeal membrane oxygenation. J Crit Care 2012;27:741 e9-18.

effect is much more pronounced with drugs that have a small Vd and for smaller patients. Extracorporeal membrane oxygenation circuit priming volumes in a child varies from 200 to 400 mL, and the circulating blood volume of an infant is 80–85 mL/kg. The dilutional effect of the circuit prime is exacerbated by the ongoing intravenous fluid requirements in the critically ill patient and by requirements for repeat blood and blood product transfusions. The degree to which ECMO itself expands the extracellular fluid compartment is debatable, and an increased drug Vd may be the result of the disease process rather than or in addition to ECMO. The prime and multiple transfusions dilute the plasma proteins and can result in decreased drug binding, increased free concentration of drug, and an apparent increase in Vd. Additional effects on plasma proteins during ECMO include binding of protein by heparin and potential denaturation of proteins passing through the membrane oxygenator. The large surface area of oxygenators can affect the Vd and drug concentrations. Dagan et al. examined circuits and showed that there was a significant decrease in drug concentration after flow through the oxygenator.[114] They found that phenytoin concentrations in the circuit decreased by 43%, whereas vancomycin and morphine decreased by 36%, phenobarbital by 17%, and gentamicin by 10%. In circuits that had been used for 5 days, the drug concentrations decreased much less: morphine by 16%, vancomycin by 11%, and phenobarbital by 6%. This suggests saturation of the binding sites over several days.[114]

Several other important factors are known to increase drug Vd, including hemodilution from priming solutions at ECMO initiation, ongoing blood product transfusions, pH alterations that affect protein binding and therefore distribution, and administration of volume to maintain circuit flows.[107] Although hemodilution can often enhance the pharmacokinetic effect of highly protein bound drugs by increasing the unbound fraction, redistribution of free drug into the tissues may result in a lower serum concentration.[107]

Much of the ECMO data evaluating Vd originate from the neonatal population. This population has a higher proportion of total body water and less adipose tissue. As a result, neonates will have a higher Vd for hydrophilic drugs (β-lactams and aminoglycosides) and a lower Vd for lipophilic drugs (fluoroquinolones and macrolides) relative to adults. There is also decreased protein binding in neonates, resulting in increased unbound drug concentrations and Vd.[116] These physiological alterations limit the use of neonatal pharmacokinetic data to guide drug dosing in critically ill adults requiring ECMO. Table 27.10 summarizes the pharmacokinetic changes during ECMO and clinical implications.[101]

DRUG CLEARANCE

Several indirect mechanisms lead to decreased drug clearance during ECMO. Preceding hypoxia and hypoperfusion may lead to a kidney insult and decrease in renal clearance. Extracorporeal membrane oxygenation can result in altered organ perfusion most prominently by the lack of pulsatility, even though tissue oxygen delivery may be adequate. However, a comparison of the half-life for gentamicin in infants who received either venoarterial ECMO or venovenous ECMO was no different.[117] Alterations in regional liver blood flow may also affect the clearance of drugs, especially those with a high extraction ratio. Decreased pulmonary blood flow during venoarterial ECMO may affect the sequestration and metabolism of many sedative and analgesic drugs by the lungs.[118] Drug removal by the ECMO circuit may reduce the bioavailability of the first dose as well as the overall clearance.[108] Decreased clearance predisposes the patient to drug toxicity, especially for drugs with a narrow therapeutic window.

The clearance of a drug is also directly affected by ECMO. Clearance can be influenced by the degree to which ECMO affects bound or unbound drug concentrations. Drug adsorption to the pump/tubing and oxygenator can also result in clearance alterations. When the ECMO circuit is changed, there can be a rapid alteration in drug concentration because the binding sites are no longer saturated, which can affect clearance. Another consideration is whether the drug is administered in the circuit or directly to the patient. When drugs are administered directly in the circuit, there can be differences in drug concentration depending on whether dosing location is before or after the oxygenator.

RENAL REPLACEMENT THERAPY

Discussion of renal replacement therapy during ECMO is complex because of the variability in techniques, including where the renal replacement circuit is located in relation to the oxygenator. This high degree of variability in techniques emphasizes the need for therapeutic drug monitoring where available, especially because adding another extracorporeal circuit can further affect the Vd, sequestration, and clearance of drugs.

REFERENCES

1. Chertow GM, Burdick E, Honour M, et al. Acute kidney injury, mortality, length of stay, and costs in hospitalized patients. J Am Soc Nephrol 2005;16:3365-70.
2. Kidney Disease: Improving Global Outcomes (KDIGO) Acute Kidney Injury Work Group. KDIGO clinical practice guidelines for acute kidney injury. Kidney Int 2012;2(suppl 1):1-138.
3. Joy MS, Matzke GR, Armstrong DK, et al. A primer on continuous renal replacement therapy for critically ill patients. Ann Pharmacother 1998;32:362-75.
4. Brivet FG, Kleinknecht DJ, Loirat P, et al. Acute renal failure in intensive care units—causes, outcome, and prognostic factors of hospital mortality; a prospective, multicenter study. French Study Group on Acute Renal Failure. Crit Care Med 1996;24:192-8.
5. Liano F, Junco E, Pascual J, et al. The spectrum of acute renal failure in the intensive care unit compared with that seen in other settings. The Madrid Acute Renal Failure Study Group. Kidney Int Suppl 1998;66:S16-24.
6. Liano F, Pascual J. Outcomes in acute renal failure. Semin Nephrol 1998;18:541-50.
7. Metnitz PG, Krenn CG, Steltzer H, et al. Effect of acute renal failure requiring renal replacement therapy on outcome in critically ill patients. Crit Care Med 2002;30:2051-8.
8. Vincent JL. Incidence of acute renal failure in the intensive care unit. Contrib Nephrol 2001:1-6.
9. Wang AY, Bellomo R, Cass A, et al. Health-related quality of life in survivors of acute kidney injury: the Prolonged Outcomes Study of the Randomized Evaluation of Normal versus Augmented Level Replacement Therapy study outcomes. Nephrology (Carlton) 2015;20:492-8.
10. Hofhuis JG, van Stel HF, Schrijvers AJ, et al. The effect of acute kidney injury on long-term health-related quality of life: a prospective follow-up study. Crit Care 2013;17:R17.
11. Bagshaw SM, Berthiaume LR, Delaney A, et al. Continuous versus intermittent renal replacement therapy for critically ill patients with acute kidney injury: a meta-analysis. Crit Care Med 2008;36:610-7.
12. Mehta RL, McDonald B, Gabbai FB, et al. A randomized clinical trial of continuous versus intermittent dialysis for acute renal failure. Kidney Int 2001;60:1154-63.
13. Schneider AG, Bellomo R, Bagshaw SM, et al. Choice of renal replacement therapy modality and dialysis dependence after acute kidney injury: a systematic review and meta-analysis. Intensive Care Med 2013;39:987-97.
14. Uchino S, Bellomo R, Morimatsu H, et al. Continuous renal replacement therapy: a worldwide practice survey. The beginning and ending supportive therapy for the kidney (B.E.S.T. kidney) investigators. Intensive Care Med 2007;33:1563-70.
15. Wald R, Shariff SZ, Adhikari NK, et al. The association between renal replacement therapy modality and long-term outcomes among critically ill adults with acute kidney injury: a retrospective cohort study. Crit Care Med 2014;42:868-77.
16. Davenport A, Will EJ, Davidson AM. Improved cardiovascular stability during continuous modes of renal replacement therapy in critically ill patients with acute hepatic and renal failure. Crit Care Med 1993;21:328-38.
17. John S, Griesbach D, Baumgartel M, et al. Effects of continuous haemofiltration vs intermittent haemodialysis on systemic haemodynamics and splanchnic regional perfusion in septic shock patients: a prospective, randomized clinical trial. Nephrol Dial Transplant 2001;16:320-7.
18. Coca SG, Singanamala S, Parikh CR. Chronic kidney disease after acute kidney injury: a systematic review and meta-analysis. Kidney Int 2012;81:442-8.
19. Ishani A, Xue JL, Himmelfarb J, et al. Acute kidney injury increases risk of ESRD among elderly. J Am Soc Nephrol 2009;20:223-8.

20. Ansari N. Peritoneal dialysis in renal replacement therapy for patients with acute kidney injury. Int J Nephrol 2011;2011:739-94.
21. Bonilla-Felix M. Peritoneal dialysis in the pediatric intensive care unit setting. Perit Dial Int 2009;29(suppl 2):S183-5.
22. Rumpf KW, Rieger J, Ansorg R, et al. Binding of antibiotics by dialysis membranes and its clinical relevance. Proc Eur Dial Transplant Assoc 1977;14:607-9.
23. Sieberth HG, Kierdorf HP. Is cytokine removal by continuous hemofiltration feasible? Kidney Int Suppl 1999:S79-83.
24. Cole L, Bellomo R, Davenport P, et al. Cytokine removal during continuous renal replacement therapy: an ex vivo comparison of convection and diffusion. Int J Artif Organs 2004;27:388-97.
25. Joannes-Boyau O, Honore PM, Perez P, et al. High-volume versus standard-volume haemofiltration for septic shock patients with acute kidney injury (IVOIRE study): a multicentre randomized controlled trial. Intensive Care Med 2013;39:1535-46.
26. Zhang P, Yang Y, Lv R, et al. Effect of the intensity of continuous renal replacement therapy in patients with sepsis and acute kidney injury: a single-center randomized clinical trial. Nephrol Dial Transplant 2012;27:967-73.
27. Briglia A, Paganini EP. Acute renal failure in the intensive care unit. Therapy overview, patient risk stratification, complications of renal replacement, and special circumstances. Clin Chest Med 1999;20:347-66, viii.
28. Clark WR, Ronco C. Continuous renal replacement techniques. Contrib Nephrol 2004;144:264-77.
29. Canada TIfSMP. ISMP Canada Safety Bulletin. In: Canada Safety Bulletin, 2004.
30. Locatelli F. Comparison of hemodialysis, hemodiafiltration, and hemofiltration: systematic review or systematic error? Am J Kidney Dis 2005;46:787-8; author reply 8-9.
31. Vanholder R, Van Laecke S, Glorieux G. The middle-molecule hypothesis 30 years after: lost and rediscovered in the universe of uremic toxicity? J Nephrol 2008;21:146-60.
32. O'Reilly P, Tolwani A. Renal replacement therapy III: IHD, CRRT, SLED. Crit Care Clin 2005;21:367-78.
33. Kraft D, Lode H. Elimination of ampicillin and gentamicin by hemofiltration. Klin Wochenschr 1979;57:195-6.
34. Shiraishi Y, Okajima M, Sai Y, et al. Elimination of teicoplanin by adsorption to the filter membrane during haemodiafiltration: screening experiments for linezolid, teicoplanin and vancomycin followed by in vitro haemodiafiltration models for teicoplanin. Anaesth Intensive Care 2012;40:442-9.
35. Joy MS, Matzke GR, Frye RF, et al. Determinants of vancomycin clearance by continuous venovenous hemofiltration and continuous venovenous hemodialysis. Am J Kidney Dis 1998;31:1019-27.
36. Reyes M, Benet LZ. Effects of uremic toxins on transport and metabolism of different biopharmaceutics drug disposition classification system xenobiotics. J Pharm Sci 2011;100:3831-42.
37. Sun H, Huang Y, Frassetto L, et al. Effects of uremic toxins on hepatic uptake and metabolism of erythromycin. Drug Metab Dispos 2004;32:1239-46.
38. Gonzalez D, Conrado DJ, Theuretzbacher U, et al. The effect of critical illness on drug distribution. Curr Pharm Biotechnol 2011;12:2030-6.
39. Czock D, Husig-Linde C, Langhoff A, et al. Pharmacokinetics of moxifloxacin and levofloxacin in intensive care unit patients who have acute renal failure and undergo extended daily dialysis. Clin J Am Soc Nephrol 2006;1:1263-8.
40. Bogard KN, Peterson NT, Plumb TJ, et al. Antibiotic dosing during sustained low-efficiency dialysis: special considerations in adult critically ill patients. Crit Care Med 2011;39:560-70.
41. Dowling TC, Briglia AE, Fink JC, et al. Characterization of hepatic cytochrome p4503A activity in patients with end-stage renal disease. Clin Pharmacol Ther 2003;73:427-34.
42. Joy MS, Frye RF, Nolin TD, et al. In vivo alterations in drug metabolism and transport pathways in patients with chronic kidney diseases. Pharmacotherapy 2014;34:114-22.
43. Nolin TD, Appiah K, Kendrick SA, et al. Hemodialysis acutely improves hepatic CYP3A4 metabolic activity. J Am Soc Nephrol 2006;17:2363-7.
44. Nolin TD, Naud J, Leblond FA, et al. Emerging evidence of the impact of kidney disease on drug metabolism and transport. Clin Pharmacol Ther 2008;83:898-903.
45. Vincent JL. Relevance of albumin in modern critical care medicine. Best Pract Res Clin Anaesthesiol 2009;23:183-91.
46. Ulldemolins M, Roberts JA, Rello J, et al. The effects of hypoalbuminaemia on optimizing antibacterial dosing in critically ill patients. Clin Pharmacokinet 2011;50:99-110.
47. Vilay AM, Churchwell MD, Mueller BA. Clinical review: drug metabolism and nonrenal clearance in acute kidney injury. Crit Care 2008;12:235.
48. Macias WL, Mueller BA, Scarim SK. Vancomycin pharmacokinetics in acute renal failure: preservation of nonrenal clearance. Clin Pharmacol Ther 1991;50:688-94.
49. Dettli L. Individualization of drug dosage in patients with renal disease. Med Clin North Am 1974;58:977-85.
50. Dettli L, Spring P. The dosage regimen of thiamphenicol in patients with kidney disease. Postgrad Med J 1974;50(suppl 5):32-5.
51. Dettli LC. Drug dosage in patients with renal disease. Clin Pharmacol Ther 1974;16:274-80.
52. Pea F, Viale P, Pavan F, et al. Pharmacokinetic considerations for antimicrobial therapy in patients receiving renal replacement therapy. Clin Pharmacokinet 2007;46:997-1038.
53. Conil JM, Georges B, de Lussy A, et al. Ciprofloxacin use in critically ill patients: pharmacokinetic and pharmacodynamic approaches. Int J Antimicrob Agents 2008;32:505-10.
54. Udy AA, Roberts JA, Lipman J. Implications of augmented renal clearance in critically ill patients. Nat Rev Nephrol 2011;7:539-43.
55. Matzke GR, Aronoff GR, Atkinson AJ Jr, et al. Drug dosing consideration in patients with acute and chronic kidney disease-a clinical update from Kidney Disease: Improving Global Outcomes (KDIGO). Kidney Int 2011;80:1122-37.
56. St Peter WL, Redic-Kill KA, Halstenson CE. Clinical pharmacokinetics of antibiotics in patients with impaired renal function. Clin Pharmacokinet 1992;22:169-210.

57. Verbeeck RK, Musuamba FT. Pharmacokinetics and dosage adjustment in patients with renal dysfunction. Eur J Clin Pharmacol 2009;65:757-73.

58. Heintz BH, Matzke GR, Dager WE. Antimicrobial dosing concepts and recommendations for critically ill adult patients receiving continuous renal replacement therapy or intermittent hemodialysis. Pharmacotherapy 2009;29:562-77.

59. Isla A, Rodriguez-Gascon A, Troconiz IF, et al. Population pharmacokinetics of meropenem in critically ill patients undergoing continuous renal replacement therapy. Clin Pharmacokinet 2008;47:173-80.

60. Lewis SJ, Mueller BA. Antibiotic dosing in critically ill patients receiving CRRT: underdosing is overprevalent. Semin Dial 2014;27:441-5.

61. Lewis SJ, Mueller BA. Antibiotic dosing in patients with acute kidney injury: "enough but not too much." J Intensive Care Med 2014.

62. Choi G, Gomersall CD, Tian Q, et al. Principles of antibacterial dosing in continuous renal replacement therapy. Crit Care Med 2009;37:2268-82.

63. Drusano GL. Antimicrobial pharmacodynamics: critical interactions of "bug and drug." Nat Rev Microbiol 2004;2:289-300.

64. Seyler L, Cotton F, Taccone FS, et al. Recommended beta-lactam regimens are inadequate in septic patients treated with continuous renal replacement therapy. Crit Care 2011;15:R137.

65. Mueller BA, Smoyer WE. Challenges in developing evidence-based drug dosing guidelines for adults and children receiving renal replacement therapy. Clin Pharmacol Ther 2009;86:479-82.

66. Jiang SP, Zhu ZY, Ma KF, et al. Impact of pharmacist antimicrobial dosing adjustments in septic patients on continuous renal replacement therapy in an intensive care unit. Scand J Infect Dis 2013;45:891-9.

67. Harris LE, Reaves AB, Krauss AG, et al. Evaluation of antibiotic prescribing patterns in patients receiving sustained low-efficiency dialysis: opportunities for pharmacists. Int J Pharm Pract 2013;21:55-61.

68. Hastings D, Patel B, Torloni AS, et al. Plasmapheresis therapy for rare but potentially fatal reaction to rituximab. J Clin Apher 2009;24:28-31.

69. Tiftik N, Kiykim A, Altintas E, et al. Therapeutic plasma exchange for multidrug intoxication: a case report. J Clin Apher 2003;18:132-3.

70. Yildirim C, Bayraktaroglu Z, Gunay N, et al. The use of therapeutic plasmapheresis in the treatment of poisoned and snake bite victims: an academic emergency department's experiences. J Clin Apher 2006;21:219-23.

71. Ibrahim RB, Liu C, Cronin SM, et al. Drug removal by plasmapheresis: an evidence-based review. Pharmacotherapy 2007;27:1529-49.

72. Ibrahim RB, Balogun RA. Medications in patients treated with therapeutic plasma exchange: prescription dosage, timing, and drug overdose. Semin Dial 2012;25:176-89.

73. Kale-Pradhan PB, Woo MH. A review of the effects of plasmapheresis on drug clearance. Pharmacotherapy 1997;17:684-95.

74. Ibrahim RB, Liu CY, Cronin SM, et al. Influence of plasma exchange on the disposition of the fourth generation cephalosporin cefepime. J Oncol Pharm Pract 2009;15:217-22.

75. McClellan SD, Whitaker CH, Friedberg RC. Removal of vancomycin during plasmapheresis. Ann Pharmacother 1997;31:1132-6.

76. Sagraves R, Bradberry JC. The effects of exchange transfusion on the pharmacokinetics of phenobarbital. Drug Intell Clin Pharm 1983;17:901-3.

77. Bozkurt F, Schollmeyer P, Keller E. Kinetics of ceftazidime during plasmapheresis. Eur J Clin Pharmacol 1987;33:197-201.

78. Fauvelle F, Lortholary O, Tod M, et al. Pharmacokinetics of ceftriaxone during plasma exchange in polyarteritis nodosa patients. Antimicrob Agents Chemother 1994;38:1519-22.

79. Bertino JS Jr, Kliegman RM, Myers CM, et al. Alterations in gentamicin pharmacokinetics during neonatal exchange transfusion. Dev Pharmacol Ther 1982;4:205-15.

80. Binimelis J, Bassas L, Marruecos L, et al. Massive thyroxine intoxication: evaluation of plasma extraction. Intensive Care Med 1987;13:33-8.

81. Kliegman RM, Bertino JS Jr, Fanaroff AA, et al. Pharmacokinetics of gentamicin during exchange transfusions in neonates. J Pediatr 1980;96:927-30.

82. Fauvelle F, Petitjean O, Tod M, et al. Clinical pharmacokinetics during plasma exchange. Therapie 2000;55:269-75.

83. Ibrahim RB, Balogun RA. Medications and therapeutic apheresis procedures: are we doing our best? J Clin Apher 2013;28:73-7.

84. Samtleben W, Mistry-Burchardi N, Hartmann B, et al. Therapeutic plasma exchange in the intensive care setting. Ther Apher 2001;5:351-7.

85. Spriet I, Bruggemann RJ, Annaert P, et al. Pharmacokinetic profile of voriconazole in a critically ill patient on therapeutic plasma exchange. Ther Drug Monit 2013;35:141-3.

86. Winters JL. Plasma exchange: concepts, mechanisms, and an overview of the American Society for Apheresis guidelines. Hematology Am Soc Hematol Educ Program 2012;2012:7-12.

87. McDonald V, Manns K, Mackie IJ, et al. Rituximab pharmacokinetics during the management of acute idiopathic thrombotic thrombocytopenic purpura. J Thromb Haemost 2010;8:1201-8.

88. Sabloff M, Wells PS. The effect of plasmapheresis on the serum activity level of dalteparin: a case report. Blood Coagul Fibrinolysis 2000;11:395-400.

89. Erstad BL. Designing drug regimens for special intensive care unit populations. World J Crit Care Med 2015;4:139-51.

90. Gattinoni L, Carlesso E, Langer T. Clinical review: extracorporeal membrane oxygenation. Crit Care 2011;15:243.

91. Noah MA, Peek GJ, Finney SJ, et al. Referral to an extracorporeal membrane oxygenation center and mortality among patients with severe 2009 influenza A(H1N1). JAMA 2011;306:1659-68.

92. Peek GJ, Mugford M, Tiruvoipati R, et al. Efficacy and economic assessment of conventional ventilatory support versus extracorporeal membrane oxygenation for severe adult respiratory failure (CESAR): a multicentre randomised controlled trial. Lancet 2009;374:1351-63.

93. Kohler K, Valchanov K, Nias G, et al. ECMO cannula review. Perfusion 2013;28:114-24.

94. Lequier L, Horton SB, McMullan DM, et al. Extracorporeal membrane oxygenation circuitry. Pediatr Crit Care Med 2013;14:S7-12.
95. White RL, Garnett WR, Poynor WJ, et al. Salicylate removal during plasma exchange in normal volunteers. Clin Pharm 1984;3:396-402.
96. Turner DA, Cheifetz IM. Extracorporeal membrane oxygenation for adult respiratory failure. Respir Care 2013;58:1038-52.
97. Allen S, Holena D, McCunn M, et al. A review of the fundamental principles and evidence base in the use of extracorporeal membrane oxygenation (ECMO) in critically ill adult patients. J Intensive Care Med 2011;26:13-26.
98. Hoie EB, Hall MC, Schaaf LJ. Effects of injection site and flow rate on the distribution of injected solutions in an extracorporeal membrane oxygenation circuit. Am J Hosp Pharm 1993;50:1902-6.
99. Roberts JA. Using PK/PD to optimize antibiotic dosing for critically ill patients. Curr Pharm Biotechnol 2011;12:2070-9.
100. Roberts JA, Roberts MS, Semark A, et al. Antibiotic dosing in the "at risk" critically ill patient: linking pathophysiology with pharmacokinetics/pharmacodynamics in sepsis and trauma patients. BMC Anesthesiol 2011;11:3.
101. Shekar K, Fraser JF, Smith MT, et al. Pharmacokinetic changes in patients receiving extracorporeal membrane oxygenation. J Crit Care 2012;27:741 e9-18.
102. Shekar K, Roberts JA, Smith MT, et al. The ECMO PK Project: an incremental research approach to advance understanding of the pharmacokinetic alterations and improve patient outcomes during extracorporeal membrane oxygenation. BMC Anesthesiol 2013;13:7.
103. Shekar K, Roberts JA, Welch S, et al. ASAP ECMO: Antibiotic, Sedative and Analgesic Pharmacokinetics during Extracorporeal Membrane Oxygenation: a multi-centre study to optimise drug therapy during ECMO. BMC Anesthesiol 2012;12:29.
104. Buck ML. Pharmacokinetic changes during extracorporeal membrane oxygenation: implications for drug therapy of neonates. Clin Pharmacokinet 2003;42:403-17.
105. Mulla H, Lawson G, von Anrep C, et al. In vitro evaluation of sedative drug losses during extracorporeal membrane oxygenation. Perfusion 2000;15:21-6.
106. Wildschut ED, Ahsman MJ, Allegaert K, et al. Determinants of drug absorption in different ECMO circuits. Intensive Care Med 2010;36:2109-16.
107. Shekar K, Roberts JA, McDonald CI, et al. Sequestration of drugs in the circuit may lead to therapeutic failure during extracorporeal membrane oxygenation. Crit Care 2012;16:R194.
108. Bhatt-Meht V, Annich G. Sedative clearance during extracorporeal membrane oxygenation. Perfusion 2005;20:309-15.
109. Shekar K, Roberts JA, McDonald CI, et al. Protein-bound drugs are prone to sequestration in the extracorporeal membrane oxygenation circuit: results from an ex vivo study. Crit Care 2015;19:164.
110. Berthoin K, Le Duff CS, Marchand-Brynaert J, et al. Stability of meropenem and doripenem solutions for administration by continuous infusion. J Antimicrob Chemother 2010;65:1073-5.
111. Mehta NM, Halwick DR, Dodson BL, et al. Potential drug sequestration during extracorporeal membrane oxygenation: results from an ex vivo experiment. Intensive Care Med 2007;33:1018-24.
112. Preston TJ, Hodge AB, Riley JB, et al. In vitro drug adsorption and plasma free hemoglobin levels associated with hollow fiber oxygenators in the extracorporeal life support (ECLS) circuit. J Extra Corpor Technol 2007;39:234-7.
113. Preston TJ, Ratliff TM, Gomez D, et al. Modified surface coatings and their effect on drug adsorption within the extracorporeal life support circuit. J Extra Corpor Technol 2010;42:199-202.
114. Dagan O, Klein J, Gruenwald C, et al. Preliminary studies of the effects of extracorporeal membrane oxygenator on the disposition of common pediatric drugs. Ther Drug Monit 1993;15:263-6.
115. Shekar K, Roberts JA, McDonald CI, et al. Protein-bound drugs are prone to sequestration in the extracorporeal membrane oxygenation circuit: results from an ex vivo study. Crit Care 2015;19:164.
116. Alcorn J, McNamara PJ. Pharmacokinetics in the newborn. Adv Drug Deliv Rev 2003;55:667-86.
117. Bhatt-Mehta V, Johnson CE, Schumacher RE. Gentamicin pharmacokinetics in term neonates receiving extracorporeal membrane oxygenation. Pharmacotherapy 1992;12:28-32.
118. Boer F. Drug handling by the lungs. Br J Anaesth 2003;91:50-60.
119. Tolwani A. Continuous renal-replacement therapy for acute kidney injury. N Engl J Med 2012;367:2505-14.
120. Robert R, Rochard E, Malin F, et al. Amikacin pharmacokinetics during continuous veno-venous hemofiltration. Crit Care Med 1991;19:588-9.
121. Armendariz E, Chelluri L, Ptachcinski R. Pharmacokinetics of amikacin during continuous veno-venous hemofiltration. Crit Care Med 1990;18:675-6.
122. Lawless S, Restaino I, Azin S, et al. Effect of continuous arteriovenous haemofiltration on pharmacokinetics of amrinone. Clin Pharmacokinet 1993;25:80-2.
123. Shearer ES, O'Sullivan EP, Hunter JM. Clearance of atracurium and laudanosine in the urine and by continuous venovenous haemofiltration. Br J Anaesth 1991;67:569-73.
124. Isla A, Arzuaga A, Maynar J, et al. Determination of ceftazidime and cefepime in plasma and dialysate-ultrafiltrate from patients undergoing continuous veno-venous hemodiafiltration by HPLC. J Pharm Biomed Anal 2005;39:996-1005.
125. Isla A, Gascon AR, Maynar J, et al. Cefepime and continuous renal replacement therapy (CRRT): in vitro permeability of two CRRT membranes and pharmacokinetics in four critically ill patients. Clin Ther 2005;27:599-608.
126. Malone RS, Fish DN, Abraham E, et al. Pharmacokinetics of cefepime during continuous renal replacement therapy in critically ill patients. Antimicrob Agents Chemother 2001;45:3148-55.
127. Evers J, Borner K, Koeppe P. Cefotiam during continuous haemofiltration. Eur J Clin Pharmacol 1993;44:509-10.
128. Davies SP, Lacey LF, Kox WJ, et al. Pharmacokinetics of cefuroxime and ceftazidime in patients with acute renal failure treated by continuous arteriovenous haemodialysis. Nephrol Dial Transplant 1991;6:971-6.

129. Traunmuller F, Schenk P, Mittermeyer C, et al. Clearance of ceftazidime during continuous venovenous haemofiltration in critically ill patients. J Antimicrob Chemother 2002;49:129-34.

130. Matzke GR, Frye RF, Joy MS, et al. Determinants of ceftazidime clearance by continuous venovenous hemofiltration and continuous venovenous hemodialysis. Antimicrob Agents Chemother 2000;44:1639-44.

131. Mariat C, Venet C, Jehl F, et al. Continuous infusion of ceftazidime in critically ill patients undergoing continuous venovenous haemodiafiltration: pharmacokinetic evaluation and dose recommendation. Crit Care 2006;10:R26.

132. Isla A, Gascon AR, Maynar J, et al. In vitro AN69 and polysulphone membrane permeability to ceftazidime and in vivo pharmacokinetics during continuous renal replacement therapies. Chemotherapy 2007;53:194-201.

133. Matzke GR, Frye RF, Joy MS, et al. Determinants of ceftriaxone clearance by continuous venovenous hemofiltration and hemodialysis. Pharmacotherapy 2000;20:635-43.

134. Weiss LG, Cars O, Danielson BG, et al. Pharmacokinetics of intravenous cefuroxime during intermittent and continuous arteriovenous hemofiltration. Clin Nephrol 1988;30:282-6.

135. Vossen MG, Gattringer KB, Jager W, et al. Single-dose pharmacokinetics of cidofovir in continuous venovenous hemofiltration. Antimicrob Agents Chemother 2014;58:1952-5.

136. Keller E, Fecht H, Bohler J, et al. Single-dose kinetics of imipenem/cilastatin during continuous arteriovenous haemofiltration in intensive care patients. Nephrol Dial Transplant 1989;4:640-5.

137. Vos MC, Vincent HH, Yzerman EP. Clearance of imipenem/cilastatin in acute renal failure patients treated by continuous hemodiafiltration (CAVHD). Intensive Care Med 1992;18:282-5.

138. Davies SP, Azadian BS, Kox WJ, et al. Pharmacokinetics of ciprofloxacin and vancomycin in patients with acute renal failure treated by continuous haemodialysis. Nephrol Dial Transplant 1992;7:848-54.

139. Wallis SC, Mullany DV, Lipman J, et al. Pharmacokinetics of ciprofloxacin in ICU patients on continuous veno-venous haemofiltration. Intensive Care Med 2001;27:665-72.

140. Lindsay CA, Bawdon R, Quigley R. Clearance of ticarcillin-clavulanic acid by continuous venovenous hemofiltration in three critically ill children, two with and one without concomitant extracorporeal membrane oxygenation. Pharmacotherapy 1996;16:458-62.

141. Markou N, Fousteri M, Markantonis SL, et al. Colistin pharmacokinetics in intensive care unit patients on continuous venovenous haemofiltration: an observational study. J Antimicrob Chemother 2012;67:2459-62.

142. Vilay AM, Grio M, Depestel DD, et al. Daptomycin pharmacokinetics in critically ill patients receiving continuous venovenous hemodialysis. Crit Care Med 2011;39:19-25.

143. Cirillo I, Vaccaro N, Balis D, et al. Influence of continuous venovenous hemofiltration and continuous venovenous hemodiafiltration on the disposition of doripenem. Antimicrob Agents Chemother 2011;55:1187-93.

144. Nicolau DP, Crowe H, Nightingale CH, et al. Effect of continuous arteriovenous hemodiafiltration on the pharmacokinetics of fluconazole. Pharmacotherapy 1994;14:502-5.

145. Yagasaki K, Gando S, Matsuda N, et al. Pharmacokinetics and the most suitable dosing regimen of fluconazole in critically ill patients receiving continuous hemodiafiltration. Intensive Care Med 2003;29:1844-8.

146. Muhl E, Martens T, Iven H, et al. Influence of continuous veno-venous haemodiafiltration and continuous veno-venous haemofiltration on the pharmacokinetics of fluconazole. Eur J Clin Pharmacol 2000;56:671-8.

147. Gattringer R, Meyer B, Heinz G, et al. Single-dose pharmacokinetics of fosfomycin during continuous venovenous haemofiltration. J Antimicrob Chemother 2006;58:367-71.

148. Boulieu R, Bastien O, Bleyzac N. Pharmacokinetics of ganciclovir in heart transplant patients undergoing continuous venovenous hemodialysis. Ther Drug Monit 1993;15:105-7.

149. Zarowitz BJ, Anandan JV, Dumler F, et al. Continuous arteriovenous hemofiltration of aminoglycoside antibiotics in critically ill patients. J Clin Pharmacol 1986;26:686-9.

150. Lehman ME, Kolb KW. Gentamicin elimination in a patient undergoing continuous ultrafiltration. Clin Pharm 1985;4:327-30.

151. Ernest D, Cutler DJ. Gentamicin clearance during continuous arteriovenous hemodiafiltration. Crit Care Med 1992;20:586-9.

152. Mueller BA, Scarim SK, Macias WL. Comparison of imipenem pharmacokinetics in patients with acute or chronic renal failure treated with continuous hemofiltration. Am J Kidney Dis 1993;21:172-9.

153. Fish DN, Teitelbaum I, Abraham E. Pharmacokinetics and pharmacodynamics of imipenem during continuous renal replacement therapy in critically ill patients. Antimicrob Agents Chemother 2005;49:2421-8.

154. Kraft MD, Pasko DA, DePestel DD, et al. Linezolid clearance during continuous venovenous hemofiltration: a case report. Pharmacotherapy 2003;23:1071-5.

155. Meyer B, Kornek GV, Nikfardjam M, et al. Multiple-dose pharmacokinetics of linezolid during continuous venovenous haemofiltration. J Antimicrob Chemother 2005;56:172-9.

156. Fiaccadori E, Maggiore U, Rotelli C, et al. Removal of linezolid by conventional intermittent hemodialysis, sustained low-efficiency dialysis, or continuous venovenous hemofiltration in patients with acute renal failure. Crit Care Med 2004;32:2437-42.

157. Mauro LS, Peloquin CA, Schmude K, et al. Clearance of linezolid via continuous venovenous hemodiafiltration. Am J Kidney Dis 2006;47:e83-6.

158. Leblanc M, Raymond M, Bonnardeaux A, et al. Lithium poisoning treated by high-performance continuous arteriovenous and venovenous hemodiafiltration. Am J Kidney Dis 1996;27:365-72.

159. van Bommel EF, Kalmeijer MD, Ponssen HH. Treatment of life-threatening lithium toxicity with high-volume continuous venovenous hemofiltration. Am J Nephrol 2000;20:408-11.

160. Hansen E, Bucher M, Jakob W, et al. Pharmacokinetics of levofloxacin during continuous veno-venous hemofiltration. Intensive Care Med 2001;27:371-5.

161. Guenter SG, Iven H, Boos C, et al. Pharmacokinetics of levofloxacin during continuous venovenous hemofiltration and

162. Isla A, Maynar J, Sanchez-Izquierdo JA, et al. Meropenem and continuous renal replacement therapy: in vitro permeability of 2 continuous renal replacement therapy membranes and influence of patient renal function on the pharmacokinetics in critically ill patients. J Clin Pharmacol 2005;45:1294-304.

163. Ververs TF, van Dijk A, Vinks SA, et al. Pharmacokinetics and dosing regimen of meropenem in critically ill patients receiving continuous venovenous hemofiltration. Crit Care Med 2000;28:3412-6.

164. Valtonen M, Tiula E, Backman JT, et al. Elimination of meropenem during continuous veno-venous haemofiltration and haemodiafiltration in patients with acute renal failure. J Antimicrob Chemother 2000;45:701-4.

165. Langgartner J, Vasold A, Gluck T, et al. Pharmacokinetics of meropenem during intermittent and continuous intravenous application in patients treated by continuous renal replacement therapy. Intensive Care Med 2008;34:1091-6.

166. Robatel C, Decosterd LA, Biollaz J, et al. Pharmacokinetics and dosage adaptation of meropenem during continuous venovenous hemodiafiltration in critically ill patients. J Clin Pharmacol 2003;43:1329-40.

167. Krueger WA, Neeser G, Schuster H, et al. Correlation of meropenem plasma levels with pharmacodynamic requirements in critically ill patients receiving continuous veno-venous hemofiltration. Chemotherapy 2003;49:280-6.

168. Hirata K, Aoyama T, Matsumoto Y, et al. Pharmacokinetics of antifungal agent micafungin in critically ill patients receiving continuous hemodialysis filtration. Yakugaku Zasshi 2007;127:897-901.

169. Bolon M, Bastien O, Flamens C, et al. Midazolam disposition in patients undergoing continuous venovenous hemodialysis. J Clin Pharmacol 2001;41:959-62.

170. Fuhrmann V, Schenk P, Jaeger W, et al. Pharmacokinetics of moxifloxacin in patients undergoing continuous venovenous haemodiafiltration. J Antimicrob Chemother 2004;54:780-4.

171. Cussonneau X, Bolon-Larger M, Prunet-Spano C, et al. Evaluation of MPA and MPAG removal by continuous venovenous hemodiafiltration and continuous hemofiltration. Ther Drug Monit 2008;30:100-2.

172. Fuhrmann V, Schenk P, Mittermayer C, et al. Single-dose pharmacokinetics of ofloxacin during continuous venovenous hemofiltration in critical care patients. Am J Kidney Dis 2003;42:310-4.

173. Lau AH, Kronfol NO. Effect of continuous hemofiltration on phenytoin elimination. Ther Drug Monit 1994;16:53-7.

174. Bauer SR, Salem C, Connor MJ Jr, et al. Pharmacokinetics and pharmacodynamics of piperacillin-tazobactam in 42 patients treated with concomitant CRRT. Clin J Am Soc Nephrol 2012;7:452-7.

175. Valtonen M, Tiula E, Takkunen O, et al. Elimination of the piperacillin/tazobactam combination during continuous venovenous haemofiltration and haemodiafiltration in patients with acute renal failure. J Antimicrob Chemother 2001;48:881-5.

176. Mueller SC, Majcher-Peszynska J, Hickstein H, et al. Pharmacokinetics of piperacillin-tazobactam in anuric intensive care patients during continuous venovenous hemodialysis. Antimicrob Agents Chemother 2002;46:1557-60.

177. Awissi DK, Beauchamp A, Hebert E, et al. Pharmacokinetics of an extended 4-hour infusion of piperacillin-tazobactam in critically ill patients undergoing continuous renal replacement therapy. Pharmacotherapy 2015;35:600-7.

178. Davies JG, Greenwood EF, Kingswood JC, et al. Quinine clearance in continuous venovenous hemofiltration. Ann Pharmacother 1996;30:487-90.

179. Armstrong DK, Hidalgo HA, Eldadah M. Vancomycin and tobramycin clearance in an infant during continuous hemofiltration. Ann Pharmacother 1993;27:224-7.

180. Thomson AH, Grant AC, Rodger RS, et al. Gentamicin and vancomycin removal by continuous venovenous hemofiltration. DICP 1991;25:127-9.

181. Matzke GR, O'Connell MB, Collins AJ, et al. Disposition of vancomycin during hemofiltration. Clin Pharmacol Ther 1986;40:425-30.

182. Santre C, Leroy O, Simon M, et al. Pharmacokinetics of vancomycin during continuous hemodiafiltration. Intensive Care Med 1993;19:347-50.

183. Reetze-Bonorden P, Bohler J, Kohler C, et al. Elimination of vancomycin in patients on continuous arteriovenous hemodialysis. Contrib Nephrol 1991;93:135-9.

184. DelDot ME, Lipman J, Tett SE. Vancomycin pharmacokinetics in critically ill patients receiving continuous venovenous haemodiafiltration. Br J Clin Pharmacol 2004;58:259-68.

185. Robatel C, Rusca M, Padoin C, et al. Disposition of voriconazole during continuous veno-venous haemodiafiltration (CVVHDF) in a single patient. J Antimicrob Chemother 2004;54:269-70.

186. Quintard H, Papy E, Massias L, et al. The pharmacokinetic profile of voriconazole during continuous high-volume venovenous hemofiltration in a critically ill patient. Ther Drug Monit 2008;30:117-9.

187. Fuhrmann V, Schenk P, Jaeger W, et al. Pharmacokinetics of voriconazole during continuous venovenous haemodiafiltration. J Antimicrob Chemother 2007;60:1085-90.

Section 6

Liver/Gastrointestinal

Chapter 28: Management and Drug Dosing in Acute Liver Failure

Andrew C. Fritschle Hilliard, Pharm.D., BCPS, BCCCP; and David R. Foster, Pharm.D., FCCP

LEARNING OBJECTIVES

1. Define acute liver failure (ALF) and describe the epidemiology of ALF.
2. Describe the pathophysiology of ALF.
3. Describe and contrast etiologies of ALF including acetaminophen, idiosyncratic drug-induced ALF, and viral infections.
4. Explain different prognostic indicators used in ALF.
5. Describe clinical presentation of patients presenting with ALF.
6. Define the mechanism of action of acetylcysteine in the management of acetaminophen toxicity.
7. Summarize the four grades of encephalopathy.
8. Compare agents used in the treatment of hepatic encephalopathy.
9. Identify the most common infectious pathogen classes in patients with ALF.
10. Describe nonpharmacologic interventions in the management of ALF.
11. Describe general principles of hepatic drug clearance and potential mechanisms of altered drug disposition in ALF.
12. Apply principles of altered drug disposition in ALF in selecting and modifying pharmacotherapy in a patient with ALF.

ABBREVIATIONS IN THIS CHAPTER

AASLD	American Association for the Study of Liver Diseases	E_H	Hepatic extraction ratio
ALF	Acute liver failure	ICP	Intracranial pressure
CL_{int}	Intrinsic hepatic drug clearance	KCH	King's College Hospital (criteria)
CPP	Cerebral perfusion pressure	MELD	Model for End-Stage Liver Disease
CTP	Child-Pugh (Child-Turcotte-Pugh) (score)	NAPQI	N-acetyl-p-benzoquinone imine
		OLT	Orthotopic liver transplantation
DILI	Drug-induced liver injury	Q_H	Hepatic blood flow

INTRODUCTION

Acute liver failure (ALF) is a rare form of severe liver disease, characterized by a rapid deterioration of liver function in individuals without known preexisting liver disease.[1,2] ALF is associated with substantial morbidity and mortality, often resulting in the need for life-sustaining therapies and potential liver transplantion for definitive treatment. Further, ALF can impact the pharmacokinetics of numerous drugs. In this chapter, the pathophysiology of ALF is reviewed, followed by an overview of ALF management, and general recommendations for drug dosing in ALF.

DEFINITIONS

Acute liver failure represents a syndrome, rather than a specific disease, and can have several causes that vary in outcome.[3] In the past, ALF has also been called fulminant hepatic failure or fulminant hepatitis. A widely used definition for ALF is acute onset (illness less than 26 weeks in duration) of coagulation abnormalities (commonly, an international normalized ratio [INR] of 1.5 or greater) and any degree of hepatic encephalopathy (which can be defined as any change in mental status) in a patient without preexisting hepatic disease.[1] Other definitions have characterized ALF as development of hepatic encephalopathy within 8 weeks of the first symptoms of liver disease (of note, the key features of the definition are the same: hepatic encephalopathy and symptoms of hepatic failure [jaundice, coagulopathy] in the absence of chronic hepatic disease).[4,5] Acute liver failure can further be subdivided into categories on the basis of the length of illness (Table 28.1); this subclassification can be useful in identifying the etiology of ALF.[4] More recently, the term *acute liver injury* has been used to describe patients with severe liver injury (INR of 2 or greater and AST [aspartate transaminase] greater than 10 times the upper limit of normal) with no evidence of encephalopathy.[6] It is important to differentiate ALF from "acute on chronic" liver failure because the treatment and prognosis of each disease can differ substantially. Acute on chronic liver failure is generally regarded as an acute deterioration of preexisting, chronic liver disease that is usually related to an identifiable precipitating event that may be unrelated to the original cause of liver disease.[7] Acute on chronic liver failure will not be discussed at length in this chapter; however, the care of patients with acute on chronic liver failure resembles that of patients with ALF.

Table 28.1 Classifications of Acute Liver Failure[4]

Term	Symptom Duration[a]
Hyperacute	< 7 days
Acute	7–21 days
Subacute	> 21 days and < 26 weeks

[a]Symptom duration from onset of jaundice to hepatic encephalopathy.

EPIDEMIOLOGY

Acute liver failure is relatively uncommon in developed countries, with about 2,000–3,000 cases in the United States per year, and is most commonly seen in young adults in their third decade.[1,4,8] The ALF Study Group collected data related to ALF epidemiology for almost a decade; during this time, 67% of ALF cases were in women, and the mean age was 38 years (range 17–79 years).[3] Of note, the etiology of ALF has a geographic distribution: in North America and Western Europe, the primary causes are acetaminophen toxicity and idiosyncratic drug hepatotoxicity, whereas in Asia and developing nations, the primary causes are infectious (particularly hepatitis B virus and hepatitis E virus). Acute liver failure is often associated with a poor outcome. The mortality rate associated with ALF can exceed 40%–50%, depending on the etiology and type of care provided, and overall 1-year survival including patients receiving a transplant is about 65%.[1,9,10] The primary causes of death in ALF are cerebral edema (as a result of increased intracranial pressure [ICP]), sepsis, and shock/multiorgan failure.[9] Ultimately, orthotopic liver transplantation (OLT) is the only definitive therapy proved to be of benefit in patients with ALF who are unable to regenerate sufficient hepatocyte mass.[1,9]

PATHOPHYSIOLOGY

Specific mechanisms of disease vary for different ALF causes. However, common to most etiologies is the presence of massive hepatocyte loss resulting in rapid loss of hepatic metabolic and immune function.[2,8] The liver has the capacity to regenerate lost mass; however, ALF occurs when loss of hepatic cells exceeds the liver's ability to regenerate.[11] Precipitating factors for hepatocyte loss vary by etiology (see text that follows) and include both direct injury and immunologic injury.[12] With respect to immunologic injury, innate immune-mediated injury is triggered early, which may be followed by adaptive immune responses.[12]

The pattern of hepatocyte death may follow a pattern of necrosis, apoptosis, or both.[11] Necrosis involves depletion of adenosine triphosphate (ATP), leading to cell lysis and secondary inflammation, whereas apoptosis is an ATP-dependent programmed cell death.[11] Although once thought to be separate entities in ALF, necrosis and apoptosis may share initiating factors and signaling pathways and may thus occur as alternating patterns of hepatocyte destruction.[11] Mitochondrial permeability transition (a process leading to mitochondrial swelling) may be a common event causing both patterns of hepatocyte destruction, where the pattern of death depends on whether ATP is depleted (necrosis) or preserved (apoptosis).[11] Apoptosis may be the predominant mode of hepatocyte destruction in ALF caused by viral and toxic etiologies.[12] Necrosis is often related to metabolic injury (leading to ATP depletion) and can be caused by ischemia/reperfusion and acute drug-induced hepatotoxicity.[13]

The acute and massive loss of hepatocytes in ALF leads to the release of ammonia, alanine, lactate, and proinflammatory cytokines from the splanchnic circulation, including tumor necrosis factor alpha, interleukin (IL)-1 beta, and IL-6.[10,12] This inflammatory response is likely key to the systemic inflammation associated with ALF. Furthermore, the systemic inflammation can contribute to cerebral edema by decreasing cerebrovascular tone.[10,12] Release of intracellular materials from hepatocytes may lead to the polymerization of proteins that impairs hepatic microcirculation.[10] Increased gut permeability may lead to increased absorption of luminal endotoxin, which, in conjunction with reduced hepatic endotoxin clearance, can further propagate the condition of systemic inflammation.[10]

Acute liver failure leads to a syndrome that may include many physiologic derangements, including hepatic encephalopathy, cerebral edema, coagulopathy, oliguria/acute renal failure, portal hypertension, acidosis, systemic vasodilation with hypotension, hypoglycemia, respiratory failure, and impaired platelet and white blood cell function.[5,10] More than half of patients with ALF meet the criteria for systemic inflammatory syndrome.[5] In short, the profound hepatic dysfunction associated with ALF often precipitates the development of multiple organ dysfunction syndrome.[10] As indicated previously, the primary causes of death in ALF are cerebral edema, sepsis, and shock/multiorgan failure.[3,14] Other causes of death include cardiac arrhythmia/arrest, respiratory failure, and infection (bacterial and fungal).[3,14] Of note, despite the high prevalence of coagulopathy in ALF, mortality secondary to hemorrhage is rare in ALF.[3]

ETIOLOGY

The causes of ALF include several toxic, infectious, metabolic, and vascular insults to the liver.[10] As indicated previously, the frequency of the various etiologies of ALF follows a geographic distribution. The most common etiology of ALF in North America and Western Europe is acetaminophen toxicity. In the ALF Study Group registry, acetaminophen accounted for almost 40% of all cases of ALF.[14] Idiosyncratic drug reactions (nonacetaminophen, 13% of cases) and viral hepatitis (hepatitis A virus infections and hepatitis B virus infections, collectively 11% of cases), were the next most common causes.[14] In contrast, viral infections (hepatitis A virus, hepatitis B virus, and hepatitis E virus) are the most predominant causes of ALF in the developing world.[2] In up to 15% of ALF cases, there is no determinate cause.[3] Determining the etiology of ALF is important because this assists in determining the appropriate therapy, helps rule out contraindications to transplantation, and can help predict prognosis.[15]

Acetaminophen

As indicated earlier, acetaminophen is the most common cause of ALF in developed countries, accounting for greater than 25,000 hospitalizations and 400–500 deaths per year in the United States.[3,16] It is likely that some cases of ALF with no recognizable cause may also be attributed to acetaminophen toxicity because acetaminophen adducts (produced by the binding of an active acetaminophen metabolite to cysteine residues) have been detected in some of these cases.[17,18] Acetaminophen-related ALF is dose related. At therapeutic doses, greater than 90% of an acetaminophen dose is metabolized in the liver by a combination of glucuronidation and sulfonation (with the resulting metabolites excreted in the urine), about 2% of a dose is excreted unchanged in the urine, and 5%–10% of the dose is metabolized by cytochrome P450 (CYP) 2E1.[16] The metabolism of acetaminophen by CYP2E1 results in the formation of N-acetyl-p-benzoquinone imine (NAPQI), an extremely reactive metabolite.[19] At normal acetaminophen doses, the small amount of NAPQI that is formed is rapidly conjugated by hepatic glutathione and excreted in the urine. At supratherapeutic doses, sulfation and glucuronidation pathways become saturated, and more acetaminophen is metabolized to NAPQI by CYP2E1, eventually resulting in the depletion of hepatic glutathione.[16,19] When hepatic glutathione stores are depleted by about 70%–80%, NAPQI begins to form protein adducts through covalent binding to cysteine residues, leading to hepatocyte injury.[13] Glutathione depletion may contribute to additional injury because of oxidative stress, and hepatocyte death stimulates the innate immune system, which can also exacerbate hepatic injury.[16,19] In addition to acetaminophen dose, other factors that may increase the risk of acetaminophen-related ALF after acetaminophen overdose include malnutrition, advanced age, concomitant use of CYP2E1 inducers, concomitant use of drugs that deplete glutathione stores (e.g., sulfamethoxazole/trimethoprim), and chronic alcoholism (chronic ethanol ingestion can induce CYP2E1; in contrast, acute ethanol ingestion may offer some protection against acetaminophen-induced ALF).[19]

Acetaminophen toxicity can occur as a result of both intentional and unintentional overdoses. In the United States, around 37% of acetaminophen ALF cases are caused by intentional overdose, whereas 57% are caused by accidental toxicity.[14] Patients with unintentional overdose are more likely to have used multiple acetaminophen-containing products.[20] A single acute ingestion (total consumption within 8 hours) of 7.5–10 g or greater in adults or 150 mg/kg in children younger than 6 years may result in hepatotoxicity (although these estimates may be conservative).[18,19] In data collected by the ALF Study Group on acetaminophen-related ALF, the median acetaminophen dose ingested was 13.2 g/day (range 2.6–75 g/day); 83% of the patients had ingested greater than 4 g/day, which is considered the toxic breakpoint.[14]

Idiosyncratic Drug-Induced ALF (Non-acetaminophen)

Drug-induced liver injury (DILI) is a recognized complication of more than 1,000 drugs and supplements and has an annual incidence of 1 in 10,000–100,000.[21] Drug-induced liver injury is the second most common cause of ALF in the United States, representing about 11-13% of all ALF cases.[14,22] However, less than 10% of all DILI progresses to ALF; for example, in a study conducted by the Drug-Induced Liver Injury Network, only 6% of all DILI cases resulted in transplantation or death.[2,23] In a more recent study from the same network that evaluated

660 patients with idiosyncratic DILI, almost 10% of all patients died or required a transplant (5% and 4.5%, respectively) within 6 months of DILI.[24] The incidence of DILI-related ALF is about one or two cases per 1 million people per year, or 1 in 30,000–100,000 prescriptions.[2,25] Drug-induced liver injury–related ALF is idiosyncratic and unpredictable and can vary in both severity and time course.[2,25] Furthermore, DILI-related ALF can be independent of the dose, route, or duration of therapy with the offending agent.[25] It often follows a subacute course and can progress to ALF despite discontinuation of the precipitating drug.[2] Mechanistically, it is possible that many causes of DILI-related ALF are a result of individual differences in drug metabolism (e.g., because of genetic differences) that lead to the formation of a toxic metabolite.[20] Acute liver failure can be caused by either the offending agent itself or a metabolite. Damage may result from direct injury or stress, initiation of an immune response, or changes in mitochondrial function, ultimately leading to mitochondrial permeability transition and necrosis/apoptosis.[26] Conventional hypersensitivity is seen in less than one-third of patients with DILI, and the liver can show either cholestatic or hepatocellular patterns of injury (the latter is associated with a worse prognosis).[2] In general, the onset of DILI-associated ALF evolves more slowly than the onset observed with acetaminophen.[25] Spontaneous recovery is often slow with DILI-related ALF. Overall transplant-free survival rates are around 27%, and up to 42% of patients require a transplant.[25] Transplant-free survival may be predicted by the degree of liver dysfunction (serum bilirubin, INR, and prognostic scores [see Prognostic Indicators in ALF section]); other factors that may be related to outcome include presence of jaundice, elevated serum aminotransferases, and advanced age.[2,22]

A wide variety of drugs can cause DILI-related ALF, and geographic differences exist in causative agents. In Western nations, conventional medications are commonly implicated, whereas in Asian countries, natural products and dietary supplements are commonly implicated.[26] In the ALF Study Group registry, more than 60 individual agents were identified as potential causes of ALF (Box 28.1).[22] The most commonly reported drug classes associated with ALF are antimicrobials (representing almost half of all cases), followed by nonsteroidal anti-inflammatory drugs, antiretroviral drugs, anticancer drugs/biologics, and dietary supplements/illicit substances.[20]

Viral Infections

Viral infections are a relatively infrequent cause of ALF in developed nations and have gradually been declining as a cause of ALF.[2] In the United States, hepatitis A virus and hepatitis B virus are the most common viral etiologies of ALF; about 7% of ALF cases are caused by hepatitis B virus and 4% of cases by hepatitis A virus.[14] Only 1% of cases of hepatitis A virus and hepatitis B virus infections ultimately progress to ALF.[20] Prognostic factors that may predict a poor outcome for ALF caused by hepatitis A virus or hepatitis B virus include ALT (alanine aminotransferase) less than 2,600 U/L, serum creatinine greater than 2 mg/dL, and need for intubation, vasopressors, or both.[20] Hepatitis B–related ALF is probably initiated by an immune response and can manifest as either a primary infection or a secondary reactivation in chronic carriers (reactivation can be spontaneous or occur after immunosuppression/cancer chemotherapy).[15,20] The liver damage related to hepatitis A virus infection is likely a result of an excessive immune response associated with a dramatic decrease in viral load.[15] Hepatitis B–related ALF is often associated with a poor prognosis and results in death or transplantation in up to 80% of cases.[3,15] In contrast, hepatitis A virus-related ALF is generally associated with a better prognosis than is hepatitis B virus.[3,15]

In developing countries, hepatitis E virus is an important cause of ALF, particularly in pregnant women. Hepatitis E virus is spread through enteric transmission, and large waterborne epidemics are possible in developing regions.[15,20] Other less common viral causes of ALF are possible, particularly during immunosuppression, including herpes simplex viruses 1 and 2, adenovirus, varicella zoster virus, and parvovirus B19.[15,20]

Other Causes

In addition to the more common etiologies of ALF described earlier, there are many miscellaneous causes of ALF. These include ischemic hepatitis (i.e., "shock liver"), autoimmune hepatitis, Wilson disease, specific toxic insults (e.g., because of mushroom poisoning), the HELLP syndrome (hemolysis, elevated liver enzymes, low platelets)/fatty liver of pregnancy, and the Budd-Chiari syndrome (acute hepatic vein thrombosis).[14,27] Finally, in many ALF cases, there is no definite etiology; in the ALF Study Group registry, around 17% of all ALF cases were described as having an indeterminate etiology.[14]

PROGNOSTIC INDICATORS IN ALF

Estimating a patient's prognosis in ALF can be important because this may relate to the decision to proceed with OLT. However, in contrast to chronic liver diseases, the relative infrequency of ALF in conjunction with the heterogeneity of disease associated with ALF has made it difficult to develop prognostic indicators. As a result, to date, there is no single reliable prognostic scoring system used to grade the severity or prognosis of ALF, although several prognostic scoring systems have been used to help predict the need for OLT.[1] The most commonly used prognostic models include Clichy's criteria, the King's College Hospital (KCH) criteria, and the Model for End-Stage

Liver Disease (MELD) (Table 28.2). The Child-Pugh (Child-Turcotte-Pugh; CTP) score is not used for prognostic determinations in ALF, but it may assist in drug dosing in ALF (see text that follows).[32] Clichy's criteria considers plasma factor V concentrations, encephalopathy grade, and patient age; use of Clichy's criteria is restricted in part because of the limited availability of factor V concentration measurement, the fact that the model was developed from patients with ALF with hepatitis B virus infection, and evidence that Clichy's criteria may be less

---

Box 28.1. Drugs Associated with Drug-Induced ALF[a]

I. Antimicrobial Agents
A. Antituberculosis drugs 18.8%
  Isoniazid alone 11.3%
  Isoniazid combined with two of three: rifampin, pyrazinamide, and ethambutol 4.5%
  Rifampin and pyrazinamide with or without ethambutol 2.3%
  Dapsone 0.075%
B. Sulphur-containing drugs 9.0%
  Trimethoprim/sulfamethoxazole alone 4.5%
  Trimethoprim/sulfamethoxazole in combination with azithromycin, statin, or antiretroviral drugs 2.3%
  Sulfasalazine 2.3%
C. Other antibiotics 14.3%
  Nitrofurantoin alone 8.3%
  Nitrofurantoin with a statin 0.75%
  Misc: amoxicillin, doxycycline, ciprofloxacin, clarithromycin, cefepime 5.3%
D. Antifungal agents 4.5%
  Terbinafine 2.3%
  Itraconazole 0.75%
  Ketoconazole alone 0.75%
  Ketoconazole with ezetimibe 0.75%
E. Antiretroviral drugs 3.0%
  Stavudine with didanosine 1.5%
  Lamivudine with stavudine and nelfinavir 0.75%
  Abacavir 0.75%

II. Central Nervous System Drugs
A. Antiepileptic drugs 8.3%
  Phenytoin 6.0%
  Carbamazepine 2.3%
  Valproic acid 1.5%
B. Psychotropic agents
  Quetiapine 0.75%
  Nefazodone 0.75%
  Fluoxetine 0.75%
  Venlafaxine 0.75%
D. Anesthetics 1.5%
  Halothane 0.75%
  Isoflurane 0.75%

III. Other Agents
A. Antimetabolites and enzyme inhibitors 8.3%
  Disulfiram 3.0%
  Propylthiouracil 3.8%
  Allopurinol 0.75%
  Melphalan 0.75%
B. Nonsteroidal anti-inflammatory drugs (NSAIDs) 5.3%
  Bromfenac 3%
  Diclofenac 1.5%
  Etodolac 0.75%
C. Biological agents and leukotriene inhibitors 3.0%
  Gemtuzumab 0.75%
  Zafirlukast 0.75%
  Interferon beta 0.75%
  Bacille-Calmette-Guérin (BCG) 0.75%
D. Statins and ezetimibe 4.5%
  Cerivastatin 1.5%
  Simvastatin (± ezetimibe) 1.5%
  Atorvastatin 1.5%
E. Other drugs 6.0%
  Troglitazone 3.0%
  Oxyiminoalkanoic acid derivative 0.75%
  Methyldopa 3.0%
  Hydralazine 0.75%

IV. Complementary and Alternative Medicine (CAM) and Illicit Substances
  Unspecified herbal preparations 2.3%
  Usnic acid 1.5%
  Thermoslim (contains saw palmetto) 0.75%
  Herbal mixture (contains blue-green algae) 0.75%
  Ma-Huang 0.75%
  Horny goat weed 0.75%
  Black cohosh 0.75%
  Hydroxycut 0.75%
  Uva-ursi 0.75%
  Cocaine 0.75%
  Ecstasy 0.75%

[a] Cases were identified over a 10.5-year period by the ALF Study Group. Numbers represent the proportion of drug-induced ALF cases caused by individual agents/classes (out of 133 total cases of drug-induced ALF).

Adapted from: Reuben A, Koch DG, Lee WM. Acute Liver Failure Study Group. Drug-induced acute liver failure: results of a U.S. multicenter, prospective study. Hepatology 2010;52:2065-76.

accurate than KCH criteria.[33] The KCH criteria are more widely used than are the Clichy criteria and have separate approaches for patients with either acetaminophen or non–acetaminophen-related ALF. The KCH criteria consider both the etiology and the clinical parameters of ALF.[29] Although the KCH criteria have a high specificity and positive predictive value (70%–100%) for identifying patients likely to have a poor prognosis, they have a low negative predictive value for poor outcome (25%–94%) (i.e., not meeting the criteria does not necessarily predict survival).[1,34,35] The MELD score was originally developed to predict the survival of patients undergoing TIPS (transjugular intrahepatic portosystemic shunts) and is used in some centers to identify patients who should be listed for transplantation.[33,36] The MELD is a continuous score that incorporates serum creatinine, serum bilirubin, and INR (Table 28.2). Although MELD has performed better than KCH and Clichy's criteria in some studies comparing MELD with KCH and/or Clichy's criteria in ALF, this has not consistently been the case.[33,37-39] Furthermore, it is unclear what, if any, MELD score should serve as the cutoff value indicating the need for transplantation in ALF (although scores of 30–35 are often reported as cutoffs, MELD scores can fluctuate substantially in ALF, and patients with higher MELD scores may survive without transplantation).[33,39-41]

Clinical predictors of poor outcome in patients with ALF are likely as important as (if not more important than) prognostic scoring systems in predicting prognosis and guiding treatment decisions. These include etiology (specifically, idiosyncratic drug injury, acute hepatitis [and other non-hepatitis A virus infections], autoimmune hepatitis, mushroom poisoning, Wilson disease, and Budd-Chiari syndrome) and encephalopathy grade on admission (grade III or IV, see Table 28.3).[1] Similarly, in some studies, common intensive care prognostic models (e.g., the Acute Physiology and Chronic Health Evaluation [APACHE] II and APACHE III) have been better predictors of prognosis in ALF than have the liver-specific models mentioned previously.[30,42,43] Ultimately, no single scoring system has been shown to perform reliably as an indicator of prognosis in ALF, and both methodological flaws and reporting limitations are common in existing studies.[44] Therefore, the American Association for the Study of Liver Diseases (AASLD) does not recommend relying entirely on scoring systems to guide decisions regarding prognosis and need for transplantation in ALF.[1]

CLINICAL PRESENTATION

Initial clinical presentation of ALF is multifactorial, varying according to the underlying etiology of the organ compromise and the time of presentation to the health care system. Early signs of ALF may include malaise, nausea, vomiting, anorexia, abdominal pain, dehydration, and fever. Initial signs of ALF are often nonspecific.[9,45] As the metabolic and detoxification function of the liver becomes compromised in the later stages of ALF, it is anticipated that the patient will have consistent clinical features of acute loss of hepatocellular function, systemic inflammatory response, and multiorgan system failure (acute renal failure is a common manifestation of ALF).[1] Clinical manifestations of ALF can be classified into three groups, based on time from the development of jaundice to the evolvement of hepatic encephalopathy. Stages may be classified as hyperacute (less than 7 days), acute (7–21 days), and subacute (3–26 weeks) (Table 28.1).[9]

MANAGEMENT OF ALF

General Considerations

The foundation for the management and treatment of ALF is largely supportive care with an emphasis on prevention or progression of secondary complications. Unfortunately, no single therapy is available to improve, reverse, or prevent further evolution of ALF from all etiologies. Hospitalization with transfer to the intensive care unit is often an appropriate escalation in care for those admitted with significant hepatocellular insufficiency because rapid deterioration in neurologic status may occur, prompting the need for rapid interventions by the medical team.[46] If treatment exists for the specific etiology of ALF, initiation of therapy should be prompt, followed by close monitoring of fluid status, hemodynamics, and metabolic abnormalities and surveillance of infection—considerations appropriate for all presentations of ALF. Laboratory monitoring for all patients should include evaluation of prothrombin time/INR, complete blood cell counts, electrolytes, lactate, creatinine, blood urea nitrogen, ammonia, acetaminophen concentration, toxicology screen, viral hepatitis serologies, and autoimmune markers. Serum aminotransferases and total bilirubin should also be included in the monitoring of these patients; however, there is poor correlation between changes in these liver-specific laboratory values and prognosis.[1]

Pharmacologic Treatment

Acetylcysteine

Acetylcysteine, a hepatoprotective agent, is an established antidote for acetaminophen toxicity. Acetylcysteine exerts its effects by restoring hepatic glutathione stores through the replenishment of cysteine, enhancing the sulfation pathway of acetaminophen elimination, and may result in a reduction reaction of NAPQI back to acetaminophen.[19] Acetylcysteine is available in both intravenous and oral preparations. The oral formulation of acetylcysteine undergoes extensive first-pass metabolism by the liver, resulting in a low yield of available drug. However, acetylcysteine

Table 28.2 Prognostic Models for ALF

Prognostic Model	Model Parameters Indicating Poor Prognosis (i.e., need for liver transplantation)	Comments
Clichy's criteria[28]	Poor prognosis in patients with grade 3 or grade 4 encephalopathy and: • Factor V concentrations < 20% for patients < 30 years • Factor V concentrations < 30% for patients > 30 years	• Derived from patients with ALF with hepatitis B infection • May be limited by availability of factor V concentrations
King's Hospital criteria[1,29,30]	*Acetaminophen-induced ALF* Poor prognosis • Arterial pH < 7.3 (regardless of stage of hepatic encephalopathy) (according to AASLD, consider arterial pH < 7.3 OR arterial lactate > 3.0 mmol/L after adequate fluid resuscitation)[1] • OR • PTT > 100 s (INR > 6.5) AND serum creatinine > 3.4 mg/dL in patients with grade 3 or 4 hepatic encephalopathy *Non–acetaminophen-induced ALF* Poor prognosis • PTT > 100 s (INR > 6.5) regardless of stage of hepatic encephalopathy) • OR • Any THREE of the following criteria: • Age < 10 or > 40 years • Jaundice for > 7 days before development of hepatic encephalopathy • PTT > 50 s (INR > 3.5) • Serum bilirubin ≥ 17 mg/dL • AND serum creatinine > 3.4 mg/dL • According to AASLD, also consider unfavorable etiology such as Wilson disease, idiosyncratic drug reaction, seronegative hepatitis[1]	• Good positive predictive value or poor outcome, but poor negative predictive value
Model for End-Stage Liver Disease (MELD)[31]	• MELD = 3.78 × ln[serum bilirubin (mg/dL)] + 11.2 × ln[INR] + 9.57 × ln[serum creatinine (mg/dL)] + 6.43 × etiology (0: cholestatic or alcoholic, 1: otherwise) • If patients have had dialysis twice per week in the previous 7 days, the serum creatinine value is set at 4.0 mg/dL • Laboratory values < 1.0 are set as 1.0 (to avoid negative values)	• Unclear what cutoff value should be used to determine candidates for transplantation, not developed or validated for ALF

AASLD = American Association for the Study of Liver Diseases; ALF = acute liver failure; PTT = partial thromboplastin time.

undergoes deacetylation in the liver to produce cysteine, which may be of benefit given that cysteine is the rate-limiting factor in glutathione production. In contrast, intravenous administration of acetylcysteine bypasses first-pass metabolism and may subsequently result in lower glutathione concentrations than oral administration.[47] The U.S. Food and Drug Administration (FDA)-approved recommendations for oral administration of acetylcysteine require a minimum treatment duration of 72 hours. The oral dosage regimen consists of a 140-mg/kg loading dose followed by maintenance dosing of 70 mg/kg every 4 hours for 18 doses or a total cumulative dose of 1330 mg/kg. Intravenous administration of acetylcysteine is provided over a minimum of 21 hours in three doses.

Administration should include an initial loading dose of 150 mg/kg (maximum of 15 g) infused over 60 minutes, followed by a dose of 50 mg/kg (maximum of 5 g) infused over 4 hours, and ending with a third dose of 100 mg/kg (maximum of 10 g) infused over 16 hours.[18] The most commonly reported adverse effects of the intravenous form include the dose-dependent anaphylactoid reactions of tachycardia, hypotension, edema, rash, pruritus, nausea, vomiting, bronchospasms, and angioedema. The incidence of adverse events noted with the intravenous form is reduced substantially when acetylcysteine is administered orally.[47] Although a systematic review did not provide conclusive evidence to support one route of acetylcysteine administration over another, the intravenous route of administration remains the preferred route for most acute ingestions.[48]

Greatest success with administration of acetylcysteine for the prevention of hepatic toxicity and subsequent ALF is seen when administration occurs within 8 hours of toxic acetaminophen ingestion. As the delay in acetylcysteine therapy extends beyond 8 hours of acetaminophen poisoning, antidotal effects decrease, and risk of ALF increases. Despite decreased efficacy when acetylcysteine is administered further from the time of an acute toxic acetaminophen ingestion, initiation of acetylcysteine regardless of post-ingestion time is typically favored because the potential benefit of administration outweighs the risk associated with its use. Hepatotoxicity risk after acetaminophen ingestion can be assessed by plotting the serum acetaminophen concentration and the corresponding hours post-ingestion on the Rumack-Matthew nomogram (Figure 28.1).[18] To use this tool effectively, a random serum acetaminophen concentration must be obtained between 4 hours and 24 hours of ingestion. If the time of ingestion is unknown, the Rumack-Matthew nomogram cannot be used to assess the need for treatment and the potential risk of hepatotoxicity. Therefore, an elevated serum acetaminophen concentration is typically treated regardless of post-ingestion time because the benefits of acetylcysteine vastly outweigh the risk of administration. If a serum acetaminophen concentration is obtained, the hour of ingestion is known, and the post-ingestion time fits within the targeted time interval of 4–24 hours, the concentration can be plotted on the Rumack-Matthew nomogram to assess the need for initiating acetylcysteine. The treatment line, also known as the parallel line at 150 mcg/mL 4 hours post-ingestion on the nomogram, is the most commonly used guideline for acetylcysteine initiation after toxic ingestion of acetaminophen.[18]

Administering acetylcysteine may also provide beneficial effects after hepatic injury in non–acetaminophen-induced ALF and alcoholic hepatitis.[47] Efficacy of acetylcysteine administration in these clinical presentations is unrelated to detoxification. Presumed beneficial mechanisms of action in these clinical scenarios include scavenging of free radicals and replenishment of glutathione stores during oxidative stress, production of nitric oxide resulting in vasodilation and hepatic perfusion, and anti-inflammatory properties through inhibition of proinflammatory factors.[18,47] In the treatment of non–acetaminophen-induced ALF, administration of oral and intravenous acetylcysteine has shown increased transplant-free survival rates and decreased length of hospitalization. For the treatment of severe

Table 28.3 Grades of Encephalopathy[1,38]

Grade	Definition
I	Changes in behavior with minimal change in level of consciousness
II	Gross disorientation, drowsiness, possible asterixis, inappropriate behavior
III	Marked confusion; incoherent speech, sleeping most of the time but arousable to vocal stimuli
IV	Comatose, unresponsive to pain, decorticate or decerebrate posturing

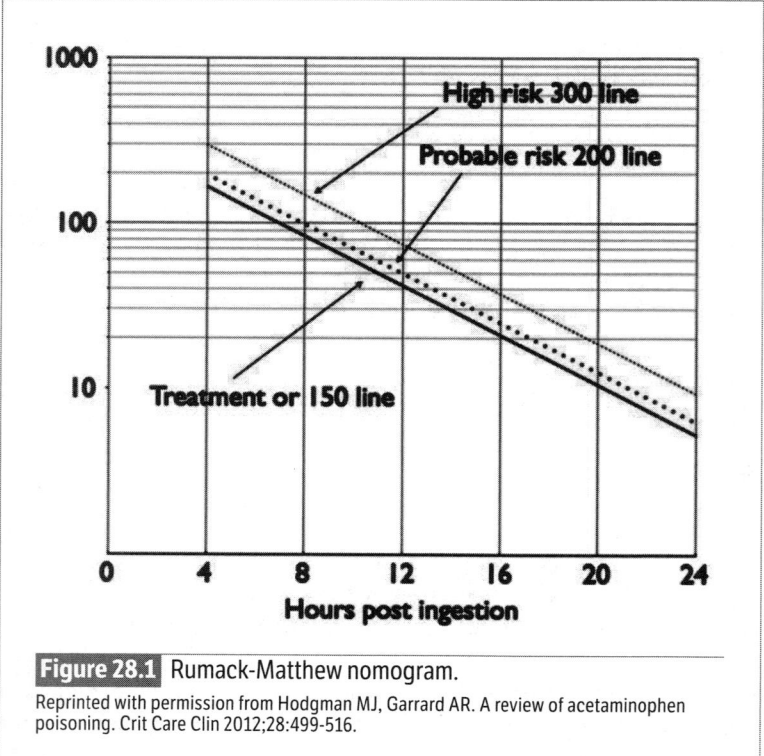

Figure 28.1 Rumack-Matthew nomogram.
Reprinted with permission from Hodgman MJ, Garrard AR. A review of acetaminophen poisoning. Crit Care Clin 2012;28:499-516.

alcoholic hepatitis, acetylcysteine has also shown theoretical benefits secondary to the antioxidant and anti-inflammatory effects. Again, despite varying data regarding benefit for acetylcysteine in non–acetaminophen-induced ALF and alcoholic hepatitis, initiation of acetylcysteine is typically favored because the potential benefits of administration outweigh the risks associated with its use.

Management of Secondary Complications

Hepatic Encephalopathy

The hallmark complication of ALF, hepatic encephalopathy, is related to cerebral edema and intracranial hemorrhage (ICH). As the severity of hepatic encephalopathy increases, denoted by grade (see Table 28.3), the rate of cerebral edema and ICH increases. These detrimental effects of hepatic encephalopathy are a result of hyperammonemia. Pharmacologic management of hepatic encephalopathy and less invasive medical interventions (excluding electroencephalogram, mechanical ventilation, and artificial liver systems) can typically bridge patients with grade I and II hepatic encephalopathy. As patients progress to grade III and IV hepatic encephalopathy, intubation and subsequent mechanical ventilation become mandatory to provide supportive care until the symptoms improve or resolve.[1]

Pharmacologic therapies for the management of hepatic encephalopathy mitigate their action through lowering of ammonia, with a focus on the ammonia-producing bacteria of the colon. Disaccharides are considered the first-line pharmacologic agents of choice for lowering the production and absorption of ammonia, with lactulose being the most commonly used agent. Lactulose is metabolized by the gut flora into acetic and lactic acids, producing an acidic, non-survival environment for the bacteria. In addition, the metabolism of lactulose inhibits the diffusion of ammonia into the systemic circulation and the subsequent conversion of ammonia to ammonium. Lactulose for hepatic encephalopathy can be administered by enteral access or per rectum and is typically titrated to 2–4 semisoft stools per day. Despite mechanistic belief of efficacy, conflicting data exist regarding substantial benefit in the treatment of hepatic encephalopathy compared with placebo. Currently, there is insufficient evidence to dispute the initiation of lactulose therapy; therefore, lactulose (or other laxative agents discussed in the following text) should be administered to all patients with hepatic encephalopathy.[49]

Despite the long-standing use of disaccharide therapy in hepatic encephalopathy, recent evidence is challenging its role as the first-line treatment option for hepatic encephalopathy. Polyethylene glycol, an osmotic laxative with gut catharsis activity, was hypothesized to resolve hepatic encephalopathy more effectively than lactulose in the Hepatic Encephalopathy: Lactulose vs Polyethylene Glycol 3350-Electrolyte Solution (HELP) study. Efficacy was evaluated by an improvement in one or more grades of hepatic encephalopathy at 24 hours after the administration of pharmacologic intervention. Therapies evaluated include lactulose 20–30 g orally or 300 g per rectum for a minimum of three doses in 24 hours compared with polyethylene glycol 4 L orally over 4 hours. Patient demographics were similar in each treatment group, including severity of liver failure. A statistically significant improvement in one or more grades of hepatic encephalopathy was noted in the polyethylene glycol treatment arm compared with the lactulose therapy treatment arm (91% vs. 52%; $p<0.01$). Use of polyethylene glycol was also shown to have a shorter time to hepatic encephalopathy resolution (1 day vs. 2 days; $p=0.01$). However, patients who received polyethylene glycol had a nonstatistically significant shorter duration of hospital stay; therefore, polyethylene glycol may provide more rapid improvement in hepatic encephalopathy, but the long-term benefits of this agent, in place of conventional disaccharide therapy, remain unknown. In addition, the dosing scheme used in the HELP study may be unrealistic for long-term adherence.[50]

Oral antimicrobials have been evaluated as an alternative treatment option for the management of hepatic encephalopathy. Similar to the goal with disaccharides, the goal with antimicrobial therapy in hepatic encephalopathy is the inhibition of ammonia production by intestinal bacteria. Agents evaluated for possible efficacy include neomycin, metronidazole, vancomycin, and, most recently, rifaximin. Use of neomycin, metronidazole, and vancomycin has decreased substantially in the treatment of hepatic encephalopathy because of toxicities and emerging resistance.[51] Neomycin administration has been associated with increased risk of nephrotoxicity and ototoxicity, and neurotoxicity has been associated with metronidazole.[51] Because of the emergence of vancomycin-resistant enterococci, use of vancomycin for hepatic encephalopathy is limited to cases of resistance.[51] Rifaximin has optimal pharmacokinetic and pharmacodynamic properties because it has minimal systemic absorption and high intraluminal and fecal drug concentration with a broad spectrum of activity against gram-positive, gram-negative, anaerobic, and aerobic organisms.[49,52] Compared with therapy for hepatic encephalopathy with disaccharides, rifaximin has shown varying results. A prospective, double-blind, randomized controlled trial of 120 patients compared rifaximin plus lactulose with lactulose alone in the treatment of overt hepatic encephalopathy.[53] No significant difference was noted between treatment groups with respect to severity of liver failure, etiology, grade of hepatic encephalopathy, or previous episodes of hepatic encephalopathy. There was a statistically significant rate of reversal of hepatic encephalopathy within 10 days of therapy in the group receiving rifaximin plus lactulose compared with the group receiving lactulose alone. In addition, patients in the combination therapy group had a statistically significant shorter duration of hospital admission and decreased rate of mortality. Therefore, it can be concluded that rifaximin is at least as efficacious as, if not superior to, lactulose, but use may be restricted by severity of illness because of the higher cost of this agent than of laxative therapy.[53]

Cerebral Edema/Intracranial Hypertension

Cerebral edema and ICH are the most serious complications of ALF and are the main cause of morbidity and mortality in ALF. However, the underlying mechanism of cerebral edema and ICH is not well known. It is hypothesized that this adverse consequence of ALF is related to osmotic disturbances because of hyperammonemia and loss of cerebral blood flow autoregulation.[1] Risk factors for developing cerebral edema and ICH include grade III or IV encephalopathy (Table 28.3), serum ammonia concentrations greater than 200 micromoles/L, and need for vasopressor or renal replacement therapies.[9]

Universal interventions should be applied to patients with high-grade hepatic encephalopathy. Recommendations include elevation of the head of the bed by 30 degrees, endotracheal intubation, management of hypertension, and minimization of painful stimulation or agitation. Placement of ICP monitoring may be considered in these patients if patients are at a center with expertise in this area.[9] Monitoring of ICP allows for evaluation of cerebral hypoperfusion through calculation of cerebral perfusion pressure (CPP; mean arterial pressure minus ICP), with the goal of maintaining a CPP of at least 50–60 mm Hg. Episodes of cerebral hypoperfusion, denoted by a CPP less than 50–60 mm Hg, place the patient at an increased risk for developing cerebral ischemia and secondary long-term cognitive detriments. Even though ICP monitoring can provide the clinician with a more clear understanding of the patient's cerebral edema and ICH status, ICP devices have not shown improvements in patient survival rates compared with patient survival rates without this invasive monitoring, and the devices are associated with greater risk (infection and hemorrhage) to the patient.[1]

Prevention strategies, as well as interventions in the management of ICP, mimic those identified for the treatment of elevated ICP in the trauma population. If an ICP monitor is present, the ICP should be maintained at 20–25 mm Hg with mean arterial pressure greater than 70 mm Hg to allow for achievement of a CPP greater than 50 mm Hg. Achievement and maintenance of a target CPP often require a balancing act of increasing the mean arterial pressure to the safest possible degree while minimizing the ICP. Vasopressor therapy may be necessary to assist in the elevation of the mean arterial pressure, with norepinephrine typically being the most appropriate first-line agent. To achieve goal ICP, osmotic therapy may be considered. Administration of intravenous mannitol has been shown to decrease elevated ICP in patients with ALF; however, use of mannitol in severe ICH has shown minimal to no benefit. Despite weaker evidence for use in more severe cases, mannitol remains the first-line therapy for ICH in ALF, according to the AASLD ALF management guidelines.[1] Mannitol should be administered as an intravenous bolus of 0.5–1 g/kg. Additional doses may be administered if the patient's serum osmolality remains less than 320 mOsm/L.[1,9] When additional doses of mannitol are contraindicated because of serum osmolality, administration of hypertonic sodium chloride may be considered. Hypertonic sodium chloride has shown similar efficacy to mannitol in the management of ICH in ALF.[9] The AASLD guidelines recommend prophylactic administration of hypertonic sodium chloride in patients at highest risk of developing cerebral edema—outlined as those with hyperammonemia, grade III or IV hepatic encephalopathy, acute renal failure, or administration of vasopressor therapy.[1] Hypertonic sodium chloride should be administered by intravenous bolus administration at a frequency of every 2–3 hours. While administering hypertonic sodium chloride, it is important to monitor serum sodium often with the goal of achieving a concentration of 145–155 mmol/L.[46] If ICP remains elevated despite an adequate challenge of mannitol, hypertonic saline, or both, barbiturate agents may be considered.[1] A barbiturate coma induced by pentobarbital administration of 3–5 mg/kg intravenous load followed by 1–3 mg/kg/hour has been correlated with improvement in ICP in patients who are refractory to conventional therapy of mannitol or hypertonic sodium chloride.[46] Despite a benefit in decreasing ICP, barbiturate administration is often limited by hypotension, which subsequently results in a decreased CPP. The final pharmacologic agents that may be considered are corticosteroids. Although corticosteroids have shown benefit in ICH, their use is limited to elevations in ICH secondary to brain tumors and some infectious pathologies. Therefore, there is no clinical benefit to administering corticosteroids in patients with ALF despite the presence of ICH.[1]

Interventions outside pharmacologic therapies have been evaluated for the management of ICH, including induction of hyperventilation and hypothermia. Despite perceived mechanistic benefit, both interventions have failed to provide substantial improvement; therefore, the AASLD guidelines do not recommend the induction of hyperventilation and hypothermia in the management of ICH in ALF. Hyperventilation, denoted by a partial pressure of carbon dioxide of 25–30 mm Hg, provides restoration in cerebrovascular autoregulation and subsequent improvement in ICP. Despite this benefit, the duration of effects provided by hypoventilation is short-lived. Hypothermia has been evaluated as a method to control and prevent ICH as well as prevent cerebral edema.[1] The mechanisms through which hypothermia has been proposed to prevent cerebral edema include hyperemia, alteration in metabolism of ammonia and glucose, and reduction in cerebral metabolism and blood flow. However, most data evaluating the benefit of hypothermia are derived from animal models, with only limited experience in human subjects.[1,54] To date, data evaluations are lacking to recommend hypothermia as a treatment modality for the management of ICH in ALF.

Seizure prophylaxis has been evaluated in the management of cerebral edema and ICH because it is known that seizure activity can increase the ICP as well as result in cerebral hypoxia and subsequent edema. Despite several trials evaluating the role of seizure prophylaxis in ALF, clinical studies are inconclusive for a benefit in this population; seizure prophylaxis is therefore not recommended by the AASLD management guidelines.[1] Although prophylactic administration of antiepileptics is not recommended, monitoring of epileptiform discharge should be conducted by electroencephalogram for the following indications: grade III or IV hepatic encephalopathy, sudden change in neurologic status, myoclonus, or during titration of barbiturate therapy for management of cerebral edema.[46] If seizure activity does present, prompt control of the seizure and initiation of maintenance therapy should be considered in accordance to standard epilepsy treatment with phenytoin or an equivalent antiepileptic.[1]

Infection

Despite impairment of host-defense mechanisms in patients with ALF, there is lack of evidence to suggest empiric initiation of antibacterial or antifungal therapy.[1,45] However, surveillance monitoring for signs and symptoms of an infectious source should be implemented because etiologies of the ALF may mask symptoms of systemic infection—particularly fever in the presence of acetaminophen-induced ALF. Prompt collection of blood cultures and early evaluation of chest radiographs should occur at the earliest signs of infection or neurologic deterioration. The most common site of infection is the lungs, followed by the urinary tract and the bloodstream. Infectious organisms most commonly isolated from this population include gram-negative enteric bacilli, gram-positive cocci, and *Candida* spp.[9] Empiric antimicrobial administration should be considered in patients when surveillance cultures denote a significant infecting organism, worsening hepatic encephalopathy, hypotension nonresponsive to traditional interventions, and presence of systemic inflammatory response syndrome criteria. Initial therapy should provide a broad spectrum of antimicrobial coverage, covering *Staphylococcus, Streptococcus, Escherichia coli,* and *Enterobacter* spp., and should consider local rates of susceptibilities. In patients who are OLT candidates, there may be a lower threshold to initiate empiric antimicrobial therapy because a recent or active infection may reduce the success of transplantation or delay the OLT procedure.[9,46]

Coagulopathy

Coagulopathy commonly presents with the development of ALF and is typically denoted by the laboratory findings of thrombocytopenia, prolonged prothrombin time/INR, or both. This disorder arises as a result of inadequate synthesis of fibrinolytic proteins, anticoagulant proteins, and precoagulation factors as well as enhanced consumption of clotting factors and dysfunction in platelet activity.[9,45,46] This disruption in the coagulation pathway results in a mismatch of hypercoagulable and coagulopathic states, but often, these differing hematologic states balance each other.[9] Therefore, the frequency of spontaneous, clinically relevant bleeding episodes is low, with a reported incidence of less than 10%.[46] If a bleeding episode occurs, it commonly presents in the mucosa of the stomach, lungs, or gastrointestinal (GI) tract. Therefore, patients admitted to the intensive care unit with the presence of ALF should receive either histamine-2 receptor blocking agents or proton pump inhibitors, both considered first-line agents, for stress ulcer prophylaxis of the GI tract.[1,9] Sucralfate may be used as a second-line option for patients with existing contraindications to first-line therapy.

Patients with ALF may have a vitamin K deficiency. Because of this deficiency and the coagulation abnormalities, it is recommended to empirically administer vitamin K to these patients.[1,46] The AASLD guidelines recommend administering vitamin K 5–10 mg subcutaneously, typically for 3 days. However, subcutaneous vitamin K is known to have erratic absorption in patients with ALF, so use of the intravenous or oral formulations is usually preferred. Beyond administering vitamin K, complete correction or reversal of coagulopathies and associated abnormal laboratory values is not recommended for all patients presenting with ALF. Administration of fresh frozen plasma (FFP), platelets, recombinant factor VIIa, or cryoprecipitate to reverse coagulopathy should be reserved for patients with an active bleed or for patients requiring invasive interventions, such as the placement of an ICP monitor for management of cerebral edema and ICH.[9] When reversal is required, FFP is typically the initial agent used to correct the coagulation abnormality. Administration of recombinant factor VIIa should be reserved for patients whose reversal with FFP has failed. Timing of administration of recombinant factor VIIa in relation to planned intervention is crucial for efficacy because this agent has a short terminal half-life. It is recommended interventions be done 20–30 minutes after administration. Cryoprecipitate should be reserved for the patient's demonstration of hypofibrinogenemia, denoted by a serum fibrin concentration less than 100 mg/dL. Furthermore, transfusion of platelets should be reserved for cessation of active bleeding in patients with a platelet count of less than 10,000/mm^3 to 50,000/mm^3.[9,46]

General Supportive Care

The management of metabolic derangements, nutrition, and renal failure in the ALF population mimics standard care for other critically ill patients. Information regarding these topics can be found in Chapter 3, "Electrolytes," Chapter 4, "Nutrition Support," and Chapter 26, "Acute Kidney Injury—Prevention and Management."

Nonpharmacologic Management

Extracorporal Liver Support

Extracorporal liver support systems, or liver assist devices, have been developed to mimic the function of the liver in patients with ALF, acute on chronic liver failure, and end-stage liver disease.[9,55] Using a concept similar to the function of external devices used in renal replacement therapy, extracorporal liver support systems may serve as a bridge therapy until recovery or transplantation. Many systems have been developed and can be classified into nonbiological and biological systems. Activity of the nonbiological systems is provided through the elimination of albumin-bound water-insoluble molecules (including, but not limited to, bilirubin, bile acids, fatty acids) using high-flux membrane extracorporal liver support systems. Biological extracorporal liver support systems differ because of the use of living hepatocytes, which provide detoxification as well as synthetic and metabolic activity.[55] Despite the potential efficacy of extracorporal liver support systems in ALF, randomized controlled trials have failed to show long-term benefits. An additional limitation to the use of these systems is their lack of availability in many health care institutions. Further development and research of these devices is needed to warrant the routine implementation of these devices in the management of ALF.[1,55]

Liver Transplantation

The management of ALF with irreversible injury is limited to OLT because this intervention serves as the only definitive treatment option.[9] Acute liver failure accounts for about 5%–6% of OLT performed in the United States.[56,57] The timing of referral for OLT provides some complexity in the management of ALF; referral should be made in enough time to allow for assessment of candidacy but should not be delayed to the extent that the patient's level of critical illness impedes the patient's surviving the procedure. Acute liver failure is one of the few conditions that allows for status 1A (urgent) placement on the United Network for Organ Sharing.[1] Calculation of the patient's MELD score, as well as evaluation of relative and absolute contraindications to transplantation, must be completed in the consideration of listing for transplantation. Relative contraindications include age older than 65, severe malnutrition, other organ failure, previous abdominal surgery, poor functional status, and poor medical compliance. Severe cardiopulmonary disease, irreversible cerebral injury, sepsis or active infection, HIV, extrahepatic malignancy, vascular anomaly or thrombosis, active alcohol or illicit drug use, and psychosocial issues are commonly considered contraindications to OLT.[56] Survival rate 1 year after OLT in patients with ALF (75%) is less than in those who receive a transplant for chronic liver failure (87%).[1,56] However, patients who receive OLT for ALF tend to have better long-term survival (survival beyond the first year). Therefore, urgent OLT should be considered in those with prognostic indicators indicating low probability of survival.[1]

DRUG DOSING IN ALF

The liver plays an integral role in the pharmacokinetics of numerous drugs, and impaired hepatic function can affect drug metabolism, biliary excretion, and plasma protein binding.[58] Unfortunately, most data regarding the impact of hepatic dysfunction come from studies of chronic liver diseases, and information is limited on the impact of ALF on drug pharmacokinetics and drug dosing modifications. Furthermore, existing studies often group patients with different etiologies and severity of liver disease (that may be associated with a broad range of pharmacokinetic changes).[59] Despite this lack of information, the rapid loss of liver function and massive necrosis/apoptosis associated with ALF can be expected to have clinically important effects on drug pharmacokinetics that may warrant changes in drug dosing.[60] Patients with ALF may also have acute renal failure, which can reduce the clearance of renally eliminated drugs. Ultimately, ALF can significantly affect several key pharmacokinetic processes, including absorption, distribution, metabolism, and elimination.[60] In the section that follows, we review the basic principles of hepatic drug clearance and discuss potential mechanisms of altered drug pharmacokinetics that may warrant changes in drug therapy.

Principles of Hepatic Drug Clearance

Hepatic drug clearance is a function of the hepatic blood flow (Q_H) and the hepatic extraction ratio (E_H) of a given drug.[58] Intrinsic hepatic drug clearance (CL_{int}) represents the metabolism of unbound drug (i.e., it is independent of Q_H and extent of protein binding) by the liver.[61] The E_H represents the efficiency with which the liver clears a drug from the circulation, and using E_H, drugs can be classified as having high (E_H greater than 0.6), intermediate (E_H 0.3–0.6), or low (E_H less than 0.3) E_H values (Table 28.4).[58,61] The primary determinants of drug metabolism are Q_H, the extent of plasma protein binding, and CL_{int}. The metabolism of drugs with high E_H is limited by liver blood flow and is relatively insensitive to changes in plasma protein binding and the activity of drug-metabolizing enzymes. In contrast, the metabolism of drugs with low E_H is more dependent on alterations in hepatic enzyme function (i.e., CL_{int}) and plasma protein binding, and less dependent on Q_H. Drugs with intermediate E_H values can be affected to some extent by changes in Q_H, plasma protein binding, and CL_{int}. In addition to affecting hepatic clearance, E_H affects the bioavailability of enterally administered drug; drugs with high E_H tend to undergo substantial first-pass metabolism, whereas drugs with low E_H are generally not subject to substantial first-pass metabolism by the liver.[62]

Potential Mechanisms of Altered Drug Disposition in ALF

Many pathological changes during ALF can contribute to altered drug disposition, making prediction of pharmacokinetics difficult. Potential physiologic changes leading to pharmacokinetic changes include (but are not limited to) a reduction in hepatocyte cell mass, alterations in hepatic perfusion (including portal venous perfusion and arterial perfusion), alterations in hepatic enzyme and hepatic transporter function, alterations in hepatic protein synthesis, and alterations in renal function associated with ALF.[63] A discussion of how various pharmacokinetic processes may be affected by ALF is presented in the following section.

Alterations in Drug Absorption

Acute liver failure can alter the oral bioavailability of enterally administered drugs by several mechanisms. Alterations in intestinal permeability caused by the inflammation associated with ALF may affect drug absorption from the intestine, although these changes are not well characterized, and may be affected by several mechanisms (i.e., alterations in passive permeability, alterations in mucosal transporter function, etc.). Similarly, enteral absorption can be influenced by alterations in gastric motility that may be present in ALF.[60] More importantly, ALF may be associated with changes in hepatic first-pass metabolism. Under normal conditions, after oral administration, high E_H drugs are extensively (greater than 60%) removed from the liver by first-pass

Table 28.4 Hepatic Extraction Ratios of Selected Drugs Used in the Intensive Care Unit[a]

Low E_H (< 0.3)	Intermediate E_H (0.3–0.6)	High E_H (> 0.6)
Acetaminophen	Amiodarone	Buspirone
Alprazolam	Amitriptyline	Chlorpromazine
Carbamazepine	Atorvastatin	Cyclosporine
Ceftriaxone	Azathioprine	Doxepin
Chlordiazepoxide	Carvedilol	Fluvastatin
Clarithromycin	Ciprofloxacin	Imipramine
Clindamycin	Clomipramine	Isosorbide dinitrate
Diazepam	Clozapine	Labetalol
Diphenhydramine	Codeine	Lovastatin
Flurazepam	Diltiazem	Metoprolol
Glipizide	Erythromycin	Midazolam
Isoniazid	Felodipine	Morphine
Lamotrigine	Fluphenazine	Nicardipine
Lansoprazole	Haloperidol	Nitroglycerine
Lansoprazole	Itraconazole	Perphenazine
Levetiracetam	Lidocaine	Propranolol
Lorazepam	Nifedipine	Quetiapine
Methadone	Nortriptyline	Sertraline
Methylprednisone	Olanzapine	Sirolimus
Metoclopramide	Omeprazole	Tacrolimus
Metronidazole	Paroxetine	Trimipramine
Mycophenolate mofetil	Pravastatin	Venlafaxine
Oxazepam	Ranitidine	Verapamil
Phenobarbital	Simvastatin	Zaleplon
Phenytoin		
Prednisolone		
Prednisone		
Rifampin		
Risperidone		
Temazepam		
Theophylline		
Tiagabine		
Tolbutamide		
Topiramate		
Trazadone		
Triazolam		
Valproic acid		
Zolpidem		

[a]Table is intended to provide examples of E_H for some commonly encountered drugs and is not an exhaustive list.

E_H = hepatic extraction ratio.
Adapted from: Delco F, Tchambaz L, Schlienger R, et al. Dose adjustment in patients with liver disease. Drug Saf 2005;28:529-45.

metabolism (i.e., bioavailability less than 40%), whereas low E_H drugs are not significantly removed by first-pass metabolism (first-pass removal of 30% or less).[61] A reduction in the drug-metabolizing capacity of the liver during ALF is expected to result in an increase in the enteral bioavailability of high E_H drugs.[58] Similarly, alterations in blood flow from the intestine to the liver may also contribute to increased enteral bioavailability, although these changes are not as well characterized in ALF as in chronic hepatic diseases. Therefore, intravenous administration of high E_H drugs may be preferred to enteral administration. If enteral administration of high E_H drugs is used, initial doses should be lowered (see text that follows). Examples of high E_H drugs are shown in Table 28.4. The enteral bioavailability of low E_H drugs is less likely to be affected by ALF.[61]

Alterations in Drug Distribution

Alterations in plasma protein concentrations in ALF can affect the volume of distribution of drugs that are highly protein bound (i.e., drugs with 90% or greater protein binding).[62] Potential mechanisms for decreased plasma protein binding include impaired hepatic protein synthesis, accumulation of exogenous compounds that can inhibit protein binding (e.g., bilirubin), and potential qualitative changes in albumin.[58,60] Reductions in plasma albumin in ALF can lead to higher concentrations of free drug for agents that are highly bound to albumin.[58] This may be clinically important because the unbound drug is generally responsible for generating a pharmacologic effect.[61] Furthermore, changes in the concentration of unbound drug resulting in changes in volume of distribution may lead to alterations in clearance.[62] Simultaneous increases in unbound fraction and decreases in metabolism (see text that follows) of highly bound drugs cleared by the liver can result in toxicity.[62] Because the time course of ALF is variable and the half-life of albumin is relatively long (i.e., about 21 days), reductions in plasma albumin are not as predictable in ALF as in chronic liver diseases. Volume of distribution may also be influenced by third spacing (because of ascites, edema, or both); this may be particularly important for hydrophilic drugs (e.g., aminoglycosides).[60]

Table 28.5 Child-Pugh (CTP) Score[a,32]

Variable	Points Awarded for Observed Findings		
	1 Point	2 Points	3 Points
Encephalopathy grade	Absent	1–2	3–4
Ascites	Absent	Slight	Moderate
Serum bilirubin (mg/dL)	<2	2–3	>3
Serum albumin (g/dL)	>3.5	2.8–3.5	<2.8
Prothrombin time (seconds prolonged)	<4	4–6	>6

[a]A (mild): 5–6 points; B (moderate): 7–9 points; C (severe): 10–15 points.

Alterations in Drug Metabolism and Clearance

In general, hepatic drug metabolism is likely impaired in patients with ALF, although most available data come from chronic liver diseases. Hepatic metabolism may be impaired because of several mechanisms. Hepatic transporters mediate the transport of some drugs in or out of hepatocytes and into the bile canaliculus. Transporter expression and activity may be altered in acute and chronic liver diseases; however, a detailed discussion of transporter alterations is beyond the scope of this chapter.[60] Alterations in hepatic enzymatic capacity (including alterations in hepatic enzyme expression and loss of hepatocytes) can substantially affect hepatic drug metabolism.[60] The effect of ALF on drug metabolism may partly depend on whether the drug is a high, intermediate, or low extraction drug.[60] As indicated earlier, E_H describes the efficiency of drug removal by the liver and is dependent on Q_H, CL_{int}, and plasma protein binding.[61] Intrinsic drug clearance is an indication of the liver's ability to clear unbound drug from the blood and depends on hepatic metabolic enzyme activity and the function of hepatic transporters.[58] Therefore, ALF may result in a reduction in E_H because of a reduction in the expression and activity of drug-metabolizing enzymes and may further affect metabolism as a result of changes in Q_H.[60] The hepatic drug clearance of low E_H drugs tends to be sensitive to changes in enzyme activity and protein binding.[60] High E_H drugs are more sensitive to alterations in Q_H.[60] Although specific data regarding hepatic enzyme activity in ALF are lacking, data in chronic liver diseases such as cirrhosis can offer insight into probable alterations. Cytochrome P450 enzymes are likely more affected in cirrhosis than are phase II metabolizing enzymes.[63,64] The extent to which liver disease affects drug metabolism depends on several factors, including the metabolic pathway involved, extent of injury, and time course of injury.[59] Results of studies in cirrhosis have been variable; however, in general, the activity and expression of CYP3A, CYP1A2, and CYP2C19 appear to be most susceptible to the effects of chronic liver disease, whereas CYP2D6 and CYP2C9 may be more preserved.[59,64] In a study evaluating CYP3A activity in cirrhosis, CYP3A activity was correlated with CTP and MELD scores.[65] In this study of patients with severe cirrhosis (CTP class C or MELD of 15 or higher), the unbound clearance of midazolam (a CYP3A substrate) was

Table 28.6 Examples of Drugs with Dosing Guidelines Based on CTP Score[a,b]			
Drug	**Dosage Recommendation**		
	Mild Disease (CTP class A, score 5–6)	Moderate Disease (CTP class B, score 7–9)	Severe Disease (CTP class C, score 10–15)
Caspofungin		35 mg/day (70-mg loading dose if indicated)	Not recommended
Clarithromycin			Reduce dose by 50%
Clindamycin			Monitor hepatic function
Esomeprazole			Maximum 20 mg/day
Eszopiclone			Initiate 1 mg/day
Metronidazole			Reduce dose by 50%
Rifampin		Monitor hepatic function	Monitor hepatic function
Sirolimus	Reduce dose by 33%	Reduce dose by 33%	Reduce dose by 33%
Tigecycline			100-mg loading dose; then 25 mg every 12 hours
Venlafaxine		Reduce dose by 50%	Reduce dose by at least 50%
Voriconazole	Reduce dose by 50%	Reduce dose by 50%	Not recommended

[a]This is an abbreviated list and does not contain all drugs with dosing guidelines based on Child-Pugh (CTP) score.

[b]CTP score was not designed for use in ALF and has not been validated in ALF. Proposed approaches for patients with ALF include calculating an individual patient's CTP score or assuming that the patient has severe disease (CTP class C, score 10–15).

Adapted from: Budingen FV, Gonzalez D, Tucker AN, et al. Relevance of liver failure for anti-infective agents: from pharmacokinetic alterations to dosage adjustments. Ther Adv Infect Dis 2014;2:17-42; and Spray JW, Willett K, Chase D, et al. Dosage adjustment for hepatic dysfunction based on Child-Pugh scores. Am J Health Syst Pharm 2007;64:690, 2-3.

14% of the corresponding midazolam clearance in control subjects.[65] Although caution should be used in extrapolating these results to ALF, it is likely that ALF is associated with a reduction in CYP function and expression, given the extensive hepatocyte necrosis and apoptosis that is characteristic of ALF. In one of the few pharmacokinetic studies conducted in ALF, the plasma half-life of antipyrine was significantly prolonged in patients after acetaminophen overdose (antipyrine is a substrate for several CYP enzymes, including CYP1A2, CYP2C9, and CYP3A4).[66,67] Similarly, in a study that included eight subjects with acute hepatitis (out of 18 total subjects with liver disease), antipyrine clearance was decreased compared with controls, and this was most pronounced in patients with encephalopathy.[68] Of note, an in vivo test of CYP1A2 as a measure of liver function (LiMAx test) showed decreased CYP1A2 function in patients with ALF, with lower function in patients with ALF without spontaneous recovery than in patients with ALF with spontaneous recovery.[69] For low E_H drugs, changes in protein binding can also affect metabolism (see earlier text). Specifically, low E_H drugs with high protein binding may be sensitive to alterations in protein binding that may be present in ALF.[60]

Phase II enzymes may also be affected by ALF, although they are generally thought to be less affected than phase I enzymes in chronic liver diseases.[60] For example, the metabolism of benzodiazepines eliminated by phase II reactions (e.g., oxazepam, temazepam, lorazepam) may be less likely to have reduced clearance than benzodiazepines metabolized by phase I reactions (e.g., midazolam, diazepam).[70] In general, sulfonation reactions are more affected than glucuronidation.[60] Acute liver failure is often associated with renal dysfunction, which affects the renal clearance of drugs, and should be accounted for when selecting a dosing regimen.

Guidelines for Drug Dosing in ALF

The relative paucity of data regarding pharmacokinetic changes in ALF, in combination with the variability in the presentation of ALF, limits the ability to develop specific dosing guidelines. However, several generalizations may be made. First, when available, serum drug concentrations should be monitored to assist in drug dosing in ALF, and when possible, monitoring of free drug concentrations may be preferred (to monitoring of total concentrations).[62] Unfortunately, serum concentration monitoring is available for only a minority of drugs used clinically.

For some drugs, dosing recommendations based on the CTP score may be available; however, these recommendations are generally based on chronic liver diseases, not ALF.[62] The CTP classification assigns points according to the presence of ascites and encephalopathy, as well as serum bilirubin,

Table 28.7 Summary of Potential Pharmacokinetic Changes in Acute Liver Failure

Pharmacokinetic Parameter	Potential Change	Recommendation
Enteral bioavailability	• May be increased, particularly with high E_H drugs	• Consider parenteral formulation if available • Consider lower dose - A conservative approach is to assume 100% bioavailability of high E_H drugs, and dose using the formula: adjusted initial dose = (normal dose × bioavailability in normal liver function)/100[a]
Volume of distribution	• Increases in free concentrations of drugs highly bound to albumin • Potential increases in volume of distribution of hydrophilic drugs in the setting of ascites/edema	• Consider monitoring free drug concentrations, if available • Account for changes in protein binding when interpreting total drug concentrations • Consider higher loading doses for hydrophilic drugs (e.g., aminoglycosides) in the setting of ascites

Clearance	• Impaired hepatic drug metabolism by CYP enzymes
	• High E_H drugs are more sensitive to alterations in hepatic blood flow (e.g., during shock)
	• Low E_H drugs are more sensitive to alterations in CYP activity and protein binding
		• Consider therapeutic drug monitoring, if available
		• For drugs with guidelines based on CTP score, consider using clinical characteristics to estimate a CTP score and follow guidelines for severe disease[b]
		• In the absence of dosing guidelines based on CTP score, the following guidelines may be considered:
		  - For high E_H drugs administered orally: initial maintenance dose = (normal dose × bioavailability in normal liver function)/100[a]
		  - For high E_H drugs administered intravenously: initial maintenance dose = normal dose[a]
		  - For low E_H drugs with low binding to albumin (< 90% binding): initial dose = normal initial dose,[a] maintenance dose should be reduced to 50% of normal in patients with calculated CTP class A, reduced to 25% of normal dose in calculated CTP class B; for calculated CTP class C, avoid drugs without proven safety in this population, or initiate low dose and monitor therapy closely[a]
		  - For low E_H drugs with high binding to albumin (≥ 90% binding): monitor therapy closely[a]
		  - For intermediate E_H drugs, initial dose is the low range of normal dose; maintenance dose should be adjusted on the basis of guidelines for low E_H drugs
		• Closely monitor patients for efficacy and signs of toxicity
		• Adjust doses as necessary on the basis of renal function

[a]Adapted from: Delco F, Tchambaz L, Schlienger R, et al. Dose adjustment in patients with liver disease. Drug Saf 2005;28:529-45; and Perianez-Parraga L, Martinez-Lopez I, Ventayol-Bosch P, et al. Drug dosage recommendations in patients with chronic liver disease. Rev Esp Enferm Dig 2012;104:165-84.
[b]The CTP (Child-Pugh) score was not developed for use in acute liver failure.
E_H = hepatic extraction ratio.

albumin, and prothrombin time (Table 28.5).[32] The patient is classified as having mild, moderate, or severe disease. Although the CTP score was not developed for the intent of drug dosing, the FDA has included its use in a guidance statement for pharmacokinetic studies in hepatic impairment, and dosing guidelines based on the CTP score are included in the labeling of some drugs (see Table 28.6 for examples). In the absence of dosing recommendations specific to ALF, guidelines based on the CTP score may be used as an initial guide to dose drugs in ALF (i.e., either using patient characteristics to calculate a CTP score or assuming the patient has severe disease). For drugs with no dosing guidelines based on CTP scores, doses may be adjusted on the basis of a drug's E_H and protein binding (see Table 28.7).[70,71]

It is likely that drugs with a high E_H will have an increased enteral bioavailability in ALF; in these cases, administering lower doses (and gradually titrating doses on the basis of response and toxicity) or using parenteral administration may be warranted. If enteral administration of a drug with high E_H is required, a conservative approach is to assume 100% bioavailability of these agents and to dose on the basis of the following formula: adjusted initial dose = (normal dose × bioavailability in normal liver function)/100.[70] Acute liver failure is often associated with acute renal failure, which may warrant a dose adjustment of drugs that are cleared through the kidneys. Furthermore, management of ALF and acute renal failure may require the use of extracorporeal support systems (e.g., molecular adsorbent recirculating systems, renal replacement therapy). Information regarding drug dosing in renal failure and during use of extracorporeal support systems is found in Chapter 41, "Drug Dosing in Special ICU Populations." In all cases, patients should be closely monitored for signs of both efficacy and toxicity. A summary of the guidelines for drug dosing in ALF is presented in Table 28.7.

REFERENCES

1. Lee WM, Larson AM, Stravitz RT. AASLD Position Paper: The Management of Acute Liver Failure: Update 2011. 2011:1-79. Available at www.aasld.org/sites/default/files/guideline_documents/alfenhanced.pdf. Accessed June 2015.
2. Bernal W, Auzinger G, Dhawan A, et al. Acute liver failure. Lancet 2010;376:190-201.
3. Lee WM, Squires RH Jr, Nyberg SL, et al. Acute liver failure: summary of a workshop. Hepatology 2008;47:1401-15.
4. Bernal W, Wendon J. Acute liver failure. N Engl J Med 2013;369:2525-34.
5. Whitehouse T, Wendon J. Acute liver failure. Best Pract Res Clin Gastroenterol 2013;27:757-69.
6. Acute Liver Failure Study Group [homepage on the Internet]. Available at www.utsouthwestern.edu/labs/acute-liver/clinical-trials/patient-enrollment.html. Accessed August 27, 2015.
7. Olson JC, Kamath PS. Acute-on-chronic liver failure: concept, natural history, and prognosis. Curr Opin Crit Care 2011;17:165-9.
8. Sundaram V, Shaikh OS. Acute liver failure: current practice and recent advances. Gastroenterol Clin North Am 2011;40:523-39.
9. Wang DW, Yin YM, Yao YM. Advances in the management of acute liver failure. World J Gastroenterol 2013;19:7069-77.
10. Larsen FS, Bjerring PN. Acute liver failure. Curr Opin Crit Care 2011;17:160-4.
11. Rutherford A, Chung RT. Acute liver failure: mechanisms of hepatocyte injury and regeneration. Semin Liver Dis 2008;28:167-74.
12. Chung RT, Stravitz RT, Fontana RJ, et al. Pathogenesis of liver injury in acute liver failure. Gastroenterology 2012;143:e1-e7.
13. Malhi H, Gores GJ, Lemasters JJ. Apoptosis and necrosis in the liver: a tale of two deaths? Hepatology 2006;43:S31-44.
14. Ostapowicz G, Fontana RJ, Schiodt FV, et al. Results of a prospective study of acute liver failure at 17 tertiary care centers in the United States. Ann Intern Med 2002;137:947-54.
15. Ichai P, Samuel D. Epidemiology of liver failure. Clin Res Hepatol Gastroenterol 2011;35:610-7.
16. Chun LJ, Tong MJ, Busuttil RW, et al. Acetaminophen hepatotoxicity and acute liver failure. J Clin Gastroenterol 2009;43:342-9.
17. Khandelwal N, James LP, Sanders C, et al.; Acute Liver Failure Study G. Unrecognized acetaminophen toxicity as a cause of indeterminate acute liver failure. Hepatology 2011;53:567-76.
18. Hodgman MJ, Garrard AR. A review of acetaminophen poisoning. Crit Care Clin 2012;28:499-516.
19. Bunchorntavakul C, Reddy KR. Acetaminophen-related hepatotoxicity. Clin Liver Dis 2013;17:587-607, viii.
20. Lee WM, Seremba E. Etiologies of acute liver failure. Curr Opin Crit Care 2008;14:198-201.
21. Grant LM, Rockey DC. Drug-induced liver injury. Curr Opin Gastroenterol 2012;28:198-202.
22. Reuben A, Koch DG, Lee WM. Acute Liver Failure Study Group. Drug-induced acute liver failure: results of a U.S. multicenter, prospective study. Hepatology 2010;52:2065-76.
23. Chalasani N, Bonkovsky HL, Fontana R, et al. Features and outcomes of 899 patients with drug-induced liver injury: the DILIN Prospective Study. Gastroenterology 2015;148:1340-52 e7.
24. Fontana RJ, Hayashi PH, Gu J, et al. Idiosyncratic drug-induced liver injury is associated with substantial morbidity and mortality within 6 months from onset. Gastroenterology 2014;147:96-108 e4.
25. Lee WM. Drug-induced acute liver failure. Clin Liver Dis 2013;17:575-86, viii.
26. Suk KT, Kim DJ. Drug-induced liver injury: present and future. Clin Mol Hepatol 2012;18:249-57.
27. Taylor RM, Tujios S, Jinjuvadia K, et al. Short and long-term outcomes in patients with acute liver failure due to ischemic hepatitis. Dig Dis Sci 2012;57:777-85.
28. Bernuau J, Goudeau A, Poynard T, et al. Multivariate analysis of prognostic factors in fulminant hepatitis B. Hepatology 1986;6:648-51.
29. O'Grady JG, Alexander GJ, Hayllar KM, et al. Early indicators of prognosis in fulminant hepatic failure. Gastroenterology 1989;97:439-45.
30. Cox NR, Mohanty SR. Acute liver failure. Hosp Physician 2009:7-15.
31. Ge PL, Du SD, Mao YL. Advances in preoperative assessment of liver function. Hepatobiliary Pancreat Dis Int 2014;13:361-70.
32. U.S. Food and Drug Administration (FDA). Guidance for Industry: Pharmacokinetics in Patients with Impaired Hepatic Function: Study Design, Data Analysis, and Impact on Dosing and Labeling. Available at www.fda.gov/downloads/drugs/guidancecomplianceregulatoryinformation/guidances/ucm072123.pdf. Accessed August 27, 2015.
33. Polson J. Assessment of prognosis in acute liver failure. Semin Liver Dis 2008;28:218-25.
34. Shakil AO, Kramer D, Mazariegos GV, et al. Acute liver failure: clinical features, outcome analysis, and applicability of prognostic criteria. Liver Transpl 2000;6:163-9.
35. Anand AC, Nightingale P, Neuberger JM. Early indicators of prognosis in fulminant hepatic failure: an assessment of the King's criteria. J Hepatol 1997;26:62-8.
36. Malinchoc M, Kamath PS, Gordon FD, et al. A model to predict poor survival in patients undergoing transjugular intrahepatic portosystemic shunts. Hepatology 2000;31:864-71.

37. Lee HS, Choi GH, Joo DJ, et al. Prognostic value of model for end-stage liver disease scores in patients with fulminant hepatic failure. Transplant Proc 2013;45:2992-4.

38. Conn HO, Leevy CM, Vlahcevic ZR, et al. Comparison of lactulose and neomycin in the treatment of chronic portal-systemic encephalopathy. A double blind controlled trial. Gastroenterology 1977;72:573-83.

39. Dhiman RK, Jain S, Maheshwari U, et al. Early indicators of prognosis in fulminant hepatic failure: an assessment of the Model for End-Stage Liver Disease (MELD) and King's College Hospital criteria. Liver Transpl 2007;13:814-21.

40. Yantorno SE, Kremers WK, Ruf AE, et al. MELD is superior to King's College and Clichy's criteria to assess prognosis in fulminant hepatic failure. Liver Transpl 2007;13:822-8.

41. Parkash O, Mumtaz K, Hamid S, et al. MELD score: utility and comparison with King's College criteria in non-acetaminophen acute liver failure. J Coll Physicians Surg Pak 2012;22:492-6.

42. Fikatas P, Lee JE, Sauer IM, et al. APACHE III score is superior to King's College Hospital criteria, MELD score and APACHE II score to predict outcomes after liver transplantation for acute liver failure. Transplant Proc 2013;45:2295-301.

43. Guler N, Unalp O, Guler A, et al. Glasgow coma scale and APACHE-II scores affect the liver transplantation outcomes in patients with acute liver failure. Hepatobiliary Pancreat Dis Int 2013;12:589-93.

44. Wlodzimirow KA, Eslami S, Chamuleau RA, et al. Prediction of poor outcome in patients with acute liver failure—systematic review of prediction models. PLoS One 2012;7:e50952.

45. Pyleris E, Giannikopoulos G, Dabos K. Pathophysiology and management of acute liver failure. Ann Gastroenterol 2010;23:257-65.

46. Stravitz RT, Kramer AH, Davern T, et al. Intensive care of patients with acute liver failure: recommendations of the U.S. Acute Liver Failure Study Group. Crit Care Med 2007;35:2498-508.

47. Bass S, Zook N. Intravenous acetylcysteine for indications other than acetaminophen overdose. Am J Health Syst Pharm 2013;70:1496-501.

48. Brok J, Buckley N, Gluud C. Interventions for paracetamol (acetaminophen) overdose. Cochrane Database Syst Rev 2006;2:CD003328.

49. Sharma P, Sharma BC. Management of overt hepatic encephalopathy. J Clin Exp Hepatol 2015;5:S82-7.

50. Rahimi RS, Singal AG, Cuthbert JA, et al. Lactulose vs polyethylene glycol 3350—electrolyte solution for treatment of overt hepatic encephalopathy: the HELP randomized clinical trial. JAMA Intern Med 2014;174:1727-33.

51. Patidar KR, Bajaj JS. Antibiotics for the treatment of hepatic encephalopathy. Metab Brain Dis 2013;28:307-12.

52. XIFAXAN(R) oral tablets, rifaximin oral tablets [product information]. Morrisville, NC: Salix Pharmaceuticals, 2010.

53. Sharma BC, Sharma P, Lunia MK, et al. A randomized, double-blind, controlled trial comparing rifaximin plus lactulose with lactulose alone in treatment of overt hepatic encephalopathy. Am J Gastroenterol 2013;108:1458-63.

54. Vaquero J. Therapeutic hypothermia in the management of acute liver failure. Neurochem Int 2012;60:723-35.

55. Faybik P, Krenn CG. Extracorporeal liver support. Curr Opin Crit Care 2013;19:149-53.

56. Alqahtani SA. Update in liver transplantation. Curr Opin Gastroenterol 2012;28:230-8.

57. Findlay JY. Patient selection and preoperative evaluation for transplant surgery. Anesthesiol Clin 2013;31:689-704.

58. Verbeeck RK. Pharmacokinetics and dosage adjustment in patients with hepatic dysfunction. Eur J Clin Pharmacol 2008;64:1147-61.

59. Rodighiero V. Effects of liver disease on pharmacokinetics. An update. Clin Pharmacokinet 1999;37:399-431.

60. Budingen FV, Gonzalez D, Tucker AN, et al. Relevance of liver failure for anti-infective agents: from pharmacokinetic alterations to dosage adjustments. Ther Adv Infect Dis 2014;2:17-42.

61. Lin S, Smith BS. Drug dosing considerations for the critically ill patient with liver disease. Crit Care Nurs Clin North Am 2010;22:335-40.

62. Nguyen HM, Cutie AJ, Pham DQ. How to manage medications in the setting of liver disease with the application of six questions. Int J Clin Pract 2010;64:858-67.

63. McLean AJ, Morgan DJ. Clinical pharmacokinetics in patients with liver disease. Clin Pharmacokinet 1991;21:42-69.

64. Villeneuve JP, Pichette V. Cytochrome P450 and liver diseases. Curr Drug Metab 2004;5:273-82.

65. Albarmawi A, Czock D, Gauss A, et al. CYP3A activity in severe liver cirrhosis correlates with Child-Pugh and model for end-stage liver disease (MELD) scores. Br J Clin Pharmacol 2014;77:160-9.

66. Engel G, Hofmann U, Heidemann H, et al. Antipyrine as a probe for human oxidative drug metabolism: identification of the cytochrome P450 enzymes catalyzing 4-hydroxyantipyrine, 3-hydroxymethylantipyrine, and norantipyrine formation. Clin Pharmacol Ther 1996;59:613-23.

67. Forrest JA, Roscoe P, Prescott LF, et al. Abnormal drug metabolism after barbiturate and paracetamol overdose. Br Med J 1974;4:499-502.

68. Andreasen PB, Ranek L. Liver failure and drug metabolism. Scand J Gastroenterol 1975;10:293-7.

69. Lock JF, Kotobi AN, Malinowski M, et al. Predicting the prognosis in acute liver failure: results from a retrospective pilot study using the LiMAx test. Ann Hepatol 2013;12:556-62.

70. Delco F, Tchambaz L, Schlienger R, et al. Dose adjustment in patients with liver disease. Drug Saf 2005;28:529-45.

71. Perianez-Parraga L, Martinez-Lopez I, Ventayol-Bosch P, et al. Drug dosage recommendations in patients with chronic liver disease. Rev Esp Enferm Dig 2012;104:165-84.

Chapter 29
Acute Gastrointestinal Bleeding: Prophylaxis and Treatment

Salmaan Kanji, Bsc. Pharm, Pharm.D.; and David Williamson, B. Pharm, M.Sc., Ph.D., BCPS

LEARNING OBJECTIVES

1. Differentiate between the typical presentation of upper and lower gastrointestinal (GI) bleeding.
2. Identify risk factors for clinically relevant GI bleeding in the intensive care unit.
3. Identify measures for the primary prevention of both upper and lower GI bleeding.
4. Individualize the reversal of drug-associated bleeding according to the likely offending agent.
5. Understand the role of acid-suppressive therapy and other hemostatic agents in the acute management of clinically significant GI bleeding.
6. Identify strategies for the secondary prevention of GI bleeding using risk stratification tools.
7. Understand the role of *Helicobacter pylori* screening and treatment in the setting of peptic ulcer disease.
8. Consider the risks and benefits of reintroducing anticoagulation, antiplatelet therapies, and NSAIDs.

ABBREVIATIONS IN THIS CHAPTER

COX-2	Cyclooxygenase-2	NSAID	Nonsteroidal anti-inflammatory drug
FFP	Fresh frozen plasma	PCC	Prothrombin complex concentrate
H_2RB	Histamine-2 receptor blocker	PPI	Proton pump inhibitor
ICU	Intensive care unit	SRMD	Stress-related mucosal disease
LMWH	Low-molecular-weight heparin		

INTRODUCTION

Acute upper and lower gastrointestinal bleeding (GI) are common conditions that require admission to the intensive care unit (ICU) or complicate the stay of patients admitted for other ailments. Despite advances in endoscopic and pharmacologic therapies, morbidity and mortality associated with upper and lower GI bleeding remain significant.[1,2] In addition, the epidemiology of GI bleeding is evolving, given that a decrease in the incidence of upper GI bleeding and an increase in the incidence of lower GI bleeding have occurred in recent years.[3]

Peptic ulcer disease remains the most common cause of GI bleeding. Nonsteroidal anti-inflammatory drugs (NSAIDs) and aspirin use as well as *Helicobacter pylori* infection are the primary causes.[4,5] Lower GI bleeding is not as well studied as upper GI bleeding and remains likely underreported because many patients with bleeding remain without medical evaluation.[6] Three levels of bleeding, ranging from occult to moderate to severe, show the gravity of the disease.[7] Diverticular disease is the most common cause of lower GI bleeding. In the critically ill, mesenteric ischemia and ischemic colitis are also common. Admission to the ICU for upper and lower GI bleeding is determined by the presence of hypotension, respiratory failure, cardiac ischemia, and new neurological dysfunction.

CLINICAL PRESENTATION AND PATHOPHYSIOLOGY

Upper GI Bleeding

Upper GI bleeding is defined as bleeding originating from the esophagus, stomach, or duodenum.[7] Clinically important upper GI bleeding has been defined as macroscopic bleeding causing hemodynamic instability or necessitating blood transfusions. The most common presentations for upper GI bleeding are hematemesis, vomiting of fresh blood or coffee ground–like matter, and melena, which are black and tarry stools. Hematochezia, the passage of fresh blood with stools, may also be present in upper GI bleeding, most often when the bleeding is clinically significant. Common causes of upper GI bleeding include duodenal and gastric ulcer disease, erosive gastritis, esophageal variceal hemorrhage, and Mallory-Weiss tears (Box 29.1). In critically ill patients, stress-related mucosal disease (SRMD) is a common cause of ICU-acquired GI bleeding. Because significant bleeding reduces intravascular volume, it commonly presents with systemic symptoms such as resting tachycardia and hypotension or postural changes in blood pressure.[8]

The pathophysiology of upper GI bleeding varies according to cause. Peptic ulcer disease is mainly caused by *H. pylori* infection.[9] This gram-negative bacteria causes inflammation of the gastric and duodenal mucosa, which renders the mucosa more vulnerable to ulceration that can progress to the submucosa and damage arterial walls.[7,10] The NSAIDs inhibit cyclooxygenase and modify prostaglandin production, thereby reducing the protection provided by the mucosa. In much the same way as *H. pylori*, NSAID use enables the formation of mucosal ulcerations. Whereas *H. pylori* is responsible for more duodenal than gastric ulcers, NSAIDs have a more predominant effect on the stomach than on the duodenum.[7] In the presence of both pathologic factors, the risk of ulceration seems to be additive.[11] In addition, drugs that inhibit platelet aggregation (e.g., selective serotonin reuptake inhibitors or the coagulation cascade) increase the risk of GI bleeding in patients with preexisting mucosal damage.[12]

Stress-related mucosal disease develops when critical illness induces a reduction in cardiac output, catecholamine-induced vasoconstriction, and proinflammatory cytokine release. The ensuing splanchnic hypoperfusion induces an imbalance between oxygen delivery and demand, inducing mucosal ischemia and a reduction in the capacity to neutralize hydrogen ions. A reduction in motility as well as a reduction in protective mucus production also contribute to the development of SRMD (Figure 29.1).[13] The initial mucosal injury can remain superficial and lead to occult blood loss from the bleeding of mucosal capillaries. In certain cases, the injury can evolve to larger vessels and cause severe bleeding.

Mallory-Weiss tears are longitudinal lacerations to the mucosa of the stomach cardia or at the gastroesophageal junction that are caused by a sudden increase in intra-abdominal pressure, which is most often caused by vomiting.[14] Initially described in patients with acute alcohol ingestion, Mallory-Weiss tears are often described in other conditions associated with repeated vomiting (i.e., chemotherapy, gastroenteritis). Esophageal varices develop as the result of portal hypertension secondary to liver cirrhosis and can be life threatening. Because the management and outcomes are different from those for other causes of upper GI bleeding, this subject is beyond the scope of this chapter and will be covered with liver diseases (Chapter 28).

Lower GI Bleeding

Lower GI bleeding is defined as bleeding from the gut distal to the ligament of Treitz. Hematochezia is the most common feature, but melena can also be present, especially in patients with bleeds originating from the distal small bowel and colon. The most common causes of lower GI bleeding are colonic diverticulosis, colorectal malignancy, inflammatory bowel disease, anorectal disease, mesenteric ischemia, and ischemic colitis.[2,15,16] Colonic diverticulosis develops with age as the colonic wall weakens, creating protrusions, usually at the insertion of the vasa recta artery.[17] Bleeding is secondary to the rupture of this artery and spontaneously resolves in many cases. However, in 3%–5% of cases, bleeding can be important.[18] Clinically significant bleeding secondary to diverticular disease has been associated with diabetes, hypertension, anticoagulation, and ischemic heart disease.[18] Mesenteric ischemia and ischemic colitis arise from an imbalance between oxygen supply and demand in the small bowel and colon. Thrombosis, emboli, and vasoconstriction caused by medications such as vasopressors are responsible for mesenteric ischemia.[7] The main causes of mesenteric ischemia are arterial embolism, arterial thrombosis, small vessel occlusion, and venous thrombosis. Atherosclerosis and cardiac disease (valvular disease, atrial arrhythmias, ventricular dilatation) are important risk factors.[19] A hypercoagulable state, hypovolemia, and previous arterial emboli are also associated with mesenteric ischemia.[20] Ischemic colitis is caused by reduced perfusion to the colon, and bleeding occurs as the result of mucosal necrosis. Colon carcinomas represent an important proportion of rectal bleeding in older patients. These tumors tend to bleed much more slowly.[21] Crohn disease, ulcerative colitis, hemorrhoids, and anal fissures are other common causes of lower GI bleeding.

Box 29.1. Causes of Upper GI Bleeding

Common
Peptic ulcer disease (gastric and duodenal ulcers) (28%–59%)

Variceal bleeding (6%–14%)

Gastritis/duodenitis (9%–31%)

Esophagitis (4%–18%)

Mallory-Weiss tears (4%–7%)

Less common
Malignancy (2%–4%)

No diagnosis (8%–25%)

Others

Adapted from: van Leerdam ME. Epidemiology of acute upper gastrointestinal bleeding. Best Pract Res Clin Gastroenterol 2008;22:209-24.

Epidemiology

The reported incidence of upper GI bleeding leading to hospitalization varies from 37 to 172 per 100,000 adults.[1,22] Differences in reported incidents are attributable to variations in studied populations and study periods. Duodenal and gastric ulcers represent the most common etiologies of upper GI bleeds, followed by Mallory-Weiss tears and esophagitis.[22] The reported incidence of lower GI bleeding in the general population varies from 22 to 87 per 100,000 adults.[2,22]

Peptic Ulcer Disease

The hospitalization rates for peptic ulcer bleeding have been declining in recent years because of reduced *H. pylori* infection rates and increased use of proton pump inhibitors (PPIs).[23,24] In the United States, the age/sex-adjusted incidence of peptic ulcer bleeding decreased from 41.8 to 35.7 per 100,000 between 2001 and 2009.[25] In Spain, the incidence of hospitalization for upper GI bleeding decreased from 54.6 in 1996 to 25.8 per 100,000 person-years in 2006.[23]

Stress-Related Mucosal Disease

Endoscopic studies suggest that most critically ill patients develop gastric erosions related to SRMD during the ICU stay.[26] However, the incidence of clinically important upper GI bleeding, defined as the presence of hematemesis, bloody GI aspirate, or melena, is 1.5%–2.8% in the critically ill.[27,28] In patients with risk factors such as mechanical ventilation and coagulopathy, the incidence increases to 3.7%.[28] Nevertheless, these data were published 15–20 years ago, and because the treatment of critically ill patients has evolved during the past decades, the incidence of SRMD is declining.[29] Contemporary studies tend to suggest a decline in the incidence of clinically important upper GI bleeding.[29,30]

Mallory-Weiss Syndrome

Mallory-Weiss tears are a common cause of upper GI bleeding and represent 3%–12% of cases.[14,22] However, most cases resolve spontaneously, and clinically significant bleeding is rare.[14]

Lower GI Bleeding

The incidence of lower GI bleeding requiring hospitalization, for both acute and occult bleeding, is reported to be 20–33 per 100,000 in studies from the United States and Spain.[2,31] A recent population-based study of patients undergoing colonoscopy in Iceland reported a crude incidence of 87 per 100,000 per year.[15]

RISK FACTORS

The risk of upper GI bleeding is significantly increased in older age. Studies have reported a 4-fold increase in the risk in patients 75 years and older.[32] Nonsteroidal anti-inflammatory drugs are a major risk factor for upper GI bleeding caused by peptic ulcers. Although all NSAIDs are associated with an increased risk of upper GI bleeding, traditional NSAIDs are associated with a greater risk of upper GI bleeding than are cyclooxygenase-2 (COX-2) selective inhibitors.[33] Among the traditional NSAIDs, ibuprofen seems to have the best safety profile, whereas ketorolac has the worst.[33] As previously mentioned, *H. pylori* also plays an important role in the pathogenesis and risk of developing upper GI bleeding.

In patients with GI bleeding, risk factors identifiable on admission that are associated with an increased risk of developing acritical illness include coagulopathy, hypotension, neurologic dysfunction, and an Acute Physiology and Chronic Health Evaluation II (APACHE II) score greater than 15.[34] When comparing upper and lower GI bleeding, male sex and NSAID use have been associated with an increased risk of upper GI bleeding, whereas the number of comorbidities and a recent diagnosis were associated with an increased risk of lower GI bleeding.[31]

Peptic Ulcer Disease

H. pylori and NSAIDs are the two main causes of peptic ulcer disease. As rates of *H. pylori*–associated peptic ulcer disease have declined, some studies have reported an increase in low-dose-aspirin–associated disease.[35] Several demographic and lifestyle risk factors have been associated with complicated peptic ulcer disease. Older age, male sex, significant alcohol consumption, tobacco use, comorbidities, and psychological stress have been linked, although not always consistently across studies, to an increased risk of complicated peptic ulcer disease.[36,37] Serotonin reuptake inhibitors have also been associated with a modest increase in upper GI bleeding, which significantly increases in the presence of NSAID use.[38] Patients at high risk of NSAID-associated GI bleeding are those with a history of complicated ulcer and two other risk factors (age older than 65 years, high-dose NSAID therapy, and concurrent use of aspirin, corticosteroids, or anticoagulants).[39] Patients with one risk factor or a history of uncomplicated ulcer are considered at moderate risk.

Stress-Related Mucosal Disease

Historically, SRMD has been associated with head trauma (Cushing ulcers) and major burns (Curling ulcers). In the critically ill, the risk of SRMD has been associated with respiratory failure and coagulopathy. The presence of both factors has been associated with a 3.7% incidence of GI bleeding compared with 0.1% in patients without these risk factors.[28] Other factors commonly associated with SRMD include hypotension, sepsis, surgery, hepatic failure, and renal failure.[13,27] Receiving enteral nutrition is an independent protective factor, even in the presence of ranitidine.[27]

Mallory-Weiss Syndrome

Mallory and Weiss first described the condition in 1929 in the setting of acute alcohol ingestion.[40] Other factors that have been associated with Mallory-Weiss tears include NSAID use, anticoagulation, and the presence of hiatal hernia.[41]

Lower GI Bleeding

As the incidence of diverticulosis and ischemia increases with age, so does the incidence of lower GI bleeding.[2] In a recent study, the age-standardized incidence rate of acute lower GI bleeding increased from 18 per 100,000 per year in patients 25–39 years of age to 187 and 690 per 100,000 per year in patients 60–79 and 80–105 years of age, respectively.[15] Male sex has been inconsistently associated with an increased risk of lower GI bleeding.[2,31] The presence of comorbidities and the use of NSAIDs, antiplatelet agents including aspirin, and anticoagulants have also been associated with an increased risk of lower GI bleeding.[42] Rebleeding occurs more often in older patients and those exposed to NSAIDs and nonaspirin antiplatelet agents.[13] Finally, independent risk factors for clinically significant (compared with nonsignificant) bleeding include age, non-hemorrhoidal bleeding, and combined use of aspirin and warfarin.[15]

OUTCOMES

The consequences and complications associated with upper and lower GI bleeding are broad and include anemia, emergency surgery, cardiac ischemia, and hospitalization, as well as an increased risk of death.[43] The mortality associated with upper GI bleeding has been declining in recent years.[9] A recent database study from the United States reported a 2.45% case fatality for upper GI bleeding.[25] Intensive care unit–acquired GI bleeding in mechanically ventilated patients has been associated with an increased risk of death.[43] Clinically important upper GI bleeding in critically ill patients has also been associated with an increase in length of stay secondary to bleeding of 3.8–7.9 days.[43]

Many risk factors are associated with unfavorable outcomes in patients with an upper GI bleed, including increasing age, APACHE II score, comorbid conditions, liver disease, hypotension or shock on presentation, hospitalization, and rebleeding.[1,32,44,45] Rebleeding occurs in 7%–16% of patients after endoscopic treatment and has a major influence on the outcomes of upper GI bleeding.[1,10] The reported mortality rate in patients with recurrent bleeding is greater than 30%.[46]

The mortality risk appears to be similar when comparing peptic ulcer disease with non-ulcer causes of upper GI hemorrhage.[47,48] In the specific case of Mallory-Weiss syndrome, age older than 65 years and comorbidities are independently associated with an increased risk of mortality.[48]

In patients with lower GI bleeding, the reported mortality is 2.2%–8.8%.[16,31,49,50] When patients with lower GI bleeding were compared with those with upper GI bleeding, one study reported a greater risk of mortality (8.8% vs. 5.5%) and an increased length of hospitalization (11.6 vs. 7.7 days).[31] Risk factors for unfavorable outcomes in patients with a lower GI bleed include advanced age, hemodynamic instability, comorbid conditions, already being hospitalized, and use of certain drugs such as aspirin and NSAIDs.[2]

PREVENTION OF GI BLEEDING

Stress Ulcer Prophylaxis

Although clinically significant GI bleeding rarely occurs in critically ill patients, strategies to prevent stress ulcers have long been advocated in high-risk patients.[51,52] Stress ulcer prophylaxis is aimed at reducing the risk of clinically important upper GI bleeding and consequently improving outcomes such as length of stay in critically ill patients. Stress ulcer prophylaxis is recommended in patients with risk factors for SRMD, notably coagulopathy and mechanical ventilation for more than 48 hours.[51,52] Several pharmacologic agents have been advocated for preventing stress ulcers, including antacids, sucralfate, histamine-2 receptor blockers (H_2RBs), and PPIs.[53] Antacids, titrated to obtain a gastric pH above 3.5, reduced GI bleeding.[54] Frequent administration and the risk of drug interactions significantly limit antacid use. Sucralfate, which protects the gastric mucosa by forming a cytoprotective barrier, reduces ulcerations compared with placebo.[26] Histamine-2 receptor blockers reduce gastric acid and secretions by competitively inhibiting histamine binding to parietal cell receptors. In a pivotal clinical trial, H_2RBs reduced the relative and absolute risks of clinically important GI bleeding by 66% and 2.1%, respectively, compared with sulcralfate.[55] Proton pump inhibitors increase gastric pH by inactivating the parietal cell H^+/K^+ ATPase enzyme. Although no large and adequately powered studies compare PPIs with H_2RBs, a recent meta-analysis suggests that PPIs are more effective at reducing the risk of clinically significant GI bleeding.[56] In North America, observational studies have shown that PPIs are the most commonly used agents in critically ill patients.[57] Although H_2RBs and PPIs reduce the risk of clinically significant GI bleeding, a corresponding impact on mortality has not been shown.[58]

The use of stress ulcer prophylaxis is not without risks. Using H_2RBs and PPIs in critically ill patients may be associated with infectious complications, particularly *Clostridium difficile*–associated diarrhea and nosocomial pneumonia. Given that gastric acid contents are protective against bacterial survival in the stomach, there is evidence that alkalizing agents such as PPIs and H_2RBs promote bacterial overgrowth.[59,60] However, evidence from randomized controlled trials supporting these associations is limited because nosocomial infections, and especially *C. difficile* infections, are rarely reported. In a recent meta-analysis comparing PPIs with H$_2$RBs, investigators of eight trials reported on the risk of ventilator-associated pneumonia and found no difference in the risk of nosocomial pneumonia.[10] However, no studies reported on the risk of *C. difficile* infections. Several observational studies have assessed the association between PPI or H$_2$RB use and the risk of developing nosocomial pneumonia and *C. difficile*–associated diarrhea. Some studies of critically ill patients have reported an independent increased risk of nosocomial pneumonia with PPI use, whereas others have not found this association.[61-65] Different patient populations, differing definitions of nosocomial pneumonia, and residual confounding may account for these different findings. The risk of *C. difficile*–associated diarrhea is increased with PPI use in several observational studies, but not in others.[66-71] Variations in endemicity, susceptibility of populations, and presence of other risk factors such as the use of broad-spectrum antibiotics may explain these contrasting results.[72] In addition, patients taking H$_2$RBs seem to be at lower risk of contracting *C. difficile*–associated diarrhea compared with those taking PPIs.[73]

Because using H$_2$RBs and PPIs for stress ulcer prophylaxis has been questioned for efficacy and safety reasons, enteral nutrition alone has been suggested as a potential alternative to acid-suppressive therapies.[74] Studies have suggested that enteral nutrition improves mucosal blood flow and may increase gastric pH.[75] Because of observational data, some authors suggest using enteral nutrition as the only stress ulcer prophylaxis in most critically ill patients (excluding trauma and burn patients).[74] However, no randomized controlled trials have directly compared enteral nutrition with H$_2$RBs or PPIs.

Prevention of Drug-Induced/Associated GI Bleeding

Because NSAID, COX-2 inhibitor, and aspirin users have an increased risk of GI bleeding, mucosal protection strategies are used to prevent the development of peptic ulceration. Proton pump inhibitors, high-dose H$_2$RBs, and misoprostol all reduce the risk of peptic ulcers.[75] The COX-2 inhibitors are associated with a lower incidence of peptic ulcers than are the NSAIDs. However, the combined use of low-dose aspirin and COX-2 inhibitors is associated with the same risk of GI bleeding as the use of NSAIDs. In addition, this protective effect of COX-2 inhibitors is undermined by an increased risk of myocardial infarction.[76] Hence, recent recommendations for preventing NSAID-related ulcer complications consider both the GI risk (low, moderate, or high) and the cardiovascular risk (requirement of aspirin for preventing serious cardiovascular events). Risk factors for NSAID GI toxicity include age older than 65 years, high-dose NSAID therapy, a history of uncomplicated ulcer, and concurrent use of aspirin, corticosteroids, or anticoagulants. Patients with a history of a complicated ulcer (especially recent) or more than two risk factors are considered at high GI bleeding risk. Patients with one or two risk factors are considered at moderate GI bleeding risk. Patients with no risk factors are considered at low GI bleeding risk.

In patients at high cardiovascular risk, naproxen has been advocated as the NSAID of choice in combination with a PPI or misoprostol.[39] In patients who are also at high GI risk, avoiding NSAIDs and COX-2 inhibitors is recommended. In patients at low cardiovascular risk, using an NSAID alone is acceptable if the risk of GI bleeding is low. However, a PPI or misoprostol is suggested in patients at moderate GI risk. Finally, in patients at low cardiovascular risk and high risk of GI toxicity, avoiding NSAIDs, if possible, or using a COX-2 inhibitor combined with a PPI or misoprostol is recommended.[39]

APPROACH TO DIAGNOSIS

Data gathered from the history, physical assessment, and laboratory tests dictate the need for resuscitation, describe the severity of bleeding, identify the potential sources of bleeding, and facilitate the triage of further diagnostic or therapeutic interventions.[9] The initial assessment begins with an evaluation of hemodynamic stability. Patients presenting with hypotension, evidence of end-organ ischemia, or large volumes of blood loss need immediate resuscitation. In the clinical setting, most patients who present with upper GI bleeding have hematemesis or melena. Those presenting with melena or hematochezia are typically thought to have lower GI bleeding.

Upper GI Bleeding

Presentation with frank hematemesis typically suggests more severe bleeding than presentation with coffee ground emesis. Melena usually indicates upper GI bleeding, but it can also occur with bleeding from the distal small bowel or the proximal colon. Hematochezia usually indicates GI bleeding from the colon, but it can occur with massive upper GI bleeding. The history obtained from the patient or family member can also be valuable. Patients with a history of GI bleeding typically bleed from the same lesion. The approach to diagnosis and management may also be affected by a patient history of liver disease (and knowledge of existing varices or portal hypertension), peptic ulcer disease and its previous investigations, previous *H. pylori* treatment, malignancy, or alcohol abuse. A medication history specifically looking for use of NSAIDs, aspirin, anticoagulants, antiplatelet agents, and corticosteroids helps identify risk and potential causative factors. Patients taking iron supplements or bismuth-containing products may present with black stools, which can be mistaken for melena.

Patients presenting with hemodynamic instability need immediate resuscitation with crystalloid fluids and blood products. Patients may also present with orthostatic hypotension, confusion, tachycardia, supraventricular tachyarrhythmias, and cold or mottled extremities. The symptoms reported immediately preceding the acute event can also help predict the source of bleeding. Epigastric or right upper quadrant pain can be indicative of peptic ulcer bleeding, whereas reflux, dysphagia, and odynophagia may predict esophageal ulceration. Intractable vomiting, retching, or even coughing can precede hemorrhage from a Mallory-Weiss tear, and cachexia or significant involuntary weight loss may suggest malignancy.[77] Laboratory tests should include a complete blood cell count, serum electrolytes and chemistries, liver function tests, and coagulation studies. Initial hemoglobin values usually appear normal as patients are losing whole blood. With resuscitation and time, hemoglobin concentrations usually drop within 24 hours.

Lower GI Bleeding

Patients with lower GI bleeding typically present with hematochezia or (rarely) melena if they have right-sided colonic bleeding. Patient histories, physical assessments, and laboratory investigations play a similar role in suspected upper GI bleeding. The goals of initial assessment are to assess the severity of bleeding, triage the patient to the appropriate care setting, initiate resuscitation, and consider the potential source of bleeding. After resuscitation, diagnostic and potentially therapeutic interventions such as colonoscopy may be warranted.

INITIAL MANAGEMENT

Airway and Vascular Access

All patients with GI bleeding and hemodynamic instability should be admitted to the ICU for resuscitation, cardiac monitoring, and pulse oximetry. All patients should receive supplemental oxygen, and patients with decreased levels of consciousness, ongoing hematemesis, or respiratory distress may need endotracheal intubation. Intubation not only helps facilitate endoscopy, but also protects against the risk of aspiration. All patients should receive either a central venous catheter or two large-bore peripheral venous catheters for resuscitation.

Fluid Resuscitation and Blood Transfusion

Hemodynamic stabilization before endoscopy improves patient outcomes. Bleeding and/or hypotensive patients should receive intravenous crystalloid fluids such as normal saline or lactated Ringer solution (i.e., boluses of 500 mL over 30 minutes or less) while being typed and cross-matched for blood transfusions. The frequency and number of fluid boluses should be evaluated in the context of blood pressure response, acknowledging that over-resuscitation may also be harmful. Crystalloid resuscitation causes a dilution of the blood remaining in the vascular space and may result in increased bleeding from clot destabilization and dilution of factors that allow new clot formation.[78] Smaller, more frequent, boluses are more likely to result in the smallest effective volume administered to achieve hemodynamic stabilization.

Beyond evidence of massive hemorrhage, the decision to transfuse blood should be directed by measured hemoglobin concentrations. A randomized controlled trial of 921 adults with acute upper GI bleeding suggested that a restrictive transfusion practice is associated with improved outcomes compared with a liberal transfusion practice.[79] Patients in this trial were randomized to receive blood transfusions when hemoglobin concentrations fell below 7 g/dL (conservative arm) or 9 g/dL (liberal arm). Of note, patients with massive hemorrhage, low risk of further bleeding, acute coronary syndrome, or significant cardiovascular disease were excluded. About one-half of the patients in the study had peptic ulcer disease, whereas one-fourth had variceal bleeding. The conservative transfusion strategy was associated with a lower mortality (hazard ratio 0.55; 95% confidence interval, 0.33–0.92), less rebleeding, and fewer complications. All patients in this study underwent early endoscopy. In addition to blood, transfusion of fresh frozen plasma (FFP) is indicated for patients with significant coagulopathy (i.e., international normalized ratio [INR] greater than 1.5). Similarly, platelet transfusions are indicated for patients presenting with thrombocytopenia (i.e., platelet count less than 50,000/mm^3).[80]

Reversal of Drug-Associated Bleeding

Whenever possible, drugs implicated in causing or facilitating GI bleeding should be discontinued. In some cases, the effects of these drugs should be reversed (Table 29.1). The original indication for the drug in question, however, must be considered, and the risks and benefits of discontinuation/reversal must be considered. In some cases, consultation with a specialist may be warranted to fully assess the risks versus the benefits (i.e., reversal of a low-molecular-weight heparin [LMWH] for treatment of pulmonary embolism). Anti-inflammatory drugs such as NSAIDs and aspirin should be held to prevent further irritation to exposed ulcers and/or blood vessels.

If safe to do so, vitamin K antagonists (i.e., warfarin) should be reversed with FFP rather than vitamin K because the onset of activity with vitamin K can be delayed as long as 6–24 hours.[81] Prothrombin complex concentrates (PCCs) are also an alternative to FFP and may be considered together with vitamin K as an alternative to FFP. Four-factor

Table 29.1 Antidotes and Reversal Strategies for Drug-Associated Bleeding

Drug Associated with Bleeding	Antidote or Reversal Strategy	Comments
NSAID	Discontinue (or hold) NSAID therapy	
Aspirin, clopidogrel, other antiplatelet agents	Platelet transfusion ± DDAVP (0.3 mcg/kg IV over 30 min)	Minimal evidence supporting this practice. Risks and benefits of reversal must be considered
Warfarin	FFP (15–30 mL/kg IV) OR PCC[a] (i.e., Octaplex: four-factor PCC containing factors II, VII, IX, and X) AND vitamin K (5–10 mg IV over 20–60 min)	If only three-factor PCC is available (containing factors II, IX, X), it should be supplemented with FFP and vitamin K
Heparin and LMWH (i.e., enoxaparin, dalteparin, tinzaparin)	Heparin infusion: Protamine IV dose is based on the amount of heparin received in the past 2–2½ hr	1 unit of protamine neutralizes ~100 units of heparin. Maximal dose is 50 mg. The effect of LMWH is only 60%–75% reversed with protamine
	1–1.5 mg per 100 units of heparin (< 30 min since heparin)	
	0.5–0.75 mg per 100 units of heparin (30–120 min since heparin)	
	0.25–0.375 mg per 100 units of heparin (more than 2 hr since heparin)	
	Enoxaparin: 1 mg of protamine for every 1 mg of enoxaparin	
	Dalteparin and tinzaparin: 1 mg of protamine for every 100 anti-Xa units	
Direct factor Xa inhibitors (rivaroxaban, apixaban, edoxaban)	Four-factor PCC[a] (i.e., Octaplex; 50 units/kg) or activated PCC (i.e., FEIBA; 25–100 units/kg IV). If only three-factor PCC is available, it should be supplemented with FFP	Optimal dose has not been established. Recommended dosing is based on case reports
Direct thrombin inhibitors (i.e., dabigatran)	Activated PCC (i.e., FEIBA; 25–100 units/kg IV)	Optimal dose has not been established. Recommended dosing is based on case reports

[a]Octaplex dosing is based on the INR (INR < 4: 25 units/kg to a maximum of 2,500 units; INR = 4–6: 35 units/kg to a maximum of 3,500 units; INR > 6: 50 units/kg to max of 5,000 units).

DDAVP = desmopressin; FFP = fresh frozen plasma; IV = intravenous(ly); LMWH = low-molecular-weight heparin; NSAID = nonsteroidal anti-inflammatory drug; PCC = prothrombin complex concentrate.

PCCs such as Octaplex or Kcentra contain clotting factors II, VII, IX, and X and are prepared from human plasma. Although vitamin K administered intravenously is rarely associated with anaphylactic reactions, the onset of activity is faster than with other routes of administration and is more desirable in acute or major bleeding.

Anticoagulation with heparin or LMWH can be reversed with protamine sulfate, which binds to and inactivates heparin molecules that are subsequently cleared by the reticular endothelial system. Anaphylactic reactions, hypotension, and bronchospasm can occur because of histamine release, but these adverse effects are rare and typically transient. Furthermore, in the absence of heparin or at excessive doses, protamine has weak antiplatelet and anticoagulant activity. The clinical importance of these effects in patients who are bleeding is not well established, but they are easily avoided using the maximum dose of 50 mg.[82] The time elapsed since the last exposure to heparin should also be considered because less protamine is required if some of the heparin has already been eliminated.

Reversal of anticoagulation from unfractionated heparin is more predictable than from LMWH because protamine sulfate only partly reverses the effects of LMWH. Some studies suggest that protamine sulfate reverses only 60% of the antifactor Xa (anti-Xa) activity of LMWH.[83]

Reversal of anticoagulation from new oral anticoagulants (i.e., dabigatran, rivaroxaban, and apixaban) is a greater challenge as we wait for antidotes that are currently being developed and evaluated in clinical trials. Rivaroxaban and apixaban are inhibitors of factor Xa, and dabigatran is a direct thrombin inhibitor. Dabigatran has the longest half-life at 14–17 hours, whereas the half-lives of rivaroxaban and apixaban are 7–11 hours and 8–14 hours, respectively. Idarucizumab, a monoclonal antibody with a greater affinity for dabigatran than thrombin, may be the first antidote approved for use. Initial evidence suggests that idarucizumab rapidly and completely reverses the effects of dabigatran.[84] Andexanet, a recombinant, modified factor Xa molecule, is currently being evaluated for the reversal of anticoagulation from factor Xa inhibitors such as rivaroxaban and apixaban.[85] Phase III trials are currently under way. Although these agents represent promising options for patients who are bleeding, rapid reversal strategies are still required until these agents become available. Several prohemostatic agents or coagulation factor concentrates have been suggested, but human evidence is limited for the efficacy of these treatments. The PCCs (e.g., Octaplex and Kcentra) and the activated PCCs (e.g., FEIBA) can be tried to reverse the effects, with the choice of agent dependent on availability.[86] The PCCs appear to be less effective than the activated PCCs in reversing anticoagulation with dabigatran compared with rivaroxaban in healthy volunteers and ex vivo studies.[87,88] Evidence for activated factor VIIa is less compelling. Human evidence is limited to describe the efficacy and safety of these products in this setting.

Platelet transfusions are commonly administered in the setting of GI bleeding if patients are on antiplatelet agents, but this practice is not evidence based. The role of platelet transfusion is not well defined, but platelets may be indicated in patients on antiplatelet therapy (i.e., aspirin or clopidogrel). The risks of reversal must be considered according to the original indication of the drug (i.e., prevention of acute coronary syndrome or maintenance of stent patency).[89] Desmopressin has also been used in this setting because its presumed mechanism of action is the release of von Willebrand factor from endothelial cells, which in turn can stabilize platelets and promote binding to the endothelium. Bleeding times are shortened with desmopressin in healthy volunteers taking aspirin or ticlopidine, but evidence in patients who are bleeding is limited.[90,91]

Hemostatic Medications

Early initiation of acid-suppressive therapy in upper GI bleeding serves two purposes: (1) neutralization of gastric acid can improve the stabilization of blood clots and (2) continued therapy reduces rebleeding rates, hospital lengths of stay, and the need for blood transfusions, particularly in peptic ulcer disease treated endoscopically (Table 29.2).[92,93] The role of acid-suppressive therapy before endoscopy in undifferentiated bleeding is a source of controversy because of conflicting findings in clinical trials. A meta-analysis of six randomized controlled trials suggests that although there is no evidence that PPI therapy before endoscopy affects outcomes like mortality, rebleeding, or need for surgery, it reduces the stigmata of recent hemorrhage and subsequently the need for endoscopic therapy during the index endoscopy.[94] Proton pump inhibitors are preferred to H_2RAs and traditionally have been initiated as high-dose continuous infusions. Recent evidence suggests that high-dose continuous infusions are associated with no better outcomes than intermittent dosing strategies (i.e., intravenous pantoprazole or esomeprazole 40 mg twice daily).[95] However, some still advocate for high-dose therapy in patients with high-risk stigmata (i.e., Rockall scores greater than 6).[96] There is no evidence for the use of acid-suppressive therapy in the acute management of lower GI bleeding.

Tranexamic acid is an antifibrinolytic agent often used in surgical settings as a hemostatic drug. A recent systematic review suggests that, in the absence of acid-suppressive therapy and endoscopic treatment, a mortality benefit is associated with tranexamic acid. This effect did not occur, however, when only studies with patients who received conventional therapy were retained.[97] Given that acid-suppressive therapy plus endoscopic intervention (when indicated) is the standard of care, tranexamic acid currently has no role in the treatment of upper GI bleeding.

Prokinetic agents such as erythromycin and metoclopramide have also been studied in upper GI bleeding. Prokinetic therapy before endoscopy improves gastric emptying of blood, clots, and food to improve visualization at the time of endoscopy. Results from a meta-analysis of small trials suggest that both erythromycin and metoclopramide reduce the need for repeat endoscopy but that they affect other clinical outcomes.[98] There are more trials with erythromycin than with metoclopramide. Meta-analyses of erythromycin studies consistently show a reduced need for second endoscopy, but these meta-analyses also show inconsistent effects on other meaningful clinical outcomes compared with placebo.[99,100] Despite these limitations, erythromycin may be considered before endoscopy in patients with upper GI bleeding.

Vasopressin, somatostatin, and their synthetic analogs (terlipressin and octreotide, respectively) are vasoactive medications that reduce splanchnic blood flow. They are used to achieve hemostasis in variceal hemorrhage. Theoretically, the same mechanism would be beneficial in other sources of GI bleeding, but evidence is limited to support their use at this time. However, small, low-quality studies suggest a possible benefit of octreotide in reducing rebleeding rates from lower GI bleeding caused by angiodysplasia. Similar evidence suggests that octreotide leads to a reduction in bleeding time with endoscopically treated peptic ulcers but not for other causes of nonvariceal hemorrhage.[101-103]

Role of Endoscopy/Colonoscopy and Other Invasive Interventions

Early endoscopy (within 24 hours) is advocated for most patients to identify the source of bleeding, to assist in the triage of further interventions and patient management, and for use therapeutically to achieve hemostasis. For diagnosis, endoscopy is the definitive test. Endoscopic findings are typically described using the Forrest classification (class Ia: spurting hemorrhage; class Ib: oozing hemorrhage; class IIa: nonbleeding visible vessel; class IIb: adherent clot; class IIc: flat pigmented spot; class III: clean ulcer base).[104] The lesion's appearance can help determine both the patient's risk of rebleeding and the need for specific interventions. Although early endoscopy is recommended for most patients with hematemesis, its impact on the outcome is controversial. Studies describing its effect on resource use and patient outcome are conflicting.[105-108] Endoscopic treatments aimed at controlling bleeding may include injection of epinephrine, thermal coagulation, use of hemostatic clips or fibrin sealants, argon plasma coagulation, or a combination of these therapies.[109] Standard approaches to therapy usually involve a combination of treatments, depending on the location of the lesion and the endoscopist's preference.

Colonoscopy is the definitive test for lower GI bleeding once upper GI bleeding has been ruled out. Colonoscopy is used to visualize and assess the source and severity of bleeding, obtain samples for pathology, and provide therapeutic intervention. Urgent colonoscopy often is done without mechanical bowel preparation, which limits the ability to visualize the source of bleeding. If a patient is hemodynamically stable after resuscitation, colonoscopy is often delayed to allow time for adequate bowel preparation (i.e., enteral administration of 4 L of polyethylene glycol).[110] Similar to early endoscopy for upper GI bleeding, early colonoscopy has been associated with better triage of patients, improved resource use, and a reduction in the risk of rebleeding. However, these findings have not been consistent in clinical trials.[111-113] Other diagnostic tests such as radionuclide imaging and angiography can also be used to identify sources of bleeding. These noninvasive or minimally invasive tests require active bleeding at the time of the study to detect the source. These strategies are typically reserved for patients in whom colonoscopy is either not feasible because of severe bleeding or nondiagnostic with persistent or intermittent bleeding.[114]

In the past, surgery was the mainstay of treatment for both upper and lower GI bleeding. However, early

Table 29.2 Drug Therapy for Hemostasis and Prevention of Rebleeding

Indication	Drug Therapy	Comment
Hemostasis	*High-dose IV PPI therapy:* Pantoprazole 80 mg IV bolus, followed by 8 mg/hr for 72 hr or	Intermittent dosing is noninferior to high-dose therapy, although some still advocate the high-dose regimens for patients presenting with high-risk stigmata
	Esomeprazole 80 mg IV bolus, followed by 8 mg/hr for 72 hr	
	Intermittent-dose IV PPI therapy: Pantoprazole 40 mg IV BID	
	Esomeprazole 40 mg IV BID	
	Tranexamic acid 10 mg/kg IV QID or 1 g IV QID	Tranexamic acid most likely to be of benefit if endoscopy not available or delayed. Many different dosing regimens have been studied for a variety of indications. Others in addition to the recommendation here may also be appropriate
	Erythromycin 3 mg/kg IV over 20–30 min given 30–90 min before endoscopy	Erythromycin can enhance gastric emptying to facilitate endoscopy and may reduce the need for repeat endoscopy
	Octreotide 50–100 mcg IV bolus, followed by 25 mcg/hr for up to 3 days or until resolution of bleeding	According to small, low-quality studies, octreotide may reduce the risk of rebleeding in angiodysplasia-related GI bleeding. Similar small studies suggest a reduction in the duration of bleeding of endoscopically treated peptic ulcers
Prevention of rebleeding	*Oral PPI Therapy:* Pantoprazole 40 mg BID	Some evidence suggests that once-daily dosing is appropriate for patients at low risk of rebleeding (i.e., Rockall score < 6)
	Esomeprazole 40 mg QD	
	Lansoprazole 30 mg BID	
	Rabeprazole 20 mg BID	
	Omeprazole 20 mg BID	
	Dexlansoprazole 30 mg BID	

BID = twice daily; PPI = proton pump inhibitor; QD = once daily; QID = four times daily.

endoscopic intervention has significantly reduced the need for more invasive operations. Now, surgery is usually reserved for failed endoscopic therapies with persistent bleeding, hemodynamic instability caused by persistent or recurrent bleeding despite aggressive resuscitation, or visceral perforation. Interventional angiography with transarterial embolization is another option recommended ahead of surgery for persistent or recurrent bleeding despite endoscopy/colonoscopy.

PREVENTION OF REBLEEDING

Risk factors associated with upper GI rebleeding include the presence of hemodynamic instability, hemoglobin nadirs of less than 10 g/L, active bleeding at the time of endoscopy, larger ulcer sizes, and ulcers in the posterior duodenal bulb or high lesser gastric curvature.[115]

Risk Stratification

Risk assessment using endoscopic, clinical, and laboratory findings can be useful in predicting the risk of rebleeding in patients presenting with acute upper GI bleeding. The two most commonly used scoring tools are the Rockall and Blatchford scores. The Rockall score incorporates risk factors such as age, presence of shock, comorbidities, and endoscopic findings (Table 29.3). A score of 2 or less is associated with a low risk of further bleeding or death.[116] The advantages of the Blatchford score are that it does not require endoscopic findings and that it can be used earlier (Table 29.4). This score incorporates laboratory findings, vital signs, comorbidities, melena, and syncope. Scores range from 0 to 23, where a score of zero means that a patient has a low likelihood of requiring urgent endoscopy.[117]

Acid-Suppressive Therapies

A twice-daily intravenous PPI is part of the initial treatment of all patients presenting with upper GI bleeding. This therapy should be continued post-endoscopic treatment. In patients at high risk of rebleeding (i.e., Rockall score 6 or greater), the intravenous PPI may be changed to a twice-daily oral formulation 72 hours post-endoscopy.[96] Patients at a lower risk of rebleeding may continue acid-suppressive therapy with only once-daily dosing of a PPI.[118] Histamine-2 receptor blockers have also been studied in this setting, but they are inferior to PPIs.[119]

Role of *H. pylori* Screening and Treatment in Peptic Ulcer Disease

Antimicrobial treatment of *H. pylori*–infected individuals with upper GI bleeding is associated with a significant reduction in ulcer relapse. Relapse rates in untreated infected individuals with duodenal ulcers are 65%–95%, whereas successful eradication with antibiotics reduces the risk of relapse to less than 10%.[120] A meta-analysis comparing *H. pylori* eradication with antisecretory therapy alone suggests that five patients need to be treated to prevent recurrent bleeding episodes.[121]

All patients presenting with upper GI bleeding should be tested for *H. pylori*. The American College of Gastroenterology recommends antral biopsy for urease testing as the test of choice in patients undergoing endoscopy.[118,122] Other options include histology and culture. The advantage of bacterial culture is that, if isolated, antimicrobial sensitivities can be measured. The challenges are that it is not routinely available and that it is technically difficult. Patients who do not undergo endoscopy should be tested by noninvasive means such as breath testing or fecal antigen testing.[118,122] Urea breath testing is an attractive noninvasive option in which patients are given a labeled carbon isotope by mouth; as the *H. pylori* lyse urea to produce carbon dioxide (CO_2) and ammonia, the tagged CO_2 can be detected in breath samples. Regardless of the test used, the positive predictive value is high (0.85–0.99), but the negative predictive value is low (0.45–0.75), particularly in the setting of acute upper GI bleeding.[118] High false-negative results occur in the context of acute bleeding, PPI

Table 29.3 Rockall Score for Stratifying Risk				
Score	**0**	**1**	**2**	**3**
Age (yr)	< 60	60–79	> 79	
Comorbidity			Congestive heart failure, ischemic heart disease, major comorbidity	Kidney failure, liver failure, metastatic cancer
Hemodynamic status	No shock	Heart rate > 100 beats/min	Systolic blood pressure < 100 mm Hg	
Diagnosis	Mallory-Weiss tear	All other diagnoses	GI malignancy	
Major stigmata of recent hemorrhage			Blood, adherent clot, spurting vessel	
Scores of 3 or more are associated with mortality.				

use, and preexisting antimicrobial therapy. Guideline recommendations suggest that negative *H. pylori* diagnostic tests in the acute setting should be repeated.[118] The association between *H. pylori* and duodenal ulcers has traditionally been stronger than that between *H. pylori* and gastric ulcers, with original reports describing the prevalence of *H. pylori* infection with duodenal ulcers at 80%–95%. With such a high prevalence, empiric treatment of *H. pylori* with duodenal ulcers was common without diagnostic testing. Recent reports in the United States and parts of Europe suggest that this association is becoming less common (i.e., 50%–75%).[123] Given this observation, it is prudent to confirm the diagnosis before treatment rather than treat empirically.[124]

Many treatment regimens have been investigated for eradicating *H. pylori*. All of them involve a combination of antimicrobials with an antisecretory agent. Recommended therapies are provided in Table 29.5.[122] Clarithromycin-based triple therapy and bismuth-based quadruple therapy have eradication rates of 70%–80%.[122] The therapy durations recommended in the United States are usually longer (10–14 days) than those in other parts of the world (7–10 days). Data from meta-analyses suggest that eradication rates are higher with longer durations of therapy.[125] This may be because antimicrobial resistance, particularly with clarithromycin and metronidazole, is increasing and is associated with treatment failure.[126,127] Thus, it seems prudent to recommend longer durations of therapy. Treatment durations of less than 7 days are clearly inferior and are not recommended. Confirmation of eradication 4 weeks after treatment is strongly recommended, given the emergence of resistance and the availability of inexpensive, noninvasive testing (stool and breath testing).[122]

REINTRODUCTION OF ANTICOAGULATION, ANTIPLATELET THERAPY, AND NSAIDS

Patients presenting with drug-associated GI bleeding may be ineligible for permanent discontinuation of the offending drug. Patients taking NSAIDs for mild pain syndromes may be able to address their pain with non-NSAID alternatives (e.g., acetaminophen and other non-narcotic

Table 29.4 Blatchford Score for Stratifying Risk[a]

Risk Factor	Parameter	Score
Systolic blood pressure (mm Hg)	100–109	1
	90–99	2
	< 90	3
Heart rate (beats/min)	> 100	1
Melena	Present	1
Syncope	Present	2
Comorbidity	Hepatic disease	2
	Heart failure	2
Blood urea nitrogen (mmol/L)	6.5–8.0	2
	8.0–10.0	3
	10.0–25.0	4
	> 25	6
Hemoglobin (g/L) for men	12.0–12.9	1
	10.0–11.9	3
	< 10.0	6
Hemoglobin (g/L) for women	10.0–11.9	1
	< 10	6

[a]A score of 0 means the patient has a low likelihood of needing urgent endoscopy.

Table 29.5 Recommended *H. pylori* Treatment Regimens

Regimen	Duration (days)	Eradication Rates (%)
Any PPI[a] BID AND Clarithromycin 500 mg BID AND Amoxicillin 1000 mg BID	10–14	70–85
Any PPI BID AND Clarithromycin 500 mg BID AND Metronidazole 500 mg BID	10–14	70–85
Bismuth subsalicylate 525 mg QID AND Tetracycline 500 mg QID AND Metronidazole 250 mg QID AND Ranitidine 150 mg BID OR any PPI QD-BID	10–14	75–90
[b]Any PPI BID AND amoxicillin 1000 mg BID for 5 days, followed by any PPI BID AND clarithromycin 500 mg BID AND tinidazole 500 mg BID for another 5 days	10	> 90

[a]PPI therapy may include pantoprazole 40 mg BID, lansoprazole 30 mg BID, omeprazole 20 mg BID, rabeprazole 20 mg BID, or esomeprazole 40 mg QD (note: esomeprazole is a delayed-release formulation and is dosed QD).
[b]The efficacy of sequential therapy has not been shown in North America.
PPI = proton pump inhibitor.
Adapted from: Chey WD, Wong BC; Practice Parameters Committee of the American College of Gastroenterology. American College of Gastroenterology guideline on the management of *Helicobacter pylori* infection. Am J Gastroenterol 2007;102:1808-25.

analgesics), but patients on antiplatelet or anticoagulant therapy for cardiovascular or stroke prophylaxis will likely need to reinitiate therapy at some point after the bleeding episode resolves.

In NSAID-induced bleeding where anti-inflammatory therapy needs to be reintroduced, options may include reinitiating the NSAID in combination with a PPI or changing the NSAID to a COX-2 inhibitor either alone or in combination with a PPI. Other combination therapies including misoprostol, sucralfate, and H_2RAs have been studied, but they are either poorly tolerated or inferior to PPIs.[128,129] Adding a PPI to an NSAID reduces the risk of recurrent bleeding, as does changing from an NSAID to a COX-2 inhibitor. The combination of a COX-2 inhibitor and a PPI is associated with the greatest risk reduction.[118] Even in lower GI bleeding, discontinuing NSAID therapy has been associated with reduced rebleeding rates.[42]

Discontinuation or prolonged delays in reinitiating low-dose aspirin after a GI bleeding event are associated with significant cardiovascular morbidity. Discontinuation of prophylactic aspirin is associated with a 3-fold increase in major cardiac events, most of which occur 7–10 days after discontinuation.[130] It is recommended that aspirin therapy be reintroduced as soon as the perceived risks of bleeding no longer outweigh the cardiovascular risks of withholding prophylaxis.[129] Analyses of randomized controlled data suggest that immediately reintroducing aspirin post-endoscopy is associated with negligible increases in rebleeding rates, whereas discontinuing aspirin is associated with an increased mortality at 8 weeks.[118]

In patients who present with dual antiplatelet therapy or with a thienopyridine (e.g., clopidogrel, ticlopidine, or prasugrel), the decision about when to reinitiate is more complicated. Clinical practice guidelines suggest that antiplatelet therapy should be reinitiated as soon as possible post-endoscopy, provided there is no longer a suggestion of ongoing bleeding (usually 3–7 days post-endoscopy). Consultation with a cardiology specialist before endoscopy is recommended to fully assess the risks of withholding antiplatelet therapy.[128] The risk of GI bleeding with clopidogrel is greater than with aspirin plus a PPI, and dual antiplatelet therapy has a 2- to 3-fold increase in the risk of GI bleeding compared with aspirin alone.[118,131] Adding a PPI to clopidogrel is associated with up to a 50% reduction in the risk of major bleeding, but this may also increase the risk of adverse cardiovascular events. All PPIs inhibit the cytochrome P450 (CYP) 2C19 necessary to activate clopidogrel to its active form. Pharmacokinetic studies confirm this interaction, but clinical studies fail to consistently show a meaningful clinical impact. Given the inconclusive nature of these data, clinical practice guidelines recommend concomitant PPI use in all patients on antiplatelet therapy for secondary prophylaxis of GI bleeding.[131] The concerns of PPI use and clopidogrel do not extend to prasugrel because this drug does not require activation by CYP2C19.[132]

Data regarding the optimal time and how to resume anticoagulation therapy are scant. Resumption of anticoagulant therapy with warfarin has been studied in patients with atrial fibrillation after a GI bleeding event. A retrospective cohort study of more than 1,300 patients with atrial fibrillation who were recovering from major GI bleeding found that reinitiating warfarin within 7–30 days after the GI bleed was associated with a reduced risk of thromboembolism and mortality compared with delaying reinitiation beyond 30 days.[133]

CONCLUSION

Gastrointestinal bleeding is associated with significant morbidity and mortality, regardless of whether it occurs in the community or in the hospital. Although endoscopy is the cornerstone for diagnostic and therapeutic purposes, drug therapy continues to play an important role in reversal of anticoagulation, achievement of hemostasis, and prevention of rebleeding. This field is actively evolving, with ongoing trials evaluating hemostatic drugs like tranexamic acid and novel antidotes for newer anticoagulants as well as acid-suppressive therapy in the context of early endoscopy. Clinical pharmacists play an important role in assessing patients who are bleeding for providing antidotal therapies, selecting hemostatic agents, and promoting adherence to preventive drug therapy.

REFERENCES

1. van Leerdam ME. Epidemiology of acute upper gastrointestinal bleeding. Best Pract Res Clin Gastroenterol 2008;22:209-24.
2. Longstreth GF. Epidemiology and outcome of patients hospitalized with acute lower gastrointestinal hemorrhage: a population-based study. Am J Gastroenterol 1997;92:419-24.
3. Lanas A, Remacha B, Sainz R, et al. Study of outcome after targeted intervention for peptic ulcer resistant to acid suppression therapy. Am J Gastroenterol 2000;95:513-9.
4. Lewis JD, Bilker WB, Brensinger C, et al. Hospitalization and mortality rates from peptic ulcer disease and GI bleeding in the 1990s: relationship to sales of nonsteroidal anti-inflammatory drugs and acid suppression medications. Am J Gastroenterol 2002;97:2540-9.
5. Sanchez-Delgado J, Gene E, Suarez D, et al. Has H. pylori prevalence in bleeding peptic ulcer been underestimated? A meta-regression. Am J Gastroenterol 2011;106:398-405.
6. Talley NJ, Jones M. Self-reported rectal bleeding in a United States community: prevalence, risk factors, and health care seeking. Am J Gastroenterol 1998;93:2179-83.
7. Feinman M, Haut ER. Lower gastrointestinal bleeding. Surg Clin North Am 2014;94:55-63.
8. Gralnek IM, Barkun AN, Bardou M. Management of acute bleeding from a peptic ulcer. N Engl J Med 2008;359:928-37.

9. Lau JY, Barkun A, Fan DM, et al. Challenges in the management of acute peptic ulcer bleeding. Lancet 2013;381:2033-43.

10. Wilkins T, Khan N, Nabh A, et al. Diagnosis and management of upper gastrointestinal bleeding. Am Fam Physician 2012;85:469-76.

11. Huang JQ, Sridhar S, Hunt RH. Role of Helicobacter pylori infection and non-steroidal anti-inflammatory drugs in peptic-ulcer disease: a meta-analysis. Lancet 2002;359:14-22.

12. Jiang HY, Chen HZ, Hu XJ, et al. Use of selective serotonin reuptake inhibitors and risk of upper gastrointestinal bleeding: a systematic review and meta-analysis. Clin Gastroenterol Hepatol 2015;13:42-50 e3.

13. Stollman N, Metz DC. Pathophysiology and prophylaxis of stress ulcer in intensive care unit patients. J Crit Care 2005;20:35-45.

14. Lecleire S, Antonietti M, Ducrotte P. [Mallory-Weiss syndrome: diagnosis and treatment]. Presse Med 2010;39:640-4.

15. Hreinsson JP, Gumundsson S, Kalaitzakis E, et al. Lower gastrointestinal bleeding: incidence, etiology, and outcomes in a population-based setting. Eur J Gastroenterol Hepatol 2013;25:37-43.

16. Gayer C, Chino A, Lucas C, et al. Acute lower gastrointestinal bleeding in 1,112 patients admitted to an urban emergency medical center. Surgery 2009;146:600-6; discussion 6-7.

17. Strate LL, Modi R, Cohen E, et al. Diverticular disease as a chronic illness: evolving epidemiologic and clinical insights. Am J Gastroenterol 2012;107:1486-93.

18. Lewis M; NDSG. Bleeding colonic diverticula. J Clin Gastroenterol 2008;42:1156-8.

19. Acosta S. Mesenteric ischemia. Curr Opin Crit Care 2015;21:171-8.

20. Sise MJ. Acute mesenteric ischemia. Surg Clin North Am 2014;94:165-81.

21. Triadafilopoulos G. Management of lower gastrointestinal bleeding in older adults. Drugs Aging 2012;29:707-15.

22. Hreinsson JP, Kalaitzakis E, Gudmundsson S, et al. Upper gastrointestinal bleeding: incidence, etiology and outcomes in a population-based setting. Scand J Gastroenterol 2013;48:439-47.

23. Lanas A, Garcia-Rodriguez LA, Polo-Tomas M, et al. The changing face of hospitalisation due to gastrointestinal bleeding and perforation. Aliment Pharmacol Ther 2011;33:585-91.

24. Hermansson M, Ekedahl A, Ranstam J, et al. Decreasing incidence of peptic ulcer complications after the introduction of the proton pump inhibitors, a study of the Swedish population from 1974-2002. BMC Gastroenterol 2009;9:25.

25. Laine L, Yang H, Chang SC, et al. Trends for incidence of hospitalization and death due to GI complications in the United States from 2001 to 2009. Am J Gastroenterol 2012;107:1190-5; quiz 6.

26. Eddleston JM, Pearson RC, Holland J, et al. Prospective endoscopic study of stress erosions and ulcers in critically ill adult patients treated with either sucralfate or placebo. Crit Care Med 1994;22:1949-54.

27. Cook D, Heyland D, Griffith L, et al. Risk factors for clinically important upper gastrointestinal bleeding in patients requiring mechanical ventilation. Canadian Critical Care Trials Group. Crit Care Med 1999;27:2812-7.

28. Cook DJ, Fuller HD, Guyatt GH, et al. Risk factors for gastrointestinal bleeding in critically ill patients. Canadian Critical Care Trials Group. N Engl J Med 1994;330:377-81.

29. Krag M, Perner A, Wetterslev J, et al. Stress ulcer prophylaxis in the intensive care unit: is it indicated? A topical systematic review. Acta Anaesthesiol Scand 2013;57:835-47.

30. Faisy C, Guerot E, Diehl JL, et al. Clinically significant gastrointestinal bleeding in critically ill patients with and without stress-ulcer prophylaxis. Intensive Care Med 2003;29:1306-13.

31. Lanas A, Garcia-Rodriguez LA, Polo-Tomas M, et al. Time trends and impact of upper and lower gastrointestinal bleeding and perforation in clinical practice. Am J Gastroenterol 2009;104:1633-41.

32. Blatchford O, Davidson LA, Murray WR, et al. Acute upper gastrointestinal haemorrhage in west of Scotland: case ascertainment study. BMJ 1997;315:510-4.

33. Masso Gonzalez EL, Patrignani P, Tacconelli S, et al. Variability among nonsteroidal antiinflammatory drugs in risk of upper gastrointestinal bleeding. Arthritis Rheum 2010;62:1592-601.

34. Inayet N, Amoateng-Adjepong Y, Upadya A, et al. Risks for developing critical illness with GI hemorrhage. Chest 2000;118:473-8.

35. Musumba C, Jorgensen A, Sutton L, et al. The relative contribution of NSAIDs and Helicobacter pylori to the aetiology of endoscopically-diagnosed peptic ulcer disease: observations from a tertiary referral hospital in the UK between 2005 and 2010. Aliment Pharmacol Ther 2012;36:48-56.

36. Lau JY, Sung J, Hill C, et al. Systematic review of the epidemiology of complicated peptic ulcer disease: incidence, recurrence, risk factors and mortality. Digestion 2011;84:102-13.

37. Levenstein S, Rosenstock S, Jacobsen RK, et al. Psychological stress increases risk for peptic ulcer, regardless of Helicobacter pylori infection or use of nonsteroidal anti-inflammatory drugs. Clin Gastroenterol Hepatol 2015;13:498-506 e1.

38. Anglin R, Yuan Y, Moayyedi P, Tse F, et al. Risk of upper gastrointestinal bleeding with selective serotonin reuptake inhibitors with or without concurrent nonsteroidal anti-inflammatory use: a systematic review and meta-analysis. Am J Gastroenterol 2014;109:811-9.

39. Lanza FL, Chan FK, Quigley EM; Practice Parameters Committee of the American College of Gastroenterology. Guidelines for prevention of NSAID-related ulcer complications. Am J Gastroenterol 2009;104:728-38.

40. Mallory GK, Weiss S. Hemorrhages from lacerations of the cardiac orifice of the stomach due to vomiting. Am J Med Sci 1929;178:506-12.

41. Kortas DY, Haas LS, Simpson WG, et al. Mallory-Weiss tear: predisposing factors and predictors of a complicated course. Am J Gastroenterol 2001;96:2863-5.

42. Nagata N, Niikura R, Aoki T, et al. Effect of proton-pump inhibitors on the risk of lower gastrointestinal bleeding associated with NSAIDs, aspirin, clopidogrel, and warfarin. J Gastroenterol 2015 Feb 21. [Epub ahead of print]

43. Cook DJ, Griffith LE, Walter SD, et al. The attributable mortality and length of intensive care unit stay of clinically important gastrointestinal bleeding in critically ill patients. Crit Care 2001;5:368-75.

44. Imperiale TF, Dominitz JA, Provenzale DT, et al. Predicting poor outcome from acute upper gastrointestinal hemorrhage. Arch Intern Med 2007;167:1291-6.

45. Jairath V, Thompson J, Kahan BC, et al. Poor outcomes in hospitalized patients with gastrointestinal bleeding: impact of baseline risk, bleeding severity, and process of care. Am J Gastroenterol 2014;109:1603-12.

46. Rockall TA, Logan RF, Devlin HB, et al. Risk assessment after acute upper gastrointestinal haemorrhage. Gut 1996;38:316-21.

47. Marmo R, Del Piano M, Rotondano G, et al. Mortality from nonulcer bleeding is similar to that of ulcer bleeding in high-risk patients with nonvariceal hemorrhage: a prospective database study in Italy. Gastrointest Endosc 2012;75:263-72, 72 e1.

48. Ljubicic N, Budimir I, Pavic T, et al. Mortality in high-risk patients with bleeding Mallory-Weiss syndrome is similar to that of peptic ulcer bleeding. Results of a prospective database study. Scand J Gastroenterol 2014;49:458-64.

49. Rios A, Montoya MJ, Rodriguez JM, et al. Severe acute lower gastrointestinal bleeding: risk factors for morbidity and mortality. Langenbecks Arch Surg 2007;392:165-71.

50. Arroja B, Cremers I, Ramos R, et al. Acute lower gastrointestinal bleeding management in Portugal: a multicentric prospective 1-year survey. Eur J Gastroenterol Hepatol 2011;23:317-22.

51. ASHP Therapeutic Guidelines on Stress Ulcer Prophylaxis. ASHP Commission on Therapeutics and approved by the ASHP Board of Directors on November 14, 1998. Am J Health Syst Pharm 1999;56:347-79.

52. Dellinger RP, Levy MM, Rhodes A, et al. Surviving sepsis campaign: international guidelines for management of severe sepsis and septic shock: 2012. Crit Care Med 2013;41:580-637.

53. Plummer MP, Blaser AR, Deane AM. Stress ulceration: prevalence, pathology and association with adverse outcomes. Crit Care 2014;18:213.

54. Hastings PR, Skillman JJ, Bushnell LS, et al. Antacid titration in the prevention of acute gastrointestinal bleeding: a controlled, randomized trial in 100 critically ill patients. N Engl J Med 1978;298:1041-5.

55. Cook D, Guyatt G, Marshall J, et al. A comparison of sucralfate and ranitidine for the prevention of upper gastrointestinal bleeding in patients requiring mechanical ventilation. Canadian Critical Care Trials Group. N Engl J Med 1998;338:791-7.

56. Alhazzani W, Alenezi F, Jaeschke RZ, et al. Proton pump inhibitors versus histamine 2 receptor antagonists for stress ulcer prophylaxis in critically ill patients: a systematic review and meta-analysis. Crit Care Med 2013;41:693-705.

57. Barletta JF, Kanji S, MacLaren R, et al.; American-Canadian consortium for intensive care drug utilization I. Pharmacoepidemiology of stress ulcer prophylaxis in the United States and Canada. J Crit Care 2014;29:955-60.

58. Krag M, Perner A, Wetterslev J, et al. Stress ulcer prophylaxis versus placebo or no prophylaxis in critically ill patients. A systematic review of randomised clinical trials with meta-analysis and trial sequential analysis. Intensive Care Med 2014;40:11-22.

59. Thorens J, Froehlich F, Schwizer W, et al. Bacterial overgrowth during treatment with omeprazole compared with cimetidine: a prospective randomised double blind study. Gut 1996;39:54-9.

60. Wang K, Lin HJ, Perng CL, et al. The effect of H2-receptor antagonist and proton pump inhibitor on microbial proliferation in the stomach. Hepatogastroenterology 2004;51:1540-3.

61. MacLaren R, Reynolds PM, Allen RR. Histamine-2 receptor antagonists vs proton pump inhibitors on gastrointestinal tract hemorrhage and infectious complications in the intensive care unit. JAMA Intern Med 2014;174:564-74.

62. Miano TA, Reichert MG, Houle TT, et al. Nosocomial pneumonia risk and stress ulcer prophylaxis: a comparison of pantoprazole vs ranitidine in cardiothoracic surgery patients. Chest 2009;136:440-7.

63. Bateman BT, Bykov K, Choudhry NK, et al. Type of stress ulcer prophylaxis and risk of nosocomial pneumonia in cardiac surgical patients: cohort study. BMJ 2013;347:f5416.

64. Mallow S, Rebuck JA, Osler T, et al. Do proton pump inhibitors increase the incidence of nosocomial pneumonia and related infectious complications when compared with histamine-2 receptor antagonists in critically ill trauma patients? Curr Surg 2004;61:452-8.

65. Beaulieu M, Williamson D, Sirois C, et al. Do proton-pump inhibitors increase the risk for nosocomial pneumonia in a medical intensive care unit? J Crit Care 2008;23:513-8.

66. Buendgens L, Bruensing J, Matthes M, et al. Administration of proton pump inhibitors in critically ill medical patients is associated with increased risk of developing Clostridium difficile-associated diarrhea. J Crit Care 2014;29:696 e11-5.

67. Dial S, Alrasadi K, Manoukian C, et al. Risk of Clostridium difficile diarrhea among hospital inpatients prescribed proton pump inhibitors: cohort and case-control studies. CMAJ 2004;171:33-8.

68. Barletta JF, Sclar DA. Proton pump inhibitors increase the risk for hospital-acquired Clostridium difficile infection in critically ill patients. Crit Care 2014;18:714.

69. Pepin J, Saheb N, Coulombe MA, et al. Emergence of fluoroquinolones as the predominant risk factor for Clostridium difficile-associated diarrhea: a cohort study during an epidemic in Quebec. Clin Infect Dis 2005;41:1254-60.

70. Beaulieu M, Williamson D, Pichette G, et al. Risk of Clostridium difficile-associated disease among patients receiving proton-pump inhibitors in a Quebec medical intensive care unit. Infect Control Hosp Epidemiol 2007;28:1305-7.

71. Debast SB, Vaessen N, Choudry A, et al. Successful combat of an outbreak due to Clostridium difficile PCR ribotype 027 and recognition of specific risk factors. Clin Microbiol Infect 2009;15:427-34.

72. Stevens V, Dumyati G, Brown J, et al. Differential risk of Clostridium difficile infection with proton pump inhibitor use by level of antibiotic exposure. Pharmacoepidemiol Drug Saf 2011;20:1035-42.

73. Kwok CS, Arthur AK, Anibueze CI, et al. Risk of Clostridium difficile infection with acid suppressing drugs and antibiotics: meta-analysis. Am J Gastroenterol 2012;107:1011-9.

74. Hurt RT, Frazier TH, McClave SA, et al. Stress prophylaxis in intensive care unit patients and the role of enteral nutrition. JPEN J Parenter Enteral Nutr 2012;36:721-31.

75. Rostom A, Dube C, Wells G, et al. Prevention of NSAID-induced gastroduodenal ulcers. Cochrane Database Syst Rev 2002;4:CD002296.

76. Coxib and traditional NSAID Trialists' (CNT) Collaboration; Bhala N, Emberson J, et al. Vascular and upper gastrointestinal effects of non-steroidal anti-inflammatory drugs: meta-analyses of individual participant data from randomised trials. Lancet 2013;382:769-79.
77. Dworzynski K, Pollit V, Kelsey A, et al.; Guideline Development G. Management of acute upper gastrointestinal bleeding: summary of NICE guidance. BMJ 2012;344:e3412.
78. Bougle A, Harrois A, Duranteau J. Resuscitative strategies in traumatic hemorrhagic shock. Ann Intensive Care 2013;3:1.
79. Villanueva C, Colomo A, Bosch A, et al. Transfusion strategies for acute upper gastrointestinal bleeding. N Engl J Med 2013;368:11-21.
80. Razzaghi A, Barkun AN. Platelet transfusion threshold in patients with upper gastrointestinal bleeding: a systematic review. J Clin Gastroenterol 2012;46:482-6.
81. Choudari CP, Rajgopal C, Palmer KR. Acute gastrointestinal haemorrhage in anticoagulated patients: diagnoses and response to endoscopic treatment. Gut 1994;35:464-6.
82. Levy JH, Tanaka KA. Anticoagulation and reversal paradigms: is too much of a good thing bad? Anesthesia and analgesia 2009;108:692-4.
83. Warkentin TE, Crowther MA. Reversing anticoagulants both old and new. Can J Anaeth 2002;49:S11-25.
84. Pollack CV Jr, Reilly PA, Eikelboom J, et al. Idarucizumab for dabigatran reversal. N Engl J Med 2015 June 22. [Epub ahead of print]
85. Mo Y, Yam FK. Recent advances in the development of specific antidotes for target-specific oral anticoagulants. Pharmacotherapy 2015;35:198-207.
86. Lazo-Langner A, Lang ES, Douketis J. Clinical review: clinical management of new oral anticoagulants: a structured review with emphasis on the reversal of bleeding complications. Crit Care 2013;17:230.
87. Levine M, Goldstein JN. Emergency reversal of anticoagulation: novel agents. Curr Neurol Neurosci Rep 2014;14:471.
88. Marlu R, Hodaj E, Paris A, et al. Effect of non-specific reversal agents on anticoagulant activity of dabigatran and rivaroxaban: a randomised crossover ex vivo study in healthy volunteers. Thromb Haemost 2012;108:217-24.
89. ASGE Standards of Practice Committee; Anderson MA, Ben-Menachem T, et al. Management of antithrombotic agents for endoscopic procedures. Gastrointest Endosc 2009;70:1060-70.
90. Flordal PA, Sahlin S. Use of desmopressin to prevent bleeding complications in patients treated with aspirin. Br J Surg 1993;80:723-4.
91. Mannucci PM, Vicente V, Vianello L, et al. Controlled trial of desmopressin in liver cirrhosis and other conditions associated with a prolonged bleeding time. Blood 1986;67:1148-53.
92. Green FW Jr, Kaplan MM, Curtis LE, et al. Effect of acid and pepsin on blood coagulation and platelet aggregation. A possible contributor prolonged gastroduodenal mucosal hemorrhage. Gastroenterology 1978;74:38-43.
93. Leontiadis GI, Sreedharan A, Dorward S, et al. Systematic reviews of the clinical effectiveness and cost-effectiveness of proton pump inhibitors in acute upper gastrointestinal bleeding. Health Technol Assess 2007;11:iii-iv, 1-164.
94. Sreedharan A, Martin J, Leontiadis GI, et al. Proton pump inhibitor treatment initiated prior to endoscopic diagnosis in upper gastrointestinal bleeding. Cochrane Database Syst Rev 2010;7:CD005415.
95. Sachar H, Vaidya K, Laine L. Intermittent vs continuous proton pump inhibitor therapy for high-risk bleeding ulcers: a systematic review and meta-analysis. JAMA Intern Med 2014;174:1755-62.
96. Cheng HC, Wu CT, Chang WL, et al. Double oral esomeprazole after a 3-day intravenous esomeprazole infusion reduces recurrent peptic ulcer bleeding in high-risk patients: a randomised controlled study. Gut 2014;63:1864-72.
97. Bennett C, Klingenberg SL, Langholz E, et al. Tranexamic acid for upper gastrointestinal bleeding. Cochrane Database Syst Rev 2014;11:CD006640.
98. Barkun AN, Bardou M, Martel M, et al. Prokinetics in acute upper GI bleeding: a meta-analysis. Gastrointest Endosc 2010;72:1138-45.
99. Bai Y, Guo JF, Li ZS. Meta-analysis: erythromycin before endoscopy for acute upper gastrointestinal bleeding. Aliment Pharmacol Ther 2011;34:166-71.
100. Szary NM, Gupta R, Choudhary A, et al. Erythromycin prior to endoscopy in acute upper gastrointestinal bleeding: a meta-analysis. Scand J Gastroenterol 2011;46:920-4.
101. Bon C, Aparicio T, Vincent M, et al. Long-acting somatostatin analogues decrease blood transfusion requirements in patients with refractory gastrointestinal bleeding associated with angiodysplasia. Aliment Pharmacol Ther 2012;36:587-93.
102. Brown C, Subramanian V, Wilcox CM, et al. Somatostatin analogues in the treatment of recurrent bleeding from gastrointestinal vascular malformations: an overview and systematic review of prospective observational studies. Dig Dis Sci 2010;55:2129-34.
103. Imperiale TF, Birgisson S. Somatostatin or octreotide compared with H2 antagonists and placebo in the management of acute nonvariceal upper gastrointestinal hemorrhage: a meta-analysis. Ann Intern Med 1997;127:1062-71.
104. Forrest JA, Finlayson ND, Shearman DJ. Endoscopy in gastrointestinal bleeding. Lancet 1974;2:394-7.
105. Bjorkman DJ, Zaman A, Fennerty MB, et al. Urgent vs. elective endoscopy for acute non-variceal upper-GI bleeding: an effectiveness study. Gastrointest Endosc 2004;60:1-8.
106. Sarin N, Monga N, Adams PC. Time to endoscopy and outcomes in upper gastrointestinal bleeding. Can J Gastroenterol 2009;23:489-93.
107. Tsoi KK, Chiu PW, Chan FK, et al. The risk of peptic ulcer bleeding mortality in relation to hospital admission on holidays: a cohort study on 8,222 cases of peptic ulcer bleeding. Am J Gastroenterol 2012;107:405-10.
108. Wysocki JD, Srivastav S, Winstead NS. A nationwide analysis of risk factors for mortality and time to endoscopy in upper gastrointestinal haemorrhage. Aliment Pharmacol Ther 2012;36:30-6.
109. Laine L, McQuaid KR. Endoscopic therapy for bleeding ulcers: an evidence-based approach based on meta-analyses of randomized controlled trials. Clin Gastroenterol Hepatol 2009;7:33-47; quiz 1-2.

110. Church J, Kao J. Bedside colonoscopy in intensive care units: indications, techniques, and outcomes. Surg Endosc 2014;28:2679-82.

111. Green BT, Rockey DC, Portwood G, et al. Urgent colonoscopy for evaluation and management of acute lower gastrointestinal hemorrhage: a randomized controlled trial. Am J Gastroenterol 2005;100:2395-402.

112. Laine L, Shah A. Randomized trial of urgent vs. elective colonoscopy in patients hospitalized with lower GI bleeding. Am J Gastroenterol 2010;105:2636-41; quiz 42.

113. Small RL, Ryburn JA, Wendel JF. Low levels of nucleotide diversity at homoeologous Adh loci in allotetraploid cotton (Gossypium L.). Mol Biol Evol 1999;16:491-501.

114. Lhewa DY, Strate LL. Pros and cons of colonoscopy in management of acute lower gastrointestinal bleeding. World J Gastroenterol 2012;18:1185-90.

115. Garcia-Iglesias P, Villoria A, Suarez D, et al. Meta-analysis: predictors of rebleeding after endoscopic treatment for bleeding peptic ulcer. Aliment Pharmacol Ther 2011;34:888-900.

116. Rockall TA, Logan RF, Devlin HB, et al. Selection of patients for early discharge or outpatient care after acute upper gastrointestinal haemorrhage. National Audit of Acute Upper Gastrointestinal Haemorrhage. Lancet 1996;347:1138-40.

117. Blatchford O, Murray WR, Blatchford M. A risk score to predict need for treatment for upper-gastrointestinal haemorrhage. Lancet 2000;356:1318-21.

118. Barkun AN, Bardou M, Kuipers EJ, et al. International consensus recommendations on the management of patients with nonvariceal upper gastrointestinal bleeding. Ann Intern Med 2010;152:101-13.

119. Levine JE, Leontiadis GI, Sharma VK, et al. Meta-analysis: the efficacy of intravenous H2-receptor antagonists in bleeding peptic ulcer. Aliment Pharmacol Ther 2002;16:1137-42.

120. Hopkins RJ, Girardi LS, Turney EA. Relationship between Helicobacter pylori eradication and reduced duodenal and gastric ulcer recurrence: a review. Gastroenterology 1996;110:1244-52.

121. Gisbert JP, Khorrami S, Carballo F, et al. Meta-analysis: Helicobacter pylori eradication therapy vs. antisecretory non-eradication therapy for the prevention of recurrent bleeding from peptic ulcer. Aliment Pharmacol Ther 2004;19:617-29.

122. Chey WD, Wong BC; Practice Parameters Committee of the American College of Gastroenterology. American College of Gastroenterology guideline on the management of Helicobacter pylori infection. Am J Gastroenterol 2007;102:1808-25.

123. Ciociola AA, McSorley DJ, Turner K, et al. Helicobacter pylori infection rates in duodenal ulcer patients in the United States may be lower than previously estimated. Am J Gastroenterol 1999;94:1834-40.

124. Chiorean MV, Locke GR III, Zinsmeister AR, et al. Changing rates of Helicobacter pylori testing and treatment in patients with peptic ulcer disease. Am J Gastroenterol 2002;97:3015-22.

125. Calvet X, Garcia N, Lopez T, et al. A meta-analysis of short versus long therapy with a proton pump inhibitor, clarithromycin and either metronidazole or amoxycillin for treating Helicobacter pylori infection. Aliment Pharmacol Ther 2000;14:603-9.

126. Meyer JM, Silliman NP, Wang W, et al. Risk factors for Helicobacter pylori resistance in the United States: the surveillance of H. pylori antimicrobial resistance partnership (SHARP) study, 1993-1999. Ann Intern Med 2002;136:13-24.

127. Osato MS, Reddy R, Reddy SG, et al. Pattern of primary resistance of Helicobacter pylori to metronidazole or clarithromycin in the United States. Arch Intern Med 2001;161:1217-20.

128. Abraham NS, Hlatky MA, Antman EM, et al. ACCF/ACG/AHA 2010 expert consensus document on the concomitant use of proton pump inhibitors and thienopyridines: a focused update of the ACCF/ACG/AHA 2008 expert consensus document on reducing the gastrointestinal risks of antiplatelet therapy and NSAID use. A report of the American College of Cardiology Foundation Task Force on Expert Consensus Documents. J Am Coll Cardiol 2010;56:2051-66.

129. Rostom A, Moayyedi P, Hunt R; Canadian Association of Gastroenterology Consensus G. Canadian consensus guidelines on long-term nonsteroidal anti-inflammatory drug therapy and the need for gastroprotection: benefits versus risks. Aliment Pharmacol Ther 2009;29:481-96.

130. Biondi-Zoccai GG, Lotrionte M, Agostoni P, et al. A systematic review and meta-analysis on the hazards of discontinuing or not adhering to aspirin among 50,279 patients at risk for coronary artery disease. Eur Heart J 2006;27:2667-74.

131. Bhana A, Petersen I, Baillie KL, et al.; The Mhapp Research Programme C. Implementing the World Health Report 2001 recommendations for integrating mental health into primary health care: a situation analysis of three African countries: Ghana, South Africa and Uganda. Int Rev Psychiatry 2010;22:599-610.

132. Collet JP, Hulot JS, Abtan J, et al. Prasugrel but not high dose clopidogrel overcomes the lansoprazole neutralizing effect of P2Y12 inhibition: Results of the randomized DOSAPI study. Eur J Clin Pharmacol 2014;70:1049-57.

133. Qureshi W, Mittal C, Patsias I, et al. Restarting anticoagulation and outcomes after major gastrointestinal bleeding in atrial fibrillation. Am J Cardiol 2014;113:662-8.

Section 7

Acute Pulmonary Disease

Chapter 30: Pulmonary Arterial Hypertension

Steven E. Pass, Pharm.D., FCCP, FCCM, FASHP, BCPS;
and Joseph E. Mazur, Pharm.D., BCPS

LEARNING OBJECTIVES

1. Discuss the epidemiology of pulmonary hypertension (PH) and pulmonary arterial hypertension (PAH).
2. Differentiate the different pathophysiologic mechanisms of PAH.
3. Discuss how molecular, cellular, and genetic mechanisms may play a future role in treatment of the critically ill patient.
4. Summarize the diagnosis and classification of PAH.
5. Detail the differing diagnostic scenarios and noninvasive/invasive tools that may be deployed for diagnosing PAH.
6. Review the medications used to treat PAH.
7. Evaluate the treatment options for patients with PAH in the intensive care unit (ICU).
8. Discuss the role of combination therapy in the treatment of PAH and considerations for the critically ill patient.
9. Summarize the adjunctive therapies used in PAH treatment and the level of evidence behind them.
10. Compare the different treatment guidelines published for the practitioner, and assess the evidence-based recommendations that can be used for ICU patients.
11. Explain the management of acutely decompensated patients with PH/PAH who develop right ventricular failure.
12. Discuss specific clinical pearls for treating patients in the ICU with PH/PAH as it relates to monitoring and adverse effect considerations.

ABBREVIATIONS IN THIS CHAPTER

CCB	Calcium channel blocker	BREATHE	Protocolised trial of invasive and non-invasive weaning off ventilation
CrCl	Creatinine clearance		
ETA	Endothelin type A	CHEST	Crystalloid versus Hydroxyethyl Starch Trial
ETB	Endothelin type B		
ICU	Intensive care unit	FREEDOM-C	Oral treprostinil for the treatment of pulmonary arterial hypertension in patients receiving background endothelin receptor antagonist and phosphodiesterase type 5 inhibitor therapy
mPAP	Mean pulmonary artery pressure		
NYHA	New York Heart Association		
PAH	Pulmonary arterial hypertension		
PDE-5	Phosphodiesterase type 5		
PGI_2	Prostaglandin I2/prostacyclin	PATENT	Pulmonary Arterial Hypertension sGC-Stimulator Trial
PH	Pulmonary hypertension		
PVR	Pulmonary vascular resistance	SERAPHIN	Study with an Endothelin Receptor Antagonist in Pulmonary Arterial Hypertension to Improve Clinical Outcome
RHC	Right heart catheterization		
RV	Right ventricle/ventricular		
Study Names			
ARIES	Ambrisentan in Pulmonary Arterial Hypertension, Randomized, Double-Blind, Placebo-Controlled, Multicenter, Efficacy	TRIUMPH	Translational Research Investigating Underlying Disparities in Acute Myocardial Infarction Patients' Health Status

INTRODUCTION

Pulmonary arterial hypertension (PAH) is a progressive disease caused by a narrowing of the blood vessels in the pulmonary vasculature. Pulmonary arterial hypertension is a rare subset of pulmonary hypertension (PH) that is differentiated from other types of PH as a primary process or in association with another condition.[1] Pulmonary arterial hypertension is diagnosed by right heart catheterization (RHC) showing precapillary PH with a mean pulmonary artery pressure (mPAP) of 25 mm Hg or greater and a pulmonary capillary wedge pressure of less than 15 mm Hg.[2] According to the patient's clinical condition, PAH can be divided into various categories on the basis of severity of illness: stable and satisfactory, stable and not satisfactory, and unstable and deteriorating.[2]

Management of PAH in the intensive care unit (ICU) may consist of diagnostic evaluation for patients with suspected PAH, treatment modifications for patients with PAH on chronic therapies, or a combination of worsening signs and symptoms in patients with PAH complicated with infection/sepsis, medication nonadherence respiratory failure, pulmonary embolism, or arrhythmias. The primary focus of therapy in the ICU setting consists of maintaining or improving pulmonary pressures, optimizing right ventricular (RV) function and hemodynamics, providing enhanced awareness, continuing chronic therapies, and managing the underlying cause of ICU admission. Because of the complexity of PAH treatment and the difficulties with managing this disease in the ICU setting, it is important that clinicians be familiar with its pathophysiology and potential complications and the medications used for treatment.

The critical care pharmacist plays a vital role as part of the interdisciplinary team, with an increasing number of patients being admitted to the ICU on chronic PAH treatments. With the recent approval of several pharmacologic modalities for treating PAH, the pharmacist can ascertain patient-specific adverse effects, guide prescribers on the complexity of the pharmacokinetics/pharmacodynamics for each agent, and be a stakeholder for patient education on the intravenous, inhalation, subcutaneous, and oral therapies. The purpose of this chapter is to clarify the classification of PAH versus that of PH, describe tools used for diagnosis and monitoring, and detail pharmacotherapy options with a focus on treatment in the ICU.

EPIDEMIOLOGY

Before the advent of new therapies for PAH treatment, the median survival for this disease entity was very poor. Older data from the Patient Registry for Primary Pulmonary Hypertension also indicated poor survival for patients with the diagnosis of primary PH, with a median survival of 2.8 years (95% confidence interval, 1.9–3.7 years).[3] Newer PAH registries indicate better survival rates than previously, but ultimately, not an overly improved prognosis, despite the newer agents and combination treatment options currently available. The most recent Registry to Evaluate Early- and Long-term Pulmonary Arterial Hypertension Disease Management in the United States (REVEAL registry) showed an improvement in survival after 1 year, an older patient population (mean age of 53 years), a higher proportion of women (1.7:1), and a higher proportion of blacks (4.3:1).[4]

Pulmonary hypertension is more prevalent than PAH because the most common cause of PH in the United States is left heart failure. Pulmonary arterial hypertension is a rarer entity, but if left untreated, it has a high mortality rate leading to RV failure and death.[4] Overall, PAH tends to affect younger women more than males.[6] Retrospective studies show that in-hospital mortality is higher in critically ill patients with PAH admitted to the ICU, ranging from 9% overall to 17% in patients with RV failure.[7,8]

PATHOPHYSIOLOGY

The targeted proven therapies for treatment of PAH have centered on three major pathways: the prostacyclin pathway, the endothelial pathway, and the nitric oxide pathway (Figure 30.1). In the prostacyclin pathway, endothelial cells form arachidonic acid that produces endogenous prostacyclin (prostaglandin I2 or PGI_2). Prostaglandin I2 has many effects, including antithrombotic, anti-inflammatory, and vasodilatory effects. Epoprostenol, the first prostacyclin analog developed for PAH therapy, is the gold standard for treatment to which other therapies are benchmarked.[9]

Another pathway contributing to PAH involves the endothelial pathway. Endothelin receptors are located on pulmonary artery smooth muscle cells and are divided into endothelin type A (ETA) and endothelin type B (ETB). Endothelin type A receptors have a higher affinity for endothelin-1, and activation leads to vasoconstriction and proliferation of vascular smooth muscle. Endothelin type B receptors can also produce these effects, but they indirectly produce vasodilation by PGI_2 and nitric oxide release from endothelial cells. The vasoconstrictive and smooth muscle effects of endothelin-1 negatively affect vessel tone and fibroblast activation. Endothelin-1 is the one subtype of naturally occurring peptides that might have the most significant impact on lung vascular remodeling.[10,11]

The nitric oxide and cyclic guanosine monophosphate (cGMP) pathways are intertwined and center on nitric oxide being produced from L-arginine. Cyclic GMP and soluble guanylate cyclase (sGC) have smooth muscle relaxing effects, thought to be a result of inhibiting phosphodiesterase type 5 (PDE-5) or activating sGC, which keeps smooth muscle relaxed and averts the vasoconstrictor and platelet activation seen in PAH. Nitric oxide may independently have a positive effect on relaxation of smooth muscle.[12] Nitric oxide and cGMP are key secondary targets for patient therapy.

The dysfunction and pathways described previously combine to result in intimal hyperplasia, medial thickening, and advanced remodeling and fibrosis. This, together with inflammatory and progenitor cells, has been postulated to contribute to the remodeling process of pulmonary vasculature. This progressive increase in pulmonary vascular resistance (PVR) creates an increased RV afterload and right heart failure.[9] The platelet dysfunction and thrombotic mechanisms are also a hallmark when describing PAH. Many vasoconstrictive substances have been implicated as a cause: von Willebrand factor, plasminogen activator inhibitor type 1, thromboxane A_2, platelet-derived growth factor, transforming growth factor β, and endothelial growth factor.[9,13,14] Promising advances

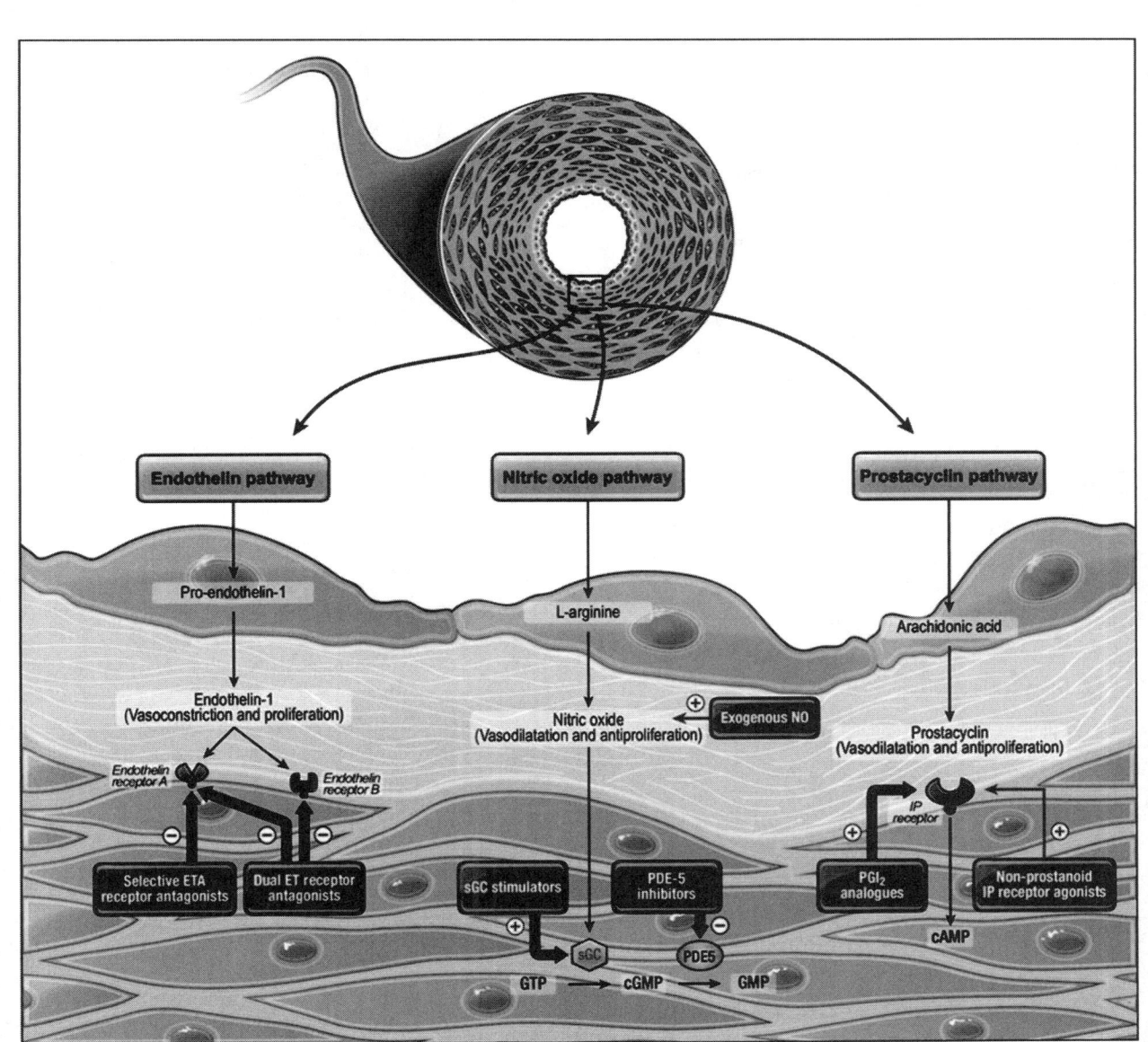

Figure 30.1 Established vasomotor pathways targeted by current and emerging therapies in pulmonary arterial hypertension.[a]

[a]The three major pathways (ET-1, nitric oxide, and prostacyclin) involved in the regulation of pulmonary vasomotor tone are shown. These pathways represent the targets of all currently approved PAH therapies. Endothelial dysfunction results in decreased production of endogenous vasodilatory mediators (nitric oxide and prostacyclin) and the up-regulation of ET-1, which promotes vasoconstriction and smooth muscle cell proliferation. The ET-1 pathway can be blocked by either selective or nonselective ET-1 receptor antagonists; the nitric oxide pathway can be manipulated by direct administration of exogenous nitric oxide, inhibition of PDE-5, or stimulation of sGC; and the prostacyclin pathway can be enhanced by the administration of prostanoid analogs or non-prostanoid IP receptor agonists.

ET = endothelin; ETA = endothelin type A; IP = prostaglandin I2; NO = nitric oxide; PDE-5 = phosphodiesterase type 5; PGI2 = prostaglandin I2/prostacyclin; sGC = soluble guanylate cyclase.

Adapted with permission from: Lippincott Williams & Wilkins/Wolters Kluwer Health: Humbert M, Lau EM, Montani D, et al. Advances in therapeutic interventions for patients with pulmonary arterial hypertension. Circulation 2014;130:2189-208.

Table 30.1 Updated Classification of Pulmonary Hypertension
1. Pulmonary arterial hypertension
1.1 Idiopathic PAH
1.2 Heritable PAH
1.2.1 BMPR2
1.2.2 ALK-1, ENG, SMAD9, CAV1, KCNK3
1.2.3 Unknown
1.3 Drug and toxin induced
1.4 Associated with:
1.4.1 Connective tissue disease
1.4.2 Human immunodeficiency virus (HIV) infection
1.4.3 Portal hypertension
1.4.4 Congenital heart diseases
1.4.5 Schistosomiasis
1' Pulmonary veno-occlusive disease and/or pulmonary capillary hemangiomatosis
1" Persistent pulmonary hypertension of the newborn (PPHN)
2. Pulmonary hypertension due to left heart disease
2.1 Left ventricular systolic dysfunction
2.2 Left ventricular diastolic dysfunction
2.3 Valvular disease
2.4 Congenital/acquired left heart inflow/outflow tract obstruction and congenital cardiomyopathies
3. Pulmonary hypertension due to lung diseases and/or hypoxia
3.1 Chronic obstructive pulmonary disease
3.2 Interstitial lung disease
3.3 Other pulmonary diseases with mixed restrictive and obstructive pattern
3.4 Sleep-disordered breathing
3.5 Alveolar hypoventilation disorders
3.6 Chronic exposure to high altitude
3.7 Developmental lung diseases
4. Chronic thromboembolic pulmonary hypertension (CTEPH)
5. Pulmonary hypertension with unclear multifactorial mechanisms
5.1 Hematologic disorders: chronic hemolytic anemia, myeloproliferative disorders, splenectomy
5.2 Systemic disorders: sarcoidosis, pulmonary histiocytosis, lymphangioleiomyomatosis
5.3 Metabolic disorders: glycogen storage disease, Gaucher disease, thyroid disorders
5.4 Others: tumoral obstruction, fibrosing mediastinitis, chronic renal failure, segmental PH

Republished with permission from: Journal of the American College of Cardiology, from: Simmoneau G, Gatzoulis MA, Adatia I, et al. Updated clinical classification of pulmonary hypertension. J Am Coll Cardiol 2013; 62:D34-41. Permission conveyed through Copyright Clearance Center, Inc.

in the genetic, molecular, and cellular mechanisms of PAH have led to novel targets as potential drug therapies.

Data analyses for the past 20 years link familial PAH in 80%–85% of families with a PAH family history to a gene coding bone morphogenetic protein receptor type 2 (*BMPR2*). The *BMPR2* mutations have shown a high risk of PAH development, and the importance of this *BMPR2* pathway to vascular remodeling is a focus of current research.[9] Additional genetic components related to PAH include mutations to activating A receptor type II–like kinase 1 (*ALK1*), endoglin (*ENG*), and SMAD family member 9 (*SMAD9*) genes.[15] Further research in this area may lead to the next generation of targets for PAH pharmacologic therapies.

CLASSIFICATION

Various iterations in the classification of PH have evolved from 1998 to 2015, with the most recent consensus being reached at the 5th World Symposium in Nice, France.[16] This symposium established a categorical clinical classification of PH according to similar hemodynamic characteristics and similar pathological findings in order to standardize management.[16] This resulted in five groups of PH disorders (Table 30.1): group 1 (PAH), group 2 (PH caused by left heart disease), group 3 (PH caused by chronic lung disease, hypoxia, or both), group 4 (chronic thromboembolic PH), and group 5 (PH caused by unclear multifactorial mechanisms).[17] Apart from the PH group classifications, patients can be categorized into four World Health Organization (WHO) functional classes according to their functional status and symptoms, adapted from the New York Heart Association (NYHA) classification system (Table 30.2).

The advantage for a standardized PH classification schematic is that clinicians and researchers can use similar terminology when making diagnoses and treating patients. In addition, the U.S. Food and Drug Administration (FDA) and the European Medicines Agency can do the same for new product labeling.[17]

Pharmacists can play an important role in determining the classification of PH by obtaining a thorough medication history (including herbal supplements and over-the-counter products). Identifying definite, likely, or possible risk factors from patients with PAH who have been

Table 30.2 World Health Organization (WHO) Functional Classification for Patients with Pulmonary Arterial Hypertension	
Class	Description
I	Patients with pulmonary hypertension but without resulting limitation of physical activity; ordinary physical activity does not cause undue dyspnea or fatigue, chest pain, or near syncope
II	Patients with pulmonary hypertension resulting in slight limitation of physical activity; they are comfortable at rest; ordinary physical activity causes undue dyspnea or fatigue, chest pain, or near syncope
III	Patients with pulmonary hypertension resulting in marked limitation of physical activity; they are comfortable at rest; less-than-ordinary physical activity causes undue dyspnea or fatigue, chest pain, or near syncope
IV	Patients with pulmonary hypertension with an inability to carry out any physical activity without symptoms; these patients manifest signs of right heart failure; dyspnea and/or fatigue can even be present at rest; discomfort is increased by any physical activity

Republished with permission from: American Journal of Cardiology, from: Waxman AB, Zamanian RT. Pulmonary arterial hypertension: new insights into the optimal role of current and emerging prostacyclin therapies. Am J Cardiol 2013;111(suppl):1A-16A; permission conveyed through Copyright Clearance Center, Inc.

on medications or other toxins is key to the class 1 diagnosis. Agents linked with a definite cause of PAH include aminorex, fenfluramine, dexfenfluramine, toxic rapeseed oil, benfluorex, and SSRIs (selective serotonin reuptake inhibitors) taken during pregnancy after 20 weeks' gestation. Agents identified as likely contributing to PAH include amphetamines, L-tryptophan, methamphetamines, and dasatinib. Agents possibly linked to PAH include cocaine, phenylpropanolamine, St. John's wort, various chemotherapeutic agents, interferon α and β, and amphetamine-like drugs.[18]

DIAGNOSIS

Medical History

Obtaining a personalized medical history from either the patient or the family member is key to eliciting drug or toxin exposure, familial history of PAH, and disease states contributory to PAH, which could entail connective tissue disorders (e.g., scleroderma), HIV, portal hypertension, congenital heart disease, or schistosomiasis.[5]

Physical Examination

Patients in the ICU with PAH may present with signs and symptoms of RV failure, the most common of which are lower extremity edema, dyspnea on exertion, and angina. Patients who are syncopal have a worsening prognosis because this may reflect a low cardiac output state. Clinicians monitor for various cardiac abnormalities such as an accentuated second heart sound, a tricuspid regurgitation, or a systolic murmur. These symptoms, in whole or in part, occur at rest and may indicate a patient with advanced PAH.[5]

Blood Tests and Immunology

Routine blood tests comprising basic metabolic profiles, hematology, and thyroid function tests should be obtained for patients admitted to the ICU. Workup of thrombotic abnormalities includes obtaining antiphospholipid antibodies, lupus anticoagulant, and anticardiolipin antibodies. If liver involvement is suspected, liver function tests and hepatitis serologies should be obtained, together with HIV testing.[2] There is some debate regarding the role of obtaining circulating biomarkers such as brain natriuretic peptide (BNP) concentrations or troponins and what they mean prognostically.[2] It has been suggested that with various therapy goals in mind, achieving the lowest possible or personal best BNP or N-terminal pro–B-type natriuretic peptide (NT-proBNP) is appropriate.[19]

Chest Radiographs

Chest radiographs are a routine part of the workup for PAH. In most patients presenting with idiopathic PAH, the chest radiograph is abnormal. "Pruning" or loss of the peripheral blood vessels is described. Right ventricular hypertrophy or dilation cannot easily be distinguished on a chest radiograph.[5]

Electrocardiogram

Electrocardiogram (ECG), also part of the diagnostic algorithm for PAH, is used to assess RV hypertrophy and strain, as well as right atrial dilation. The ECG has a sensitivity of 55% and a specificity of 70% as a screening tool for patients with PH. Atrial arrhythmias (e.g., atrial fibrillation or flutter) are common in patients with a diagnosis of advanced PAH.[5]

Echocardiography

The significance of echocardiography is that it can provide the clinician with a rough estimate of right heart size (including the RV and atrium), RV function, and possible PAH. Various equations can measure pulmonary artery systolic pressures. Although not always accurate, pulmonary artery systolic pressure can be elevated in disease states such as cirrhosis, hyperthyroidism, heart failure, kidney disease, and increased blood pressure.[20] Transthoracic echocardiography serves as the most important noninvasive tool to assess PH in both ICU and non-ICU settings.[21]

Pulmonary Function Tests

Making the diagnosis of PAH in critically ill patients with the aid of pulmonary function tests is often not a practical option, but if feasible, it may help identify interstitial lung disease or chronic obstructive pulmonary disease. The diffusing capacity for carbon monoxide is about 60%–80% of predicted in patients with idiopathic PAH.[5] The degree of hypoxemia in patients with PAH centers on ventilation-perfusion mismatch, with decreased mixed venous oxygen saturation (Svo_2) values stemming from low output cardiac states.

Exercise Testing

The 6-minute walk test is a common end point marker in efficacy trials for PAH therapies.[5] The 6-minute walk test is a practical simple test that requires a 100-ft hallway but no exercise equipment or advanced training for technicians.[22] This test has been correlated with workload, heart rate, oxygen saturation, and dyspnea response. Cardiopulmonary testing (with an upright bicycle or treadmill) is used to grade PH severity in the outpatient setting. Treadmill testing is also an option in the ambulatory workup of PH, but it may not be an appropriate testing determination of PH in the hospital inpatient setting.[21] These tests are not only used for diagnosis but also to assess disease progression.

Cardiac Catherization—RHC

The gold standard for diagnosing and classifying severity of PAH is an RHC, with or without concomitant vasoreactivity testing. Key parameters that are elicited through an RHC include right atrial pressure, pulmonary capillary wedge pressures, and RV pressure. A pulmonary capillary wedge pressure greater than 15 mm Hg excludes the diagnosis of PAH, whereas an mPAP of 25 mm Hg or greater at rest defines PAH. The gold standard for cardiac output measurement is the direct Fick method (which directly measures oxygen uptake); however, the indirect Fick method (which estimates oxygen values from tables) is not reliable. After RHC is performed and a diagnosis of PAH is made, vasoreactivity testing can be done to see whether patients are classified as either responders or non-responders to determine whether they are candidates for calcium channel blocker (CCB) therapy.[5]

Vasoreactivity Challenge

The three main agents for acute vasodilator challenges are intravenous epoprostenol, intravenous adenosine, and inhaled nitric oxide. A positive acute response is defined as a reduction in mPAP of 10 mm Hg or greater to an absolute value of mPAP of 40 mm Hg or less with an increased or unchanged cardiac output (class I, level of evidence C).[2]

Patients admitted to the ICU are often in a decompensated state of RV failure whereby pharmacologic treatments must be titrated to improve RV function and ameliorate adverse effects (e.g., dyspnea or exercise intolerance). Patients may also be admitted for the vasodilator challenge, which may elicit better symptomatic and prognostic information. Patients classified as being in an unstable and deteriorating state have worsening WHO functional class, a poor 6-minute walk of less than 300 m, a peak VO_2 of less than 12 mL/minute/kg, rising BNP/NT-proBNP plasma concentrations, evidence of pericardial effusion, tricuspid annular planar systolic excursion less than 1.5 cm, right atrial pressure greater than 15 mm Hg, or a cardiac index of 2.0 L/minute/m^2 or less.[23] The agents and doses used for pulmonary vasoreactivity testing are intravenous epoprostenol (2–12 ng/kg/minute for 10 minutes), intravenous adenosine (50–350 mcg/kg/minute for 2 minutes), or inhaled nitric oxide (10–20 ppm for 5 minutes).[5]

TREATMENT

Calcium Channel Blockers

Calcium channel blockers decrease calcium influx into the smooth muscle cells of the arterial wall and the myocardial cells by inhibiting L-type voltage-dependent sodium channels. This also represents a possible mechanism of PAH development.[24] The concept of CCB responders versus non-responders is relevant when considering CCB as an agent to treat patients with PAH because about 5% of patients will benefit from CCB treatment long term. Two studies have shown that CCB may be useful in patients with PAH. Rich and colleagues studied CCB therapy in 47 patients with PAH. These authors found a 20% reduction in mPAP and PVR (with nifedipine and diltiazem in 72% of patients), with 15 patients (32%) defined as pressure responders (significant improvement in mPAP and PVR index). In another study by the same lead author, 17 of 64 patients (27%) had a 20% reduction in mPAP and PVR when treated with nifedipine 20 mg or diltiazem 60 mg, with a 94% survival at 5 years (compared with 55% in patients who did not respond to therapy.[25,26] Advanced therapies with acute vasoactive agents such as adenosine, epoprostenol, and nitric oxide have replaced CCB as the preferred agents in clinical trials. This is primarily due to the significant adverse effects of the CCBs, which include negative inotropy (diltiazem and verapamil), hypotension (seen with all agents with escalating doses from CCB trials), edema, nausea, headache, and acute hospitalization.

Overall, CCB efficacy is limited in patients with PAH, and these agents are contraindicated in most patients given the presence of decompensated right/left heart failure or bradycardia.[27] Therefore, CCBs have been relegated to possible last-line therapies, but they are a viable option for patients who may not respond to other therapies.

Implications for the Critical Care Practitioner

Although not widely recommended, CCB agents may be used in the early stages of PAH because of their availability and ease of administration. Patients should be closely monitored for changes in blood pressure and heart rate as well as other potential adverse effects. Critical care monitoring flowsheets and medication administration records should be closely monitored to determine the accuracy and efficacy of dosing and the potential need for alterations in therapy.

Epoprostenol Analogues

The mainstay of PAH therapy in the critically ill patient has traditionally been epoprostenol. Epoprostenol is a prostacyclin PGI_2 analog with unique pharmacologic properties, including direct vasodilation of the pulmonary vasculature and platelet aggregation inhibition. Epoprostenol has shown symptomatic and hemodynamic improvements in patients with severe primary PH, survival benefits longer term in patients with NYHA function class III or IV, and mortality benefits in subsets of patients with PH caused by scleroderma.[28,29] In a 12-week, prospective, randomized trial of 81 patients with severe primary PH (NYHA functional class III or IV), 41 patients treated with intravenous epoprostenol at a mean dose of approximately 9 ng/kg/minute showed exercise capacity improvements (6-minute walk test) and hemodynamic improvements (pulmonary artery pressures, PVR) compared with conventional therapies. The most noteworthy finding showed improved survival at 12 weeks in the epoprostenol group, with eight patients dying in the conventional group (p=0.003) after adjustment of variables.[28] Newer trials have shown similar results in both hemodynamic and survival improvement with epoprostenol.

Epoprostenol is FDA labeled for the treatment of PAH in WHO group 1 patients to improve exercise capacity.[30] The recommended starting dose is 2 ng/kg/minute intravenously, and the dose is slowly titrated in increments of 0.5–2 ng/kg/minute every 15 minutes to a maximum tolerated dose. The most common adverse effects are nausea, vomiting, jaw pain, headache, flushing, erythema, anxiety, musculoskeletal aches/pain, and photosensitivity.[30] Epoprostenol can also be administered by the inhalational route; however, this has not been well studied in PAH. A typical dosing strategy is to administer 50–85 mcg/kg/minute by nebulizer and then taper to the maximum effect. Another strategy is to nebulize at a fixed concentration of 10–20 mcg/mL at a rate of 0.2–0.3 mL/minute.[31]

Implications for the Critical Care Practitioner

Epoprostenol requires close monitoring because of the effects on decreasing blood pressure, heart rate, increased risk of bleeding, short half-life (4–5 minutes), and unstable nature (specifically the *Flolan* product).[24] Administration of epoprostenol is through a central line with a 0.22-micron filter; however, a peripheral line may be used on a short-term basis until central access can be established. There are infectious risks from pulmonary artery catheterization, as well as central and peripheral line infections, with the most common pathogens being *Staphylococcus aureus* and *Micrococcus* spp.[32] The pharmacist should have a good understanding of the different infusion pumps (for home use), priming rates and volumes needed, typical dosage titrations required for acute therapy in the ICU, risks associated with interrupted PGI_2 therapy, adverse effects and their potential treatments to optimize titration, compounding, distributing process for timely administration, diluents required for admixture (sterile diluent for Flolan and either 0.9% sodium chloride or sterile water for Veletri), and strategies for transitioning to alternative therapy such as treprostinil.[30,33]

There are critical elements about epoprostenol management that place the pharmacist at the forefront of care. These center on the use of correct and constant dosing weights, expertise of shelf lives of the various products used, and practical coordination of backup cartridges/intravenous bags if the patient is in the ICU for greater than 24 hours. Patient dosing weights need to be based on original weights for the patient (and rates that patients have been titrated to in the outpatient setting) and may need to be verified by home infusion nurses/pharmacists or other providers. Errors can occur with nanogram per kilogram per minute conversions to microgram per kilogram per minute conversions by hospital-based pumps, so the patient-pharmacist interaction and medication reconciliation on admission is paramount. Backup cartridges (if patients are stable to mix their own infusions) or infusion bags need to be stored appropriately and made available to the nursing units, which requires interdisciplinary collaboration. This change can be seen with the newer *Veletri* agent and the need for every 24- to 72-hour changes, instead of more frequent 8-hour switches with the older product. Finally, titration of the agent epoprostenol needs to be managed by experienced physicians because hemodynamic instability can occur if lines are primed, agents are abruptly discontinued, or the patient's baseline condition worsens.

Transitioning from intravenous epoprostenol to oral or subcutaneous dosage forms of other classes has been described in case reports in the literature with success, with recommendations not specific regarding whether these can be done in an acute critical care situation.[33] Other transitions from subcutaneous to intravenous to inhalational have been described.

Conversion from epoprostenol to treprostinil is accomplished by initiating treprostinil while simultaneously decreasing epoprostenol. The treprostinil package insert recommends a seven-step process (Table 30.3).[34]

Treprostinil

Treprostinil is a tricyclic benzidine analog of epoprostenol that has a comparatively longer half-life (4–4.5 hours) and is more stable in solution than epoprostenol.[34] Treprostinil is FDA labeled to improve exercise capacity in WHO group 1 patients with PAH. Treprostinil has several routes of administration, including intravenous, subcutaneous, inhalational, and oral.

The efficacy of this agent has been shown in several clinical trials. A double-blind, randomized trial of the subcutaneous infusion was compared with placebo in 470 patients with PAH.[35] Treprostinil dosed at 1.25 ng/kg/minute titrated to effect to a maximum of 22.5 ng/kg/minute over 12 weeks resulted in improved 6-minute walk distance, Borg dyspnea score, pulmonary hemodynamics, and quality of life.[36] The TRIUMPH-1 study was a randomized controlled trial of the addition of inhaled treprostinil or placebo to oral therapy with bosentan or sildenafil in 235 patients with NYHA class III or IV PAH.[37] Treprostinil was initiated at a dose of three inhalations four times daily titrated to a maximum of nine inhalations four times daily. Patients in the treprostinil group had a mean increase of 19 m in the 6-minute walk distance and increased quality of life. Two randomized controlled trials (FREEDOM C and FREEDOM C2) investigated the oral dosage form of treprostinil to bosentan or sildenafil in patients with PAH.[38,39] The FREEDOM C trial randomized 350 patients to 1 mg of oral treprostinil twice daily to a maximum of 16 mg twice daily or matching placebo. The FREEDOM C2 trial randomized 310 patients to 0.25 mg of oral treprostinil twice daily (mean dose 3.1 mg twice daily) or matching placebo. Neither trial showed a difference in the primary outcome of the 6-minute walk distance. A third trial of monotherapy with oral treprostinil at a starting dose of 0.25–1 mg twice daily to a maximum dose of 12 mg twice daily or placebo showed a difference in 6-minute walk distance and the combined end point of 6-minute walk distance and Borg dyspnea score.[40]

Dosing of treprostinil varies by the route of administration. The initial dosing of intravenous treprostinil (Remodulin) is typically 1.25 ng/kg/minute, but this should be reduced to 0.625 ng/kg/minute in severe hepatic insufficiency. The infusion rate should be increased in increments of 1.25 ng/kg/minute per week for the first 4 weeks of treatment and then 2.5 ng/kg/minute per week for the remaining duration of infusion to clinical response.[34] In the ICU setting, the dosing titration may be more rapid, with a starting dose of 1–3 mg/kg/minute, gradually increased by 1–2 ng/kg/minute two or three times weekly. The dosing of the inhalational form (Tyvaso) is rarely initiated in the ICU because of the difficulties with the required inhalation system. In these cases, the patient should be transitioned to intravenous therapy. The inhalational form of treprostinil in the outpatient setting is typically initiated as three inhalations four times daily spaced at least 4 hours apart and is increased by three inhalations every 1–2 weeks to a maximum of nine inhalations four times daily.[41]

Oral treprostinil therapy may also be initiated in the outpatient setting. The dosing of Orenitram is 0.25 mg twice daily or 0.125 mg three times daily administered with food. The dose is increased in increments of 0.25 or 0.5 mg twice daily or 0.125 mg three times daily every 3–4 days to achieve optimal clinical response.[42] Oral treprostinil should be avoided in severe hepatic insufficiency and used with caution because tablets may lodge in diverticuli. The most common adverse effects with treprostinil are hypotension, jaw pain, chest pain, flushing, cough, headache, dizziness, throat irritation, nausea, and diarrhea. If

Table 30.3 Seven-Step Process for Conversion of Epoprostenol to Treprostinil

Step	Flolan Dose	Remodulin Dose
1	Unchanged	Initiate at 10% of starting Flolan dose
2	Decrease Flolan to 80% of starting dose	Increase to 30% of starting Flolan dose
3	Decrease Flolan to 60% of starting dose	Increase to 50% of starting Flolan dose
4	Decrease Flolan to 40% of starting dose	Increase to 70% of starting Flolan dose
5	Decrease Flolan to 20% of starting dose	Increase to 90% of starting Flolan dose
6	Decrease Flolan to 5% of starting dose	Increase to 110% of starting Flolan dose
7	Discontinue Flolan	Continue at 110% and increase in 5%–10% increments as needed

Adapted from: Treprostinil (Orenitram) [package insert]. Research Triangle Park, NC: United Therapeutics, 2014.

administered in the ICU setting, the extended-release tablets cannot be split, crushed, or chewed.

Implications for the Critical Care Practitioner

Diluents required for the intravenous treprostinil admixture include the sterile diluent, 0.9% sodium chloride, or sterile water. Subcutaneous administration may lead to infusion-site reactions, which occur with a prevalence of about 10%. This has prompted some patients to be transitioned to the intravenous or inhalation route. Strategies to reduce these reactions include avoiding sensitive areas, relocating to a new infusion site (abdomen, thighs, posterior upper arms, etc.), and using topical agents (ice, topical agents such as lidocaine, corticosteroids, antihistamines, or calcineurin inhibitors), and oral nonsteroidal agents, antihistamines, or GABA [γ-aminobutyric acid] analogs.[43]

The conversion for patients being switched from intravenous treprostinil to intravenous epoprostenol is approximately 1.25:1, respectively.[44] Dosing of the subcutaneous formulation requires re-titration if the infusion is stopped for more than 4–6 hours, and the oral formulation requires re-titration if more than two consecutive doses are missed. The adverse effect profile of treprostinil is different from that of epoprostenol. With the treprostinil half-life being 4 hours versus 4–6 minutes with epoprostenol, this offers the theoretical advantage of not causing the major rapid pulmonary vasoconstriction and emergency situations that would be seen in sudden discontinuation.

Iloprost

Iloprost is another example of a prostacyclin analog that is administered as an inhalation, but it can also be given by the intravenous route (although not available in the United States). Iloprost is FDA labeled for the treatment of PAH (WHO group 1) to improve a composite end point consisting of exercise tolerance, symptoms (NYHA class), and lack of deterioration. Data behind the efficacy of inhaled iloprost centers on the Aerosolized Iloprost Randomized Study (AIR) trial, which randomized patients to receive up to 30 mcg per day (2.5 or 5 mcg inhaled six to nine times per day) or placebo.[45] Patients who received iloprost showed improvements in 6-minute walk distance, symptom improvement (NYHA class), decreased PVR, less dyspnea, and improved quality of life.

Iloprost is initially dosed at 2.5 mcg administered as six to nine inhalations per day at least 2 hours apart by the I-neb AAD system.[46] If the 2.5-mcg dose is well tolerated, the dose can be increased to 5 mcg. Patients with severe hepatic impairment (Child-Pugh class B or C) should have the dosing interval increased to 3–4 hours. Renal dosing adjustments are not required. The adverse effect profile of iloprost is similar to that of epoprostenol and treprostinil, with the most common adverse effects of hypotension, bronchospasm, cough, jaw pain, and headache.[46] There are no significant drug interactions; however, concurrent use with antihypertensive agents, anticoagulants, and platelet inhibitors should be closely monitored.

Implications for the Critical Care Practitioner

Doses should be reduced (and may need to be avoided) if the systolic blood pressure (SBP) is less than 85 mm Hg or if pulmonary edema develops. There are several limitations to administration of inhaled iloprost, including the feasibility of inhalations administered six to nine times per day, inability to mix with other medications, and inability to administer if a patient requires mechanical ventilation. Patients on mechanical ventilation may receive iloprost by ultrasonic nebulizer; however, this strategy has not been well studied. Therefore, patients admitted to the ICU may need conversion to other agents or discontinuation of therapy if unresponsive to self-inhalation techniques.

Endothelin Receptor Antagonists

Endothelin-1 causes vasoconstriction and cell proliferation through activation of the ETA and ETB receptors on smooth muscle cells.[47] Endothelin type A mediates vasoconstriction, whereas ETB mediates vasodilation through release of nitric oxide.[10] The mechanism of action for the endothelin receptor antagonists is selective ETA antagonism with minimal effect on ETB.

Several clinical trials have shown the efficacy of the endothelin receptor antagonists. The BREATHE-1 trial was a double-blind, placebo-controlled, multicenter study of bosentan in 213 patients with PAH.[48] Patients were randomized to one of three groups: bosentan 62.5 mg twice daily increased to 125 mg after 4 weeks of treatment (n=74), bosentan 62.5 mg twice daily increased to 250 mg after 4 weeks of treatment (n=70), or placebo (n=69). The primary outcome of 6-minute walking distance was increased overall by 44 m in bosentan-treated patients (27 m in the bosentan 125-mg group and 46 m in the bosentan 250-mg group), which was a statistically significant difference compared with a decrease of 8 m in the placebo group. Patients treated with bosentan also showed improvements in secondary clinical end points monitored, including Borg dyspnea score, change in WHO functional class, and clinical worsening defined as the sum of death, hospitalization for PAH, discontinuation of therapy for PAH, and need for epoprostenol.

The SERAPHIN trial was a phase III, multicenter, double-blind, randomized, placebo-controlled, event-driven study of macitentan in 742 patients with PAH.[49] Patients were randomly assigned to one of three treatment groups: macitentan 3 mg daily, macitentan 10 mg daily, or placebo. The primary outcome of the time from the initiation of treatment to the first occurrence of a composite end point of death, atrial septostomy, lung transplantation, initiation of treatment with intravenous or subcutaneous prostanoids, or worsening of PAH was seen in 31.4% of patients in the macitentan 10-mg group, 38% of patients in the macitentan 3-mg group, and 46.4% of patients in the placebo group.

The ARIES-1 and ARIES-2 trials were concurrent, double-blind, placebo-controlled trials that randomized patients with PAH to placebo or ambrisentan 5 or 10 mg (ARIES-1) or placebo or ambrisentan 2.5 or 5 mg (ARIES-2).[50] All ambrisentan groups showed an increase in the primary outcome of 6-minute walk test distance compared with placebo (ARIES-1: 31 m and 51 m for ambrisentan 5 mg and 10 mg, respectively; ARIES-2: 32 m and 59 m for ambrisentan 2.5 mg and 5 mg, respectively).

All three of the currently available endothelin receptor antagonists are FDA labeled for the treatment of PAH in WHO group 1 patients to improve exercise ability and to decrease clinical worsening.[51-53] Ambrisentan is initiated at a dose of 5 mg daily, which can be increased to 10 mg daily if tolerated. Bosentan is initiated at 62.5 mg twice daily, which can be increased to 125 mg twice daily. Macitentan is dosed at 10 mg daily (higher doses are not recommended). Renal adjustment is not needed for bosentan or macitentan; however, ambrisentan is not recommended for patients with a creatinine clearance (CrCl) less than 20 mL/minute/1.73 m^2. All three agents should be avoided in moderate to severe hepatic impairment.

The most common adverse effects with the endothelin receptor antagonists are anemia, nasal congestion, sinusitis, fluid retention, headache, bronchitis, and urinary tract infections. The major drug interactions vary between agents; however, all three agents have increases in serum concentrations when administered with strong cytochrome P450 (CYP) 3A4 (and CYP2C9 with bosentan) inhibitors and decreases in serum concentrations when administered with strong CYP3A4 inducers. All three agents are pregnancy category X and should be avoided in females who are or may become pregnant.

Implications for the Critical Care Practitioner

The endothelin receptor antagonists are associated with an increase in peripheral and pulmonary edema, increased bleeding risks, and increases in liver function tests; patients should be closely monitored for signs and symptoms of these potentially serious effects. Decreases in hemoglobin concentrations of more than 0.8 mg/dL are considered significant and warrant further investigation to determine the causality. Medications in this class should not be crushed; however, bosentan tablets can be split or dissolved in water. If oral or tube administration is not possible, conversion to an intravenous alternative (typically epoprostenol) may be required. With oral agents in this class, it is rare to initiate them in the ICU. Typically, the more critical treatment decision is when to discontinue or hold endothelin receptor antagonists when a patient presents with significant hypotension.[31]

PDE-5 Inhibitors

Nitric oxide induces the formation of intracellular cGMP, which leads to relaxation of the pulmonary vascular smooth muscle and dilation of the pulmonary arterioles.[54] The isoenzyme that is primarily responsible for the breakdown of cGMP is PDE-5. Inhibitors of PDE-5 increase cGMP concentrations and allow for prolonged action of cGMP. Clinical studies with both sildenafil and tadalafil have shown the efficacy of the PDE-5 inhibitors in reducing clinical worsening, improving 6-minute walk test, and improving quality of life, but with no reduction in mortality.[55-57]

Sildenafil (Revatio) is FDA labeled for the treatment of PAH in WHO group 1 adults to improve exercise ability and delay clinical worsening.[58] The oral dose is 5 or 20 mg three times daily, spaced at least 4–6 hours apart. The intravenous dose is 2.5 or 10 mg three times daily administered as a bolus. No dose adjustments are recommended for renal or hepatic impairment. The Viagra formulation of sildenafil is not FDA labeled for use in PAH, but several studies and case series have shown an improvement in pulmonary hemodynamics at doses of 25–100 mg per day.[56,59]

Tadalafil is FDA labeled for the treatment of PAH in WHO group 1 adults to improve exercise ability.[60] The dose is 40 mg once daily, and doses should not be divided. For patients with mild to moderate renal impairment (CrCl 31–80 mL/minute/1.73 m^2) or hepatic impairment, the dose should be decreased to 20 mg daily. Use of tadalafil should be avoided for severe renal impairment (CrCl less than 30 mL/minute/1.73 m^2) or hepatic cirrhosis.

The most common adverse effects associated with the PDE-5 inhibitors are epistaxis, headache, flushing, erythema, dyspepsia, rhinitis, hypotension, priapism, and visual or hearing loss.[58,60] Significant drug interactions include the CYP3A4 inhibitors, amlodipine, α-receptor blocking agents, and organic nitrates. For patients who may require nitrate administration for chest pain, it is recommended to avoid these agents for at least 24–48 hours after the last dose. Blood pressure should be closely monitored in these patients.

Implications for the Critical Care Practitioner

Phosphodiesterase type 5 inhibitors may cause hypotension and a resultant increase in heart rate; patients should be closely monitored for signs and symptoms of these potentially serious effects. Sildenafil is available as an oral suspension; however, tablets of all PDE-5 inhibitors can be crushed for feeding tube administration. Others forms of sildenafil (e.g., Viagra) may be used for PAH if needed due to institutional formulary restrictions.

sGC Stimulator

Riociguat is a novel agent for the treatment of PAH. The mechanism of action is through stimulation of sGC and increased binding to nitric oxide to sGC, leading to an increase in synthesis of cGMP by the nitric oxide–sGC–cGMP pathway.[61] The beneficial effects of cGMP in PAH include vasodilation, inhibition of smooth cell proliferation, prevention of fibrosis, and antithrombotic and anti-inflammatory effects.[61]

Riociguat has shown efficacy in two major trials: PATENT-1 and CHEST-1. The PATENT-1 trial was a phase III randomized controlled study of 443 patients with PAH.[62] Patients with symptomatic PAH who received riociguat 2.5 mg three times daily showed a 30-m increase their 6-minute walk test from baseline compared with a decrease of 6 m in the placebo group. The CHEST-1 trial was a phase III, multicenter, randomized, double-blind, placebo-controlled study of 261 patients with inoperable chronic thromboembolic PH.[63] Patients who received riociguat 1 mg three times daily showed a 39-m increase their 6-minute walk test from baseline compared with a decrease of 6 m in the placebo group.

Riociguat is FDA labeled for the treatment of WHO group 1 PAH to improve exercise capacity, improve WHO functional class, and delay clinical worsening.[64] It is also FDA labeled for persistent or recurrent chronic thromboembolic PH (WHO group 4) after surgical treatment or inoperable chronic thromboembolic PH to improve exercise capacity and WHO functional class.[64] The starting dose is 1 mg three times daily, but this may be reduced to 0.5 mg three times a day for patients with low blood pressure at initiation, or those who develop low blood pressure after initiation. Doses are titrated in increments of 0.5 mg to a maximum of 2.5 mg three times daily. No dosage adjustments are required for renal or hepatic insufficiency, but use is not recommended for a CrCl less than 15 mL/minute/1.73 m², hemodialysis, or severe hepatic impairment (Child-Pugh class C). Riociguat is contraindicated in pregnancy (pregnancy category X).

The most common adverse effects of riociguat are headache, dyspepsia/gastritis, dizziness, nausea, diarrhea, hypotension, vomiting, anemia, gastroesophageal reflux, and constipation.[64] Significant drug interactions include azole antifungals, protease inhibitors, nitrates, and PDE-5 inhibitors, all of which may lead to increased hypotensive effects requiring riociguat dose reductions.

Implications for the Critical Care Practitioner

Riociguat may increase the risk of bleeding, hypotension, and pulmonary edema; patients should be closely monitored for signs and symptoms of these potentially serious effects. There are few data regarding the ability to split or crush the tablet, but the manufacturer recommends to avoid this because of teratogenic concerns. If doses are held for more than 3 consecutive days, patients will require re-titration to their chronic dosage schedule. For patients with a current history of smoking, higher doses may be required in the ICU setting because of an increase in serum concentrations secondary to abrupt discontinuation of smoking (50%–60% serum concentration reduction in smokers).[64]

Supportive Therapies

In addition to the vasodilators, there are several adjunctive therapies that may be beneficial in PAH therapy and are recommended in the most recent guidelines.[2] As discussed previously, patients with PAH are at an increased risk of thromboembolism and may benefit from anticoagulation. Use of anticoagulants in this setting is somewhat controversial; however, warfarin is recommended, titrated to an INR (international normalized ratio) of 1.5–2.5 if no bleeding contraindications exist.[2] Diuretics are recommended in patients with PAH with signs of RV failure and fluid retention; however, no specific recommendations are made regarding choice of agents.[2] Digoxin may improve cardiac index (short-term effect), but it is most commonly used for patients with PAH who develop atrial tachycardia in order to slow the ventricular rate. These strategies may be used in the ICU setting unless contraindicated due to the underlying critical illness.

Treatment of the Critically Ill Patient with PAH

Pulmonary arterial hypertension in itself can cause the acute RV decompensation. This is of particularly concern when patients are admitted to the ICU on several pharmacologic therapies. The RV adapts poorly to sudden increases in afterload, and this can result in decreased contractility and hemodynamic collapse.[65] Right ventricular dysfunction can result from excess RV afterload, inadequate RV preload, decreased RV contractility, or altered systemic vasodilation.[31] In the ICU setting, additional triggers such as sepsis, trauma, anemia, pulmonary embolism, medication nonadherence, interruption of chronic therapy, and arrhythmias can quickly overwhelm the effectiveness of any RV compensatory mechanisms.[65]

Overall treatment goals are to manage fluids judiciously, reduce venous filling pressures, and normalize cardiac output (Figure 30.2).[66] Fluid management should consist of maintaining net negative fluid balance in patients with RV failure and PAH. This may require the use of diuretic therapy or renal replacement therapies as indicated. For maintenance of blood pressure and cardiac output, various agents are preferred. Dobutamine is a β_1-agonist that decreases right and left ventricular afterload and improves cardiac output. This agent has adverse effects related to tachyarrhythmias, which can be problematic in low cardiac output states. Another option is milrinone, a phosphodiesterase type 3 inhibitor. In addition to milrinone's inotropic properties, it acts as a pulmonary vasodilator and improves RV function and decreases PVR.[67]

If vasoconstrictors are indicated due to the systemic vasodilation caused by dobutamine, then norepinephrine (predominantly an α_1-vasoconstrictor at increasing dosages starting at 5–10 mcg/minute) is the vasopressor of choice. Other options for vasopressors include phenylephrine and vasopressin; dopamine and epinephrine are considered last-line options because of the increased potential for adverse effects. Inhalational formulations of phosphodiesterase inhibitors such as milrinone have not been studied in these patients.[68]

Patients with acutely decompensated PAH require immediate stabilization to improve oxygenation, optimize preload, decrease afterload, and improve RV contractility, all while maintaining therapeutic pulmonary pressures. They also require interventions to their maintenance regimens to dose adjust for end-organ complications such as renal or hepatic dysfunction. Patients with newly diagnosed advanced PAH require centers with expertise in PH management. If further treatments are required after advance treatments and combinations are used, lung or heart-lung transplantation, or the use of bridge therapies with venovenous and venoarterial extracorporeal membrane oxygenation, may be indicated.

Most PH centers have developed treatment algorithms for patients admitted with worsening heart failure. If patients are currently maximized on diuretics, inotropes, intravenous prostacyclins, PDE-5 inhibitors, and endothelin receptor antagonists, inhaled nitric oxide or inhaled prostaglandins (epoprostenol) can be used as last therapeutic options.

MONITORING OF THE CRITICALLY ILL PATIENT WITH PAH

Monitoring of the ICU patient with PAH is important for several reasons, including the evaluation of treatment strategies, potential adverse effects of therapy, and clinical worsening. Although the use of pulmonary artery catheters has declined in the ICU, these devices are important for measuring hemodynamic parameters in patients with PAH, including RA pressure, left atrial pressure, cardiac output, and Svo_2. Echocardiography may be useful in settings where more invasive monitoring is unavailable. Together with cardiac and pulmonary hemodynamic monitoring, patients should have their renal and hepatic function, tissue perfusion/oxygenation, neurohormonal markers, and markers of fluid balance (e.g., daily weight and fluid input and output) monitored very closely (Table 30.4).[65] Cardiac biomarkers, such as troponin and natriuretic peptides, may also be useful given that increases in these values are associated with worsening outcomes in PAH.[68]

PRACTICAL CONSIDERATIONS FOR THE CRITICAL CARE PHARMACIST

The treatment of patients with PAH in the ICU can pose a challenge, and recent data analyses point out that they constitute a complex patient population receiving high-risk

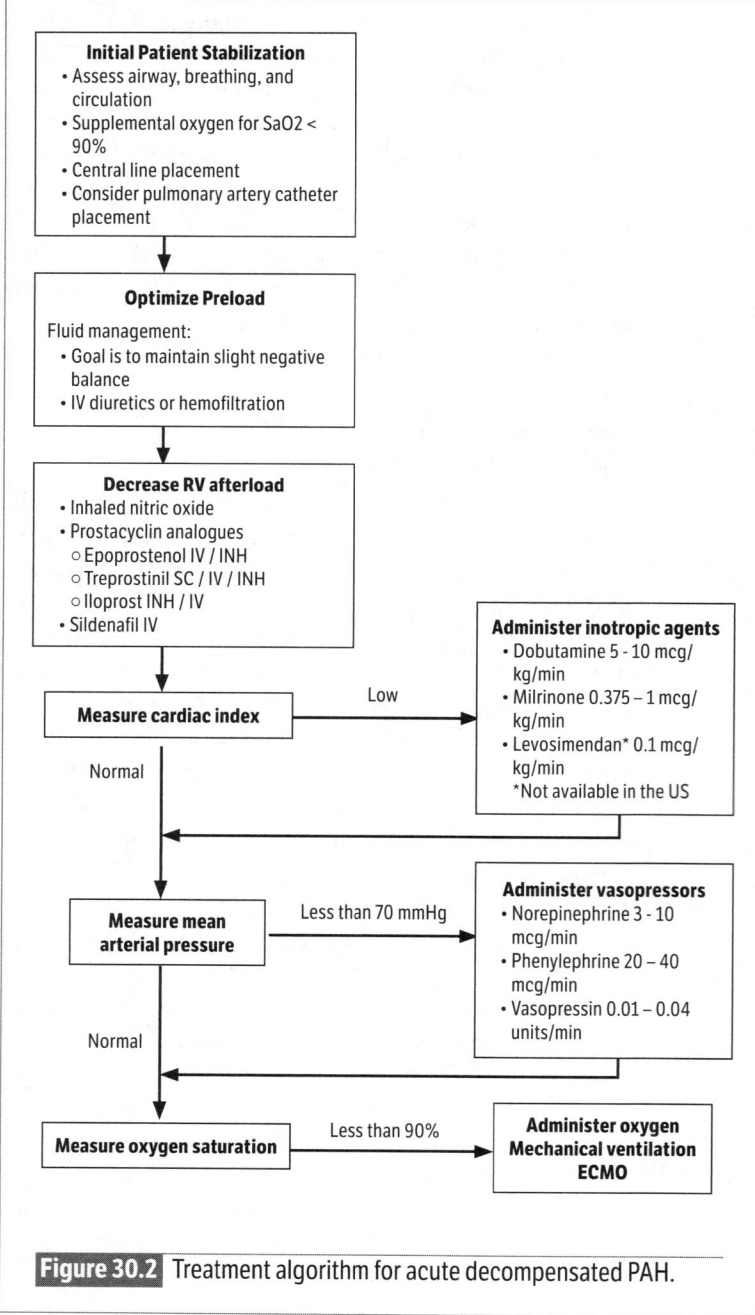

Figure 30.2 Treatment algorithm for acute decompensated PAH.

medications. A national survey emphasized serious or potentially serious intravenous prostacyclin administration errors.[43] There are four major considerations regarding the role of the pharmacist and potential areas of intervention for the critically ill patient with PAH. First, the stability of the patient is of paramount importance. Depending on overall patient status (especially RV failure, septic shock, and cardiogenic shock), intravenous, inhalational, or oral therapies may require adjustment or discontinuation. The RV adapts poorly to sudden increases in afterload, and this can result in decreased contractility and hemodynamic collapse.[65] Right ventricular dysfunction can result from excess RV afterload, inadequate RV preload, decreased RV contractility, or altered systemic vasodilaton.[31] In the ICU setting, additional triggers such as sepsis, trauma, anemia, pulmonary embolism, medication nonadherence, interruption of chronic therapy, and arrhythmias can quickly overwhelm the effectiveness of any RV compensatory mechanism.[65]

Because of the short half-life of these agents, most patients should be kept on intravenous prostacyclin without interruption. This includes careful medication reconciliation, often requiring a call to the company providing the parenteral prostacyclin to confirm original dosing weight, rate of administration, and vial concentration. The next decision may involve the provision and decision to use patients' home infusion pumps or may involve whether to convert the patient to a hospital-based pump where therapies can be prepared and supplied solely from the pharmacy department. Second, there are concerns for the oral or enteral agents with respect to how they can be administered in the mechanically ventilated patient or NPO (nothing by mouth) patient. Among the PDE-5 inhibitors and endothelin antagonists, only sildenafil has a commercially available suspension and is an intravenous alternative, with the five other agents available as tablets or capsules with limited ability to administer enterally or parenterally (Table 30.5).[69] Inhalation treatments such as inhaled iloprost may pose a problem in dosing frequency with a patient on either invasive or noninvasive mechanical ventilation. Of note, when these PAH medication classes were FDA labeled for use in the United States, studies assessing their safety in the critically ill ICU patient were not done. This requires clinical judgment and individualization of therapy when dosing patients with PAH. Third, practitioners need to understand and be well-versed when patients present to the ICU with infected

continued on page 623

Table 30.4 Recommended Monitoring of the Critically Ill Patient with Severe Pulmonary Arterial Hypertension

Parameter	Modality	Treatment Goal
Renal function	Urinary catheter	Maintain kidney function and diuresis. In general a net negative fluid balance is required
	Serum creatinine; I & O	
Hepatic function	AST, ALT, bilirubin	Reduce hepatic congestion
		Maintain hepatic perfusion
Cardiac function	Central venous line (central venous pressure, $SCVO_2$)	Improvement in cardiac function demonstrated by an increase in cardiac output with improvement (reduction) in right atrial pressures
	Pulmonary arterial catheter (RA pressure, cardiac index, PAPm, PVR, SVO_2)	$SCVO_2 > 70\%$, $SVO_2 > 65\%$
	Echocardiography	Improve LV filling
Tissue perfusion / oxygenation	Lactate	< 2 mmol/L
Neurohormonal markers	Brain natriuretic peptides (BNP or NT-proBNP)	Reduction in BNP levels
Myocardial perfusion	Systemic blood pressure (noninvasive or invasive)	Ensure adequate systemic diastolic pressure (> 60 mm Hg)
	ECG	Avoid/treat tachycardia/tachyarrhythmia
	Troponin	Optimize myocardial perfusion (negative troponin)

ALT = alanine aminotransferase; AST = aspartate aminotransferase; BNP = brain natriuretic peptide; ECG = electrocardiogram; LV = left ventricle; NT-proBNP = N-terminal fragment of brain natriuretic peptide; PAPm = mean pulmonary arterial pressure; PVR = pulmonary vascular resistance; RA = right atrial; $SCVO_2$ = central venous oxygen saturation; SVO_2 = mixed venous oxygen saturation.

Reprinted with permission from: Hoeper MM, Granton J. Intensive care unit management of patients with severe pulmonary hypertension and right heart failure. Am J Respir Crit Care Med 2011;184:1114-24.

Table 30.5 Vasodilator Agents for PAH

Drug Class	Generic (Brand) Name	Route	Dosing	Adverse Effects	Major Drug Interactions	Monitoring	Clinical Notes
Prostacyclin analogs	Epoprostenol (Flolan/Veletri)	IV/	IV: 2 ng/kg/min; increase every 15 minutes to effect	Flushing, headache, nausea, hypotension, chest pain, jaw pain	• Antihypertensives • Anticoagulants • Platelet inhibitors • Digoxin	• Blood pressure • Heart rate • Bleeding	• Requires in-line 0.22-micron filter • Reconstitute Flolan with sterile diluent only and Veletri with sterile water or 0.9% sodium chloride • Reconstituted solutions only good for 8 hours (Flolan) or 48 hours (Veletri)
		INH	INH: 50 mcg/kg/min; taper to maximum effect				
	Treprostinil (Remodulin)	SC/IV	1.25 ng/kg/min; increase by 1.25 ng/kg/min every week for 4 weeks; then by 2.5 ng/kg/min per week	Hypotension, jaw pain, chest pain, flushing, nausea	• Antihypertensives • Anticoagulants • Platelet inhibitors • CYP2C8 inhibitors or inducers • Diuretics	• Blood pressure • Heart rate • Bleeding	• Reconstitute with sterile diluent, sterile water, or 0.9% sodium chloride • Reduce dose to 0.625 ng/kg/min in severe hepatic insufficiency
	(Tyvaso)	INH	Three to nine inhalations QID	Cough, headache, nausea, dizziness, flushing, throat irritation, diarrhea, pharyngolaryngeal pain			• Requires Tyvaso inhalation system
	(Orenitram)	Oral	0.25 mg BID or 0.125 mg TID (max 21 mg BID)	Headache, nausea, and diarrhea			• Use with caution in diverticulosis • Avoid use in severe hepatic insufficiency • Requires re-titration if two or more doses missed
	Iloprost (Ventavis)	INH	2.5–5 mcg six to nine times per day	Hypotension, bronchospasm, pulmonary edema	• Antihypertensives • Anticoagulants • Platelet inhibitors	• Blood pressure • Heart rate • Bleeding	• Requires I-neb AAD system or nebulizer • Avoid use if SBP < 85 mm Hg • Administer no more than every 2 hours • Reduce dosing intervals to 3–4 hours in Child-Pugh class B or C
Endothelin receptor antagonists	Ambrisentan (Letairis)	Oral	5–10 mg daily	Peripheral edema, nasal congestion, sinusitis, flushing	• Cyclosporine	• Peripheral edema • Pulmonary edema • Hematocrit • LFTs	• Tablets should not be crushed • Contraindicated in idiopathic pulmonary fibrosis • REMS program required for females • Not recommended for CrCl < 20 mL/min/1.73 m^2
	Bosentan (Tracleer)	Oral	62.5–125 mg BID	Fluid retention, hepatotoxicity	• Ritonavir • Cyclosporine • Glyburide • CYP 2C9 or 3A4 inhibitors	• Peripheral edema • Pulmonary edema • Hematocrit • LFTs	• Tracleer access program required • Avoid in moderate to severe hepatic failure • No renal adjustment recommended
	Macitentan (Opsumit)	Oral	10 mg daily	Anemia, pharyngitis, headache, bronchitis, urinary tract infections	• CYP3A4 inducers or inhibitors	• Peripheral edema • Pulmonary edema • Hematocrit • LFTs	• Tablets should not be crushed • REMS program required for females • No renal adjustment recommended

Table 30.5 Vasodilator Agents for PAH (continued)

Drug Class	Generic (Brand) Name	Route	Dosing	Adverse Effects	Major Drug Interactions	Monitoring	Clinical Notes
PDE-5 inhibitors	Sildenafil (Revatio)	Oral	5 or 20 mg TID	Epistaxis, headache, flushing, erythema, dyspepsia, rhinitis, hypotension, priapism, hearing or visual loss	• CYP3A4 inhibitors • Amlodipine • -Blockers • Organic nitrates	• Blood pressure • Heart rate	• Available as oral suspension • Avoid use with other nitrates • No renal adjustment recommended
		IV	2.5 or 10 mg TID				
	Tadalafil (Adcirca)	Oral	40 mg daily				• Divided doses not recommended • CrCl 31–80 mL/min/1.73 m²: start at 20 mg daily • CrCl < 30 mL/min/1.73 m²: avoid use • Avoid use in severe hepatic cirrhosis
Soluble guanylate cyclase stimulator	Riociguat (Adempas)	Oral	1–2.5 mg TID	Headache, dyspepsia, gastritis, dizziness, nausea, diarrhea, hypotension, vomiting, anemia, constipation, gastroesophageal reflux	• Strong CYP inhibitors • P-glycoprotein inhibitors • Nitrates • PDE-5 inhibitors	• Peripheral edema • Blood pressure • Bleeding	• Requires re-titration if more than 3 days missed • REMS program required for females • Avoid use in severe hepatic impairment, CrCl < 15 mL/min/1.73 m², and hemodialysis

BID = twice daily; INH = inhalational; IV = intravenous; LFT = liver function test; PDE-5 = phosphodiesterase type 5; QID = four times daily; REMS = Risk Evaluation and Mitigation Strategies; SBP = systolic blood pressure; SC = subcutaneous; TID = three times daily.

Adapted from: Epoprostenol (Flolan) [package insert]. Research Triangle Park, NC: GlaxoSmithKline, March 2011; Epoprostenol (Veletri) [package insert]. South San Francisco, CA: Actelion Pharmaceuticals US, June 2012; Treprostinil (Remodulin) [package insert]. Research Triangle Park, NC: United Therapeutics, 2014; Jing ZC, Keyur P, Pulido T, et al. Efficacy and safety of oral treprostinil monotherapy for the treatment of pulmonary arterial hypertension: a randomized, controlled trial. Circulation 2013;127:624-33; Treprostinil (Tyvaso) [package insert]. Research Triangle Park, NC: United Therapeutics, 2014; Olschewski H, Simmoneau G, Galie N, et al. Inhaled iloprost for severe pulmonary hypertension. N Engl J Med 2002;347:322-9; Galie N, Olschewski H, Oudiz RJ, et al. Ambrisentan for the treatment of pulmonary arterial hypertension: results of the Ambrisentan in Pulmonary Arterial Hypertension, Randomized, Double-Blind, Placebo-Controlled, Multicenter, Efficacy (ARIES) study 1 and 2. Circulation 2008;117:3010-9; Bosentan (Tracleer) [package insert]. South San Francisco, CA: Actelion Pharmaceuticals US, October 2012; Macitentan (Opsumit) [package insert]. South San Francisco, CA: Actelion Pharmaceuticals US, February 2015; Wang RC, Jiang FM, Zheng QL, et al. Efficacy and safety of sildenafil treatment in pulmonary arterial hypertension: a systematic review. Respir Med 2014;108:531-7; Ghofrani HA, Wiedemann R, Rose F, et al. Sildenafil for treatment of lung fibrosis and pulmonary hypertension: a randomized trial. Lancet 2002;360:895-900; Ghofrani HA, D'Armini AM, Grimminger F, et al. Riociguat for the treatment of chronic thromboembolic pulmonary hypertension. N Engl J Med 2013;369:319-29.

---

continued from page 621

Hickman or PICC (peripherally inserted central catheter) lines and know how to convert to other therapies with the correct priming volumes. Fourth, anticoagulation of the patient with PAH in the ICU, treatment of pregnant patients with PAH, and the decision about mechanical ventilation in the decompensated patient all require the interdisciplinary team to weigh in on these decisions.

Finally, there should be consideration of administrative oversight from an interdisciplinary perspective on keeping these patients with PAH safe when being admitted to inpatient settings. This could take the form of protocol/guideline development as it relates to acute vasoactive trials while in the ICU, policies on the criteria of when patients should be transitioned from home intravenous/subcutaneous pumps, electronic medical record assimilation of order sets, and, finally, the integration of home-based infusion services and their roles in educating patients in the institutional setting.

REFERENCES

1. Rich S. What is pulmonary arterial hypertension? Pulm Circ 2012;2:271-2.
2. Galie N, Hoeper MM, Humbert M, et al. Guidelines for the diagnosis and treatment of pulmonary hypertension. Eur Heart J 2009;30:2493-537.
3. D'Alonzi GE, Barst RJ, Ayres SM, et al. Survival in patients with primary pulmonary hypertension. Results from a national prospective registry. Ann Intern Med 1991;115:343-9.
4. Badesch DB, Raskob GE, Elliott CG, et al. Pulmonary arterial hypertension – baseline characteristics from the REVEAL registry. Chest 2010;137:376-87.
5. Rich JD, Rich S. Clinical diagnosis of pulmonary hypertension. Circulation 2014;130;1820-30.
6. Rich S. Clinical insights into the pathogenesis of primary pulmonary hypertension. Chest 1998;114(3 suppl):237S-41S.
7. Muzevich KM, Chohan H, Grinnan DC. Management of pulmonary vasodilator therapy in patients with pulmonary arterial hypertension during critical illness. Crit Care 2014;18:1-10.

8. Campo A, Mathai SC, Le Pavec J, et al. Outcomes of hospitalisation for right heart failure in pulmonary arterial hypertension. Eur Respir J 2011;38:359-67.

9. Humbert M, Lau EM, Montani D, et al. Advances in therapeutic interventions for patients with pulmonary arterial hypertension. Circulation 2014;130:2189-208.

10. Shao D, Park JE, Wort SJ. The role of endothelin-1 in the pathogenesis of pulmonary arterial hypertension. Pharmacol Res 2011;63:504-11.

11. Rubin LJ. Endothelin receptor antagonists for the treatment of pulmonary artery hypertension. Life Sci 2012;91:517-21.

12. Humbert M, Sitbon O, Simmoneau G. Treatment of pulmonary arterial hypertension. N Engl J Med 2004;351:1425-36.

13. Tuder RM, Stacher E, Robinson J, et al. Pathology of pulmonary hypertension. Clin Chest Med 2013;34:639-50.

14. Herve P, Humbert M, Sitbon O, et al. Pathobiology of pulmonary hypertension – the role of platelets and thrombosis. Clin Chest Med 2001;22:451-8.

15. Austin ED, Loyd JE. The genetics of pulmonary arterial hypertension. Circ Res 2014;115:189-200.

16. Lau EM, Humbert M. A critical appraisal of the updated 2014 Nice Pulmonary Hypertension Classification System. Can J Cardiol 2014;31:1-8.

17. Galie N, Corris PA, Frost A, et al. Updated treatment algorithm of pulmonary arterial hypertension. J Am Coll Cardiol 2013;62:D60-72.

18. Simmoneau G, Gatzoulis MA, Adatia I, et al. Updated clinical classification of pulmonary hypertension. J Am Coll Cardiol 2013; 62:D34-41.

19. Hoeper MM, Bogaard HJ, Condliffe R, et al. Definitions and diagnosis of pulmonary hypertension. J Am Coll Cardiol 2013;62:D42-50.

20. Shah SJ. Pulmonary hypertension. JAMA 2012;308:1366-74.

21. Montani D, Gunther S, Dorfmuller P, et al. Pulmonary arterial hypertension. Orphanet J Rare Dis 2013;8:1-28.

22. ATS statement: guidelines for the six-minute walk test. Am J Respir Crit Care Med 2002;166:111-7.

23. ACCF/AHA 2009 expert consensus document on pulmonary hypertension. J Am Coll Cardiol 2009;53;1573-619.

24. Montani D, Chaumais MC, Guignabert C, et al. Targeted therapies in pulmonary arterial hypertension. Pharm Ther 2014;141:172-91.

25. Rich S, Kaufman E. High dose titration of calcium channel blocking agents for primary pulmonary hypertension: guidelines for short-term drug testing. J Am Coll Cardiol 1991;18:1323-71.

26. Rich S, Kaufman E, Levy PS. The effect of high doses of calcium-channel blockers on survival in primary pulmonary hypertension. N Engl J Med 1992;327:76-81.

27. Badesch DB, Abman SH, Simmoneau G, et al. Medical therapy for pulmonary arterial hypertension. Updated ACCP evidence-based clinical practice guidelines. Chest 2007;131:1917-28.

28. Barst RJ, Rubin LJ, Long WA, et al. A comparison of continuous intravenous epoprostenol (prostacyclin) with conventional therapy for primary pulmonary hypertension. N Engl J Med 1996;334:296-301.

29. Badesch DB, Tapson VF, McGoon MD, et al. Continuous intravenous epoprostenol for pulmonary hypertension due to scleroderma spectrum of disease – a randomized, controlled trial. Ann Intern Med 2000;132:425-34.

30. Epoprostenol (Flolan) [package insert]. Research Triangle Park, NC: GlaxoSmithKline, March 2011.

31. Jentzer JC, Mathier MA. Pulmonary hypertension in the intensive care unit. J Intensive Care Med 2015; May 5. [Epub ahead of print]

32. Doran AK, Ivy DD, Barst RJ, et al.; and the Scientific Leadership Council of the Pulmonary Hypertension Association. Guidelines for the prevention of central venous catheter-related blood stream infections with prostanoid therapy for pulmonary arterial hypertension. Int J Clin Pract Suppl 2008;160:5-9.

33. Epoprostenol (Veletri) [package insert]. South San Francisco, CA: Actelion Pharmaceuticals US, June 2012.

34. Treprostinil (Remodulin) [package insert]. Research Triangle Park, NC: United Therapeutics, 2014.

35. Simmoneau G, Barst RJ, Galie N, et al. Continuous subcutaneous infusion of treprostinil, a prostacyclin analogue, in patients with pulmonary arterial hypertension. Am J Respir Crit Care Med 2002;165:800-4.

36. Tapson VF, Gomberg-Maitland M, McLaughlin VV, et al. Safety and efficacy of IV treprostinil for pulmonary arterial hypertension: a prospective, multicenter, open-label, 12-week trial. Chest 2006;129:683-8.

37. McLaughlin VV, Benza RL, Rubin LJ, et al. Addition of inhaled treprostinil to oral therapy for pulmonary arterial hypertension: a randomized controlled clinical trial. J Am Coll Cardiol 2010;55:1915-22.

38. Tapson VF, Torres F, Kermeen F, et al. Oral treprostinil for the treatment of pulmonary arterial hypertension in patients on background endothelin receptor antagonist and/or phosphodiesterase type 5 inhibitor therapy (the FREEDOM-C study): a randomized controlled trial. Chest 2012;142:1383-90.

39. Tapson VF, Jing ZC, Xu KF, et al. Oral treprostinil for the treatment of pulmonary arterial hypertension in patients receiving background endothelin receptor antagonist and phosphodiesterase type 5 inhibitor therapy (the FREEDOM-C2 study): a randomized controlled trial. Chest 2013;144:952-8.

40. Jing ZC, Keyur P, Pulido T, et al. Efficacy and safety of oral treprostinil monotherapy for the treatment of pulmonary arterial hypertension: a randomized, controlled trial. Circulation 2013;127:624-33.

41. Treprostinil (Tyvaso) [package insert]. Research Triangle Park, NC: United Therapeutics, 2014.

42. Treprostinil (Orenitram) [package insert]. Research Triangle Park, NC: United Therapeutics, 2014.

43. Mathier MA, McDevitt S, Saggar R, Subcutaneous treprostinil in pulmonary arterial hypertension: practical considerations. J Heart Lung Transplant 2010;29:1210-7.

44. Minai OA, Parambil J, Dweik RA, et al. Impact of switching from epoprostenol to IV treprostinil on treatment satisfaction and quality of life in patients with pulmonary hypertension. Respir Med 2013;107:458-65.

45. Olschewski H, Simmoneau G, Galie N, et al. Inhaled iloprost for severe pulmonary hypertension. N Engl J Med 2002;347:322-9.

46. Iloprost (Ventavis) [package insert]. South San Francisco, CA: Actelion Pharmaceuticals US, November 2013.
47. Spieker LE, Noll G, Ruschitzka FT, et al. Endothelin receptor antagonists in congestive heart failure: a new therapeutic principle for the future? J Am Coll Cardiol 2001;37:1493-505.
48. Rubin LJ, Badesch DB, Barst RJ, et al. Bosentan therapy for pulmonary arterial hypertension. N Engl J Med 2002;346:896-903.
49. Pulido T, Adzerikho I, Channick RN, et al. Macitentan and morbidity and mortality in pulmonary arterial hypertension. N Engl J Med 2013;369:809-18.
50. Galie N, Olschewski H, Oudiz RJ, et al. Ambrisentan for the treatment of pulmonary arterial hypertension: results of the Ambrisentan in Pulmonary Arterial Hypertension, Randomized, Double-Blind, Placebo-Controlled, Multicenter, Efficacy (ARIES) study 1 and 2. Circulation 2008;117:3010-9.
51. Bosentan (Tracleer) [package insert]. South San Francisco, CA: Actelion Pharmaceuticals US, October 2012.
52. Macitentan (Opsumit) [package insert]. South San Francisco, CA: Actelion Pharmaceuticals US, February 2015.
53. Ambrisentan (Letairis) [package insert]. Foster City, CA: Gilead Sciences, January 2014.
54. Jackson G, Benjamin N, Jackson N, et al. Effects of sildenafil on human hemodynamics. Am J Cardiol 1999;83:13C-20C.
55. Galie N, Ghofrani HA, Torbicki A, et al. Sildenafil citrate therapy for pulmonary arterial hypertension. N Engl J Med 2005;353:2148-57.
56. Galie N, Brundage BH, Ghofrani HA, et al. Tadalafil therapy for pulmonary arterial hypertension. Circulation 2009;119:2894-903.
57. Wang RC, Jiang FM, Zheng QL, et al. Efficacy and safety of sildenafil treatment in pulmonary arterial hypertension: a systematic review. Respir Med 2014;108:531-7.
58. Sildenafil (Revatio) [package insert]. New York: Pfizer Labs, January 2014.
59. Ghofrani HA, Wiedemann R, Rose F, et al. Sildenafil for treatment of lung fibrosis and pulmonary hypertension: a randomized trial. Lancet 2002;360:895-900.
60. Tadalafil (Adcirca) [package insert]. Indianapolis: Eli Lilly, 2014.
61. Dasgupta A, Bowman L, D'Arsigny C, et al. Soluble guanylate cyclase: a new therapeutic target for pulmonary arterial hypertension and chronic thromboembolic pulmonary hypertension. Clin Pharmacol Ther 2015;97:88-102.
62. Ghofrani HA, Galie N, Grimminger F, et al. Riociguat for the treatment of pulmonary arterial hypertension. N Engl J Med 2013;369:330-40.
63. Ghofrani HA, D'Armini AM, Grimminger F, et al. Riociguat for the treatment of chronic thromboembolic pulmonary hypertension. N Engl J Med 2013;369:319-29.
64. Riociguat (Adempas) [package insert]. Whippany, NJ: Bayer HealthCare Pharmaceuticals, September 2014.
65. Hoeper MM, Granton J. Intensive care unit management of patients with severe pulmonary hypertension and right heart failure. Am J Respir Crit Care Med 2011;184:1114-24.
66. Zamanian RT, Kudelko KT, Sung YK, et al. Current clinical management of pulmonary arterial hypertension. Circ Res 2014;115:131-47.
67. Poor HD, Venetuolo CE. Pulmonary hypertension in the intensive care unit. Prog Cardiovasc Dis 2012;55:187-98.
68. Bangash MN, Kong ML, Pearse RM. Use of inotropes and vasopressor agents in critically ill patients. Brit J Pharmacol 2012;165:2015-33.
69. Bauer SR, Tonelli AR. Beyond the evidence: treating pulmonary hypertension in the intensive care unit. Crit Care 2014;18:524.

Chapter 31: Critical Care Management of Asthma and Chronic Obstructive Pulmonary Disease

Amanda Zomp, Pharm.D., BCPS; Katherine Bidwell, Pharm.D., BCPS; and Stephanie Mallow Corbett, Pharm.D., FCCM

LEARNING OBJECTIVES

1. Summarize the economic impact of acute asthma and COPD on the healthcare system.
2. Evaluate and compare pathophysiologic differences between asthma and COPD.
3. Identify criteria for ICU admission for acute asthma and COPD.
4. Recommend goals/treatment strategies of asthma management in critically ill patients.
5. Recommend goals/treatment strategies of COPD management in critically ill patients.
6. Explain the therapeutic approach to Asthma-COPD overlap syndrome.

ABBREVIATIONS IN THIS CHAPTER

ACOS	Asthma-COPD overlap syndrome	ICS	Inhaled corticosteroids
COPD	Chronic obstructive pulmonary disease	ICU	Intensive care unit
ED	Emergency department	LABA	Long-acting β-agonist
FEV_1	Forced expiratory volume in 1 second	MDI	Metered dose inhaler
FVC	Forced vital capacity	NIV	Noninvasive ventilation
GINA	Global Initiative for Asthma	PEEPi	Intrinsic positive end-expiratory pressure
GOLD	Global Initiative for Chronic Obstructive Lung Disease	PEFR	Peak expiratory flow rate
		SABA	Short-acting β-agonist

INTRODUCTION

Acute respiratory failure secondary to asthma or chronic obstructive pulmonary disease (COPD) commonly requires frequent and prolonged admission to an intensive care unit (ICU). Although mortality has improved over time in patients with asthma, COPD is now the third leading cause of death in the United States.[1] In addition, there has been increased awareness and focus on asthma COPD overlap syndrome (ACOS). Much of the published literature on these topics has targeted epidemiology, pathophysiology, clinical diagnosis, and outpatient and emergency department (ED) therapeutic management, with limited focus on ICU therapeutic management. Although this chapter will briefly review the epidemiology, pathophysiology, and clinical diagnosis of these diseases, further detailed mechanisms and pathways are beyond the scope of this chapter and may be found in several exceptional texts, guidelines, and reviews. The primary focus of this chapter will be on the evidence-based approach to ICU management of asthma, COPD, and ACOS.

OVERVIEW OF ASTHMA AND COPD

Epidemiology

Asthma and COPD are significant contributors to morbidity and mortality internationally and have a considerable impact on health care costs. The overall economic impact in the United States is reportedly $56 and $49.9 billion annually for asthma and COPD, respectively.[1,2]

Asthma, which tends to develop early in life, is genetically and environmentally influenced. The Centers for Disease Control and Prevention (CDC) statistics indicate that 25.7 million people in the United States are given a diagnosis of asthma, increasing steadily from 3.1% in 1980 to 8.4% of the population in 2010.[2] This increase in asthma diagnosis in 2010 had a minimal impact on ED visits and hospitalizations, accounting for 1.8 million visits and 439,000 admissions, respectfully. Mortality is usually preventable, as shown by the steady decrease in CDC mortality rates despite similar hospitalizations since 2001. This is secondary to the successful reversibility of airway inflammation with early treatment.

Despite decreasing mortality, the health care impact remains substantial. One-fourth of all ED visits are secondary to asthma exacerbations, and 5%–10% reportedly require ICU admission.[3,4] Childhood respiratory infections including respiratory syncytial virus and parainfluenza virus may influence the development of asthma.[5] Environmental factors that influence the development of asthma include allergens, tobacco smoke, air pollution, and some occupational exposures. Risk of mortality is heightened in pediatric patients, females, black Americans, and those with lower socioeconomic status.[2]

Chronic obstructive pulmonary disease has been diagnosed in about 14.2 million people nationally, varies drastically by state, and was associated with 1.5 million ED visits, 715,000 hospitalizations, and 133,965 deaths in 2009.[1,6,7] It is reportedly the third leading cause of mortality, with a rate of 40.8 per 100,000 deaths in 2010, preceded by cancer and cardiovascular disease.[8] Chronic obstructive pulmonary disease exacerbations resulting in hospitalizations reportedly account for 40%–75% of associated COPD health care costs.[9] Upward of 20% of COPD hospitalizations may result in ICU admission.[10] Smoking and age are the greatest risk factors for developing COPD, and patients with COPD typically present with several comorbidities including, but not limited to, coronary artery disease, congestive heart failure, diabetes with neuropathy, atrial fibrillation/flutter, and lung cancer.[9]

There is increasingly more literature regarding ACOS.[11] The prevalence has been difficult to characterize because often patients with characteristics of a secondary disease were excluded from clinical trials, and in clinical trials that were inclusive, different definitions were used to characterize these patients.[11-15] In trials that have investigated overlap syndrome, the prevalence of asthma in COPD cohorts ranged from 15% to 55%.[11] Patients with ACOS are reportedly younger and experience a greater frequency and severity of exacerbations.[13] A large multicenter population-based survey using standardized definitions to classify asthma, COPD, and overlap syndrome showed that patients with ACOS have worse general health status, increased exacerbation risk, and more hospitalizations than do those with COPD alone.[15]

Pathophysiology

Acute respiratory failure requiring ICU admission is characterized by the inability to maintain homeostasis secondary to hypercapnia and hypoxemia.[16] Severe asthma and COPD exacerbations can induce acute respiratory failure, but through different pathophysiologic pathways. Asthma is defined by the Global Initiative for Asthma (GINA) as "a heterogeneous disease, usually characterized by chronic airway inflammation."[5] It is an immunohistopathologic process mediated by cytokine release and chemokines that trigger and regulate transcription factors that induce inflammatory response.[5] The immunologic findings in sudden-onset and fatal asthma differ from those in slow or late-onset asthma, such that neutrophils in bronchial epithelium are more predominant in sudden-onset compared to eosinophils in late-onset. Occupational asthma and smokers also have a predominance of neutrophils. Mast cell activation and epithelial cell injury, together with sub-basement membrane thickening, bronchial smooth muscle hypertrophy and hyperplasia, and increased mucus secretions, contribute to airway structural changes and resultant inflammation.[5] These factors influence the severity of asthma according to the degree of obstruction of airflow caused by bronchial smooth muscle contraction, bronchial inflammation-associated mucosal edema, and mucus plugging.[17,18]

In allergic asthma, the degree of cross-linking of immunoglobulin E (IgE) antibodies by allergen influences the development and severity. This type of bronchoconstriction is induced through mast cell activation and release of histamine, tryptase, cysteinyl-leukotrienes, and prostaglandin D_2.[5,19-21] Macrophages may further release cytokines and inflammatory mediators after allergen activation.[5,22] Airway obstruction results in a decrease in forced expiratory volume in 1 second (FEV_1), which in turn leads to air trapping and increasing functional residual capacity and a decreased forced vital capacity (FVC). Thus, a decreased FEV_1/FVC ratio, with partial bronchodilator reversibility, is characteristic of asthma. Research is emerging showing inflammatory volatility, in which selective treatment based on phenotype may target improved therapeutic response. Some encouraging research efforts have been focused on leukotriene modifiers and anti-IgE, and continued investigations are under way.[5,23]

Chronic obstructive pulmonary disease has been defined by the Global Initiative for Chronic Obstructive Lung Disease (GOLD) guidelines as "a common preventable and treatable disease, characterized by airflow limitation that is usually progressive and associated with an enhanced chronic inflammatory response in the airways and the lung to noxious particles or gases."[24] Chronic obstructive pulmonary disease typically develops later in life, is characterized by a limitation in expiratory flow and hyperinflation that is not completely reversible, and is usually confounded by several comorbidities. Chronic obstructive pulmonary disease can resemble aspects of both emphysema (alveolar damage) and chronic bronchitis (airway inflammation). The repeated exposure to noxious stimuli activates neutrophils and macrophages, which leads to airway remodeling, mucous hypersecretion, and impaired ciliary function resulting in carbon dioxide (CO_2) retention. In smokers, cytotoxic T lymphocytes also contribute to the inflammatory response. The progression of lung damage is affected by the release of various cytokines and oxidative stress. An increase in proteases is evident in patients with COPD. Proteases may induce breakdown in connective tissue, impairing gas exchange through the mediation of elastin damage and resulting in hypoxemia and hypercapnia.[24] Patients with severe COPD have weak diaphragm tone and diaphragmatic dysfunction, requiring ribcage and abdominal muscles to be recruited during inspiration and end-expiration, respectively. The resultant paradoxical breathing leads to a rise in gastric pressure contributing to intrinsic positive end-expiratory pressure (PEEPi).[24,25] Increased airflow limitation can trigger a COPD exacerbation, resulting in an increased work of breathing, air-trapping, a reduction of chest wall and lung compliance, and PEEPi, which over time will result in respiratory muscle fatigue, increased dead space ventilation, and worsening gas exchange.[24,26] Increased hypoxemia is also affected by ventilation/perfusion mismatch. Similar to patients with asthma, patients with COPD develop decreased FEV_1 and FVC and a resultant decreased FEV_1/FVC ratio, mildly to non-reversible with bronchodilators. Patients with COPD also develop increases in residual volume and total lung capacity. Genetic risk factors are thought to contribute to the development and magnitude of inflammatory response, although there are limited and mixed data regarding the genomes identified.[24] α1-Antitrypsin deficiency has been the most widely studied genetic disease, with focused efforts to target treatment optimization according to genetic predisposition.[24]

The pathophysiology of patients with severe asthma exacerbations alone differs from that of patients with severe COPD exacerbations, but several characteristics are shared in ACOS. Patients with ACOS have variable airflow obstruction that is not completely reversible.[11,15,27] In addition, these patients experience increased bronchial hyper-responsiveness. Louie et al. proposed two clinical phenotypes: (1) asthma with partly reversible airflow obstruction and (2) COPD with emphysema accompanied by reversible or partly reversible airflow obstruction.[28] These phenotypes may then present independently or in a combined fashion represented by eosinophilic bronchiolitis or neutrophilic bronchiolitis.[28] Airway inflammation is predominantly a result of neutrophil activation. Cytotoxic T lymphocytes, alveolar macrophages, and proteases have also been implicated in ACOS.[23,28] Some genetic similarities have also been described that influence bronchial hyper-responsiveness and FEV_1/FVC.[29]

Triggers of Acute Severe Exacerbations

Several triggers are shared in patients with acute severe exacerbations of both asthma and COPD. Among them, medication noncompliance because of educational gap, lack of access to medications, or patient adherence is a leading cause of severe exacerbations. Upper respiratory infections and pneumonia, together with environmental factors such as allergens, are also associated with an increased risk of severe exacerbations.[1,2] In addition, exercise can induce bronchospasm and hyperinflation,[5,24] and severe stress has been associated with exacerbations, although the exact mechanism is not well understood.[5]

Patients with additional comorbidities such as cardiovascular disease or other chronic lung disease, those requiring greater than two canisters of short-acting β-agonist (SABA) per month, and those with two or more hospitalizations or three or more ED visits for asthma in the past year have a higher likelihood of severe asthma exacerbations. Severe COPD exacerbations may be precipitated by pulmonary thromboembolism, ischemic heart disease, acute heart failure, arrhythmias, alcohol consumption, inactivity, history of reflux or heartburn, and COPD exacerbations themselves.[30]

Severe asthma exacerbations may be drug induced secondary to concomitant diseases requiring the use of medications that can disrupt airway patency and increase airway resistance.[16] β-Adrenergic blockers, nonsteroidal anti-inflammatory agents including aspirin, and steroid taper have been associated with bronchospasm.

Clinical Presentation

A life-threatening asthma exacerbation is characterized by an inability to speak, a reduced peak expiratory flow rate (PEFR) of less than 25% of a patient's personal best, and a failed response to frequent bronchodilator administration and intravenous steroids.[18,31] Often, PEFR and bedside spirometry cannot be performed in these patients. However, if performed, values generally show an FEV_1 or a PEFR less than 25% predicted.[31] Vital sign abnormalities include tachycardia (greater than 120 beats/minute), tachypnea (greater than 30 breaths/minute), and hypotension as intravascular volume depletion worsens secondary to insensible fluid loss.[31,32] Arterial blood gas may show an acute respiratory alkalosis with normal oxygenation in patients with an asthma exacerbation.[33] In more severe cases, patients will develop a mild or acute respiratory acidosis with a widening A-a gradient indicative of respiratory failure.[34] It is important that these patients be recognized promptly because they are exhausting their accessory muscles, resulting in excessive CO_2 retention. Patients with hypercapnia have wider degrees of pulsus paradoxus, whereas low pulsus paradoxus is indicative of severe hyperinflation, which can result in extracardiac tamponade.[31,35,36] Arrhythmias are common in patients with asthma[31,37] and may be induced secondary to electrolyte abnormalities during management of acute exacerbations with high-dose β-agonist agents.[38] Some patients may develop a pneumothorax or pneumomediastinum, likely because of increases in intrathoracic pressure, and warrant the need for chest tube placement for decompression.[5]

Severe COPD exacerbation may develop acutely or for a period of days. Patients generally develop worsening dyspnea, increasing cough, or an increase or change in sputum production from baseline as a result of increased inflammation. Physically, patients tend to appear in acute distress. Presentation with fatigue, weight loss, and anorexia is common in patients with severe COPD.[24,39] Tachypnea, tachycardia, and decreased blood pressure secondary to PEEPi are common vital sign abnormalities. Respiratory acidosis also develops in acute exacerbations. Use of accessory inspiratory muscles is indicative of increased severity, and paradoxical breathing is associated with a poor prognosis, leading to impending respiratory failure and arrest.[24,40] Patients with severe hypoxemia may present cyanotic and/or comatose. Development of hypercapnic respiratory failure with preserved ventilation/perfusion match indicates the need for mechanical ventilation.[26]

ICU ADMISSION

Severity of illness warranting ICU admission for asthma may include presentation of dyspnea refractory to aggressive bronchodilator therapy, pneumonia, pneumothorax, PEFR less than 40% predicted personal best or lack of adequate response despite aggressive treatment, hypercarbia (partial pressure of carbon dioxide in the blood [Paco$_2$] greater than 45 mm Hg), hypoxemia (partial pressure of oxygen in the blood [Pao$_2$] less than 60 mm Hg on room air) requiring oxygen supplementation, or a combination of these factors. A history of several ED visits and tracheal intubation secondary to asthma are additional risk factors for asthma-related mortality. In addition, the absence of wheezing implying minimal air movement, use of accessory muscles, a decrease in systolic blood pressure during inspiration by greater than 15 mm Hg, bradycardia, diaphoresis, cyanosis, anxiety, and inability to talk imply severe obstruction.[31,41-43]

The severity of COPD may be assessed using the staging criteria developed by the American Thoracic Society and GOLD, which classifies patients into four categories: stage I (mild), stage II (moderate), stage III (severe), and stage IV (very severe) according to the level of obstruction as defined by FEV$_1$.[24] In addition to baseline COPD severity, frequent exacerbations that require hospitalization, several comorbidities, and previous need for mechanical ventilation are risk factors for more severe exacerbations. Early warning scores have also been developed to assist in the triage for ICU admission and taking into consideration parameters associated with poor prognosis.[44] Factors influencing ICU admission include severe dyspnea refractory to initial aggressive therapy, mental status changes, persistent or worsening hypoxemia, persistent or worsening respiratory acidosis, hemodynamic instability, and the need for mechanical ventilation.[24,26] The treatment algorithms for severe asthma and COPD exacerbations are shown in Figure 31.1 and Figure 31.2, respectively. Comparative therapeutic management of severe exacerbations for patients with asthma and COPD admitted to the ICU is outlined in Table 31.1.

Supportive respiratory care can be provided in different levels according to patient needs. Critically ill patients may require oxygen

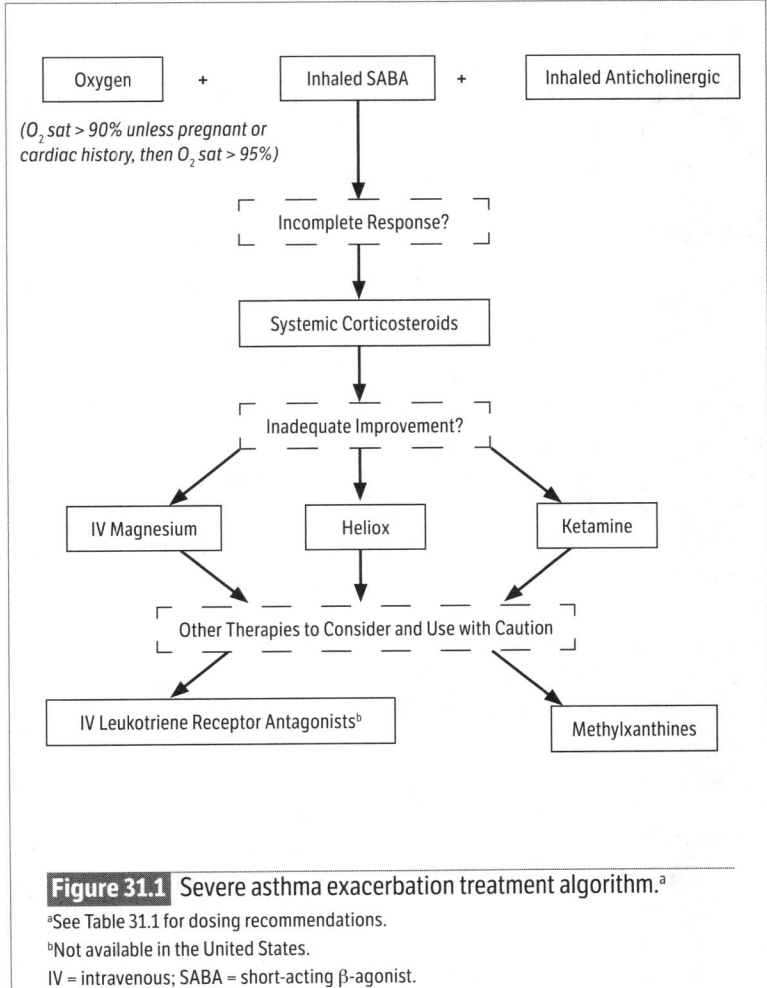

Figure 31.1 Severe asthma exacerbation treatment algorithm.[a]
[a]See Table 31.1 for dosing recommendations.
[b]Not available in the United States.
IV = intravenous; SABA = short-acting β-agonist.

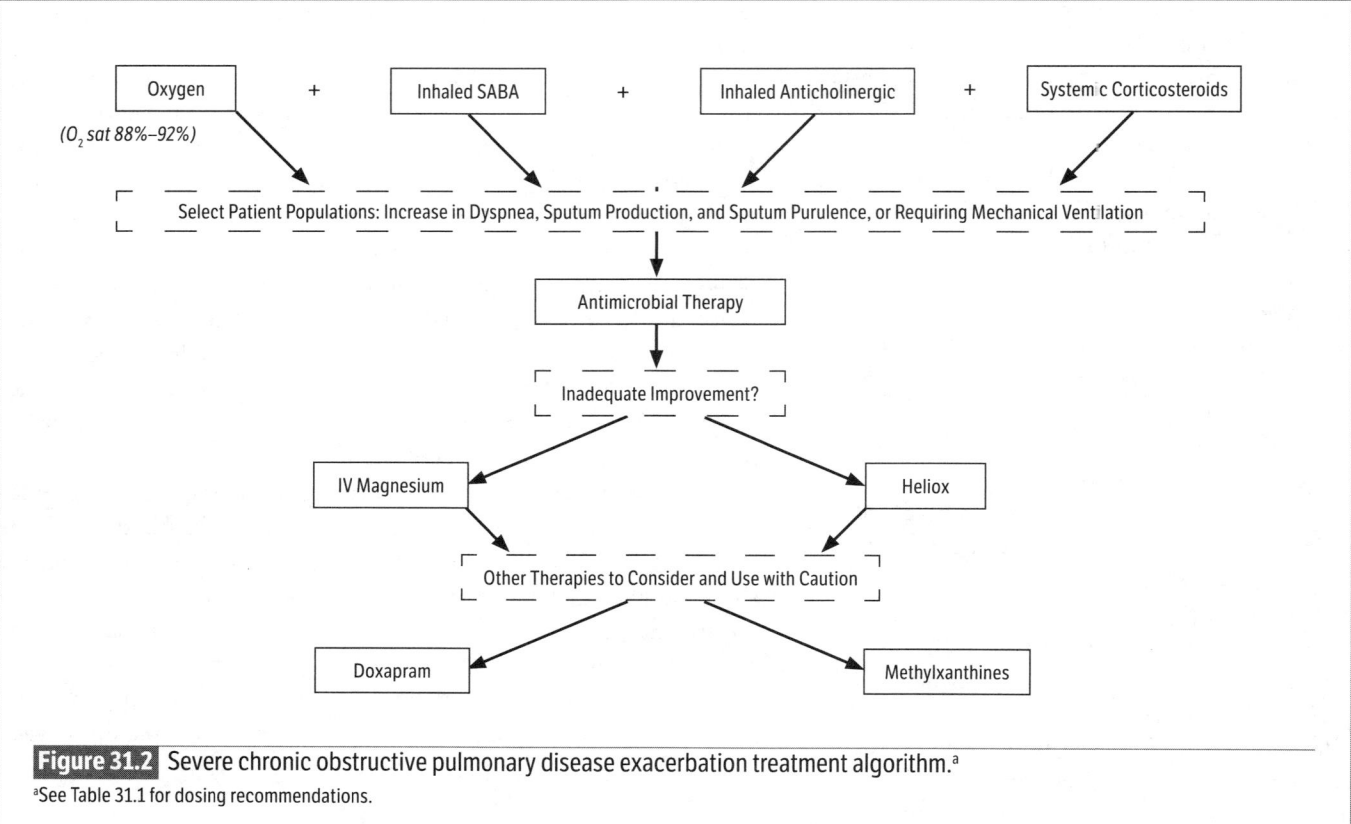

Figure 31.2 Severe chronic obstructive pulmonary disease exacerbation treatment algorithm.[a]
[a]See Table 31.1 for dosing recommendations.

therapy, noninvasive ventilation (NIV), or invasive mechanical ventilation. This section will provide a brief overview of these supportive therapy options.

Oxygen

Oxygen therapy is an important component in the management of severe asthma and COPD exacerbations. Patients experiencing severe exacerbations of either etiology often present with hypoxemia and require supplemental oxygen. The current asthma guidelines recommend the administration of oxygen by nasal cannula or mask in order to achieve oxygen saturation (Sao_2) values greater than 90%. Other patient populations such as pregnant women and individuals with a cardiac history may have higher oxygen requirements, so an Sao_2 of greater than 95% is often desired in these patients.[71] In COPD, the target oxygen saturation is 88%–92%, which is partly based on data analyses that show patients who received oxygen therapy titrated to a saturation of 88%–92% had lower mortality than those administered high-flow oxygen therapy.[72] Caution is advised with oxygen supplementation in patients with COPD, however, because many of these patients rely on a slight level of hypoxemia as a trigger for their respiratory drive secondary to chronic hypercapnia.[45] In addition, it is important to monitor the degree of oxygen supplementation in these patients, because too much oxygen may also increase ventilation/perfusion mismatch by inducing vasodilation to areas not previously well ventilated, decrease respiratory rate centrally (O_2 retainers are very sensitive to O_2), and perpetuate the Haldane effect.

Inhaled medications are often administered through nebulizers with the use of oxygen to enhance drug delivery to the lower airways, especially in patients with severe airway restriction. It is important to monitor the fractional concentration of oxygen administered to these critically ill patients, given that this may be more harmful than beneficial to these patients. A study by Chien et al. found that patients who received 100% oxygen had elevations in $Paco_2$, and patients with more severe airway obstructions often had more hypercarbia, thereby increasing their risk of respiratory depression secondary to CO_2 retention.[47,73]

Noninvasive Ventilation

Noninvasive ventilation may be an option for patients with severe COPD exacerbation, although its potential benefit in asthma exacerbations remains unclear.[3,74] In patients with hypercapnia and acute respiratory failure secondary to COPD exacerbation, NIV improves mortality and respiratory acidosis and decreases the need for intubation and treatment failures.[75,76] Noninvasive ventilation also decreases complications associated with invasive mechanical ventilation in patients with COPD, such as ventilator-associated pneumonia and hospital length of stay.[76] In a recent evaluation of the addition of NIV to standard medical therapy in patients admitted to an ICU for a severe asthma exacerbation, a clear benefit of NIV when added to standard medical therapy was not shown. Overall, the results suggested that adding NIV to standard therapy in patients with asthma reduces inhaled bronchodilator requirements, accelerates improvement in lung function, and reduces hospital length of stay, but larger studies are needed to further evaluate these findings.[74]

Although NIV may be appropriate for some patients experiencing a severe asthma exacerbation, data analyses are insufficient for the current guidelines to provide a recommendation regarding its use in severe exacerbations. The GINA guidelines currently recommend proceeding with intubation as soon as it is deemed medically necessary and intubation should not be delayed by the administration of alternative therapies, including NIV.[5,71]

In patients with COPD, however, NIV should be considered for those with respiratory acidosis and severe dyspnea with increased work of breathing or clinical signs of respiratory muscle fatigue. These may include respiratory accessory muscle use, paradoxical motion of the abdomen, or retraction of the intercostal spaces.[40] The use of NIV for severe COPD exacerbation is a level A recommendation from the GOLD guidelines.[24]

Mechanical Ventilation

Patients experiencing worsening respiratory failure during a severe exacerbation despite standard medical therapy often require endotracheal intubation and respiratory support with mechanical ventilation. Currently, there are no parameters to suggest when intubation should occur in severe asthma exacerbation; instead, the decision should be based on clinical judgment.[42,71] Indications for intubation in patients with asthma may include worsening hypoxemia and hypercarbia, hemodynamic instability, altered mental status, and increased work of breathing.[42,71] Patients with near-fatal asthma can be challenging to intubate and can often have high ventilator requirements because of the high airway resistance and mucus plugging in the distal airways.[3] The GINA guidelines recommend a ventilator strategy of permissive hypercapnia or controlled hypoventilation, which provides adequate oxygenation and ventilation but decreases the risk of barotrauma secondary to high airway pressures.[5,71]

Patients with severe COPD exacerbation who are unable to tolerate NIV or whose NIV therapy fails may be candidates for invasive mechanical ventilation. Other indications for invasive mechanical ventilation include the inability to clear respiratory secretions, respiratory or cardiac arrest, diminished consciousness, massive aspiration, severe hemodynamic instability without response to fluids and vasoactive medications, and severe ventricular arrhythmias.[77] The decision to institute invasive mechanical ventilation in patients with a severe COPD exacerbation should be made depending on the reversibility of the cause of exacerbation, the patient's wishes, the appropriate resources, the availability of providers with knowledge about ventilator management, and a risk assessment of complications related to invasive ventilation. These complications include ventilator-associated pneumonia, barotrauma, and inability to wean from mechanical ventilation.[24]

ASTHMA
Treatment Goals

The main treatment goals for a severe asthma exacerbation are to correct significant hypoxemia using supplemental oxygen and to rapidly reverse airflow obstruction with the administration of inhaled SABAs and systemic corticosteroids.[5,71] Although reducing the risk of future exacerbations is also an important treatment goal, this section will focus on the critical care therapeutic management of life-threatening asthma exacerbations (Figure 31.1).

Pharmacologic Interventions

Bronchodilators

The current asthma guidelines recommend that all patients experiencing an asthma exacerbation receive a SABA by repeated administration with either a metered dose inhaler (MDI) or nebulization immediately on presentation, which should be continued until resolution of acute symptoms.[18,43,47,71] Short-acting β-agonists stimulate the $β_2$-receptors on smooth muscle cells and cause relaxation of respiratory smooth muscle. This relaxation leads to bronchodilation and a decrease in airway obstruction.[42,47] Selective SABAs (albuterol, levalbuterol, pirbuterol) are recommended in acute exacerbation to decrease the risk of cardiotoxicity that can be associated with high doses of SABAs.[18,71] Albuterol is the most common bronchodilator administered during severe asthma exacerbations. Dosing and monitoring recommendations are provided in Table 31.1. Theoretically, levalbuterol may have fewer cardiovascular adverse effects than albuterol and may be preferable in severe asthma exacerbations when frequent or large doses are required. However, several studies have failed to show a significant difference in heart rate elevation after the administration of albuterol and levalbuterol.[18,71,78-81] In addition, the efficacy of levalbuterol when administered as a continuous nebulization has not yet been evaluated.[18,71,81]

In critically ill patients, it is preferable that SABAs be administered as a nebulizer rather than by an MDI to provide a continuous delivery of medication to the obstructed airways.[47] Patients who require ICU admission may have severe airway edema and increased mucus production, which can further worsen airway obstruction.[47] Administering β-agonists by nebulizer either intermittently or continuously should improve the likelihood that bronchodilators are delivered to the lower airways during an acute exacerbation.[47] Several studies have evaluated the effects of continuous versus intermittent nebulization on pulmonary function in patients presenting to the ED. A meta-analysis of eight studies, most of which enrolled only adults, found that patients who received continuous nebulization of SABAs in the ED had an improvement in their pulmonary function tests (PEFR and FEV_1) after 2–3 hours of therapy. Patients with severe acute exacerbations were found to specifically benefit from continuous nebulization of SABAs, but additional studies are needed to confirm these findings.[46]

Studies have found that systemic β-agonists, such as intravenous or subcutaneous epinephrine or terbutaline, are not more efficacious than inhaled β-agonists in the management of an acute asthma exacerbation, and it is possible that they are associated with more cardiovascular adverse effects. Critically ill patients may benefit from systemic administration of β-agonists if they lack a good response to inhaled SABA therapy or if they are unable to receive inhaled medications, although data evaluations have not shown improved outcomes with this approach.[42] Long-acting β-agonists (LABAs) in combination with inhaled glucocorticoids have been shown to be effective in preventing asthma exacerbations, but their use in the treatment of severe acute exacerbations has not been demonstrated.

Inhaled Anticholinergic Agents

Inhaled anticholinergic medications such as ipratropium bromide cause bronchodilation by selectively binding to the muscarinic receptors on smooth muscle cells in the airways and reducing bronchoconstriction.[47] Administration of ipratropium in addition to a SABA is recommended to promote additional bronchodilation through a different pathway. Studies have not found a significant benefit when ipratropium is continued after the initial doses are given in the ED, but it is often common practice to continue the administration of ipratropium with a SABA in critically ill patients.[18] Targeting different sites and mechanisms of airway bronchodilation with different medications may benefit patients who experience severe bronchoconstriction and require ICU admission for an acute asthma exacerbation.[47]

Corticosteroids

Systemic corticosteroids are recommended in patients who have an incomplete response to the initial administration of an inhaled SABA, and they should be continued during hospital admission.[18,71] Corticosteroids decrease airway obstruction during an asthma exacerbation by decreasing inflammation, increasing the number of $β_2$-receptors and increasing their responsiveness to β-agonists, reducing airway edema, and suppressing certain proinflammatory cytokines by interfering with the regulation of their transcription.[42,47,82] A meta-analysis evaluating the use of corticosteroids in patients presenting to the ED found that patients who received corticosteroids had an increase in PEFR at the end of treatment.[48] There was often a delay in the improvement of pulmonary function after the administration of corticosteroids in these studies, so it is recommended that corticosteroids be initiated within the first hour of presentation.[47,48] An additional meta-analysis evaluated the effects of varying doses of corticosteroids in hospitalized patients and found that there was no added benefit to improvement in pulmonary function when doses of methylprednisolone greater than 60–80 mg per day were used. However, none of the studies that were reviewed included patients who required mechanical ventilation or ICU admission.[83] The exact dose of corticosteroids a patient should receive during an acute exacerbation is not known at this time, but studies have indicated that doses of prednisone greater than 100 mg per day do not provide a significant benefit.[49] It is recommended that patients receive 60–80 mg per day of prednisone or methylprednisolone during acute exacerbations, followed by a decrease in dose once the patient has signs of improvement in pulmonary function. Corticosteroids should be tapered in patients who require treatment for longer than 1 week unless they only require a 10-day course of systemic corticosteroids and are also on an inhaled corticosteroid (ICS).[3,5]

Studies have indicated that an ICS may prevent hospital admissions for acute asthma exacerbations compared with placebo, but their role in acute exacerbations is less clear. It is possible that adding an ICS to systemic corticosteroids during an acute exacerbation will improve outcomes, but no data suggest that an ICS alone should be used during an acute exacerbation. In addition, the optimal dosing, delivery, and frequency of ICS administration during an exacerbation are currently unknown and require further evaluation.[84]

Intravenous Magnesium Sulfate

In patients with severe and life-threatening asthma exacerbations, intravenous magnesium sulfate may be beneficial.[18,71] Magnesium is thought to cause bronchodilation by inhibiting calcium channels on smooth muscle, which causes relaxation of smooth muscle.[3,82] Magnesium may also have anti-inflammatory effects by interfering with the activation and release of neutrophils in patients with asthma.[85,86] A meta-analysis of 14 studies found that patients who received magnesium sulfate as a single intravenous dose of 1.2 or 2 g had improved lung function and decreased hospital admissions when inhaled SABAs and systemic corticosteroids did not provide a sufficient response.[87] A study by Silverman et al. evaluated the addition of 2 g of intravenous magnesium sulfate to nebulized albuterol and intravenous methylprednisolone therapy in patients who presented to the ED with a severe acute asthma exacerbation defined by an initial FEV_1 of 30% or less of predicted. There was no difference in the rate of hospital admissions between the groups, but patients who received magnesium had a significantly higher FEV_1 after 240 minutes of the protocol (48.2% of predicted vs. 43.5% of predicted, p<0.05). These investigators further evaluated changes in FEV_1 in patients according to their severity on admission and found that patients with an initial FEV_1 of less than 20% of predicted had the best response after magnesium administration, whereas patients with an FEV_1 of 25%–30% did not appear to benefit as much from intravenous magnesium.[57] Although it may seem that magnesium could particularly benefit patients experiencing a severe or life-threatening asthma exacerbation, the meta-analysis by Kew et al. was unable to detect a significant difference between three severity subgroups.[87] Additional studies with clearly defined groups of severity are needed to further determine whether there is a role for intravenous magnesium in the management of severe asthma exacerbations.

Ketamine

Ketamine is an anesthetic agent with bronchodilatory properties that may reduce airway resistance in patients with an acute asthma exacerbation.[47,59] Ketamine may prevent reuptake of norepinephrine, and the increase in norepinephrine concentrations may stimulate $β_2$-receptors, which will result in increased bronchodilation.[59] Early studies found that ketamine reduced bronchospasm in patients when it was used as an anesthetic agent, and it was especially beneficial in patients with a history of severe pulmonary disorders.[59] Several case studies evaluating the use of ketamine in mechanically ventilated patients with severe asthma exacerbations found that ketamine decreased bronchoconstriction and improved oxygenation in these patients.[59] Heshmati and colleagues evaluated the use of ketamine in 11 patients with status asthmaticus who did not respond to standard medical therapy (β-agonists, corticosteroids, and theophylline) and who had not improved after 24 hours of mechanical ventilation.[60] These patients received a 1 mg/kg loading dose of ketamine followed by a continuous infusion at a rate of 1 mg/kg/hour for 2 hours. The investigators found significant improvements in mean peak airway pressures, mean $Paco_2$, and mean Pao_2 after completion of the 2-hour infusion, but the lack of a control group does not allow for evaluation of the effects of ketamine on ventilator days or other important variables.[60] Although data are still limited, ketamine may be beneficial in patients with asthma that is refractory to other standard treatments. In addition, ketamine has been recommended for rapid sequence intubation in patients with asthma secondary to its bronchodilatory effects compared with other agents that have potential for bronchoconstriction, although improved outcomes have not been published.[88,89–91]

Heliox

Heliox is a mixture of about 70%–80% helium and 20%–30% oxygen that results in a very low-density gas that may decrease airway resistance and result in an improvement in airflow and ventilation in patients experiencing an acute asthma exacerbation.[47,61] A review of 10 studies of heliox administration in nonintubated patients found that heliox was no more effective than oxygen or air delivery in these patients.[62] However, patients with moderate to severe impairment experienced a significant increase in pulmonary function with heliox, so it is possible that heliox provides the most benefit in patients who are experiencing severe airflow resistance during an exacerbation.[47,62]

Heliox may be more beneficial as a drug-delivery agent because heliox-driven albuterol may result in the deposition of albuterol into the distal airways of severely restricted patients.[47] A 2002 study by Kress et al. found that patients who received albuterol nebulized with an 80:20 mixture of heliox had an improvement in respiratory function compared with those who only received albuterol nebulized with oxygen.[61] A meta-analysis by Rodrigo and colleagues found that patients who received a SABA nebulized with heliox had a 17.2% increase in mean percentage of change in PEFR from baseline compared with patients who received a β-agonist nebulized with oxygen. They also found that the greatest improvement in PEFR secondary to heliox-driven β-agonist nebulization seemed to occur in the studies that evaluated patients with acute severe exacerbations.[63] The asthma guidelines currently state that heliox may be beneficial in patients with impending respiratory failure, but its use should not delay intubation in any patient if intubation is needed.[71]

Therapies to Use with Caution

Methylxanthines

Methylxanthines such as theophylline and aminophylline are no longer recommended by the asthma guidelines because they appear not to provide any additional benefit when administered with adequate doses of a SABA. In addition, methylxanthines have several adverse effects associated with their use, including potential arrhythmias.[47] If a patient is maintained on a methylxanthine at home before being admitted for an acute exacerbation, blood levels should be monitored often.

Intravenous Leukotriene Receptor Antagonists

Leukotrienes are inflammatory mediators that play a significant role in airway disease by causing bronchoconstriction, increased mucous production, recruitment of other inflammatory mediators, and proliferation of airway smooth muscle cells.[47] Leukotriene receptor antagonists such as montelukast can promote bronchodilation by reversing the bronchoconstriction and airway inflammation that is caused by leukotriene mediators.[47,69] A study evaluating the use of intravenous montelukast in patients with acute asthma, although not yet available in the United States, found that patients who received 7 mg of intravenous montelukast in addition to the standard treatment for an asthma exacerbation had a significant improvement in their FEV_1 compared with patients who only received standard medical therapy.[69] Although the onset of bronchodilation after intravenous montelukast administration is not as fast as the onset of bronchodilation after inhaled SABAs, it does seem to provide an improvement in bronchodilation within 10–20 minutes of administration and appears to last up to 24 hours.[69,70] Additional studies are needed to determine the role of leukotriene receptor antagonists in the management of severe asthma exacerbations.

Special Population Considerations—Pregnancy

Asthma is a common respiratory condition that affects women during pregnancy. It is estimated that 20% of pregnant women with asthma experience exacerbations that require medical interventions, and up to 6% of those require hospital admission for treatment of their severe exacerbation.[92,93] Worsening of asthma symptoms occurs most often in the second and third trimesters, with a peak of exacerbations late in the second trimester.[93,94] Exacerbations rarely occur during the labor and delivery part of pregnancy.[93] According to Chan et al., ICU admission should be considered for pregnant women who have either an FEV_1 of less than 25% or an FEV_1 that does not improve more than 10% after treatment with a sufficient dose of an inhaled SABA.[93]

Inhaled SABAs are the mainstay of treatment in pregnant patients with severe asthma exacerbations. Albuterol continues to be the preferred agent in these patients and is generally considered safe to use in pregnancy.[94] Patients should receive a continuous nebulization of albuterol at a dose of 0.5–1 mg/hour.[93] Systemic epinephrine should be avoided in these patients because of the increase in uterine vasoconstriction associated with its use. If a systemic β-agonist is needed to improve asthma symptoms in severe exacerbations, it is recommended that subcutaneous terbutaline be used instead of epinephrine.[93,95] Patients should also receive systemic corticosteroids, either methylprednisolone or prednisone, at the time of SABA initiation. Enzymes within the placenta metabolize a large percentage of these maternal corticosteroids, so there should be minimal exposure to the fetus during the treatment for asthma exacerbations.[96] However, there is still the potential for impaired fetal growth development because of exposure to corticosteroids, but the risk of these adverse effects should be weighed against the benefit of corticosteroids to the mother. Intravenous magnesium sulfate can also be administered to pregnant patients to provide additional bronchodilation during an acute exacerbation.[93]

Pregnant patients should be administered supplemental oxygen to maintain oxygen saturations of at least 95%. If patients experience continued hypoxia despite oxygen supplementation, significant respiratory acidosis, maternal fatigue, or other signs of an increased work of breathing, intubation and mechanical ventilation should be considered.[93] Permissive hypercapnia should also be used in pregnant patients experiencing an asthma exacerbation as it is used in non-pregnant patients. There is concern about using permissive hypercapnia in pregnant patients because of the potentially negative effects of elevated Pco_2 on uterine blood flow as well as the potential for developing fetal respiratory acidosis.[93] However, as with other therapies, the benefit of permissive hypercapnia to the mother and her survival must be weighed against the potential adverse effects to the fetus.

COPD MANAGEMENT

Treatment Goals

The treatment goals for an acute exacerbation of COPD are two-fold. The first is to provide supportive care and resolve the acute exacerbation with minimal impact on the patient's lung function, and the second is to prevent future exacerbations.[97] Both of these goals are important in the treatment of patients with COPD and are therefore common end points used in clinical trials. This chapter will primarily focus on the resolution of the exacerbation of COPD in the critically ill patient and successful discharge from the ICU (Figure 31.2), but it is important to note the therapies that are associated with prolonged time to next exacerbation as well.

Pharmacologic Interventions

Bronchodilators

Short-acting inhaled β-agonists with or without short-acting inhaled anticholinergic agents are the preferred agents for bronchodilation in COPD exacerbation. Short-acting bronchodilators are often used in increasing doses and frequencies to provide symptomatic relief.[45] Dosing and monitoring recommendations are provided in Table 31.1. Despite their widespread acceptance, the use of these agents is a level of evidence C recommendation in the GOLD guidelines because of the lack of controlled trials examining their efficacy in COPD exacerbation management.[24] A meta-analysis of 12 studies comparing the delivery of short-acting bronchodilators by MDI and nebulization found no difference in efficacy in patients with an acute airflow obstruction ($p>0.05$). Similar results were seen in the subgroup analysis of patients with COPD exacerbation. Most studies used spacers with MDIs, although they may not be necessary for

Table 31.1 Comparison of Pharmacologic Management of Asthma and COPD in the ICU

Pharmacologic Treatment	Asthma	COPD
Inhaled Short-Acting β-Agonists[11,24,42,45,46]		
Recommendation	Recommended in all patients	SABA preferred agent for bronchodilation; nebulization may be more convenient
Dosing	Nebulization: 0.5–5 mg q20min by nebulizer for three doses, followed by 2.5–10 mg q1–4hr as needed or 10–15 mg administered over 1 hr by continuous nebulization MDI: 4–8 puffs (18 mcg/puff) q20min for up to 4 hr, followed by 4–8 puffs q1–4hr as needed	MDI: 2 puffs q2–4hr Nebulization: 2.5 mg q2–4hr
Outcome	Improvement in PEFR and FEV_1 after 2–3 hr of continuous nebulization	No data in exacerbation Stable COPD: Improve FEV_1, symptoms
Monitoring	Heart rate, serum potassium	Heart rate, serum potassium
Inhaled Short-Acting Anticholinergics[11,24,45,47]		
Recommendation	Recommended in addition to an inhaled SABA	Recommended in addition to SABA for bronchodilation; nebulization may be more convenient
Dosing	Nebulization: 0.5 mg q20min for at least three doses and then 0.5 mg q6hr as needed during ICU admission	MDI: 2 puffs q2–4hr Nebulizer: 0.5 mg q2–4hr
Outcome	Studies have not indicated a benefit when it is continued after initial doses in the ED but likely beneficial to target several mechanisms of bronchodilation in ICU patients	No data in exacerbation Stable COPD: Combination β-agonist and anticholinergic further improved FEV_1 and symptoms
Monitoring	Dry mouth	Dry mouth
Systemic Corticosteroids[3,48,49,50-53]		
Recommendation	Administer to all patients soon after initiation of SABA therapy	Likely beneficial; use lowest effective dose
Dosing	60–80 mg per day of prednisone or methylprednisolone	Lowest effective dose (range prednisone 40 mg daily – methylprednisolone 0.5 mg/kg q6hr); prefer enteral therapy for maximum 10 days
Outcome	Improvement in PEFR	Shorter duration of mechanical ventilation, fewer failures of NIV
Monitoring	Hyperglycemia	Hyperglycemia
Antimicrobial Therapy[54-56]		
Recommendation	Possibly beneficial if cause of exacerbations is expected to be from an infectious source	Likely beneficial; choice based on local susceptibility patterns Common antibiotic classes used may include fluoroquinolones, macrolides, β-lactam/β-lactamase combinations, tetracyclines, and cephalosporins (third or fourth generation)
Dosing	Ceftriaxone 1 g q24 hr and azithromycin 500 mg q24 hr (add oseltamivir if exacerbation occurs during influenza season)	Dose adjust according to renal/hepatic function; 5- to 10-day course
Outcome	May reduce mortality if initiated within 12 hr; data are limited	Lower mortality, shorter duration of MV, shorter hospital LOS, reduced need for additional antibiotics, improved FEV_1
Monitoring	Culture results, resistance patterns	Resistance patterns
Intravenous Magnesium Sulfate[57,58]		
Recommendation	Recommended in patients with severe exacerbations unresponsive to first-line therapies	Not routinely recommended
Dosing	Magnesium sulfate 2 g IV dose in addition to a nebulized SABA and IV corticosteroids	Magnesium sulfate 2 g IV dose

Table 31.1 Comparison of Pharmacologic Management of Asthma and COPD in the ICU (continued)

Pharmacologic Treatment	Asthma	COPD
Outcome	Increase in FEV_1 after administration, especially in patients with an initial FEV_1 < 20% at presentation	Increase in FEV_1 after β-agonist administration, improved PEFR
Monitoring	Hypotension, vasodilation, flushing, hypermagnesemia	Hypotension, vasodilation, flushing, hypermagnesemia
Ketamine[31,59,60]		
Recommendation	Not enough data to support regular use	No recommendation
Dosing	Bolus doses of 0.2–1 mg/kg, followed by infusions of 0.5–1 mg/kg/hr (largest dose was 2.5 mg/kg/hr)	N/A
Outcome	Potential improvement in FEV_1, peak airway pressure, Pao_2 and $Paco_2$	N/A
Monitoring	Dysphoria, heart rate, blood pressure, oral and respiratory secretions, intracranial pressure	N/A
Heliox[48,61-65]		
Recommendation	May benefit patients in severe respiratory distress as a last treatment option before intubation; also beneficial as the delivery system for inhaled β-agonists	May be considered as adjunct in select patient populations (high auto-PEEP, try to prevent intubation)
Dosing	Heliox as either 70:30 or 80:20 ratios of helium to oxygen	Heliox as either 70:30 or 80:20 ratios of helium to oxygen
Outcome	Increase in mean PEFR compared with oxygen administration of albuterol nebulization. Greatest change in patients with severe asthma exacerbation	Potential for reduced hypercapnia, reduced auto-PEEP, reduced systolic pressure variation
Monitoring	Few adverse effects; inconsistent delivery in non-commercially available delivery system	Inconsistent delivery in non-commercially available delivery system
Methylxanthines[66-68]		
Recommendation	Not recommended but may continue in patients who are maintained on them at home	Second-line therapy if lack of response to short-acting inhaled bronchodilators
Dosing		Aminophylline 6 mg/kg IV load; then 0.5–0.9 mg/kg/hr IV infusion
Outcome	Benefits outweighed by risk of adverse effects	No benefit in clinical outcomes, FEV_1, FVC, or ventilation/perfusion, but increase in AEs
Monitoring	Plasma concentration, heart rate, respiratory rate	Plasma concentrations, heart rate, respiratory rate
Intravenous Leukotriene Receptor Antagonists[69,70]		
Recommendation	May benefit patients with severe asthma but not currently available for use in the United States	No recommendation
Dosing	One dose of IV montelukast 7 mg in addition to standard treatment (inhaled SABA, IV steroids)	N/A
Outcome	Improvement in FEV_1 compared with patients who only received standard therapy	N/A
Monitoring	Headache and mood changes	N/A

AE = adverse effect; COPD = chronic obstructive pulmonary disease; FEV_1 = forced expiratory volume in 1 second; FVC = forced vital capacity; ICU = intensive care unit; IV = intravenous; LOS = length of stay; MDI = metered dose inhaler; MV = mechanical ventilation; N/A = not applicable; NIV = noninvasive ventilation; PEEP = peak end-expiratory pressure; PEFR = peak expiratory flow rate; q = every; SABA = short-acting β-agonist.

adequate drug delivery.[98] Nebulization may be a more convenient route of delivery for critically ill patients or those who are unable to hold their breath after actuation of an MDI because of severe dyspnea.[24]

Long-acting β-agonists and anticholinergic agents have been shown to reduce exacerbations,[24] but their role in an acute exacerbation remains unclear. An unblinded randomized controlled pilot study compared indacaterol (a LABA) daily with salbutamol (a SABA) three times a day, in addition to standard therapy, in 29 patients admitted to the ED. The authors found that the patients in the indacaterol group had more improvement in pulmonary function (FEV_1, PEFR) and Po_2/Fio_2 (fraction of inspired oxygen) ratio than did the patients in the traditional salbutamol therapy group.[99] The results of this study suggest that LABAs have a role in COPD exacerbation. However, this study did not include critically ill patients, and the administration of LABAs to critically ill patients may not always be feasible because LABAs are primarily available as dry powder inhalers that are not compatible with ventilators or may be difficult to use for patients with severe respiratory distress.

Corticosteroids

The use of corticosteroids in COPD exacerbations is a mainstay of therapy to decrease the systemic and local inflammation. The use of systemic corticosteroids in COPD exacerbation is recommended by the GOLD guidelines (level of evidence A).[24] Corticosteroids have been associated with improved FEV_1, decreased treatment failures, and reduced hospital length of stay.[100-102]

Unfortunately, the optimal dose and duration of corticosteroids remains under debate, especially in the critically ill population. The dose recommended by the GOLD guidelines is 40 mg of prednisone equivalent daily (preferably oral) for 5 days; however, this recommendation is largely based on studies that do not include critically ill patients. A randomized, double-blind trial including 83 patients 18 years and older with COPD exacerbation requiring hospitalization and ventilator support (invasive or NIV) compared methylprednisolone 0.5 mg/kg intravenously every 6 hours for 72 hours, 0.5 mg/kg every 12 hours on days 4–6, and 0.5 mg/kg daily on days 7–10 with placebo. The investigators found that the steroid arm had a shorter duration of mechanical ventilation (p=0.04), shorter length of ICU stay (p=0.09), fewer failures of NIV (p=0.004), and more hyperglycemia (p=0.04). This study was not powered to detect differences in length of stay or mortality.[50] Another study of 217 critically ill patients 40 years and older with COPD exacerbation requiring mechanical ventilation compared open-label enteral prednisone 1 mg/kg daily for a maximum of 10 days with a control group. No significant differences in ICU mortality, NIV failure, duration of mechanical ventilation, or ICU length of stay were identified, although the study did not meet power. There was an increase in hyperglycemia in the steroid group (p=0.015).[51] A cohort study by Kiser et al. compared high-dose (more than 240 mg/day) and lower-dose (240 mg/day or less) methylprednisolone in 17,239 patients with COPD exacerbation admitted to an ICU. Patients who received higher-dose methylprednisolone had longer ICU and hospital length of stay, higher hospital costs, longer duration of mechanical ventilation, and more hyperglycemia and fungal infections. There was no difference in mortality between the two groups.[52]

A recent meta-analysis included trials evaluating systemic corticosteroid use in ICU and non-ICU patient populations. The results showed improvement in treatment success in the overall population in the corticosteroid group. Treatment success was defined to include the following: (1) clinical improvement as assessed by a questionnaire; (2) improvement in FEV_1 or blood gases; (3) reduction in length of hospital stay in acute care patients and lack of need for intubation in patients on NIV or reduced mortality for mechanically ventilated, critically ill patients. No difference was seen in mortality, although only 9 of the 12 articles included mortality as an end point. The number of hyperglycemic episodes was higher in the corticosteroid group. Despite the overall benefit in the ICU subgroup, the use of corticosteroids had no effect on treatment success.[53] This result should be interpreted with caution, however, because this analysis included only two clinical trials with different study designs, as evidenced by high heterogeneity in this subgroup ($I^2 = 77.4\%$).

An additional consideration in the critically ill population is whether the possibility of altered bioavailability of corticosteroids secondary to hypoxemia or fluid overload should affect the route of administration of these drugs. Inhaled corticosteroids may provide an additional alternative route because they improve lung function and reduce the frequency of COPD exacerbations,[24] but data regarding their utility in the management of COPD exacerbation are currently lacking.

According to currently available evidence, corticosteroid therapy seems to be beneficial in patients with COPD exacerbation. The two available studies of ICU patients used different dosing strategies for corticosteroids, and the optimal dose remains unknown. It would be reasonable to use the lowest effective dose of corticosteroid with consideration for a relative maximum dose of methylprednisolone 0.5 mg/kg intravenously every 6 hours (2 mg/kg/day). Oral or enteral therapy is preferred if this route of administration is possible, and the duration of therapy should be limited to a maximum of 10 days to minimize adverse effects.[24]

Antimicrobial Therapy

Chronic obstructive pulmonary disease exacerbation caused by an infection may be of a bacterial or viral etiology.[24] Bacteria represent 40%–50% of COPD exacerbations.

The most commonly seen bacteria are *Haemophilus influenzae*, *Streptococcus pneumoniae*, and *Moraxella catarrhalis*. In a recent study evaluating the etiology of COPD exacerbation in patients with severe COPD, the most common bacterial pathogen isolated was *Pseudomonas aeruginosa*. There was also a notable percentage of isolates (6%) with *Staphylococcus aureus*, and patients with more frequent exacerbations had a higher likelihood of having Enterobacteriaceae.[103] Atypical bacteria (*Chlamydia pneumoniae* and *Mycoplasma pneumoniae*) make up 5%–10% of COPD exacerbations. Viruses are the causative pathogen in 30%–40% of COPD exacerbations. The most commonly seen virus is rhinovirus, followed by parainfluenza, influenza, respiratory syncytial virus, coronavirus, and adenovirus.[104,105]

Unfortunately, because of inconsistencies in clinical trial design, including the definition of COPD exacerbation, exclusion of subjects with pneumonia, and lack of placebo-controlled arm, the routine use of antibiotics for COPD exacerbation is controversial. A meta-analysis found that antibiotics in COPD exacerbation were beneficial and decreased the incidence of treatment failure, but they had no effect on mortality or hospital length of stay.[104] An ongoing clinical trial is evaluating the need for antibiotic therapy in moderate exacerbation of COPD in an attempt to answer this controversial question.[106] Therapy with antibiotics is currently recommended by the GOLD guidelines for patients who have the three cardinal symptoms: increase in dyspnea, sputum production, and sputum purulence (level B recommendation).[24] In patients with severe COPD exacerbation, particularly those who require either noninvasive or invasive ventilation, the indication for antibiotic therapy is slightly clearer. A randomized controlled trial was conducted to evaluate the use of ofloxacin in patients with COPD exacerbation requiring mechanical ventilation. The results of this study showed a reduction in mortality in the ofloxacin group compared with placebo of 4% versus 22%, respectively (p=0.01), as well as a significant reduction in the need for additional antibiotics, duration of mechanical ventilation, and length of hospital stay.[54] Another study compared amoxicillin/clavulanic acid with placebo in patients with COPD exacerbation. The results of a subgroup analysis of patients with severe COPD at baseline showed a significant improvement in FEV_1 after antibiotic treatment (p<0.01).[55] The use of antibiotics in patients with COPD exacerbation requiring mechanical ventilation (invasive or noninvasive) is a level B recommendation in the GOLD guidelines.[24]

Although the ideal treatment remains to be determined, the evidence supports the use of antibiotic therapy in critically ill patients with severe COPD exacerbations. Table 31.1 outlines antibiotic considerations according to common pathogens; however, therapy should be selected according to local susceptibility patterns of antibiotics to target the aforementioned pathogens, with consideration for coverage of *Pseudomonas* spp. and Enterobacteriaceae in certain patients. The length of therapy recommended by the guidelines is 5–10 days (level of evidence D).

Heliox

As mentioned earlier in this chapter, heliox is a mixture of helium and oxygen that results in a lower-density gas and may reduce resistance in the airways where airflow is turbulent. However, because COPD largely affects the small airways in the lungs, where flow is laminar rather than turbulent, the effect of heliox theoretically may not be as pronounced as in patients with asthma. A prospective study of 25 mechanically ventilated patients with COPD exacerbation evaluated the effect of heliox on respiratory and hemodynamic parameters at baseline, during heliox treatment, and after heliox treatment. The results showed a significant improvement in PEEPi, trapped lung volume, and cardiac performance. The authors concluded that heliox may be a useful adjunct for patients with severe COPD exacerbation and high PEEPi causing systolic pressure variations.[64] A review of the use of heliox for COPD exacerbation mentions successful case reports/case series of heliox improving hypercapnia and avoiding intubation. In mechanically ventilated patients, small studies had conflicting results, with some showing improved work of breathing and decreased auto-PEEP and others showing an inconsistent or lack of benefit. Overall, the author did not recommend the use of heliox because of a lack of robust data and limited availability of the heliox delivery system.[65]

Heliox was also studied as a driving gas for administering the SABA salbutamol and budesonide with the hypothesis that it would be beneficial for drug delivery to the small airways and alveoli. This prospective, randomized trial found no difference in Pao_2, $Paco_2$, FEV_1, or FVC, which suggests a limited benefit of using heliox to improve drug delivery in COPD exacerbation, although the sample size was small (n=30).[107] Heliox may be a beneficial adjunct therapy in select patient populations, such as those with high auto-PEEP or impending hypercapnic respiratory failure, but more evidence is needed before heliox can be a routinely recommended therapy.

Intravenous Magnesium Sulfate

Magnesium may be beneficial in COPD exacerbation because of its bronchodilatory effect, which is thought to be due to bronchial smooth muscle relaxation. In a review of four randomized trials, the authors found that intravenous magnesium had no significant effect on bronchodilation, but they did note an improvement in FEV_1 after an inhaled SABA was administered in the magnesium group compared with the control group, and magnesium use after SABA administration was associated with an increased PEFR.[58] The use of magnesium is not currently recommended by the guidelines, and further investigative controlled trials are needed before its use can be routinely recommended.

Therapies to Use with Caution

Methylxanthines

Intravenous methylxanthines may be considered in patients with an inadequate response to short-acting inhaled bronchodilators and are considered second-line therapy. This is a level B recommendation from the GOLD guidelines.[24] Studies examining the use of intravenous aminophylline in COPD exacerbation did not find any significant benefit in clinical outcomes (including dyspnea and length of hospital stay), FEV_1, FVC, or ventilation/perfusion. However, these studies did find a statistically significant increase in adverse effects with aminophylline, including nausea/vomiting, tremor, tachycardia, and diarrhea.[66-68] According to the currently available data, methylxanthines should not be routinely used for COPD exacerbation.

Doxapram

Doxapram is a respiratory stimulant that has been used to treat respiratory failure in COPD exacerbation. It works by stimulating respiration by acting on central and peripheral chemoreceptors and causing an increased tidal volume. A review of randomized trials found that doxapram may be slightly better than placebo in improving oxygenation and correcting respiratory acidosis. When doxapram was compared with NIV, the results were conflicting, with one study showing better blood gases in the NIV group and another showing no difference.[108] Current evidence does not support the use of doxapram and other respiratory stimulants, and their use is not recommended by the current guidelines.[24]

ASTHMA-CHRONIC OBSTRUCTIVE PULMONARY DISEASE OVERLAP SYNDROME

Patients with ACOS have a higher rate of exacerbation and likely a higher disease severity.[15] A joint project by GINA and GOLD sought to provide treatment guidance according to the differentiating features of ACOS; however, therapeutic management in ICU patients has not been delineated.[11] Given the characteristics of ACOS, patients should be treated with systemic corticosteroids, SABAs, and short-acting inhaled anticholinergics. Because ACOS features resemble those of asthma and COPD, it is likely that these patients will also benefit from other bronchodilator therapies mentioned in this chapter, although data are insufficient to provide recommendations at this time. Patients with ACOS exacerbation should also be assessed for infectious causes of their exacerbation and should be treated accordingly using clinical judgment. Targeted recommendations for ACOS exacerbation require further investigation.

REFERENCES

1. American Lung Association. Chronic Obstructive Pulmonary Disease (COPD) Fact Sheet. March 8, 2015. Available at www.lung.org/lung-disease/copd/resources/fact-figures/COPD-Fact-Sheet.html.

2. Centers for Disease Control and Prevention (CDC). Asthma Facts – CDC's National Asthma Control Program Grantees. Atlanta: CDC, July 2013. Available at www.cdc.gov/asthma/pdfs/asthma_facts_program_grantees.pdf. Accessed September 10, 2015.

3. Louie S, Morrissey BM, Kenyon NJ, et al. The critically ill asthmatic—from ICU to discharge. Clin Rev Allergy Immunol 2012;43:30-44.

4. Pendergraft TB, Stanford RH, Beasley R, et al. Rates and characteristics of intensive care unit admissions and intubations among asthma-related hospitalizations. Ann Allergy Asthma Immunol 2004;9:29-35.

5. Global Initiative for Asthma. Global Strategy for Asthma Management and Prevention. 2014. Available at www.ginasthma.org.

6. Criner GJ, Bourbeau J, Diekemper RL, et al. Prevention of acute exacerbations of chronic obstructive pulmonary disease: American College of Chest Physicians and Canadian Thoracic Society Guideline. Chest 2015;147:894-942.

7. Kosacz NM, Punturieri A, Croxton TL, et al. Chronic obstructive pulmonary disease among adults – United States, 2011. MMWR Morb Mortal Wkly Rep 2012;61:938-43.

8. Centers for Disease Control and Prevention (CDC). COPD Death Rates in the United States. Available at www.cdc.gov/copd/data.htm. Accessed September 10, 2015.

9. Hillas G, Perlikos F, Tsiligianni I, et al. Managing comorbidities in COPD. Int J Chron Obstruct Pulmon Dis 2015;10:95-109.

10. Makhoul N, Khamisy-Farah R, Farah R. Length of stay and outcome of hospitalized chronic obstructive pulmonary disease patients, differences between general medical ward and intensive care unit: a cohort study. West Indian Med J 2013;62:738-43.

11. Global Initiative for Asthma, Global Initiative for Chronic Obstructive Lung Disease. Diagnosis of Diseases of Chronic Airflow Limitation: Asthma, COPD and Asthma-COPD Overlap Syndrome (ACOS). 2014. Available at www.ginasthma.org.

12. Menezes AM, Victora CG, Perez-Padilla R; et al. The Platino project: methodology of a multicenter prevalence survey of chronic obstructive pulmonary disease in major Latin American cities. BMC Med Res Methodol 2004;4:15.

13. Hardin M, Silverman EK, Barr RG, et al. The clinical features of the overlap between COPD and asthma. Respir Res 2011;12:127.

14. Marsh SE, Travers J, Weatherall M, et al. Proportional classifications of COPD phenotypes. Thorax 2008;63:761-7.

15. Menezes AM, Montes de Oca M, Perez-Padilla R, et al. Increased risk of exacerbation and hospitalization in subjects with an overlap phenotype: COPD-asthma. Chest 2014;145:297-304.

16. Herlihy A, Mallow Corbett S, Sessler CN. Drug-induced acute respiratory failure. In: Papadopoulos J, Cooper B, Kane-Gill S, et al., eds. Drug-Induced Complications in the Critically Ill Patient: A Guide for Recognition and Treatment. Mount Prospect, IL: Society of Critical Care Medicine, 2012:87-105.

17. Rajaram S. Life-threatening asthma. In: Parrillo J, Dellinger R, eds. Critical Care Medicine: Principles of Diagnosis and Management in the Adult, 4th ed. St. Louis: Mosby, 2013:645-61.
18. National Asthma Education and Prevention Program. Expert panel report 3 (EPR-3): guidelines for the diagnosis and management of asthma-summary report 2007. J Allergy Clin Immunol 2007;120(5 suppl):S94-138.
19. Boyce JA. The role of mast cells in asthma. Prostaglandins Leukot Essent Fatty Acids 2003;69:195-205.
20. Galli SJ, Kalesnikoff J, Grimbaldeston MA, et al. Mast cells as "tunable" effector and immunoregulatory cells: recent advances. Annu Rev Immunol 2005;23:749-86.
21. Robinson DS. The role of the mast cell in asthma: induction of airway hyperresponsiveness by interaction with smooth muscle? J Allergy Clin Immunol 2004;114:58-65.
22. Peters-Golden M. The alveolar macrophage: the forgotten cell in asthma. Am J Respir Cell Mol Biol 2004;31:3-7.
23. Gibson PG. Why inflammatory phenotyping is necessary for successful drug evaluation in asthma and COPD. Eur Respir J 2013;42:891-2.
24. Global Initiative for Chronic Obstructive Lung Disease. Global Strategy for the Diagnosis, Management, and Prevention of Chronic Obstructive Pulmonary Disease. Global Initative for Chronic Obstructive Lung Disease; 2015 Available at www.goldcopd.org/uploads/users/files/GOLD_Report_2015_Feb18.pdf.
25. Barbera JA, Roca J, Ferrer A, et al. Mechanisms of worsening gas exchange during acute exacerbations of chronic obstructive pulmonary disease. Eur Respir J 1997;10:1285-91.
26. Dominguez-Cherit G, Posadas-Calleja J. Chronic obstructive pulmonary disease. In: Parrillo J, Dellinger R, eds. Critical Care Medicine: Principles of Diagnosis and Management in the Adult, 4th ed. St. Louis: Mosby, 2013:662-73.
27. Gibson PG, Simpson JL. The overlap syndrome of asthma and COPD: what are its features and how important is it? Thorax 2009;64:728-35.
28. Louie S, Zeki AA, Schivo M, et al. The asthma-chronic obstructive pulmonary disease overlap syndrome: pharmacotherapeutic considerations. Expert Rev Clin Pharmacol 2013;6:197-219.
29. Chang J, Mosenifar Z. Differentiating COPD from asthma in clinical practice. J Intensive Care Med 2007;22:300-9.
30. Hurst JR, Vestbo J, Anzueto A, et al. Susceptibility to exacerbation in chronic obstructive pulmonary disease. N Engl J Med 2010;363:1128-38.
31. Schivo M, Phan C, Louie S, et al. Critical asthma syndrome in the ICU. Clin Rev Allergy Immunol 2015;48:31-44.
32. Albertson TE, Schivo M, Gidwani N, et al. Pharmacotherapy of critical asthma syndrome: current and emerging therapies. Clin Rev Allergy Immunol 2015;48:7-30.
33. Mountain RD, Heffner JE, Brackett NC Jr, et al. Acid-base disturbances in acute asthma. Chest 1990;98:651-5.
34. Nowak RM, Tomlanovich MC, Sarkar DD, et al. Arterial blood gases and pulmonary function testing in acute bronchial asthma. predicting patient outcomes. JAMA 1983;249:2043-6.
35. Mountain RD, Sahn SA. Clinical features and outcome in patients with acute asthma presenting with hypercapnia. Am Rev Respir Dis 1988;138:535-9.
36. Molfino NA, Nannini LJ, Martelli AN, et al. Respiratory arrest in near-fatal asthma. N Engl J Med 1991;324:285-8.
37. Warnier MJ, Rutten FH, Kors JA, et al. Cardiac arrhythmias in adult patients with asthma. J Asthma 2012;49:942-6.
38. Kokot F, Hyla-Klekot L. Drug-induced abnormalities of potassium metabolism. Pol Arch Med Wewn 2008;118:431-4.
39. Schols AM, Soeters PB, Dingemans AM, et al. Prevalence and characteristics of nutritional depletion in patients with stable COPD eligible for pulmonary rehabilitation. Am Rev Respir Dis 1993;147:1151-6.
40. Clinical indications for noninvasive positive pressure ventilation in chronic respiratory failure due to restrictive lung disease, COPD, and nocturnal hypoventilation—a consensus conference report. Chest 1999;116:521-34.
41. Pollart SM, Compton RM, Elward KS. Management of acute asthma exacerbations. Am Fam Physician 2011;84:40-7.
42. Mannam P, Siegel MD. Analytic review: management of life-threatening asthma in adults. J Intensive Care Med 2010;25:3-15.
43. Camargo CA Jr, Rachelefsky G, Schatz M. Managing asthma exacerbations in the emergency department: summary of the national asthma education and prevention program expert panel report 3 guidelines for the management of asthma exacerbations. J Emerg Med 2009;37(2 suppl):S6-S17.
44. Eccles SR, Subbe C, Hancock D, et al. CREWS: improving specificity whilst maintaining sensitivity of the national early warning score in patients with chronic hypoxaemia. Resuscitation 2014;85:109-11.
45. Bourdet S, Williams D. Chronic obstructive pulmonary disease. In: DiPiro J, Talbert R, Yee G, et al., eds. Pharmacotherapy: A Pathophysiologic Approach, 6th ed. New York: McGraw-Hill, 2005:537-56.
46. Camargo CA Jr, Spooner CH, Rowe BH. Continuous versus intermittent beta-agonists in the treatment of acute asthma. Cochrane Database Syst Rev 2003;4:CD001115.
47. Papiris SA, Manali ED, Kolilekas L, et al. Acute severe asthma: new approaches to assessment and treatment. Drugs 2009;69:2363-91.
48. Rowe BH, Spooner C, Ducharme FM, et al. Early emergency department treatment of acute asthma with systemic corticosteroids. Cochrane Database Syst Rev 2001;1:CD002178.
49. Lazarus SC. Clinical practice. Emergency treatment of asthma. N Engl J Med 2010;363:755-64.
50. Alia I, de la Cal MA, Esteban A, et al. Efficacy of corticosteroid therapy in patients with an acute exacerbation of chronic obstructive pulmonary disease receiving ventilatory support. Arch Intern Med 2011;171:1939-46.
51. Abroug F, Ouanes-Besbes L, Fkih-Hassen M, et al. Prednisone in COPD exacerbation requiring ventilatory support: an open-label randomised evaluation. Eur Respir J 2014;43:717-24.
52. Kiser TH, Allen RR, Valuck RJ, et al. Outcomes associated with corticosteroid dosage in critically ill patients with acute exacerbations of chronic obstructive pulmonary disease. Am J Respir Crit Care Med 2014;189:1052-64.

53. Abroug F, Ouanes I, Abroug S, et al. Systemic corticosteroids in acute exacerbation of COPD: a meta-analysis of controlled studies with emphasis on ICU patients. Ann Intensive Care 2014;4:32.
54. Nouira S, Marghli S, Belghith M, et al. Once daily oral ofloxacin in chronic obstructive pulmonary disease exacerbation requiring mechanical ventilation: a randomised placebo-controlled trial. Lancet 2001;358:2020-5.
55. Allegra L, Blasi F, de Bernardi B, et al. Antibiotic treatment and baseline severity of disease in acute exacerbations of chronic bronchitis: a re-evaluation of previously published data of a placebo-controlled randomized study. Pulm Pharmacol Ther 2001;14:149-55.
56. Sandrock CE, Norris A. Infection in severe asthma exacerbations and critical asthma syndrome. Clin Rev Allergy Immunol 2015;48:104-13.
57. Silverman RA, Osborn H, Runge J, et al. IV magnesium sulfate in the treatment of acute severe asthma: a multicenter randomized controlled trial. Chest 2002;122:489-97.
58. Shivanthan MC, Rajapakse S. Magnesium for acute exacerbation of chronic obstructive pulmonary disease: a systematic review of randomised trials. Ann Thorac Med 2014;9:77-80.
59. Lau TT, Zed PJ. Does ketamine have a role in managing severe exacerbation of asthma in adults? Pharmacotherapy 2001;21:1100-6.
60. Heshmati F, Zeinali MB, Noroozinia H, et al. Use of ketamine in severe status asthmaticus in intensive care unit. Iran J Allergy Asthma Immunol 2003;2:175-80.
61. Kress JP, Noth I, Gehlbach BK, et al. The utility of albuterol nebulized with heliox during acute asthma exacerbations. Am J Respir Crit Care Med 2002;165:1317-21.
62. Rodrigo G, Pollack C, Rodrigo C, et al. Heliox for nonintubated acute asthma patients. Cochrane Database Syst Rev 2006;4:CD002884.
63. Rodrigo GJ, Castro-Rodriguez JA. Heliox-driven beta2-agonists nebulization for children and adults with acute asthma: a systematic review with meta-analysis. Ann Allergy Asthma Immunol 2014;112:29-34.
64. Lee DL, Lee H, Chang HW, et al. Heliox improves hemodynamics in mechanically ventilated patients with chronic obstructive pulmonary disease with systolic pressure variations. Crit Care Med 2005;33:968-73.
65. Hess DR. Heliox and noninvasive positive-pressure ventilation: a role for heliox in exacerbations of chronic obstructive pulmonary disease? Respir Care 2006;51:640-50.
66. Rice KL, Leatherman JW, Duane PG, et al. Aminophylline for acute exacerbations of chronic obstructive pulmonary disease. A controlled trial. Ann Intern Med 1987;107:305-9.
67. Duffy N, Walker P, Diamantea F, et al. Intravenous aminophylline in patients admitted to hospital with non-acidotic exacerbations of chronic obstructive pulmonary disease: a prospective randomised controlled trial. Thorax 2005;60:713-7.
68. Barbera JA, Reyes A, Roca J, et al. Effect of intravenously administered aminophylline on ventilation/perfusion inequality during recovery from exacerbations of chronic obstructive pulmonary disease. Am Rev Respir Dis 1992;145:1328-33.
69. Camargo CA Jr, Gurner DM, Smithline HA, et al. A randomized placebo-controlled study of intravenous montelukast for the treatment of acute asthma. J Allergy Clin Immunol 2010;125:374-80.
70. Camargo CA Jr, Smithline HA, Malice MP, et al. A randomized controlled trial of intravenous montelukast in acute asthma. Am J Respir Crit Care Med 2003;167:528-33.
71. National Heart, Lung, and Blood Institute (NHLBI). National Asthma Education and Prevention Program: Expert Panel Report 3. Guidelines for the Diagnosis and Management of Asthma. 2007. Report No. 07-4051. Available at www.nhlbi.nih.gov/files/docs/guidelines/asthgdln.pdf.
72. Austin MA, Wills KE, Blizzard L, et al. Effect of high flow oxygen on mortality in chronic obstructive pulmonary disease patients in prehospital setting: randomised controlled trial. BMJ 2010;341:c5462.
73. Chien JW, Ciufo R, Novak R, et al. Uncontrolled oxygen administration and respiratory failure in acute asthma. Chest 2000;117:728-33.
74. Gupta D, Nath A, Agarwal R, et al. A prospective randomized controlled trial on the efficacy of noninvasive ventilation in severe acute asthma. Respir Care 2010;55:536-43.
75. Ram FS, Picot J, Lightowler J, et al. Non-invasive positive pressure ventilation for treatment of respiratory failure due to exacerbations of chronic obstructive pulmonary disease. Cochrane Database Syst Rev 2004;3:CD004104.
76. Brochard L, Mancebo J, Wysocki M, et al. Noninvasive ventilation for acute exacerbations of chronic obstructive pulmonary disease. N Engl J Med 1995;333:817-22.
77. Conti G, Antonelli M, Navalesi P, et al. Noninvasive vs. conventional mechanical ventilation in patients with chronic obstructive pulmonary disease after failure of medical treatment in the ward: a randomized trial. Intensive Care Med 2002;28:1701-7.
78. Nelson HS, Bensch G, Pleskow WW, et al. Improved bronchodilation with levalbuterol compared with racemic albuterol in patients with asthma. J Allergy Clin Immunol 1998;102(6 pt 1):943-52.
79. Datta D, Vitale A, Lahiri B, et al. An evaluation of nebulized levalbuterol in stable COPD. Chest 2003;124:844-9.
80. Lam S, Chen J. Changes in heart rate associated with nebulized racemic albuterol and levalbuterol in intensive care patients. Am J Health Syst Pharm 2003;60:1971-5.
81. Phipps P, Garrard CS. The pulmonary physician in critical care. 12: acute severe asthma in the intensive care unit. Thorax 2003;58:81-8.
82. Rowe BH, Edmonds ML, Spooner CH, et al. Corticosteroid therapy for acute asthma. Respir Med 2004;98:275-84.
83. Manser R, Reid D, Abramson M. Corticosteroids for acute severe asthma in hospitalised patients. Cochrane Database Syst Rev 2001;1:CD001740.
84. Edmonds ML, Camargo CA Jr, Pollack CV Jr, et al. Early use of inhaled corticosteroids in the emergency department treatment of acute asthma. Cochrane Database Syst Rev 2003;3:CD002308.
85. Rowe BH, Bretzlaff JA, Bourdon C, et al. Intravenous magnesium sulfate treatment for acute asthma in the emergency department: a systematic review of the literature. Ann Emerg Med 2000;36:181-90.

86. Cairns CB, Kraft M. Magnesium attenuates the neutrophil respiratory burst in adult asthmatic patients. Acad Emerg Med 1996;3:1093-7.
87. Kew KM, Kirtchuk L, Michell CI. Intravenous magnesium sulfate for treating adults with acute asthma in the emergency department. Cochrane Database Syst Rev 2014;5:CD010909.
88. Stollings JL, Diedrich DA, Oyen LJ, et al. Rapid-sequence intubation: a review of the process and considerations when choosing medications. Ann Pharmacother 2014;48:62-76.
89. Burburan SM, Xisto DG, Rocco PR. Anaesthetic management in asthma. Minerva Anestesiol 2007;73:357-65.
90. Eames WO, Rooke GA, Wu RS, et al. Comparison of the effects of etomidate, propofol, and thiopental on respiratory resistance after tracheal intubation. Anesthesiology 1996;84:1307-11.
91. Mace SE. Challenges and advances in intubation: rapid sequence intubation. Emerg Med Clin North Am 2008;26:1043-68, x.
92. Bain E, Pierides KL, Clifton VL, et al. Interventions for managing asthma in pregnancy. Cochrane Database Syst Rev 2014;10:CD010660.
93. Chan AL, Juarez MM, Gidwani N, et al. Management of critical asthma syndrome during pregnancy. Clin Rev Allergy Immunol 2015;48:45-53.
94. Elsayegh D, Shapiro JM. Management of the obstetric patient with status asthmaticus. J Intensive Care Med 2008;23:396-402.
95. Hanania NA, Belfort MA. Acute asthma in pregnancy. Crit Care Med 2005;33(10 suppl):S319-24.
96. Murphy VE, Fittock RJ, Zarzycki PK, et al. Metabolism of synthetic steroids by the human placenta. Placenta 2007;28:39-46.
97. Martinez FJ, Han MK, Flaherty K, et al. Role of infection and antimicrobial therapy in acute exacerbations of chronic obstructive pulmonary disease. Expert Rev Anti Infect Ther 2006;4:101-24.
98. Turner MO, Patel A, Ginsburg S, et al. Bronchodilator delivery in acute airflow obstruction. A meta-analysis. Arch Intern Med 1997;157:1736-44.
99. Segreti A, Fiori E, Calzetta L, et al. The effect of indacaterol during an acute exacerbation of COPD. Pulm Pharmacol Ther 2013;26:630-4.
100. Davies L, Angus RM, Calverley PM. Oral corticosteroids in patients admitted to hospital with exacerbations of chronic obstructive pulmonary disease: a prospective randomised controlled trial. Lancet 1999;354:456-60.
101. Maltais F, Ostinelli J, Bourbeau J, et al. Comparison of nebulized budesonide and oral prednisolone with placebo in the treatment of acute exacerbations of chronic obstructive pulmonary disease: a randomized controlled trial. Am J Respir Crit Care Med 2002;165:698-703.
102. Niewoehner DE, Erbland ML, Deupree RH, et al. Effect of systemic glucocorticoids on exacerbations of chronic obstructive pulmonary disease. Department of Veterans Affairs Cooperative Study Group. N Engl J Med 1999;340:1941-7.
103. Domenech A, Puig C, Marti S, et al. Infectious etiology of acute exacerbations in severe COPD patients. J Infect 2013;67:516-23.
104. Vollenweider DJ, Jarrett H, Steurer-Stey CA, et al. Antibiotics for exacerbations of chronic obstructive pulmonary disease. Cochrane Database Syst Rev 2012;12:CD010257.
105. Eldika N, Sethi S. Role of nontypeable haemophilus influenzae in exacerbations and progression of chronic obstructive pulmonary disease. Curr Opin Pulm Med 2006;12:118-24.
106. Rohde GG, Koch A, Welte T; ABACOPD study group. Randomized double blind placebo-controlled study to demonstrate that antibiotics are not needed in moderate acute exacerbations of COPD—the ABACOPD study. BMC Pulm Med 2015;15:5.
107. Yongjiu X, Longxiang S, Bingchao H, et al. Heliox as a driving gas to atomize inhaled drugs on acute exacerbation of chronic obstructive pulmonary disease: a prospective clinical study. Chin Med J 2014;127:29-35.
108. Greenstone M, Lasseron T. Doxapram for ventilator failure due to exacerbations of chronic obstructive pulmonary disease. Cochrane Database Syst Rev 2003;1:CD000223.

Section 8

Cardiovascular Critical Care

Chapter 32: Acute Decompensated Heart Failure

*Jo E. Rodgers, Pharm.D., FCCP, BCPS-AQ Cardiology; and
Brent N. Reed, Pharm.D., FAHA, BCPS-AQ Cardiology*

LEARNING OBJECTIVES

1. Describe the pathophysiology, epidemiology, and etiology of acute decompensated heart failure (ADHF).
2. Identify prognostic factors (hemodynamic subsets) that can be used to stratify patients with ADHF by risk for unfavorable outcomes.
3. Recommend an initial diuretic strategy to treat individual patients with ADHF experiencing volume overload, including the role of intravenous vasodilators for acute dyspnea relief.
4. Evaluate therapeutic options for treating patients with ADHF demonstrating refractoriness to intravenous diuretic therapy, including the role of adjunct diuretics, vasopressin receptor antagonists, and ultrafiltration.
5. Differentiate the role of vasodilators and inotropes for the management of ADHF.
6. Advocate for the appropriate use of guideline-driven medical therapies during ADHF episodes, including when to continue and discontinue such therapies.
7. Recognize the role of cardiac transplantation and various types of mechanical circulatory support (intra-aortic balloon pump, temporary and permanent ventricular assist devices, and extracorporeal membrane oxygenation) in ADHF management.

ABBREVIATIONS IN THIS CHAPTER

ACE	Angiotensin-converting enzyme	LVAD	Left ventricular assist device
ADHF	Acute decompensated heart failure	MCS	Mechanical circulatory support
BNP	B-type or brain natriuretic peptide	PA	Pulmonary artery
GDMT	Guideline-directed medical therapy	PCWP	Pulmonary capillary wedge pressure
GI	Gastrointestinal	RV	Right ventricular
IABP	Intra-aortic balloon pump	VAD	Ventricular assist device
LV	Left ventricular		

INTRODUCTION

Acute decompensated heart failure (ADHF) is a clinical diagnosis characterized by the emergence of new or worsening signs and/or symptoms of heart failure. Most ADHF cases require escalated medical care, although prompt management may prevent the need for admission to an intensive care unit. Patients with ADHF may present with signs and symptoms consistent with volume overload, reduced tissue perfusion, or both, regardless of whether the exacerbation occurs in the context of heart failure with reduced ejection fraction (formerly known as *systolic dysfunction*) or heart failure with preserved ejection fraction (formerly known as *diastolic dysfunction*). An exacerbation of ADHF may also be classified by the ventricular chamber affected (i.e., right heart failure, left heart failure, or biventricular failure). Cardiogenic shock is differentiated from ADHF by the presence of systemic hypoperfusion, which often manifests clinically as end-organ dysfunction.

The number of patients with heart failure is expected to increase by almost 50% by 2030.[1] Heart failure represents up to 3% of all hospitalizations in the United States, resulting in more than 3 million hospitalizations annually; in patients older than 65 years, heart failure represents the most common reason for hospital admission.[2] Following hospital discharge, the risk of early readmission for heart failure remains unacceptably high and has been highlighted as a key quality measure with significant financial implications.[3] Consequently, patients with ADHF should receive extensive postdischarge care and planning in addition to the acute interventions necessary to improve symptoms, restore hemodynamic stability, and reduce the risk of in-hospital morbidity and mortality.

The pathophysiology of ADHF depends in part on the underlying etiology of chronic heart failure. Insulting factors that can destabilize a patient with chronic heart failure include those that increase fluid retention and thus signs and symptoms of congestion (e.g., excess fluid intake, nonadherence to diet or diuretic therapy), enhance the excess neurohormonal activation responsible for chronic heart failure (e.g., nonadherence to inhibitors of the renin-angiotensin-aldosterone system or sympathetic nervous system), and impair cardiac output (e.g., acute myocardial infarction, arrhythmias). In addition, patients may present with progressive worsening of cardiac output, despite guideline-directed medical therapy (GDMT); these patients should be evaluated for advanced therapies (e.g., cardiac transplantation). Often, the reason for an acute exacerbation is multifactorial, and patients with more advanced heart failure can experience acute decompensation after even a relatively mild insult.

CLINICAL PRESENTATION

Hemodynamic Subsets

Classification by Signs and Symptoms

The diagnosis of ADHF should be based primarily on signs and symptoms.[3] Volume overload is the most common presentation of ADHF, and the sign and symptom that best correlate with volume status are jugular venous distension and orthopnea, respectively.[4] Although an S3 gallop is very specific for volume overload, pulmonary crackles and lower extremity edema have low specificity and sensitivity.[3]

Medical management of ADHF is determined by differentiating whether the patient has signs and symptoms of fluid overload or hypoperfusion.[4,5] Patients with volume overload may present with pulmonary congestion (orthopnea, dyspnea with minimal exertion), systemic congestion (gastrointestinal [GI] discomfort, ascites, and peripheral edema), or both. In contrast, hypoperfusion commonly presents as extreme fatigue with hypotension, narrow pulse pressure, worsening renal function, cool extremities, or poor mentation. Gastrointestinal symptoms (e.g., nausea, vomiting, early cachexia) may result from GI edema secondary to volume overload or hypoperfusion of the GI tract. In patients with both volume overload and hypoperfusion, low-output symptoms may not be obvious until congestion is optimally managed.

Classification by Hemodynamic Monitoring

As shown in the Evaluation Study of Congestive Heart Failure and Pulmonary Artery Catheterization Effectiveness (ESCAPE), routine placement of a pulmonary artery (PA) catheter does not affect survival and is therefore not indicated in a broad population of patients with ADHF.[6] However, invasive hemodynamic monitoring with a PA catheter may be considered in patients who have respiratory distress or hypoperfusion and in whom cardiac filling pressures cannot be readily ascertained. In addition, invasive monitoring may be considered in select patients who are persistently symptomatic despite standard therapies; have uncertain fluid or hemodynamic status, low systolic blood pressure or symptomatic hypotension, worsening renal function, or a requirement for intravenous vasoactive therapy; or are being evaluated for mechanical circulatory support (MCS) or cardiac transplantation. Of importance, in each of these cases, the level of evidence for invasive hemodynamic monitoring remains expert opinion.[7] Nonetheless, it may assist in classifying patients into a hemodynamic subset as well as selecting appropriate medical therapy.

Hemodynamic monitoring is typically performed with a flow-directed PA catheter (also known as a Swan-Ganz catheter) placed percutaneously through a central vein. The catheter is advanced through the right atrium and ventricle and into the PA. At the proximal end of the catheter, a balloon may be periodically inflated to "wedge" the balloon in a pulmonary capillary, yielding the PA occlusion pressure or *pulmonary capillary wedge pressure* (PCWP). In the absence of certain cardiac structural abnormalities (e.g., mitral valve disease) or pulmonary disease, this pressure estimates the left atrial or pulmonary venous pressure and left ventricular (LV) end-diastolic pressure. The PCWP reflects preload and is a useful marker of volume status; an elevated PCWP indicates volume overload, whereas a reduced PCWP indicates intravascular volume depletion or inadequate filling pressures. According to the Frank-Starling curve, a PCWP of 6–12 mm Hg is desirable in normal patients, whereas a PCWP of 15–18 mm Hg is commonly required in patients with heart failure to ensure adequate stroke volume.

Cardiac output may also be measured with a PA catheter; 4–6 L/minute/m^2 is considered normal. A more useful clinical parameter is cardiac index (CI), which is the cardiac output normalized for body surface area; 2.8–4.2 L/minute/m^2 is considered normal, although a CI of 2.2 L/minute/m^2 in patients with ADHF is usually acceptable. A mixed venous oxygen saturation (SVO_2), which reflects the percentage of oxygen bound to hemoglobin returning to the right side of the heart, may be obtained from the tip of the PA catheter. The SVO_2 represents net oxygen delivery and consumption at the tissue level; 60%–80% is normal, and a low number indicates impaired peripheral blood flow. Because the use of PA catheters has declined since publication of the ESCAPE trial, the SVO_2 may also obtained from internal jugular or subclavian catheters.

Finally, systemic vascular resistance may be calculated using parameters obtained from a PA catheter. Systemic vascular resistance represents the sum of forces impeding the ejection of blood from the left ventricle (i.e., afterload) and is therefore inversely related to cardiac output; 800–1200 dyne/sec/cm^5 is considered normal. Vasoconstriction increases vascular resistance, whereas vasodilation reduces it. An elevated systemic vascular resistance is common in untreated heart failure and can be managed with intravenous or oral arterial vasodilators. In contrast, a low resistance is consistent with vasodilatory shock (e.g., sepsis) as well as end-stage heart failure.

Patients with ADHF may be classified into four hemodynamic subsets on the basis of a CI above or below 2.2 L/minute/m^2 and a PCWP above or below 18 mm Hg (Table 32.1). Patients in the wet-warm (subset II; volume overload but with adequate peripheral perfusion) and wet-cold (subset IV; volume overload and hypoperfusion) profiles have a 2- and 2.5-fold greater risk of death at 1 year, respectively, compared with dry-warm patients.[4,8] In patients with volume overload (subset II), intravenous administration of agents that reduce preload (e.g., loop diuretics, nitroglycerin) is the most appropriate initial therapy. In patients with hypoperfusion (subset III), therapy may differ depending on initial presentation. If the PCWP is significantly below 15 mm Hg, diuretic therapy should be held and fluid restriction liberalized to increase LV filling pressure, consequently improving CI. In select cases, intravenous fluids may be required. For patients in whom CI remains low despite an optimal Frank-Starling relationship (i.e., end-stage heart failure refractory to GDMT), intravenous inotropic therapy is indicated. Patients with both volume overload and hypoperfusion (subset IV) have the worst prognosis. Therapy usually involves a combination of the agents used in subsets II and III (i.e., a combination of diuretics and vasodilators or inotropes) to achieve therapeutic goals. Careful monitoring and individualization of drug therapy is imperative in this population (Table 32.1).

Laboratories

Plasma B-type or brain natriuretic peptide (BNP) and N-terminal pro-BNP concentrations are positively correlated with the presence of volume overload and heart failure

Table 32.1 Management Strategy by Hemodynamic Subset

Subset	Management
Subset I PCWP 15–18 mm Hg[a] CI > 2.2 L/min/m^2	Optimize GDMT and device therapy for chronic heart failure

Subset II:
 Fluid Overload
 PCWP > 18 mm Hg,
 CI > 2.2 L/min/m^2
	Intravenous loop diuretic therapy (dose ≥ chronic oral daily dose)
	 If diuresis is inadequate to relieve symptoms:
	     a) increase intravenous loop diuretic dose
	     b) add second diuretic (e.g., thiazide)
	 In the absence of symptomatic hypotension, intravenous vasodilators (nitroglycerin, nesiritide, nitroprusside) for relief of dyspnea

Subset III:
 Hypoperfusion
 PCWP 15–18 mm Hg[a]
 CI < 2.2 L/min/m^2
	If PCWP < 15 mm Hg, hold diuretic therapy and liberalize fluid restriction and/or administer intravenous fluids to achieve a PCWP of 15–18 mmHg
	 If end-stage heart failure refractory to GDMT and device therapy, intravenous inotropic therapy (temporary, short-term):
	     a) to maintain systemic perfusion and preserve end-organ performance
	     b) to "bridge" to MCS or cardiac transplantation
	 If ineligible for MCS or cardiac transplantation, long-term inotropic therapy may be used as palliative therapy

Subset IV: **Fluid overload and hypoperfusion** PCWP > 18 mm Hg, CI < 2.2 L/min/m^2	Intravenous diuretic therapy and intravenous inotropic therapy as described for Subset II and III

[a] In the absence of cardiac dysfunction, normal range for PCWP is 5–12 mm Hg; higher filling pressures (i.e., 15–18 mm Hg) are necessary in patients with heart failure to optimize CI.

CI = cardiac index; GDMT = guideline-directed medical therapy; MCS = mechanical circulatory support.

severity. These assays are useful in the differential diagnosis of dyspnea, because a BNP concentration less than 100 pg/mL has a 96% predictive value for excluding heart failure.[9] In addition, an elevated BNP concentration before discharge is associated with an increased risk of poor long-term outcomes.[9] Of importance, any pathophysiologic process that increases right heart pressures elevates BNP; concentrations may also be mildly elevated with advanced age, female sex, and renal dysfunction and reduced in obesity.[4] The utility of serial BNP measurement in managing chronic heart failure remains the subject of ongoing research.

Several factors are prognostic for outcomes in patients with ADHF. According to data compiled from the Acute Decompensated Heart Failure National Registry (ADHERE), elevated blood urea nitrogen, low systolic blood pressure, and elevated serum creatinine concentrations were associated with the highest risk of in-hospital mortality; patients with all three features have a 20% risk of in-hospital mortality.[10] Hyponatremia, elevations in troponin I, ischemic etiology, and poor functional capacity are also negative prognostic factors.[11] In the Organized Program to Initiate Lifesaving Treatment in Hospitalized Patients with Heart Failure (OPTIMIZE-HF) registry, low blood pressure and poor renal function were negative prognostic markers for readmission or death, whereas use of standard heart failure therapies or placement of an implantable cardioverter-defibrillator at discharge was associated with an improved prognosis.[12]

VOLUME MANAGEMENT

Loop Diuretics

Intravenous loop diuretics are recommended for patients with ADHF and evidence of significant volume overload. Furosemide, bumetanide, and torsemide may be used for this purpose, although furosemide is the most widely used agent. After an intravenous bolus, loop diuretics reduce preload within 5–15 minutes through functional venodilation and later (after more than 20 minutes) by sodium and water excretion. In patients receiving chronic loop diuretic therapy before admission, intravenous loop diuretics should be administered at a dose that equals or exceeds the chronic oral daily dose. According to the results of the Diuretic Optimization Strategies Evaluation (DOSE) trial, initial loop diuretic therapy may be administered as either intermittent boluses or continuous infusion[7,13] because no differences occurred in the coprimary end points of patient global assessment of symptoms and mean change in serum creatinine when either intermittent bolus versus continuous infusion administration or high versus low dose were compared. However, high doses (2.5 times the oral dose before admission, without accounting for bioavailability) showed greater net fluid loss and change in weight at 72 hours as well as a transient increase in renal dysfunction.[13]

Among the available loop diuretic agents, bioavailability is the primary difference between oral formulations (Table 32.2), whereas intravenous formulations differ by drug concentration. The latter may be clinically relevant when these agents are administered by continuous infusion, in which case furosemide can be associated with considerable added volume. In light of the DOSE trial, continuous infusions are less often used but may occasionally be necessary to administer very high total daily doses when the dose-response ceiling of bolus administration has been reached.

The rate of diuresis should be closely monitored, with careful measurement of fluid intake and output as well as body weight determined at the same time each day. After a single intravenous bolus of loop diuretic, 250–500 mL of fluid loss should occur within 4 hours. Common 24-hour goals for fluid loss are 1–2 L net negative, although some

Table 32.2 Loop Diuretics Used in Acute Decompensated Heart Failure

Loop Diuretics	Oral Bioavailability	Initial Intravenous Daily Dose(s)[a,b]	Usual Dose (maximum dose/day)	Ceiling Dose Based on Creatinine Clearance	Half-life
Furosemide (Lasix)	10%–100% (mean 50%)	20–40 mg once or twice	20–160 mg/day (600 mg)	> 50 mL/min: 80–160 mg 20–50: 160 mg < 20: 400 mg	0.3–3.4 hr
Bumetanide (Bumex)	80%–90%	0.5–1 once or twice	0.5–4 mg/day (10 mg)	> 50 mL/min: 1–2 mg 20–50: 2 mg < 20: 8–10 mg	0.3–1.5 hr
Torsemide (Demadex)	80%–100%	10–20 mg once	10–80 mg/day (200 mg)	> 50 mL/min: 20–40 mg 20–50: 40 mg < 20: 100 mg	3–4 hr

[a]Equivalent oral dose: furosemide 40–80 mg = torsemide 20 mg = bumetanide 1 mg.
[b]For diuretic-naive patients.

patients may experience and tolerate greater net fluid loss. Of importance, select patients (e.g., those with poor renal function, low albumin) may only tolerate being net negative less than 1 L/day. Vital signs, daily serum electrolytes, blood urea nitrogen, and serum creatinine should be closely monitored. Dietary sodium and fluid restriction is also warranted. Of importance, the goal PCWP is 15–18 mm Hg in patients with ADHF because of the higher preload necessary to optimize cardiac output (i.e., because of a flatter Frank-Starling curve). Cardiac output may also decline with excess PCWP; thus, improved renal function and enhanced diuresis may occur as elevated filling pressures resolve. This phenomenon may also occur because of reduced renal congestion. An acute reduction in venous return may compromise effective preload in patients with diastolic dysfunction, patients with intravascular depletion, or those in whom the CI is significantly dependent on adequate filling pressure. Of importance, intravascular volume depletion may occur in the setting of rapid diuresis, despite total body volume overload; thus, daily diuresis goals must be highly individualized. Although most patients tolerate a 2 L/day net negative diuresis, some end-stage patients, especially those who are malnourished, may only tolerate ½–1 L/day net negative diuresis. Ototoxicity may be avoided by avoiding rapid infusion rates (greater than 4 mg/minute intravenous bolus) and minimizing other ototoxic agents, such as aminoglycosides. In addition, dose-related adverse effects include hypotension, renal impairment, and electrolyte wasting.

Diuretic Resistance

Adjunct Diuretics

Occasionally, patients have a suboptimal response to high doses of loop diuretics. In patients with ADHF, both pharmacokinetic and pharmacodynamic mechanisms may lead to diuretic resistance.[14] First, delayed absorption may result in concentrations that fail to reach the threshold necessary for producing effective diuresis. In addition, compensatory sodium reabsorption in the distal convoluted tubule may occur as a result of loop diuretic administration; over time, chronic administration of loop diuretics may lead to hypertrophic remodeling of the nephron, which may also increase sodium reabsorption. Finally, reduced cardiac output may limit renal perfusion as well as renal drug delivery.

Several strategies have been hypothesized to overcome diuretic resistance. First, higher doses of loop diuretics may be administered to achieve concentrations near the peak of the concentration-response curve. As suggested in Table 32.2, the single dose above which additional response is unlikely to occur (i.e., the *ceiling dose*) depends on renal function. A second approach for overcoming diuretic resistance is using a continuous intravenous infusion. Although no advantages of initial continuous infusion administration were seen in the DOSE trial, investigators did not enroll patients with diuretic resistance; thus, it is unknown how continuous infusion compares with bolus administration in this population. A third strategy includes adding a second diuretic with a different mechanism of action, such as a thiazide-type diuretic (e.g., oral metolazone, hydrochlorothiazide, or chlorthalidone; or intravenous chlorothiazide; Table 32.3), to produce a synergistic diuretic effect. Sequential nephron blockade with a loop and thiazide diuretic should generally be reserved for hospitalized patients because severe electrolyte and volume depletion may occur. Given the cost associated with intravenous chlorothiazide, oral thiazide diuretics should be considered first line.

Intravenous Vasodilators

In the absence of symptomatic hypotension, intravenous venodilators such as nitroglycerin and nesiritide may be used in addition to diuretics to aid in acute dyspnea

Table 32.3 Thiazide Diuretics Used in Acute Decompensated Heart Failure

Thiazide Diuretics	Oral Bioavailability	Initial Daily Dose(s)	Duration
Hydrochlorothiazide (PO) (Microzide)	65%–75%	25–50 mg once to twice	5–15 hr
Chlorothiazide (IV) (Diuril)	N/A	250–500 mg once to four times	0.75–2 hr
Chlorthalidone (PO) (Hygroton)	65%	12.5–25 mg once	24–72 hr
Metolazone (PO) (Zaroxolyn)	40%–65%	2.5–10 mg once to twice	8–14 hr

IV = intravenous; N/A = not applicable; PO = oral.

relief.[7,15] Intravenous vasodilator therapy will be discussed in detail later in this chapter.

Dopamine

Despite mounting evidence that dopamine imparts no benefit in patients with ADHF, its use remains common in select scenarios. As in other critical care settings, lower doses of dopamine (less than 3 mcg/kg/minute) were once theorized to improve renal impairment in the setting of ADHF because of the activation of renal dopaminergic receptors[16]; however, this has since been discredited in several randomized controlled trials.[17,18] When added to low-dose furosemide (5 mg/hour) in the Dopamine in Acute Decompensated Heart Failure (DAD-HF) trial, dopamine at doses of 5 mcg/kg/minute provided the same degree of diuresis as high-dose furosemide (20 mg/hour) with no deleterious impact on renal function.[16] However, in the second Dopamine in Acute Decompensated Heart Failure (DAD-HF II) trial, no differences were demonstrated when the same combination of low-dose furosemide and dopamine was compared with low-dose furosemide alone, suggesting that dopamine had no impact on diuresis or other renal outcomes.[17] A similar lack of benefit was shown in the Renal Optimization Strategies Evaluation (ROSE) trial, when patients with ADHF and renal impairment were randomized to low-dose dopamine (2 mcg/kg/minute) or placebo in a randomized controlled fashion.[18]

Anecdotal reports of improved renal function with dopamine in practice are likely a result of its inotropic effects in ADHF, which have been observed even at low doses.[19] However, using dopamine for this purpose is unlikely to provide any additional benefit over traditional inotropes and it may increase tachyarrhythmias by comparison. Although low-dose dopamine is still included as a recommendation for augmenting diuresis in clinical practice guidelines, this recommendation may change when the results of DAD-HF II and ROSE are integrated into future editions.[7]

Vasopressin Receptor Antagonists

Reduced cardiac output may lead to excess stimulation of arterial baroreceptors, which results in enhanced arginine vasopressin secretion and water retention. Consequently, many patients with heart failure present with some degree of hypervolemic hyponatremia, although its prevalence and severity varies. Hyponatremia is commonly mild, asymptomatic, and self-limited, but patients may present with lethargy, confusion, respiratory arrest, cerebral edema, seizures, coma, or death. Indeed, hyponatremia has been associated with increased mortality in this population.[20] The primary strategy for managing hyponatremia in heart failure is to manage volume overload with fluid restriction and diuretic administration. Although a combination of hypertonic saline and loop diuretic therapy has been associated with improved hyponatremia without a deleterious impact on volume status, this strategy is not commonly used.[21] Vasopressin antagonists are therefore an alternative for patients with severe hyponatremia who are refractory to initial measures or who develop neurologic symptoms. Of importance, rapid correction of hyponatremia (greater than 12 mmol/L within 24 hours) should be avoided.[22]

Tolvaptan is an oral inhibitor of vasopressin-2 V_2 receptors in renal tubules, where it prevents the formation of aquaporins and thus inhibits free water reabsorption; it is indicated for managing hypervolemic and euvolemic hyponatremia associated with heart failure and other select diseases. Conivaptan, an intravenous inhibitor of V_2 and V_{1a} receptors in vascular smooth muscle, is only indicated for euvolemic hyponatremia. Despite being available orally, tolvaptan should be initiated in the hospital to allow for close monitoring and to avoid an overly rapid rise in serum sodium. Of note, hyponatremia recurs after discontinuing therapy with tolvaptan, suggesting it has no impact on underlying pathophysiology.[23] In the Efficacy of Vasopressin Antagonism in Heart Failure Outcome Study with Tolvaptan (EVEREST) trial, patients hospitalized with New York Heart Association class III–IV heart failure were randomized to treatment with tolvaptan or placebo. Tolvaptan was associated with improvement in hyponatremia, diuresis, and some symptoms of congestion; however, global clinical status at discharge, mortality, or heart failure readmissions were unchanged.[24,25] Consequently, vasopressin antagonists should be reserved for patients with ADHF and volume overload who have persistent severe hyponatremia and are at risk of having cognitive symptoms despite water restriction and optimization of GDMT.[7]

Ultrafiltration

Ultrafiltration had previously emerged as an alternative strategy for rapid volume removal, given that salt and water may be eliminated at rates of up to 500 mL/hour. Because of its isotonic method of volume removal, ultrafiltration was surmised to provide a safe and effective approach to improving congestion while avoiding the adverse effects of diuretic therapy, such as hemodynamic perturbations, electrolyte loss, and renal impairment. In patients with ADHF and volume overload, the Ultrafiltration versus Intravenous Diuretics for Patients Hospitalized for Acute Decompensated Congestive Heart Failure (UNLOAD) trial suggested that ultrafiltration improved weight loss and net fluid loss compared with intravenous diuretics, as well as reduced readmissions and urgent office or emergency department visits.[26] However, in the Cardiorenal Rescue Study in Acute Decompensated Heart Failure (CARRESS-HF) trial, a more recent study of patients with ADHF, persistent congestion, and renal impairment; an algorithm of stepped pharmacologic therapy (i.e., loop diuretics, thiazide-type diuretics, vasodilators, and inotropes) was superior to ultrafiltration at preserving renal function with a similar amount of weight loss.[27] Ultrafiltration was also associated with a higher rate of adverse events, including infections and bleeding complications. Consequently, ultrafiltration may be considered to alleviate congestive symptoms and fluid weight in patients with obvious volume overload or in those refractory to medical therapy.[7]

HEMODYNAMIC SUPPORT

Vasodilators

Vasodilators may exert benefit in patients with ADHF through several mechanisms. First, venous dilatation can improve refractory congestive symptoms by helping mobilize fluid and enhancing diuresis. In addition, dilating the venous vasculature may improve end-organ function by relieving the deleterious impact of excess venous congestion on the liver, kidneys, and GI tract. For patients whose congestion impairs the Frank-Starling relationship, enhanced volume removal with vasodilators in conjunction with diuretic therapy may restore optimal preload conditions. For vasodilators with effects on the arterial vasculature, reducing the excess systemic vascular resistance imparted by the sympathetic nervous system and renin-angiotensin-aldosterone system can confer improved LV performance as a result of reduced afterload. Although reductions in systemic vascular resistance can significantly reduce blood pressure in patients with normal LV function, improved LV performance as the result of reduced afterload in patients with impaired LV function may lead to minimal changes in mean arterial pressure.

Although oral vasodilators such as long-acting nitrates (e.g., isosorbide dinitrate), hydralazine, and angiotensin-converting enzyme (ACE) inhibitors are often used in patients with ADHF, the focus of this chapter will be the continuous infusions unique to this setting. Intravenous vasodilators used in ADHF include nitroglycerin, sodium nitroprusside, and nesiritide, each of which differs slightly in pharmacologic and pharmacokinetic effects (summarized in Table 32.4). Nitroglycerin acts almost exclusively as a venous dilator except at high doses (greater than 100 mcg/minute). Consequently, nitroglycerin is usually reserved for relieving venous congestion and improving refractory congestive symptoms. Sodium nitroprusside and nesiritide act as both venous and arterial vasodilators throughout their respective dosing ranges and may therefore improve LV performance through beneficial reductions in afterload, in addition to improving venous congestion. Although BNP should expectedly produce increased urine output through natriuresis, clinical trials (discussed below) do not suggest that this additional property of nesiritide imparts any clinically meaningful effect. From a pharmacokinetic standpoint, the effects of nitroglycerin and nitroprusside may be seen within minutes, whereas the onset of nesiritide may be delayed by up to 15–20 minutes. Nesiritide also has a longer half-life, which may make it more problematic in patients who develop hypotension.

The presence of relative hypotension (i.e., systolic blood pressure less than 90 mm Hg) precludes vasodilator use in many patients with ADHF. As discussed previously, invasive hemodynamic monitoring with a PA catheter can confirm reduced cardiac output in the setting of an elevated systemic vascular resistance, where vasodilator use may

Table 32.4 Intravenous Vasodilators Used in Acute Decompensated Heart Failure

Agent	Mechanism of Action	Vascular Effects	Onset	Half-life	Dosing	Disadvantages
Nesiritide (Natrecor)	Recombinant BNP	Venous and arterial vasodilator	15 min	15–20 min	2 mcg/kg bolus (optional); then 0.01 mcg/kg/min Infusions of up to 0.03 mcg/kg/min have been used	Hypotension Slower onset Longer half-life Cost
Nitroglycerin	Exogenous NO donor	Primarily venous; arterial at high doses	Immediate	< 4 min	Initiate at 5–10 mcg/min Effective range 25–200 mcg/min	Hypotension Tachyphylaxis
Sodium nitroprusside (Nipride)	Exogenous NO donor	Venous and arterial vasodilator	Immediate	2 min	Initiate at 0.1–0.2 mcg/kg/min Effective range 0.5–3 mcg/kg/min	Hypotension Accumulation of toxic metabolites in severe hepatic and/or renal impairment

BNP = B-type or brain natriuretic peptide; NO = nitric oxide.

still be beneficial despite low systemic pressures. With the exception of nesiritide, prospective studies of vasodilator use in ADHF are limited. In the Acute Decompensated Heart Failure National Registry (ADHERE) assessing the in-hospital mortality of patients with ADHF, nitroglycerin and nesiritide were associated with lower mortality than inotropes but were similar when compared with each other.[28] In a single-center retrospective study, patients receiving short-term use of sodium nitroprusside demonstrated improved hemodynamic parameters as well as reduced all-cause mortality compared with patients who did not receive nitroprusside although the latter was likely a result of increased chronic vasodilator use among patients transitioned from intravenous sodium nitroprusside.[29]

In contrast to nitroglycerin and sodium nitroprusside, nesiritide has been the subject of several large randomized controlled trials in ADHF. In the Vasodilation in the Management of Acute CHF (VMAC) trial, which compared nitroglycerin and nesiritide in patients with ADHF and congestive symptoms, nesiritide conferred significant improvements in PCWP after several hours, but the differences had mostly dissipated by 48 hours.[15] Some, but not all, subjective symptoms of congestion were initially improved with nesiritide compared with nitroglycerin, but were no different at study conclusion. A randomized controlled trial known as the Acute Study of Clinical Effectiveness of Nesiritide in Decompensated Heart Failure (ASCEND) indicated that patients receiving nesiritide did no better or worse when the agent was added to standard therapies.[30] Similarly, in the ROSE trial, adding low-dose nesiritide (0.005 mcg/kg/minute) to standard therapy had no impact on urine output or other clinical outcomes in patients with ADHF and renal impairment.[18]

With respect to disadvantages, all three agents share hypotension as their most common adverse effect. In addition, tachyphylaxis often occurs with prolonged infusions of nitroglycerin (e.g., more than 12–72 hours) and less commonly with sodium nitroprusside. Sodium nitroprusside is associated with the unique risk of cyanide or thiocyanate toxicity in severe hepatic or renal dysfunction, although the risk is low in patients with ADHF given the lower doses and shorter durations commonly used in this setting. Its other disadvantages are of a practical nature; sodium nitroprusside commonly requires admission to an intensive care unit and placement of an arterial line for monitoring. Nesiritide is associated with rates of hypotension comparable to nitroglycerin and nitroprusside, but its long half-life may make it more problematic in patients with ADHF. In addition, given its lack of benefit compared with older agents, the cost of nesiritide precludes its use in most patients.

In the absence of symptomatic hypotension, intravenous nitroglycerin, sodium nitroprusside, or nesiritide may be considered as an adjuvant to diuretic therapy for relief of dyspnea in patients admitted with ADHF, especially in those whose symptoms are potentially life threatening.[7] In addition, their use should be preferentially considered over inotropes in patients with low cardiac output and normal or elevated blood pressure because these patients may benefit from improved ventricular performance as a result of reduced afterload. In the latter scenario, assessing invasive hemodynamic parameters with a PA catheter should be strongly considered before initiating vasodilators. Given the tenuous hemodynamic status of most patients with ADHF, nitroglycerin and sodium nitroprusside should be initiated at low doses and titrated no faster than every 5–15 minutes, depending on patient response. For nesiritide, bolus administration can be omitted in patients at risk of hypotension. Among the three agents, nitroglycerin may be more favorable for patients with marginal blood pressure because its mostly venous vasodilatory effects may not impart significant reductions in systemic arterial pressure. Sodium nitroprusside and, to a lesser degree, nesiritide, should be considered for patients with hypertension or those whose hemodynamics suggest systemic perfusion is likely to improve with reduced systemic vascular resistance. Given its minimal benefit over older agents and greater cost, nesiritide offers few practical advantages over nitroglycerin or sodium nitroprusside. As with the nitroprusside study described earlier, the ultimate goal should be to transition from intravenous to oral therapies, specifically a GDMT with similar hemodynamic properties.[29]

Inotropes

Positive inotropic agents enhance tissue perfusion through increased myocardial contractility. Because of their effect on cardiac output, inotropes can also reverse the end-organ abnormalities that often complicate ADHF (e.g., cardiorenal syndrome). However, they do not impart a mortality benefit in ADHF and in fact may increase the risk of death as well as adverse effects. Dobutamine and milrinone are the two most commonly used agents in ADHF and will therefore be the focus of this chapter. Digoxin also has inotropic properties; however, the role of digoxin is primarily for the management of chronic heart failure in the outpatient setting.

Although dobutamine and milrinone increase myocardial contractility, they differ in many aspects (summarized in Table 32.5). Dobutamine exerts its inotropic effects primarily by stimulating myocardial β_1 receptors. Some vasodilation may occur at lower doses because of dobutamine's effects on β_2 receptors in vascular smooth muscle, although this may be counteracted by corresponding improvements in cardiac output or its effects on peripheral α_1 receptors at higher doses. Milrinone increases intracellular concentrations of cyclic adenosine monophosphate by inhibiting phosphodiesterase type 3, which confers enhanced contractility in myocardial tissue as well as relaxation of vascular smooth muscle in pulmonary and systemic arterial beds. As a result of these combined effects, milrinone is often called an inodilator.

Milrinone is often recommended in patients receiving chronic β-blockers because it bypasses β receptors, although there is no evidence to suggest it confers a clinically meaningful benefit over dobutamine in this regard. In fact, some small studies suggest that chronic β-blocker use influences adrenergic receptor regulation, thereby preserving the potential for pharmacologic action by dobutamine.[31] Studies are underway to address whether the pharmacologic activity of inotrope use in patients receiving β-blockers before admission depends on the inotrope selected and the β-blocker the patient had been receiving. Similarly, whether patients should continue receiving β-blockers in the setting of inotrope therapy also remains an area of controversy. Given the benefits of continuing β-blockers during an ADHF episode (as well as the worsened clinical outcomes associated with their discontinuation),[32,33] some clinicians may prefer to continue β-blockers when initiating inotrope therapy.

Regarding pharmacokinetic properties, dobutamine has a fairly rapid onset of action and a short half-life; thus, it can be titrated rapidly depending on patient response. A notable exception occurs in patients who have been receiving dobutamine for extended periods (greater than 24 hours) because down-regulation of β-adrenergic receptors may make rapid weaning difficult.[34] In this latter scenario, therapy may need to be slowly tapered in a stepwise fashion depending on patient tolerance. Comparatively, milrinone has a slower onset of action and a longer half-life. Milrinone is primarily eliminated by renal clearance, and its half-life can be especially prolonged in patients with significant renal impairment. Consequently, it should be used with caution in patients with renal impairment and, if selected, initiated at lower doses and titrated more slowly.

As with vasodilators, few randomized controlled trials have assessed intravenous inotropes in ADHF. As previously discussed, when retrospectively compared with other vasoactive therapies in ADHERE, inotrope use portended an increase in mortality even when adjusted for differences in baseline characteristics.[28] The arrhythmogenic potential of inotropic therapy serves as a pharmacologically plausible explanation for an increased risk of mortality, but this impact has not been confirmed in prospective studies. Only milrinone has been the subject of a large, prospective, randomized controlled trial; the Outcomes of a Prospective Trial of Intravenous Milrinone for Exacerbations of Chronic Heart Failure (OPTIME-CHF) showed that its routine use did not confer improved clinical outcomes and, instead, increased the risk of hypotension and atrial arrhythmias.[35] Of note, patients with an indication for inotropic therapy (e.g., cardiogenic shock) were excluded from the trial; thus, it assessed only the routine use of milrinone in a diverse population with ADHF.

The decision to initiate inotrope therapy may be based on clinical features or invasive hemodynamic parameters. Whereas some clinicians prefer to initiate inotropes empirically when patients are refractory to other therapies or when unexpected responses occur (e.g., worsening renal function, ongoing congestion), others prefer invasive hemodynamic monitoring to confirm the presence of low cardiac output. As previously described, routine placement of a PA catheter does not improve outcomes in patients with ADHF, but its use is common when confirming the need for inotrope therapy and guiding dose titration.[6]

Inotropes may improve cardiac output and therefore end-organ perfusion, but their potential benefit must be weighed against the risk of significant adverse effects. Both dobutamine and milrinone increase the sensitivity of the myocardium to catecholamines and other potentially arrhythmogenic stimuli. The commonly held notion that milrinone increases the risk of atrial arrhythmias whereas dobutamine increases the risk of ventricular arrhythmias has not been conclusively shown in the literature. Both

Table 32.5 Positive Inotropic Agents Used in Acute Decompensated Heart Failure

Agent	Mechanism of action	Clinical Effects	Onset	Half-life	Dosing
Dobutamine (Dobutrex)	β-Adrenergic stimulation	Increased contractility by $β_1$ stimulation Mild vasodilation as the result of $β_2$ stimulation	< 10 min	2–5 min	Initiate at 1–2 mcg/kg/min Usual range of 2–10 mcg/kg/min
Milrinone (Primacor)	PDE3 inhibition	Increased contractility by enhanced cAMP in myocardial cells Pulmonary and systemic vasodilation as a result of enhanced cAMP in vascular smooth muscle	5–15 min	2–3 hr (prolonged in renal impairment)	Initiate at 0.1–0.2 mcg/kg/min[a] Usual range of 0.3–0.8 mcg/kg/min

cAMP = cyclic adenosine monophosphate; PDE3 = phosphodiesterase type 3.
[a]Bolus dosing listed in labeling but not used in practice

agents likely increase the risk of arrhythmias to a comparable degree. With respect to distinguishing adverse effects, milrinone is associated with higher rates of hypotension as well as rare cases of thrombocytopenia.

Inotropic agents are warranted as temporary or short-term therapy to maintain systemic perfusion and preserve end-organ function, or as a "bridge" to MCS or cardiac transplantation. For patients who are ineligible for advanced therapies, long-term inotropic therapy may be used as part of a palliative approach.[7] As with vasodilators, inotrope administration requires frequent blood pressure monitoring as well as continuous monitoring for arrhythmias. Long-term use of intravenous inotropes for reasons other than those outlined previously is potentially harmful. Dobutamine can be titrated every 5–15 minutes depending on response, whereas milrinone should be titrated more slowly because of its slower onset of action and longer half-life (e.g., every 6–12 hours, or up to every 12 hours in patients with renal impairment). Tapering should occur gradually with both agents and be guided by patient response. Initiating agents that optimize ventricular loading conditions (e.g., ACE inhibitors or other oral vasodilators) may assist with inotrope weaning.

The decision regarding which inotrope to choose is often both clinician- and patient-dependent. An individual patient's response is often unpredictable, and switching between therapies is common. In the setting of right ventricular (RV) failure, both therapies exert similar inotropic effects, although the vasodilating effects of milrinone may be helpful in patients with elevated pulmonary pressures. The systemic vasodilating effects of milrinone may be problematic in patients with low blood pressure. Therefore, dobutamine is usually preferred in patients with marginal blood pressure, although it, too, can lower blood pressure at low doses. Dobutamine may also be preferred in patients with renal impairment, although milrinone is not absolutely contraindicated. In fact, if renal impairment improves with enhanced tissue perfusion, higher doses may be required.

Dopamine

The role of dopamine as an adjunct to diuretics has been discussed previously. Its use may also be considered for patients in whom a decrease in blood pressure with dobutamine or milrinone is problematic because dopamine provides positive inotropic effects without systemic vasodilation; this feature may make it particularly useful in patients with mixed shock syndromes (e.g., combined cardiogenic and septic shock). However, its impact on α and β receptors can be highly variable in individual patients, making dose titration a challenge. Therefore, many clinicians prefer the combined use of dobutamine and a vasopressor with more predictable hemodynamic effects (e.g., norepinephrine) in this setting because titration of one or the other on the basis of patient response is more straightforward.

MANAGING CHRONIC THERAPIES DURING AN ACUTE DECOMPENSATION

In the absence of hemodynamic instability or other contraindications, guidelines recommend that GDMT be continued.[7] During hospitalization, every effort should be made to optimize standard heart failure therapy, although the timing of such is critical. β-Blockers should generally be continued during a hospitalization unless recent dose initiation or up-titration is thought to be the etiology of decompensation. In such cases, β-blockers may be dose reduced or temporarily held. Otherwise, discontinuation is discouraged because it has been associated with worse outcomes in both the prospective Beta-Blocker Continuation versus Interruption in Patients with Congestive Heart Failure Hospitalized for a Decompensation Episode (B-CONVINCED) trial and the retrospective OPTIMIZE-HF registry.[32,33] For patients not receiving β-blockers, the Initiation Management Predischarge Process for Assessment of Carvedilol Therapy in Heart Failure (IMPACT-HF) trial showed that initiating β-blockers before discharge improved use at 90 days without increasing adverse effects.[36] Guidelines recommend initiating β-blockers after optimal volume status has been achieved and after intravenous diuretics, vasodilators, and inotropic agents have been discontinued, although caution should be exercised in patients recently requiring inotropic therapy.[7]

In the setting of renal dysfunction, ACE inhibitors, angiotensin receptor blockers, and aldosterone antagonists may also need to be temporarily held, especially with coexisting oliguria or hyperkalemia. Therapies that can cause worsening renal function (e.g., ACE inhibitors) should be initiated or titrated cautiously during aggressive diuresis. If an aldosterone antagonist is initiated in the setting of aggressive diuresis, serum potassium concentrations should be monitored closely as diuretic therapy is weaned or transitioned to a chronic oral regimen. Elevated serum digoxin concentrations may warrant dose reduction or temporary discontinuation, especially in the setting of declining renal function. Permanent discontinuation is generally discouraged because an association between digoxin withdrawal and worsening heart failure is well documented.[37,38] Digoxin discontinuation may be appropriate if serum concentrations cannot be maintained in a desirable range (0.5–0.9 ng/mL) because of fluctuating renal function.

TEMPORARY MCS

Many different temporary MCS modalities are available for patients with rapidly deteriorating ADHF or those refractory to pharmacologic support (Table 32.6). In general, indications for temporary MCS include cardiogenic shock with potentially recoverable cardiac function, hemodynamic support in high-risk patients undergoing cardiovascular procedures, or as a bridge to definitive therapy (e.g., durable MCS, cardiac transplantation).[7,39] Three commonly used types of devices include the intra-aortic balloon pump (IABP), temporary ventricular assist device (VAD), and extracorporeal membrane oxygenation (Table 32.6). The role of extracorporeal membrane oxygenation is discussed separately (see page 656).

Patients for whom temporary MCS should be avoided include those with advanced peripheral vascular disease (particularly aortic disease for IABP and Impella), irreversible complications (e.g., anoxic brain injury after cardiac arrest), or patients who are otherwise ineligible for definitive therapies. The thrombotic risks of each device warrant systemic anticoagulation, although temporary IABP support without anticoagulation has been reported.[40] Consequently, MCS should generally be avoided in patients with bleeding diathesis or other contraindications to anticoagulation. Other complications of temporary MCS include infection and vascular injury.

Intra-aortic Balloon Pump

An IABP consists of an elongated balloon affixed to the end of a catheter that is inserted into a large peripheral artery and advanced until the balloon rests in the descending aorta (between the aortic arch and the splanchnic arteries). An IABP provides hemodynamic support by inflating during diastole, which enhances diastolic pressure and thus coronary perfusion, and by deflating during systole, which exerts a vacuum-like effect to reduce LV afterload, thereby improving cardiac output. According to the results of the second Intraaortic Balloon Pump in Cardiogenic Shock (IABP-SHOCK II) trial, the indiscriminant use of IABP in patients with cardiogenic shock has not been associated with improved outcomes.[41] Thrombocytopenia may result from prolonged IABP use, which can be further worsened by concomitant anticoagulation therapy.

Temporary VADs

Temporary VADs include the percutaneously placed Impella (Abiomed, Danvers, MA) and TandemHeart (CardiacAssist, Pittsburgh, PA) devices and the surgically implanted CentriMag device (Thoratec Corp., Pleasanton, CA) (Table 32.6). Each provides continuous blood flow, although the Impella device facilitates flow by an axial mechanism, whereas the TandemHeart and the CentriMag both facilitate centrifugal flow. Unique complications of each device relate primarily to the implantation technique or the mechanism for facilitating blood flow. The axial flow mechanism of the Impella device confers an increased risk of hemolysis. Transseptal placement required for the TandemHeart device is associated with complications related to perforation and shunt formation. Finally, the CentriMag device is associated with risks related to the invasive surgical procedure required for its placement (e.g., tissue injury). A more detailed discussion of the hemodynamic complications of VADs, including RV failure, appears in the Durable MCS section.

ADVANCED CARDIOVASCULAR THERAPIES

Patients with end-stage heart failure may be eligible for durable MCS or cardiac transplantation. To be considered candidates for these advanced therapies, patients must undergo rigorous evaluation. Although cardiac transplantation remains the most optimal long-term strategy for

Table 32.6 Temporary Mechanical Circulatory Support Devices

Device	Implantation Technique	Technical Aspects	Augmented CO (max)
Intra-aortic balloon pump	Percutaneously inserted into a large artery and advanced into the descending thoracic aorta	Provides systolic and diastolic support by counterpulsation	1 L/min
Impella	Percutaneously inserted into a large artery and advanced across the aortic valve into the left ventricle	Facilitates continuous axial flow; pumps blood from LV to ascending aorta by rotating impeller pump	2.5 L/min (Impella 2.5) or 5.0 L/min (Impella 5.0)
TandemHeart	Extracorporeal pump with a percutaneously placed inflow cannula advanced transseptally from the right to left atrium	Facilitates continuous centrifugal flow; pumps blood from LA to systemic circulation or RA to pulmonary circulation	5 L/min
CentriMag	Extracorporeal pump with surgically-placed inflow and outflow cannulae that bypass the affected ventricle	Facilitates continuous centrifugal flow; pumps blood from LA to systemic circulation or RA to pulmonary circulation	10 L/min

CO = cardiac output; LA = left atrium; LV = left ventricle; RA = right atrium; RV = right ventricle.

end-stage heart failure, limited donor availability as well as advances in durable MCS technology have led to sustained growth of VAD implantation.

Durable MCS

Indications for durable MCS include patients being evaluated for cardiac transplantation ("bridge to candidacy"), those awaiting a suitable donor ("bridge to transplantation"), or as a permanent strategy ("destination therapy"). Relative contraindications to durable MCS include high perioperative risk, anatomic abnormalities expected to affect device function, irreversible pulmonary hypertension, comorbid conditions expected to limit survival, and inability to manage the device or pharmacologic therapy.[7] Durable MCS can be distinguished as providing LV, RV, or biventricular support, although left ventricular assist device (LVAD) implantation is most commonly used in practice and will be the focus of this chapter.

The two LVADs currently approved in the United States are the HeartMate II (Thoratec) and the HeartWare (HeartWare, Framingham, MA) ventricular assist systems. The HeartMate II is approved for both bridge to transplantation and destination therapy, whereas the HeartWare is currently approved only for bridge to transplantation. Both devices consist of an inflow cannula inserted into the apex of the left ventricle, a pumping unit, an outflow cannula inserted into the ascending aorta, and a subcutaneously placed driveline that connects the device to an external controller and power supply. The HeartMate II and the HeartWare are capable of producing up to 10 L/minute of continuous blood flow; blood flow is facilitated by axial flow in the HeartMate II and by centrifugal flow in the HeartWare.

Although a variety of parameters reported by the LVAD controller can help in troubleshooting complications, only pump speed can be adjusted directly. All LVADs are preload-dependent and afterload-sensitive; thus, the flow reported by the LVAD may indicate changes in hemodynamic status. Low blood flow may indicate hypovolemia or bleeding. High flows may represent systemic vasodilation, which could be an early sign of sepsis. Pulsatility index (PI) is a unique parameter that reflects the alterations in blood flow provided by contraction of the native left ventricle and negatively correlates with the degree of support required of the LVAD. Low PI may therefore represent low preload (e.g., hypovolemia or excess pump speed) or worsening LV function. High PI is uncommon except when LV function has improved. Finally, spikes in the power required by the LVAD to facilitate blood flow can indicate pump thrombosis.

A particularly challenging issue in a subset of patients with an LVAD is new-onset RV failure, often because of delayed resolution of pulmonary hypertension secondary to volume overload accompanied by an increase in venous return imparted by the LVAD. In addition, unloading of the left ventricle by the device may cause a leftward shift in the ventricular septum, which may further compromise RV geometry. Inotrope therapy can be used to improve RV contractility. The pulmonary vasodilation exerted by milrinone may be helpful in coexisting pulmonary hypertension, although systemic vasodilation may make dobutamine a better choice in select patients. Selective pulmonary vasodilators, such as phosphodiesterase type 5 inhibitors or inhaled epoprostenol, may be helpful for reducing RV afterload. Aggressive volume removal and/or temporary reductions in LVAD speed may be required to alleviate excess RV preload. In refractory cases, temporary placement of an RV assist device or extracorporeal membrane oxygenation may be required.

The most significant challenge in patients with an LVAD is preventing device thrombosis while mitigating bleeding risk. Antithrombotic regimens often consist of both antiplatelet and anticoagulant therapy (usually aspirin and vitamin K antagonists). Antithrombotic management is complicated by acquired von Willebrand syndrome, which occurs as a result of shear stress imparted by the LVAD.[42] In addition, bleeding at specific sites (e.g., intestinal mucosa) is thought to occur as a result of the loss of pulsatile flow with continuous-flow LVADs.[42] Nonetheless, hemorrhagic complications may require a temporary decrease in anticoagulation therapy or cessation. Blood transfusion may be required for critical bleeding events, and leukocyte-reduced blood should be selected in patients undergoing bridge to transplantation to reduce the risk of allosensitization. Pump thrombosis is a potentially life-threatening complication requiring urgent evaluation. Consensus on the treatment of thrombosis is lacking; available modalities have included enhanced antiplatelet or anticoagulation therapy, thrombolytics, and, in severe cases, pump exchange or urgent transplantation.[43]

Other complications of LVADs include infections and arrhythmias. Even mild infections thought to be localized to the driveline site or pump pocket (for HeartMate II) should be treated with aggressive empiric antimicrobial therapy to prevent seeding of the device. Patients with preexisting atrial fibrillation are treated similarly after LVAD implantation. Preexisting ventricular arrhythmias may not resolve after LVAD implantation and may in fact become worse for a time after surgery. If efforts to address hypovolemia (e.g., fluids, lower LVAD speed) are not effective for reducing arrhythmia burden, drug therapy (e.g., amiodarone, β-blockers) should be considered.

Cardiac Transplantation

The immediate postoperative treatment of cardiac transplant recipients is focused on bridging the patient to organ recovery, which can be delayed by prolonged ischemic time as well as reperfusion injury. Because of denervation of the implanted donor heart, inotropic and chronotropic therapy is especially important in the perioperative period. A variety of inotropic agents (e.g., dobutamine, milrinone, epinephrine, isoproterenol) may be employed in this setting. Delays in myocardial recovery often impair the relationship between preload and stroke volume; thus, the donor heart may be especially reliant on chronotropy to maintain cardiac output. Heart rate targets in excess of 90 beats/minute are often advocated, and additional pharmacologic therapy (e.g., albuterol, theophylline) or temporary pacing may be required in patients whose heart rate remains low despite chronotropic therapy (e.g., isoproterenol).[44] Vasopressors may also be required to maintain peripheral perfusion (mean arterial pressure greater than 65 mm Hg). Preventing excess preload (central venous pressure less than 12 mm Hg) with the use of diuretics and venous vasodilators is necessary to prevent right heart overload. As with LVAD implantation, efforts to aggressively manage pulmonary hypertension are necessary to prevent acute right heart failure. Elevated pulmonary pressures that remain refractory to volume removal may require the use of selective pulmonary vasodilators.

After the immediate postoperative treatment of cardiac transplant recipients, achieving an appropriate degree of immunosuppression becomes the emphasis of drug therapy management. For patients with inadequate immunosuppression, the most common manifestation of acute graft rejection is ADHF, and patients are initially treated similarly to those with native heart failure. Other manifestations of acute graft rejection include myocardial ischemia, arrhythmias, and cardiac arrest, and each complication is acutely managed similarly in transplant recipients to those with native disease. Until graft dysfunction can be differentiated as being acute cellular rejection or antibody-mediated rejection in nature, aggressive corticosteroid use is often selected as an empiric immunosuppressive approach. Specific strategies for managing acute cellular rejection or antibody-mediated rejection differ by center.[44-46] In addition to corticosteroids, therapeutic approaches for acute cellular rejection often include antithymocyte globulin, whereas consensus on managing antibody-mediated rejection is less clear.[45] Therapeutic modalities for antibody-mediated rejection include corticosteroids, plasmapheresis, intravenous immunoglobulin G, and upstream anti-immunoglobulin therapies, such as rituximab and bortezomib.[46]

PHARMACIST'S ROLE

Several studies have shown the positive role that pharmacists can play in managing patients with chronic heart failure. Given the growing emphasis on transitions of care and preventing heart failure readmissions, it is likely that many of these interventions will increasingly affect patients with ADHF. The PHARM (Pharmacist in Heart Failure Assessment Recommendation and Monitoring) study was the first randomized controlled trial to show the role of a clinical pharmacist in managing patients with chronic heart failure (n=192). Patients randomized to pharmacist intervention had a significant reduction in the combined primary end point, all-cause mortality and hospitalization or emergency department visit for heart failure (odds ratio 0.22, p=0.005), primarily because of a reduction in heart failure hospitalization.[47] A more recent study showed higher rates of initiation or dose titration of select GDMTs with pharmacist-led 30-minute medication optimization compared with usual care. However, there was no difference in the primary end point, all-cause mortality, or heart failure related hospitalization.[48] Multidisciplinary disease management programs, specialized heart failure clinics, and home-based interventions involving pharmacists have been associated with a wide range of benefits, including reduced heart failure readmissions and emergency department visits as well as improved adherence and symptoms.[49] Pharmacists can provide a variety of services on the multidisciplinary team, including serving as experts on patient counseling.[50] Finally, a recent systematic review of multidisciplinary teams involving a pharmacist showed reductions in all-cause and heart failure hospitalizations. Lack of impact on mortality may have occurred because of limitations in study design (size, duration of follow-up).[51] The American Heart Association recently published a statement describing transitional care interventions and outcomes and discussing implications and recommendations for research and clinical practice to enhance patient-centered outcomes.[52] This statement acknowledges that of the transition of care programs for patients with heart failure (n=20), 75% used a collaborative, multidisciplinary team that included pharmacists.

CONCLUSION

Optimal management of ADHF requires pharmacists to effectively identify prognostic factors that allow stratification on the basis of potential lack of benefit or propensity for adverse events from ADHF therapies. Initial intravenous diuretic regimens should target prompt dyspnea relief, as should adjunctive strategies for managing refractoriness to diuretics. Select patients warrant intravenous vasodilator and/or inotropic therapy, and appropriate patient selection is critical for safe and effective use of these therapies. In addition to playing a key role in ensuring the optimal use of intravenous therapies, pharmacists should advocate for the appropriate use of GDMTs yet appreciate when referral for cardiac transplantation or MCS is necessary.

REFERENCES

1. Go AS, Mozaffarian D, Roger VL, et al.; American Heart Association Statistics Committee and Stroke Statistics Subcommittee. Executive summary: heart disease and stroke statistics—2014 update: a report from the American Heart Association. Circulation 2014;129:399-410.
2. Nieminen MS, Harjola VP. Definition and epidemiology of acute heart failure syndromes. Am J Cardiol 2005;96:5G-10G.
3. Lindenfeld J, Albert NM, Boehmer JP, et al. HFSA 2010 Comprehensive Heart Failure Practice Guideline. J Card Fail 2010;16:e1-194.
4. Nohria A, Mielniczuk LM, Stevenson LW. Evaluation and monitoring of patients with acute heart failure syndromes. Am J Cardiol 2005;9:32G-40G.
5. Nohria A, Lewis E, Stevenson LW. Medical management of advanced heart failure. JAMA 2002;287:628-40.
6. Binanay C, Califf RM, Hasselblad V, et al.; ESCAPE Investigators and ESCAPE Study Coordinators. Evaluation study of congestive heart failure and pulmonary artery catheterization effectiveness: the ESCAPE trial. JAMA 2005;294:1625-33.
7. Yancy CW, Jessup M, Bozkurt B, et al.; American College of Cardiology Foundation; American Heart Association Task Force on Practice Guidelines. 2013 ACCF/AHA guideline for the management of heart failure: a report of the American College of Cardiology Foundation/American Heart Association Task Force on Practice Guidelines. J Am Coll Cardiol 2013;62:e147-239.
8. Forrester JS, Diamond G, Chatterjee K, et al. Medical therapy of acute myocardial infarction by application of hemodynamic subsets (first of two parts). N Engl J Med 1976;295:1356-62.
9. Maisel A, Mueller C, Adams K Jr, et al. State of the art: using natriuretic peptide levels in clinical practice. Eur J Heart Fail 2008;10:824-39.
10. Fonarow GC, Adams KF Jr, Abraham WT, et al.; ADHERE Scientific Advisory Committee, Study Group, and Investigators. Risk stratification for in-hospital mortality in acutely decompensated heart failure: classification and regression tree analysis. JAMA 2005;293:572-80.
11. Gheorghiade M, Zannad F, Sopko G, et al.; International Working Group on Acute Heart Failure Syndromes. Acute heart failure syndromes: current state and framework for future research. Circulation 2005;112:3958-68.
12. O'Connor CM, Abraham WT, Albert NM, et al. Predictors of mortality after discharge in patients hospitalized with heart failure: an analysis from the Organized Program to Initiate Lifesaving Treatment in Hospitalized Patients with Heart Failure (OPTIMIZE-HF). Am Heart J 2008;156:662-73.
13. Felker GM, Lee KL, Bull DA, et al.; NHLBI Heart Failure Clinical Research Network. Diuretic strategies in patients with acute decompensated heart failure. N Engl J Med 2011;364:797-805.
14. Cleland JG, Coletta A, Witte K. Practical applications of intravenous diuretic therapy in decompensated heart failure. Am J Med 2006;119(12 suppl 1):S26-36.
15. Publication Committee for the VMAC Investigators (Vasodilatation in the Management of Acute CHF). Intravenous nesiritide vs nitroglycerin for treatment of decompensated congestive heart failure: a randomized controlled trial. JAMA 2002;287:1531-40.
16. Giamouzis G, Butler J, Starling RC, et al. Impact of dopamine infusion on renal function in hospitalized heart failure patients: results of the Dopamine in Acute Decompensated Heart Failure (DAD-HF) trial. J Card Fail 2010;16:922-30.
17. Triposkiadis FK, Butler J, Karayannis G, et al. Efficacy and safety of high dose versus low dose furosemide with or without dopamine infusion: the Dopamine in Acute Decompensated Heart Failure II (DAD-HF II) trial. Int J Cardiol 2014;172:115-21.
18. Chen HH, Anstrom KJ, Givertz MM, et al.; NHLBI Heart Failure Clinical Research Network. Low-dose dopamine or low-dose nesiritide in acute heart failure with renal dysfunction: the ROSE acute heart failure randomized trial. JAMA 2013;310:2533-43.
19. Ungar A, Fumagalli S, Marini M, et al. Renal, but not systemic, hemodynamic effects of dopamine are influenced by the severity of congestive heart failure. Crit Care Med 2004;32:1125-9.
20. Lee WH, Packer M. Prognostic importance of serum sodium concentration and its modification by converting-enzyme inhibition in patients with severe chronic heart failure. Circulation 1986;73:257-67.
21. Licata G, Di Pasquale P, Parrinello G, et al. Effects of high-dose furosemide and small-volume hypertonic saline solution infusion in comparison with a high dose of furosemide as bolus in refractory congestive heart failure: long-term effects. Am Heart J 2003;145:459-66.
22. Adrogué HJ, Madias NE. Hyponatremia. N Engl J Med 2000;342:1581-9.
23. Schrier RW, Gross P, Gheorghiade M, et al.; SALT Investigators. Tolvaptan, a selective oral vasopressin V2-receptor antagonist, for hyponatremia. N Engl J Med 2006;355:2099-112.
24. Gheorghiade M, Konstam MA, Burnett JC Jr, et al.; Efficacy of Vasopressin Antagonism in Heart Failure Outcome Study with Tolvaptan (EVEREST) Investigators. Short-term clinical effects of tolvaptan, an oral vasopressin antagonist, in patients hospitalized for heart failure: the EVEREST Clinical Status Trials. JAMA 2007;297:1332-43.
25. Konstam MA, Gheorghiade M, Burnett JC Jr, et al.; Efficacy of Vasopressin Antagonism in Heart Failure Outcome Study with Tolvaptan (EVEREST) Investigators. Effects of oral tolvaptan in patients hospitalized for worsening heart failure: the EVEREST Outcome Trial. JAMA 2007;297:1319-31.
26. Costanzo MR, Guglin ME, Saltzberg MT, et al.; UNLOAD Trial Investigators. Ultrafiltration versus intravenous diuretics for patients hospitalized for acute decompensated heart failure. J Am Coll Cardiol 2007;49:675-83.
27. Bart BA, Goldsmith SR, Lee KL, et al.; Heart Failure Clinical Research Network. Ultrafiltration in decompensated heart failure with cardiorenal syndrome. N Engl J Med 2012;367:2296-304.
28. Abraham WT, Adams KF, Fonarow GC, et al.; ADHERE Scientific Advisory Committee and Investigators; ADHERE Study Group. In-hospital mortality in patients with acute decompensated heart failure requiring intravenous vasoactive medications: an analysis from the Acute Decompensated Heart Failure National Registry (ADHERE). J Am Coll Cardiol 2005;46:57-64.

29. Mullens W, Abrahams Z, Francis GS, et al. Sodium nitroprusside for advanced low-output heart failure. J Am Coll Cardiol 2008;52:200-7.

30. O'Connor CM, Starling RC, Hernandez AF, et al. Effect of nesiritide in patients with acute decompensated heart failure. N Engl J Med 2011;365:32-43.

31. Metra M, Nodari S, D'Aloia A, et al. Beta-blocker therapy influences the hemodynamic response to inotropic agents in patients with heart failure: a randomized comparison of dobutamine and enoximone before and after chronic treatment with metoprolol or carvedilol. J Am Coll Cardiol 2002;40:1248-58.

32. Jondeau G, Neuder Y, Eicher JC, et al.; B-CONVINCED Investigators. B-CONVINCED: beta-blocker continuation vs. interruption in patients with congestive heart failure hospitalized for a decompensation episode. Eur Heart J 2009;30:2186-92.

33. Fonarow GC, Abraham WT, Albert NM, et al.; OPTIMIZE-HF Investigators and Coordinators. Influence of beta-blocker continuation or withdrawal on outcomes in patients hospitalized with heart failure: findings from the OPTIMIZE-HF program. J Am Coll Cardiol 2008;52:190-9.

34. Teng JK, Kwan CM, Lin LJ, et al. Down-regulation of beta-adrenergic receptors on mononuclear leukocytes induced by dobutamine treatment in patients with congestive heart failure. Eur Heart J 1993;14:1349-53.

35. Cuffe MS, Califf RM, Adams KF Jr, et al.; Outcomes of a Prospective Trial of Intravenous Milrinone for Exacerbations of Chronic Heart Failure (OPTIME-CHF) Investigators. Short-term intravenous milrinone for acute exacerbation of chronic heart failure: a randomized controlled trial. JAMA 2002;287:1541-7.

36. Gattis WA, O'Connor CM, Gallup DS, et al.; IMPACT-HF Investigators and Coordinators. Predischarge initiation of carvedilol in patients hospitalized for decompensated heart failure: results of the Initiation Management Predischarge: Process for Assessment of Carvedilol Therapy in Heart Failure (IMPACT-HF) trial. J Am Coll Cardiol 2004;43:1534-41.

37. Packer M, Gheorghiade M, Young JB, et al. Withdrawal of digoxin from patients with chronic heart failure treated with angiotensin-converting-enzyme inhibitors. RADIANCE Study. N Engl J Med 1993;329:1-7.

38. Uretsky BF, Young JB, Shahidi FE, et al. Randomized study assessing the effect of digoxin withdrawal in patients with mild to moderate chronic congestive heart failure: results of the PROVED trial. PROVED Investigative Group. J Am Coll Cardiol 1993;22:955-62.

39. Rihal CS, Naidu SS, Givertz MM, et al.; Society for Cardiovascular Angiography and Interventions (SCAI); Heart Failure Society of America (HFSA); Society of Thoracic Surgeons (STS); American Heart Association (AHA), and American College of Cardiology (ACC). 2015 SCAI/ACC/HFSA/STS Clinical Expert Consensus Statement on the Use of Percutaneous Mechanical Circulatory Support Devices in Cardiovascular Care: Endorsed by the American Heart Association, the Cardiological Society of India, and Sociedad Latino Americana de Cardiologia Intervencion; Affirmation of Value by the Canadian Association of Interventional Cardiology-Association Canadienne de Cardiologie d'intervention. J Am Coll Cardiol 2015; 65:e7-e26.

40. Pucher PH, Cummings IG, Shipolini AR, et al. Is heparin needed for patients with an intra-aortic balloon pump? Interact Cardiovasc Thorac Surg 2012;15:136-9.

41. Thiele H, Zeymer U, Neumann FJ, et al.; IABP-SHOCK II Trial Investigators. Intra-aortic balloon support for myocardial infarction with cardiogenic shock. N Engl J Med 2012;367:1287-96.

42. Stewart GC, Givertz MM. Mechanical circulatory support for advanced heart failure: patients and technology in evolution. Circulation 2012;125:1304-15.

43. Goldstein DJ, John R, Salerno C, et al. Algorithm for the diagnosis and management of suspected pump thrombus. J Heart Lung Transplant 2013;32:667-70.

44. Costanzo MR, Dipchand A, Starling R, et al.; International Society of Heart and Lung Transplantation Guidelines. The International Society of Heart and Lung Transplantation Guidelines for the care of heart transplant recipients. J Heart Lung Transplant 2010;29:914-56.

45. Lindenfeld J, Miller GG, Shakar SF, et al. Drug therapy in the heart transplant recipient: part I: cardiac rejection and immunosuppressive drugs. Circulation 2004;110:3734-40.

46. Chih S, Tinckam KJ, Ross HJ. A survey of current practice for antibody-mediated rejection in heart transplantation. Am J Transplant 2013;13:1069-74.

47. Gattis WA, Hasselblad V, Whellan DC, et al. Reduction in heart failure events by the addition of a clinical pharmacist to the heart failure management team: results of the Pharmacist in Heart Failure Assessment Recommendation and Monitoring (PHARM) Study. Arch Intern Med 1999;159:1939-45.

48. Lowrie R, Mair FS, Greenlaw N, et al. Heart failure optimal outcomes from pharmacy study I. Pharmacist intervention in primary care to improve outcomes in patients with left ventricular systolic dysfunction. Eur Heart J 2012;33:314-24.

49. Milfred-LaForest SK, Chow SL, DiDomenico RJ, et al. Clinical Pharmacy Services in Heart Failure: an opinion paper from the Heart Failure Society of America and American College of Clinical Pharmacy Cardiology Practice and Research Network. Pharmacotherapy 2013;33:529-48.

50. Wiggins BS, Rodgers JE, DiDomenico RJ, et al. Discharge counseling for patients with heart failure or myocardial infarction: a best practices model developed by members of the American College of Clinical Pharmacy's Cardiology Practice and Research Network based on the Hospital to Home (H2H) Initiative. Pharmacotherapy 2013;33:558-80.

51. Koshman SL, Charrois TL, Simpson SH, et al. Pharmacist care of patients with heart failure: a systematic review of randomized trials. Arch Intern Med 2008;168:687-94.

52. Albert NM, Barnason S, Deswal A, et al.; American Heart Association Complex Cardiovascular Patient and Family Care Committee of the Council on Cardiovascular and Stroke Nursing, Council on Clinical Cardiology, and Council on Quality of Care and Outcomes Research. Transitions of care in heart failure: a scientific statement from the American Heart Association. Circ Heart Fail 2015;8:384-409.

Chapter 33: Management of Acute Coronary Syndrome

Zachary A. Stacy, Pharm.D., M.S., FCCP, BCPS; and
Paul P. Dobesh, Pharm.D., FCCP, BCPS-AQ Cardiology

LEARNING OBJECTIVES

1. Review the pathophysiology and presentation of patients with an acute coronary syndrome (ACS).
2. Describe the role of anti-ischemic therapy in the management of ACS.
3. Compare and contrast the antiplatelets and anticoagulants routinely used in ACS.

ABBREVIATIONS IN THIS CHAPTER

ACS	Acute coronary syndrome	LMWH	Low-molecular-weight heparin
ACT	Activated clotting time	MI	Myocardial infarction
AT	Antithrombin	NSTE	Non–ST-segment elevation
CABG	Coronary artery bypass grafting	PCI	Percutaneous coronary intervention
CK	Creatine kinase	STEMI	ST-segment elevation myocardial infarction
cTnI	Cardiac troponin I		
cTnT	Cardiac troponin T	TIMI	Thrombolysis In Myocardial Infarction
CV	Cardiovascular	UFH	Unfractionated heparin
DAPT	Dual antiplatelet therapy	Groups and Organizations	
GRACE	Global Registry of Acute Coronary Events	ACCF/AHA	American College of Cardiology Foundation/American Heart Association
HIT	Heparin-induced thrombocytopenia	ESC	European Society of Cardiology
ICH	Intracranial hemorrhage		

INTRODUCTION

Cardiovascular (CV) disease is the leading cause of death in the United States. An acute coronary syndrome (ACS), including unstable angina and myocardial infarction (MI), are the most common cause of CV death.[1-3] An estimated 15.5 million Americans older than 20 years have coronary artery disease. The overall prevalence of MI is 2.8% in U.S. adults (4.0% in men vs. 1.8% in women).[3] The complexity of the disease combined with the rapidly evolving literature can be overwhelming to practitioners. The primary purpose of this chapter is to discuss important considerations in disease assessment and medication evaluation in ACS management.

PATHOPHYSIOLOGY

Mechanism of Plaque Rupture and Thrombus Formation

An ACS event begins with the rupture of an unstable coronary atherosclerotic plaque.[14] This rupture exposes the plaque contents to the circulating blood. The thrombogenic contents, including collagen and tissue factor, promote platelet adhesion and activation. Platelet-derived vasoactive substances such as adenosine diphosphate (ADP) and thromboxane A_2 (TXA_2) promote additional platelet activation and vasoconstriction. Platelet activation also results in a conformational change to the glycoprotein IIb/IIIa surface receptor. Platelet aggregation involves the crosslinking of activated platelets through the surface glycoprotein IIb/IIIa receptor with fibrinogen. Simultaneously, the extrinsic clotting cascade is activated, leading to the production of thrombin (factor IIa) and ultimately fibrin (factor Ia).

Disease Assessment

Patients with suspected ACS should have a comprehensive workup that evaluates chest pain history, cardiac markers, and electrocardiographic (ECG) findings.[1,2]

Risk Scoring

Several risk assessment scores have been developed and validated to encourage the timely diagnosis and treatment of patients presenting with an ACS. A score can easily and objectively risk-stratify patients with non-specific ischemic symptoms. Most clinical prediction algorithms use a combination of clinical history, physical examination, cardiac markers, and ECG. These scoring systems are not designed to assess whether a patient's signs and symptoms are caused by ACS, but to estimate their in-hospital, 6-month, and 3-year mortality. Three common examples of validated risk assessment scores include the Thrombolysis In Myocardial

Table 33.1 Predictive Risk Scores[4-6]

PURSUIT Score (0–18 points)			TIMI Score (0–7 points)		
Age	50	8	Age ≥ 65 years	Yes	1
	60	9		No	0
	70	11	> 3 CAD risk factors	Yes	1
	80	12		No	0
Sex	Male	1	Known CAD > 50%	Yes	1
	Female	0		No	0
Worst CCS class in past 6 weeks	No angina/CCS I or II	0	Aspirin use in past 7 days	Yes	1
	CCS III or IV	2		No	0
Signs of heart failure	Yes	2	Recent (< 24 hr) severe angina	Yes	1
	No	0		No	0
ST depression	Yes	1	Elevated cardiac markers	Yes	1
	No	0		No	0
			ST deviation > 0.5 mm	Yes	1
				No	0

GRACE Score (0–258 points)									
Killip Class	Points	SBP (mm Hg)	Points	Heart Rate (beats/min)	Points	Age	Points	Creatinine (mg/dL)	Points
I	0	< 80	58	< 50	0	< 30	0	0–0.39	1
II	20	80–99	53	50–69	3	30–39	8	0.4–0.79	4
III	39	100–119	43	70–89	9	40–49	25	0.8–1.19	7
IV	59	120–139	34	90–109	15	50–59	41	1.20–1.59	10
		140–159	24	110–149	24	60–69	58	1.6–1.99	13
		160–199	10	150–199	38	70–79	75	2–3.99	21
		> 200	0	> 200	46	80–89	91	> 4	28
						> 90	100		

CAD = coronary artery disease; CCS = Canadian Cardiovascular Society; GRACE = Global Registry of Acute Coronary Events; PURSUIT = Platelet Glycoprotein IIb-IIIa in Unstable Angina: Receptor Suppression Using Integrilin Therapy; SBP = systolic blood pressure; TIMI = thrombolysis in myocardial infarction (score).

Table 33.2 PQRST Pain Assessment in Patients Having an ACS Event

Precipitative	Nonexertional; may occur at rest
Palliative	No relief with rest or organic nitrates
Quality	Stabbing or crushing
Region	Substernal; anterior midline
Radiation	Either arm or shoulder, back, upper abdomen, and lower jaw
Severity	7–10 on a 10-point scale
Temporal	> 20 min

Infarction (TIMI), Platelet Glycoprotein IIb-IIIa in Unstable Angina: Receptor Suppression Using Integrilin Therapy (PURSUIT), and Global Registry of Acute Coronary Events (GRACE) scores (Table 33.1). The TIMI score uses seven variables, all of which carry the same magnitude of risk, to predict death, MI, or target vessel revascularization at 14 days.[4] The PURSUIT score uses five variables to predict short-term outcomes at 30 days, whereas the GRACE score uses eight variables to predict in-hospital mortality and MI.[5,6] An updated GRACE score (GRACE 2.0) has been created to simplify and strengthen the predictability of the clinical tool (substitutes Killip class for diuretic use, and serum creatinine with a history of renal dysfunction).[7] Patients with an ACS can be assigned a low, moderate, or high-risk score to aid in their prognosis and care. No prediction tool has been proven superior to another, so many clinicians use the TIMI risk score for ease and convenience.

Chest Pain Story

Chest pain is the most common symptom reported in patients experiencing an ACS event.[1,2] Because chest pain is subjective, the PQRST [pain characteristics in low back pain syndrome] pain assessment method can be used to accurately and comprehensively acquire the classic characteristics of the event (Table 33.2). The chest pain associated with an ACS event is not typically precipitated by exertion and often occurs at rest. In addition, rest or organic nitrate administration does not typically result in the palliation of ACS chest pain. Patients may qualify the chest pain as a stabbing and/or crushing pain. This pain typically begins at the anterior midline and may radiate to either arm or shoulder, the back, or the lower jaw. Pain reported below the lower jaw and above the umbilicus is possible during or immediately after an ACS event. Patients often report the pain as severe, equivalent to a score of 7/10. Finally, the absence of pain relief from rest and organic nitrates usually results in episodes lasting more than 20 minutes. Although these characteristics describe the classic chest pain symptoms, women, patients with diabetes, and older adult patients may have an atypical presentation. Other associated symptoms that may occur during an ACS event include diaphoresis, shortness of breath, distress, nausea, and vomiting.

Cardiac Markers

Patients with severe or prolonged myocardial ischemia will develop myocardial necrosis. Myocardial infarction is associated with elevations in both specific and non-specific cardiac markers. These biochemical markers are important in the evaluation, diagnosis, and triage of patients with chest pain (Table 33.3). Accurate interpretation of clinically relevant biomarkers requires an understanding of both their biology and their kinetics. Creatine kinase (CK) is composed of three isoenzymes: CK-MB, CK-MM, and CK-BB. Although CK is found in many tissues throughout the body, the distribution of the isoenzymes varies significantly. About 20% of total CK in the cardiac muscle is CK-MB compared with only 2%–5% of total CK in the skeletal muscle. The total CK is not cardiac-specific, and elevations can been observed in patients with cardiac, skeletal, and cerebral injuries. The CK-MB is the most cardiac-specific isoenzyme because of its relatively low distribution in non-cardiac tissues. Elevations in both total CK and CK-MB can be observed after cardiac and non-cardiac injuries. The CK-MB/total CK ratio or CK-MB relative index can be used to differentiate cardiac disease from non-cardiac disease.[8] A CK-MB greater than 5% of the total CK is suggestive of an ACS event. The CK isoenzymes share a similar kinetic pattern including an initial rise in 4–9 hours, a peak in 24 hours, and normalization in 24–48 hours. Because of advances in troponin assays, CK and CK-MB are no longer recommended in the diagnosis of ACS. If measured in this setting, several CK-MB and total CK measurements should be considered to avoid a false-negative result early (within 0–4 hours) after the onset of chest pain.

Table 33.3 Kinetic Profiles of Cardiac Biomarkers[8-10]

Cardiac Biomarker	Normal Range	Time to Onset	Time to Peak	Time to Normalization
Myoglobin		1–2 hr	4–12 hr	24 hr
Creatine kinase		4–9 hr	24 hr	48–72 hr
Creatine kinase-MB		4–9 hr	24 hr	48–72 hr
Troponin I		4–9 hr	12–24 hr	Within 14 days
Troponin T		4–9 hr	12–24 hr	Within 14 days

False-positive results can be observed in patients with muscle disorders, chronic renal failure, hypothyroidism, pulmonary edema, and congestive heart failure.[1,2]

Myoglobin is a small protein found in high concentrations in both cardiac and skeletal muscles. Although non-specific for cardiac disease, the kinetic profile of myoglobin aids in its clinical utility. Myoglobin is released within 1–2 hours after muscle injury. A peak myoglobin concentration is achieved within 4–12 hours and is rapidly cleared from the blood within 24 hours. Myoglobin has a high negative predictive value and poor specificity, making it more clinically useful to rule out ACS, rather than confirming the diagnosis.[8]

Troponin is a three-protein complex (troponin C [TnC], troponin T [TnT], and troponin I [TnI]) used in the contractile apparatus of muscles. Although cardiac and skeletal muscles both contain TnT and TnI, the amino acid sequence is unique enough to differentiate cardiac troponin (cTnC, cTnT, and cTnI) from skeletal troponin. The troponin subunits share a similar kinetic pattern including an initial rise in 4–9 hours, a peak in 12–24 hours, and normalization within 14 days. Several cTnT or cTnI measurements should be considered to avoid a false-negative result early (within 0–4 hours) after the onset of chest pain. Troponin is routinely measured at baseline, 8 hours, and 16 hours to assist in the diagnosis of ACS. The European Society of Cardiology (ESC) and the American College of Cardiology (ACC) Joint Committee have defined MI as an elevated cardiac troponin above the 99th percentile of the healthy reference population.[9]

Troponin has several ideal features, including biologic, kinetic, and prognostic, which makes it a valuable test in the clinical assessment of ACS. First, cTnT and cTnI is found in relatively high concentrations within the myocardium and is absent within non-cardiac tissue and in the blood of healthy individuals. Second, troponin is released rapidly after myocardial injury, aiding in a timely diagnosis. Third, the magnitude of troponin elevation has been correlated with the risk of death after an ACS event. In addition, troponin may be helpful in identifying an optimal management strategy. Finally, the technology to measure cTnT and cTnI has seen several clinically significant advances. The likelihood of a false-positive and negative result with troponin is less than with myoglobin and CK-MB. Most assays are highly sensitive and specific, and point-of-care troponin testing can produce a qualitative and quantitative result in about 15 minutes. False positives can be observed in patients with other cardiac disease states including advanced heart failure, myocarditis, and pericarditis. Some non-cardiac disease states may also result in a false-positive troponin including chronic obstructive pulmonary disease, pulmonary embolism, and chronic renal failure. In renal failure, an elevated cTnT is observed more often than is cTnI because of cTnT's instability in the serum and higher clearance during dialysis.[10]

ECG Findings

Myocardial ischemia and infarction can be detected using a 12-lead ECG. The ECG can help clinicians understand the presence, extent, and severity of ischemia. Ischemic episodes can be observed on the ECG within minutes of the index event. An ECG should be ordered and interpreted within 10 minutes on arrival to an emergency department.[1] Typical ECG findings indicative of ischemia include T-wave inversion, ST-segment depression, and ST-segment elevation. Comparison of a baseline ECG can be helpful in assessing whether ischemic changes are

Table 33.4 ECG Changes During Ischemia and Infarction[11]

ECG Leads	ECG Change	Vessel	Location
V_2–V_4	Poor R-wave progression	Left anterior descending artery (diagonal branch)	Anterior wall
	ST-segment elevation		
	T-wave inversion		
II, III, and aVF	T-wave inversion	Right coronary artery (posterior descending branch)	Inferior wall
	ST-segment elevation		
I, aVL, V_5, and V_6	ST-segment elevation	Left coronary artery (circumflex branch)	Lateral wall
V_1–V_4	Tall R-waves	Left coronary artery (circumflex branch)	Posterior wall
	ST-segment depression	Right coronary artery (posterior descending branch)	
	Upright T-waves		
V_1 and V_2	R-wave disappearance	Left anterior descending artery (septal branch)	Septal wall
	ST-segment elevation		
	T-wave inversion		

new or old. Changes within specific groupings of ECG leads can suggest the location of the occluded coronary lesion (Table 33.4).[11]

Patients with unstable angina and non–ST-segment elevation (NSTE) may present with T-wave inversion and ST-segment depression, and in some instances, the ECG may remain normal. However, the diagnosis of ST-segment elevation myocardial infarction (STEMI) requires the presence of ST-segment elevation. The ESC and ACC guidelines have defined the amplitude change needed for ST-segment elevation as 0.2 mV in men and 0.15 mV in women (leads V_2 and V_3) or 0.1 mV in any other ECG lead. Pathologic Q waves may also occur several hours to days after an MI. A Q wave appears when electrical activity is absent and rarely disappears despite aggressive pharmacologic and reperfusion strategies.[1,2,11]

The presence of a left bundle branch block (LBBB), which may occur in 7% of patients, makes interpreting the ECG more difficult during periods of ischemia.[12] The baseline ST-segment and T-wave morphology seen with LBBB can mask or mimic the ECG findings during an infarction. A new LBBB is always pathological and may be a sign of MI. The Sgarbossa criteria can be used in patients with a new LBBB and suggestion of an infarct. A Sgarbossa score of 3 or greater has a specificity of 90% for detecting an infarct.[13]

ROLE OF GUIDELINES

Guidelines

Several groups have written guidelines for the management of ACS, including the ACC and the American Heart Association (AHA). The 2013 STEMI and 2014 NSTE ACC/AHA guidelines use both a class and a level system to describe the magnitude and strength of the recommendation. A class I recommendation signifies that the potential benefits outweigh any perceived risks, whereas a class III recommendation implies that the procedure or treatment has no benefit or may be harmful. A level A recommendation is derived from several randomized controlled trials or a meta-analysis, whereas a level C recommendation is based on case studies or expert opinion.[1,2]

Other expert groups have either written or endorsed guidelines (e.g., Society for Cardiovascular Angiography and Interventions, Society of Thoracic Surgeons, ESC). Although other consensus statements and guidelines exist, the ACC/AHA guidelines are considered the gold standard for preventing ACS and treating patients with ACS in the United States.

Core Measures

The ACS core measures represent standards of care that have a clear morbidity and mortality benefit. The acute MI set consists of seven measures (Table 33.5) involving care at admission and on discharge. This quality initiative allows patients, accrediting agencies, and reimbursement groups to evaluate institutions on the basis of performance and quality.[15]

ANTI-ISCHEMIC THERAPY

Oxygen

Historically, oxygen has routinely been administered to all patients with suspected ACS on arrival to the hospital.

Table 33.5 Acute MI Core Measures[15]

Performance Measure No.	Performance Measure Name	Description
AMI-1	Aspirin at arrival	Aspirin administered within 24 hr before or after hospital arrival
AMI-3	ACEI or ARB for LVSD	ACEI or ARB prescribed at hospital discharge in patients with a left ventricular ejection fraction < 40%
AMI-5	β-Blocker prescribed at discharge	β-Blocker prescribed at hospital discharge
AMI-7	Median time to fibrinolysis	Median time from arrival to administration of fibrinolytic therapy in patients with ST-segment elevation
AMI-7a	Fibrinolytic therapy received within 30 min of hospital arrival	Fibrinolytic therapy administered ≤ 30 min from hospital arrival in patients with ST-segment elevation
AMI-8	Median time to primary PCI	Median time from hospital arrival to PCI in patients with ST-segment elevation
AMI-8a	Primary PCI received within 90 min of hospital arrival	PCI performed ≤ 90 min from hospital arrival in patients with ST-segment elevation

ACEI = angiotensin-converting enzyme inhibitor; ARB = angiotensin receptor blocker; LVSD = left ventricular systolic dysfunction; MI = myocardial infarction; PCI = percutaneous coronary intervention.

Evidence for this practice is seeded by weak studies performed in non-human models. Oxygen administration has become routine practice because of the hypothesis that supplemental oxygen improves coronary perfusion pressures and reduces myocardial necrosis. However, hyperoxia appears to have some detrimental effects such as reflex vasoconstriction, increased peripheral and systemic vascular resistance, and cardiotoxicity from oxygen free radicals.[16] Consequently, guidelines now recommend supplemental oxygen during the first 6 hours after arrival in patients with respiratory distress, hypoxic signs and symptoms, or an oxygen saturation less than 90% (American College of Cardiology Foundation [ACCF]/AHA] NSTE class I, level of evidence [LOE] C and STEMI class I, LOE B).[1,2]

Nitrates

The selection and role of nitrate administration in the management of ACS is highly dependent on the formulation's pharmacokinetic profiles. Nitroglycerin forms free radical nitric oxide, which activates guanylate cyclase, resulting in an increase of guanosine 3',5'-monophosphate (cyclic GMP) resulting in smooth muscle vasodilation. In general, nitrates should be considered for symptomatic relief because they have no long-term mortality benefit.[17,18]

Sublingual nitrates are recommended for symptomatic relief in the management of acute chest pain. However, patients experiencing an ACS event may not receive any symptomatic relief from sublingual administration. Most patients with acute chest pain will receive up to 3 sublingual nitroglycerin 0.4-mg tablets administrated 5 minutes apart (ACCF/AHA NSTE and STEMI class I, LOE C).[1,2] The sublingual tablets are quickly dissolved and absorbed through buccal absorption with a mean Cmax (maximum concentration) of 6-7 minutes. In the acute setting, nitrates dilate both normal and atherosclerotic coronary arteries to enhance coronary blood flow to the myocardium. In vessels that are almost 100% occluded, additional vasodilation likely has little to no benefit.

In the setting of acute chest pain, intravenous nitroglycerin administration may provide additional benefit by decreasing preload and left ventricular end-diastolic volume. Ultimately, these hemodynamic changes provide a reduction in myocardial oxygen demand. Continued use of intravenous nitroglycerin typically occurs in patients who have had an ACS event with ongoing hypertension or symptoms of heart failure (ACCF/AHA NSTE class I, LOE B and STEMI class I, LOE C).[1,2] Extreme caution should be taken in patients who are normotensive, and intravenous nitroglycerin should be avoided in patients with hypotension (systolic blood pressure less than 90 mm Hg). Nitroglycerin should also be avoided in patients with ventricular dysfunction who are preload-dependent. Typically, intravenous nitroglycerin is initiated at 5 mcg/minute with dosage adjustments of 5 to 10 mcg/minute up to a maximum dose of 200 mcg/minute. Tolerance can develop with intravenous nitroglycerin within 12 to 24 hours. Clinicians should reassess the need for and effectiveness of intravenous nitroglycerin every 6–12 hours.

β-Blockers

β-Blockers are routinely used in both acute and chronic management of ACS. β-Adrenergic inhibitors reduce blood pressure, heart rate, and contractility, which ultimately reduces cardiac demand. Inhibition of norepinephrine on cardiac tissue reduces the need for oxygen-rich blood supply. In general, β-blockers should be selected on the basis of their selectivity and binding properties. Patients experiencing an ACS event should receive a $β_1$-selective agent without intrinsic sympathomimetic activity.

β-Blockers have been proven safe and effective in most patients with ACS.[19] β-Blockers should be initiated within the first 24 hours in patients without heart failure, low-output state, and cardiogenic shock (ACCF/AHA NSTE class I, LOE A and STEMI class I, LOE B).[1,2] The use of β-blockers in patients with other contraindications including a PR interval greater than 0.24 second, second- or third-degree heart block, or severe airway disease should also be avoided. The use of intravenous β-blockers should be avoided in patients in shock or with risk factors for cardiogenic shock, including age older than 70 years, heart rate greater than 110 beats/minute or less than 60 beats/minute, systolic blood pressure less than 120 mm Hg, and late presentation (ACCF/AHA NSTE class III, LOE B and STEMI class IIa, LOE B).[1,2] Patients with stable heart failure and an ejection fraction less than 40% should be initiated on metoprolol succinate, bisoprolol, or carvedilol before discharge. These agents have a proven mortality benefit in patients with systolic heart failure.

Several early trials showed benefits with the use of early β-blockers on infarct size, recurrent chest pain, reinfarction, and death.[20-23] More recently, the Clopidogrel and Metoprolol in Myocardial Infarction Trial (COMMIT) study was designed to evaluate the use of β-blockers in the management of acute MI.[19] Patients presenting with STEMI were randomized to receive intravenous metoprolol (n=22,929) or placebo (n=22,923). Patients randomized to receive β-blocker therapy were initiated on intravenous metoprolol (up to 15 mg) and then converted to oral metoprolol succinate (up to 200 mg daily). The use of early β-blocker therapy resulted in significantly fewer reinfarctions (2.0% vs. 2.5%; p=0.001) and ventricular fibrillation events (2.5% vs. 3.5%; p=0.001) but increased the risk of cardiogenic shock (5.0% vs. 3.9%; p<0.00001). The risks of β-blocker use were highest during hospital admission days 0–1, and the benefits of β-blocker therapy were seen more gradually over time. These data analyses influenced the core measures to eliminate the β-blocker requirement at admission and support the use of β-blockers; then, the hemodynamic status was stable.[15]

Calcium Channel Blockers

Calcium channel blockers provide vasodilation, a reduction in heart rate, and a reduction in myocardial contractility. The calcium channel blockers need to be considered by class. Although the dihydropyridines provide vasodilation and a reduction in blood pressure, the class may cause reflex tachycardia.[24] Clinically, it would be prudent to administer concomitant β-blockers with dihydropyridine calcium channel blockers, especially nifedipine. The non-dihydropyridine calcium channel blockers decrease blood pressure, heart rate, and myocardial contractility. Clinically, the non-dihydropyridine calcium channel blockers should be avoided in patients with pulmonary edema or heart failure because of their negative inotropic effects.

Non-dihydropyridine calcium channel blockers can be used in patients with persistent chest pain and a contraindication to β-blockers (ACCF/AHA NSTE class I, LOE B).[1,2] Patients with significant left ventricular dysfunction, PR interval greater than 0.24 second, or second- or third-degree heart block should not receive a non-dihydropyridine calcium channel blocker such as verapamil or diltiazem. Calcium channel blockers may be beneficial in patients with chest pain secondary to coronary artery spasm (ACCF/AHA NSTE class I, LOE C).[2] The ACCF/AHA guidelines make no formal recommendations regarding the use of calcium channel blockers in the management of STEMI.[1]

Verapamil and diltiazem have provided reductions in reinfarction rates in patients without left ventricular dysfunction in some trials. The DAVIT-II (Danish Verapamil Infarction Trial) found no difference in mortality in patients receiving verapamil compared with placebo after 18 months (11.1% vs. 13.8%; p=0.11).[25] Reinfarction rates were lower with verapamil (11.0%) than with placebo (13.2%; p=0.04). In a subgroup analysis, verapamil was associated with lower mortality in patients without heart failure (7.7% vs. 11.8%; p=0.02). Diltiazem was studied in patients who had experienced a non–Q-wave MI.[26] No difference in overall mortality was seen between diltiazem and placebo (3.1% vs. 3.8%; p=0.373). Reinfarction rates were lower with diltiazem (5.2%) than with placebo (9.3%; p=0.0297).

Morphine

Opioid analgesics are used for their potent analgesic and anxiolytic properties. In addition, opioid analgesics provide modest reductions in vascular resistance, heart rate, and systolic blood pressure. These hemodynamic properties are beneficial in patients experiencing cardiac chest pain.[27-29]

In patients with chest pain despite antianginal therapy, intravenous morphine sulfate 2–4 mg may be administered (ACCF/AHA NSTE class IIb, LOE B and STEMI class I, LOE C).[1,2] Morphine administration can be repeated every 5–15 minutes for persistent chest pain with blood pressure monitoring. The use of morphine should not preclude the use of other anti-ischemic agents aimed at increasing coronary supply and reducing demand. The most critical adverse effects with morphine are hypotension and respiratory depression. Naloxone 0.4–2.0 mg should be readily available to prevent respiratory and circulatory depression.

ANTITHROMBOTIC THERAPY

The thrombotic nature of most ACS events makes timely and appropriate antithrombotic therapy critical to optimal treatment of these patients. Antithrombotic therapy is composed of antiplatelet and anticoagulant agents. Although platelets dominate the pathophysiological process in arterial thrombosis, the central role of thrombin in both platelet activation and coagulation makes both types of therapy necessary in the patient with ACS.[30,31]

Of note, not all agents have been investigated across the spectrum of ACS, or in different management strategies. The choice of antiplatelet and anticoagulant therapy, as well as dose, may change depending on the patient's ACS diagnosis and management approach (Table 33.6).

Antiplatelet Therapy

Aspirin

Aspirin has been the cornerstone of antiplatelet therapy in patients with ACS for several decades. Early and maintained aspirin therapy has shown the ability to reduce death and MI in patients across the spectrum of ACS.[32] Although there is little controversy about using an initial dose of 162–325 mg chewed and swallowed for rapid platelet inhibition, even for patients on chronic aspirin, the daily dose of aspirin after the initial loading dose use of aspirin remains an issue of discussion.

Aspirin acetylates a specific hydroxyl group of serine 530 on cyclooxygenase (COX)-1 enzyme, which inhibits the binding of arachidonic acid and subsequent creation of TXA_2 in platelets and prostacyclin (PGI_2) in endothelial cells.[33] Aspirin-induced inhibition of TXA_2 and PGI_2 produces opposing effects on hemostasis. In platelets, TXA_2 stimulates the platelet release reaction, causing platelet aggregation as well as producing potent vasoconstriction. In contrast, vascular endothelium-derived PGI_2 serves as a protective factor by preventing platelet activation and providing vascular smooth muscle dilation.[33,34] Aspirin's ability to inhibit platelet aggregation, even with a short half-life (15–20 minutes), is because of the irreversible binding

continued on page 669

Table 33.6 Antithrombotic Drug Use and Dosing Across the Spectrum of ACS and Management Strategy

Drug	NSTE ACS — Early Invasive Strategy	NSTE ACS — Ischemia-Driven Strategy	STEMI — Primary PCI	STEMI — Fibrinolytic Reperfusion
Antiplatelet Therapy				
Aspirin	LD: 162–325 mg MD: 81 mg QD	LD: 162–325 mg MD: 81 mg QD	LD: 162–325 mg MD: 81 mg QD	LD: 162–325 mg MD: 81 mg QD
P2Y$_{12}$ inhibitors				
Clopidogrel	LD: 600 mg MD: 75 mg QD	LD: 300 mg MD: 75 mg QD	LD: 600 mg MD: 75 mg QD	LD: 300 mg Age > 75 years: No loading dose given MD: 75 mg QD
Prasugrel	LD: 60 mg MD: 10 mg QD Weight < 60 kg: MD: 5 mg QD	LD: 30 mg[a] MD: 10 mg QD[a] Weight < 60 kg: MD: 5 mg QD[a] Age ≥ 75 years: MD: 5 mg QD[a]	LD: 60 mg MD: 10 mg QD Weight < 60 kg: MD: 5 mg QD	No recommendation
Ticagrelor	LD: 180 mg MD: 90 mg BID	LD: 180 mg MD: 90 mg BID	LD: 180 mg MD: 90 mg BID	No recommendation
Cangrelor	30-mcg/kg IV bolus, followed by 4-mcg/kg/min IV infusion for at least 2 hr or duration of PCI	No recommendation	30 mcg/kg IV bolus, followed by 4 mcg/kg/min IV infusion for at least 2 hr or duration of PCI	No recommendation
GP IIb/IIIa inhibitor				
Abciximab	0.25-mg/kg IV bolus, followed by 0.125-mcg/kg/min IV infusion of 12 hr after PCI	No recommendation	0.25 mg/kg IV bolus, followed by 0.125 mcg/kg/min (maximum 10 mcg/min) IV infusion of 12 hr after PCI, OR 0.25 mg/kg IC bolus only	No recommendation
Eptifibatide	180-mcg/kg IV bolus × 2 given 10 min apart, followed by 2 mcg/kg/min IV infusion initiated after first bolus and continued for 18–24 hr after PCI CrCl < 50 mL/min/1.73 m^2: Reduce infusion by 50% Hemodialysis: Avoid use	No recommendation	180 mcg/kg IV bolus × 2 given 10 min apart, followed by 2 mcg/kg/min IV infusion initiated after first bolus and continued for 18–24 hr after PCI CrCl < 50 mL/min/1.73 m^2: Reduce infusion by 50% Hemodialysis: Avoid use	No recommendation
Tirofiban	25-mcg/kg IV bolus, followed by 0.15 mcg/kg/min CrCl < 30 mL/min/1.73 m^2: Reduce infusion by 50%	No recommendation	25 mcg/kg IV bolus, followed by 0.15 mcg/kg/min CrCl < 30 mL/min/1.73 m^2: Reduce infusion by 50%	No recommendation

Table 33.6 Antithrombotic Drug Use and Dosing Across the Spectrum of ACS and Management Strategy *(continued)*

Drug	NSTE ACS — Early Invasive Strategy	NSTE ACS — Ischemia-Driven Strategy	STEMI — Primary PCI	STEMI — Fibrinolytic Reperfusion
Anticoagulant Therapy				
Bivalirudin	0.10-mg/kg IV bolus, followed by 0.25 mg/kg/hr IV infusion continued until completion of PCI	No recommendation	0.75 mg/kg IV bolus, followed by 1.75 mg/kg/hr IV infusion until completion of PCI CrCl < 30 mL/min/1.73 m²: Reduce infusion to 1 mg/kg/hr	No recommendation
Enoxaparin	1 mg/kg SC every 12 hr until PCI. A 0.3-mg/kg IV bolus should be given if PCI occurs before two SC doses have been given, or if the last dose was given 8–12 hr before PCI. An initial 30-mg IV bolus can be given. CrCl < 30 mL/min/1.73 m²: 1 mg/kg SC every 24 hr	1 mg/kg SC every 12 hr for duration of hospitalization. An initial 30 mg IV bolus can be given. CrCl < 30 mL/min/1.73 m²: 1 mg/kg SC every 24 hr	0.5 mg/kg one time IV bolus[a]	30-mg IV bolus, followed by 1 mg/kg SC every 12 hr for up to 8 days or hospital discharge. SC doses should be initiated within 15 min of the IV bolus. The first two SC doses should be capped at 100 mg CrCl < 30 mL/min/1.73 m²: 30-mg IV bolus, followed by 1 mg/kg SC every 24 hr. The first SC dose should be capped at 100 mg Age ≥ 75 years: No IV bolus. Initiate at 0.75 mg/kg SC every 12 hr. The first two SC doses should be capped at 75 mg. CrCl < 30 mL/min/1.73 m² AND age ≥ 75 years: No IV bolus. Initiate at 1 mg/kg every 24 hr. The first dose should be capped at 100 mg
Fondaparinux	2.5 mg SC QD until PCI At time of PCI: No GP IIb/IIIa: IV UFH 85 units/kg[b] With GP IIb/IIIa: IV UFH 60 units/kg[b]	2.5 mg SC QD for up to 8 days or duration of hospitalization	No recommendation	2.5 mg IV first dose, followed by 2.5 mg SC next day for up to 8 days or hospital discharge
Unfractionated heparin	60 units/kg (maximum 4,000 units) IV bolus, followed by 12 units/kg/hr (initial maximum 1000 units/hr)[b]	60 units/kg (maximum 4,000 units) IV bolus, followed by 12 units/kg/hr (initial maximum 1,000 units/hr)	No GP IIb/IIIa: 70 to 100 units/kg IV bolus to achieve a therapeutic ACT[b] GP IIb/IIIa: 50–70 units/kg IV bolus to achieve a therapeutic ACT[b]	60 units/kg (maximum 4000 units) IV bolus, followed by 12 units/kg/hr (initial maximum 1,000 units/hr)

Table 33.6 Antithrombotic Drug Use and Dosing Across the Spectrum of ACS and Management Strategy (continued)

Drug	NSTE ACS Early Invasive Strategy	Ischemia-Driven Strategy	STEMI Primary PCI	Fibrinolytic Reperfusion
Fibrinolytics				
Alteplase (t-PA)	No recommendation	No recommendation	No recommendation	15 mg IV bolus, followed by a 0.75-mg/kg IV infusion for 30 min (50 mg maximum), followed by a 0.5-mg/kg IV infusion for 60 min (35 mg maximum)
Reteplase (r-PA)	No recommendation	No recommendation	No recommendation	10 units IV × two doses given 30 min apart
Tenecteplase (TNK)	No recommendation	No recommendation	No recommendation	Single weight-based IV bolus: < 60 kg: 30 mg 60–69 kg: 35 mg 70–79 kg: 40 mg 80–89 kg: 45 mg ≥ 90 kg: 50 mg

[a]Not mentioned in the ACC/AHA guidelines, but evidence exists.
[b]Additional IV boluses of UFH may be needed to maintain a therapeutic ACT.

ACS = acute coronary syndromes; ACT = activated clotting time; BID = twice daily; CrCl = creatinine clearance; GP = glycoprotein; IC = intracoronary; IV = intravenous(ly); LD = loading dose; MD = maintenance dose; NSTE = non–ST-segment elevation; PCI = percutaneous coronary intervention; QD = once daily; SC = subcutaneous(ly); STEMI = ST-segment elevation myocardial infarction; UFH = unfractionated heparin

continued from page 666

to the COX-1 enzyme in platelets, whereas vascular endothelial cells have the ability to regenerate new COX and sustain normal function.[33,35] A single dose of 100 mg will eliminate TXA_2 production.[36] Doses below 100 mg result in dose-dependent effects on TXA_2 and COX inhibition, with daily dosing resulting in a cumulative effect.[34-36]

The Antithrombotic Trialists' Collaboration showed the protective effects of aspirin in patients with a high risk of vascular events.[37] Aspirin provided a significant reduction in nonfatal MI, nonfatal stroke, or vascular death in patients presenting with unstable angina and acute MI. Aspirin doses of 75–1,500 mg daily were evaluated with no significant difference in efficacy between lower doses (75–150 mg), medium doses (160–325 mg), and higher doses (500–1,500 mg). Higher doses were associated with increased GI irritation. In the Clopidogrel and Aspirin Optimal Dose Usage to Reduce Recurrent Events–Seventh Organization to Assess Strategies in Ischemic Syndromes (CURRENT–OASIS 7) trial, aspirin doses of 300–325 mg daily provided no efficacy benefit over doses of 75–100 mg daily, with significantly more GI bleeding with the higher-dose regimen.[38] The Clopidogrel in Unstable Angina to Prevent Recurrent Events (CURE) trial showed an aspirin dose-dependent increase in major bleeds in clopidogrel plus aspirin therapy with a 4.9% rate in daily aspirin doses greater than 200 mg.[39] Low doses of aspirin may selectively bind platelet COX, resulting in the inhibition of TXA_2 with the advantage of leaving vascular endothelial PGI_2 production intact.[35,36] Although the current ACC/AHA guidelines provide a class I, LOE A recommendation for post-loading doses of 81–325 mg daily, a daily maintenance dose of 81 mg daily is considered reasonable (class IIa, LOE B).[1,2]

$P2Y_{12}$ Inhibitors

Currently, four $P2Y_{12}$ inhibitors are available for use in patients with ACS.[40-43] Clopidogrel is an orally administered, selective, irreversible inhibitor of the $P2Y_{12}$ receptor. Similar to its predecessor ticlopidine, clopidogrel is a thienopyridine prodrug that requires hepatic activation. The active metabolite of clopidogrel is responsible for binding to the $P2Y_{12}$ receptor leading to platelet inhibition. The active metabolite of clopidogrel has a reactive thiol group, which forms a disulfide bond with the cysteine residues on the $P2Y_{12}$ receptor, creating an irreversible inhibition of the $P2Y_{12}$ receptor for the life of the platelet.[44,45] This ultimately leads to prevention of ADP-mediated platelet activation and aggregation. Because of this irreversible binding, it is recommended that clopidogrel therapy be withheld for 5 days before coronary artery bypass grafting (CABG) or other major surgery to allow time for new uninhibited platelets to be created.[1,2]

Clopidogrel has been extensively studied in patients with ACS. In the CURE trial, patients with NSTE ACS receiving a 300-mg loading dose of clopidogrel followed by 75 mg daily had a significant reduction in CV death, MI, and stroke compared with those receiving aspirin alone (9.3% vs. 11.4%; p<0.001).[39] The results of the CURE trial created a paradigm change by making dual antiplatelet therapy (DAPT) the standard of care in patients with NSTE ACS. Data analyses from the COMMIT and the Clopidogrel as Adjunctive Reperfusion Therapy-Thrombolysis in Myocardial Infarction 28 (CLARITY-TIMI 28) showed similar benefits of DAPT with aspirin and clopidogrel over the use of aspirin alone in patients presenting with STEMI. Using DAPT with clopidogrel typically comes at the risk of a statistically significant absolute increase in major bleeding of about 1%, but without a significant increase in life-threatening bleeding, intracranial hemorrhage (ICH), or fatal bleeding.[39,46,47] Therefore, clopidogrel is currently the only $P2Y_{12}$ inhibitor with evidence across the spectrum of ACS (NSTE ACS and STEMI) and can be used regardless of the management strategy selected (ischemia-driven, early invasive, fibrinolysis, or primary percutaneous coronary intervention [PCI]).[1,2] Despite the wealth of data and experience using clopidogrel as part of DAPT, three main controversies raise questions about the widespread use of clopidogrel in all patients with ACS. These issues include concern about drug interactions, variability in the antiplatelet response, and cytochrome P450 (CYP) 2C19 polymorphisms.

Clopidogrel requires a two-step activation by several CYP enzymes (2C19, 3A4, 1A2, 2B6), with more than 50% of metabolism being because of CYP2C19.[45,48] Because of the significant role of CYP219 metabolism in creating the active clopidogrel metabolite, drug interactions that reduce the amount of active clopidogrel have become an issue of concern. Although the clopidogrel prescribing information makes a general statement about the potential for inhibitors of CYP2C19 to reduce concentrations in the active metabolite and a reduction in platelet inhibition, most of the controversy surrounds the concomitant use of proton pump inhibitors (PPIs). Package labeling recommends avoiding the concomitant use of clopidogrel with omeprazole and esomeprazole and suggests considering less potent CYP2C19 inhibitor PPIs such as dexlansoprazole, lansoprazole, and pantoprazole that have had less impact on platelet function in pharmacodynamic studies.[49] In a pharmacodynamic evaluation, there was a significant increase in platelet reactivity with 7 days of clopidogrel with omeprazole compared with clopidogrel alone, suggesting less active clopidogrel when combined with a PPI.[50] This concern grew when several observational cohort trials also suggested worse clinical outcomes in patients receiving a PPI with clopidogrel.[51,52] Despite complex matching and propensity scoring in these analysis, they are unable to account for the potential that patients receiving PPIs may be sicker patients.[53] In contrast, a post hoc analysis of prospectively designed studies showed no difference in adverse clinical outcomes in patients receiving PPIs with clopidogrel compared with those receiving clopidogrel alone.[54] The only prospectively designed study to answer this question was discontinued early because of funding issues. Despite this flaw, there was no signal of an increase in the risk of CV events in patients receiving clopidogrel and omeprazole compared with clopidogrel alone (p=0.98).[55] Therefore, the clinical relevance of the PPI and clopidogrel drug interaction may be limited.

Probably the most significant area of controversy surrounding clopidogrel use is the variability in platelet inhibition. Although several different testing methods and definitions have been used, data analyses show that up to 40% of patients (5%–44%) do not obtain adequate platelet inhibition, which has been termed *nonresponsiveness*.[56,57] Several studies have shown that patients who are identified as nonresponsive to clopidogrel have significantly more adverse CV outcomes than those who achieve an adequate response.[56-58] Although patients who have an adequate antiplatelet response to clopidogrel seem to rarely have adverse CV events, and those who are nonresponders are more likely to have events, most patients classified as nonresponders also do not have CV events. Therefore, platelet function testing has a much stronger negative than positive predictive value (predicting who will not have events compared with predicting those who will). Nevertheless, platelet function testing in existing studies and practice does not follow these results and tries to decide how to manage nonresponders. Current trials have not provided guidance on the utility of a tailored strategy with antiplatelet selection (switching to prasugrel) or dosing (clopidogrel 150 mg instead of 75 mg daily) in patients determined to be nonresponsive on the basis of platelet reactivity testing results.[59,60] Of note, these studies have only been conducted in patients undergoing elective PCI or low-risk ACS; higher-risk ACS patients who have more adverse CV events would be expected to have the most benefit from alternative $P2Y_{12}$ strategies.

Clopidogrel's reliance on CYP2C19 for most of its metabolism to the active compound has made polymorphism of this enzyme a suspected culprit in the genesis of clopidogrel nonresponsiveness. Although more than 20 genetic polymorphisms have been identified for CYP2C19, the most significant include *CYP2C19*2* and *CYP2C19*3* because these polymorphisms result in the loss of the functional allele.[40,45] Studies have shown a reduction in the formation of clopidogrel's active metabolite-based *CYP2C19* genotype. Although some studies have also shown an increase in CV events in patients with *CYP2C19* polymorphisms, not all studies confirm these findings.[61] Studies have tried to correlate the antiplatelet effect of clopidogrel and *CYP2C19* polymorphisms. Results from these studies have shown that identifying *CYP2C19* status explains only 12%–15% of the variability in clopidogrel response.[62,63] Therefore, many patients with "wild-type" *CYP2C19* will still not achieve adequate antiplatelet response to clopidogrel. At this time, genetic testing is not the answer to explaining poor antiplatelet response to clopidogrel therapy.

Prasugrel was developed to overcome some of the limitations and concerns with clopidogrel. Although prasugrel is a thienopyridine similar to ticlopidine and clopidogrel that requires hepatic activation, the conversion of prasugrel to its active compound requires only a single step with several CYP enzymes able to contribute. Therefore, the formation of prasugrel to its active compound is faster and more efficient than that of clopidogrel. No significant CYP drug interactions have been reported with prasugrel.[64] In pharmacodynamic studies, prasugrel provides both faster and more potent platelet inhibition than clopidogrel.[65-67] Pharmacodynamic data analyses show that patients found to be nonresponders to clopidogrel consistently become responders when given prasugrel.[65-67] Because prasugrel also forms an irreversible disulfide bond with the $P2Y_{12}$ receptor and the level of platelet inhibition is greater, a 7-day hold is recommended for patients needing CABG or other major surgery.[1,2]

The efficacy and safety of prasugrel was assessed in patients with NSTE ACS and STEMI undergoing PCI in the Trial to Assess Improvement in Therapeutic Outcomes by Optimizing Platelet Inhibition with Prasugrel Thrombolysis In Myocardial Infarction 38 (TRITON-TIMI 38).[68] The regimen of a prasugrel loading dose of 60 mg followed by 10 mg daily provided a significant reduction in CV death, MI, and stroke (9.9% vs. 12.1%; p<0.001) as well as stent thrombosis (1.1% vs. 2.4%; p<0.001) compared with a 300-mg loading dose of clopidogrel followed by 75 mg daily. Prasugrel had an exaggerated benefit in patients with diabetes mellitus, who typically have higher platelet reactivity. Although patients without diabetes mellitus had a significant 14% relative reduction in the primary end point with the use of prasugrel over clopidogrel (p=0.02), patients with diabetes mellitus had a significant 30% relative reduction with the use of prasugrel (p<0.001).[69] Although using a 300-mg loading dose of clopidogrel could be considered a criticism of the trial, pharmacodynamic data analyses show that this regimen of prasugrel still provides significantly better platelet inhibition than does double-dose clopidogrel (600-mg load and 150 mg daily).[69]

Because of the more potent platelet inhibition of prasugrel compared with clopidogrel, major bleeding was significantly higher for patients receiving prasugrel compared with clopidogrel (2.4% vs. 1.8%; p<0.001).[70] Although the absolute numbers were low, there was also an increase in the incidence of life-threatening (0.9% vs. 1.4%; p=0.01) and fatal (0.1% vs. 0.4%; p=0.002) bleeding with the use of prasugrel. To identify which patients were at higher risk of bleeding with prasugrel, a post hoc analysis was performed on the TRITON-TIMI 38 database. In this analysis, patients with weight less than 60 kg, age older than 75 years, or a history of transient ischemic attack (TIA) or stroke had higher rates of bleeding using prasugrel relative to clopidogrel than did the overall study group. Therefore, when considering the efficacy and safety together as a net clinical benefit (death, MI, stroke, and major bleeding), the optimal patient for receiving prasugrel would weigh more than 60 kg, be younger than 75 years, and have no history of TIA or stroke. This patient population made up 80% of patients in the TRITON-TIMI 38 trial, and these patients had a 20% significant benefit of receiving prasugrel over clopidogrel (10.2% vs. 12.5%; p<0.001).[71] Prasugrel is generally not recommended in patients older than 75 years because of excess fatal bleeding, except in patients presenting with diabetes mellitus or STEMI. Despite the higher risk of bleeding, the profound benefit of prasugrel compared with clopidogrel in patients with diabetes mellitus or STEMI outweighs this risk. Patients weighing less than 60 kg are recommended to receive a maintenance dose of 5 mg daily instead of the typical 10-mg daily dose. Because patients with a history of TIA or stroke were the only group in which the risk of bleeding with prasugrel outweighed the benefits, prasugrel is contraindicated in this patient population.

In contrast to the thienopyridines, ticagrelor is a cyclopentyltriazolopyrimidine and is not a prodrug that requires hepatic conversion in order to provide its antiplatelet effect. Ticagrelor is structurally an adaptation of adenosine triphosphate (ATP), which is a known $P2Y_{12}$ receptor antagonist. Although the thienopyridines bind irreversibly to the $P2Y_{12}$ receptor for the life of the platelet by a disulfide bond, ticagrelor has shown both reversible and noncompetitive binding to the $P2Y_{12}$ receptor at a site different from that of the endogenous agonist ADP.[72] Similar to prasugrel, loading and maintenance doses of ticagrelor provide both faster and more potent platelet inhibition than clopidogrel.[73-75] Data analyses supporting crushed ticagrelor tablet administration show that this may offer advantages in critical care patients.[76] Pharmacodynamic data analyses show that patients found to be nonresponders to clopidogrel consistently become responders when given ticagrelor.[75] The reversible binding of ticagrelor requires twice-daily dosing for sustained $P2Y_{12}$ receptor inhibition. Twice-daily CV medications have poorer adherence than once-daily medications.[150] Although ticagrelor produces greater platelet inhibition than clopidogrel, patients who missed a single dose of ticagrelor had platelet inhibition similar to those receiving clopidogrel at 24 hours.[74] Therefore, patients missing a single dose retain a pharmacodynamic response similar to that with clopidogrel. Despite the reversible binding, platelet function recovery to the level of clopidogrel at 5 days still takes about 3 days with ticagrelor. Even with the faster return of platelet function after discontinuing ticagrelor, a 5-day hold is still recommended before CABG or major surgery. This recommendation is based on the similar rates of major bleeding in the Platelet Inhibition and Patient Outcomes (PLATO) trial for clopidogrel and ticagrelor when the agents were held for 5 days before CABG surgery.[1,2,77]

Although ticagrelor does not require hepatic activation to induce its antiplatelet effect, it is metabolized to an active metabolite and many inactive metabolites by CYP3A4 and CYP3A5.[78] Therefore, CYP3A4 inhibitors have the potential to increase the risk of bleeding, and inducers may reduce its efficacy. Currently, strong CYP3A4 inhibitors and inducers should not be coadministered with ticagrelor.[42] Moderate CYP3A4 inhibitors such as diltiazem and amiodarone may have a proportional effect on ticagrelor exposure, but they are not contraindicated.[79] Because some statins have significant CYP3A4 metabolism, coadministration of ticagrelor with more than 40 mg of simvastatin or lovastatin could increase the risk of myopathy and should be avoided. Ticagrelor is also a substrate and inhibitor of P-glycoprotein. Therefore, new steady-state digoxin concentrations should be monitored when initiating ticagrelor therapy.[80] P-glycoprotein inhibitors such as cyclosporine increase the exposure of ticagrelor, but no dose adjustment is needed.[42]

In addition to its antiplatelet effects, ticagrelor has been shown in preclinical studies to interfere with adenosine metabolism and increase adenosine concentrations by inhibition of adenosine uptake by erythrocytes. This interaction probably occurs through inhibition of the sodium-independent equilibrative nucleoside transporter 1 (ENT-1).[81-83] Erythrocyte ENT-1 is responsible for uptake of adenosine into the cell, where it is metabolized by several mechanisms. The ability of ticagrelor to inhibit adenosine's uptake by ENT-1 is likely because of the similar chemical structure of the two molecules. This interaction produces an increase in adenosine exposure. The quantifiable impact of the increased adenosine exposure is not fully understood, but it may offer clinical advantages and disadvantages to ticagrelor. Studies have shown that ticagrelor can augment both endogenous and exogenous adenosine-induced coronary blood flow in a canine model as well as in healthy volunteers.[81,82] This increase in coronary blood flow may provide a clinical advantage by producing sustained and elevated adenosine concentrations in ischemic tissues leading to improved perfusion. Increased adenosine exposure may also explain some of the unique adverse effects shown with ticagrelor (i.e., dyspnea, ventricular pauses, and gout) that are not typically seen with the thienopyridine $P2Y_{12}$ inhibitors. It has been shown that continuous infusions of adenosine can produce dyspnea without bronchospasm.[84] Continuous infusions of adenosine have also shown the ability to produce sinoatrial nodal pauses, compared with the more common occurrence of atrioventricular (AV) block produced by bolus doses of adenosine.[85] The increase in gout may be explained by the fact that uric acid is a breakdown product of purine (adenosine) metabolism.

The efficacy and safety of ticagrelor has been shown in patients with NSTE ACS and STEMI in the PLATO trial.[77] The regimen of a ticagrelor loading dose of 180 mg followed by 90 mg twice daily provided a significant reduction in CV death, MI, and stroke (9.8% vs. 11.7%; p<0.001), as well as stent thrombosis (1.3% vs. 1.9%; p=0.009), compared with a 300- or 600-mg loading dose of clopidogrel followed by 75 mg daily. The loading dose of clopidogrel did not affect the study results. Of interest, there was not only a significant reduction in MI, as typically shown in these trials, but also a significant reduction in CV mortality (4.0% vs. 5.1%; p=0.001), which is rarely shown with DAPT. It is unknown whether this reduction in CV mortality is the result of the more potent antiplatelet effect of ticagrelor compared with clopidogrel or the result of improved adenosine-induced coronary perfusion. Using ticagrelor as part of DAPT did increase the risk of major bleeding compared with clopidogrel (4.5% vs. 3.8%; p=0.03) without an increase in life-threatening bleeding, ICH, or fatal bleeding. The incidence of dyspnea, Holter monitor–detected bradycardia, and gout was also significantly higher in patients receiving ticagrelor compared with clopidogrel. Most cases of dyspnea are mild to moderate in severity and resolve in 1–2 weeks. Patients with a history of heart failure, chronic obstructive pulmonary disease, or other causes of dyspnea are not at higher risk of developing ticagrelor-related dyspnea.[86] Although patients at risk of bradycardia (known sick sinus syndrome, second- or third-degree AV conduction block, or previously documented syncope suspected to be because of bradycardia unless treated with a pacemaker) were not enrolled in the PLATO trial, there was no difference in symptomatic events.[77] The proposed mechanism behind these unique adverse effects is ticagrelor's competition with adenosine for ENT-1 and its delayed adenosine metabolism. This mechanism is supported by the lack of a sustained impact of these adverse effects. Because of the elevation in adenosine produced as a result of the acute ischemia of an ACS event in local tissues, the adverse effects of dyspnea and ventricular pauses are typically seen early in ticagrelor therapy. When the ischemic stimulus is reduced during the next 30 days, the rates of these adverse effects are reduced, and the need to discontinue therapy is rare.

Ticagrelor is contraindicated in patients receiving a chronic dose of aspirin greater than 100 mg daily. This recommendation is based on results from a subanalysis of the PLATO trial.[87] In this analysis, the benefit of ticagrelor appeared to be attenuated in patients enrolled in North America, specifically the United States. Actually, patients in the United States enrolled in the PLATO trial had a numerical increase in the primary end point with the use of ticagrelor compared with clopidogrel (11.9% vs. 9.5%; p=0.1459), as well as in each of the individual components of the composite end point. This effect may have been a result of the higher maintenance dose of aspirin used in the United States compared with the rest of the world. Patients in the United States were more likely to take a median maintenance aspirin dose of at least 300 mg daily (53.6%) compared with the rest of the world (1.7%). Patients enrolled in the United States who received a maintenance aspirin dose of at least 300 mg daily had an increase in the risk of ischemic events with the use of ticagrelor compared with clopidogrel (hazard ratio [HR] 1.62; 95% confidence interval [CI], 0.99–2.64) but a reduction in ischemic events if a maintenance dose of aspirin was 100 mg daily or less (HR 0.73; 95% CI, 0.40–1.33). The finding that the aspirin dose affected ischemic outcomes in patients receiving ticagrelor was not just a U.S. phenomenon. In patients in the rest of the world, it was also shown that aspirin dose influenced ischemic outcomes, with patients receiving a lower maintenance dose of aspirin having benefit with ticagrelor compared with clopidogrel (HR 0.78; 95% CI, 0.69–0.87) that seemed to be lost with a higher maintenance dose of aspirin (HR 1.23; 95% CI, 0.71–2.14). Consequently, a maintenance dose of aspirin 75–100 mg daily is recommended in order for ticagrelor to show the benefits of ticagrelor over clopidogrel.[88]

Cangrelor is currently the only available intravenously administered $P2Y_{12}$ inhibitor. As with ticagrelor, cangrelor is structurally derived from ATP and provides reversible inhibition of the $P2Y_{12}$ receptor by binding in a different location for ADP. Even with loading doses, oral $P2Y_{12}$ inhibitors take a minimum of 1–2 hours to obtain maximum platelet inhibition and 4–7 days for platelet recovery after discontinuation. Cangrelor achieves maximum platelet inhibition within about 2 minutes of an intravenous bolus dose, with restoration of normal platelet reactivity within 1–2 hours of cessation of the infusion.[89,90] Cangrelor has an elimination half-life of less than 9 minutes and is eliminated by ATPases in the blood. Therefore, hepatic or renal dysfunction is unlikely to affect the pharmacokinetics of cangrelor. The fast return to normal platelet function may provide safety advantages for cangrelor over other $P2Y_{12}$ inhibitors in the context of bleeding or transition to CABG surgery.[91]

The CHAMPION PHOENIX trial evaluated a strategy of pre-PCI cangrelor (30-mcg/kg bolus dose, followed by a 4-mcg/kg per minute continuous infusion) and post-PCI clopidogrel compared with only post-PCI clopidogrel (300- or 600-mg loading dose, followed by 75 mg daily).[92] Patients with ACS constituted 44% of the total patients undergoing PCI in the trial (26% NSTE ACS and 18% STEMI). At 48 hours, cangrelor provided a significant reduction in death, MI, ischemia-driven revascularization, and stent thrombosis compared with clopidogrel (4.7% vs. 5.9%; p=0.005), without an increase in major bleeding (minor bleeding was higher with cangrelor). Because the chemical structure of cangrelor is similar to that of ticagrelor, dyspnea was reported more with the use of cangrelor, but the shorter drug exposure time likely contributed to a lower incidence (1.2%) and discontinuation rate (0.1%) with cangrelor than with ticagrelor in the PLATO trial (13.8% and 0.9%, respectively). The utility of cangrelor in patients preloaded with clopidogrel is unknown, as is how it might compare with faster-acting prasugrel and ticagrelor.

Cangrelor may interfere with the binding of the active metabolites of clopidogrel and prasugrel. Studies have shown that when clopidogrel is given with cangrelor, the ability of the thienopyridines to irreversibly inhibit platelet function is reduced.[93] It is thought that the reversible inhibitor cangrelor directly prevents the binding of the short-lived, but irreversible active metabolites.[94] Once the infusion is discontinued, no impact on the pharmacodynamic effect of clopidogrel was seen. This same interaction would be expected with prasugrel. Therefore, it is important that if cangrelor is used, the loading dose of the thienopyridine not be given until the cangrelor infusion has been discontinued.

Glycoprotein IIb/IIIa Inhibitors

Because binding of fibrinogen to the platelet glycoprotein (GP) IIb/IIIa receptor represents the final common step in platelet aggregation, inhibition of this interaction represents an ideal target for pharmacotherapy. Three GP IIb/IIIa inhibitors are currently available for use, with all agents available intravenously only. Abciximab is a chimeric human-murine monoclonal antibody Fab fragment that blocks GP IIb/IIIa receptor-fibrinogen binding. Abciximab has irreversible binding to the GP IIb/IIIa receptor, with platelet function recovery occurring over about 48 hours after discontinuation of the infusion.[95] Unbound abciximab is eliminated rapidly, with less than 5% being detectable in plasma 2 hours after a bolus. Because of the strong binding of abciximab to the GP IIb/IIIa receptor, the drug/receptor ratio is about 2:1. Therefore, platelet transfusions can absorb the excess abciximab and would be effective in the management of a major bleeding episode.[2,95]

Eptifibatide and tirofiban are commonly called "small-molecule" GP IIb/IIIa inhibitors because they are peptide and nonpeptide inhibitors of the GP IIb/IIIa receptor, respectively, and have a much small molecular weight than abciximab. These agents have reversible binding of the GP IIb/IIIa receptor. Therefore, platelet function recovery occurs in 2–4 hours after discontinuation of the infusion.[95] The reversible binding of the small-molecule agents requires that they overwhelm the ability of fibrinogen to bind to the GP IIb/IIIa receptor with high concentrations and a drug/receptor ratio that is around 500–1,000:1. Consequently, platelet transfusion would be unable to absorb excess drug and would not be helpful in the management of bleeding with eptifibatide or tirofiban.[2,95]

In addition to bleeding, GP IIb/IIIa inhibitors can cause thrombocytopenia in about 1% of patients receiving abciximab and 0.5% of patients receiving eptifibatide and tirofiban. Because GP IIb/IIIa inhibitors should be administered with a heparin, it is important to differentiate GP IIb/IIIa inhibitor–induced thrombocytopenia from heparin-induced thrombocytopenia (HIT). Thrombocytopenia from a GP IIb/IIIa inhibitor occurs more rapidly (within hours), and the platelet count nadir is typically lower (about 20,000) than in HIT. Unlike patients with HIT, if thrombocytopenia occurs with abciximab, platelet transfusion can be administered. Although the efficacy of platelet transfusion for thrombocytopenia from eptifibatide or tirofiban may be limited, it would unlikely be harmful in HIT.

Glycoprotein IIb/IIIa inhibitors have been extensively studied in patients with ACS.[96-101] Many of the initial studies were conducted before the standard use of DAPT. In the Intracoronary Stenting and Antithrombotic Regimen: Rapid Early Action for Coronary Treatment (ISAR-REACT 2) trial, patients receiving a 600-mg loading dose of clopidogrel and undergoing PCI for NSTE ACS had a significant reduction in CV events with a GP IIb/IIIa inhibitor (abciximab) compared with placebo.[102] Of interest, the benefit was only shown in patients who had a positive troponin (13.1% vs. 18.3%; p=0.02), with no difference in patients without elevated troponins (4.6% in both groups). Therefore, GP IIb/IIIa inhibitors provide added benefit in the setting of early DAPT, but they should be reserved for high-risk patients with a positive troponin.[2]

Only one clinical outcome trial has compared the GP IIb/IIIa inhibitors. In the TARGET (Treatment Approaches in Renal Cancer Global Evaluation Trial) study, patients undergoing PCI had significantly more CV events at 30 days with tirofiban than with abciximab (7.6% vs. 6.0%; p=0.38).[101] All the benefits of abciximab over tirofiban were realized in the 63% of patients with NSTE ACS in the trial (9.3% vs. 6.3%; p<0.05). These results led to the investigation and use of a higher-dose tirofiban regimen. Although subsequent trials have shown no differences between high-dose tirofiban and abciximab, all trials to date have evaluated surrogate end points (ST-segment resolution, myocardial perfusion), and no comparative clinical outcome trials have been conducted.[103-105]

Anticoagulant Therapy

Although many antiplatelet agents are given to patients with ACS, a single anticoagulant agent is usually selected. To date, anticoagulant therapy has been targeted either against factor IIa (thrombin) directly or its production by inhibiting factor Xa. Unfractionated heparin (UFH) has been used in the treatment of patients with ACS for several decades. Unfractionated heparin provides its anticoagulant effect by first binding to antithrombin (AT) and increasing its potency by 1,000-fold.[106] The UFH-AT complex inhibits several clotting factors, with most of the impact coming from inhibition of factor Xa and thrombin. Because of the size of the UFH molecule, it inhibits these two factors in an equal ratio.

According to experience, UFH can be used across the spectrum of ACS and regardless of the management strategy.[1,2] The recommended dosing of UFH has changed several times during its history in an attempt to maximize efficacy and minimize bleeding. Currently, the recommended dose of UFH is a bolus of 60 units/kg (maximum total dose of 4,000 units) and an initial infusion rate of 12 units/kg/hour (maximum 4,000 units/hour). Because of the unpredictable interpatient variability of the anticoagulant response of UFH, therapy needs to be monitored with an activated partial thromboplastin time (aPTT). The aPTT should be measured every 6 hours until two consecutive readings are within the therapeutic range, as determined by the individual institution's protocol, and then every 24 hours for the duration of UFH therapy. If a dose adjustment is made, the same monitoring schedule should be reinitiated. Platelet counts should also be monitored daily or every other day for HIT. Although HIT typically presents 5 days or more after UFH exposure, it can occur within hours if the patient has been exposed to heparin in the past 3 months.[107] If HIT is suspected, UFH should be discontinued, and anticoagulation with an intravenous direct thrombin inhibitor should be provided.

Compared with UFH, low-molecular-weight heparins (LMWHs) provide a predictable anticoagulant dose response, no need for routine therapeutic monitoring, and a lower incidence of HIT.[106] As with UFH, LMWH must also bind to AT to provide its anticoagulant activity, with more impact against factor Xa than thrombin (3–4:1 ratio). Even though the risk of HIT is lower with LMWH than with UFH, the monitoring of platelet counts is still warranted. Because of the 90% cross-reactivity between HIT antibodies from LMWH and UFH, LMWH is not considered a safe alternative in patients who develop HIT from UFH.[107] Although other LMWHs are available, enoxaparin is the most widely studied agent and is the only LMWH discussed in the ACC/AHA guidelines.[1,2] The dosing of enoxaparin varies depending on the diagnosis and management strategy selected. Therefore, careful attention needs to be maintained to prevent inappropriate dosing and to maximize efficacy and safety. Although most patients receiving an LMWH do not require therapeutic monitoring, an anti-factor Xa (anti-Xa) level may be desired in certain patient populations. Groups in which anti-Xa monitoring may be helpful are pediatric patients, pregnant patients, patients with obesity (greater than 190 kg), and patients with severe renal insufficiency.[106] The target peak anti-Xa level would be 0.3–0.7 IU/mL, obtained 4 hours after the third dose. Although pediatric and pregnant patients rarely have ACS, it is more common in patients with obesity and severe renal insufficiency. Because patients with ACS typically receive anticoagulant therapy for a few days, the utility of anti-Xa monitoring in these patients may be limited.

Fondaparinux is currently the only pentasaccharide available for use. Fondaparinux must also bind to AT, with its anticoagulant activity specifically targeted against factor Xa, with no activity against thrombin.[106] Fondaparinux also provides a predictable anticoagulant dose response and no need for therapeutic monitoring. Although there are case reports of thrombocytopenia with fondaparinux, the incidence is thought to be extremely rare. Given the lack of antibody cross-reactivity, it is reasonable to consider fondaparinux in patients with a history of HIT.[107] Given the long half-life of fondaparinux, the dose in patients with ACS is 2.5 mg subcutaneously once daily. Fondaparinux is contraindicated in patients with a creatinine clearance of less than 30 mL/minute/1.73 m^2 because of the significant degree of renal elimination. There can also be accumulation in patients with a creatinine clearance of 30–60 mL/minute/1.73 m^2, but this is typically not a factor with the short duration of therapy in patients with ACS.[108]

As with LMWH, most patients do not require therapeutic monitoring, although it may be desired in certain special populations. A chromogenic assay of anti-Xa calibrated with fondaparinux produces reliable and reproducible results.[109-111] Fondaparinux needs to be used to form the standard curves to measure fondaparinux concentrations.[106] Results obtained using an LMWH standard curve are less accurate, and standard curves using UFH are completely inaccurate and should not be used.[109,112] Peak plasma concentrations are typically achieved within 3 hours after dosing.[113]

Bivalirudin is an intravenously administered direct thrombin inhibitor. Therefore, bivalirudin does not have to first bind to AT to provide its anticoagulant effect. By not having to bind to AT, bivalirudin can inhibit not only free or soluble thrombin, similar to UFH and LMWH, but also fibrin-bound thrombin.[106] Fibrin-bound thrombin is still enzymatically active, but the bulky AT-anticoagulant complexes are unable to gain access. The clinical benefit of bivalirudin's inhibition of this larger pool of thrombin is difficult to quantify. Bivalirudin is only used in patients with ACS who receive PCI and can be monitored with an activated clotting time (ACT) in the catheterization laboratory. Bivalirudin initiated before the patient arrives in the cardiac catheterization laboratory is sometimes monitored with an aPTT, but appropriate goals and subsequent dose adjustments based on aPTT results are not well established.

ANTITHROMBOTIC THERAPY IN NSTE ACS

Treatment of patients with NSTE ACS consists of two initial strategies (Figure 33.1). One approach is the early invasive strategy, where the intent is to take the patient to the cardiac catheterization laboratory for angiography and perform PCI (usually with stenting), if necessary. The other approach is termed an *ischemia-driven strategy*, which has also been called the non-invasive strategy, medical management, or a conservative approach. In this strategy, the intent is to treat the patient medically without PCI. If the patient has no relief or has a recurrence of ischemia, the patient is evaluated with angiography, and PCI is performed if the patient is a candidate.

Regardless of the management strategy selected, all patients should receive an initial dose of chewable aspirin 162–325 mg as soon as possible, followed by 81 mg daily.[1,2] A clopidogrel loading dose, followed by maintenance doses, could be substituted in patients with a hypersensitivity or GI intolerance to aspirin. Aspirin desensitization may be considered in cases of hypersensitivity after the patient has stabilized. Dual antiplatelet therapy with a $P2Y_{12}$ inhibitor should be administered to all patients without a contraindication. If DAPT is administered before the management approach has been decided, a 300- or 600-mg loading dose of clopidogrel or a 180-mg loading dose of ticagrelor should be given.[1,2] These agents are preferred because they have shown efficacy in both an ischemia-driven and an early invasive management strategy.[39,77,114]

Early Invasive Strategy

Compared with primary PCI in the setting of STEMI, the need for immediate reperfusion in the setting of NSTE ACS has not been proved to improve clinical outcomes. The optimal timing of coronary angiography has not been determined. Although some institutions may prefer an early (within 24 hours) or a delayed (25–72 hours) approach, most studies evaluating an early invasive strategy for NSTE ACS have deferred angiography and potential revascularization for 12–72 hours.[2] This provides time to optimize and maximize pharmacotherapy.

An initial chewable aspirin dose should have been given even before the management strategy has been determined. If the patient for some reason has not received aspirin, the patients not on chronic aspirin should receive a dose of 325 mg as soon as possible before PCI, and those on chronic aspirin should receive a dose of 81–325 mg (class I, LOE B).[2] Doses of aspirin after PCI should be 81 mg daily (class IIa, LOE B).[2]

Patients undergoing PCI should be given a loading dose of a $P2Y_{12}$ inhibitor before the procedure (class 1, LOE A recommendation).[2] If clopidogrel is selected, the loading dose should be 600 mg instead of 300 mg. This is based on data analyses showing that a 600-mg loading dose provides more potent platelet inhibition as well as faster platelet inhibition. Pharmacodynamic studies have shown that the 300-mg loading dose provides maximal platelet inhibition in 6–8 hours.[115] Despite these pharmacodynamic data with a 300-mg loading dose, data evaluations

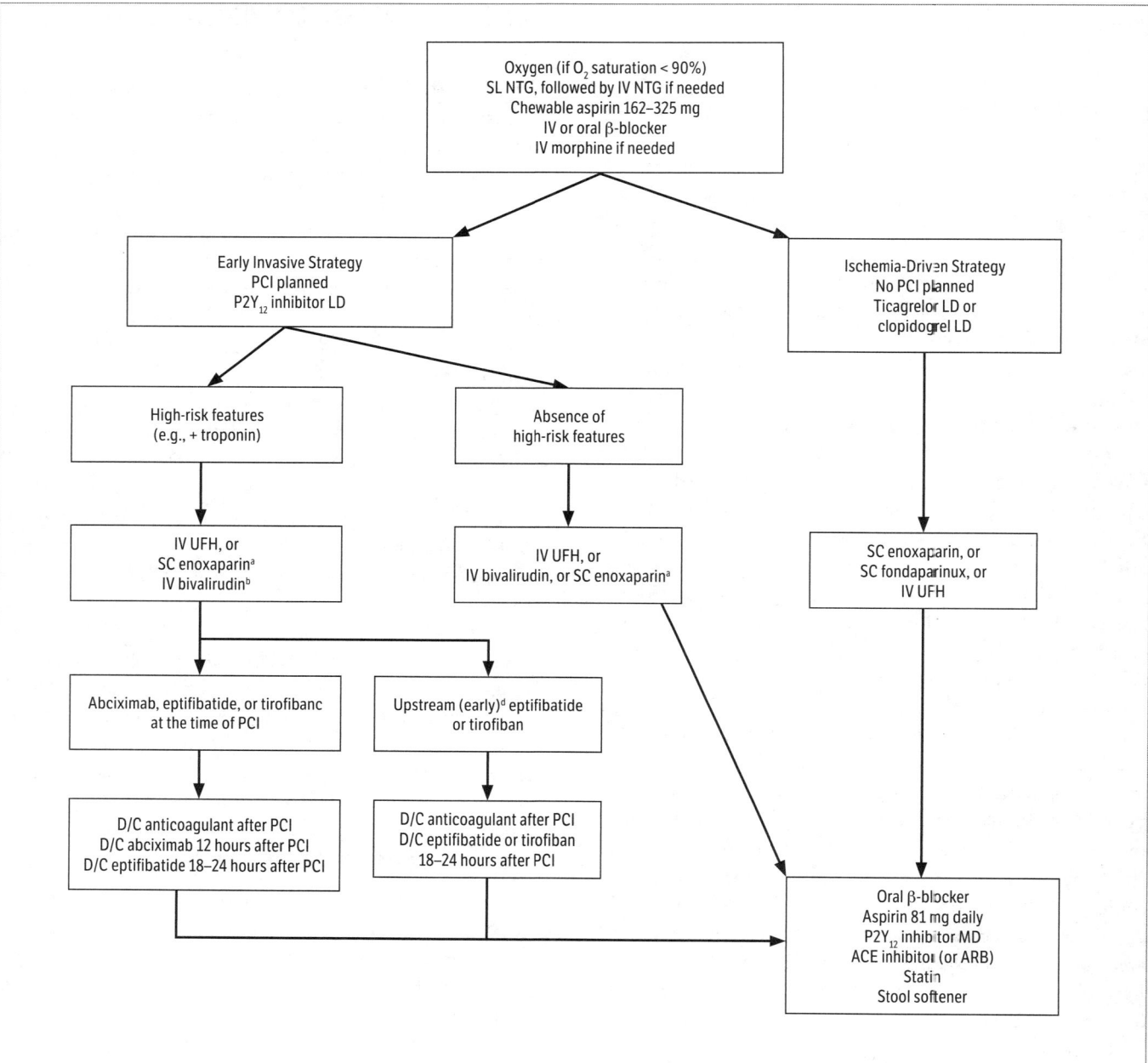

Figure 33.1 Treatment algorithm for management of non–ST-segment elevation acute coronary syndrome.

aIf the last dose of enoxaparin is given within 8 hours of PCI, no additional anticoagulant is needed. If the last dose of enoxaparin is given 8–12 hours before PCI, an additional IV bolus dose of 0.3 mg/kg of enoxaparin should be given at the time of PCI.
bBivalirudin should not be used in this setting if a glycoprotein IIb/IIIa inhibitor is being used because the patient has high-risk features (e.g., positive troponin).
cData for high-dose tirofiban in this setting are based on surrogate end point data.
dUse of upstream or early glycoprotein IIb/IIIa inhibitor therapy may be preferred only in patients who have not, or will not, receive a loading dose of an oral $P2Y_{12}$ inhibitor or cangrelor before PCI.

ACE = angiotensin-converting enzyme; ARB = angiotensin receptor blocker; D/C = discontinue; IV = intravenous; LD = loading dose; MD = maintenance dose; NTG = nitroglycerin; PCI = percutaneous coronary intervention; SC = subcutaneous; SL = sublingual; UFH = unfractionated heparin.

from the CREDO (Clopidogrel for the Reduction of Events During Observation) trial suggest that there is no benefit in clinical outcomes unless the 300-mg loading dose is given 15 hours before PCI.[116] A 600-mg loading dose can achieve maximum platelet inhibition within 2–4 hours.[117] Using a 600-mg loading dose has also shown a significant reduction in CV events compared with a 300-mg loading dose in patients with ACS undergoing PCI.[118] Although a 900-mg loading dose has also been evaluated, there was no increase in platelet inhibition compared with a 600-mg dose.[119] It appears that there is a saturation of conversion to active compound, and no improved efficacy would be expected. Given the superior efficacy shown in the TRITON-TIMI 38 and PLATO trials, prasugrel and ticagrelor, respectively, are recommended to be used over clopidogrel (class IIa, LOE B).[2,68,77]

The role of GP IIb/IIIa inhibitors has become more complex in the past decade. Currently, use of these agents should be reserved for patients with high-risk features such as an elevated troponin.[2,102] Once the decision to use a GP IIb/IIIa inhibitor is made, the timing of initiating the agent also needs to be considered. One approach is to provide an upstream GP IIb/IIIa inhibitor, which is initiating the agent early, several hours or even days before PCI. The other approach is waiting to administer the GP IIb/IIIa inhibitor at the time of PCI. These approaches have been compared in the EARLY-ACS (Early Glycoprotein IIb/IIIa Inhibition in Non-ST-segment Elevation Acute Coronary Syndrome) trial.[120] In this trial, upstream GP IIb/IIIa inhibitor use did not improve clinical outcomes but did produce more major bleeding. Therefore, there seems to be limited justification for this approach. One instance when the upstream approach may be rational is when patients with high-risk features are not planned to receive $P2Y_{12}$ therapy until the time of PCI. The delayed use of $P2Y_{12}$ inhibitors is occasionally employed by clinicians or institutions that prefer to know when the coronary anatomy is amendable to PCI and when CABG surgery has been ruled out. The justification follows that this avoids the need to wait 5–7 days for platelet recovery from $P2Y_{12}$ inhibitor therapy.

Anticoagulant therapy with UFH in patients with NSTE ACS using an invasive approach is a class I, LOE C recommendation.[2] Enoxaparin was compared with UFH in patients with NSTE ACS with an invasive approach in the SYNERGY (Superior Yield of the New Strategy of Enoxaparin, Revascularization and Glycoprotein IIb/IIIa Inhibitors) trial.[121] The overall results of the trial showed no difference between the agents in the incidence of death or MI and showed an increase in major bleeding in patients receiving enoxaparin. Of interest, 39% of patients in the trial received both agents sometime during the study. It obviously becomes difficult to determine how two agents are different if patients receive both agents. When patients who received only UFH or enoxaparin throughout the study are analyzed, there is a significant reduction in death and MI with the use of enoxaparin compared with UFH, without an increase in major bleeding. Patients who have received their last subcutaneous dose 8–12 hours before PCI, or have received less than two subcutaneous doses of enoxaparin, should receive an additional 0.3-mg/kg intravenous bolus dose at the time of PCI to ensure adequate anticoagulant effect (class I, LOE B).[2,121]

Although fondaparinux is discussed in the ACC/AHA NSTE ACS guidelines, use in the United States with PCI is limited. In the Organization to Assess Strategies in Acute Ischemic Syndromes (OASIS)-5 trial, patients undergoing PCI receiving fondaparinux have significantly higher rates of catheter thrombosis than do patients receiving enoxaparin.[122,123] Therefore, using fondaparinux alone in patients undergoing PCI is a class III, LOE B recommendation.[2] If patients are receiving fondaparinux and need to receive PCI, additional anticoagulant therapy with UFH is required. The dose of UFH at the time of PCI differs depending on whether the patient is taking a GP IIb/III inhibitor (85 units/kg) or not (60 units/kg). Additional doses of UFH may need to be given during the procedure passed on the ACT. Therefore, in patients for whom it is expected that PCI will be needed, fondaparinux is typically avoided.

Bivalirudin is also an alternative for anticoagulant therapy in patients with NSTE ACS with an early invasive approach (class I, LOE B).[2] Evidence for using bivalirudin in these patients comes from the Acute Catheterization and Urgent Intervention Triage Strategy (ACUITY) trial.[124] Compared with many other ACS trials of AT, the ACUITY trial used a quadruple composite end point (death, MI, unplanned revascularization for ischemia, and major bleeding) and a fairly liberal definition for major bleeding. Consequently, a 5-cm bruise was counted as equal to a death or MI as an end point event. Regardless, patients receiving a heparin (UFH or LMWH) and a GP IIb/IIIa inhibitor had efficacy and safety similar to patients receiving bivalirudin and a GP IIb/IIIa inhibitor. Therefore, the ACUITY trial showed that bivalirudin and a GP IIb/IIIa inhibitor therapy should not be used together because of a lack of any benefit, and this approach would significantly increase costs compared with a heparin and a GP IIb/IIIa inhibitor. The group receiving bivalirudin alone with only a "bailout" GP IIb/IIIa inhibitor had a reduction in the primary end point compared with a heparin and a GP IIb/IIIa inhibitor, which was driven by a reduction in major bleeding (3.0% vs. 5.7%; $p<0.001$). Although rescue or bailout GP IIb/IIIa is commonly used, this has never been prospectively evaluated.

The ability to use bivalirudin on its own without a GP IIb/IIIa inhibitor can significantly reduce the cost of antithrombotic therapy and has led to increased bivalirudin use in patients with NSTE ACS and an early invasive approach. However, using bivalirudin in this setting is not without controversy. The ischemic end points in the trial trended higher with bivalirudin alone than with a heparin and a GP IIb/IIIa inhibitor by 0.5%, which grew to 1% when higher-risk troponin-positive patients were evaluated.[124,125] Given the known benefit of GP IIb/IIIa inhibitor in patients who are troponin positive from the ISAR-REACT 2 trial, questions remain whether bivalirudin alone should be used in all patients. Although the ISAR-REACT 4 trial tried to compare bivalirudin alone with a heparin and a GP IIb/IIIa inhibitor in these higher-risk patients, the trial overestimated the suggested difference (4.6% vs. 1% seen in ACUITY) and was underpowered.[126] Even in the ISAR-REACT 4 trial, patients with higher troponin concentrations (greater than 0.12 mcg/L) show a 2.3% benefit in patients receiving the GP IIb/IIIa inhibitor. This was a subgroup analysis of the overall data and was not powered to show significance. More recent analyses have also suggested that bivalirudin alone does not provide significant benefit over UFH alone.[127-129] Despite these questions, the availability of generic bivalirudin makes the cost of bivalirudin alone even more attractive.

Ischemia-Driven Strategy

As previously mentioned, chewable aspirin should have been administered at a dose of 162–325 mg as soon as possible on presentation, followed by 81 mg daily. Although some clinicians may believe that DAPT is given only in patients receiving PCI and stents for prevention of stent thrombosis, DAPT is also indicated in patients who do not undergo PCI. The role of DAPT became evident after the results of the CURE trial.[39] The support for this regimen of clopidogrel with aspirin in patients not receiving PCI comes from the fact that about 80% of the patients in the CURE trial were treated with an ischemia-driven approach. The 300-mg loading dose of clopidogrel is supported by the results of the CURRENT–OASIS 7 trial.[118] In this trial, a higher loading dose of clopidogrel 600 mg provided no additional benefit over a 300-mg loading dose in the patients with NSTE ACS undergoing an ischemia-driven approach. In the PLATO trial, the benefit of ticagrelor over clopidogrel as part of DAPT was consistent regardless of whether the patient was treated with PCI (HR 0.84) or with an ischemia-driven approach (HR 0.85).[77] Prasugrel was compared with clopidogrel in patients with NSTE ACS using an ischemia-driven approach in the TRILOGY-ACS (Targeted Platelet Inhibition to Clarify the Optimal Strategy to Medically Manage Acute Coronary Syndromes) trial, with no difference in efficacy or safety between the agents.[130] The ACC/AHA guidelines provide a class I, LOE B recommendation for using clopidogrel (300-mg loading dose followed by 75 mg daily) or ticagrelor (180-mg loading dose followed by 90 mg twice daily) as part of DAPT with an ischemia-driven approach.[2] Up to 1 year of DAPT is recommended in patients with an ischemia-driven approach for NSTE ACS. A class IIa, LOE B recommendation is given for the use of ticagrelor over clopidogrel according to the results of the PLATO trial.[2,77] Although prasugrel provides no efficacy or safety differences compared with clopidogrel, the higher cost of prasugrel makes its selection unreasonable.

Triple antiplatelet therapy with a GP IIb/IIIa inhibitor has no role in patients with an ischemia-driven approach. Abciximab provided no benefit over placebo with an ischemia-driven approach in the Global Utilization of Streptokinase and Tissue Plasminogen Activator for Occluded Coronary Arteries (GUSTO) IV trial.[131] There was also no benefit of eptifibatide or tirofiban in the subgroup of patients with an ischemia-driven approach from the PURSUIT and PRISM-PLUS (Platelet Receptor Inhibition in Ischemic Syndrome Management in Patients Limited by Unstable Signs and Symptoms) trials, respectively.[97,98]

Anticoagulant therapy is also provided for the duration of hospitalization. Using UFH is reasonable and has a class 1, LOE B recommendation for use for 48 hours.[2] Enoxaparin has shown a significant reduction in CV events without an increase in major bleeding compared with UFH with an ischemia-driven approach in the ESSENCE (Efficacy and Safety of Subcutaneous Enoxaparin in Non–Q wave Coronary Events) and TIMI – 11b trials.[132,133] The use of enoxaparin is given a class 1, LOE A recommendation in the ACC/AHA guidelines because of these results.[2] In patients with an ischemia-driven approach, enoxaparin is dosed 1 mg/kg subcutaneously every 12 hours. Patients with severe renal insufficiency should receive the same dose given every 24 hours. Although an initial 30-mg intravenous loading dose can be given, it is uncertain whether this provides any clinical benefit.[2,133]

Fondaparinux had similar efficacy and less major bleeding than enoxaparin with an ischemia-driven approach in the OASIS-5 trial.[122] Although this mainly European-based trial had some external validity issues that may explain the difference in bleeding, it seems reasonable to prefer fondaparinux in patients considered to have a higher risk of bleeding (class 1, LOE B).[2] Bivalirudin has not been evaluated outside the setting of PCI and therefore would not be considered an option with an ischemia-driven approach.

ANTITHROMBOTIC THERAPY

Because of the extensive thrombus with almost 100% occlusion of the infarct-related coronary artery, patients with STEMI need immediate reperfusion therapy. Reperfusion should typically occur within 12 hours of symptom onset, but the sooner the better. Irreversible myocardial cell death occurs within 1–2 hours of symptom onset with completion of the area of infarct within 6–12 hours. Patients with ongoing ischemia and a large area of myocardium at risk or patients with hemodynamic instability may benefit from reperfusion therapy between 12 and 24 hours. Regardless of the reperfusion therapy selected,

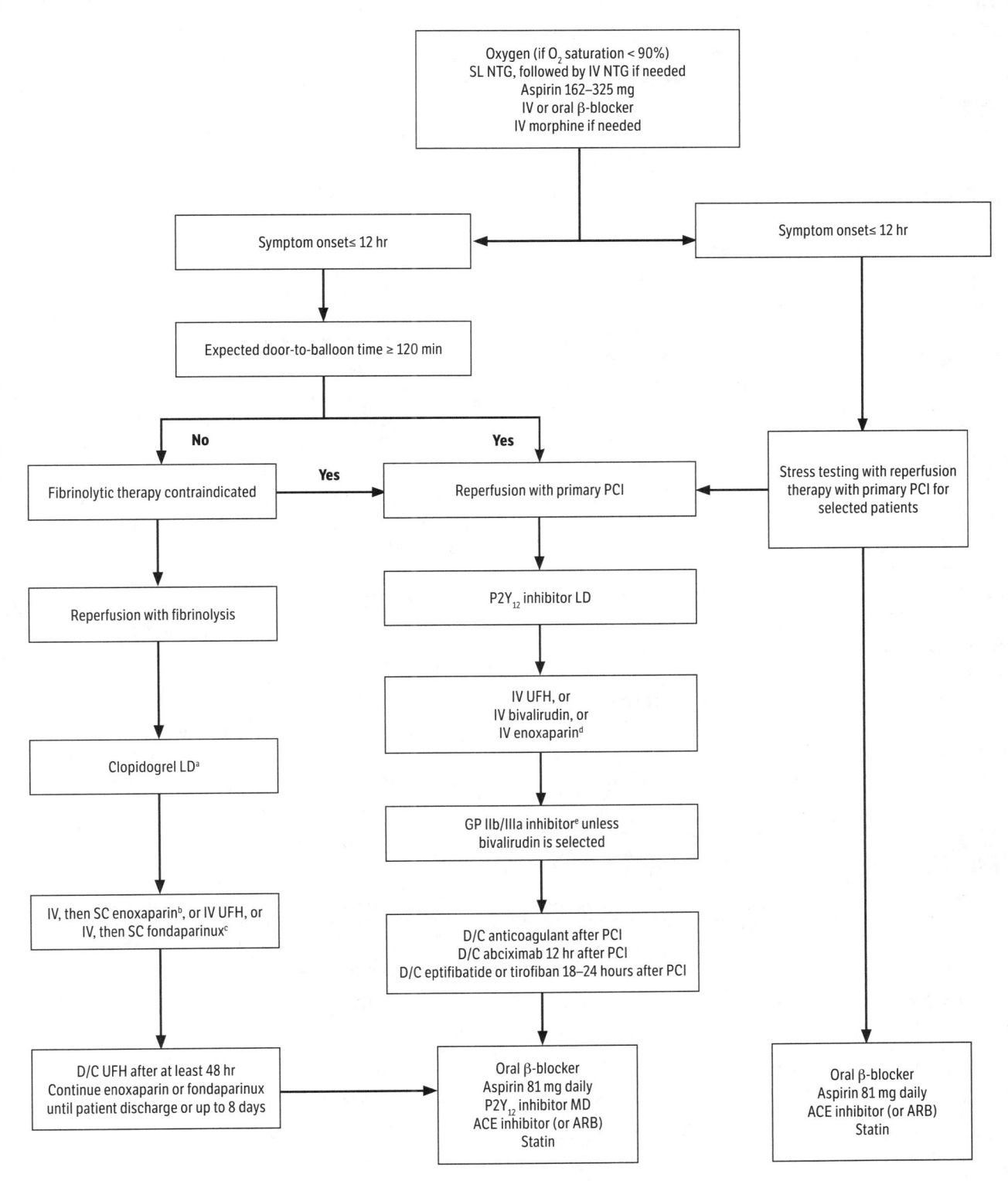

Figure 33.2 Treatment algorithm for management of ST-segment elevation myocardial infarction.

[a]A clopidogrel loading dose has not been evaluated in patients > 75 years receiving fibrinolysis; therefore, the risk of bleeding in these patients is unknown.
[b]The first subcutaneous dose of enoxaparin should follow within 15 min of the intravenous dose in this setting.
[c]The first subcutaneous dose of fondaparinux is given 24 hr after the intravenous dose in this setting.
[d]Enoxaparin is not mentioned in this setting in the current guidelines.
[e]Abciximab has the highest level of evidence for use in this setting.

antithrombotic therapy is critical to optimize outcomes (Figure 33.2). Although selection and dosing of appropriate antithrombotic agents may be similar to management of NSTE ACS, there are important differences to consider (Table 33.7).

Primary PCI

Patients who can receive timely reperfusion with a door-to-balloon time of 120 minutes or less should receive primary PCI.[1] In this setting, primary PCI has shown better vessel patency and has less risk of reocclusion and ICH that comes with the use of fibrinolytic therapy.

Management of oral antiplatelet therapy in patients with STEMI with primary PCI is the same as in those with NSTE ACS with an early invasive approach. An initial loading dose of chewable aspirin is indicated (class I, LOE B), with a maintained dose of 81 mg daily being preferred (class IIa, LOE B).[1] If clopidogrel is the $P2Y_{12}$ inhibitor being used, a 600-mg loading dose should be used to provide more rapid platelet inhibition. A 60-mg loading dose of prasugrel or a 180-mg loading dose of ticagrelor can also be used because these agents both showed significant benefit over clopidogrel in the patients with STEMI in the TRITION-TIMI 38 and PLATO trials, respectively.[70,77] All $P2Y_{12}$ inhibitors, even prasugrel, should be administered as soon as possible before the patient arrives in the cardiac catheterization laboratory. Because of the high-risk nature of patients with STEMI, GP IIb/IIIa inhibitors have shown a reduction in ischemic events in patients undergoing primary PCI. Although most of the clinical evidence exists with abciximab (class IIa, LOE A), eptifibatide and high-dose tirofiban are also listed as options because of surrogate end point data (class IIa, LOE B) and the fact that most of the abciximab data were generated before aggressive use of $P2Y_{12}$ inhibitor loading doses.[1] Intracoronary abciximab (0.25-mg/kg bolus only) has also shown benefit and may be considered (class IIb, LOE B).[1,134-136] Because about 90% of a total dose of abciximab is given in the bolus anyway, this approach may be all that is needed while $P2Y_{12}$ inhibitor therapy takes effect. This approach requires more study before it should completely replace standard dosing of abciximab. This should not be tried with boluses of small-molecule GP IIb/IIIa inhibitors because most of their total doses are provided during the infusions.

There are decades of experience with the use of UFH as anticoagulant therapy in patients undergoing primary PCI for STEMI (class I, LOE C).[1] Because of how rapid PCI needs to occur in the treatment of STEMI and because anticoagulant therapy is not typically needed postprocedure, bolus doses are all that may be required. If a GP IIb/IIIa inhibitor is also being given, a bolus dose of 50–70 units/kg intravenously is recommended to achieve a therapeutic ACT of 200–250 seconds. If a GP IIb/IIIa inhibitor is not being used, a higher dose of 70–100 units/kg intravenously is recommended to achieve a therapeutic ACT of 250–300 seconds with the HemoTec device or 300–350 seconds with the Hemochron device.

Bivalirudin use in primary PCI is supported by the HORIZONS (Harmonizing Outcomes with Revascularization and Stents) trial.[137] Using bivalirudin alone had similar

Table 33.7 $P2Y_{12}$ Inhibitor Comparisons[40-43]

Property	Clopidogrel	Prasugrel	Ticagrelor	Cangrelor
Brand name	Plavix	Effient	Brilinta	Kengreal
Drug class	Thienopyridine	Thienopyridine	Cyclopentyltriazolopyrimidine	ATP analog
Absorption	≥ 50%	80%	36%	100%
Tmax	2 hr	30 min	60 min	2 min
Onset of action	75 mg: 3–5 days 300 mg: 6–8 hr 600 mg: 2–4 hr	10 mg: 3 days 60 mg: 30–60 min	90 mg: 2–3 days 180 mg: 60 min	2 min
Metabolism	Hepatic (2C19, 3A4, 1A2, 2B6)	Hepatic (2B6, 3A4, 2C9, 2C19)	Hepatic (3A4, 2C9)	ATPases in vascular endothelium
Prodrug	Yes	Yes	No	No
Active metabolite	Oxo-clopidogrel	R-138727	AR-C12490XX	None
$P2Y_{12}$ binding	Irreversible	Irreversible	Reversible	Reversible
Half-life	6 hr	7 hr	12 hr	3–5 min
Platelet recovery	~5 days	~7 days	~3 days	1–2 hr

efficacy with significantly less major bleeding than did using a heparin and a GP IIb/IIIa inhibitor (4.9% vs. 8.3%; p<0.001). Patients receiving bivalirudin alone had a significant increase in the rate of acute stent thrombosis (1.3% vs. 0.3%). As with the ACUITY trial, this probably represents the lack of adequate antiplatelet therapy with the rapid use of PCI in STEMI and the inability of clopidogrel and bivalirudin to provide protection in this acute time interval.[124] As in the ACUITY trial, GP IIb/IIIa inhibitors were reserved for bailout therapy only. As previously discussed, the lack of benefit of bivalirudin alone compared with UFH alone has raised questions about the role of bivalirudin.[128,129] Of note, a definitive study has yet to be completed to answer this question. Using bivalirudin in primary PCI for STEMI is a class I, LOE B recommendation.[1]

Although a 2.5-mg intravenous dose followed by subcutaneous dosing of fondaparinux was evaluated in the OASIS-6 trial, fondaparinux is not commonly used in primary PCI.[138] There was no difference in the rates of death or MI with the use of fondaparinux compared with UFH in 31% of patients undergoing primary PCI in the OASIS-6 trial. As in the OASIS-5 trial, there was an increase in catheter thrombosis in patients receiving fondaparinux.[123,138] Therefore, if fondaparinux is used in primary PCI, UFH must be given at the time of PCI as with NSTE ACS and an early invasive management. Because of how rapidly PCI should occur in STEMI, there seems to be little utility to fondaparinux in this setting. Although enoxaparin is not given a recommendation for or against use in the ACC/AHA guidelines, the ATOLL (STEMI Treated with Primary Angioplasty and Intravenous Lovenox or Unfractionate Heparin) trial suggests outcomes similar to those with UFH, and a meta-analysis supports a reduction in mortality compared with UFH with a one-time intravenous dose of enoxaparin 0.5 mg at the time of PCI.[139,140]

Reperfusion with Fibrinolysis

Fibrinolytic Therapy

Fibrinolytic agents represent the only available pharmacotherapy able to break down a thrombus and open occluded vessels. This is achieved by the agents acting as a tissue plasminogen activator that increases the conversion of plasminogen to the proteolytic enzyme plasmin. Plasmin is then able to cleave fibrin and fibrinogen, hopefully opening the infarct-related artery. Fibrin specificity is a pharmacologic property that may provide benefits. Currently used agents rank in fibrin specificity as tenecteplase > alteplase > reteplase.[141] Agents that are more fibrin-specific may have an efficacy and safety advantage. A more fibrin-specific agent would be expected to have better efficacy because the occluding thrombus is mainly composed of fibrin, and activity on free fibrinogen would not provide benefit. This may be especially true in an "older" thrombus that is more than 2 hours old in which more fibrin would be incorporated in the thrombus. There may also be less bleeding with a fibrin-specific agent because fewer fibrin degradation products, which have antithrombotic activity, are formed by not breaking down both fibrin and fibrinogen. This may also allow more free fibrinogen available for use for potential bleeding episodes. It remains to be determined whether the fibrin specificity of a fibrinolytic agent affects clinical outcomes. The significantly less major bleeding (not ICH), need for transfusion, and reduced mortality in patients presenting within 4–6 hours after symptom onset with the use of tenecteplase compared with alteplase suggest the potential for fibrin specificity to affect outcomes, but this is not definitive.[142] Although alteplase had been the fibrinolytic of choice for more than a decade, the newer bolus-only agents provide easier use and less potential for dosing errors.

Despite the worldwide experience with fibrinolytic therapy, there are limitations that must be considered. Regardless of the fibrinolytic agent used, patency (TIMI grade 2 and 3 flow) is restored in 60%–85% of patients, but only 50%–60% of patients achieve full myocardial reperfusion (TIMI grade 3 flow).[143,144] Even if optimal myocardial blood flow is achieved, fibrinolytic therapy has a reocclusion rate of 10%–15%. Fibrinolytic therapy is associated with a higher rate of ICH than is antithrombotic therapy or primary PCI (see Box 33.1). The incidence of ICH has been estimated to occur in 1 in 150–200 treated patients; however, the incidence was slightly higher in the GUSTO-III trial, occurring in about 1 in 100 treated patients.[142,145,146] Patients with ICH on fibrinolytic therapy is typically a catastrophic event, resulting in death or disabling stroke.

Adjunctive Antithrombotic Therapy

As with all other management strategies for ACS, patients receiving fibrinolysis for STEMI should also receive a loading dose of chewable aspirin (class I, LOE A), followed by 81 mg daily (class IIa, LOE B).[1] Using DAPT with fibrinolysis is more limited than with other areas of ACS management. Clopidogrel is the only $P2Y_{12}$ inhibitor to be studied with the use of fibrinolytics; therefore, prasugrel and ticagrelor should not be used.[46,47] In the CLARITY-TIMI 28 trial, DAPT with clopidogrel and aspirin provided significant benefit over aspirin alone in patients with STEMI receiving fibrinolysis as primary reperfusion therapy (15% vs. 21.7%; p<0.001), without an increase in major bleeding or ICH.[47] Of note, a 300-mg loading dose of clopidogrel was used in this trial, and a 600-mg loading dose has not been investigated and should not be used. Because of concerns about ICH, patients older than 75 years were not evaluated in the CLARITY-TIMI 28 trial. Therefore, patients older than 75 should not receive a loading dose of clopidogrel and should be initiated on 75 mg daily.

> **Box 33.1 Absolute and Relative Contraindications for Fibrinolytic Therapy in STEMI**
>
> **Absolute contraindications**
> - Prior intracranial hemorrhage at any time
> - Prior ischemic stroke within 3 months
> - Known malignant intracranial neoplasm (primary or metastatic)
> - Known structural cerebral vascular lesion (arteriovenous malformation)
> - Suspected aortic dissection
> - Active bleeding (excluding menses) or bleeding diathesis
> - Significant closed-head or facial trauma within 3 months
> - Intracranial or intraspinal surgery within 2 months
> - Severe uncontrolled hypertension unresponsive to emergency therapy
>
> **Relative contraindications**
> - History of chronic, severe, poorly controlled hypertension
> - Significant hypertension on presentation (systolic blood pressure > 180 mm Hg or diastolic blood pressure > 110 mm Hg)
> - Prior ischemic stroke more than 3 months ago
> - Dementia
> - Traumatic or prolonged cardiopulmonary resuscitation (more than 10 minutes)
> - Major surgery within 3 weeks
> - Internal bleeding within 2–4 weeks
> - Noncompressible vascular punctures
> - Pregnancy
> - Active peptic ulcer disease
> - Oral anticoagulant therapy
> - Known intracranial pathology not mentioned in absolute contraindications

Using half-dose fibrinolytic therapy with a GP IIb/IIIa inhibitor has been studied extensively.[147] Although initial studies showed significant improvement in patency of the infarct-related artery and myocardial perfusion with this combination, no improvement in mortality was shown.[148] Although the combination did produce a reduction in MI, this did not lead to a reduction in mortality at 1 year and came at the cost of significantly higher major bleeding. Therefore, this combination is no longer recommended.

Many of the initial trials evaluating the efficacy and safety of fibrinolytic therapy used UFH as the anticoagulant. Because of this experience, UFH has a class I, LOE C recommendation from the ACC/AHA for use for 48 hours, or until revascularization, if needed.[1] Enoxaparin is also recommended for use in patients with STEMI receiving fibrinolysis (class I, LOE A).[1] In the ExTRACT-TIMI 25 (Enoxaparin and Thrombolysis Reperfusion for Acute Myocardial Infarction Treatment, Thrombolysis in Myocardial Infarction-Study 25) trial, enoxaparin provided a significant reduction in death and MI compared with UFH (9.9% vs. 12.0%; $p<0.001$).[149] Although there was an increase in major bleeding with the use of enoxaparin compared with UFH (2.1% vs. 1.4%; $p<0.001$), there was no difference in ICH. Dosing of enoxaparin in this setting typically requires a 30-mg intravenous loading dose, with subcutaneous dosing to begin within 15 minutes after the intravenous dose is given. Careful attention is needed when dosing enoxaparin in this setting because initial subcutaneous doses are capped, and dosing is different for patients 75 years or older and those with severe renal insufficiency. Enoxaparin therapy should be given for the duration of hospitalization, or up to 8 days or the need for revascularization.

According to the results of the OASIS-6 trial, fondaparinux is given initially as a 2.5-mg intravenous dose followed by 2.5 mg subcutaneously the following day (class I, LOE B).[1,138] In the OASIS-6 trial, fondaparinux had efficacy (HR 0.96) and safety (HR 0.95) similar to UFH in patients with STEMI receiving fibrinolytic therapy. Similar to enoxaparin, fondaparinux should be given for the duration of hospitalization, or up to 8 days or the need for revascularization. Anticoagulant therapy with bivalirudin has not been adequately investigated and is not recommended with the use of fibrinolytic therapy.

Follow-up angiography is recommended for patients receiving reperfusion therapy with fibrinolytic therapy. If the results of fibrinolytic therapy are found incomplete or unsuccessful, PCI is indicated. In patients receiving UFH, an additional bolus dose of UFH will likely be needed to achieve a therapeutic ACT as directed with primary PCI. If the patient is receiving enoxaparin, an additional 0.3-mg/kg intravenous bolus dose should be given if the last subcutaneous dose was more than 8–12 hours before PCI, similar to patients with NSTE ACS with an early invasive approach.[1] As with other areas of PCI in ACS management, patients receiving fondaparinux need to receive UFH, with the dose depending on the additional use of a GP IIb/IIIa inhibitor.

ROLE OF THE PHARMACIST

Acute coronary syndromes represent a significant health burden to patients with CV disease. Patients should be aggressively treated to reduce future ischemic events and improve survival. The role of the pharmacist is more valuable than ever in ACS as the number of medication options increases and drug regimens become more complex. The pharmacist must consider the clinical characteristics of the patient experiencing an ACS event when selecting an agent and regimen and should monitor the safety and efficacy of medications. New pharmacologic controversies involving clinical response to medications, intensity and duration of therapies, drug-drug interactions, and adverse effects provide an opportunity for pharmacists to educate health care clinicians and further enhance patient care.

REFERENCES

1. O'Gara PT, Kushner FG, Ascheim DD, et al. 2013 ACCF/AHA guideline for management of ST-elevation myocardial infarction. A report from the American College of Cardiology Foundation/American Heart Association task force on practice guidelines. Circulation 2013;127:e363-e425.
2. Amsterdam EA, Wenger NK, Brindis RG, et al. 2014 AHA/ACC guideline for the management of patients with non-ST-elevation acute coronary syndrome. A report of the American College of Cardiology/American Heart Association task force on practice guidelines. Circulation 2014;130:e344-e426.
3. Mozaffarian D, Benjamin EJ, Go AS, et al.; on behalf of the American Heart Association Statistics Committee and Stroke Statistics Subcommittee. Heart disease and stroke statistics—2015 update: a report from the American Heart Association. Circulation 2015;131:e29-e322.
4. Antman EM, Cohen M, Bernink PJ, et al. The TIMI risk score for unstable angina/non-ST elevation MI: a method for prognostication and therapeutic decision making. JAMA 2000;284:835-42.
5. Boersma E, Pieper KS, Steyerberg EW, et al. Predictors of outcome in patients with acute coronary syndromes without persistent ST-segment elevation. Results from an international trial of 9461 patients. The PURSUIT Investigators. Circulation 2000;101:2557-67.
6. Granger CB, Goldberg RJ, Dabbous O, et al. Predictors of hospital mortality in the Global Registry of Acute Coronary Events. Arch Intern Med 2003;163:2345-53.
7. Pieper KS, Gore JM, FitzGerald G, et al. Validity of a risk-prediction tool for hospital mortality: the Global Registry of Acute Coronary Events. Am Heart J 2009;157:1097-105.
8. Pierce GF, Jaffe AS. Increased creatinine kinase MB in the absence of acute myocardial infarction. Clin Chem 1986;32:2044-51.
9. Thygesen K, Alpert JS, White HD, et al. Joint ESC/ACCF/AHA/WHF Task Force for the redefinition of myocardial infarction. Eur Heart J 2007;28:2525-38.
10. Tanindi A, Cemri M. Troponin elevation in conditions other than acute coronary syndromes. Vasc Health Risk Manag 2011;7:597-603.
11. Birnbaum Y, Nikus K, Kligfield P, et al. The role of the EKG in diagnosis, risk estimation, and catheterization laboratory activation in patients with acute coronary syndromes: a consensus document. Ann Noninvasive Electrocardiol 2014;19:412-25.
12. Go AS, Barron HV, Rundle AC, et al. Bundle-branch block and in-hospital mortality in acute myocardial infarction. National Registry of Myocardial Infarction 2 Investigators. Ann Intern Med 1998;129:690-7.
13. Sgarbossa EB, Pinski SL, Barbagelata A, et al. Electrocardiographic diagnosis of evolving acute myocardial infarction in the presence of left bundle-branch block. GUSTO-1 (Global Utilization of Streptokinase and Tissue Plasminogen Activator for Occluded Coronary Arteries) Investigators. N Engl J Med 1996;334:481-7.
14. Libby P, Theroux P. Pathophysiology of coronary artery disease. Circulation 2005;111:3481-8.
15. Specifications Manual for the National Hospital Inpatient Quality Measures. Acute Coronary Syndromes. Discharges 1-1-2015 through 9-30-15. Version 4.4a. Available at https://osstatic.outcome.com/online_doc_qi/StrokePMT/measure/MeasureDesc_StrokeCM.pdf. Accessed October 19, 2015.
16. Finamore SR, Kennedy L. Understanding the role of oxygen in acute coronary syndromes. J Emerg Nurs 2013;39:e45-9.
17. ISIS-4 (Fourth International Study of Infarct Survival) Collaborative Group. ISIS-4: a randomised factorial trial assessing early oral captopril, oral mononitrate, and intravenous magnesium sulphate in 58,050 patients with suspected acute myocardial infarction. ISIS-4 (Fourth International Study of Infarct Survival) Collaborative Group. Lancet 1995;345:669-85.
18. Gruppo Italiano per lo Studio della Sopravvivenza nell'infarto Miocardico. GISSI-3: effects of lisinopril and transdermal glyceryl trinitrate singly and together on 6-week mortality and ventricular function after acute myocardial infarction. Lancet 1994;343:1115-22.
19. Chen ZM, Pan HC, Chen YP, et al. Early intravenous then oral metoprolol in 45 852 patients with acute myocardial infarction: randomised placebo-controlled trial COMMIT (ClOpidogrel and Metoprolol in Myocardial Infarction Trial) collaborative group. Lancet 2005;366:1622-32.
20. Beta-blocker Heart Attack Trial Research Group. A randomized trial of propranolol in patients with acute myocardial infarction, I: mortality results. JAMA 1982;247:1707-14.
21. Roberts R, Rogers WJ, Mueller HS, et al. Immediate versus deferred beta-blockade following thrombolytic therapy in patients with acute myocardial infarction: results of the Thrombolysis In Myocardial Infarction (TIMI) II-B Study. Circulation 1991;83:422-37.
22. First International Study of Infarct Survival Collaborative Group. Randomised trial of intravenous atenolol among 16 027 cases of suspected acute myocardial infarction: ISIS-1. Lancet 1986;2:57-66.
23. Ibanez B, Macaya C, Sanchez-Brunete V, et al. Effect on early metoprolol on infarct size in ST-segment elevation myocardial infarction patients undergoing primary percutaneous coronary intervention: the effect of metoprolol in cardioprotection during an acute myocardial infarction (METOCARD-CNIC) trial. Circulation 2013;128:1495-503.
24. Khoynezhad A, Dobesh PP, Stacy ZA, et al. The role of intravenous dihydropyridine calcium channel blockers in the perioperative management of patients undergoing coronary artery bypass surgery. Curr Vasc Pharmacol 2008;6:186-94.
25. Effect of verapamil on mortality and major events after acute myocardial infarction (the Danish Verapamil Infarction Trial II–DAVIT II). Am J Cardiol 1990;66:779-85.
26. Gibson RS, Boden WE, Theroux P, et al. Diltiazem and reinfarction in patients with non-Q-wave myocardial infarction. Results of a double-blind, randomized, multicenter trial. N Engl J Med 1986;315:423-9.
27. Conti R. Intravenous morphine and chest pain. Clin Cardiol 2011;34:464-5.
28. Meine TJ, Roe MT, Chen AY, et al. Association of intravenous morphine use and outcomes in acute coronary syndromes: results from the CRUSADE Quality Improvement Initiative. Am Heart J 2005;149:1043-9.
29. Iakobishvili Z, Cohen E, Garty M, et al. Use of intravenous morphine for acute decompensated heart failure in patients with and without acute coronary syndromes. Acute Card Care 2011;13:76-80.

30. Fuster V, Badimon L, Badimon JJ, et al. The pathogenesis of coronary artery disease and the acute coronary syndromes (first of two parts). N Engl J Med 1992;326:242-50.

31. Fuster V, Badimon L, Badimon JJ, et al. The pathogenesis of coronary artery disease and the acute coronary syndromes (second of two parts). N Engl J Med 1992;326:310-8.

32. Baigent C, Blackwell L, Collins R, et al. Aspirin in the primary and secondary prevention of vascular disease: collaborative meta-analysis of individual data from randomised trials. Lancet 2009;373:1849-60.

33. Vane JR, Botting RM. The mechanism of action of aspirin. Thromb Res 2003;110:255-8.

34. Burch JW, Stanford N, Majerus PW. Inhibition of platelet prostaglandin synthetase by oral aspirin. J Clin Invest 1978;61:314-9.

35. Awtry EH, Loscalzo J. Aspirin. Circulation 2000;101:1206-18.

36. Patrignani P, Filabozzi P, Patrono C. Selective cumulative inhibition of platelet thromboxane production by low-dose aspirin in healthy subjects. J Clin Invest 1982;69:1366-72.

37. Antithrombotic Trialists' Collaboration. Collaborative meta-analysis of randomised trials of antiplatelet therapy for prevention of death, myocardial infarction, and stroke in high risk patients. BMJ 2002;324:71-86.

38. The CURRENT – OASIS 7 Investigators. Dose comparisons of clopidogrel and aspirin in acute coronary syndrome. N Engl J Med 2010;363:930-42.

39. Yusuf S, Zhao F, Mehta SR, et al. Effects of clopidogrel in addition to aspirin in patients with acute coronary syndromes without ST-segment elevation. N Engl J Med 2001;345:494-502.

40. Ferri N, Corsini A, Bellosta S. Pharmacology of the new $P2Y_{12}$ receptor inhibitors: insights on pharmacokinetic and pharmacodynamic properties. Drugs 2013;73:1681-709.

41. Dobesh PP. Pharmacokinetics and pharmacodynamics of prasugrel, a thienopyridine P2Y12 inhibitor. Pharmacotherapy 2009;29:1089-102.

42. Dobesh PP, Oestreich JH. Ticagrelor: pharmacokinetics, pharmacodynamics, clinical efficacy, and safety. Pharmacotherapy 2014;34:1077-90.

43. Oestreich JH, Dobesh PP. Cangrelor for treatment during percutaneous coronary intervention. Future Cardiol 2014;10:201-13.

44. Jiang X, Samant S, Lesko L. Clinical pharmacokinetics and pharmacodynamics of clopidogrel. Clin Pharmacokinet 2015;54:147-66.

45. Sangkuhl K, Klein T, Altman R. Clopidogrel pathway. Pharmacogenet Genomics 2010;20:463-5.

46. Chen ZM, Jiang LX, Chen YP, et al. Addition of clopidogrel to aspirin in 45,852 patients with acute myocardial infarction: randomised placebo-controlled trial. Lancet 2005;366:1607-21.

47. Sabatine MS, Cannon CP, Gibson CM, et al.; for the CLARITY – TIMI 28 Investigators. Addition of clopidogrel to aspirin and fibrinolytic therapy for myocardial infarction with ST-segment elevation. N Engl J Med 2005;352:1179-89.

48. Kazui M, Nishiya Y, Ishizuka T, et al. Identification of the human cytochrome P450 enzymes involved in the two oxidative steps in the bioactivation of clopidogrel to its pharmacologically active metabolite. Drug Metab Div 2010;38:92-9.

49. Sanofi Pharmaceuticals. Plavix_ US Prescribing Information [CLO-FPLR-SL-DEC13]. 2013. Available at http://products.sanofi.us/plavix/plavix.html. Accessed August 25, 2015.

50. Gilard M, Arnaud B, Cornily JC, et al. Influence of omeprazole on the antiplatelet action of clopidogrel associated with aspirin. The randomized, double-blind OCLA (Omeprazole CLopidogrel Aspirin) study. J Am Coll Cardiol 2008;51:256-60.

51. Juurlink DN, Gomes T, Ko DT, et al. A population-based study of the drug interaction between proton pump inhibitors and clopidogrel. CMAJ 2009;180:713-8.

52. Ho PM, Maddox TM, Wang L, et al. Risk of adverse outcomes associated with concomitant use of clopidogrel and proton pump inhibitors following acute coronary syndrome. JAMA 2009;301:937-44.

53. Charlot M, Ahlehoff O, Norgaard ML, et al. Proton-pump inhibitors are associated with increased cardiovascular risk independent of clopidogrel use. A nationwide cohort study. Ann Intern Med 2010;153:378-86.

54. O'Donoghue ML, Braunwald E, Antman EM, et al. Pharmacodynamic effect and clinical efficacy of clopidogrel and prasugrel with or without a proton-pump inhibitor: an analysis of two randomised trials. Lancet 2009;374:989-97.

55. Bhatt DL, Cryer BL, Contant CF, et al.; for the COGENT Investigators. Clopidogrel with or without omeprazole in coronary artery disease. N Engl J Med 2010;363:1909-17.

56. Bonello L, Tantry US, Marcucci R, et al. Consensus and future directions on the definition on high on-treatment platelet reactivity to adenosine diphosphate. J Am Coll Cardiol 2010;56:919-33.

57. Tantry US, Bonello L, Aradi D, et al. Consensus and update on the definition of on-treatment platelet reactivity to adenosine diphosphate associated with ischemia and bleeding. J Am Coll Cardiol 2013;62:2261-73.

58. Angiolillo DJ, Fernandez-Ortiz A, Bernardo E, et al. Variability in individual responsiveness to clopicogrel. Clinical implications, management, and future perspectives. J Am Coll Cardiol 2007;49:1505-16.

59. Price MJ, Berger PB, Teirstein PS, et al.; for the GRAVITAS Investigators. Standard- vs high-dose clopidogrel based on platelet function testing after percutaneous coronary intervention. The GRAVITAS randomized trial. JAMA 2011;305:1097-105.

60. Trenk D, Stone GW, Gawaz M, et al. A randomized trial of prasugrel versus clopidogrel in patients with high platelet reactivity on clopidogrel after elective percutaneous coronary intervention with implementation of drug-eluting stents: results of the TRIGGER-PCI (Testing platelet reactivity in patients undergoing elective stent placement on clopidogrel to guide alternative therapy with prasugrel) study. J Am Coll Cardiol 2012;59:2159-64.

61. Scott SA, Sangkuhl K, Gardner EE, et al. Clinical pharmacogenetics implementation consortium guidelines for cytochrome P450-2C19 (CYP2C19) genotype and clopidogrel therapy. Clin Pharmacol Ther 2011;90:328-32.

62. Shuldiner AR, O'Connell JR, Bliden KP, et al. Association of cytochrome P450 2C19 genotype with the antiplatelet effect and clinical efficacy of clopidogrel therapy. JAMA 2009;302:849-57.

63. Hochholzer W, Trenk D, Fromm MF, et al. Impact of cytochrome P450 2C19 loss-of-function polymorphism and of major demographic characteristics on residual platelet function after loading and maintenance treatment with clopidogrel in

64. Rehmel JL, Eckstein JA, Farid NA, et al. Interactions of two major metabolites of prasugrel, a thienopyridine antiplatelet agent, with the cytochromes P450. Drug Metab Dispos 2006;34:600-7.
65. Jernberg T, Payne CD, Winters KJ, et al. Prasugrel achieves greater inhibition of platelet aggregation and a lower rate of nonresponders compared with clopidogrel in aspirin-treated patients with stable coronary artery disease. Eur Heart J 2006;27:1166-73.
66. Brandt JT, Payne CD, Wiviott SD, et al. A comparison of prasugrel and clopidogrel loading doses on platelet function: magnitude of platelet inhibition is related to active metabolite formation. Am Heart J 2007;153:66 e9-16.
67. Weerakkody GJ, Jakubowski JA, Brandt JT, et al. Comparison of speed of onset of platelet inhibition after loading doses of clopidogrel versus prasugrel in healthy volunteers and correlation with responder status. Am J Cardiol 2007;100:331-6.
68. Wiviott SD, Braunwald E, McCabe CH, et al.; for the TRITON-TIMI 38 Investigators. Prasugrel versus clopidogrel in patients with acute coronary syndromes. N Engl J Med 2007;357:2001-15.
69. Wiviott SD, Braunwald E, Angiolillo DJ, et al.; for the TRITON-TIMI 38 Investigators. Greater clinical benefit of more intense oral antiplatelet therapy with prasugrel in patients with diabetes mellitus in the trial to assess improvement in therapeutic outcomes by optimizing platelet inhibition with prasugrel – Thrombolysis in Myocardial Infarction 38. Circulation 2008;118:1626-36.
70. Wiviott SD, Trenk K, Frelinger AL, et al.; for the PRINCIPLE-TIMI 44 Investigators. Prasugrel compared with high-loading- and maintenance-dose clopidogrel in patients with planned percutaneous coronary intervention. The Prasugrel in Comparison to Clopidogrel for Inhibition of Platelet Activation and Aggregation-Thrombolysis in Myocardial Infarction 44 Trial. Circulation 2007;116:2923-32.
71. Wiviott SD, Desai N, Murphy SA, et al. Efficacy and safety of intensive antiplatelet therapy with prasugrel from TRITON – TIMI 38 in a core clinical cohort defined by worldwide regulatory agencies. Am J Cardiol 2011;108:905-11.
72. van Giezen JJ, Berntsson P, Zachrisson H, et al. Comparison of ticagrelor and thienopyridine P2Y(12) binding characteristics and antithrombotic and bleeding effects in rat and dog models of thrombosis/hemostasis. Thromb Res 2009;124:565-71.
73. Husted S, Emanuelsson H, Heptinstall S, et al. Pharmacodynamics, pharmacokinetics, and safety of the oral reversible P2Y12 antagonist AZD6140 with aspirin in patients with atherosclerosis: a double-blind comparison to clopidogrel with aspirin. Eur Heart J 2006;27:1038-47.
74. Gurbel PA, Bliden KP, Butler K, et al. Randomized double-blind assessment of the ONSET and OFFSET of the antiplatelet effects of ticagrelor versus clopidogrel in patients with stable coronary artery disease: the ONSET/OFFSET study. Circulation 2009;120:2577-85.
75. Gurbel PA, Bliden KP, Butler K, et al. Response to ticagrelor in clopidogrel nonresponders and responders and effect of switching therapies: the RESPOND study. Circulation 2010;121:1188-99.
76. Parodi G, Xanthopoulou I, Bellandi B, et al. Ticagrelor crushed tablets administered in STEMI patients. The MOJITO study. J Am Coll Cardiol 2015;65:511-2.
77. Wallentin L, Becker RC, Budaj A, et al.; for the PLATO Investigators. Ticagrelor versus clopidogrel in patients with acute coronary syndromes. N Engl J Med 2009;361:1045-57.
78. Teng R, Oliver S, Hayes MA, et al. Absorption, distribution, metabolism, and excretion of ticagrelor in healthy subjects. Drug Metab Dispos 2010;38:1514-21.
79. Teng R, Butler K. Effect of the CYP3A inhibitors, diltiazem and ketoconazole, on ticagrelor pharmacokinetics in healthy volunteers. J Drug Asses. 2013;2:30-9.
80. Teng R, Butler K. A pharmacokinetic interaction study of ticagrelor and digoxin in healthy volunteers. Eur J Clin Pharmacol 2013;69:1801-8.
81. van Giezen JJ, Sidaway J, Glaves P, et al. Ticagrelor inhibits adenosine uptake in vitro and enhances adenosine-mediated hyperemia responses in a canine model. J Cardiovasc Pharmacol Ther 2012;17:164-72.
82. Wittfeldt A, Emanuelsson H, Brandrup-Wognsen G, et al. Ticagrelor enhances adenosine-induced coronary vasodilatory responses in humans. J Am Coll Cardiol 2013;61:723-7.
83. Armstrong D, Summers C, Ewart L, et al. Characterization of the adenosine pharmacology of ticagrelor reveals therapeutically relevant inhibition of equilibrative nucleoside transporter 1. J Cardiovasc Pharmacol Ther 2014;19:209-19.
84. Scirica BM, Cannon CP, Emanuelsson H, et al. The incidence of bradyarrhythmias and clinical bradyarrhythmic events in patients with acute coronary syndromes treated with ticagrelor or clopidogrel in the PLATO (Platelet Inhibition and Patient Outcomes) trial: results of the continuous electrocardiographic assessment substudy. J Am Coll Cardiol 2011;57:1908-16.
85. Camm AJ, Garratt CJ. Adenosine and supraventricular tachycardia. N Engl J Med 1991;325:1621-9.
86. Storey RF, Becker RC, Harrington RA, et al. Characterization of dyspnoea in PLATO study patients treated with ticagrelor or clopidogrel and its association with clinical outcomes. Eur Heart J 2011;32:2945-53.
87. Mahaffey KW, Wojdyla DM, Carroll K, et al.; for the PLATO Investigators. Ticagrelor compared with clopidogrel by geographic region in the Platelet Inhibition and Patient Outcomes (PLATO) trial. Circulation 2011;124:544-54.
88. Gaglia MA, Waksman R. Overview of the 2010 Food and Drug Administration cardiovascular and renal drugs advisory committee meeting regarding ticagrelor. Circulation 2011;123:451-6.
89. Akers WS, Oh JJ, Oestreich JH, et al. Pharmacokinetics and pharmacodynamics of a bolus and infusion of cangrelor: a direct, parenteral P2Y12 receptor antagonist. J Clin Pharmacol 2010;50:27-35.
90. Storey RF, Oldroyd KG, Wilcox RG. Open multicentre study of the P2T receptor antagonist AR-C69931MX assessing safety, tolerability and activity in patients with acute coronary syndromes. Thromb Haemost 2001;85:401-7.
91. Carney EF. Antiplatelet therapy: can cangrelor bridge the gap to cardiac surgery? Nat Rev Cardiol 2012;9:128.
92. Bhatt DL, Stone GW, Mahaffey KW, et al.; for the CHAMPION PHOENIX Investigators. Effect of platelet inhibition with cangrelor during PCI on ischemic events. N Engl J Med 2013;368:1303-13.
93. Dovlatova NL, Jakubowski JA, Sugidachi A, et al. The reversible P2Y antagonist cangrelor influences the ability of the active

94. Steinhubl SR, Oh JJ, Oestreich JH, et al. Transitioning patients from cangrelor to clopidogrel: pharmacodynamic evidence of a competitive effect. Thromb Res 2008;121:527-34.

95. Dobesh PP, Latham KA. Advancing the battle against acute ischemic syndromes: a focus on the GP IIb-IIIa inhibitors. Pharmacotherapy 1998;18:663-85.

96. EPILOG Investigators. Platelet glycoprotein IIb/IIIa receptor blockade and low-dose heparin during percutaneous coronary revascularization. N Engl J Med 1997;336:1689-96.

97. The PRISM-PLUS Study Investigators. Inhibition of the platelet glycoprotein IIb/IIIa receptor with tirofiban in unstable angina and non-Q-wave myocardial infarction. N Engl J Med 1998;338:1488-97.

98. The PURSUIT Trial Investigators. Inhibition of platelet glycoprotein IIb/IIIa with eptifibatide in patients with acute coronary syndromes. N Engl J Med 1998;339:436-43.

99. EPISTENT Investigators. Randomized placebo-controlled and balloon-angioplasty-controlled trial to assess safety of coronary stenting with use of platelet glycoprotein IIb/IIIa receptor blockade. Lancet 1998;352:87-92.

100. ESPRIT Investigators. Novel dosing regimen of eptifibatide in planned coronary stent implantation (ESPRIT): a randomized, placebo-controlled trial. Lancet 2000;356:2037-44.

101. The TARGET Investigators. Comparison of two platelet glycoprotein IIb/IIIa inhibitors, tirofiban and abciximab, for the prevention of ischemic events with percutaneous coronary revascularization. N Engl J Med 2001;344:1888-94.

102. Kastrati A, Mehilli J, Neumann FJ, et al.; for the ISAR-REACT 2 Trial Investigators. Abciximab in patients with acute coronary syndromes undergoing percutaneous coronary intervention. JAMA 2006;295:1531-8.

103. Valgimigli M, Percoco G, Barbieri D, et al. The additive value of tirofiban administered with high-dos bolus in the prevention of ischemic complications during high-risk coronary angioplasty: the ADVANCE trial. J Am Coll Cardiol 2004;44:14-9.

104. Bolognese L, Falsini G, Liistro F, et al. Randomized comparison of upstream tirofiban versus downstream high bolus dose tirofiban or abciximab on tissue-level perfusion and troponin release in high-risk acute coronary syndromes treated with percutaneous coronary interventions: the EVEREST trial. J Am Coll Cardiol 2006;47:522-8.

105. Valgimigli M, Campo G, Percoco G, et al.; for the MULTISTRATEGY Investigators. Comparison of angioplasty with infusion of tirofiban or abciximab with implantation of sirolimus-eluting or uncoated stents for acute myocardial infarction: the MULTISTRATEGY randomized trial. JAMA 2008;299:1788-99.

106. Garcia DA, Baglin TP, Weitz JI, et al. Parenteral anticoagulants. Chest 2012;141(suppl 2):e24S-e43S.

107. Linkins LA, Dans AL, Moores LK, et al. Treatment and prevention of heparin-induced thrombocytopenia Chest 2012;141(suppl 2):e495S-e530S.

108. Turpie AGG, Lensing WA, Fuji T, et al. Pharmacokinetic and clinical data supporting the use of fondaparinux 1.5 mg once daily in the prevention of venous thromboembolism in renally impaired patients. Blood Coagul Fibrinolysis 2009;20:114-21.

109. Smogorzewska A, Brandt JT, Chandler WL, et al. Effect of fondaparinux on coagulation assays. Results of the College of American Pathologists proficiency testing. Arch Pathol Lab Med 2006;130:1605-11.

110. Depasse F, Gerotziafas GT, Busson J, et al. Assessment of three chromogenic and one clotting assay for the measurement of synthetic pentasaccharide fondaparinux (Arixtra) anti-Xa activity. J Thromb Haemost 2004;2:346-8.

111. Klaeffling C, Piechottka G, Daemgen-Von BG, et al. Development and clinical evaluation of two chromogenic substrate methods for monitoring fondaparinux sodium. Ther Drug Monit 2006;28:375-81.

112. Depasse F, Gilbert M, Goret V, et al. Anti-Xa monitoring: inter-assay variability. Thromb Haemost 2000;84:1122-3.

113. Donat F, Duret JP, Santoni A, et al. The pharmacokinetics of fondaparinux sodium in healthy volunteers. Clin Pharmacokinet 2002;41(suppl 2):39-45.

114. Mehta SR, Yusuf S, Peters RJ, et al.; for the CURE Investigators. Effects of pretreatment with clopidogrel and aspirin followed by long-term therapy in patients undergoing percutaneous coronary intervention: the PCI-CURE study. Lancet 2001;358:527-33.

115. Price MJ, Coleman JL, Steinhubl SR. Onset and offset of platelet inhibition after high-dose clopidogrel loading and standard daily therapy measured by a point-of-care assay in healthy volunteers. Am J Cardiol 2006;98:681-4.

116. Steinhubl SR, Berger PB, Brennan DM, et al.; for the CREDO Investigators. Optimal timing for the initiation of pre-treatment with 300 mg clopidogrel before percutaneous coronary intervention. J Am Coll Cardiol 2006;47:939-43.

117. Hochholzer W, Trenk D, Frundi D, et al. Time dependence of platelet inhibition after a 600-mg loading dose of clopidogrel in a large, unselected cohort of candidates for percutaneous coronary intervention. Circulation 2005;111:2560-4.

118. Mehta SR, Tanguay JF, Eikelboom JW, et al.; for the CURRENT – OASIS 7 Investigators. Double-dose versus standard-dose clopidogrel and high-dose versus low-dose aspirin in individuals undergoing percutaneous coronary intervention for acute coronary syndromes (CURRENT-OASIS 7): a randomised factorial trial. Lancet 2010;376:1233-43.

119. von Beckerath N, Taubert D, Pogatsa-Murry G, et al. Absorption, metabolization, and antiplatelet effects of 300-, 600-, and 900-mg loading doses of clopidogrel: results of the ISAR-CHOICE (Intracoronary Stenting and Antithrombotic Regimen: Choose Between 3 High Oral Doses for Immediate Clopidogrel Effect) trial. Circulation 2005;112:2946-50.

120. Giugliano RP, White JA, Bode C, et al.; for the EARLY ACS Investigators. Early versus delayed, provisional eptifibatide in acute coronary syndromes. N Engl J Med 2009;360:2176-90.

121. The SYNERGY Trial Investigators. Enoxaparin vs unfractionated heparin in high-risk patients with non-ST-segment elevation acute coronary syndromes managed with an intended early invasive strategy. JAMA 2004;292:45-54.

122. Yusuf S, Mehta SR, Chrolavicius S, et al.; for the OASIS-5 Investigators. Comparison of fondaparinux and enoxaparin in acute coronary syndromes. N Engl J Med 2006;354:1464-76.

123. Mehta SR, Granger CB, Eikelboom JW, et al. Efficacy and safety of fondaparinux versus enoxaparin in patients with acute coronary syndromes undergoing percutaneous coronary

124. Stone GW, McLaurin BT, Cox DA, et al.; for the ACUITY Investigators. Bivalirudin for patients with acute coronary syndromes. N Engl J Med 2006;355:2203-16.

125. Stone GW, White HD, Ohman EM, et al.; for the ACUITY Investigators. Bivalirudin in patients with acute coronary syndromes undergoing percutaneous coronary intervention: a subgroup analysis from the Acute Catheterization and Urgent Intervention Triage strategy (ACUITY) trial. Lancet 2007;369:907-19.

126. Kastrati, A, Neumann FJ, Schulz S, et al.; for the ISAR – REACT 4 Trial Investigators. Abciximab and heparin versus bivalirudin for non-ST-elevation myocardial infarction. N Engl J Med 2011;365:1980-9.

127. Kastrati A, Neumann FJ, Mehilli J, et al.; for the ISAR – REACT 3 Trial Investigators. Bivalirudin versus unfractionated heparin during percutaneous coronary intervention. N Engl J Med 2008;359:688-96.

128. Shahzad A, Kemp I, Mars C, et al.; for the HEAT – PPCI trial investigators. Unfractionated heparin versus bivalirudin in primary percutaneous coronary intervention (HEAT – PPCI): an open-label, single centre, randomised controlled trial. Lancet 2014;384:1849-58.

129. Schulz S, Richardt G, Laugwitz KL, et al.; for the BRAVE 4 Investigators. Prasugrel plus bivalirudin vs. clopidogrel plus heparin in patients with ST-segment elevation myocardial infarction. Eur Heart J 2014;35:2285-94.

130. Roe MT, Armstrong PW, Fox KA, et al.; for the TRILOGY ACS Investigators. Prasugrel versus clopidogrel for acute coronary syndromes without revascularization. N Engl J Med 2012;367:1297-309.

131. The GUSTO IV Investigators. Effect of glycoprotein IIb/IIIa receptor blocker abciximab on outcomes in patients with acute coronary syndromes without early coronary revascularization: the GUST IV – ACS randomised trial. Lancet 2001;357:1915-24.

132. Cohen M, Demers C, Gurfinkle EP, et al.; for the ESSENCE Study Group. A comparison of low-molecular-weight heparin with unfractionated heparin for unstable coronary artery disease. N Engl J Med 1997;337:447-52.

133. Antman EM, McCabe CH, Gurfinkle EP, et al.; for the TIMI 11B Investigators. Enoxaparin prevents deaths and cardiac ischemic events in unstable angina/non-Q-wave myocardial infarction: results of the Thrombolysis in Myocardial Infarction (TIMI 11B) trial. Circulation 1999;100:1593-601.

134. Thiele H, Schindler K, Friedenberger J, et al. Intracoronary compared with intravenous bolus abciximab application in patients with ST-elevation myocardial infarction undergoing primary percutaneous coronary intervention: the Randomized Leipzig Immediate Percutaneous Coronary Intervention Abciximab IV Versus IC in ST-Elevation Myocardial Infarction Trial. Circulation 2008;118:49-57.

135. Bertrand OF, Rodés-Cabau J, Larose E, et al.; for the EASY – MI Study Investigators. Intracoronary compared to intravenous abciximab and high-dose bolus compared to standard dose inpatients with ST-segment elevation myocardial infarction undergoing transradial primary percutaneous coronary intervention: a two-by-two factorial placebo-controlled randomized study. Am J Cardiol 2010;105:1520-7.

136. Stone GW, Maehara A, Godlewski J, et al.; for the INFUSE – AMI Investigators. Intracoronary abciximab and aspiration thrombectomy in patients with large anterior myocardial infarction: the INFUSE – AMI randomized trial. JAMA 2012;307:1817-26.

137. Stone GW, Witzenbichler B, Guagliumi G, et al.; for the HORIZONS – AMI Trial Investigators. Bivalirudin during primary PCI in Acute Myocardial Infarction. N Engl J Med 2008;358:2218-30.

138. The OASIS-6 Trial Group. Effects of fondaparinux on mortality and reinfarction in patients with acute ST-segment elevation myocardial infarction: the OASIS-6 randomized trial. JAMA 2006;295:1519-30.

139. Montalescot G, Zeymer U, Silvain J, et al.; for the ATOLL Investigators. Intravenous enoxaparin or unfractionated heparin in primary percutaneous coronary intervention for ST-elevation myocardial infarction: the international randomised open-label ATOLL trial. Lancet 2011;378:693-703.

140. Navarese EP, De Luca G, Castriota F, et al. Low-molecular-weight heparin use. Unfractionated heparin in the setting of percutaneous coronary intervention for ST-elevation myocardial infarction: a meta-analysis. J Thromb Haemost 2011;9:1902-15.

141. Ross AM. New plasminogen activators: a clinical review. Clin Cardiol 1999;22:165-71.

142. The ASSENT-2 Investigators. Single-bolus tenecteplase compared with front-loaded alteplase in acute myocardial infarction: the ASSENT-2 double-blind randomised trial. Lancet 1999;354:716-22.

143. The GUSTO Angiographic Investigators. The effects of tissue plasminogen activator, streptokinase, or both on coronary-artery patency, ventricular function, and survival after acute myocardial infarction. N Engl J Med 1993;329:1615-22.

144. Bode C, Smalling RW, Berg G, et al. Randomized comparison of coronary thrombolysis achieved with double-bolus reteplase (recombinant plasminogen activator) and front-loaded, accelerated alteplase (recombinant tissue plasminogen activator) in patients with acute myocardial infarction. Circulation 1996;94:891-8.

145. Gore JM, Granger CB, Simoons ML, et al. Stroke after thrombolysis: mortality and functional outcomes in the GUSTO-I trial. Circulation 1995;92:2811-8.

146. The GUSTO III Investigators. A comparison of reteplase with alteplase for acute myocardial infarction. N Engl J Med 1997;337:1118-23.

147. Dobesh PP, Kasiar JB. Administration of glycoprotein IIb-IIIa inhibitors in patients with ST-segment elevation myocardial infarction. Pharmacotherapy 2002;22:864-88.

148. The GUSTO V Investigators. Reperfusion therapy for acute myocardial infarction with fibrinolytic therapy or combination reduced fibrinolytic therapy and platelet glycoprotein IIb/IIIa inhibition: the GUSTO V randomised trial. Lancet 2001;357:1905-14.

149. Antman EM, Morrow DA, McCabe CH, et al.; for the ExTRACT – TIMI 25 Investigators. Enoxaparin versus unfractionated heparin with fibrinolysis for ST-elevation myocardial infarction. N Engl J Med 2006;354:1477-88.

150. Bae JP, Dobesh PP, Klepser DG, et al. Adherence and dosing frequency of common medications for cardiovascular patients. AM J Manag Care 2012;18:139-46.

Chapter 34: Management of Cardiac Arrest

Toby C. Trujillo, Pharm.D., FCCP, FAHA, BCPS-AQ Cardiology

LEARNING OBJECTIVES

1. Discuss the epidemiology, etiology, and most common causes of cardiac arrest.
2. Define each component of the "chain of survival," and apply this concept to a patient with cardiac arrest.
3. Discuss the importance of electrical defibrillation and its effect on survival for a patient with ventricular fibrillation (VF) or pulseless ventricular tachycardia (PVT).
4. Given an individual patient who presents with sudden cardiac arrest, develop an appropriate treatment plan for VF, PVT, pulseless electrical activity, or asystole depending on the underlying patient-specific cause.
5. Compare and contrast the different sympathomimetic agents used to treat VF or PVT.
6. Discuss the role of vasopressin for a patient with cardiac arrest.
7. Describe the role of antiarrhythmic agents in a patient with VF or PVT.
8. Describe the role of therapeutic hypothermia to optimize outcomes in patients with cardiac arrest.
9. Discuss treatment strategies that pertain to post-resuscitative care after a cardiac arrest.
10. Formulate a monitoring plan for the post-resuscitation phase of cardiac arrest.

ABBREVIATIONS IN THIS CHAPTER

ACLS	Advanced cardiac life support	PEA	Pulseless electrical activity
AED	Automated external defibrillator	PVT	Pulseless ventricular tachycardia
AHA	American Heart Association	ROSC	Return of spontaneous circulation
CPP	Coronary perfusion pressure	SCA	Sudden cardiac arrest
CPR	Cardiopulmonary resuscitation	SCD	Sudden cardiac death
EMS	Emergency medical services	VF	Ventricular fibrillation
MI	Myocardial infarction	VT	Ventricular tachycardia

OVERVIEW OF SUDDEN CARDIAC DEATH/ SUDDEN CARDIAC ARREST

Introduction/Definitions

Sudden cardiac death (SCD) is defined by the World Health Organization as an unexpected death that occurs within 1 hour from symptom onset in a witnessed event, or within 24 hours from the last time the patient was observed as being alive and without symptoms in unwitnessed circumstances.[1] A key aspect of the definition is the duration of symptoms preceding the terminal event. Although often interchanged with SCD, sudden cardiac arrest (SCA) is a distinct event. Sudden cardiac arrest is defined as the cessation of cardiac function leading to circulatory collapse that is reversed by cardiopulmonary resuscitation (CPR) or defibrillation.[1] The cessation of cardiac mechanical activity as confirmed by the absence of signs of circulation (e.g., a detectable pulse, unresponsiveness, and apnea) in SCD typically occurs when a triggering activity takes place in vulnerable substrate that results in a life-terminating cardiac rhythm such as ventricular fibrillation (VF), pulseless electrical activity (PEA), or asystole. In many cases of SCA/SCD, preexisting heart disease may or may not have been known to be present, but the time and mode of death are unexpected. These definitions incorporate key elements of natural, rapid, and unexpected.[2]

Epidemiology of SCA

Sudden cardiac death accounts for more than 50% of the deaths from cardiovascular disease; therefore, SCD/SCA represents a significant and challenging burden from a public health perspective.[1] Current estimates are that 600,000 people in the United States experience SCA, and the survival rate for these events in the community is only 6%. Survival for in-hospital cardiac arrest is better, but still low at 24%.[3-5] Unfortunately, these survival rates have not meaningfully improved during the past 30 years despite significant efforts at improving treatment options and public awareness.[6,7] The estimates of SCA and SCD are challenging to ascertain, given the variability seen with different data sources, but death certificate data suggest that SCD accounts for 15%–20% of the total mortality in the United States and other industrialized countries.[8] However, death certificate data may overestimate the prevalence of SCD.[9,10] In a prospective evaluation of deaths in one county in Oregon, SCD was implicated in 5.6% of annual mortality.[7] As previously mentioned, despite advances in the management of coronary heart disease, the outcomes of patients with SCA are still suboptimal, although the prognosis varies significantly according to the initial rhythm and location of presentation. The risk of experiencing SCA is increased by several factors (see Table 34.1).[8-11] For example, the incidence increases dramatically with age and with underlying cardiac disease. In addition, men are 2–3 times more likely than women to experience SCA.[8] Among the 161,808 postmenopausal women who participated in the Women's Health Initiative and were followed for an average of 10.8 years, the incidence rate of SCD was 2.4 per 10,000 women per year, and almost one-half of women who experienced SCD had no prior clinically recognized coronary heart disease.[13]

Etiology/Clinical Presentation

Typical signs and symptoms of a patient presenting with SCD/SCA are consistent with lack of circulation because of the cessation of cardiac mechanical activity. Anxiety, crushing chest pain, nausea, vomiting, and diaphoresis can precede an arrest when the causative event is cardiac in nature. After an arrest, individuals are unresponsive and apneic, with no detectable pulse or blood pressure.[14] Most SCD occurs in adults, with less than 1% of patients being younger than 35 years. Coronary heart disease is the most common cardiac pathology of SCD, affecting about 70%–75% of individuals, with the presence of underlying cardiomyopathies the second most common pathology at 10%–15%. The actual percentage may vary by sex and region of the world, though, with coronary heart disease being the primary underlying pathology in only 50% of women and an estimated 50%–60% of individuals in Japan.[8] Unfortunately, in many patients (about two-thirds), cardiac arrest is the first clinical sign of coronary artery disease with no preceding signs or symptoms.[12,15]

In the adult population, cardiac arrest is typically the result of an underlying arrhythmia. Historically, VF and pulseless ventricular tachycardia (PVT) have been the most common initial rhythm, accounting for 70% of SCAs, but their incidence is now 20%–25%.[15] At the same time, the incidence of PEA or asystole as the first recorded rhythm has increased from 21% to 31% and from 17% to 28%, respectively,

Table 34.1 Causes of Sudden Cardiac Death[12]

Coronary heart disease	Ischemia secondary to arthrosclerotic heart disease
	Anomalous coronary
	Coronary vasospasm
Cardiomyopathies	Ischemic cardiomyopathy
	Nonischemic/idiopathic dilated cardiomyopathy
	Hypertrophic cardiomyopathy
	Takotsubo cardiomyopathy
	Infiltrative sarcoid heart disease
	Infiltrative amyloid heart disease
	Arrhythmogenic right ventricular dysplasia/cardiomyopathy
	Left ventricular noncompaction
	Myocarditis
	Valvular heart disease
	Congenital heart disease
Electrophysiologic	Long QT syndrome
	Short QT syndrome
	Brugada syndrome
	Catecholaminergic polymorphic VT
	Idiopathic VF
	Ventricular preexcitation
Metabolic	Hyper/hypokalemia
	Hypomagnesemia
	Hypocalcemia
	Severe acidosis
Noncardiac	Intracranial hemorrhage
	Pulmonary embolus
	Epileptic seizure

VF = ventricular fibrillation; VT = ventricular tachycardia.

during the past 2 decades.[15,16] The decline in VT/ventricular tachycardia (VF) and the increase in PEA and asystole as the initial rhythm identified in SCA may result from the confluence of several environmental, clinical, pharmacologic, or interventional factors. Several of these likely include the increasing role of implantable pacemakers and defibrillators in the treatment of patients with heart failure (HF), as well as the use of effective pharmacotherapy for HF such as angiotensin-converting enzyme inhibitors and β-blockers.[15] Part of this changing pattern may also be because of an increased proportion of arrests occurring in the home, where the arrest is less likely to be witnessed. In addition, these patients are more likely to be older with several comorbidities that lead to precipitants of PEA (respiratory, metabolic, vascular) as opposed to VF or PVT.[8] Nonetheless, this declining incidence is particularly troubling because survival rates are substantially higher with shockable rhythms such as VF and PVT than with non-shockable rhythms such as PEA and asystole. Survival rates with VF/PVT are 15%–23% versus 0%–5% with asystole.[7]

GENERAL APPROACH TO MANAGEMENT

In patients with SCA/SCD, the ultimate goal is the long-term survival of a neurologically intact patient. Intermediate goals that facilitate this ultimate objective include (1) early CPR and defibrillation, (2) increased coronary perfusion pressure (CPP) and cerebral blood flow, (3) return of spontaneous circulation (ROSC), (4) survival to hospital admission, (5) stabilization of the patient, and (6) prevention of future SCD episodes. The 2010 American Heart Association (AHA) guidelines for CPR and emergency cardiovascular care emphasize high-quality CPR and attempted defibrillation for pulseless VT/VF, as well as advances in post-cardiac arrest interventions to optimize outcomes.[6,17]

A three-phase model for treating SCA from either VT or PVT highlights the impact of time on the likelihood of success for CPR of defibrillation. The model postulates that the first 5 minutes after an arrest is the electric phase, and rapid defibrillation should be a top priority because it will likely be successful at producing a perfusing rhythm. In fact, data analyses indicate that survival can exceed 60% with proper defibrillation in the electric phase. The second or circulatory phase takes place 5–10 minutes after SCA, and the delivery of chest compressions should take priority, followed by defibrillation. The supporting concepts are that chest compressions are necessary to restore some blood flow to the myocardium in this phase to increase the chances of successful defibrillation. The third or metabolic phase postulates that after 10 minutes, the use of chest compressions and defibrillation is insufficient to improve survival, and some form of metabolic resuscitation may be needed. Overall, the model highlights the need to quickly identify patients with SCA and provide life-saving interventions as soon as possible.[15]

Cardiopulmonary Resuscitation

Cardiopulmonary resuscitation is an attempt to restore spontaneous circulation by performing chest compressions (to restore threshold blood flows, particularly to the heart and brain) with or without ventilations. Two theories exist on how CPR may restore some level of blood flow.[16] The first, the cardiac pump theory, simply states that active compression of the heart between the sternum and the vertebrae creates forward flow. Echocardiography, however, has revealed that left ventricular size does not always change with compressions and that the mitral valve may, in fact, be open.[16] The second, the thoracic pump theory, postulates that blood flow is restored through changes in intrathoracic pressure and the differential compressibility of the arteries and veins. In this model, the heart merely acts as a passive conduit for flow. However, both models likely contribute to the mechanism of blood flow with CPR.

An important consideration regarding survival is the quality of the CPR delivered because high-quality CPR continues to be emphasized in the latest AHA guidelines.[6] Manual chest compressions should be delivered such that the sternum is depressed at least 2 inches 100–120 times per minute. The upper limit is a new recommendation based on one study showing that higher rates lead to inadequate chest compression. Ideally, half of the time is spent in compression, and interruptions in the delivery of compressions should be minimized. If ventilation is being delivered simultaneously, caution should be used not to overinflate the thoracic cavity.[6] The delivery of suboptimal CPR is more common than desired, especially when rescuers are fatigued.[18,19] Conversely, when high-quality CPR is delivered, the chance for survival is increased.[20] Several devices are available that provide prompts and/or feedback in "real time"; however, data showing improvement in survival are lacking.[21,22] In addition, mechanical devices designed to improve hemodynamics have been studied, but inconsistent results limit their applicability in routine practice.[23]

The evolution of resuscitation techniques has a long history, with the first landmark article, released in 1960, describing the use of chest compressions and ventilation in 20 patients, with three patients receiving defibrillation for VF. All 20 patients had ROSC, with 14 patients surviving long term.[23] Resuscitation techniques have been studied for many years. Research began to accrue, and the AHA published the first guidelines for cardiac arrest in 1966.[24] Resuscitation techniques have evolved over the years since culminating in the most recent guidelines, published in full in 2010 with updates provided in 2015.[6] The "chain of survival" continues to be the focal point for the approach to treating SCA/SCD and continues to highlight the need for timely interventions. The 2010 guidelines, together with the 2015 update, list five links in the chain of survival:

(1) Immediate recognition of cardiac arrest and activation of emergency medical services (EMS)

(2) Early CPR with an emphasis on chest compressions

(3) Rapid defibrillation

(4) Effective advanced life support

(5) Integrated post-cardiac arrest care

Although all five links in the chain of survival are important, the most crucial appear to be the first three, particularly early CPR with good chest compressions.[6] The available literature supports this assessment because CPR has been shown to prolong the time VF is present as well as increase the chances that defibrillation will terminate VF.[6] Successful defibrillation during witnessed VF arrests decreases rapidly from the onset of collapse, with survival rates decreasing 7%–10% per minute in the absence of CPR.[25] If immediate CPR is added, the decrease in survival is more gradual, reduced to 3%–4% per minute after arrest onset.[26] Additional studies have shown that when properly combined, CPR and defibrillations can increase survival rates above 50% of out-of-hospital cardiac arrest.[27] Although CPR is critical to increase survival, it is unlikely to terminate VF alone and lead to restoration of a perfusing rhythm. As such, the 2010 AHA guidelines specifically emphasize the integration of early CPR and defibrillation, especially mentioning the use of automated external defibrillators (AEDs), which is reinforced in the 2015 update (see Figure 34.1).[22,28] Although CPR and defibrillation are crucial, delivering advanced cardiac life support (ACLS) and effective post-resuscitative care is also a key component in the chain of survival. In fact, the growing importance of post-arrest care reflects that optimizing many organ systems may help improve outcomes.[29]

Basic Life Support

The 2010 AHA guidelines, and subsequently the 2015 update, introduced major changes in recommendations for how basic life support should be delivered. The old pneumonic for rescuers—"ABC," representing airway, breathing, and circulation—was replaced with "CAB," representing circulation, airway, and breathing.[30] The changes reflected the challenges of lay rescuers when trying to assess for respirations using the look, listen, and feel approach, as well as the potential for agonal respirations being mistaken for normal breathing. Assessing a pulse may also be challenging for a lay rescuer. As such, the guidelines were revised to ensure that rescuers delivered timely chest compressions and defibrillation, interventions that are known to increase survival. When first encountering a patient with presumed cardiac arrest, the initial action is to determine the patient's responsiveness. If there is no response, the rescuer should immediately activate the emergency medical response system. Once emergency medical response is contacted, the rescuer should either secure or call for an AED and immediately start CPR with chest compressions. Health care providers at this point should assess for a pulse before CPR but take no more than 10 seconds to do so. If one is not detected within this short time, chest compressions should be initiated immediately.[30] The importance of timely chest compressions has previously been highlighted, and the prompt provision of chest compressions (high-quality CPR) is thus of paramount importance and should be provided regardless of the rescuer's skill or experience. The most recent basic life support algorithm calls for initiating CPR, with rhythm check every 2 minutes, shocking if indicated with an AED, with continued repetition. Once chest compressions have been initiated, a trained rescuer should incorporate rescue breaths into the process because opening the airway has the potential to improve oxygenation and allow for better attempts at ventilation. Rescue breaths and airway management should in no way impede or delay the delivery of compressions and defibrillation, however. A trained rescuer can deliver rescue breaths, either by mouth to mouth or, preferentially, by bag-mask ventilation, delivering a breath over 1 second, using enough volume to elicit a visible chest rise and using a compression/ventilation ratio of 30:2.[22,29] If no AED is available, cycles of chest compression and rescue breaths should continue (with pulse checks every 2 minutes) until the arrival of EMS or the ROSC. If an AED is available, the rhythm should be analyzed to determine whether defibrillation is advised (see Figure 34.1). If so, one shock should be delivered with the immediate resumption of chest compressions, followed by rescue breaths. The rhythm can be reevaluated and an additional shock delivered, if appropriate, after an additional 2 minutes of high-quality CPR plus rescue breaths. This algorithm should be repeated until help arrives or until the rhythm is no longer "shockable." If the rhythm is not shockable, chest compressions and rescue breath cycles should be continued until help arrives or until the patient attains ROSC. Ongoing education of health care providers and especially the public is needed to continue to improve outcomes in SCA. The problem of poor-quality CPR being delivered was previously highlighted, and more importantly, only 20%–30% of adults with out-of-hospital cardiac arrest receive bystander CPR.[30] This has led to further educational interventions in an attempt to increase the quality and delivery of CPR, and EMS dispatchers often try to give instructions over the telephone when EMS is activated. Recent data analyses have shown that delivering hands-only CPR is as effective at improving survival as delivering CPR combined with rescue breaths.[30,31] This finding is important because bystanders are reluctant to consider mouth to mouth, although one data set cites panic as a reason not to pursue bystander CPR rather than actual reluctance.[31]

Advanced Cardiac Life Support

The transition from basic life support to ACLS triggers the implementation of more advanced interventions. Advanced cardiac life support providers can use an advanced airway (endotracheal tube, laryngeal mask airway) to more adequately provide ventilation to the patient. When this occurs, the rescuers no longer need to provide the cycles of 30:2 compression to ventilation. Instead, continuous chest compressions are recommended without pauses for ventilations, and the rescuer providing the ventilations needs to deliver a breath once every 6–8 seconds. If capable, ACLS providers may implement more advanced metrics of monitoring that may assist in determining the success of resuscitation efforts. The available literature suggests that the monitoring of end-tidal carbon dioxide ($ETCO_2$), CPP, and $Scvo_2$ (central venous oxygen saturation) can provide valuable information regarding the success of resuscitation, and the 2010 guidelines strongly recommend $ETCO_2$ monitoring during CPR if at all possible.[28]

If the cardiac rhythm is deemed non-shockable, it is likely to be either asystole or PEA, and ACLS providers must quickly consider whether reversible causes are present (see Table 34.2). If the person is in VF or PVT, one shock should be delivered (appropriate to the available electrical device), with the immediate resumption of chest compressions (using 30 compressions to two breaths for five cycles, or 2 minutes of continuous compressions with assisted ventilations) before rechecking the rhythm or pulse. If there is still a shockable rhythm, one shock should be delivered, and at this time, pharmacologic intervention can be considered. Although drug therapy with primarily vasopressors and antiarrhythmic agents is still a recommended component of advanced resuscitation efforts, the current literature suggests that these interventions will have minimal impact on overall long-term survival (see Figure 34.1). Vasopressors are typically recommended to be initiated after a first unsuccessful attempt at defibrillation, with antiarrhythmic therapy an option for consideration after two failed attempts at defibrillation. Chest compressions for 2 minutes (five cycles of chest compressions to breaths) should be performed in between attempts at defibrillation. This algorithm will repeat until a pulse is obtained with effective circulation, the rhythm changes, or resuscitation efforts cease.[22,28] Despite its limited role in improving outcomes compared with the delivery of high-quality CPR and defibrillation, drug therapy still has a role in ACLS, and pharmacists should be well versed in using these agents during SCA.

Drug Administration Considerations in Cardiac Arrest

Although specific medications such as vasopressors and antiarrhythmic agents play only a secondary role in the overall ACLS effort, ensuring the appropriate preparation of these agents together with appropriate dose and frequency of administration is an important consideration for the multidisciplinary cardiac arrest team. Properly trained pharmacists can perform any role on this team; however, managing crash cart medications and drug therapy overall is perhaps best suited for the skills a pharmacist can bring to this multidisciplinary team. Specific recommendations have been developed to define the role of pharmacists as part of the ACLS team, as well as the training needed for individuals to fulfill their role successfully.[32] Appropriate training will allow pharmacists to anticipate drug therapy needs during the management of cardiac arrest and ensure that dose, frequency, and drug selection are appropriate according to the AHA guidelines. In addition, pharmacists who are members of an in-hospital cardiac arrest team can facilitate the gathering of pertinent information related to drug therapy administration in the field by emergency medical personnel (EMS). Drug therapy in the field typically will consist of routine ACLS medications but may also include more unique agents such as thrombolytic therapy for ST-elevation myocardial infarction (MI). Identifying the drugs, doses, and timing of doses delivered will facilitate the continuation of resuscitation efforts in the hospital.[33]

Considerations regarding the route of administration to deliver medications include the ease of obtaining access, ability to effectively deliver drug therapy into the central circulation, and minimization of any interruptions in chest compressions during CPR. A peripheral intravenous line is often the easiest to attain during resuscitation attempts. Drug administered through this line can be followed by a 20-mL bolus of intravenous fluid and elevation of the arm to facilitate drug entry into the central circulation.[32] Although delivering medication through a central line would be preferred with respect to attaining rapid access to the central circulation and at higher concentrations, obtaining central line access during CPR is often not feasible. If a central line is already in place, it should be used for drug administration.[33] Intraosseous cannulation is preferred if intravenous access is not available, and many studies have documented the success of this route in both the adult and pediatric populations.[26,34] Pharmacokinetic data available indicate that similar responses occur with intraosseous and intravenous administration with respect to area under the curve and peak concentrations.[35] Several devices are available to achieve rapid intraosseous access and can easily be placed on the first attempt more than 80% of the time.[33] If neither intravenous nor intraosseous access can be obtained, some medications can be administered through an endotracheal tube. These medications include epinephrine, vasopressin, lidocaine, atropine, and naloxone. No data currently exist with amiodarone. The absorption through alveoli is rapid, but this results in lower plasma concentrations when the same dose is administered intravenously. Therefore, when medications are given by the endotracheal route, a dose of 2–2.5 times the recommended intravenous dose should be used and diluted in 5–10 mL of sterile water or 0.9% normal saline.[33]

MANAGEMENT OF SPECIFIC RHYTHM DISORDERS

Ventricular Fibrillation/Pulseless Ventricular Tachycardia

Nonpharmacologic Therapy—Defibrillation

Electrical defibrillation is the only effective method of restoring a perfusing cardiac rhythm in either VF or PVT; therefore, it is a crucial link in the chain of survival, especially for a witnessed arrest.[22,26] As previously discussed, the probability of successful defibrillation is directly related to the time interval between the onset of VF and the delivery of the first shock.[26] In one study, each 1-minute reduction in the time to defibrillation resulted in a 23% relative improvement in survival (odds ratio [OR] 0.77 [95% confidence interval {CI}, 0.73–0.81]).[36] As discussed previously, CPR delivery before defibrillation may increase

Table 34.2 Potential Causes and Interventions for Cardiac Arrest[22,28]

Suspected Condition	Clues	Intervention	Comments
H's			
Hypovolemia	History, flat neck veins	IV bolus fluids	Most common cause of PEA. All patients should receive fluid bolus
Hypoxia	Cyanosis, blood gases, airway problems	100% oxygen	All patients should be adequately ventilated; check endotracheal tube placement
Hydrogen ion acidosis	History of bicarbonate-responsive preexisting acidosis	Buffers (sodium bicarbonate 1 mEq/kg IV x 1)	
Hyper/hypokalemia	History of renal failure, diabetes, recent dialysis, dialysis fistulas, medications	Calcium/potassium administration	Sodium bicarbonate for hyperkalemia (IIb/C); add $D_{50}W$ and insulin if ECG changes are present
Hypoglycemia	History of diabetes	Dextrose	
Hypothermia	History of exposure to cold, central body temperature	Rewarming, oxygen, IV fluids	
T's			
Toxins (overdose)	Bradycardia, history of ingestion, empty bottles at the scene, pupils, neurologic examination	Alkalinize urine if appropriate; calcium chloride if appropriate	Question family members for possible overdose in patient with no other clear cause of PEA
Tamponade (cardiac)	History (trauma, renal failure, thoracic malignancy), no pulse with CPR, vein distention, impending tamponade-tachycardia, hypotension, low pulse pressure changing to sudden bradycardia as terminal event	Needle aspiration of fluid	
Tension pneumothorax	History (asthma, ventilator, chronic obstructive pulmonary disease, trauma), no pulse with CPR, neck vein distention, tracheal deviation	Needle decompression; chest tube	
Thrombosis (cardiac; MI or pulmonary; PE)	History, ECG, enzymes	Various	Fibrinolytics reasonable if presumed or known PE (IIa/B)
Trauma	History, examination	Various	

CPR = cardiopulmonary resuscitation; $D_{50}W$ = dextrose 50% in water; IV = intravenous(ly); MI = myocardial infarction; PE = pulmonary embolism; PEA = pulseless electrical activity.

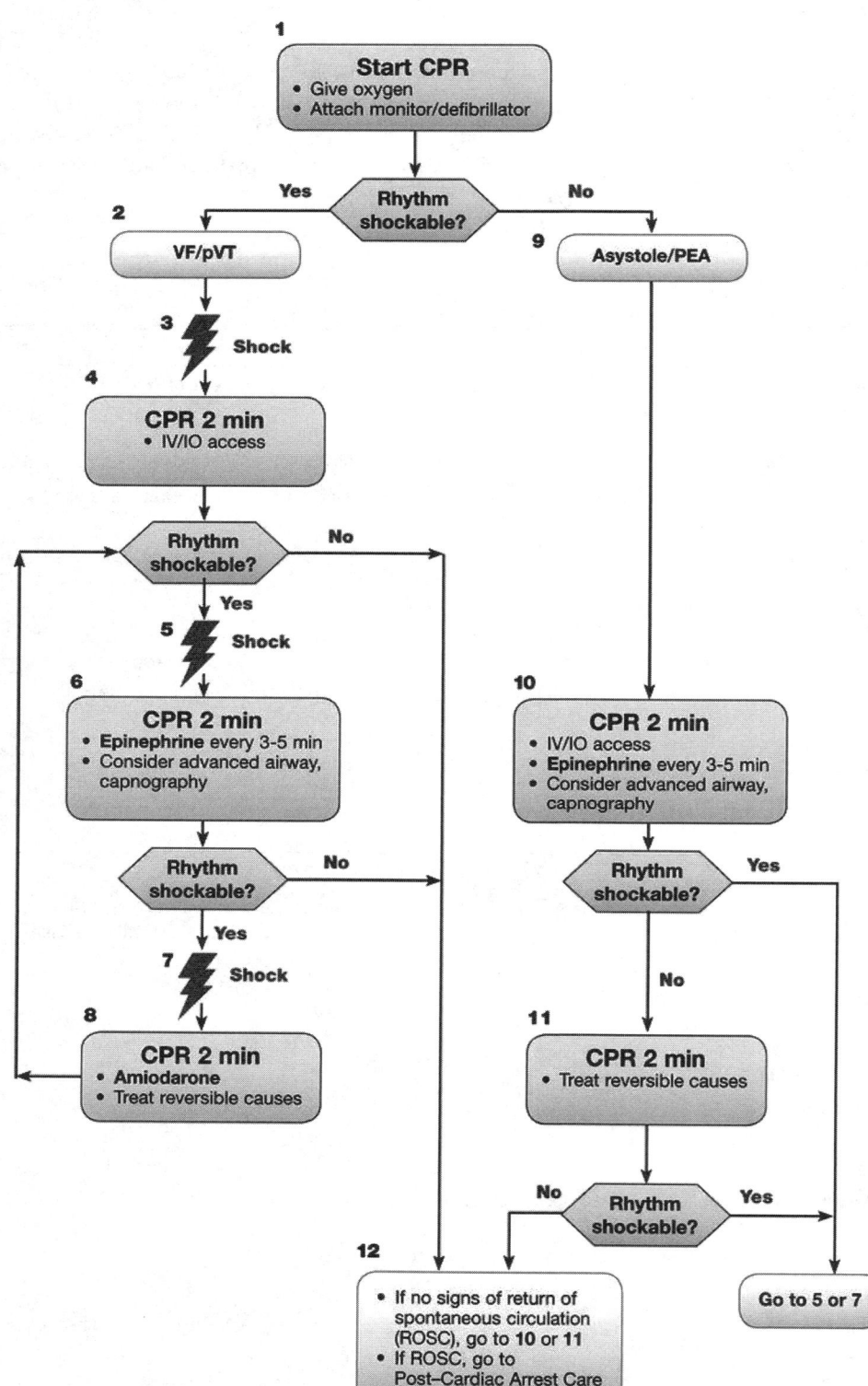

Figure 34.1 Adult cardiac arrest algorithm—2015 update.

CPR = cardiopulmonary resuscitation; IV/IO = intravenous/intraosseous; PEA = pulseless electrical activity.

Reproduced with permission from: Wolters Kluwer Health, Inc. Part 7: Adult Advanced Cardiovascular Life Support: 2015 American Heart Association Guidelines Update for Cardiopulmonary Resuscitation and Emergency Cardiovascular Care. Link MS, Berkow LC, Kudenchuk PJ, et al.

the chances of success, especially if the time from arrest is greater than 5 minutes.[26] For in-hospital cardiac arrest, if an AED is available, CPR should begin while the AED is being placed. With out-of-hospital cardiac arrest, there is growing evidence that CPR before defibrillation is beneficial. Clinical trials indicate that CPR before defibrillation increased ROSC, survival to discharge, and 1-year survival.[26,37,38] In one trial, the provision of about 90 seconds of CPR before defibrillation was associated with an increased rate of hospital survival (27% vs. 17%; p=0.01).[37] Higher survival rates were reported in patients with response intervals greater than 5 minutes when 3 minutes of CPR was administered before defibrillation (22% vs. 4%; p=0.006).[38] Additional studies have indicated that total survival is increased when each defibrillation was preceded by 200 uninterrupted chest compressions (57% [19 of 33] vs. 20% [18 of 92], p=0.001) as well as neurologically normal survival (48% [16 of 33] vs. 15% [14 of 92], p=0.001).[39] Finally, one study noted improved in-hospital survival (from 22% to 44%, p=0.0024) in patients with witnessed VF using a modified resuscitation protocol that included 200 preshock chest compressions.[40] However, not all published studies support the premise of CPR before defibrillation.[41,42] Given the overall positive results, the 2010 AHA guidelines and 2015 update continue to offer that EMS personnel may give 2 minutes of chest compressions before attempting defibrillation. Recommendations are similar for individuals in the metabolic phase, although the chances of achieving ROSC are much lower.

The 2010 AHA guidelines and 2015 update continue to recommend one shock for VF or PVT with the immediate resumption of chest compressions.[22,26] This revision from previous versions where stacked multiple shocks were initially given is largely because of the prolonged time noted (about 55 seconds) to deliver three stacked shocks without providing adequate chest compressions.[42] The defibrillation attempt should be with 360 J (monophasic defibrillator) or 150–200 J (biphasic defibrillator). An AED, if available, should be used as soon as possible, with the electrode pads placed in an anterolateral position on the patient. After defibrillation is attempted, CPR should be immediately restarted and continued for 2 minutes without checking a pulse. The omission of the pulse check after defibrillation is again a paradigm shift in the algorithm that is related to myocardial stunning with resultant poor perfusion and diminished cardiac output immediately after electrical therapy.[26] After 2 minutes of chest compressions, the rhythm and pulse should be rechecked. If there is still evidence of VF or PVT, repeat single-discharge defibrillation should be attempted with the addition of pharmacologic therapy. Once an airway is achieved, patients should be ventilated with 100% oxygen. Laryngeal mask airways and esophageal-tracheal combination tubes represent several available airway adjuncts, but the preferred airway is an endotracheal tube placed with direct laryngoscopy. Other interventions are also being evaluated as nonpharmacologic therapy. Additional nonpharmacologic therapy where there is evolving evidence includes placing a left ventricular assist device, performing angiography and percutaneous coronary intervention during suspected MI, and using ECMO (extracorporeal membrane oxygenation). These procedures have improved outcomes in some series, but the logistics of widespread implementation is daunting.[43-45] Although there are no conclusive human data regarding these interventions, they raise interesting concepts worthy of discussion and evaluation.

Pharmacologic Therapy

Vasopressors

No placebo-controlled trials have shown that administering vasopressors in SCA increases the rate of neurologically intact survival at discharge. However, the available evidence indicates that vasopressors can increase the rate of ROSC (see Table 34.3). As such, vasopressors continue to be the first pharmacologic agents administered in the setting of cardiac arrest. The primary goal of vasopressor therapy is to augment the low coronary and cerebral perfusion pressures encountered during CPR. Chest compressions can provide some degree of blood flow but only an estimated 25% of that encountered under basal conditions.[46] When CPP remains below 15 mm Hg, the ROSC is unlikely, which is likely to be encountered even with properly performed chest compressions.[47,48] Vasopressor therapy works to increase CPP and arterial pressure through its vasoconstrictive properties. Epinephrine and vasopressin are the two main vasopressor agents to consider, as stated in the 2010 AHA guidelines, although the 2015 update provides alternative recommendations on vasopressin that will subsequently be addressed.[22] Other agents that are pure α_1-agonists (phenylephrine and methoxamine) or agents with more potent α_1 activity (norepinephrine) have also been investigated in the setting of SCA, generally compared with epinephrine, though. When pure α_1-agonists were compared with epinephrine, no differences in long-term survival between the agents were noted.[49-51] Comparisons between epinephrine and norepinephrine generally have not revealed differences in ROSC, survival to hospital admission, or, most importantly, long-term survival.[52,53] Given the decades-long experience in managing SCA and the lack of strong outcome data suggesting that alternative catecholamine derivatives improve outcome, epinephrine continues to be a drug of first choice (together with vasopressin) for the treatment of VF, PVT, asystole, and PEA. Epinephrine is an α- and β-receptor agonist causing both vasoconstriction and increased inotropic/chronotropic activity on the heart. Its effectiveness, however, is primarily through its α effects.[54]

Although epinephrine is a first-line recommendation for pharmacologic therapy, few adequately randomized controlled trials evaluate it in the setting of

Table 34.3 Evidence-Based Recommendations[22,28]

Recommendations	Recommendation Grades[a]
Immediate bystander CPR	
High-quality CPR should be performed with minimal interruption in chest compressions and defibrillation as soon as possible	Class I, LOE A
Epinephrine	
1 mg IV/IO should be administered every 3–5 min in patients with cardiac arrest	Class IIb, LOE A
Vasopressin	
40 units IV/IO may replace either the first or the second dose of epinephrine in patients with cardiac arrest	Class IIb, LOE A
Amiodarone	
300 mg IV/IO can be followed by 150 mg IV/IO in patients with VF/PVT unresponsive to CPR, shock, and a vasopressor	Class IIb, LOE B
Lidocaine	
Lidocaine can be considered in patients with VF/PVT as an alternative if amiodarone is not available. The initial dose is 1–1.5 mg/kg IV. Additional doses of 0.5–0.75 mg/kg can be administered at 5- to 10-min intervals to a maximum dose of 3 mg/kg if VF/PVT persists	Class IIb, LOE B
Magnesium	
Magnesium is recommended for VF/PVT that is caused by torsades de pointes. 1–2 g diluted in 10 mL of D_5W should be administered IV/IO push over 15 min	Class IIb, LOE C
Routine administration of magnesium sulfate in cardiac arrest is not recommended	Class III, LOE A
Fibrinolysis	
Fibrinolytic therapy should not be used routinely in cardiac arrest	Class III, LOE B
When PE is presumed or known to be the cause, empiric fibrinolytic therapy can be considered	Class IIa, LOE B
Hypothermia	
Comatose adult patients with ROSC after out-of-hospital VF cardiac arrest should be cooled to 32°C–34°C (89.6°F–93.2°F) for 12–24 hr	Class I, LOE B
Induced hypothermia can be considered for comatose adult patients with ROSC after in-hospital cardiac arrest of any initial rhythm or after out-of-hospital cardiac arrest with an initial rhythm of PEA or asystole	Class IIb, LOE B

D_5W = dextrose 5% in water IO = intraosseous(ly) LOE = level of evidence; PVT = pulseless ventricular tachycardia; ROSC = return of spontaneous circulation.

[a]Key for evidence-based classifications:

Class of recommendations:

Class I: High-level prospective studies support the action or therapy, and the benefit substantially outweighs the potential for harm. The treatment should be administered.

Class IIa: The weight of evidence supports the action or therapy, and the therapy is considered acceptable and useful. It is reasonable to administer the treatment.

Class IIb: The evidence documents only short-term benefits, or weakly positive or mixed results. Class IIb recommendations are identified by terms such as "may be useful" or "can be considered."

Class III: The risk outweighs the benefit for a particular treatment. The treatment should not be administered and may be harmful.

Levels of Evidence (LOEs):

Level A: Data derived from multiple randomized clinical trials or meta-analyses

Level B: Data derived from a single randomized trial or nonrandomized studies

Level C: Only consensus opinion of experts, case studies, or standard of care

out-of-hospital SCA versus placebo. Available evidence as such comes from less robust trial designs. In one study, patients were randomized to receive standard ACLS with intravenous drug administration or standard ACLS without intravenous drug administration.[55] Of the 851 patients analyzed, VF/PVT was the initial rhythm in 34%. Intravenous medications administered included epinephrine (79%), atropine (46%), and amiodarone (17%). A significant increase in ROSC (40% vs. 25%, $p<0.001$) and hospital admission (43% vs. 29%, greater than $p<0.001$) was noted in patients who received intravenous therapy. This difference was primarily observed in patients with initial rhythms other than VF/PVT. The role of epinephrine in contributing to these outcomes was not assessed. In one small randomized controlled trial comparing epinephrine with placebo in 534 patients, ROSC (23.5% vs.

8.4%, p<0.001) and survival to hospital admission (25.4% vs. 13%, greater than p<0.001) were significantly higher with epinephrine, but there was no difference in survival to hospital discharge (4% vs. 1.9%, p=0.15).[56] However, contrasting results were observed in one large prospective registry study of more than 400,000 patients, which failed to show a survival benefit with epinephrine.[57] Despite a significant improvement in ROSC with epinephrine (adjusted OR [95% CI] 2.36 [2.22–2.5]), both 1-month survival (adjusted OR [95% CI] 0.46 [0.42–0.51]) and survival with good neurologic function (adjusted OR [95% CI] 0.31 [0.26–0.36]) were lower in patients who received epinephrine. These findings were confirmed through various sensitivity analyses accounting for in-hospital epinephrine use and CPR duration.

Disparate results for epinephrine may be related to its underlying pharmacology. Epinephrine causes α_1-mediated vasoconstriction that increases coronary perfusion and may also promote ventricular defibrillation. But the same α_1-mediated vasoconstriction may lead to decreased perfusion of other vital organs.[58] In addition, β_1-agonist effects may lead to increased myocardial metabolic demands, impaired oxygen delivery, and increased lactate production in the post-resuscitation period.[59]

Despite these potential concerns, the larger controversy during the past 10–15 years is the appropriate dose of epinephrine in the management of SCA. The rationale for higher doses (5–10 mg) compared with standard doses is the lack of tissue responsiveness when acidosis is present. Three separate studies in the 1990s comparing high-dose epinephrine (7–10 mg or 0.2 mg/kg) with standard-dose epinephrine (1 mg) found no differences in immediate survival, ROSC, or survival to hospital discharge.[52,60-61] A subsequent meta-analysis, however, found a higher ROSC with high-dose epinephrine, but no overall mortality benefit was seen.[62] In the largest study to date with out-of-hospital SCA caused by VF, PEA, or asystole, 3,327 patients were randomized to a high-dose strategy (5 mg of epinephrine) versus a standard-dose strategy (1 mg).[63] Repeated doses could be administered up to a total of 15 mg for epinephrine. The rates of ROSC and survival to hospital admission were higher in the high-dose strategy, but neurologic outcome and survival to hospital discharge were similar between groups. Despite the improving rate of ROSC in SCA in several trials, no studies have shown a difference in survival. Possible reasons include the post-resuscitation adverse effects associated with higher doses such as myocardial dysfunction, tachycardia, and hypertension. As such, a 1-mg dose of epinephrine administered by intravenous or intraosseous injection every 3–5 minutes during cardiac arrest is reasonable to consider.[28] Higher doses may be administered to treat specific disorders such as β-blocker or calcium channel blocker overdose. In addition, higher doses can be considered if indicated through arterial diastolic pressure (or CPP) monitoring.

Vasopressin

Vasopressin, also known as antidiuretic hormone, is a neuropeptide hormone that increases blood pressure and systemic vascular resistance through potent vasoconstriction. The vasoconstrictive properties are primarily because of its effects on the V1 receptor. Stimulation of the V2 receptors on the renal collecting duct causes an antidiuretic effect and hence the name "antidiuretic hormone," which vasopressin is sometimes called. As a potential initial option for vasopressor therapy, vasopressin has several theoretical advantages over epinephrine. The metabolic acidosis that often accompanies cardiac arrest can blunt the vasoconstrictive effect of adrenergic agents such as epinephrine, but not with vasopressin. Vasopressin, because it does not act on β_1-adrenergic receptors, lacks the potential to raise myocardial oxygen demand in the post-resuscitative phase. Vasopressin has a more gradual onset and sustained effect than epinephrine, leading, in theory, to sustained peripheral vasoconstriction. Vasopressin also may have a beneficial effect on renal blood flow by stimulating V2 receptors in the kidney, causing vasodilation and increased water reabsorption. With respect to splanchnic blood flow, however, vasopressin has a detrimental effect compared with epinephrine.[64] Advancing the idea that vasopressin may improve outcomes in SCA compared with epinephrine is the fact that measuring the vasopressin levels in patients undergoing CPR has shown a high correlation between the levels of endogenous vasopressin released and the potential for ROSC.[64] In fact, in one study, plasma vasopressin concentrations were about 3 times as high in survivors as in non-survivors, suggesting that vasopressin is released as an adjunct vasopressor to epinephrine in life-threatening events such as cardiac arrest.[65] Vasopressin appeared in the resuscitation guidelines after 2000 after animal and small human studies appeared to confirm its potential to increase CPP, improving the ROSC.

Despite the favorable trajectory of vasopressin in the realm of SCA, clinical trials have not consistently shown superior results compared with epinephrine (see Table 34.4). Three large randomized trials that enrolled individuals with SCA to receive vasopressin 40 units intravenously × 1 dose or epinephrine 1 mg resulted in similar outcomes between the two groups with respect to ROSC, survival to discharge, and neurologic outcome.[66-68]

In one large trial of out-of-hospital arrest, no significant differences were noted in ROSC, hospital admission rate, or discharge rate.[66] However, when patients were stratified according to their initial rhythm, those with asystole had a significantly higher rate of hospital admission (29% vs. 20%; p=0.02) and discharge (4.7% vs. 1.5%; p=0.04) with vasopressin than with epinephrine. In addition, a subgroup analysis of 732 patients who required additional epinephrine therapy despite the two doses of study drug had significant benefits in ROSC (37% vs.

Table 34.4 Investigative Trials with Vasopressin in Cardiac Arrest

Author	Initial Rhythm	Intervention	n	Initial Resuscitation Vasopressin	Initial Resuscitation Epinephrine
Wenzel et al. (66)	VF/PVT: 40% PEA: 16% Asystole: 45%	Vasopressin 40 units vs. epinephrine 1 mg for two doses as initial drug treatment	1,186	145/589 (25%)	167/597 (28%)
Lindner et al. (67)	VF: 100%	Vasopressin 40 units vs. epinephrine 1 mg for initial drug treatment	40	16/20 (80%)	11/20 (55%)
Stiell et al. (68)	VF/PVT: 21% PEA: 48% Asystole: 31%	Vasopressin 40 units vs. epinephrine 1 mg for initial drug treatment	200	62/104 (60%)	57/96 (59%)
Callaway et al. (69)	VF: 15% PEA: 22% Asystole: 50%	Vasopressin 40 units or placebo as soon as possible after the first dose of epinephrine 1 mg	325	52/167 (31%)	48/158 (30%)
Gueugniaud et al. (70)	VF: 9% PEA: 8% Asystole: 83%	Epinephrine 1 mg followed by vasopressin 40 units (< 10 s apart) vs. epinephrine alone for two doses	2,894	413/1,442 (29%)	428/1,452 (30%)
Mentzelopoulos et al. (71)	VF/PVT: 14% PEA: 25% Asystole: 61%	Vasopressin 20 units + epinephrine 1 mg + methylprednisolone 40 mg (vasopressin + epinephrine were repeated during each of four subsequent CPR cycles vs. epinephrine 1 mg) vs. epinephrine 1 mg	100	39/48 (81%)a	27/52 (52%)
Mukoyama et al. (72)	VF: 24% Asystole/PEA: 76%	Vasopressin 40 units vs. epinephrine 1 mg for a maximum of four doses	336	51/178 (29%)	42/158 (27%)
Ong et al. (73)	VF/PVT: 8% PEA: 20% Asystole: 72%	Vasopressin 40 units vs. epinephrine 1 mg	727	119/374 (32%)	106/353 (30%)

26%; p=0.002), hospital admission rate (26% vs. 16%; p=0.002), and discharge rate (6.2% vs. 1.7%; p=0.002) with vasopressin. There was a trend, however, toward a poorer neurologic state or coma among the patients who survived to discharge and received vasopressin. A systematic review and analysis was conducted stemming from the data at the time looking at five randomized controlled trials comparing vasopressin and epinephrine in SCA.[74] No statistically significant differences were observed between the two agents with respect to ROSC, death, or neurologic impairment in survivors. Further subgroup analysis by presenting rhythm also failed to show any differences between vasopressin and epinephrine.

Given the evidence to date, several investigations tested the hypothesis of combined therapy (vasopressin plus epinephrine) versus epinephrine alone.[69,70] In one trial, patients who had received more than one dose of epinephrine during CPR for out-of-hospital SCA were randomized to vasopressin (40 units, n=167) or placebo (n=158). No differences were found between groups with respect to ROSC, nor was response according to initial cardiac rhythm different between groups.[70] The second trial was also of patients with out-of-hospital arrest who were randomized to either successive doses of vasopressin 40 units and epinephrine 1 mg (n=1,442) or epinephrine 1 mg and placebo (n=1,452). No statistically significant differences in survival to hospital admission were seen between the combination groups and the epinephrine-only group (20.7% vs. 21.3%), or in ROSC (28.6% vs. 29.5%), or survival to hospital discharge (37.5% vs. 51.5%).[69] One study evaluated a multidrug regimen that also included corticosteroids for patients with in-hospital cardiac arrest.[71]

In this study, patients were randomized to receive either epinephrine alone or 20 units of vasopressin plus 1 mg of epinephrine and 40 mg of methylprednisolone (followed by hydrocortisone in the post-resuscitative phase). Vasopressin 20 units plus epinephrine 1 mg was repeated during each of four subsequent CPR cycles. This study marks the first to include corticosteroids as part of drug therapy during CPR. The rationale is based on the hemodynamic effects of steroids alone with their potential to affect the intensity of the post-resuscitation systemic inflammatory response and organ dysfunction. Significant benefits were observed in ROSC (81% vs. 52%, p=0.003) and survival to hospital discharge (19% vs. 4%, p=0.02) with combination therapy including corticosteroids. Future studies are required to determine the role of vasopressin and corticosteroids for cardiac arrest.

In lieu of the conflicting results across many randomized controlled trials, a meta-analysis was performed to further define the role of vasopressin.[75] Six studies were chosen for analysis (four out-of-hospital arrests and two in-hospital arrests) including 4,745 patients. No significant improvements were noted with vasopressin therapy in ROSC (OR [95% CI] 1.25 [0.9–1.74]), long-term survival (OR [95% CI] 1.13 [0.71–1.78]), or favorable neurologic outcome (OR [95% CI] 0.87 [0.49–1.52]). When patients were stratified according to the presence of VF/PVT as their initial rhythm, the incidence of ROSC (OR [95% CI] 1.18 [0.82–1.69]) and long-term survival (OR [95% CI] 0.95 [0.66–1.37]) was similar with vasopressin. Of note, in patients with asystole, vasopressin was associated with superior long-term survival rates relative to control (OR [95% CI] 1.8 [1.04–3.12]).

In summary, existing evidence has not consistently shown an advantage of vasopressin to epinephrine in patients with SCA. As such, in the 2010 guidelines, one single dose of vasopressin 40 units given intravenously/intraosseously can be considered as an alternative to either the first or the second dose of epinephrine. Because repeated doses of vasopressin seem to lack benefit, they are not recommended. However, one major change in the 2015 update was the removal of vasopressin from the ACLS cardiac arrest algorithm recognizing the equivalence of effects with epinephrine.[22,28] This change is likely to generate some controversy, given the data supporting the use of vasopressin in SCA and the time and resources it may take to effectively remove vasopressin as an option to use in SCA, including the education of health care professionals. Although vasopressin is no longer an option in the 2015 updated recommendations, the available scientific data nonetheless support the recommendations in the 2010 guidelines. In addition, future prospective trials are needed to validate the role of vasopressin in certain subpopulations (e.g., asystole) or when combined with corticosteroids.

Antiarrhythmics

Administering antiarrhythmic agents is considered second line to using vasopressor therapy after unsuccessful defibrillation attempts. Conceptually, antiarrhythmic agents prevent the development or recurrence of VF and PVT by raising the defibrillation threshold. Despite their inclusion in the resuscitation guidelines, evidence is lacking that using antiarrhythmic agents improves survival to hospital discharge. Current guidelines recommend using a single agent, if possible, to mitigate the potential for adverse effects if the patient is resuscitated.[76]

Historically, lidocaine was considered the preferred antiarrhythmic agent for SCA because of its perceived lower risk of adverse events compared with procainamide, as well as available animal studies showing lidocaine's ability to raise the defibrillation threshold and prevent post-MI VF.[33,77] Only one retrospective analysis associated lidocaine use with improved hospital admission rates in patients with out-of-hospital SCA.[78] However, other published trials have not identified a benefit for lidocaine with respect to ROSC, or survival to hospital admission or discharge.[77,79] Given the lack of evidence to support a benefit for lidocaine to improve outcomes, it is currently recommended only when amiodarone is not available.

Amiodarone is the recommended antiarrhythmic in patients with VF or PVT who are unresponsive to CPR, defibrillation, and vasopressor therapy. Amiodarone is useful for both atrial and ventricular arrhythmias because of its many actions on sodium, potassium, and calcium channels as well as its β_1-adrenergic receptors. Amiodarone is classified as a class III antiarrhythmic, but it has electrophysiologic characteristics of all four Vaughan Williams classifications. Available clinical trial data showing that amiodarone improves the rate of ROSC and survival to hospital admission make it the first-line antiarrhythmic agent in patients with SCA having VF or PVT.

Initial evidence supporting the use of amiodarone came in 1999 with publication of the ARREST trial.[80] Five hundred four patients with out-of-hospital SCA secondary to VF or PVT were randomized in a double-blind fashion to receive either amiodarone 300 mg or placebo after having received epinephrine 1 mg and three unsuccessful defibrillation attempts. Recipients of amiodarone were more likely to be resuscitated and survive to hospital admission (44% vs. 34%, p=0.03), but there was no difference in survival to hospital discharge (13.4% vs. 13.2%, p=NS). A subsequent trial (known as the ALIVE trial) compared amiodarone 5 mg/kg with lidocaine 1.5 mg/kg in patients with out-of-hospital cardiac arrest caused by VF.[81] After three unsuccessful defibrillations as well as a single dose of epinephrine (1 mg), followed by another defibrillation attempt, patients received randomized antiarrhythmic therapy. Amiodarone was associated with a relative improvement of 90% in survival to hospital admission compared with lidocaine (22.8% vs. 12%; OR 2.17 [95% CI, 1.21–3.83]; p=0.009). Similar to the ARREST trial, there was no difference in survival to hospital discharge (amiodarone 5% vs. lidocaine 3%; p=0.34). Survival to hospital admission was highly dependent on the time from initiation of resuscitation efforts, with amiodarone having no benefit over lidocaine when antiarrhythmic therapy was administered more than 24 minutes from initiation of resuscitation. Amiodarone and lidocaine have also been compared in patients after in-hospital cardiac arrest. In a multicenter, retrospective review, 194 patients with VF or PVT who received amiodarone (n=74), lidocaine (n=79), or both (n=41) were evaluated.[82] The survival rates at 24 hours were 55%, 63%, and 50% for patients receiving amiodarone, lidocaine, or both, respectively (p=0.39). There was no difference in survival to hospital discharge (amiodarone 39%; lidocaine 45%; both 42%; p=0.72). After adjusting for multiple covariates, Cox regression analysis revealed higher survival to 24 hours (hazard ratio [HR] [95% CI] 3.15 [1.68–5.92], p<0.001) and hospital discharge (HR [95% CI] 3.25 [1.22–8.65], p=0.02) in patients who received lidocaine than in those who received amiodarone. The mean initial dose of amiodarone, though, was 190 mg, and only 25% of patients received the recommended dose of 300 mg.

Adverse effects of amiodarone encountered in cardiac arrest include hypotension and bradycardia.[22,28] Amiodarone's adverse hemodynamic effects are primarily attributed to vasoactive solvents, namely polysorbate 80 and benzyl alcohol. A formulation of amiodarone exists that does not contain these solvents, and adverse hemodynamic effects appear to be minimized.[83] Nevertheless, administering a vasoconstrictor before amiodarone can potentially prevent hypotension.

Amiodarone should be administered as a 300-mg bolus after unsuccessful defibrillation and the administration of one dose of epinephrine. A supplemental dose of 150 mg by intravenous bolus can be considered if resuscitation attempts are still unsuccessful. If ROSC is achieved, a 1-mg/minute intravenous infusion for 6 hours should be implemented, followed by a maintenance infusion of 0.5 mg/minute. If amiodarone is unavailable, lidocaine can be administered at a dose of 1–1.5 mg/kg. Additional doses of 0.5–0.75 mg/kg can be considered up to a maximum dose of 3 mg/kg if VF or PVT persists. If ROSC is achieved, a maintenance infusion of 1–4 mg/minute is recommended, with a reduction to 1–2 mg/minute in patients with underlying hepatic dysfunction.[22,76]

Magnesium

Severe hypomagnesemia has been associated with VF/PVT, but routine administration of magnesium during a cardiac arrest has shown no benefit in clinical outcome. Three randomized placebo-controlled trials failed to identify a benefit for magnesium to improve outcomes in SCA caused by VF in the prehospital, intensive care unit, or emergency department environments.[84-86]

Two observational trials, though, have noted an improvement in ROSC in patients with arrests associated with torsades de pointes who received a 1- to 2-g bolus of magnesium by intravenous push.[87,88] Therefore, magnesium administration should only be administered to these patients.

Thrombolysis

Myocardial infarction or pulmonary embolism is often the underlying cause for many SCAs because such thrombolytics have been evaluated during CPR in the management of SCA. Earlier smaller studies have shown some benefit with their use, but in the two largest randomized controlled trials, no difference was noted. In the first, 233 patients with PEA were randomized to receive either tissue plasminogen activator (tPA) or placebo.[79] The proportion of patients with ROSC was 21.4% and 23.3% for tPA- and placebo-treated patients, respectively. There was no significant difference in hemorrhage rates. The second study randomized patients with out-of-hospital cardiac arrest to receive either tenecteplase or placebo.[78] After a blinded review by the data and safety monitoring board, the criteria for futility were met, and enrollment was terminated. A total of 1,050 patients were analyzed, and both ROSC (tenecteplase, 55% vs. placebo, 55%; p=0.96) and survival to hospital discharge (tenecteplase, 15.1% vs. placebo, 17.5%, p=0.33) were similar between groups. Furthermore, the incidence of intracranial hemorrhage was significantly greater with tenecteplase than with placebo (2.7% vs. 0.4%, p=0.006). Given these results, fibrinolytic therapy should not be used routinely in cardiac arrest; however, when pulmonary embolism is presumed (or known) to be the cause, fibrinolytics can be considered.[22]

Therapies with No Role or Potential Harm

Sodium bicarbonate has historically been used to correct acidosis in the setting of SCA. Cardiac arrest produces acidemia secondary to low blood flow and hypoxemia. Important considerations include that acidosis impairs receptor responsiveness to adrenergic agents, may impair defibrillation, impairs myocardial contractility, and reduces the rate of ROSC and short-term survival. As such, it was thought that correcting acidosis using buffering agents might improve outcomes. However, using sodium bicarbonate during resuscitation efforts is now recognized to have no positive effect and may, in fact, have deleterious effects. One prospective randomized controlled trial of 502 patients with out-of-hospital cardiac arrest secondary to VF or asystole provided mixed results. Administering 250 mL of a buffer solution resulted in no improvements in ROSC or survival to discharge.[33] A second prospective controlled trial of 874 out-of-hospital patients with

SCA administered a 1-mEq/kg dose of bicarbonate or placebo showed no difference in survival in the trial overall; however, in patients with prolonged arrest (greater than 15 minutes), there was a trend for increased survival (32.8% vs. 15.4%) with bicarbonate administration.[89] In contrast, several data sources suggest that bicarbonate administration results in worse outcomes.[90-93] Exogenous administration of sodium bicarbonate has several potential disadvantages, including inducing extracellular alkalosis, exacerbating alkalemia, and inhibiting the release of oxygen. It may also lead to hyperosmolality and hypernatremia. Given these potential drawbacks and the preponderance of data suggesting harm, the routine use of sodium bicarbonate is strongly discouraged. However, sodium bicarbonate may still be considered in specific situations, which will be discussed later.[33]

Outside the management of hyperkalemia, the exogenous administration of calcium in the management of SCA is rarely needed. Clinical trials have found variable effects on ROSC, and no trials have shown a benefit on survival either to hospital admission or to discharge. As such, routine administration is not recommended.[90] Although atropine is present in previous versions of the ACLS guidelines, the 2010 update withdrew atropine as a recommendation in the management of VF/PVT. Removal was based on the lack of any high-quality evidence defining a benefit for atropine in SCA.[33]

PEA and Asystole

Pulseless electrical activity is defined as the absence of a detectable pulse and the presence of some type of electrical activity other than VF or PVT. Available studies indicate that patients with PEA actually have mechanical cardiac contractions, but they are too weak to produce a palpable pulse or blood pressure. Although PEA is still classified as a "rhythm of survival," the success rate of treatment is much lower than the rates seen with VF/PVT.[94] Asystole is commonly the end-stage terminal rhythm that is observed in attempted but unsuccessful resuscitation for VF/PVT or PEA. It is typically viewed as a confirmation of death as opposed to a rhythm to be treated, given that the survival rate is only 1 or 2 patients in 100.

Nonpharmacologic Therapy

Both PEA and asystole are considered non-shockable rhythms, and when they are identified in the course of resuscitation, high-quality CPR should be resumed immediately for 2 minutes before checking a rhythm again. Although defibrillation has no role in managing these rhythms, the most important intervention in PEA arrest is to identify and treat the underlying cause. Many conditions that inhibit effective cardiac contraction may lead to PEA arrest, and correcting these conditions is vital to improving survival. Suspected causes should be investigated while the patient receives high-quality CPR. The "Hs and Ts" (see Table 34.2) are the most common causes of PEA/asystole arrest, and if identified, rapid management of these conditions should ensue. Airway management should also be a priority in managing asystole/PEA arrest, given that hypoxemia is likely an underlying factor.[22,28,33]

Pharmacologic Therapy

Vasopressors

The primary pharmacologic agents that can be considered in treating asystole or PEA are epinephrine and vasopressin, although similar to patients with VT/VF, the use of vasopressin is no longer recommended in PEA/asystole according to the 2015 AHA guideline update. Although no studies evaluate these therapies solely in patients with asystole or PEA, these rhythms represent those of most patients included in clinical trials.[57] In an observational trial where the first documented rhythm was PEA or asystole, epinephrine was associated with a significant improvement in ROSC, but 1-month survival and survival with good neurologic function were lower with epinephrine.[57] In contrast, in a subgroup analysis of a randomized controlled trial comparing epinephrine with placebo, higher rates of ROSC and survival to hospital admission were observed with epinephrine in patients with non-shockable rhythms.[95]

Vasopressin has also had variable results in currently available studies. In a post hoc subgroup analysis of patients with out-of-hospital arrest and asystole as the first identified rhythm, survival rates to hospital admission (29% vs. 20%, p=0.02) and discharge (4.7% vs. 1.5%, p=0.04) were significantly higher with vasopressin than with epinephrine.[66] There was, however, a nonstatistically significant increase in coma/vegetative state with vasopressin (40% vs. 0%, p=0.14). Similar findings were cited in a meta-analysis of randomized controlled trials comparing vasopressin with control.[72] Patients with asystole who were administered the study drug within 20 minutes had higher rates of ROSC (OR [95% CI] 1.7 [1.17–2.47]) and long-term survival (OR [95% CI] 2.84 [1.19–6.79]). However, one randomized controlled trial that evaluated combination therapy with vasopressin and epinephrine reported no advantage with vasopressin in patients with asystole.[71] In fact, a post hoc subgroup analysis of patients with PEA as the initial rhythm showed a lower survival rate (0% vs. 5.8%, p=0.02) with combination therapy than with epinephrine alone.

Similar to the management of VF/PVT, epinephrine 1 mg intravenously/intraosseously is recommended in the management of PEA/asystole. In the 2010 AHA guidelines, vasopressin 40 units intravenously/intraosseously could replace the first or second dose of epinephrine, although as previously mentioned, this is removed from the 2015 update. However, as in VT/VF, the scientific literature available would still support vasopressin as an option for use.[22,28]

Atropine

Similar to the management of VF/PVT, one agent that is no longer recommended in the setting of PEA or asystole is atropine.[28] Atropine is an antimuscarinic agent that blocks the depressant effect of acetylcholine on both heart rate and atrioventricular nodal conduction, thus decreasing parasympathetic tone. No prospective controlled trials show benefit from atropine for the treatment of asystole or PEA, and conflicting evidence exists across retrospective and observational reports. Therefore, atropine should not routinely be administered in this setting.

Acid/Base

As discussed previously, sodium bicarbonate was once given routinely to reduce the detrimental effects associated with acidosis (e.g., reduced myocardial contractility), enhance the effect of epinephrine, and improve the rate of defibrillation, but few clinical data support its use, and in fact, routine muse maybe harmful.[89,96] Sodium bicarbonate can be used in special circumstances, which may more likely be encountered with PEA/asystolic arrest (i.e., underlying metabolic acidosis, hyperkalemia, salicylate overdose, or tricyclic antidepressant overdose); however, the dosage should be guided by laboratory analysis, if possible. Tromethamine (THAM) is an alternative buffering agent that acts as a proton acceptor, but there is a dearth of clinical experience with this agent in cardiac arrest, and outcome studies are not currently available.[28]

POST-RESUSCITATION CARE

General Measures

During the past decade, there has been increasing recognition that systematic post-cardiac arrest care is vital to increasing the likelihood of survival and increasing quality of life.[29] Survivors of SCA have a high mortality rate within the first 24 hours as the unstable myocardium tries to mitigate any ischemia and reperfusion injury. As patients convalesce beyond 24 hours, they are susceptible to sepsis and multiorgan dysfunction that may lead to shock, all the while being at risk of SCA recurrence.[97] The four main components of postcardiac arrest syndrome highlighting succinct pathophysiologic processes and potential areas for treatment include postcardiac arrest brain injury, myocardial dysfunction, systemic ischemia/reperfusion response, and persistent precipitating pathology. Management of multiorgan dysfunction and potential central nervous system injury during post-arrest care has the potential to reduce mortality.[29,97] After ROSC, adequate airway and oxygenation must be ensured. Additional post-arrest measures include appropriate fluid resuscitation and correction of electrolyte and acid-base imbalances. Appropriate intensive care unit measures include raising the head of the bed to 30 degrees (if this can be tolerated hemodynamically) to reduce the risk of aspiration, ventilator-associated pneumonia, and cerebral edema. Because the most common cause of cardiac arrest is ischemia, a rapid search for electrocardiographic (ECG) changes consistent with acute MI should be undertaken as soon as possible in the post-arrest time interval.[98] If an acute MI is present, urgent revascularization should be enacted immediately. Hemodynamic instability may be present post-arrest, necessitating the implementation of vasoactive drug therapy to improve cardiac output and/or address inappropriate vasodilation. Few data exist regarding which vasoactive agents are preferred in the post-cardiac arrest period. Reasonable goals for adequate hemodynamic status include a mean arterial pressure greater than 65 mm Hg and a venous oxygen saturation greater than 70%.[29]

Therapeutic Hypothermia

Targeted temperature management has become a vital intervention to improve outcomes in patients who are resuscitated from SCA but remain comatose. Temperature elevations after SCA can impair neurologic recovery, potentially through the release of inflammatory cytokines. Restoring blood flow after cardiac arrest can lead to several chemical cascades and destructive enzymatic reactions that can result in cerebral injury. These reactions include free radical production, excitatory amino acid release, and calcium shifts, which ultimately lead to mitochondrial damage and apoptosis.[99] Case series and clinical studies that showed an association between pyrexia of 37.6°C and higher and worsening survival laid the foundation for investigating induced hypothermia as a therapeutic intervention in SCA survivors. Hypothermia can protect from cerebral injury by suppressing these chemical reactions, thereby reducing the production of free radicals.[33] Various animal models have shown improved functional recovery and reduced cerebral deficits with the induction of mild therapeutic hypothermia.[100]

The first success with hypothermia was described in two pivotal trials.[101,102] In the first study, resuscitated patients after VF cardiac arrest who remained comatose were randomized to undergo therapeutic hypothermia, targeting a temperature of 32°C–34°C (89.6°F–93.2°F), for 24 hours or no intervention.[101] The primary end point was neurologic outcome within 6 months of cardiac arrest. Secondary end points were mortality (within 6 months) and complication rate within 7 days. A favorable neurologic outcome was achieved in 55% of patients in the hypothermia group as opposed to 39% in the normothermia group (p=0.009). In addition, mortality rates were improved significantly in the hypothermia group (41% vs. 55%; p=0.02). The incidence of complications (e.g., bleeding, pneumonia, sepsis, and renal failure) did not differ between the two groups (73% for the hypothermia group and 70% for the normothermia group; p=0.70). Entry criteria in the second trial were similar to those in the previous trial, but the target temperature for hypothermia was 33°C (91.4°F), which was maintained for 12 hours.[102] The primary outcome measure was survival to hospital discharge with good neurologic function. Forty-nine percent of patients in the hypothermia group had good neurologic function on discharge (either to home or to a rehabilitation facility) compared with 26% of patients in the normothermia group (p=0.046). Mortality rates were similar between the two groups (51% for the hypothermia group and 68% for the normothermia group; p=0.145). Hypothermia was associated with a lower cardiac index, higher systemic vascular resistance, and hyperglycemia.

Data on therapeutic hypothermia have continued to accumulate since the publication of these landmark trials. These include studies of arrests caused by rhythms other than VF. Two nonrandomized trials found benefit for therapeutic hypothermia in improving neurologic function in patients presenting with PEA/asystolic arrest.[103,104] An additional study showed that therapeutic hypothermia (combined with percutaneous coronary intervention, tight glycemic control, and seizure control) doubled the 1-year survival rate (reportedly with good brain function) from 26% to 56%.[105] The implementation of therapeutic hypothermia in clinical practice (i.e., outside the context of a clinical trial) has also been evaluated. A review of this topic found significant variation in reported protocols but showed that survival and neurologic outcomes benefit from post-arrest hypothermia and "are robust when compared over a wide range of studies of actual implementation" (OR [95% CI] 2.5 [1.8–3.3]).[106] No method for achieving targeted temperature control has been shown to be the most appropriate for use. Main methods currently in use include cold-water immersion, endovascular cooling catheters, and surface-cooling devices.[29] After the cooling period, patients should undergo a controlled rewarming period at 0.5°C–1°C every hour until normal core temperature is reached.

After a review of the available data to date, the current guidelines recommend that unconscious adult patients with spontaneous circulation after out-of-hospital cardiac arrest be cooled to 32°C–36°C for at least 24 hours.[29,107] This is particularly true of VF arrest (class I recommendation; level of evidence B). There is less robust evidence for other arrests, but according to the guidelines, hypothermia should be considered for comatose adult patients with ROSC after in-hospital cardiac arrest with any rhythm and/or out-of-hospital cardiac arrest with an initial rhythm of PEA (class IIb recommendation; level of evidence B).

Pharmacists play an important role in optimizing outcomes with patients receiving therapeutic hypothermia post-SCA. Ensuring that adequate analgesia and sedation therapy is being provided as well as that neuromuscular blocking agents are being used appropriately are areas where pharmacists can have a direct impact on optimizing care. Several complications such as coagulopathy, dysrhythmias, hyperglycemia, increased incidence of pneumonia, and sepsis may occur as a result of induced hypothermia, and appropriate interventions should be at the forefront of daily assessment and development of pharmacotherapy plans for these patients. In addition, hypothermia can have profound effects on drug distribution and elimination.[108] Although the duration of hypothermia is typically short, careful monitoring during this period is necessary, particularly with vasoactive agents.

CONCLUSIONS

Despite the available treatments for patients with SCA, survival remains low. Interventions that prevent the occurrence of SCA in the first place are likely the most effective means of reducing mortality. When SCA occurs, high-quality CPR is crucial to the success of any subsequent ACLS interventions. In patients with VF/PVT as the initial cardiac rhythm, defibrillation should be implemented rapidly with minimal interruptions to chest compressions in order to optimize outcomes. In the setting of unsuccessful defibrillation attempts, pharmacologic therapy can increase the ROSC and survival to hospital admission but, unfortunately, does not translate to improved long-term survival. Implementing high-quality post-arrest care, including therapeutic hypothermia, increases the likelihood of long-term survival with good neurologic recovery.

REFERENCES

1. Yousuf O, Chrispin J, Tomaselli GF, et al. Clinical management and prevention of sudden cardiac death. Circ Res 2015;116:2020-40.

2. Sandroni C, Nolan J, Cavallaro F, et al. In-hospital cardiac arrest: incidence, prognosis and possible measures to improve survival. Intensive Care Med 2007;33:237-45.

3. Strategies to Improve Cardiac Arrest Survival: A Time to Act. Available at www.iom.edu/CardiacArrestSurvival. Accessed August 30, 2015.

4. Daya MR, Schmicker RH, May S, et al. Current Burden of Cardiac Arrest in the United States. Available at http://iom.nationalacademies.org/~/media/Files/Report%20Files/2015/ROC.pdf. Accessed August 30, 2015

5. Chan PS. Public health burden of in-hospital cardiac arrest. Available at http://iom.nationalacademies.org/~/media/Files/Report%20Files/2015/GWTG.pdf. Accessed August 30, 2015.

6. Travers AH, Rea TD, Bobrow BJ, et al. Part 4: CPR overview: 2010 American Heart Association guidelines for cardiopulmonary resuscitation and emergency cardiovascular care. Circulation 2010;122:S676-S684.

7. Sasson C, Rogers MA, Dahl J, et al. Predictors of survival from out-of-hospital cardiac arrest: a systematic review and meta-analysis. Circ Cardiovasc Qual Outcomes 2010;3:63-81.

8. Hayashi M, Shimizu W, Albert CM. The spectrum of epidemiology underlying sudden cardiac death. Circ Res 2015;116:1887-906.

9. Weil MH, Tang W. Rhythms and outcomes of cardiac arrest. Crit Care Med 2010;38:310.

10. Nichol G, Thomas E, Callaway CW, et al. Regional variation in out-of-hospital cardiac arrest incidence and outcome. JAMA 2008;300:1423-31.

11. Weil MH, Fries M. In hospital cardiac arrest. Crit Care Med 2005;33:2825-30.

12. Bertoia ML, Allison MA, Manson JE, et al. Risk factors for sudden cardiac death in postmenopausal women. J Am Coll Cardiol 2012;60:2674.

13. Chugh SS, Jui J, Gunson K, et al. Current burden of sudden cardiac death: multiple source surveillance versus retrospective death certificate based review in a large U.S. community. J Am Coll Cardiol 2004;44:1268.

14. Myerburg RJ, Castellanos A. Emerging paradigms of the epidemiology and demographics of sudden cardiac arrest. Heart Rhythm 2006;3:235-9.

15. Myerburg RJ, Castellanos A. Cardiac arrest and sudden cardiac death. In: Mann DL, Zipes DP, Libby P, et al., eds. Braunwald's Heart Disease: A Textbook of Cardiovascular Medicine, 10th ed. Philadelphia: Elsevier, 2014:821-60.

16. Patil KD, Halperin HR, Becker LB. Cardiac arrest. Resuscitation and reperfusion. Circ Res 2015;116:2041-9.

17. Cooper JA, Cooper JD, Cooper JM. Cardiopulmonary resuscitation: history, current practice, and future direction. Circulation 2006;114:2839-49.

18. Berg MD, Schexnayder SM, Chameides L, et al. Part 13: pediatric basic life support: 2010 American Heart Association guidelines for cardiopulmonary resuscitation and emergency cardiovascular care. Circulation 2010;122:S862-S875.

19. Soar J, Edelson DP, Perkins GD. Delivering high quality cardiopulmonary resuscitation in hospital. Curr Opin Crit Care 2011;17:225-30.

20. Christenson J, Andrusiek D, Everson Stewart S, et al. Chest compression fraction determines survival in patients with out-of-hospital ventricular fibrillation. Circulation 2009;120:1241-7.

21. Cave DM, Gazmuri RJ, Otto CW, et al. Part 7: CPR techniques and devices: 2010 American Heart Association guidelines for cardiopulmonary resuscitation and emergency cardiovascular care. Circulation 2010;122:S720-S728.

22. Neumar RW, Shuster M, Callaway CW, et al. Part 1: executive summary. 2015 American Heart Association guidelines update for cardiopulmonary resuscitation and emergency cardiovascular care. Circulation 2015;132(suppl 2):S315-367.

23. Kouwenhoven WB, Jude JR, Knickerbocker GG. Closed chest cardiac massage. JAMA 1960;173:1064-7.

24. Cardiopulmonary resuscitation. JAMA 1966;198:372-9.

25. Larsen MP, Eisenberg MS, Cummins RO, et al. Predicting survival from out-of-hospital cardiac arrest: a graphic model. Ann Emerg Med 1993;22:1652-8.

26. Link MS, Atkins DL, Passman RS, et al. Part 6: electrical therapies: automated external defibrillators, defibrillation, cardioversion, and pacing: 2010 American Heart Association guidelines for cardiopulmonary resuscitation and emergency cardiovascular care. Circulation 2010;122:S706-S719.

27. Rea TD, Helbock M, Perry S, et al. Increasing use of cardiopulmonary resuscitation during out-of-hospital ventricular fibrillation arrest: survival implications of guideline changes. Circulation 2006;114:2760-5.

28. Neumar RW, Otto CW, Link MS, et al. Part 8: adult advanced cardiovascular life support: 2010 American Heart Association guidelines for cardiopulmonary resuscitation and emergency cardiovascular care. Circulation 2010;122:S729-S767.

29. Peberdy MA, Callaway CW, Neumar RW, et al. Part 9: postcardiac arrest care: 2010 American Heart Association guidelines for cardiopulmonary resuscitation and emergency cardiovascular care. Circulation 2010;122:S768-S786.

30. Berg RA, Hemphill R, Abella BS, et al. Part 5: adult basic life support: 2010 American Heart Association guidelines for cardiopulmonary resuscitation and emergency cardiovascular care. Circulation 2010;122:S685-S705.

31. Swor R, Khan I, Domeier R, et al. CPR training and CPR performance: do CPR trained bystanders perform CPR? Acad Emerg Med 2006;13:596-601.

32. Dager W, Bolesta S, Brophy G, et al. An opinion paper outlining recommendations for training, credentialing, documenting, and justifying critical care pharmacy services. Pharmacotherapy 2011;31:135e-75e.

33. Hesch KA. Cardiac arrest and advanced cardiac life support. In: Pharmacotherapy Self-Assessment Program (PSAP) 2014. Critical and Urgent Care. Kansas City, MO: American College of Clinical Pharmacy, 2014:3-24.

34. Weiser G, Hoffmann Y, Galbraith R, et al. Current advances in intraosseous infusion—a systematic review. Resuscitation 2012;83:20-6.

35. Hoskins SL, do Nascimento P Jr, Lima RM, et al. Pharmacokinetics of intraosseous and central venous drug delivery during cardiopulmonary resuscitation. Resuscitation 2012;83:107-12.

36. Weisfeldt ML, Becker LB. Resuscitation after cardiac arrest: a 3 phase time sensitive model. JAMA 2002;288:3035-8.

37. Cobb LA, Fahrenbruch CE, Walsh TR, et al. Influence of cardiopulmonary resuscitation prior to defibrillation in patients with out-of-hospital ventricular fibrillation. JAMA 1999;281:1182-8.

38. Wik L, Hansen TB, Fylling F, et al. Delaying defibrillation to give basic cardiopulmonary resuscitation to patients with out-of-hospital ventricular fibrillation: a randomized trial. JAMA 2003;289:1389-95.

39. Kellum MJ, Kennedy KW, Ewy GA. Cardiocerebral resuscitation improves survival of patients with out-of-hospital cardiac arrest. Am J Med 2006;119:335-40.

40. Garza AG, Gratton MC, Salomone JA, et al. Improved patient survival using a modified resuscitation protocol for out-of-hospital cardiac arrest. Circulation 2009;119:2597-605.

41. Koike S, Tanabe S, Ogawa T, et al. Immediate defibrillation or defibrillation after cardiopulmonary resuscitation. Prehosp Emerg Care 2011;15:393-400.

42. Valenzuela TD, Roe DJ, Nichol G, et al. Outcomes of rapid defibrillation by security officers after cardiac arrest in casinos. N Engl J Med 2000;343:1206-9.

43. Tuseth V, Salem M, Pettersen R, et al. Percutaneous left ventricular assist in ischemic cardiac arrest. Crit Care Med 2009;37:1365-72.

44. Sunde K. Experimental and clinical use of ongoing mechanical cardiopulmonary resuscitation during angiography and percutaneous coronary intervention. Crit Care Med 2008;36:S405-S408.

45. Varon J, Acosta P. Extracorporeal membrane oxygenation in cardiopulmonary resuscitation: are we there yet? Crit Care Med 2008;36:2685-6.

46. Chamberlain D, Frenneaux M, Fletcher D. The primacy of basics in advanced life support. Curr Opin Crit Care 2009;15:198-202.

47. Robinson LA, Brown CG, Jenkins J, et al. The effect of norepinephrine versus epinephrine on myocardial hemodynamics during CPR. Ann Emerg Med 1989;18:336-40.

48. Paradis NA, Martin GB, Rivers EP, et al. Coronary perfusion pressure and the return of spontaneous circulation in human cardiopulmonary resuscitation. JAMA 1990;263:1106-13.

49. Larabee TM, Liu KY, Campbell JA, et al. Vasopressors in cardiac arrest: a systematic review. Resuscitation 2012;83:932-9.

50. Ornato JP. Use of adrenergic agonists during CPR in adults. Ann Emerg Med 1993;22:411-6.

51. Brown C, Wiklund L, Bar-Joseph G, et al. Future directions for resuscitation research. IV. Innovative advanced life support pharmacology. Resuscitation 1996;33:163-77.

52. Callaham M, Madsen CD, Barton CW, et al. A randomized clinical trial of high dose epinephrine and norepinephrine vs standard dose epinephrine in prehospital cardiac arrest. JAMA 1992;268:2667-72.

53. Lindner KH, Ahnefeld FW, Grunert A. Epinephrine versus norepinephrine in prehospital ventricular fibrillation. Am J Cardiol 1991;67:427-8.

54. Attaran RR, Ewy GA. Epinephrine in resuscitation: curse or cure? Future Cardiol 2010;6:473-82.

55. Olasveengen TM, Sunde K, Brunborg C, et al. Intravenous drug administration during out-of-hospital cardiac arrest: a randomized trial. JAMA 2009;302:2222-9.

56. Jacobs IG, Finn JC, Jelinek GA, et al. Effect of adrenaline on survival in out-of-hospital cardiac arrest: a randomised double-blind placebo controlled trial. Resuscitation 2011;82:1138-43.

57. Hagihara A, Hasegawa M, Abe T, et al. Prehospital epinephrine use and survival among patients with out-of-hospital cardiac arrest. JAMA 2012;307:1161-8.

58. Ristagno G, Tang W, Huang L, et al. Epinephrine reduces cerebral perfusion during cardiopulmonary resuscitation. Crit Care Med 2009;37:1408-15.

59. Rivers EP, Wortsman J, Rady MY, et al. The effect of the total cumulative epinephrine dose administered during human CPR on hemodynamic, oxygen transport, and utilization variables in the postresuscitation period. Chest 1994;106:1499-507.

60. Woodhouse SP, Cox S, Boyd P, et al. High dose and standard dose adrenaline do not alter survival compared with placebo, in cardiac arrest. Resuscitation 1995;30:243-9.

61. Brown CG, Martin DR, Pepe PE, et al. A comparison of standard-dose and high-dose epinephrine in cardiac arrest outside the hospital. The Multicenter High-Dose Epinephrine Study Group. N Engl J Med 1992;327:1051-5.

62. Vandycke C, Martens P. High dose versus standard dose epinephrine in cardiac arrest—a meta-analysis. Resuscitation 2000;45:161-6.

63. Gueugniaud PY, Mols P, Goldstein P, et al.; European Epinephrine Study Group. A comparison of repeated high doses and repeated standard doses of epinephrine for cardiac arrest outside the hospital. N Engl J Med 1998;339:1595-601.

64. Wenzel V, Raab H, Dunser MW. Role of arginine vasopressin in the setting of cardiopulmonary resuscitation. Best Pract Res Clin Anaesthesiol 2008;22:287-97.

65. Lindner KH, Haak T, Keller A, et al. Release of endogenous vasopressors during and after cardiopulmonary resuscitation. Heart 1996;75:145-50.

66. Wenzel V, Krismer AC, Arntz HR, et al. A comparison of vasopressin and epinephrine for out-of-hospital cardiopulmonary resuscitation. N Engl J Med 2004;350:105-13.

67. Lindner KH, Dirks B, Strohmenger HU, et al. Randomised comparison of epinephrine and vasopressin in patients with out-of-hospital ventricular fibrillation. Lancet 1997;349:535-7.

68. Stiell IG, Hebert PC, Wells GA, et al. Vasopressin versus epinephrine for in hospital cardiac arrest: a randomised controlled trial. Lancet 2001;358:105-9.

69. Callaway CW, Hostler D, Doshi AA, et al. Usefulness of vasopressin administered with epinephrine during out-of-hospital cardiac arrest. Am J Cardiol 2006;98:1316-21.

70. Gueugniaud PY, David JS, Chanzy E, et al. Vasopressin and epinephrine vs. epinephrine alone in cardiopulmonary resuscitation. N Engl J Med 2008;359:21-30.

71. Mentzelopoulos SD, Zakynthinos SG, Tzoufi M, et al. Vasopressin, epinephrine, and corticosteroids for in-hospital cardiac arrest. Arch Intern Med 2009;169:15-24.

72. Mukoyama T, Kinoshita K, Nagao K, et al. Reduced effectiveness of vasopressin in repeated doses for patients undergoing prolonged cardiopulmonary resuscitation. Resuscitation 2009;80:755-61.

73. Ong ME, Tiah L, Leong BS, et al. A randomised, double-blind, multicenter trial comparing vasopressin and adrenaline in patients with cardiac arrest presenting to or in the emergency department. Resuscitation 2012;83:953-60.

74. Aung K, Htay T. Vasopressin for cardiac arrest: a systematic review and meta-analysis. Arch Intern Med 2005;165:17-24.

75. Mentzelopoulos SD, Zakynthinos SG, Siempos I, et al. Vasopressin for cardiac arrest: meta-analysis of randomized controlled trials. Resuscitation 2012;83:32-9.

76. Ong ME, Pellis T, Link MS. The use of antiarrhythmic drugs for adult cardiac arrest: a systematic review. Resuscitation 2011;82:665-70.

77. Harrison EE. Lidocaine in prehospital countershock refractory ventricular fibrillation. Ann Emerg Med 1981;10:420-3.

78. Herlitz J, Ekstrom L, Wennerblom B, et al. Lidocaine in out-of-hospital ventricular fibrillation. Does it improve survival? Resuscitation 1997;33:199-205.

79. Weaver WD, Fahrenbruch CE, Johnson DD, et al. Effect of epinephrine and lidocaine therapy on outcome after cardiac arrest due to ventricular fibrillation. Circulation 1990;82:2027-34.

80. Kudenchuk PJ, Cobb LA, Copass MK, et al. Amiodarone for resuscitation after out-of-hospital cardiac arrest due to ventricular fibrillation. N Engl J Med 1999;341:871-8.

81. Dorian P, Cass D, Schwartz B, et al. Amiodarone as compared with lidocaine for shock-resistant ventricular fibrillation. N Engl J Med 2002;346:884-90.

82. Rea RS, Kane Gill SL, Rudis MI, et al. Comparing intravenous amiodarone or lidocaine, or both, outcomes for inpatients with pulseless ventricular arrhythmias. Crit Care Med 2006;34:1617-23.

83. Somberg JC, Timar S, Bailin SJ, et al. Lack of hypotensive effect with rapid administration of a new aqueous formulation of intravenous amiodarone. Am J Cardiol 2004;93:576-81.

84. Allegra J, Lavery R, Cody R, et al. Magnesium sulfate in the treatment of refractory ventricular fibrillation in the prehospital setting. Resuscitation 2001;49:245-9.

85. Fatovich DM, Prentice DA, Dobb GJ. Magnesium in cardiac arrest (the magic trial). Resuscitation 1997;35:237-41.

86. Thel MC, Armstrong AL, McNulty SE, et al. Randomised trial of magnesium in in-hospital cardiac arrest. Lancet 1997;350:1272-6.

87. Manz M, Pfeiffer D, Jung W, et al. Intravenous treatment with magnesium in recurrent persistent ventricular tachycardia. New Trends Arrhythmias 1991;7:437-42.

88. Tzivoni D, Banai S, Schuger C, et al. Treatment of torsade de pointes with magnesium sulfate. Circulation 1988;77:392-7.

89. Vukmir RB, Katz L; Sodium Bicarbonate Study Group. Sodium bicarbonate improves outcome in prolonged prehospital cardiac arrest. Am J Emerg Med 2006;24:156-61.

90. van Walraven C, Stiell IG, Wells GA, et al. Do advanced cardiac life support drugs increase resuscitation rates from in hospital cardiac arrest? The OTAC Study Group. Ann Emerg Med 1998;32:544-53.

91. Skovron ML, Goldberg E, Suljaga-Petchel K, et al. Factors predicting survival for six months after cardiopulmonary resuscitation: multivariate analysis of a prospective study. Mt Sinai J Med 1985;52:271-5.

92. Roberts D, Landolfo K, Light R, et al. Early predictors of mortality for hospitalized patients suffering cardiopulmonary arrest. Chest 1990;97:413-9.

93. Delooz HH, Lewi PJ. Are inter-center differences in EMS-management and sodium-bicarbonate administration important for the outcome of CPR? The Cerebral Resuscitation Study Group. Resuscitation 1989;17(suppl):S161-72.

94. Nadkarni VM, Larkin GL, Peberdy MA, et al. First documented rhythm and clinical outcome from in-hospital cardiac arrest among children and adults. JAMA 2006;295:50-7.

95. Sutton RM, Berg RA, Helfaer MA. Epinephrine for resuscitation from cardiac arrest: a double-edged sword? Crit Care Med 2009;37:1518-20.

96. Bjerneroth G. Tribonat—a comprehensive summary of its properties. Crit Care Med 1999;27:1009-13.

97. Neumar RW, Nolan JP, Adrie C, et al. Postcardiac arrest syndrome: epidemiology, pathophysiology, treatment, and prognostication. A consensus statement from the International Liaison Committee on Resuscitation (American Heart Association, Australian and New Zealand Council on Resuscitation, European Resuscitation Council, Heart and Stroke Foundation of Canada, InterAmerican Heart Foundation, Resuscitation Council of Asia, and the Resuscitation Council of Southern Africa); the American Heart Association Emergency Cardiovascular Care Committee; the Council on Cardiovascular Surgery and Anesthesia; the Council on Cardiopulmonary, Perioperative, and Critical Care; the Council on Clinical Cardiology; and the Stroke Council. Circulation 2008;118:2452-83.

98. Anyfantakis ZA, Baron G, Aubry P, et al. Acute coronary angiographic findings in survivors of out-of-hospital cardiac arrest. Am Heart J 2009;157:312-8.

99. Nolan JP, Morley PT, Vanden Hoek TL, et al. Therapeutic hypothermia after cardiac arrest: an advisory statement by the advanced life support task force of the International Liaison Committee on Resuscitation. Circulation 2003;108:118-21.

100. Safar P, Xiao F, Radovsky A, et al. Improved cerebral resuscitation from cardiac arrest in dogs with mild hypothermia plus blood flow promotion. Stroke 1996;27:105-13.

101. Hypothermia After Cardiac Arrest Study Group. Mild therapeutic hypothermia to improve the neurologic outcome after cardiac arrest. N Engl J Med 2002;346:549-56.

102. Bernard SA, Gray TW, Buist MD, et al. Treatment of comatose survivors of out-of-hospital cardiac arrest with induced hypothermia. N Engl J Med 2002;346:557-63.

103. Holzer M, Mullner M, Sterz F, et al. Efficacy and safety of endovascular cooling after cardiac arrest: cohort study and Bayesian approach. Stroke 2006;37:1792-7.

104. Arrich J. Clinical application of mild therapeutic hypothermia after cardiac arrest. Crit Care Med 2007;35:1041-7.

105. Sunde K, Pytte M, Jacobsen D, et al. Implementation of a standardized treatment protocol for post resuscitation care after out-of-hospital cardiac arrest. Resuscitation 2007;73:29-39.

106. Sagalyn E, Band RA, Gaieski DF, et al. Therapeutic hypothermia after cardiac arrest in clinical practice: review and compilation of recent experiences. Crit Care Med 2009;37:S223-S226.

107. Gaieski DF, Abella BS, Goyal M. CPR and post arrest care: overview, documentation, and databases. Chest 2012;141:1082-9.

108. Arpino PA, Greer DM. Practical pharmacologic aspects of therapeutic hypothermia after cardiac arrest. Pharmacotherapy 2008;28:102-11.

Chapter 35: Acute Management of Arrhythmias

James E. Tisdale, Pharm.D., FCCP, FAPhA, FAHA, BCPS

LEARNING OBJECTIVES

1. Describe features, epidemiology, pathophysiology, etiologies, risk factors, and morbidity and mortality associated with sinus bradycardia and atrioventricular (AV) blocks.
2. Design patient-specific drug therapy and/or nonpharmacologic treatment plans for critically ill patients with sinus bradycardia or AV blocks.
3. Describe features, epidemiology, pathophysiology, etiologies, risk factors, and morbidity and mortality associated with paroxysmal supraventricular tachycardias (PSVTs).
4. Describe and differentiate between AV node reentrant tachycardia, AV reciprocating tachycardia, and atrial tachycardia.
5. Design patient-specific drug therapy and/or nonpharmacologic treatment plans for critically ill patients with PSVT without preexcitation.
6. Design patient-specific drug therapy and/or nonpharmacologic treatment plans for critically ill patients with PSVT with preexcitation.
7. Describe features, epidemiology, pathophysiology, etiologies, risk factors, and morbidity and mortality associated with atrial fibrillation (AF).
8. Design patient-specific drug therapy and/or nonpharmacologic treatment plans for critically ill patients with AF.
9. Design patient-specific drug therapy plans for prophylaxis of AF after coronary artery bypass graft surgery and noncardiac thoracic surgery.
10. Describe features, epidemiology, pathophysiology, etiologies, risk factors, and morbidity and mortality associated with monomorphic ventricular tachycardia (VT) with a pulse.
11. Design patient-specific drug therapy and/or nonpharmacologic treatment plans for critically ill patients with monomorphic VT with a pulse.
12. Describe features, epidemiology, pathophysiology, etiologies, risk factors, and morbidity and mortality associated with torsades de pointes (TdP).
13. Design patient-specific drug therapy and/or nonpharmacologic treatment plans for critically ill patients with TdP.

ABBREVIATIONS IN THIS CHAPTER

AF	Atrial fibrillation	HIE	Hyperinsulinemia-euglycemia
AT	Atrial tachycardia	ICU	Intensive care unit
AV	Atrioventricular	LQTS	Long QT syndrome
AVNRT	Atrioventricular node reentrant tachycardia	MI	Myocardial infarction
		PSVT	Paroxysmal supraventricular tachycardia
AVRT	Atrioventricular reciprocating tachycardia	SNPs	Single nucleotide polymorphisms
CABG	Coronary artery bypass graft	TEE	Transesophageal echocardiogram
CAST	Cardiac Arrhythmia Suppression Trial	TdP	Torsades de pointes
DCC	Direct current cardioversion	U.S.	United States
HF	Heart failure	VT	Ventricular tachycardia
HFrEF	Heart failure with reduced ejection fraction	WPW	Wolff-Parkinson-White (syndrome)

Box 35.1. Class of Recommendation and Levels of Evidence

In tables and figures, references are made to class of recommendation and levels of evidence. Those are defined as follows:

- Class I, IIa, IIb, or III = class of treatment recommendation from evidence-based and/or expert consensus-based treatment guidelines.
- Class I: Benefit >>> Risk; procedure/treatment should be administered.
- Class IIa: Benefit >> Risk; It is reasonable to perform procedure/administer treatment.
- Class IIb: Benefit ≥ Risk; Procedure/treatment may be considered.
- Class III: Risk ≥ Benefit: Procedure/treatment should not be performed/administered because it is not helpful and/or may be harmful.
- LOE = Level of evidence from evidence-based and/or expert consensus-based treatment guidelines.
- LOE A – Multiple populations evaluated; data derived from multiple randomized clinical trials or meta-analyses.
- LOE B – Limited populations evaluated; data derived from a single randomized trial or nonrandomized studies.
- LOE C – Very limited populations evaluated; only consensus opinion of experts, case studies, or standard of care.

SUPRAVENTRICULAR ARRHYTHMIAS

Bradycardias

Features

Normal heart rate is generally defined as 60–100 beats/minute. Sinus bradycardia is defined as a heart rate less than 60 beats/minute with otherwise normal sinus rhythm (Figure 35.1).[1] Atrioventricular (AV) node block (also known as AV block) is defined as delay in impulse conduction in the AV node or the bundle of His.[1] Atrioventricular block is categorized as first, second, or third degree, depending on the location of the conduction delay and the electrocardiogram (ECG) manifestation. First-degree AV block is defined as a PR interval greater than 0.2 second with 1:1 AV conduction (Figure 35.2). Second-degree AV block occurs when a proportion of impulses are not conducted through the AV node to the ventricles. Second-degree AV block occurs in two primary patterns. Mobitz type I second-degree AV block (also known as Wenckebach) is defined as a repeating pattern with a constant PP interval but with a progressively prolonging PR

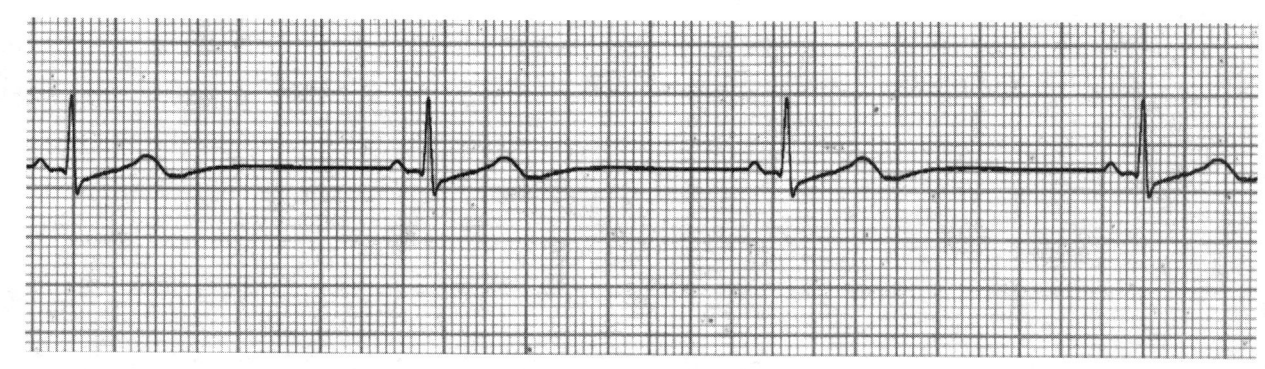

Figure 35.1 Sinus bradycardia.

Reprinted with permission from: Tisdale JE. Review of cardiac arrhythmias and rhythm interpretation. In: Wiggins BS, Sanoski CA. Emergency Cardiovascular Pharmacotherapy. A Point-of-Care Guide. Bethesda, MD: American Society of Health-System Pharmacists, 2012:27.

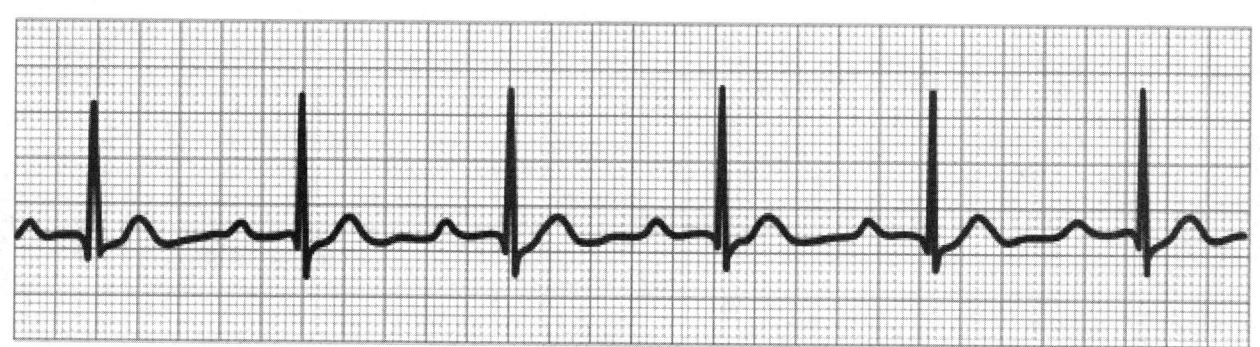

Figure 35.2 First-degree atrioventricular block.

Reprinted with permission from: Tisdale JE. Review of cardiac arrhythmias and rhythm interpretation. In: Wiggins BS, Sanoski CA. Emergency Cardiovascular Pharmacotherapy. A Point-of-Care Guide. Bethesda, MD: American Society of Health-System Pharmacists, 2012:29.

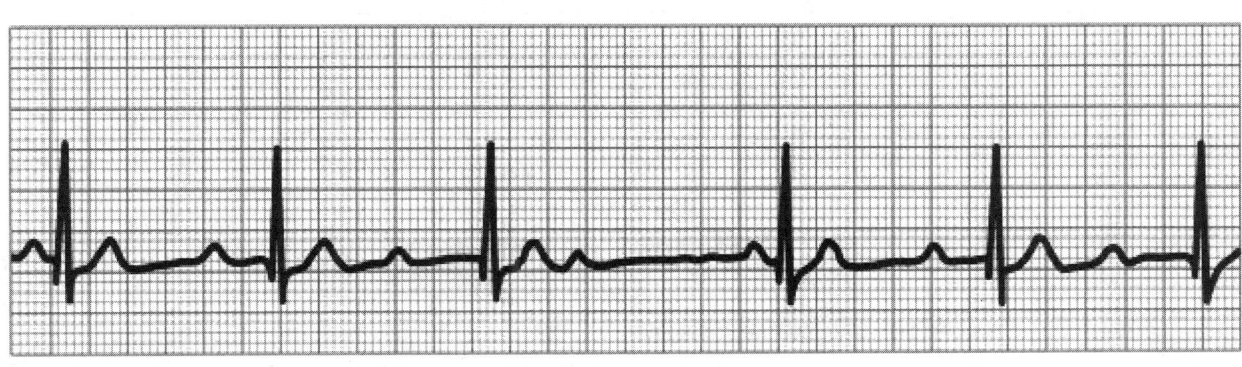

Figure 35.3 Second-degree atrioventricular block, Mobitz type I (Wenckebach).

Reprinted with permission from: Tisdale JE. Review of cardiac arrhythmias and rhythm interpretation. In: Wiggins BS, Sanoski CA. Emergency Cardiovascular Pharmacotherapy. A Point-of-Care Guide. Bethesda, MD: American Society of Health-System Pharmacists, 2012:29.

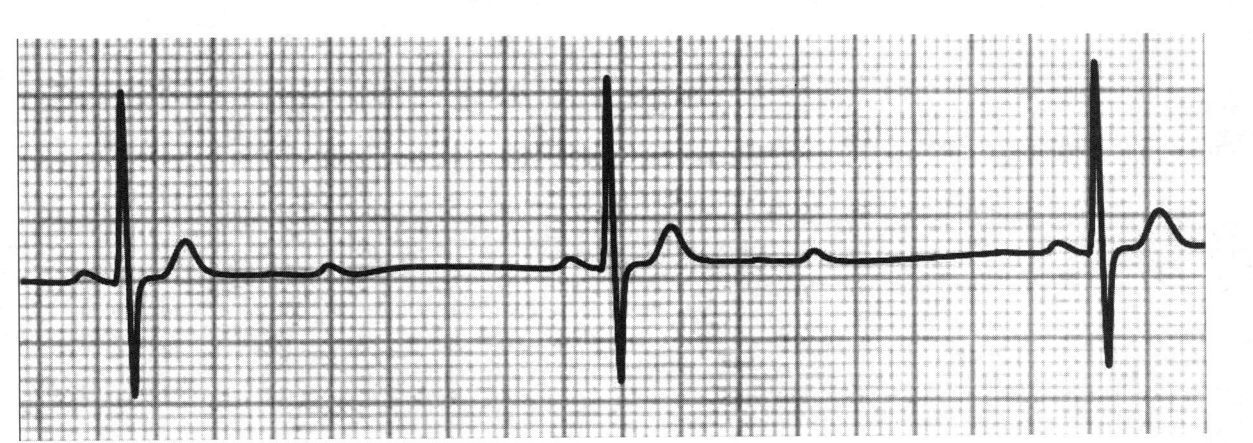

Figure 35.4 Second-degree atrioventricular block, Mobitz type II.

Reprinted with permission from: Tisdale JE. Review of cardiac arrhythmias and rhythm interpretation. In: Wiggins BS, Sanoski CA. Emergency Cardiovascular Pharmacotherapy. A Point-of-Care Guide. Bethesda, MD: American Society of Health-System Pharmacists, 2012:29.

interval until the impulse resulting in atrial depolarization (represented by the P wave) fails to be conducted through the AV node to the ventricles (Figure 35.3). Mobitz type II AV block is defined as a consistent PR interval until the impulse resulting in atrial depolarization (represented by the P wave) abruptly fails to be conducted (Figure 35.4). Third-degree AV block, also known as "complete heart block," represents AV dissociation, during which the AV node is impermeable to impulse conduction. Therefore, atrial and ventricular depolarization/contraction occur independently (Figure 35.5). QRS complexes may be narrow, reflecting block within the AV node, or wide, reflecting conduction block in the His-Purkinje system.

Epidemiology

Prevalence of the disease known as "sick sinus syndrome," which is associated with sinus bradycardia, is about 1 in 600 individuals older than 65 years.[1] Prevalence of Mobitz type II second-degree AV block is about 0.003%.[2] Prevalence of third-degree AV block is about 0.02%–0.04% in the general adult population.[2,3] In a study encompassing 1991–1998, sinus node dysfunction accounted for 13.2% of hospital discharges associated with arrhythmias in older adult patients; third-degree AV block accounted for 5.8%, and Mobitz type I second-degree AV block accounted for 1.4%.[4]

Clinically relevant bradycardia, excluding transient episodes, accounts for about 10% of the arrhythmias in patients in intensive care units (ICUs).[5,6] Of bradycardia episodes occurring in ICUs, third-degree AV block constitutes about 31%, with the remainder including asystole (28%), sinus bradycardia (6%), second-degree AV block (6%), junctional bradycardia (6%), and various others.[5]

Pathophysiology

Sick sinus syndrome resulting in sinus bradycardia occurs because of the development of fibrotic tissue in the

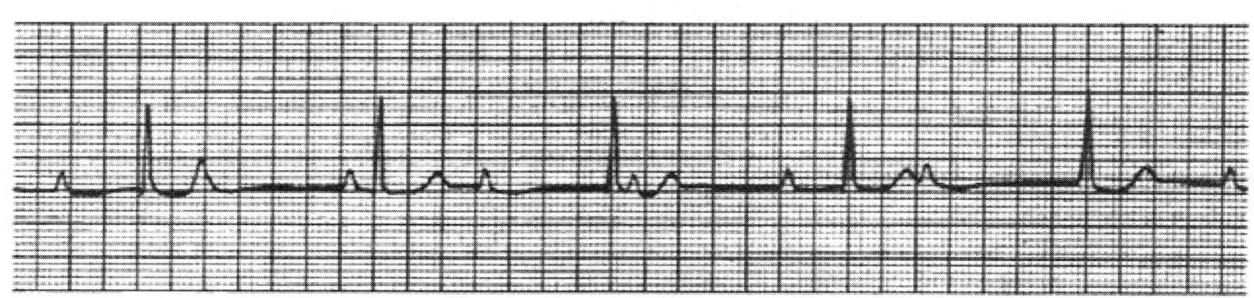

Figure 35.5 Third-degree atrioventricular block (AV dissociation).

Reprinted with permission from: Tisdale JE. Review of cardiac arrhythmias and rhythm interpretation. In: Wiggins BS, Sanoski CA. Emergency Cardiovascular Pharmacotherapy. A Point-of-Care Guide. Bethesda, MD: American Society of Health-System Pharmacists, 2012:29.

AV = Atrioventricular

sinoatrial node, replacing normal sinoatrial node tissue.[1] Idiopathic AV block may be caused by degenerative changes within the AV node.

Etiologies

Sinus node dysfunction may occur as a result of disease or drug therapy. Disease-associated sinus bradycardia may occur as a result of myocardial ischemia or myocardial infarction (MI), particularly involving the right coronary artery, a branch of which provides blood supply to the sinus node (and the inferior wall of the left ventricle); hypothyroidism; heart failure (HF); hypothermia; pericarditis; infiltrative diseases such as sarcoidosis, amyloidosis, or hemochromatosis; increased intracranial pressure; neurocardiac syncope; carotid sinus hypersensitivity; autoimmune diseases such as systemic lupus erythematosus, rheumatoid arthritis, or scleroderma; electrolyte imbalances such as hypo- or hyperkalemia; myotonic muscular dystrophy; surgical trauma such as during valve replacement, heart transplantation, or correction of congenital heart disease; and vasovagal responses during coughing, micturition, defecation, or vomiting. In critically ill patients, bradycardia associated with hyperkalemia is not uncommon.[6] Other causes of sinus bradycardia in patients in the ICU can include sleep apnea, increased intracranial pressure, and enhanced parasympathetic activity during endotracheal suctioning or emesis.[6]

Idiopathic degeneration of the sinus node can occur with aging, sometimes leading to the condition known as sick sinus syndrome. In some cases, sick sinus syndrome occurs as a result of familial sinus node disease because of mutations in genes encoding cardiac sodium channels, the hyperpolarization activated "funny" (I_f) current, and others. Drug therapy that may cause sinus bradycardia includes adrenergic β-receptor blockers (β-blockers); non-dihydropyridine calcium channel blockers (diltiazem, verapamil); amiodarone; dronedarone; flecainide; propafenone; sotalol; digoxin; clonidine; anesthetics such as dexmedetomidine, halothane, ketamine, and propofol; and several others.[7]

Similar to sinus node dysfunction, AV block may be caused by diseases or drug therapy. Atrioventricular block may occur as a result of myocardial ischemia or MI; infiltrative diseases such as sarcoidosis and amyloidosis; Hodgkin diseases; multiple myeloma; infectious processes such as Chagas disease, myocarditis, rheumatic fever, and endocarditis; rheumatic diseases such as rheumatoid arthritis, scleroderma, and Reiter syndrome; neuromuscular diseases such as myotonic muscular dystrophy; electrolyte disturbances such as hypo- or hyperkalemia; surgical trauma; and accidental damage during catheter ablation. Drug therapy that may cause AV block includes β-blockers, diltiazem, verapamil, amiodarone, dronedarone, adenosine, flecainide, propafenone, sotalol, digoxin, clonidine, paclitaxel, and several others.[7] Atrioventricular block occurring in ICU patients can be a result of sleep apnea, increased intracranial pressure, or enhanced parasympathetic activity during endotracheal suctioning, emesis, or endoscopy.[6]

Morbidity and Mortality

First-degree AV block does not usually result in bradycardia and is therefore rarely symptomatic. Bradycardia caused by sinus node dysfunction or second- or third-degree AV block can result in dizziness, fatigue, light-headedness, syncope, chest pain (in patients with underlying ischemic heart disease), and shortness of breath and other symptoms of HF (in patients with underlying left ventricular dysfunction). The average lengths of ICU stay and hospital stay in older adult patients with a principal hospital discharge diagnosis of sinus node dysfunction are 1.1 days and 5.3 days, respectively; for those with a discharge diagnosis of third-degree AV block, 1.5 days and 5.6 days, respectively; and for those with a discharge diagnosis of Mobitz type I second-degree AV block, 1.1 days and 4.8 days, respectively.[4] Bradycardia is rarely a direct cause of mortality.

Treatment

The potential for drug-induced sinus bradycardia or AV block must be considered. If the patient is receiving therapy with any drugs that may cause bradycardia, they should be discontinued. A treatment algorithm for management of bradycardia is presented in Figure 35.6.[8] Symptomatic or hemodynamically unstable bradycardia should be managed acutely with intravenous atropine, which increases heart rate by anticholinergic activity.[8] Several studies have reported that atropine improves heart rate and associated symptoms in patients with sinus bradycardia and/or AV block. In a study of 61 patients with bradycardia associated with MI (n=32 with sinus bradycardia, n=29 with AV block or junctional rhythm), atropine administration increased the heart rate from 46 ± 14 beats/minute to 79 ± 12 beats/minute ($p<0.001$).[10] In a small study in which 15 patients received atropine for intraoperative bradycardia (defined as heart rate less than 50 beats/minute or less than 60 beats/minute with a concomitant decrease in blood pressure), atropine increased heart rate to 70 beats/minute or more in a mean time of 270 seconds (range 30–490).[11] However, response to atropine is not universal. Brady et al.[12] assessed the response to atropine administered prehospital by emergency medical services personnel in 131 patients with bradycardia (AV block, n=45; sinus bradycardia, n=35; junctional bradycardia, n=38; idioventricular bradycardia, n=13). Complete response associated with atropine (defined as heart rate greater than 60 beats/minute and return of systolic blood pressure to greater than 90 mm Hg) occurred in 27.5%; partial response (defined as transient increase in heart rate to greater than 60 beats/minute and systolic blood pressure greater than 90 mm Hg, or an increase in heart rate of 10 or more beats/minute or systolic pressure of 10 mm Hg or greater that was either transient or maintained) occurred in 19.8% of patients. In 49.6% of patients, there was no response, whereas an adverse response (development of more than six ventricular premature depolarizations per minute or development of ventricular tachycardia [VT] or ventricular fibrillation) occurred in 2.3%.[12]

Atropine should be administered in doses of 0.5 mg intravenously every 3–5 minutes to a maximum recommended dose of 3 mg. In patients with symptomatic or hemodynamically unstable bradycardia unresponsive to atropine,

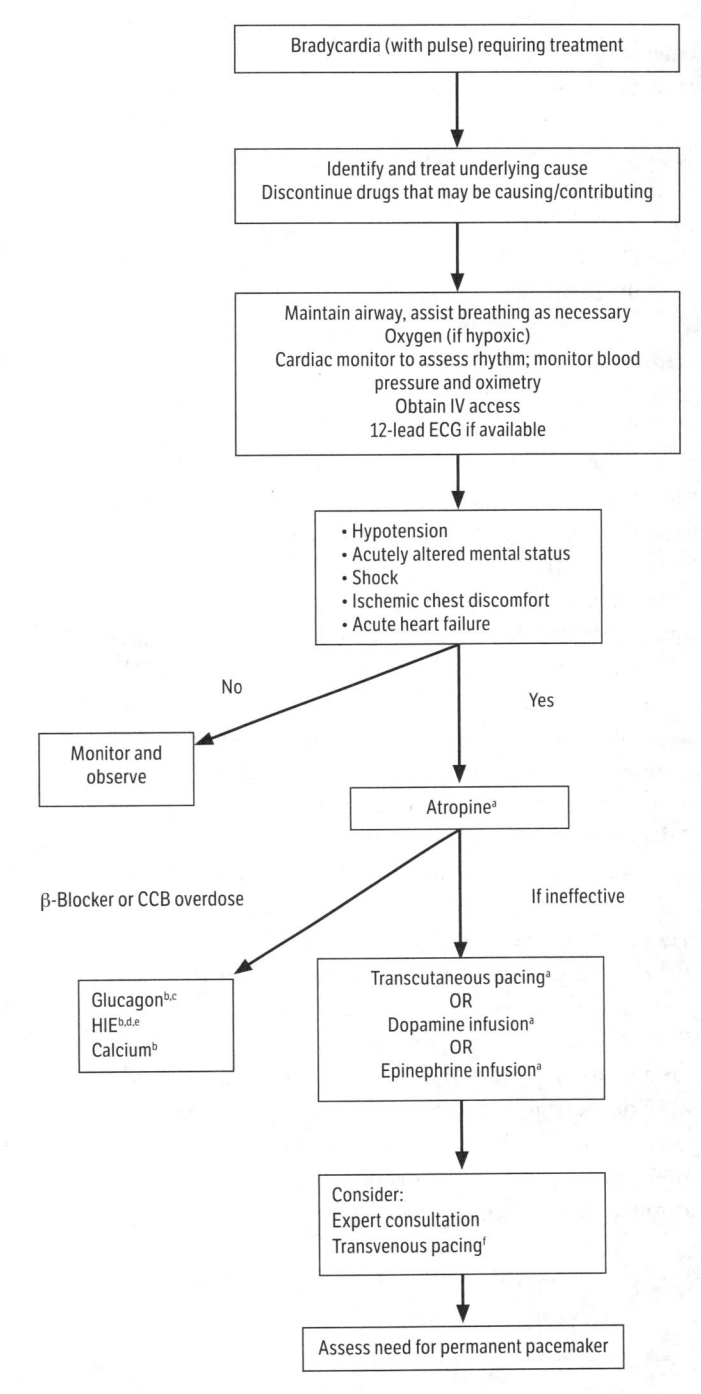

Figure 35.6 Treatment algorithm for critically ill patients with bradycardias.

[a] Class IIa, level of evidence (LOE) B.[8]
[b] Class IIb, LOE C.[8,9]
[c] Glucagon may be recommended for management of β-blocker overdose, but evidence is insufficient to recommend it for management of CCB overdose.[9]
[d] Class IIb, LOE B.[8,9]
[e] HIE has a class IIb recommendation, level of evidence B for calcium channel blocker overdose, and a class IIb recommendation, level of evidence C for β-blocker overdose.[9]
CCB = calcium channel blocker; ECG = electrocardiogram; HIE = hyperinsulinemia-euglycemia therapy; IV = intravenous(ly).
[f] Class IIa, LOE C[8]

and in whom transcutaneous or transvenous pacing is unavailable or ineffective, or while awaiting placement of a pacemaker, alternative drug therapy includes dopamine 2–10 mcg/kg/minute, titrated to response, or epinephrine 2–10 mcg/minute, titrated to response.[8] Dopamine and epinephrine increase heart rate through agonism of adrenergic β_1-receptors. Atropine, dopamine, and epinephrine should be used cautiously in patients with myocardial ischemia or MI because increasing heart rate and myocardial oxygen demand may enhance ischemia and extend the infarct.

Temporary transcutaneous or transvenous pacing may be used to maintain an adequate heart rate until underlying etiologies for bradycardia can be corrected or a permanent pacemaker, when necessary, can be implanted. Long-term management of sick sinus syndrome or AV block that is not associated with correctable conditions requires implantation of a permanent pacemaker.

If symptomatic or hemodynamically unstable bradycardia is because of a presumed or documented overdose of β-blockers, appropriate treatment with intravenous glucagon, calcium, and/or hyperinsulinemia-euglycemia (HIE) therapy may be initiated.[9,13] Glucagon may be administered as an intravenous bolus dose of 3–10 mg (0.05–0.15 mg/kg), followed by a continuous infusion of 3–5 mg/hour (0.05–0.10 mg/kg/hour), titrated to achieve an adequate hemodynamic response.[12] Evidence supporting the efficacy of glucagon for management of β-blocker overdose is derived primarily from case reports.[9] Calcium 0.3 mEq/kg may be administered, either as calcium gluconate (10%) 0.6 mL/kg or calcium chloride (10%) 0.2 mL/kg over 5–10 minutes, followed by an infusion of 0.3 mEq/kg/hour.[9] Although recommended, evidence supporting calcium infusion for β-blocker overdose is somewhat limited.[9] Some evidence suggests that HIE is a reasonable option for patients with β-blocker overdose and shock refractory to other treatments.[9] Hyperinsulinemia-euglycemia may be administered as regular insulin 1-international unit/kg bolus followed by continuous infusion of 0.5–1 international units/kg/hour. The infusion dose may be titrated every 30 minutes to achieve the desired response. Because of the potential for insulin-associated electrolyte shifts, close monitoring of serum electrolyte concentrations during HIE therapy is recommended. Intravenous dextrose 25 g may be administered with the initial insulin bolus to maintain euglycemia (blood glucose 100–250 mg/dL), followed by continuous dextrose infusion at 0.5 g/kg/hour.[9,13] In refractory cases of β-blocker or calcium channel blocker overdose, lipid emulsion infusions have been administered with some success.[9,14,15]

If symptomatic or hemodynamically unstable bradycardia is because of a presumed or documented overdose of diltiazem or verapamil, evidence supporting the efficacy of specific antidotes is lacking.[9] Several case reports describe administration of HIE for management of calcium channel blocker overdose and suggest that HIE, at doses described previously, is a reasonable therapeutic option.[9] More limited evidence, also from case reports, is available to support calcium administration for management of calcium channel blocker overdose; calcium administration may be considered for patients with calcium channel blocker overdose and shock that are refractory to other treatments.[9] Evidence is insufficient to recommend glucagon for management of calcium channel overdose.[9]

Paroxysmal Supraventricular Tachycardia (AV node reentrant tachycardia, AV reciprocating tachycardia [including Wolff-Parkinson-White {syndrome} {WPW}], atrial tachycardia)

Features

The term *paroxysmal supraventricular tachycardia* (PSVT) refers to a group of arrhythmias that require atrial or AV

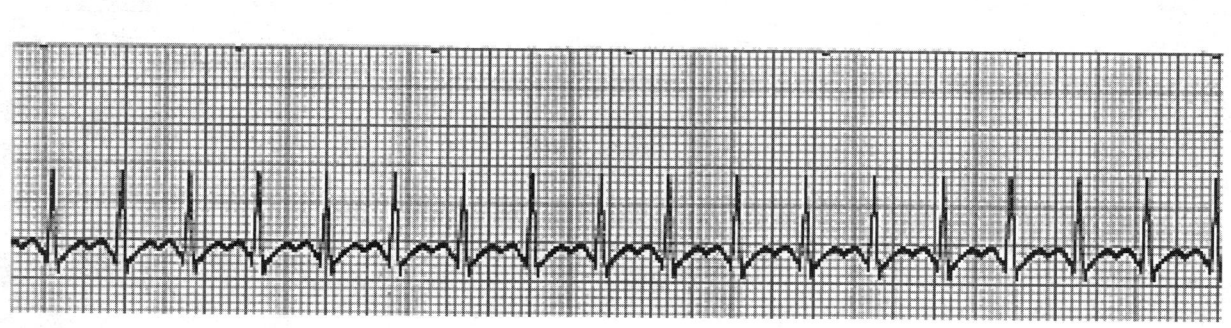

Figure 35.7 Atrioventricular nodal reentrant tachycardia.

Reprinted with permission from: Tisdale JE. Review of cardiac arrhythmias and rhythm interpretation. In: Wiggins BS, Sanoski CA. Emergency Cardiovascular Pharmacotherapy. A Point-of-Care Guide. Bethesda, MD: American Society of Health-System Pharmacists, 2012:35.

nodal tissue for their initiation and maintenance.[16] Arrhythmias included within the term *PSVT* include AV node reentrant tachycardia (AVNRT), atrioventricular reentrant tachycardia (AVRT), and atrial tachycardia (AT).[17] In patients with AVNRT or AVRT, heart rates are 150–250 beats/minute, and the rhythm is regular.[18] Heart rates in patients with focal AT are typically 150–250 beats/minute, whereas in multifocal atrial tachycardia, heart rates are generally 100–150 beats/minute.[18] Focal AT is a regular rhythm; multifocal AT is irregular, but it can be distinguished from atrial fibrillation (AF) by the presence of P waves, which are absent in AF.[18] A rhythm strip depicting AVNRT, the most common form of PSVT, is provided in Figure 35.7.

Epidemiology

The incidence of PSVT is about 35 cases per 100,000 individuals annually; the prevalence of PSVT is about 2.25 per 1,000 individuals.[19] Atrioventricular node reentrant tachycardia constitutes about 60% of PSVT cases.[16] Around 30% of PSVT cases are AVRT, with the remaining 10% occurring because of AT.[16] Atrial tachycardia can be focal or multifocal.

The onset of AVNRT can occur at any age, but it occurs most often during the fourth or fifth decades of life.[20] In one analysis, the mean age of onset of PSVT was 57 years.[18] Atrioventricular reciprocating tachycardia commonly occurs in pediatric populations.[20]

Around 0.1%–2% of patients hospitalized in ICUs develop PSVT.[21-23] Paroxysmal supraventricular tachycardia accounts for about 7% of arrhythmias occurring in ICUs and for about 8% of tachyarrhythmias occurring in ICUs.[5]

Pathophysiology

Atrioventricular node reentrant tachycardia has traditionally been thought of as a reentrant arrhythmia occurring within the AV node, which is functionally divided into two pathways. In most patients, antegrade AV nodal conduction occurs through the slower pathway, and retrograde conduction from ventricles back to atria occurs through the faster pathway.[17] In a small proportion of patients (5%–10%), conduction occurs in the opposite direction, where antegrade conduction occurs over the fast pathway and retrograde conduction occurs over the slow pathway.[17] However, it is now recognized that in many patients, a component of the reentrant circuit may exist outside the AV node in perinodal tissue.[17]

Atrioventricular reentrant tachycardia is an arrhythmia in which one pathway of the reentrant circuit is within the AV node, and the other involves an accessory pathway, which is an extranodal pathway that connects the atria and ventricles across the ridge that separates atria from ventricles.[17] In 90%–95% of patients with AVRT, conduction during the arrhythmia is orthodromic, with antegrade conduction through the AV node and retrograde conduction through the accessory pathway[16]; conduction in the opposite direction is called antidromic. Perhaps the best-known condition that can lead to AVRT is WPW, the accessory pathway for which is known as the bundle of Kent. In patients with WPW, preexcitation is demonstrated on an ECG during sinus rhythm, which is evidence of antegrade conduction by the accessory pathway.[16] The degree of preexcitation evident on the ECG depends on the relative conduction from the atria to the ventricle through the AV node as opposed to via the accessory pathway.[17]

Focal AT occurs as a result of regular atrial activation from a single atrial focus; multifocal AT occurs as a result of atrial activation from multiple foci.[17]

Etiologies

Paroxysmal supraventricular tachycardia is often idiopathic, occurring in relatively young individuals with no history or evidence of structural heart disease. Atrial tachycardia may occur in patients with congenital or acquired heart disease. Atrioventricular reciprocating tachycardia may occur in patients with accessory pathways because of hypertrophic cardiomyopathy or Ebstein's anomaly.[17] Atrial tachycardia may be precipitated by drugs such as β-receptor agonists including albuterol and terbutaline; excessive use of caffeine; theophylline; or digitalis glycoside toxicity.[7]

Risk Factors

About two-thirds of patients who develop PSVT are female.[19] Age older than 65 years and female sex are independent risk factors for PSVT.[19] Other risk factors for PSVT have not been identified.

Morbidity and Mortality

Symptoms associated with PSVT are related primarily to heart rate and include palpitations, dizziness, and light-headedness. Other symptoms can include shortness of breath and chest pain. Around 15% of patients have syncope.[17] If rapid PSVT persists for weeks to months, a reversible tachycardia-induced cardiomyopathy may result.[24] The average lengths of ICU stay and hospital stay in older adult patients with a principal hospital discharge diagnosis of PSVT are 0.8 days and 4.2 days, respectively.[4]

Wolff-Parkinson-White syndrome is associated with sudden cardiac death in 0.15%–0.39% of patients.[16] Sudden cardiac death in WPW usually occurs in patients who also have AF, which may be initiated by rapid AVRT. If AF develops in patients having WPW with an accessory pathway with a short antegrade refractory period, AF can result in a rapid ventricular response that may degenerate into ventricular fibrillation.[17] Patients with WPW who are at increased risk of sudden death include those with very short (less than 250 milliseconds) preexcited RR intervals during AF, multiple accessory pathways, history of symptomatic tachycardias, and Ebstein's anomaly.[17]

Treatment

Paroxysmal supraventricular tachycardia that is hemodynamically unstable, or for which adenosine therapy is not desired, should be treated with synchronized direct current cardioversion (DCC).[8] If time permits, the patient should be sedated for cardioversion. The initial recommended DCC dose is 50–100 joules (J) biphasic shock for a regular PSVT; if irregular, the dose should be 120–200 J biphasic shock, or 200 J monophasic shock.[8]

For patients with AVNRT that is hemodynamically stable, vagal maneuvers should be administered in an attempt to terminate the arrhythmia before initiation of drug therapy.[17] Vagal maneuvers stimulate parasympathetic nervous system activity, increasing serum acetylcholine concentrations, which inhibits AV nodal conduction, facilitating termination of the arrhythmia. Vagal maneuvers alone may terminate PSVT in up to 25% of cases.[8] The simplest vagal maneuver in a conscious patient is cough, which stimulates the vagus nerve. Unilateral carotid sinus massage may also be tried; however, carotid sinus massage should not be done in patients with a history of stroke or transient ischemic attack, or in those in whom carotid bruits are detected on auscultation. Conscious patients can also be instructed to do the Valsalva maneuver, during which one bears down against a closed glottis. If vagal maneuvers are unsuccessful at restoring sinus rhythm, or if they only transiently restore sinus rhythm, drug therapy should be administered subsequently.

Intravenously administered AV node-inhibiting drugs are the primary pharmacologic option for termination of AVNRT. In patients with AVNRT, AV node-inhibiting drugs interrupt the AV node reentrant circuit and terminate the arrhythmia. Drugs that may be used for termination of hemodynamically stable AVNRT are presented in Table 35.1. Adenosine, which is the drug therapy of choice, should be administered after vagal maneuvers have failed. Adenosine directly inhibits AV node conduction and successfully terminates AVNRT in about 90% of patients.[25] Adenosine is also sometimes administered to assist with the diagnosis of narrow QRS complex tachycardias.[17] If the rhythm is AVNRT, adenosine administration usually terminates the arrhythmia; if the arrhythmia is atrial flutter, AV nodal inhibition by adenosine often slows the rate of the arrhythmia enough to uncover the typical flutter waves. Carotid sinus massage may also be used for this purpose.

Drugs for the termination of hemodynamically stable AVRT are presented in Table 35.2. In patients with AVRT and preexcitation, adenosine should be avoided because it may provoke AF with a rapid ventricular response.[17] Algorithms for managing PSVT without preexcitation and PSVT with preexcitation are presented in Figure 35.8 and Figure 35.9.

Long-term management of AVNRT and AVRT consists primarily of catheter ablation, which is considered first-line therapy.[17]

Atrial Fibrillation

Features

Atrial fibrillation is a supraventricular tachyarrhythmia characterized on ECG by absence of distinct repeating P waves, an undulating baseline representing chaotic atrial electrical activity, and an irregularly irregular rhythm (Figure 35.10).[26] During AF, atrial depolarization is not occurring, and therefore, coordinated atrial contraction is absent. Paroxysmal AF is defined as that which terminates spontaneously or with intervention within 7 days of onset and is associated with recurring episodes of variable frequency and duration. Persistent AF is continuous AF that lasts longer than 7 days. Long-standing persistent AF is continuous AF that lasts longer than 12 months. The term *permanent AF* is applied when the patient and clinician arrive at a joint decision to terminate further attempts to reestablish and/or maintain sinus rhythm.[26] In about 50% of patients with acute AF in the ICU, the rhythm spontaneously reverts to normal sinus rhythm within 48 hours.[27]

Epidemiology

Atrial fibrillation is often described as the most common arrhythmia encountered in clinical practice. Estimates regarding the prevalence of AF in the United States (U.S.) in 2010 were 2.7–6.1 million patients.[28,29] The prevalence of AF is expected to continue to rise and to reach 5.6–12 million patients by 2050.[29] The prevalence of AF increases with advancing age. In individuals 50–59 years of age, the prevalence of AF is about 0.5%, doubling with each subsequent decade to a prevalence of about 9% in individuals 80–89 years of age.[30] The incidence of AF in men ranges from 20.6 per 100,000 people 15–44 years of age to 1,077 per 100,000 in those 85 years and older.[2] In women, the incidence of AF is 6.6 per 100,000 from 15 to 44 years of age and 1,204 per 100,000 in those 85 years and older.[2] About 45% of patients with AF are men.[2]

Atrial fibrillation is a common arrhythmia in critically ill patients. The overall incidence of AF in patients during stays in medical ICUs and/or surgical ICUs is 7.2%–10.5%.[21,22,31,32] New-onset AF in medical ICUs/surgical ICUs occurs in 4.5%–7.2% of patients.[22,31,32] New-onset AF associated with sepsis AF occurs in 4%–14% of patients.[33-35] The incidence of AF increases according to the severity of sepsis; in one analysis, the incidence of new-onset AF was 8% (range 0%–14%), 10% (4%–23%), and 23% (6%–46%) in patients with sepsis, severe sepsis, and septic shock, respectively.[35]

continued on page 716

Table 35.1 Drugs for Termination of Paroxysmal Supraventricular Tachycardia in Critically Ill Patients

Drug	Mechanism	Dose	Adverse Effects
Adenosine[a]	Direct AV node inhibition	6 mg IV rapid push followed by 20 mL NS flush. If no response in 1–2 min, administer 12 mg rapid IV push followed by 20 mL NS flush	Chest discomfort Flushing Sinus pauses Bronchospasm (contraindicated in patients with asthma)
Diltiazem[a,b]	Direct AV node inhibition	15–20 mg (0.25 mg/kg) IV over 2 min. If necessary, in 15 min, give an additional 20–25 mg (0.35 mg/kg) over 2 min. Maintenance infusion 5–15 mg/hr	Bradycardia Hypotension HF precipitation/exacerbation (contraindicated in patients with HFrEF)
Verapamil[a,b]	Direct AV node inhibition	2.5–5.0 mg IV bolus over 2 min (over 3 min in older patients). If no response and no adverse effects, give repeated doses of 5–10 mg IV every 30 min to a total dose of 20 mg Alternative regimen: 5 mg IV bolus every 15 min to a total dose of 30 mg	Bradycardia Hypotension HF precipitation/ exacerbation (contraindicated in patients with HFrEF)
β-Blockers[a]	AV node inhibition by inhibition of β-receptors	Esmolol 500 mcg/kg IV over 1 min; then 50 mcg/kg/min continuous IV infusion. If inadequate response, give second loading dose of 500 mcg/kg IV and increase maintenance infusion to 100 mcg/kg/min. Increment dose increases in this manner as necessary to maximum infusion of 300 mcg/kg/min Metoprolol tartrate 5 mg IV over 1–2 min; repeat as required every 5 min to maximum dose of 15 mg Propranolol 0.5–1 mg IV over 1 min; repeat as required up to a total dose of 0.1 mg/kg	Bradycardia Hypotension
Ibutilide[c]	Slows conduction in accessory pathway in preexcited PSVT	1 mg IV over 10 min; if < 60 kg, 0.01 mg/kg; repeat initial dose if necessary 10 min after first dose	QT interval prolongation, torsades de pointes, nonsustained ventricular tachycardia
Procainamide[c]	Slows conduction in accessory pathway in preexcited PSVT	17 mg/kg IV administered at rate of 20–50 mg/min; terminate loading infusion if hypotension, QRS complex increases ≥ 50%, or arrhythmia is terminated. Maintenance IV infusion 1–4 mg/min	Hypotension Heart failure Torsades de pointes
Flecainide[c,d]	Slows conduction in accessory pathway in preexcited PSVT	2 mg/kg IV over 10 min	Heart failure Rapid atrial flutter Hypotension Ventricular proarrhythmia – avoid in patients with structural heart disease

| Table 35.1 | Drugs for Termination of Paroxysmal Supraventricular Tachycardia in Critically Ill Patients (continued) |

Drug	Mechanism	Dose	Adverse Effects
Digoxin[a]	Vagal stimulation, direct AV node inhibition	4–6 mcg/kg IV over 5 min 1–1.5 mcg/kg IV every 4–8 hr to a total loading dose of 8–12 mcg/kg	Bradycardia Nausea, vomiting Anorexia AV block Ventricular arrhythmias
Amiodarone[a,c]	β-Blocker Calcium channel blocker	150 mg IV over 10 min and repeated if necessary, followed by 1 mg/min continuous IV infusion for 6 hr, followed by 0.5 mg/min. Total dose should not exceed 2.2 g over 24 hr	Bradycardia Hypotension Phlebitis QT interval prolongation Torsades de pointes

[a]Contraindicated in patients with Wolff-Parkinson-White syndrome or other preexcitation syndromes.
[b]Verapamil and diltiazem should only be administered to patients with narrow complex arrhythmias and should never be administered to patients with wide complex arrhythmias.
[c]Avoid in patients with QTc interval > 440 ms (> 500 ms in patients with ventricular conduction abnormalities).
[d]Flecainide not available intravenously in the United States.
AV = atrioventricular; AVNRT = atrioventricular node reentrant tachycardia; HF = heart failure; HFrEF = heart failure with reduced ejection fraction; IV = intravenous(ly); NS = normal saline; PSVT = paroxysmal supraventricular tachycardia.

continued from page 714

Atrial fibrillation occurs commonly after thoracic surgery. The incidence of AF after coronary artery bypass graft (CABG) surgery is 30%–47%[36-39]; the incidence is in the lower end of that range in patients undergoing isolated CABG and higher in patients undergoing both CABG and valve replacement surgery. Atrial fibrillation also occurs commonly in patients undergoing noncardiac thoracic surgery, specifically pulmonary resection and esophagectomy. The incidence of AF after pulmonary resection is 12%–30% after lobectomy and 23%–67% after pneumonectomy.[40,41] Atrial fibrillation occurs in 13%–46% of patients after esophagectomy.[41,42] The average time of onset of AF after both CABG and noncardiac thoracic surgery is 2–3 days.[43,44]

Pathophysiology

Atrial fibrillation occurs as a result of structural and/or electrophysiological abnormalities that provoke abnormal impulse formation in the atria or pulmonary veins and subsequent impulse propagation by atrial reentry.[26] Atrial fibrillation requires a trigger for initiation, which is most commonly ectopic impulses generated in the left atrial myocardial sleeves that extend back into the pulmonary veins. Once triggered, AF is propagated by several simultaneously active atrial reentrant circuits associated with increased dispersion of atrial conduction and refractoriness.

Etiologies

Etiologies of AF include conditions/diseases that promote atrial hypertrophy, fibrosis, dilation, ischemia, or infiltration. Inflammation and oxidative stress may play a role in development of AF, as well as activation of the autonomic nervous system and the renin-angiotensin-aldosterone system. Several risk factors for AF exist, which contribute to these etiologies.

Drugs may provoke AF.[7,45] It has long been recognized that heavy alcohol intake is associated with AF. Consumption of 35 or more drinks per week was associated with a hazard ratio for AF of 1.45 (1.02–2.04) in men.[46] Drugs that could contribute to new-onset AF in ICU patients include adenosine, dobutamine, aminophylline, milrinone, and high-dose methylprednisolone administered in pulse doses.[45]

Risk Factors

Risk factors for AF include older age, hypertension, diabetes mellitus, MI, valvular heart disease, HF, obesity, obstructive sleep apnea, smoking, and hyperthyroidism.[26] Some genetic variants have been associated with AF, and familial clusters of AF have been identified, indicating that, for some patients, a genetic predisposition to AF may exist.[26]

In critically ill patients with sepsis, risk factors for development of new-onset AF include older age, white race, acute organ dysfunction, mechanical ventilation, admission to the ICU, right heart catheterization, diagnosis of endocarditis, presence of a respiratory tract infection, and CABG surgery.[35,47] In patients with severe sepsis, additional risk factors for new-onset AF include obesity, HF, metastatic or hematologic malignancy, prior stroke, respiratory failure, renal failure, hematologic failure, abdominal or skin or soft tissue infection source, primary bacteremia, and infection with gram-positive bacteria or fungus.[33] Factors associated with a lower risk of new-onset AF in patients with severe sepsis include female sex, black or Hispanic race, hypertension, diabetes mellitus, acidosis, and urinary tract source of infection.[33] Reasons for these factors associated with a lower risk of new-onset AF in patients with severe sepsis are unknown.

Risk factors for AF after CABG surgery include age older than 60 years, male sex, previous AF, PR interval greater than 200 milliseconds, diabetes mellitus, hypertension, and left ventricular ejection fraction less than 40%.[48] A risk score for prediction of post-CABG AF has been developed using these risk factors; each risk factor receives 1 point, with the exception of age older than 60 years (2 points) and history of AF (3 points). The risk of AF after bypass surgery using this risk score is as follows: score = 0–1: AF risk 7.5%–8.5%; score = 2: AF risk 12%–20%; score = 3: AF risk 20%–28%; score = 4: AF risk 33%–34%; score = 5: AF risk 40%–45%; score of 6 or higher: AF risk 42%–67%.[48] In addition, some patients may have a genetic predisposition to develop postoperative AF; several SNPs (single nucleotide polymorphisms) have been independently associated with post-CABG AF.[49] However, incorporating genetic information into the earlier-mentioned AF risk score did not improve its performance.[48] Preoperative plasma concentrations of B-type natriuretic peptide (BNP; greater than 31 pg/mL) and N-terminal-proBNP (NT-proBNP; greater than 74 pg/mL) are predictive of the development of post-CABG AF.[50]

Risk factors for AF after noncardiac thoracic surgery include lobectomy, bilobectomy, pneumonectomy, resection of mediastinal tumor or thymectomy, and esophagectomy; segmentectomy and multiple wedge resections were not associated with an increased risk of postoperative AF.[51] Other independent risk factors for AF after noncardiac thoracic surgery include male sex, age 50–59 years, age older than 60–69 years, age 70 years and older, history of HF, history of arrhythmias, history of peripheral vascular disease, and intraoperative transfusions.[44] Independent risk factors for AF occurring after pulmonary resection for lung cancer include pneumonectomy, bilobectomy, older age, male sex, and clinical stage II or greater.[52] Preoperative plasma BNP concentration greater than 30 pg/mL and preoperative plasma NT-proBNP concentration greater than 113 pg/mL are independent risk factors for AF after noncardiac thoracic surgery.[53,54] A prediction rule for AF after major noncardiac thoracic surgery was developed and includes male sex (1 point), preoperative heart rate of 72 beats/minute or greater (1 point), age 55–74 years (3 points), and age 75 years or older (4 points).[52] The risk of postoperative AF ranges from 0% (0 points) to 55% (6 points).[55]

Morbidity and Mortality

Symptoms of AF are generally related to heart rate and include palpitations, dizziness, fatigue, light-headedness, shortness of breath, syncope, and exacerbation of HF symptoms. If the heart rate is sufficiently rapid, patients may be hemodynamically unstable with hypotension, acute chest pain, and/or cardiogenic shock. Atrial fibrillation is associated with a 2- to 7-fold increase in the risk of stroke, depending on the presence of other stroke risk factors. Atrial fibrillation is also associated with an increased risk of thromboembolism events other than stroke. The risk of new HF is increased about 3-fold in patients with AF. Atrial fibrillation is associated with a doubling in the incidence of dementia and a doubling in the risk of overall mortality.[26]

Hemodynamic instability occurs in 37% of patients who develop new-onset AF in an ICU.[32] Around 10% of patients with preexisting AF who develop AF in the ICU are hemodynamically unstable.[32] New-onset AF in critically ill patients doubles the length of ICU stay as well as the total duration of hospital stay.[31] In-hospital mortality and 60-day mortality are significantly greater in critically ill patients who develop new-onset AF.[22,31] Atrial fibrillation in critically ill patients may be associated with thromboembolism[23]; in one study of 108 ICU patients who developed supraventricular arrhythmias (79% of which were AF), 12 patients (11%) developed arterial thromboembolic events.[23] These events included five strokes, three mesenteric infarctions, two limb ischemia, and two MIs.

In critically ill patients with sepsis, AF is associated with prolonged duration of ICU stay,[35] prolonged duration of total hospital stay,[34] and a higher risk of ICU mortality, in-hospital mortality, and 28-day mortality.[34,35] In addition, patients with sepsis who develop AF have a higher risk of requiring mechanical ventilation and a subsequently longer duration of mechanical ventilation.[34] In patients with severe sepsis, AF is associated with an increased risk of in-hospital stroke and in-hospital mortality.[33]

Post-CABG AF is associated with symptoms, hypotension, HF, increased need for inotropic medications, acute kidney injury, increased use of the intra-aortic balloon pump, prolonged ventilation, readmission to the ICU, and increased need for tracheostomy.[56] In addition, post-CABG AF is associated with an increased risk of perioperative stroke.[44] Post-CABG AF leads to prolonged length of ICU, step-down unit, and total hospital stay.[43,57] Furthermore, AF is the most common cause of hospital readmission after CABG surgery.[58] Post-CABG AF is associated with an increased risk of short- and long-term mortality.[59]

Atrial fibrillation after noncardiac thoracic surgery is associated with symptoms, hemodynamic instability,[60] and stroke.[44,61] Atrial fibrillation after noncardiac thoracic surgery is associated with increased duration of ICU and total hospital stays and higher use of health care resources.[41] Post-noncardiac thoracic surgery AF is associated with an increased risk of postoperative mortality, though it is unclear whether the mortality is directly associated with AF or whether AF is a marker for more severe illness.[41,44]

Table 35.2 Drugs for Ventricular Rate Control in Critically Ill Patients with Atrial Fibrillation

Drug	Mechanism	Dose	Adverse Effects
β-Blockers[a]	AV node inhibition by inhibition of β-receptors	Esmolol 500 mcg/kg IV over 1 min; then 50 mcg/kg/min continuous IV infusion. If inadequate response, give second loading dose of 500 mcg/kg IV and increase maintenance infusion to 100 mcg/kg/min. Increment dose increases in this manner as necessary to maximum infusion of 300 mcg/kg/min	Bradycardia Hypotension
		Metoprolol tartrate 2.5–5 mg IV over 2 min; up to a total of three doses	
		Propranolol 1 mg IV over 1 min; up to three doses at 2-min intervals	
Diltiazem[a]	Direct AV node inhibition	0.25 mg/kg IV bolus over 2 min; then 5–15 mg/hr continuous IV infusion	Bradycardia Hypotension HF precipitation/exacerbation (contraindicated in patients with HFrEF)
Verapamil[a]	Direct AV node inhibition	0.075–0.15 mg/kg IV bolus over 2 min; may give an additional 10 mg after 30 min if no response; then 0.005 mg/kg/min continuous infusion	Bradycardia Hypotension HF precipitation/exacerbation (contraindicated in patients with HFrEF)
Digoxin[a]	Vagal stimulation, direct AV node inhibition	0.25 mg IV with repeat dosing to a maximum of 1.5 mg over 24 hr	Bradycardia Nausea, vomiting Anorexia AV block Ventricular arrhythmias
Amiodarone[a,b]	β-Blocker Calcium channel blocker	300 mg IV over 1 hr; then 10–50 mg/hr over 24 hr	Bradycardia Hypotension Phlebitis QT interval prolongation Torsades de pointes

[a]Contraindicated in patients with Wolff-Parkinson-White syndrome or other preexcitation syndromes.
[b]Avoid in patients with QTc interval > 440 ms (> 500 ms in patients with ventricular conduction abnormalities).

Treatment

A broad scheme for management of AF in the critically ill patient is presented in Figure 35.11. Atrial fibrillation that is hemodynamically unstable resulting in hypotension, acutely altered mental status, signs of shock, ischemic chest discomfort, or acute HF should be treated with synchronized DCC.[8] If time permits, the patient should be sedated for cardioversion. The initial recommended DCC dose is 120–200 J biphasic shock or 200 J monophasic shock.[8]

The goals of drug therapy for AF in critically ill patients are ventricular rate control, conversion to sinus rhythm, and prevention of thromboembolism. Drug therapy options for ventricular rate control for critically ill patients with AF are presented in Table 35.2 and include β-blockers, diltiazem, verapamil, digoxin, and amiodarone, all administered intravenously. Intravenous β-blockers have been shown to be effective for achieving ventricular rate control in patients with acute AF.[62-64] Diltiazem was effective in controlling ventricular rate in 83% of patients with acute AF.[65] The efficacy of β-blockers and calcium channel blockers for acute ventricular rate control is about equivalent,[62-64] though diltiazem may achieve ventricular rate control more rapidly than metoprolol.[64] Intravenous diltiazem was found to achieve ventricular rate control in a higher proportion of patients with acute AF than digoxin or

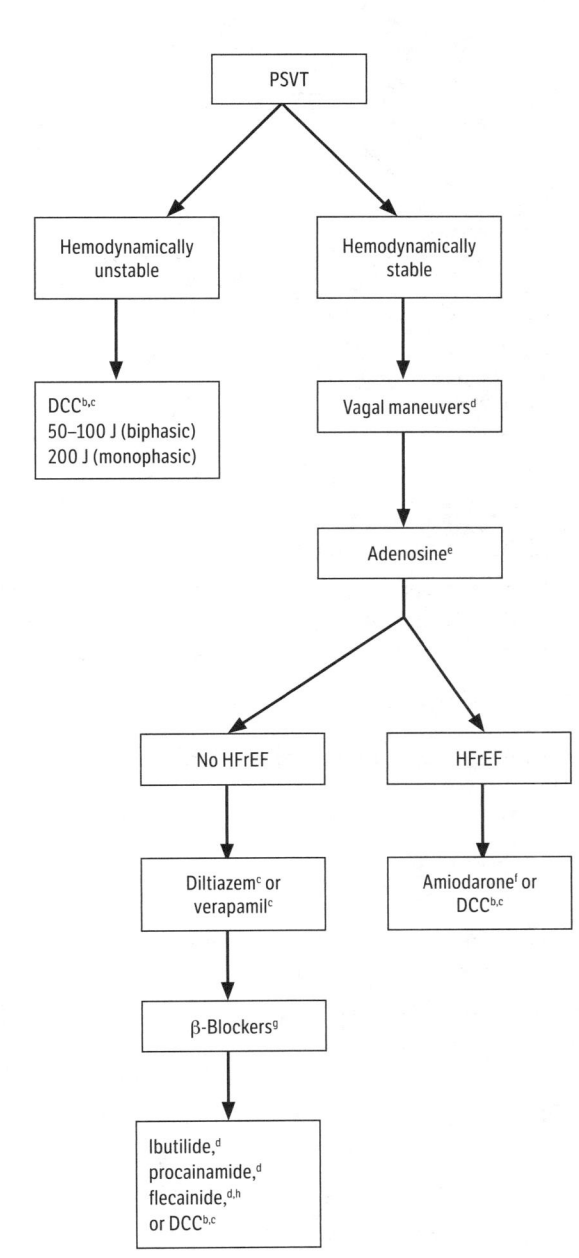

Figure 35.8 Treatment algorithm for critically ill patients with paroxysmal supraventricular tachycardia without preexcitation.[a]

[a]All drugs administered intravenously.
[b]If possible, establish IV access before cardioversion and administer sedation if the patient is conscious.
[c]Class IIa, LOE B.[8]
[d]Class of recommendation or level of evidence (LOE) not provided in the treatment guidelines.[8,17]
[e]Class I, LOE B.[8,17]
[f]Class IIb, LOE C.[17]
[g]Class IIa, LOE C.[8]
[h]Flecainide not available intravenously in the United States.
DCC = direct current cardioversion (synchronized); HFrEF = heart failure with reduced ejection fraction; PSVT = paroxysmal supraventricular tachycardia.

amiodarone, and rate control was achieved in a shorter time with diltiazem than with digoxin or amiodarone as well.[66,67] Intravenous diltiazem achieves ventricular rate control significantly more rapidly than intravenous verapamil and may also be associated with less propensity to cause profound hypotension.[68] Digoxin administered alone is not a particularly effective agent for ventricular rate control in patients with acute AF, and its onset of action is slow, requiring several hours.[26,67,69] Intravenous amiodarone has been shown to be more effective than digoxin for lowering ventricular rate in patients with acute AF, but it is not as effective as intravenous diltiazem.[66,70] A treatment algorithm for ventricular rate control in patients with acute AF is presented in Figure 35.12, which is based on treatment guidelines for AF not associated with surgery,[26] post-CABG AF,[26] and AF after noncardiac thoracic surgery.[44] If adequate ventricular rate control cannot be achieved using maximally tolerated doses of drugs administered as recommended in Figure 35.12, combinations of drugs may be used. For example, unless patients have acute decompensated HF and/or heart failure with reduced ejection fraction (HFrEF), the combination of digoxin and β-blockers or calcium channel blockers can be used, keeping in mind that there is a drug interaction between verapamil and digoxin requiring administration of about 50% of the usual digoxin dose.

For patients with AF and WPW or other preexcitation syndromes, administration of diltiazem, verapamil, digoxin, or amiodarone is contraindicated because these drugs can accelerate the ventricular rate.[26] In this situation, intravenous procainamide or ibutilide should be administered to slow the ventricular rate or restore sinus rhythm.[26]

Drug therapy options for conversion of AF to sinus rhythm in critically ill patients, which are presented in Table 35.3, include ibutilide, dofetilide, flecainide, propafenone, and amiodarone. These drugs slow atrial conduction velocity and/or prolong atrial refractoriness, promoting disruption of reentrant circuits and restoration of sinus rhythm.

A treatment algorithm for conversion of AF to sinus rhythm is presented in Figure 35.13. Within each category, there is no designated first-line drug therapy; medications should be selected on the basis of usual time required for AF conversion, adverse effect profile, and other patient-specific considerations. Direct current cardioversion is generally more effective than drugs for conversion of AF to sinus rhythm. However, patients who undergo elective DCC must be sedated and/or anesthetized to avoid the discomfort associated with delivery of an electrical shock to the chest. Therefore, it is important that patients undergoing elective DCC not eat within about 8–12 hours before the procedure to avoid aspiration of stomach contents during the period of sedation/anesthesia. This must be considered when deciding whether to administer elective DCC or drug therapy for conversion of AF to sinus rhythm. If a patient presents with AF requiring nonemergency conversion to sinus rhythm and the patient has eaten a meal that day, pharmacologic conversion must be performed, or DCC must be postponed to the following day to allow for a period of fasting before the procedure.

Dofetilide is effective for conversion of AF to sinus rhythm in up to 30% of patients (compared with the 1.2% efficacy rate associated with placebo).[71] About 70% of dofetilide-associated AF conversions occur within 24 hours, and about 25% require 36 hours.[71] The primary adverse effect associated with dofetilide is torsades de pointes (TdP), which occurs in about 0.8% of patients with normal left ventricular function and about 3.3% of patients with HFrEF.[72] To minimize the risk of TdP, the dofetilide dose should be carefully adjusted in patients with chronic kidney disease or acute kidney injury (see Table 35.3). Ibutilide is effective for the conversion of AF to sinus rhythm in 30%–50% of patients.[73,74] The average time to conversion to sinus rhythm after ibutilide administration is 27 minutes.[74] The primary adverse effect associated with ibutilide is TdP, which occurs in up to 8% of patients.[74] However, the incidence of TdP in patients requiring one dose of ibutilide 1 mg is only 1.7%–2.5%; the TdP incidence rises when a second dose of 1 mg is administered.[74] A single oral dose of flecainide or propafenone has been shown to be effective for restoration of sinus rhythm.[75,76] In outpatients with AF, this approach is successful at terminating AF in 58%–94% of patients, depending on the duration of AF. The average time to conversion is 110–287 minutes.[75,76] The efficacy of this approach in hospitalized critically ill patients is unknown, but it may be reasonable to try this approach in patients who can take oral medications and who do not have contraindications to flecainide or propafenone (Table 35.3; Figure 35.13). Intravenous amiodarone may be effective for conversion of AF to sinus rhythm, with conversion times of 8–24 hours.[77]

Anticoagulation of hospitalized critically ill patients with AF is desirable but may be challenging because many critically ill patients may have absolute or relative contraindications to anticoagulation.[78] Critically ill patients may

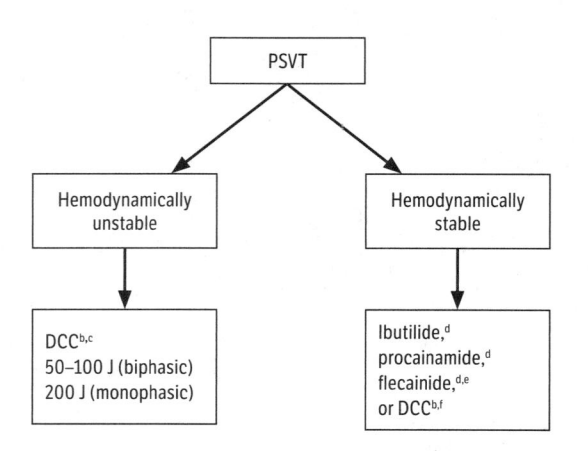

Figure 35.9 Treatment algorithm for critically ill patients with paroxysmal supraventricular tachycardia with preexcitation.[a]

[a]All drugs administered intravenously.
[b]If possible, establish IV access before cardioversion and administer sedation if the patient is conscious.
[c]Class IIa, level of evidence (LOE) B.[8]
[d]Class I, LOE B.[17]
[e]Flecainide not available intravenously in the United States.
[f]Class I, LOE C.[17]

DCC = direct current cardioversion (synchronized); PSVT = paroxysmal supraventricular tachycardia.

be at increased risk of anticoagulation-associated bleeding as a result of several factors, including stroke, hemorrhage, thrombocytopenia, acute kidney injury, liver failure, acute respiratory distress syndrome, trauma, and recent surgery.[78] Therefore, decisions regarding anticoagulation should be made with careful consideration of the potential benefits versus risks. For a critically ill patient with a history of AF who is experiencing AF in the ICU and who was receiving outpatient therapy with oral anticoagulation,

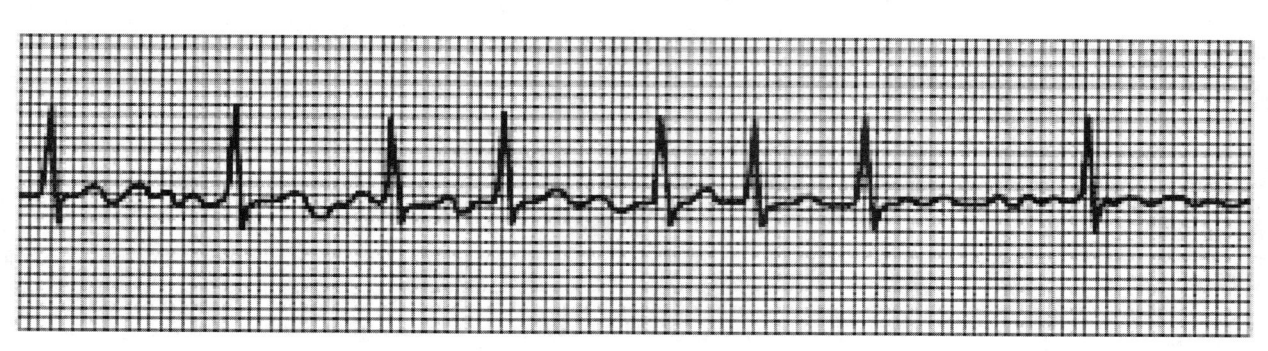

Figure 35.10 Atrial fibrillation.

Reprinted with permission from: Tisdale JE. Review of cardiac arrhythmias and rhythm interpretation. In: Wiggins BS, Sanoski CA. Emergency Cardiovascular Pharmacotherapy. A Point-of-Care Guide. Bethesda, MD: American Society of Health-System Pharmacists, 2012:32.

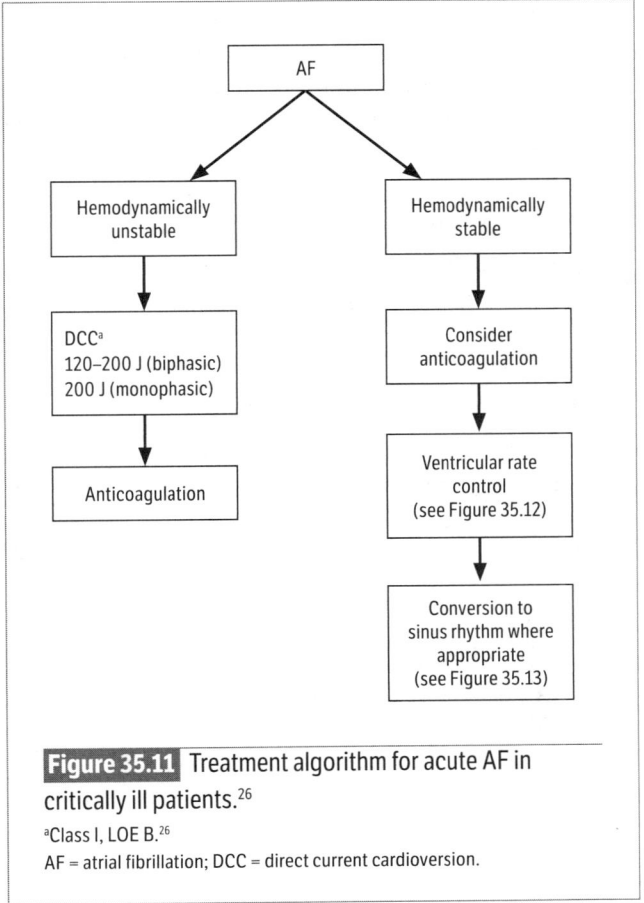

Figure 35.11 Treatment algorithm for acute AF in critically ill patients.[26]
aClass I, LOE B.[26]
AF = atrial fibrillation; DCC = direct current cardioversion.

anticoagulation should be continued whenever possible and appropriate. It may be reasonable to discontinue oral anticoagulation and initiate intravenous heparin or subcutaneous low-molecular-weight heparin therapy during the hospitalization. For critically ill patients with new-onset AF, the decision regarding the need for long-term anticoagulation will likely be deferred to postdischarge follow-up. During the period of hospitalization, anticoagulation is desirable if the bleeding risk is acceptable.

Patients with AF that is hemodynamically unstable should undergo immediate DCC (Figure 35.11), after which anticoagulation should be initiated in appropriate patients. Anticoagulation should be considered for patients with hemodynamically stable AF as well, particularly for patients undergoing elective DCC. If AF has been present for longer than 48 hours, anticoagulation should be initiated for patients with an acceptable bleeding risk. Bridging therapy with unfractionated heparin or low-molecular-weight heparin is recommended for patients with AF and a mechanical heart valve undergoing procedures requiring interruption of oral anticoagulation.[26] For patients with AF less than 48 hours' duration and high risk of thromboembolism who require conversion to sinus rhythm, intravenous unfractionated heparin, subcutaneous low-molecular-weight heparin, or a factor Xa or direct thrombin inhibitor is recommended as soon as possible before or immediately after cardioversion, followed by long-term anticoagulation.[26] For patients with AF less than 48 hours' duration who are at low risk of thromboembolism, intravenous heparin, subcutaneous low-molecular-weight heparin, a new oral anticoagulant, or no antithrombotic may be considered for cardioversion, with no need for postcardioversion anticoagulation.[26] For patients with AF greater than 48 hours' duration who require conversion to sinus rhythm, conversion to sinus rhythm should be deferred if an atrial thrombus is identified on transesophageal echocardiogram (TEE), and anticoagulation should be initiated and continued for 3–4 weeks before repeating the TEE.[26]

In view of symptoms, morbidity, and prolonged length of ICU and total hospital stay associated with postoperative AF, prophylaxis may be reasonable in high-risk patients.[26,44,79] For patients undergoing CABG surgery with or without valve replacement who are at high risk of AF, preoperative administration of β-blockers and/or amiodarone is reasonable. β-Blockers have been shown to significantly reduce the incidence of post-CABG AF; in a Cochrane systematic review, the odds ratio (95% confidence interval) for post-CABG AF associated with β-blockers was 0.35 (0.26–0.49).[79] β-Blockers should not be discontinued before CABG surgery because preoperative β-blocker discontinuation increases the risk of postoperative AF. Oral amiodarone has also been shown to reduce the incidence of post-CABG AF[39] and is recommended in patients at high risk of AF.[26] Other drugs that may be considered for prophylaxis of post-CABG AF in patients at high risk include sotalol[26,80] and colchicine.[26,81] Drugs for prevention of post-CABG AF are presented in Table 35.4.

Pharmacologic prophylaxis of AF after noncardiac thoracic surgery is also recommended for intermediate- or high-risk patients.[44] As with post-CABG AF, patients taking β-blockers before noncardiac thoracic surgery should continue to take them postoperatively.[44] Intravenous diltiazem has been shown to reduce the incidence of AF after noncardiac thoracic surgery.[61] Amiodarone reduces the incidence of AF after pulmonary resection[40,82] as well as after esophagectomy.[42] Atorvastatin has been shown to reduce the incidence of AF after noncardiac thoracic surgery,[83] as has intravenous magnesium.[84] Drugs for prevention of AF after noncardiac thoracic surgery are presented in Table 35.5.

VENTRICULAR ARRHYTHMIAS

Ventricular Tachycardia

Features

In this section, VT with a pulse will be discussed. Pulseless VT will be discussed in the chapter titled Management of Cardiac Arrest. For this chapter, VT refers to monomorphic VT, a tachyarrhythmia of ventricular origin for which the QRS complexes appear the same (i.e., have a single consistent morphology) (Figure 35.14).

Ventricular tachycardia may be nonsustained or sustained.[85] Nonsustained VT is defined as three or more consecutive complexes in duration, at a rate of greater than 100 beats/minute, and which terminates spontaneously in less than 30 seconds.[85] Sustained VT also occurs at a rate greater than 100 beats/minute, but it is greater than 30 seconds in duration or requires termination because of hemodynamic compromise in less than 30 seconds.[85]

Epidemiology

The incidence of VT is variable and dependent on the etiology and underlying comorbidities. Around 2%–4% of patients having an acute MI develop sustained VT.[86] Most of these patients experience VT within 48 hours of the MI, whereas a small proportion may develop VT later than 48 hours. Nonsustained VT occurs in 20%–80% of patients with HF.[87]

The overall incidence or prevalence of VT in critically ill patients in ICUs has not been studied widely. In an epidemiologic study conducted in a 10-bed ICU in a university hospital in South America from August 1971 to April 1983, 502 of 2,820 patients (17.8%) developed "rapid ventricular arrhythmia."[88] Reinelt et al.[5] reported that VT occurred in 54 of 756 patients (7.1%) in a medical-cardiology ICU at a university hospital during an almost 3-year period. A total of 135 episodes of VT (49% of all episodes of tachycardias) occurred in these 54 patients.

Pathophysiology

Ventricular tachycardia is usually triggered by a ventricular premature depolarization and is sustained by ventricular reentry.

Etiologies

In about 80% of cases, VT occurs in the setting of structural heart disease, primarily coronary heart disease and/or left ventricular dysfunction/cardiomyopathy.[2,85] In the absence of structural heart disease, right ventricular outflow tract VT is the most common type.[89] Other etiologies of VT include electrolyte abnormalities such as hypokalemia, hypoxia, and, rarely, drugs.[90] Flecainide and propafenone can induce an incessant VT characterized by wide QRS complexes having a sinusoidal appearance.[91,92] Flecainide was associated with

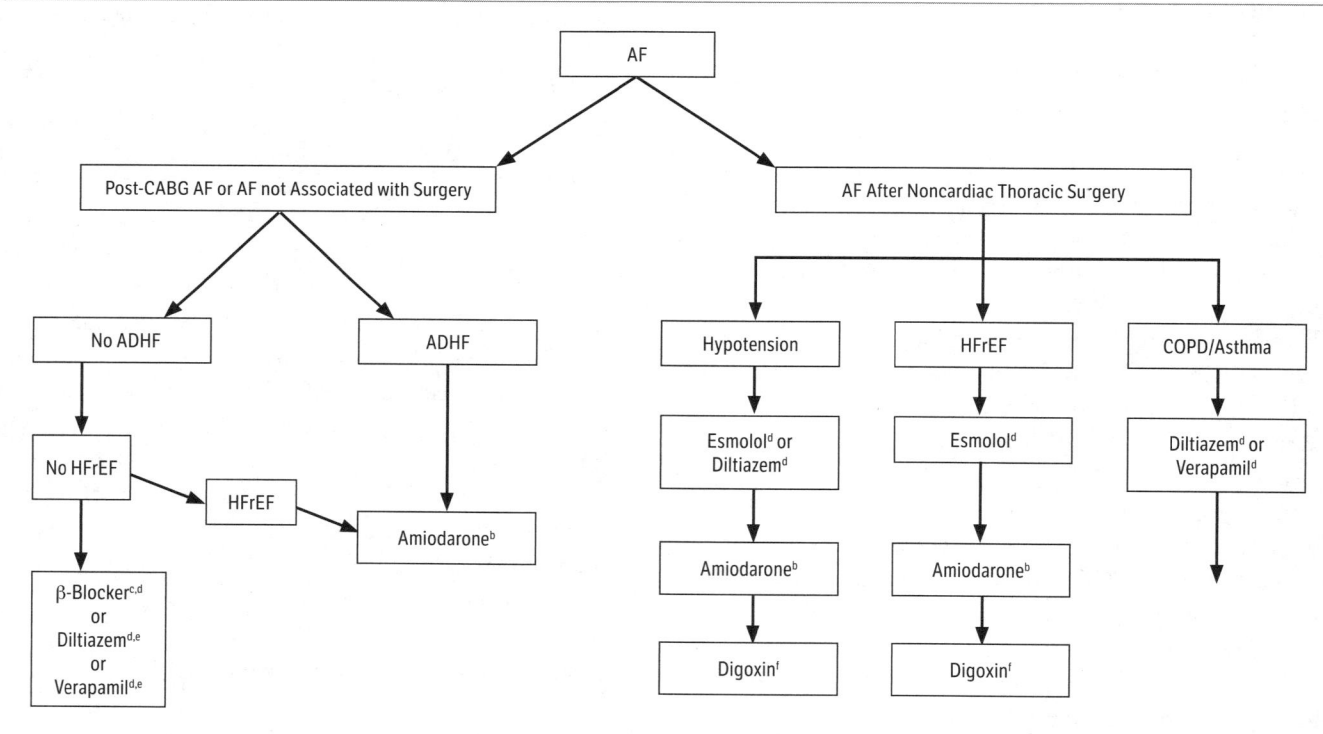

Figure 35.12 Treatment algorithm for acute ventricular rate control in critically ill patients with hemodynamically stable AF.[a]

[a]Drugs administered intravenously.
[b]Class IIa, LOE B.[26,44]
[c]Esmolol, metoprolol, or propranolol.
[d]Class I, LOE B.[26,44]
[e]Diltiazem is generally preferred to verapamil because of a lower potential for profound hypotension.[68]
[f]Class IIb, LOE B.[26,44]

ADHF = acute decompensated heart failure; CABG = coronary artery bypass graft; COPD = chronic obstructive pulmonary disease.

increased mortality, because of presumed ventricular proarrhythmia, in patients after MI in the CAST study (Cardiac Arrhythmia Suppression Trial).[93] In this study and its follow-up,[94] the Vaughan-Williams class IC drugs encainide and moricizine were also associated with increased mortality caused by presumed ventricular proarrhythmia; therefore, flecainide and, by extension, propafenone are contraindicated in patients with any history of coronary heart disease.

Ibutilide has been associated with episodes of nonsustained VT in about 5% of patients.[95]

Risk Factors

Independent predictors of sustained VT after an acute MI include lower baseline systolic blood pressure, in-hospital use of intravenous lidocaine for post-MI VT prophylaxis, higher Killip class, faster heart rate, and advanced age.[86]

Table 35.3 Drugs for Conversion to Sinus Rhythm in Critically Ill Patients with Atrial Fibrillation

Drug	Mechanism	Dose	Adverse Effects
Amiodarone[a,b]	Na channel inhibition, I_{Kr} inhibition	150 mg IV over 10 min; then 1 mg/min continuous IV infusion for 6 hr, followed by 0.5 mg/min or 600–800 mg orally daily in divided doses to a total load of up to 10 g; then 200 mg orally once daily as maintenance	Bradycardia Hypotension Phlebitis QT interval prolongation Torsades de pointes
Dofetilide[b]	I_{Kr} inhibition	CrCl > 60 mL/min: 500 mcg orally twice daily CrCl 40–60 mL/min: 250 mcg CrCl 20–40 mL/min: 125 mcg orally twice daily CrCl < 20 mL/min: contraindicated	QT interval prolongation, torsades de pointes
Ibutilide[b]	I_{Kr} inhibition	1 mg IV over 10 min; may repeat 1 mg once, if necessary, 10 min after first dose If weight < 60 kg, use 0.01 mg/kg	QT interval prolongation Torsades de pointes Nonsustained ventricular tachycardia
Flecainide[b,c,d]	Na channel inhibition	2 mg/kg IV over 10 min or 200–300 mg orally × 1	Heart failure Rapid atrial flutter Hypotension Ventricular proarrhythmia – avoid in patients with structural heart disease
Propafenone[c,d]	Na channel inhibition	2 mg/kg IV over 10 min or 450–600 mg orally × 1	Heart failure Rapid atrial flutter Hypotension Ventricular proarrhythmia – avoid in patients with structural heart disease
Procainamide[b]	Slows conduction in accessory pathway in patients with AF due to WPW	17 mg/kg IV administered at rate of 20–50 mg/min; terminate loading infusion if hypotension, QRS complex increases ≥ 50%, or arrhythmia is terminated. Maintenance IV infusion 1–4 mg/min	Hypotension Heart failure QT interval prolongation Torsades de pointes

[a]Contraindicated in patients with WPW or other preexcitation syndromes.
[b]Avoid in patients with QTc interval > 440 ms (> 500 ms in patients with ventricular conduction abnormalities).
[c]Flecainide and propafenone are not available intravenously in the United States.
[d]β-Blocker, diltiazem, or verapamil should be administered ≥ 30 min before administration of flecainide or propafenone.
CrCl = creatinine clearance; I_{Kr} = rapid component of delayed rectifier potassium current; Na = sodium; WPW = Wolff-Parkinson-White (syndrome).

Female sex and β-blocker use within 2 weeks prior may be protective.[86]

Morbidity and Mortality

Post-MI VT portends a negative prognosis. In patients who experience VT after an acute MI who do not have HF or cardiogenic shock, the hazard ratio for 30-day mortality is 12.9 (7.8–21.3) and, for 1-year mortality, 2.5 (1.7–3.6).[86] Ventricular tachyarrhythmias in critically ill patients are associated with an increased risk of mortality (relative risk 1.47 [1.29–1.67]).[88]

Treatment

Ventricular tachycardia that is hemodynamically unstable should be treated with synchronized DCC.[8] If time permits, the patient should be sedated for cardioversion. The initial recommended DCC dose is 100 J monophasic or biphasic waveform.[8]

Drugs for treatment of hemodynamically stable VT are presented in Table 35.6. Drugs for VT termination include procainamide, amiodarone, sotalol, and lidocaine, all administered intravenously. In a randomized study, intravenous procainamide was significantly more effective at terminating spontaneous sustained monomorphic VT than lidocaine (12 of 15 patients [80%] vs. 3 of 14 patients [21%] with VT successfully terminated, p<0.01).[96] Procainamide terminated 38 of 48 VT episodes (79%) compared with 6 of 31 VT episodes (19%) terminated with lidocaine.[96] Intravenous amiodarone was shown to be effective for management of

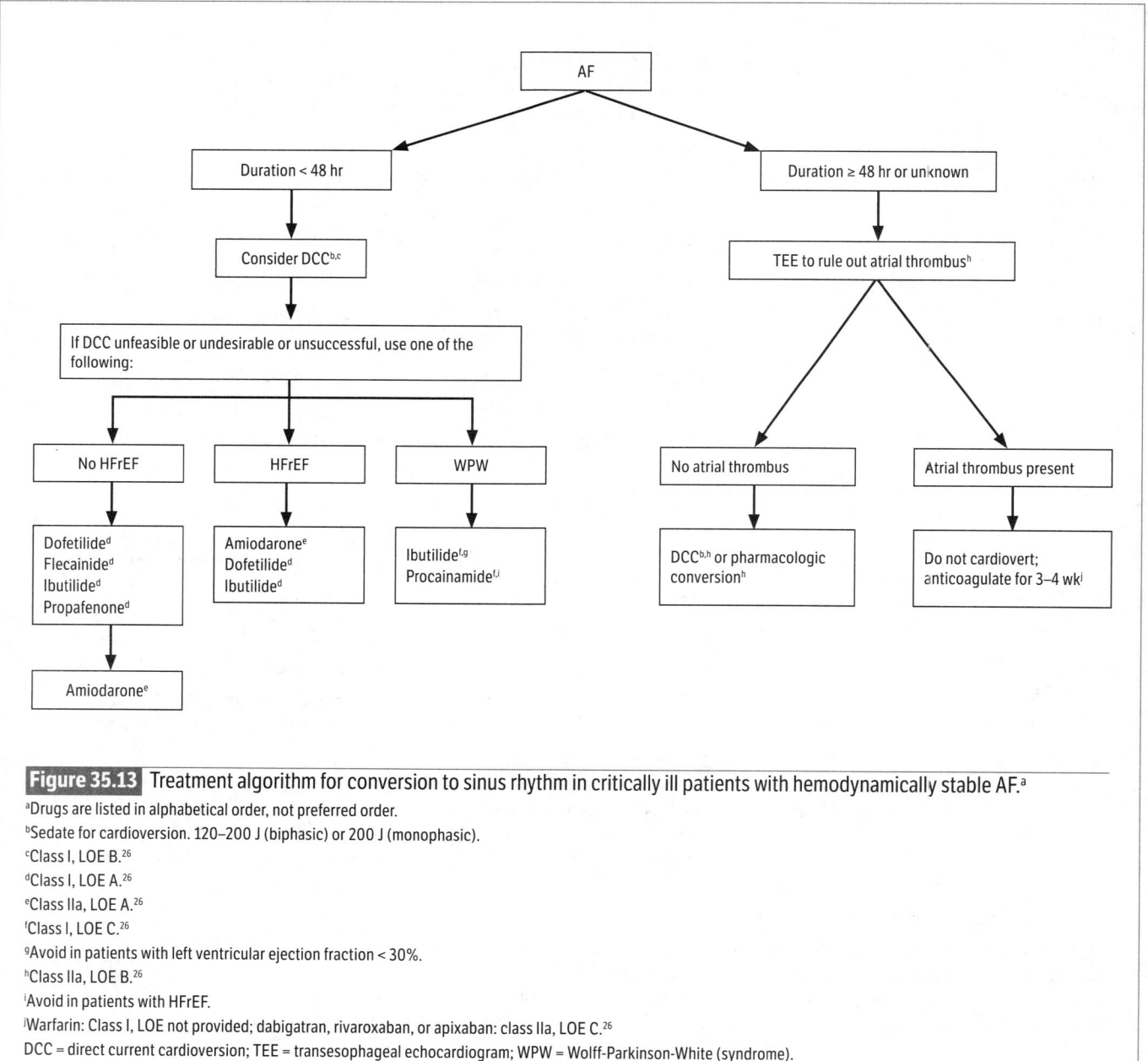

Figure 35.13 Treatment algorithm for conversion to sinus rhythm in critically ill patients with hemodynamically stable AF.[a]

[a]Drugs are listed in alphabetical order, not preferred order.
[b]Sedate for cardioversion. 120–200 J (biphasic) or 200 J (monophasic).
[c]Class I, LOE B.[26]
[d]Class I, LOE A.[26]
[e]Class IIa, LOE A.[26]
[f]Class I, LOE C.[26]
[g]Avoid in patients with left ventricular ejection fraction < 30%.
[h]Class IIa, LOE B.[26]
[i]Avoid in patients with HFrEF.
[j]Warfarin: Class I, LOE not provided; dabigatran, rivaroxaban, or apixaban: class IIa, LOE C.[26]
DCC = direct current cardioversion; TEE = transesophageal echocardiogram; WPW = Wolff-Parkinson-White (syndrome).

life-threatening ventricular arrhythmias in a double-blind dose-ranging study.[97] Intravenous amiodarone was also found to be more effective than lidocaine for termination of incessant, shock-resistant VT (VT terminated in 78% of amiodarone-treated patients vs. 27% of lidocaine-treated patients, p<0.05).[98] In addition, intravenous amiodarone has been shown to be effective for terminating sustained hypotensive VT refractory to therapy with procainamide, lidocaine, and bretylium.[99] Evidence supports the efficacy of intravenous sotalol for termination of hemodynamically stable monomorphic VT.[100] Like procainamide and amiodarone, intravenous sotalol was found to be more effective than lidocaine for termination of spontaneous sustained VT in a randomized, double-blind study; VT termination rates in the sotalol and lidocaine groups were 69% and 18%, respectively (p=0.003).[101] Because of the superior efficacy of procainamide, amiodarone, and sotalol, lidocaine should be considered a second-line therapy for termination of monomorphic VT.[8] Intravenous procainamide and sotalol should be avoided in patients with HFrEF because of negative inotropic activity and an increased risk of TdP. A treatment algorithm for termination of ventricular tachycardia is presented in Figure 35.15. For patients who do not respond to maximally tolerated doses of drugs recommended in Figure 35.15, elective DCC may be necessary.

Torsades de Pointes

Features

Torsades de pointes is a polymorphic VT associated with prolongation of the QT interval.[102] The term *torsades de pointes* means "twisting of the points" and was originally named because of the ECG appearance of the "points" of the QRS complex twisting around the isoelectric baseline (Figure 35.16).[103] Torsades de pointes is also characterized on ECG by a short-long-short RR interval pattern immediately preceding the onset of the arrhythmia.[102] Heart rates during TdP range from 160 to 240 beats/minute.[102] Although TdP often terminates spontaneously, it can degenerate into ventricular fibrillation and cause sudden cardiac death. QT interval prolongation and TdP may be congenital (congenital long QT syndrome [LQTS]) or acquired. Acquired QT interval prolongation and TdP is usually caused by drugs.[90]

Epidemiology

Thirteen forms of the congenital LQTS have been identified.[104] Overall, congenital LQTS occurs in about 1 in 2,000 live births.[2] The incidence of TdP in patients with congenital LQTS is variable, about 14%–21% among patients younger than 12 years, 25% among patients 12–18 years of age, and 16%–39% among patients 18–40 years of age.[104]

The overall incidence of drug-induced TdP in the general population is unknown. A population-based study in Sweden found an annualized incidence of TdP of 4 per 100,000.[105] Extrapolation of that incidence to the population of the U.S. suggests that around 12,000–13,000 cases of drug-induced TdP may occur annually.[90] However, a more recent study conducted in Berlin estimated the annual incidence of drug-induced LQTS/TdP in that city to be 2.5 per million in men and 4 per million in women.[106] Extrapolation of those estimates to the U.S. population suggests a lower incidence of drug-induced LQTS/TdP, about 400 cases annually in men and 640 cases per women, for an annual number of just more than 1,000 cases. The incidence of drug-induced TdP in the U.S. requires further study. The risk of TdP associated with individual QT interval–prolonging drugs is 2%–12%.[90]

QT interval prolongation is prevalent in critically ill patients. In a study conducted during a 1-year period in 1,159 consecutive patients admitted to two cardiac ICUs at a large academic medical center, Bazett's corrected QT (QTc) interval prolongation was present in 28% of patients on admission, and 18% had a QTc interval greater than 500 milliseconds.[107] Of these, 35% and 42%, respectively, were subsequently prescribed QT interval–prolonging

Table 35.4	Drugs for Prophylaxis of Post-CABG AF	
Drug	**Dose**	**Guideline Recommendation[26]**
Amiodarone[a]	10 mg/kg orally initiated 6 days before surgery and continued for 6 days postoperatively[39]	Class IIa, LOE A
Sotalol[a]	80–120 mg orally twice daily initiated 24–48 hr before surgery and continued 4 days postoperatively[80]	Class IIb, LOE B
Colchicine	1.0 mg orally twice daily on postoperative day 3, followed by 0.5 mg orally twice daily for 1 mo	Class IIb, LOE B
	In patients < 70 kg: 0.5 mg orally twice daily, followed by 0.25 mg orally twice daily for 1 mo[81]	

[a]Avoid in patients with QTc interval > 440 ms (> 500 ms in patients with ventricular conduction abnormalities).

drugs, despite being admitted with QTc interval prolongation.[107] Pickham et al. reported that 24% of patients in adult ICU and progressive care units developed QTc interval prolongation.[108] In a prospective cohort study of patients admitted to a mixed medical-surgical ICU, 52% had a QTc interval greater than 500 milliseconds during the ICU stay.[109] The prevalence of QTc interval prolongation in critically ill patients is high because of a preponderance of risk factors, including comorbid conditions and frequent use of QT interval–prolonging medications.[107]

The incidence of TdP in critically ill patients in ICUs has not been widely studied. Pickham et al. reported one case of TdP among 154 patients (0.6%) in adult ICUs and progressive care units during a 2-month period.[108] This represented 1 of 16 cardiac arrests (6%) in these units during this time.

Pathophysiology

Torsades de pointes occurs as a result of prolongation of ventricular repolarization and increased heterogeneity (dispersion) of ventricular repolarization.[85,110] Drugs that induce TdP usually inhibit the rapid component of the delayed rectifier potassium current (I_{Kr}), resulting in prolonged ventricular repolarization and corresponding prolongation of the QTc interval.[110,111] Torsades de pointes is likely triggered by early afterdepolarizations, the propensity for which is increased in the setting of prolonged ventricular repolarization.[112] After triggered initiation, TdP is propagated by reentry.

Etiologies

As described, TdP may be congenital or acquired. Congenital LQTS leading to TdP is caused by mutations in up to 13 different genes, but more than 92% of cases are accounted for by mutations in *KCNQ1*, *KCNH2*, and *SCNA5*, which encode the slow component of the delayed rectifier potassium channel (I_{Ks}), I_{Kr}, and sodium channels, respectively.[113] Acquired TdP is most commonly caused by drugs. Medications that may cause TdP include those from a variety of drug classes, including antiarrhythmic agents, antibiotics and other anti-infectives, antipsychotics, antidepressants, and many others.[90] A good resource for up-to-date lists of drugs that may prolong the QT interval and cause TdP is maintained on the website *crediblemeds.org*, which is maintained by AZCERT (Arizona Center for Education and Research on Therapeutics). Drugs that may cause TdP are listed in Table 35.7. Many of these drugs are used in the ICU, including antibiotics, antiarrhythmics, antiemetics, and others. In particular, intravenous haloperidol has commonly been used in ICUs for delusional agitation. Intravenous haloperidol has been associated with a high incidence of TdP in critically ill patients in some series, particularly in association with higher doses.[114] Because of a lack of evidence of efficacy and the risk of QTc interval prolongation and TdP associated with intravenous haloperidol, the drug is no longer recommended for management of delirium in adult patients in the ICU.[115]

Table 35.5 Drugs for Prophylaxis of AF After Noncardiac Thoracic Surgery

Drug	Dose	Guideline Recommendation[44]
Diltiazem	0.25 mg/kg IV over 30 min; then 0.1 mg/kg/hr continuous IV infusion for 18–24 hr[61]	Class IIa, LOE B
	On morning of postoperative day 1, initiate 120 mg orally twice daily for 14 days[61]	
Amiodarone[a]	Pulmonary resection: 300 mg IV bolus initiated immediately after surgery and transfer to ICU; then 600 mg orally twice daily for 3–5 days[82]	Class IIa, LOE A
	Esophagectomy: 43.75 mg/hr IV continuous infusion for 96 hr, initiated at time of induction of anesthesia[42]	Class IIb, LOE B
Atorvastatin	20–40 mg orally once daily[83]	Class IIb, LOE C
Magnesium[b]	Magnesium sulfate 2 g IV administered over 20 min at time of thoracotomy and 2 g IV administered over 20 min 6 hr later[84]	Class IIb, LOE C

[a]Avoid in patients with QTc interval > 440 ms (> 500 ms in patients with ventricular conduction abnormalities).
[b]When serum magnesium concentration is low or total body magnesium depletion is suspected.

Risk Factors

Risk factors for drug-induced TdP have been widely described. Drug-induced TdP is substantially dependent on risk factors and is a particularly rare occurrence in the absence of risk factors. In an analysis of 144 published articles describing 249 patients who experienced TdP induced by noncardiac drugs, almost 100% of the patients had at least one risk factor, and 71% of the patients had two or more risk factors.[116]

Risk factors for drug-induced TdP are listed in Box 35.2. The risk of TdP increases markedly when the QTc interval is prolonged to beyond 500 milliseconds.[117] More than 90% of TdP cases occur when the QTc interval is greater than 500 milliseconds, and TdP rarely occurs when the QTc interval is less than 500 milliseconds.[118] The risk of TdP also may be increased when the QTc interval is prolonged greater than 60 milliseconds from pretreatment

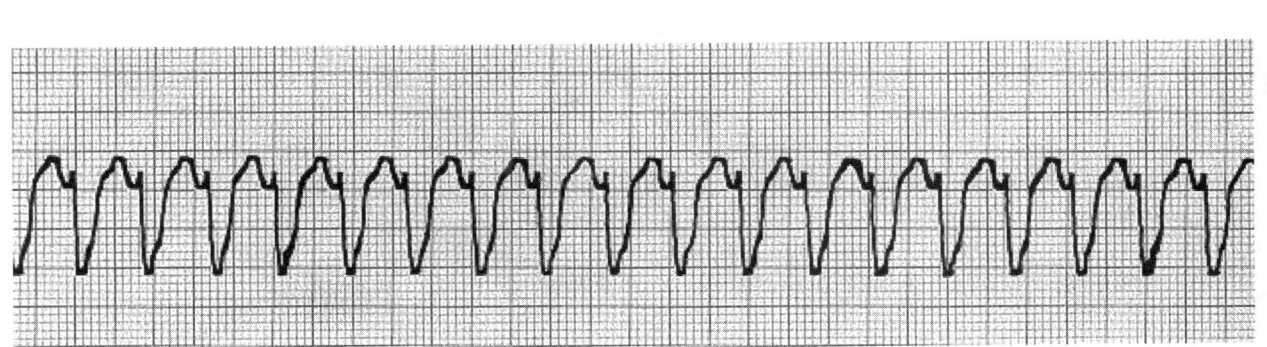

Figure 35.14 Ventricular tachycardia.

Reprinted with permission from: Tisdale JE. Review of cardiac arrhythmias and rhythm interpretation. In: Wiggins BS, Sanoski CA. Emergency Cardiovascular Pharmacotherapy. A Point-of-Care Guide. Bethesda, MD: American Society of Health-System Pharmacists, 2012:36.

Table 35.6 Drugs for Termination of Hemodynamically Stable VT in Critically Ill Patients

Drug	Dose	Adverse Effects
Amiodarone[a]	150 mg IV given over 10 min and repeated if necessary, followed by a continuous IV infusion of 1 mg/min for 6 hr; then 0.5 mg/min. Total dose should not exceed 2.2 g over 24 hr	Bradycardia, hypotension, phlebitis, QT interval prolongation
Lidocaine	Loading dose of 1.0–1.5 mg/kg IV; repeat if necessary at 0.5–0.75 mg/kg every 5–10 min up to maximum total dose of 3 mg/kg. Then administer continuous IV infusion at 1–4 mg/min	Slurred speech, mental status changes, seizures
Procainamide[a,b]	20–50 mg/min continuous IV infusion until VT terminated, hypotension occurs, or QRS duration prolonged by 50%, or total cumulative dose of 17 mg/kg administered. Alternative loading regimen: 100 mg IV every 5 min until VT is terminated or other conditions described above are met	Bradycardia, hypotension, torsades de pointes
Sotalol[a,b]	1.5 mg/kg IV administered by slow infusion over 5 hr	Bradycardia, hypotension, torsades de pointes

[a]Avoid in patients with QTc interval > 440 ms (> 500 ms in patients with ventricular conduction abnormalities).
[b]Avoid in patients with heart failure and/or QT interval prolongation.
VT = ventricular tachycardia.

value.[118] Women are at a higher risk of TdP than men, possibly as a result of proarrhythmic effects of estradiol in women[119] or protective effects of testosterone in men.[120] Hypokalemia, hypomagnesemia, and hypocalcemia increase the risk of TdP; hypokalemia was present in 28% of TdP associated with noncardiac drugs.[116] Low extracellular potassium concentrations enhance drug-induced I_{Kr} inhibition.[121] Older age is a risk factor for TdP for reasons that are uncertain, but this could be related to declining serum testosterone concentrations in men and low serum progesterone concentrations in postmenopausal women.[119,120] Heart failure with reduced ejection fraction is a prominent risk factor for drug-induced TdP; the incidence of TdP associated with drugs such as ibutilide and dofetilide is 2–3 times higher in patients with HFrEF than in patients with normal left ventricular function.[72,122]

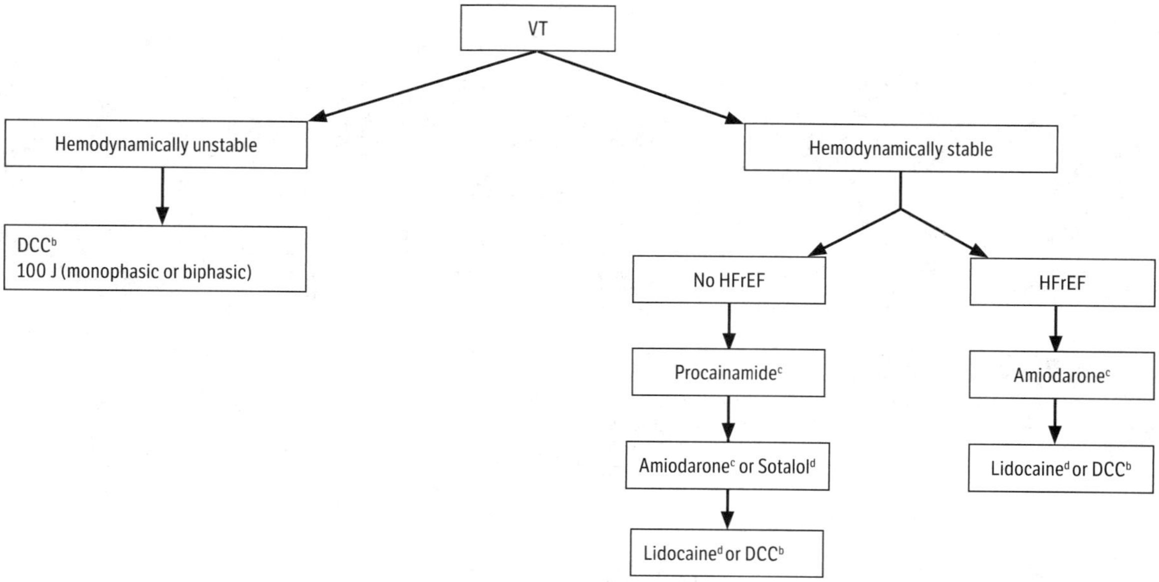

Figure 35.15 Treatment algorithm for termination of VT in critically ill patients.[a]

[a]All drugs administered intravenously.
[b]Class IIb, LOE C.[8]
[c]Class IIa, LOE B.[8]
[d]Class IIb, LOE B.[8]
DCC = direct current cardioversion (synchronized); VT = ventricular tachycardia.

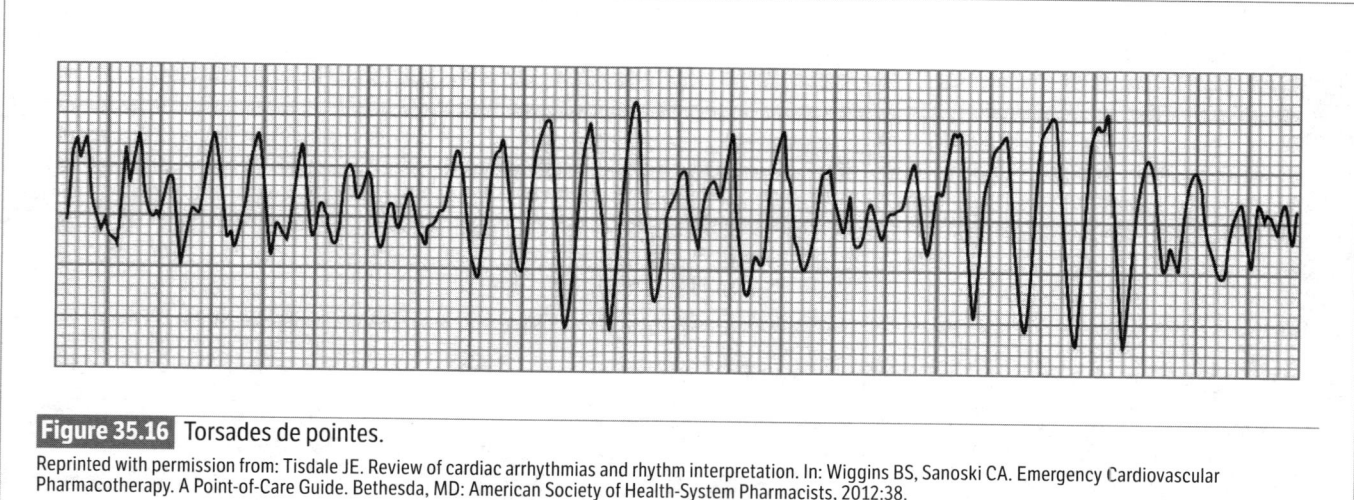

Figure 35.16 Torsades de pointes.

Reprinted with permission from: Tisdale JE. Review of cardiac arrhythmias and rhythm interpretation. In: Wiggins BS, Sanoski CA. Emergency Cardiovascular Pharmacotherapy. A Point-of-Care Guide. Bethesda, MD: American Society of Health-System Pharmacists, 2012:38.

Some patients who develop drug-induced TdP may have an underlying genetic predisposition. Polymorphisms of genes associated with the congenital LQTS may be present in 10%–15% of patients with drug-induced TdP.[123]

Risk factors for QTc interval prolongation in critically ill patients have been identified and incorporated into a QTc interval prolongation risk score, in which 1, 2, or 3 points was assigned to each risk factor.[124] Independent risk factors for QTc interval prolongation in critically ill patients were similar to those associated with TdP and included age 68 years or older (1 point), female sex (1 point), taking a loop diuretic (1 point), serum potassium of 3.5 mEq/L or less (2 points), admission QTc interval of 450 milliseconds or greater (2 points), acute MI (2 points), HFrEF (3 points), receiving one QTc interval–prolonging agent (3 points), and receiving two or more QTc interval–prolonging drugs (3 points). In addition, sepsis was an independent risk factor for QTc interval prolongation (3 points).[124] A risk score in the intermediate (7–10) or high (11 or more) range predicted critically ill patients at highest risk of developing QTc interval prolongation.[124]

Morbidity and Mortality

Drug-induced TdP occurring in the ICU may be associated with prolonged duration of hospital stay.[114] Torsades de pointes may remain hemodynamically stable, or it may be hemodynamically unstable and rapidly degenerate into ventricular fibrillation and cause cardiac arrest/sudden cardiac death.

Prevention and Treatment

In critically ill patients receiving drugs that may cause TdP, clinicians must be attentive to methods of reducing the risk of TdP. QTc interval–prolonging drugs should be avoided, whenever possible, in patients with a pretreatment QTc

Table 35.7 Drugs That May Cause Torsades de Pointes

Drug Class	Drug(s)
Anesthetic	Propofol
	Sevoflurane
Antiarrhythmic	Amiodarone
	Disopyramide
	Dofetilide
	Dronedarone
	Flecainide
	Ibutilide
	Procainamide
	Quinidine
	Sotalol
Antibiotic	Azithromycin
	Ciprofloxacin
	Clarithromycin
	Erythromycin
	Levofloxacin
	Moxifloxacin
Anticancer	Arsenic trioxide
	Vandetanib
Antiemetic	Droperidol
	Ondansetron
Antidepressant	Citalopram
	Escitalopram
Antifungal	Fluconazole
	Pentamidine
Antimalarial	Chloroquine
	Halofantrine
Antipsychotic	Chlorpromazine
	Haloperidol
	Pimozide
	Thioridazine
Cholinesterase inhibitor	Donepezil
Miscellaneous	Cocaine
	Methadone

Box 35.2. Risk Factors for Drug-Induced TdP

- QTc interval > 500 ms
- Increase in QTc interval ≥ 60 ms from pretreatment value
- Female sex
- Age > 65 yr
- HFrEF
- Recent myocardial infarction
- Hypokalemia
- Hypomagnesemia
- Hypocalcemia
- Treatment with diuretics
- Bradycardia
- Sequential bilateral bundle branch block
- Elevation in serum concentration of QTc interval–prolonging drug because of drug interaction or inadequate dose adjustment for kidney disease
- Rapid intravenous injection of QTc interval–prolonging drug
- Possible genetic predisposition
- History of drug-induced TdP

HFrEF = heart failure with reduced ejection fraction; TdP = torsades de pointes.

interval greater than 450 milliseconds. If a patient receiving a QTc interval–prolonging drug has a QTc interval increase of 60 milliseconds or greater from pretreatment value, the dose should be reduced or the drug discontinued whenever possible. Drugs with the potential to cause TdP should be discontinued if the QTc interval is prolonged to greater than 500 milliseconds. Serum potassium, magnesium, and calcium concentrations should be maintained within the normal range. When possible, avoid use of drugs with the potential to cause TdP in patients with HFrEF, particularly if the left ventricular ejection fraction is less than 20%. Doses of renally eliminated QTc interval–prolonging drugs should be adjusted in patients with acute kidney injury or chronic kidney disease. When possible, avoid using combinations of drugs that prolong the QTc interval. Avoid concomitant use of cytochrome P450 (CYP) system inhibitors and QTc interval–prolonging drugs that are CYP substrates. Avoid administering drugs with the potential to cause TdP in patients with a history of drug-induced TdP and in those with a diagnosis of the congenital LQTS. Critically ill patients receiving therapy with a QTc interval–prolonging drug should be maintained on continuous telemetry monitoring, and the QTc interval should be documented every 8–12 hours.[102]

A treatment algorithm for management of TdP in critically ill patients is presented in Figure 35.17. Patients with TdP that is hemodynamically unstable should undergo asynchronous defibrillation, rather than synchronized cardioversion, because synchronization of shocks in polymorphic arrhythmias is often impossible.[8] In patients with TdP that is hemodynamically stable, intravenous magnesium is recommended, primarily on the basis of two observational studies.[125,126] In patients who do not respond to intravenous magnesium, isoproterenol or overdrive pacing may be used if patients have TdP that is associated with bradycardia or that appears to be precipitated by pauses in rhythm. Elective defibrillation may be used in refractory cases that are hemodynamically stable.[8] Refractory TdP associated with sotalol has been successfully managed using hemodialysis[127] or peritoneal dialysis.[128]

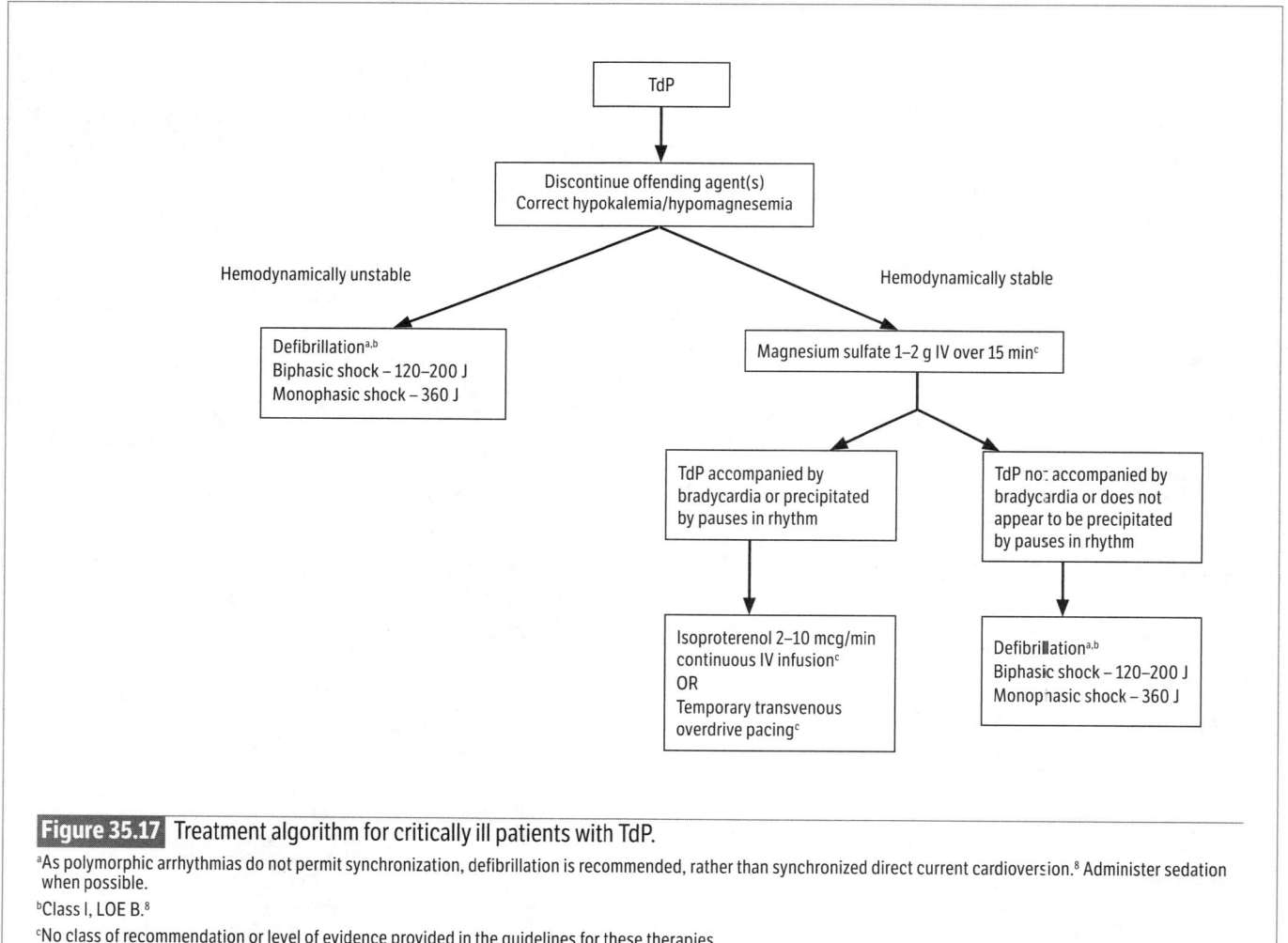

Figure 35.17 Treatment algorithm for critically ill patients with TdP.

[a]As polymorphic arrhythmias do not permit synchronization, defibrillation is recommended, rather than synchronized direct current cardioversion.[8] Administer sedation when possible.
[b]Class I, LOE B.[8]
[c]No class of recommendation or level of evidence provided in the guidelines for these therapies.
TdP = torsades de pointes.

REFERENCES

1. Mangrum JM, DiMarco JP. The evaluation and management of bradycardia. N Engl J Med 2000;342:703-9.
2. Mozaffarian D, Benjamin EJ, Go AS, et al.; on behalf of the American Heart Association Statistics Committee and Stroke Statistics Subcommittee. Heart disease and stroke statistics—2015 update: a report from the American Heart Association. Circulation 2015;131:e29-e322.
3. Kojic EM, Hardarson T, Sigfusson N, et al. The prevalence and prognosis of third-degree atrioventricular conduction block: the Reykjavik study. J Intern Med 1999;246:81-6.
4. Baine WB, Yu W, Weis KA. Trends and outcomes in the hospitalization of older Americans for cardiac conduction disorders or arrhythmias, 1991-1998. J Am Geriatr Soc 2001;49:763-70.
5. Reinelt P, Karth GD, Geppert A, et al. Incidence and type of cardiac arrhythmias in critically ill patients: a single center experience in a medical-cardiological ICU. Intensive Care Med 2001;27:1466-73.
6. Reising S, Kusumoto F, Goldschlager N. Life-threatening arrhythmias in the intensive care unit. J Intensive Care Med 2007;22:3-13.
7. Tisdale JE. Supraventricular arrhythmias. In: Tisdale JE, Miller DA, eds. Drug-Induced Diseases: Prevention, Detection and Management, 2nd ed. Bethesda, MD: American Society of Health-System Pharmacists, 2010:445-84.
8. Neumar RW, Otto CW, Link MS, et al. Part 8: adult advanced cardiovascular life support: 2010 American Heart Association Guidelines for Cardiopulmonary Resuscitation and Emergency Cardiovascular Care. Circulation 2010;122(suppl 3):S729-S767.
9. Vanden Hoek TL, Morrison LJ, Shuster M, et al. Part 12: cardiac arrest in special situations. 2010 American Heart Association guidelines for cardiopulmonary resuscitation and emergency cardiovascular care. Circulation 2010;122(suppl):S829-S861.
10. Chadda KD, Lichstein E, Gupta PK, et al. Bradycardia-hypotension syndrome in acute myocardial infarction. Reappraisal of the overdrive effects of atropine. Am J Med 1975;59:158-64.
11. Smith I, Monk TG, White PF. Comparison of transesophageal atrial pacing with anticholinergic drugs for the treatment of sinus bradycardia. Anesth Analg 1994;78:245-52.
12. Brady WJ, Swart G, DeBehnke DJ, et al. The efficacy of atropine in the treatment of hemodynamically unstable bradycardia and atrioventricular block: prehospital and emergency department considerations. Resuscitation 1999;41:47-55.
13. Kerns W II. Management of β-adrenergic blocker and calcium channel antagonist toxicity. Emerg Med Clin North Am 2007;25:309-31.
14. Barton CA, Johnson NB, Mah ND, et al. Successful treatment of a massive metoprolol overdose using intravenous lipid emulsion and hyperinsulinemia/euglycemia therapy. Pharmacotherapy 2015;35:e56-60.
15. Sebe A, Dişel NR, Akpinar AA, et al. Role of intravenous lipid emulsions in the management of calcium channel blocker and β-blocker overdose: 3 years experience of a university hospital. Postgrad Med 2015;127:119-24.
16. Delecrétaz E. Supraventricular tachycardia. N Engl J Med 2006;354:1039-51.
17. Blomström-Lundqvist C, Scheinman MM, Aliot EM, et al. ACC/AHA/ESC guidelines for the management of patients with supraventricular arrhythmias—executive summary: a report of the American College of Cardiology/American Heart Association Task Force on Practice Guidelines, and the European Society of Cardiology Committee for Practice Guidelines (Writing Committee to Develop Guidelines for the Management of Patients With Supraventricular Arrhythmias.). J Am Coll Cardiol 2003;42:1493-531.
18. Link MS. Evaluation and initial treatment of supraventricular tachycardia. N Engl J Med 2012;367:1438-48.
19. Orejarena LA, Vidaillet H, DeStefano F, et al. Paroxysmal supraventricular tachycardia in the general population. J Am Coll Cardiol 1998;31:150-7.
20. Ganz LI, Friedman PL. Supraventricular tachycardia. N Engl J Med 1995;332:162-73.
21. Annane D, Sébille V, Duboc D, et al. Incidence and prognosis of sustained arrhythmias in critically ill patients. Am J Respir Crit Care Med 2008;178:20-5.
22. Goodman S, Shirov T, Weissman C. Supraventricular arrhythmias in intensive care unit patients: short and long-term consequences. Anesth Analg 2007;104:880-6.
23. Champion S, Lefort Y, Gaüzère BA, et al. CHADS2 and CHA2DS2-VASc scores can predict thromboembolic events after supraventricular arrhythmia in the critically ill patients. J Crit Care 2014;29:854-8.
24. Wu EB, Chia HM, Gill JS. Reversible cardiomyopathy after radiofrequency ablation of lateral free-wall pathway-mediated incessant supraventricular tachycardia. Pacing Clin Electrophysiol 2000;23:1308-10.
25. DiMarco JP, Miles W, Akhtar M, et al. Adenosine for paroxysmal supraventricular tachycardia: dose ranging and comparison with verapamil. Assessment in placebo-controlled, multicenter trials. The Adenosine for PSVT Study Group. Ann Intern Med 1990;113:104-10.
26. January CT, Wann LS, Alpert JS, et al. 2014 AHA/ACC/HRS guideline for the management of patients with atrial fibrillation: a report of the American College of Cardiology/American Heart Association Task Force on Practice Guidelines and the Heart Rhythm Society. J Am Coll Cardiol 2014;64:e1-76.
27. Khoo C, Lip GYH. Acute management of atrial fibrillation. Chest 2009;135:849-59.
28. Go AS, Hylek EM, Phillips KA, et al. Prevalence of diagnosed atrial fibrillation in adults: national implications for rhythm management and stroke prevention: the AnTicoagulation and Risk Factors in Atrial Fibrillation (ATRIA) Study. JAMA 2001;285:2370-5.
29. Miyasaka Y, Barnes ME, Gersh BJ, et al. Secular trends in incidence of atrial fibrillation in Olmsted County, Minnesota, 1980 to 2000, and implications on the projections for future prevalence [published correction appears in Circulation. 2006;114:e498]. Circulation 2006;114:119-25.
30. Kannel WB, Wolf PA, Benjamin EJ, et al. Prevalence, incidence, prognosis, and predisposing conditions for atrial fibrillation: population-based estimates. Am J Cardiol 1998;82(8A):2N-9N.
31. Chen AY, Sokol SS, Kress JP, et al. New-onset atrial fibrillation is an independent predictor of mortality in medical intensive care unit patients. Ann Pharmacother 2015;49:523-7.

32. Kanji S, Williamson DR, Yaghchi BM, et al. Epidemiology and management of atrial fibrillation in medical and noncardiac surgical adult intensive care unit patients. J Crit Care 2012;27:326.e1-8.
33. Walkey AJ, Wiener RS, Ghobrial JM, et al. Incident stroke and mortality associated with new-onset atrial fibrillation in patients hospitalized with severe sepsis. JAMA 2011;306:2248-55.
34. Christian SA, Schorr C, Ferchau L, et al. Clinical characteristics and outcomes of septic patients with new-onset atrial fibrillation. J Crit Care 2008;23:532-6.
35. Kuipers S, Klein Klouwenberg PMC, Cremer OL. Incidence, risk factors and outcomes of new-onset atrial fibrillation in patients with sepsis: a systematic review. Crit Care 2014;18:688.
36. Guarnieri T, Nolan S, Gottlieb SO, et al. Intravenous amiodarone for the prevention of atrial fibrillation after open heart surgery: the Amiodarone Reduction in Coronary Heart (ARCH) trial. J Am Coll Cardiol 1999;34:343-7.
37. Giri S, White CM, Dunn AB, et al. Oral amiodarone for prevention of atrial fibrillation after open heart surgery, the Atrial Fibrillation Suppression Trial (AFIST): a randomized placebo-controlled trial. Lancet 2001;357:830-6.
38. Connolly SJ, Cybulsky I, Lamy A, et al. Double-blind, placebo-controlled, randomized trial of prophylactic metoprolol for reduction of hospital length of stay after heart surgery: the beta-Blocker Length of Stay (BOLS) study. Am Heart J 2003;145:226-32.
39. Mitchell LB, Exner DV, Wyse DG, et al. Prophylactic oral amiodarone for the prevention of arrhythmias that begin early after revascularization, valve replacement, or repair: PAPABEAR: a randomized controlled trial. JAMA 2005;294:3093-100.
40. Tisdale JE, Wroblewski HA, Wall DS, et al. A randomized trial evaluating amiodarone for prevention of atrial fibrillation after pulmonary resection. Ann Thorac Surg 2009;88:886-95.
41. Tisdale JE, Wroblewski HA, Kesler KA. Prophylaxis of atrial fibrillation after noncardiac thoracic surgery. Semin Thorac Surg 2010;22:310-20.
42. Tisdale JE, Wroblewski HA, Wall DS, et al. A randomized, controlled study of amiodarone for prevention of atrial fibrillation after transthoracic esophagectomy. J Thorac Cardiovasc Surg 2010;140:45-51.
43. Hogue CW, Creswell LL, Gutterman DD, et al. Epidemiology, mechanisms and risks. American College of Chest Physicians guidelines for the management of postoperative atrial fibrillation after cardiac surgery. Chest 2005;128:9S-16S.
44. Frendl G, Sodickson AC, Chung MK, et al. 2014 AATS guidelines for the prevention and management of perioperative atrial fibrillation and flutter for thoracic surgical procedures. J Thorac Cardiovasc Surg 2014;148:e153-e193.
45. Kaakeh Y, Overholser BR, Lopshire JC, et al. Drug-induced atrial fibrillation. Drugs 2012;72:1617-30.
46. Mukamal KJ, Tolstrup JS, Friberg J, et al. Alcohol consumption and risk of atrial fibrillation in men and women: the Copenhagen City Heart Study. Circulation 2005;112:1736-42.
47. Walkey AJ, Greiner MA, Heckbert SR, et al. Atrial fibrillation among Medicare beneficiaries hospitalized with sepsis: incidence and risk factors. Am Heart J 2013;165:949-955.e3.
48. Kolek MJ, Muehlschlegel D, Bush WS, et al. Genetic and clinical risk prediction model for postoperative atrial fibrillation. Circ Arrhythm Electrophysiol 2015;8:25-31.
49. Body SC, Collard CD, Shernan SK, et al. Variation in the 4q25 chromosomal locus predicts atrial fibrillation after coronary artery bypass graft surgery. Circ Cardiovasc Genet 2009;2:499-506.
50. Gibson PH, Croal BL, Cuthbertson BH, et al. Use of preoperative natriuretic peptides and echocardiographic parameters in predicting new-onset atrial fibrillation after coronary artery bypass grafting: a prospective comparative study. Am Heart J 2009;158:244-51.
51. Vaporciyan AA, Correa AM, Rice DC, et al. Risk factors associated with atrial fibrillation after noncardiac thoracic surgery: analysis of 2588 patients. J Thorac Cardiovasc Surg 2004;127:779-86.
52. Onaitis M, D'Amico T, Zhao Y, et al. Risk factors for atrial fibrillation after lung cancer surgery: analysis of the Society of Thoracic Surgeons general thoracic surgery database. Ann Thorac Surg 2010;90:368-74.
53. Amar D, Zhang H, Shi W, et al. Brain natriuretic peptide and risk of atrial fibrillation after thoracic surgery. J Thorac Cardiovasc Surg 2012;144:1249-53.
54. Gurgo AM, Ciccone AM, D'Andrilli A, et al. Plasma NT-proBNP levels and the risk of atrial fibrillation after major lung resection. Minerva Cardioangiol 2008;56:581-5.
55. Passman RS, Gingold DS, Amar D, et al. Prediction rule for atrial fibrillation after major noncardiac thoracic surgery. Ann Thorac Surg 2005;79:1698-703.
56. Mathew JP, Parks R, Savino JS, et al. Atrial fibrillation following coronary artery bypass surgery: predictors, outcomes, and resource utilization. JAMA 1996;276:300-6.
57. Aranki SF, Shaw DP, Adams DH, et al. Predictors of atrial fibrillation after coronary artery surgery: current trends and impact on hospital resources. Circulation 1996;94:390-7.
58. Lahey SJ, Campos CT, Jennings B, et al. Hospital readmission after cardiac surgery: does "fast track" cardiac surgery result in cost saving or cost shifting? Circulation 1998;98(suppl):II-35–II-40.
59. Phan K, Ha HS, Phan S, et al. New-onset atrial fibrillation following coronary artery bypass surgery predicts long-term mortality: a systematic review and meta-analysis. Eur J Cardiothorac Surg 2015; Jan 18; doi: 10.1093/ejcts/ezu551.
60. Barbetakis N, Vassiliadis M. Is amiodarone a safe antiarrhythmic to use in supraventricular tachyarrhythmias after lung cancer surgery? BMC Surg 2004;4:7.
61. Amar D, Roistacher N, Rusch VW, et al. Effects of diltiazem prophylaxis on the incidence and clinical outcome of atrial arrhythmias after thoracic surgery. J Thorac Cardiovasc Surg 2000;120:790-8.
62. Platia EV, Michelson EL, Porterfield JK, et al. Esmolol versus verapamil in the acute treatment of atrial fibrillation or atrial flutter. Am J Cardiol 1989;63:925-9.
63. Abrams J, Allen J, Allin D, et al. Efficacy and safety of esmolol vs propranolol in the treatment of supraventricular tachyarrhythmias: a multicenter double-blind clinical trial. Am Heart J 1985;110:913-22.
64. Demircan C, Cikriklar HI, Engindeniz Z, et al. Comparison of the effectiveness of intravenous diltiazem and metoprolol in the

management of rapid ventricular rate in atrial fibrillation. Emerg Med J 2005;22:411-4.

65. Ellenbogen KA, Dias VC, Plumb VJ, et al. A placebo-controlled trial of continuous intravenous diltiazem infusion for 24-hour heart rate control during atrial fibrillation and atrial flutter: a multicenter study. J Am Coll Cardiol 1991;18:891-7.

66. Siu CW, Lau CP, Lee WL, et al. Intravenous diltiazem is superior to intravenous amiodarone or digoxin for achieving ventricular rate control in patients with acute uncomplicated atrial fibrillation. Crit Care Med 2009;37:2174-9.

67. Tisdale JE, Padhi ID, Goldberg AD, et al. A randomized, double-blind comparison of intravenous diltiazem and digoxin for atrial fibrillation after coronary artery bypass surgery. Am Heart J 1998;135:739-47.

68. Phillips BG, Gandhi AJ, Sanoski CA, et al. Comparison of intravenous diltiazem and verapamil for the acute treatment of atrial fibrillation and atrial flutter. Pharmacotherapy 1997;17:1238-45.

69. Jordaens L, Trouerbach J, Calle P, et al. Conversion of atrial fibrillation to sinus rhythm and rate control by digoxin in comparison to placebo. Eur Heart J 1997;18:643-8.

70. Hofmann R, Steinwender C, Kammler J, et al. Effects of a high dose intravenous bolus amiodarone in patients with atrial fibrillation and a rapid ventricular rate. Int J Cardiol 2006;110:27-32.

71. Singh S, Zoble RG, Yellen L, et al. Efficacy and safety of oral dofetilide in converting to and maintaining sinus rhythm in patients with chronic atrial fibrillation or atrial flutter. The Symptomatic Atrial Fibrillation Investigative research on Dofetilide (SAFIRE-D) study. Circulation 2000;102:2385-90.

72. Torp-Pedersen C, Moller M, Bloch-Thomsen PE, et al. Dofetilide in patients with congestive heart failure and left ventricular dysfunction. Danish Investigations of Arrhythmia and Mortality on Dofetilide Study Group. N Engl J Med 1999;341:857-65.

73. Ellenbogen KA, Clemo HF, Stambler BS, et al. Efficacy of ibutilide for termination of atrial fibrillation and atrial flutter. Am J Cardiol 1996;78(suppl 1):42-5.

74. Stambler BS, Wood MA, Ellenbogen KA, et al. Efficacy and safety of repeated doses of ibutilide for rapid conversion of atrial flutter or fibrillation. Circulation 1996;94:1613-21.

75. Alboni P, Botto GL, Baldi N, et al. Outpatient treatment of recent-onset atrial fibrillation with the "pill-in-the-pocket" approach. N Engl J Med 2004;351:2384-91.

76. Khan IA. Single oral loading dose of propafenone for pharmacological cardioversion of recent-onset atrial fibrillation. J Am Coll Cardiol 2001;37:542-7.

77. Slavik RS, Tisdale JE, Borzak S. Pharmacologic conversion of atrial fibrillation: a systematic review of the evidence. Prog Cardiovasc Dis 2001;44:121-52.

78. Crawford TC, Oral H. Cardiac arrhythmias: management of atrial fibrillation in the critically ill patient. Crit Care Clin 2007;23:855-72.

79. Crystal E, Garfinkle MS, Connolly SS, et al. Interventions for preventing post-operative atrial fibrillation in patients undergoing heart surgery. Cochrane Database Syst Rev 2004;4:CD003611.

80. Gomes JA, Ip J, Santoni-Rugiu F, et al. Oral d,l sotalol reduces the incidence of postoperative atrial fibrillation in coronary artery bypass surgery patients: a randomized double-blind, placebo-controlled study. J Am Coll Cardiol 1999;34:334-9.

81. Imazio M, Brucato A, Ferrazzi P, et al. Colchicine reduces postoperative atrial fibrillation: results of the Colchicine for the Prevention of the Postpericardiotomy Syndrome (COPPS) atrial fibrillation substudy. Circulation 2011;124:2290-5.

82. Riber LP, Christensen TD, Jensen HK, et al. Amiodarone significantly decreases atrial fibrillation in patients undergoing surgery for lung cancer. Ann Thorac Surg 2012;94:339-46.

83. Amar D, Zhang H, Heerdt PM, et al. Statin use is associated with a reduction in atrial fibrillation after noncardiac thoracic surgery independent of C-reactive protein. Chest 2005;128:3421-7.

84. Terzi A, Furlan G, Chiavacci P, et al. Prevention of atrial tachyarrhythmias after non-cardiac thoracic surgery by infusion of magnesium sulfate. Thorac Cardiovasc Surg 1996;44:300-3.

85. Zipes DP, Camm AJ, Borggrefe M, et al. ACC/AHA/ESC 2006 guidelines for management of patients with ventricular arrhythmias and the prevention of sudden cardiac death: a report of the American College of Cardiology/American Heart Association Task Force and the European Society of Cardiology Committee for Practice Guidelines (Writing Committee to Develop Guidelines for Management of Patients With Ventricular Arrhythmias and the Prevention of Sudden Cardiac Death). J Am Coll Cardiol 2006;48:e247-e346.

86. Al-Khatib SM, Stebbins AL, Califf RM, et al. Sustained ventricular arrhythmias and mortality among patients with acute myocardial infarction: Results from the GUSTO-III trial. Am Heart J 2003;145:515-21.

87. Saltzman HE. Arrhythmias and heart failure. Cardiol Clin 2014;32:125-33.

88. Artucio H, Periera M. Cardiac arrhythmias in critically ill patients: epidemiologic study. Crit Care Med 1990;18:1383-8.

89. Lemery R, Brugada P, Bella PD, et al. Nonischemic ventricular tachycardia: clinical course and long-term follow-up in patients without clinically overt heart disease. Circulation 1989;79:990-9.

90. Tisdale JE. Ventricular arrhythmias. In: Tisdale JE, Miller DA, eds. Drug-Induced Diseases: Prevention, Detection and Management, 2nd ed. Bethesda, MD: American Society of Health-System Pharmacists, 2010:485-515.

91. Sellers TD, DiMarco JP. Sinusoidal ventricular tachycardia associated with flecainide acetate. Chest 1984;85:647-9.

92. Buss J, Neuss H, Bilgin Y, et al. Malignant ventricular tachyarrhythmias in association with propafenone treatment. Eur Heart J 1985;6:424-8.

93. Echt DS, Liebson PR, Mitchell LB, et al. Mortality and morbidity in patients receiving encainide, flecainide, or placebo: the Cardiac Arrhythmia Suppression Trial. N Engl J Med 1991;324:781-8.

94. The Cardiac Arrhythmia Suppression Trial II Investigators. Effect of the antiarrhythmic agent moricizine on survival after myocardial infarction. N Engl J Med 1992;327:227-33.

95. Kowey PR, VanderLugt JT, Luderer JR. Safety and risk/benefit analysis of ibutilide for acute conversion of atrial fibrillation/flutter. Am J Cardiol 1996;78(suppl 8A):46-52.

96. Gorgels AP, van den Dool A, Hofs A, et al. Comparison of procainamide and lidocaine in terminating sustained

monomorphic ventricular tachycardia. Am J Cardiol 1996;78:43-6.

97. Scheinman MM, Levine JH, Cannom DS, et al. Dose-ranging study of intravenous amiodarone in patients with life-threatening ventricular tachyarrhythmias. The Intravenous Amiodarone Multicenter Investigators Group. Circulation 1995;92:3264-72.

98. Somberg JC, Bailin SJ, Haffajee CI, et al. Intravenous lidocaine versus intravenous amiodarone (in a new aqueous formulation) for incessant ventricular tachycardia. Am J Cardiol 2002;90:853-9.

99. Levine JH, Massumi A, Scheinman MM, et al. Intravenous amiodarone for recurrent sustained hypotensive ventricular tachyarrhythmias. Intravenous Amiodarone Multicenter Trial Group. J Am Coll Cardiol 1996;27:67-75.

100. deSouza IS, Martindale JL, Sinert R. Antidysrhythmic drug therapy for the termination of stable, monomorphic ventricular tachycardia: a systematic review. Emerg Med J 2015;32:161-7.

101. Ho DS, Zecchin RP, Richards DA, et al. Double-blind trial of lignocaine versus sotalol for acute termination of spontaneous sustained ventricular tachycardia. Lancet 1994;344:18-23.

102. Drew BJ, Ackerman MJ, Funk M, et al.; on behalf of the American Heart Association Acute Cardiac Care Committee of the Council on Clinical Cardiology, the Council on Cardiovascular Nursing, and the American College of Cardiology Foundation. Prevention of torsade de pointes in hospital settings: a scientific statement from the American Heart Association and the American College of Cardiology Foundation. Circulation 2010;121:1047-60.

103. Dessertenne F. La tachycardie ventriculaire á deux foyers opposes variables. Arch Mal Coeur Vaiss 1966;59:263-72.

104. Goldenberg I, Zareba W, Moss AJ. The long QT syndrome. Curr Probl Cardiol 2008;33:629-94.

105. Darpö. B. Spectrum of drugs prolonging QT interval and the incidence of torsades de pointes. Eur Heart J Suppl 2001;3(suppl K):K70-K80.

106. Sarganas G, Garbe E, Klimpel A, et al. Epidemiology of symptomatic drug-induced long QT syndrome and torsade de pointes in Germany. Europace 2014;16:101-8.

107. Tisdale JE, Wroblewski HA, Overholser BR, et al. Prevalence of QT interval prolongation in patients admitted to cardiac care units and frequency of subsequent administration of QT-interval prolonging drugs. Drug Saf 2012;35:459-70.

108. Pickham D, Helfenbein E, Shinn JA, et al. High prevalence of corrected QT interval prolongation in acutely ill patients is associated with mortality: results of the QT in Practice (QTIP) study. Crit Care Med 2012;40:394-9.

109. Hoogstraaten E, Rijkenberg S, van der Voort PHJ. Corrected QT-interval prolongation and variability in intensive care patients. J Crit Care 2014;29:835-9.

110. Choudhuri I, Pinninti M, Marwali MR, et al. Polymorphic ventricular tachycardia – part I: structural heart disease and acquired causes. Curr Probl Cardiol 2013;38:463-96.

111. Antzelevich C, Shimizu W. Cellular mechanisms underlying the long QT syndrome. Curr Opin Cardiol 2002;17:43-51.

112. Belardinelli L, Antzelevich C, Vos MA. Assessing predictors of drug-induced torsades de pointes. Trends Pharmacol Sci 2003;24:619-25.

113. Priori SG, Wilde AA, Horie M, et al. HRS/EHRA/APHRS expert consensus statement on the diagnosis and management of patients with inherited primary arrhythmia syndromes. Heart Rhythm 2013;10:1932-63.

114. Sharma ND, Rosman HS, Padhi ID, et al. Torsades de pointes associated with intravenous haloperidol in critically ill patients. Am J Cardiol 1998;81:238-40.

115. Barr J, Fraser GL, Puntillo K, et al. Clinical practice guidelines for the management of pain, agitation, and delirium in adult patients in the intensive care unit. Crit Care Med 2013;41:263-306.

116. Zeltser D, Justo D, Halkin A, et al. Torsade de pointes due to noncardiac drugs: most patients have easily identifiable risk factors. Medicine 2003;82:282-90.

117. Moss AJ, Schwartz PJ, Crampton RS, et al. The long QT syndrome. Prospective longitudinal study of 328 families. Circulation 1991;84:1136-44.

118. U.S. Department of Health and Human Services (DHHS), Food and Drug Administration, Center for Drug Evaluation and Research (CDER), Center for Biologics Evaluation and Research (CBER). Guidance for Industry. E14 Clinical Evaluation of QT/QTc Interval Prolongation and Proarrhythmic Potential for Non-Antiarrhythmic Drugs. Rockville, MD: DHHS, 2005.

119. Odening KE, Choi BR, Liu GX, et al. Estradiol promotes sudden cardiac death in transgenic long QT type 2 rabbits while progesterone is protective. Heart Rhythm 2012;9:823-32.

120. Rautaharju PM, Zhou SH, Wong S, et al. Sex differences in the evolution of the electrocardiographic QT interval with age. Can J Cardiol 1992;8:690-5.

121. Yang T, Roden DM. Extracellular potassium modulation of drug block of I_{Kr}. Implications for torsade de pointes and reverse use-dependence. Circulation 1996;93:407-11.

122. Stambler BS, Beckman KJ, Kadish AH, et al. Acute hemodynamic effects of intravenous ibutilide in patients with or without reduced left ventricular function. Am J Cardiol 1997;80:458-63.

123. Yang P, Kanki H, Drolet B, et al. Allelic variants in long-QT disease genes in patients with drug-associated torsades de pointes. Circulation 2002;105:1943-8.

124. Tisdale JE, Jaynes HA, Kingery JR, et al. Development and validation of a risk score to predict QT interval prolongation in hospitalized patients. Circ Cardiovasc Qual Outcomes 2013;6:479-87.

125. Manz M, Pfeiffer D, Jung W, et al. Intravenous treatment with magnesium in recurrent persistent ventricular tachycardia. New Trends Arrhythmias 1991;7:437-42.

126. Tzivoni D, Banai S, Schuger C, et al. Treatment of torsade de pointes with magnesium sulfate. Circulation 1988;77:392-7.

127. Singh SN, Lazin A, Cohen A, et al. Sotalol-induced torsades de pointes successfully treated with hemodialysis after failure of conventional therapy. Am Heart J 1991;121:601-2.

128. Tang S, Lo CY, Lo WK, et al. Sotalol-induced torsade de pointes in a CAPD patient—successful treatment with intermittent peritoneal dialysis (letter). Perit Dial Int 1997;17:207-8.

Chapter 36

Pharmacologic Challenges During Mechanical Circulatory Support in Adults

Amy L. Dzierba, Pharm.D., FCCM, BCPS; and Erik Abel, Pharm.D., BCPS

LEARNING OBJECTIVES

1. Describe the different types of mechanical circulatory support (MCS) in an adult patient.
2. Explain altered pharmacokinetics and pharmacodynamics of medications during MCS.
3. State dosing recommendations of common medications used during extracorporeal membrane oxygenation on the basis of current literature.

ABBREVIATIONS IN THIS CHAPTER

ECLS	Extracorporeal life support	VA-ECMO	Venovenous extracorporeal membrane oxygenation
ECMO	Extracorporeal membrane oxygenation		
IABP	Intra-aortic balloon pump	VV-ECMO	Venoarterial extracorporeal membrane oxygenation
LVAD	Left ventricular assist device		
MCS	Mechanical circulatory support	VAD	Ventricular assist device
PVC	Polyvinyl chloride		

INTRODUCTION

Mechanical circulatory support (MCS) is a broad-reaching description of the advanced technology and capability available today to support patients with acute or chronic hemodynamic compromise when conventional therapies have failed or are unsustainable. As MCS has evolved, so has its implementation into clinical practice. As will be discussed later in this chapter, the options for MCS largely depend on the primary organ system needing support—cardiovascular/cardiopulmonary versus pulmonary only. Long-term cardiovascular support with durable implantable ventricular assist devices (VADs) and the total artificial heart provide a management option in end-stage heart failure beyond the traditional construct of palliative care versus transplantation. However, short-term cardiac support allows options to provide acute cardiovascular MCS for temporary support with intra-aortic balloon pumps (IABPs), paracorporeal/extracorporeal VADs, or extracorporeal life support (ECLS)/extracorporeal cardiopulmonary resuscitation (ECPR) by venoarterial (VA) extracorporeal membrane oxygenation (ECMO).[1-5] However, ECLS by venovenous (VV) ECMO has grown significantly as a promising modality of therapy for patients with severe acute pulmonary failure.[3,6]

Early descriptions of MCS were documented in the early 19th century and further described in the 1930s.[7] However, these therapies were first applied to human subjects in 1953 by J. Gibbon Jr using a heart-lung machine for atrial septal defect repair and in 1954 by C. Walton Lillehei, M.D., to successfully perform cardiac surgery using controlled cross-circulation and a bubble oxygenator.[8,9] Many notable events have been pioneered to bring us to the advances in MCS we see today (Table 36.1).

Although thoracic organ transplantation is commonly considered the gold standard treatment for end-stage heart or lung disease, growing comorbidities, psychosocial concerns, and lack of donor organ availability have driven the advancement of MCS, particularly for cardiovascular support. As MCS has advanced, implantable VADs have evolved from large pulsatile devices to smaller, more durable continuous flow devices. Other advances have allowed exploration into further application of MCS for other populations. In the severely critically ill patient with cardiac or cardiopulmonary compromise, the growing application of ECLS has shown that MCS may have a role in hemodynamic support

Table 36.1 Timeline of Landmarks and Advances in Mechanical Circulatory Support

1950s	Membrane oxygenators were first developed
1972	Hill and colleagues used ECMO for respiratory failure for 75 hours
1975	NIH initiates study of ECMO for adult respiratory failure
1975	First NIH-sponsored multicenter trial of temporary LVADs for acute heart failure
1976	Bartlett and colleagues reported the first successful use of ECMO in neonates
1994	HeartMate LVAD (Thermo Cardiosystems, Inc.) FDA approved for BTT
2002	HeartMate XVE for destination therapy approved by FDA
2006	Polymethylpentene oxygenator (Quadrox D, Maquet Cardiovascular) approved by the FDA
2009	Expansion of ECLS for pulmonary failure secondary to the H1N1 influenza epidemic

BTT = bridge to transplantation; DT = destination therapy; ECLS = extracorporeal life support; ECMO = extracorporeal membrane oxygenation; LVAD = left ventricular assist device; NIH = National Institutes of Health.

beyond the operating room or in end-stage heart failure. Extracorporeal membrane oxygenation and ECLS are forms of mechanical respiratory and circulatory support that have considerably evolved during the past decade.[10] With new developments in this technology, use in adults has been growing rapidly, a trend that was initially seen after the 2009 influenza A (H1N1) pandemic.[11,12] The growing use of MCS and increasing complexity of available devices, in addition to the complicated pathophysiology and pharmacotherapeutic support requirements of these patients, deliver an undeniable need for the critical care clinician to understand the principles and ramifications of MCS.

INDICATIONS AND TYPES OF MCS

The type of MCS, as well as the intent and potential duration, depends on several factors, including patient acuity, comorbidities, and prognosis. The progression and options for support can be dynamic, given a patient's clinical progress and etiology of hemodynamic compromise. As a general construct, the options for support can be divided according to the primary organ dysfunction (respiratory vs. cardiac) and can further be divided into temporary versus long-term MCS (Table 36.2). For some cardiac indications, a patient may be optimized and go directly to long-term MCS. All forms of MCS are considered a "bridge" or intervention to a progressive improvement in a patient's clinical status—be it a "bridge" to recovery from the acute pulmonary or cardiac disease; a "bridge" from a temporary to a durable MCS device; or a "bridge" from chronic MCS to transplantation or palliative care. Particularly in relation to long-term MCS, the intent should be declared before the time of implantation with the understanding that during long-term support, clinical factors (new improvement or deterioration) may influence change in the intent of support (Figure 36.1). For long-term MCS, the intent of the "bridge" has been defined by INTERMACS (Interagency Registry for Mechanically Assisted Circulatory Support) as described in Table 36.3.

Resource use and the fundamental oath of *primum non nocere* (first, do no harm) are notwithstanding when it comes to patient selection. As such, MCS strategies must consider contraindications that account for complications during MCS and therapies required during support, in addition to the reversibility of the patient's disease state and likely prognosis when considering comorbidities (Table 36.4 and Table 36.5).

GENERAL DEVICE OVERVIEW AND SETTINGS

The MCS devices available for clinical use can vary among institutions; however, for some devices, availability can also differ according to enrollment and participation criteria for clinical trials as well as indication approval/availability by country.[19] In general, each device is connected to a controller that mediates the speed or vacuum/rate of the respective pump, and the speed most directly dictates power consumption of the respective pump (other factors may also play a role in power consumption). Aside from IABPs, a list of MCS devices can be found in Table 36.6. Although somewhat proprietary to each device, almost all MCS devices require some level of anticoagulation, which will be discussed later in the chapter.

IABP Counterpulsation[20]

An IABP is generally placed by femoral arterial catheter (in some scenarios, it can also be placed by left brachial, axillary, or subclavian arteries) and advanced into the descending thoracic aorta. The IABP is an intervention that can provide selective systolic afterload reduction while enabling diastolic augmentation of blood pressures, all contributing to sustaining an increased mean arterial pressure. Intra-aortic balloon pump deflation provides systolic afterload reduction to ease cardiac work (does not directly increase cardiac output). Subsequently, IABP inflation enables diastolic augmentation of systemic mean arterial blood pressures through displacement of blood to increase mean arterial perfusion pressure. The timing of IABP inflation and deflation can be set to trigger from electrocardiogram, pacemaker, or arterial line pressures or can be manually set. Patients with aortic valve

Table 36.2 Indications and Associated Types of MCS

Primary Dysfunction	Indications	Potential Means of MCS
Respiratory	• Hypoxic and/or hypercapnic respiratory failure owing to any cause (ARDS, BTT, primary graft dysfunction after lung transplantation) • Severe air leak syndromes	• VV-ECMO • AV CO_2R (hypercapnic respiratory failure only, in limited use)

Cardiac; temporary MCS	• Cardiogenic shock secondary to one of the below causes and refractory to standard therapies:
	  1. Post-cardiotomy
	  2. Myocarditis
	  3. Nonischemic cardiomyopathy
	  4. Pulmonary embolism
	• Extracorporeal cardiopulmonary resuscitation
	• Bridge to VAD or heart or heart & lung transplantation
	• Primary graft failure after heart transplantation
	• Prevention or treatment of right ventricular failure after LVAD implantation
	• Pulmonary hypertension
		• Intra-aortic balloon pump
		• VA-ECMO
		• Extracorporeal VAD
		• Percutaneous VAD
		• Paracorporeal VAD

Cardiac; long-term MCS	• Class IV, ACC/AHA stage D heart failure symptoms, EF < 25% • Refractory cardiogenic shock (INTERMACS category 1) • Dependent on IABP or other form of temporary MCS 7 days • Intermittent/continuous inotropic therapy (INTERMACS category 2–3) for more than 14 days • Evidence of poor cardiac output with low cardiac index (< 2.3 L/min), elevated filling pressures (PCWP > 20 mm Hg) and hypotension with SBP < 90 mm Hg • Cardiopulmonary exercise testing with peak VO_2 < 14 mL/kg/min with cardiac limitation and/or poor prognostic indicators with other parameters	• Durable implantable LVAD or heart assist system • Total artificial heart

ACC/AHA = American College of Cardiology/American Heart Association; ARDS = acute respiratory distress syndrome; AV CO_2R = arterial venous carbon dioxide removal; ECMO = extracorporeal membrane oxygenation; EF = ejection fraction; IABP = intra-aortic balloon pump; INTERMACS = Interagency Registry for Mechanically Assisted Circulatory Support; MCS = mechanical circulatory support; PCWP = pulmonary capillary wedge pressure; SBP = systolic blood pressure; VAD = ventricular assist device; VA-ECMO = venoarterial extracorporeal membrane oxygenation; VV-ECMO = venovenous extracorporeal membrane oxygenation; VO_2 = oxygen consumption.

regurgitation/insufficiency may not benefit from this means of afterload reduction because of worsening regurgitation during diastole. Patients with tachyarrhythmias and/or irregular heart rates may have less-than-optimal IABP synchronization. The level of support from an IABP coincides with the timing of inflation/deflation per related heartbeat. For example, 1:1 is one inflation/deflation per every heartbeat (maximal support), and 1:4 is one inflation/deflation for every fourth heartbeat (less support). Blood flow stagnation associated with decreasing of IABP support increases the thrombotic risk and may warrant anticoagulation. Immobility is a predominant limitation to this form of MCS that is particularly seen when the IABP is placed femorally.

Percutaneous VADs

Currently, a handful of MCS devices can be used for temporary support. In the United States, such devices include the TandemHeart pVAD (Cardiac Assist, Pittsburgh, PA) and the Impella (Abiomed, Danvers, MA). Future developments may include newer or modified percutaneous devices to provide left ventricular support that is more robust, but these are also being developed to provide less invasive right ventricular support.[21] These devices are currently used predominantly in cardiogenic shock or as temporary support during high-risk interventional or electrophysiological cardiac procedures. The TandemHeart pVAD device (Cardiac Assist, Pittsburgh, PA) can be used as an MCS device capable of providing up to 8 L/minute of support by centrifugal pump (continuous non-pulsatile blood flow). Depending on the manner of configuration, it is capable of providing left ventricular support by atrial transseptal puncture cannulation, or using an alternative cannula (Protek Duo), it may also be set up to provide right ventricular support or enable VV-ECLS.[22] Another device, the Impella (Abiomed), comes in differing platforms enabling 2.5, 3.5, or 5.0 L/minute of non-pulsatile blood flow support to the left ventricle.[23-26] These devices are

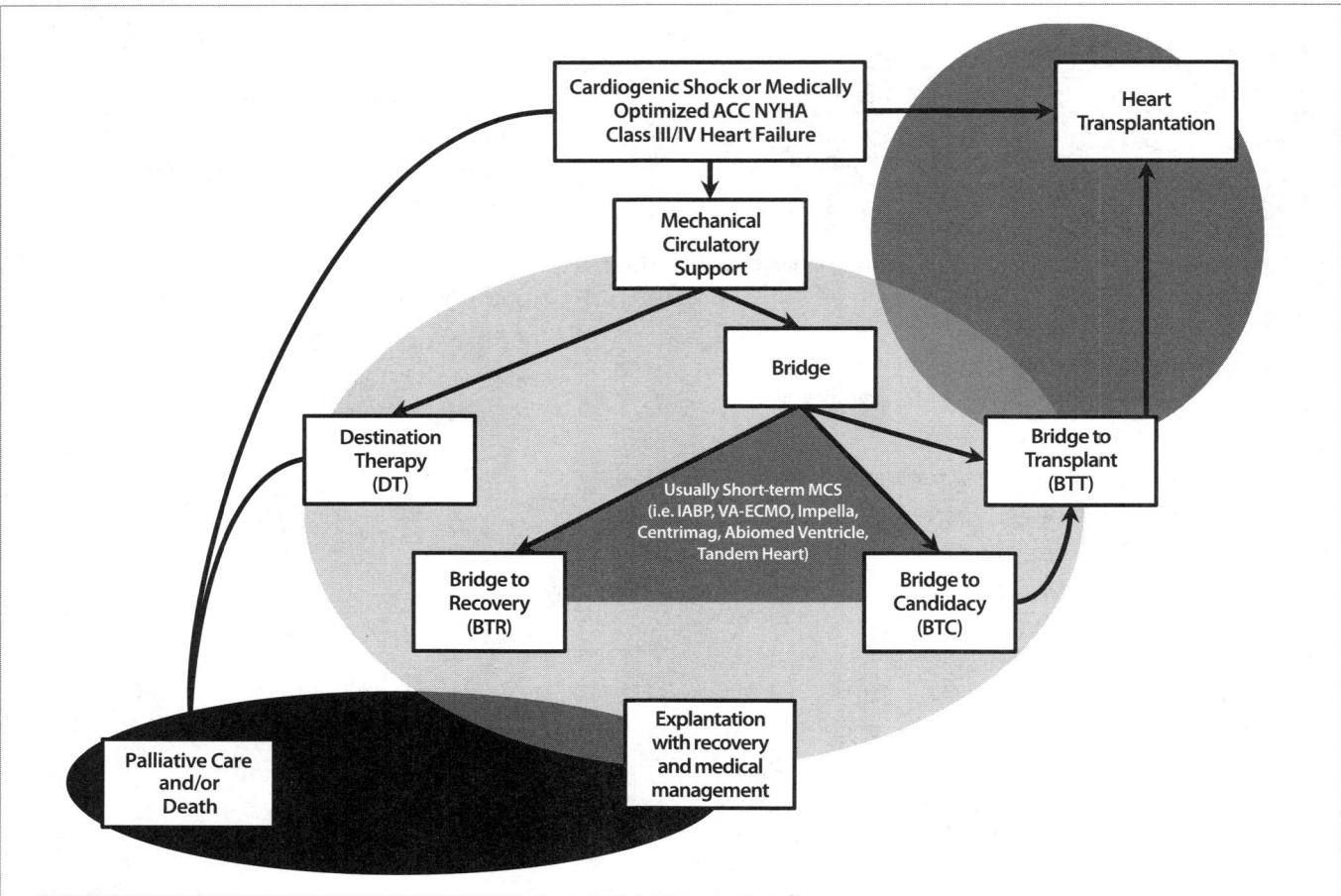

Figure 36.1 Dynamic progression of heart failure advanced therapies.
ACC NYHA = American College of Cardiology, New York Heart Association; IABP = intra-aortic balloon pump; VA-ECMO; venoarterial extracorporeal membrane oxygenation.

placed into the aorta across the aortic valve percutaneously for the 2.5- or 3.5-L/minute platforms or by surgical placement if using the 5.0-L/minute platform. As it resides in the left ventricular cavity, blood is suctioned into the inflow port and through the outflow port in the ascending aorta. The anticoagulation regimen for this device is a common topic of debate and medication safety discussion because it requires a heparinized dextrose purge solution (ranging from D_5W to $D_{50}W$) to lubricate and cool the rotary motor and minimize blood-motor interface. Management can be complicated by migration and malposition of the catheter/cannula within the left ventricle, leading to arrhythmias and hemolysis. Specific contraindications to this device include mechanical aortic valve, moderate to severe aortic stenosis, moderate to severe aortic insufficiency, and severe peripheral vascular disease. More recently the Impella RP (Abiomed) was introduced to the market as a temporary MCS device that can provide support to those with acute right ventricular dysfunction/failure. Configured slightly different than the other Impella devices, the Impella RP is placed in the femoral vein and advanced to reside with the inflow area within the inferior vena cava and outflow within the pulmonary artery. A pulmonary artery catheter is commonly used concurrently,

Table 36.3 Classification of Long-term MCS with Ventricular Assist Devices

Destination therapy	Formal designation for patients who meet the criteria for long-term mechanical support but who are not a transplant candidate because of relative or absolute contraindications
BTT	Formal designation for patients eligible to be listed as candidates for heart transplantation
Bridge to candidacy OR bridge to recovery	Designation used to describe the approach to temporary MCS when short-term LVADs are used to support a patient until a long-term prognosis can be determined, which may include explantation with recovery, implantation of long-term durable LVAD support, heart transplantation, or palliative care

BTT = bridge to transplantation; LVAD = left ventricular assist device; MCS = mechanical circulatory support

however, cardiac outputs are favored to be calculated by Fick method rather than thermodilution because of the heat generated by the pump and subsequent interference. A heparin purge solution is still required with this device.

Extracorporeal or Paracorporeal VADs

Various extracorporeal VADs are available, although some common examples include the Thoratec CentriMag Blood Pump (Thoratec Corporation, Pleasanton, CA), BVS 5000 Ventricular Support System (Abiomed), and AB5000 Circulatory Support System (Abiomed). The CentriMag Blood Pump provides up to 9 L/minute of continuous non-pulsatile blood flow by a magnetically levitated impeller. Although commonly used for a longer duration, this device is approved by the U.S. Food and Drug Administration (FDA) for up to 6 hours of MCS as a bridge to decision for other advanced therapies, but it is also approved by the FDA for use as a right VAD for up to 30 days for patients in cardiogenic shock caused by acute right ventricular failure.[27,28] The BVS 5000 (Abiomed) can be used for temporary unilateral (left or right) or biventricular support. This device is a more simplistic VAD with two sac-like chambers that fill semi-passively by gravitational force and that are subsequently emptied by an air-driven pump to deliver up to 6 L/minute of pulsatile blood flow by displacement. The filling chamber should be watched closely for signs of thrombus development.[29] The AB5000 Circulatory Support System (Abiomed) can also be configured for use as temporary unilateral (left or right) or biventricular support. This device rests in a paracorporeal manner on the chest of the patient and, through vacuum assistance, can provide up to 6 L/minute of pulsatile blood flow.[30]

Table 36.4 Potential Complications of MCS[13-18]

- Mechanical (circuit/pump) complications
- Bleeding and transfusion
  - Hemorrhagic stroke
  - Gastrointestinal bleeding
  - Pulmonary hemorrhage
  - Acquired von Willebrand factor deficiency
- Postoperative right heart failure
- Thrombosis
  - Embolic stroke
  - TIA
  - Systemic embolization
  - Venous thrombosis
- Mechanical hemolysis and hemolysis-induced end-organ damage
- Arrhythmias
- New infections
- Cannula/conduit displacement

TIA = transient ischemic attack.

Table 36.5 Comorbidities and Prognostic Considerations to Consider Before Initiating MCS

Temporary MCS	Long-term MCS
• Active systemic infection, particularly bacteremia	• Active systemic infection
• Prolonged ventilation > 10 days or with high airway pressure and/or high F_{IO_2} > 7 days	• End-organ or multisystem organ failure including impending renal or hepatic failure
• Established multisystem organ failure	• Right ventricular failure
• Contraindications to anticoagulation	• Moderate to severe valvular disease
• Refusal to receive blood products	• Neurologic deficits or psychosocial limitations impairing ability to manage device (e.g., daily activities, rehabilitation potential, cognitive function according to neurocognitive evaluation)
• Ungrafted severe burns	
• Quadriplegia	• Severe pulmonary disease
• Bone marrow transplant recipients	• Coexisting terminal disease
• Inadequate CPR > 5 minutes or prolonged CPR > 30 minutes	• Refractory or uncontrolled ventricular tachyarrhythmias
• Intracranial hemorrhage	• Known bleeding or clotting disorder
• Evidence of neurologic insult	• Visual or hearing impairment
• Profound metabolic acidosis with pH < 7.1	• Social support network
• Requirement of prolonged neuromuscular blockade infusion	• Insurance/financial means to support long-term care needs
• Requirement of prolonged high-dose vasoactive drugs	
• Not a transplant candidate and presenting with either primary/idiopathic pulmonary hypertension or end-stage cardiopulmonary disease	
• Specific to VA-ECMO or IABP: tachyarrhythmias and aortic valve regurgitation	

CPR = cardiopulmonary resuscitation; F_{IO_2} = fraction of inspired oxygen; IABP = intra-aortic balloon pump; VA-ECMO = venoarterial extracorporeal membrane oxygenation.

Durable Implantable VADs and Total Artificial Hearts

Ongoing developments have continued to enable prolonged MCS to patients. Early durable VADs, such as the HeartMate XVE, were quite large with large-bore drivelines and mediated pulsatile flow by an electrically controlled pusher plate that displaced blood and required minimal anticoagulation. However, the life span of this device was limited by the wear and tear on the metal bearings in the motor as well as the potential acquired dysfunction of the integrated porcine valves within the inflow and outflow cannula/conduits. This device has since been replaced in therapy with newer continuous-flow, non-pulsatile VADs (either axial or centrifugal flow), which has facilitated much longer pump life. Although requiring full anticoagulation, these newer devices such as the HeartMate II (Thoratec, Pleasanton, CA) and HeartWare HVAD (HeartWare, Framingham, MA), have provided acceptable risk profiles for thrombosis and bleeding in clinical trials. Simplistically, these devices are implanted

Table 36.6 MCS Devices

Temporary Circulatory Support Devices

Device	Impella 2.5, 3.5, 5.0, RP	Tandem Heart	Abiomed BVS 5000	CentriMag	Abiomed Ventricle	Extracorporeal Membrane Oxygenation (ECMO)
Flow type: Support duration Location	Non-pulsatile; axial flow; short term; percutaneous	Centrifugal; short term; extracorporeal	Pulsatile; short term; extracorporeal	Non-pulsatile; centrifugal, short extracorporeal	Pulsatile; intermediate term; paracorporeal	Centrifugal; short term; extracorporeal
Mechanics	Axial rotor spins	Three rotating cones	Two blood sacs; mimics native heart	Spinning impeller	Blood sac; pneumatic drive	Continuous flow extracorporeal pump connected in circuit to a membrane oxygenator
Volume	N/A	10 mL	100 mL	N/A	100 mL	1 L
Support range	Up to 2.5, 3.5, and 5.0 L/min, respectively	Up to 4 L/min; depends on catheter size	Up to 6 L/min	Up to 9.9 L/min	Up to 6 L/min	2–6 L/min Do not run at < 500 mL/min

Long-term Circulatory Support Devices

Device	HeartMate II	HeartWare (HVAD)	SynCardia Total Artificial Heart (TAH)	HeartMate III[a]
Flow type: Support duration Location	Non-pulsatile; axial flow; long-term; implanted	Non-pulsatile; centrifugal flow; long-term; implanted	Pulsatile; long-term; implanted; replaces native ventricles	Partial artificial pulsatility; magnetically levitated centrifugal flow; long-term; implanted
Mechanics	Axial rotor spins 8,000–15,000 rpm	Impeller spins 2,000–3,000 rpm	Replaces both native ventricles; pneumatic drive	Axial rotor spins 8,000–15,000 rpm
Volume	125 mL total	45 mL	70 mL max	125 mL total
Support range	Flow estimated; range 3–10 L/min	Up to 10 L/min	Up to 9 L/min	Flow estimated; range 3–10 L/min

[a]Currently in clinical trials.

by placing an inflow cannula/conduit into the apex of the left ventricle, which pulls blood through the pump to exit through the outflow graft that is attached to the ascending aorta. Although these devices provide selective support of the left ventricle, the care management must also facilitate appropriate medical management of right ventricular support to enable successful patient treatment.[31] For implantable devices, the connection to the power source and controller is enabled by a driveline that is usually tunneled through the abdomen to an exit site. In select patients, a total artificial heart may be considered, particularly in patients with biventricular heart failure who are listed for heart transplantation. The HeartMate II (Thoratec) can deliver up to 10 L/minute of blood flow by an axial rotor that spins at 8,000–15,000 rpm. The device controller provides alarms regarding flow disturbances, pump failure, low power, power or connection disruptions, and controller malfunction. The HeartWare HVAD (HeartWare) provides up to 10 L/minute by a centrifugal flow impeller spinning at 2,000–3,000 rpm.

ECLS or ECMO

Similar to cardiopulmonary bypass, ECLS/ECMO drains venous blood through large-bore cannulas, pumped through an oxygenator (usually by means of a centrifugal, non-pulsatile pump), where it is oxygenated and cleared of carbon dioxide and then actively pumped back into the body. The modality of support depends on the means of vascular cannulation. Venovenous cannulation removes deoxygenated venous blood from the vena cava and returns blood near the right atrium after circulating through the oxygenator and circuit; it requires the heart circulate blood to maintain end-organ perfusion. Venoarterial cannulation is more complex. With peripheral cannulation, the venous inflow cannula removes blood from the vena cava by the femoral vein and delivers oxygenated blood by femoral or axillary artery outflow cannula to the descending aorta, resulting in retrograde flow to the ascending aorta. Central cannulation, commonly seen post-cardiotomy, removes blood from the right atrium and delivers oxygenated blood into the ascending aorta immediately distal to the coronary sinus. Femoral cannulation of VA-ECMO can increase the risk of lower limb ischemia obstruction of distal blood flow. This may be avoided by placing a distal perfusion catheter to either the femoral artery or a distal site such as the posterior tibial or dorsalis pedis arteries. Because of the low-flow state within the heart, VA-ECMO can be associated with a risk of intracardiac and/or aortic root thrombus.

Considerations of which populations may be considered for VV-ECMO versus VA-ECMO are outlined in Table 36.2. Beyond anticoagulation considerations, ECMO/ECLS presents considerably more pharmacologic challenges, as will be outlined in the following section. Extracorporeal membrane oxygenation/ECLS has evolved significantly, with almost 250 centers registered with the Extracorporeal Life Support Organization, allowing for variation in circuit setup and management. Although the components required are fundamentally the same (pump, oxygenator, circuit tubing, and cannula), variation in pharmacologic interactions has been described among different proprietary constituents of these ECMO/ECLS circuits.

PHARMACOLOGIC CHALLENGES WITH MCS

Drug-Circuit Interactions and Considerations—Overview

When administering a drug, there is a balance between the dose administered and the elicited response, with the goal of providing a therapeutic effect while minimizing toxicity. This relationship between the drug dose and response may be altered in critically ill patients as a result of pharmacokinetic and pharmacodynamic changes.[32] The use of ECMO can lead to additional pharmacokinetic alterations.[33] Providing optimal dosing regimens for patients receiving ECMO requires a working knowledge of pharmacokinetic and pharmacodynamic alterations propelled by drug, disease, and extracorporeal factors (Figure 36.2). Despite improvements in this technology and resurgence of its application for respiratory failure, there remains a paucity of evidence and understanding of pharmacotherapy in patients receiving MCS. Almost all of the data that have been published on changes in pharmacokinetics during MCS have been with ECMO, with few or no data published regarding pharmacokinetic changes in patients with heart failure having VADs.

The elimination of drugs from the body is highly dependent on clearance and volume of distribution.[34] The liver and the kidneys serve as the two major organ systems

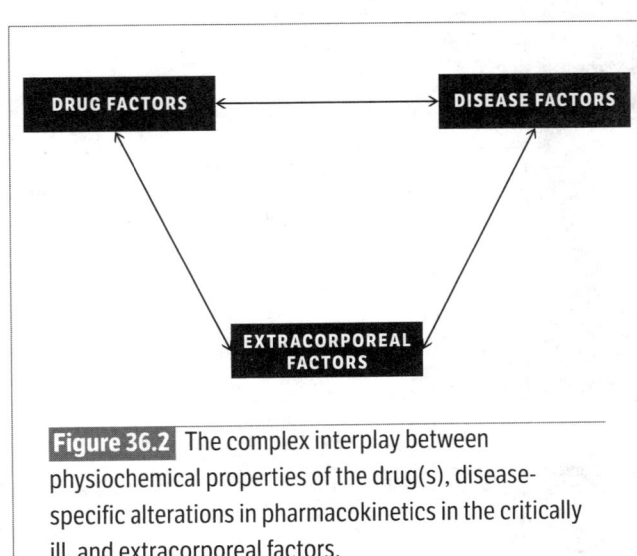

Figure 36.2 The complex interplay between physiochemical properties of the drug(s), disease-specific alterations in pharmacokinetics in the critically ill, and extracorporeal factors.

responsible for drug elimination. Additional losses of drugs through the skin and gastrointestinal tract or biliary excretion can serve as minor pathways of drug elimination. Organ impairment or failure, altered plasma protein binding, increases in circulating volume, and perfusion abnormalities are often encountered in critically ill patients, resulting in changes in absorption, distribution, metabolism, and elimination of the drugs, creating challenges in drug dosing. In addition, patients receiving ECMO may have an array of pathophysiological changes, including acute kidney injury and decreased hepatic blood flow, leading to changes in drug clearance; however, these changes from ECMO may be difficult to ascertain in the already critically ill patient.

Changes in volume of distribution owing to ECMO may be caused by hemodilution, sequestration of drugs as a result of circuit-related factors, decreased circulating albumin, or alterations in protein binding from pH aberrations. Priming solutions (plasma, saline, or albumin) that are used on initiation of ECMO increase the patient's circulating volume and may lead to pharmacologic alterations with hydrophilic drugs, resulting in potentially decreased plasma concentrations.[35,36] In addition, the dilution of plasma proteins, notably albumin, may affect highly protein bound drugs, leading to potential toxicities as a result of an increased proportion of unbound fraction of the drug.[37]

Data concerning drug sequestration within the ECMO circuit are limited. The membrane oxygenator and polyvinyl chloride (PVC) tubing are two circuit components that provide a large surface area for dug sequestration, leading to potential drug loss over time.[38,39] Some studies have shown that both the PVC tubing and the membrane oxygenators absorb drugs to a similar extent, whereas others have shown significant differences.[39-45] Results from a simulated circuit showed an average of 80% loss of fentanyl in the circuit without oxygenators at 120 minutes, with only an additional 5% loss when a Quadrox D oxygenator was added.[39] Up to 40% of morphine was lost in all circuits, and no differences were noted in those with and without oxygenators.[39] A saturation point may exist, leading to liberation of sequestered drug back into the circulation; however, this concept has not been studied.

Understanding the physicochemical properties of drugs can assist in determining the relationship between the dose administered and the anticipated concentration achieved in the blood.[41] The octanol-water partition coefficient is a common way to report a drug's measure of lipophilicity.[43] Log P, the logarithm of the ratio of the concentrations of the unionized solute in the solvents, may be used to understand the behavior of drug molecules.[43] Therefore, drugs with high log P values (around 2.0) will have a propensity to be very soluble in organic materials such as the plastic tubing used in the ECMO circuit.[44] However, to date, there has been no characterization of the drug-circuit interaction beyond 24 hours, and as such, little speculation can be made regarding the adsorptive capacity of the circuit over longer periods of ECMO support.

Overall, data are sparse relating to drug dosing in adult patients receiving ECMO. However, extrapolations from ex vivo studies may be useful to anticipate alterations in the pharmacokinetics of a drug that may occur during ECMO. In addition, some generalizations can be made with hydrophilic versus lipophilic drugs. Lipophilic drugs tend to be more affected by the ECMO circuitry and may require higher-than-expected dosing regimens to achieve the same therapeutic effect without ECMO (Figure 36.3).

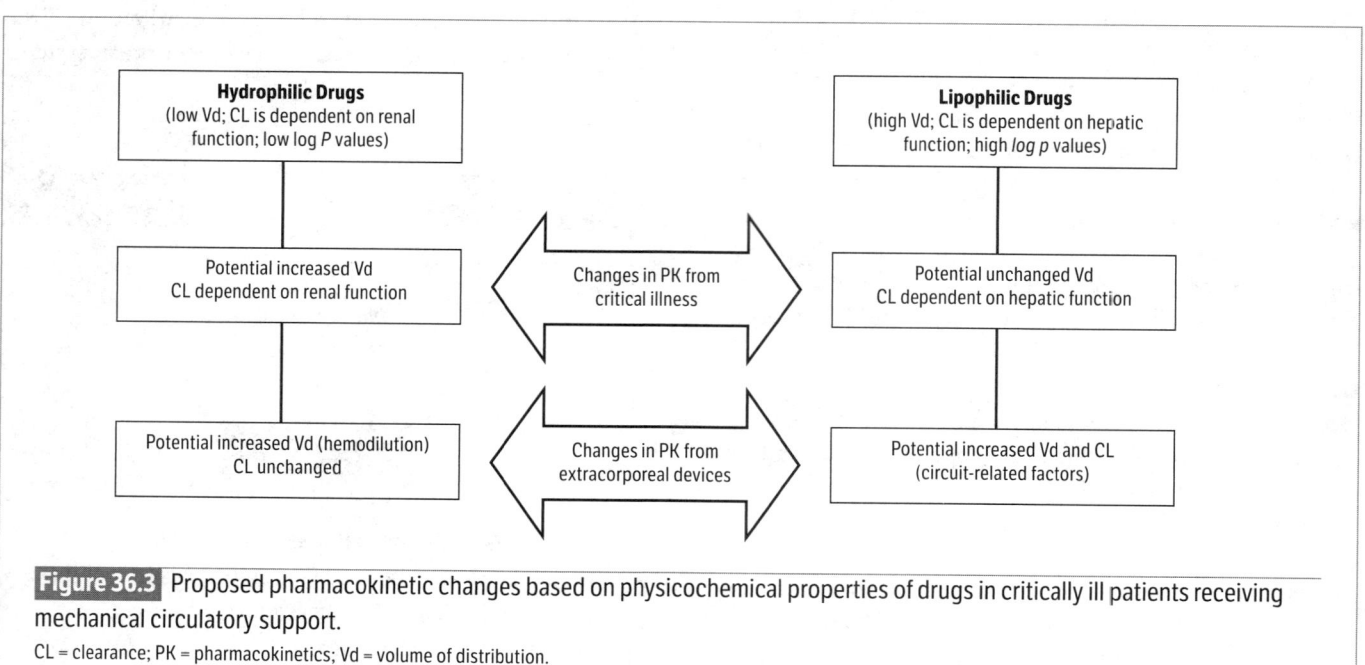

Figure 36.3 Proposed pharmacokinetic changes based on physicochemical properties of drugs in critically ill patients receiving mechanical circulatory support.

CL = clearance; PK = pharmacokinetics; Vd = volume of distribution.

Drug-Circuit Interactions and Considerations—Analgesia and Sedation

The provision of analgesia and sedation is common practice for mechanically ventilated patients in the ICU to provide comfort and maintain patient safety. Medication selection should be based on the patient's needs, with titration to a predetermined goal in accordance with recently published guidelines.[45] The use of analgesia and sedation during ECMO contributes to the reduction in oxygen consumption, facilitates patient-ventilator synchrony, diminishes patient stress and discomfort, and prevents patient-initiated device dislodgement or removal.[10]

Results from several investigations using ex vivo models have shown a loss of analgesics and sedatives within the ECMO circuit.[42,46,47] These studies using neonatal ECMO circuits composed of PVC tubing and silicone rubber membrane oxygenators established an early loss of commonly used sedatives.[42,46,47] One investigation observed up to a 68% loss of midazolam and a 98% loss of propofol within 40–120 minutes.[42] Steady morphine concentrations have been observed over time, with only about 20% drug loss over 6–24 hours.[46,47] However, in contrast, significant reductions in fentanyl concentrations have been observed within 3 hours.[46] Reductions of up to 30% from the original concentration of lorazepam have also been detected.[47] An adult ECMO in vitro circuit using PVC tubing with a hollow polymethylpentene fiber membrane oxygenator showed up to a 93% decrease in dexmedetomidine concentrations at 24 hours.[48] A more recent study used ex vivo ECMO circuits to measure concentrations of morphine, fentanyl, and midazolam throughout a 24-hour period.[44] At 24 hours, average drug recovery relative to baseline from both the circuits and the controls was lower with the lipophilic drugs, including fentanyl 3%, midazolam 13%, and morphine 103%.[44] Of interest, in the first hour of the ECMO run, up to 70% and 50% of fentanyl and midazolam, respectively, were lost in the circuit, and fentanyl was undetectable at 24 hours.[44] Because of the lack of sequestration of morphine in the ECMO circuit, it would seem to be a preferred agent for prolonged periods of ECMO; however, the risks of accumulation, especially in patients with renal injury; the profound hypotensive effects; and the deliriogenic effects make morphine an unattractive agent for prolonged sedation.[45]

Adult patients receiving ECMO for respiratory failure appear to have increased requirements of analgesia and sedation over time.[49,50] A small, single-center, retrospective study showed an increase in the daily dose of midazolam on average by 18 mg (p=0.001) and morphine on average by 29 mg (p=0.02).[50] Patients receiving VV-ECMO had a significantly higher daily midazolam dose requirement than did patients receiving VA-ECMO (p=0.005).[50]

Despite these studies showing an increased need for analgesics and sedatives during ECMO, it remains unknown whether the increased requirements clinically observed are a result of circuit-related factors alone or whether other factors such as tolerance, age, or organ function are contributors.[47] To date, data are sparse to guide the appropriate dosing of analgesics and sedatives in adult patients receiving ECMO with newer technology. Furthermore, there is a lack of outcomes data associated with these observational experiences. One approach to achieving adequate deep sedation in patients receiving ECMO would be to start with continuous infusions of both an analgesic and a sedative, anticipating requirements that exceed standard doses. In addition, establishing daily sedative goals with the potential for sedative interruption, anticipating significant dose reductions at ECMO discontinuation, and monitoring for signs of withdrawal and delirium should be considered.

Drug-Circuit Interactions and Considerations—Anti-infective Agents

Infections are commonly encountered in critically ill patients. Source control in addition to timely and appropriate antimicrobials remains the cornerstone to the success of the treatment for a critically ill patient.[51] Most antimicrobial dosing regimens are established in healthy adults with normal physiology; however, significant changes in rate of clearance and volume of distribution may have profound effects on drug concentrations in the critically ill patient on ECMO.[52] The changes in clearance and volume of distribution could result in substantial drug losses, leading to therapeutic failures, development of resistance, and worse outcomes. Monitoring of drug concentrations is not possible with many anti-infective agents; therefore, clinicians must rely on knowledge of a drug's physiochemical properties, pharmacokinetic characteristics, and published experience to guide appropriate dosing. Until recently, there has been very little in the literature on the effects of antimicrobial dosing in the critically ill adult patient receiving ECMO.

Vancomycin

Vancomycin pharmacokinetics has been described in adult patients receiving ECMO.[53,54] Using a population pharmacokinetic model for vancomycin, a significant decrease in clearance and increases in volume of distribution were observed in a mixed population receiving ECMO.[53] A more recent study compared the pharmacokinetics of vancomycin in adult patients receiving continuous infusion vancomycin with and without the use of ECMO.[54] All patients received a 35-mg/kg loading dose over 4 hours, followed by a continuous infusion aimed to target a serum concentration of 20–30 mg/L.[54] Throughout the first 24 hours of the study, there were no differences in clearance or volume of distribution between the two groups.

In addition, an ex vivo study showed very little loss of vancomycin using modern adult ECMO circuitry.[44] Current dosing of vancomycin in critically ill adult patients receiving ECMO appears to be no different than critically ill patients not receiving ECMO; however, because therapeutic drug monitoring is widely available, concentrations should be routinely monitored to ensure adequate therapy.

Aminoglycosides

Aminoglycosides have concentration-dependent killing, often used in conjunction with other gram-negative antimicrobial agents to treat life-threatening infections in adult patients. As a class, these agents are hydrophilic, with a low molecular weight, low protein binding, and a small volume of distribution. The study of aminoglycoside pharmacokinetic alterations with ECMO is largely limited to the neonatal population. These studies have consistently observed a significant increase in volume of distribution and a decrease in clearance leading to an extension of the dosing interval in this population, despite the variability in trial design and methodology.[55-58] No studies currently address the pharmacokinetic changes of aminoglycosides in the adult patient receiving ECMO; however, because of the highly hydrophilic nature of this class, no changes in clearance as a result of sequestration would be expected. Therapeutic drug monitoring is readily available for this class of anti-infectives, thereby ensuring effective concentrations to treat the infection while limiting nephrotoxicity.

Penicillins/Extended-Spectrum Penicillins/Cephalosporins/Carbapenems

There is no adult literature on changes in pharmacokinetic parameters in adult patients receiving ECMO with the penicillin, extended-spectrum penicillin, or cephalosporin antimicrobial classes. These classes of anti-infectives are commonly used in the treatment of gram-negative infections in the critically ill patient population. They have time-dependent bactericidal effects and are therefore most effective when concentrations are maintained above the minimum inhibitory concentration for at least 40% of the dosing interval. Substantial increases in meropenem clearance were observed in two patients receiving ECMO for treatment of severe respiratory failure secondary to pneumonia.[59] Only when the dose of meropenem was administered as a high-dose infusion (6.5 g every 24 hours) were optimal concentrations attained.[59] Supporting this concept, a recent ex vivo ECMO study observed a 24-hour average drug recovery relative to baseline from the circuits and controls for meropenem to be 20% and 42%, respectively.[44] Increases in volume of distribution and clearance of meropenem have been observed in the critically ill patient with sepsis not receiving ECMO, leading to suboptimal drug concentrations.[36,60] Mechanical circulatory support can induce a systemic inflammatory-like response, independently from sepsis, augmenting clearance and volume of distribution. In addition, significant meropenem degradation has been observed at ambient temperatures (37°C); this may therefore lead to inaccurate conclusions of the effects of ECMO circuitry on increased clearance. Dosing regimens in the adult patients receiving one of these anti-infective classes should account for these significant changes in pharmacokinetics while the patients are receiving ECMO, resulting in higher doses with more frequent dosing intervals, extended infusions, or continuous infusions.

Antifungals

Few studies have been published on the pharmacokinetic changes of antifungal agents in adult patients receiving ECMO. Significant drug sequestration of voriconazole has been observed in an ex vivo model.[46] The authors observed a 71% loss of voriconazole at 24 hours.[46] One case report observed undetectable voriconazole serum concentrations despite dose increases (8 mg/kg) in an adult patient receiving ECMO.[61] However, in another case report, voriconazole concentrations were sustained with an increased dose.[62] Given the relatively high lyophilic nature of voriconazole, it would not be surprising to have decreased plasma concentrations with recommended doses; however, there are no current recommendations on dosing regimens in critically ill patients receiving ECMO. Conflicting case reports have been published on caspofungin, observing either no effect on pharmacokinetic parameters or an increase in clearance.

Others

The results of a case series in adult patients receiving linezolid and ECMO showed alterations in linezolid pharmacokinetics.[63] Two of the three patients had no changes in volume of distribution, with one patient with cystic fibrosis having a substantial decrease in volume of distribution, and all three patients had an increased clearance.[63] The hydrophilic nature of this drug and the documented variability of linezolid serum concentrations in critically ill patients potentially caused by augmented renal clearance may influence these pharmacokinetic alterations to a greater extent than sequestration from the ECMO circuit.[64] One case reports no pharmacokinetic changes in a patient receiving ECMO.[65] Many tigecycline classes of anti-infectives are used in the critically ill patient receiving ECMO; however, no data have been published in adult patients thus far.

COMPLICATIONS OF MCS

Complications of MCS can be multifactorial, which, in some cases, may partly be a result of the comorbidities of the patient population. Nonetheless, there are commonalities largely related to neurologic events, bleeding, thrombosis, hemolysis, device malfunction, or infection (see Table 36.6).

BLEEDING, THROMBOSIS, AND ANTICOAGULATION

Fundamentally, successful MCS depends on the function of the MCS device and its impact on the intrinsic rheologic properties of blood and particularly its influence on key interactions in thrombosis and hemostasis. Many proprietary MCS devices (predominantly VADs) provide device-specific anticoagulation recommendations, although the translation of these recommendations into practice is sometimes limited by clinical processes, variance in coagulation assays, coagulation assay availability, and interpretation. Nonetheless, anticoagulation strategies for MCS are without robust data, but often, they are standardized within a given institution. For temporary MCS, the most widely used form of systemic anticoagulation is heparin, and in some centers, aspirin and other antiplatelet agents are also integrated (see Table 36.7 for examples). In addition, some centers have used alternative parenteral anticoagulation with direct thrombin inhibitors (e.g., bivalirudin or argatroban), even in the absence of active concerns for heparin-induced thrombocytopenia.[66-68] For long-term MCS, recommendations are largely proprietary and device-specific, with the commonalities in the antithrombotic regimens being aspirin, warfarin with variable patient/institutional targets, and variable use of parenteral anticoagulation among institutions for perioperative anticoagulation bridging (see Table 36.7 for examples). Nonetheless, the safety and efficacy of apixaban, dabigatran, rivaroxaban, enoxaparin, or other anticoagulants in patients with MCS devices has not been established.

Coagulopathies that may occur because of MCS include fibrinolysis and acquired von Willebrand syndrome, thereby increasing bleeding risk. The development of acquired von Willebrand syndrome has been described in both ECLS and VAD populations.[69-72] Procedural- and surgical-related bleeding commonly are sources of major bleeding; however, some of the most common other sources include significant epistaxis or gastrointestinal bleeding. In some scenarios, this may be isolated to the identified arteriovenous malformations or angiodysplasias that are thought to be related to decreases in pulse pressure concomitantly with increased continuous flow pressures within the capillary bed, leading to the exposure of existing arteriovenous malformations or the development of new ones.[72,73]

In contrast, there remains potential increased thrombotic risk secondary to infection as well as hemolysis. Infection, particularly bacteremias, is sometimes a forgotten thrombotic risk factor not well characterized in MCS. The complex interaction of the inflammatory and coagulation cascades existing in sepsis can be further complicated in patients undergoing MCS.[74] Because the circulatory dynamics are somewhat compensated for in MCS patients with sepsis, the first presenting symptom of sepsis is sometimes hemoglobinuria or hemolysis. Hemolysis or pump thrombosis can have varying presentations including pump-related alarms (often indicating low flow and/or power elevations), which may also coincide with hyperkalemia, new non-hemorrhagic anemia, or urine color changes (may appear as hematuria, but in severe cases, can be tea-colored, brown, or black). It is also important to recognize that hemolysis may occur because of several other factors within the MCS circuit (Figure 36.4). At a minimum, at least low levels of mechanical hemolysis can be expected with most forms of MCS. However, worsening hemolysis may potentiate further ramifications that commonly appreciated.[77] Through hemolysis, hemoglobin is liberated from the red blood cells into circulation, together with other intracellular enzymes and electrolytes. Circulating plasma-free hemoglobin is usually scavenged by haptoglobin, thus limiting downstream effects. However, in severe hemolysis when haptoglobin cannot maintain this balance, plasma-free hemoglobin may facilitate a prothrombotic state. This state may be enabled through direct platelet activation by plasma-free hemoglobin as well as scavenging of endothelial derived nitric oxide that, under normal circumstances, minimizes thrombotic interactions of the endothelium and platelets.[78] Further end-organ damage may be mediated by hemolysis such as acute kidney injury.[79,80] Although more investigation is still needed on the optimal detection and management, current recommendations indicate further workup for hemolysis and device thrombosis if lactate dehydrogenase (LDH) is 2.5–3 times the upper limit of normal (normal range 140–280 IU/L) or if the plasma-free hemoglobin is greater than 40 mg/dL (normal 0–10 mg/dL).[81,82]

Coagulation and Testing During MCS

Expected changes in the coagulation are expected during MCS, including activation and amplification of the coagulation cascade and activation of platelets—all largely because of continual interaction with an artificial surface. Differing attempts for advancement have been made to lessen this effect such as altering the surface of the device (as seen in the Heartmate XVE) or enhancing the biocompatibility of the tubing by adding bonded surfaces to the inner lining.

Currently, the only available guidelines for MCS anticoagulation are the 2014 ELSO Anticoagulation Guidelines and the 2013 International Society of Heart and Lung Transplantation (ISHLT) Guidelines for Mechanical Circulatory Support, both of which provide general recommendations on the management according to the available

Table 36.7 Example of Initial Post-MCS Insertion Antithrombotic Regimen[a]

	LVAD	Aspirin	Heparin Infusion (once hemostasis achieved)[b]	Initial Warfarin INR Goal
Long-term MCS Devices	Heartmate II Heartmate III	POD 0: 325 mg x 1 Ongoing: 81 mg daily	• By POD2: Initiate "Heparin – no dose escalation at 5 units/kg/hr" • By POD3: Increase to "Heparin Sliding Scale" titrating to institutional goals	2–3
	HeartWare	POD 0: 325 mg × 1 Ongoing: 325 mg daily	• Within 12 hr postop: Initiate "Heparin – no dose escalation at 5 units/kg/hr" • By POD1: Increase to "Heparin Sliding Scale" titrating to institutional goals	2–3
Temporary MCS Devices	IABP	If indicated by concurrent ischemic heart disease	• If indicated for acute coronary syndrome (ACS) management – according to institutional protocol • As level of IABP support decreases, anticoagulation may warranted	N/A
	Impella	81 mg daily	• Different protocols exist and wide degree of interpretation of manufacturer recommendation – many remaining medication safety concerns • Purge solution: Heparin 25,000/1,000 mL D10W – titrated by device to goal purge pressure • Within 1 hr post-procedural: Initiate separate "Heparin Sliding Scale" at 6 units/kg/hr and titrate to institutional goals • Increased monitoring is recommended if Impella purge solution infusion rates have changed considerably (i.e., increased or decreased by 4 mL/hr)	N/A
	TandemHeart	POD 0: 325 mg × 1 Ongoing: 81 mg daily	• Within 6 hr Postop: Initiate "Heparin – no dose escalation at 5 units/kg/hr" • By POD1/post-procedural day 1: Increase to "Heparin Sliding Scale" titrating to institutional goals	N/A
	CentriMag Abiomed ventricle Abiomed BVS 5000	POD 0: 325 mg × 1 Ongoing: 81 mg daily	• Within 12 hr Postop: Initiate "Heparin – no dose escalation at 5 units/kg/hr" • By POD1: • Increase to "Heparin Cardiac Sliding Scale" titrating to institutional goals	N/A
	ECMO	If indicated by concurrent ischemic heart disease Insufficient data to support or refute role otherwise	• Within 6 hr postop: Initiate "Heparin Sliding Scale" at 12 units/kg/hr"-titrating to institutional goals • Consider more conservative dosing approach in patients post-cardiotomy	N/A

[a]See also https://evidencebasedpractice.osumc.edu/Documents/Guidelines/VAD.pdf.
[b]Monitoring and adjustments should be made at routine feasible time windows that adhere to both blood conservation considerations and safe, assertive antithrombotic management.

evidence.[2,83] In both acute and chronic management, monitoring coagulation parameters is imperative to navigating the delicate balance between bleeding and thrombotic complications. Nonetheless, the science surrounding the optimal management and monitoring of antithrombotics and hemostatics remains quite uncertain—as evidenced by considerable variability in practice and gaps in supporting evidence. Heparin therapy has been the mainstay for anticoagulation in the acute setting for many disease states, including those in the MCS population. One of the most common areas of clinical debate and uncertainty revolves around heparin therapy in MCS. The debate is at least 3-fold surrounding the monitoring assays (ACT [activated clotting time], activated partial thromboplastin time [aPTT], and anti-factor Xa [anti-Xa]); the definition of "therapeutic range," particularly with aPTT and anti-Xa; and the role of antithrombin. Debate exists largely because of the lack of consistent evidence to guide therapy and the inability to directly translate the evidence into practice among institutions. The best example of this is the definition of a heparin therapeutic range. Years ago, Chiu and colleagues established heparin therapeutic ranges for aPTT monitoring in an animal model deriving a ratio-based goal of aPTT of 1.5–2.5 times the baseline aPTT.[84] Some guidelines and institutions still apply this in practice, which results in common aPTT goals of 40–60 seconds or 60–80 seconds. However, concerns about data with this ratio-based heparin therapeutic goal approach were published by Brill-Edwards and colleagues, where protamine titrations of heparinized samples had considerable sensitivity variation among aPTT reagents, thus refuting ratio-based aPTT goals for heparin monitoring.[85] Today, many laboratories use a modified Brill-Edwards method with an anti-Xa correlation curve to derive an institution-specific aPTT therapeutic range for heparin monitoring. Fundamentally, this presents inherent limitations in translating heparin anticoagulation goals between institutions.

Recent interest in anti-Xa monitoring of heparin also stimulated similar interest within the MCS population, and so far, anti-Xa and aPTT monitoring have shown discordance.[86] Anti-Xa activity may be a potential option, but they are not well validated in all populations, particularly the MCS population. As previously mentioned, all MCS types induce at least minimal levels of mechanical hemolysis. Of note, the presence of hyperbilirubinemia or hemolysis has been shown to influence the chromogenic anti-Xa assay, potentially representing the activity as falsely low.[87] Overall, anticoagulation management and monitoring during MCS remains a conundrum. The roles of common laboratory tests used in monitoring and decision-making regarding anticoagulation, thrombosis, and hemostasis can be found in Table 36.8.

Management of Device-Related Severe Hemolysis and Thrombosis

Severe hemolysis and pump thrombosis are of serious concern with MCS devices and require thorough troubleshooting to further complications, although in some scenarios, operative intervention or device change-out is required. In MCS, hemolysis and device thrombosis are commonly discussed in similar contexts, largely because of the associated clinical progression that is commonly seen as the pathogenesis continues from thrombus initiation to complete thrombosis (see Figure 36.5). The workup for confirmation of device thrombosis commonly entails evaluating the device and cardiac function for contributing factors including documentation and alarm history for suction events, power spikes, speed changes, volume status, and arrhythmias. Additional considerations include urinalysis and blood cultures; imaging to evaluate cannula(e) position and obstruction/thrombus by echocardiography or computed tomography (CT); and imaging to evaluate right ventricular function, gas exchange evaluation of the oxygenator for ECLS, or the echocardiographic ramp study in the scenario of left ventricular assist devices (LVADs).[88] The ramp study can provide an indirect evaluation of a potential intra-device thrombus because the VAD itself cannot be viewed internally by imaging. The ramp study evaluates for decreases in left ventricular end-diastolic dimension by echocardiogram during simultaneous increases in LVAD speeds and correlating power consumption. If thrombus were likely, potential obstruction within the VAD would be evidenced by lacking augmentation of VAD flows as well as minimal decreases in left ventricular end-diastolic dimension despite increasing VAD speeds. Additional investigation into compliance with anticoagulation regimen and goals should be assessed, together with quantifiable hemolysis laboratory values to evaluate the degree of elevation (e.g., LDH and plasma-free hemoglobin).

Although manipulation of the cannulae or changing of the oxygenator can be accomplished with a somewhat lower risk in temporary MCS or ECLS, the management decision for implanted durable MCS devices (LVADs) is more complex. The most definitive option for device thrombosis is surgical change-out of the device. However, surgical intervention comes with many other risks, most notably the risk of bleeding because of reoperation (particularly with a redo sternotomy). Some centers have tried to standardize the thought process for evaluation and treatment of suspected LVAD thrombosis.[81] Therefore, in some scenarios, medical treatment of hemolysis and/or partial pump thrombosis may be pursued to avoid

continued on page 750

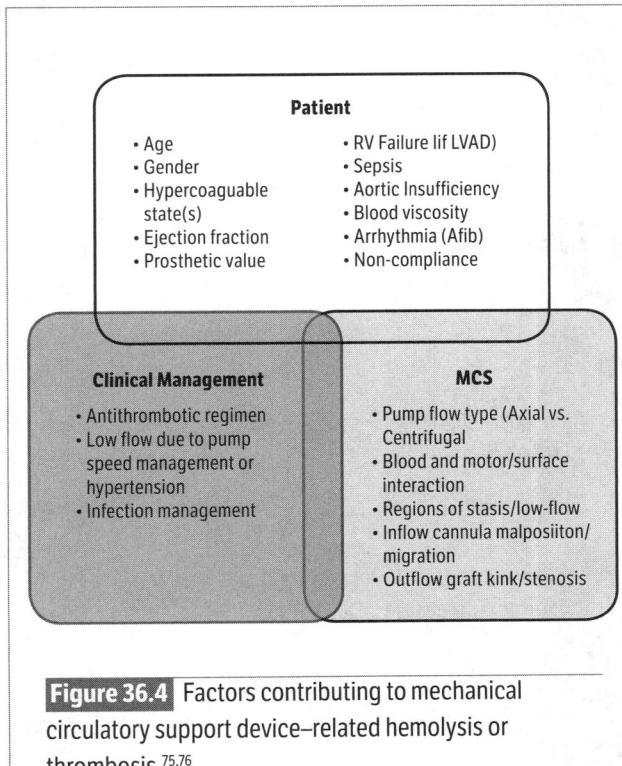

Figure 36.4 Factors contributing to mechanical circulatory support device–related hemolysis or thrombosis.[75,76]

Table 36.8 Antithrombotic and Hemostasis Monitoring: Roles and Limitations in MCS

Monitoring Value	Acute	Chronic	Management Role
CBC with platelets	X	X	• Evaluate trends of anemia • Provide signals of infections • Ensure adequate platelets for hemostasis, and indicators of potential HIT • *MCS commonly associated with platelet consumption and thrombocytopenia*
PT/INR	X	X	• Marker of extrinsic pathway and hepatic synthetic function • Used for therapeutic monitoring of warfarin during long term MCS • *Unreliable marker of coagulation in patients with cirrhosis, patients on DTI therapy, or those with congestive hepatopathy*
aPTT	X		• Commonly used for heparin or DTI therapeutic monitoring • *Varying reagent sensitivities among laboratories and may vary annually within an insitution limiting generalizable goals* • *Unreliable marker of coagulation in patients with cirrhosis, those with congestive hepatopathy, or those with lupus anticoagulant/antiphospholipid antibodies*
ACT	X		• Crude point-of-care whole blood coagulation assay that can be used to monitor heparin or DTI therapy • *Varying proprietary sensitivity among brands and variable sensitivity among high- vs. low-range cartridges* • *Lack of assay specificity limits translation guidance toward a focused therapeutic intervention*
Fibrinogen	X		• A protein required in clot formation and particularly a clot with adequate tensile strength • *Provides information on available concentrations; however, does not indicate confirmation of presence of fibrinolysis*
Antithrombin activity	X		• Anti-inflammatory protein that enables many actions, but predominantly thought of contextually in relation to how it enables indirect anticoagulation by heparin and its role in heparin resistance • *Role unclear in MCS, particularly adult ECMO* • *Assays vary in functional use and interpretation* • *Mutations in AT may exist not necessary detected by the assay*
Anti-Xa activity	X		• Commonly used for heparin therapeutic monitoring • Reflective of heparin concentration/activity • *Chromogenic assay that may be influenced by other substances or disease states (i.e., hyperbilirubinemia, hemolysis, and hypertriglyceridemia)*
Thromboelastography (TEG or ROTEM)	X		• Functional assay having coagulation kinetics and/or defects • Commonly used to guide hemostasis interventions after cardiopulmonary bypass • *Not widely available* • *Not easily interpretable*
Lactate dehydrogenase (LDH)	X	X	• Quantitative marker of degree of hemolysis • Readily available in most laboratories • Elevations have been shown to correlate well with LVAD thrombosis • *Not specific to hemolysis because it may also be elevated in liver disease or in patients with shocked liver but can be validated by testing pfHgb*

Table 36.8 Antithrombotic and Hemostasis Monitoring: Roles and Limitations in MCS *(continued)*

Monitoring Value	Acute	Chronic	Management Role
Plasma-free hemoglobin (pfHgB)	X		• Quantitative marker of degree of hemolysis • *Not readily available in all laboratories*
Haptoglobin	X		• Qualitative marker of hemolysis • Available in most laboratories • *Does not indicate degree of hemolysis, and most forms of MCS produce at least low concentrations of hemolysis*
Hypercoagulable state workup	X		• May include protein C or S deficiency, anticardiolipin antibodies, lupus anticoagulant with prothrombin mutation, factor V Leiden, heparin-induced thrombocytopenia • *May be reasonable to rule out in some clinical scenarios, although low yield*
Liver function tests (AST, ALT, total bilirubin)	X		• May provide indicators of underlying coagulopathy, ongoing hemolysis, or congestive hepatopathy

DTI = direct thrombin inhibitor.

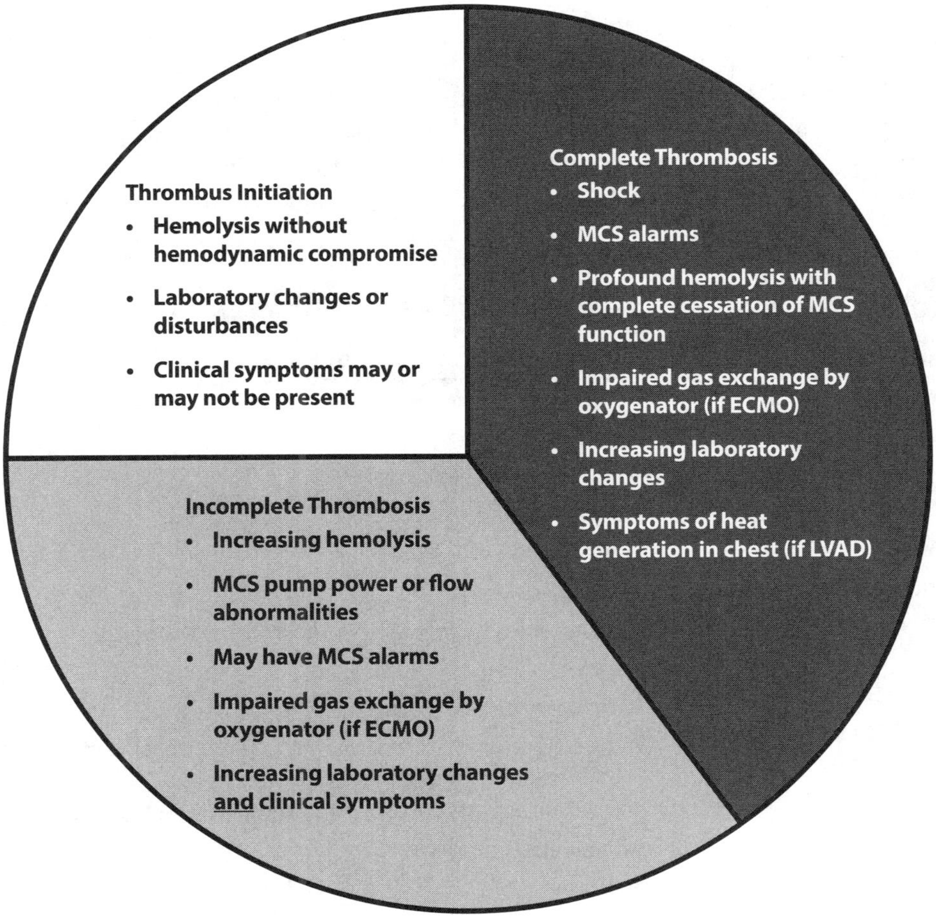

Figure 36.5 Progression of device-related hemolysis and thrombosis in MCS.[75]

Thrombus Initiation
- Hemolysis without hemodynamic compromise
- Laboratory changes or disturbances
- Clinical symptoms may or may not be present

Incomplete Thrombosis
- Increasing hemolysis
- MCS pump power or flow abnormalities
- May have MCS alarms
- Impaired gas exchange by oxygenator (if ECMO)
- Increasing laboratory changes <u>and</u> clinical symptoms

Complete Thrombosis
- Shock
- MCS alarms
- Profound hemolysis with complete cessation of MCS function
- Impaired gas exchange by oxygenator (if ECMO)
- Increasing laboratory changes
- Symptoms of heat generation in chest (if LVAD)

continued from page 747

unnecessary surgery or extreme surgical risk. Although this strategy may be successful if the process is identified early, published data of the attempts with alteplase, glycoprotein IIb/IIIa inhibitors, or direct thrombin inhibitors have not shown it to be largely successful.[89]

INFECTION TREATMENT AND PREVENTION IN PATIENTS WITH MCS

The consequence and management of infections in patients with MCS create many clinical challenges beyond the pharmacologic challenges described earlier in this chapter. The presence of indwelling or implanted prosthetic material lends itself to greater infectious complexities, and in the case of long-term devices, the driveline care must be consistent and meticulous to avoid seeding infectious risk at this abdominal wound. Infections in these long-term MCS devices have been characterized by ISHLT (Table 36.9).

Furthermore, before placement of the device or for surgical procedures occurring after device placement, antibiotic coverage for surgical prophylaxis for MCS-related or non–MCS-related surgical procedures should account for the site of procedure, previous infections (if VAD), proximity to driveline site or VAD pocket, and any other potential exposure or bacteremia secondary to the procedure. In some circumstances, this requires broader prophylactic antibiotic coverage.[91]

Beyond the immediate pericperative/periprocedural period of up to 48 hours after device placement, evidence neither supports nor refutes the use of ongoing prophylactic antibiotics owing to indwelling cannulae for MCS, and practice patterns have considerable variability.[92,93] Nonetheless, consideration for appropriate antimicrobial stewardship practices should be advocated. However, if an infection is identified or suspected, antibiotic coverage should account for the site of suspected infection, previous pathogens and susceptibilities, proximity to driveline site or VAD pocket, and any other potential exposure or bacteremia. Once the source is identified and controlled, treatment duration largely depends on the nature of the infection. However, if the infection is VAD-related or VAD-specific, prolonged (greater than 4 weeks) antimicrobial therapy is commonly used. In addition, because LVAD change-out is not without considerable risk, long-term oral antibiotic suppression therapy may be considered for some infections.

FUTURE DIRECTIONS

Mechanical circulatory support has shown considerable advances through the years; however, the pharmacotherapeutic challenges remain complex and require familiarity among the clinical care team to provide optimal outcomes. Advances in the future, including transcutaneous power supplies and smaller devices, may help eliminate some of these obstacles. However, ongoing research is needed to help refine recommendations for anticoagulation in MCS, particularly

Table 36.9 ISHLT Definitions of Infections in Patients with VADs[90]

Infection Type	Defined Areas Affected
VAD-specific infections	• Pump and/or cannula infections
	• Pocket infections
	• Percutaneous driveline infections
	○ Superficial infection
	○ Deep infection
VAD-related infections	• Infective endocarditis
	• Bloodstream infections that may be VAD related or non-VAD related
	• Mediastinitis
	○ Sternal wound infection SSI-organ space
	○ VAD pocket infection (continuous with mediastinum or already situated in the mediastinum depending on the device used)
	○ Non-VAD: Other causes of mediastinitis, perforation of the esophagus
Non-VAD infections	• Lower respiratory tract infection
	• Cholecystitis
	• *Clostridium difficile* infection
	• Urinary tract infection

SSI = surgical site infection.

for the ideal management of sedation, analgesia, and antibiotic dosing in ECLS. Although some data can assist in our management today, every opportunity should be taken to provide a more individualized approach through guided therapy with therapeutic drug monitoring and with dosing tailored to known pharmacokinetic alterations. Various organizations are have been involved in the regulation, registry development, and advancement of MCS therapy. For further information, please see the following:

- ELSO: Extracorporeal Life Support Organization
- INTERMACS: Interagency Registry for Mechanically Assisted Circulatory Support
- ISHLT: International Society of Heart and Lung Transplantation

REFERENCES

1. Peura JL, Colvin-Adams M, Francis GS, et al. Recommendations for the use of mechanical circulatory support: device strategies and patient selection: a scientific statement from the American Heart Association. Circulation 2012;126:2648-67.
2. Feldman D, Pamboukian SV, Teuteberg JJ, et al. International Society for Heart and Lung Transplantation. The 2013 International Society for Heart and Lung Transplantation Guidelines for mechanical circulatory support: executive summary. J Heart Lung Transplant 2013;32:157-87.
3. ELSO Guidelines for Cardiopulmonary Extracorporeal Life Support. Extracorporeal Life Support Organization, Version 1.3. Ann Arbor, MI: ELSO, November 2013. www.elsonet.org.
4. ELSO Adult Cardiac Failure Supplement to the ELSO General Guidelines. Extracorporeal Life Support Organization. Available at http://elsonet.org/resources/guidelines. Accessed August 1, 2015.
5. ELSO ECPR Supplement to the ELSO General Guidelines. Extracorporeal Life Support Organization. Available at http://elsonet.org/resources/guidelines. Accessed August 1, 2015.
6. ELSO Adult Respiratory Failure Supplement to the ELSO General Guidelines. Extracorporeal Life Support Organization. Available at http://elsonet.org/resources/guidelines. Accessed August 1, 2015.
7. Kirklin JK, Frazier OH, eds. ISHLT Monograph Series: Mechanical Circulatory Support. New York: Elsevier, 2006:77-104.
8. Annich GM, Lynch WR, MacLaren G, et al., eds. Extracorporeal Cardiopulmonary Support in Critical Care, 4th ed. Ann Arbor, MI: Extracorporeal Life Support Organization, 2012.
9. Cohn LH, ed. Cardiac Surgery in the Adult, 4th ed. New York: McGraw-Hill, 2012.
10. Brodie D, Bacchetta M. Extracorporeal membrane oxygenation for ARDS in adults. N Engl J Med 2011;365:1905-14.
11. Peek GJ, Mugford M, Tiruvoipati R, et al. Efficacy and economic assessment of conventional ventilatory support versus extracorporeal membrane oxygenation for severe adult respiratory failure (CESAR): a multicentre randomised controlled trial. Lancet 2009;374:1351-63.
12. Pham T, Combes A, Rozé H, et al. Extracorporeal membrane oxygenation for pandemic influenza A(H1N1)-induced acute respiratory distress syndrome: a cohort study and propensity-matched analysis. Am J Respir Crit Care Med 2013;187:276-85.
13. John R. Gastrointestinal bleed after left ventricular assist device implantation: incidence, management, and prevention. Ann Cardiothorac Surg 2014;3:475-9.
14. McIlvennan CK, Magid KH, Ambardekar AV, et al. Clinical outcomes after continuous-flow left ventricular assist device: a systematic review. Circ Heart Fail 2014;7:1003-13.
15. Kirklin JK, Naftel DC, Kormos RL, et al. Fifth INTERMACS annual report: risk factor analysis from more than 6,000 mechanical circulatory support patients. J Heart Lung Transplant 2013;32:141-56.
16. Starling RC, Moazami N, Silvestry SC, et al. Unexpected abrupt increase in left ventricular assist device thrombosis. N Engl J Med 2014;370:33-40.
17. Kalogeropoulos AP, Kelkar A, Weinberger JF, et al. Validation of clinical scores for right ventricular failure prediction after implantation of continuous-flow left ventricular assist devices. J Heart Lung Transplant 2015 [Epub ahead of print].
18. Matthews JC, Koelling TM, Pagani FD, et al. The right ventricular failure risk score a pre-operative tool for assessing the risk of right ventricular failure in left ventricular assist device candidates. J Am Coll Cardiol 2008;51:2163-72.
19. Ensor CR, Paciullo CA, Cahoon WD Jr, et al. Pharmacotherapy for mechanical circulatory support: a comprehensive review. Ann Pharmacother 2011;45:60-77.
20. Webb CA, Weyker PD, Flynn BC. Management of intra-aortic balloon pumps. Semin Cardiothorac Vasc Anesth 2014;27:1-16.
21. Myat A, Patel N, Tehrani S, et al. Percutaneous circulatory assist devices for high-risk coronary intervention. J Am Coll Cardiol Interv 2015;8:229-44.
22. Kar B, Gregoric ID, Basra SS, et al. The percutaneous ventricular assist device in severe refractory cardiogenic shock. J Am Coll Cardiol 2011;57:688-96.
23. Impella 2.5 Instructions for Use & Clinical Reference Manual. Available at www.abiomed.com/assets/AIC_2-5_IFU_Rev_G.pdf. Accessed March 6, 2015.
24. Impella 5.0 Instructions for Use & Clinical Reference Manual. Available at www.abiomed.com/assets/2011/01/AIC-5.0-Manual_US.pdf. Accessed March 6, 2015.
25. Impella LD Instructions for Use & Clinical Reference Manual. Available at www.abiomed.com/assets/2011/01/AIC-LD-Manual_US.pdf. Accessed March 6, 2015.
26. Impella CP Instructions for Use & Clinical Reference Manual. Available at www.abiomed.com/assets/0048-9001-rF-CP-IFU.pdf. Accessed March 6, 2015.
27. De Robertis F, Birks EJ, Barlow P, et al. End-stage cardiac failure managed with Levitronix CentriMag short-term ventricular assist device (VAD). J Heart Lung Transplant 2005;24(2 suppl 1):559.
28. 2nd Generation CentriMag System Operating Manual. Available at www.thoratec.com/_assets/download-tracker/centrimag/PL-0047%20Rev%2006%20Thor_US%20Operating%20Manual%20-%202nd%20Gen%20CentriMag%20System.pdf. Accessed March 6, 2015.

29. Abiomed BVS5000 BI-Ventricular Support System Operator's Manual. Available at www.abiomed.com/assets/2010/11/BVS5000_Operators_Manual_P.pdf. Accessed March 6, 2015.

30. AB5000 Circulatory Support System Operator's Manual. Available at www.abiomed.com/assets/2010/11/0015_9000_rL.pdf. Accessed March 6, 2015.

31. Lahm T, McCaslin CA, Wozniak TC, et al. Medical and surgical treatment of acute right ventricular failure. J Am Coll Cardiol 2010;56:1435-46.

32. Smith BS, Yogaratnam D, Levasseur-Franklin KE, et al. Introduction to drug pharmacokinetics in the critically ill patient. Chest 2012;141:1327-36.

33. Shekar K, Fraser JF, Smith MT, et al. Pharmacokinetic changes in patients receiving extracorporeal membrane oxygenation. J Crit Care 2012;27:741.

34. Buxton IO, Benet LZ. Chapter 2. Pharmacokinetics: the dynamics of drug absorption, distribution, metabolism, and elimination. In: Brunton LL, Chabner BA, Knollmann BC, eds. Goodman & Gilman's The Pharmacological Basis of Therapeutics, 12e. New York: McGraw-Hill, 2011. Available at http://accessmedicine.mhmedical.com/content.aspx?bookid=374&Sectionid=41266207. Accessed March 6, 2015.

35. Smith BS, Yogaratnam D, Levasseur-Franklin KE, et al. Introduction to drug pharmacokinetics in the critically ill patient. Chest 2012;141:1327-36.

36. Roberts JA, Lipman J. Pharmacokinetic issues for antibiotics in the critically ill patient. Crit Care Med 2009;37:840-51.

37. Buck ML. Pharmacokinetic changes during extracorporeal membrane oxygenation: implications for drug therapy of neonates. Clin Pharmacokinet 2003;42:403-17.

38. Preston TJ, Ratliff TM, Gomez D, et al. Modified surface coatings and their effect on drug adsorption within the extracorporeal life support circuit. J Extra Corpor Technol 2010;42:199-202.

39. Preston TJ, Hodge AB, Riley JB, et al. In vitro drug adsorption and plasma free hemoglobin levels associated with hollow fiber oxygenators in the extracorporeal life support (ECLS) circuit. J Extra Corpor Technol 2007;39:234-7.

40. Rosen DA, Rosen KR, Silvasi DL. In vitro variability in fentanyl absorption by different membrane oxygenators. J Cardiothorac Anesth 1990;4:332-5.

41. Wildschut ED, Ahsman MJ, Allegaert K, et al. Determinants of drug absorption in different ECMO circuits. Intensive Care Med 2010;36:2109-16.

42. Mulla H, Lawson G, von Anrep C, et al. In vitro evaluation of sedative drug losses during extracorporeal membrane oxygenation. Perfusion 2000;15:21-6.

43. Poole SK, Poole CF. Separation methods for estimating octanol-water partition coefficients. J Chromatogr B Analyt Technol Biomed Life Sci 2003;797:3-19.

44. Shekar K, Roberts JA, McDonald CI, et al. Sequestration of drugs in the circuit may lead to therapeutic failure during extracorporeal membrane oxygenation. Crit Care 2012;16:R194.

45. Barr J, Fraser GL, Puntillo K, et al. Clinical practice guidelines for the management of pain, agitation, and delirium in adult patients in the intensive care unit. Crit Care Med 2013;41:263-306.

46. Mehta NM, Halwick DR, Dodson BL, et al. Potential drug sequestration during extracorporeal membrane oxygenation: results from an ex vivo experiment. Intensive Care Med 2007;33:1018-24.

47. Bhatt-Mehta V, Annich G. Sedative clearance during extracorporeal membrane oxygenation. Perfusion 2005;20:309-15.

48. Wagner D, Pasko D, Phillips K, et al. In vitro clearance of dexmedetomidine in extracorporeal membrane oxygenation. Perfusion 2013;28:40-6.

49. Shekar K, Roberts JA, Ghassabian S, et al. Sedation during extracorporeal membrane oxygenation—why more is less. Anaesth Intensive Care 2012;40:1067-9.

50. Shekar K, Roberts JA, Mullany DV, et al. Increased sedation requirements in patients receiving extracorporeal membrane oxygenation for respiratory and cardiorespiratory failure. Anaesth Intensive Care 2012;40:648-55.

51. Dellinger RP, Levy MM, Rhodes A, et al. Surviving Sepsis Campaign: international guidelines for management of severe sepsis and septic shock: 2012. Crit Care Med 2013;41:580-637.

52. Smith BS, Yogaratnam D, Levasseur-Franklin KE, et al. Introduction to drug pharmacokinetics in the critically ill patient. Chest 2012;141:1327-36.

53. Mulla H, Pooboni S. Population pharmacokinetics of vancomycin in patients receiving extracorporeal membrane oxygenation. Br J Clin Pharmacol 2005;60:265-75.

54. Donadello K, Roberts JA, Cristallini S, et al. Vancomycin population pharmacokinetics during extracorporeal membrane oxygenation therapy: a matched cohort study. Crit Care 2014;18:632.

55. Bhatt-Mehta V, Johnson CE, Schumacher RE. Gentamicin pharmacokinetics in term neonates receiving extracorporeal membrane oxygenation. Pharmacotherapy 1992;12:28-32.

56. Southgate WM, DiPiro JT, Robertson AF. Pharmacokinetics of gentamicin in neonates on extracorporeal membrane oxygenation. Antimicrob Agents Chemother 1989;33:817-9.

57. Cohen P, Collart L, Prober CG, et al. Gentamicin pharmacokinetics in neonates undergoing extracorporeal membrane oxygenation. Pediatr Infect Dis J 1990;9:562-6.

58. Dodge WF, Jelliffe RW, Zwischenberger JB, et al. Population pharmacokinetic models: effect of explicit versus assumed constant serum concentration assay error patterns upon parameter values of gentamicin in infants on and off extracorporeal membrane oxygenation. Ther Drug Monit 1994;16:552-9.

59. Shekar K, Roberts JA, Ghassabian S, et al. Altered antibiotic pharmacokinetics during extracorporeal membrane oxygenation: cause for concern? J Antimicrob Chemother 2013;68:726-7.

60. Tröger U, Drust A, Martens-Lobenhoffer J, et al. Decreased meropenem levels in intensive care unit patients with augmented renal clearance: benefit of therapeutic drug monitoring. Int J Antimicrob Agents 2012;40:370-2.

61. Ruiz S, Papy E, Da Silva D, et al. Potential voriconazole and caspofungin sequestration during extracorporeal membrane oxygenation. Intensive Care Med 2009;35:183-4.

62. Spriet I, Annaert P, Meersseman P, et al. Pharmacokinetics of caspofungin and voriconazole in critically ill patients during extracorporeal membrane oxygenation. J Antimicrob Chemother 2009;63:767-70.

63. De Rosa FG, Corcione S, Baietto L, et al. Pharmacokinetics of linezolid during extracorporeal membrane oxygenation. Int J Antimicrob Agents 2013;41:590-1.

64. Zoller M, Maier B, Hornuss C, et al. Variability of linezolid concentrations after standard dosing in critically ill patients: a prospective observational study. Crit Care 2014;18:R148.

65. Veinstein A, Debouverie O, Grégoire N, et al. Lack of effect of extracorporeal membrane oxygenation on tigecycline pharmacokinetics. J Antimicrob Chemother 2012;67:1047-8.

66. Pieri M, Agracheva N, Bonaveglio E, et al. Bivalirudin versus heparin as an anticoagulant during extracorporeal membrane oxygenation: a case-control study. J Cardiothorac Vasc Anesth 2013;27:30-4.

67. Ranucci M, Ballotta A, Kandil H, et al.; Surgical and Clinical Outcome Research Group. Bivalirudin-based versus conventional heparin anticoagulation for postcardiotomy extracorporeal membrane oxygenation. Crit Care 2011;15:R275.

68. Beiderlinden M, Treschan T, Görlinger K, et al. Argatroban in extracorporeal membrane oxygenation. Artif Organs 2007;31:461-5.

69. Heilmann C, Geisen U, Beyersdorf F, et al. Acquired von Willebrand syndrome in patients with extracorporeal life support (ECLS). Intensive Care Med 2012;38:62-8.

70. Meyer AL, Malehsa D, Budde U, et al. Acquired von Willebrand syndrome in patients with a centrifugal or axial continuous flow left ventricular assist device. JACC Heart Fail 2014;2:141-5.

71. Crow S, Chen D, Milano C, et al. Acquired von Willebrand syndrome in continuous-flow ventricular assist device recipients. Ann Thorac Surg 2010;90:1263-9; discussion 1269.

72. Suarez J, Patel CB, Felker GM, et al. Mechanisms of bleeding and approach to patients with axial-flow left ventricular assist devices. Circ Heart Fail 2011;4:779-84.

73. Achneck HE, Sileshi B, Parikh A, et al. Pathophysiology of bleeding and clotting in the cardiac surgery patient: from vascular endothelium to circulatory assist device surface. Circulation 2010;122:2068-77.

74. Levi M, Schultz M, van der Poll T. Disseminated intravascular coagulation in infectious disease. Semin Thromb Hemost 2010;36:367-77.

75. Blitz A. Pump thrombosis—a riddle wrapped in a mystery inside an enigma. Ann Cardiothorac Surg 2014;3:450-71.

76. Tchantchaleishvili V, Sagebin F, Ross RE, et al. Evaluation and treatment of pump thrombosis and hemolysis. Ann Cardiothorac Surg 2014;3:490-5.

77. Vermeulen Windsant IC, Hanssen SJ, Buurman WA, et al. Cardiovascular surgery and organ damage: time to reconsider the role of hemolysis. J Thorac Cardiovasc Surg 2011;142:1-11.

78. Helms CC, Marvel M, Zhao W, et al. Mechanisms of hemolysis-associated platelet activation. J Thromb Haemost 2013;11:2148-54.

79. Qian Q, Nath KA, Wu Y, et al. Hemolysis and acute kidney failure. Am J Kidney Dis 2010;56:780-4.

80. Concepcion B, Korbet SM, Schwartz MM. Intravascular hemolysis and acute renal failure after mitral and aortic valve repair. Am J Kidney Dis 2008;52:1010-5.

81. Goldstein DJ, John R, Salerno C, et al. Algorithm for the diagnosis and management of suspected pump thrombus. J Heart Lung Transplant 2013;32:667-70.

82. Shah P, Mehta VM, Cowger JA, et al. Diagnosis of hemolysis and device thrombosis with lactate dehydrogenase during left ventricular assist device support. J Heart Lung Transplant 2014;33:102-4.

83. ELSO Anticoagulation Guidelines 2014. Extracorporeal Life Support Organization. Available at http://elsonet.org/resources/guidelines. Accessed August 1, 2015.

84. Chiu HM, Hirsh J, Yung WL, et al. Relationship between the anticoagulant and antithrombotic effects of heparin in experimental venous thrombosis. Blood 1977;49:171-84.

85. Brill-Edwards P, Ginsberg JS, Johnston M, et al. Establishing a therapeutic range for heparin therapy. Ann Intern Med 1993;119:104-9.

86. Adatya S, Uriel N, Yarmohammadi H, et al. Anti-factor Xa and activated partial thromboplastin time measurements for heparin monitoring in mechanical circulatory support. JACC Heart Fail 2015;3:314-22.

87. Kostousov V, Nguyen K, Hundalani SG, et al. The influence of free hemoglobin and bilirubin on heparin monitoring by activated partial thromboplastin time and anti-Xa assay. Arch Pathol Lab Med 2014;138:1503-6.

88. Uriel N, Morrison KA, Garan AR, et al. Development of a novel echocardiography ramp test for speed optimization and diagnosis of device thrombosis in continuous-flow left ventricular assist devices: the Columbia ramp study. J Am Coll Cardiol 2012;60:1764-75.

89. Jennings DL, Weeks PA. Thrombosis in continuous-flow left ventricular assist devices: pathophysiology, prevention, and pharmacologic management. Pharmacotherapy 2015;35:79-98.

90. Hannan MM, Husain S, Mattner F, et al. International Society for Heart and Lung Transplantation. Working formulation for the standardization of definitions of infections in patients using ventricular assist devices. J Heart Lung Transplant 2011;30:375-84.

91. Acharya MN, Som R, Tsui S. What is the optimum antibiotic prophylaxis in patients undergoing implantation of a left ventricular assist device? Interact Cardiovasc Thorac Surg 2012;14:209-14.

92. Bratzler DW, Dellinger EP, Olsen KM, et al. American Society of Health-System Pharmacists (ASHP); Infectious Diseases Society of America (IDSA); Surgical Infection Society (SIS); Society for Healthcare Epidemiology of America (SHEA). Clinical practice guidelines for antimicrobial prophylaxis in surgery. Surg Infect (Larchmt) 2013;14:73-156.

93. Glater-Welt LB, Schneider JB, Zinger MM, et al. Nosocomial bloodstream infections in patients receiving extracorporeal life support: variability in prevention practices: a survey of the Extracorporeal Life Support Organization members. J Intensive Care Med 2015 Feb 10.

Section 9

Other Urgencies and Emergencies

Chapter 37: Hypertensive Crisis

Jeremy Flynn, Pharm.D., FCCP, FCCM; Melissa Nestor, Pharm.D., BCPS; and Komal Pandya, Pharm.D., BCPS

LEARNING OBJECTIVES

1. Understand the basic underlying pathophysiology of hypertensive crisis within the context of underlying disease states and etiologies.
2. List the possible organ system dysfunctions that are possible with hypertensive crisis.
3. Describe management options that are preferred and those that should be used with caution.
4. Understand disease- and etiology-specific treatment options.

ABBREVIATIONS IN THIS CHAPTER

ACEI	Angiotensin-converting enzyme inhibitor	ICU	Intensive care unit
APH	Acute postoperative hypertension	MAP	Mean arterial pressure
aSAH	Aneurysmal subarachnoid hemorrhage	RAAS	Renin-angiotensin-aldosterone system
DBP	Diastolic blood pressure	SBP	Systolic blood pressure
ICH	Intracerebral hemorrhage		

INTRODUCTION

Epidemiology

Hypertension is extremely common with a prevalence of about 25%–30% and affects an estimated 80 million adults in the United States and more than 970 million adults worldwide. Compared with other dietary, lifestyle, and metabolic risk factors, hypertension is the leading cause of death in women and the second leading cause of death in men, behind smoking. In the United States, there is a higher prevalence of hypertension in black populations than in white, Hispanic, and Asian populations. In addition, the prevalence of hypertension in all population groups increases with age.[1] The Seventh Report of the Joint National Committee on Prevention, Detection, Evaluation, and Treatment of High Blood Pressure (JNC-7) classified patients according to systolic blood pressure (SBP) and diastolic blood pressure (DBP) values ([prehypertension (SBP 120–139 mm Hg or DBP 80–89 mm Hg], stage 1 hypertension [SBP 140–159 mm Hg or DBP 90–99 mm Hg], and stage 2 hypertension [SBP of 160 mm Hg or greater or DBP of 100 mm Hg or greater]) and recommended that patients with a diagnosis of stage 1 or 2 hypertension receive pharmacologic management if lifestyle modifications have failed to achieve blood pressure goals.[2] The 2014 report relaxes treatment initiation for the general population 60 years and older to a threshold of SBP of 140 mm Hg or greater or DBP of 90 mm Hg or greater in the absence of other risk factors such as chronic kidney disease, diabetes mellitus, and cerebrovascular disease.[3] Although much of the morbidity and mortality associated with hypertension is attributed to processes developing over time, patients may also present with in hypertensive crisis, placing them at risk of impending or progressive organ damage. Hypertensive crisis has been estimated to occur in 1% of adults with a history of hypertension annually; however, the true incidence may be higher, especially given that one investigation showed that 23% of hypertensive crisis cases requiring emergency department management occurred in patients with no history of hypertension.[4]

Pathophysiology

Acute blood pressure elevation in hypertensive crisis may be caused by a variety of underlying etiologies, and it may occur in patients with a history of hypertension or in those without. Several different causes of hypertensive crisis exist including, but not limited to, history of essential hypertension, renal disease, pregnancy, endocrine disorders, drug-induced hypertension, autonomic dysfunction, and disorders of the central nervous system.[5] With respect to patients with essential hypertension, situations such as inadequately controlled hypertension, medication nonadherence, and lack of consistent medical follow-up are common patient-specific scenarios that lead from essential hypertension to hypertensive crises. Although the overall precipitating causes may differ, the underlying pathology of hypertensive crisis can be defined by how it affects the regulation of hemodynamic parameters. Systolic blood pressure is determined by cardiac output, a product of stroke volume and heart rate, and systemic vascular resistance, a function of peripheral vascular resistance and renal vascular resistance.[6] Marked hypertension is often associated with increased levels of vasoactive substances, such as norepinephrine, antidiuretic hormone, and the renin-angiotensin-aldosterone system (RAAS), or by direct pressure-related effects on the vasculature.

Increased blood pressure caused by an increased systemic vascular resistance can be mediated by an increase in circulating endogenous catecholamines. Vasoconstriction and increased heart rate mediated by increased norepinephrine and epinephrine, whether as a primary disease process or as a secondary response, can contribute to hypertensive crisis.[7] Renin is typically released from the kidneys as a response to a perceived decreased arterial blood volume, and once in circulation, it catalyzes the conversion of angiotensinogen, a liver-derived zymogen, to angiotensin I. Circulating angiotensin I is converted by angiotensin-converting enzyme to active angiotensin II, which has several mechanisms by which it affects blood pressure by augmenting circulating blood volume and inducing vasoconstriction. Angiotensin II acts directly on vascular smooth muscle to induce vasoconstriction, thus increasing systemic vascular resistance. Increased circulating blood volume is influenced by angiotensin II because it enhances the release of aldosterone, increasing sodium reabsorption as well as increasing secretion of antidiuretic hormone. Angiotensin II also plays a role in smooth muscle cell growth and migration, but the role of this effect in acute hypertensive crisis remains unclear.[8] In sustained or severe hypertension, stressed vascular endothelium may be overwhelmed and unable to balance vasoconstrictive processes with compensatory nitric oxide and prostacyclin, continuing the cycle of ongoing hypertension. This loss of endothelial function is not well understood; however, proinflammatory processes and pressure-related endothelial damage are likely involved in furthering vasoconstriction.[9]

CLINICAL PRESENTATION

Hypertensive crises can be subdivided into hypertensive urgency and emergency. Presence of end-organ damage is the distinction between the two, with end-organ damage being present with hypertensive emergency. Clinical presentation varies from patient to patient. Organ dysfunction is uncommon with DBPs less than 130 mm Hg (except in children and in pregnancy). One recent study by Zampaglione and colleagues found single-organ involvement in 83%, two-organ involvement in 14%, and three- or more organ involvement in only 3% of hypertensive emergencies (Table 37.1).[4] In another study examining the prevalence of various end-organ complications in patients with hypertensive crisis, neurologic complications—specifically cerebral infarctions—were the most prevalent, followed by acute heart failure and acute myocardial infarction.[10] Standard treatment of a hypertensive crisis in the intensive care unit (ICU) involves continuous blood pressure monitoring and parenteral administration of an antihypertensive agent.[2,11,12]

Blood Pressure

Hypertensive emergencies are characterized by severe elevations in blood pressure (greater than 180/120 mm Hg) complicated by evidence of impending or progressive target organ dysfunction. Examples include hypertensive encephalopathy, intracerebral hemorrhage, acute myocardial infarction, acute left ventricular failure with pulmonary edema, unstable angina pectoris, dissecting aortic

Table 37.1 End-Organ Damage Associated with Hypertensive Emergency

End-Organ Damage Type	Cases (%)
Cerebral infarction	24.5
Intracerebral or subarachnoid bleed	4.5
Hypertensive encephalopathy	16.3
Acute pulmonary edema	22.5
Acute congestive heart failure	14.3
Acute myocardial infarction or unstable angina	12.0
Aortic dissection	2.0
Eclampsia	2.0

Data from: Zampaglione B, Pascale C, Marchisio M, et al. Hypertensive urgencies and emergencies. Prevalence and clinical presentation. Hypertension 1996;27:144-7.

aneurysm, and eclampsia. Hypertensive urgencies are situations associated with severe elevations in blood pressure without progressive target organ dysfunction. Examples include upper levels of hypertension associated with severe headache, shortness of breath, epistaxis, or severe anxiety. Most of these patients present as nonadherent or inadequately treated patients with hypertensive emergencies, often with little or no evidence of target organ damage.[4,11]

Optic Fundi

Retinopathy is a hallmark symptom of hypertensive crisis and is present in many patients on presentation. Typical findings on optic examination include hard exudates, hemorrhages, and papilledema. Retinal hemorrhages are a result of necrosis of the capillary and precapillary arteriolar walls. This endothelial necrosis leads to leakage and deposition of plasma proteins in the posterior retina, which manifests as hard exudates. Papilledema is defined as a swelling of the optic disc and, in the past, was associated with a poor prognosis; however, this finding is no longer a prognostic indicator. With blood pressure management, retinal lesions may be reversed.[4,11-13]

Cardiovascular

Hypertensive crisis can result in acute heart failure and lead to pulmonary edema. This can be attributed to increases in preload and afterload. Acute heart failure is the presenting symptom in 11%–15% of patients. Common cardiovascular findings in these patients may include underlying ischemic heart disease, acute myocardial infarction, angina symptoms, and left ventricular hypertrophy. Aortic dissection is less common, but when it does occur, it is life threatening.[2,11,13]

Neurologic

Neurologic symptoms are often the presenting complaint in hypertensive crisis. More than 60% of patients present with headaches, and up to 28% experience dizziness.[4] Cerebrovascular events occur in 7% of patients with hypertensive crisis and include transient or focal cerebral ischemia as well as cerebral and subarachnoid hemorrhage. Hypertensive encephalopathy is characterized by headache, nausea, vomiting, and blurred vision. Other symptoms may include impaired cognition, generalized seizures, and cortical blindness. Hypertensive encephalopathy is likely to arise from loss of autoregulation in cerebral vessels as the result of severe increases in SBP. Normally, cerebral blood flow is maintained constant despite fluctuations in a range of perfusion pressures. With chronic hypertension, adaptive processes allow cerebral blood flow to be maintained at a higher perfusion pressures and thereby prohibit or attenuate the severity of hypertensive encephalopathy during sudden increases in blood pressure. At very high pressures, this autoregulatory process breaks down. This may occur when the blood pressure is greater than 160/100 mm Hg in previously normotensive patients. In patients with chronic hypertension, it rarely develops until the blood pressure is greater than 200/120 mm Hg. Pathologic findings include cerebral microinfarctions, petechial hemorrhages, and cerebral edema. As the blood pressure is reduced, fluid extravasation decreases, and cerebral autoregulation gradually normalizes. In patients with chronic hypertension, autoregulation may take time to reestablish. Therefore, depending on the clinical scenario, blood pressure should be lowered slowly in severely hypertensive subjects with chronic hypertension to avoid precipitating cerebral ischemia.[4,11-14]

Renal

Renal involvement is also a common complication. Nonnephrotic–range proteinuria is commonly associated with elevated serum creatinine concentrations. Increased serum creatinine (greater than 2.3 mg/dL) occurs in 31% of patients at presentation. Overt nephrotic syndrome is uncommon. Urinalysis may be useful in differentiating if kidney injury is acute versus chronic in nature. Hypokalemic metabolic alkalosis may develop as a result of volume depletion and secondary hyperaldosteronism. Plasma renin activity and aldosterone are increased in most cases.[4,13,15]

Hematologic

Microangiopathic hemolytic anemia, thrombocytopenia, increased fibrin degradation, and increased fibrinogen are commonly seen. Erythrocyte sedimentation rate is often elevated because of renal failure and anemia.[16]

DIAGNOSTIC CONSIDERATIONS AND CLINICAL EVALUATION

Early triage to emergency departments to initiate appropriate therapeutic interventions for these patients is critical to affecting morbidity and mortality. Patients presenting with hypertensive crisis may represent up to 25% of all patient visits to busy urban emergency departments.[2] Evaluation of patients with hypertension involves assessment of lifestyle, identification of risk factors and comorbidities that may affect prognosis and guide treatment, identification of potential causes of high blood pressure, and assessment for the presence of target organ damage and cerebrovascular disease. Patient evaluation is made through ascertaining medical history, physical examination, routine laboratory tests, and other diagnostic procedures. The physical examination should include an appropriate measurement of blood pressure with verification in the contralateral arm; examination of the optic fundi; calculation of BMI (body mass index); auscultation for carotid, abdominal, and femoral bruits; palpation of the thyroid gland; thorough examination of the heart and lungs; examination of the abdomen for enlarged kidneys, masses, distended urinary bladder, and abnormal aortic pulsation; palpation of the lower extremities for edema and pulses; and neurologic assessment.[12,14,16]

Patients with hypertensive crisis should be admitted to an ICU for continuous hemodynamic monitoring and administration of intravenous antihypertensive agents. According to the JNC-7 guidelines, the initial goal of therapy in hypertensive emergencies is to reduce the mean arterial blood pressure by no more than 20%–25% (within minutes to 1 hour) and then, if stable, to an SBP of 160 mm Hg and/or a DBP of 100–110 mm Hg during the next 2–6 hours. More aggressive blood pressure reductions may precipitate and perpetuate renal, cerebral, or coronary ischemia. This recommendation is based on the body's ability to autoregulate tissue perfusion in the brain, heart, and kidneys. If this level of blood pressure reduction is well tolerated, further gradual reductions toward a goal blood pressure can be executed in the next 24–48 hours. There are exceptions to this treatment strategy. There is no clear evidence from clinical trials that patients with an acute ischemic stroke benefit from the use of immediate intravenous antihypertensive treatment unless it is lowered to enable the use of thrombolytic agents. In addition, patients with aortic dissection should have their SBP lowered to less than 120 mm Hg as quickly as possible, if tolerated. It is imperative to ensure appropriate monitoring for signs or symptoms of ischemia-related end-organ system deterioration that may accompany changes in SBP, DBP, or mean arterial pressure (MAP).[12,14,16]

The JNC-7 criteria for accurate blood pressure measurements require that two readings be taken 5 minutes apart with the patient at rest in a seated and standing position.[2] Recall that there is a statistical tendency for repeat measurements to regress toward the mean of measurements. A study of 195 consecutive patients with hypertension in an emergency department validated this mathematical principle and documented a mean decline of 11.6 mm Hg in repeated DBP readings. Unexpectedly high blood pressure readings should be repeated because a measurement error can occur from the misapplication of the sphygmomanometer cuff, use of an inappropriately sized cuff, or operator error. In addition, consider whether the hypertension is reactive in nature. If the hypertension is caused by anxiety, pain, or use of sympathomimetics (such as decongestants or cocaine) or by withdrawal states (e.g., withdrawal from alcohol or antihypertensive medication), addressing the underlying condition is an imperative part of management. Urine toxicology for cocaine can be helpful in select, high-risk patient populations.

A thorough patient history is needed to determine concomitant disease states and home blood pressure readings, if possible. Furthermore, elucidating the patient's home medications and medication adherence is essential. This history should include prescription medications, over-the-counter medications, and recreational drugs as well as any supplements because any of these may contribute to the patient's clinical picture.[11]

Neurologically, patients should be evaluated for any symptoms associated with ischemic or hemorrhagic stroke or hypertensive encephalopathy. A funduscopic optical examination to assess for papilledema, hemorrhage, or exudates within the eye may be indicated. A thorough cardiovascular assessment is also necessary. Crucial components include auscultation for new murmurs associated with aortic insufficiency or dissection as well as checking for mitral regurgitation, which could be associated with ischemia. A gallop could indicate acute heart failure. The lung fields should be auscultated to check for crackles suggestive of pulmonary edema.

Laboratory tests should be assessed to validate physical examination findings. These should include serum electrolytes, serum creatinine, and a complete blood cell count with peripheral smear. A 12-lead electrocardiogram should be ascertained to determine myocardial ischemia or left ventricular hypertrophy. A chest radiograph could help determine the presence of pulmonary edema, widened mediastinum, or cardiac enlargement. A urine analysis may be helpful in assessing for casts and proteinuria. More extensive testing for identifiable causes of hypertensive crisis are not usually indicated unless blood pressure control is not achieved or unless the clinical and routine laboratory evaluation strongly suggests an identifiable secondary cause (i.e., vascular bruits, symptoms of catecholamine excess, unprovoked hypokalemia).

In addition, two emerging risk factors may be evaluated, particularly in those with cerebrovascular disease but without other risk factor abnormalities: (1) high-sensitivity C-reactive protein, a marker of inflammation; and (2) homocysteine. Current data do not highlight the role of these factors in the management of hypertensive crisis, but they may come to play a role in chronic management and risk assessment.

General Therapeutic Approach

In patients with hypertensive urgencies, blood pressure is lowered over 24–48 hours, usually with oral medication. Some patients with hypertensive urgencies may respond to treatment with an oral, short-acting agent such as captopril, labetalol, or clonidine together with a period of observation. However, there is no evidence to suggest that failure to aggressively lower blood pressure in these patients while admitted to the emergency department is associated with any increased short-term risk to these patients. Furthermore, they may benefit from adjustment in their current antihypertensive therapy or reinstitution of medications if nonadherence is a problem. Patients should be discharged from the emergency department with a confirmed follow-up visit within 24–48 hours postdischarge. The term *urgency* may lead to overly aggressive antihypertensive treatment with intravenous drugs or even oral agents to rapidly lower blood pressure. However, this practice is not without risk. Oral loading doses of antihypertensive agents may lead to accumulation of drug, which may result in hypotension after discharge from the emergency department. Patients who continue to be nonadherent often return to the emergency department within weeks.[13,14,16]

Patients with hypertensive emergency require immediate control of the blood pressure to attenuate end-organ damage. Blood pressure in patients with hypertensive emergencies should be treated in a controlled fashion in an ICU. Continuous blood pressure monitoring should be considered in these patients to assist in appropriate titration of therapeutic agents. Type of monitoring may vary from blood pressure cuff to more invasive intra-arterial blood pressure monitoring. Choice of monitoring mechanism is complex and may depend on the type of patient, cause of hypertensive crisis, and agents used to control hemodynamics. Once therapeutic end points have been achieved, the patient can be initiated on a regimen of oral maintenance antihypertensive therapy.

Medical Therapies

Calcium Channel Antagonists

Calcium channel antagonist agents or calcium channel blockers have clinical application in a variety of cardiovascular disease states. Although there are six known types of calcium channels, only the L- and T-type channels are thought to have effects relevant to cardiovascular disease.[17] The clinical role of T-type calcium channel antagonism remains undefined and is an area for further research.[18] L-type calcium channel antagonists can be subdivided into three major subclasses: dihydropyridines (nicardipine and clevidipine), phenylalkylamines (verapamil), and benzothiazepines (diltiazem).

L-type calcium channels are widespread in a variety of tissues including the cardiovascular system, neuronal, and secretory tissue. Calcium channel antagonists inhibit calcium influx during depolarization and result in end effects such as decreased vascular constriction, decreased atrioventricular nodal conduction, and negative inotropy—though these are strongly influenced by calcium channel antagonist structure and subclass. The classical targets for calcium channel antagonists are the Ca_v1 L-type receptors found on myocardial and vascular smooth muscle, which can reach the receptor either by the open channel or though the lipid membrane of a closed channel. Verapamil and diltiazem are charged at physiologic pH, enter calcium channels in the open state, and have increased activity on cardiac L-type channels. This results in the decreased atrioventricular node transduction and negative inotropy associated with these agents. In contrast, dihydropyridine agents are more lipophilic, exerting their action on closed or inactive calcium channels with a higher affinity for vascular calcium channels.[19] For this reason, we will now focus on dihydropyridine calcium channel antagonists, of which two are currently available in intravenous formulations: nicardipine and clevidipine.

Nicardipine

Nicardipine is a dihydropyridine calcium channel antagonist, indicated for short-term management of hypertension. Nicardipine exerts its antihypertensive action by selective dilation of arterial and coronary vascular smooth muscle with no significant venodilatory effects. A fairly quick onset of action of 5–15 minutes is observed with a duration of antihypertensive effects of 4–6 hours and a terminal half-life of 14 hours, prolonged in patients with hepatic impairment (Table 37.2). Nicardipine has linear kinetics, is highly (greater than 95%) protein bound, and is metabolized by the liver by the cytochrome P450 (CYP) enzymes, primarily by CPY2C8, CYP2D6, and CYP3A4. No pharmacokinetic differences have been seen between younger individuals and those older than 65 years. Nicardipine is contraindicated in patients with advanced aortic stenosis.[11,20]

Nicardipine should be initiated at 5 mg/hour and increased by 2.5 mg/hour every 15 minutes until goal blood pressure is attained, with a maximum of 15 mg/hour. Once goal blood pressure is achieved, a taper of 3–5 mg/hour every 15 minutes should be tried, as tolerated. Nicardipine is available as a premixed infusion of either 0.1 or 0.2 mg/mL (in either dextrose or saline solutions) or as a concentrated solution (2.5 mg/mL), which is recommended to be diluted to a concentration of 0.1 mg/mL in buffered solutions for a pH of 3.7–4.7 and 3.5, respectively.[21,22] Although typically well tolerated, adverse events associated with nicardipine are typically those associated with vasodilation such as headache, hypotension, and tachycardia. To avoid potential peripheral vein irritation, manufacturers recommend changing infusion sites every 12 hours.

Clevidipine

Clevidipine is a third-generation dihydropyridine calcium channel antagonist, also indicated for short-term management of hypertension. Clevidipine exerts its antihypertensive action by a selective effect of arterioles, with minimal effects on venous capacitance vessels and cardiac preload. Clevidipine has a rapid onset of action, about 2–4 minutes, with a terminal half-life of about 15 minutes because it is metabolized by esterases predominantly in the blood and extravascular tissues (Table 37.2). Clevidipine is highly protein bound (greater than 99%), and although data are limited, no drug-drug interactions are likely because it is hydrolyzed by esterases, and neither clevidipine nor its metabolites are expected to interfere with CYP enzymes

Table 37.2 Medications Used for the Management of Hypertensive Crisis

Medication	Mechanism of Action	Dosing	Adverse Effects	Utility in Hypertensive Crisis
Nicardipine	Dihydropyridine calcium channel antagonist	Continuous infusion Typical initial dose: 5 mg/hr Titrate by: 2.5 mg/hr every 15 min Dosing range: 5–15 mg/hr	Headache Tachycardia Contraindicated: Advanced aortic stenosis	Wide range of utility as first-line continuous infusion agent for many populations with hypertensive crisis
Clevidipine	Dihydropyridine calcium channel antagonist	Continuous infusion Typical initial dose: 1–2 mg/hr Titrate by: Double dose as quickly as 90-s intervals initially, lengthening to every 5–10 min as goal BP obtained Dosing range: Average of 21 mg/hr per 24-hr period (1,000 mL) recommended Limited data > 32 mg/hr	Minimal-modest reflex tachycardia Elevated triglycerides (in lipid vehicle) Contraindicated: Severe aortic stenosis Soybean or egg allergy	May have application in many populations with hypertensive crisis, studied specifically in: Neurologic injury (ICH, aSAH, ischemic stroke) Postoperative hypertension
Enalaprilat	Angiotensin-converting enzyme inhibitor	Typical initial dose: 1.25 mg IV q6hr Dosing range: Up to 5 mg/dose reported	Hyperkalemia Angioedema Contraindicated: Pregnancy History of angioedema	Advantageous for maintenance therapy, but long duration of action (12–24 hr) limits utility for acute intervention; not first-line agent
Sodium nitroprusside	Nitric oxide donor Arteriolar and venous dilator	Continuous infusion Dosing range: 0.3–10 mcg/kg/min Titrate by: 0.25–0.5 mcg/kg/min every 2–5 min	Significant hypotension Cyanide toxicity Methemoglobinemia	Aortic dissection Avoid in acute coronary syndromes
Nitroglycerin	Converted to nitric oxide Venous dilation >>> arteriolar	Continuous infusion Dosing range: 2–200 mcg/min Titrate by: 5 mcg/min every 3–5 min --OR-- Dosing range: 0.2–2 mcg/kg/min Titrate by: 0.2–0.5 mcg/kg/min every 3–5 min	Hypotension Reflex tachycardia Headache (> 60% of patients)	
Hydralazine	Exact mechanism unclear Arteriolar dilator through inhibition of calcium release from sarcoplasmic reticulum	10–20 mg IV or IM every 4–6 hr	Unpredictable response in blood pressure Systemic lupus erythematosus	Unpredictable antihypertensive effects; therefore, not first line

Table 37.2 Medications Used for the Management of Hypertensive Crisis (continued)

Medication	Mechanism of Action	Dosing	Adverse Effects	Utility in Hypertensive Crisis
Esmolol	Cardioselective β_1-adrenergic receptor antagonist	Loading dose: 0.5–1 mg/kg IV over 1 min Continuous infusion: 50–300 mcg/min Titrate by: 25–50 mcg/kg/min every 5–10 min	Hypotension Bradycardia	Postoperative hypertension Acute coronary syndrome
Labetalol	Combined α_1- and nonselective β-adrenergic receptor antagonist	Incremental bolus dosing: 10–80 mg at 10-min intervals until target BP achieved Loading dose: 10–20 mg IV Continuous infusion: 0.5–1 mg/min Titrate by: 0.5–1 mg/min every 30 min	Hypotension Bradycardia Fatigue	Widely used as first-line agent for bolus treatment in many populations with hypertensive crisis
Phentolamine	Competitive antagonist of peripheral α_1- and α_2-receptors	Loading dose: 5–15 mg IV Continuous infusion: 1–40 mg/hr Titrated hourly	Chest pain Tachycardia Flushing Headache	Situations of catecholamine access: Pheochromocytoma Cocaine overdose Amphetamine overdose Clonidine withdrawal
Fenoldapam	Peripheral dopamine type 1 receptor agonist	Continuous infusion: 0.1–1.6 mcg/kg/min Titrate by: 0.05–0.1 mcg/kg/min every 15 min	Headache Flushing Tachycardia Dizziness	

aSAH = aneurysmal subarachnoid hemorrhage; BP = blood pressure; ICH = intracerebral hemorrhage; IM = intramuscularly; IV = intravenously; q = every.

at therapeutic concentrations. No dose adjustments are recommended in the setting of hepatic or renal impairment, though it may be prudent to initiate dosing at the lower end of the recommended range in the older adult population. Clevidipine is generally well tolerated, showing minimal to modest reflex tachycardia and an increase in serum triglyceride concentrations in some study populations (decreased with the discontinuation of clevidipine).[23]

It is recommended to initiate clevidipine at a dose of 1–2 mg/hour, with a doubling of the dose at short (90 seconds) intervals initially, lengthening to every 5–10 minutes as goal blood pressure is attained. Clinical experience is limited with doses above 32 mg/hour. Clevidipine is available for intravenous use in a 20% lipid emulsion (2 kcal/mL) and, like similar formulations, contraindicated in patients with allergies to soybeans/soy products or eggs/egg products. Because of the lipid vehicle, doses greater than 1,000 mL/day (an average of 21 mg/hour/day) are not recommended. In addition, there is limited experience with treatment courses exceeding 72 hours in duration. Caloric intake and triglyceride concentrations should be assessed for patients receiving clevidipine. Clevidipine may be infused by central or peripheral venous access, and because of the risk of bacterial growth in the lipid medium, the vial must be changed every 12 hours.[23,24]

Angiotensin-Converting Enzyme Inhibitors

Enalaprilat

Enalaprilat is the active form of the prodrug enalapril and is the only angiotensin-converting enzyme inhibitor (ACEI) available in an intravenous formulation. Like all ACEIs, enalaprilat prevents the conversion of angiotensin I to angiotensin II as part of the RAAS. This system is vital in maintaining blood pressure, electrolyte balance, and volume status. Renin, released by juxtaglomerular cells in the afferent arterioles in response to decreased renal perfusion and/or sodium load, cleaves angiotensinogen to angiotensin I, which is then converted to angiotensin II by angiotensin-converting enzyme, the target for ACEI agents. Angiotensin II stimulates G-protein angiotensin II type 1 receptors, resulting in arteriolar constriction, including marked efferent arteriole constriction, release of aldosterone and antidiuretic hormone, and increased sympathetic nervous system activity, and it has a role in cardiac mitogenesis and remodeling. Angiotensin-converting enzyme inhibitors also prevent the breakdown of substance P and bradykinin, a vasodilator.[25,26]

Enalaprilat may be given in hypertensive crisis with an initial dose of 1.25 mg intravenously every 6 hours, given as a slow intravenous push over 5 minutes, with antihypertensive effects seen as quickly as 10–15 minutes after infusion, a maximal onset in 0.5–1 hour, and duration of action of 12–24 hours (Table 37.2).[27,28] Although this is advantageous in maintenance therapy, allowing for daily dosing of oral enalapril, this long duration of action may be detrimental in patients experiencing hypotension after drug administration. Also of note is that the baseline degree of RAAS activity may affect patient response to enalaprilat. The degree of blood pressure lowering in patients with hypertensive crisis has been correlated with plasma renin concentration, with a higher degree of response in patients having a high degree of RAAS activity.[29]

Enalaprilat is primarily excreted unchanged in the urine (61%) and feces (33%), with a recommended lower initial dose of 0.625 mg in patients with a CrCl of less than 30 mL/minute/1.73 m^2 and care taken in patients on hemodialysis. Renal impairment is associated with enalaprilat use, mediated by its overall hypotensive effects and specifically alteration of angiotensin II–mediated efferent arteriolar vasoconstriction, more often observed in patients with baseline renal compromise. In addition, enalaprilat should be used with caution in patients with aortic stenosis or hyperkalemia, and it is contraindicated in pregnant patients and patients with a history of hereditary or idiopathic angioedema.[26,28,30] Reported adverse effects with enalaprilat include cough, angioedema, and hypotension. The inhibition of bradykinin and substance P is thought to relate to the incidence of ACEI-associated cough. Angioedema is a relatively rare (0.1%–0.3% incidence) but potentially life-threatening adverse effect of ACEI therapy, typically manifesting with edema of the face, tongue, and throat with reports of death from laryngeal edema reported. Elevated bradykinin is also thought to be associated with angioedema, more commonly seen in women and black patients than in non-black patients.[26,31,32]

Vasodilators

Sodium Nitroprusside

Functionally, sodium nitroprusside is a nitric oxide donor that is converted to a free radical that activates endovascular guanyl cyclase. This results in myosin dephosphorylation and subsequent vascular smooth muscle relaxation. Sodium nitroprusside acts on arteriolar and venous smooth muscle, thereby reducing both preload and afterload. Unpredictable decreases in blood pressure are often seen in patients with hypovolemia or diastolic dysfunction because of sodium nitroprusside effects on preload. In patients with left ventricular failure, decreases in preload may result in a decreased cardiac index, whereas reductions in afterload prohibit the reflexive tachycardia that would normally occur with a drop in cardiac output.[11]

Sodium nitroprusside infusion is typically initiated as a continuous intravenous infusion with a starting infusion rate of 0.3–0.5 mcg/kg/minute, with increases in increments of 0.5 mcg/kg/minute to achieve hemodynamic targets (Table 37.2).[11] The treatment duration should be as short as possible, and to avoid doses exceeding 2 mcg/kg/minute. The dosage requirement in older adult patients is typically lower than in younger patients. The exact mechanism of this increased sensitivity is unknown but is thought to be related to diminished baroreceptor reflex activity, resistance of cardiac adrenergic receptors to catecholamine stimulation, or variations in the direct vasodilating effects of sodium nitroprusside.[33] It has an immediate onset and duration of effect of 2–3 minutes. Tachyphylaxis may develop while using this agent. More severe toxicity associated with sodium nitroprusside is a result of the release of cyanide with interference with cellular respiration. Sodium nitroprusside is metabolized into cyanogen, which is converted to thiocyanate by the enzyme thiosulfate sulfurtransferase. It contains 44% cyanide by weight.[11] Cyanide is released non-enzymatically from sodium nitroprusside, the amount generated being dependent on the dose of sodium nitroprusside administered. Cyanide toxicity may manifest as an unexplained cardiac arrest, coma, encephalopathy, convulsions, hyperreflexia, blurred vision, tinnitus, and irreversible focal neurologic changes. Because free cyanide radicals may bind and inactivate tissue cytochrome oxidase, thereby preventing oxidative phosphorylation, increased cyanide concentrations may also cause tissue anoxia, anaerobic metabolism, and lactic acidosis. Patients receiving sodium nitroprusside with symptoms of central nervous system dysfunction, cardiovascular instability, and increasing metabolic acidosis should be assessed for cyanide toxicity.[34] The current laboratory monitoring methods for cyanide toxicity may be insensitive, given that the accuracy of laboratory results relies on proper storage conditions of blood samples. However, if clinical suspicion of toxicity is high, initiating treatment can be considered before receiving laboratory results. In addition, a rise in serum thiocyanate concentrations is a late-occurring event and is not directly related to cyanide toxicity. Red blood cell cyanide concentrations may be a more reliable method of monitoring for cyanide toxicity, but this is not currently widely available. A red blood cell cyanide concentration above 40 nmol/mL correlates with detectable metabolic changes. Cyanide toxicity is unusual until the total dose exceeds 300 mg or the infusion rate is above 20 mcg/kg/minute, although toxic cyanide concentrations have been seen at various infusion rates. In general, the risk of toxicity increases incrementally with increasing doses.[34] Concentrations greater than 200 nmol/mL are associated with severe clinical symptoms, and concentrations greater than 400 nmol/mL are considered lethal. To avoid potential toxicity, the treatment duration with sodium nitroprusside should be as short as possible, and the infusion rate should be no greater than 2 mcg/kg/minute. The concentrations should be maintained below 10 mg/dL to avoid thiocyanate toxicity. When toxicity is confirmed or suspected, sodium nitroprusside administration should be discontinued. An infusion of thiosulfate may be used in patients receiving higher dosages (4–10 mcg/kg/minute) of sodium nitroprusside.[35] For sodium nitroprusside infusions of 4–10 mcg/kg/minute or greater or infusions longer than 30 minutes, thiosulfate can be coadministered at a 10:1 sodium nitroprusside/thiosulfate ratio to avoid cyanide toxicity.

Furthermore, sodium nitroprusside comprises a ferrous ion center complexed with five cyanide moieties, which may react with methemoglobin and produce cyanomethemoglobin. Normal methemoglobin concentrations can bind the cyanide released from 18 mg of sodium nitroprusside. The total dose of sodium nitroprusside required to cause 10% methemoglobinemia is greater than 10 mg/kg (greater than 10 mcg/kg/minute for more than 16 hours).[11]

Other methods of cytotoxicity may arise through the release of nitric oxide, with hydroxyl radical and peroxynitrite generation leading to lipid peroxidation. Sodium nitroprusside activates guanylate cyclase, which stimulates the formation of cyclic guanosine monophosphate that relaxes smooth muscle.[35]

Thiocyanate is also toxic; however, it is 100-fold less toxic than cyanide. It is eliminated by renal excretion, with a half-life of 3–7 days.[11] Sodium nitroprusside infusions of 2–5 mcg/kg/minute for 7–14 days may be needed to generate thiocyanate toxicity. Nonspecific symptoms of thiocyanate toxicity include fatigue, tinnitus, nausea, and vomiting; clinical signs include hyperreflexia, confusion, psychosis, and miosis.[35]

Normally, adults can detoxify 50 mg of sodium nitroprusside using existing stores of sulfur, but malnutrition, surgery, diuretic use, or other factors can reduce this capacity. Cyanide is metabolized in the liver to thiocyanate and requires thiosulfate to occur. Thiocyanate is 100 times less toxic than cyanide. Thiocyanate is excreted through the kidneys. Cyanide removal therefore requires adequate liver function, adequate renal function, and adequate bioavailability of thiosulfate. Cyanide is known to interfere with cellular respiration. Friederich and colleagues showed that lipid peroxidation in the substantia nigra of rats occurs after the administration of sodium nitroprusside. Lipid peroxidation has also been shown in hepatocytes. In addition, sodium nitroprusside causes concentration- and time-dependent ototoxicity.[34]

As an alternative to thiosulfate, hydroxycobalamin (vitamin B_{12a}) received marketing approval in 2006 from the U.S. Food and Drug Administration (FDA) for the treatment of known or suspected cyanide poisoning at a starting dose of 5 g administered by intravenous infusion over 15 minutes.[11,16]

Nitroglycerin

Nitroglycerin is primarily a venodilator; however, arteriodilation of vascular smooth muscle can occur at high doses. Regarding mechanism of action, nitroglycerin is converted to nitric oxide, which activates guanylate cyclase and stimulates the production of cyclic GMP. This produces venous smooth muscle relaxation and reduction in preload.[36] In volume-depleted patients, a reduction in preload reduces cardiac output, which may be undesirable in patients with compromised myocardial, cerebral, or renal perfusion. Severe hypotension and reflex tachycardia have been reported in these patients quickly after initiating a nitroglycerin infusion. For the treatment of hypertensive crisis, nitroglycerin is initiated at a rate of 5 mcg/minute by continuous intravenous infusion. The dose may be titrated in increments of 5 mcg/minute every 3–5 minutes to an infusion rate of 20 mcg/minute. If blood pressure response is inadequate to this infusion rate, the dose may be increased by 10 mcg/minute every 3–5 minutes, up to a maximum rate of 200 mcg/minute (Table 37.2). If a weight-based dosing algorithm is used, the usual starting dose is 0.2 mcg/kg/minute. The dose may be increased in increments of 0.2–0.5 mcg/kg/minute every 3–5 minutes to a maximum dose of 2 mcg/kg/minute. Onset of action of nitroglycerin is within 2–5 minutes, and the duration of action is 5–10 minutes, with a half-life of 1–3 minutes.[11] Tolerance of the hemodynamic effects of nitroglycerin limits its clinical utility.[37] Headache is the most common adverse effect, and methemoglobinemia is a rare complication of prolonged infusions.[2] It can also cause hypotension and reflex tachycardia. Administration of low-dose nitroglycerin (approximately equal to 60 mcg/minute) as an adjunct to other intravenous antihypertensive agents may be useful for patients with hypertensive emergencies associated with acute coronary syndromes or acute pulmonary embolism.[38]

Hydralazine

Hydralazine is a peripheral, direct-acting vasodilator that relaxes arteriolar smooth muscle by inhibiting calcium ion release from the sarcoplasmic reticulum. The specific mechanism of action is not well understood, but proposed mechanisms include inhibition of calcium release caused by inositol trisphosphate and reducing calcium turnover.[39] There is also a potential for direct myocardial effect from increased influx of calcium into the sarcolemma that may be a result of the stimulation of β-adrenergic receptors.[40] Other proposed mechanisms of action include membrane hyperpolarization and inhibition of oxidase formation.[41] The arteriodilation reduces cardiac afterload and may improve cardiac function in patients with heart failure.

The initial dose of hydralazine is a 10-mg bolus by slow intravenous administration every 4–6 hours as needed to attain target blood pressure (Table 37.2). Repeated bolus doses generally should not exceed 20 mg, although they may be increased to 40 mg. Blood pressure begins to decrease within 10–30 minutes, and the fall can last from 2–4 hours.[11] Hydralazine may also be given intramuscularly, which may be advantageous in patients with poor vasculature making it difficult to obtain intravenous access. The onset of action post-intravenous administration is 10–20 minutes, and its duration of action of 1–4 hours. After intramuscular or intravenous administration, a latency period of 5–15 minutes is followed by a progressive and often precipitous fall in blood pressure that can last up to 12 hours post-administration. Although the circulating half-life of the drug is only about 3 hours, the context-sensitive half-life of activity on blood pressure is about 100 hours.[42] Although the mechanism behind this finding is unclear, it may be a result of active metabolites, arteriolar endothelial tissue binding, or a prolonged effect on endothelium-derived relaxing factor. Because of its prolonged and unpredictable antihypertensive effects and its inability to be titrated efficiently, hydralazine is best avoided in the management of hypertensive crises and is not usually considered a first-line agent for the management of hypertensive crisis.

Adrenergic-Receptor Antagonists

Esmolol

Esmolol is a cardioselective $β_1$-adrenergic antagonist with a rapid onset of action and a short duration of action. It is a negative inotrope and chronotrope. Because it is a $β_1$-cardioselective drug, it pairs well with a direct-acting α-adrenergic vasodilator such as phentolamine because esmolol possesses no direct vasodilatory actions. A loading dose of esmolol can be given as a 0.5- to 1-mg/kg loading dose over 1 minute, followed by initiation of an infusion at 50 mcg/kg/minute (Table 37.2). The bolus dose can be repeated. The infusion can be titrated in 25- to 50-mcg/kg/minute increments as needed to a maximum of 300 mcg/kg/minute.[43] The onset of action is about 1 minute with a terminal half-life of 9 minutes and a duration of action of 10–20 minutes. The drug is rapidly metabolized by erythrocyte esterases; thus, concomitant anemia may prolong the duration of effect.[16,43,44]

One significant indication for esmolol is to attenuate the sympathetic discharge seen with severe postoperative hypertension, given that cardiac output, heart rate, and blood pressure are increased.[45] Esmolol is also safe in the setting of myocardial ischemia.[46] Patients should be closely monitored for bradycardia, which may occur more often in older adults. If bradycardia occurs, the infusion should be discontinued, and the effects of esmolol on heart rate are eliminated within 20 minutes. Esmolol reduces cardiac index and may worsen or exacerbate the symptoms of patients with acute heart failure. Patients with reactive airway disease should be monitored for exacerbation, though several studies have shown that esmolol, being a cardioselective drug, is well tolerated in patients with pulmonary disease.[47] Contraindications to esmolol use include concurrent β-blocker therapy, bradycardia, and acute decompensated heart failure. Accidental overdoses of esmolol caused by dilution errors have been reported, which have resulted in fatalities attributed to bolus doses of 625–2500 mg (12.5–50 mg/kg). Premixed injection solutions are available and may help mitigate such dosage errors.

Labetalol

Labetalol is a combined $α_1$- and nonselective β-adrenergic receptor antagonist. Pharmacodynamically, its action is primarily mediated by β-blockade, with an α- to β-receptor activity ratio of 1:7 when given intravenously.[15] Unlike cardioselective β-blockers, which decrease cardiac output, labetalol maintains cardiac output because $α_1$-blockade minimizes the reductions in cardiac output seen with β-blockade alone. It also reduces peripheral vascular resistance without diminishing peripheral blood flow, thereby maintaining cerebral, renal, and coronary blood flow. Given that labetalol has little effect on cerebral circulation, it is not associated with increased ICP. Because it is a nonselective β-blocker, labetalol should be used with caution in patients with reactive airway disease or chronic obstructive pulmonary disease. It may exacerbate or precipitate acute decompensated heart failure and should not be used in patients with second- or third-degree atrioventricular block or bradycardia.[48]

Labetalol can be given as an intravenous bolus, with incrementally larger doses should repeat dosing be required, until the desired hemodynamic state is achieved. The patient is less likely to respond if no response is observed after a cumulative dose of 300 mg is given (Table 37.2). An intravenous loading dose of labetalol 10–20 mg typically precedes either an infusion or ongoing bolus doses of labetalol. As a single bolus dose, labetalol has an onset of action of 2–5 minutes, with a duration of action of 2–4 minutes.[16] Incremental bolus doses of 20–80 mg every 10 minutes can be continued until the target blood pressure is attained. Labetalol may also be administered as a continuous intravenous infusion initiated at 0.5–1 mg/minute, adjusted by 0.5–1 mg/minute every 30 minutes until the target blood pressure is attained. Intravenous bolus doses of 1–2 mg/kg have resulted in clinically significant decreases in blood pressure; these should therefore be avoided, if possible. The duration of effect with repeated sequential bolus doses or infusions is 2–4 hours, with an elimination half-life of 5.5 hours.

Phentolamine

Phentolamine is a competitive antagonist of peripheral α_1- and α_2-receptors and antagonizes the effects of epinephrine and norepinephrine at these receptors, resulting in vasodilation. Furthermore, it has positive inotropic and chronotropic effects on the heart as a result of its α_2-blockade. It is generally used to treat hypertensive emergencies induced by catecholamine excess. Examples of such disorders include pheochromocytoma, interactions between monoamine oxidase inhibitors and other drugs or food, cocaine toxicity, amphetamine overdose, and clonidine withdrawal.[11,49] Phentolamine is initiated as an intravenous bolus dose of 5–15 mg (Table 37.2). Its onset of action is 1–2 minutes, with a duration or action of 10–30 minutes. It should be used with caution in those with coronary artery disease because it can potentiate angina symptoms or myocardial infarction. Tachycardia, flushing, and headache are also commonly occurring adverse effects. The compensatory tachycardia can be ameliorated by administering an intravenous β-blocker.[2]

Fenoldopam

Fenoldopam is a dopamine type 1 receptor agonist in the periphery with no activity on dopamine type 2 receptors.[50] It is 10 times more potent at renal dopamine type 1 receptors than dopamine. Agonism of postsynaptic dopamine type 1 receptors results in vasodilation of peripheral arteries as well as the renal and mesenteric vasculature.

Fenoldopam is typically initiated as a continuous intravenous infusion with a starting rate of 0.1–0.3 mcg/kg/minute. The infusion rate may be titrated in increments of 0.05–0.1 mcg/kg/minute every 15 minutes until the target hemodynamics are achieved, to a maximal infusion rate of 1.6 mcg/kg/minute (Table 37.2).[11] Data are limited regarding the use of fenoldopam in patients older than 65 years. Fenoldopam should be initiated cautiously in the older adult, usually starting at the low end of the dosing range. The onset of action is less than 5 minutes with a half-life of 9.8 minutes.[2,15,50] Adverse effects associated with fenoldopam include headache, flushing, tachycardia, and dizziness. A dose-related increase in intraocular pressure is also possible; thus, fenoldopam should be administered with caution in patients with narrow-angle glaucoma. The drug formulation contains sodium metabisulfate, which should be avoided in patients with an allergy to sulfites.[50]

The overall effect of this vasodilation is a lowering of blood pressure and total peripheral resistance while preserving renal blood flow. Fenoldopam has been shown to improve creatinine clearance, urine flow rates, and sodium excretion in patients with severe hypertension with both normal and impaired renal function. The effects of fenoldopam on renal function were assessed in a meta-analysis involving patients from 16 randomized controlled trials. Authors evaluated the renal-protective properties of fenoldopam in a variety of settings. Fenoldopam was associated with a lower risk of the need for renal replacement and in-hospital death.[51]

SPECIAL CONSIDERATIONS

Hypertension in Pregnancy

Hypertension, although common in the general population, is also a complication in 10% of pregnancies worldwide. Although the etiologies of hypertension are multifactorial, the American College of Obstetricians and Gynecologists has streamlined hypertension during pregnancy to four categories: (1) preeclampsia-eclampsia, (2) chronic hypertension, (3) chronic hypertension with superimposed preeclampsia, and (4) gestational hypertension.[52] Of these, preeclampsia is the most commonly seen etiology of hypertension in pregnancy and is most often associated with hypertensive emergency. Preeclampsia typically develops after 20 weeks of gestation and may manifest through the postpartum period. Diagnostic criteria for preeclampsia include elevated blood pressure of 140/90 mm Hg or greater (on two separate occasions) or confirmed persistent blood pressure of 160/110 mm Hg or greater, and concomitant proteinuria or any of thrombocytopenia, renal insufficiency, impaired liver function, pulmonary edema, or cerebral/visual symptoms (Table 37.3). Hypertensive urgency in the pregnant patient is defined as an SBP of 180 mm Hg or greater and/or a DBP of 120 mm Hg or greater without progressive end-organ damage. Hypertensive emergency in the pregnant patient is defined as persistent (15 minutes or more) hypertension (SBP of 160 mm Hg or greater and/or DBP of 110 mm Hg or greater) in a pregnant or postpartum patient with preeclampsia or eclampsia. Blood pressure criteria for hypertensive emergency are set at lower levels because peripartum patients may develop complications of hypertensive crisis, such as myocardial infarction, stroke, hypertensive encephalopathy, and pulmonary edema, at lower levels of hypertension compared with the general population.[53,54]

For pregnant patients presenting with hypertensive crisis, initial clinical goals of patient stabilization and prevention of end-organ damage remain at the forefront, but

Table 37.3 Special Considerations for Hypertensive Crisis Management

Population	Hypertensive Crisis Criteria	Blood Pressure Goal	Medication Considerations
Aortic dissection	Pathological finding on imaging. No specific diagnostic criteria related to hemodynamics	HR < 60 beats/min, SBP < 120 mm Hg. DBP reduction by 10%–15% or < 110 mm Hg. Prefer to achieve within 5–20 min	Preferred initial agent: esmolol
Acute coronary syndromes	None specified outside general population	None specified outside general population	Preferred agent: nitroglycerin. Alternatives: IV β-blockers but may cause shock in patients > 70 years, HR. Avoid sodium nitroprusside, enalaprilat
Pheochromocytoma	None specified outside general population	None specified outside general population	Use α-adrenoceptor blocking agents (phentolamine). Adjunctive β-adrenoceptor blockers and calcium channel antagonists may be used
Pregnancy	Persistent hypertension (SBP ≥ 160 mm Hg and/or DBP ≥ 110 mm Hg) in a pregnant or postpartum patient with eclampsia or preeclampsia	Reduction in MAP of 15%–25% -and/or- Goal SBP 140–150 mm Hg. Goal DBP 90–100 mm Hg	Fast-acting and titratable agents allow for closer control. Avoid esmolol unless necessary because it crosses placenta. Avoid enalaprilat (contraindicated in second/third trimester of pregnancy)
Intracranial hemorrhage	SBP > 200 mm Hg or DBP > 150 mm Hg OR SBP > 150 mm Hg or MAP > 130 mm Hg with possibility of increased ICP	Guideline recommendation: "Aggressive reduction of blood pressure with frequent monitoring" -Consider goal SBP < 180 mm Hg. "Acute lowering of SBP to 140 is probably safe" -Current data do support a goal SBP < 140 mm Hg in ICH	Common first-line intermittent therapy: labetalol, hydralazine. Common first-line CI: nicardipine/clevidipine, labetalol
Ischemic stroke	SBP > 220 mm Hg or DBP > 120 mm Hg	Reduction in SBP recommended. Initial lowering of SBP by 15% and follow neurologic status. SBP lowering < 120 mm Hg may be associated with poor outcome	In patients post-thrombolysis with tPA: Goal SBP < 180 mm Hg & DBP < 120 mm Hg. Labetalol (bolus & CI) and nicardipine typical first-line agents for BP lowering

Table 37.3 Special Considerations for Hypertensive Crisis Management *(continued)*

Population	Hypertensive Crisis Criteria	Blood Pressure Goal	Medication Considerations
Subarachnoid hemorrhage	Unsecured aneurysm, SBP > 160 mm Hg (associated with higher rebleed rate)	SBP < 160 mm Hg	Labetalol, nicardipine, clevidipine typical first-line agents
		Optimal magnitude of BP decrease not established	CI nicardipine may achieve BP goal faster than bolus labetalol dosing
Postoperative hypertension	Lack of consensus	Lack of consensus	Labetalol, nicardipine, clevidipine, sodium nitroprusside, nitroglycerin are typical first-line agents
	SBP ≥ 180–200 mm Hg (≥ 140 mm Hg in neurosurgical patients)	Cardiac surgery: BP > 140/90 mm Hg or a	
	DBP ≥ 110 mm Hg (≥ 95 mm Hg in neurosurgical patients)	MAP of at least 105 mm Hg	Avoid hydralazine, enalaprilat if possible
	MAP ≥ 20% from baseline		
	Cardiac surgery: BP > 140/90 mm Hg or a		Addressing reversible causes: pain, anxiety, hypothermia
	MAP of at least 105 mm Hg		
Acute pulmonary embolism	Lack of consensus	SBP ≥ 160 mm Hg	Nitroglycerin if evidence of acute severe pulmonary congestion
	SBP ≥ 160 mm Hg		
	MAP ≥ 120 mm Hg		

CI = continuous infusion; HR = heart rate; ICP = intracranial pressure; tPA = tissue plasminogen activator.

in addition, preservation of adequate uteroplacental perfusion must be considered. For patients with hypertensive urgency, blood pressure should be lowered slowly over 24–48 hours, and oral antihypertensive agents are typically used. For patients with hypertensive emergency, immediate blood pressure intervention should be made, with goals of reducing MAP by 15%–25% and/or a goal SBP range of 140–150 mm Hg and a DBP range of 90–100 mm Hg. In addition to antihypertensive medications, other interventions may be considered such as administration of magnesium for associated eclampsia, support of end-organ dysfunction, and consideration of fetal delivery. A recent Cochrane review showed no preferred agent for the treatment of hypertensive emergency in pregnancy, though—as with all hypertensive crisis treatment options—intravenous agents that are short acting and titratable are preferred.[55]

Commonly used agents include intravenous hydralazine and labetalol as first-line options with safety evidence established in pregnant patients, though limited comparative data exist. Nicardipine may also be used in pregnant patients, with a recent meta-analysis showing increased success of blood pressure control in patients receiving nicardipine compared with labetalol, with a more favorable fetal adverse event profile warranting further investigation.[56] Sodium nitroprusside may be considered as a last-line agent, though accumulation of cyanide or thiocyanate limits its use. Enalaprilat should be avoided because ACEI agents and angiotensin receptor blocking agents are contraindicated in the second and third trimesters of pregnancy. Esmolol should be avoided unless necessary by another compelling indication (such as aortic dissection) because it crosses the placenta and is associated with fetal bradycardia and persistent β-blockade (Figure 37.1).[57]

Neurologic Injury

Intracerebral Hemorrhage

Elevated blood pressure is commonly seen in patients with hemorrhagic stroke. The newly published 2015 guidelines for the management of spontaneous intracerebral hemorrhage (ICH) from the American Heart Association/American Stroke Association (AHA/ASA) contain updated recommendations for blood pressure management. For patients with ICH having an SBP between 150 and 220 mm Hg, the guidelines now state that lowering the SBP to 140 mm Hg is safe and can be effective for improving functional outcome, provided there are no contraindications to acute blood pressure treatment. This is a stronger recommendation for an SBP goal of 140 mm Hg in ICU patients than the previous 2010 guideline. For patients with an SBP greater than 220 mm Hg, the guidelines state that it may be reasonable to consider aggressive reduction in blood pressure, but they do not provide a specific target or goal at this time (Table 37.3).[58] Much of this is based on data from the Intensive Blood Pressure Reduction in Acute Cerebral Hemorrhage Trial (INTERACT1) and the Antihypertensive Treatment in Acute Cerebral Hemorrhage (ATACH) and the second Intensive Blood Pressure Reduction in Acute Cerebral Hemorrhage Trial (INTERACT2) investigations.[59-61] The phase III ATACH II trial is currently enrolling patients to investigate early intensive compared with standard blood pressure control in patients with spontaneous ICH, which may help further guide care in these patients.[62] One area where specific blood pressure recommendations remain unclear from a guideline perspective is in patients with oral anticoagulant–associated ICH. Patients with oral anticoagulant–associated ICH present with challenges similar to those in patients with spontaneous ICH, but they also carry consideration for urgent reversal of anticoagulation. Oral anticoagulant therapy not only increases the risk of ICH in general but is also associated with an increased rate of hematoma enlargement.[63] A recent review of a large cohort of patients with oral anticoagulant–associated ICH shows decreased hematoma expansion in patients with an SBP less than 160 mm Hg within 4 hours after hospital admission.[64] There is no evidence assessing intensive treatment with an SBP goal of less than 140 mm Hg in the setting of oral anticoagulant–associated ICH, though this may be an appropriate goal for this population.

Currently, no specific medication agents are recommended as first-line agents from guideline recommendations (Figure 37.2). It is stated, however, that for patients with an SBP greater than 220 mm Hg, aggressive management of blood pressure reduction with a continuous intravenous infusion should be considered.[58] Despite no guideline-endorsed agents of choice, some data suggest certain optimal agents for blood pressure management in ICH. Typical first-line agents for intermittent administration include labetalol and hydralazine, with calcium channel antagonists, sodium nitroprusside, and labetalol as continuous infusion when required.[65] Many direct comparisons between agents are small and retrospective and suggest overall similar lowering of MAP and clinical outcomes in patients with labetalol versus nicardipine, with differences dependent on route of administration (i.e., intravenous vs. intermittent bolus) meriting further investigation.[66,67] The ongoing ATACH II trial will hopefully shed more light on characterizing nicardipine use in this population. Open-label, single-agent investigations using nicardipine and clevidipine show efficacy in maintaining blood pressure goals in patients with ICH and tolerable safety profiles.[68,69] Sodium nitroprusside has fallen out of favor because of its unfavorable adverse effect profile and the availability of newer agents, and, according to one large database review, it may be associated with higher mortality than nicardipine in patients with ICH.[69]

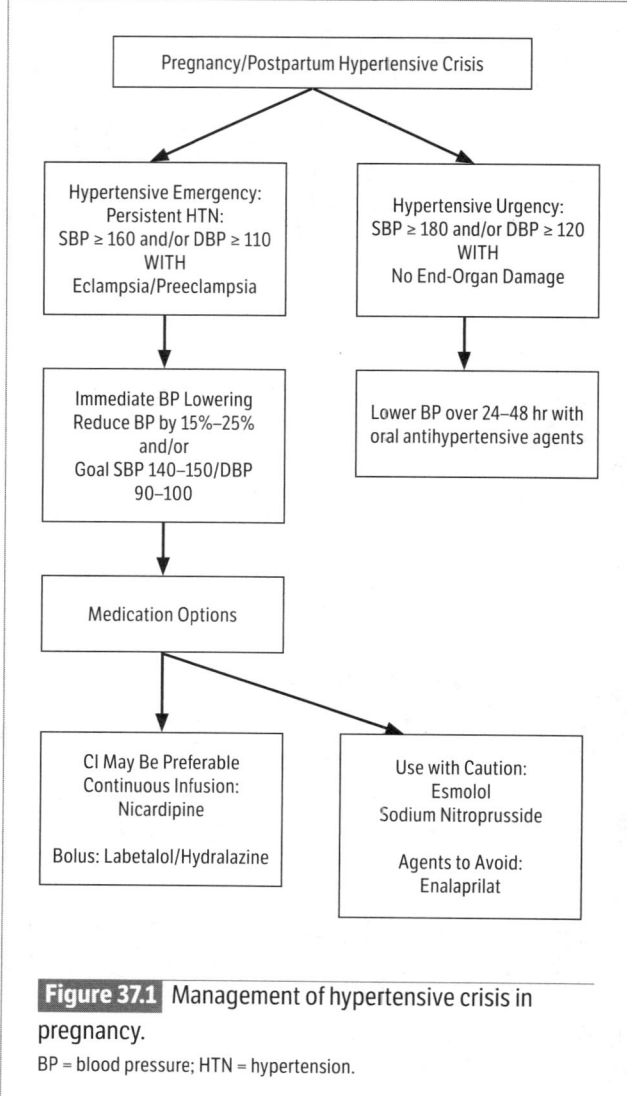

Figure 37.1 Management of hypertensive crisis in pregnancy.
BP = blood pressure; HTN = hypertension.

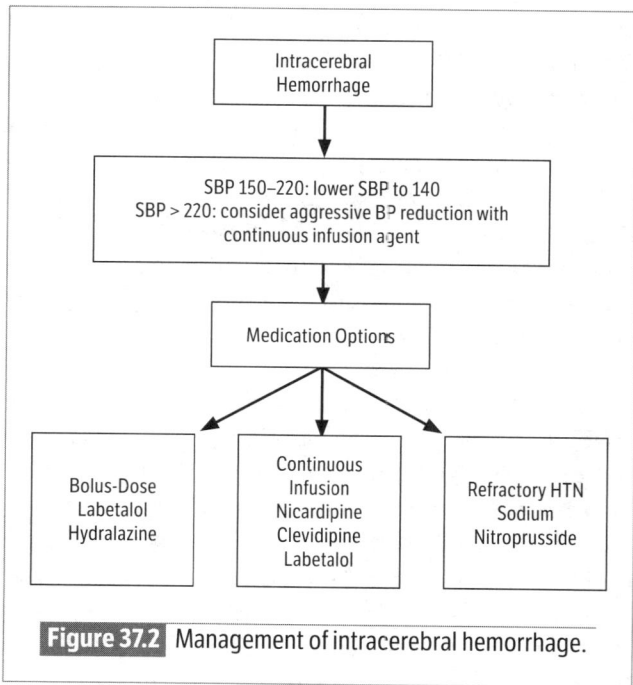

Figure 37.2 Management of intracerebral hemorrhage.

Ischemic Stroke

As in hemorrhagic stroke, elevated blood pressure may be observed in patients with ischemic stroke, which is often higher in those with preexisting hypertension, and management of extreme hypertension must be balanced with maintaining cerebral perfusion to vulnerable tissue. Although an absolute blood pressure target in the acute phase is as yet undefined, elevated blood pressure in patients with ischemic stroke has been associated with poorer outcomes. Observational data show a U-shaped relationship between blood pressure parameters and outcome measures, such as early neurologic deterioration, poor neurologic outcome, and mortality, with poor outcomes associated with extremes of both hypotension (120/70 mm Hg or less) and hypertension (200/110 mm Hg or greater).[70,71] The AHA/ASA Guidelines for the Early Management of Patients with Acute Ischemic Stroke recommend limited blood pressure intervention in the initial 24-hour period after ischemic stroke unless blood pressure is 220/120 mm Hg or greater or there is a concomitant indication for intervention such as myocardial infarction or aortic dissection. Although an absolute numerical target for blood pressure management of hypertension in acute ischemic stroke has yet to be defined, guideline-based treatment calls for an SBP reduction by 15% in concert with clinician judgment in patients with hypertension in early acute ischemic stroke.[72] The more recent China Antihypertensive Trial in Acute Ischemic Stroke (CATIS) found that acute blood pressure lowering by 10%–25% in patients with non-recombinant tissue plasminogen activator with SBP 140–220 mm Hg during the first 24 hours of acute ischemic stroke may be safe; however, further investigation is needed before early intervention for patients with a blood pressure of 220/110 mm Hg or less becomes part of routine management in the early phase of ischemic stroke (Table 37.3).[73]

One subset of patients with ischemic stroke with clearly defined blood pressure goals consists of patients eligible for antifibrinolytic therapy with recombinant tissue plasminogen activator.[72,74] Retrospective evaluations of recombinant tissue plasminogen activator in ischemic stroke use suggest that any protocol deviations with thrombolytic use, including blood pressure control, as well as hyperglycemia and baseline coagulation, are associated with an increased incidence of hemorrhage.[75-77] Blood pressure control in patients receiving recombinant tissue plasminogen activator should be monitored closely to ensure mitigation not only of hemorrhagic events, but also as a component of overall progress toward optimal outcomes.[78,79] For patients eligible for recombinant tissue plasminogen activator therapy, blood pressure should be maintained greater than 185/110 mm Hg before administration using medical therapy (labetalol, nicardipine) as needed. After administration of recombinant tissue plasminogen activator, blood pressure should be monitored frequently to maintain a goal of 180/105 mm Hg or greater for 24 hours.[72]

Although recommendations can be made for blood pressure thresholds for treatment of extreme hypertension in ischemic stroke and management of post–recombinant tissue plasminogen activator administration, evidence-based data recommending the specific agents of choice for initial management of hypertension are limited and littered with conflicting findings.[66,80,81] The BEST (Beta-Blocker Evaluation in Survival Trial) study found no benefit to administering atenolol or propranolol within 48 hours of ischemic stroke; however, labetalol is often used as a first-choice agent for treatment of hypertension in the ischemic stroke population.[65,82] In INWEST (Intravenous Nimodipine West European Stroke Trial), subjects receiving intravenous nimodipine had poorer outcomes, though whether this was related to specific properties of nimodipine itself or the pronounced effect seen in DBP is unclear.[80] Retrospective evaluations of the use of continuous infusion nicardipine, another calcium channel antagonist, support its use as an alternative to other antihypertensive agents such as labetalol without evidence of drug class–mediated deleterious effects, though prospective data in ischemic stroke are needed. The pharmacodynamic profile of the only intravenous ACEI, enalaprilat, limits the use of this class of agents in acute hypertension in ischemic stroke.[73,83] Although no specific agents are specified in the AHA/ASA Guidelines

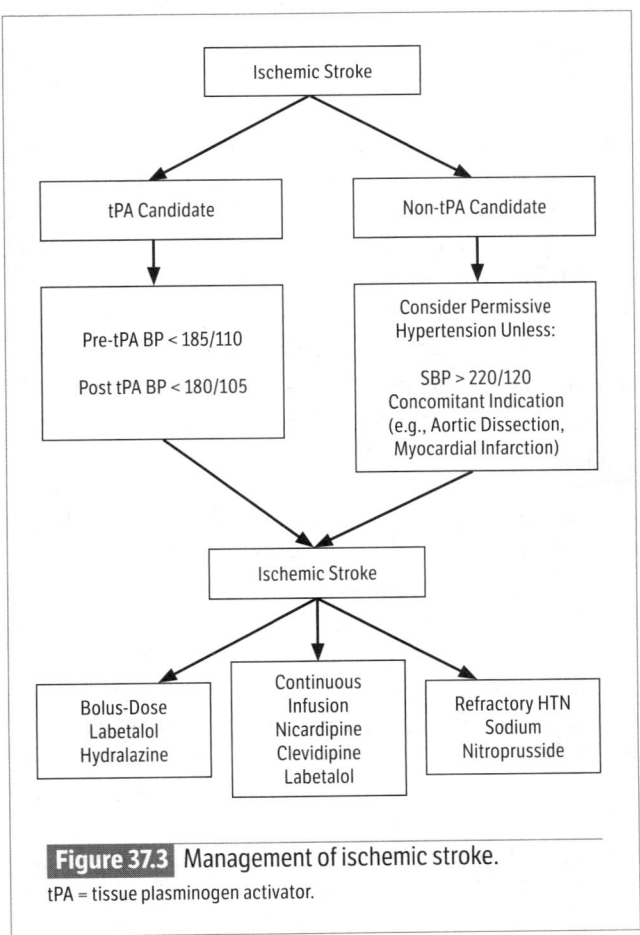

Figure 37.3 Management of ischemic stroke.
tPA = tissue plasminogen activator.

for the Early Management of Patients with Acute Ischemic Stroke, a general approach to management of hypertension is described, based largely on clinical opinion and agents used in recombinant tissue plasminogen activator investigations. Labetalol is recommended as the first-line agent of choice for intermittent bolus administration together with nicardipine for continuous infusion. Although not specified in the 2013 guidelines, clevidipine may be considered according to institutional availability and preference. The guidelines do mention consideration of other agents such as hydralazine and enalaprilat when clinically appropriate and consideration of sodium nitroprusside in patients with uncontrolled hypertension with the agents previously mentioned or a DBP greater than 140 mm Hg (Figure 37.3).[72]

Subarachnoid Hemorrhage

Patients presenting with aneurysmal subarachnoid hemorrhage (aSAH) may have a variety of blood pressure management needs throughout their treatment process because altered autoregulation, concern for rebleeding events, and delayed neurologic defects are just a few processes in aSAH that may be affected by blood pressure alterations. Rebleeding in aneurysm rupture is associated with increased mortality and morbidity, with peak rebleeding seen within the first 24 hours after aneurysm rupture, often within the first 6–12 hours.[84,85] Early surgical or endovascular intervention has helped attenuate the incidence of in-hospital rebleeding in aSAH; however, rebleeding may occur, and due consideration should be given to management of hypertension before aneurysm obliteration. Systolic blood pressures greater than 160 mm Hg and MAPs less than 70 mm Hg or greater than 130 mm Hg have been associated with rebleeding and poor outcome in aSAH (Table 37.3).[86,87] The AHA/ASA Guidelines for the Management of Aneurysmal Subarachnoid Hemorrhage recommend that acute hypertension be controlled, particularly before definitive aneurysmal intervention, with a recommendation that "a decrease in systolic blood pressure to less than 160 mm Hg is reasonable."[88] There are no specified blood pressure parameter recommendations post-intervention within the guideline, but close attention should be paid to blood pressure monitoring after intervention.

Although there is some evidence specific to the aSAH population regarding antihypertensive selection, the AHA/ASA guidelines make no specific endorsements for particular agents. One retrospective investigation shows efficiency in achieving blood pressure goals with improved time within goal MAP, decreased needs for additional antihypertensive agents, and number of treatment failures with continuous infusion nicardipine similar to that with bolus-dose labetalol.[89] It has also been shown that continuous infusion labetalol versus continuous infusion nicardipine has similar maintenance of blood pressure goals in patients with aSAH and ICH, though with a faster time to goal MAP with nicardipine.[67] A prospective evaluation of nicardipine and sodium nitroprusside infusions for acute blood pressure control has been done in patients with aSAH and ICH. Overall blood pressure control was similar between both treatment groups, with similar time spent within target blood pressure range but with overall fewer adjustments to infusion doses and requirements of additional as-needed medication in patients receiving nicardipine.[90] An open-label pilot study of five patients also suggests that clevidipine can successfully be used for acute blood pressure management in aSAH, though larger investigations are warranted.[91] Although firm recommendations regarding antihypertensive agent selection cannot be made at this time, institutional blood pressure goals and medication availability should be considered. Given the risk of early rebleeding and the recommended SBP goals of 160 mm Hg or less, continuous infusion preparations may yield less blood pressure variability, which may correlate with improved overall patient outcomes, though there is scant evidence at best to support this at this time (Figure 37.4).

Postoperative Hypertension

Hypertension is a common occurrence in postoperative patients, and though commonly seen, no specific criteria exist for diagnosis. Acute postoperative hypertension (APH) typically has an early onset, within 2 hours after surgery, and typically abates within 6 hours or less, though may persist beyond that period. Factors predisposing patients include preoperative conditions such as hypertension, diabetes mellitus, and renal disease; postoperative

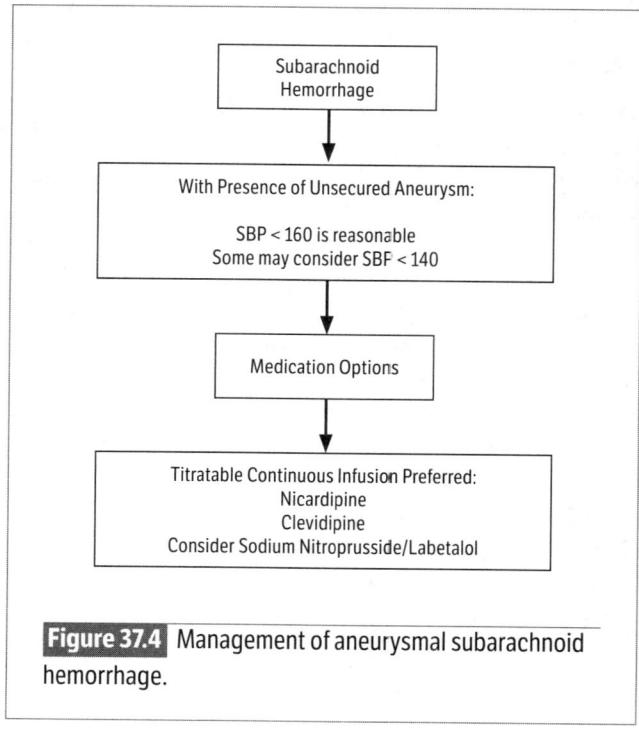

Figure 37.4 Management of aneurysmal subarachnoid hemorrhage.

factors such as pain, anxiety, and emergence from anesthesia; and intraoperative factors such as type of surgery performed, duration of procedure, and anesthetic agents used. Although many factors play a role in APH, preoperative hypertension is highly associated with the development of postoperative hypertension and should be considered in the perioperative workup.[92-94] Although several risk factors exist for APH, activation of the sympathetic nervous system with elevation of plasma catecholamines appears to be higher in patients with APH. It does not appear that the RAAS plays a significant role in the development of postoperative hypertension, at least in the cardiac surgery population, though data suggest that the RAAS does play a role in other patient populations.[95-97] Although the full pathophysiology of APH has yet to be fully described, interventions should be made to prevent serious sequelae such as hemorrhagic stroke or cerebral ischemia, cardiovascular complications, pulmonary edema, or complications related to surgical site and bleeding.

At this time, there is a lack of consensus regarding both the definition of APH and the optimal treatment goals for patients with non-cardiac surgery. Definitions for APH in non-cardiac surgery as defined by clinical investigations range from blood pressure measurements of SBP of 180–200 mm Hg or greater (140 mm Hg or greater in neurosurgical postoperative investigations), DBP of 110 mm Hg or greater (95 mm Hg or greater in neurosurgical postoperative investigations), MAP of 20% or greater of baseline value, or some combination thereof (Table 37.3).[98-100] Treatment interventions should include mitigation of causes of APH such as hypothermia and shivering, optimization of ventilatory parameters, adequate analgesia and sedation as needed, management of volume status, and other reversible causes. Once these are optimized, antihypertensive medication can be considered for treatment of APH with goal blood pressure lowering at surgeon/anesthesiologist discretion in non-cardiac surgery. Because most APH is transient, short-acting agents, such as labetalol, as well as agents that are easily titratable, such as nicardipine, clevidipine, and sodium nitroprusside, can be considered. Agents with less uniform responses to therapy or with long durations of action, such as hydralazine and enalaprilat, are not routinely recommended for use in APH and should be used with caution, if at all.

A few key studies have compared various intravenous agents for the management of APH. One multicenter, prospective, randomized study that sought to compare the safety and efficacy of nicardipine with that of sodium nitroprusside in both cardiac and non-cardiac surgical patients found that both agents were equally effective.[101] Patients receiving nicardipine appeared to have more rapid control of APH. Furthermore, the total number of dose titrations to achieve target blood pressure was fewer in the group receiving nicardipine. No difference occurred in rates of adverse events. In a randomized, double-blind, placebo-controlled trial completed by investigators in the ESCAPE-2 (Endovascular Treatment for Small Core and Proximal Occlusion Ischemic Stroke) trial, researchers sought to determine the safety and efficacy of clevidipine in treating APH after cardiac surgery. Clevidipine was associated with lower rates of treatment failure than placebo with no difference of adverse events.

The ECLIPSE (Evaluation of Clevidipine in the Perioperative Treatment of Hypertension Assessing Safety Events) trial compared the efficacy of clevidipine with that of sodium nitroprusside, nitroglycerin, and nicardipine for the management of acute hypertension post–cardiac surgery. This study was a multicenter, prospective, open-label, randomized, parallel comparison study. The primary end point of this trial was a composite end point of safety assessed by the incidence of all-cause mortality, stroke, myocardial infarction, and renal dysfunction. Mortality was significantly higher in the treatment group receiving sodium nitroprusside versus clevidipine. Clevidipine was also more effective than nitroglycerin or sodium nitroprusside in maintaining blood pressure within target ranges. There was no difference in efficacy between clevidipine and nicardipine unless the target blood pressure range was narrowed (Figure 37.5).[102]

Pheochromocytoma

Pheochromocytomas are catecholamine-producing tumors arising from the chromaffin cells of the adrenal gland, though 10%–15% of tumors may be extra-adrenal. Although the prevalence in patients with hypertension is only 0.2%–0.4%, pheochromocytoma is often on the differential diagnosis for patients with acute, otherwise unexplained hypertensive crisis. Of note, patients with pheochromocytoma may also be normotensive or only moderately hypertensive (Table 37.3). About one-fourth of pheochromocytomas are hereditary, and typical symptoms such as headache, sweating, and palpitation are caused by tumor-secreted catecholamines. In most cases, catecholamines are released intermittently, typically both epinephrine and norepinephrine with a predominance of norepinephrine. For patients with pheochromocytoma with hypertensive crisis, management with an α-receptor antagonist such as phentolamine is the recommended initial treatment. After initiation of α-receptor blockade, β-receptor antagonists, such as esmolol, may be required for additional mediation of epinephrine-mediated effects or tachycardia induced by α-receptor antagonism. Surgical resection is often used for definitive treatment of patients with pheochromocytoma, though around 10% of cases are malignant, requiring additional interventions with chemotherapy and radiation. Preoperative initiation of α-blockade with phenoxybenzamine is recommended with the addition of β-receptor antagonists as needed. There is some evidence using calcium channel antagonists in the preoperative period, but data regarding use in pheochromocytoma-induced hypertensive crisis are scarce. Clinical judgment on a case-by-case basis is recommended in patients with pheochromocytoma with hypertensive crisis not responding adequately to α- and β-receptor antagonism.[103,104]

Aortic Dissection

Aortic dissection, although present in only 2% of patients presenting with hypertensive crisis, is rapidly fatal and can be considered a surgical emergency.[4] Elevated blood pressures in conjunction with atherosclerosis within the aorta can result in tears within the intimal layer of the blood vessel. These tears permit the development of a false lumen within the wall of the aorta. As blood is ejected from the left ventricle and into the aorta, the resulting high pulsatile pressure separates the aortic wall into two layers. Therefore, clinically, patients with dissection present with symptoms of retrosternal or interscapular chest pain that radiates down the back. Dissection can result in impeded blood flow to branches of blood vessels from the aorta, leading to end-organ ischemia. Diagnosis is usually confirmed by transesophageal echocardiography, CT (computed tomography), or MRI (magnetic resonance imaging).

There are three major classification systems for aortic dissection (Table 37.4). The Stanford system is the most classically used by surgeons because it is a simple guide to determine whether the patient is a surgical emergency. A type A dissection according to the Stanford system would likely be considered a surgical emergency. These patients may present with symptoms associated with malperfusion of the brain and coronary arteries. Conversely, type B dissections may present with symptoms of malperfusion of the spinal cord, liver, small intestines, kidneys, or lower extremities. Several different patient-specific features have been seen among patients presenting with dissection. Disease states such as hypertension, hyperlipidemia, diabetes, and Marfan syndrome have been associated with increasing risk. Furthermore, pregnancy, cocaine abuse, a history of cardiac surgery, or the presence of a bicuspid aortic valve may also be associated with dissection.[105]

To avoid propagation of intimal dissection, patients presenting with aortic dissection require immediate intravenous antihypertensive treatment as soon dissection is suspected.[15] An exception to this would be a subset of patients who may present as hypotensive as a result of their dissection. Progression of the dissection depends on the degree of blood pressure elevation as well as the velocity of left ventricular ejection. For this reason, therapeutic interventions aimed at both heart rate and blood pressure are used for these cases. Emergency intervention usually involves rapid intravenous administration of β-blocking agents such as esmolol in an attempt to reduce heart rate to less than 60 beats/minute.[43] Vasodilating agents such as nicardipine or sodium nitroprusside may be added to β-blocking agents to achieve an

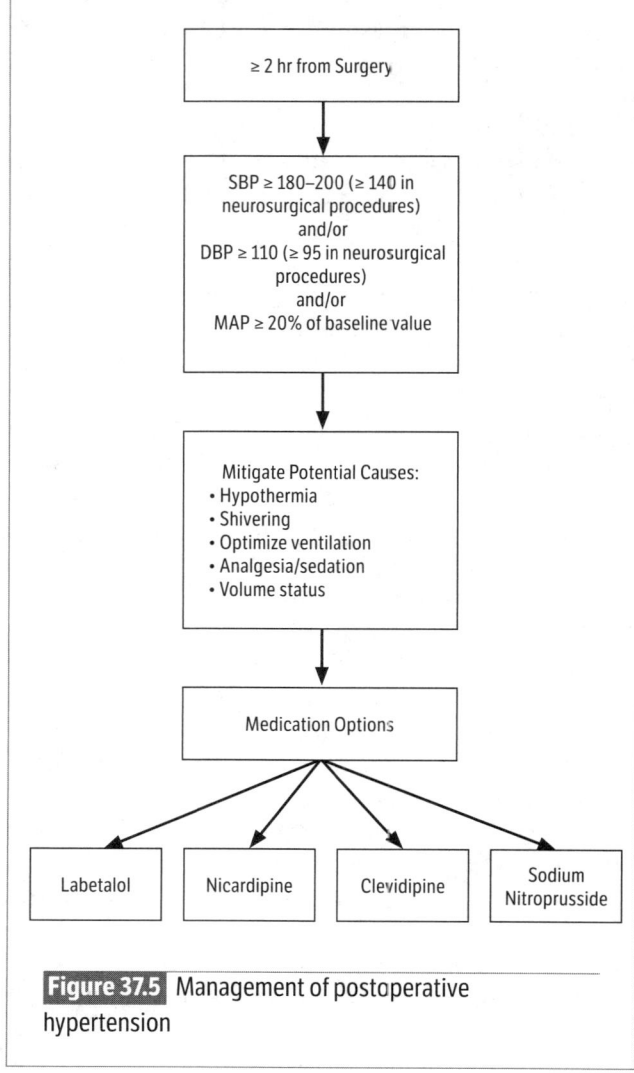

Figure 37.5 Management of postoperative hypertension

Table 37.4 Classification Systems of Aortic Dissection

Stanford
- Type A: ascending aorta affected
- Type B: ascending aorta not affected

De Bakey
- Type 1: entire aorta affected
- Type 2: ascending aorta affected
- Type 3: descending aorta affected

Svensson
- Class 1: classic dissection with true and false lumen
- Class 2: intramural hematoma or hemorrhage
- Class 3: subtle dissection without hematoma
- Class 4: atherosclerotic penetrating ulcer
- Class 5: iatrogenic or traumatic dissection

SBP less than 120 mm Hg. The DBP should be reduced by 10%–15%, or at least to less than 110 mm Hg. These interventions and targets are ideally obtained within 20 minutes (ideally within 5–10 minutes) of presentation to the health care setting.[106] Although esmolol is not FDA approved for hypertensive crisis with aortic dissection, it has been used to treat hypertension associated with acute aortic dissection (Figure 37.6). In sequence of administration, β-blocking agent administration should precede the initiation of any antihypertensive agent that may cause reflexive tachycardia or position inotropy to avoid exacerbating the dissection. These hemodynamic end points should be maintained as long as the patient remains symptomatically stable or until the patient can be taken to the operating room for more definitive management of the dissection.[107]

Acute Coronary Syndromes

Hypertensive crisis can negatively affect both the structure and the function of the left ventricle as well as coronary circulation. The RAAS is activated, resulting in systemic vasoconstriction and increased myocardial oxygen demand and subsequent left ventricular hypertrophy. Coronary blood flow is negatively affected by both this hypertrophy and the endothelial destruction within the capillaries as a result of acute rises in blood pressure. Therefore, patients with hypertensive crisis can present with acute coronary syndromes (Table 37.3).

In patients with coronary artery disease presenting with an acute coronary syndrome, the theoretical "coronary steal" (i.e., redistribution of oxygenated blood away from non-vasodilating areas of ischemia toward nonischemic myocardium with dilated coronary arteries) results in reduced coronary perfusion pressure to further exacerbate and potentiate injury.[108] A study by Mann and colleagues examined the effects of sodium nitroprusside on regional myocardial blood flow in patients with coronary artery disease. These investigators found that sodium nitroprusside significantly reduced regional myocardial specific blood flow and increased coronary artery vascular resistance. This effect was seen regardless of the presence of collateralization.[109] Therefore, sodium nitroprusside should not routinely be administered to patients with hypertensive emergency in the setting of acute coronary syndromes because it has been associated with increased mortality. This was especially prominent when it was administered within 9 hours of onset of chest pain in patients with acute coronary syndrome and elevated left ventricular filling pressure.

Nitroglycerin decreases preload and myocardial oxygen consumption by decreasing left ventricular end-diastolic volume and myocardial wall tension, making it the preferred agent in the setting of hypertensive crisis complicated by myocardial ischemia.[2] However, before the administration of any nitrate medication, the medical team should determine whether the patient has been taking a phosphodiesterase type 5 (PDE-5) inhibitor because the combination can cause profound hypotension for up to 48 hours after the last dose of a PDE-5 inhibitor. In one study, standing SBP fell below 85 mm Hg in more patients receiving tadalafil than in placebo (p<0.05), with no difference in the response to sublingual nitroglycerin. Within 48 hours after the last dose of a PDE-5 inhibitor, ischemic chest pain can be treated with β-blockers, calcium channel blockers, morphine, oxygen, and aspirin while avoiding nitrates.[110]

Intravenous β-blocking agents are also an option for these patients. A meta-analysis of patients receiving β-blockers post–acute coronary syndrome found a 14% risk reduction in mortality through 7 days and a 23% reduction in long-term mortality. In-hospital β-blocker administration can reduce myocardial infarct size and rates of mortality, postinfarction ischemia, and nonfatal acute myocardial infarction.[111] These agents may also be beneficial for non–ST-segment elevation myocardial infarction. The Clopidogrel and Metoprolol in Myocardial Infarction Trial (COMMIT) study randomized patients to receive early treatment with intravenous metoprolol or placebo after acute myocardial infarction. Investigators found that although early intravenous metoprolol in this setting reduced the risks of reinfarction and ventricular fibrillation, it increased the risk of cardiogenic shock.[112] This finding was especially observed within the 24 hours after admission. Although oral β-blocker therapy is still recommended, the authors cautioned against initiating intravenous β-blocker therapy. Rather, the authors purported that intravenous β-blockage should only be initiated after the post–myocardial infarction hemodynamic status has stabilized.[111] Contraindications to β-blockers include moderate to severe left ventricular dysfunction with pulmonary

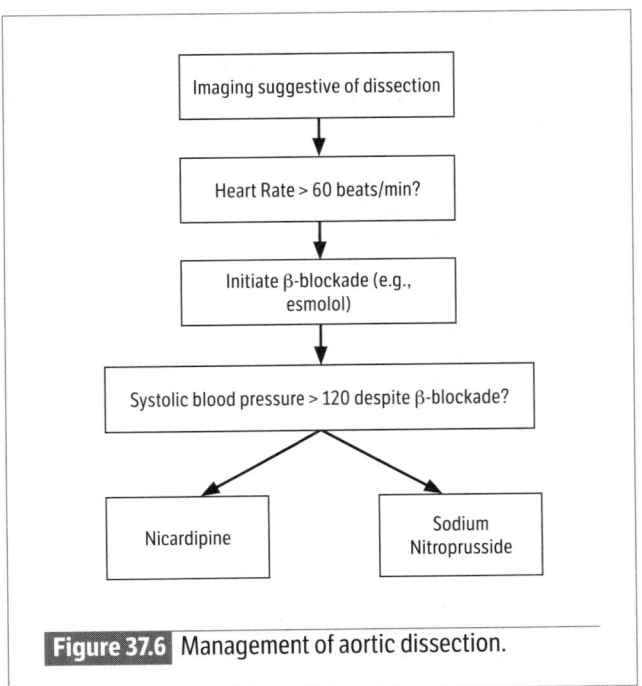

Figure 37.6 Management of aortic dissection.

edema, hypotension, second- or third-degree heart block, bradycardia, and reactive airways disease.[48]

Enalaprilat would appear to be an ideal agent in managing hypertensive crisis when a patient presents with acute coronary syndrome, given the activation of RAAS that is seen. However, the Cooperative New Scandinavian Enalapril Survival Study II (CONSENSUS II) showed a trend toward increased mortality when enalaprilat was administered within 24 hours of acute myocardial infarction. Of note, this observation may have occurred because of hypotension after drug administration. However, it may be considered a favorable option in patients with hypertensive emergency in the setting of left ventricular failure, given that ACEI agents are a key intervention in the management of heart failure (Figure 37.7).[113]

Cocaine Intoxication

Cocaine is an illicit drug derived from the leaves of the coca plant (*Erythroxylum coca*) and is predominantly found in the Andes mountain range of South America. Historically, natives of this region would chew the leaves of the coca plant to relieve fatigue. Cocaine was extracted and used for medicinal purposes as an ophthalmic anesthetic during eye surgery in the 1880s. Subsequently, cocaine was widely used in the United States. It was an ingredient in the recipe for the original Coca-Cola. Legislation to make cocaine and illegal substance dates back to the early 20th century; however, cocaine remains a common drug of abuse.

Cocaine has three distinct mechanisms of action. It is an indirect sympathomimetic that blocks the presynaptic reuptake of biogenic amines at adrenergic receptors. This mechanism has been seen in neurons containing serotonin, dopamine, norepinephrine, and epinephrine. Overall, this results in vasoconstriction in both cardiac and peripheral vasculature.[114,115] This sympathomimetic activity is also seen in its stimulation of α- and β-adrenergic receptors, resulting in increased myocardial demand and impaired perfusion. The euphoric properties of cocaine are a result of inhibition of serotonin reuptake in the central nervous system. Cocaine is also a sodium channel blocker, resulting in slowed nerve conduction and an anesthetic effect. In severe overdose, cardiac sodium channel blockade manifests as prolongation of the QRS complex on electrocardiogram and clinically as negative inotropy. Finally, cocaine increases the concentration of the excitatory amino acids glutamate and aspartate in the central nervous system, particularly in the nucleus accumbens.

Symptoms of acute ingestion or overdose vary by organ system affected. With the cardiovascular system, arterial vasoconstriction is seen in addition to a prothrombotic state.[114,115] It can cause tachycardia, hypertension, increased myocardial oxygen demand, and increased vascular shearing forces. Cocaine causes dose-dependent coronary vasoconstriction and is associated with cardiac ischemia.[116-118]

The negative inotropic effects shown by high doses of cocaine may cause acute depression of left ventricular function and acute decompensated heart failure. Cocaine can also cause supraventricular and ventricular dysrhythmias through several mechanisms. Aortic dissection and rupture rarely occur as a result of acute intoxication.[119,120] Furthermore, coronary artery aneurysms are relatively common in these patients and may be another potential cause of myocardial infarction.[121-123]

When clinically evaluating a patient presenting with suspected cocaine intoxication or overdose, capillary blood glucose, acetaminophen concentrations, and salicylate concentrations should be ascertained to rule out hypoglycemia and possible common co-ingestions. The patient's core temperature should be evaluated, and concomitant hyperthermia should be treated, if needed. Cocaine is rapidly metabolized and detectable in blood and urine only briefly after use. Benzoylecgonine is the major metabolite in cocaine that can be detected in the urine for several days after intermittent use and up to 10 days after heavy use. Benzoylecgonine can also be found in the blood, saliva, hair, and meconium of patients with suspected overdose. Because patients may have packed their body cavities with cocaine in an attempt to transport the drug, radiographs may be warranted to ensure their removal to avoid possible continued absorption. Patients with overdose who experience chest pain should prompt electrocardiogram measurements to evaluate for any conduction system abnormalities. Serum biomarkers to detect the presence of circulating troponin, myoglobin, creatine kinase (CK), or CK-MB may be warranted in the setting of chest pain and abnormal electrocardiogram.

Patients with cocaine-related unstable angina, non–ST-segment elevation myocardial infarction, or ST-segment elevation myocardial infarction are treated in a manner similar to other patients with acute coronary syndrome. The most important exception to this is the administration of medications with unopposed α-blockade. Administration of such agents can cause coronary artery vasoconstriction, systemic hypertension, and increased severity and duration of cocaine toxicity. Furthermore, there are theoretical concerns of coronary artery vasoconstriction and systemic hypertension, which can result from unopposed α-adrenergic stimulation. In addition, mortality rates in patients with cocaine-associated myocardial

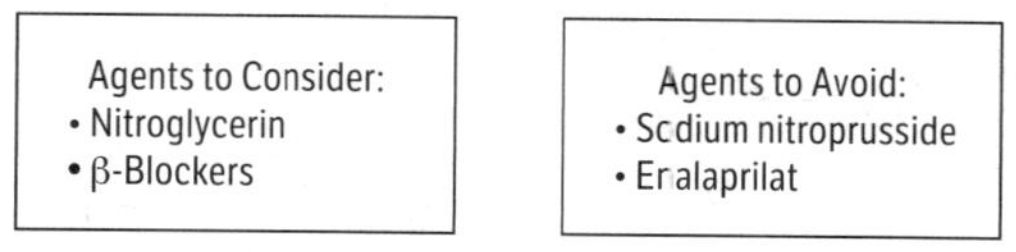

Agents to Consider:	Agents to Avoid:
• Nitroglycerin	• Sodium nitroprusside
• β-Blockers	• Enalaprilat

Figure 37.7 Management of hypertensive crisis associated with acute coronary syndromes.

infarction are low; thus, the usual benefit from β-blockers after myocardial infarction may be lost.

In addition to treatment with antihypertensive agents, patients who may have recently used cocaine may have significant psychomotor agitation, which may contribute to their hypertensive crisis. Adequate sedation with benzodiazepines may be needed in addition to the aforementioned management strategies (Figure 37.8).

Acute Pulmonary Embolism

Almost 50% of patients with an acute pulmonary embolism are hypertensive as a result of accompanying dyspnea, anxiety, or chest pain. Administration of supplemental oxygen, afterload reduction, preload reduction, and diuresis are the mainstay therapeutic interventions in the management of hypertensive crisis caused by acute pulmonary embolism. Blood pressure reduction decreases myocardial oxygen demand and may also enhance cardiac output. Nitroglycerin and sodium nitroprusside are the intravenous antihypertensives most commonly used in this setting. In one single-group, nonrandomized, open-label, standard therapy controlled study, high-dose nitroglycerin infusions were used to aggressively lower blood pressure (SBP of 160 mm Hg or greater or MAP of 120 mm Hg or greater) in patients with acute pulmonary embolism with acute decompensated heart failure refractory to initial antihypertensive therapy (Table 37.3).[124] Study investigators used bolus doses of intravenous nitroglycerin (2 mg intravenously every 3 minutes up to 10 doses) and adjusted dosing to desired symptomatic response. High-dose nitroglycerin administration resulted in fewer ICU admissions, fewer endotracheal intubations, and fewer troponin-level elevations compared with standard therapy. Only one patient in the intervention group developed symptomatic hypotension compared with none in the standard treatment arm. Fewer patients in the high-dose nitroglycerin treatment arm had troponin elevations or biomarker evidence of myocardial infarction. Overall, rapid blood pressure management in patients with acute severe pulmonary congestion as a result of their acute pulmonary embolism may result in the avoidance of endotracheal intubation.[2,107]

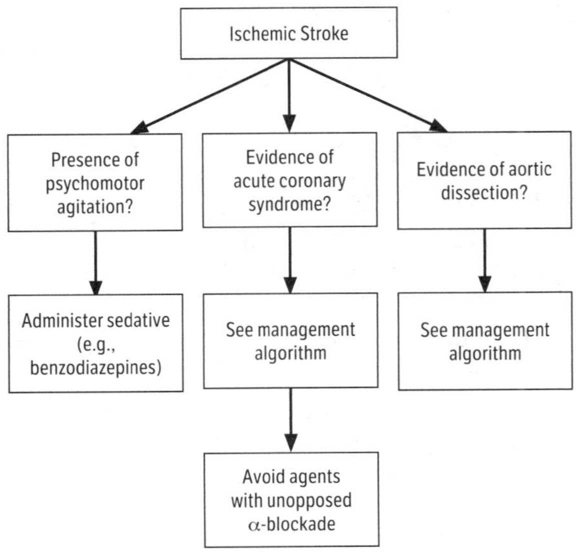

REFERENCES

1. Mozaffarian D, Benjamin EJ, Go AS, et al. Heart disease and stroke statistics—2015 update: a report from the American Heart Association. Circulation 2015;131:e29-322.
2. Chobanian AV, Bakris GL, Black HR, et al. The Seventh Report of the Joint National Committee on Prevention, Detection, Evaluation, and Treatment of High Blood Pressure: the JNC 7 report. JAMA 2003;289:2560-72.
3. James PA, Oparil S, Carter BL, et al. 2014 evidence-based guideline for the management of high blood pressure in adults: report from the panel members appointed to the Eighth Joint National Committee (JNC 8). JAMA 2014;311:507-20.
4. Zampaglione B, Pascale C, Marchisio M, et al. Hypertensive urgencies and emergencies. Prevalence and clinical presentation. Hypertension 1996;27:144-7.
5. Vaughan CJ, Delanty N. Hypertensive emergencies. Lancet 2000;356:411-7.
6. Houston MC. Pathophysiology, clinical aspects, and treatment of hypertensive crises. Prog Cardiovasc Dis 1989;32:99-148.
7. Floras JS. Epinephrine and the genesis of hypertension. Hypertension 1992;19:1-18.
8. Weir MR, Dzau VJ. The renin-angiotensin-aldosterone system: a specific target for hypertension management. Am J Hypertens 1999;12:205s-13s.
9. Ault MJ, Ellrodt AG. Pathophysiological events leading to the end-organ effects of acute hypertension. Am J Emerg Med 1985;3:10-5.
10. Martin JF, Higashiama E, Garcia E, et al. Hypertensive crisis profile. Prevalence and clinical presentation. Arq Bras Cardiol 2004;83:131-6; 25-30.
11. Rhoney D, Peacock WF. Intravenous therapy for hypertensive emergencies, part 1. Am J Health Syst Pharm 2009;66:1343-52.
12. Flanigan JS, Vitberg D. Hypertensive emergency and severe hypertension: what to treat, who to treat, and how to treat. Med Clin North Am 2006;90:439-51.
13. Aggarwal M, Khan IA. Hypertensive crisis: hypertensive emergencies and urgencies. Cardiol Clin 2006;24:135-46.
14. Varon J, Marik PE. The diagnosis and management of hypertensive crises. Chest 2000;118:214-27.
15. Kitiyakara C, Guzman NJ. Malignant hypertension and hypertensive emergencies. J Am Soc Nephrol 1998;9:133-42.
16. Varon J, Marik PE. Clinical review: the management of hypertensive crises. Crit Care 2003;7:374-84.

Figure 37.8 Management of hypertensive crisis associated with cocaine overdose.

17. Triggle DJ. Calcium channel antagonists: clinical uses--past, present and future. Biochem Pharmacol 2007;74:1-9.
18. Richard S. Vascular effects of calcium channel antagonists: new evidence. Drugs 2005;65(suppl 2):1-10.
19. Opie LH. Calcium channel antagonists. Part I. Fundamental properties: mechanisms, classification, sites of action. Cardiovasc Drugs Ther 1987;1:411-30.
20. Curran MP, Robinson DM, Keating GM. Intravenous nicardipine: its use in the short-term treatment of hypertension and various other indications. Drugs 2006;66:1755-82.
21. Cardene I.V. [package insert]. Deerfield, IL: Baxter Healthcare, July 2014.
22. Handbook on Injectable Drugs, 16th ed. Bethesda, MD: American Society of Health-System Pharmacists, 2011.
23. Deeks ED, Keating GM, Keam SJ. Clevidipine: a review of its use in the management of acute hypertension. Am J Cardiovasc Drugs 2009;9:117-34.
24. Cleviprex [package insert]. Graz, Austria: Fresenius Kabi, August 2013.
25. White CM. Pharmacologic, pharmacokinetic, and therapeutic differences among ACE inhibitors. Pharmacotherapy 1998;18:588-99.
26. Breckenridge A. Angiotensin converting enzyme inhibitors. Br Med J (Clin Res Ed) 1988;296:618-20.
27. Given BD, Taylor T, Hollenberg NK, et al. Duration of action and short-term hormonal responses to enalapril (MK 421) in normal subjects. J Cardiovasc Pharmacol 1984;6:436-41.
28. Todd PA, Goa KL. Enalapril. A reappraisal of its pharmacology and therapeutic use in hypertension. Drugs 1992;43:346-81.
29. Hirschl MM, Binder M, Bur A, et al. Impact of the renin-angiotensin-aldosterone system on blood pressure response to intravenous enalaprilat in patients with hypertensive crises. J Hum Hypertens 1997;11:177-83.
30. Enalaprilat [package insert]. Lake Forest, IL: Hospira, March 2010.
31. Vasekar M, Craig TJ. ACE inhibitor-induced angioedema. Curr Allergy Asthma Rep 2012;12:72-8.
32. Agostoni A, Cicardi M, Cugno M, et al. Angioedema due to angiotensin-converting enzyme inhibitors. Immunopharmacology 1999;44:21-5.
33. Wood M, Hyman S, Wood AJ. A clinical study of sensitivity to sodium nitroprusside during controlled hypotensive anesthesia in young and elderly patients. Anesth Analg 1987;66:132-6.
34. Friederich JA, Butterworth JF IV. Sodium nitroprusside: twenty years and counting. Anesth Analg 1995;81:152-62.
35. Hall VA, Guest JM. Sodium nitroprusside-induced cyanide intoxication and prevention with sodium thiosulfate prophylaxis. Am J Crit Care 1992;1:19-25; quiz 6-7.
36. Ignarro LJ. After 130 years, the molecular mechanism of action of nitroglycerin is revealed. Proc Natl Acad Sci USA 2002;99:7816-7.
37. Hirai N, Kawano H, Yasue H, et al. Attenuation of nitrate tolerance and oxidative stress by an angiotensin II receptor blocker in patients with coronary spastic angina. Circulation 2003;108:1446-50.
38. Varon J. Treatment of acute severe hypertension: current and newer agents. Drugs 2008;68:283-97.
39. Gurney AM, Allam M. Inhibition of calcium release from the sarcoplasmic reticulum of rabbit aorta by hydralazine. Br J Pharmacol 1995;114:238-44.
40. Azuma J, Sawamura A, Harada H, et al. Mechanism of direct cardiostimulating actions of hydralazine. Eur J Pharmacol 1987;135:137-44.
41. Munzel T, Kurz S, Rajagopalan S, et al. Hydralazine prevents nitroglycerin tolerance by inhibiting activation of a membrane-bound NADH oxidase. A new action for an old drug. J Clin Invest 1996;98:1465-70.
42. O'Malley K, Segal JL, Israili ZH, et al. Duration of hydralazine action in hypertension. Clin Pharmacol Ther 1975;18:581-6.
43. Gray RJ. Managing critically ill patients with esmolol. An ultra short-acting beta-adrenergic blocker. Chest 1988;93:398-403.
44. Singh PP, Dimich I, Sampson I, et al. A comparison of esmolol and labetalol for the treatment of perioperative hypertension in geriatric ambulatory surgical patients. Can J Anaesth 1992;39:559-62.
45. Smerling A, Gersony WM. Esmolol for severe hypertension following repair of aortic coarctation. Crit Care Med 1990;18:1288-90.
46. Mooss AN, Hilleman DE, Mohiuddin SM, et al. Safety of esmolol in patients with acute myocardial infarction treated with thrombolytic therapy who had relative contraindications to beta-blocker therapy. Ann Pharmacother 1994;28:701-3.
47. Sheppard D, DiStefano S, Byrd RC, et al. Effects of esmolol on airway function in patients with asthma. J Clin Pharmacol 1986;26:169-74.
48. Grossman E, Ironi AN, Messerli FH. Comparative tolerability profile of hypertensive crisis treatments. Drug Saf 1998;19:99-122.
49. Phillips RA, Greenblatt J, Krakoff LR. Hypertensive emergencies: diagnosis and management. Prog Cardiovasc Dis 2002;45:33-48.
50. Murphy MB, Murray C, Shorten GD. Fenoldopam: a selective peripheral dopamine-receptor agonist for the treatment of severe hypertension. N Engl J Med 2001;345:1548-57.
51. Landoni G, Biondi-Zoccai GG, Tumlin JA, et al. Beneficial impact of fenoldopam in critically ill patients with or at risk for acute renal failure: a meta-analysis of randomized clinical trials. Am J Kidney Dis 2007;49:56-68.
52. Hypertension in pregnancy. Report of the American College of Obstetricians and Gynecologists' Task Force on Hypertension in Pregnancy. Obstet Gynecol 2013;122 1122-31.
53. Vadhera RB, Simon M. Hypertensive emergencies in pregnancy. Clin Obstet Gynecol 2014;57:797-805.
54. Too GT, Hill JB. Hypertensive crisis during pregnancy and postpartum period. Semin Perinatol 2013;37:280-7.
55. Duley L, Meher S, Jones L. Drugs for treatment of very high blood pressure during pregnancy. Cochrane Database Syst Rev 2013;7:Cd001449.
56. Nooij LS, Visser S, Meuleman T, et al. The optimal treatment of severe hypertension in pregnancy: update of the role of nicardipine. Curr Pharm Biotechnol 2014;15:64-9.

57. Podymow T, August P. Update on the use of antihypertensive drugs in pregnancy. Hypertension 2008;51:960-9.
58. Hemphill JC III, Greenberg SM, Anderson CS, et al. Guidelines for the management of spontaneous intracerebral hemorrhage: a guideline for healthcare professionals from the American Heart Association/American Stroke Association. Stroke 2015;46:2032-60.
59. Anderson CS, Huang Y, Wang JG, et al. Intensive blood pressure reduction in acute cerebral haemorrhage trial (INTERACT): a randomised pilot trial. Lancet Neurol 2008;7:391-9.
60. Antihypertensive treatment of acute cerebral hemorrhage. Crit Care Med 2010;38:637-48.
61. Anderson CS, Heeley E, Huang Y, et al. Rapid blood-pressure lowering in patients with acute intracerebral hemorrhage. N Engl J Med 2013;368:2355-65.
62. Qureshi AI, Palesch YY. Antihypertensive treatment of acute cerebral hemorrhage (ATACH) II: design, methods, and rationale. Neurocrit Care 2011;15:559-76.
63. Flibotte JJ, Hagan N, O'Donnell J, et al. Warfarin, hematoma expansion, and outcome of intracerebral hemorrhage. Neurology 2004;63:1059-64.
64. Kuramatsu JB, Gerner ST, Schellinger PD, et al. Anticoagulant reversal, blood pressure levels, and anticoagulant resumption in patients with anticoagulation-related intracerebral hemorrhage. JAMA 2015;313:824-36.
65. Mayer SA, Kurtz P, Wyman A, et al. Clinical practices, complications, and mortality in neurological patients with acute severe hypertension: the Studying the Treatment of Acute hyperTension registry. Crit Care Med 2011;39:2330-6.
66. Liu-Deryke X, Janisse J, Coplin WM, et al. A comparison of nicardipine and labetalol for acute hypertension management following stroke. Neurocrit Care 2008;9:167-76.
67. Ortega-Gutierrez S, Thomas J, Reccius A, et al. Effectiveness and safety of nicardipine and labetalol infusion for blood pressure management in patients with intracerebral and subarachnoid hemorrhage. Neurocrit Care 2013;18:13-9.
68. Koga M, Arihiro S, Hasegawa Y, et al. Intravenous nicardipine dosing for blood pressure lowering in acute intracerebral hemorrhage: the Stroke Acute Management with Urgent Risk-factor Assessment and Improvement-Intracerebral Hemorrhage study. J Stroke Cardiovasc Dis 2014;23:2780-7.
69. Graffagnino C, Bergese S, Love J, et al. Clevidipine rapidly and safely reduces blood pressure in acute intracerebral hemorrhage: the ACCELERATE trial. Cerebrovasc Dis 2013;36:173-80.
70. Castillo J, Leira R, Garcia MM, et al. Blood pressure decrease during the acute phase of ischemic stroke is associated with brain injury and poor stroke outcome. Stroke 2004;35:520-6.
71. Leonardi-Bee J, Bath PM, Phillips SJ, et al. Blood pressure and clinical outcomes in the International Stroke Trial. Stroke 2002;33:1315-20.
72. Jauch EC, Saver JL, Adams HP Jr, et al. Guidelines for the early management of patients with acute ischemic stroke: a guideline for healthcare professionals from the American Heart Association/American Stroke Association. Stroke 2013;44:870-947.
73. He J, Zhang Y, Xu T, et al. Effects of immediate blood pressure reduction on death and major disability in patients with acute ischemic stroke: the CATIS randomized clinical trial. JAMA 2014;311:479-89.
74. Tissue plasminogen activator for acute ischemic stroke. The National Institute of Neurological Disorders and Stroke rt-PA Stroke Study Group. N Engl J Med 1995;333:1581-7.
75. Katzan IL, Furlan AJ, Lloyd LE, et al. Use of tissue-type plasminogen activator for acute ischemic stroke: the Cleveland area experience. JAMA 2000;283:1151-8.
76. Tanne D, Bates VE, Verro P, et al. Initial clinical experience with IV tissue plasminogen activator for acute ischemic stroke: a multicenter survey. The t-PA Stroke Survey Group. Neurology 1999;53:424-7.
77. Tanne D, Kasner SE, Demchuk AM, et al. Markers of increased risk of intracerebral hemorrhage after intravenous recombinant tissue plasminogen activator therapy for acute ischemic stroke in clinical practice: the Multicenter rt-PA Stroke Survey. Circulation 2002;105:1679-85.
78. Tomii Y, Toyoda K, Nakashima T, et al. Effects of hyperacute blood pressure and heart rate on stroke outcomes after intravenous tissue plasminogen activator. J Hypertens 2011;29:1980-7.
79. Ahmed N, Wahlgren N, Brainin M, et al. Relationship of blood pressure, antihypertensive therapy, and outcome in ischemic stroke treated with intravenous thrombolysis: retrospective analysis from Safe Implementation of Thrombolysis in Stroke-International Stroke Thrombolysis Register (SITS-ISTR). Stroke 2009;40:2442-9.
80. Ahmed N, Nasman P, Wahlgren NG. Effect of intravenous nimodipine on blood pressure and outcome after acute stroke. Stroke 2000;31:1250-5.
81. Liu-DeRyke X, Levy PD, Parker D Jr, et al. A prospective evaluation of labetalol versus nicardipine for blood pressure management in patients with acute stroke. Neurocrit Care 2013;19:41-7.
82. Barer DH, Cruickshank JM, Ebrahim SB, et al. Low dose beta blockade in acute stroke ("BEST" trial): an evaluation. Br Med J (Clin Res Ed) 1988;296:737-41.
83. Schrader J, Luders S, Kulschewski A, et al. The ACCESS study: evaluation of acute candesartan cilexetil therapy in stroke survivors. Stroke 2003;34:1699-703.
84. Inagawa T, Kamiya K, Ogasawara H, et al. Rebleeding of ruptured intracranial aneurysms in the acute stage. Surg Neurol 1987;28:93-9.
85. Naidech AM, Janjua N, Kreiter KT, et al. Predictors and impact of aneurysm rebleeding after subarachnoid hemorrhage. Arch Neurol 2005;62:410-6.
86. Ohkuma H, Tsurutani H, Suzuki S. Incidence and significance of early aneurysmal rebleeding before neurosurgical or neurological management. Stroke 2001;32:1176-80.
87. Claassen J, Vu A, Kreiter KT, et al. Effect of acute physiologic derangements on outcome after subarachnoid hemorrhage. Crit Care Med 2004;32:832-8.
88. Connolly ES Jr, Rabinstein AA, Carhuapoma JR, et al. Guidelines for the management of aneurysmal subarachnoid hemorrhage: a guideline for healthcare professionals from the American Heart Association/American Stroke Association. Stroke 2012;43:1711-37.

89. Woloszyn AV, McAllen KJ, Figueroa BE, et al. Retrospective evaluation of nicardipine versus labetalol for blood pressure control in aneurysmal subarachnoid hemorrhage. Neurocrit Care 2012;16:376-80.

90. Roitberg BZ, Hardman J, Urbaniak K, et al. Prospective randomized comparison of safety and efficacy of nicardipine and nitroprusside drip for control of hypertension in the neurosurgical intensive care unit. Neurosurgery 2008;63:115-20; discussion 20-1.

91. Varelas PN, Abdelhak T, Corry JJ, et al. Clevidipine for acute hypertension in patients with subarachnoid hemorrhage: a pilot study. Int J Neurosci 2014;124:192-8.

92. Gal TJ, Cooperman LH. Hypertension in the immediate postoperative period. Br J Anaesth 1975;47:70-4.

93. Haas CE, LeBlanc JM. Acute postoperative hypertension: a review of therapeutic options. Am J Health Syst Pharm 2004;61:1661-73; quiz 74-5.

94. Weant KA, Flynn JD, Smith KM. Postoperative hypertension. Orthopedics 2004;27:1159-61.

95. Wallach R, Karp RB, Reves JG, et al. Pathogenesis of paroxysmal hypertension developing during and after coronary bypass surgery: a study of hemodynamic and humoral factors. Am J Cardiol 1980;46:559-65.

96. Breslow MJ, Jordan DA, Christopherson R, et al. Epidural morphine decreases postoperative hypertension by attenuating sympathetic nervous system hyperactivity. JAMA 1989;261:3577-81.

97. Olsen KS, Pedersen CB, Madsen JB, et al. Vasoactive modulators during and after craniotomy: relation to postoperative hypertension. J Neurosurg Anesthesiol 2002;14:171-9.

98. Orlowski JP, Vidt DG, Walker S, et al. The hemodynamic effects of intravenous labetalol for postoperative hypertension. Cleve Clin J Med 1989;56:29-34.

99. Dimich I, Lingham R, Gabrielson G, et al. Comparative hemodynamic effects of labetalol and hydralazine in the treatment of postoperative hypertension. J Clin Anesth 1989;1:201-6.

100. Goldberg ME, Clark S, Joseph J, et al. Nicardipine versus placebo for the treatment of postoperative hypertension. Am Heart J 1990;119:446-50.

101. Halpern NA, Goldberg M, Neely C, et al. Postoperative hypertension: a multicenter, prospective, randomized comparison between intravenous nicardipine and sodium nitroprusside. Crit Care Med 1992;20:1637-43.

102. Aronson S, Dyke CM, Stierer KA, et al. The ECLIPSE trials: comparative studies of clevidipine to nitroglycerin, sodium nitroprusside, and nicardipine for acute hypertension treatment in cardiac surgery patients. Anesth Analg 2008;107:1110-21.

103. Mazza A, Armigliato M, Marzola MC, et al. Anti-hypertensive treatment in pheochromocytoma and paraganglioma: current management and therapeutic features. Endocrine 2014;45:469-78.

104. McMillian WD, Trombley BJ, Charash WE, et al. Phentolamine continuous infusion in a patient with pheochromocytoma. Am J Health Syst Pharm 2011;68:130-4.

105. Golledge J, Eagle KA. Acute aortic dissection. Lancet 2008;372:55-66.

106. Elliott WJ. Hypertensive emergencies. Crit Care Clin 2001;17:435-51.

107. Rhoney D, Peacock WF. Intravenous therapy for hypertensive emergencies, part 2. Am J Health Syst Pharm 2009;66:1448-57.

108. P. Braunwald's Heart Disease: A Textbook of Cardiovascular Medicine, 10th ed. Philadelphia: Elsevier, 2015.

109. Mann T, Cohn PF, Holman LB, et al. Effect of nitroprusside on regional myocardial blood flow in coronary artery disease. Results in 25 patients and comparison with nitroglycerin. Circulation 1978;57:732-8.

110. Kloner RA, Hutter AM, Emmick JT, et al. Time course of the interaction between tadalafil and nitrates. J Am Coll Cardiol 2003;42:1855-60.

111. Chae C. Clinical Trials in Cardiovascular Disease: A Companion to Braunwald's Heart Disease. Philadephia: Saunders, 1999.

112. Chen ZM, Pan HC, Chen YP, et al. Early intravenous then oral metoprolol in 45,852 patients with acute myocardial infarction: randomised placebo-controlled trial. Lancet 2005;366:1622-32.

113. Swedberg K, Held P, Kjekshus J, et al. Effects of the early administration of enalapril on mortality in patients with acute myocardial infarction. Results of the Cooperative New Scandinavian Enalapril Survival Study II (CONSENSUS II). N Engl J Med 1992;327:678-84.

114. Lange RA, Cigarroa RG, Flores ED, et al. Potentiation of cocaine-induced coronary vasoconstriction by beta-adrenergic blockade. Ann Intern Med 1990;112:897-903.

115. Kalsner S. Cocaine sensitization of coronary artery contractions: mechanism of drug-induced spasm. J Pharmacol Exp Ther 1993;264:1132-40.

116. Hollander JE, Hoffman RS, Gennis P, et al. Prospective multicenter evaluation of cocaine-associated chest pain. Cocaine Associated Chest Pain (COCHPA) Study Group. Acad Emerg Med 1994;1:330-9.

117. McCord J, Jneid H, Hollander JE, et al. Management of cocaine-associated chest pain and myocardial infarction: a scientific statement from the American Heart Association Acute Cardiac Care Committee of the Council on Clinical Cardiology. Circulation 2008;117:1897-907.

118. Hollander JE, Hoffman RS, Burstein JL, et al. Cocaine-associated myocardial infarction. Mortality and complications. Cocaine-Associated Myocardial Infarction Study Group. Arch Intern Med 1995;155:1081-6.

119. Hsue PY, Salinas CL, Bolger AF, et al. Acute aortic dissection related to crack cocaine. Circulation 2002;105:1592-5.

120. Dean JH, Woznicki EM, O'Gara P, et al. Cocaine-related aortic dissection: lessons from the International Registry of Acute Aortic Dissection. Am J Med 2014;127:878-85.

121. Satran A, Bart BA, Henry CR, et al. Increased prevalence of coronary artery aneurysms among cocaine users. Circulation 2005;111:2424-9.

122. Waller B. Hurst's The Heart, 13th ed. New York: McGraw-Hill, 2010.

123. Glickel SZ, Maggs PR, Ellis FH Jr. Coronary artery aneurysm. Ann Thorac Surg 1978;25:372-6.

124. Levy P, Compton S, Welch R, et al. Treatment of severe decompensated heart failure with high-dose intravenous nitroglycerin: a feasibility and outcome analysis. Ann Emerg Med 2007;50:144-52.

Medication Withdrawal in the Intensive Care Unit

Colgan T. Sloan, Pharm.D., BCPS; Robert French, M.D., MPH; Nicholas B. Hurst, M.D., M.S.; Stephen R. Karpen, Pharm.D.; and Mazda Shirazi, M.D., Ph.D.

LEARNING OBJECTIVES

1. Identify medications that, if discontinued, may complicate the care of patients in the intensive care unit (ICU).
2. Discuss the diagnosis of medication withdrawal in ICU patients.
3. Review treatment strategies for ICU patients thought to have medication withdrawal.

ABBREVIATIONS IN THIS CHAPTER

GABA	γ-Amino butyric acid	SNRI	Serotonin and norepinephrine reuptake inhibitor
ICU	Intensive care unit		
NRT	Nicotine replacement therapy	SSRI	Selective serotonin reuptake inhibitor

INTRODUCTION

Medication withdrawal is a potentially serious complication in all patients taking chronic medications; some medication classes pose a greater risk of withdrawal. We identified popular medications with clinically relevant withdrawal syndromes. It must be stressed that the evidence base for many of the recommendations in this chapter is of moderate to low quality. Many of the recommendations from this chapter are based on limited evidence and expert opinion; we implore readers to apply these recommendations judiciously to patient care. The many contributing factors to the paucity of high-quality evidence in this area include underrecognition by clinicians, methodological limitations (e.g., small sample size, nonrandomized, retrospective), and ethical concerns with treating potentially life-threatening withdrawal syndromes with substandard comparators. The ICU team should diligently identify medications with a withdrawal concern and anticipate how to address these, being wary not to overlook iatrogenic causes of medication withdrawal. In reviewing medications that may have pertinent withdrawal symptoms, we hope to raise awareness about this potentially overlooked aspect of patient care within the intensive care unit (ICU).

BACLOFEN WITHDRAWAL

Background

Baclofen (4-amino-3(p-chlorophenyl)butyric acid) is structurally similar to the inhibitory neurotransmitter γ-amino butyric acid (GABA). Baclofen is an agonist at the GABA-B receptors located in the dorsal horns of the spinal cord and elsewhere in the central nervous system (CNS) (see Figure 38.1). Although its mechanism of action in the treatment of muscular spasticity is not entirely known, baclofen is believed to suppress the release of excitatory neurotransmitters involved in monosynaptic and polysynaptic stretch reflexes, resulting in reduced muscle tone and vasospasm.[1]

Baclofen is used orally or intrathecally in the treatment of chronic muscular spasticity caused by neurologic injury and neuromuscular disorders such as spinal cord injury, multiple sclerosis cerebral palsy, and traumatic brain injury. Oral baclofen has been used in the treatment of alcohol abuse disorder and other addiction disorders; it too is abused.[2]

Intrathecal baclofen is administered using a programmable metallic infusion pump that is surgically implanted, typically in the lower abdomen. The pump stores and releases the programmed amount of baclofen through a flexible catheter into the intrathecal space.[3,4] Long-term administration causes down-regulation of GABA-B receptors.[5] Interrupting intrathecal baclofen administration because of problems with the pump or the catheter can lead to an acute life-threatening withdrawal state that is characterized by delirium, autonomic instability, hyperthermia, and muscular spasticity. Patients who have a baclofen pump are therefore technology-dependent.

Diagnosis

Baclofen withdrawal is a clinical diagnosis. Neuropsychiatric symptoms include auditory, visual, and tactile hallucinations; delusions; confusion; agitation; disorientation; fluctuation of consciousness; insomnia; anxiety; depersonalization; and formal thought disorder.[6] Other signs and symptoms include rebound spasticity, autonomic instability, hyperthermia, and pruritus.[7,8] Withdrawal should be considered when suggestive symptoms occur in a patient who is receiving chronic oral baclofen therapy, abuses oral baclofen, has an intrathecal baclofen pump, or, in the absence of a reliable medication history, has a history of or examination findings suggestive of chronic muscle spasticity. In a review of published case reports, the latency until onset of withdrawal symptoms was 1–4 days after the cessation of oral baclofen and 12–24 hours after the cessation of intrathecal baclofen.[6] A differential diagnosis is presented in Table 38.1.

Management

Definitive management of acute baclofen withdrawal involves resuming baclofen therapy. Management of withdrawal from intrathecal baclofen is therefore more complicated than management of withdrawal from oral baclofen.

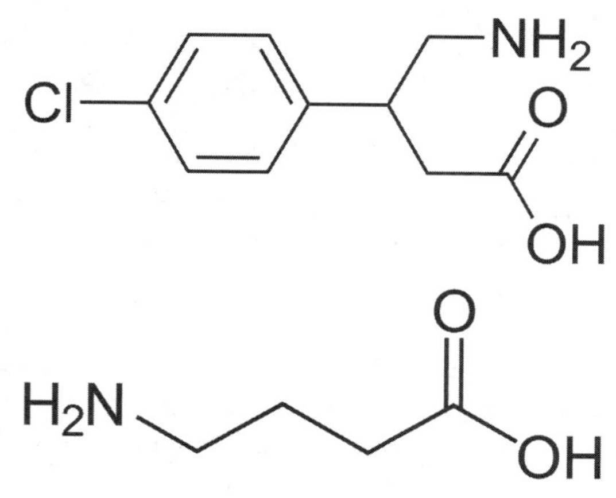

The pump should be interrogated by a physician familiar with intrathecal infusion pumps. Pump-related problems include programming errors, battery exhaustion, and low residual volume. Forty percent of withdrawal states are the result of catheter-related problems; therefore, the integrity of the catheter should be investigated by abdominal radiograph or catheterogram. Catheter-related problems include migration kinking, breakage, and leaks where the catheter meets the pump.[14]

A variety of medications, and combinations of medications, have been used to control symptoms during the interval between presentation and restoration of intrathecal baclofen delivery. Evidence supporting any specific therapeutic action is lacking. Enteral baclofen is often used; however, it is generally considered ineffective because adequate CNS concentrations cannot be attained.[15-17] Propofol and benzodiazepines are both GABA-A receptor agonists and therefore potentially bypass the down-regulated CNS GABA-B receptors.[12,15,18,19] Baclofen has been used to treat withdrawal in a patient with chronic use of γ-hydroxybutyrate (GHB).[20] Sodium oxybate (Xyrem), a U.S. Food and Drug Administration (FDA)-approved medication with the same chemical structure as GHB, as a treatment for baclofen withdrawal has not been reported. Given the FDA's REMS (Risk Evaluation and Mitigation Strategies) in place for sodium oxybate, clinicians will not likely have access to sodium oxybate.[21] Cyproheptadine has been used to control serotonergic findings.[12,16]

Cases in which intrathecal baclofen is interrupted because of the removal of an infected pump are particularly problematic because intrathecal baclofen cannot readily be resumed. Such cases have resulted in withdrawal states lasting more than 1 month, only to be resolved once the infection clears and the pump is replaced.[15,22] In one study, intrathecal baclofen administered using an indwelling lumbar

Figure 38.1 Baclofen (top); γ-amino butyric acid (bottom).
Reprinted from: Wikipedia Commons (https://commons.wikimedia.org/wiki/File:Baclofen.svg; https://commons.wikimedia.org/wiki/File:Gamma-Aminobutters%C3%A4ure_-_gamma-aminobutyric_acid.svg).

Table 38.1 Differential Diagnosis for Baclofen Withdrawal[9-13]

Autonomic dysreflexia
Malignant hyperthermia
Neuroleptic malignant syndrome
Serotonin syndrome
Sympathomimetic toxicity
Alcohol withdrawal
Benzodiazepine withdrawal
Sepsis
Dystonia
Seizure

drain catheter in conjunction with a patient-controlled analgesia pump was used to treat acute withdrawal that occurred after the removal of a catheter because of its proximity to an infection site; this patient was ultimately weaned to oral medication.[8] Intrathecal baclofen through a temporary, externalized, intrathecal catheter was used to prevent withdrawal in a case where the pump and catheter were removed because of infection at the site of the pump.[23]

SELECTIVE SEROTONIN/NOREPINEPHRINE REUPTAKE INHIBITOR WITHDRAWAL

Background

Selective serotonin reuptake inhibitors (SSRIs) and serotonin and norepinephrine reuptake inhibitors (SNRIs) are among the most prescribed pharmaceuticals in the United States. Data from the Centers for Disease Control and Prevention in 2011 showed that 1 in 10 Americans reported taking an antidepressant medication.[24] The SSRIs and SNRIs are considered first-line treatment for depression.[25] They work by modulating the neurotransmission of serotonin and norepinephrine, resulting in increased availability of these molecules at the synaptic cleft and thereby affecting mood. The exact mechanism of this effect is unknown.

Case reports describing withdrawal reactions after cessation of these agents began to appear in the medical literature in the 1990s.[26,27] These reports described a range of symptoms including extrapyramidal effects, shocklike sensations, dizziness, light-headedness, and delirium. Psychological symptoms such as anxiety, irritability, and insomnia were also described. Collectively, these are termed the *antidepressant discontinuation syndrome*. These symptoms have been described to occur after both abrupt cessation and gradual taper. Onset of symptoms usually occurs a few days after cessation and can last for weeks.[28] Agents with longer half-lives or active metabolites tend to be less likely to cause the syndrome.[29]

More severe reactions have also been reported in the literature. In one case report, a patient developed refractory hypertension after stopping citalopram that resolved on reinitiation.[30] Another patient had strokelike symptoms and a pill-rolling tremor post-surgically that was attributed to discontinuing milnacipran the night before. After a negative workup, the patient's milnacipran was reinitiated, and the symptoms resolved.[31] These cases show the importance of including SSRI/SNRI withdrawal syndrome in the differential of critically ill patients.

Diagnosis

Selective serotonin reuptake inhibitor/SNRI discontinuation syndrome is a clinical diagnosis. Diagnostic criteria have been proposed.[32] These criteria consider both the physical and psychological effects of discontinuation. The diagnosis should be considered in a patient with symptoms of discontinuation syndrome who has been taking an SSRI/SNRI for at least 1 month followed by an abrupt cessation or decrease in dose.

Other etiologies in the critically ill patient should be considered because many of the symptoms are nonspecific. Conversely, in many cases, the symptoms can be attributed to other etiologies such as ICU delirium, sepsis, or stroke, and consideration of SSRI/SNRI discontinuation syndrome may be overlooked (see Table 38.2).

Management

General supportive care is indicated for all cases of discontinuation syndrome. Definitive management of SSRI/SNRI discontinuation syndrome involves resuming therapy with the previous agent or another in the same class, unless contraindicated.[33] The lowest dose that the patient tolerated before the onset of symptoms should be initiated. If the ultimate goal is discontinuation of therapy, a more gradual taper may be tried. Alternatively, switching to another agent with a longer half-life, such as fluoxetine, which has the added

Table 38.2 Diagnostic Criteria for SSRI/SNRI Discontinuation

Criterion	Description
A	Dose reduction or complete cessation after ≥ 1 month of use
B	Development of two or more of the following within 1–7 days of criterion A • Dizziness, light-headedness, vertigo, feeling faint • Shocklike sensations or paresthesias • Anxiety • Diarrhea • Fatigue • Gait instability • Headache • Insomnia • Irritability • Nausea and/or emesis • Tremor • Visual disturbances
C	Criterion B symptoms cause clinically significant distress or impairment
D	Symptoms not better explained by other cause

Adapted from: Black K, Shea C, Dursun S, et al. Selective serotonin reuptake inhibitor discontinuation syndrome: proposed diagnostic criteria. J Psychiatry Neurosci 2000;25:255-61.

SNRI = serotonin and norepinephrine reuptake inhibitor; SSRI = selective serotonin reuptake inhibitor.

benefit of an active metabolite, may aid in preventing recrudescence of the discontinuation syndrome.[34]

NICOTINE WITHDRAWAL
Background

Nicotine is the primary component of tobacco and tobacco products responsible for addiction and withdrawal. The underlying pharmacology of its addiction and withdrawal profile is multifactorial and complex. The nicotinic cholinergic receptor (nAChR) is the primary target of nicotine and is found in both the central and peripheral nervous systems.[35] The nAChR is a ligand-gated ion channel structurally composed of five pore-forming subunits. In mammalian neuronal cells, homo- and heteropentameric receptors are composed of $\alpha_2-\alpha_{10}$ and $\beta_2-\beta_4$ subunits. Ligands of the receptor, such as nicotine, bind at the subunit interfaces, with the relative ion permeability dictated by the specific subunits composing the receptor.[36] The $\alpha_4\beta_2$-receptor subtypes are thought to be primarily responsible for nicotine dependence in people.[35] Agonism of central nAChRs results in the release of dopamine in the mesolimbic area, corpus striatum, frontal cortex, and other areas thought to play a role in drug-induced reward.[37] With chronic stimulation, the amount of nAChRs in the brain is increased. This up-regulation is thought to be because of receptor desensitization.[38] Thus, pharmacologically, nicotine binding may alleviate symptoms of withdrawal.

Diagnosis

It is estimated that 20%–46% of patients admitted to the ICU are smokers and have the potential to have nicotine withdrawal symptoms during their stay.[39] Symptoms generally begin 1–2 days after cessation and peak within the first week. In the outpatient setting, symptoms of nicotine withdrawal classically include irritability, anxiety, dysphoria, restlessness, insomnia, increased appetite, and weight gain. Nicotine withdrawal in the ICU setting has been studied significantly less. In hospitalized but not critical patients, nicotine withdrawal has been reported to include bradycardia, irritability, anxiety, agitation, confusion, and hallucinations.[40] A history of smoking is a risk factor for developing delirium, and there is an increased risk of agitation, an increased risk of self-removal of tubes and catheters, and an increased need for sedatives, analgesics, neuroleptics, and physical restraints with nicotine abstinence in smokers in the ICU.[41,42] Management of these symptoms in the ICU patient has not been well studied.

Management

The mainstay of therapy for the treatment of nicotine withdrawal in the outpatient setting is nicotine replacement therapy (NRT). Nicotine replacement therapy has been shown to be safe and useful in this population and provides no increased risk of stroke, arrhythmia, angina, myocardial infarction, or death.[43-45] It remains unclear whether these conclusions hold true in the critical patient. A retrospective case-control review showed an increased risk of mortality in critically ill patients when NRT was used.[46] An increase in mortality was also seen in critical care cardiovascular smokers receiving NRT compared with smokers not receiving NRT and nonsmokers. We recommend withholding NRT during the ICU stay but continuing NRT after hospital discharge.[47] A prospective observational study of NRT in the ICU showed no difference in hospital and ICU mortality, hospital length of stay, and 28-day mechanical ventilator– and ICU-free days in active tobacco users receiving NRT compared with those not receiving NRT. Of interest, NRT was associated with more days with a positive CAM-ICU (confusion assessment method for the ICU) score, but a lower median RASS (Richmond Agitation-Sedation Scale) score. Furthermore, higher cumulative doses of opioids and benzodiazepines were required in patients taking NRT, but less dexmedetomidine and haloperidol were required.[48] Finally, a study of 423 smokers in a mixed medical and surgical ICU assessed the use of transdermal NRT. Therapy in this study consisted of a median dose of 20 mg/day beginning a median of 2.3 days after ICU admission and continuing for a median of 6 days. Use of NRT was more likely to occur in patients previously receiving more than 2 sedatives than in smokers not receiving NRT. Unadjusted survivor length in the ICU was greater in the NRT group, but the hazard ratio for ICU and in-hospital mortality was no different between groups after covariate adjustment.[49]

Many dosage forms are available for using NRT (gum, nasal spray, inhalers, tablets, transdermal patches); however, the transdermal route may be preferred in the ICU patient because of ease of use and consistency in nicotine delivery in this population. Nicotine patches deliver 7, 14, or 21 mg over 24 hours. Most studies report use of the 21-mg patch, but several studies do not specify the dose or dosage form used during NRT. Doses of up to 44 mg/day have safely been used.[50] If NRT therapy is tried, we recommend that the 21- or 14-mg/day patch be used; if an accurate smoking history can be obtained, patients smoking more than 10 cigarettes per day should start with the 21-mg/day patch (those smoking 10 or fewer cigarettes per day use the 14-mg/day patch initially).[51] Of note, the patch dosing recommendations are not derived from an ICU population, and individual patient assessment is prudent.

The use of varenicline and bupropion cannot be recommended at this time; these medications have been shown to increase smoking cessation but not to relieve symptoms of nicotine withdrawal.[52] Further studies of their use in the critical care setting are required; ICU clinicians should note that small studies found a decreased risk of mortality in patients with acute subarachnoid hemorrhage but an increased risk of mortality in the cardiothoracic ICU population.[47,52,53] Dexmedetomidine and clonidine have been investigated for their role in smoking cessation; however, clinical studies on their safety and efficacy, especially in the critical care population, are lacking.[54,55]

OPIOID WITHDRAWAL

Background

Opioids are the class of pharmaceuticals that bind to opioid receptors to produce an opium-like effect. Four subtypes of receptors have been identified—μ, κ, δ, and nociceptin/orphanin FQ—which themselves have subtypes.[56,57] Signal transduction is mediated by G protein–coupled receptors that work through a variety of mechanisms, with the end effect of decreased neuronal transmission. Opioid receptors are found throughout the CNS. The receptors in the locus ceruleus are thought to mediate the withdrawal syndrome through increased release of norepinephrine when the opioid-induced inhibition is removed.[58]

The prototypic opioid, morphine, is one of the oldest xenobiotics used as medicinal therapy (see Figure 38.2). Several derivatives and functionally similar compounds now constitute the opioid class of pharmaceuticals. Although some compounds are structurally dissimilar to morphine, as a class, opioids are used primarily in the treatment of acute and chronic pain and are the most commonly used psychoactive substance in the world.[59] Many formulations exist, together with several routes of administration including oral, intravenous, transdermal, and intranasal.

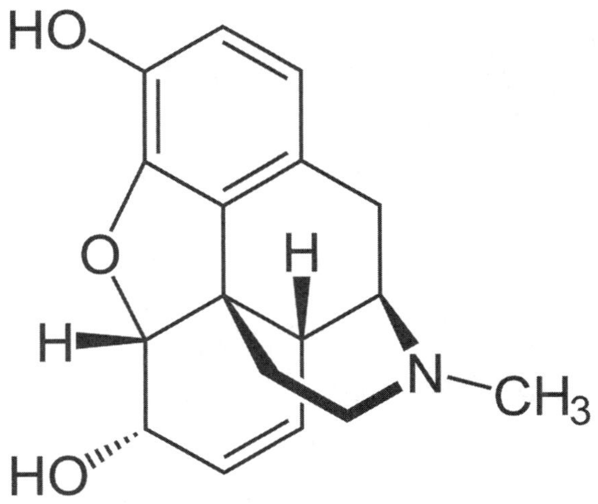

Figure 38.2 Morphine.
Reprinted from: Wikipedia Commons (https://commons.wikimedia.org/wiki/File:Morphin_-_Morphine.svg).

Diagnosis

Opioid withdrawal is a clinical diagnosis. The withdrawal syndrome is a collection of signs and symptoms that occur after cessation of an opioid agonist. The opioid toxidrome consists of respiratory depression, CNS depression, miosis, bradycardia, and decreased gut motility.[60] The withdrawal syndrome predictably consists of the opposite of these symptoms, including irritability, insomnia, mydriasis, tachycardia, vomiting, and diarrhea. There can also be diaphoresis, piloerection, and yawning. The *Diagnostic and Statistical Manual of Mental Disorders* (*DSM-5*) lists criteria for the diagnosis of opioid withdrawal, as shown in Table 38.3.[61] Clinicians in the ICU may find the *DSM-5* criteria difficult to apply directly, given the many dynamic comorbid disease processes present in many ICU patients. Intensive care unit staff must be aware of iatrogenic opioid withdrawal symptoms; we recommend tracking a patient's analgesia and sedative use for a fixed time interval (e.g., 12 or 24 hours) to identify appreciable decreases in use, which may indicate a patient's increased risk of withdrawal. Long-term, high-dose, continuous administration

Table 38.3 Diagnostic Criteria for Opioid Withdrawal

Criterion	Description
A	Reduction in dose or complete cessation of opioid after prolonged or heavy use OR Administration of an opioid antagonist after a period of opioid use
B	Presence of at least three of the following signs/symptoms developing within minutes to days of criterion A: • Dysphoric mood • Nausea or vomiting • Muscle aches • Lacrimation or rhinorrhea • Pupillary dilation, piloerection, or sweating • Diarrhea • Yawning • Fever • Insomnia
C	Criterion B symptoms cause clinically significant distress or impairment
D	Symptoms not better explained by other cause

Adapted from: Diagnostic and Statistical Manual of Mental Disorders (DSM-5). Substance-Related and Addictive Disorders. Arlington, VA: American Psychiatric Publishing, 2013.

of opioids is likely to place patients at increased risk of withdrawal later in their hospital stay. Intensive care unit clinicians should try to identify these at-risk patients before withdrawal symptoms start.

Severity and onset of withdrawal vary and are influenced by the dose of opioid and the duration of use. There is some evidence that route of administration also plays a role. In a retrospective analysis of heroin users who underwent acute withdrawal after inpatient admission for treatment, injection users had increased severity using the clinical opiate withdrawal scale.[62] Onset of withdrawal varies depending on the half-life of the opioid. Agents having a longer half-life result in a later onset of withdrawal symptoms.[63]

A less common, but more severe complication reported in the literature is takotsubo cardiomyopathy. A 60-year-old woman who stopped taking sustained-release morphine when her prescription ran out sought care when she began to have withdrawal symptoms. She developed chest pain and underwent cardiac catheterization, which did not reveal coronary disease. Echocardiography showed apical hypokinesis with basal hypercontractility and a reduced ejection fraction.[64] Cases have also been reported after withdrawal of heroin, methadone, and buprenorphine.[65-67]

Of importance, opioid withdrawal can occur in a variety of situations and not just in the heroin user. The rise in use of prescription opioids has resulted in a rise in abuse of these medications as well.[68] Many patients are receiving chronic opioid therapy in the treatment of chronic pain and are therefore subject to the potential for withdrawal.

Management

Many methods are available in the management of opioid withdrawal. Definitive management is resuming opioid therapy. In non-intubated patients, simply resuming the patient's prehospital opioid medication regimen in those using opioids for chronic pain may stave off withdrawal symptoms. If avoiding withdrawal is the primary concern, lower opioid doses are usually sufficient to attenuate withdrawal symptoms, compared with analgesia dosing. In the critically ill, mechanically ventilated patient, opioids are commonly used for pain management, and they greatly reduce the risk of opioid withdrawal during the acute ICU admission.

Administering a long-acting opioid agonist such as methadone to act as a maintenance therapy is another option. Although this strategy when allowing the withdrawal syndrome to occur may be medically undesirable (e.g., in the pregnant mother), it has other complicating factors. Methadone can cause corrected QT (QTc) prolongation leading to fatal dysrhythmias.[69] The potential for synergistic effects on the QT interval in the critically ill patient who may already be undergoing pharmacotherapy with agents that can prolong the QT makes this of particular concern. Legal concerns also make methadone potentially problematic. In some states, treating opioid withdrawal syndrome with methadone is only permissible as an adjunct to a primary medical or surgical problem. Table 38.4 provides dosing recommendations for opioid withdrawal management using methadone over 2 weeks. Twice-daily dosing is recommended to mitigate the risk of overdose on methadone initiation during days 1–4.[70]

When opioid administration is not desired or is expected to be ineffective, such as after administering an opioid antagonist like naloxone, an α_2-adrenergic agonist can be used. These agents act at the α_2-adrenergic receptor, resulting in a decrease in neuronal transmission in a fashion similar to opioids. In this way, they decrease sympathetic outflow and reduce the withdrawal symptoms. Because they inhibit adrenergic tone, there is a risk of hypotension and bradycardia when using these agents. Clonidine, the most common medication of this class, is used with a dosing regimen of 0.1–0.2 mg orally every 4–6 hours (see Figure 38.3). A Cochrane review from 2014 found the α_2-adrenergic agonists clonidine and lofexidine to be superior to placebo in the treatment of opioid withdrawal.[71] There is growing interest in the use of dexmedetomidine for opioid withdrawal syndrome. It is similar to clonidine but is available as a titratable intravenous infusion with a greater affinity for the α_2-receptor.[72] Its use has been described in both adults and pediatric populations, and it has been shown to be safe in the critically ill.[73-75] Given the limited data, dexmedetomidine has been recommended as adjunctive therapy until more research has been conducted to better define doses and limitations.[76]

BENZODIAZEPINE WITHDRAWAL

Background

Benzodiazepines represent a class of medications commonly used for their anticonvulsant, anxiolytic, muscle-relaxant, and sedative properties.[77,78] Benzodiazepines achieve these effects through binding of the GABAA receptor, binding

Table 38.4 Methadone for Opioid Withdrawal Management

Days 1–4	15 mg by mouth twice daily
Days 5–8	35 mg by mouth once daily
Day 9	30 mg by mouth once daily
Day 10	25 mg by mouth once daily
Day 11	20 mg by mouth once daily
Day 12	15 mg by mouth once daily
Day 13	10 mg by mouth once daily
Day 14	5 mg by mouth once daily
Day 15	Stop

Adapted from: World Health Organization (WHO). Clinical Guidelines for Withdrawal Management of Drug Dependence in Closed Setting. Geneva: WHO, 2009.

between the α and β subunits.[79] Unlike other sedative-hypnotics (e.g., barbiturates), benzodiazepines require GABA to exert their functional effects. With long-term exposure to benzodiazepines and other GABAA agonists, GABA receptors may be down-regulated, making the neuronal cell more excitable, potentiating serious withdrawal syndromes.[79]

Diagnosis

Hallmark symptoms of benzodiazepine withdrawal include, but are not limited to, headaches, tremors, seizures, hallucinations, tachycardia, hypertension, diaphoresis, perceptual changes, and other findings common to critically ill patients not having benzodiazepine withdrawal.[80] The usual course of benzodiazepine withdrawal follows three phases: first, there is a "rebound" of the symptom originally treated (e.g., insomnia, anxiety) lasting 1–4 days, depending on the pharmacokinetic properties of the individual agent; second, there is "full-blown" withdrawal, which may last up to 14 days; and third, there is a reemergence of the disease process originally treated.[80] A clinical diagnosis may be made on the basis of a patient's presentation, what is known of the patient's medical history, and evaluation of the patient's medication list or a controlled substance prescription database, when available. Severe withdrawal symptoms are more likely to be realized in patients using short-acting benzodiazepines; longer-acting benzodiazepines often contain active metabolites and result in a self-titrating effect.[80] Patients with long-term use of benzodiazepines for several years may have a higher incidence of withdrawal symptoms; in one study, 27%–45% of diazepam or lorazepam users, for an average of 3.5 years, experienced withdrawal symptoms.[81-83]

Management

Commonly used sedation strategies in the ICU—as-needed administration of benzodiazepines or continuous infusions of propofol—attenuate the effects of benzodiazepine withdrawal, given their activation of the GABAA receptor.[84] Current guidelines regarding pain and agitation state that "sedation strategies using nonbenzodiazepine sedatives (either propofol or dexmedetomidine) may be preferred to sedation with benzodiazepines (either midazolam or lorazepam) to improve clinical outcomes in mechanically ventilated adult ICU patients."[85] Clinicians are advised to avoid continuous infusions of benzodiazepines; however, the phrasing of the guideline statement may lead clinicians to eschew any use of benzodiazepines for fear of worsening the delirium. Isolated, judicious use of as-needed benzodiazepine doses is highly unlikely to result in clinically relevant withdrawal symptoms. Given the pharmacologic differences between benzodiazepines and barbiturates, barbiturates are an effective strategy for patients with benzodiazepine withdrawal syndromes refractory to the simple reintroduction of benzodiazepines.[86] Clinicians are cautioned to use barbiturates judiciously given the unfavorable safety profile of barbiturates relative to benzodiazepines. Table 38.5 provides a suggested regimen using diazepam for high-dose benzodiazepine withdrawal, defined as patients using greater than 50 mg/day of diazepam, or equivalent benzodiazepines. It is recommended to reduce doses on the basis of a patient's tolerability; if a patient has withdrawal symptoms, experts recommend staying at the current dose of the taper until the patient tolerates the dose before further reduction and recommend against increasing the dose. For this reason, no precise time interval is recommended in Table 38.5; doses are reported as milligrams of diazepam, but equivalent benzodiazepine doses may certainly be substituted as indicated.

Table 38.6 is a compilation of suggested dose equivalents for oral benzodiazepines. Dose equivalency is an inexact science, and clinicians must account for interpatient variability together with differences in absorption, onset, protein binding, duration, and presence of pertinent active metabolite(s), together with the intended use of

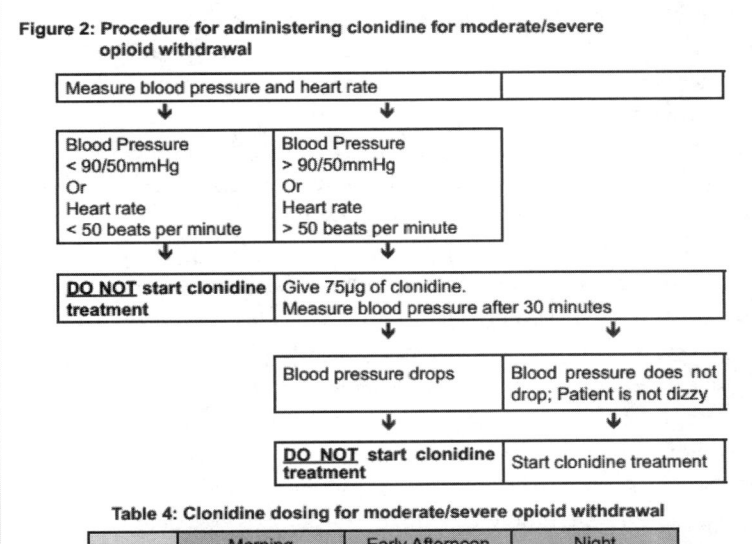

Figure 38.3 Procedure for administering clonidine for moderate/severe opioid withdrawal.

Reprinted from: World Health Organization (WHO). Clinical Guidelines for Withdrawal Management of Drug Dependence in Closed Setting. Geneva: WHO, 2009.

Table 38.5 High-Dose Benzodiazepine Reduction Schedule[a]

	Morning	Afternoon	Evening	Nighttime
Start of taper	10	10	10	10
First reduction	10	5	5	10
Second reduction	5	—	5	10
Third reduction	—	—	—	10
Fourth reduction	—	—	—	5

[a]Doses reported in milligrams of diazepam.

benzodiazepines.[70,79,87,88] Appropriate monitoring is warranted with the administration of any benzodiazepine, regardless of the proposed equipotency (note the listed ranges for various benzodiazepine equivalents).

α_2-AGONIST WITHDRAWAL

Background

α_2-Adrenergic agonists and imidazoline derivatives (e.g., clonidine, guanfacine, tizanidine, dexmedetomidine) are treatments for a variety of medical diagnoses, including essential hypertension, attention-deficit/hyperactivity disorder, nasal congestion, Gilles de la Tourette syndrome, opioid withdrawal, spasticity, sedation, open-angle glaucoma, ocular hypertension, and tension-type headaches. This class of medications may be administered by oral (immediate- and extended-release formulations), intravenous, transdermal, and topical (nasal and ophthalmologic) routes.[89] α_2-Adrenergic receptors are found in the central and peripheral nervous systems; the central effects of presynaptic agonism inhibit sympathetic outflow, resulting in bradycardia and hypotension.[90]

Individual agents differ in their affinity for imidazoline and α_2-receptors, centrally and peripherally. The effects of each receptor subtype, together with the interplay between central α_2 and imidazoline receptors' contributions to hypotension, have not been fully elucidated. Dexmedetomidine has high affinity for the α_{2A}-receptor, which is thought to provide the sedative effects of this and other α_2-agonists.[91]

Although structurally dissimilar, α_2-agonists (particularly clonidine) attenuate the untoward effects of opioid withdrawal.[92] Along these same lines, the opioid-receptor antagonist naloxone reverses some effects of clonidine overdose.[93] This effective overlap is hypothesized to stem from the similar effects of opioids and α_2-agonists on potassium efflux in the locus ceruleus.[94]

Diagnosis

Abrupt tapering or cessation of centrally acting α_2-adrenergic agonists can induce withdrawal symptoms,

Table 38.6 Oral Benzodiazepine Approximate Equipotent Doses[70,79,87,88]

Alprazolam	0.5–1 mg
Chlordiazepoxide	25–50 mg
Clonazepam	0.5 mg
Diazepam	10 mg
Lorazepam	1–2 mg
Midazolam	5 mg

Adapted from: World Health Organization (WHO). Clinical Guidelines for Withdrawal Management of Drug Dependence in Closed Setting. Geneva: WHO, 2009.

including rebound hypertension, insomnia, delirium, irritability, tremor, and palpitations.[90,95-100] Neuroleptic malignant syndrome, malignant hyperthermia, and serotonin syndrome are examples of potentially medication-induced symptoms that can easily be confused with α_2-agonist withdrawal.[99] Expanding beyond medication-induced causes, withdrawal can easily be overlooked in critically ill patients, given the nonspecific symptoms associated with an increase in sympathomimetic activity. Withdrawal symptoms from oral clonidine are expected to present within 16–72 hours of cessation.[99,100]

A case of clonidine prescribed to alleviate withdrawal symptoms that resulted in a prolonged stay in the ICU secondary to iatrogenic clonidine withdrawal highlights the need to keep α_2-agonist withdrawal in the differential diagnosis.[99] A patient on an intrathecal clonidine pump failure had severe withdrawal, which resulted in stress-induced cardiomyopathy, highlighting the serious consequences of clonidine withdrawal.[101] Reports of dexmedetomidine withdrawal exist in the literature with features similar to clonidine and other α_2-agonist withdrawal.[96,97] These cases are associated with prolonged use of dexmedetomidine and can be managed through modalities described in the next section.

Management

α_2-Agonists may be used for opioid withdrawal; conversely, morphine administration attenuates hypertension-associated α_2-agonist withdrawal in rats.[71,102] Because opioids are commonly administered in the ICU setting for analgesia,[85] this theoretically may blunt some of the effects seen with α_2-agonist withdrawal. More studies in humans are needed before opioids can be recommended solely for α_2-agonist withdrawal. Given the safety concerns with opioids, regardless of a patient's sex, we do not recommend using opioids solely to manage α_2-agonist withdrawal.[103] Mild cases of α_2-agonist withdrawal may be managed nonpharmacologically with monitoring and supportive care. Cases increasing in severity may be managed either indirectly (with supportive measures) or directly (administration of the recently withdrawn agent or another α_2-agonist).[96,97] We are unaware of any reports using dexmedetomidine to manage withdrawal of an α_2-agonist agent and do not recommend this approach at present. Clonidine has the largest body of literature regarding its withdrawal, partly because of its widespread use but also because of the pharmacokinetic properties relative to other α_2-agonists (e.g., shorter half-life than guanfacine). The longer half-life agents are thought to self-taper and are hypothesized to have less severe withdrawal symptoms as a result.[100]

CONCLUSION

The intent of this chapter was to provide a brief overview of the diagnosis, management, and potential treatments for patients with medication withdrawal; we recognize that this does not list all the potential medications that patients may withdraw from. Together with resource use, safety, cost, and other considerations, clinicians are encouraged to weigh the risks and benefits of withdrawal management in the ICU. An interdisciplinary approach to determining a patient's actual medication use, with a well-trained clinical pharmacist readily available, is invaluable in identifying patients with potential medication withdrawal early in their ICU stay. Clinicians are encouraged to consider iatrogenic withdrawal syndromes in addition to prehospital medication withdrawal manifesting in the ICU. Medication withdrawal is rarely the cause for a patient's ICU admission; however, if withdrawal is not identified, or is left untreated, it can further complicate the care of ICU patients. All members of the interdisciplinary ICU team should be aware of these potentially serious medical issues.

REFERENCES

1. Coffey JR, Cahill D, Steers W, et al. Intrathecal baclofen for intractable spasticity of spinal origin: results of a long-term multicenter study. J Neurosurg 1993;2:226-32.
2. Nasti JJ, Brakoulias V. Chronic baclofen abuse and withdrawal delirium. Aust N Z J Psychiatry 2011;1:86-7.
3. Khurana SR, Garg DS. Spasticity and the use of intrathecal baclofen in patients with spinal cord injury. Phys Med Rehabil Clin North Am 2014;3:655-69, ix.
4. Shellock FG, Crivelli R, Venugopalan R. Programmable infusion pump and catheter: evaluation using 3-tesla magnetic resonance imaging. Neuromodulation 2008;3:163-70.
5. Kroin JS, Bianchi GD, Penn RD. Intrathecal baclofen down-regulates GABAB receptors in the rat substantia gelatinosa. J Neurosurg 1993;4:544-9.
6. Leo RJ, Baer D. Delirium associated with baclofen withdrawal: a review of common presentations and management strategies. Psychosomatics 2005;6:503-7.
7. Ben Smail D, Hugeron C, Denys P, et al. Pruritus after intrathecal baclofen withdrawal: a retrospective study. Arch Phys Med Rehabil 2005;3:494-7.
8. Duhon BS, MacDonald JD. Infusion of intrathecal baclofen for acute withdrawal. Technical note. J Neurosurg 2007;4:878-80.
9. McAllen KJ, Schwartz DR. Adverse drug reactions resulting in hyperthermia in the intensive care unit. Crit Care Med 2010;38(6 suppl):S244-52.
10. Rolland B, Jaillette E, Carton L, et al. Assessing alcohol versus baclofen withdrawal syndrome in patients treated with baclofen for alcohol use disorder. J Clin Psychopharmacol 2014;1:153-6.
11. Ross JC, Cook AM, Stewart GL, et al. Acute intrathecal baclofen withdrawal: a brief review of treatment options. Neurocrit Care 2011;1:103-8.
12. Salazar ML, Eiland LS. Intrathecal baclofen withdrawal resembling serotonin syndrome in an adolescent boy with cerebral palsy. Pediatr Emerg Care 2008;10:691-3.
13. Specchio N, Carotenuto A, Trivisano M, et al. Prolonged episode of dystonia and dyskinesia resembling status epilepticus following acute intrathecal baclofen withdrawal. Epilepsy Behav 2011;3:321-3.
14. Watve SV, Sivan M, Raza WA, et al. Management of acute overdose or withdrawal state in intrathecal baclofen therapy. Spinal Cord 2012;2:107-11.
15. Douglas AF, Weiner HL, Schwartz DR. Prolonged intrathecal baclofen withdrawal syndrome. Case report and discussion of current therapeutic management. J Neurosurg 2005;6:1133-6.
16. Saveika JA, Shelton JE. Cyproheptadine for pediatric intrathecal baclofen withdrawal: a case report. Am J Phys Med Rehabil 2007;12:994-7.
17. Shirley KW, Kothare S, Piatt JH Jr, et al. Intrathecal baclofen overdose and withdrawal. Pediatr Emerg Care 2006;4:258-61.
18. Ackland GL, Fox R. Low-dose propofol infusion for controlling acute hyperspasticity after withdrawal of intrathecal baclofen therapy. Anesthesiology 2005;3:663-5.
19. Cruikshank M, Eunson P. Intravenous diazepam infusion in the management of planned intrathecal baclofen withdrawal. Dev Med Child Neurol 2007;8:626-8.
20. LeTourneau JL, Hagg DS, Smith SM. Baclofen and gamma-hydroxybutyrate withdrawal. Neurocrit Care 2008;3:430-3.
21. U.S. Food and Drug Administration (FDA). REMS@FDA, Available at www.accessdata.fda.gov/scripts/cder/rems/index.cfm. Accessed March 15, 2015.

22. Hansen CR, Gooch JL, Such-Neibar T. Prolonged, severe intrathecal baclofen withdrawal syndrome: a case report. Arch Phys Med Rehabil 2007;11:1468-71.
23. Bellinger A, Siriwetchadarak R, Rosenquist R, et al. Prevention of intrathecal baclofen withdrawal syndrome: successful use of a temporary intrathecal catheter. Reg Anesth Pain Med 2009;6:600-2.
24. Pratt LA, Brody DJ, Quiping G. Antidepressant Use in Persons Aged 12 and Over: United States, 2005–2008. NCHS Data Brief, No. 76. Hyattsville, MD: National Center for Health Statistics, 2011.
25. Rosenbaum JF, Fava M, Hoog SL, et al. Selective serotonin reuptake inhibitor discontinuation syndrome: a randomized clinical trial. Biol Psychiatry 1998;2:77-87.
26. Haddad P. The SSRI discontinuation syndrome. J Psychopharmacol 1998;3:305-13.
27. Leiter FL, Nierenberg AA, Sanders KM, et al. Discontinuation reactions following sertraline. Biol Psychiatry 1995;10:694-5.
28. Fava GA, Gatti A, Belaise C, et al. Withdrawal symptoms after selective serotonin reuptake inhibitor discontinuation: a systematic review. Psychother Psychosom 2015;2:72-81.
29. Renoir T. Selective serotonin reuptake inhibitor antidepressant treatment discontinuation syndrome: a review of the clinical evidence and the possible mechanisms involved. Front Pharmacol 2013;16:4-45.
30. Astorne Figari WJ, Herrmann S, et al. New onset hypertension following abrupt discontinuation of citalopram. Clin Nephrol 2014;3:202-4.
31. Williams GW, Gandhi SJ, Altamirano A. An acute neurological syndrome with cerebrovascular and parkinsonian clinical features associated with perioperative SNRI withdrawal. J Neurosurg Anesthesiol 2013;3:353-4.
32. Black K, Shea C, Dursun S, et al. Selective serotonin reuptake inhibitor discontinuation syndrome: proposed diagnostic criteria. J Psychiatry Neurosci 2000;3:255-61.
33. Schatzberg AF, Blier P, Delgado PL, et al. Antidepressant discontinuation syndrome: consensus panel recommendations for clinical management and additional research. J Clin Psychiatry 2006;67(suppl 4):27-30.
34. Stork CM. Chapter 75 Serotonin reuptake inhibitors and atypical antidepressants. In: Hoffman RS, Howland MA, Lewin N, et al., eds. Goldfrank's Toxicologic Emergencies, 10th ed. Pages 1018-28. New York: McGraw-Hill, 2014.
35. Benowitz NL. Drug therapy. Pharmacologic aspects of cigarette smoking and nicotine addition. N Engl J Med 1988;20:1318-30.
36. Changeux JP, Edelstein SJ. Nicotinic Acetylcholine Receptors: From Molecular Biology to Cognition. New York: Odile Jacob, 2005.
37. Pomerleau OF, Pomerleau CS. Neuroregulators and the reinforcement of smoking: towards a biobehavioral explanation. Neurosci Biobehav Rev 1984;4:503-13.
38. West RJ, Russell MA. Cardiovascular and subjective effects of smoking before and after 24 h of abstinence from cigarettes. Psychopharmacology (Berl) 1987;1:118-21.
39. Clark BJ, Moss M. Secondary prevention in the intensive care unit: does intensive care unit admission represent a "teachable moment"? Crit Care Med 2011;6:1500-6.
40. Rigotti NA, Munafo MR, Stead LF. Smoking cessation interventions for hospitalized smokers: a systematic review. Arch Intern Med 2008;18:1950-60.
41. Dubois MJ, Bergeron N, Dumont M, et al. Delirium in an intensive care unit: a study of risk factors. Intensive Care Med 2001;8:1297-304.
42. Lucidarme O, Seguin A, Daubin C, et al. Nicotine withdrawal and agitation in ventilated critically ill patients. Crit Care 2010;2:R58.
43. Joseph AM, Norman SM, Ferry LH, et al. The safety of transdermal nicotine as an aid to smoking cessation in patients with cardiac disease. N Engl J Med 1996;24:1792-8.
44. Kimmel SE, Berlin JA, Miles C, et al. Risk of acute first myocardial infarction and use of nicotine patches in a general population. J Am Coll Cardiol 2001;5:1297-302.
45. Tzivoni D, Keren A, Meyler S, et al. Cardiovascular safety of transdermal nicotine patches in patients with coronary artery disease who try to quit smoking. Cardiovasc Drugs Ther 1998;3:239-44.
46. Lee AH, Afessa B. The association of nicotine replacement therapy with mortality in a medical intensive care unit. Crit Care Med 2007;6:1517-21.
47. Paciullo CA, Short MR, Steinke DT, et al. Impact of nicotine replacement therapy on postoperative mortality following coronary artery bypass graft surgery. Ann Pharmacother 2009;7:1197-202.
48. Cartin-Ceba R, Warner DO, Hays JT, et al. Nicotine replacement therapy in critically ill patients: a prospective observational cohort study. Crit Care Med 2011;7:1635-40.
49. Gillies MA, McKenzie CA, Whiteley C, et al. Safety of nicotine replacement therapy in critically ill smokers: a retrospective cohort study. Intensive Care Med 2012;10:1683-8.
50. Tran-Van D, Herve Y, Labadie P, et al. [Restlessness in intensive care unit: think to the nicotinic withdrawal syndrome]. Ann Fr Anesth Reanim 2004;6:604-6.
51. Healthcare GC. NicoDerm CQ label [package insert]. 2006. Accessed 2/22/15 URL: http://www.accessdata.fda.gov/drugsatfda_docs/label/2006/020165s023lbl.pdf.
52. Wilby KJ, Harder CK. Nicotine replacement therapy in the intensive care unit: a systematic review. J Intensive Care Med 2014;1:22-30.
53. Seder DB, Schmidt JM, Badjatia N, et al. Transdermal nicotine replacement therapy in cigarette smokers with acute subarachnoid hemorrhage. Neurocrit Care 2011;1:77-83.
54. Franks P, Harp J, Bell B. Randomized, controlled trial of clonidine for smoking cessation in a primary care setting. JAMA 1989;21:3011-3.
55. Gourlay S, Forbes A, Marriner T, et al. A placebo-controlled study of three clonidine doses for smoking cessation. Clin Pharmacol Ther 1994;1:64-9.
56. Benich JJ III. Opioid dependence. Prim Care 2011;1:59-70, vi.
57. Nelson LS, Olsen D. Chapter 38 Opioids. In: Hoffman RS, Howland MA, Lewin N, et al., eds. Goldfrank's Toxicologic Emergencies, 10th ed. Pages 492-509. New York: McGraw-Hill, 2014.
58. Tetrault JM, O'Connor PG. Substance abuse and withdrawal in the critical care setting. Crit Care Clin 2008;4:767-88, viii.

59. Rehni AK, Jaggi AS, Singh N. Opioid withdrawal syndrome: emerging concepts and novel therapeutic targets. CNS Neurol Disord Drug Targets 2013;1:112-25.

60. Holstege CP, Borek HA. Toxidromes. Crit Care Clin 2012;4:479-98.

61. Diagnostic and Statistical Manual of Mental Disorders (DSM-5). Substance-Related and Addictive Disorders. Arlington, VA: American Psychiatric Publishing, 2013.

62. Smolka M, Schmidt LG. The influence of heroin dose and route of administration on the severity of the opiate withdrawal syndrome. Addiction 1999;8:1191-8.

63. Gordon D, Dahl J. Opioid withdrawal, #95, 2nd ed. J Palliat Med 2011;8:965-6.

64. Sarcon A, Ghadri JR, Wong G, et al. Takotsubo cardiomyopathy associated with opiate withdrawal. QJM 2014;4:301-2.

65. Maruyama S, Nomura Y, Fukushige T, et al. Suspected takotsubo cardiomyopathy caused by withdrawal of bupirenorphine in a child. Circ J 2006;4:509-11.

66. Revelo AE, Pallavi R, Espana-Schmidt C, et al. "Stoned" people can get stunned myocardium: a case of heroin withdrawal precipitating Tako-Tsubo cardiomyopathy. Int J Cardiol 2013;3:e96-8.

67. Saiful FB, Lafferty J, Jun CH, et al. Takotsubo cardiomyopathy due to iatrogenic methadone withdrawal. Rev Cardiovasc Med 2011;3:164-7.

68. Patel G. The management of substance abuse in the critically ill. Dis Mon 2014;8:429-41.

69. Stringer J, Welsh C, Tommasello A. Methadone-associated Q-T interval prolongation and torsades de pointes. Am J Health Syst Pharm 2009;9:825-33.

70. World Health Organization (WHO). Clinical Guidelines for Withdrawal Management of Drug Dependence in Closed Setting. Geneva: WHO, 2009.

71. Gowing L, Farrell MF, Ali R, et al. Alpha2-adrenergic agonists for the management of opioid withdrawal. Cochrane Database Syst Rev 2014;3:CD002024.

72. Giovannitti JA Jr, Thoms SM, Crawford JJ. Alpha-2 adrenergic receptor agonists: a review of current clinical applications. Anesth Prog 2015;1:31-9.

73. Honey BL, Benefield RJ, Miller JL, et al. Alpha2-receptor agonists for treatment and prevention of iatrogenic opioid abstinence syndrome in critically ill patients. Ann Pharmacother 2009;9:1506-11.

74. Oschman A, McCabe T, Kuhn RJ. Dexmedetomidine for opioid and benzodiazepine withdrawal in pediatric patients. Am J Health Syst Pharm 2011;13:1233-8.

75. Upadhyay SP, Mallick PN, Elmatite WM, et al. Dexmedetomidine infusion to facilitate opioid detoxification and withdrawal in a patient with chronic opioid abuse. Indian J Palliat Care 2011;3:251-4.

76. Albertson TE, Chenoweth J, Ford J, et al. Is it prime time for alpha2-adrenocepter agonists in the treatment of withdrawal syndromes? J Med Toxicol 2014;4:369-81.

77. Poyares D, Guilleminault C, Ohayon MM, et al. Chronic benzodiazepine usage and withdrawal in insomnia patients. J Psychiatr Res 2004;3:327-34.

78. Vicens C, Fiol F, Llobera J, et al. Withdrawal from long-term benzodiazepine use: randomised trial in family practice. Br J Gen Pract 2006;533:958-63.

79. Lee DC. Chapter 74 Sedative-Hypnotics. In: Hoffman RS, Howland MA, Lewin N, et al., eds. Goldfrank's Toxicologic Emergencies, 10th ed. Pages 1002-1017. New York: McGraw-Hill, 2014.

80. Petursson H. The benzodiazepine withdrawal syndrome. Addiction 1994;11:1455-9.

81. Onyett SR. The benzodiazepine withdrawal syndrome and its management. J R Coll Gen Pract 1989;321:160-3.

82. Tyrer P, Rutherford D, Huggett T. Benzodiazepine withdrawal symptoms and propranolol. Lancet 1981;8219:520-2.

83. Murphy SM, Tyrer P. A double-blind comparison of the effects of gradual withdrawal of lorazepam, diazepam and bromazepam in benzodiazepine dependence. Br J Psychiatry 1991;511-6.

84. Yip GM, Chen ZW, Edge CJ, et al. A propofol binding site on mammalian GABAA receptors identified by photolabeling. Nat Chem Biol 2013;11:715-20.

85. Barr J, Fraser GL, Puntillo K, et al. Clinical practice guidelines for the management of pain, agitation, and delirium in adult patients in the intensive care unit. Crit Care Med 2013;1:263-306.

86. Kawasaki SS, Jacapraro JS, Rastegar DA. Safety and effectiveness of a fixed-dose phenobarbital protocol for inpatient benzodiazepine detoxification. J Subst Abuse Treat 2012;3:331-4.

87. Ashton C. Benzodiazepines: How They Work and How to Withdraw (The Ashton Manual), Available at www.benzo.org.uk/manual/bzcha01.htm#4.

88. Farinde A. Benzodiazepine Equivalency Table. Available at http://emedicine.medscape.com/article/2172250-overview. Accessed March 2, 2015.

89. Hutchison TA, Shahan DR, Anderson ML. DRUGDEX System. Micromedex 2.0 [Internet database]. Greenwood Village, CO: Thomson Reuters (Healthcare). Updated periodically.

90. Reid JL, Wing LM, Dargie HJ, et al. Clonidine withdrawal in hypertension. Changes in blood-pressure and plasma and urinary noradrenaline. Lancet 1977;8023:1171-4.

91. Bhana N, Goa KL, McClellan KJ. Dexmedetomidine. Drugs 2000;2:263-8; discussion 69-70.

92. Gold MS, Redmond DE Jr, Kleber HD. Clonidine blocks acute opiate-withdrawal symptoms. Lancet 1978;8090:599-602.

93. Farsang C, Kapocsi J, Vajda L, et al. Reversal by naloxone of the antihypertensive action of clonidine: involvement of the sympathetic nervous system. Circulation 1984;3:461-7.

94. Aghajanian GK, Wang YY. Common alpha 2- and opiate effector mechanisms in the locus coeruleus: intracellular studies in brain slices. Neuropharmacology 1987;7B:793-9.

95. Karol DE, Muzyk AJ, Preud'homme XA. A case of delirium, motor disturbances, and autonomic dysfunction due to baclofen and tizanidine withdrawal: a review of the literature. Gen Hosp Psychiatry 2011;1:84 e1-2.

96. Kukoyi A, Coker S, Lewis L, et al. Two cases of acute dexmedetomidine withdrawal syndrome following prolonged infusion in the intensive care unit: report of cases and review of the literature. Hum Exp Toxicol 2013;1:107-10.

97. Miller JL, Allen C, Johnson PN. Neurologic withdrawal symptoms following abrupt discontinuation of a prolonged dexmedetomidine infusion in a child. J Pediatr Pharmacol Ther 2010;1:38-42.

98. Reid JL, Campbell BC, Hamilton CA. Withdrawal reactions following cessation of central alpha-adrenergic receptor agonists. Hypertension 1984;6(5 pt 2):II71-5.

99. Shaw M, Matsa R. Clonidine withdrawal induced sympathetic surge. BMJ Case Rep 2015; Jun 2;2015.

100. Wilson MF, Haring O, Lewin A, et al. Comparison of guanfacine versus clonidine for efficacy, safety and occurrence of withdrawal syndrome in step-2 treatment of mild to moderate essential hypertension. Am J Cardiol 1986;9:43E-49E.

101. Lee HM, Ruggoo V, Graudins A. Intrathecal clonidine pump failure causing acute withdrawal syndrome with "stress-induced" cardiomyopathy. J Med Toxicol 2015 Sep 14. [Epub ahead of print]

102. Thoolen MJ, Timmermans PP, van Zwieten PA. The influence of continuous infusion and sudden withdrawal of azepexole (B-HT 933) on blood pressure and heart rate in the spontaneously hypertensive and normotensive rat. Suppression of the withdrawal responses by morphine. J Pharmacol Exp Ther 1981;3:786-91.

103. Kaplovitch E, Gomes T, Camacho X, et al. Sex differences in dose escalation and overdose death during chronic opioid therapy: a population-based cohort study. PloS One 2015;8:e0134550.

Chapter 39 Endocrine Disorders

Robert L. Talbert, Pharm.D.

LEARNING OBJECTIVES

1. Describe the epidemiology, pathophysiology, clinical presentation (signs and symptoms), and management of myxedema coma, thyroid storm, adrenal insufficiency, hypercortisolism, and pheochromocytoma.
2. Outline nonpharmacologic and pharmacologic management of the disease states described above.

ABBREVIATIONS IN THIS CHAPTER

ACTH	Adrenocorticotropin hormone	TSH	Thyroid-stimulating hormone
CS	Cushing syndrome	T3	Triiodothyronine
FT4	Free thyroxine	T4	Thyroxine

THYROID DISORDERS

Myxedema Coma

Definition and Epidemiology

Myxedema coma is the term given to the most severe presentation of profound hypothyroidism, which is often fatal despite therapy. Decompensation of the patient with hypothyroidism into a coma may be precipitated by a few drugs (e.g., amiodarone, lithium, and sunitinib), systemic illnesses (e.g., pneumonia), and other causes. Myxedema coma typically presents in older women in the winter months and is associated with signs of hypothyroidism, hypothermia, hyponatremia, hypercarbia, and hypoxemia. Treatment must be initiated promptly in an intensive care unit setting. Although thyroid hormone therapy is critical to survival, it remains uncertain whether it should be administered as thyroxine (T4), triiodothyronine (T3), or both. Adjunctive measures, such as ventilation, warming, fluids, antibiotics, vasopressors, and corticosteroids, may be essential for survival. Mortality in myxedema coma is estimated to be as high as 25%–65%, and early recognition is key to survival.[1] The most typical precipitating factor is discontinuation of thyroid hormone replacement therapy, but this entity may be confused with other disease states such as hepatotoxicity. Careful attention to nonspecific complaints, myxedematous changes (e.g., puffiness and slowed mentation), and signs of dysfunction of any organ system, especially in older female patients, may lead to the ultimate correct diagnosis. Any history of thyroid disease and evidence of a surgical scare indicating thyroid surgery would be important. Myxedema coma must be recognized and treated emergently, usually before laboratory confirmation. Ventilatory support and thyroid hormone replacement are the two most important therapeutic maneuvers in the treatment of myxedema coma.[2] In critical illness, thyroid function tests can be difficult to interpret, and some of these situations are summarized in Figure 39.1.

Pathophysiology

The underlying cause is a profound lack of T3 and T4; however, reduced deiodinase activity limiting the conversion of T4 to T3 may be a contributing factor. Some authors prefer intravenous T3, but others consider treatment with T3 or T4 equivalent. Controversy exists whether the combination of T3 and T4 is better than single-agent therapy. An important drug-induced presentation for myxedema coma is the concurrent use of amiodarone.[3,4] It is thought that amiodarone interferes with the extrathyroidal production of T3 from T4.

Clinical Presentation and Laboratory Diagnosis

Typical signs and symptoms of hypothyroidism (dry skin, brittle nails, weight gain, and lethargy as well as hypothermia, hyponatremia, hypercarbia, hypoxemia, and altered mental status) must be present. The recent development of rating scales may aid in the rapid diagnosis of impending and frank myxedema coma. The scoring systems include a composite of alterations of thermoregulatory system, central nervous system (CNS), cardiovascular system, gastrointestinal (GI) system, and metabolic system and presence or absence of a precipitating event.[5] In the scale developed by Chiong et al., six variables were created for the screening tool: heart rate, temperature, Glasgow Coma Scale, thyroid-stimulating hormone (TSH), free thyroxine (FT4), and precipitating factors. The screening tool has a sensitivity and specificity of about 80%; however, this study was based on a small number of patients, and validation with a larger population is needed. The screening tool for assessing myxedema coma is presented in Table 39.1.

Typical laboratory abnormalities include low FT4 and high TSH in primary myxedema coma and low TSH in secondary myxedema coma. In a series of 10 patients, Chiong et al. found TSH to range from about 10 mU/mL to 140 mU/L. The FT4 concentrations ranged from undetectable to 1.7 ng/dL.[5] Although this is a small study, it makes the point that interpretation of thyroid tests must be done in the context of the patient's clinical findings and with the understanding that concurrent disease states can influence thyroid tests and interpretation (see Figure 39.1).

Treatment

The mainstay of treatment is intravenous T3 or T4. Given that T3 is several times more potent than T4 and that T4 needs to be converted for the greater activity, T3 is the preferred drug. Although there are no randomized trials of intravenous T3, some authors recommend that T3 doses be normally administered at least 4 hours—and not

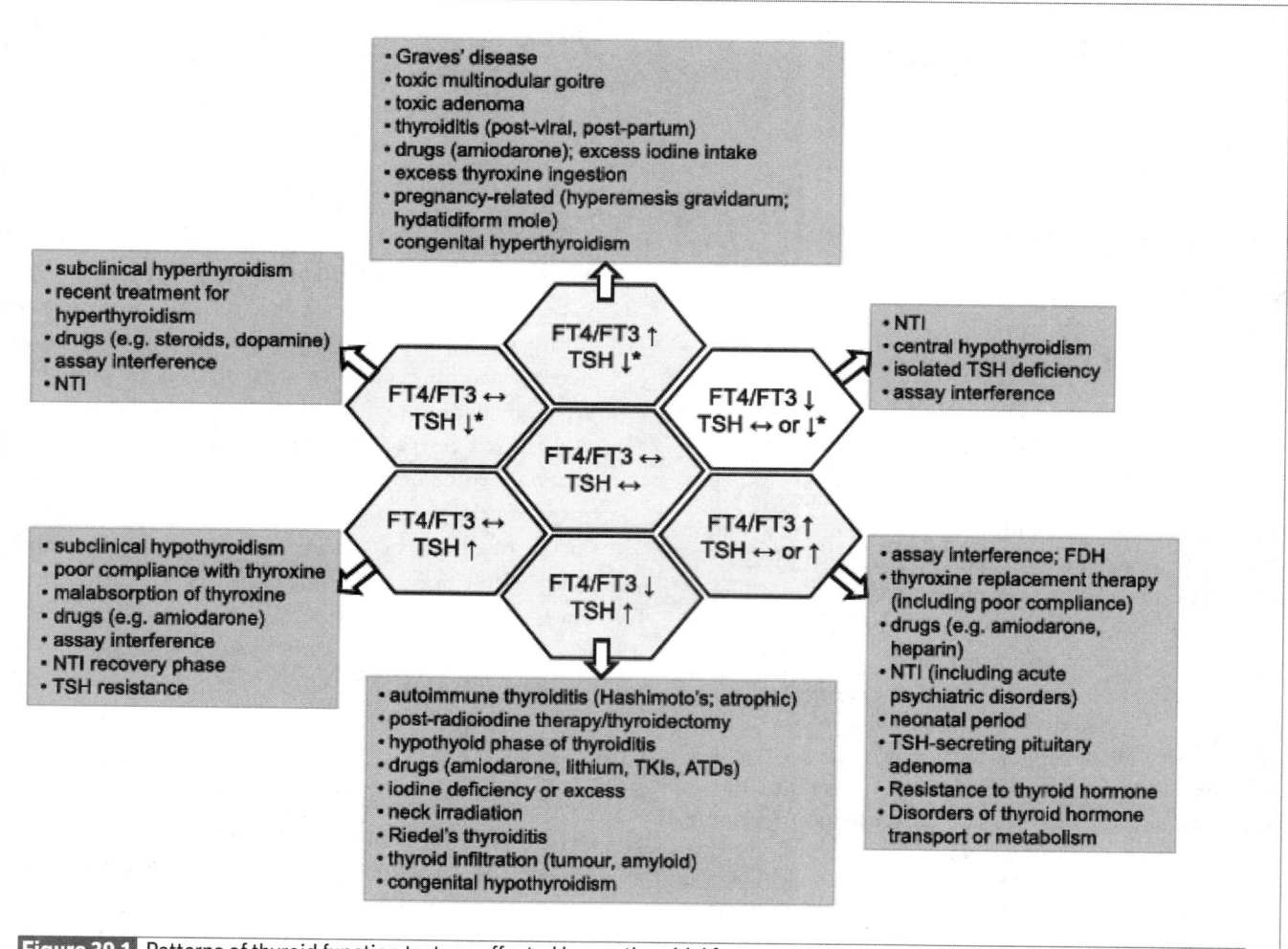

Figure 39.1 Patterns of thyroid function tests as affected by nonthyroidal factors.

ATD = antithyroid drug; FDH = familial dysalbuminemic hyperthyroxinemia; FT3 = free triiodothyronine; FT4 = free thyroxine; NTI = non-thyroidal illness; TKI = tyrosine kinase inhibitor; TSH = thyroid-stimulating hormone.

more than 12 hours—apart. An initial intravenous dose of T3 is 25–50 mcg for emergency treatment and then a daily dose of 10–20 mcg. If the patient has underlying cardiovascular disease, this dose may be excessive. According to the author's experience, oral dosing of T3 or T4 should be avoided because the bioavailability appears to be reduced, and normal absorption may not occur until several days after therapy is initiated. Once the clinical condition is stabilized, oral therapy may be resumed or initiated.

Glucocorticoid support is empirically administered if adrenal gland failure has occurred simultaneously and to help stabilize blood pressure. Hydrocortisone 100 mg intravenously every 8 hours is the standard approach. Some patients require intravenous vasopressor support, and norepinephrine is a logical choice. Ventilatory support as needed may be required in some patients. Addressing other precipitating factors such as underlying infection and sepsis is also an important aspect of care. Because many patients present with hypothermia, warming should be considered with very low body temperatures (less than 95°F).

Assessment of Outcomes

The two most important parameters to gauge the success of treatment are improving mental status as measured by the Glasgow Coma Scale and increasing levels of thyroid hormones and reduction in TSH.

Thyroid Storm (Thyroid Crisis)

Definition and Epidemiology

Thyroid storm, also known as thyroid crisis, is thyrotoxicosis in the extreme. It is considered a medical emergency and presents with many of the typical symptoms associated with hyperthyroidism, except that thyroid storm must have the component of altered mental status. The most common trigger for thyroid storm is discontinuation or irregular use of antithyroidal agents.

Although the prevalence of thyroid storm is imprecise because of the rare nature of this disorder, recent retrospective cohort studies suggest a prevalence of about 0.2 per 100,000 population.[6] Reports and reviews from 2 decades ago suggested that mortality with thyroid storm ranged from 20% to 100%, but more recent reports have found mortality rates ranging from 9.5% to 11%. This disparity is most likely because of better and earlier recognition of patients at risk of thyroid storm and more aggressive and earlier treatment. The most common cause of death is heart failure or multiorgan failure (see Tables 39.2 and 39.3).

Pathophysiology

The underlying pathophysiology is similar to thyrotoxicosis and is mediated by thyroid-stimulating autoantibodies

Table 39.1 Myxedema Coma Screening Tool

Criterion		Score
GCS		
0–10		4
11–13		3
14		2
15		0
TSH		
> 30 mU/L		2
15–30 mU/L		1
Low FT4[a]		1
Hypothermia (< 95°F)		1
Bradycardia (< 60 beats/min)		1
Precipitating event[b]		1
Total Score	**Category**	**Recommendation**
8–10		Proceed with treatment
5–7	Likely	Treat if there are no other plausible causes
< 5	Unlikely	Consider other diagnosis

[a]FT4 < 0.6 ng/dL.
[b]Events included burns, carbon monoxide retention, GI hemorrhage, infection/sepsis, medications, stroke, surgery, and trauma.
FT4 = free thyroxine; GCS = Glasgow Coma Scale (score); TSH = thyroid-stimulating hormone.
Adapted from: Chiong YV, Bammerlin E, Mariash CN. Development of an objective tool for the diagnosis of myxedema coma. Transl Res 2015;166:233-43.

Table 39.2 Thyroid Storm: Drugs and Doses

Drug	Dosing	Comment
Propylthiouracil	500–1,000 mg PO load; then 250 mg q4hr	Blocks new hormone synthesis
		Blocks T4–T3 conversion
		Should not be used in children because of hepatoxicity
Methimazole	60–80 mg/day PO in divided doses	Blocks new hormone synthesis
Propranolol	60–80 mg PO q4hr	Use with caution in decompensated systolic heart failure
		Blocks T4–T3 conversion at high doses
		Alternative drug: esmolol infusion
Sodium iodide	Up to 2 g/day PO in single or divided doses	Do not start until 1 hr after antithyroid drugs
		Blocks new hormone synthesis
		Blocks thyroid hormone release
Lugol solution	5–10 drops TID PO in water or juice	IBID
SSKI	1 or 2 drops TID PO in water or juice	IBID
Dexamethasone	5–20 mg/day PO or IV in divided doses	Prophylaxis against relative adrenal insufficiency
Prednisone	25–100 mg/day PO in divided doses	Prophylaxis against relative adrenal insufficiency
		Exists as a prodrug and methylprednisone or hydrocortisone may be better choices
Methylprednisolone	20–80 mg IV in divided doses	Prophylaxis against relative adrenal insufficiency
Hydrocortisone	300 mg IV load; then 100 mg q8hr	Prophylaxis against relative adrenal insufficiency
		May block conversion of T4 to T3
Acetaminophen	325–500 mg TID-QID PO not to exceed 2 g/day	Should be used instead of NSAID. NSAID may displace
		Thyroid hormone from plasma proteins thereby increasing free fraction

IV = intravenous(ly); NSAID = nonsteroidal anti-inflammatory agent; PO = orally; q = every; TID = three times daily; QID = four times daily.
Modified from: DiPiro JT, Talbert RL, Yee GC, et al., eds. Pharmacotherapy: A Pathophysiologic Approach, 9th ed. New York: McGraw-Hill, 2014:1191-216.

directed against the thyrotropin receptor on the surface of the thyroid cell. Binding of these immunoglobins to the receptor activates downstream G-protein signaling and adenylate cyclase in the same manner as TSH. Because the thyroid hormones T3 and T4 bind to receptors in many tissues in the body, the symptoms and clinical presentation can affect many organ systems.

Clinical Presentation and Laboratory Diagnosis

Compared with thyrotoxicosis, the presenting symptoms are qualitatively similar but more severe (see Table 39.4). In addition to the common signs and symptoms of thyrotoxicosis, multiorgan system failure may be seen in thyroid storm, and altered mental status is a required feature for the diagnosis. Other notable differences between thyrotoxicosis and thyroid storm are GI and hepatic dysfunction (63% vs. 0%), the occurrence of atrial fibrillation (52% vs. 0%), and heart failure (33% vs. 0%).[7] In addition to signs, symptoms, and laboratory features, two notable clinical rating scales have been useful in earlier and more valid identification of thyroid storm. The Burch-Wartofsky score and the Akamizu criteria have been used for identifying thyroid storm.[8,9] The American Thyroid Association guidelines recommend a scale based on thermoregulatory dysfunction, cardiovascular features, GI-hepatic dysfunction, CNS dysfunction, and precipitant history (Table 39.5).

Precipitating factors for thyroid storm include infection, trauma, surgery, radioactive iodine treatment, and withdrawal of antithyroid drugs or lack of treatment. Although clinical decompensation lasts an average of 72 hours, it may persist for up to 8 days.

Table 39.3 Laboratory Measurements in Thyroid Storm

Very low or undetectable TSH
Elevated free thyroxine
Elevated bilirubin
Elevated transaminases

Treatment

Treatment measures that should be instituted promptly include (1) suppression of thyroid hormone formation and release, (2) provision of antiadrenergic therapy, (3) administration of corticosteroids to preserve vasomotor tone, and (4) treatment of associated complications or coexisting factors that may have precipitated the storm such as infection requiring antimicrobial treatment. Of the thioamides, propylthiouracil is preferred because it blocks new hormone formation and the peripheral conversation of T4 to T3. Methimazole has a theoretical advantage because of its longer duration of action. Because methimazole is teratogenic, it should not be used in patients who are pregnant or thought to be pregnant. If patients cannot take orally administered medications, the tablets can be crushed into a suspension and instilled by gastric or rectal tube; oral therapy is not possible. All iodine therapy should be administered 1–2 hours after propylthiouracil or methimazole has been given to prevent iodine-stimulated thyroid hormone synthesis.

Esmolol infusion would be most useful in patients with systolic heart failure for whom the state of compensation is unknown because the drug has a very short half-life and is rapidly cleared on discontinuation. Propranolol can be given orally or intravenously, but recall that it has a large first-pass effect with oral administration, and the intravenous dose is small (0.5–1 mg) in comparison. The target heart rate with antiadrenergic therapy is usually 90–100 beats/minute.

Assessment of Outcomes

Signs and symptoms of thyroid storm may begin to resolve within 8–12 hours, but the return to entirely normal heart rate, mental status, and so forth may take as long as 1–2 weeks. Thyroid-stimulating hormone will continue to be suppressed for weeks after clinical improvement; however, FT4 concentrations should normalize in 1–2 weeks.

Table 39.4 Signs and Symptoms of Thyroid Storm

Symptoms	Signs
Altered mental status and/or coma	Fever (temperature often > 39.4°C or 103°F)
Anxiety	Tachycardia
Palpitations	Tachypnea
Emotional liability	Dehydration
Heat intolerance	Vomiting
Nausea	Diarrhea
Psychosis	Hypotension
Lethargy	

Once the patient has become clinically sound, doses of the thionamides can be reduced to maintenance levels and corticosteroids tapered and discontinued within a few days of clinical stability. Rigorous follow-up is necessary to prevent relapses, and precipitating factors should be avoided.

PHEOCHROMOCYTOMA

Definition and Epidemiology

Pheochromocytomas are catecholamine-producing neuroendocrine tumors that can be adrenal or extra-adrenal in origin. In patients with an established mutation or hereditary syndrome, the condition may manifest at a younger age than in those with sporadic disease. Pheochromocytoma can be associated with certain genetic syndromes such as MEN 2 (multiple endocrine neoplasia type 2), NF (neurofibromatosis), and VHL (von Hippel-Lindau) syndrome. Pheochromocytoma is diagnosed with biochemical confirmation of hormonal excess followed by anatomical localization (CT [computed tomography] or MRI [magnetic resonance imaging]).

Pheochromocytoma occurs in 2–8 patients in 1,000,000, with about 1,000 cases diagnosed yearly in the United States. It mainly occurs in young or middle-aged adults, though it presents earlier in hereditary syndrome. About 15% are extra-adrenal (located in any orthosympathetic tissue); of these, 9% are in the abdomen, and 1% are located elsewhere. Some extra-adrenal pheochromocytomas are probably actually paragangliomas, but the distinction is only possible after surgical resection. Pheochromocytoma has an estimated prevalence of 0.1%–0.6% in individuals with hypertension; it is therefore a rare disease.

Pathophysiology

These tumors secrete high amounts of catecholamines, mainly epinephrine, plus norepinephrine to a lesser extent.

Clinical Presentation and Laboratory Diagnosis

The classic symptoms of pheochromocytoma are headache, palpitation, anxiety, and diaphoresis, and the tumor can occur at any age with equal sex distribution. Signs and symptoms of pheochromocytomas often include the following:

- High blood pressure
- Rapid or forceful heartbeat
- Profound sweating
- Severe headache
- Tremors
- Paleness in the face
- Shortness of breath

Table 39.5 Point Scale for the Diagnosis of Thyroid Storm

Criteria	Points
Temperature (°F)	
99.0–99.9	5
100.0–100.9	10
101.0–101.0	15
102.0–102.9	20
103.0–103.9	25
≥ 104.0	30
Cardiovascular, tachycardia (beats per minute)	
100–109	5
110–119	10
120–129	15
130–139	20
≥ 140	25
Atrial fibrillation	
Absent	0
Present	10
Heart failure	
Absent	0
Mild	5
Moderate	10
Severe	20
GI-hepatic dysfunction	
Absent	0
Moderate (diarrhea, abdominal pain, nausea/vomiting	10
Severe (jaundice)	20
CNS disturbance	
Absent	0
Mild (agitation)	10
Moderate (delirium, psychosis, extreme lethargy)	20
Severe (seizure, coma)	30
Precipitant history	
Positive	0
Negative	10
Scores totaled	
> 45	Thyroid storm
25–44	Impending storm
< 25	Storm unlikely

Modified from: Bahn et al. Hyperthyroidism and other causes of thyrotoxicosis; management guidelines of the American Thyroid Association anc American Association of Clinical Endocrinologists. Thyroid 2011;21:593-646

Less common signs or symptoms may include the following:

- Anxiety or sense of doom
- Abdominal pain
- Constipation
- Weight loss

These signs and symptoms often occur in brief spells of 15–20 minutes. Spells can occur several times a day or less often. Blood pressure may be within the normal range or remain elevated between episodes.

Diagnosis depends on biochemical evidence of excessive production of catecholamines. This is straightforward when test results are orders of magnitude above the concentrations expected in healthy individuals and those with essential hypertension. Equivocal results pose a management dilemma.

Evidence now indicates that initial screening for pheochromocytoma should include measurements of plasma-free metanephrines or urinary fractionated metanephrines. Liquid chromatography/mass spectrometry offers several advantages over other analytic methods and is the method of choice when measurements include methoxytyramine, the O-methylated metabolite of dopamine. The plasma test offers advantages over the urine test, although it is rarely implemented correctly, rendering the urine test preferable for mainstream use. To ensure optimal diagnostic sensitivity for the plasma test, reference intervals must be established for blood samples collected after 30 minutes of supine rest and after an overnight fast when measurements include methoxytyramine. Similarly, collected blood samples during screening, together with use of age-adjusted reference intervals, further minimize false-positive results. Extents and patterns of increases in plasma normetanephrine, metanephrine, and methoxytyramine can additionally help predict size and adrenal versus extra-adrenal locations of tumors, as well as the presence of metastases and underlying germline mutations of tumor susceptibility genes.[10]

One diagnostic test used in the past for a pheochromocytoma was to administer clonidine, a centrally acting α_2-agonist used to treat high blood pressure. Clonidine mimics catecholamines in the brain, causing it to reduce the activity of the sympathetic nerves controlling the adrenal medulla. A healthy adrenal medulla will respond to the clonidine suppression test by reducing catecholamine production; lack of a response is evidence of pheochromocytoma.

Treatment

Surgical resection of the tumor is the treatment of first choice, by either open laparotomy or laparoscopy. Given the complexity of perioperative management, and the potential for catastrophic intra- and postoperative complications, such surgery should be performed only at centers experienced in the management of this disorder. In addition to the surgical expertise that such centers can provide, they have the necessary endocrine and anesthesia resources. It may also be necessary to carry out adrenalectomy, a complete surgical removal of the affected adrenal gland(s). Either surgical option requires prior treatment with the non-specific and irreversible α-adrenoceptor blocker phenoxybenzamine or a short-acting α-antagonist (e.g., prazosin, terazosin, or doxazosin).[11] Phenoxybenzamine is lipophilic and may have blood pressuring–lower effects for up to 7 days after dosing. Initial doses in adults are 10–20 mg/day and up to 20–40 mg/day for maintenance. Bioavailability is 20%–30%, and variation from patient to patient is to be expected. An alternative rapid-acting α_1-antagonist is phentolamine. The initial dose is 5 mg intravenously/intramuscularly 1–2 hours before surgery, and repeated dosing if needed is 5 mg intravenously/intramuscularly every 2–4 hours. Unfortunately, the manufacturer has discontinued production of phentolamine, and currently, there is a shortage. Before surgery, the patient is conventionally prepared with α-adrenergic blockade (over 10–14 days), and subsequently, additional β-adrenergic blockade is required to treat any associated tachyarrhythmias. In preoperative assessment, it is obligatory to monitor arterial blood pressure. Doing so permits the surgery to proceed while minimizing the likelihood of severe intraoperative hypertension (as might occur when the tumor is manipulated). Some authorities would recommend that a combined α/β-blocker such as labetalol also be given to slow the heart rate. Regardless, a β_1-receptor selective β-blocker such as atenolol must never be used in the presence of a pheochromocytoma because of the risk of such a treatment leading to unopposed α-agonism and, thus, severe and potentially refractory hypertension. Studies have shown that labetalol is effective in the treatment of essential hypertension, renal hypertension, pheochromocytoma, pregnancy hypertension, and hypertensive emergencies.[12] The patient with pheochromocytoma is invariably volume depleted. The chronically elevated adrenergic state characteristic of an untreated pheochromocytoma leads to near-total inhibition of renin-angiotensin activity, resulting in excessive fluid loss in the urine and thus reduced blood volume. Hence, once the pheochromocytoma has been resected, thereby removing the major source of circulating catecholamines, a situation arises where there is both very low sympathetic activity and volume depletion. This can result in profound hypotension. Therefore, it is usually advised to "salt load" patients with pheochromocytoma before their surgery. This may consist of simple interventions such as consumption of high-salt food preoperatively, direct salt replacement, or administration of intravenous saline solution.

Assessment of Outcomes

The signs and symptoms of catecholamine excess (elevated heart rate and blood pressure, anxiety, etc.) should abate soon after surgery. As mentioned previously, blood pressure should be monitored closely, and a significant decrease in blood pressure should be anticipated because of the volume-depleted state. Normal saline or lactated Ringer solution should be titrated to maintain mean arterial pressure in a near-normal range.

ADRENAL DISORDERS

Adrenal Insufficiency (Addison Disease)

Definition and Epidemiology

Primary adrenal insufficiency or Addison disease most often involves destruction of all regions of the adrenal gland, leading to deficiencies in cortisol, aldosterone, and various androgens with elevation in corticotropin-releasing hormone and adrenocorticotropin hormone (ACTH). In developed countries, the most common cause is autoimmune destruction of the adrenal gland, whereas tuberculosis is more commonly the cause in developing countries. In chronic adrenal insufficiency, adrenal crisis (AC) occurred in 8.3 crises per 100 patient-years. Precipitating causes were mainly GI infection, fever, and emotional stress (20% for each), but other stressful events (e.g., major pain, surgery, strenuous physical activity, heat, pregnancy) or unexplained sudden onset of AC (7%) were also documented. Given that corticosteroids are metabolized primarily through cytochrome P450 (CYP) 3A4, many drugs (e.g., carbamazepine, phenytoin) can increase the replacement doses needed. Patients with a previous AC were at a higher risk of crisis (odds ratio 2.85; 95% confidence interval [CI], 1.5–5.5; p<0.01). However, no further risk factors could be identified. Ten patients died during follow-up; in four cases, death was associated with AC (0.5 AC-related deaths per 100 patient-years).[13]

Another common cause of adrenal insufficiency is withdrawal of corticosteroid therapy, which is related to duration and amount of corticosteroid use. Stratified by administration form, percentages of patients with adrenal insufficiency ranged from 4.2% for nasal administration (95% CI, 0.5–28.9) to 52.2% for intra-articular administration (95% CI, 40.5–63.6). Stratified by disease, percentages ranged from 6.8% for asthma with inhalation corticosteroids only (95% CI, 3.8–12.0) to 60.0% for hematological malignancies (95% CI, 38.0–78.6). The risk also varied according to dose, from 2.4% (95% CI, 0.6–9.3) (low dose) to 21.5% (95% CI, 12.0–35.5) (high dose), and according to treatment duration, from 1.4% (95% CI, 0.3–7.4) (less than 28 days) to 27.4% (95% CI, 17.7–39.8) (more than 1 year) in patients with asthma.[14]

Pathophysiology

As described earlier, autoimmune destruction of the adrenal gland leading to deficiencies of cortisol, aldosterone, and androgens is the most common etiology in developed countries. Secondary adrenal insufficiency is usually a result of destruction of the pituitary gland caused by tumors or surgery. The principal difference is that aldosterone secretion remains intact so that normal potassium concentrations are observed, and ACTH is low or absent in contrast to primary adrenal insufficiency.

Clinical Presentation and Laboratory Diagnosis

The signs and symptoms of adrenal insufficiency are presented in Table 39.6. Common laboratory tests for

Table 39.6 Signs and Symptoms of Adrenal Insufficiency

Signs	Symptoms
Weight loss	Weakness
Increased pigmentation	Malaise
Hypotension (postural)	Myalgias
Fever	Anorexia
Decreased body hair	Vomiting
Vitiligo	Salt craving
Features of hypopituitarism (amenorrhea, cold intolerance)	Memory impairment
	Depression

Table 39.7 Laboratory Testing in Adrenal Insufficiency

Test	Change
Serum cortisol	Decreased and lack of change with stimulation
ACTH	Increased in primary adrenal insufficiency; decreased/undetectable in secondary adrenal insufficiency
Potassium	Increased in primary adrenal insufficiency; normal in secondary adrenal insufficiency
Others may include insulin hypoglycemia test, metyrapone test, and CRH stimulation test	

ACTH = adrenocorticotropin hormone; CRH = corticotropin-releasing hormone.

diagnosis are presented in Table 39.7. In critically ill patients, laboratory monitoring and interpretation of tests can be somewhat difficult. It is important to consider the clinical presentation together with relevant laboratory tests to determine the best course of action for each patient.

Treatment

Adrenal crisis (Addison disease) is a medical emergency, and intravenous corticosteroids and volume resuscitation are of the utmost importance. Intravenous hydrocortisone 100 mg intravenous bolus should be followed by an infusion of 10 mg/hour. Some authors recommend 100 mg every 8 hours. Hydrocortisone is the preferred agent because it has both corticosteroid and mineralocorticoid activity (hydrocortisone 50 mg = fludrocortisones 0.1 mg). Once the patient has been stabilized, the dose may be tapered to 50 mg every 6–8 hours.

All patients will be in a volume-depleted state. Concurrent administration of normal saline or lactated Ringer solution at high flow rates will help restore a normal volume status and support blood pressure.[15] Mineralocorticoid support with fludrocortisone 0.1 mg can be used in persisting hyperkalemia.

Assessment of Outcomes

Improved vasomotor tone after corticosteroid replacement will resolve hypotension, improve glycemic control, and maintain normal electrolyte status.

Adrenal Excess (Cushing Syndrome)

Definition and Epidemiology

Cushing syndrome (CS) results from the effects of supraphysiologic concentrations of glucocorticoids originating either from exogenous administration or less commonly from endogenous overproduction by the adrenal glands. Cushing syndrome has an incidence of 10–15 people per 1 million; however, studies of patients with diabetes, obesity, hypertension, and osteoporosis found a high prevalence of CS among these populations. Cushing syndrome is associated with high mortality if untreated, and the patient may survive only 4–5 years. The clinical manifestations of CS range from the distinctive clinical features (purple striae, facial plethora, proximal myopathy) to common conditions such as hypertension, obesity, and diabetes. Clinical practice guidelines recommend biochemical tests to screen patients for CS; however, the sensitivity and specificity of these tests vary, so a careful analysis must be performed to avoid misdiagnosis.

Pathophysiology

Cushing syndrome can be ACTH-dependent (80% of cases) or ACTH-independent. About 85% of ACTH-dependent cases are caused by a pituitary adenoma. Overproduction of ACTH causes bilateral adrenal hyperplasia. Adrenocorticotropin hormone can also be produced by ectopic ACTH-secreting tumors and non-neoplastic corticotropin hypersecretion, perhaps because of excess production of CRH (corticotropin-releasing hormone), accounting for the most cases of ACTH-dependent CS. Ectopic ACTH production can be caused by non-adrenal tumors such as small cell lung carcinoma.

Clinical Presentation and Laboratory Diagnosis

The clinical presentation and tests for laboratory diagnosis are presented in Table 39.8 and Table 39.9.

Treatment

The mainstay of treatment in CS when hypercortisolism is caused by a pituitary adenoma (called Cushing disease) is surgical removal of the pituitary adenoma. If hypercortisolism is caused by adrenal adenoma or carcinoma, surgical removal of the affected adrenal gland or total removal in adrenal carcinoma is necessary if possible. Transsphenoidal surgery is used for Cushing disease to remove the pituitary tumor overproducing ACTH, and it is successful in about

Table 39.8 Signs and Symptoms of Cushing Syndrome

Signs	Symptoms
~90% have central obesity and facial rounding	Myopathies in 65%
Facial plethora	Muscle weakness in 58%
Moon facies	
Buffalo hump	
Hypertension in 75%–85%	
Psychiatric features in ~50%	
Purple striae	

Table 39.9 Laboratory Tests in Cushing Syndrome

Test	Change in Cushing Syndrome
Plasma cortisol	Increased[a]
Urine cortisol	Increased
Saliva cortisol	Increased
Plasma ACTH	Increased

[a]Depending on the exact cause of hypercortisolism, hyperplasia, adenoma, or carcinoma, cortisol may be suppressed with dexamethasone administration. Low-dose dexamethasone will suppress cortisol in hyperplasia but not in adrenal adenoma or carcinoma.

Table 39.10 Drugs for Control of Cushing Syndrome

Drug	Usual Range	Comments
Aminoglutethimide	1 g/day divided evenly q6hr	Maximum: 2 g/day
Cyproheptadine	24–34 mg/day divided four times daily	Maximum: 32 mg/day
Ketoconazole	200–1,200 mg/day divided twice daily	Maximum: 1,600 mg/day; CYP3A4 substrate and inhibitor (strong)
Metyrapone	1–2 g/day divided every 4–6 hr	Maximum: 6 g/day; CYP3A4 inducer
Mifepristone	600–1,200 mg/day	Maximum: 1,200 mg/day not to exceed 20 mg/kg/day
Mitotane	1–4 g/day	Maximum 3 g TID; take with food to decrease GI effects

q = every; TID = three times daily.

90% of cases. After surgery, corticosteroid support will be needed, and the typical starting dosing is hydrocortisone 100 mg every 8 hours and gradual reduction for about 3 weeks. Adjunctive radiation may also be used if the entire tissue source cannot be removed. Pharmacologic therapy is palliative only but may useful for control of symptoms. Table 39.10 outlines the drugs used in CS. A combination regimen of ketoconazole and metyrapone is commonly used because these agents have synergistic mechanisms of action. Aminoglutethimide has fallen out of favor as a first-line drug because of adverse effects and high relapse rates. Drugs used for CS are not curative and are often used to prepare patients for surgery. Monotherapy is rarely used, and most patients will require combination therapy for better control of symptoms and laboratory parameters of CS.

Assessment of Outcomes

Blood pressure should return to a near-normal level in a few days unless the patient has coexisting essential hypertension. Psychiatric symptoms should dissipate over days to weeks. Cortisol concentrations should drop abruptly with tumor removal, and patients will require long-term glucocorticoid support. Other pituitary hormones are likely to be affected as well, and thyroid supplementation will likely be needed. Other pituitary hormones may need to be replaced depending on the patient's age. Adult patients usually need only glucocorticoid and thyroid hormone support.

REFERENCES

1. Wartofsky L. Myxedema coma. Endocrinol Metab Clin North Am 2006;35:687-98, vii-viii.
2. Mitchell JM. Thyroid disease in the emergency department. Thyroid function tests and hypothyroidism and myxedema coma. Emerg Med Clin North Am 1989;7:885-902.
3. Agarwal V, Parikh V, Otterbeck PE, et al. Myxedema coma induced by short-term amiodarone therapy. Am J Med Sci 2014;347:258-9.
4. Chakraborty S, Fedderson J, Gums JJ, et al. Amiodarone-induced myxedema coma – a case and review of the literature. Arch Med Sci 2014;10:1263-7.
5. Chiong YV, Bammerlin E, Mariash CN. Development of an objective tool for the diagnosis of myxedema coma. Transl Res 2015;166:233-43.
6. Wartofsky L. Clinical criteria for the diagnosis of thyroid storm. Thyroid 2012;22:659-60.
7. Angell TE, Lechner MG, Nguyen CT, et al. Clinical features and hospital outcomes in thyroid storm: a retrospective cohort study. J Clin Endocrinol Metab. 2015;100:451-9.
8. Akamizu T, Satoh T, Isozaki O, et al. Diagnostic criteria, clinical features, and incidence of thyroid storm based on nationwide surveys. Thyroid 2012;22:661-79.
9. Burch HB, Wartofsky L. Life-threatening thyrotoxicosis. Thyroid storm. Endocrinol Metab Clin North Am 1993;22:263-77.
10. Garrahy A, Casey R, Wall D, et al. A review of the management of positive biochemical screening for phaeochromocytoma and paraganglioma: a salutary tale. Int J Clin Pract 2015;69:802-9.
11. van der Zee PA, de Boer A. Pheochromocytoma: a review on preoperative treatment with phenoxybenzamine or doxazosin. Neth J Med 2014;72:190-201.
12. MacCarthy EP, Bloomfield SS. Labetalol: a review of its pharmacology, pharmacokinetics, clinical uses and adverse effects. Pharmacotherapy 1983;3:193-219.
13. Charmandari E, Nicolaides NC, Chrousos GP. Adrenal insufficiency. Lancet 2014;383:2152-67.
14. Broersen LH, Pereira AM, Jorgensen JO, et al. Adrenal insufficiency in corticosteroids use: systematic review and meta-analysis. J Clin Endocrinol Metab 2015;100:2171-80.
15. Aulinas A, Casanueva F, Goni F, et al. Adrenal insufficiency and adrenal replacement therapy. Current status in Spain. Endocrinol Nutr 2013;60:136-43.

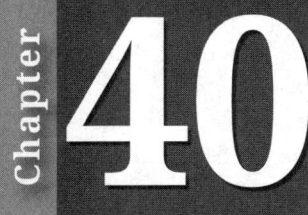

Oncologic Emergencies

Ali McBride, Pharm.D., M.S., BCPS, BCOP; Michelle Nadeau, Pharm.D., BCPS; and Cory M. Vela, Pharm.D.

LEARNING OBJECTIVES

1. Define tumor lysis syndrome (TLS).
2. Identify patient- and tumor-related risk factors for developing TLS.
3. Describe preventive and treatment interventions for managing TLS.
4. Summarize the signs and symptoms of hypercalcemia of malignancy (HCM).
5. Review and evaluate treatment options for HCM.
6. Understand the pathophysiology of syndrome of inappropriate diuretic hormone (SIADH) in the setting of malignancy.
7. Describe management strategies for cancer-related SIADH.
8. Identify the signs and symptoms of superior vena cava syndrome (SVCS).
9. Summarize treatment options in patients with a diagnosis of SVCS.
10. Review the incidence, prognosis, and management of malignant spinal cord compression.

ABBREVIATIONS IN THIS CHAPTER

AVP	Arginine vasopressin	SIADH	Syndrome of inappropriate diuretic hormone
cAMP	Cyclic adenosine monophosphate	SVC	Superior vena cava
HCM	Hypercalcemia of malignancy	SVCS	Superior vena cava syndrome
MSCC	Malignant spinal cord compression	TLS	Tumor lysis syndrome
PTH	Parathyroid hormone		

INTRODUCTION

Cancer treatments may lead to an increase in critical care conditions, in some cases necessitating urgent care and acute monitoring. These conditions often develop in many different manifestations but can often lead to critical if not urgent issues for patients with cancer. These disease states require rapid interventions because of their acute manifestation and potential onset of death or irreparable damage to the patient. Oncologic emergencies are defined as an acute condition caused by cancer or its treatment.

Oncologic emergencies are classified into specific categories: structural or obstructive emergencies, defined by the mass or size of a tumor in a space-occupying area (i.e., superior vena cava syndrome [SVCS], spinal cord compression); metabolic or hormonal emergencies (i.e., hypercalcemia and syndrome of inappropriate diuretic hormone [SIADH]); and secondary complications arising from treatment effects such as treatment-related oncologic emergencies (i.e., tumor lysis syndrome [TLS]).

TUMOR LYSIS SYNDROME

Definition/Pathophysiology

The destruction of tumor cells either spontaneously or in response to chemotherapy results in TLS.[1] Tumor lysis syndrome is most commonly associated with hematologic lymphomas and leukemias, including Burkitt lymphoma and acute lymphoblastic leukemia, but it has also been associated with low-grade lymphomas and solid tumors

(Table 40.1).[2] The massive efflux of the intracellular components from these malignant cells, including proteins, metabolites, and nucleic acids, overwhelms normal homeostatic processes and can lead to life-threatening electrolyte abnormalities including hyperuricemia, hyperphosphatemia, hyperkalemia, and secondary hypocalcemia.[1]

Hyperuricemia occurs as a direct consequence of the release of nucleic acid by-products when tumor cells are lysed. The DNA is metabolized to pyrimidine and purine nucleotides, and the latter is converted to hypoxanthine. Xanthine oxidase then mediates the conversion of hypoxanthine to xanthine and the conversion of xanthine to uric acid.[3,4] Under normal homeostatic processes, renal excretory mechanisms facilitate the clearance of uric acid; uric acid is filtered by the glomerulus, reabsorbed by the proximal tubule, and then secreted by the distal tubule.[5] However, renal excretory capacities become saturated in the setting of TLS, resulting in the precipitation of uric acid crystals within the tubular infrastructure, obstruction with decreased urine flow, vasoconstriction, and acute kidney injury.[6]

Tumor cells harbor intracellular phosphates at 4 times the concentration of normal cells.[7] The rapid release of phosphate from tumor cells in response to chemotherapy and the potential for concomitant uric acid nephropathy overwhelm normal renal excretory capacities for phosphate. The resultant hyperphosphatemia can manifest clinically as nausea, vomiting, lethargy, or mental status changes.[1,2,7]

Hypocalcemia occurs secondary to hyperphosphatemia and the formation of calcium phosphate precipitates. Calcium phosphate precipitates can deposit within various tissue beds, including the cardiac vasculature and the kidneys, thereby potentiating the risk of acute kidney injury and serious cardiac arrhythmias. Hypocalcemia can also cause neuromuscular irritability and seizures.[1]

Tumor cells also harbor high concentrations of potassium, and the rapid release of potassium from lysing tumor cells can overwhelm normal metabolic processes. In the setting of hyperuricemia-induced acute kidney injury and calcium phosphate nephropathy, renal clearance of potassium is compensated, thereby increasing serum concentrations of potassium.[3] Elevated potassium can present as nausea, vomiting, or muscle weakness and can also cause serious electrocardiographic (ECG) changes, specifically peaked T waves and widening of the QRS complex. Hyperkalemia can also manifest as ventricular arrhythmias, which can lead to sudden cardiac death when coupled with secondary hypocalcemia.[1,2,7]

Tumor lysis syndrome is classified as laboratory or clinical TLS as defined by the Cairo and Bishop criteria. Laboratory TLS (LTLS) requires at least a 25% change from baseline for two or more of the following laboratory parameters: hyperuricemia (greater than 8.0 mg/dL), hyperphosphatemia (greater than 4.5 mg/dL), hyperkalemia (greater than 6.0 mmol/L), and hypocalcemia (corrected calcium less than 7.0 mg/dL). These metabolic changes are expected to occur simultaneously at least 3 days before or 7 days after initiating treatment as part of the definition of LTLS (Table 40.2). Clinical TLS is defined by the presence of at least one clinical manifestation of TLS including renal insufficiency, arrhythmias, and seizures in addition to LTLS.[2,8]

Table 40.1 Risk Factors for Tumor Lysis Syndrome (TLS)

Characteristic	Risk Factor
Tumor-specific	Tumor type (i.e., aggressive lymphoma, acute lymphoblastic leukemia and acute myeloid leukemia)
	Bulky tumor mass
	Extensive tumor infiltration/metastasis
	Elevated LDH
	Cell-lysis potential
	Sensitivity of tumor to chemotherapy
Patient-specific	Baseline renal dysfunction
	Elevated uric acid
	Hypotension
	Dehydration/oliguria

Table 40.2 Cairo-Bishop Definition of Laboratory and Clinical Tumor Lysis Syndrome

Cairo-Bishop Definitions of Tumor Lysis Syndrome (TLS)	
Laboratory TLS (LTLS)[a]	
Hyperuricemia	Uric acid > 8.0 mg/dL
Hyperkalemia	Potassium > 6.0 mmol/L
Hyperphosphatemia	Phosphorus > 4.5 mg/dL
Hypocalcemia	Corrected calcium < 7.0 mg/dL
Clinical Tumor Lysis Syndrome (CTLS)[b]	
Seizures	
Cardiac arrhythmias	
Elevated serum creatinine (> 1.5 × ULN)	
Death	

[a]LTLS requires two or more metabolic abnormalities occurring within the same 24-hr window either 3 days before or up to 7 days after initiating chemotherapy.

[b]CTLS requires the presence of LTLS plus one of the clinical manifestations.

ULN = upper limit of normal.

Incidence/Epidemiology

Tumor lysis syndrome typically occurs in response to the treatment of hematologic malignancies, specifically high-grade lymphomas—most commonly, Burkitt lymphoma and acute lymphoblastic leukemia—but it has also been associated with low-grade lymphomas, including indolent non-Hodgkin lymphoma, Hodgkin lymphoma, chronic lymphocytic leukemia, and multiple myeloma and solid tumors with high tumor burden including metastatic breast cancer, small cell lung cancer, melanoma, and non–small cell lung cancer.[2,3,8,9]

Tumor lysis syndrome can also occur spontaneously in the absence of treatment. Spontaneous TLS is usually observed in the setting of Burkitt lymphoma but has also been associated with other hematologic malignancies and solid tumors. Although the risk factors for developing spontaneous TLS are not clearly defined, spontaneous TLS is typically associated with a poor prognosis compared with classic TLS.[2,3,5] Workup of TLS should be considered when there is a malignancy with unexplained reason of acute kidney failure.

Risk factors for TLS include both tumor- and patient-specific factors. Tumor-specific risk factors include tumor burden, which is related to the bulkiness of the tumor mass, and the extent of tumor infiltration and/or metastasis and cell lysis potential, which is related to lactate dehydrogenase concentrations, the rate of cell proliferation, and the sensitivity of the tumor to chemotherapy including Burkitt lymphoma, lymphoblastic lymphoma, and B-cell acute lymphoblastic leukemia. The intensity of chemotherapy is also grouped with tumor-related factors when assessing the risk of TLS; the higher the intensity of the chemotherapy, the greater the potential for tumor cell lysis. Patient-specific factors can also determine the risk of TLS and include baseline nephropathy, dehydration, and hypotension, all of which can result in decreased urine flow and increase the propensity for uric acid and/or calcium phosphate precipitation (Table 40.1).[1,2,8]

Assessment of risk factors allows for stratification of patients according to predicted risk of TLS and can direct the management strategy of TLS. Most risk assessment models center on the underlying malignancy and stratify patients as high, intermediate, or low risk depending on the presence and/or degree of tumor-related manifestations and baseline patient-specific characteristics.[2,8]

The risk stratification model proposed by Cairo et al. stratifies patients according to the underlying malignancy (Table 40.3) and extent of metastasis/bulkiness of the disease, type of chemotherapy, and preexisting renal dysfunction, among other factors. This model, however, does not directly outline treatment recommendations for each stratification group, thereby creating challenges when applying it to clinical practice for the management of TLS.[2,8]

MANAGEMENT OF TLS

The goal of managing TLS is to prevent the potentially serious renal, neurologic, and cardiac sequelae that can result from TLS. The initiation of preventive and treatment interventions is directed by the initial risk assessment of patients at risk of these serious complications.

Prophylaxis

Hydration/Urine Output Goals

All patients at risk of TLS and without contraindications to aggressive fluid therapy should be initiated on intravenous hydration therapy. Fluids should be initiated at least 24–48 hours before chemotherapy and continued through the completion of chemotherapy. The role of fluids in the setting of TLS is 2-fold: (1) dilute the extracellular space to reduce serum concentrations of potassium, phosphate, and uric acid; and (2) increase renal blood flow and filtration, promote high urine output, and prevent the accumulation of nephrotoxic calcium phosphate and uric acid precipitates within the kidneys.[2,5,7,10]

Fluid therapy should be titrated as needed to achieve a target urine output of 80–100 mL/m^2/hour or maintained at 1–2 times fluid maintenance requirements. Loop diuretics can be considered if target urine outputs are not achieved with continuous hydration therapy.[2,7,10]

Historically, urine alkalinization with sodium bicarbonate was recommended as part of the management of TLS. Although mechanistically, urine alkalinization increases the

Table 40.3 Incidence of Tumor Lysis Syndrome by Risk Category

Malignancy	Incidence (%)
High risk	
Acute lymphocytic leukemia (ALL)	5.2-23
Acute myeloid leukemia (AML) with WBC>75,000	18
B-cell ALL	26.4
Burkitt's lymphoma	14.9
Intermediate risk	
AML with WBC=25,000-50,000	6
Diffuse large B-cell lymphoma	6
Low risk	
AML with WBC<25,000	1
Chronic lymphocytic leukemia (CLL)	0.33

Adapted from Wilson et al.

WBC=white blood cell

renal clearance of uric acid, the solubility of uric acid precursors, including hypoxanthine and xanthine, is decreased. The risk of xanthine nephropathy increases, particularly in the setting of the concomitant use of allopurinol, which acts as a competitive inhibitor of xanthine oxidase and prevents the conversion of hypoxanthine and xanthine to uric acid, ultimately increasing the concentration of these uric acid precursors. Furthermore, urine alkalinization decreases the solubility of calcium phosphate, thereby exacerbating the underlying risks associated with calcium phosphate precipitation. Therefore, given the risk of xanthine and calcium phosphate precipitation, sodium bicarbonate is no longer recommended for the prevention of TLS.[1,3,5,7,10,11]

Allopurinol

Allopurinol is readily used in combination with fluid therapy for preventing TLS. By blocking xanthine oxidase, allopurinol decreases the conversion of hypoxanthine and xanthine to uric acid (Figure 40.1). The role of allopurinol in managing TLS, however, is limited to prevention, given its negligible effects on existing uric acid.[1,5,7,10,11]

The recommended dose of allopurinol is 100 mg/m^2 orally every 8 hours or 10 mg/kg/day orally divided every 8 hours. Allopurinol is converted to oxypurinol, which is an active metabolite that also serves as a xanthine oxidase inhibitor.[2,10] The onset of action of xanthine oxidase activity, however, for both allopurinol and oxypurinol, is delayed; therefore, normalization of uric acid concentrations may be prolonged, ultimately delaying the initiation of chemotherapy.[10]

Allopurinol should be dose reduced by 50% for patients with renal insufficiency. The concomitant use of allopurinol and purine analogs (i.e., mercaptopurine, azathioprine) and purine-based chemotherapy should be avoided because allopurinol may prevent the degradation of these purine analogs and increase treatment-related toxicities (i.e., bone marrow suppression). Alternatively, purine analogs can be dose reduced by 70% when used concomitantly with allopurinol.[2]

Allopurinol is usually well tolerated but has been associated with hypersensitivity reactions including, but not limited to, Stevens-Johnson syndrome and toxic epidermal necrolysis. These reactions may manifest as fever and rash and may have a delayed onset. In addition, the risk of obstructive uropathy is inherent with the use of allopurinol, given the increased concentrations of xanthine and hypoxanthine, and should be closely monitored for the duration of therapy.[1,2,3,5,7,10]

Treatment

Rasburicase

Rasburicase, a recombinant urate oxidase, has become the mainstay of therapy for treatment of TLS given its ability to readily degrade existing uric acid (Figure 40.1). Rasburicase enzymatically converts uric acid to allantoin, a formulation of uric acid that is highly soluble and readily excreted by the kidney.[2,3,5,10]

Rasburicase is U.S. Food and Drug Administration approved for managing TLS in patients with leukemia, lymphoma, and solid tumors with baseline hyperuricemia or expected hyperuricemia after initiating chemotherapy. The initial recommended dose of rasburicase was 0.15–0.2 mg/kg as a daily 30-minute intravenous infusion, given up to 7 days; however, new recommendations have amended this to include rasburicase 0.1–0.2 mg/kg as a single dose for managing TLS.[11] Abbreviated dosing strategies are equivocal for fixed- and flat-dosing schedules, including rasburicase 6- and 3-mg dosing, and although this scheduling has not been incorporated into the guidelines, the flat-dose scheduling is often

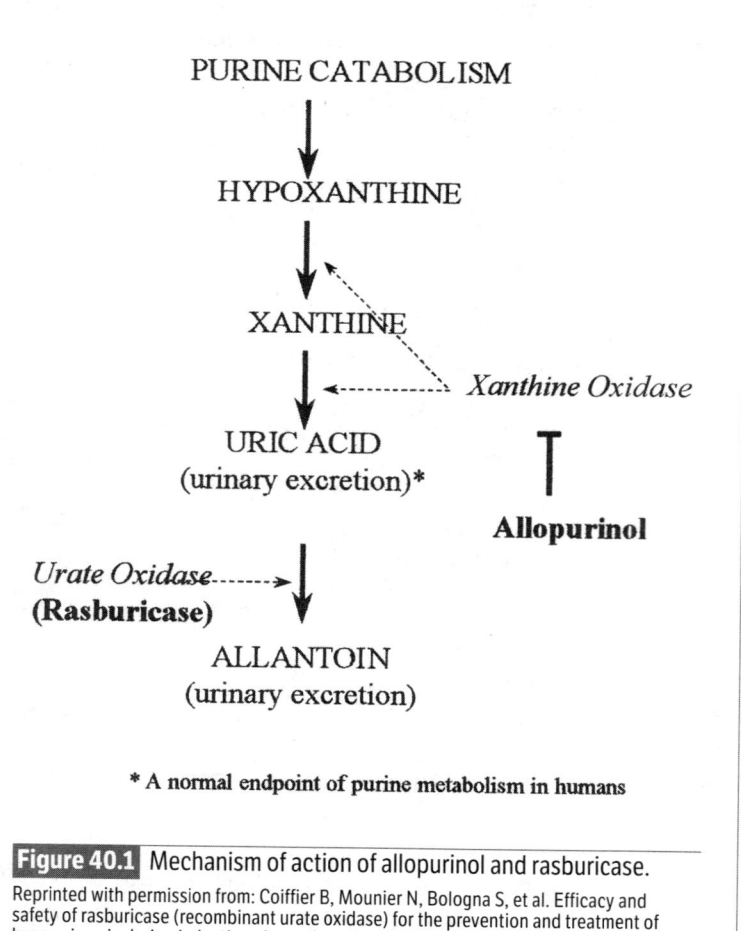

Figure 40.1 Mechanism of action of allopurinol and rasburicase.

Reprinted with permission from: Coiffier B, Mounier N, Bologna S, et al. Efficacy and safety of rasburicase (recombinant urate oxidase) for the prevention and treatment of hyperuricemia during induction chemotherapy of aggressive non-Hodgkin's lymphoma: results of the GRAAL1 (Groupe d'Etude des Lymphomes de l'Adulte Trial on Rasburicase Activity in Adult Lymphoma) study. J Clin Oncol 2003;23:4402-6.

used in clinical practice.[12-16] Treatment duration depends on reducing uric acid concentrations and achieving uric acid control.[2,10] Given the comparative efficacy of weight-based dosing in normalizing elevated uric acid concentrations and the high cost of rasburicase, fixed dosing serves as a cost strategy for managing TLS.[12-16]

Rasburicase, as an enzyme, continues to degrade uric acid in blood samples and can lead to falsely low readings of uric acid. The samples should therefore be collected in pre-chilled tubes and maintained on ice en route to the laboratory to ensure an accurate analysis of uric acid concentrations.[2,17]

Rasburicase is usually well tolerated with the exception of hypersensitivity reactions that can manifest as pruritus and dermatologic reactions. Of note, all patients should be screened for glucose-6-phosphate-dehydrogenase (G6PD) deficiency before treatment with rasburicase. Patients with G6PD deficiency are unable to metabolize the hydrogen peroxide by-products produced by the conversion of uric acid to allantoin and are at increased risk of hemolytic anemia and methemoglobinemia. Glucose-6-phosphate dehydrogenase deficiency is most commonly observed among patient populations of Mediterranean, Southeast Asian, and African American descent.[2,17]

Electrolyte Monitoring/Management

Monitoring is recommended for the duration of the risk of TLS. Consensus guidelines recommend increasing the frequency of electrolyte monitoring, including uric acid, phosphate, potassium, and calcium, depending on the risk of TLS: every 4–6 hours, every 8–12 hours, and once daily for high-, intermediate-, and low-risk TLS, respectively. Continuous cardiac monitoring is recommended for patients at high risk of TLS. In addition, parameters to assess for renal function, including serum creatinine and urine output, should be monitored continuously. The correction of electrolyte abnormalities is recommended before initiating chemotherapy. In addition, prompt therapeutic interventions are recommended for any symptomatic manifestations of these biochemical derangements.[1-3,5,7,8]

Hyperphosphatemia

Hydration is usually sufficient to correct elevated phosphate concentrations. Oral phosphate binders, including aluminum hydroxide, lanthanum carbonate, and sevelamer hydroxide, can be considered for treating hyperphosphatemia, although their efficacy is limited by the slow onset of action required to achieve target phosphate concentrations. Phosphate binders inhibit the absorption of phosphate through the gastrointestinal tract.

Hypocalcemia

Treatment of asymptomatic hypocalcemia is not recommended. Instead, it is more appropriate to correct the underlying cause of hyperphosphatemia. However, symptomatic hypocalcemia manifesting as severe cardiac arrhythmias or seizures should be treated with intravenous calcium gluconate.

Hyperkalemia

The goal of treating hyperkalemia in the setting of TLS is to prevent cardiac sequelae. An oral ion-exchange resin, sodium polystyrene sulfonate, can be considered for patients with asymptomatic hyperkalemia, although efficacy is limited by the slow onset of action and limited therapy duration, given the risk of colonic necrosis with repeated doses. Symptomatic hyperkalemia requires prompt intervention; insulin (with glucose), β-agonists, and sodium bicarbonate will facilitate the intracellular shift of potassium from plasma, and are all treatment modalities that can be considered.

Elimination of exogenous potassium sources should also be considered. In addition, any medications known to inhibit renal secretion of potassium should be discontinued, including potassium supplements, potassium-sparing diuretics, aldosterone antagonists, and nonsteroidal anti-inflammatory agents.

Careful monitoring for ECG changes is indicated, and calcium gluconate can be considered for cardiac arrhythmias for membrane stabilization.

Renal Replacement Therapy

Renal replacement therapy is recommended as a definitive treatment modality for TLS, and it should be considered for TLS-induced kidney injury in the setting of severe metabolic instabilities despite prophylactic measures. Continuous renal replacement therapy includes hemodialysis, hemofiltration, and hemodiafiltration and is the preferred method of dialysis to allow for continuous and targeted removal of solutes released by lysing tumor cells. Dialysis should be continued until renal function is fully recovered, which may require weeks of therapy.[1-3,5,7,8]

HYPERCALCEMIA

Hypercalcemia of malignancy (HCM) is often an acute manifestation, with outcomes that yield a poor prognosis with a correlated high mortality rate. Hypercalcemia of malignancy has been reported to occur in around 10%–20% of patients with cancer. Outcomes for patients with a diagnosis of HCM are reported to range from only 2 months to 6 months from the initial diagnosis, with up to half of the patients dying within 1 month.[2] The incidence of HCM is low at initial presentation of a cancer diagnosis, but it increases with progression of disease.[18] Hypercalcemia of malignancy is associated with several disease states including breast cancer, multiple myeloma, squamous cell carcinoma of the lung, squamous cell carcinoma of head and neck, renal cell carcinoma, lymphoma, and other malignancies including ovarian cancer, pancreatic cancer, and unknown primary cancer.[18] Many pathophysiologic mechanisms may contribute to HCM (Figure 40.2).

Cancer-associated hypercalcemia is classified into four different types: local osteolytic hypercalcemia, humoral HCM, 1,25(OH)-secreting lymphomas, and ectopic hyperparathyroidism.[19] Local osteolytic hypercalcemia is caused by an increase in bone resorption by osteoclasts, leading to local destruction of the bone by the tumor. In turn, this releases the calcium deposits of the bone into the serum. Certain tumors, including solid cancers, non-Hodgkin lymphoma, and blast phase chronic myeloid leukemia, secrete parathyroid hormone (PTH)-related protein, which can mimic PTH by stimulating the type 1 PTH receptor.[20,21] Parathyroid hormone–related protein is a monomeric amino acid peptide sequence that mimics PTH protein structure. The protein is normally secreted by neuroendocrine, epithelia, and mesodermal tissue. Another known cause of HCM, although to a lesser extent, is by lymphoma tumors, which may directly secrete 1,25-dihydroxyvitamin D (calcitriol).[22] The release of calcitriol leads to increased activation of osteoclast bone resorption and calcium reabsorption in the intestine. The last cause of HCM, the ectopic secretion of PTH by tumors, has been reported in case studies but is rarely observed.[23]

Signs and Symptoms

Signs of HCM may often vary depending on patient characteristics and tolerance. Patients' calcium concentrations may be at higher concentrations of the normal calcium range without symptoms of hypercalcemia. These symptoms often vary in nature, but they bring to light the mnemonic "stones, bones, abdominal moans, and psychic groans" used to guide most symptoms that reflect hypercalcemia (Table 40.4).

Patients may have neuromuscular adverse effects, which can include fatigue, confusion, and muscle weakness, constipation, and tetany. Gastrointestinal adverse effects can include nausea, vomiting, abdominal pain, appetite suppression and cachexia, and pancreatitis. Renal effects commonly seen are polydipsia, nocturia and polyuria, and nephrolithiasis caused by hypercalciuria from the kidneys. Renal adverse effects can also include dehydration and nephrocalcinosis. Cardiovascular adverse effects can be noted on ECG readings including a shortened QT interval as well as hypertension, with rare report of arrhythmias. Bone pain is also common in patients with malignancy because of the release of calcium of the bone by osteoclasts.[19]

Diagnosis

Diagnoses of hypercalcemia are often based on the total serum calcium concentration. Because 40%–45% of serum calcium is bound to proteins, predominantly albumin, the serum calcium concentration must be corrected in the presence of hypoalbuminemia or hyperalbuminemia.[19] Measuring the serum ionized calcium concentration can also be useful and does not need to be corrected for abnormalities in albumin concentrations.

Although malignancy is often clinically evident and diagnosed before it leads to symptomatic hypercalcemia, it is still important to distinguish cancer-related hypercalcemia from hypercalcemia as the result of primary hyperparathyroidism or other causes (e.g., excess vitamin A or D, medications, thyrotoxicosis).[22] It is also possible that more than one etiology is present. Thus, determining the reason for hypercalcemia is essential to treating the underlying cause. Hypercalcemia presents with the same general symptomology according to condition of severity, but a differential diagnosis can be done by ruling out other causes through a careful history and laboratory testing (e.g., intact PTH concentrations or PTH-related protein secretion).

Treatment

Managing hypercalcemia largely depends on its severity, which generally correlates with the measured serum calcium concentration.[19] Regardless of the degree of severity, it is crucial that patients minimize any factors that may contribute to raising the serum calcium concentrations. This may involve avoiding certain medications (e.g., thiazide diuretic, calcium or vitamin D supplements), maintaining sufficient fluid intake, or remaining ambulatory.[19,23]

For asymptomatic patients with mild hypercalcemia, removal of any contributing factors may be enough to correct the issue. If patients are symptomatic or their total serum calcium is closer to 12 mg/dL, normal saline hydration can be initiated (Table 40.5). The rate of hydration can be 200–500 mL/hour going up to 4–6 L/day. However, factors such as the patient's current level of dehydration and any comorbidities like congestive heart failure or renal insufficiency should be considered. In addition to tracking the serum calcium, electrolytes and urine output should be monitored, and care should be taken to make sure the patient does not become fluid overloaded. Although loop diuretics are commonly paired with saline hydration therapy to increase the excretion of calcium, evidence for their efficacy outside the setting of fluid overload is more limited.[19]

Patients with moderate hypercalcemia can be initiated on intravenous bisphosphonate therapy in addition to general supportive measures and saline hydration. Bisphosphonates inhibit osteoclast-mediated resorption and the release of calcium from the bone. They are given intravenously for hypercalcemia because of their poor absorption profile when taken orally. Zoledronic acid (4 mg intravenously given over 15 minutes) and pamidronate (given over 4–6 hours, see Table 40.4) are commonly used for this indication.[23,24] Serum calcium decreases within 24–48 hours after administration, and the maximum effect can

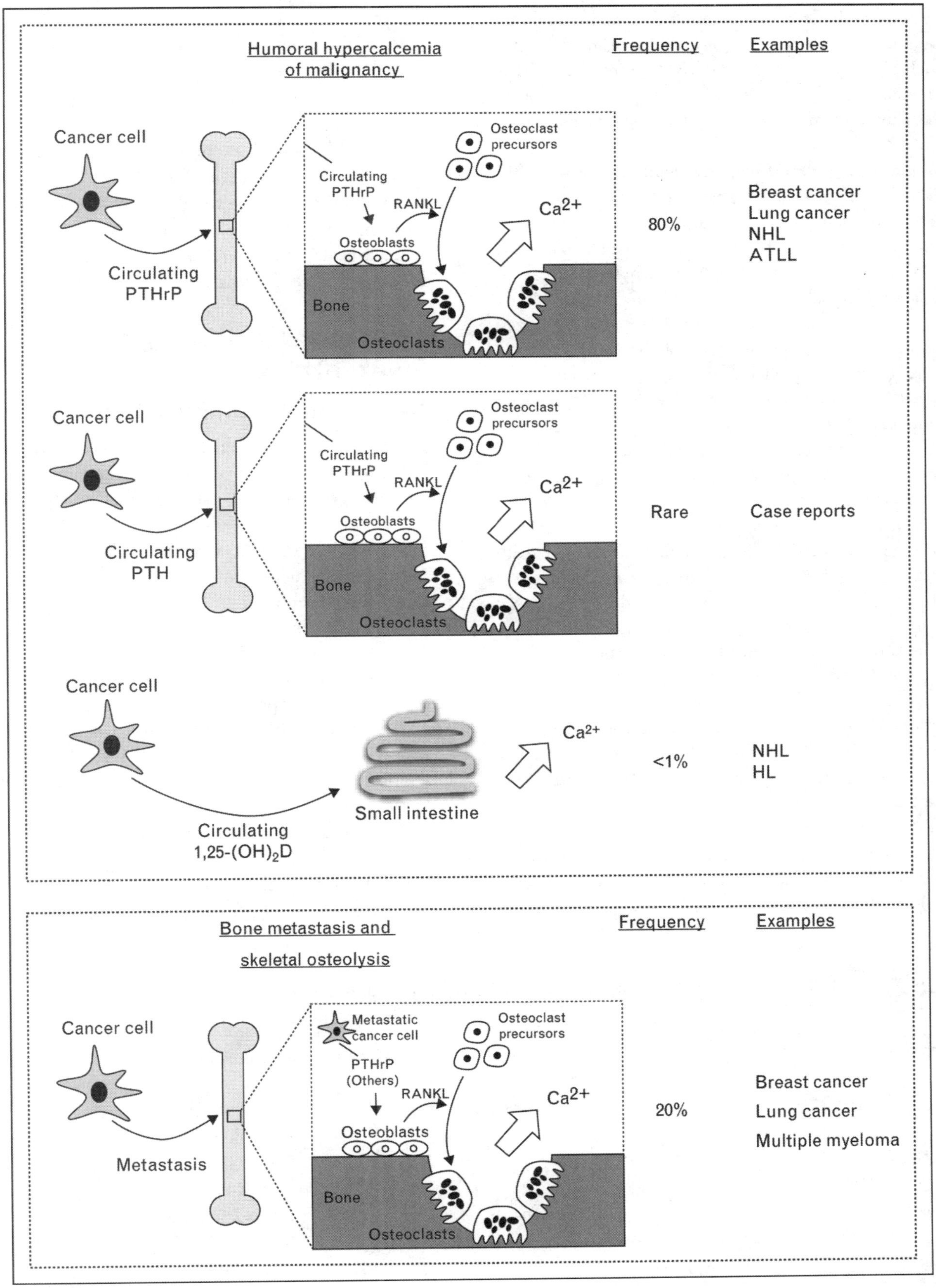

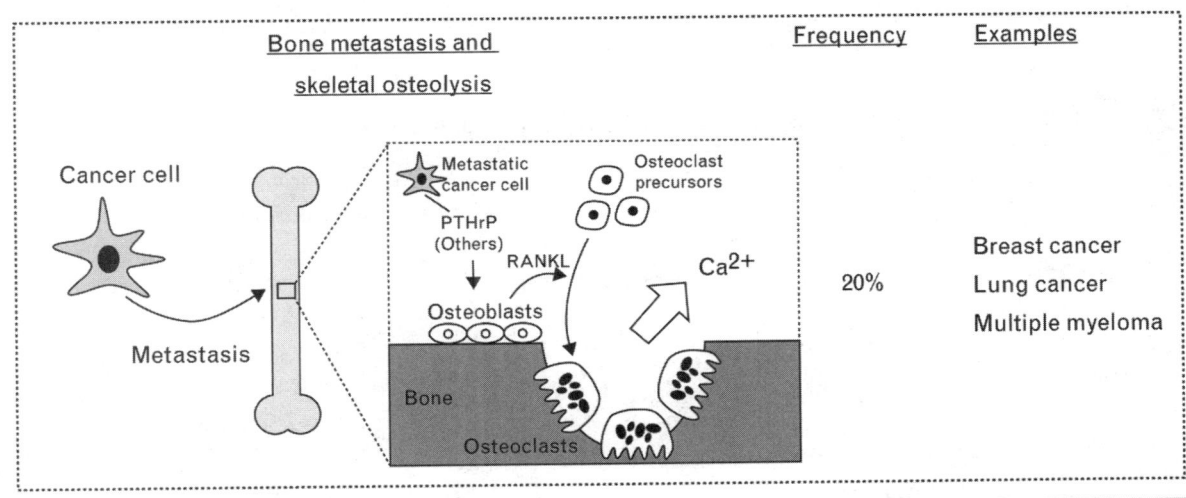

Figure 40.2 Etiology of hypercalcemia of malignancy.
Reprinted with permission from: Clines GA Mechanisms and treatment of hypercalcemia of malignancy. Curr Opin Endocrinol Diabetes Obes 2011;18:339-46.

be seen within 3–7 days. Although zoledronic acid has a significantly higher response rate in some studies and can be given for a shorter period, this must be weighed against its much higher cost compared with pamidronate.[25] With both medications, serum creatinine and other serum electrolytes should be monitored as well as the serum calcium concentration.

For severe hypercalcemia, treatment should be initiated immediately with normal saline hydration, a bisphosphonate, and calcitonin. Although it has a more transient and smaller magnitude of effect than do bisphosphonates, calcitonin is given in this setting because of its quicker onset of action (decreases seen within 2 hours after administration) compared with bisphosphonates.[26] It antagonizes PTH, thereby decreasing osteoclast activity and promoting renal excretion of calcium, and is given at an initial dose of 4 international units/kg twice daily as either an intramuscular or a subcutaneous injection. Prolonged exposure to calcitonin can increase the risk of tachyphylaxis, and often, a maximum threshold of 2–3 days in considered for use in treatment.[27]

In patients who are refractory to bisphosphonate therapy or who have marked renal insufficiency, denosumab may provide another option for treating HCM. Denosumab decreases osteoclast formation and activation by binding to the receptor activator of nuclear factor-κB ligand (RANKL) and preventing its interaction with the receptor activator of nuclear factor-κB (RANK) on the osteoclast cell surface.[17] It is given as a subcutaneous injection of 120 mg every 4 weeks. During the first month of therapy, additional doses of 120 mg are given on days 8 and 15. A response is typically seen within 9 days, but a complete response may not occur until 3 weeks after administration.

Other therapies that can aid in managing hypercalcemia but that are used less commonly include glucocorticoids, which decrease calcitriol production; gallium nitrate, which inhibits bone resorption and promotes formation; cinacalcet, which is a calcimimetic that sensitizes the calcium-sensing receptor on the parathyroid gland and in turn lowers PTH synthesis; and dialysis.[19] However, all of these therapies are limited by either efficacy or adverse effects.

Of note, although these measures all decrease the serum calcium concentration, the cause of the hypercalcemia must ultimately be addressed. For hypercalcemia caused by malignancy, treatment of the cancer should be implemented as appropriate to prevent further recurrences of hypercalcemia and provide for a more sustained response.

SYNDROME OF INAPPROPRIATE DIURETIC HORMONE

Definition/Pathophysiology

Hyponatremia is defined as total body water excess in relation to serum sodium and is the most common electrolyte disorder associated with malignancy. Hyponatremia can further be classified as mild (less than 135 mmol/L), moderate (less than 130 mmol/L), or profound (less than 125 mmol/L) depending on serum sodium concentrations. The presentation of hyponatremia is a spectrum of clinical symptoms ranging from mild nausea and vomiting to severe neurological deficits including the potential for seizure, coma, or respiratory arrest. Hyponatremia is considered a poor prognostic factor and is associated with significant mortality and morbidity, including increased length of hospital stay. Syndrome of inappropriate diuretic hormone is the most common cause of cancer-related hyponatremia.[28,29]

Ectopic production of arginine vasopressin (AVP) by tumor cells serves as the underlying mechanism for SIADH in the setting of malignancy. Under normal physiologic controls, AVP functions to regulate fluid and

Table 40.4 Clinical Signs and Symptoms Associated with Hypercalcemia

Renal "Stones"	Skeleton "Bones"	Gastrointestinal "Moans"	Psychic "Groans"	Cardiovascular	Other
Nephrolithiasis	Bone pain	Nausea, vomiting	Impaired concentration	Hypertension	Itching
Nephrogenic diabetes insipidus	Arthritis	Anorexia	Confusion	Shortened QT interval	Keratitis
Dehydration	Osteoporosis	Constipation	Fatigue	Cardiac arrhythmias	
Nephrocalcinosis	Osteitis fibrosis cystica in hyperparathyroidism	Abdominal pain	Muscle weakness	Vacular calcification	
		Pancreatitis	Coma		
		Peptic ulcer disease			

Table 40.5 Current Treatments for Hypercalcemia of Malignancy

Agent	Dosage	Indication	Mechanism of Action	Adverse Effects
IV infusion of saline	4–6 L/day	Hydration	Increase calciuria	Volume expansion, hypokalemia, hypomagnesemia, may exacerbate CHF, dehydration if used before intravascular volume is restored
Furosemide	20–60 mg up to 500 mg/day	Loop diuretic	Increase in diuresis and calciuria	Hypokalemia, hypomagnesemia
Pamidronate	15–90 mg IV in 4–6 hr	Bisphosphonate	Inhibits osteoclast action and bone resorption	Nephrotoxicity, hypocalcemia
Zoledronic acid	4 mg IV over 15 min	Bisphosphonate	Inhibits osteoclast action and bone resorption	Nephrotoxicity, hypocalcemia
Denosumab	120 mg SC, dosing schedule of day 1, 8, 15, 29; then monthly	RANKL inhibitor	Inhibits osteoclast recruitment, maturation, and activation and slows bone resorption	Hypocalcemia
Calcitonin	200–500 IU/day	Hormone	Inhibits vitamin D conversion to calcitriol	Nausea, vomiting, escape phenomenon
Prednisone	40–100 mg/day	Corticosteroid	Decrease in Ca^{2+} absorption, increase in calciuria	Iatrogenic Cushing syndrome
Hemodialysis	Ca^{2+}-free dialysate		Dialysis of Ca^{2+} from the circulation	Dialysis related

CHF = congestive heart failure; IV = intravenous(ly); RANKL = receptor activator of nuclear factor kappa-B ligand; SC = subcutaneously.

electrolyte balance and maintain effective plasma osmolality. Arginine vasopressin is stimulated in response to plasma hyperosmolality or hypovolemia. In the setting of increased effective plasma osmolality, osmoreceptors are activated within the hypothalamus, stimulating the release of AVP from the posterior pituitary. Arginine vasopressin then binds to V_2 receptors within the basolateral membrane of collecting tubules of the kidney and stimulates the production of cyclic adenosine monophosphate (cAMP). Cyclic adenosine monophosphate mediates the synthesis of aquaporin-2 water channels, which are inserted within the walls of the collecting-duct of the kidney to ultimately increase water permeability and reabsorption and reestablish normal serum osmolality. Corrected serum osmolality then serves as a negative feedback for continued AVP secretion and activity.[28,30-32]

Decreased effective blood volume also serves as a stimulus for increased AVP. Baroreceptors within the vasculature of the heart sense circulating blood volume, and in the setting of hypovolemia, AVP is released, which binds to V_1 receptors within blood vessels and causes vasoconstriction in an effort to increase systemic vascular resistance. In the setting of malignancy, production of AVP is ectopic and secreted in the absence of plasma hyperosmolality or hypovolemia, thereby creating a dilutional hyponatremia with increased total body weight and maintained serum sodium concentrations.

Incidence/Risk Factors

Syndrome of inappropriate diuretic hormone is most commonly associated with small cell lung cancer with an incidence of 11%–15%.[31] Syndrome of inappropriate diuretic hormone has also been reported among other subtypes of lung cancer including adenocarcinomas, squamous cell carcinomas, and large cell carcinomas, although incidence is limited to case reports. Head and neck cancer is the second most common malignancy associated with SIADH, particularly head and neck cancers of squamous cell histology. The incidence of SIADH among other cancer types is rare but has been reported for cervical, breast, and prostate cancer and hematologic malignancies including Hodgkin lymphoma, non-Hodgkin lymphoma, chronic lymphocytic leukemia, and multiple myeloma.[28,31-33]

Beyond the ectopic production of AVP by these specific cancer types, many chemotherapy agents used in treating malignancy may cause SIADH. Chemotherapy agents including the vinca alkaloids, specifically vincristine and vinblastine; platinum agents, including cisplatin and carboplatin; and alkylating agents, including cyclophosphamide and melphalan, potentiate the hyponatremic effects of SIADH by increasing the production of AVP. Immunomodulator agents including interferon and aldesleukin have also been reported to cause hyponatremic effects consistent with SIADH.[28,31,34] Syndrome of inappropriate diuretic hormone may also be related to the supportive care interventions used for palliation of patients with cancer, including analgesic medications, specifically opioids and nonsteroidal anti-inflammatory agents, antidepressants, and aggressive hydration therapy required with specific chemotherapy agents to mitigate potentially toxic adverse effects.[31,35]

Clinical Presentation/Symptoms

The clinical presentation of SIADH is a wide spectrum of neurological symptoms. The severity of the neurological symptoms is related to the acuity of the change in the plasma sodium concentration, degree of the hyponatremia, and ability of the adaptive mechanisms within the brain to respond to and compensate for changes in effective plasma osmolality. Normal compensatory mechanisms will respond to decreased plasma osmolality related to hyponatremia by increasing the transit of water and limiting the transit of organic solutes into the cerebral space to effectively maintain the normal total brain volume. These compensatory mechanisms become overwhelmed in the setting of acute or severe hyponatremia and cannot provide for timely correction of hyponatremia, thereby increasing the risk of cerebral edema and irreversible neurological damage. Symptom severity is determined by the degree of cerebral edema; mild hyponatremia is characterized by headache, weakness, and decreased concentration, whereas profound hyponatremia is characterized by altered mental status, hallucinations, seizures, obtundation, and respiratory arrest.[28,29,31]

Management of SIADH

The goal of managing SIADH in the setting of malignancy is to prevent the potentially serious neurological complications caused by severe hyponatremia. Optimal management of tumor-related SIADH is treatment of the underlying malignancy. Given the delayed therapeutic effects of chemotherapy to correct hyponatremia related to SIADH, other treatment modalities can be considered to optimize sodium/water balance. Hypertonic (3%) saline is recommended for treating symptomatic SIADH and can be administered as a continuous infusion at a rate of 1–2 mL per kilogram of body weight per hour or as 150-mL boluses every 20 minutes with repeat 150-mL infusions continued only until symptoms have resolved or serum sodium has increased by 5 mmol/L. Careful and periodic monitoring of changes in serum sodium is recommended to reduce the risk of overcorrection, including osmotic demyelination, which can be characterized by severe lethargy, motor weakness and paralysis, confusion, behavioral changes, and even coma.[30] After the first hour of therapy, it is recommended to discontinue the hypertonic saline if the serum sodium concentration has increased by 5 mmol/L and symptoms have improved and to transition to treatment aimed at the underlying cause of SIADH with continuous monitoring of serum sodium for the first 24 hours. Correction of sodium should be limited to 10 mmol/L for the first 24 hours and 8 mmol/L every 24 hours thereafter to decrease the risk of osmotic demyelination. If symptoms do not improve despite a serum sodium increase of 5 mmol/L within the first hour of therapy, hypertonic saline can be titrated to increase serum sodium by an additional 1 mmol/L not to exceed 130 mmol/L (even if symptoms persist); however, other causes of hyponatremia should be investigated.[28,29,31] Various formulas are available for calculating the initial rate of hypertonic saline. The mostly widely accepted formula, the Adrogue-Madias model, aims to achieve a 1-mmoL/L/hour increase in serum sodium, although correction speed may surpass that predicted by the equation, thereby necessitating careful monitoring.[29-30]

All patients with asymptomatic SIADH and without contraindications to aggressive fluid restriction should be limited to 500 mL below the average daily urine output. Fluid restriction is an effective therapeutic strategy for correcting hyponatremia in the setting of SIADH, although compliance may be challenging, ultimately necessitating the initiation of other pharmacotherapeutic interventions for tumor-related SIADH (Table 40.6). Demeclocycline is a tetracycline derivative that inhibits the formation of cAMP, thereby blocking the downstream-mediated effects of AVP on the kidneys. At the recommended dose of 600 mg orally once daily, demeclocycline is generally well tolerated, although higher doses have been associated with renal toxicity.[28,29,31,36]

Arginine vasopressin receptor antagonists block the binding of AVP to the V_2 receptors within the renal collecting ducts, thereby increasing water excretion. Conivaptan and tolvaptan are the two vasopressin antagonists available. Conivaptan is a nonselective vasopressin antagonist that binds to both V_{1A} and V_2 receptors and is indicated for treating euvolemic or hypervolemic hyponatremia. The recommended dose of conivaptan is 20 mg administered as an intravenous infusion over 30 minutes, followed by a continuous infusion of 20 mg/day, although the treatment is limited to 2–4 days. Tolvaptan is an oral, selective vasopressin antagonist that binds specifically to V_2 receptors. Tolvaptan is indicated for treating symptomatic euvolemic or hypervolemic hyponatremia that has not responded to a trial of fluid restriction. The recommended starting dose of tolvaptan is 15 mg orally once daily, which can be titrated to 30 and 60 mg, depending on the serum sodium response. Both conivaptan and tolvaptan require careful

Table 40.6 Therapeutic Treatment Options for Syndrome of Inappropriate Antidiuretic Hormone Secretion

Treatment	Mechanism of Action	Administration/Use	Monitoring	Adverse Effects
Hypertonic saline (3%)	Functions as electrolyte replacement for the treatment of symptomatic hyponatremia	Given as 1–2 mL/kg/hr or as 150-mL boluses every 20 min until symptoms have resolved or serum sodium increases by 5 mmol/L	Serum sodium; recommended to stop therapy if serum sodium increases by 5 mmol/L or more within the first hour; correction should be limited to 10 mmol/L within the first 24 hr and 8 mmol/L every 24 hr thereafter	Central pontine myelinolysis; Overhydration; Pulmonary edema; Congestive heart failure
Aggressive fluid restriction	Prevents further fluid accumulation and promotes fluid loss to correct hypervolemia	Restrict all fluid intake, intravenous or oral, to a total volume that is 500 mL lower than the patient's 24-hr urine output	Electrolytes; renal function panel; close supervision of intake	Dehydration; Serum creatinine elevations
Demeclocycline	Inhibits formation of cAMP and subsequent AVP binding to prevent water reabsorption	Demeclocycline 600–1,200 mg orally once daily	Serum sodium; renal function panel; liver function panel; anaphylaxis	Serum creatinine elevations; Hepatic toxicity
Conivaptan	V_{1A} and V_2 AVP receptor antagonist promotes excretion of water	Conivaptan IV 20 mg, over 30 min, followed by conivaptan IV 20–40 mg over 24 hr for 2–4 days	Serum sodium; renal function panel; urine output; liver function panel; concomitant use with CYP3A4 inhibitors; blood pressure	Hypotension; Hypokalemia; Injection-site reactions
Tolvaptan	V_{1A} and V_2 AVP receptor antagonist promotes excretion of water	Tolvaptan 15 mg orally once daily, may increase to a maximum of 60 mg orally once daily for no more than 30 days	Serum sodium; renal function panel; urine output; liver function panel; concomitant use with CYP3A4 inhibitors; blood pressure	Nausea; Xerostomia; Increased thirst; Hepatic toxicity

AVP = arginine vasopressin; cAMP = cyclic adenosine monophosphate.

monitoring of serum sodium to minimize the risk of overcorrection and osmotic demyelination. Although mechanistically, the AVP receptor antagonists serve as a targeted therapy for tumor-related SIADH, consensus guidelines do not recommend the routine use of vasopressin receptor antagonists for treating SIADH. Use of AVP receptor antagonists in the setting of malignancy is limited to case reports and case series.[29,36]

SUPERIOR VENA CAVA SYNDROME

The superior vena cava (SVC) is a vessel originating from the confluence of the brachiocephalic veins and ending at the superior right atrium. Superior vena cava syndrome arises when the SVC becomes completely or partly obstructed or compressed, resulting in reduced venous drainage from the head, neck, and upper extremities to the right side of the heart. It is estimated that 15,000 cases of SVCS occur in the United States each year.[37] Malignancies are the most common underlying factor identified in the development of SVCS; however, other factors can cause this condition.[37] The most common malignancies associated with SVCS include lymphoma, lung cancer, breast cancer, and other mediastinal metastatic lesions.[38] Additional nonmalignant causes of SCVS account for 35% of cases and are attributed to the frequent use of central venous catheters and thrombosis.[37,39]

Diagnosis

The diagnosis of SVCS is largely clinical, and the signs and symptoms of SVCS are highly variable. The clinical presentation of each patient depends on the degree of SVC narrowing and speed of compression or obstruction.[38,40]

Most commonly, the onset of SVCS is slow and progressively worsens over several weeks, which allows the body to create collateral veins to provide alternative routes of venous drainage back to the right atrium. In rare cases, SCVS has been reported to develop quickly in rapidly growing tumors and thrombosis.[41] Early signs of SVCS include facial swelling, extremity edema, distended neck and chest veins, dyspnea, non-productive cough, and hoarseness.[11] Those with advanced symptoms of SVCS present with respiratory distress, cyanosis of the face or upper torso, engorged conjunctivae, mental status changes, coma, or seizures.[39] In addition, patients presenting with declining cognitive function should receive a neurological evaluation to rule out brain metastases.

Imaging of the mediastinum region has a widely accepted role in the diagnosis of SVCS. Computed tomography (CT) scan is the most useful radiographic study and should be completed with contrast material.[37,39] Magnetic resonance imaging (MRI) is an acceptable alternative in patients who cannot tolerate contrast medium.[37] Imaging studies can aid in identifying the underlying cause of the SVCS (i.e., external compression, thrombosis).[40]

Treatment

Initial treatment options in managing SVCS largely depend on the severity of symptoms present on diagnosis and the underlying condition. In most cases, SVCS is not considered a medical emergency because the onset is rarely sudden and provides the body time to compensate by directing blood through the azygous system.[40] Because of the slow onset of symptoms, it is considered safe and appropriate to obtain biopsies and imaging studies in an attempt to apply effective therapy. Patients who present with neurological dysfunction or airway compromise may require emergency treatment with an endovascular stent. Nonspecific measures commonly used for the primary management of SVCS aim to decrease intracranial pressure by elevating the head of the bed and administering diuretics.[42] Glucocorticoids may be useful in shrinking tumors caused by lymphoma, but they offer no benefit in lung cancer.[38]

Patients who warrant immediate treatment or whose chemotherapy or radiation therapy has failed may benefit from the placement of an endovascular stent that should not disrupt further diagnostic evaluations and may improve symptoms within 24–48 hours.[42-44] Intravascular thrombus associated with a central venous catheter can be appropriately treated through catheter removal in conjunction with administration of an anticoagulant to minimize clot embolization.[40] In addition, endovascular stent placement can be considered for thrombus associated with an indwelling catheter.[43]

Cases of SVCS as a result of malignancy, newly diagnosed or preexisting, can effectively be managed by chemotherapy or radiation. Lymphoma, small cell lung cancer, and germ cell tumors are generally chemosensitive and are appropriately managed through the administration of systemic chemotherapy. Radiation therapy is the treatment of choice for SVCS caused by non–small cell lung cancer and other metastatic solid tumors that have well-defined borders and are less chemosensitive.[38,45]

NEUROLOGICAL

Spinal Cord Compression

The incidence of malignant spinal cord compression (MSCC) is estimated to be 1 in 12,700 patients with cancer, or 5%, annually.[46,47] Although any metastatic or locally advanced cancer has the potential to induce MSCC, certain cancers have a stronger probability than do others.[46] Malignancies of the prostate, breast, and lung have been associated with 15%–20% of MSCC cases in adults.[48-50] In addition, non-Hodgkin lymphoma, multiple myeloma, and renal cell carcinoma each account for 5%–10% of cases; remaining cases are attributed to colorectal cancer, cancer of unknown primary origin, and sarcoma.[46,51] Compression of the spinal cord can occur anywhere along the spine; however, most commonly, MSCC is associated with the thoracic spine (70%), followed by the lumbosacral spine (20%) and the cervical spine (10%).[38] Furthermore, it is not uncommon to have involvement along the spine at several locations, which is more commonly seen in breast and prostate cancers.[38]

Malignant spinal cord compression is often defined as compression of the spinal cord and/or cauda equina caused by extradural metastatic or locally advanced malignancy.[38,52] Several phases are involved in the development of MSCC, the first consisting of tumor enlargement resulting in compression of the extradural space. Research suggests that the spread of metastatic disease occurs from direct arterial embolization by malignant cells.[53] Continued expansion of malignant tumors resulting in worsening compression obstructs the venous plexus and leads to edema formation. Subsequent production of inflammatory cytokines increases blood flow and continues to increase the formation of edema.[38] Early-stage spinal cord injury originates from edema formation. As the MSCC progresses, the edema induces a state of ischemia-hypoxia and, if left untreated, results in irreversible damage to the spinal cord.[38]

Diagnosis

Signs and symptoms of MSCC include pain and deficits in motor, sensory, and autonomic function.[52] Up to 95% of patients with MSCC present with back pain at the time of diagnosis for a median of several weeks before presentation, which may precede a cancer diagnosis.[52] Patients describe a localized pain that progressively worsens over several weeks.[46] A distinguishing feature of MSCC from other types of back pain is the increase in pain when in a supine or relaxing position compared with when upright as a result of distension of the epidural venous plexus.[42]

Deficits in motor function are the most noticeable symptom of MSCC and are present in 60%–85% of patients at the time of diagnosis.[46,50] A total of two-thirds of patients diagnosed with MSCC are non-ambulatory at the time of diagnosis.[46,50] Early identification of motor function weakness is important because pretreatment neurological status is the most important predictor of post-treatment function.[39,46,50]

The prevalence of sensory deficits is estimated to occur in 40%–90% of patients with MSCC, although patients tend to be less aware of sensory deficits than of motor function deficits.[46,50] It is thought that sensory levels are located one to five segments below the site of spinal cord compression.[50]

Complications involving autonomic dysfunction include decreased anal sphincter tone, decreased perianal sensibility, and distended bladder with postvoid residual volumes greater than 150 mL.[38,50] Isolated incidents of any of these symptoms are not indicative of the development of MSCC. Autonomic dysfunction, specifically urinary retention, is present on diagnosis in about 50% of MSCC cases and is an unfavorable prognostic factor.[38,52]

Because of symptoms that are not unique to MSCC, patients should undergo imaging studies to rule out other causes of their symptoms or to confirm a diagnosis of MSCC. The gold standard for the diagnosis of MSCC is an MRI, which provides a sensitivity of 93%, specificity of 97%, and accuracy of 95% and aids in the preparation of radiation fields.[40,52,53] Use of an MRI for imaging lesions in one study altered radiation fields and affected treatment choices in 40% of patients.[54] As discussed previously, involvement of more than one area of the spinal cord is common; therefore, imaging studies should include the entire spine.[38] When an MRI is contraindicated or unavailable, CT myelography is considered an acceptable alternative.[52]

Treatment

The primary treatment goals in MSCC include pain control and the preservation and/or restoration of neurological functioning. Corticosteroids are considered the first-line treatment for most patients with MSCC because they decrease edema, have tumoricidal effect in certain types of cancer, and are associated with resolution of neurological deficits.[38,52,53] Although the most effective loading dose, maintenance dose, and treatment duration are controversial, one randomized study stratified patients to receive 96 or 16 mg of dexamethasone daily in combination with radiotherapy.[55] Better outcomes were not associated with higher doses, but they were associated with greater rates of adverse effects. Administration practices may vary between institutions, but common corticosteroid loading and maintenance doses include high doses (dexamethasone 100 mg loading dose, followed by 96 mg daily) or moderate doses (dexamethasone 10 mg loading dose, followed by 16 mg daily).[53]

The optimal dose and treatment regimen of radiotherapy in managing MSCC lack consistency as well. Radiotherapy should involve the malignant area of the spine as well as one or two vertebral bodies above and below the site of compression. The most commonly used radiotherapy schedule in the United States provides a total of 30 Gray in 10 fractions because higher doses have not been associated with better outcomes.[53,56] Lower doses and fewer fractions could be appropriately considered in patients who have a poor prognosis or more comorbidities.

Given recent surgical advances, patients who have a favorable performance score may benefit from decompression surgery. Those who can withstand a surgical procedure may achieve immediate decompression as well as spinal reconstruction to provide stabilization.[53] A randomized trial determined that direct decompressive surgery plus radiotherapy was superior to radiotherapy alone for improving and regaining the ability to walk, increasing overall survival and functional ability, maintaining continence, and reducing opioid analgesic use.[57] Weaknesses of this study include the lack of generalizability to every tumor type seen in practice and the inclusion of patients with only one area of spinal cord involvement. As a result, eligible patients should be compared with those included in this study to determine the best treatment modality for their primary tumor causing MSCC.

SUMMARY

As more treatment options emerge and people live longer with cancer, it is important to quickly and accurately identify the oncologic emergencies with which patients may present. Tumor lysis syndrome has the potential to result in nephrotoxicity, neurological defects, and myocardial events if no appropriate measures are taken. Hypercalcemia of malignancy occurs in up to 20% of patients with cancer and is a poor prognostic feature. Measures for treating HCM all work to decrease the serum calcium concentration; however, the underlying malignancy should be addressed to prevent recurrence. Clinical presentation of hyponatremia has a large spectrum of symptoms, and SIADH is usually the cause of cancer-related hyponatremia. Although the treatment of hyponatremia largely revolves around fluid restriction, it is important to address cancer-related treatment options. Superior vena cava syndrome can present as a gradual or rapid onset, with the former allowing sufficient time to decide how best to treat the patient. Therapies can range from removing the central venous catheter to placing an endovascular stent. Patients with MSCC often present with pain and decreased neurological functioning. Treatment strategies are aimed at decreasing inflammation and targeting the primary tumor as quickly as possible to restore normal functioning. Early identification of oncologic emergencies with appropriate treatment has the potential to prevent the further complications and improve the patient's quality of life.

REFERENCES

1. Howard SC, Jones DP, Pui CH. The tumor lysis syndrome. N Engl J Med 2011;364:1844-54.
2. Coiffier B, Altman A, Pui CH, et al. Guidelines for the management of pediatric and adult tumor lysis syndrome: an evidence-based review. J Clin Oncol 2008;26:2767-78.
3. Wilson FP, Berns JS. Tumor lysis syndrome: new challenges and recent advances. Adv Chronic Kidney Dis 2014;21:18-26.
4. Cairo MS, Bishop M. Tumor lysis syndrome: new therapeutic strategies and classification. Br J Haematol 2004;127:3-11.
5. Rampello E, Fricia T, Malaguarnera M. The management of tumor lysis syndrome. Nat Clin Pract Oncol 2006;3:438-47.
6. Abu-Alfa AK, Younes A. Tumor lysis syndrome and acute kidney injury: evaluation, prevention and management. Am J Kidney Dis 2010;55:1-13.
7. Davidson MD, Thakkar S, Hix JK, et al. Pathophysiology, clinical consequences, and treatment of tumor lysis syndrome. Am J Med 2004;116:546-54.
8. Cairo MS, Coiffier B, Reiter A, et al. Recommendations for evaluation of risk and prophylaxis of tumor lysis syndrome (TLS) in adults and children with malignant disease: an expert TLS panel consensus. Br J Haematol 2010;149:578-86.
9. McBride A, Westervelt P. Recognizing and managing the expanded risk of tumor lysis syndrome in hematologic and solid malignancies. J Hematol Oncol 2012;5:1-11.
10. Will A, Tholouli E. The clinical management of tumor lysis syndrome in haematological malignancies. Br J Haematol 2011;154:3-13.
11. Cairo MS, Coiffier B, Reiter A, et al. Recommendations for the evaluation of risk and prophylaxis of tumour lysis syndrome (TLS) in adults and children with malignant diseases: an expert TLS panel consensus. Br J Haematol 2010;149:578-86.
12. Knoebel RW, Lo M, Crank CW. Evaluation of a low, weight-based dose of rasburicase in adult patients for the treatment or prophylaxis of tumor lysis syndrome. J Oncol Pharm Pract 2011;17:147-54.
13. Vines AN, Shanholtz CB, Thompson JL. Fixed-dose rasburicase 6 mg for hyperuricemia and tumor lysis syndrome in high-risk cancer patients. Ann Pharmacother 2010;44:1529-37.
14. Trifilio S, Gordon L, Singhal S, et al. Reduced-dose rasburicase (recombinant xanthine oxidase) in adult cancer patients with hyperuricemia. Bone Marrow Transplant 2006;37:997-1001.
15. Reeves DJ, Bestul DJ. Evaluation of a single fixed dose of rasburicase 7.5 mg for the treatment of hyperuricemia in adults with cancer. Pharmacotherapy 2008;28:685-90.
16. McBride A, Lathan SC, Boehmer L, et al. A comparative evaluation of single fixed-dosing and weight-based dosing of rasburicase for tumor lysis syndrome. Pharmacotherapy 2013;33:295-303.
17. Hochberg J, Cairo MS. Rasburicase: future directions in tumor lysis management. Expert Opin Biol Ther 2008;8:1595-604.
18. Vassilopoulo-Sellin R, Newman BM, Taylor SH, et al. Incidence of hypercalcemia in patients with malignancy referred to a comprehensive cancer center. Cancer 1993;71:1309-12.
19. Stewart AF. Clinical practice. Hypercalcemia associated with cancer. N Engl J Med. 2005;352:373-9.
20. Ikeda K, Ohno H, Hane M, et al. Development of a sensitive two-site immunoradiometric assay for parathyroid hormone-related peptide: evidence for elevated levels in plasma in patients with adult T-cell leukemia/lymphoma and B-cell lymphoma. J Clin Endocrinol Metab 1994;79:1322-7.
21. Seymour JF, Grill V, Martin TJ, et al. Hypercalcemia in the blast phase of chronic myeloid leukemia associated with elevated parathyroid hormone-related protein. Leukemia 1993;7:1672-5.
22. Seymour JF, Gagel RF. Calcitriol: the major humoral mediator of hypercalcemia in Hodgkin's disease and non-Hodgkin's lymphoma. Blood 1993;82:1383-94.
23. Mundy GR. Metastasis to bone: causes, consequences and therapeutic opportunities. Nat Rev Cancer 2002;2:584-93.
24. Nussbaum SR, Gaz RD, Arnold A. Hypercalcemia and ectopic secretion of parathyroid hormone by an ovarian carcinoma with rearrangement of the gene for parathyroid hormone. N Engl J Med 1990;323:1324-8.
25. Major P, Lortholary A, Hon J et al. Zoledronic acid is superior to pamidronate in the treatment of hypercalcemia of malignancy: a pooled analysis of two randomized, controlled clinical trials. J Clin Oncol 2001;19:558-67.
26. Wisnewski LA. Salmon calcitonin in the acute management of hypercalcemia. Calcif Tissue Int 1990;46:256.
27. Vaughn CB, Vaitkevicius VK. The effects of calcitonin in hypercalcemia in patients with malignancy. Cancer 1974;34:1268.
28. Raftopoulos H. Diagnosis and management of hyponatremia in cancer patients. Support Cancer Care 2007;15:1341-7.
29. Spasovski G, Vanholder R, Allolio B, et al. Clinical practice guideline on diagnosis and treatment of hyponatremia 2014;170:1-47.
30. Ellison DH, Berl T. The syndrome of inappropriate antidiuresis. N Engl J Med 2007;356:2064-72.
31. Castillo JJ, Vincent M, Justice E. Diagnosis and management of hyponatremia in cancer patients. Oncologist 2012;17:756-65.
32. Sorensen JB, Anderson MK, Hansen HH. Syndrome of inappropriate secretion of antidiuretic hormone in malignant disease. J Intern Med 1995;238:97-110.
33. Rosner MH, Dalkin AC. Electrolyte disorders associated with cancer. Adv Chronic Kidney Dis 2014;21:7-17.
34. Berghmans T. Hyponatremia related to medical anticancer treatment. Support Care Cancer 1996;4:341-50.
35. Liamis G, Milionis H, Elisaf M. A review of drug-induced hyponatremia. Am J Kidney Dis 2008;52:144-53.
36. Onitilo AA, Kio E, Suhail AR. Tumor-related hyponatremia. Clin Med Res 2007;5:228-37.
37. Lewis MA, Hendrickson AW, Moynihan TJ. Oncologic emergencies: pathophysiology, presentation, diagnosis, and treatment. CA Cancer J Clin 2011;61:287-314.

38. Gucalp R, Dutcher J. Chapter 276. Oncologic emergencies. In: Longo DL, Fauci AS, Kasper DL, et al., eds. Harrison's Principles of Internal Medicine, 18e. New York: McGraw-Hill, 2012. Available at http://accesspharmacy.mhmedical.com.proxy.lib.ohio.
39. Colen FN. Oncologic emergencies: superior vena cava syndrome, tumor lysis syndrome, and spinal cord compression. J Emerg Nurs 2008;34:535-7.
40. Cervantes A, Chirivella I. Oncological emergencies. Ann Oncol 2004;15(suppl 4):iv299-306.
41. Halfdanarson TR, Hogan WJ, Moynihan TJ. Oncologic emergencies: diagnosis and treatment. Mayo Clin Proc 2006;81:835-48.
42. Krimsky WS, Behrens RJ, Kerkvliet GJ. Oncologic emergencies for the internist. Cleve Clin J Med 2002;69:209-22.
43. Lanciego C, Chacon JL, Julian A, et al. Stenting as first option for endovascular treatment of malignant superior vena cava syndrome. AJR Am J Roentgenol 2001;177:585-93.
44. Yim CD, Sane SS, Bjarnason H. Superior vena cava stenting. Radiol Clin North Am 2000;38:409-24.
45. Yu JB, Wilson JD, Detterbeck FC. Superior vena cava syndrome—a proposed classification system and algorithm for management. J Thorac Oncol 2008;3:811-4.
46. Schiff D. Spinal cord compression. Neurol Clin 2003;21:67-86.
47. Loblaw DA, Laperriere NJ, Mackillop WJ. A population-based study of malignant spinal cord compression in Ontario. Clin Oncol (R Coll Radiol) 2003;15:211-7.
48. Helweg-Larsen S, Hansen SW, Sorensen PS. Second occurrence of symptomatic metastatic spinal cord compression and findings of multiple spinal epidural metastases. Int J Radiat Oncol Biol Phys 1995;33:595-8.
49. Maranzano E, Latini P, Ceccaglini F, et al. Radiation therapy in spinal cord compression: a prospective analysis of 105 consecutive patients. Cancer 1991;67:1311-7.
50. Schiff D, O'Neill BP, Suman VJ. Spinal epidural metastasis as the initial manifestation of malignancy: clinical features and diagnostic approach. Neurology 1997;49:452-6.
51. Abraham JL, Banffy MB, Harris MB. Spinal cord compression in patients with advanced metastatic cancer: "all I care about is walking and living my life." JAMA 2008;299:937-46.
52. Prasad D, Schiff D. Malignant spinal-cord compression. Lancet Oncol 2005;6:15-24.
53. Cole JS, Patchell RA. Metastatic epidural spinal cord compression. Lancet Neurol 2008;7:459-66.
54. Colletti PM, Siegel HJ, Woo MY, et al. The impact of treatment planning of MRI of the spine in patients suspected of vertebral metastasis: an efficacy study. Comput Med Imaging Graph 1996;20:159-62.
55. Graham PH, Capp A, Delaney G, et al. Clin Oncol (R Coll Radiol) 2006;18:70-6.
56. Lewis MA, Hendrickson AW, Moynihan TJ. Oncologic emergencies: pathophysiology, presentation, diagnosis, treatment. CA Cancer J Clin 2011;61:287-314.
57. Patchell RA, Tibbs PA, Regine WF, et al. Direct decompressive surgical resection in the treatment of spinal cord compression caused by metastatic cancer: a randomized trial. Lancet 2005;366:643-8.

Section 10

Miscellaneous

Chapter 41

Drug Dosing in Special Intensive Care Unit Populations

Jeffrey F. Barletta, Pharm.D., FCCM

LEARNING OBJECTIVES

1. Compare and contrast the different descriptors used to characterize body mass.
2. Describe the pharmacokinetic changes that occur with morbid obesity.
3. List the steps to take when calculating a dosing regimen for the morbidly obese patient.
4. Develop a pharmacotherapy plan for a critically ill patient who is morbidly obese.
5. Describe the pharmacokinetic changes that occur with pregnancy.
6. List the medications that should not be considered in the critically ill pregnant patient.
7. Develop a pharmacotherapy plan for a critically ill patient who is pregnant.
8. Describe the pharmacokinetic changes that occur with therapeutic plasma exchange.
9. Develop a pharmacotherapy plan for a critically ill patient who is undergoing therapeutic plasma exchange therapy.
10. Describe the pharmacokinetic changes that occur with molecular adsorbent recirculating system therapy.
11. Develop a pharmacotherapy plan for a critically ill patient who is undergoing molecular adsorbent recirculating system therapy.

ABBREVIATIONS IN THIS CHAPTER

AdjBW	Adjusted body weight	MARS	Molecular adsorbent recirculating system
BMI	Body mass index	MIC	Minimum inhibitory concentration
IBW	Ideal body weight	TBW	Total body weight
ICU	Intensive care unit	VTE	Venous thromboembolism
LBW	Lean body weight		
LMWH	Low-molecular-weight heparin		

INTRODUCTION

Drug dosing in the intensive care unit (ICU) can be extremely challenging because of the pharmacokinetic variability that exists in this population compared with patients in a non-ICU setting. Even within the ICU, several special populations present unique challenges because of their pharmacokinetic differences and the relative lack of outcomes data available. This chapter is designed to address drug dosing in four such special populations: patients with extremes in size, pregnant patients, patients undergoing therapeutic plasma exchange, and patients receiving molecular adsorbent recirculating system (MARS) therapy. Although several other special populations could be included in this chapter (e.g., renal replacement therapies, hepatic failure, extracorporeal membrane oxygenation), the reader is referred to that specific section in this book.

OBESITY

Body Composition and Size Descriptors

Body size and shape (also known as *habitus*) refer to physical attributes of individuals such as height, weight, and body proportions. Measurement of these attributes is termed *anthropometry*. Epidemiologic studies during several decades in the United States have shown a general increase in these measures as well as variability within each measure.[1-4] Data analyses from 2011 to 2012 have shown that 69% of the U.S. population are overweight, 35% are obese, and 6.4% are morbidly obese.[5] With respect to weight, the morbidly obese population presents the greatest challenge with drug dosing because these patients are typically not well represented in pharmacokinetic studies that lead to recommended dosages in product labels. Of interest, several studies have shown an obesity paradox whereby mortality is lower in critically ill patients with extremes in body size.[6-8] These findings may be confounded by the presence of malnutrition near the time of ICU admission.[9]

Several sophisticated methods exist to quantitatively assess fat mass, fat-free mass, and body water.[10] Examples include bioelectrical impedance analysis, dual energy x-ray absorptiometry, and computerized tomography. However, these techniques are primarily used in the realm of research and are not routinely used in the clinical setting. Nevertheless, the metabolic aspects of these measurements can influence the pharmacokinetics of medications. For example, when mass is added to or lost from the body, there is a concomitant gain or loss (about 25% of that change) of lean tissue that is metabolically active.[11] Furthermore, there are different types of adipose tissue, and variability in metabolic activity exists. White adipose tissue is responsible for nutrient and energy storage, but brown adipose tissue has energy-dissipating activity and is thought to be protective against body fat accumulation.[12,13]

The descriptor used by the World Health Organization to characterize size is body mass index (BMI) (Table 41.1). However, BMI is not routinely used for medication dosing. Instead, when weight-based dosing is indicated, the patient's measured or reported actual (total) body weight (TBW) or some adjustment from TBW is used. These adjustments can include ideal body weight (IBW), lean body weight (LBW), fat-free mass, or some other form of adjusted body weight (AdjBW). Adjusted body weight calculations commonly use a correction factor to add some portion of the difference between TBW and IBW to the IBW (Table 41.2). It is important to understand the differences and limitations with each weight measure because variance with the calculated dose of more than 100% can be noted. Ideal body weight is sometimes used as a surrogate for LBW and presumes drug distribution into lean (i.e., non-adipose) tissue. The most common formula used to estimate IBW was proposed by Devine and was thought to have originated from life insurance tables published in 1959 (Table 41.2).[16] In fact, the proper terminology was actually "desirable" weight, which later became synonymous with "ideal" weight—the weight associated with the lowest mortality.[18] Of note, IBW estimations are based on height alone; therefore, the value does not change with increasing weight. As such, it can be argued that LBW is a better representation of fat-free mass. One formula for LBW commonly cited in the literature is the James equation.[19] This formula yields increasing weight estimations as a patient gains TBW, up to a point. Specifically, the estimation of LBW begins to decrease as TBW continues to increase (e.g., above 100–110 kg in average-height females and above 120–130 kg in average-height males).[20] The James equation therefore tends to underestimate LBW at extremes in weight. In lieu of these limitations, an alternative formula was proposed by Janmahasatian et al.[17] With this equation, LBW estimates continue to rise as body weight increases and may therefore better reflect the increase in lean tissue that can also

Table 41.1 World Health Organization Definitions for Size Descriptors

Body Mass Index (kg/m²)	Considered:
< 18.5	Underweight
18.5–24.9	Healthy weight
25–29.9	Pre-obese (also called overweight)
30–34.9	Obese class I
35–39.9	Obese class II
≥ 40	Obese class III (also called morbidly obese)

Data from: World Health Organization (WHO). Global Strategy on Diet, Physical Activity and Health. Available at www.who.int/dietphysicalactivity/childhood_what/en/. Accessed June 26, 2015.

Table 41.2 Equations for Estimating Body Size Descriptors

Size Descriptor	Equation
Body mass index (kg/m²)	$TBW/height(m)^2$
Body surface area (m²)[14]	$\sqrt{[(height(cm) \times TBW)/3600]}$
Body surface area (m²)[15]	$TBW^{0.425} \times height(cm)^{0.725} \times 0.007184$
Ideal body weight (kg)[16]	Males: 50 kg + 2.3 kg/in. for height > 5 ft
	Females: 45.5 kg + 2.3 kg/in. for height > 5 ft
Lean body weight (kg)[17]	Males: $(9270 \times TBW)/(6680 + 216 \times BMI)$
	Females: $(9270 \times TBW)/(8780 + 244 \times BMI)$
Adjusted body weight (kg)	$CF(TBW - IBW) + IBW$

CF = correction factor (usually = 0.4); IBW = ideal body weight (kg); TBW = total body weight (kg).

occur with increases in adiposity. Therefore, this formula should be used when estimating LBW or fat-free mass in clinical practice, particularly in more extreme forms of obesity. However, this formula can be cumbersome at the bedside; thus, it is recommended to use some form of automated dosing program (e.g., spreadsheet program) to avoid calculation errors. Another descriptor commonly used as an alternative is AdjBW using a "correction factor." These formulas, which originated from pharmacokinetic experiments with aminoglycoside dosing, use a correction factor to account for some fraction of the difference between TBW and IBW. The most common correction factor in the pharmacokinetic literature is 0.4; however, a wide degree of variability has been reported, with correction factors of 0.14–0.98 for various drugs.[21] Some have argued that a correction factor of 0.25 may better estimate LBW, given that there is about a 25% increase in lean tissue as fat mass is gained. However, there are no clinical trials comparing these methods.

Although there may be a preferred weight measure for a particular drug, each of the aforementioned size descriptors is limited by its inability to assess the ratio of fat mass to fat-free mass. This permits assumptions about body composition that may not be entirely accurate. The importance of this is shown in the following example. Suppose a loading dose is needed for a medication in three male patients, all 40 years of age, all 70 inches tall, and all weighing 100 kg. The first patient is very muscular with very little fat mass, the second has obesity, and the third has substantial fluid retention. All would receive the same dose based on all weight descriptors (i.e., TBW, IBW, LBW, etc.), but there are clearly differences in body composition that could influence volume of distribution and/or clearance and the resultant drug concentrations.

Pharmacokinetic Considerations

The two independent pharmacokinetic parameters commonly used to describe drug disposition in the body are volume of distribution and clearance. Volume of distribution is a theoretical parameter used to describe the size of the compartment into which a drug will distribute. This is the most influential parameter when a single dose of medication is administered such as a loading dose. In general, drugs with a smaller volume of distribution tend to be hydrophilic drugs and remain in the extracellular space with little distribution into adipose tissue. Drugs with larger volumes of distribution are often more lipophilic and distribute into adipose tissue and other areas of the body.

The second pharmacokinetic factor used to describe drug disposition is clearance. Studies evaluating the impact of obesity on clearance have produced mixed results. Some studies have shown an increase in clearance, largely because of increased kidney size and blood flow, whereas others have shown no difference. One challenge related to clearance in the patient with obesity is which weight to use in formulas for estimating creatinine clearance. One study compared measured creatinine clearance with calculated estimates using the Cockcroft-Gault formula and different measures for weight (TBW, IBW, AdjBW with correction factors of 0.3 and 0.4, LBW).[22] Total body weight overestimated true clearance by almost 2-fold, whereas IBW underestimated clearance by around 23%. Lean body weight using the formula from Janmahasatian et al.[17] provided the most accurate estimations of measured creatinine clearance. Strengths of this study are that it included hospitalized patients as opposed to healthy volunteers, though patients admitted to an ICU were excluded.

When considering the pharmacokinetic differences that exist in patients with obesity versus nonobese patients, the concept of dose proportionality must be examined. Dose proportionality suggests that as weight increases (from standard size to a nonstandard size), pharmacokinetic parameters such as volume of distribution and clearance increase by the same ratio. For example, assume that a drug is given as a 1-mg/kg dose with a volume of distribution of 50 L and a clearance of 100 mL/minute according to studies of middle-aged adults with normal size, shape, and weight. Next, assume that the same drug is given to a group of patients with morbid obesity who have the same age and height but who weigh twice as much. If the resultant volume of distribution and clearance are 100 L and 200 mL/minute, the concept of dose proportionality will apply because a doubling in weight is associated with a doubling in volume of distribution and clearance and no change in volume of distribution or clearance relative to weight (i.e., liters per kilogram or liters per hour per kilogram). In that setting, TBW would be the most appropriate measure to use for weight-based dosing. In contrast, if the volume of distribution and clearance do not change in proportion to the observed differences in TBW, another weight measure such as LBW or AdjBW using some correction factor may better reflect the changes that occur. In general, few drugs that are renally eliminated have characteristics of dose proportionality.

Calculating a Dose in the Patient with Morbid Obesity

Although several factors must be considered when calculating a dosing regimen for the critically ill patient with morbid obesity, a few overarching principles exist (Box 41.1). These factors should be assessed in conjunction with the stepwise approach presented in the paragraphs that follow. With that in mind, the first step is to assess the degree of obesity in the individual patient. When dealing with mild to moderate forms of obesity (i.e., BMI 25–35 kg/m^2), published dosing recommendations are usually appropriate because these patients were likely included in the trials that led to the dosing in the product label.

As BMI approaches and exceeds 40 kg/m² (i.e., morbid obesity), drug dosing is more complicated because these patients were often excluded from dosing studies or represented in such small numbers that a meaningful conclusion cannot be drawn. In these instances, the clinician should evaluate clinical trials with that medication conducted in patients with morbid obesity. It is important to assess whether the degree of obesity presented in the trials is similar to that of the individual patient at hand, especially if dealing with more extreme forms of obesity (i.e., BMI greater than 50 kg/m²).

If clinical trials do not exist or if the patient does not fit the profile of the patients in the clinical investigations, the clinician should search for pharmacokinetic trials of patients with obesity and assess whether dose proportionality exists. For medications that are weight based (i.e., milligrams per kilogram of body weight), the clinician must weigh the benefits and risks of using TBW versus LBW or some correction factor AdjBW. For medications that are non–weight based (i.e., milligrams per dose), the clinician may choose to administer a dose on the higher end of the recommended dosing range. If pharmacokinetic trials specific to patients with obesity do not exist, some generalizations can be made regarding pharmacokinetic parameters. Drugs that have a small volume of distribution typically do not distribute extensively into adipose tissue. Weight-based dosing, particularly for loading doses, can be performed using LBW. Drugs with a large volume of distribution would be anticipated to require loading doses based on TBW or AdjBW, but there are exceptions to this generalization. For example, digoxin has an average volume of distribution of around 500 L but is proportional to IBW (according to the Devine equations) and not TBW.[23] This is because digoxin has a high affinity for cardiac and skeletal muscle, and adipose tissue is not an active reservoir. Clinicians must therefore use caution when making assumptions based on volume of distribution, especially when it is high.

In some situations, when clinical and pharmacokinetic trials do not exist, it may be necessary to extrapolate dosing information from similar drugs (i.e., drugs in the same structural class) or consider an alternative agent. Other important factors to consider are the adverse effect profile of the medication and the method for administering and titrating to effect. For some medications (especially those with dose-dependent adverse effects), it may be preferable to use a series of smaller doses that can be rapidly titrated to effect versus a single, large loading dose or maintenance doses that may be based on TBW (even when TBW may be the preferred weight measure for dosing). This method is commonly used for sedatives and analgesics in the postoperative setting. Finally, the ability to do therapeutic drug monitoring may be considered when selecting an agent and used whenever available. This allows the clinician to rapidly assess whether pharmacokinetic and pharmacodynamic goals are being met and to adjust the dosing regimen as necessary.

Medication-Specific Recommendations

Analgesics

Even though opioid medications are highly lipophilic compounds, LBW is the most appropriate weight measurement for dosing them. One study evaluated analgesic response with a fixed 4-mg dose of morphine and reported no significant differences between individuals who were nonobese, individuals with obesity, and individuals with morbid obesity.[24] Similarly, studies with fentanyl have shown a nonlinear relationship between dosing requirements and TBW. Dosing regimens based on TBW could therefore lead to excessive dosing in patients with morbid obesity.[25,26] Remifentanil pharmacokinetics were evaluated in one study where the volume of distribution and the clearance were more closely related to lean body mass than to TBW.[27] A second study evaluated sufentanil and showed a linear correlation between the volume of distribution and the degree of obesity, with a prolonged half-life in patients with obesity.[28] This suggests that TBW should be used for loading doses, but LBW or IBW for maintenance dosing.

In summary, available data analyses suggest that dosing adjustments with opioids are unnecessary in patients with obesity and that the same strategy as used in nonobese patients can be sought. Because opioid doses in adult patients are typically non–weight based, incremental doses that can be rapidly titrated to effect (similar to what is

---

Box 41.1. Practical Considerations When Calculating Drug Regimens in Critically Ill Patients with Morbid Obesity

Seek consistency with the weight measure that is used for weight-based dosing and for all dosing-related calculations (e.g., creatinine clearance calculations).

Use dosing calculators or computer programs to assist with calculations from complex formulas.

When evaluating the literature for data to assist with dosing, verify the weight of the actual patient in question is within the range of weights included in the clinical trial.

The degree of variability in pharmacokinetic parameters (such as volume of distribution and clearance) is much greater in critically ill patients than in the non–critically ill population.

When no outcomes data are available, clinicians should evaluate pharmacokinetic studies to assess for dose proportionality.

When there are no comparative pharmacokinetic data, the clinician must balance the risk of adverse effects using a higher dose (or dosing based on TBW) with the risk of treatment failure using lower doses (or dosing based on LBW).

In some cases, even when TBW may be the most appropriate measure for weight-based dosing, the adverse effect profile may preclude its use in favor of smaller doses that can be rapidly titrated to effect.

LBW = lean body weight; TBW = total body weight.

used in a recovery room setting) are recommended. In all cases, the degree of underlying pain, age of the patient, presence of ventilatory support, and likelihood that tolerance is occurring should be used to guide therapy.

Sedatives

Sedation strategies that use non-benzodiazepine medications are preferred in mechanically ventilated, critically ill patients because of their association with reduced durations of mechanical ventilation and shorter ICU lengths of stay.[29] Propofol is the most widely used sedative because of its favorable pharmacokinetic profile, including a rapid onset and short duration of effect.[30] Several pharmacokinetic models have been developed to evaluate propofol pharmacokinetics and pharmacodynamics in patients with morbid obesity. Servin et al. reported that both clearance and volume of distribution were correlated with TBW (r=0.76 and 0.61 for clearance and volume of distribution, respectively).[31] Others have developed allometric models using TBW or some form of AdjBW to better characterize propofol dosing.[32-34] Nevertheless, despite these data implying that TBW is the preferred weight measure for weight-based dosing, several studies have shown obesity to be an independent predictor of propofol-related adverse effects.[35,36] Therefore, because of the hemodynamic concerns with large doses of propofol and the fact that propofol can rapidly be titrated to effect, either LBW or some correction factor AdjBW should be used for initial dosing calculations.

There are no data evaluating the impact of obesity on dexmedetomidine pharmacokinetics in the ICU. Pharmacokinetic studies with dexmedetomidine have shown a large volume of distribution (greater than 100 L), and one study noted clearance to be correlated with weight.[37] Nevertheless, because of concerns with adverse effects such as bradycardia and hypotension, either LBW or AdjBW should be used for weight-based calculations, with titration to the desired level of sedation.

Benzodiazepines are highly lipophilic compounds, and marked differences in pharmacokinetic variables have been detected in individuals with obesity compared with nonobese individuals. In one study with midazolam, both volume of distribution and elimination half-life were significantly greater in the obese cohort (volume of distribution 2.66 vs. 1.74 L/kg; half-life 5.94 vs. 2.27 hours).[38] The observed increase in half-life was presumed to be caused by the large volume of distribution because no difference was noted in total clearance (472 vs. 530 mL/minute). Therefore, LBW should be used to calculate doses for continuous infusions, but TBW can be considered for single doses (because of increased volume of distribution). A safer approach, though, would be to use LBW or a series of smaller intravenous doses until the desired effect is achieved.

Neuromuscular Blocking Agents

Most neuromuscular blocking agents are polar, hydrophilic compounds, which suggests that distribution into adipose tissue is limited and that LBW is the preferred weight measure for both loading and maintenance doses. This was confirmed in several pharmacokinetic studies evaluating the neuromuscular blocking agents vecuronium, rocuronium, atracurium, and cisatracurium, where a longer duration of action was seen when doses were calculated according to TBW.[39-42] Succinylcholine, however, should be dosed according to TBW because of the strong correlation between pseudocholinesterase activity and BMI.[43] Furthermore, research has shown a substantial number of patients with poorer intubating conditions when either IBW or LBW was used rather than TBW.[44]

Anticoagulants

Anticoagulant dosing can be particularly challenging because of the deleterious effects associated with doses that are too low and the increased risk of bleeding when doses are too high. Several studies have evaluated the pharmacokinetics of anticoagulants in obesity when used for both venous thromboembolism (VTE) prophylaxis and treatment.

Prophylaxis

In most hospitalized patients, the choice of an anticoagulant for VTE prophylaxis is between a low-molecular-weight heparin (LMWH) and low-dose unfractionated heparin. There is no class I evidence to provide guidance on the preferred agent, but one study of more than 24,000 bariatric surgery patients showed the adjusted rates of VTE to be lower in patients who received LMWH (0.25%) compared with those who received unfractionated heparin (0.68%).[45] No significant difference in hemorrhage rates occurred. Other studies have evaluated prophylactic dosing of LMWH in obesity, most of which are specific to the bariatric surgery population and not the critically ill. Overall, it appears that higher doses are necessary to achieve antifactor Xa (anti-Xa) concentrations in the recommended range, but the exact dose is less clear. Scholten et al., who conducted a pre-post study using enoxaparin 40 mg every 12 hours (compared with 30 mg every 12 hours) in bariatric surgery patients, reported significantly fewer VTE events (0.6% vs. 5.4%, p<0.01).[46] This is one of the few prospective studies that used VTE events as the primary outcome measure. Other investigators have evaluated a BMI-stratified or weight-based approach. In one study, patients with a BMI of 50 kg/m^2 or less received enoxaparin 40 mg every 12 hours, whereas those with a BMI greater than 50 kg/m^2 received 60 mg every 12 hours.[47] The incidence of subtherapeutic anti-Xa levels was slightly lower in the 60-mg dosing cohort (21% vs. 14%), indicating that a higher dose was required when the BMI exceeded 50 kg/m². However, supratherapeutic anti-Xa levels were somewhat higher (0% vs. 17%). A second study evaluated a BMI-stratified approach for dosing enoxaparin in bariatric surgery.[48] In this study, twice-daily enoxaparin was administered in 30-mg doses for patients with a BMI less than 40 kg/m², 40 mg for BMI 41–49 kg/m², 50 mg for BMI 50–59 kg/m², and 60 mg when BMI exceeded 59 kg/m². No episodes of VTE were recorded, and 5 of 170 (2.9%) had a bleeding event (40-mg dose, n=4; 60-mg dose, n=1). Ludwig et al. evaluated a weight-based approach for dosing enoxaparin in surgical ICU patients using 0.5 mg/kg twice daily.[49] The mean BMI for this cohort was 46.4 kg/m², and 30% had BMIs greater than 45 kg/m². Overall, 91% of patients had anti-Xa levels in the therapeutic range, and only one patient had minor bleeding. Finally, Bickford et al. evaluated a similar regimen (enoxaparin 0.5 mg/kg twice daily) in a cohort of trauma patients.[50] Target anti-Xa levels were achieved in 86% of patients. Overall, the cumulative data suggest that higher-than-standard doses are required for the obese population. However, the specific dose requires further study. The only dosing regimen associated with outcomes data (i.e., VTE rates) is 40 mg every 12 hours, but higher doses may be necessary, particularly in patients with more extreme forms of obesity.

No comparative trials have evaluated subcutaneous unfractionated heparin dosing in individuals with morbid obesity. One study showed heparin activity (measured by anti-Xa and anti-IIa activity) to be related to abdominal skinfold thickness.[51] In fact, a relative decrease in anti-Xa activity of around 33% was noted when abdominal skinfold thickness increased from 10 mm to 20 mm. Higher doses can therefore be considered.

Treatment

Several pharmacokinetic studies have evaluated weight-based dosing of LMWHs, but few include a large number of patients with more extreme forms of obesity.[52] One retrospective study of patients with morbid obesity (BMI greater than 40 kg/m²) reported lower initial doses of enoxaparin based on TBW (0.8 mg/kg every 12 hours) but anti-Xa levels that were either at or above the recommended range in 84% of patients.[53] A subgroup analysis from the ESSENCE (Efficacy and Safety of Subcutaneous Enoxaparin in Unstable Angina and Non-Q-Wave MI) and TIMI (Thrombolysis in Myocardial Infarction) 11B trials showed no difference in efficacy (composite of death, myocardial infarction, or urgent revascularization) or major hemorrhage between patients with and without obesity when enoxaparin was dosed according to TBW, but the average weight and BMI for the cohort with obesity were only 94 kg and 33.8 kg/m², respectively.[54] In contrast, a second study showed that bleeding rates may be higher in patients with more extreme forms of obesity.[55] This study used a large, national, quality improvement database in which 19,061 patients with acute coronary syndromes were stratified into four cohorts according to TBW (100 kg or less, 101–120 kg, 121–150 kg, and greater than 150 kg). Major bleeding rates followed a U-shaped pattern, being highest in patients who weighed 100 kg or less and greater than 150 kg. Of interest, 80% of patients who weighed more than 150 kg received a lower dose than recommended based on TBW (1 mg/kg). When bleeding rates were compared between patients who received recommended doses (0.95–1.05 mg/kg) and reduced doses (less than 0.95 mg/kg), recommended doses were associated with a 2.4-fold increase in bleeding. Nevertheless, published recommendations suggest that LMWHs should be dosed using TBW without a dose-capping strategy.[52] Given the potential for bleeding, particularly when weight exceeds 150 kg, using some correction factor AdjBW with anti-Xa monitoring may be a safer approach.

In many situations, the safest strategy to obtain therapeutic anticoagulation in a patient with morbid obesity is to administer a continuous infusion of unfractionated heparin. Unfractionated heparin offers the advantage of a shorter half-life, an effect that subsides more rapidly on discontinuation and offers more efficient reversal with protamine, should a bleeding event occur. Nevertheless, issues still exist regarding unfractionated heparin dosing in obesity. Unfractionated heparin has a volume of distribution that is similar to the blood volume, thereby suggesting IBW or LBW as the most appropriate weight descriptor for dosing. However, the published nomograms commonly used in clinical practice are based on TBW.[56] In one study, activated partial thromboplastin time (aPTT) values were significantly higher in patients with morbid obesity (BMI greater than 40 kg/m²) who received initial heparin doses of 80 units/kg and 18 units/kg/hour based on TBW compared with their non-morbidly obese counterparts (BMI of 40 kg/m² or less), who received similar initial, weight-based doses.[57] A second report described heparin dosing in a patient weighing 388 kg with suspected pulmonary embolism.[58] This is the heaviest patient in the literature for whom heparin dosing is described. In this case report, a therapeutic aPTT was ultimately reached with a dose of 9.4 units/kg/hour based on TBW. Of interest, this translates to a dose of 18.7 units/kg/hour (a common initial dose in most nomograms) based on an AdjBW. Therefore, given the association between heparin doses using TBW and supratherapeutic aPTTs, a strategy using AdjBW with a correction factor of 0.3 or 0.4 is suggested.

Antimicrobial Agents

Dosing of antimicrobial agents requires careful consideration of the pharmacokinetic alterations that occur with obesity and whether these alterations infringe on the ability to reach agent-specific pharmacodynamic goals (Table 41.3). With respect to pharmacodynamics, antibiotics are classified as either concentration- or time-dependent. With concentration-dependent antibiotics, the goal is to achieve the highest possible concentration (balancing efficacy and safety) above the minimum inhibitory concentration (MIC) for that organism. Time-dependent antibiotics, however, require maximizing the time that drug concentrations remain above the MIC. For most antibiotics, obesity is associated with an increase in both volume of distribution and clearance. These changes can lead to lower peak concentrations (important for concentration-dependent antibiotics) and prolonged periods of subtherapeutic concentrations (important for time-dependent antibiotics). The exact degree of variability depends on the specific antibiotic in question, and careful assessment for dose proportionality is required. Furthermore, the implications of this variability on clinical outcomes depend on several factors such as the pharmacodynamic characteristics of the antibiotic, the MIC of the infecting organism, the site of the infection, and the presence of host-immune factors.

Surgical Prophylaxis

Several studies have evaluated antimicrobial dosing in obesity in the setting of surgical prophylaxis.[59-62] In one study, a 2-g dose of cefazolin was compared with a 3-g dose in patients who underwent bariatric surgery.[60] Using cefazolin serum concentrations, pharmacokinetic variables were assessed, and a pharmacodynamic model was developed. In the patient cohort with a BMI greater than 50 kg/m², the time that the free (unbound) drug concentration was above the MIC (where MIC was 8 mcg/mL) was 4.1 hours for the 2-g dose and 4.8 hours for the 3-g dose. It was concluded that both regimens would provide sufficient antibiotic exposure for most surgical procedures. In contrast, Brill et al. used a microdialysis technique to compare unbound cefazolin concentrations in subcutaneous adipose tissue, together with serum concentrations, in a group of bariatric surgery patients with morbid obesity (average BMI was 47 ± 6 kg/m²) versus nonobese controls (average BMI was 28 ± 3 kg/m²).[59] After a 2-g dose, no difference was noted in the area under the curve (AUC) with serum concentrations, but subcutaneous adipose tissue concentrations were significantly lower in patients with morbid obesity. A Monte Carlo simulation model showed serum concentrations below those required to reach pharmacodynamic goals after 180 minutes, particularly with organisms having a higher MIC. In lieu of these results, together with a relatively safe adverse effect profile, a 3-g dose is recommended. If dosing consistency is a priority (between patients with and without obesity), a 2-g dose can be administered, but measures are necessary to ensure the dose is repeated intraoperatively after 2–3 hours.

Similar results have been reported with cefoxitin. In a microdialysis study using subcutaneous adipose tissue from patients undergoing elective abdominal or pelvic surgery, cefoxitin concentrations were markedly reduced in patients with obesity.[62] In fact, tissue penetration (measured as $AUC_{tissue}/AUC_{plasma}$) was only 22% of that reported in normal-weight patients, even though patients with obesity received a higher dose (2 g vs. 1 g). Suboptimal pharmacodynamics with cefoxitin have also been described in non–critically ill patients with normal body habitus.[61] Using cefoxitin in patients with morbid obesity (at least using standard dosing regimens) can be questioned.

Table 41.3 Pharmacodynamic Goals for Commonly Used Antibiotics in the ICU

Antimicrobial	Pharmacodynamic Parameter That Best Describes Activity	Threshold for Efficacy
Penicillins	fT > MIC	> 50%
Cephalosporins	fT > MIC	> 50%–70%
Carbapenems	fT > MIC	> 40%
Aminoglycosides	fCmax/MIC	> 8–10:1
Fluoroquinolones	AUC/MIC	Gram-negative: > 125:1
		Gram-positive: > 30:1
Vancomycin	AUC/MIC	> 400:1
Linezolid	fT > MIC	> 40%–80%
	AUC/MIC	> 80–120:1

fT > MIC = percentage of time the free concentration (fT) is above the minimum inhibitory concentration (MIC); fCmax/MIC = ratio of maximum free concentration (fCmax) to MIC; AUC/MIC = ratio of area under the curve (AUC) to MIC.

Data from: Adembri C, Fallani S, Cassetta MI, et al. Linezolid pharmacokinetic/pharmacodynamic profile in critically ill septic patients: intermittent versus continuous infusion. Int J Antimicrob Agents 2008;31:122-9; DeRyke CA, Kuti JL, Nicolau DP. Reevaluation of current susceptibility breakpoints for Gram-negative rods based on pharmacodynamic assessment. Diagn Microbiol Infect Dis 2007;58:337-44; Roberts JA, Lipman J. Pharmacokinetic issues for antibiotics in the critically ill patient. Crit Care Med 2009;37:840-51; quiz 59.

Treatment

Penicillins, Cephalosporins, and Carbapenems

β-Lactams are one of the more commonly prescribed classes of antimicrobials in the critically ill, and data evaluations describing their pharmacokinetics in obesity are beginning to accumulate, although they are still limited. In general, both volume of distribution and clearance are increased in patients with obesity and thereby have the potential to decrease their time above the MIC. One study evaluated β-lactam pharmacokinetics (piperacillin/tazobactam, cefepime, ceftazidime, and meropenem) in a cohort of critically ill patients with and without obesity.[63] Overall, marked variability was noted, and a substantial number of patients both with and without obesity did not attain adequate serum concentrations with standard dosing regimens. This highlights the influence that critical illness may have on drug pharmacokinetics and the limitations with extrapolating data from non-ICU settings. A second report evaluated only piperacillin/tazobactam dosing in patients with morbid obesity admitted to a trauma/surgical ICU.[64] In this study, pharmacodynamic goals were successfully reached (up to the susceptibility breakpoint of 16 mg/L) using a standard dose of 4.5 g every 6 hours infused over 30 minutes. Cefepime dosing has been described in patients with morbid obesity who underwent bariatric surgery.[65] Using patient-specific pharmacokinetic data, pharmacodynamic models were developed for two dosing scenarios: 2 g every 12 hours and 2 g every 8 hours. The time above the MIC fell below the goal of 60% when the MIC was greater than 4 mg/L for the every-12-hour regimen and greater than 8 mg/L for the every-8-hour regimen. Cefepime should therefore be administered using a dose of 2 g every 8 hours.

Most studies evaluating carbapenem pharmacokinetics in obesity were conducted in the non-ICU population, but one study assessed meropenem dosing in nine critically ill patients with morbid obesity.[66] Meropenem volume of distribution was slightly larger than the averages reported in nonobese patients (38 L vs. 22–29 L), but clearance was similar (10.5 L/hour vs. 9.3–11.5 L/hour). Pharmacodynamic modeling showed that standard dosing (1 g every 8 hours over 30 minutes) could attain target pharmacodynamic goals when MICs were 2 or lower. A second study reported doripenem pharmacokinetics in 10 non-ICU patients with morbid obesity.[67] In this study, obesity was associated with both higher volumes of distribution and clearance compared with those previously reported in nonobese patients. However, these changes did not lead to the inability to reach pharmacodynamic targets because standard dosing (500 mg intravenously every 8 hours over 60 minutes) was sufficient for MICs of 2 or less. Finally, ertapenem pharmacokinetics were evaluated in 30 healthy volunteers whose weight ranged from normal (i.e., BMI less than 25 kg/m^2) to morbidly obese (average BMI was 43 kg/m^2).[68] Area under the curve was significantly lower in individuals with obesity than in those with normal weight. Standard dosing (1 g daily) failed to reach pharmacodynamic targets in any of the patients (obese and nonobese). Of interest, one study compared clinical outcomes in colorectal surgery patients who received either ertapenem or cefotetan, and surgical site infections were greater in both treatment groups when the BMI exceeded 30 kg/m^2 than in patients whose BMIs were below 30 kg/m^2 (ertapenem 27% vs. 13%; cefotetan 42% vs. 26%).[69] In summary, it appears that standard doses of both meropenem and doripenem can be used in patients with morbid obesity, but use of ertapenem should be reconsidered, based on its inability to reach pharmacodynamic goals and the higher incidence of clinical failure in patients with obesity.

Fluoroquinolones

Even though fluoroquinolones are one of the more commonly used classes of antimicrobials in the critically ill, data describing their dosing in obesity are limited. One study reported increases of 23% for volume of distribution and 29% for renal clearance in a cohort of healthy volunteers with obesity (vs. nonobese controls) who received ciprofloxacin.[70] A second report described a patient weighing 226 kg who received ciprofloxacin 800 mg intravenously every 12 hours and achieved a peak serum concentration within the desired therapeutic range.[71] In contrast, one study of healthy volunteers reported no differences in either volume of distribution or clearance after a weight-based ciprofloxacin dose of 2.85 mg/kg.[72] Levofloxacin pharmacokinetics were described in one study that included hospitalized patients with obesity and ambulatory volunteers.[73] In this study, wide variability occurred, but both volume of distribution (liters) and clearance (milliliters per minute) were similar to that reported in the package labeling. Dosage adjustments therefore appear to be unnecessary. Nevertheless, pharmacodynamic goals can be difficult to reach with levofloxacin, even in normal-sized individuals.[74] Caution is warranted when using levofloxacin in patients with morbid obesity, especially when treating gram-negative organisms with an MIC of 1 or greater.

Aminoglycosides

Several studies have evaluated aminoglycosides in obesity, and both volume of distribution and clearance values tend to increase. However, there is much variability regarding the extent of that change, and it is not proportional to weight gain. One review noted an increase of 9%–58% for volume of distribution and 15%–91% for clearance in patients with obesity compared with nonobese controls.[75] Aminoglycoside doses in patients with obesity should be determined using AdjBW with a correction factor of 0.4, recognizing that a range of correction factors have been reported.[75] Intervals are more often chosen according to the estimated half-life.

An important factor when considering an aminoglycoside as a potential option in the morbidly obese population is whether the required dose for attaining optimal peak concentrations is within the individual clinician's range of comfort. With large-dose (e.g., 7 mg/kg AdjBW) and extended-interval (e.g., 24 hours for normal renal function) aminoglycoside dosing strategies, it is not uncommon for calculated initial doses to exceed 1 g (for gentamicin or tobramycin) in patients with morbid obesity, which could prompt the use of a dose-capping strategy. Dose capping has the potential to prolong the time to reach goal peak concentrations while waiting for concentrations to be measured/reported and could possibly affect the clinical outcome. For this reason, other appropriate antibiotics should be considered as first-line therapy for treating gram-negative infections in patients with morbid obesity.

Vancomycin

Vancomycin is one of the more challenging antibiotics to dose in obesity because of the many factors that influence its clearance beyond size and calculated creatinine clearance.[76] Several studies have shown that vancomycin pharmacokinetics correlate best with TBW, which is the weight descriptor recommended in published guidelines.[77,78] However, this does not imply dose proportionality, and clinicians must evaluate the specific differences identified in both volume of distribution and clearance in patients with morbid obesity. For example, Bauer et al. reported a volume of distribution of 52 L in a cohort of patients with morbid obesity (average weight 165 kg) compared with 46 L in those with normal weight (average weight 68 kg),[79] with clearance values of 197 mL/minute and 77 mL/minute, respectively. In this example, the principles of dose proportionality would apply for clearance but not for volume of distribution. Blouin et al. found a volume of distribution of 43 L in patients with morbid obesity (average weight 165 kg) versus 29 L in normal-weight patients (average weight 75 kg),[80] with clearance values of 188 mL/minute and 81 mL/minute, respectively. Similarly, the concept of dose proportionality is valid for clearance but not for volume of distribution. Adane et al. evaluated vancomycin pharmacokinetic parameters in a cohort of patients with morbid obesity (median weight 148 kg) with confirmed *Staphylococcus aureus* infections.[81] Population mean volumes of distribution were 0.51 L/kg based on TBW (0.76 L/kg based on AdjBW with a 0.4 correction factor), and clearance was 6.54 L/hour. Scatterplots had better correlation of volume of distribution and clearance with TBW than with AdjBW.

Several papers have linked vancomycin-induced nephrotoxicity to exposure and AUC, but nephrotoxicity may also be influenced by weight.[82] In one study, weight in excess of 101 kg was significantly associated with nephrotoxicity (hazard ratio 3.17 [1.18–8.53], p=0.022) together with trough value and ICU residence.[83] This could be related to more extensive vancomycin exposure because the mean trough values were only slightly higher (12.5 vs. 9.8 mg/L, p=0.03).

In summary, some disparity exists in the available pharmacokinetic data regarding the relationship between weight and volume of distribution. This would be most relevant for calculating a loading dose because volume of distribution is the primary determinant of concentration. Given the concern with dose-related adverse drug events, a conservative approach would be to use AdjBW for weight-based calculations, especially because loading doses are typically 25–30 mg/kg. However, maintenance doses and the resultant AUCs are largely influenced by clearance; therefore, TBW may be the more appropriate weight descriptor. Regardless of the weight descriptor chosen to calculate the initial regimen, therapeutic drug monitoring should be used with adjustments as necessary. Measuring two serum concentration samples with an individualized pharmacokinetic assessment may be superior to a trough-only monitoring method in these patients.[84]

Linezolid

Linezolid is more commonly used for methicillin-resistant *S. aureus* in critically ill patients, but data in patients with obesity are limited. Studies have shown lower serum concentrations in patients with morbid obesity, but substantial differences in clinical cure have not been recognized.[85-87] However, one case report described failure with linezolid in a patient weighing 265 kg (BMI 82 kg/m^2). In this report, peak and trough concentrations were only 4.13 and 1.27 mcg/mL, respectively.[88] Therefore, standard dosing regimens (600 mg intravenously every 12 hours) can be considered when the BMI is 50 kg/m^2 or less, but caution should be used in patients with more extreme forms of obesity or with organisms having a high MIC.

Daptomycin

The daptomycin product label recommends TBW as the measure for weight-based dosing, even in patients who are obese.[89] However, pharmacokinetic studies have not shown dose proportionality with parameters such as volume of distribution and clearance.[90,91] Higher concentrations have been noted with daptomycin (after weight-based dosing) in patients with obesity compared with nonobese patients, which may in fact be advantageous because of concentration-dependent killing. Adverse effects, however, may be more prevalent because several studies have reported increased creatinine phosphokinase concentrations when daptomycin was dosed as milligrams per kilogram using TBW in obesity.[92,93] This has prompted some to suggest consideration for LBW or some correction factor AdjBW in this population.[94,95]

CONSIDERATIONS FOR UNDERWEIGHT PATIENTS

Few data exist to evaluate drug dosing in patients who are markedly underweight. In general, standard drug doses or doses on the lower end of the dosing range should be appropriate. One precaution, though, pertains to anticoagulant medications. Fixed doses of medications such as LMWH, when used for VTE prophylaxis, can yield concentrations more consistent with therapeutic anticoagulation than with prophylaxis. In fact, the product label for enoxaparin cites increased exposure when weight is less than 45 kg for women and 57 kg for men.[96] Bleeding rates may be higher if standard doses are administered. Bleeding rates may also be higher with weight-based dosing of anticoagulants. A large registry trial of patients with acute VTE who received either LMWH or unfractionated heparin reported bleeding rates of 8.3% and 3.9% when TBW was less than 50 kg and between 50 and 100 kg, respectively (odds ratio [95% confidence interval] 2.2 [1.2–4.0]).[97] This difference occurred primarily because of minor bleeding.

A second complication that can occur in underweight patients is the presence of cachexia. Cachexia is a weight-loss syndrome characterized as an involuntary weight loss of 5% or more (or a BMI less than 20 kg/m²) plus at least three of the following: decreased muscle strength, fatigue, anorexia, low fat-free mass, and/or abnormal biochemistry.[98] It is not synonymous with age-related muscle loss, starvation, malabsorption, or other conditions where TBW may be low. Pharmacokinetic alterations encountered with cachexia include decreased volume of distribution, altered protein binding (because of hypoalbuminemia), and reduced metabolism.[99] Although most of these data are in the cancer and HIV populations, there are implications for medications administered in the ICU. Critical care clinicians should be cognizant of these alterations and calculate their medication regimens accordingly.

PREGNANCY

Critically ill obstetric patients present many challenges to the ICU team because of their unique physiology and specific medical disorders that occur during pregnancy and the postpartum period.[100,101] The most common reasons for ICU admission are hemorrhage and hypertension, but about 20%–30% of obstetric ICU patients present with non-obstetric causes for ICU admission such as sepsis.[102] One of the overarching considerations when caring for a pregnant woman is to consider the benefits and risks of medications for both mother and fetus. That said, the mother's life and safety are the top priority, and medications should not be withheld because of fetal concerns.[102] Fetal compromise is often the result of maternal decompensation.[103] For many disease processes, the initial assessment during the acute phase of illness is no different from that of a nonpregnant patient. For example, treatment of severe sepsis or septic shock should be consistent with the recommendations from the Surviving Sepsis Campaign guidelines.[102,104] In fact, these guidelines have been endorsed by the Royal College of Obstetricians & Gynaecologists.[105,106] Aggressive fluid resuscitation should be sought with early administration of broad-spectrum antimicrobial therapy. If fluids alone cannot maintain adequate tissue perfusion, vasopressor therapy with norepinephrine should be implemented. Although norepinephrine has been associated with uterine contractions and decreased uterine blood flow, its benefit on maternal resuscitation outweighs any risks.[107,108]

Pharmacokinetic Considerations

Pregnancy induces physiologic changes in virtually every organ system, which can substantially affect drug pharmacokinetics.[100,101] The most significant change is the increase in blood volume, which is about 50% greater than in a nonpregnant patient.[109] This results in a larger volume of distribution, particularly for hydrophilic medications or medications with a small volume of distribution. In addition, the increase in blood volume leads to a dilutional hypoalbuminemia whereby albumin concentrations can decrease by 20%–30%.[100] Activity of the cytochrome P450 (CYP) system is increased, specifically isoenzymes CYP3A4, CYP2D6, and CYP2C9. Glomerular filtration increases by about 50%; thus, medications that are predominantly renally eliminated require a dosage adjustment. Of interest, one report suggested that only 1.29% of published pharmacokinetic studies provide data for pregnant women.[110] Careful assessment and monitoring is necessary.

Medication Classification in Pregnancy

Most clinicians are familiar with the categories used by the U.S. Food and Drug Administration to characterize the relative safety of medications used during pregnancy. This system consists of five categories (A, B, C, D, and X), which represent the overall ratio of benefit-risk for use. One misconception is that these categories solely represent risk and increase proportionally from category A to X. For example, isotretinoin is commonly prescribed for acne and is labeled pregnancy category X because of its well-known association with birth defects. Phenytoin is labeled pregnancy category D because of congenital fetal malformation. The difference between the two drugs is not that one has a higher risk of fetal harm, but the benefit to be gained with its use (i.e., treatment of a life-threatening seizure vs. treatment of acne). Examples of medications that should be avoided in pregnancy (because of safer alternatives) are listed in Table 41.4.

Effective June 30, 2015, a new rule was implemented for labeling regarding pregnancy and lactation.[111] The old categories (A, B, C, D, and X) were removed together with the subsections "pregnancy," "labor and delivery," and "nursing mothers." These subsections were replaced by "pregnancy," "lactation," and "females and males of reproductive potential." Under the new rule, the pregnancy subsection is more thorough and includes information regarding available registries of data (if existent), a summary of the risks, a statement regarding systemic absorption, and information to assist health care providers in making prescribing decisions about the medication (e.g., dose adjustments during pregnancy and the postpartum period, disease-associated maternal/fetal risk, maternal and fetal adverse reactions, and the effect of the drug on labor and delivery).

Medication-Specific Recommendations

Vasopressors

Most data surrounding vasopressor therapy are in the setting of blood pressure management during spinal anesthesia for cesarean delivery. Ephedrine and phenylephrine have been the two preferred medications for this indication. Historically, ephedrine had been preferred because of animal studies showing better preservation of uteroplacental blood flow and concerns with the use of pure α-agonists.[112,113] However, better fetal acid-base status with phenylephrine has been cited in several reports.[114,115] In lieu of these data, several groups (including the American Society of Anesthesiologists) have recommended phenylephrine as first-line therapy for spinal anesthesia-induced hypotension except in the setting of maternal bradycardia, where ephedrine may be preferred.[116-119]

Table 41.4 Commonly Used Medications in Critical Care That Should Be Avoided in Pregnancy

Medication	Alternative	Comments
ACE inhibitors/angiotensin II receptor blockers	Labetalol, hydralazine, nicardipine, nifedipine	ACE inhibitors are associated with fetal renal failure and teratogenic effects and are contraindicated
Echinocandins	Amphotericin B	Teratogenic effects have been reported in animal studies. Human data are nonexistent
Esmolol	Labetalol	Esmolol has the potential to cause fetal bradycardia
Fluconazole	Amphotericin B	Doses > 300 mg are considered teratogenic
Fluoroquinolones	β-Lactams, cephalosporins, macrolides. Specific agent will be based on clinical situation	Concerns exist for abnormal fetal development (particularly from animal studies), but fluoroquinolones can be considered when multidrug-resistant organisms are encountered
Sodium nitroprusside	Nicardipine	Concerns for fetal cyanide toxicity limit the use of sodium nitroprusside
Tetracyclines	β-Lactams, cephalosporins, macrolides. Specific agent will be based on clinical situation	Tetracyclines bind calcium and cause permanent discoloration of teeth
Trimethoprim/sulfamethoxazole	β-Lactams, cephalosporins. Specific agent will be based on clinical situation	Teratogenic effects noted with use in first trimester. Sulfonamides may be harmful in third trimester
Valproate	Levetiracetam	Valproate should be considered a last resort in status because of its association with links to spina bifida
Voriconazole	Amphotericin B	Voriconazole is teratogenic in animals. Data in humans are limited to one observation (with a good outcome)
Warfarin	Low-molecular-weight heparin	Warfarin is associated with teratogenic effects and is contraindicated

For the treatment of severe sepsis or shock, the choice of a specific vasopressor should be no different from in a nonpregnant patient. Restoring maternal perfusion pressure is of greatest importance and should override concerns for uterine vasoconstriction. Norepinephrine is therefore the agent of choice. If hypotension persists despite norepinephrine, second-line agents include epinephrine and vasopressin. Data analyses describing these agents in pregnancy are sparse. Epinephrine crosses the placenta and can inhibit contractions. Case reports have described the use of epinephrine in the setting of anaphylaxis during pregnancy.[120] In one report, an epinephrine infusion was administered for 3.5 hours, and no fetal adverse effects were reported.[121]

Antimicrobial Therapy

Early, appropriate antimicrobial therapy is crucial in the care of the critically ill, infected patient. Similar to therapy for nonpregnant patients, broad-spectrum therapy should be implemented as soon as possible. Empiric antibiotic selection should address safety to the infant, especially during the first trimester when major organogenesis takes place. However, little safety information is available for many of the newer anti-infective agents—those commonly considered for empiric therapy in the ICU. Antibiotics such as β-lactams and macrolides have substantial data, and their use in pregnancy is generally well accepted.[122] One large population-based, multisite, case-control study of more than 18,000 participants confirmed the safety of penicillins, cephalosporins, and macrolides, but sulfonamides and nitrofurantoin were associated with birth defects.[123] Tetracyclines readily cross the placenta and, when used beyond the second trimester, bind calcium and cause permanent discoloration of teeth.[122]

Fluoroquinolones are often avoided during pregnancy because of concerns with abnormal fetal cartilage development. An additional concern pertains to their mechanism of action (inhibition of DNA synthesis) and theoretical mutagenic and carcinogenic potential. These concerns originate from animal models with doses that are substantially higher than those used in the clinical arena.[124] In humans, most studies have not shown an association with fluoroquinolones and fetal harm. Ciprofloxacin has been the most extensively studied. Therefore, although routine use of fluoroquinolones is not recommended, they can be considered when multidrug-resistant organisms are encountered.[124]

Vancomycin is often considered for resistant gram-positive infections, but there is little information regarding its transplacental passage to the fetus. One study measured maternal and cord blood vancomycin levels at delivery after three different dosing regimens: 1 g every 12 hours, 15 mg/kg every 12 hours, and 20 mg/kg every 8 hours.[125] Maternal and cord blood vancomycin concentrations were therapeutic in 32% and 9% with a 1-g dose every 12 hours, 50% and 33% with a 15-mg/kg dose every 12 hours, and 83% and 83% with a 20-mg/kg dose every 8 hours. No adverse effects were noted. These data analyses show significant passage of vancomycin to the fetus, but higher doses are required to reach therapeutic levels. Although vancomycin use is generally considered safe, therapeutic drug monitoring should be used.[126]

The treatment of fungal infections in obstetric patients can be challenging because of the limited therapeutic options and the high morbidity and mortality associated with these infections. Fluconazole is widely considered for empiric therapy; however, several reports have shown significant teratogenic risk, particularly with doses used to treat systemic infections (i.e., greater than 300 mg/day).[127] Because voriconazole has been shown to be teratogenic in animal studies, it should not be considered. Similarly, the echinocandins have been studied in animal models, and teratogenic effects were recognized. There are no data in humans. Amphotericin B is the safest antifungal drug in pregnancy and considered the agent of choice. Although nephrotoxicity is an important limitation, its incidence is similar to that reported in nonpregnant patients.[127] Liposomal amphotericin B can also be considered safe in pregnancy, but limited data exist with other lipidic derivatives. These products should only be considered when other polyenes are unavailable.

Antihypertensive Medications

Various antihypertensive agents can be considered to manage hypertension during pregnancy, but this discussion will focus on managing acute hypertensive crises in critically ill pregnant women. Intravenous hydralazine and labetalol have long been considered first-line agents because of their favorable adverse effect profile and extensive clinical experience in the critical care setting.[128] Several groups, including the European Society of Cardiology, have recommended labetalol over hydralazine in pregnant patients.[129,130] In fact, hydralazine is no longer listed as a first-line option because of concerns with more perinatal adverse effects. In one meta-analysis, hydralazine was associated with several adverse outcomes compared with alternative therapy (e.g., labetalol and nifedipine), including more maternal hypotension, placental abruption, adverse effects on fetal heart rate, cesarean section, maternal oliguria, and low Apgar scores.[131]

The calcium channel blockers nifedipine and nicardipine are potential options, and both are safe and effective during pregnancy.[132,133] In fact, nifedipine is listed as either a first- or a second-line agent, according to many guideline groups.[128,130] Nifedipine should be administered orally (vs. sublingually); thus, administration in the critically ill patient may not be possible. Of note, pregnant patients often receive concomitant magnesium therapy, and isolated reports of profound hypotension or neuromuscular blockade with nifedipine exist.[133]

Several antihypertensive agents should be avoided. Agents that act on the renin-angiotensin system (e.g., angiotensin-converting enzyme [ACE] inhibitors, angiotensin II receptor blockers) are contraindicated because of increased fetal mortality and morbidity, including oligohydramnios, renal dysgenesis calvarial hypoplasia, and fetal growth restriction.[133] These agents should not be used. Esmolol has the potential to cause fetal bradycardia, and loop diuretics are controversial because of theoretical concerns for reduced plasma volume. Sodium nitroprusside should be reserved for severe, life-threatening emergencies when other agents have failed because of its potential for cyanide and thiocyanate toxicity for both mother and fetus.

Sedatives and Analgesics

Data describing sedative and analgesic use specific to pregnancy are limited, but in general, recommendations from evidence-based guidelines should apply.[134] For example, validated sedation scoring systems should be used, and light levels of sedation should be maintained. Non-benzodiazepine medications are preferred to benzodiazepines because of their association with shorter lengths of ICU stay. Propofol is the most commonly used regimen in the ICU, and its use has been described in the operating room during cesarean sections. Overall, propofol rapidly crosses the placenta but seems to have no major neonatal adverse effects.[135-138] Reports characterizing the safety of propofol for longer-term sedation are limited. Case reports have described propofol use ranging from 10 to 48 hours.[139-141] Although significant teratogenic events were not evident, neonatal respiratory depression (postdelivery) can occur.

Dexmedetomidine is a second, non-benzodiazepine option commonly considered in the ICU, but no studies describe its use in critically ill, pregnant women. Limited experiences with dexmedetomidine near the time of cesarean section have resulted in the delivery of healthy infants.[142,143] Fetal bradycardia has not been reported, but more rigorous evaluation is necessary, particularly with higher doses of dexmedetomidine. Dexmedetomidine may increase the frequency of uterine contraction, which may preclude its use in some pregnant ICU patients.

Studies conducted in the 1970s suggested that benzodiazepines contribute to malformations such as facial clefts when used during the first trimester, but later studies (that were better controlled) have refuted this association.[144] However, benzodiazepines do readily cross the placenta; therefore, neonatal respiratory depression may occur if used before delivery. High doses of intravenous lorazepam may lead to propylene glycol toxicity, given that its clearance is reduced in neonates.[145] Nevertheless, as with all medications used in the ICU during pregnancy, risk-benefit must be assessed, and therapy should not be withheld if necessary (e.g., treatment of status).

Data with opioid analgesics during pregnancy in the ICU setting are limited, with most data in reference to maternal illicit substance abuse or opioid dependency.[146] In general, several reports have shown that short-term use of morphine or fentanyl is considered safe. As with all opioids, though, respiratory depression can occur with higher doses or more prolonged use near the end of pregnancy. Overall, the general principles of pain management used in nonpregnant patients can be applied to pregnant ICU patients. These include using validated pain scales, not relying on vital signs alone to assess pain, and avoiding morphine in renal failure.

Anticoagulants

Pregnancy is associated with a hypercoagulable state that is caused by a combination of physical and hormonal factors, together with changes in the balance of procoagulant versus anticoagulant factors.[147,148] Critically ill pregnant patients should receive VTE prophylaxis with either LMWH or unfractionated heparin. Neither crosses the placenta, and both are safe.[148,149] Low-molecular-weight heparin may be preferred to unfractionated heparin because of its increased bioavailability and lower risk of maternal osteoporosis and heparin-induced thrombocytopenia.[150] Dosing recommendations for LMWH are similar to those recommended in nonpregnant patients (e.g., enoxaparin 40 mg subcutaneously daily).[148,150] In some cases, though, twice-daily dosing may be necessary because of changes in renal excretion and protein binding. With unfractionated heparin, higher doses have been recommended by the American College of Obstetricians and Gynecologists: 5,000–7,500 units subcutaneously during the first trimester, 7,500–10,000 units subcutaneously during the second trimester, and 10,000 units subcutaneously during the third trimester, each every 12 hours.[148] Of note, multidose vials of both LMWH and unfractionated heparin contain benzyl alcohol, which has been reported to cause gasping syndrome in neonates. Either preservative-free formulations or single-dose syringes are advised.[151]

For treatment of acute VTE, either LMWH or unfractionated heparin is acceptable.[148,150,152] Unfractionated heparin may be preferable because of its rapid onset and the ability to make frequent dosing adjustments.[108,147,152] Inadequate anti-Xa levels have occurred with standard weight-based dosing of LMWH, which is worrisome in the setting of pulmonary embolism. If LMWH is chosen for initial therapy, twice-daily dosing should be considered.[147,152] Warfarin, which has well-known fetal teratogenic effects, should not be used.

For patients with heparin-induced thrombocytopenia, either argatroban or fondaparinux can be considered. No fetal adverse effects have been reported with these agents in case reports.[153-157]

Medications for Postpartum Hemorrhage

Postpartum hemorrhage is an obstetric emergency and one of the most common causes of maternal morbidity and mortality.[158,159] Oxytocin is widely regarded as the drug of choice and works by inducing fast and long-acting contractions of the myometrium. After intravenous administration, uterine contractions have been reported within 1 minute.[158] Administration methods (bolus vs. infusion) vary depending on the organization, but rapid administration may lead to peripheral vasodilation, hypotension, and an increase in cardiac output.[158,160] As such, the American College of Obstetricians and Gynecologists recommends 10–40 units in 1 L of normal saline or lactated Ringer solution administered by continuous infusion.[161]

If oxytocin is ineffective, ergot alkaloids (e.g., methylergonovine) are second line. These agents, which produce strong α-adrenergic stimulation, are contraindicated in patients with hypertension, preeclampsia, or a history of myocardial infarction. An alternative to ergot alkaloids is carboprost, a prostaglandin analog. Because carboprost causes bronchospasm, it should not be used in patients with asthma or respiratory insufficiency.

Other agents that have recently been considered include recombinant factor VII and tranexamic acid. Data analyses assessing the efficacy of recombinant factor VII are primarily through case reports, case series, and registry data; there are no randomized controlled trials.[162-166] One systematic review reported that recombinant factor VII was effective in stopping or reducing bleeding in 85% of cases.[164] Collectively, the most common dose was about 80–90 mcg/kg.

There is one randomized controlled trial evaluating the benefit of tranexamic acid in 144 women with postpartum hemorrhage.[167] Women with blood loss exceeding 800 mL after vaginal delivery were randomized to receive tranexamic acid (4-g load over 1 hour, followed by 1 g/hour for 6 hours) or not. Blood loss at 6 hours post-enrollment was lower with tranexamic acid (median 173 vs. 221 mL, p=0.041), as was duration of bleeding and progression to severe hemorrhage. A second trial is ongoing that is anticipated to enroll 20,000 women.[168] Of note, this trial will use a lower dose: 1 g followed by an additional 1 g if bleeding continues.

In summary, both recombinant factor VII and tranexamic acid could be useful therapies for postpartum hemorrhage; however, the current data are not robust enough to recommend them as early options. These agents can be considered when bleeding fails to resolve after traditional therapies. Further studies are needed to establish the safest and most cost-effective dose for each therapy.

THERAPEUTIC PLASMA EXCHANGE

Therapeutic plasma exchange or plasmapheresis is an extracorporeal procedure wherein plasma is separated from the cellular components of blood and all solutes in plasma are removed. To maintain normal plasma volume, replacement solutions, which are typically albumin or fresh frozen plasma, are infused. By removing and discarding plasma, any medication or solute present in plasma is thereby lost. In the ICU, therapeutic plasma exchange may be used to treat a vast array of disorders such as thrombocytopenic purpura, myasthenia gravis, Guillain-Barré syndrome, chronic inflammatory demyelinating polyneuropathy, Goodpasture syndrome, rapidly progressive glomerulonephritis, and acute antibody-mediated renal allograft rejection.[169,170]

Elimination through plasma exchange is a passive process that follows linear kinetics.[171] A single exchange of 1 plasma volume will remove around 63% of all solutes, whereas an exchange of 1.5 times the plasma volume will remove around 78%.[172] In general, a drug is more likely to be removed if it has a small volume of distribution (i.e., less than 0.2 L/kg) or a high degree of protein binding (i.e., greater than 80%).[169] This differs from renal replacement therapies, where drugs with high protein binding are not effectively removed. One of the most influential factors, even more important than drug pharmacokinetics, is the time between dose administration and therapeutic plasma exchange initiation. Several studies have shown a strong correlation of drug removal when therapeutic plasma exchange was initiated shortly after dose administration.[169,173] In fact, for some drugs—even those with a small volume of distribution—removal can be minimized by allowing for an adequate distribution time before initiating therapeutic plasma exchange.[174] Distribution half-life can therefore be an important parameter to assess in these instances. Exchanges at the end of a dosing interval will lead to a smaller loss of drug than exchanges occurring just after a dose.

Agent-Specific Recommendations

Several pharmacokinetic studies have evaluated the effect of therapeutic plasma exchange on drug removal. Most of the available data are not with medications commonly used in the ICU. For a review of these medications, the reader is referred elsewhere.[169,171,175]

Cephalosporins

Several papers have described cephalosporin dosing in patients undergoing therapeutic plasma exchange.[174,176-178] One report described cefepime removal after a single 2-g dose administered over 30 minutes and given 2 hours before the plasma exchange.[174] Cefepime has a volume of distribution of around 0.2–0.3 L/kg, and its degree of protein binding is less than 20%.[173] Despite a low volume of distribution, the amount of drug removed was only about 4%, indicating that supplemental doses are not required, provided the drug is administered at least 2 hours before plasma exchange.

The pharmacokinetic profile of ceftazidime is similar to that of cefepime, with a volume of distribution of 0.23 L/kg and protein binding of less than 20%.[173] In one report, a single dose of ceftazidime 2 g was administered 15–120 minutes before plasma exchange.[177] The amount of drug removal ranged from 2% to 9%, with greater extraction occurring with shorter intervals between drug administration and the procedure. It is therefore recommended to administer ceftazidime at least 2 hours before therapeutic plasma exchange.[173]

Ceftriaxone has a small volume of distribution (0.1–0.2 L/kg), but unlike cefepime or ceftazidime, it is highly protein bound (90%–95%).[173] One study assessed ceftriaxone concentrations when administered immediately and 6 hours before plasma exchange.[178] Drug removal was greater when ceftriaxone was given immediately before the exchange (23% mg vs. 17%). A second study compared ceftriaxone concentrations after a 2-g dose administered 3 hours versus 15 hours before a plasma exchange.[176] The fraction of drug removed was significantly greater with early administration (12.7% vs. 5.7%, p<0.05). Ceftriaxone should therefore be administered at least 15 hours before therapeutic plasma exchange.

Vancomycin

Few reports describe the impact of vancomycin removal after therapeutic plasma exchange.[179-183] The results have been inconsistent, with two reports showing minimal removal (less than 10%)[179,181] and three reports showing considerable removal (i.e., up to 49%).[180,182,183] This disparity could be a result of the timing of the dose relative to the plasma exchange because little information was provided in this respect. Given these results, administering vancomycin after therapeutic exchange seems reasonable. Therapeutic drug monitoring should be used accordingly.

Tobramycin

Data regarding the influence of therapeutic plasma exchange on tobramycin removal are limited to four patients.[184-186] In these cases, the fraction of drug eliminated was only 4.3%–10.9%, but serum concentrations were markedly reduced. It is unclear whether this was secondary to the plasma exchange procedure or to endogenous aminoglycoside clearance. Nevertheless, administering tobramycin after therapeutic plasma exchange or at least 2 half-lives before the procedure is appropriate.[173]

Digoxin

Digoxin has an extremely large volume of distribution (5–8 L/kg), and after the distribution phase, less than 1% remains in the plasma. Analyses of case reports have shown that only 1%–2% of digoxin is removed after a single plasma exchange.[187,188] Therapeutic plasma exchange is therefore anticipated to have minimal influence on digoxin removal, provided it is done post-distribution.

Phenytoin

Phenytoin has a volume of distribution of about 0.65 L/kg in patients without kidney disease and is highly protein bound (90%). Theoretically, plasma exchange should have a marked influence on its kinetics; however, analyses of case report data show otherwise. Most data analyses show that only about 3%–5% of phenytoin total body stores were removed after a plasma exchange. The largest documented removal of phenytoin was from a report wherein 10% of total body stores of phenytoin were removed, and plasma concentrations were reduced by 3.2 mcg/mL.[189] Clinicians should use therapeutic drug monitoring to modify the dosing regimen as needed.

MOLECULAR ADSORBENT RECIRCULATING SYSTEM

Liver failure is associated with the accumulation of several toxic metabolites, many of which are highly bound to albumin. Molecular adsorbent recirculating system (MARS) therapy is a liver support system that removes protein-bound and water-soluble toxins through albumin dialysis. Molecular adsorbent recirculating system therapy is used in conjunction with continuous renal replacement therapy wherein blood is pumped through a specialized high-flux filter, and protein-bound and water-soluble substances pass through the membrane into the albumin-enriched dialysate (Figure 41.1).[190] The albumin dialysate passes through a low-flux dialysis filter (against a bicarbonate-based dialysate) to remove water-soluble substances and then through two adsorption columns (one with uncoated charcoal and the second with an anion exchanger resin adsorber) to remove albumin-bound toxins. The regenerated albumin solution can then bind new toxins from the blood.

Drug dosing in patients receiving MARS therapy is complex because clinicians have to account for not only the drug removal with the MARS system itself, but also the clearance provided by the renal replacement therapy. It can be anticipated that drugs with both high and low degrees of protein binding will be removed. Few data describe the effect of MARS therapy on drug removal. One case report described the impact of MARS therapy on teicoplanin, a large glycopeptide (molecular weight 1,500–1,900 Da) that is about 90% protein bound.[191] In this report, teicoplanin concentrations decreased by 73% after the first cycle of MARS therapy and 84% after the second cycle, with the duration of MARS therapy at 9 hours and 16 hours, respectively, and most drug removal occurring during the first 4 hours. A second report described moxifloxacin and meropenem removal using an in vitro model.[192] The concentration for both medications decreased by 50% within 60 minutes post-MARS initiation. Drug removal was recognized with each component of MARS (i.e., the MARS flux dialyzer, the low-flux dialyzer, the charcoal column,

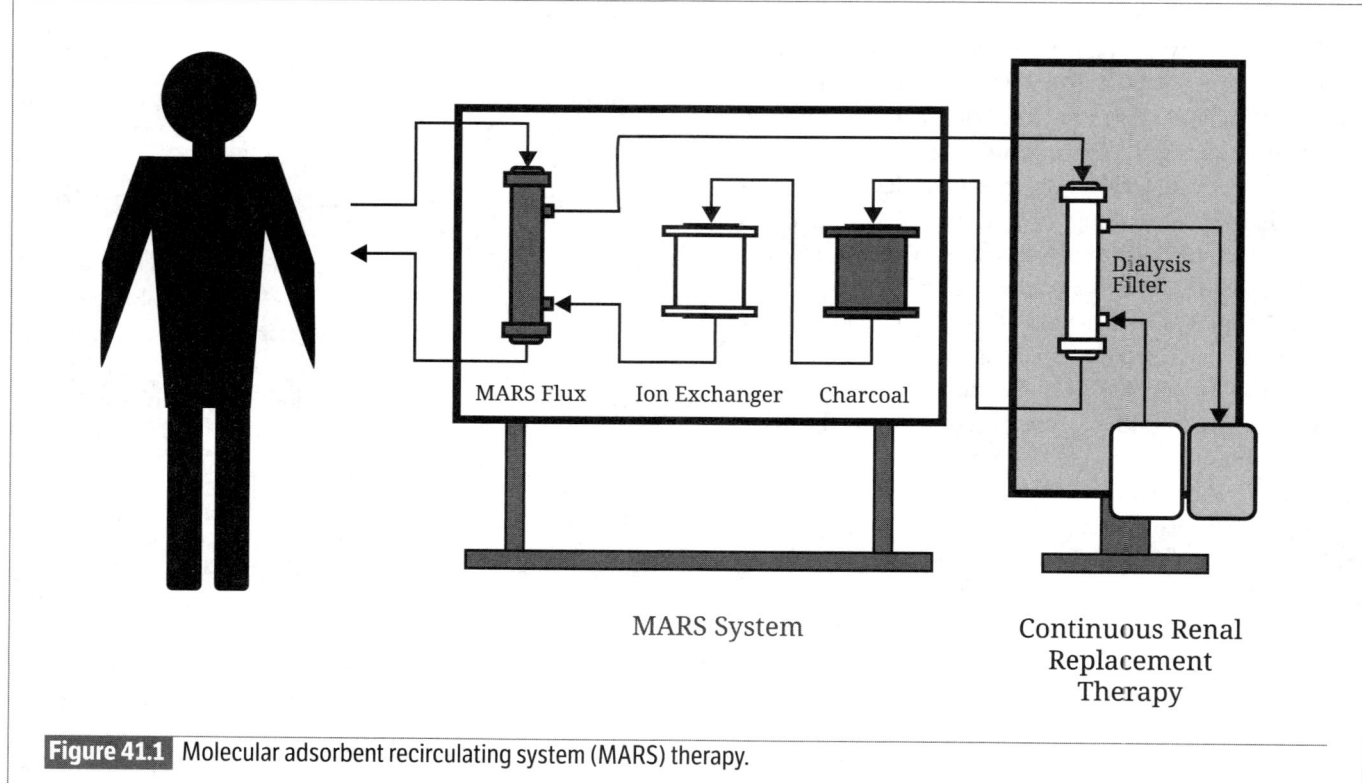

Figure 41.1 Molecular adsorbent recirculating system (MARS) therapy.

and the anion exchanger) for both medications. Piperacillin/tazobactam pharmacokinetics were described in one patient receiving MARS for acetaminophen-induced liver failure.[193] After administering a single dose of 4.5 g over 3 hours (with concomitant MARS therapy), piperacillin concentrations decreased from 173 mcg/mL to 116 mcg/mL, a decrease of around 33%. In fact, the calculated half-life was 3.7-fold shorter than that previously reported with CVVHD (continuous venovenous hemodialysis) alone, indicating additional drug removal by MARS.

CONCLUSION

There are variable degrees of evidence to guide clinicians with drug doses in special populations. For many of these populations, though, the data are limited to case reports or small case series. Clinicians must appreciate the pharmacokinetic variability that exists and base decisions after a careful assessment of risk-benefit. Medication regimens should be individualized and a "one-size-fits-all" approach avoided. Therapeutic drug monitoring should be used whenever applicable.

REFERENCES

1. Centers for Disease Control and Prevention (CDC). Behavioral Risk Factor Surveillance System. Available at www.cdc.gov/obesity/downloads/dnpao-state-obesity-prevalence-map-2012.pdf. Accessed June 26, 2015.
2. Flegal KM, Carroll MD, Ogden CL, et al. Prevalence and trends in obesity among US adults, 1999-2008. JAMA 2010;303:235-41.
3. Godoy R, Goodman E, Levins R, et al. Anthropometric variability in the USA: 1971-2002. Ann Hum Biol 2005;32:469-86.
4. World Health Organization (WHO). Global Health Observatory Data Repository. Overweight/Obesity: Mean Body Mass Index Trends. Available at http://apps.who.int/gho/data/node.main.A904. Accessed June 26, 2015.
5. Ogden CL, Carroll MD, Kit BK, et al. Prevalence of childhood and adult obesity in the United States, 2011-2012. JAMA 2014;311:806-14.
6. Pickkers P, de Keizer N, Dusseljee J, et al. Body mass index is associated with hospital mortality in critically ill patients: an observational cohort study. Crit Care Med 2013;41:1878-83.
7. Prescott HC, Chang VW, O'Brien JM Jr, et al. Obesity and 1-year outcomes in older Americans with severe sepsis. Crit Care Med 2014;42:1766-74.
8. Wacharasint P, Boyd JH, Russell JA, et al. One size does not fit all in severe infection: obesity alters outcome, susceptibility, treatment, and inflammatory response. Crit Care 2013;17:R122.
9. Robinson MK, Mogensen KM, Casey JD, et al. The relationship among obesity, nutritional status, and mortality in the critically ill. Crit Care Med 2015;43:87-100.
10. Thibault R, Genton L, Pichard C. Body composition: why, when and for who? Clin Nutr 2012;31:435-47.
11. Heymsfield SB, Gonzalez MC, Shen W, et al. Weight loss composition is one-fourth fat-free mass: a critical review and critique of this widely cited rule. Obes Rev 2014;15:310-21.

12. Chechi K, Nedergaard J, Richard D. Brown adipose tissue as an anti-obesity tissue in humans. Obes Rev 2014;15:92-106.
13. Karastergiou K, Smith SR, Greenberg AS, et al. Sex differences in human adipose tissues – the biology of pear shape. Biol Sex Differ 2012;3:13.
14. Mosteller RD. Simplified calculation of body-surface area. N Engl J Med 1987;317:1098.
15. Du Bois D, Du Bois EF. Clinical calorimetry. Tenth paper. A formula to estimate the approximate surface area if height and weight be known. Arch Intern Med 1916;17:863.
16. Devine BJ. Case number 25: gentamicin therapy. Drug Intell Clin Pharm 1974;8:650-5.
17. Janmahasatian S, Duffull SB, Ash S, et al. Quantification of lean bodyweight. Clin Pharmacokinet 2005;44:1051-65.
18. Pai MP, Paloucek FP. The origin of the "ideal" body weight equations. Ann Pharmacother 2000;34:1066-9.
19. James WP. Research on Obesity. London: Her Majesty's Stationery Office, 1976.
20. Green B, Duffull SB. Caution when lean body weight is used as a size descriptor for obese subjects. Clin Pharmacol Ther 2002;72:743-4.
21. Pai MP. Drug dosing based on weight and body surface area: mathematical assumptions and limitations in obese adults. Pharmacotherapy 2012;32:856-68.
22. Demirovic JA, Pai AB, Pai MP. Estimation of creatinine clearance in morbidly obese patients. Am J Health Syst Pharm 2009;66:642-8.
23. Abernethy DR, Greenblatt DJ, Smith TW. Digoxin disposition in obesity: clinical pharmacokinetic investigation. Am Heart J 1981;102:740-4.
24. Patanwala AE, Holmes KL, Erstad BL. Analgesic response to morphine in obese and morbidly obese patients in the emergency department. Emerg Med J 2014;31:139-42.
25. Shibutani K, Inchiosa MA Jr, Sawada K, et al. Accuracy of pharmacokinetic models for predicting plasma fentanyl concentrations in lean and obese surgical patients: derivation of dosing weight ("pharmacokinetic mass"). Anesthesiology 2004;101:603-13.
26. Shibutani K, Inchiosa MA Jr, Sawada K, et al. Pharmacokinetic mass of fentanyl for postoperative analgesia in lean and obese patients. Br J Anaesth 2005;95:377-83.
27. Egan TD, Huizinga B, Gupta SK, et al. Remifentanil pharmacokinetics in obese versus lean patients. Anesthesiology 1998;89:562-73.
28. Schwartz AE, Matteo RS, Ornstein E, et al. Pharmacokinetics of sufentanil in obese patients. Anesth Analg 1991;73:790-3.
29. Fraser GL, Devlin JW, Worby CP, et al. Benzodiazepine versus nonbenzodiazepine-based sedation for mechanically ventilated, critically ill adults: a systematic review and meta-analysis of randomized trials. Crit Care Med 2013;41(9 suppl 1):S30-8.
30. Gill KV, Voils SA, Chenault GA, et al. Perceived versus actual sedation practices in adult intensive care unit patients receiving mechanical ventilation. Ann Pharmacother 2012;46:1331-9.
31. Servin F, Farinotti R, Haberer JP, et al. Propofol infusion for maintenance of anesthesia in morbidly obese patients receiving nitrous oxide. A clinical and pharmacokinetic study. Anesthesiology 1993;78:657-65.
32. Cortinez LI, Anderson BJ, Penna A, et al. Influence of obesity on propofol pharmacokinetics: derivation of a pharmacokinetic model. Br J Anaesth 2010;105:448-56.
33. Cortinez LI, De la Fuente N, Eleveld DJ, et al. Performance of propofol target-controlled infusion models in the obese: pharmacokinetic and pharmacodynamic analysis. Anesth Analg 2014;119:302-10.
34. van Kralingen S, Diepstraten J, Peeters MY, et al. Population pharmacokinetics and pharmacodynamics of propofol in morbidly obese patients. Clin Pharmacokinet 2011;50:739-50.
35. Shearin AE, Patanwala AE, Tang A, et al. Predictors of hypotension associated with propofol in trauma patients. J Trauma Nurs 2014;21:4-8.
36. Wani S, Azar R, Hovis CE, et al. Obesity as a risk factor for sedation-related complications during propofol-mediated sedation for advanced endoscopic procedures. Gastrointest Endosc 2011;74:1238-47.
37. Valitalo PA, Ahtola-Satila T, Wighton A, et al. Population pharmacokinetics of dexmedetomidine in critically ill patients. Clin Drug Investig 2013;33:579-87.
38. Greenblatt DJ, Abernethy DR, Locniskar A, et al. Effect of age, gender, and obesity on midazolam kinetics. Anesthesiology 1984;61:27-35.
39. Leykin Y, Pellis T, Lucca M, et al. The effects of cisatracurium on morbidly obese women. Anesth Analg 2004;99:1090-4, table of contents.
40. Leykin Y, Pellis T, Lucca M, et al. The pharmacodynamic effects of rocuronium when dosed according to real body weight or ideal body weight in morbidly obese patients. Anesth Analg 2004;99:1086-9, table of contents.
41. Schwartz AE, Matteo RS, Ornstein E, et al. Pharmacokinetics and pharmacodynamics of vecuronium in the obese surgical patient. Anesth Analg 1992;74:515-8.
42. van Kralingen S, van de Garde EM, Knibbe CA, et al. Comparative evaluation of atracurium dosed on ideal body weight vs. total body weight in morbidly obese patients. Br J Clin Pharmacol 2011;71:34-40.
43. Bentley JB, Borel JD, Vaughan RW, et al. Weight, pseudocholinesterase activity, and succinylcholine requirement. Anesthesiology 1982;57:48-9.
44. Lemmens HJ, Brodsky JB. The dose of succinylcholine in morbid obesity. Anesth Analg 2006;102:438-42.
45. Birkmeyer NJ, Finks JF, Carlin AM, et al. Comparative effectiveness of unfractionated and low-molecular-weight heparin for prevention of venous thromboembolism following bariatric surgery. Arch Surg 2012;147:994-8.
46. Scholten DJ, Hoedema RM, Scholten SE. A comparison of two different prophylactic dose regimens of low molecular weight heparin in bariatric surgery. Obes Surg 2002;12:19-24.
47. Borkgren-Okonek MJ, Hart RW, Pantano JE, et al. Enoxaparin thromboprophylaxis in gastric bypass patients: extended duration, dose stratification, and antifactor Xa activity. Surg Obes Relat Dis 2008;4:625-31.
48. Singh K, Podolsky ER, Um S, et al. Evaluating the safety and efficacy of BMI-based preoperative administration of low-molecular-weight heparin in morbidly obese patients undergoing Roux-en-Y gastric bypass surgery. Obes Surg 2012;22:47-51.

49. Ludwig KP, Simons HJ, Mone M, et al. Implementation of an enoxaparin protocol for venous thromboembolism prophylaxis in obese surgical intensive care unit patients. Ann Pharmacother 2011;45:1356-62.

50. Bickford A, Majercik S, Bledsoe J, et al. Weight-based enoxaparin dosing for venous thromboembolism prophylaxis in the obese trauma patient. Am J Surg 2013;206:847-51; discussion 51-2.

51. Kroon C, de Boer A, Kroon JM, et al. Influence of skinfold thickness on heparin absorption. Lancet 1991;337:945-6.

52. Nutescu EA, Spinler SA, Wittkowsky A, et al. Low-molecular-weight heparins in renal impairment and obesity: available evidence and clinical practice recommendations across medical and surgical settings. Ann Pharmacother 2009;43:1064-83.

53. Deal EN, Hollands JM, Riney JN, et al. Evaluation of therapeutic anticoagulation with enoxaparin and associated anti-Xa monitoring in patients with morbid obesity: a case series. J Thromb Thrombolysis 2011;32:188-94.

54. Spinler SA, Inverso SM, Cohen M, et al. Safety and efficacy of unfractionated heparin versus enoxaparin in patients who are obese and patients with severe renal impairment: analysis from the ESSENCE and TIMI 11B studies. Am Heart J 2003;146:33-41.

55. Spinler SA, Ou FS, Roe MT, et al. Weight-based dosing of enoxaparin in obese patients with non-ST-segment elevation acute coronary syndromes: results from the CRUSADE initiative. Pharmacotherapy 2009;29:631-8.

56. Raschke RA, Reilly BM, Guidry JR, et al. The weight-based heparin dosing nomogram compared with a "standard care" nomogram. A randomized controlled trial. Ann Intern Med 1993;119:874-81.

57. Barletta JF, DeYoung JL, McAllen K, et al. Limitations of a standardized weight-based nomogram for heparin dosing in patients with morbid obesity. Surg Obes Relat Dis 2008;4:748-53.

58. Myzienski AE, Lutz MF, Smythe MA. Unfractionated heparin dosing for venous thromboembolism in morbidly obese patients: case report and review of the literature. Pharmacotherapy 2010;30:324.

59. Brill MJ, Houwink AP, Schmidt S, et al. Reduced subcutaneous tissue distribution of cefazolin in morbidly obese versus non-obese patients determined using clinical microdialysis. J Antimicrob Chemother 2014;69:715-23.

60. Ho VP, Nicolau DP, Dakin GF, et al. Cefazolin dosing for surgical prophylaxis in morbidly obese patients. Surg Infect (Larchmt) 2012;13:33-7.

61. Moine P, Fish DN. Pharmacodynamic modelling of intravenous antibiotic prophylaxis in elective colorectal surgery. Int J Antimicrob Agents 2013;41:167-73.

62. Toma O, Suntrup P, Stefanescu A, et al. Pharmacokinetics and tissue penetration of cefoxitin in obesity: implications for risk of surgical site infection. Anesth Analg 2011;113:730-7.

63. Hites M, Taccone FS, Wolff F, et al. Case-control study of drug monitoring of beta-lactams in obese critically ill patients. Antimicrob Agents Chemother 2013;57:708-15.

64. Sturm AW, Allen N, Rafferty KD, et al. Pharmacokinetic analysis of piperacillin administered with tazobactam in critically ill, morbidly obese surgical patients. Pharmacotherapy 2014;34:28-35.

65. Rich BS, Keel R, Ho VP, et al. Cefepime dosing in the morbidly obese patient population. Obes Surg 2012;22:465-71.

66. Cheatham SC, Fleming MR, Healy DP, et al. Steady-state pharmacokinetics and pharmacodynamics of meropenem in morbidly obese patients hospitalized in an intensive care unit. J Clin Pharmacol 2014;54:324-30.

67. Kays MB, Fleming MR, Cheatham SC, et al. Comparative pharmacokinetics and pharmacodynamics of doripenem and meropenem in obese patients. Ann Pharmacother 2014;48:178-86.

68. Chen M, Nafziger AN, Drusano GL, et al. Comparative pharmacokinetics and pharmacodynamic target attainment of ertapenem in normal-weight, obese, and extremely obese adults. Antimicrob Agents Chemother 2006;50:1222-7.

69. Itani KM, Jensen EH, Finn TS, et al. Effect of body mass index and ertapenem versus cefotetan prophylaxis on surgical site infection in elective colorectal surgery. Surg Infect (Larchmt) 2008;9:131-7.

70. Allard S, Kinzig M, Boivin G, et al. Intravenous ciprofloxacin disposition in obesity. Clin Pharmacol Ther 1993;54:368-73.

71. Caldwell JB, Nilsen AK. Intravenous ciprofloxacin dosing in a morbidly obese patient. Ann Pharmacother 1994;28:806.

72. Hollenstein UM, Brunner M, Schmid R, et al. Soft tissue concentrations of ciprofloxacin in obese and lean subjects following weight-adjusted dosing. Int J Obes Relat Metab Disord 2001;25:354-8.

73. Cook AM, Martin C, Adams VR, et al. Pharmacokinetics of intravenous levofloxacin administered at 750 milligrams in obese adults. Antimicrob Agents Chemother 2011;55:3240-3.

74. Kuti JL, Shore E, Palter M, et al. Tackling empirical antibiotic therapy for ventilator-associated pneumonia in your ICU: guidance for implementing the guidelines. Semin Respir Crit Care Med 2009;30:102-15.

75. Pai MP, Bearden DT. Antimicrobial dosing considerations in obese adult patients. Pharmacotherapy 2007;27:1081-91.

76. del Mar Fernandez de Gatta Garcia M, Revilla N, Calvo MV, et al. Pharmacokinetic/pharmacodynamic analysis of vancomycin in ICU patients. Intensive Care Med 2007;33:279-85.

77. Grace E. Altered vancomycin pharmacokinetics in obese and morbidly obese patients: what we have learned over the past 30 years. J Antimicrob Chemother 2012;67:1305-10.

78. Rybak M, Lomaestro B, Rotschafer JC, et al. Therapeutic monitoring of vancomycin in adult patients: a consensus review of the American Society of Health-System Pharmacists, the Infectious Diseases Society of America, and the Society of Infectious Diseases Pharmacists. Am J Health Syst Pharm 2009;66:82-98.

79. Bauer LA, Black DJ, Lill JS. Vancomycin dosing in morbidly obese patients. Eur J Clin Pharmacol 1998;54:621-5.

80. Blouin RA, Bauer LA, Miller DD, et al. Vancomycin pharmacokinetics in normal and morbidly obese subjects. Antimicrob Agents Chemother 1982;21:575-80.

81. Adane ED, Herald M, Koura F. Pharmacokinetics of vancomycin in extremely obese patients with suspected or confirmed *Staphylococcus aureus* infections. Pharmacotherapy 2015;35:127-39.

82. Carreno JJ, Kenney RM, Lomaestro B. Vancomycin-associated renal dysfunction: where are we now? Pharmacotherapy 2014;34:1259-68.

83. Lodise TP, Patel N, Lomaestro BM, et al. Relationship between initial vancomycin concentration-time profile and nephrotoxicity among hospitalized patients. Clin Infect Dis 2009;49:507-14.

84. Hong J, Krop LC, Johns T, et al. Individualized vancomycin dosing in obese patients: a two-sample measurement approach improves target attainment. Pharmacotherapy 2015;35:455-63.

85. Bhalodi AA, Papasavas PK, Tishler DS, et al. Pharmacokinetics of intravenous linezolid in moderately to morbidly obese adults. Antimicrob Agents Chemother 2013;57:1144-9.

86. Meagher AK, Forrest A, Rayner CR, et al. Population pharmacokinetics of linezolid in patients treated in a compassionate-use program. Antimicrob Agents Chemother 2003;47:548-53.

87. Stein GE, Schooley SL, Peloquin CA, et al. Pharmacokinetics and pharmacodynamics of linezolid in obese patients with cellulitis. Ann Pharmacother 2005;39:427-32.

88. Muzevich KM, Lee KB. Subtherapeutic linezolid concentrations in a patient with morbid obesity and methicillin-resistant Staphylococcus aureus pneumonia: case report and review of the literature. Ann Pharmacother 2013;47:e25.

89. Cubicin [package insert]. Lexington, MA: Cubist Pharmaceuticals, 2014.

90. Dvorchik BH, Damphousse D. The pharmacokinetics of daptomycin in moderately obese, morbidly obese, and matched nonobese subjects. J Clin Pharmacol 2005;45:48-56.

91. Pai MP, Norenberg JP, Anderson T, et al. Influence of morbid obesity on the single-dose pharmacokinetics of daptomycin. Antimicrob Agents Chemother 2007;51:2741-7.

92. Bhavnani SM, Rubino CM, Ambrose PG, et al. Daptomycin exposure and the probability of elevations in the creatine phosphokinase level: data from a randomized trial of patients with bacteremia and endocarditis. Clin Infect Dis 2010;50:1568-74.

93. Bookstaver PB, Bland CM, Qureshi ZP, et al. Safety and effectiveness of daptomycin across a hospitalized obese population: results of a multicenter investigation in the southeastern United States. Pharmacotherapy 2013;33:1322-30.

94. Ng JK, Schulz LT, Rose WE, et al. Daptomycin dosing based on ideal body weight versus actual body weight: comparison of clinical outcomes. Antimicrob Agents Chemother 2014;58:88-93.

95. Polso AK, Lassiter JL, Nagel JL. Impact of hospital guideline for weight-based antimicrobial dosing in morbidly obese adults and comprehensive literature review. J Clin Pharm Ther 2014;39:584-608.

96. Lovenox [package insert]. Bridgewater, NJ: Sanofi US, 2013.

97. Barba R, Marco J, Martin-Alvarez H, et al. The influence of extreme body weight on clinical outcome of patients with venous thromboembolism: findings from a prospective registry (RIETE). J Thromb Haemost 2005;3:856-62.

98. Evans WJ, Morley JE, Argiles J, et al. Cachexia: a new definition. Clin Nutr 2008;27:793-9.

99. Trobec K, Kerec Kos M, von Haehling S, et al. Pharmacokinetics of drugs in cachectic patients: a systematic review. PLoS One 2013;8:e79603.

100. Anderson GD. Pregnancy-induced changes in pharmacokinetics: a mechanistic-based approach. Clin Pharmacokinet 2005;44:989-1008.

101. Yeomans ER, Gilstrap LC III. Physiologic changes in pregnancy and their impact on critical care. Crit Care Med 2005;33(10 suppl):S256-8.

102. ACOG Practice Bulletin No. 100: critical care in pregnancy. Obstet Gynecol 2009;113(2 pt 1):443-50.

103. Fernandez-Perez ER, Salman S, Pendem S, et al. Sepsis during pregnancy. Crit Care Med 2005;33(10 suppl):S286-93.

104. Dellinger RP, Levy MM, Rhodes A, et al. Surviving sepsis campaign: international guidelines for management of severe sepsis and septic shock: 2012. Crit Care Med 2013;41:580-637.

105. Royal College of Obstetricians & Gynaecologists. Bacterial Sepsis in Pregnancy. Green-top Guidelines No. 64a. 2012. Available at https://www.rcog.org.uk/globalassets/documents/guidelines/gtg_64a.pdf. Accessed July 20, 2015.

106. Royal College of Obstetricians & Gynaecologists. Bacterial Sepsis Following Pregnancy. Green-top Guidelines No. 64b. 2012. Available at https://www.rcog.org.uk/globalassets/documents/guidelines/gtg_64b.pdf. Accessed July 20, 2015.

107. Barton JR, Sibai BM. Severe sepsis and septic shock in pregnancy. Obstet Gynecol 2012;120:689-706.

108. Ko R, Mazur JE, Pastis NJ, et al. Common problems in critically ill obstetric patients, with an emphasis on pharmacotherapy. Am J Med Sci 2008;335:65-70.

109. Pritchard JA. Changes in the blood volume during pregnancy and delivery. Anesthesiology 1965;26:393-9.

110. McCormack SA, Best BM. Obstetric pharmacokinetic dosing studies are urgently needed. Front Pediatr 2014;2:9.

111. U.S. Food and Drug Administration (FDA). Drug Development and Approval Process: Pregnancy and Lactation Labeling. Available at www.fda.gov/Drugs/DevelopmentApprovalProcess/DevelopmentResources/Labeling/ucm093307.htm. Accessed June 26, 2015.

112. James FM III, Greiss FC Jr, Kemp RA. An evaluation of vasopressor therapy for maternal hypotension during spinal anesthesia. Anesthesiology 1970;33:25-34.

113. Ralston DH, Shnider SM, DeLorimier AA. Effects of equipotent ephedrine, metaraminol, mephentermine, and methoxamine on uterine blood flow in the pregnant ewe. Anesthesiology 1974;40:354-70.

114. Lee A, Ngan Kee WD, Gin T. A quantitative, systematic review of randomized controlled trials of ephedrine versus phenylephrine for the management of hypotension during spinal anesthesia for cesarean delivery. Anesth Analg 2002;94:920-6, table of contents.

115. Ngan Kee WD, Lee A, Khaw KS, et al. A randomized double-blinded comparison of phenylephrine and ephedrine infusion combinations to maintain blood pressure during spinal anesthesia for cesarean delivery: the effects on fetal acid-base status and hemodynamic control. Anesth Analg 2008;107:1295-302.

116. Practice guidelines for obstetric anesthesia: an updated report by the American Society of Anesthesiologists Task Force on Obstetric Anesthesia. Anesthesiology 2007;106:843-63.

117. Loubert C. Fluid and vasopressor management for cesarean delivery under spinal anesthesia: continuing professional development. Can J Anaesth 2012;59:604-19.

118. Nag DS, Samaddar DP, Chatterjee A, et al. Vasopressors in obstetric anesthesia: a current perspective. World J Clin Cases 2015;3:58-64.

119. Ngan Kee WD. Prevention of maternal hypotension after regional anaesthesia for caesarean section. Curr Opin Anaesthesiol 2010;23:304-9.

120. Hepner DL, Castells M, Mouton-Faivre C, et al. Anaphylaxis in the clinical setting of obstetric anesthesia: a literature review. Anesth Analg 2013;117:1357-67.

121. Gei AF, Pacheco LD, Vanhook JW, et al. The use of a continuous infusion of epinephrine for anaphylactic shock during labor. Obstet Gynecol 2003;102:1332-5.

122. Lamont HF, Blogg HJ, Lamont RF. Safety of antimicrobial treatment during pregnancy: a current review of resistance, immunomodulation and teratogenicity. Expert Opin Drug Saf 2014;13:1569-81.

123. Crider KS, Cleves MA, Reefhuis J, et al. Antibacterial medication use during pregnancy and risk of birth defects: National Birth Defects Prevention Study. Arch Pediatr Adolesc Med 2009;163:978-85.

124. Yefet E, Salim R, Chazan B, et al. The safety of quinolones in pregnancy. Obstet Gynecol Surv 2014;69:681-94.

125. Onwuchuruba CN, Towers CV, Howard BC, et al. Transplacental passage of vancomycin from mother to neonate. Am J Obstet Gynecol 2014;210:352 e1-4.

126. Nahum GG, Uhl K, Kennedy DL. Antibiotic use in pregnancy and lactation: what is and is not known about teratogenic and toxic risks. Obstet Gynecol 2006;107:1120-38.

127. Pilmis B, Jullien V, Sobel J, et al. Antifungal drugs during pregnancy: an updated review. J Antimicrob Chemother 2015;70:14-22.

128. Committee Opinion No. 623: emergent therapy for acute-onset, severe hypertension during pregnancy and the postpartum period. Obstet Gynecol 2015;125:521-5.

129. Regitz-Zagrosek V, Blomstrom Lundqvist C, Borghi C, et al. ESC guidelines on the management of cardiovascular diseases during pregnancy: the Task Force on the Management of Cardiovascular Diseases during Pregnancy of the European Society of Cardiology (ESC). Eur Heart J 2011;32:3147-97.

130. Al Khaja KA, Sequeira RP, Alkhaja AK, et al. Drug treatment of hypertension in pregnancy: a critical review of adult guideline recommendations. J Hypertens 2014;32:454-63.

131. Magee LA, Cham C, Waterman EJ, et al. Hydralazine for treatment of severe hypertension in pregnancy: meta-analysis. BMJ 2003;327:955-60.

132. Nij Bijvank SW, Duvekot JJ. Nicardipine for the treatment of severe hypertension in pregnancy: a review of the literature. Obstet Gynecol Surv 2010;65:341-7.

133. Vidaeff AC, Carroll MA, Ramin SM. Acute hypertensive emergencies in pregnancy. Crit Care Med 2005;33(10 suppl):S307-12.

134. Barr J, Fraser GL, Puntillo K, et al. Clinical practice guidelines for the management of pain, agitation, and delirium in adult patients in the intensive care unit. Crit Care Med 2013;41:263-306.

135. Dailland P, Cockshott ID, Lirzin JD, et al. Intravenous propofol during cesarean section: placental transfer, concentrations in breast milk, and neonatal effects. A preliminary study. Anesthesiology 1989;71:827-34.

136. Gin T, Yau G, Gregory MA. Propofol during cesarean section. Anesthesiology 1990;73:789.

137. Gregory MA, Gin T, Yau G, et al. Propofol infusion anaesthesia for caesarean section. Can J Anaesth 1990;37:514-20.

138. Jauniaux E, Gulbis B, Shannon C, et al. Placental propofol transfer and fetal sedation during maternal general anaesthesia in early pregnancy. Lancet 1998;352:290-1.

139. Bacon RC, Razis PA. The effect of propofol sedation in pregnancy on neonatal condition. Anaesthesia 1994;49:1058-60.

140. Bloor GK, Jones MJ, Turner DA. Absence of clinically significant neonatal respiratory depression after prolonged maternal propofol administration. Anaesthesia 1987;42:1233-4.

141. Hilton G, Andrzejowski JC. Prolonged propofol infusions in pregnant neurosurgical patients. J Neurosurg Anesthesiol 2007;19:67-8.

142. Abu-Halaweh SA, Al Oweidi AK, Abu-Malooh H, et al. Intravenous dexmedetomidine infusion for labour analgesia in patient with preeclampsia. Eur J Anaesthesiol 2009;26:86-7.

143. Palanisamy A, Klickovich RJ, Ramsay M, et al. Intravenous dexmedetomidine as an adjunct for labor analgesia and cesarean delivery anesthesia in a parturient with a tethered spinal cord. Int J Obstet Anesth 2009;18:258-61.

144. McElhatton PR. The effects of benzodiazepine use during pregnancy and lactation. Reprod Toxicol 1994;8:461-75.

145. De Cock RF, Knibbe CA, Kulo A, et al. Developmental pharmacokinetics of propylene glycol in preterm and term neonates. Br J Clin Pharmacol 2013;75:162-71.

146. Bulloch MN, Carroll DG. When one drug affects 2 patients: a review of medication for the management of nonlabor-related pain, sedation, infection, and hypertension in the hospitalized pregnant patient. J Pharm Pract 2012;25:352-67.

147. Stone SE, Morris TA. Pulmonary embolism during and after pregnancy. Crit Care Med 2005;33(10 suppl):S294-300.

148. James A. Practice bulletin no. 123: thromboembolism in pregnancy. Obstet Gynecol 2011;118:718-29.

149. Fuller KP, Turner G, Polavarapu S, et al. Guidelines for use of anticoagulation in pregnancy. Clin Lab Med 2013;33:343-56.

150. Bates SM, Greer IA, Middeldorp S, et al. VTE, thrombophilia, antithrombotic therapy, and pregnancy: Antithrombotic Therapy and Prevention of Thrombosis, 9th ed: American College of Chest Physicians Evidence-Based Clinical Practice Guidelines. Chest 2012;141(2 suppl):e691S-736S.

151. Shapiro NL. Pregnancy. In: Dager WE, Gulseth MP, Nutescu EA, eds. Anticoagulation Therapy: A Point-of-Care Guide. Bethesda, MD: American Society of Health-System Pharmacists, 2011:343-67.

152. Greer IA. Thrombosis in pregnancy: updates in diagnosis and management. Hematology Am Soc Hematol Educ Program 2012;2012:203-7.

153. Ekbatani A, Asaro LR, Malinow AM. Anticoagulation with argatroban in a parturient with heparin-induced thrombocytopenia. Int J Obstet Anesth 2010;19:82-7.

154. Harenberg J. Treatment of a woman with lupus and thromboembolism and cutaneous intolerance to heparins using fondaparinux during pregnancy. Thromb Res 2007;119:385-8.

155. Mazzolai L, Hohlfeld P, Spertini F, et al. Fondaparinux is a safe alternative in case of heparin intolerance during pregnancy. Blood 2006;108:1569-70.

156. Young SK, Al-Mondhiry HA, Vaida SJ, et al. Successful use of argatroban during the third trimester of pregnancy: case report and review of the literature. Pharmacotherapy 2008;28:1531-6.

157. Elsaigh E, Thachil J, Nash MJ, et al. The use of fondaparinux in pregnancy. Br J Haematol 2015;168:762-4.

158. Bohlmann MK, Rath W. Medical prevention and treatment of postpartum hemorrhage: a comparison of different guidelines. Arch Gynecol Obstet 2014;289:555-67.

159. Girard T, Mortl M, Schlembach D. New approaches to obstetric hemorrhage: the postpartum hemorrhage consensus algorithm. Curr Opin Anaesthesiol 2014;27:267-74.

160. Van de Velde M, Diez C, Varon AJ. Obstetric hemorrhage. Curr Opin Anaesthesiol 2015;28:186-90.

161. ACOG Practice Bulletin: Clinical Management Guidelines for Obstetrician-Gynecologists No. 76, October 2006: postpartum hemorrhage. Obstet Gynecol 2006;108:1039-47.

162. Ahonen J. The role of recombinant activated factor VII in obstetric hemorrhage. Curr Opin Anaesthesiol 2012;25:309-14.

163. Barillari G, Frigo MG, Casarotto M, et al. Use of recombinant activated factor VII in severe post-partum haemorrhage: data from the Italian Registry: a multicentric observational retrospective study. Thromb Res 2009;124:e41-7.

164. Franchini M, Franchi M, Bergamini V, et al. The use of recombinant activated FVII in postpartum hemorrhage. Clin Obstet Gynecol 2010;53:219-27.

165. Kobayashi T, Nakabayashi M, Yoshioka A, et al. Recombinant activated factor VII (rFVIIa/NovoSeven(R)) in the management of severe postpartum haemorrhage: initial report of a multicentre case series in Japan. Int J Hematol 2012;95:57-63.

166. Phillips LE, McLintock C, Pollock W, et al. Recombinant activated factor VII in obstetric hemorrhage: experiences from the Australian and New Zealand Haemostasis Registry. Anesth Analg 2009;109:1908-15.

167. Ducloy-Bouthors AS, Jude B, Duhamel A, et al. High-dose tranexamic acid reduces blood loss in postpartum haemorrhage. Crit Care 2011;15:R117.

168. Shakur H, Elbourne D, Gulmezoglu M, et al. The WOMAN Trial (World Maternal Antifibrinolytic Trial): tranexamic acid for the treatment of postpartum haemorrhage: an international randomised, double blind placebo controlled trial. Trials 2010;11:40.

169. Ibrahim RB, Balogun RA. Medications in patients treated with therapeutic plasma exchange: prescription dosage, timing, and drug overdose. Semin Dial 2012;25:176-89.

170. Linenberger ML, Price TH. Use of cellular and plasma apheresis in the critically ill patient. Part II. Clinical indications and applications. J Intensive Care Med 2005;20:88-103.

171. Ibrahim RB, Liu C, Cronin SM, et al. Drug removal by plasmapheresis: an evidence-based review. Pharmacotherapy 2007;27:1529-49.

172. Linenberger ML, Price TH. Use of cellular and plasma apheresis in the critically ill patient: part 1: technical and physiological considerations. J Intensive Care Med 2005;20:18-27.

173. Kintzel PE, Eastlund T, Calis KA. Extracorporeal removal of antimicrobials during plasmapheresis. J Clin Apher 2003;18:194-205.

174. Ibrahim RB, Liu CY, Cronin SM, et al. Influence of plasma exchange on the disposition of the fourth generation cephalosporin cefepime. J Oncol Pharm Pract 2009;15:217-22.

175. Kale-Pradhan PB, Woo MH. A review of the effects of plasmapheresis on drug clearance. Pharmacotherapy 1997;17:684-95.

176. Bakken JS, Cavalieri SJ, Gangeness D, et al. Influence of therapeutic plasmapheresis on elimination of ceftiaxone. Antimicrob Agents Chemother 1993;37:1171-3.

177. Bozkurt F, Schollmeyer P, Keller E. Kinetics of ceftazidime during plasmapheresis. Eur J Clin Pharmacol 1987;33:197-201.

178. Fauvelle F, Lortholary O, Tod M, et al. Pharmacokinetics of ceftriaxone during plasma exchange in polyarteritis nodosa patients. Antimircob Agents Chemother 1994;38:1519-22.

179. Brophy DF, Mueller BA. Vancomycin removal by plasmapheresis. Ann Pharmacother 1996;30:1038.

180. Foral MA, Heineman SM. Vancomycin removal during a plasma exchange transfusion. Ann Pharmacother 2001;35:1400-2.

181. McClellan SD, Whitaker CH, Friedberg RC. Removal of vancomycin during plasmapheresis. Ann Pharmacother 1997;31:1132-6.

182. Osman BA, Lew SQ. Vancomycin removal by plasmapheresis. Pharmacol Toxicol 1997;81:245-6.

183. Sirvent AE, Borras-Blasco J, Enriquez R, et al. Extracorporeal removal of vancomycin by plasmapheresis. Ann Pharmacother 2006;40:2279-80.

184. Ouellette SM, Visconti JA, Kennedy MS. A pharmacokinetic evaluation of the effect of plasma exchange on tobramycin disposition. Clin Exp Dial Apheresis 1983;7:225-33.

185. Appelgate R, Schwartz D, Bennett WM. Removal of tobramycin during plasma exchange therapy. Ann Intern Med 1981;94:820-1.

186. Kale-Pradhan PB, Dehoorne-Smith ML, Jaworski DA, et al. Evaluation of plasmapheresis on the removal of tobramycin. Pharmacotherapy 1995;15:673-6.

187. Keller F, Hauff A, Schultze G, et al. Effect of repeated plasma exchange on steady state kinetics of digoxin and digitoxin. Arzneimittelforschung 1984;34:83-6.

188. Keller F, Kreutz G, Vohringer HF, et al. Effect of plasma exchange on the steady-state kinetics of digoxin and digitoxin. Clin Pharmacokinet 1985;10:514-23.

189. Liu E, Rubenstein M. Phenytoin removal by plasmapheresis in thrombotic thrombocytopenic purpura. Clin Pharmacol Ther 1982;31:762-5.

190. Mitzner SR, Stange J, Klammt S, et al. Extracorporeal detoxification using the molecular adsorbent recirculating system for critically ill patients with liver failure. J Am Soc Nephrol 2001;12(suppl 17):S75-82.

191. Weiler S, Falkensammer G, Seger C, et al. Teicoplanin pharmacokinetics during albumin dialysis. Artif Organs 2011;35:969-71.

192. Roth GA, Sipos W, Hoferl M, et al. The effect of the molecular adsorbent recirculating system on moxifloxacin and meropenem plasma levels. Acta Anaesthesiol Scand 2013;57:461-7.

193. Ruggero MA, Argento AC, Heavner MS, et al. Molecular adsorbent recirculating System (MARS((R)) removal of piperacillin/tazobactam in a patient with acetaminophen-induced acute liver failure. Transpl Infect Dis 2013;15:214-8.

Chapter 42: Management of the Critically Ill Burn Patient

Claire V. Murphy, Pharm.D., BCPS; and Kate Oltrogge Pape, Pharm.D., BCPS

LEARNING OBJECTIVES

1. Describe the different types of burn injury and classify its severity based on size and depth and the associated morbidity and mortality with each class.
2. Develop a plan for fluid resuscitation in a burn injury patient while weighing the risks and benefits of a plan that includes crystalloids, colloids, hypertonic saline, and/or ascorbic acid.
3. Discuss the importance of managing the burn injury in the emergent setting, including the assessment and treatment of inhalation injury and cyanide toxicity.
4. Compare the nonpharmacologic and pharmacologic options for metabolic modulation in burn injury, including nutrition support, early surgical excision, oxandrolone, and propranolol.
5. Formulate a strategy to prevent and treat complications that may arise in the burn injury patient, including sepsis, glycemic control, and venous thromboembolism.

ABBREVIATIONS IN THIS CHAPTER

ABA	American Burn Association	TBSA	Total body surface area
REE	Resting energy expenditure	VTE	Venous thromboembolism
rhGH	Recombinant human growth hormone		
SIRS	Systemic inflammatory response syndrome		

INTRODUCTION

Each year, over 450,000 individuals suffer a burn injury that requires treatment, with over 40,000 of those requiring admission to the hospital. Burn injury can affect all ages and can be caused from a variety of mechanisms, including flames, hot liquids, and chemicals. The treatment of burns has evolved over the years with advancements in fluid resuscitation, metabolic modulation, and management of complications, leading to increased survival. The critical care pharmacist can play an important role in the management of the burn injury patient by optimizing the patient's care through recommendations on fluid resuscitation, pharmacologic metabolic modulation, and using pharmacokinetic and pharmacodynamic parameters to optimize drug therapy. The key to successful outcomes in burn injury patients are driven by a multidisciplinary team, and the American Burn Association (ABA) officially recognizes the importance of having a critically care–trained pharmacist as a member, making it a requirement for verification as a certified burn center.

EPIDEMIOLOGY OF BURN INJURY

Burn injury is defined by damage to the skin and underlying tissues caused by exposure to energy sources, including heat, chemicals, electricity, and radiation. The most common cause of burn injury is cutaneous damage from thermal energy exposure to fire or flame (43% of injuries), hot liquids (34% of injuries), or hot objects (4% of injuries). Contact with chemicals, electricity, radiation, or other causes accounts for 14% of burn injuries.[1] In children younger than 5 years, scald injury and contact with hot objects are more prevalent than in adults. Similar to general trauma injuries, males have a higher incidence of burn injury than do females. This trend is observed across all age groups except among patients 80 years and older.[1] Most burn injuries occur in adults, and children younger than 16 years account for about 29% of burn-related injuries.[1]

Although burn injury is still fairly common, associated survival has drastically increased during the past decades, with the 2004–2013 average survival rate of 96.7%.[1,2] In the past decade, mortality rates have decreased significantly from 3.4% to 2.7% for males and from 4.6% to 3.3% for females, and the average hospital length of stay has decreased by 11%.[1] Although this improvement in outcomes cannot be attributed to a single intervention, potential changes include a continued focus on burn management within specialized burn centers, advances in fluid resuscitation, early debridement and grafting, and general progress in critical care and nutritional support.[3]

REVIEW OF NORMAL SKIN STRUCTURE AND FUNCTION

The skin serves many functions, including protection from traumatic injury and infection, sensory perception, thermoregulation, and regulation of fluid homeostasis. Understanding the normal structure and functions of the skin is vital because having this understanding can aid in describing both burn severity and the expected complications.

Normal skin structure contains two layers: the epidermis and the dermis. The epidermis serves as a protective, mechanical barrier from the environment, and the dermal layer supports the epidermis. Unlike the epidermis, which has no blood vessels or other structures, the dermis contains blood vessels, connective tissues (i.e., collagen and elastic fibers), nerve endings, fibroblasts, mast cells, lymphatics, and epidermal appendages (i.e., sebaceous glands, sweat glands, apocrine glands, mammary glands, and hair follicles). The epidermal appendages within the dermal layer are responsible for re-epithelialization of the epidermis and are therefore essential for wound healing in burn injury.

METABOLIC CHANGES IN BURN INJURY

Critical illness is known to result in a severe stress response that is heightened in both severity and duration in patients with severe burn injury. The threshold defining severe burn injury, as well as the associated pathophysiologic changes, varies by age and is about 30% of the total body surface area (TBSA) burned in children (0–18 years of age), 20% in adults (18–65 years of age), and 15% in older adults (older than 65 years).[4] In patients with major burn injury, this stress response consists of an early (ebb) phase and a late (flow) phase.[5] During the first 48 hours after burn injury, the ebb phase is characterized by a massive cytokine-mediated inflammatory response and a concomitantly reduced cardiac output that both contribute to hypoperfusion and hemodynamic instability.[6,7] In addition, intravascular volume losses occur during this early phase through several avenues. An osmotically driven fluid shift occurs because of an intracellular shift of sodium through sodium-ATPase transmembrane pump disturbances.[8] Histamine released from mast cells within the injured area also damages the integrity of the endothelial junctions within the capillary bed, resulting in increased capillary permeability and significant third spacing.[5,7] These relative volume losses are further intensified by insensible fluid loss through the burn wound. Early studies found a 26% reduction in plasma volume in animal models with 30% TBSA burns 18 hours after injury.[9] The rate of volume loss peaks within the first 8–12 hours after injury and slows significantly in the following 12 hours.

The late, or flow, phase typically begins after fluid resuscitation and initial stabilization is achieved. The hypermetabolic and hyperdynamic flow phase is defined by an imbalance of catabolism and anabolism, hyperglycemia, significant proteolysis, and impaired protein synthesis.[5] Sustained increases in catecholamines accompanied by reduced growth hormone and testosterone concentrations contribute to a hypermetabolic state in which resting energy expenditure (REE) can reach up to 2 times normal rates.[6,7,10,11] Significant abnormalities occur with respect to protein and lipid catabolism, resulting in nitrogen losses, lean muscle wasting, and impaired wound healing. Increased glucagon release and GLUT-4 glucose transporter–mediated insulin resistance also contribute to significant hyperglycemia in the flow phase.[12-14] Most aspects of the flow phase peak within the first month after injury, with some hypermetabolic-associated changes, such as the increased resting metabolic rate and hyperglycemia, persisting for years.[12,13]

INITIAL CARE IN BURN INJURY

Assessment of Burn Severity

Accurate assessment of the severity of burn injury is crucial in determining treatment plans, including calculating fluid volumes recommended for resuscitation, transfer to an ABA verified burn center (Box 42.1) and operative needs. The rule of nines is a common and simple method for assessing burn size (Figure 42.1).[15] Although this method has been validated, it has been attributed to overestimation of burn size.[16] The Lund and Browder chart with a definite breakdown of body areas is associated with increased predictive accuracy (Figure 42.1). Computerized programs that incorporate three-dimensional skin structure into burn size calculations have been introduced in the past decade in an attempt to further improve accuracy and assist in documentation (i.e., Sage II, 3D Burn Vision, and BurnCase 3D).[16] Regardless of the method used to determine burn size, first-degree (also known as [aka] superficial) burns are not included in the TBSA burned.

Like in assessing burn size, determining burn depth is key in determining whether surgical excision with skin grafting is required. Burn wound depth is defined as superficial, partial, or full thickness according to the degree of involvement of the epidermis and dermis. Injury limited to the epidermal layer is considered superficial (aka first degree), whereas extension into the dermis is associated with partial thickness injury (aka second degree) (see Table 42.1). The extent of the dermal layer involved will allow for further description of partial thickness injury as either superficial or deep. Damage limited to the papillary dermis, as observed in superficial partial thickness burn injury, can heal without intervention within 2 weeks. However, injury to the basal membrane of the dermal layer associated with deep partial thickness burns precludes wound healing without surgical excision and grafting. Burn injury extending into the entire epidermis and dermis is considered a full thickness wound (aka third degree). Without surgical intervention, deep partial thickness and full thickness burn wounds will have dysfunctional spontaneous healing involving granulation, contraction, and re-epithelialization from the wound margins, which can result in significant scarring or development of a non-healing chronic wound. Therefore, surgical excision of the burn wound with autologous skin grafting is the optimal wound care plan in most cases for both deep partial thickness and full thickness burn injuries.

Box 42.1. ABA Burn Center Referral Criteria

Burn injuries that should be referred to a burn center include:
1. Partial thickness burns greater than 10% TBSA
2. Burns that involve the face, hands, feet, genitalia, perineum, or major joints
3. Full thickness burns in any age group
4. Electrical burns including lightning injury
5. Chemical burns
6. Inhalation injury
7. Burn injury in patients with preexisting comorbidities that could complicate management, prolong recovery, or affect mortality
8. Any patient with burns and concomitant trauma in which the burn injury poses the greatest risk of morbidity or mortality. If the trauma poses the greater immediate risk, the patient may be initially stabilized in a trauma center before transfer to a burn center
9. Pediatric burn patients in hospitals without qualified personnel or equipment for the care of children
10. Burn injury in patients who will require special social, emotional, or rehabilitative intervention

TBSA = total body surface area.

Risk Factors for Mortality

The Baux formula, which calculated mortality risk according to age plus TBSA injured, was the first predictive formula used to determine prognosis.[3] Previously mentioned improvements in burn care leading to better outcomes now limit the accuracy of the Baux formula, and use for prognostication should be done with caution. A systematic review of 13 studies identified three predictors of mortality in adults with burn injury: age, burn size, and lower airway inhalation injury.[17,18] Burn depth, female sex, comorbidities, and burn injury complicated by pneumonia may also increase the risk of mortality in adult patients with burn injury. Despite the significant limitations of the Baux formula, no single predictive formula has been accepted in its place as a gold standard.[17-19] Among pediatric burn injury, the strongest predictor of outcome is age younger than 4 years.[20-23] After adjusting for sex, burn size, inhalation injury, and burn etiology, a study of more than 12,000 pediatric burn admissions found that mortality risk was 2.7-fold higher for children 0–1.9 years of age and 2-fold higher for children 2–3.9 years of age than for children 4 years and older. However, children are also more likely to survive even massive burns, based on estimated lethal TBSA for 50% mortality of greater than 60% regardless of age group or burn etiology, and characteristics of burn injury may not be predictive of outcome among the pediatric burn population.[23]

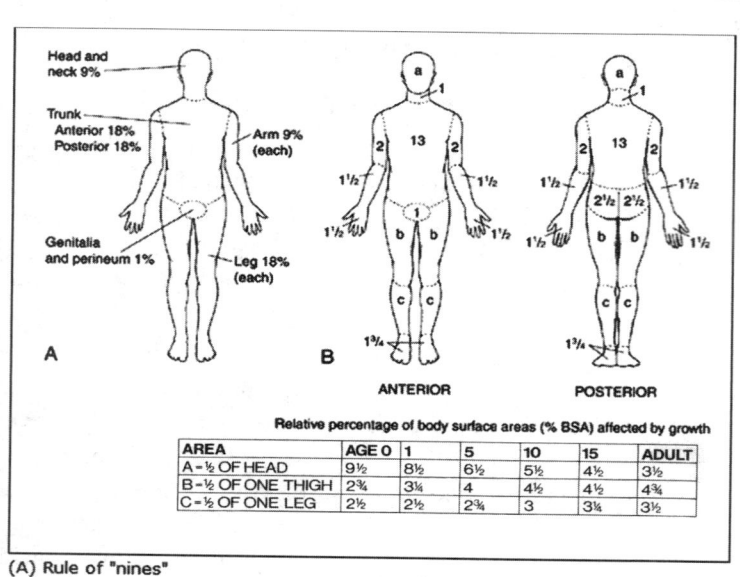

(A) Rule of "nines"
(B) Lund-Browder diagram for estimating extent of burns

Reprinted from U.S. Department of Health and Human Services. Lund-Browder chart. April 24, 2013.

Figure 42.1 Determination of burn size.

Fluid Resuscitation

During the early ebb phase, the goal of initial fluid resuscitation is adequate organ and tissue perfusion. Delayed or inadequate resuscitation can ultimately lead to the development of acute renal failure, progression of burn wound necrosis, multiorgan failure, burn shock, and increased risk of death.[24,25] Because of the large volumes required for resuscitation associated with severe burn injury, a careful balance is required to avoid both under- and over-resuscitation. In most developed countries, under-resuscitation after hospital admission is uncommon because standard calculations such as the Parkland formula are used to determine resuscitative volumes.

As in most areas of critical care, there is significant controversy regarding the optimal fluid, or fluid combination, to use for resuscitation in burn injury. Significant institutional variances exist in both formula and fluid type (e.g., crystalloid, colloid, plasma, starch, or combination) used for resuscitation because data are currently limited to support a goal standard. Although there is no standard for type of fluid or formula to use in calculating the volume needed, the most commonly used formula in the United States is the Parkland formula.[26] This formula, a crystalloid-based resuscitation model using Ringer lactate solution, is recognized by the American Burn Association (ABA) as the "consensus formula." First developed in 1968 by Baxter and Shires, the current Parkland formula consists of 4 mL/% TBSA burned per kilogram of Ringer lactate solution for resuscitation, with half of this volume administered in the first 8 hours from the time of injury, and the remaining volume infused over the following 16 hours.[9] Despite the widespread use of the Parkland formula, there are few data in humans to support its use. Other examples of crystalloid-based burn fluid resuscitation formulas are included in Tables 42.2 and 42.3.

Debate regarding the ideal crystalloid for burn resuscitation has ensued with a focus surrounding the role of balanced solutions. Although most studies have evaluated Ringer lactate solution, Gille and colleagues compared resuscitation using Ringer lactate and Ringer acetate solution in 40 patients with severe burn injury ranging from 20% to 70% TBSA burned.[27] Ringer acetate has components similar to those of Ringer lactate solution with the replacement of 27 mmol/L acetate for the 28 mmol/L of lactate found in Ringer lactate solution. The infusion rate for resuscitative fluids was based on the Parkland formula for all patients and was titrated to maintain a urine output of 0.5–1 mL/kg/hour. All patients received 20% albumin infusion after 12 hours to maintain serum albumin concentrations above 2 g/dL. Patients who received Ringer acetate and Ringer lactate solutions received similar median 24-hour resuscitative fluid volume (5,625 [25–75% interquartile range 8,450] vs. 4,900 [5,550] mL, p=0.456), and volumes administered throughout admission were similar between groups. Although patients in both groups had similar baseline burn severity and sequential organ failure assessment (SOFA) scores, those who received Ringer acetate had significant improvement in SOFA scores beginning on days 3–6 of admission. Ringer acetate was also associated with significant reductions in lactate concentrations on days 1–5 of admission. Additional clinical benefits included decreased hospital length of stay and duration of mechanical ventilation. However, the benefits observed with Ringer acetate failed to translate consistently into improved clinical outcomes, with no differences in 28- or 60-day mortality or intensive care length of stay. Further study is needed to determine the role of resuscitative crystalloids other than Ringer lactate solution in burn injury.

Table 42.1 Overview of Burn Depth

Burn Depth	Skin Structures Involved	Presentation	Sensation	Healing Time
Superficial (first degree)	Epidermis only	Dry, red, and blanches with pressure	Painful	~3–7 days
Superficial partial thickness (second degree)	Extends into superficial (papillary) dermis	Moist, red, blisters, and blanches with pressure	Painful	1–2 wk
Deep partial thickness (second degree)	Extends into deep (reticular) dermis	Moist, mottled or white, blisters and delayed blanching if at all	Painful-described as discomfort	3–4 wk, can develop scarring and contractures without surgical intervention
Full thickness (third degree)	Extends through entire dermis	Dry, leathery, white/brown	Painless	Requires excision with grafting
Fourth degree	Extends through skin and subcutaneous tissue and into underlying muscle and bone	Dry, black, charred with eschar	Painless	May require amputation with complex reconstruction

Table 42.2 Examples of Current Formulas to Estimate Resuscitation Requirements for Adult Burn Patients

Formula	Fluid	Initial Resuscitation 0–24 Hr Post-burn	24–48 Hr Post-burn
Parkland[a]	LR	4 mL/kg/% TBSA, half given over first 8 hr, remainder over following 16 hr	20%–60% of calculated plasma volume as plasma
	Plasma		D_5W to maintain urine output
Modified Parkland	LR	4 mL/kg/% TBSA, half given over first 8 hr, remainder over following 16 hr	5% albumin 0.3–1 mL/kg/% TBSA over 16 hr
Brooke	NS	1.5 mL/kg/% TBSA over 24 hr	0.5 mL/kg/% TBSA over 24 hr
	Plasma	0.5 mL/kg/% TBSA over 24 hr	0.25 mL/kg/% TBSA over 24 hr
		2,000 mL of D_5W	2,000 mL of D_5W
Modified Brooke[a]	LR	2 mL/kg/% TBSA, half given over first 8 hr, remainder over following 16 hr	No crystalloids, only D_5W to maintain urine output
	Plasma or albumin	3 mL/kg/% TBSA in children	0.3–0.5 mL/kg/% TBSA plasma or albumin
		No colloids	
Slater	LR	2 L over 24 hr (i.e., 83 mL/hr), without titration	Not described
	FFP	75 mL/hr titrated to maintain urine output goals over 36 hr	
Evans	NS	1 mL/kg/% TBSA over 24 hr	0.5 mL/kg/% TBSA over 24 hr
	Plasma	1 mL/kg/% TBSA over 24 hr	0.5 mL/kg/% TBSA over 24 hr
Haifa	LR	1 mL/kg/% TBSA over 24 hr	0.75 mL/kg/% TBSA over 24 hr
	Plasma	1.5 mL/kg/% TBSA with half given over first 8 hr, remainder over following 16 hr	0.5 mL/kg/% TBSA adjusted to urine output

[a]Many burn centers do not use colloids based on these formulas in the 24- to 48-hour period.

D_5W = dextrose 5% in water; FFP = fresh frozen plasma; LR = lactated Ringer; NS = normal saline; TBSA = total body surface area.

It is also important to remember that these formulas provide an estimate, and individual patient response should dictate ongoing resuscitative plans. Factors that can be associated with requirement of fluid volume above initially calculated amounts include concomitant injuries, electrical injury, inhalation injury, delays in resuscitation, dehydration before injury, alcohol or other substance abuse, and burn injury involving subcutaneous tissues (e.g., muscle). Over-resuscitation has become an increasing problem, and this phenomenon of excess fluid administration has been termed *fluid creep*.[28] Potential contributors to fluid creep include inaccurate estimation of burn size, improper/inadequate titration of fluids, use of additional end points for resuscitation such as cardiac index or central venous oxygen saturation, increased sedation, and analgesic infusion use.[28-31] The consequences of fluid creep include acute lung injury, intra-abdominal hypertension, abdominal compartment syndrome, and ischemic optic neuropathy.[31-35] Potential mechanisms to reduce the risk of inadequate titration that have shown reductions in 24- and 48-hour resuscitative fluid volumes include nursing and computer-directed algorithms.[36,37] The increased concern associated with fluid creep and the consequences of over-resuscitation have also led to renewed interest in the role of colloids in burn resuscitation.[38]

Although many centers have returned to using colloids in burn resuscitation, use of colloids has existed since the initial resuscitative formulas. In fact, the original Parkland formula included an infusion of plasma after 24 hours.[8,38] The theoretical benefits of colloid administration that have been shown in animal models for burn injury include increases in oncotic

Table 42.3 Examples of Current Formulas to Estimate Resuscitation Requirements for Pediatric Burn Patients

Formula	Fluid	Initial Resuscitation 0–24 Hr Post-burn	24–48 Hr Post-burn
Parkland[a]	LR	3 mL/kg/% TBSA for plus maintenance:	20%–60% of calculated plasma volume as plasma
	Plasma	-4 mL/kg/hr for 0–10 kg	D_5W to maintain urine output
		-40 mL/hr + 2 mL/kg/hr for 10–20 kg	
		-60 mL/hr = 1 mL/kg/hr for > 20 kg	
Modified Brooke[a]	LR	3 mL/kg/% TBSA in children, half given over first 8 hr, remainder over following 16 hr	No crystalloids, only D_5W to maintain urine output
	Plasma or albumin	No colloids	0.3–0.5 mL/kg/% TBSA plasma or albumin
Shriners Cincinnati	LR ± albumin	Older children:	
		4 mL/kg/% TBSA plus 1,500 mL/m² total, half given over first 8 hr, remainder over the following 16 hr	
		Younger children:	
		4 mL/kg/% TBSA plus 1500 mL/m² total	
		First 8 hr with LR with 50 mEq sodium bicarbonate	
		Second 8 hr with LR	
		Third 8 hr with 5% albumin in LR	
Galveston	LR	5,000 mL/m² burn + 2,000 mL/m² total, half given over first 8 hr, remainder over the following 16 hr	

[a]Many burn centers do not use colloids according to these formulas in the 24- to 48-hour period.
LR = lactated Ringer; TBSA = total body surface area.

pressure and subsequent improvement in intravascular fluid retention, restriction of volume losses observed in burn injury, and fluid shifts from the vascular space to the lungs and interstitium. However, significant concerns regarding the ability of colloids to remain in the intravascular space in the initial 24 hours post-injury because of increased capillary permeability and data analyses suggesting increased mortality in burn injury with colloid administration contributed to a movement away from colloid administration starting in the 1960s.[38] Not until the past decade with the documented consequences of the observed fluid creep has the potential role for colloids in burn resuscitation been reintroduced. Although most burn resuscitative formulas have historically used plasma for colloid resuscitation, several prospective studies have evaluated the role of albumin, as early as 1975.[38] The initial small randomized controlled studies consistently found that albumin administration during burn resuscitation offers a significant fluid-sparing effect.[39-42] However, most studies have failed to either evaluate or show clinical outcome benefit associated with the use of albumin. More recently, Park and colleagues evaluated 159 patients 12 years and older with greater than 20% TBSA burn who were admitted to the burn intensive care unit before and after implementation of a burn resuscitation protocol that included early use of albumin.[43] The resuscitation protocol allowed for conversion from lactated Ringer to albumin 5% continuous infusion at the same rate, if the 12-hour resuscitative fluid requirements would predict an excess of 6 mL/kg/% TBSA burn in the 24-hour resuscitative period. Although there was no difference in the total fluid volume required before and after implementing the albumin protocol, this study did show a significant clinical benefit to albumin use with a reduction in mortality (26 vs. 10%, $p<0.01$) and a decrease in duration of mechanical ventilation, vasopressor use, and incidence of abdominal compartment syndrome requiring surgical intervention. Although the role of colloids is unclear within burn resuscitation, they appear to play a role at least within patients requiring more than predicted resuscitative fluid volume.

Pharmacologic Resuscitation with Ascorbic Acid

Reactive oxygen species have been identified as a key factor in endothelial dysfunction and subsequent hypoperfusion observed in sepsis and burn injury. Reactive oxygen species production occurs through several pathways, including enzymatic induction (e.g., endothelial nitric oxide synthase), uncoupling of mitochondrial respiration, and histamine activation of xanthine oxidase. Ascorbic acid, a known antioxidant, has been shown in vitro to reduce oxidative stress-mediated endothelial dysfunction and permeability, reduce impairment of microcirculatory flow, and improve macrophage activity. Animal models have replicated these in vitro findings and also found that ascorbic acid attenuates burn-related immunosuppression, lipid peroxidation, and vascular permeability.[44-47] A single randomized controlled trial of 37 patients older than 16 years with severe burn injury (greater than 30% TBSA burns) showed that patients who received high-dose ascorbic acid had significantly lower 24-hour resuscitative fluid requirements than did control patients (3.0 ± 1.7 vs. 5.5 ± 3.1 mL/kg/% TBSA burn, p<0.01). Both groups received resuscitation using the Parkland formula calculation, which was titrated to a urine output end point of 0.5–1 mL/kg/hour, with the intervention group receiving ascorbic acid diluted 10-fold with distilled water at 66 mg/kg/hour for 24 hours concurrently with Parkland formula resuscitation (see Table 42.2). The volume associated with ascorbic acid administration was accounted for in the 24-hour fluid intake determination.[48] The difference in resuscitative volume requirements also translated to significant benefit with respect to improved Pao_2/fraction of inspired oxygen (Fio_2) ratios at 18, 24, 36, 48, and 72 hours after injury and a 9-day reduction in mechanical ventilation duration. Because of this small study, some burn centers implemented high-dose ascorbic acid resuscitation to counteract the observed fluid creep. Kahn and colleagues reported their experience with ascorbic acid (66 mg/kg/hour for 24 hours) in 17 patients compared with 16 control patients who received standard resuscitation without ascorbic acid.[49] Patients who received high-dose ascorbic acid had a significant reduction in 24-hour resuscitative fluid requirements similar to what was observed by Tanaka and colleagues (3 vs. 5.5 mL/kg/% TBSA burn, p<0.05).[48,89] Although these two small studies showed consistent benefits of high-dose ascorbic acid, concerns of osmotic diuresis and renal failure–associated calcium oxalate formation, based on animal data, were not adequately addressed in these clinical studies. Kahn and colleagues noted a higher urine output in patients receiving ascorbic acid (1.5 vs. 1 mL/kg/hour, p<0.05), which could support either osmotic diuresis or improved resuscitation and renal perfusion. However, the Kahn study failed to use standardized criteria for renal failure and did not evaluate the development of renal failure beyond the 24-hour period of ascorbic acid administration. Buehner and colleagues published a case series describing two patients treated with high-dose ascorbic acid for resuscitation of burn injury.[50] Both patients developed acute kidney injury and, on autopsy, were found to have calcium oxalate crystals within the renal tubules. To date, no studies have fully addressed the safety concerns with ascorbic acid resuscitation.

Another concern regarding high-dose ascorbic acid is the documented interference with point-of-care glucose measurements. Studies have documented significant increases in point-of-care glucose concentrations compared with serum laboratory glucose values of 10–200 mg/dL.[51,52] In addition, the interference persists beyond the discontinuation of ascorbic acid infusion, ranging from a few hours to up to 24 hours after discontinuation. Caution should be taken when monitoring glucose values during vitamin C administration and for up to 24 hours after completion of therapy.

No studies have evaluated high-dose ascorbic acid–based resuscitation in pediatric patients with burn injury. However, a single randomized controlled study compared patients who received oral antioxidant supplementation (n=17) with vitamin C (1.5 times the upper intake level), vitamin E (1.35 times the upper intake level), and zinc (2 times the recommended dietary allowance) during days 2–8 after admission with patients who received no supplementation (n=15).[53] For vitamin C, this dosing would translate to 600 mg for those 1–3 years of age, 975 mg for those 4–8 years of age, 1800 mg for those 9–13 years of age, and 2700 mg for those 14–18 years of age. Patients who received the antioxidant mixture including ascorbic acid had decreased lipid peroxidation (based on malondialdehyde concentrations) and improved wound healing. However, the clinical benefit of this intervention is limited because mortality was not evaluable on the basis of the strict inclusion criteria, and length of stay was not reported. According to the limited data showing outcomes benefits and the lack of safety data, high-dose ascorbic acid is not currently standard of care for the resuscitation of either pediatric or adult patients with burn injury.

Inhalation Injury

Up to 20% of patients hospitalized with burn injury present with inhalation injury.[54] Inhalation injury describes a group of pulmonary injuries caused by the inhalation of chemical or thermal irritants that can affect the upper or lower airways. Typically, these injuries can be further divided according to etiology: thermal injury to the upper airway above the glottis, injury throughout the pulmonary tree caused by chemical irritation, or toxicity systemically caused by carbon monoxide or cyanide inhalation. Thermal injury to the oropharynx results in pathophysiologic changes similar to those observed in cutaneous burn injury and can result in edema and ultimately airway obstruction during fluid resuscitation; therefore, the need for intubation for airway protection should be evaluated in patients at risk of inhalation injury (e.g., patients with stridor, severe facial burns, and burns greater than 50% TBSA). Injury to the lower airway is usually associated with irritation caused by by-products of incomplete combustion (e.g., sulfur dioxide, nitrogen dioxide, ammonia, chlorine, toxic aldehydes). Both epithelial and endothelial capillary cells of the airway are damaged, and significant increases in capillary permeability occur, resulting in accumulation of protein-rich fluid within the alveoli and impaired gas exchange. Additional mucociliary transport and clearance of bacteria is diminished, placing patients at higher risk of pneumonia.

Inhalation injury with concurrent cutaneous injury increases morbidity and mortality, fluid requirements for initial resuscitation, and risk of other pulmonary complications such as pneumonia.[55] Although there have been significant advances in the management of cutaneous burn injuries in the past decades, there is limited information to guide both diagnosis and treatment of inhalation injury. Currently, there are no standard diagnostic criteria for inhalation injury, and clinicians rely primarily on a history of smoke exposure in a closed space, physical examination (e.g., soot in airway, singed nasal hairs, carbonaceous sputum), fiberoptic bronchoscopy, and carboxyhemoglobin concentrations. Management focuses on supportive care with mechanical ventilation, and the only pharmacologic interventions with evidence in humans at this time are nebulized heparin and acetylcysteine.[55,56] Additional agents directed toward reducing bronchoconstriction and improving pulmonary blood flow, including nebulized β-agonists and nitric oxide, have shown potential benefits in animal models.

In addition to endothelial damage, airway obstruction occurs in inhalation injury because of the development of casts, fibrin deposition, and clot formation in the alveolar space. Nebulized heparin and acetylcysteine have been evaluated because of their potential role in reducing reactive oxygen stress and fibrin clot formation. Desai and colleagues first showed in a retrospective, observational study a significant benefit of nebulized heparin alternating with acetylcysteine with reduced requirements for reintubation and improved survival among 47 pediatric patients who received heparin 5,000 international units alternating with 20% acetylcysteine every 2 hours for 7 days after injury compared with 43 historical control patients.[57] After this study, Holt and colleagues found no benefits with nebulized heparin 5,000 international units (5,000 international units/mL) with 3 mL of 20% acetylcysteine and albuterol (2.5 mg of 0.083% solution per 3 mL) in adult patients with inhalation injury in a retrospective review.[58]

Miller and colleagues conducted a similar study in adult patients 18–80 years of age with smoke inhalation injury.[59] In this observational pre/post-intervention study, 16 patients who received 10,000 international units of nebulized heparin mixed in 3 mL of 0.9% sodium chloride every 4 hours alternating with 3 mL of 20% acetylcysteine and 0.5 mL of albuterol for 7 days were compared with 14 historical controls. Significant improvement in lung injury score (LIS) for days 2–7, pulmonary compliance, and hypoxia scores, based on the Pao_2/Fio_2 ratios, were observed in patients receiving nebulized heparin/acetylcysteine and albuterol.

Given these conflicting results, a small prospective, randomized, double-blind study compared two differing nebulized heparin strategies. Elsharnouby and colleagues compared 29 adult burn patients in the following two groups: a group receiving 5,000 international units of heparin in 3 mL of 0.9% sodium chloride nebulized alternating every 2 hours with 3 mL of 20% acetylcysteine and a group receiving 10,000 international units of heparin in 3 mL of 0.9% sodium chloride nebulized alternating every 2 hours with 3 mL of 20% acetylcysteine.[60] This study found a significant improvement in LIS scores on days 5–7 after injury as well as a significant reduction in the duration of mechanical ventilation by 8 days in the group that received 10,000 international units heparin. According to analyses of these data, when using nebulized heparin with acetylcysteine in the adult patient with inhalation injury, a higher dosing (e.g., 10,000 international units) of heparin should be used. Limited data have been reported regarding the safety of nebulized heparin and acetylcysteine. Elsharnouby and colleagues were the first to report that neither dosing strategy (5,000 or 10,000 international units of nebulized heparin) affected platelet count or coagulation parameters (activated partial thromboplastin time and thrombin clotting time), and neither strategy was associated with the development of blood-tinged secretions. Because the quality of data supporting the use of nebulized heparin with acetylcysteine in both pediatric and adult patients with inhalation injury is low, there is considerable variation in practice among burn centers with respect to nebulized heparin/acetylcysteine. A prospective, randomized, placebo-controlled, double-blind study is currently recruiting 116 patients to receive nebulization of either 25,000 international units of heparin (5 mL) or placebo (0.9% sodium chloride 5 mL) without acetylcysteine every 4 hours for up to 14 days after injury to try to provide further evidence defining the role of nebulized heparin in the management of inhalation injury.[61]

Carbon Monoxide and Cyanide Toxicity

Many fatalities at the scene occur because of carbon monoxide toxicity. Carbon monoxide is a colorless, odorless, non-irritating gas produced by incomplete combustion of carbon-containing compounds. Carbon monoxide competes with oxygen for hemoglobin binding, but it displaces oxygen and lowers oxygen delivery because of a 200- to 250-fold higher affinity for hemoglobin than for oxygen. Because of the similar absorbent spectrums of oxyhemoglobin and carboxyhemoglobin, pulse oximetry cannot distinguish between the two. The Pao_2 measurements are also limited in carbon monoxide exposure and may not reflect the degree of toxicity. Complications associated with carbon monoxide toxicity generally involve neurologic symptoms, with severity based on the measured carboxyhemoglobin concentration ranging from confusion

Table 42.4 Correlation of Carboxyhemoglobin with Symptoms of Carbon Monoxide Toxicity

Carboxyhemoglobin (%)	Presentation
5–10	Mild headache, confusion
11–20	Severe headache, flushing, visual changes
21–30	Disorientation, nausea
31–40	Irritability, dizziness, emesis
41–50	Tachypnea, tachycardia
>50	Coma, seizures, death

and headaches to coma (Table 42.4). Use of neurologic symptoms can be limited in patients with burn injury because many have received sedating medication before presentation to the emergency department. Definitive diagnosis of carbon monoxide toxicity relies primarily on laboratory confirmation of carboxyhemoglobin concentration. Carboxyhemoglobin concentrations greater than 3% in nonsmokers and greater than 10% in smokers indicate exposure to carbon monoxide.[55]

Current guidelines for the management of carbon monoxide toxicity recommend administration of 100% F_{IO_2} for patients with carboxyhemoglobin concentrations greater than 10%. Administration of 100% F_{IO_2} reduces the half-life of carboxyhemoglobin from 250 minutes at room air to 40–60 minutes. Although this can be administered by facemask in patients who are alert, patients with altered mental status should be intubated and mechanically ventilated with 100% F_{IO_2} until carboxyhemoglobin concentrations fall below 5%. Hyperbaric oxygen (HBO) can further reduce the half-life of carboxyhemoglobin, but the ABA does not currently support the use of HBO as standard of care in carbon monoxide toxicity. The hyperbaric chamber can introduce challenges into the acute phase of burn injury care because it may limit nursing and physician access to the patient during a time when frequent assessments are necessary.[62] The impact of HBO on long-term neurologic complications of carbon monoxide is controversial, but a Cochrane review of six studies found no benefit with HBO.[63] Currently, HBO should only be considered in patients whose carboxyhemoglobin concentrations remain elevated despite aggressive oxygen therapy.

Cyanide is also produced by the combustion of typical household materials, and concurrent carbon monoxide and cyanide exposure is common in house fires.[54,64] Cyanide is normally found in concentrations of 0.3–0.5 mg/L, and enzymes convert the potentially toxic cyanide to thiocyanate at a rate of 0.017 mg/kg/minute. However, in acute cyanide exposure, these enzymes are saturated, and cyanide accumulates. Cyanide inhibits cellular respiratory by interfering with the cytochrome oxidase system, ultimately resulting in hypoxia and a metabolic lactic acidosis.[65] Symptoms of cyanide toxicity closely resemble those of carbon monoxide toxicity and range from dizziness and headache to coma, seizures, and shock. It is difficult to diagnose cyanide toxicity in the burn population solely on presentation, but unfortunately, measurement of cyanide concentrations is not available at most medical centers. Therefore, clinicians should consider empiric treatment for cyanide toxicity when at least two of the following are present: (1) neurologic symptoms including altered mental status, coma, or convulsions; (2) visible soot in mouth, nares, or sputum; or (3) metabolic acidosis with an elevated lactate concentration greater than 8 mmol/L.[66]

Treatment options for cyanide toxicity (amyl nitrite perles, 10% sodium nitrite, 25% sodium thiosulfate, and hydroxocobalamin) aim to increase the metabolism and elimination of cyanide (Table 42.5). Both amyl nitrite and sodium nitrite increase cyanide elimination by first inducing methemoglobinemia. Cyanide then binds preferentially to methemoglobin, forming cyanomethemoglobin, which then essentially sequesters the cyanide.[67] As cyanide dissociates from methemoglobin, it can be metabolized through normal pathways to non-toxic thiocyanate. Although the nitrites (amyl nitrite and sodium nitrite) allow for elimination of cyanide, the induced methemoglobinemia reduces the oxygen-carrying capacity of hemoglobin, furthering the hypoxic state of patients with inhalation injury, especially in light of carbon monoxide toxicity. Therefore, both amyl nitrite and sodium nitrite are contraindicated in patients presenting with smoke inhalation.[66] Sodium thiosulfate also allows for the metabolism of cyanide to thiocyanate with minimal adverse effects by acting as a sulfhydryl donor. Hydroxocobalamin also has minimal complications and does not interfere with oxygen delivery. Hydroxocobalamin chelates cyanide, forming cyanocobalamin, which is eliminated renally.[65,66] Limited data for these agents exist, and no randomized controlled comparative studies support the use of one agent over another. The nitrites are generally avoided because of their adverse effect profile, and in cutaneous burn injury, hydroxocobalamin can make an ongoing assessment of burn wounds challenging because of significant skin and mucus membrane discoloration. Hydroxocobalamin is also known to interfere with colorimetric laboratory assays used for liver enzymes, serum creatinine, electrolytes, methemoglobin, and carboxyhemoglobin for several days after administration, further limiting its use in burn injury.

With efficacy data lacking, the decision of which agent to use is based on adverse effect profile. Therefore, sodium thiosulfate monotherapy is considered standard of care, specifically in patients with cutaneous burn injury.[65]

NUTRITION SUPPORT AND METABOLIC MODULATION

Burn injury elevates the normal metabolic rate, resulting in the loss of lean body mass and muscle wasting if there is no intervention. In both adult and pediatric patients, estimating caloric requirements with indirect calorimetry, using serial REE measurements, tends to be more accurate than using predictive equations.[11,68] Enteral nutrition should be initiated within the ebb phase because the hypermetabolic state associated with the flow phase can lead to a doubling of the normal REE. Patients should not be fed enterally if they are experiencing hypovolemic shock, showing signs of instability and hypoperfusion, or experiencing visible abdominal distension. Early enteral feeding has been shown to decrease hospital length of stay and facilitate maintenance of admission weight.[69] Because burn patients oxidize amino acids much more quickly than healthy individuals, the recommended amount of protein is 1.5–2.0 g/kg/day if renal and liver function is normal.[70] When studied in pediatric patients with severe burns (greater than 40% TBSA), enteral nutrition that was supplied predominantly as carbohydrates rather than fat improved the balance of skeletal muscle protein.[68]

Nonpharmacologic measures to reduce REE include maintaining room temperature at 30°C–32°C, providing early excision and grafting of wounds, and promptly treating infections, as well as providing proper sedation and pain control.[11] There are a variety of pharmacologic interventions to help attenuate the hypermetabolic response in burn injury and decrease catabolism, enhance lean mass accretion, and maintain protein stores. These agents include oxandrolone, recombinant human growth hormone (rhGH), and adrenergic blockers.

Oxandrolone, an anabolic androgenic steroid, promotes protein synthesis and skeletal muscle growth and decreases time for wound healing. Oxandrolone should be dosed at 10 mg twice daily in adult patients, and the dose should be reduced in older adult patients to 5 mg twice daily because of the increased risk of adverse effects. Studies have shown oxandrolone to decrease hospital length of stay and patients to regain weight and lean mass faster than placebo when initiated 5–7 days after admission.[71,72] Doses of 0.1 mg/kg twice daily in pediatric patients have also been shown to improve lean body mass, serum visceral proteins, and muscle strength while promoting weight gain and increasing mineral bone content.[11] Even when treated for up to 1 year post-burn, oxandrolone improved lean body mass at 6, 9, and 12 months after the burn, and bone mineral content was also improved.[73] Pediatric patients who received oxandrolone for 1 year post-burn also show improvements for up to 5 years after treatment in height, bone mineral content, cardiac work, and muscle strength, with the greatest improvements seen in children ages 7–18 years.[74]

Adverse effects of oxandrolone include increased hepatic transaminases, and these should be monitored weekly while on oxandrolone therapy. If significant or persistent elevations of serum liver function tests occur, oxandrolone should be discontinued. Patients should not receive oxandrolone if they are pregnant or have a history of liver disease or cancer. Alterations in cholesterol have also been noted with oxandrolone, including lowering of high-density lipoprotein cholesterol and elevations in total or low-density lipoprotein cholesterol.[75] Oxandrolone has also been associated with the formation of edema and exacerbating heart failure.[11,75]

Table 42.5 Comparison of Available Cyanide Antidotes in Burn Injury

Agent	Mechanism	Dosing	Advantages	Disadvantages
Hydroxocobalamin	Binds to cyanide, forming cyanocobalamin	5 g for adults given IV over 15 min, may repeat half dose if needed	Fast acting, minimal adverse effects, may cause increase in blood pressure, safe in hypoxic patients	Skin/urine discoloration, interference with colorimetric laboratory tests, significant cost
Amyl nitrite	Induces methemoglobin production	Inhale crushed perle for 30 s, repeat every 3–5 min until IV access	Fast acting, no IV access required	Less effective when used without sodium thiosulfate, significant hypotension, avoid in hypoxic patients
Sodium nitrite	Induces methemoglobin production	300 mg for adults given IV over 3–5 min	Fast acting	Less effective when used without sodium thiosulfate, significant hypotension, avoid in hypoxic patients
Sodium thiosulfate	Provides substrate for cyanide metabolism to thiocyanate	12.5 g for adults given IV over 20–30 min, may repeat half dose if needed	Does not induce methemoglobin, safe in hypoxic patients, longer duration of effect	Slower onset of action

IV = intravenous(ly).

Compared with rhGH in adult patients, oxandrolone at 10 mg twice daily had significantly fewer hyperglycemia complications, and similar wound healing benefits were seen between the two agents.[76] The optimal duration of oxandrolone therapy has not been clearly defined, and the safety of using oxandrolone in pediatric patients younger than 1 year has not been established.

Recombinant human growth hormone has also been used to promote anabolism in burn injury. Studies looking at administering rhGH in patients with large burns (greater than 40% TBSA) have suggested that rhGH promotes wound healing of the burn wound and donor sites in both adults and children, as well as decreases length of hospital stay.[77] Complications of using rhGH include increased rates of hyperglycemia, which can be up to 2.65 times more likely in adults and children who receive rhGH than in placebo.[77] Other safety concerns with rhGH include an increase in morbidity and mortality seen in critically ill patients without burn injury, mostly attributed to organ failure, septic shock, or infection that could not be controlled.[11]

Treatment with β-blockers in patients with severe burns reduces heart rate, which decreases supraphysiologic thermogenesis and REE.[78] When pediatric patients with severe burns are treated with propranolol, there is an attenuation of the hypermetabolic response and a reversal of the muscle-protein catabolism. Propranolol doses for children are initiated at 0.33 mg/kg every 4 hours and are titrated to achieve a 20% decrease in heart rate compared with the 24-hour heart rate immediately before treatment.[78] When used for up to 12 months post-burn, propranolol treatment in pediatric patients reduced REE, decreased accumulation of central mass and central fat, prevented bone loss, and improved lean body mass accretion.[79] Propranolol treatment in pediatric patients is relatively safe, with hypotension being the most common adverse effect.

Data to support β-blockade in adult burn patients are more limited. A retrospective cohort study compared adult burn patients who were previously on β-blockers, those who were initiated on β-blockers in the hospital, and a control group.[80] Those who were on β-blockers before admission had a significant reduction in healing time, and these patients tended to spend less time in the hospital. However, patients previously not on β-blockers who were initiated after their burn injury tended to have increased hospital and intensive care unit length of stay, as well as a higher mortality, although 60% of these patients were initiated on β-blockers for an in-hospital cardiac complication, such as ischemia or atrial fibrillation. Prospective, randomized, clinical studies are needed to truly determine the outcomes of using β-blockers in adult burn patients.

CHALLENGES IN THE MANAGEMENT OF SEPSIS AND SEPTIC SHOCK IN BURN INJURY

Recognition of Sepsis and Infection in Burn Injury

Because of the massive inflammatory response associated with severe burn injury, the traditional criteria for recognizing sepsis (e.g., leukocytosis, fever, tachypnea, and tachycardia) cannot be used. Traditional definitions for systemic inflammatory response syndrome (SIRS), sepsis, severe sepsis, and septic shock are discussed in chapter 15, "Severe Sepsis and Septic Shock." In patients with burn injury, the ABA defines sepsis as a trigger for concern for infection that must include at least three of six possible criteria, together with documented infection (Box 42.2).[81] The ABA does not recognize the term *severe sepsis*, and the criteria for septic shock include those defining sepsis plus the traditional hemodynamic parameters defined by the Surviving Sepsis Campaign. Of note, these

---

Box 42.2. ABA Consensus Definitions for the Sepsis Continuum in Patients with Burn Injury

Sepsis
Documented infection PLUS at least three of the following:
- Temperature > 39°C or < 36.5°C
- Progressive tachycardia
  - Adults > 110 beats/min
  - Children > 2 standard deviations (SD) above agespecific norms
- Progressive tachypnea
  - Adults > 25 beats/min not ventilated, or minute ventilation > 12 L/min ventilated
  - Children > 2 SD above agespecific norms
- Thrombocytopenia (only applicable at least 3 days after initial resuscitation)
  - Adults < 100,000/microliters
  - Children < 2 SD below agespecific norms
- Hyperglycemia in the absence of preexisting diagnosis of diabetes mellitus
  - Plasma glucose > 200 mg/dL before treatment
  - Insulin resistance (e.g., 25% increase in insulin requirements over 24 hr)
- Inability to continue enteral feeding for at least 24 hr
  - Abdominal distension
  - Enteral feeding intolerance
  - Uncontrollable diarrhea (> 2.5 L/day for adults or > 400 mL/day for children)

Severe Sepsis
- This term is not recognized by the ABA

Septic Shock
- Sepsis PLUS traditional hemodynamic alterations

burn-specific criteria were initially developed as an initiative of a consensus conference, and they have not yet been fully validated. Subsequently, studies have confirmed that the traditional SIRS criteria have poor predictive value for sepsis within the burn population.[82] Almost all patients with severe burn injury have traditional SIRS criteria, regardless of the suggestion of sepsis, and more than 95% of patients met SIRS criteria, even during periods of clinical stability. Although the ABA criteria have improved clinical value, additional criteria to assist in more accurately identifying sepsis in this population have been proposed. Additional factors to consider include a more stringent heart rate threshold (heart rate greater than 130 beats/minute), serum glucose concentrations greater than 150/dL or increasing glycemic variability, hemodynamic instability (mean arterial pressure less than 60 mm Hg or use of vasoactive agents), and evidence of pulmonary and additional diagnostic laboratory values (procalcitonin and serum N-terminal pro–B-type natriuretic peptide).[82-84]

Pharmacokinetic and Pharmacodynamic Considerations for Antimicrobial Agents in Burn Injury

The hypermetabolic alterations observed in severe burn injury are accompanied by significant pharmacokinetic alterations that can affect optimal drug dosing in this complex population.[85,86] Although there is published literature to aid practitioners in determining dosing adjustments for this population, there are limitations to the data, including significant variability in methodology and patient characteristics and small sample sizes. These studies have also shown that burn severity alone cannot predict the dosing alterations required to overcome the pharmacokinetic alterations. Practitioners should consider standard key criteria when optimizing drug dosing in burn patients (Box 42.3).

During the initial ebb phase, patients with severe burn injury have an initial decrease in creatinine clearance that returns to normal or above normal after fluid resuscitation is achieved.[87,88] Significant alterations in hepatic metabolism occur as well during the flow phase because of increased hepatic perfusion. Phase 1 metabolism (i.e., oxidation) is significantly decreased, and phase 2 metabolism (i.e., conjugation, glucuronidation) is either unchanged or increased. Significant increases in volume of distribution also occur as a result of fluid resuscitation, hyperdynamic circulation, and capillary leak. These alterations have an impact on pharmacokinetics, primarily for drugs that distribute into the extracellular fluid (e.g., aminoglycosides). Decreased protein synthesis, including both albumin and total protein concentrations, results in increased free concentrations of highly protein bound medications (e.g., phenytoin, valproic acid). In contrast, increases in acute phase proteins, including α_1-acid glycoprotein, can significantly lower free concentrations of drugs that bind to α_1-acid glycoprotein after burn injury (e.g., imipramine and lidocaine). Antimicrobial agents with specific dosing recommendations to overcome these pharmacokinetic changes are summarized in Table 42.6.

OTHER SUPPORTIVE THERAPY IN BURN INJURY

Glycemic Control in Burn Injury

During the flow phase of burn injury, hyperglycemia and insulin resistance are common. Both early and prolonged hyperglycemia after burn injury is associated with poor clinical outcomes in the burn population. Hyperglycemia has been shown to delay wound healing, promote lean muscle losses, and suppress immune function.[103,104] Although a significant body of research supports the benefits of glucose control within the critically ill population, limited data are available within the burn population. Van den Berghe's pivotal study supporting intensive insulin control in the surgical intensive care unit included only 8 total

---

Box 42.3. Key Considerations for Pharmacokinetics in Burn Injury

1. Burn size and depth
   - Burns of increasing severity are more likely associated with a profound hypermetabolic response
2. Age
   - Older patients are more likely to have preexisting renal and hepatic insufficiency
3. Time since burn injury
   - Depending on timing, pharmacokinetic alterations differ (i.e., ebb vs. flow phase)

Although metabolic rate can remain increased for years, early in the flow phase, the alterations are more profound

4. Creatinine clearance
   - Although calculated creatinine clearance may not be accurate in this population, it can be used to trend changes in renal function across time
5. Serum protein concentrations
   - Decreased albumin concentrations and increased α_1-acid glycoprotein may affect free drug concentrations
6. Volume status
   - Once adequately fluid resuscitated, volume of distribution will likely be increased because of added fluid volume and capillary leak
7. Presence of sepsis as defined by the ABA
   - Sepsis is known to increase hypermetabolism
8. Drug properties
   - Specifics regarding volume of distribution, protein binding, metabolism, and modes of elimination are needed to estimate response in patients with burn injury
9. Other information
   - Data from indirect calorimetry and interventions known to decrease metabolic rate (i.e. excision and grafting) can be used to augment assessment of hypermetabolism

Table 42.6 Suggested Antimicrobial Dose Adjustments in Patients with Burn Injury[86,87,89-102]

Agent	Reference	Suggested Dosing	Additional Considerations
Gram-negative Antimicrobials			
Amikacin	Weinbren 1999 Conil 2007	Extended-interval dosing using at least 20 mg/kg	Studies have identified inverse relationship between Cmax/MIC ratio and burn size
			Institutional data regarding MICs should be used to target Cmax/MIC ratio of > 8–10
Tobramycin	Arnould 2009 Vella 2014	Extended-interval dosing using at least 9 mg/kg	Institutional data regarding MICs should be used to target Cmax/MIC ratio of > 8–10
		Up to 45 days after injury: 10–13 mg/kg > 45 days after injury 8–10 mg/kg	

β-Lactams:
  Ceftazidime
  Meropenem
  Imipenem
  Piperacillin/tazobactam
	Weinbren 1999
	Bourget 1996
	Conil 2007
	Dailly 2003
	Doh 2010
		Consider both extended and continuous infusions	Higher-than-traditional recommended doses may been necessary in addition to extended infusions to achieve target time above MIC

Ciprofloxacin	Garrelts 1996 Lesne-Hulin 1999	400–600 mg IV every 8 hr	
Levofloxacin	Kiser 2006	750 mg every 24 hr	Consider alternative agents for organisms with MIC > 0.5 mcg/mL
Gram-positive Antimicrobials			
Vancomycin	Ellingsen 2011	48 hr to 14 days after injury: 25 mg/kg every 8 hr OR 20 mg/kg every 6 hr	Vancomycin has Vd twice normal and shorter half-life
			Dosing depends on institutional MICs for pertinent organism. These recommendations are based on an MIC of 1 mcg/mL
		> 14 days after injury: 20–25 mg/kg every 8 hr 15–20 mg every 6 hr	
Linezolid	Lovering 2009	Consider 600 mg every 8 hr	
Daptomycin	Mohr 2008	10–12 mg/kg daily	
Antifungals			
Fluconazole	Boucher 1998	No data	Half-life decreased by 13%, clearance increased by 30%
Caspofungin	Jullien 2012	No data	Report of two patients showed significant interpatient variability

Cmax = maximum drug concentration; MIC = minimum inhibitory concentration; Vd = volume of distribution.

burn and trauma patients from the total 1,548 randomized subjects.[105] Most burn centers aim for euglycemia for patients with burn injury, based on extrapolation of the NICE-SUGAR (Normoglycemia in Intensive Care Evaluation and Surviving Using Glucose Algorithm Regulation) study and the assumption that avoiding hyperglycemia may improve wound healing, reduce infections, and possibly reduce mortality.[13,103,106,107] Insulin itself has been extensively studied in burn injury as an anabolic agent and has shown anti-inflammatory properties. It reduces muscle catabolism and improves protein synthesis and wound healing.[108-110] In 2005, Pham and colleagues reported their experience with tight glycemic control (glucose target 90–120 mg/dL) by insulin infusion in 33 pediatric burn patients with a TBSA greater than 30% injured compared with 31 historical control patients.[107] Patients who received the intensive insulin protocol had a lower reported incidence of urinary tract infections and a higher rate of survival, despite similar baseline characteristics. In an adjusted logistic regression analysis, intensive insulin was associated with an adjusted odds ratio of 5.52 in favor of survival, although this failed to reach statistical significance (p=0.06). Although prevalence of hypoglycemia was not reported, administration of dextrose 50% for glucose less than 50 mg/dL was required on nine occasions in the tight glycemic control group, with no occurrences in the control group. Given these results, a prospective, randomized trial of pediatric patients with a TBSA greater than 30% burned compared tight glycemic control (n=49, glucose target 80–110 mg/dL) with conventional control (n=137, glucose target 140–180 mg/dL).[108] Intensive insulin was associated with significant reductions in the rate of infection and sepsis compared with conventional control. Although there were no differences between the groups in REE, intensive insulin significantly modulated the acute inflammatory response and resulted in improvement in lean muscle mass and bone density compared with control. The intensive insulin group also had a lower mortality rate than did controls, although this failed to reach statistical significance (4 vs. 11%, p=0.14). As observed in other critically ill populations, hypoglycemia is associated with increased morbidity and mortality with burn injury, and intensive insulin is associated with increased incidence of hypoglycemia.[111]

There are no randomized, prospective studies regarding glycemic control in adult patients with burn injury. A retrospective observational study showed significantly decreased rates of pneumonia and urinary tract infections with an insulin protocol targeting a blood glucose of 100–140 mg/dL in 152 adult burn injured patients with percent TBSA injured of 19% in the control group and 15% in the insulin protocol group.[106] This protocol was also deemed safe because no differences in the rate of hypoglycemia were observed. In another retrospective observational study of 46 patients with severe burns, early glycemic control also improved outcomes.[112] A standardized protocol was used for all patients, targeting a glucose of 110–150 mg/dL with sliding-scale insulin administration and insulin infusion initiation with repeated glucose concentrations greater than 200 mg/dL. Failure to achieve early glycemic control, defined as achievement of a daily average blood glucose of 150 mg/dL or less for a minimum of 2 consecutive days by post-burn day 3 was independently associated with an increase in mortality by 6.75-fold. Although data are limited in both pediatric and adult patients with burn injury, it is generally accepted that protocols to maintain euglycemia while avoiding both hyperglycemia and hypoglycemia (e.g., target glucose range 90–140 mg/dL) should be implemented as standard of care in this population.[111]

Venous Thromboembolism Prophylaxis

Clinical diagnosis of deep venous thrombosis in patients with burn injury can be challenging. Clinical signs that are common to both burn injury and deep venous thromboembolism include erythema, edema, and tenderness. Current data suggest a much lower incidence of venous thromboembolism (VTE) in patients with burn injury than in the general trauma population. Reported prevalence in burn patients is 1%–6%, whereas in trauma patients, reported prevalence is 5%–63%, depending on methods of diagnosis and means of mechanical or pharmacologic prophylaxis.[113-117] The current CHEST guidelines recommend pharmacologic prophylaxis with either low-dose unfractionated heparin or low-molecular-weight heparin agents with or without mechanical prophylaxis for trauma patients.[118] Literature is limited to establish the efficacy of varying VTE prophylaxis therapies in patients with burn injury, which forces extrapolation from data published in non-burn injury populations. Routine VTE prophylaxis with either unfractionated heparin or low-molecular-weight heparin is recommended by the ABA for patients with additional risk factors for VTE and no contraindications to treatment. Known VTE risk factors in burn injury include advanced age, male sex, alcoholism or tobacco use, morbid obesity, extensive or lower-extremity burns, concomitant lower-extremity trauma, use of a femoral or other central venous catheter, increased number of surgeries or blood transfusions, and prolonged immobility.[113,119] If contraindications to pharmacologic prophylaxis exist because of bleeding risk, patients should receive mechanical prophylaxis at least until this risk resolves. However, mechanical prophylaxis can prove to be potentially difficult in patients with leg burns, depending on location of injury. The ABA guidelines do not recommend one agent over another for pharmacologic prophylaxis, but a retrospective review showed no difference in the efficacy of unfractionated heparin versus enoxaparin.[120] This 10-year retrospective, cohort analysis compared patients who received prophylaxis with low-dose unfractionated heparin (n=600) or enoxaparin (n=511) with a primary end point of acute VTE according to ICD-9 coding. Among the enoxaparin-treated patients, 109 received 30 mg twice daily, and 402 received 40 mg once daily, whereas the patients given low-dose unfractionated heparin received 5,000 units twice daily. Five patients who received low-dose unfractionated heparin developed VTE (three with deep venous thromboembolism and two with pulmonary embolism), whereas no patients in the enoxaparin group developed VTE. Limitations of this study include twice-daily heparin dosing, significant baseline differences between groups including a higher number of VTE risk factors in the low-dose unfractionated heparin group, and retrospective study design. This is the only comparative study for low-dose unfractionated heparin and low-molecular-weight heparin in burn injury, and the ideal prophylactic agents therefore remain uncertain at this time.

Recent concerns regarding low-molecular-weight heparin dosing in the critically ill population have indicated a possible role for dose titration using anti-factor Xa (anti-Xa) concentration. Lin and colleagues evaluated 74 patients with burn injury who received enoxaparin 30 mg every 12 hours, which was then titrated by 20% increments to achieve a goal anti-Xa concentration of 0.2–0.4 units/mL.[121] Initial dose of 30 mg every 12 hours resulted in concentrations less than the targeted goal in 76% of the patients. On titration, the median dose to achieve an anti-Xa concentration within the goal range was 33% of the normal dosing at 40 mg every 12 hours. However, anti-Xa concentrations have not been correlated with clinical outcomes, and two patients with appropriate anti-Xa concentrations developed VTE in this study.[121] The calculation identified from this study for twice-daily enoxaparin dosing [dose (mg) = 22.8 + (3.3 × %TBSA/10) + (1.89 × (weight in kg)/10] was validated in a comparison of protocolized enoxaparin calculation and titration with historical controls by Faraklas and colleagues.[122] This comparison study found that use of this prophylactic enoxaparin dose calculator was associated with a significantly higher proportion of patients with an anti-Xa concentration within goal range (0.2–0.4 unit/mL) with the initial measurement and fewer patients who failed to achieve goal range before discontinuing enoxaparin therapy. However, two patients—one in the calculation group and one in the control group—developed VTE despite adequate anti-Xa concentrations. Although anti-Xa concentrations are used in some institutions for enoxaparin monitoring, additional research is needed to determine the role of anti-Xa concentrations and enoxaparin titration in the burn population, and data correlating anti-Xa concentrations and clinical outcomes are lacking.

MANAGEMENT OF SPECIAL POPULATIONS

Electrical Injury

Electrical injury accounts for 3.7% of all patients presenting with burn injuries, with higher rates among adults up to age 60 years than among children and older adults.[1] Electrical injuries are responsible for greater than 500 deaths annually in the United States.[123] The primary cause of death is cardiac or respiratory arrest.[124] Most electrical injuries occur in adults and are work related (61.1%). Although electrical injuries are rarer in children, they often occur within the home, and patients present with oropharyngeal injuries from biting on live wires.[124]

Injuries caused by electrical exposure are unique because they involve direct damage from the electricity as well as indirect injuries.[123] Direct damage results from the effect of the electrical current directly on tissues involving electrical charge (e.g., cardiac complications), as well as conversion of the energy to heat and the subsequent tissue necrosis. Indirect injuries can be caused by muscular contractions triggered by the electrical impulses or other associated trauma, depending on the circumstances surrounding the electrical exposure (e.g., spinal cord injury or traumatic brain injury secondary to fall). The extent of the electrical injury is determined by the electrical voltage and resistance within the tissues exposed (i.e., lowest amount of resistance in nerves, blood, muscles; highest amount of resistance in bones, tendons, fat). Higher voltage (greater than 1000 V) is associated with more severe injury than is lower voltage.

Electrical injury can cause multisystem dysfunction and is associated with higher complication rates than other burn injuries, including development of cardiovascular, neurovascular, cutaneous, and pulmonary complications.[1,123] Electrical exposure can result in the direct necrosis of myocardium as well as arrhythmias. The severity of the damage is proportional to voltage and is more severe with AC (alternating current) than with DC (direct current). Cardiac dysrhythmias can occur even with low voltage, but high-voltage current exposure carries a higher risk of ventricular asystole. Patients with electrical injury should initially be assessed with an electrocardiogram (ECG). Patients with a normal initial ECG are considered at low risk of late arrhythmias, whereas patients with transthoracic current, tetany, loss of consciousness, or a high-voltage source (greater than 1000 V) may need continuous telemetry.[125] Echocardiogram and monitoring of cardiac enzymes may also be warranted. Severity of cutaneous electrical burn injury is related to voltage and duration of exposure. Because of alterations in resistance as the result of moisture, minimal cutaneous damage may be visible on examination, whereas the subcutaneous tissue may have extensive necrosis. Therefore, the use of percent TBSA injured to determine resuscitative needs may grossly underestimate fluid volume requirements for patients with electrical injury. Higher-than-expected volumes may be required to maintain a goal urine output of 0.5–1 mL/kg/hour.

Patients presenting with electrical injury may have seizures, neurologic deficits, and tetanic muscle contractions. Common presenting symptoms include confusion, loss of consciousness, and difficulty with recall. In addition, tetany can result in rhabdomyolysis and subsequent renal failure. Monitoring of creatinine kinase and urine myoglobin and ensuring adequate fluid resuscitation are necessary to prevent renal insufficiency in this population.

Frostbite

Frostbite is a clinical diagnosis, and it is typically defined as the acute freezing of tissues when exposed to temperatures below the freezing point of intact skin. Historically, military personnel were considered at the greatest risk of developing frostbite. More recently, risk factors that are commonly identified include homeless people, alcohol or illicit drug consumption, and psychiatric illness.

Classification of frostbite injury is applied once the tissues have been rewarmed, and it is categorized into four degrees. First-degree frostbite injuries present with a numb central white plaque with surrounding edema. In second-degree injury, blisters form with surrounding edema and erythema. Third-degree injury is characterized by hemorrhagic blisters that result in a hard black eschar about 2 weeks later. Fourth-degree injury produces a complete necrosis and tissue loss.

Initially, patients may present with symptoms of numbness in the affected areas. Once the tissues are rewarmed, the numbness will fade, and a throbbing sensation may begin that can last for days or weeks. Pain is managed with opioids or nonsteroidal anti-inflammatory drugs (e.g., ibuprofen).

Treatment of frostbite injury begins with rewarming of the affected tissues, typically with warm water at 40°C–42°C. The temperature of the water should be carefully monitored not to reach a threshold that could potentially inflict a scald burn injury given that the patient may be unable to sense the temperature. Once the tissues have been rewarmed, the second goal of treatment is to restore arterial flow. One way to achieve this is using tissue plasminogen activator (tPA). Studies have suggested that treatment with tPA can decrease the number of amputations in patients with frostbite affecting the extremities.[126,127] Patients with frostbite injury are typically considered for tPA therapy if they present within 24 hours of injury, have evidence of vascular compromise on physical examination, and have significant injury consisting of second-degree frostbite. Patients are often excluded from tPA therapy if any of the following apply: recent surgery or major trauma, uncontrolled psychiatric illness or active withdrawal from an illicit substance or alcohol, pregnancy, recent cerebral vascular accident or brain metastasis, recent gastrointestinal bleed, severe hypertension, bleeding diathesis, or irreversible ischemia (presenting greater than 24 hours from injury). Treatment of frostbite in pediatric patients with tPA has not been evaluated. Both intraarterial and intravenous administration of tPA has been investigated. Early surgical intervention is typically not indicated in frostbite injury. The adage "Frostbite in January, amputation in July" is often used to describe frostbite injury. Rarely, escharotomy or fasciotomy may be indicated if compartment syndrome develops. However, if any surgical intervention is warranted in severe injury, it is often delayed for weeks to months post-injury.

As with any burn injury, prevention is the best way to avoid frostbite injury. Individuals should use protection from the environment with multilayer clothing that is dry and non-compressing. Awareness of warning signs such as cold, pain, and numbness should prompt individuals to seek shelter and warmth.

Chemical Burns

Chemical burns account for about 3% of admissions to burn centers every year, with almost 50% of these injuries occurring in a work-related setting, although many injuries can occur with exposure to common household chemical products.[1] Acidic agents can cause a caustic injury and typically account for less than half of chemical burn injuries.[128] Alkali substances, by contrast, can cause liquefaction destruction and tend to penetrate deeper, creating a worse burn injury. Alkali injuries tend to make up more than half of injuries caused by chemicals.[128]

Initial treatment of any chemical burn is immediate removal of the substance to prevent further tissue damage, such as removal of affected clothing and continuous irrigation with water or saline until skin pH returns to normal using litmus paper. Injuries to the eyes should be irrigated copiously and should be evaluated by an ophthalmologist. Some chemicals have specific treatment to prevent further tissue damage, such as burns caused by hydrofluoric acid. Free fluoride ions immobilize intracellular calcium and magnesium, causing extreme pain to the affected areas. Treatment with topical calcium gluconate gel to the burned areas is the mainstay of therapy to reduce the pain. Intravenous calcium gluconate, magnesium sulfate, or both may be indicated.

CONCLUSION

Patients with burn injury constitute a unique subset of the critically ill population. Pharmacists can play a key role with respect to optimizing care, from managing inhalation injury and metabolic modulation to recognizing sepsis and optimizing medication dosing on the basis of pharmacokinetic/pharmacodynamic alterations. The ABA recognizes the importance of the pharmacist in the care of this population and requires the involvement of a pharmacist with an understanding of the pharmacokinetic implications for patients with acute burn injuries for a burn center to become ABA verified.

REFERENCES

1. American Burn Association (ABA). 2014 National Burn Repository: report of data from 2004–2013 Dataset Version 10.0. American Burn Association NBR Advisory Committee, 2014.
2. Peck ME. Epidemiology of burns throughout the world. Part I. Distribution and risk factors. Burns 2011;37:1087-100.
3. LaBorde P. Burn epidemiology: the patient, the nation, the statistics, and the data resources. Crit Care Nurs Clin North Am 2004;16:13-25.
4. Jeschke MG, Herndon DN. Burns in children: standard and new treatments. Lancet 2014;383:1168-78.
5. Herndon DN. Total Burn Care, 3rd ed. Philadelphia: Saunders Elsevier, 2007.

6. Atiyeh BS, Gunn SWA, Dibo SA. Metabolic implications of severe burn injuries and their management: a systematic review of the literature. World J Surg 2008;32:1857-69.

7. Gauglitz GG, Jeschke MG. Pathophysiology of burn injury. In: Jeschke MG, ed. Handbook of Burns. New York: Springer-Verlag/Wien, 2012:131-49.

8. Butler KL, Sheridan RL. Organ responses and organ support. In: Jeschke MG, ed. Handbook of Burns. New York: Springer-Verlag/Wien, 2012:193-201.

9. Baxter CR, Shires T. Physiological response to crystalloid resuscitation of severe burns. Ann N Y Acad Sci 1968;150:874-94.

10. Hansbrough JF. Enteral nutritional support in burn patients. Gastroenterol Endosc Clin North Am 1998;3:645-67.

11. Miller JT, Btaiche IF. Oxandrolone treatment in adults with severe thermal injury. Pharmacotherapy 2009;29:213-26.

12. Ballian N, Rabiee A, Andersen DK, et al. Glucose metabolism in burn patients: the role of insulin and other endocrine hormones. Burns 2010;36:599-605.

13. Gauglitz GG, Herndon DN, Jeschke MG. Insulin resistance postburn: underlying mechanisms and current therapeutic strategies. J Burn Care Res 2008;29:683-94.

14. Vanhorebeek I, Langouche L, Van den Berghe G. Tight blood glucose control with insulin in the ICU: facts and controversies. Chest 2007;132:268-78.

15. Sjoberg F. Pre-hospital, fluid and early management, burn wound evaluation. In: Jeschke MG, ed. Handbook of Burns. New York: Springer-Verlag/Wien, 2012:105-16.

16. Haller HL, Giretzlehner M, Dirnberger J, et al. Medical documentation of burn injuries. In: Jeschke MG, ed. Handbook of Burns. New York: Springer-Verlag/Wien, 2012:117-29.

17. Colohan SM. Predicting prognosis in thermal burns with associated inhalational injury: a systematic review of prognostic factors in adult burn victims. J Burn Care Res 2010;31:529-39.

18. Sheppard NN, Hemington-Gorse S, Shelley OP, et al. Prognostic scoring systems in burns: a review. Burns 2011;37:1288-95.

19. Gomez M, Wong DT, Stewart TE, et al. The FLAMES score accurately predicts mortality in burn patients. J Trauma 2008;65:636-45.

20. Barrow RE, Spies M, Barrow LN, et al. Influence of demographics and inhalation injury on burn mortality in children. Burns 2004;30:72-7.

21. Barrow RE, Przkora R, Hawkins HK, et al. Mortality related to gender, age, sepsis, and ethnicity in severely burned children. Shock 2005;23:485-7.

22. Erickson EJ, Merrell SW, Saffle JR, et al. Differences in mortality from thermal injury between pediatric and adult patients. J Pediatr Surg 1991;26:821-5.

23. Thombs BD, Signh VA, Milner SM. Children under 4 years are at greater risk of mortality following acute burn injury: evidence from a national sample of 12,902 pediatric admissions. Shock 2006;26:348-52.

24. Barrow RE, Jeschke MG, Herndon DN. Early fluid resuscitation improves outcomes in severely burned children. Resuscitation 2000;45:91-6.

25. Pham TN, Cancio LC, Gibran NS. American Burn Association practice guidelines burn shock resuscitation. J Burn Care Res 2008;29:259-66.

26. Alvarado R, Chung KK, Cancio LC, et al. Burn resuscitation. Burns 2009;35:4-14.

27. Gille J, Klezcewski B, Malcharek M, et al. Safety of resuscitation with Ringer's acetate solution in severe burn (VolTRAB) – an observational trial. Burns 2014;40:871-80.

28. Pruitt BA. Protection from excessive resuscitation: "pushing the pendulum back." J Trauma 2000;49:567-8.

29. Endorf FW, Dries DJ. Burn resuscitation. Scand J Trauma Resusc Emerg Med 2011;19:69.

30. Saffle JR. The phenomenon of "fluid creep" in acute burn resuscitation. J Burn Care Res 2007;28:382-95.

31. Snell JA, Loh NH, Mahambrey T, et al. Clinical review: the critical care management of the burn patient. Crit Care 2013;17:241.

32. McBeth PB, Sass K, Nickerson D, et al. A necessary evil? Intra-abdominal hypertension complicating burn patient resuscitation. J Trauma Manag Outcomes 2014;8:12.

33. Medina MA, Moore DA, Cairns BA. A case series: bilateral ischemic optic neuropathy secondary to large volume fluid resuscitation in critically ill burn patients. Burns 2015;41:e19-23.

34. Ruiz-Castilla M. Barret JP, Sanz D, et al. Analysis of intra-abdominal hypertension in severe burn patients: the Vall d'Herbon experience. Burns 2014;40:719-24.

35. Strang SG, Van Lieshout EMM, Breederveld RS, et al. A systematic review on intra-abdominal pressure in severely burned patients. Burns 2014;40:9-16.

36. Fahlstrom K, Boyle C, Makic MBF. Implementation of a nurse-driven burn resuscitation protocol: a quality improvement project. Crit Care Nurse 2013;33:25-36.

37. Salinas J, Chung KK, Mann EA, et al. Computerized decision support system improves fluid resuscitation following severe burns: an original study. Crit Care Med 2011;39:2031-8.

38. Cartotto R, Callum J. A review of the use of human albumin in burn patients. J Burn Care Res 2012;33:702-17.

39. Cooper AB, Cohn SM, Zhang HS, et al. Five percent albumin for adult burn shock resuscitation: lack of effect on daily multiple organ dysfunction score. Transfusion 2006;46:80-9.

40. Goodwin CW, Dorethy J, Lam V, Pruitt BA. Randomized trial of efficacy of crystalloid and colloid resuscitation on hemodynamic response and lung water following thermal injury. Ann Surg 1983;197:520-31.

41. Jelenko C. Fluid shifts after burn injury. South Med J 1975;68:887-92.

42. Recinos PR, Hartford CA, Ziffren SE. Fluid resuscitation of burn patients comparing a crystalloid with a colloid containing solution: a prospective study. J Iowa Med Soc 1975;65:426-32.

43. Park SH, Hemmila MR, Wahl WL. Early albumin use improves mortality in difficult to resuscitate burn patients. J Trauma Acute Care Surg 2012;73:1294-7.

44. Cetinkale O, Senel O, Bulan R. The effect of antioxidant therapy on cell-mediated immunity following burn injury in an animal model. Burns 1999;25:113-8.

45. Kremer T, Harenber P, Hernekamp F, et al. High-dose vitamin C treatment reduces capillary leakage after burn plasma transfer in rats. J Burn Care Res 2010;31:470-9.

46. Matsuda T, Tanaka H, Yuasa H, et al. The effects of high-dose vitamin C therapy on postburn lipid peroxidation. J Burn Care Rehabil 1993;14:624-9.

47. Tanaka H, Lund T, Wiig H, et al. High dose vitamin C counteracts the negative interstitial fluid hydrostatic edema generation in thermally injured rats. Burns 1999;25:569-74.

48. Tanaka H, Matsuda T, Miyagantani Y, et al. Reduction of resuscitation fluid volumes in severely burned patients using ascorbic acid administration: a randomized, prospective study. Arch Surg 2000;135:326-31.

49. Kahn SA, Beers RJ, Lentz CW. Resuscitation after severe burn injury using high-dose ascorbic acid: a retrospective review. J Burn Care Res 2011;32:110-7.

50. Buehner M, Pamplin J, Studer L, et al. Oxalate nephropathy after continuous infusion of high-dose vitamin C as an adjunct to burn resuscitation. J Burn Care Res 2015. [Epub ahead of print]

51. Kahn SA, Lentz CW. Fictitious hyperglycemia: point-of-care glucose measurement is inaccurate during high-dose vitamin C infusion for burn shock resuscitation. J Burn Care Res 2015;36:e67-e71.

52. Sartor Z, Kesey J, Dissanaike S. The effects of intravenous vitamin C on point-of-care glucose monitoring. J Burn Care Res 2015;36:50-6.

53. Barbosa E, Faintuch J, Moreira EAM, et al. Supplementation of vitamin E, vitamin C, and zinc attenuates oxidative stress in burned children: a randomized, double-blind, placebo-controlled pilot study. Burn Care Res 2009;30:859-66.

54. Palmieri TL, Gamelli RL. Diagnosis and management of inhalation injury. In: Jeschke MG, ed. Handbook of Burns. New York: Springer-Verlag/Wien, 2012:163-72.

55. Dries DJ, Endorj FW. Inhalation injury: epidemiology, pathology, treatment strategies. Scand J Trauma Resusc Emerg 2013;21:31.

56. Toon MH, Maybauer MO, Greenwood JE, et al. Management of acute smoke inhalation injury. Crit Care Resusc 2010;12:53-61.

57. Desai MH, Micak R, Richardson J, et al. Reduction in mortality in pediatric patients with inhalation injury with aerosolized heparin/N-acetylcysteine therapy. J Burn Care Rehabil 1998;19:210-2.

58. Holt J, Saffle JR, Morris SE, et al. Use of inhaled heparin/N-acetylcysteine in inhalation injury: does it help? J Burn Care Res 2008;29:192-5.

59. Miller AC, Abel R, Ziad S, et al. Influence of nebulized unfractionated heparin and N-acetylcysteine in acute lung injury after smoke inhalation injury. J Burn Care Res 2009;30:249-56.

60. Elsharnouby NM, Eid HEA, Elezz NFA, et al. Heparin/N-acetylcysteine: an adjuvant in the management of burn inhalation injury, a study of different doses. J Crit Care 2014;29:182.e1-182.e4.

61. Glas GJ, Muller J, Binnekade JM, et al. HEPBURN- investigating the efficacy and safety of nebulized heparin versus placebo in burn patients with inhalation trauma: study protocol for a multi-center randomized controlled trial. Trials 2014;15:91.

62. Weaver LK. Hyperbaric oxygen in the critically ill. Crit Care Med 2011;39:1784-91.

63. Buckley NA, Juurlink DN, Isbister G, et al. Hyperbaric oxygen for carbon monoxide poisoning. Cochrane Database Syst Rev 2011;4:CD002041.

64. Gracia R, Shepherd G. Cyanide poisoning and its treatment. Pharmacotherapy 2004;24:1358-65.

65. Shepherd G. The role of hydroxocobalamin in acute cyanide poisoning. Ann Pharmacother 2008;42:661-9.

66. Lawson-Smith P, Jansen EC, Hyldegaard O. Cyanide intoxication as part of smoke inhalation – a review on diagnosis and treatment from the emergency perspective. Scand J Trauma 2011;19:14.

67. Barillo DV. Diagnosis and treatment of cyanide toxicity. J Burn Care Res 2009;30:148-52.

68. Hart DW, Wolf SE, Zhang XJ, et al. Efficacy of a high-carbohydrate diet in catabolic illness. Crit Care Med 2001;29:1318-24.

69. Venter M, Rode H, Sive A, et al. Enteral resuscitation and early enteral feeding in children with major burns – effect on McFarlane response to stress. Burns 2007;33:464-71.

70. Pereira CT, Murphy KD, Herndon, DN. Altering metabolism. J Burn Care Rehabil 2005;26:194-9.

71. Demling RH, Desanti L. Oxandrolone induced lean mass gain during recovery from severe burns is maintained after discontinuation of the anabolic steroid. Burns 2003;29:793-7.

72. Wolf SE, Edelman LS, Kemalyan N, et al. Effects of oxandrolone on outcome measures in the severely burned: a multicenter prospective randomized double-blind trial. J Burn Care Res 2006;27:131-9.

73. Murphy KD, Thomas S, Mlcak RP, et al. Effects of long-term oxandrolone administration in severely burned children. Surgery 2004;136:219-24.

74. Porro LF, Herndon DN, Rodriguez NA, et al. Five-year outcomes after oxandrolone administration in severely burned children: a randomized clinical trial of safety and efficacy. J Am Coll Surg 2012;214:489-504.

75. Orr R, Singh MF. The anabolic androgenic steroid oxandrolone in the treatment of wasting and catabolic disorders: review of efficacy and safety. Drugs 2004;64:725-50.

76. Demling RH. Comparison of the anabolic effects and complications of human growth hormone and the testosterone analog, oxandrolone, after severe burn injury. Burns 1999;25:215-21.

77. Breederveld RS, Tuinebreijer WE. Recombinant human growth hormone for treating burns and donor sites. Cochrane Database Syst Rev 2012;12:CD008990.

78. Herndon DN, Hart DW, Wolf SE, et al. Reversal of catabolism by beta-blockade after severe burns. N Engl J Med 2001;345:1223-9.

79. Herndon DN, Rodriguez NA, Diaz EC, et al. Long-term propranolol use in severely burned pediatric patients: a randomized controlled study. Ann Surg 2012;256:402-11.

80. Arabi S, Ahrns KS, Wahl WL, et al. Beta-blocker use is associated with improved outcomes in adult burn patients. J Trauma 2004;56:265-71.

81. Greenhalgh DG, Saffle JR, Holmes JH, et al. American Burn Association consensus conference to define sepsis and infection in burns. J Burn Care Res 2007;28:776-90.

82. Mann-Salinas EA, Baun MM, Meininger JC, et al. Novel predictors of sepsis outperform the American Burn Association sepsis criteria in the burn intensive care unit patient. J Burn Care Res 2013;34:31-43.

83. Paratz JD, Lipman J, Boots RJ, et al. A new marker of sepsis post burn injury? Crit Care Med 2014;42:2029-36.

84. Ren H, Li Y, Han C, et al. Serum procalcitonin as a diagnostic biomarker for sepsis in burned patients: a meta-analysis. Burns 2015;41:502-9.

85. Blanchet B, Jullien V, Vinsonneau C, et al. Influence of Burns on pharmacokinetics and pharmacodynamics of drugs used in the care of burn patients. Clin Pharmacokinet 2008;47:635-54.

86. Ortwine JK, Pogue JM, Faris J. Pharmacokinetics and pharmacodynamics of antibacterial and antifungal agents in adult patients with thermal injury: a review of current literature. J Burn Care Res 2015;36:e72-84.

87. Weinbren MJ. Pharmacokinetics of antibiotics in burn patients. J Antimicrob Chemother 1999;44:319-27.

88. Zdolsek HF, Kagedal B, Lisander B, et al. Glomerular filtration rate is increased in burn patients. Burns 2010;36:1271-6.

89. Conil JM, Georges B, Breden A, et al. Increased amikacin dosage requirements in burn patients receiving a once-daily regimen. Int J Antimicrob Agents 2007;28:226-30.

90. Arnould JG, Le Floch R, Piloget A. Which tobramycin dose is needed in the burn patient [letter to the editor]. Burns 2009;35:901-6.

91. Vella D, Walker SA, Walker SE, et al. Determination of tobramycin pharmacokinetics in burn patients to evaluate the potential utility of once-daily dosing in this population. J Burn Care Res 2014;35:e240-e249.

92. Bourget P, Lesne-Hulin A, Le Reveille R, et al. Clinical pharmacokinetics of piperacillin-tazobactam combination in patients with major burns and signs of infection. Antimicrob Agents Chemother 1996;40:139-45.

93. Dailly E, Kergueris MF, Pannier M, et al. Population pharmacokinetics of imipenem in burn patients. Fund Clin Pharmacol 2003;17:645-50.

94. Doh K, Woo H, Hur J, et al. Population pharmacokinetics of meropenem in burn patients. J Antimicrob Chemother 2010;65:2428-35.

95. Garrelts JC, Jost G, Kowalsky ST, et al. Ciprofloxacin pharmacokinetics in burn patients. Antimicrob Agents Chemother 1996;40:1153-6.

96. Lesne-Hulin A, Bourget P, Ravat F, et al. Clinical pharmacokinetics of ciprofloxacin in patients with major burns. Eur J Clin Pharmacol 1999;55:515-9.

97. Kiser TH, Hoody DW, Obritsch MD, et al. Levofloxacin pharmacokinetics and pharmacodynamics in patients with severe burn injury. Antimicrob Agents Chemother 2006;50:1937-45.

98. Ellingsen M, Walker SAN, Walker SE, et al. Optimizing initial vancomycin dosing in burn patients. Burns 2011;37:406-14.

99. Lovering AM, Le Floch R, Hovsepian L, et al. Pharmacokinetic evaluation of linezolid in patients with major thermal injuries. J Antimicrob Chemother 2009;63:553-9.

100. Mohr JF, Ostrosky-Zeichner L, Wainright DJ, et al. Pharmacokinetic evaluation of single-dose intravenous daptomycin in patients with thermal injury. Antimicrob Agents Chemother 2008;52:1891-3.

101. Boucher BA, King SR, Wandschneider HL, et al. Fluconazole pharmacokinetics in burn patients. Antimicrob Agents Chemother 1998;42:930-3.

102. Jullien V. Pharmacokinetics of caspofungin in two patients with burn injuries [letter to the editor]. Antimicrob Agents Chemother 2012;56:4550-1.

103. Gore DC, Chinkes D, Heggers J, et al. Association of hyperglycemia with increased mortality after severe burn injury. J Trauma 2001;51:540-4.

104. Gore DC, Chinkes DL, Hart DW, et al. Hyperglycemia exacerbates muscle protein catabolism in burn-injured patients. Crit Care Med 2002;30:2438-42.

105. Van den Berghe G, Wouters P, Weekers F, et al. Intensive insulin therapy in critically ill patients. N Engl J Med 2001;345:1359-67.

106. Hemmila MR, Taddonio MA, Arbabi S, et al. Intensive insulin therapy is associated with reduced infectious complications in burn patients. Surgery 2008;144:629-35; discussion 35-7.

107. Pham TN, Warren AJ, Phan HH, et al. Impact of tight glycemic control in severely burned children. J Trauma 2005;59:1148-54.

108. Jeschke MG, Kulp GA, Kraft R, et al. Intensive insulin therapy in severely burned pediatric patients: a prospective randomized trial. Am J Respir Crit Care Med 2010;182:351-9.

109. Pierre EJ, Barrow RE, Hawkins HK, et al. Effects of insulin on wound healing. J Trauma 1998;44:342-345.

110. Thomas SJ, Morimoto K, Herndon DN, et al. The effect of prolonged euglycemic hyperinsulinemia on lean body mass after severe burn. Surgery 2002;132:341-7.

111. Jeschke MG. Clinical review: glucose control in severely burned patients – current best practice. Crit Care 2013;17:232.

112. Murphy CV, Coffey R, Cook CH, et al. Early glycemic control in critically ill patients with burn injury. J Burn Care Res 2011;32:583-90.

113. Mullins F, Aian MAH, Jenkins D, et al. Thromboembolic complications in burn patients and associated risk factors. J Burn Care Res 2013;34:355-360.

114. Purdue GF, Hunt JL. Pulmonary emboli in burned patients. J Trauma 1988;28:218-20.

115. Rue LW, Cioffi WG, Rush R, et al. Thromboembolic complications in thermally injured patients. World J Surg 1992;16:1151-4; discussion 5.

116. Toker S, Hak D, Morgan SJ. Deep vein thrombosis in trauma patients. Thrombosis 2011;Article ID 505373.

117. Wahl WL, Brandt MM. Potential risk factors for deep venous thrombosis in burn patients. J Burn Care Rehabil 2001;22:128-31.

118. Gould MK, Garcia DA, Wren SM, et al. Prevention of VTE in nonorthopedic surgical patients: Antithrombotic Therapy and Prevention of Thrombosis, 9th ed: American College of Chest Physicians Evidence-Based Clinical Practice Guidelines. Chest 2012;141(2 suppl):e227S-277S.

119. Geerts WH, Bergqvist D, Pineo GF, et al. Prevention of venous thromboembolism: American College of Chest Physicians Evidence-Based Clinical Practice Guidelines (8th Edition). Chest 2008;133:381S-453S.

120. Bushwitz J, LeClaire A, He J, et al. Clinically significant venous thromboembolic complications in burn patients receiving unfractionated heparin or enoxaparin as prophylaxis. J Burn Care Res 2011;32:578-82.

121. Lin H, Faraklas I, Saffle J, et al. Enoxaparin dose adjustment is associated with low incidence of venous thromboembolic events in acute burn patients. J Trauma 2011;71:1557-61.

122. Faraklas I, Ghanem M, Brown A, Cochran A. Evaluation of an enoxaparin dosing calculator using burn size and weight. J Burn Care Res 2013;34:621-7.

123. Koumbourlis AC. Electrical injuries. Crit Care Med 2002;30:S424-S430.

124. Glatstein MM, Ayalon I, Miller E, et al. Pediatric electrical burn injuries: experience of a large tertiary care hospital and a review of electrical injury. Pediatr Emerg Care 2013;29:737-40.

125. Bailey B, Gaudreault P, Thivierge RL. Cardiac monitoring of high-risk patients after an electrical injury: a prospective multicentre study. Emerg Med J 2007;24:348-52.

126. Bruen KJ, Ballard JR, Morris SE, et al. Reduction in the incidence of amputation in frostbite injury with thrombolytic therapy. Arch Surg 2007;142:546-53.

127. Johnson AR, Jensen HL, Peltier G, et al. Efficacy of intravenous tissue plasminogen activator in frostbite patients and presentation of a treatment protocol for frostbite patients. Foot Ankle Spec 2011;4:344-8.

128. Hardwicke J, Hunter T, Staruch R, et al. Chemical burns – an historical comparison and review of the literature. Burns 2012;38:383-7.

Chapter 43: The Role of Pharmacotherapy in the Treatment of the Multiple Trauma Patient

Rita Gayed, Pharm.D.; Prasad Abraham, Pharm.D., FCCM, BCPS; and David V. Feliciano, M.D., FACS

LEARNING OBJECTIVES

1. List the components of the primary survey.
2. Explain the rationale for each component of the primary survey (ABCDE).
3. List the classes of hemorrhagic shock.
4. Describe the components and their roles in the massive transfusion protocol.
5. Evaluate the data for support of tranexamic acid in the management of traumatic hemorrhage.
6. Compare the data for anticoagulant versus antiplatelet therapy in the management of blunt cerebrovascular injury.
7. Evaluate the data for neuroprotection in traumatic brain injury (TBI) management.
8. Compare mannitol with hypertonic saline in the management of intracranial hypertension.
9. Review the data supporting the management of early seizures associated with TBI.
10. State the complications of spinal cord injury (SCI).
11. Review the evidence for steroids in SCI.
12. Differentiate the benefits of endovascular repair versus open surgical repair of blunt thoracic aortic aneurysms.
13. Review the evidence for somatostatin/octreotide in the management of enterocutaneous fistulas.
14. Review the pharmacologic treatment options for the management of short bowel syndrome.
15. Recall the evidence for the prevention of contrast-induced nephropathy.
16. Compare the evidence for low-molecular-weight heparins versus unfractionated heparin for venous thromboembolism prophylaxis in trauma patients.
17. State the pharmacokinetic challenges with low-molecular-weight heparin dosing in trauma.

ABBREVIATIONS IN THIS CHAPTER

AKI	Acute kidney injury	MTP	Massive transfusion protocol
aPTT	Activated partial thromboplastin time	PBRC	Packed red blood cell
BCVI	Blunt cerebrovascular injury	RIFLE	Risk, Injury, Failure, Loss, and End-stage Renal Disease
CT	Computed tomography		
DVT	Deep venous thrombosis	SBS	Short bowel syndrome
ECF	Enterocutaneous fistula	SCI	Spinal cord injury
GH	Growth hormone	TBI	Traumatic brain injury
IH	Intracranial hypertension	TIC	Trauma-induced coagulopathy
ICP	Intracranial pressure	TPN	Total parenteral nutrition
ICU	Intensive care unit	VTE	Venous thromboembolism
ISS	Injury severity score		

INTRODUCTION

Traumatic injury is a significant health care concern, accounting for almost 200,000 deaths in the United States in 2010, and is the No. 1 cause of death among people 1–44 years of age and the No. 3 killer overall.[1] This translates to an economic burden of around $406 billion annually related to health care costs and loss of productivity.[2] Although treatment of patients with traumatic injury is primarily surgical in nature, the clinical pharmacist plays a critical role in optimizing drug therapy because drug therapy is an essential part of the support care in these patients. This chapter will review the initial evaluation of the trauma patient, the physiologic changes related to traumatic injury, and the various types of traumatic injuries and the subsequent complications that require pharmacologic intervention.

INITIAL EVALUATION OF THE PATIENT (ADVANCED TRAUMA LIFE SUPPORT)

Initial evaluation of the trauma patient involves a systemic approach, divided into a primary and secondary survey, to stabilize the patient and identify any life-threatening conditions.

Primary Survey

The primary survey encompasses a series of steps designed to identify life-threatening injuries and immediately initiate management. It involves Airway maintenance with cervical spine protection, Breathing and ventilation, Circulation with hemorrhage control, Disability with respect to neurological status, and Exposure/environment (ABCDE).[3]

Airway Maintenance

Airway maintenance is of utmost importance for the trauma patient. Pulse oximetry is used as an adjunct to the primary survey to detect and monitor hypoxia. During airway maintenance, the patient's ability to maintain and protect the airway is assessed while maintaining cervical spine precautions. Some indications for securing a definitive airway when patients are unable to protect their own airway include unconsciousness or an obtunded neurological state (defined as a Glasgow Coma Scale [GCS] score less than 8), severe maxillofacial fractures, risk of aspiration (e.g., vomiting or bleeding), and risk of obstruction (e.g., stridor, laryngeal or tracheal injuries, neck hematoma). Concern for ventilation or oxygenation and the need for a definitive airway may arise in patients presenting with apnea; inadequate respiratory efforts such as tachypnea, hypoxia, hypercarbia, and cyanosis; severe closed head injury (with need for brief hyperventilation if acute neurological decompensation occurs); or massive blood loss and need for large-volume resuscitation. A definitive airway is defined as a cuffed endotracheal tube in the trachea, which is often achieved by rapid sequence intubation (RSI).[4] When RSI fails to secure the airway, a surgical airway becomes necessary.

Breathing and Ventilation

After airway assessment, the trauma patient is evaluated for breathing and ventilation, which includes adequate oxygenation and carbon dioxide exchange. A patent airway does not automatically ensure adequate ventilation.[5] Pulse oximetry allows noninvasive measurement of oxygenation; however, it can be inaccurate in different settings such as vasoconstriction, carbon monoxide poisoning, hypothermia, or severe anemia.[5] Therefore, an arterial blood gas is often required to assess the partial pressure of oxygen. Evaluation of breathing by inspecting chest wall movement, auscultation of breath sounds, and percussion is essential to help detect any abnormalities that need immediate attention such as a pneumo- or hemothorax. A tension pneumothorax can develop from either blunt or penetrating trauma and involves continuous air flow from the trachea, bronchi, or chest wall into the pleural space, causing a shift of the mediastinum, deviation of the trachea away from the tension, respiratory distress, increased intrathoracic pressures, decreased venous return, hypotension, and, ultimately, shock if unrecognized and untreated. Managing a pneumothorax includes inserting a chest tube. A hemothorax is the collection of blood in the pleural space caused by blunt or penetrating trauma and can lead to mediastinal shift, respiratory distress, and hypovolemic shock, prompting emergency management with tube thoracostomy and transfusion and immediate surgery.[3]

Circulation with Hemorrhage Control

One of the main concerns in the trauma patient is uncontrolled bleeding, which can lead to hemorrhagic shock and, if not detected and treated early, death secondary to organ hypoperfusion. Locations of hemorrhage include thoracic cavity, abdominal cavity, pelvic fracture (retroperitoneum), and long bones or obvious external bleeding.[3] Clinical assessment of hypovolemic shock secondary to hemorrhage includes parameters such as heart rate, pulse pressure, urine output, skin color, temperature, and mental status. Hemorrhagic shock is broken into four classes, based on estimated blood loss (Table 43.1). Managing hemorrhage in the trauma patient begins with securing two large-bore venous catheters for appropriate fluid resuscitation together with hemorrhage control. Trauma patients with hypovolemic shock can be classified as fluid rapid responders, transient responders, or nonresponders (Table 43.2).

Bleeding control can be done through applying direct pressure on the bleeding vessel for obvious bleeding. For less obvious sources, proximal pressure over the femoral artery in the groin or the brachial artery in the upper extremity can be applied.[6] A hemothorax is managed with insertion of a chest tube and operative control. Intra-abdominal bleeding in the setting of shock requires emergency laparotomy, and a pelvic fracture leading to hemorrhage is treated by pelvic stabilization or extraperitoneal packing.

Disability: Neurological Status

Once the ABCs have been completed, a neurological assessment including GCS score and pupillary examination (including size, symmetry, and reaction to light) is performed. Possible blunt trauma to the brain warrants a computed tomography (CT) scan for further evaluation.

Exposure and Environmental Control

A patient's clothing should be removed immediately to allow appropriate evaluation; however, it is important to ensure that the patient does not become hypothermic using warmed blankets, fluids, and air. Findings during this part of the assessment will drive further evaluation and intervention.

Adjuncts

Adjuncts to the primary survey include frequent monitoring of oxygenation and ventilation, vital signs, hemodynamics, and neurological status. In addition, a urinary catheter and a nasogastric/orogastric tube are inserted. Diagnostic imaging such as radiographs and CT scans is ordered as appropriate. The focused assessment with sonography for trauma (FAST) examination helps identify fluid or blood in the pericardial and peritoneal cavity. Four windows are examined using sonography: the pericardium, the spaces between the liver and the kidney (Morison pouch), the spaces between the spleen and the kidney (splenorenal recess), and the space over the bladder.[7-9] An unstable patient with a positive FAST is

Table 44.1 Classes of Hemorrhagic Shock

	Class I	Class II	Class III	Class IV
Blood loss (mL)	Up to 750	750–1,500	1,500–2,000	>2,000
Blood loss (% blood volume)	Up to 15	15–30	30–40	>40
Heart rate (beats/minute)	<100	100–120	120–140	>140
Blood pressure (mm Hg)	Normal	Normal	Decreased	Decreased
Pulse pressure (mm Hg)	Normal or increased	Decreased	Decreased	Decreased
Respiratory rate (breaths/minute)	14–20	20–30	30–40	>35
Urine output (mL/hr)	>30	20–30	5–15	Negligible
CNS/mental status	Slightly anxious	Mildly anxious	Anxious/confused	Confused/lethargic
Fluid replacement	Crystalloid	Crystalloid	Crystalloid/blood	Crystalloid and blood

American College of Surgeons Committee on Trauma. Advanced Trauma Life Support for Doctors, 8th ed. Chicago: American College of Surgeons Committee, 2008:61.

Table 44.2 Responses to Initial Fluid Resuscitation[a]

	Rapid Response	Transient Response	Minimal or No Response
Vital signs	Return to normal	Transient improvement	Remains abnormal
Estimated blood loss	Minimal (10%–20%)	Moderate and ongoing (20%–40%)	Severe (>40%)
Need for more crystalloid	Low	High	High
Need for blood	Low	Moderate to high	Immediate
Blood preparation	Type and crossmatch	Type-specific	Emergency blood release
Need for operative intervention	Possibly	Likely	Highly likely
Early presence of surgeon	Yes	Yes	Yes

[a] 2 L of isotonic solution in adults.

American College of Surgeons Committee on Trauma. Advanced Trauma Life Support for Doctors, 8th ed. Chicago: American College of Surgeons Committee, 2008:61.

transferred emergently to the operating room for definitive control of the hemorrhage.

On completion of the primary survey, the decision for early transfer to a more specialized trauma center is made, depending on the patient's injuries and the available resources.

Secondary Survey

The secondary survey follows the primary survey once the patient's ABCs have been stabilized and includes obtaining a medical history and completing a detailed physical examination. On the patient's arrival to the hospital, prehospital personnel can furnish much of the patient's history using the mnemonic AMPLE (A – allergies, M – medications currently used, P – past illness/pregnancy, L – last meal, E – events/environment related to injury).[3] The patient should always be asked about tetanus status.

The physical examination includes a complete assessment from head to toe, including the head and face, neck and spine, chest, abdomen, and musculoskeletal and peripheral vascular systems. The neurological examination includes a motor and sensory examination, and patients with altered consciousness should have a CT scan of the brain.

Adjuncts to the secondary survey include routine radiography and angiography, among others. Laboratory results should be reviewed, including base deficit and lactate concentrations, which are markers of hypoperfusion.

After completing the secondary survey, continuous reassessment of the patient is essential. If there is any clinical worsening, steps of the primary survey are repeated.

INITIAL MANAGEMENT

Physiology of Hypovolemic Shock

Hypovolemic shock is a state of inappropriate delivery of oxygen and nutrients to organs secondary to volume loss. Hallmarks of hypovolemic shock include hypoperfusion secondary to an unbalanced oxygen demand and supply at the cellular level. This leads to cellular injury, which initially can be reversible but can progress to irreversible damage if not recognized and managed early enough. Hemorrhagic shock is a type of hypovolemic shock secondary to blood loss. During early hemorrhagic shock, compensatory mechanisms including neuroendocrine and cardiovascular responses are activated to maintain hemodynamics and perfusion.[10] As the bleeding continues, however, compensatory mechanisms fail, and the patient goes into cardiovascular collapse. Decompensated hypovolemic shock leads to multiorgan dysfunction, inflammation, and microcirculatory shock. Once parenchymal and microvascular injury has ensued, volume resuscitation strategies cannot reverse the process. Reperfusion injury can further worsen the initial insult. If decompensated hemorrhagic shock is left untreated, the outcome can be fatal.

Non-trauma causes of hemorrhagic shock include antithrombotic therapy, coagulopathies, gastrointestinal (GI) bleeding, and a ruptured aneurysm. Pulmonary etiologies include lung cancer and cavitary lung disease, whereas obstetric/gynecologic causes include ruptured ectopic pregnancy, ruptured ovarian cyst, and placenta previa, among others. In the trauma patient, hemorrhage can be external and visible or can be internal. Lacerations, penetrating trauma (e.g., gunshot wounds), blunt trauma, and ruptured major vessels can all lead to life-threatening hemorrhage.[11]

A 70-kg patient is composed of 60% total body water (42 L), which can be further divided into 28 L of intracellular water (2 L of red cell volume and 26 L within muscles and organs) and 14 L of extracellular water (3 L of plasma volume and 11 L of interstitial space fluid, which mostly comprises the interstitial space matrix). The average adult blood volume is 7% of body weight, which is about 5 L in a 70-kg patient.[12]

There are four classes of hemorrhagic shock (classes I–IV), based on blood loss (Table 43.1). The physiology of hemorrhagic shock consists of three phases. Phase I describes the state of shock and active hemorrhage (from admission to the end of surgery/definitive bleeding control). Phase II is the obligatory extravascular fluid sequestration phase from the end of surgery to the time of maximal weight gain. Phase III describes the time during which fluid mobilization and diuresis occur (from maximal weight gain to positive fluid balance).[12]

Management of Hemorrhagic Shock: Fluid Resuscitation

The goals of managing hemorrhagic shock are to stop the bleeding and to restore hemodynamics to minimize hypoperfusion and associated ischemic damage to all organs. Management of hemorrhagic shock starts with establishing vascular access for fluid and blood resuscitation, which is accomplished by inserting at least two short, large-bore intravenous catheters.[10,13] Intravenous fluid resuscitation is an important strategy in restoring intravascular volume.

Resuscitation Goals

The aim of trauma resuscitation is to restore normal hemostasis by addressing shock and the resulting oxygen debt.[14] Oxygen debt is evaluated by monitoring either serum lactate or base deficit. The goal of trauma resuscitation is the normalization of either parameter.[15] Available resuscitation fluids include crystalloids (0.9% sodium chloride solution ["normal saline"], lactated Ringer, Plasmalyte ["balanced crystalloid"]) and colloids (albumin [4%–25%], hydroxyethyl starches, gelatin solutions).[15] Classically, lactated Ringer has been the resuscitation fluid of choice for trauma resuscitation, but other fluids have been used as well, with varying efficacy and safety profiles.[10]

Plasmalyte

Plasmalyte is a balanced crystalloid solution with different available formulations, designed to mimic human plasma.[15] It can be used for fluid resuscitation (filling the intravascular space) or fluid replacement (extravascular deficit).[15] Plasmalyte is different from lactated Ringer because it contains acetate as a buffer instead of lactate, which theoretically reduces carbon dioxide production. A theoretical concern with the use of Plasmalyte in trauma resuscitation is that it contains magnesium, which has undesirable hemodynamic effects (bradycardia, decreased peripheral vascular resistance).[16] To date, only one study has evaluated its use in trauma resuscitation.

Young et al. compared resuscitation with normal saline with resuscitation with Plasma-Lyte A, a calcium-free balanced crystalloid solution, in adult trauma patients (n=46) requiring blood transfusion and operative management within 60 minutes of hospital arrival and found that the mean base excess improvement from 0 to 24 hours, the primary outcome of the study, was significantly greater with Plasma-Lyte A (7.5 ± 4.7 vs. 4.4 ± 3.9 mmol/L; difference 3.1 [95% confidence interval {CI}, 0.5–5.6]; p = not available), with a higher pH at 24 hours (7.41 ± 0.06 vs. 7.37 ± 0.07; difference 0.05 [95% CI, 0.01–0.09]) and a lower chloride concentration at 24 hours (104 ± 4 vs. 111 ± 8 mEq/L; difference -7 [95% CI, -10 to -3]). There were no differences in the volumes of fluids administered, 24-hour urine output, resource use measures, or mortality.[17]

Although the concept of balanced resuscitation fluids with a physiology similar to human plasma is appealing and the clinical evidence in trauma is promising, more studies are needed to validate use in this population.

Colloids

Colloids are suspensions of molecules within a carrier solution, usually incapable of crossing a healthy semipermeable capillary membrane because of their molecular weight.[15] The use of colloids is supported by the rationale that they can expand the intravascular volume and maintain colloid oncotic pressure without causing fluid overload. This volume-sparing effect is traditionally thought to be in a 1:3 ratio of colloids to crystalloids to replete intravascular depletion.[15]

Different colloids are available, including human albumin and semisynthetic colloids including hydroxyethyl starches, gelatin products, and dextrans. Albumin is considered the reference colloid. Hydroxyethyl starch is produced by hydroxyethyl substitution of glucose molecules from maize, potatoes, or sorghum. This substitution leads to protection against hydrolysis and, hence, a prolonged intravascular volume expansion; however, it also increases the risk of accumulation in different tissues such as the skin, liver, and kidneys.[15]

Theoretically, semisynthetic colloids are a good alternative to costly albumin because they are good volume expanders, can be manufactured cheaply, and do not bear the risk of bloodborne infections; however, they have been shown to accumulate in different organs, causing adverse effects. In addition, high-molecular-weight hydroxyethyl starch products can cause coagulopathies. The use of hydroxyethyl starch solutions with molecular weights greater than 200 kD and a molar substitution ratio of more than 0.5 has been linked to higher rates of mortality, acute kidney injury (AKI), and renal replacement therapy use in patients with sepsis. The recommended maximal daily dose of hydroxyethyl starch is 33–50 mL/kg.[15]

Albumin

The SAFE trial, a multicenter, randomized, double-blind study, assessed the use of 4% albumin versus normal saline for intravascular fluid resuscitation in a mixed intensive care unit (ICU) patient population (43% surgical admissions vs. 57% medical admissions) and found no difference in 28-day mortality (relative risk [RR] of death 0.99; 95% CI, 0.91–1.09; p=0.87), new single-organ and multiorgan failure (p=0.85), ICU (p=0.44) or hospital length of stay (p=0.30), days of mechanical ventilation (0.74), or days of renal replacement therapy (p=0.41).[18] In a subgroup analysis of patients admitted with trauma, the albumin-receiving group had a trend toward higher 28-day mortality than the saline-receiving group (13.6% vs. 10.0%; p=0.06).

The SAFE trial investigators conducted a further post hoc analysis specifically targeting patients with a traumatic brain injury (TBI) because of concern for increased mortality in the albumin group.[19] This group of patients had an increased 24-month mortality if they had received albumin (33.2% vs. 20.4%; RR 1.63; 95% CI, 1.17–2.26; p=0.003). The effect was attributed to increased intracranial pressure (ICP).

The CRISTAL study, a multicenter, randomized, open-label trial (with investigators blinded to treatment assessment), included 2,857 patients from different ICUs receiving colloids (including gelatins, dextrans, hydroxyethyl starches, and 4% or 20% albumin) versus crystalloids (isotonic or hypertonic saline or lactated Ringer) for hypovolemic shock.[20] Seventy percent of patients were admitted to the ICU because of medical diagnosis, followed by about 20% admitted secondary to an emergency surgery (6.2%–7.8% admitted because of a scheduled surgery and 1.6%–2.5% admitted secondary to trauma). The primary outcome, 28-day mortality, did not differ between groups (25.4% in colloids vs. 27.0% in crystalloids; RR 0.96 [95% CI, 0.88–1.04]; p=0.26); however, 90-day mortality was higher in the crystalloid group (34.2% in crystalloids vs. 30.7% in colloids; RR 0.92 [95% CI, 0.86–0.99]; p=0.03). Other secondary outcomes, including the number of days alive without mechanical ventilation and without vasopressors at days 7 and 28, were all higher in the colloid group.

In a recent study evaluating the effects of intraoperative use of colloids on postoperative fluid needs, non-colloids (balanced electrolyte solution) plus low fresh frozen plasma (FFP)/red blood cell (RBC) ratio resuscitation (0.35 or less) were compared with the administration of colloids (human albumin) plus high FFP/RBC ratio resuscitation (greater than 0.35). Administering albumin and high FFP/RBC resuscitation did not prevent phase II fluid uptake (fluid sequestration phase). In contrast, it caused a decrease in urine output despite increased plasma volume.[21] The authors theorized that colloids reduce glomerular filtration and increase tubular reabsorption, thus increasing extracellular fluid and prolonging phase II.

Hydroxyethyl Starches

The Crystalloid versus Hydroxyethyl Starch Trial (CHEST), with 42% of patients admitted after surgery and 8% trauma patients, randomized patients 1:1 to either 6% hydroxyethyl starch (molecular weight 130 kD and molar substitution ratio of 0.4) or normal saline for fluid resuscitation and found no 90-day mortality difference (18% in hydroxyethyl starch group vs. 17% in normal saline group; 95% CI, 0.96–1.18; p=0.26).[22] More patients in the hydroxyethyl starch group required renal replacement therapy (7% vs. 5.8% in saline group; RR 1.21; 95% CI, 1.00–1.45; p=0.04), and more patients in the hydroxyethyl starch group developed renal injury (according to the RIFLE criteria) (7% vs. 5.8%; RR 1.21; 95% CI, 1.00–1.45; p=0.04). The use of hydroxyethyl starch was also associated with more adverse events such as pruritus and rash (5.3% vs. 2.8%, p<0.001).

In a recent meta-analysis evaluating outcomes with the use of hydroxyethyl starch for fluid resuscitation in a heterogeneous patient population including patients with trauma, sepsis, hypovolemic shock, and burns after excluding some biased trials, hydroxyethyl starch was associated with increased mortality (RR 1.09; 95% CI, 1.02–1.17), increased renal failure (RR 1.27; 95% CI, 1.09–1.47), and increased use of renal replacement therapy (RR 1.32; 95% CI, 1.15–1.50). Therefore, the use of hydroxyethyl starch is no longer recommended because of serious safety concerns.[23]

Given the evidence, crystalloids remain the main fluid of choice for resuscitation. In patients without head injury, albumin may be considered if the patient becomes fluid overloaded and continues to have intravascular depletion.

Trauma-Induced Coagulopathy

Trauma-induced coagulopathy (TIC) is "nonsurgical" bleeding from serosal surfaces, mucosal lesions, and wound sites.[24] Classically, TIC has been attributed to the dilutional effects of crystalloid and packed red blood cell (PRBC) resuscitation; however, research has revealed the presence of TIC, even in patients who had received very little resuscitation.[25] Accordingly, the focus has shifted from restoring circulating volume by intravenous fluid and RBCs to the concept of hemostatic resuscitation.

Of note, the incidence of TIC immediately after traumatic injury is quite high (24%–28%), contrary to the traditional belief that this is a later complication of trauma.[24,26,27] The evolution of TIC occurs in three phases.[25] The first phase constitutes the immediate activation of hemostatic pathways, including fibrinolysis and thrombosis associated with tissue injury. During the second phase, the patient receives resuscitation fluids and blood products, which lead to dilution of hemostatic factors. Phase 3 is the post-resuscitation phase, where a prothrombotic state prevails.

During TIC, there is a large consumption of coagulation factors and platelets secondary to the formation of thrombi and extravascular clots. Platelet migration to the injured vessel wall is interrupted once the hematocrit falls below 30%.[28] Part of the resulting coagulopathy is dilutional because of large volumes of intravenous fluids and blood products. Hormonal and cytokine changes lead to endothelial cell activation, which in turn results in changing the endothelial cell from antithrombotic to prothrombotic, a phenomenon that can lead to DIC (disseminated intravascular coagulopathy).

The combination of hypoxia, hypothermia, and acidosis has been termed the *bloody vicious triad* or *lethal triad* because of its deleterious effects in hypotensive trauma patients with TIC. Hypoxia, commonly seen in the hypoperfused trauma patient in hemorrhagic shock, exacerbates endothelial cell activation. Hypothermia, defined as a core body temperature less than 35°C, is a result of convection, radiation, wet clothing, insensible fluid losses from open wounds and surgical incisions, and resuscitation with crystalloids at room temperature or cold PRBCs.[24] The consequences of hypothermia include impaired platelet activation and adhesion, together with increased sequestration by the liver. Hypoperfusion leads to anaerobic metabolism, which results in acidosis. Coagulopathies are more pronounced when core temperature falls below 33°C and pH falls below 7.1.[29,30]

The diagnosis of TIC is based on laboratory values such as prothrombin time (greater than 1.5 times normal), activated thromboplastin time (greater than 1.5 times normal), an international normalized ratio (INR) greater than 1.5, thrombocytopenia (platelet count less than 50,000/mm³), and low fibrinogen concentration (less than 0.5–1 g/L).[24] Of note, these values do not account for dysfunctional platelets or hyperfibrinolysis.

Management of TIC is based on the concept of damage control resuscitation, which entails minimizing crystalloid resuscitation, allowing hypotension until arrival to the operating room, preventing coagulopathy through the early administration of blood products in a balanced ratio (massive transfusion protocol [MTP]), and addressing the acidosis, coagulopathy, and hypothermia associated with TIC.[31]

Resuscitation Volume

How much fluid resuscitation to provide the trauma patient is an important question to ask because more is not always better. Over-resuscitation is associated with concerns for increased tissue edema leading to complications such as the abdominal compartment syndrome, anastomotic leaks, acute coronary syndromes, and acute respiratory distress syndrome. There can also be increased bleeding from dislodged clots, a dilutional coagulopathy, and exacerbated hypothermia.[10,32]

The American College of Surgeons Committee on Trauma and the subcommittee and the international Advanced Trauma Life Support working group promote the concept of balanced resuscitation instead of aggressive resuscitation.[33] This can be achieved through the standard administration of warmed 1 L of crystalloids (lactated Ringer or 0.9% sodium chloride solutions) as a starting point instead of the previously recommended 2 L. The group also suggests the use of blood products.

In 1994, Bickell et al. published the results of a study evaluating patients with penetrating torso trauma with a prehospital systolic blood pressure of 90 mm Hg or less. Patients were randomized to receive traditional fluid resuscitation or delayed resuscitation in the field and emergency department before arrival to the operating room for definitive bleeding management.[34] Patients in the delayed fluid group received intravenous cannulation and no more than 100 mL before surgical intervention, and they had a survival benefit (70% vs. 62%; p=0.04), fewer complications, and a shorter hospital length of stay.

In a recent systemic review of 11 studies comparing liberal with restricted fluid resuscitation strategies in major trauma patients (defined as an injury severity score [ISS] of 16 or greater), there was an increase in mortality in the four included randomized trials (RR 1.18; 95% CI, 0.98–1.141) and in the seven included observational studies (odds ratio [OR] 1.14; 95% CI, 1.01–1.28) for patients who received a liberal fluid resuscitation strategy.[35]

Most of the available evidence for clinical benefit with hypotensive resuscitative strategies exists for penetrating trauma, with evidence lacking for other forms of trauma; therefore, the generalizability of this strategy remains controversial.

Massive Transfusion

In general, blood transfusion during hemorrhage is indicated in patients with a blood loss of 30% or greater (class III hemorrhage).[11] In addition, a hypotensive patient who does not respond to a 1- or 2-L crystalloid challenge should be considered for a blood transfusion. Massive transfusion is defined by administration of greater than 10 units of PRBCs in a 24-hour period. The goal of an MTP is to standardize the blood products the patient is receiving and to optimize quick access to the blood products needed. An example of an MTP is the combination of 6 units of FFP, 6 units of PRBCs, 6 packs of platelets, and 10 units of cryoprecipitate.[24]

There has been a shift from aggressive PRBC transfusion to transfusion of a standardized ratio of PRBCs/FFP/platelets because large amounts of PRBCs have been associated with negative outcomes, given recent military experience. In a retrospective evaluation, Borgman et al. found that trauma patients in the military who received a low FFP/PRBC ratio (1 unit of plasma to 8 units of PRBCs) had the highest mortality (65%) and that mortality decreased as the ratio became more balanced (34% mortality for a 1:2.5 ratio and 19% mortality for a 1:1.4 ratio).[36] The authors attributed these results to trauma-induced coagulopathies, which could be attenuated with increased transfusion of FFP.

Similar results were seen in a retrospective study evaluating a civilian trauma population that had received massive transfusion. Higher 30-day survival was associated with a higher plasma/PRBC ratio (1:2 or greater) than with a low plasma/RBC ratio (less than 1:2) (survival of 59.6% vs. 40.4%; p<0.01). The same observation was made for the platelet/RBC ratio (higher survival of 59.9% in the high-ratio group [1:2 or greater] vs. 40.1% in the low-ratio group [less than 1:2]).[37] Despite their potential significant influence on trauma resuscitation, both studies were criticized for their retrospective design and concern for survival bias (i.e., only patients who survive can receive more blood products, altering the ratio of blood products received).

In the recently published PROPPR trial (transfusion of plasma, platelets, and RBCs in a 1:1:1 vs. a 1:1:2 ratio and mortality in patients with severe trauma), severely injured patients with hemorrhagic shock were randomized to receive plasma, platelets, and PRBCs in a 1:1:1 ratio or a 1:1:2 ratio, in addition to all the uncontrolled local standard of care therapies, at the 12 participating level I trauma centers.[38] The primary outcome, all-cause mortality at 24 hours and at 30 days, was no different between the groups (24-hour mortality: 12.7% in 1:1:1 group vs. 17.0% group in 1:1:2 group; p=0.12, and 30-day mortality: 22.4% in 1:1:1 group vs. 26.1% in 1:1:2 group; p=0.26); however, exsanguination, the primary cause of death within the first 24 hours, was significantly lower in the 1:1:1 group (9.2% vs. 14.6% in 1:1:2 group; p=0.03). More patients in the 1:1:1 group achieved hemostasis within the first 24 hours (86% vs. 78% in the 1:1:2 group; p=0.006). No increased complications were seen in the 1:1:1 group, despite receiving higher volumes of plasma and platelets.

Triggers for initiating an MTP should be defined to allow rapid identification of trauma candidates because this has been shown to improve mortality as well as prevent patients without massive bleeding from receiving an MTP inappropriately.

The current indication for an MTP is the need to transfuse 6–10 units of PRBCs. Other clinical triggers may include multicavitary trauma, penetrating trauma, low hemoglobin, and free fluid present on the FAST examination.[39]

Components of MTP

Packed Red Blood Cells
Packed red blood cells are prepared by removing plasma from whole blood. One unit of PRBCs comes in a volume of 200–350 mL, and administration of 1 unit is usually expected to raise hemoglobin concentrations by 1 g/dL. Packed red blood cells not only help with oxygen transport, but are also thought to improve hemostasis by inducing platelet margination (migration of platelets to the injured epithelium wall).[24] Packed red blood cells lose some of their clinical effects during storage.

Fresh Frozen Plasma
Fresh frozen plasma can be separated from whole blood or obtained from donors by plasmapheresis and is stored at a temperature below 30°C. It contains proteins involved in hemostasis, including coagulation factors, anticoagulation proteins, and fibrinolysis proteins. Fresh frozen plasma pack volumes are usually between 150 mL and 250 mL. Trauma patients receive FFP therapy if they have active bleeding together with a prothrombin time or activated partial thromboplastin time (aPTT) greater than 1.5 times normal or if the INR is greater than 1.5 (dosed at 10–15 mL/kg).[24]

Platelets
Platelets, which are separated from whole blood by centrifugation or apheresis, can remain at room temperature for about 5 days. Platelets may need to be supplemented in trauma because of platelet consumption or a dysfunctional state during the acute phase. Patients with platelet counts less than 50,000 mm³ or those with a TBI and a platelet count less than 100,000 mm³ should receive platelets. Transfusing 1 unit of platelets is thought to increase the platelet count by 20,000. Patients who had been receiving antiplatelet medications such as aspirin or $P2Y_{12}$ inhibitors will have increased PRBC and platelet requirements.[24]

Fibrinogen
Fibrinogen, a plasma protein produced in the liver, is converted to fibrin during clot formation and is the first coagulation factor to become deficient during massive blood loss, necessitating replacement if concentrations fall below 0.8–1 g/L.[24] Fresh frozen plasma contains some fibrinogen as part of its coagulation factors; however, if fibrinogen concentrations are still not corrected, cryoprecipitate is administered. Cryoprecipitate is a blood product obtained from donors and prepared from plasma and contains different factors including fibrinogen, von Willebrand factor, fibronectin, and factors VIII and XIII. The fibrinogen concentration is expected to increase by 0.5 g/L for each dose of cryoprecipitate (dosed in 1 unit/10 kg; each dose about 8–10 units).

Pharmacologic Adjuncts

In addition to blood product transfusion, some adjuncts are used to restore hemostasis, including recombinant human factor VIIa, prothrombin complex concentrate, and antifibrinolytics such as tranexamic acid and aminocaproic acid.

Recombinant Human Factor VIIa
Recombinant human factor VIIa is indicated for the treatment of hemophilia. It works by activating platelet adhesion at the site of injury and has been evaluated in a study with blunt trauma patients, where it led to a decrease in PRBC transfusion and the need for MTPs.[40] A follow-up paper by the same group showed a decrease in multiorgan failure and acute respiratory distress syndrome; however, neither study showed improved survival.[41]

Other studies, including the large multicenter CONTROL trial, showed no survival benefit.[42] In addition, there remains the concern for thromboembolic events with the administration of factor VIIa. Given the concerns for thrombosis and the lack of survival benefit, factor VIIa use for trauma remains off-label and is not recommended as part of damage control resuscitation.

Prothrombin Complex Concentrate
Prothrombin complex concentrate contains different coagulation factors. The three-factor prothrombin complex concentrate products such as Bebulin and Profilnine SD contain factors II, IX, and X, whereas the four-factor products such as Kcentra and Octaplex contain factors II, VII, XI, and X and proteins S and C.[43-46] Compared with coagulation factor replacement with plasma, prothrombin complex concentrate products are thought to cause less volume overload, carry a lower risk of transfusion reactions, and be easier and faster to prepare than plasma, which requires an ABO type and screen, and thawing before transfusion. Prothrombin complex concentrate has mainly been studied for the reversal of bleeding secondary to anticoagulants, namely warfarin. There is some published evidence on its use in trauma patients comparing prothrombin complex concentrate with FFP. Despite no improvement in survival, a decrease in need for PRBC transfusion and in multiorgan failure was seen, together with a shorter mechanical ventilation time and hospital length of stay.[47]

Antifibrinolytics
Tranexamic acid, a commonly used antifibrinolytic agent, is a synthetic derivative of lysine.[39] It inhibits fibrinolysis by binding to the lysine site, inhibiting plasminogen activation and plasmin activity. The CRASH-2 trial was a randomized controlled trial performed in 274 hospitals.[48] More than 20,000 adult trauma patients with significant bleeding were randomly assigned within 8 hours of injury to receive either tranexamic acid (loading dose of 1 g over 10 minutes, followed by infusion of 1 g over 8

hours) or the matching placebo. All-cause mortality was significantly lower in the tranexamic acid group (14.5% vs. 16.0%; RR 0.91; 95% CI, 0.85–0.97; p=0.0035), and the risk of mortality secondary to bleeding was decreased as well (4.9% in the tranexamic acid group vs. 5.7%; RR 0.85; 95% CI, 0.76–0.96; p=0.0077). There were no statistically significant differences in thromboembolic events. The quoted benefit was only evident if tranexamic acid was administered within the first 3, with later administration leading to an increase in mortality.[49]

Morrison et al. investigated the use of tranexamic acid in military trauma patients in the Military Application of Tranexamic Acid in Trauma Emergency Resuscitation (MATTERs) study. This was a retrospective observational trial comparing patients who had received tranexamic acid with those who had not, as well as the subgroup of patients who required massive transfusion, defined as 10 units or greater of PRBCs.[50] Patients who received tranexamic acid had a lower unadjusted mortality than those who did not (17.4% vs. 23.9%; p=0.03), despite being more severely injured (mean [SD] ISS 25.2 [16.6] vs. 22.5 [18.5]; p<0.001). This benefit was more pronounced in the subgroup that required massive transfusion. A multivariate regression analysis found tranexamic acid to be an independent predictor of survival.

The MATTERs II study, published in 2013, retrospectively compared four groups of military trauma patients: the tranexamic acid/cryoprecipitate group, the tranexamic acid group, the cryoprecipitate group, and the patient group that received neither therapy.[51] Patients who had received both cryoprecipitate and tranexamic acid had the lowest mortality (11.6%) compared with the tranexamic acid group (18.2%) and the cryoprecipitate group (21.4%), despite higher ISS values and higher PRBC requirements, whereas the group that received neither therapy had the highest mortality rate (23.6%).

ORGAN-SPECIFIC INJURIES

Blunt Cerebrovascular Injuries

Epidemiology and Pathophysiology

Although once thought to be uncommon, blunt cerebrovascular injuries (BCVIs) are becoming increasingly recognized and detected. Data from a recent publication that evaluated the NIS (Nationwide Inpatient Sample), which is the largest all-payer hospital inpatient database in the United States, show that from 2003 through 2010, 1,283–2,652 patients were admitted annually for BCVI. This represented 0.46%–0.95% of all blunt trauma admissions, with the annual nationwide incidence increasing over time.[52] Blunt cerebrovascular injury is a devastating complication of trauma with an associated mortality rate of 40% and neurological comorbidity of up to 80%.[53] Blunt cerebrovascular injury is defined as a wall injury in the vertebral or carotid artery caused by nonpenetrating trauma.[54] The general mechanisms behind BCVI are related to hyperextension and rotation, hyperflexion, or a direct blow to the neck.[55] The resultant damage to the intimal layer of the artery results in exposure of the subendothelial collagen. This stimulates platelet aggregation as well as activation of the clotting cascade, resulting in thrombin generation and subsequent thrombosis.[56] One of the challenges with BCVI is that the neurological symptoms, particularly stroke, present in a latent manner with a time from injury to symptom onset of 10–72 hours, on average.[57,58] It is important that early screening be conducted to promptly identify and treat these patients during this latent period before potentially irreversible complications occur. To this end, criteria for the screening of these patients were initially proposed by Biffl et al. in 1999 and later modified in 2004 to create the Denver criteria.[55,59] Risk factors highlighted by the Denver criteria involve high-energy transfer mechanisms with the following associated injuries: (1) Le Fort II or III fractures; (2) cervical spine fracture patterns such as subluxation, fractures extending into the transverse foramen, and fractures of C1–C3; (3) basilar skull fractures with carotid canal involvement; (4) diffuse axonal injury with a GCS score of 6 or less; and (5) near hanging with anoxic brain injury.[59] Once identified, such patients should have their cerebral vasculature evaluated by four-vessel cerebral angiography ("gold standard") or CT angiography.[60] The severity of BCVI is graded using the following scale proposed by Biffl et al.[61]

- Grade I – intimal irregularity with less than 25% narrowing
- Grade II – dissection or intramural hematoma with greater than 25% narrowing
- Grade III – pseudoaneurysm
- Grade IV – occlusion
- Grade V – transection with extravasation

Management

Management of BCVI can involve anticoagulation, surgical intervention, or endovascular repair (with antiplatelet therapy). Most data evaluations for surgical intervention are from retrospective studies conducted more than 20 years ago and suggest that revascularization is beneficial in patients without neurological deficits compared with ligation.[62-66] With the growing experience in anticoagulation and advances in endovascular technology, the surgical approach has fallen out of favor. Antithrombotic therapy with heparin (goal of aPTT of 40–50 seconds) and transition to warfarin has historically been the gold standard for managing BCVI, as supported by several papers.[67-73] Of these, only one paper has shown significant neurological improvement with antithrombotic management.[69] The challenge with managing with heparin in particular is the added risk of hemorrhage with this therapy. Biffl et al. noted a 54% hemorrhage risk in their paper requiring transfusions and/or cessation of heparin therapy.[71] Despite the goal aPTT of 60–70 seconds at their institution, all the patients who bled had a mean maximum aPTT well outside the range at 87.2 seconds. The paper published by Parikh et al. had a target aPTT of 50–60 seconds and noted a 40% (6 of 15) significant hemorrhage risk in their patients.[73] In Memphis, Fabian et al. documented a 13% (6 of 47) bleeding risk when a goal aPTT of 40–50 seconds was used.[69] Although the risk of hemorrhage was lower with the lower aPTT goals, the lack of standardized aPTT levels, together with heparin's complex pharmacokinetic and pharmacodynamic properties, makes it a challenging drug to dose.[74] Moreover, 25% of the patients in the Memphis study could not receive anticoagulation with heparin for various reasons. The clinical dilemma is that systemic heparin appears to be beneficial for managing BCVI, but there is an added risk of hemorrhage or inability to initiate heparin therapy for one or more relative or absolute contraindications (TBI, recent surgery, solid organ hematoma, etc.).

Challenges with heparin therapy have forced clinicians to explore the role of antiplatelet therapy in treating these patients. In a retrospective analysis of 22 patients for an 8-year period, Wahl et al. evaluated 14 patients who received anticoagulation for BCVI, with seven receiving systemic heparin (goal aPTT of 40–60 seconds) and seven receiving aspirin.[75] All but one survived in each group with fair to good neurological examinations. Four of the seven patients receiving heparin developed significant bleeds requiring discontinuation of heparin and blood transfusions versus none in the aspirin group, which was statistically significant ($p<0.05$). Cothren et al. published their Denver experience of more than 400 patients in two studies and showed similar benefits of antiplatelet agents over heparin.[59,76] Although the authors concluded that both systemic heparin and either monotherapy or combination antiplatelet therapy are equivalent, a caveat was that the systemic heparin group had more grade II, III, and IV injuries. Morton et al. more recently published their experiences with antiplatelet therapy in severe BCVI, where all grade IV injuries (typically have contraindications to heparin) received aspirin as part of routine care, with the addition of clopidogrel in those with carotid artery involvement.[77] The authors reported a stroke rate of about 17% (10 of 59) versus reports of 40%–80% in untreated patients, showing the benefits of antiplatelet therapy in this high-risk population.[58,59,64] The challenge with the data comparing the efficacy of antiplatelet therapy with that of antithrombotic therapy is the lack of high-quality trials comparing these two therapies directly, which is highlighted in the Eastern Association for the Surgery of Trauma guidelines. These suggest that the evidence supports using antithrombotic therapy in those with no contraindications and reserving antiplatelet therapy for all others.[60] In addition to selecting the appropriate anticoagulant, therapy duration has not been well defined in the published literature, and only one study has discussed this issue to date. Biffl et al. evaluated 179 patients with BCVI who received repeat arteriography 7–10 days from the initial diagnosis.[78] Data showed that 57% of grade I and 8% of grade II injuries healed, allowing antithrombotic therapy to be discontinued, whereas 93% of grade III and 82% of grade IV injuries remained unchanged. Of note, 8% of grade I and 43% of grade II injuries progressed to pseudoaneurysms requiring intervention. This study highlighted the need for reimaging in order to adjust therapy according to the patient's response as well as potentially longer anticoagulation periods for more severe BCVI. Two additional studies evaluated long-term outcomes (mean follow-ups of 22 and 29 months) in BCVI; however, neither addressed the duration of anticoagulation.[79,80]

Endovascular therapy is an attractive option in treating patients with contraindications to anticoagulant therapy or with higher-grade lesions. This is particularly true in grade III lesions where pseudoaneurysms weaken the vascular wall, setting the stage for devastating complications if left untreated. To date, three papers have evaluated outcomes related to endovascular repair. The first paper, by Cothren et al., evaluated 46 patients with BCVI over an 8-year period (1996–2004), of whom 23 received antithrombotic therapy alone and 23 received endovascular stenting together with antithrombotic therapy.[81] The authors reported a complication rate of 21% (4 of 18) and a reocclusion rate of 45% (8 of 18) versus no complications in the 23 patients who did not receive stents, with one patient developing thrombosis. The authors recommended against the use of stents as a result of this study, although they did highlight that patients with stents did not receive antiplatelet therapy, which could have been a risk factor for reocclusion. Since then, two additional studies have been published with more positive findings. In the paper by Edwards et al., 55 patients who were alive at discharge and had long-term follow-up (mean 29 months) data were evaluated, of whom 41 received antithrombotic or antiplatelet therapy, whereas 14 received endovascular repair.[79] None of the patients in either group had a stroke after discharge, and the stents were patent on repeat angiography at a mean of 33 weeks. The final study by DiCocco et al. evaluated 222 patients with BCVI for 53 months. Endovascular repair for BCVI was used in 80 patients (41%), whereas medical management was used in 122 patients (59%).[80] Three strokes were present in each group after a mean follow-up of 22 months, and the authors concluded that the outcomes between both groups were similar, despite the more grade III injuries in the endovascular group (56 vs. 7). These studies support the use of endovascular repair as a mode of management for BCVI, with outcomes comparable with those of anticoagulant therapy alone.

In conclusion, anticoagulation plays a pivotal role in managing BCVI, with data analyses suggesting that both antithrombotic and antiplatelet therapy are reasonable therapeutic options, though the therapy duration remains undefined. Although the Eastern Association for the Surgery of Trauma guidelines suggest antithrombotic therapy as the preferred mode, challenges with heparin therapy have led more clinicians to use antiplatelet therapy instead. Endovascular repair should be reserved for patients with contraindications to anticoagulation.

Traumatic Brain Injury

Pathophysiology and Treatment

Traumatic brain injury is the disruption or alteration of brain function caused by external forces and represents heterogeneous disease that can occur through a variety of mechanisms and can vary in severity and duration.[82]

In addition to the primary TBI caused by trauma, secondary injury may develop hours to days after the initial injury. Pathophysiologic changes that occur include neurotransmitter release, free-radical generation, calcium-mediated damage, mitochondrial dysfunction, and inflammatory responses leading to cell necrosis, apoptosis, and autophagy.[83-86] The goal of the critical care practitioner in this setting is to prevent or minimize secondary injury as a result of the evolution of the TBI. The two main goals that should be instituted in the prehospital setting to prevent secondary injury are the avoidance of hypotension (systolic blood pressure less than 90 mm Hg) and hypoxia (Pao_2 of 60 mm Hg or less), as noted in the pivotal paper by Chesnut et al.[87] In this paper, the presence of hypotension and hypoxia increased the mortality rate from 26.9% to 57.2% and reduced the percentage of patients with a good or moderate neurological outcome from 53.9% to 20.5%. Beyond these fundamental parameters, there has been a significant amount of interest during the past 3 decades to develop "neuroprotective therapies" to reduce secondary brain injury and improve outcomes in patients with TBI. Table 43.3 summarizes the findings of the more recent trials evaluating neuroprotective therapies in TBI. Despite our growing knowledge with respect to the pathophysiology of TBI and the enthusiasm surrounding the results of the early progesterone trials, all therapeutic trials to date have had dismal results. This highlights the complexity of the pathophysiology of TBI and a lack of understanding of the secondary response. As of now, the area of TBI management requires further research.

Table 44.3 Summary of Major Clinical Trials Regarding Neuroprotection

Study Name	Sample Size	Trial Design	Intervention	Result
MRC CRASH[88,89]	10,008	Randomized controlled trial of patients with TBI with GCS < 14	Patients treated within 8 hr of injury with 48-hr infusion of methylprednisolone or placebo	Mortality higher at 2 wk (21.1% vs. 17.9%, p=0.0001) and 6 mo (25.7% vs. 22.3%, p=0.0001) in the treatment group
Dexanabinol trial[90]	846	Randomized controlled trial of patients with TBI with GCS of 2-5 and CT scan showing trauma	Patients treated with a single dose of 150 mg of dexanabinol within 6 hr of injury or placebo	Extended GCS at 6 mo showed no difference between each group (50% vs. 51% unfavorable score, p=0.78)
Magnesium trial[91]	499	Randomized controlled trial of patients with TBI with GCS of 3-12 (moderate to severe) or intracranial surgery	Patients treated within 8 hr of injury with 5 days of continuous infusion of magnesium to achieve a serum concentration of 2.5-5 mEq/L or 2-3.7 mEq/L or placebo	For the outcome of the composite end point of mortality, seizures, functional measures, and neuropsychological testing, there was no difference between treatment and placebo (55 percentile vs. 52 percentile, p=0.70)
SYNAPSE[92]	1,195	Randomized controlled trial of patients with TBI with GCS ≤ 8	Patients treated within 8 hr of injury with 5-day infusion of progesterone or placebo	Favorable Glasgow outcome score at 6 mo was not different between treatment and placebo group (50.4% vs. 50.5%; 95% CI, 0.77-1.18)
PROTECT III[93]	882	Randomized controlled trial of patients with TBI with GCS of 4-12	Patients treated within 4 hr of injury with 4-day infusion of progesterone or placebo	Favorable Glasgow outcome score at 6 mo was not different between treatment and placebo group (48.2% vs. 52.7%; 95% CI, -11.1 to 2.1)

TBI = traumatic brain injury.

Complications of TBI

Intracranial Hypertension

With no therapies to treat TBI directly, the goal is to manage intracranial hypertension (IH) and seizures. Intracranial hypertension can develop in up to 50% of patients with severe head injury, and persistent elevations are associated with poor outcomes.[94] Intracranial hypertension in TBI is the result of increased intracranial volume because of cerebral edema and hematoma in the cranial vault, which is a fixed-volume space. There are adaptive mechanisms (Monro-Kellie doctrine) such as reducing venous volume and cerebrospinal fluid within the brain that tolerate increases in intracranial volume to a degree; however, when the adaptive capacity is exceeded, IH occurs.[95] Although hemorrhage and hematoma are the result of the trauma causing the TBI, the development of cerebral edema is the result of low ATP (adenosine triphosphate) and subsequent excess intracellular sodium, calcium, and glutamate (cytogenic) as well as increased microvascular permeability (vasogenic).[96-99] Management of IH is multimodal and involves nonpharmacologic interventions such as elevation of the head of the bed, surgical decompression, and extraventricular drainage of cerebrospinal fluid as well as pharmacologic interventions such as pain/agitation control, hyperosmolar therapy, and barbiturate coma. Pain and agitation management practices are covered elsewhere, so this section will focus on hyperosmolar therapy and barbiturate coma.

Hyperosmolar Therapy

With cerebral edema being the primary pathophysiologic change that occurs in TBI, treatment with hyperosmotic therapy has become the cornerstone of IH management. Mannitol and hypertonic saline are the two agents routinely used to manage this complication, although data are limited supporting the use of either agent (Table 43.4). Mechanistically, although both create an osmotic gradient, hypertonic saline appears to possess additional hemodynamic, vasoregulatory, neurochemical, and immunomodulatory properties, though the clinical significance of this difference is unknown.[113] The hemodynamic effects of hypertonic saline have been well shown in several trials.[114-118] Mannitol has the potential to cause volume depletion in an already low-volume state, whereas hypertonic saline remains in the vascular space. Hypertonic saline provides low-volume resuscitation in addition to its osmotic capabilities, and as such, it has become the preferred agent in managing IH in TBI. A recently published meta-analysis also suggests that, although limited by the small size and number of eligible trials, hypertonic saline is superior to mannitol with respect to ICP control and ICP reductions, which further supports the use of hypertonic saline.[119] However, evidence is weak to support the type or dose of hypertonic saline. Current practice is that hypertonic saline in a continuous infusion or intermittent boluses is administered in patients with TBI to achieve a serum sodium concentration of 145–155 mEq/L; however, there is no evidence to support this practice.[120] The two studies that evaluated the use of hypertonic saline to a target serum sodium showed no response of ICPs after 24 hours and worse clinical outcomes.[107,108] Nonetheless, with the challenges of conducting prospective research in this population, this practice will likely remain standard of care for a significant time. Finally, continuous monitoring of patients while on hyperosmolar therapy is important to mitigate adverse effects. Mannitol carries with it the risk of dehydration, acute renal failure, rebound IH, hypotension, and hypernatremia, whereas hypertonic saline carries the risk of metabolic acidosis, acute renal failure, hypernatremia, hypokalemia, rebound IH, and phlebitis.[121] It is important that frequent monitoring (every 4–6 hours) of serum electrolytes and osmolality be performed to minimize the electrolyte abnormalities and that these therapies be weaned slowly (over 24–48 hours) to minimize the risk of rebound IH.[122] Central pontine myelinolysis is a theoretical concern with hypertonic saline use. No cases have been reported to date; however, to minimize this risk, it is important to avoid serum sodium concentrations greater than 155 mEq/L and serum osmolality greater than 320 mOsm/L and to wean hypertonic saline therapy off slowly.[123]

Barbiturate Coma

When routine sedation and analgesia management and nonpharmacologic options and hyperosmolar therapy fail to control IH, barbiturate coma is used as a last resort, as reflected in the Brain Trauma Foundation guidelines.[124,125] The mechanism behind barbiturate coma is metabolic suppression leading to reductions in cerebral blood flow and ICP.[126] Both pentobarbital and thiopental have been used to produce barbiturate coma, with traditional dosing involving several loading doses (10 mg/kg over 30 minutes, followed by 5 mg/kg every hour for three or four doses), followed by a continuous infusion of 1–3 mg/kg/hour, although it is not uncommon to exceed these doses because of the hypermetabolic nature of critically ill trauma patients.[127,128] Loading doses can also be combined in a 20- to 30-mg/kg single dose administered over 1–2 hours for convenience. Because of the poor correlation between serum or cerebrospinal fluid concentrations and clinical end points, barbiturates are typically titrated either to ICP control or, more routinely, electroencephalography (EEG) burst suppression, therefore requiring continuous EEG monitoring.[129] In addition, barbiturates are auto-inducers of their own metabolism; therefore, escalating doses may be required to control ICPs or maintain burst suppression.[128] Close monitoring of volume status and cardiac function is essential when using barbiturate coma because hypotension and myocardial depression are common adverse effects.[123] Some data suggest that barbiturates also compromise cerebral venous oxygenation in certain

Table 43.4 Summary of Studies with Mannitol and Hypertonic Saline for the Management of Intracranial Hypertension

MANNITOL

Study Citation	Sample Size	Trial Design	Intervention	Result
Marshall LF, et al.[100]	8	Nonrandomized open-label study of ICP response to mannitol in patients with TBI	Doses of 0.25, 0.5, and 1 g/kg given	Reduction in ICP similar in all three groups from a mean of 44 mm Hg to 17 mm Hg
James HE[101]	60	Nonrandomized open-label study of ICP response to mannitol in patients with various etiologies	Bolus or continuous infusion of mannitol. Doses ranged from 0.18 g/kg to 2.5 g/kg for the bolus dose and 2–20 g/kg over 2–100 hr in the continuous infusion group	For the bolus dose, mean dose response was 56% with mean time to reduction in ICP of 44 min and mean time to return to control ICP of 196 min. Responses were 99%–100% when mannitol dose was ≥ 1 g/kg
				For the continuous infusion dose, 16 of 18 maintained ICP at < 25 mm Hg during the treatment period
Schwartz M, et al.[102]	59	Prospective randomized trial of ICP response to mannitol or pentobarbital in patients with TBI	Mannitol at 1 g/kg (allowed repeat doses) or pentobarbital at 10 mg/kg bolus plus continuous infusion of 0.5–3 mg/kg/hr given to maintain goal ICP at < 20 mm Hg	Both agents equally effective in reducing ICP; however, pentobarbital may be harmful in patients who do not require hematoma evacuation (mortality rate 77% vs. 41%)
Muizelaar JP, et al.[103]	33	Nonrandomized open-label study of ICP response to mannitol in patients with severe TBI	Single bolus dose of mannitol 0.66 g/kg administered	Mannitol reduced ICP by 27% (mean of 16.9 mm Hg to 12.3 mm Hg) in patients with intact autoregulation but by only 4.7% (mean of 16.4 to 14.2 mm Hg) in patients without intact autoregulation
Mendelow AD, et al.[104]	55	Nonrandomized open-label study of ICP response to mannitol in patients with severe TBI	Single bolus dose of mannitol 0.25–0.5 g/kg administered	Statistically significant reductions in ICP from 21.9 mm Hg to 17.2 mm Hg as well as increases in cerebral blood flow (from 43.5 to 50.2 mL/100 g/min)
Smith HP, et al.[105]	80	Prospective randomized trial of neurological outcomes with mannitol in patients with severe TBI	Patients randomized to receive mannitol for ICP > 25 mm Hg or irrespective of ICP. Mannitol administered as an initial bolus dose of 0.75 mg/kg followed by 0.25 g/kg. Patients without ICP monitoring received mannitol q2hr until osmolality > 310 mOsm/L	No difference between the two groups with respect to neurological outcomes or mortality
Vialet R, et al.[106]	20	Prospective randomized trial of ICP response to mannitol in patients with severe TBI	Patients randomized to receive 2 mL/kg of 20% mannitol (175 mOsm) or 7.5% hypertonic saline (360 mOsm)	Mean number of episodes (13.3 vs. 6.9) and duration (67 min vs. 131 min) were higher in the mannitol group (p<0.01)

HYPERTONIC SALINE

Study Citation	Sample Size	Trial Design	Intervention	Result
Qureshi AI, et al.[107]	27	Retrospective, observational study of ICP response to hypertonic saline in patients with cerebral edema from many causes	Continuous infusion of 3% saline/acetate to target serum sodium of 145–155 mEq/L	ICP control in patients with TBI in 12 hr (14 mm Hg to 7 mm Hg). Less shift on CT noted. No reduction in ICP after 24 hr

Table 43.4 Summary of Studies with Mannitol and Hypertonic Saline for the Management of Intracranial Hypertension *(continued)*

HYPERTONIC SALINE

Study Citation	Sample Size	Trial Design	Intervention	Result
Qureshi AI, et al.[108]	82	Retrospective, case-control study of clinical outcomes to hypertonic saline in patients with severe TBI	Continuous infusion of 3% saline/acetate vs. 0.9% saline	Higher in-hospital mortality (OR 3.1), more pentobarbital use (7 vs. 2, p=0.04), and fewer neurological improvements (9 of 36 vs. 25 of 46, p=0.001) in hypertonic saline group
Horn P, et al.[109]	10	Prospective observational study of patients with TBI/SAH with refractory ICP	Bolus of 2 mL/kg of 7.5% hypertonic saline for ICP > 25 mm Hg	Lowered ICP (mean of 33 mm Hg to 19 mm Hg) and increased cerebral blood flow (68–79 mm Hg) in 1 hr
Cooper DJ, et al.[110]	229	Randomized controlled trial of clinical outcomes of patients with severe TBI treated with hypertonic saline in the prehospital setting	Received a single dose of 250 mL of either 7.5% hypertonic saline or lactated Ringer in addition to standard resuscitation	Similar neurological outcomes, hospital and 6-mo mortality in both groups
Ware ML, et al.[111]	13	Retrospective chart review	Received 30 mL of 23.4% hypertonic saline or 0.25–1.9 g/kg of 20% mannitol	Similar reductions in ICP. Longer duration of reduction in 23.4% group
Kerwin AJ, et al.[112]	22	Retrospective chart review	Received 30 mL of 23.4% hypertonic saline or 15–75 g of mannitol	Greater reductions in ICP and more patients responded to 23.4% hypertonic saline

ICP = intracranial pressure; q = every; SAH = subarachnoid hemorrhage.

patients, resulting in negative clinical outcomes. Therefore, some investigators advocate for invasive cerebral oxygenation monitoring when barbiturates are used, although this is not recommended in the Brain Trauma Foundation guidelines.[130] Additional monitoring for potential propylene-glycol toxicity during long-term or high-dose use with either serum propylene glycol concentrations or more readily available osmolar gap should be considered because this is the excipient in the formulation.

Posttraumatic Seizures

Pathophysiology

Posttraumatic seizures are a common complication of TBI, with an incidence of 11% in severe non-penetrating TBI and up to 35%–50% in penetrating TBI.[131] Traumatic brain injury leads to the disruption of neurons, glial cells, and fiber tracts. This disruption can cause the injured neurons to become hyperexcited, leading to seizures.[132] Risk factors for developing seizures include the presence of a depressed skull fracture, subdural or epidural hematoma, GCS score of less than 10 on presentation, intracerebral hematoma, cortical contusions, and loss of consciousness after the event.[133] Posttraumatic seizures are classified into two categories according to their time of onset: early (within 7 days of injury) and late (more than 7 days after injury). The data analyses available suggest that antiepileptic therapy decreases early seizures but has little effect on late seizures.[134] Early studies evaluating the use of antiepileptic agents in patients with TBI were related to the concern that initial seizures increase the risk of future seizures, based on the kindling phenomenon that has been described in epilepsy.[135,136] Although an interesting hypothesis, it appears that early seizures are pathophysiologically different from late seizures and, therefore, do not confer any additional risk to the development of long-term epilepsy.[137] Early seizures appear not to affect clinical outcomes. They can be detrimental in extending secondary injury in patients with severe TBI, however, by elevations in ICP, changes in blood pressure, changes in oxygenation, and so forth. Therefore, preventing early seizures through prophylaxis with antiepileptic agents is a reasonable approach.[138]

Antiepileptic Therapy

Four key studies related to managing early-onset seizures in TBI are reviewed in Table 43.5. Despite some differences in the population demographics, the data overall suggest that prophylaxis for early-onset seizures with either phenytoin or levetiracetam is a reasonable therapeutic option. The lack of significant adverse reactions and drug interactions, ease of dosing, and lower cost have made levetiracetam the preferred agent at many institutions for managing early seizures in patients with TBI.

Spinal Cord Injury

Epidemiology

Spinal injuries are common in trauma patients in the United States. Because of the acutely life-threatening and chronically life-changing consequences of spinal cord injury (SCI), early recognition is very important to guide management and to prevent the progression of secondary injury and further irreversible damage.

Management

The goal of therapy is to stabilize the resulting deficit and to prevent further progression and secondary injury from occurring. Initial treatment of a patient with SCI includes immobilization of the cervical spine in the field, during transport, and during early hospitalization. Airway management is a priority because many of these patients are at risk of hypoxemia from hypoventilation or from aspiration of gastric contents.[143] Equally important is hemodynamic stabilization because patients with SCI may have loss of systemic sympathetic vasomotor tone after the injury, leading to vasodilation, increased venous capacity, and hypotension, as previously noted.

Surgical management of a patient with SCI is indicated for the unstable spine with or without neurological involvement.[144] Goals of therapy include restoration of spinal stability, correction of spinal alignment, and decompression of affected neurons to permit the best neurological recovery possible. The timing of surgical intervention remains controversial because some clinicians believe that early intervention prevents complications of SCI, whereas others favor delayed surgery to ensure hemodynamic stabilization and decrease the bleeding risk, recognizing that perispinal hematomas organize about 48 hours after injury.[144]

Although the primary SCI is irreversible, different therapies to limit secondary injury or potentially reverse it have been evaluated over the years. Methylprednisolone, a glucocorticoid thought to reduce injury-induced lipid peroxidation in the spinal cord, was investigated in three large multicenter clinical trials, collectively called the National Acute Spinal Cord Injury Study (NASCIS), which focused primarily on patients with blunt SCI. In

Table 43.5 Summary of Major Trials for Seizure Prophylaxis After TBI

Study Citation	Sample Size	Trial Design	Intervention	Result
Young B, et al.[139]	244	Prospective, randomized, double-blind trial	Patients received phenytoin with a 20-mg/kg load followed by aggressive monitoring and adjust of phenytoin concentrations achieve a goal of 10–20 mg/dL or placebo	Incidence of early seizure in each group similar (3.7%, p=0.75)
Temkin NR, et al.[140]	404	Prospective, randomized, double-blind trial	Patients received phenytoin with a 20-mg/kg load followed by aggressive monitoring and adjust of phenytoin concentrations achieve a goal of 10–20 mg/dL or placebo	Early seizures occurred in 3.6% of phenytoin patients compared with 14.2% of placebo patients (p<0.001)
Temkin NR, et al.[141]	379	Prospective, randomized, double-blind, parallel-group trial	Patients randomized to receive IV phenytoin at 20 mg/kg followed by a 5-mg/kg/day dose for 7 days, valproate 20 mg/kg followed by 15 mg/kg/day for 1 or 6 mo	Phenytoin group had an early seizure rate of 1.5% compared with 4.5% for the combined valproate groups (p=0.14). There was a trend toward higher mortality in the valproate group (7.2% vs. 13.4%, p=0.07)
Inaba K, et al.[142]	813	Prospective observational	Patients at one hospital received primarily phenytoin at 20 mg/kg load plus a maintenance of 5 mg/kg/day for 7 days. Patients at the other hospital received primarily levetiracetam at 1 g IV q12hr for 7 days	Incidence of early seizure in each group similar (1.5%, p=0.997). The phenytoin group had more adverse reactions and subsequent discontinuation of drug. Levetiracetam group had a longer hospital length of stay (11.8 vs. 7.5 days, p<0.001). All other clinical end points were similar

IV = intravenous(ly).

1990, the NASCIS I trial sought to compare a group receiving a 30-mg/kg bolus of methylprednisolone followed by 5.4 mg/kg intravenously for 23 hours' infusion with a bolus of naloxone 5.4 mg/kg, followed by a continuous infusion of 4 mg/kg/hour, with a placebo group. Naloxone had been postulated to aid in SCI by blocking elevated levels of endogenous endorphins during SCI. A post hoc analysis found an improvement in motor function, sensation to pinprick, and touch in the patient group that had received methylprednisolone within less than 8 hours of injury, whereas treatment with naloxone at any time and treatment with methylprednisolone past the 8-hour mark showed no improvement.[145] The NASCIS II study published the 1-year follow-up results of the NASCIS I trial and reported an improvement in neurological recovery in patients who had received methylprednisolone within the first 8 hours at 6 weeks, 6 months, and 1 year after injury.[146]

In the 1997 NASCIS III study, methylprednisolone was compared with tirilazad, an inhibitor of lipid peroxidation, in a double-blind, randomized, multicenter clinical trial.[147,148] Intravenous methylprednisolone at 30 mg/kg was administered to 499 patients, who were then randomized to receive a 24-hour methylprednisolone infusion at 5.4 mg/kg, a 48-hour infusion at the same rate, or a tirilazad 2.5-mg/kg bolus every 6 hours for 48 hours. The group of patients receiving 48-hour methylprednisolone showed more neurological improvement at 6 weeks and 6 months than the other two groups, and this effect was statistically significant if methylprednisolone was initiated within 3–8 hours of injury.

Despite improvements in American Spinal Injury Association (ASIA) motor and sensory scores in the methylprednisolone groups in the NASCIS II and NASCIS III trials, the studies had confounders that limit the generalizability of the result. These include missing information concerning radiology, surgical intervention, and rehabilitation. In addition, post hoc analyses have failed to note the neurological improvement reported.[149-151]

Of note, the methylprednisolone groups in the NASCIS II and III studies had higher infection rates, in addition to respiratory complications and GI hemorrhage. According to the available evidence, the Consortium for Spinal Cord Medicine, Advanced Trauma Life Support, American Association of Neurological Surgeons, and Cervical Spine Injury clinical practice guidelines all conclude

Table 43.6 Review of Studies Evaluating Enteral vs. Parenteral Nutrition in the Trauma Population

Study Citation	Sample Size	Trial Design	Intervention	Result
Adams S, et al.[177]	46	Prospective, randomized. Trauma patients undergoing emergency laparotomy	TPN or enteral nutrition by jejunostomy starting on postoperative day 1. Patients treated a maximum of 14 days	No difference in complication rates between the two groups. Enteral feeding safe in the early postoperative period
Moore EE, et al.[178]	63	Prospective, randomized. Trauma patients undergoing emergency celiotomy with abdominal trauma index > 15	Control group received D_5W at 100 g/day. Treatment group received elemental feeds within 18 hr of surgery and advanced to goal in 72 hr	Nitrogen balance higher in enteral group ($p<0.001$) at day 7. Overall complication rates similar, but enteral group had fewer septic complications ($p<0.25$)
Moore FA, et al.[179]	59	Prospective, randomized. Trauma patients undergoing emergency laparotomy with abdominal trauma index > 15	TPN or enteral nutrition by jejunostomy starting within 12 hr of surgery infused at a rate to achieve positive nitrogen balance	Nutritional proteins were restored better in the enteral group. Enteral group had fewer infections (3% vs. 20%, $p=0.03$)
Kudsk KA, et al.[180]	98	Prospective, randomized. Trauma patients undergoing emergency laparotomy with abdominal trauma index > 15	TPN or enteral nutrition by jejunostomy starting within 24 hr of surgery	Fewer septic complications in enteral group. Overall fewer infections (0.25 vs. 0.67, $p<0.03$) in the enteral group
Moore FA, et al.[181]	230	Meta-analysis	None	Fewer septic complications in patients with enteral nutrition (18% vs. 35%, $p=0.01$)
Eyer SD, et al.[182]	38	Prospective, randomized. Patients with blunt trauma and ISS > 13	Patients received enteral nutrition by nasoduodenal tube either within 24 hr or after 72 hr of admission	More patients in the early group had P/F ratio < 150 ($p<0.05$). More infections in early treatment (29 vs. 14, $p<0.05$) but very liberal definition of infection

D_5W = dextrose 5%; ISS = injury severity score; TPN = total parenteral nutrition.

that data are insufficient to definitely recommend the use of any neuroprotective agent including steroids.

Because of SCI's devastating consequences, there is ongoing research for novel therapies for patients with SCI. The research focus has been on both neuroprotective and neurogenerative therapies. The target of neuroprotective therapies is decreasing neuroinflammation, reducing free radicals (e.g., thyrotropin-releasing hormone, which showed some benefit in neurological recovery in a 20-patient study), reducing excitotoxic damage to the neurons (NMDA [N-methyl-D-aspartate] antagonist gacyclidine, which did not show a clinical benefit at 1 year post-SCI), improving blood flow (e.g., calcium channel blocker nimodipine, which failed to show benefit), and establishing homeostasis of neurohormones and ions.[152-154]

Neuroprotective agents are aimed at promoting neuronal regeneration and restoration of axonal pathways to improve neurological function. GM1 ganglioside, a glycopeptide naturally found in high concentrations in the central nervous system (CNS), induces neuronal sprouting in vitro and promotes neuronal regeneration. Despite initial promising results, a recent Cochrane review found that GM1 was not beneficial.[155]

Further therapies currently being investigated include rho antagonist, anti-Nogo antibodies, acidic fibroblast growth factor, autologous activated macrophages, and autologous mesenchymal stem cells.[148]

Blunt Injuries to the Thoracic Aorta

Causes and Classification

Blunt injuries to the thoracic aorta are the second most common cause of death in trauma patients, with 80% dying before reaching a trauma center in the pre-airbag era. In the remaining patients who live to reach the hospital, 50% will die within 24 hours.[156] Deaths in patients with injuries to the thoracic aorta are partly related to severe associated injuries if patients do not receive medication to decrease shear stress on the area of injury. Arthurs et al. noted that 31% of patients with blunt aortic injuries had concomitant injuries to the brain, followed by abdominal (29%) and pelvic (15%) injuries.[157] Blunt aortic injuries anatomically involve primarily the descending aorta (up to 65%), followed by an almost equal distribution among the ascending aorta, the distal descending aorta, and those with injuries at several sites.[157] Mechanisms for aortic injury involve shear forces between the relatively mobile part of the vessel next to a fixed portion, compression of the vessel between bony structures, and profound intraluminal hypertension during the traumatic event.[158] Blunt traumatic aortic injuries are different from classic aortic dissections because they are true local tears without intramural dissection. They can be separated into two categories: (1) traumatic true aneurysms, which are partial-thickness tears (intima and part of media of aorta) with blood staying in the lumen; and (2) traumatic false aneurysms, which are full-thickness tears (intima, media, adventitia) with blood outside the lumen (extravasation with free bleeding or into a collection).[159] Blunt aortic injuries are typically diagnosed according to the mechanism of injury and CT angiography findings such as mediastinal hematoma, aortic pseudoaneurysm, variation in aortic contour, intimal flap, and thrombus.[159] Blunt aortic injuries are graded in severity as follows: grade I injury involves intimal tear only, grade II involves intramural hematoma, grade III involves disruption contained within a pseudoaneurysm, and grade IV involves frank rupture.[160]

Management

Surgical repair has long been the standard of care for managing blunt aortic injuries. One of the main challenges in the care of these trauma patients with blunt aortic injuries, as mentioned earlier, is the concomitant injuries that may delay immediate surgical intervention. As such, the Memphis group published two papers on the medical management of these patients with antihypertensive therapy (β-blockers plus vasodilators) until they are stable for surgical intervention, which set the foundation for the medical management of patients with blunt traumatic aortic injuries. The first study evaluated 71 patients for 4 years with blunt aortic injuries, of whom 52 were managed surgically and 19 were managed medically.[161] In the surgical group, seven patients died, with two of the deaths related to aneurysmal rupture. Among the medically managed group, although the mortality was higher because of concomitant injuries (9 of 19 [47%]), none of the patients died of aneurysmal rupture. The second paper evaluated 93 patients who were being assessed for suspected aortic injury.[162] Most of the patients (67) were treated with early surgical repair followed by delayed repair with medical management in the interim (15) and no intervention being tried in 11; 8, 2, and 6 patients, respectively, died in each group. None of the patients in this study died of aortic rupture. Between these two papers, the goals for hemodynamic control involved a heart rate of less than 100 beats/minute and a systolic blood pressure of between 100 mm Hg and 110 mm Hg. These papers established the therapeutic standard with respect to the goals for the medical management of blunt aortic injuries using antihypertensive agents. Also of note is that β-blockade therapy was always initiated first with either intravenous esmolol or labetalol followed by vasodilator therapy with sodium nitroprusside. Current alternatives to sodium nitroprusside such as nicardipine and clevidipine are also used in treating these patients. More recently, a study by Rabin et al. showed that grade I and II injuries were amenable to medical management, whereas grade III and IV injuries benefited from surgical intervention, which helps further clarify the role for the medical management of these patients.[163]

Historically, medical management of blunt aortic injuries was the cornerstone in patients with contraindications to immediate open surgical repair. In the past 2 decades, however, there has been a shift to endovascular repair. Although there are no randomized controlled studies directly comparing open surgical repair with endovascular repair, there has been an increasing trend toward using endovascular repair for these patients.[164] In addition to the advances in and access to newer endovascular technologies, a growing body of literature shows improved outcomes with endovascular repair compared with open surgical repair.[165] Most recently, a meta-analysis from the Eastern Association for the Surgery of Trauma documented a statistically significant reduction in rates of mortality (8% vs. 19%, p=0.04) and paraplegia (0.5% vs. 3%, p=0.01) with no differences in stroke rates (9.1% vs. 6.7%, p=0.69) or renal failure rates (8.6% vs. 9.3%, p=0.70) in patients receiving endovascular repair versus open surgical repair.[166] Of note, there was a fairly high rate of device-related complications (20%) in a 2008 study. However, with improvements in technology, more recent studies have shown only a 2.4% device complication rate during a 2.3-year period.[167,168] With the growing safety and improved outcomes with endovascular repair, the need for temporary control with medical management has decreased in patients with multisystem trauma including blunt aortic injuries. One caveat to these data is that in patients with stable injuries, repair in a delayed fashion seems to have better outcomes than early repair, so medical management can be used in the interim in this subset of patients.[169]

Traumatic Abdominal Injuries

Background

The concept of damage control laparotomy was first proposed by Stone et al. at Grady Memorial Hospital, where they showed that rapidly terminating the surgical procedure in patients with significant abdominal trauma and intraoperative metabolic failure resulted in improved outcomes.[170] The term *damage control*, however, was not coined until almost a decade later by Rotondo et al.[171] The adoption of damage control laparotomy as a surgical intervention to treat patients with blunt or penetrating abdominal trauma, in addition to advances in critical care medicine, has improved survival significantly.[172] These patients, however, often have nutritional depletion, respiratory failure, renal failure, and, occasionally, the development of enteroatmospheric in an open abdomen. Although these complications present later in the ICU stay, they are still important issues for the critical care pharmacist to be aware of and manage.

Management with Nutritional Support

Importance of nutritional support in the trauma patient stems from the 1970s, when multiorgan failure (now called multiorgan dysfunction syndrome [MODS]) evolved as a major clinical challenge in the critically ill trauma patient.[173] It was recognized then that persistent catabolism with consumption of visceral protein stores and delayed immunosuppression were risk factors for MODS. Therefore, a focus of research ensued on the optimal nutritional support for the trauma patient.[174,175] As our understanding of critically illness has evolved, we now recognize a condition termed *persistent inflammation-immunosuppression catabolism syndrome* (PICS), where the interplay between dysfunction of the immune system and protein catabolism may benefit from proper nutritional support as well.[176] In the critically ill trauma patient, provision of nutrition through the appropriate route and at the appropriate dose is an important clinical consideration. Although the mechanisms for how the GI tract affects immune function are unclear, most clinical trials and a meta-analysis support enteral nutrition as the preferred route in trauma patients (Table 43.6). With this in mind, it is important to obtain access to the GI tract as soon as possible to optimize nutritional status, even if it is trophic feeds, based on the most recent publication.[183] Although access to the GI tract can be challenging, there are a variety of nonsurgical methods for access.[184] Jejunal feedings are optimal because of challenges with delayed gastric emptying, gastroesophageal reflux, and reduced lower esophageal sphincter tone (aspiration risk); however, feeding of the stomach in critically ill trauma patients has also been shown as a reasonable approach and may be easily initiated in the ICU with perioral or transgastric techniques.[185-187] When enteral access is truly unobtainable or ill advised (GI discontinuity, open abdomen, persistent shock, etc.), it is reasonable to delay enteral nutrition (5–7 days) instead of initiating early total parenteral nutrition (TPN).[188] In summary, early enteral nutrition is an important therapy in the treatment of trauma patients, and it is reasonable to initiate even in patients with significant abdominal trauma. In addition to reducing septic complications, enteral nutrition may play a role in modulating PICS, although that has yet to be proven in clinical trials.

Complications

Enterocutaneous Fistula—Diagnosis and Management

With the increased use of damage control laparotomies and an associated temporary open abdomen, enterocutaneous fistula (ECF) and enteroatmospheric fistula have emerged as a rather challenging complication to manage.[189] Enterocutaneous fistula is defined as an abnormal communication between the bowel and the skin and is associated with the triad of sepsis, fluid, and electrolyte abnormalities and malnutrition.[190] Enterocutaneous fistula can be classified physiologically as low (less than 200 mL/day), moderate (200–500 mL/day), and high (greater than 500 mL/day) output. The incidence of ECF and enteroatmospheric fistulas in the trauma population ranges from 4.5% to 25% and is associated with significant morbidity and mortality.[191-196] A recent paper by Bradley et al. identified resection of the large bowel, large-volume resuscitation, and multiple re-explorations as common risk factors for developing an ECF in the trauma population.[197] Nutritional optimization is one key to managing ECF, and this is achieved through TPN, which also allows for minimized fistula output and improved wound care.[198] Although some have advocated for the use of enteral nutrition distal to the fistula when feasible, no trials directly compare this with parenteral nutrition.[198,199] Moreover, it is important to maintain appropriate fluid balance and electrolyte concentrations. Replacement of fluid losses from high-output fistulas should occur frequently (every 2–4 hours) to prevent dehydration and acute renal dysfunction. Hypokalemia is the most common electrolyte abnormality related to ECF, especially with those located in the upper GI tract. Therefore, incorporating potassium into the replacement fluid is mandatory. Duodenal or pancreatic fistulas tend to lose bicarbonate ions, so replacement with sodium bicarbonate is a reasonable intervention.[200]

With respect to pharmacotherapy, the only drug that has been evaluated in ECF is somatostatin and its analog octreotide. Somatostatin (and octreotide) has many effects on the GI tract, including enhanced fluid and electrolyte absorption and decreased secretion of gastric acid, pepsin, and bile.[201,202] It suppresses smooth muscle contractility and therefore delays gastric emptying and small bowel motility.[201,202] Because of its longer half-life, octreotide is used more often in the clinical setting.[203] Regarding the role of octreotide in the management of ECF, several trials have been conducted through the years (Table 43.7). Overall, it appears that most of the trials show a reduction in time to closure, but not necessarily an increase in the percentage of patients who successfully close their fistulas. Because octreotide is a rather benign drug, it is not unreasonable to use this as an adjunct for the management of ECF for 2 weeks.

Short Bowel Syndrome—Diagnosis and Management

Another untoward complication of intra-abdominal trauma is short bowel syndrome (SBS).[211,212] Short bowel syndrome is defined as a malabsorptive state after small bowel resection when the length of remnant small bowel is less than 200 cm.[213] Short bowel syndrome in trauma is very rare, occurring in about 8% of trauma patients who were referred for the evaluation of SBS in one series. Injury to the intestinal blood supply was the most common reason (81%) for SBS, followed by direct injury (19%).[214] The median length of small bowel in a human being is around 4 m and is divided into three sections: the duodenum (25–30 cm), the jejunum (160–200 cm), and the ileum (the rest).[215,216] With respect to function, carbohydrate

Table 43.7 Review of Studies Evaluating Somatostatin/Octreotide in the Management of Enterocutaneous Fistula

Study Citation	Sample Size	Trial Design	Intervention	Result
Isenmann et al.[204]	45	Prospective randomized	Somatostatin at 250 mcg/hr plus TPN vs. TPN alone	78% fistula closure in treatment vs. standard care group. Time to closure 13 days vs. 19 days (p=0.013)
Torres et al.[205]	40	Prospective randomized	Somatostatin at 250 mcg/hr plus TPN vs. TPN alone	Time to fistula output 50% and 75% reduction faster in somatostatin group (5.18 vs. 9.2 and 7.53 vs. 13.66, p<0.05)
Leandros et al.[206]	51	Prospective randomized	Somatostatin 250 mcg/hr, octreotide 100 mcg TID, standard care	Closure rate was 84%, 65%, and 27% for somatostatin, octreotide, and control, respectively (p=0.007)
Hernandez-Aranda et al.[207]	85	Prospective randomized	Octreotide 100 mcg TID, standard care	Time to closure 18 days for octreotide vs. 27 days for standard care (p=0.002). Closure rate was 65% vs. 56%
Jamil et al.[208]	33	Prospective randomized	Octreotide 100 mcg TID, standard care	No difference in time to closure. Closure rate was 100% in each group
Sancho et al.[209]	28	Prospective randomized	Octreotide 100 mcg TID, standard care	Time to closure 12 days for octreotide vs. 7 days for standard care (p=NS). Closure rate was 57% vs. 35% (p=NS)
Scott et al.[210]	19	Prospective randomized	Octreotide 100 mcg TID, standard care	Closure rate was 9% vs. 38% (p=NS)

NS = not significant; TID = three times daily

and protein metabolism occurs primarily in the duodenum and jejunum, bile salt and fat-soluble vitamin reabsorption occurs in the ileum, and fluid and electrolytes are absorbed in the ileum and colon. Therefore, SBS is caused by an extensive loss of the absorptive surface area of the small bowel.[217,218] The ability of the small bowel to maintain an adequate nutritional status in the face of such massive resection depends on the extent and location of the resection, presence of the ileocecal valve and colon, adaptation of the intestinal remnant, and nature and complications of underlying disease.[214,219] Normal absorption of nutrients occurs within the first 100 cm of the jejunum; however, in patients for whom there is significant loss of the jejunum, the ileum is able to adapt by hyperplasia.[220,221] The reverse, however, is not true, because specialized cells that manage vitamin B_{12} and bile salt reabsorption cannot be replaced by jejunal hyperplasia.[214] An additional complication in patients missing a significant portion of their ileum is large-volume diarrhea. If the colon is present, it may be able to adapt and significantly reduce water and electrolyte losses.[222] Bacteria in the colon are also able to metabolize unabsorbed carbohydrates into short-chain fatty acids and lactate, which can be absorbed and provide additional calories.[223]

In the patient with SBS, the treatment goals are to optimize nutritional intake, whether it be enteral or intravenous, and manage fluid and electrolyte abnormalities as a result of profound diarrhea. Management of fluid and electrolyte losses will vary according to the sections of small bowel still available; therefore, a key understanding of the functional anatomy of the small bowel is important. Dehydration caused by water and sodium losses can be a result of significant resection of the jejunum (less than 100 cm remaining) in patients with a jejunostomy and should be managed aggressively with appropriate replacement of output with normal saline.[224,225] Additional electrolyte abnormalities such as hypomagnesemia and hypocalcemia tend to be prevalent in the setting of resection of the jejunum as well, as the duodenum and proximal jejunum are absorption sites for these electrolytes.[226] These losses are further exacerbated by their binding to unabsorbed long-chain fatty acids in patients who lack a terminal ileum because the terminal ileum is responsible for the reabsorption of bile salts and fat.[227] The loss of calcium in the GI tract is also of concern because this facilitates the absorption of oxalate, which leads to the development of nephrolithiasis.[228] Replacement of magnesium and calcium should be a key intervention in this group. Of note, calcium is administered orally at 800–1,200 mg daily in divided doses to replace losses and to bind to oxalate present in the GI tract to form insoluble calcium oxalate that is readily eliminated from the body.[229] Replacement of fat-soluble vitamins (A, D, E) is important as well, with the exception of vitamin K because the colon synthesizes most of the supply. Therefore, patients with intact colons do not need replacement.[230-233] The loss of the terminal ileum also results in the inability to absorb vitamin B_{12}, so supplementation is required in these patients.

The many approaches to managing diarrhea include the following: (1) reduce transit time through the GI tract, (2) decrease secretions by the GI tract, and (3) increase the absorptive capacity of the small bowel. Reductions in transit time can be accomplished by opioid or opioid-like agents such as loperamide, codeine, diphenoxylate/atropine, and tincture of opium.[234] One study suggests that loperamide is more efficacious than codeine at reducing the output of an ileostomy; however, the various therapies can be combined for additive effects.[235] Octreotide has been evaluated for reducing the jejunal and ileal output or diarrhea in several small studies, and the overall results show a reduction in ostomy output, at least in the short term (Table 43.8). With respect to increasing absorptive capacity, the two therapeutic options are growth hormone (GH) and teduglutide. Growth hormone is a trophic factor that is thought to increase intestinal absorption. The data presented in Table 43.9 suggest that the overall GH used short term (4 weeks) increases overall intestinal absorption, reduces fecal weight or output, and increases patient weight. Of note, high-carbohydrate diets are necessary to see the benefits of GH therapy, together with concurrent supplementation of glutamine. Teduglutide is a novel GLP (glucagon-like peptide)-2 analog that appears to modulate the expansion of the intestinal mucosa by stimulating crypt cell growth and reducing enterocyte apoptosis.[252] The data presented in Table 43.9 show significant reductions of TPN volume in patients who received teduglutide treatment for 24 weeks, and teduglutide has received U.S. Food and Drug Administration approval for the treatment of patients with SBS.

Acute Kidney Injury

Background

Acute kidney injury is a common complication in the trauma population, especially in patients experiencing significant blood loss and the resulting hypoperfusion.[257] Less severe AKI has been reported at an incidence as high as 30% in the trauma patient.[258] There is a higher in-hospital mortality risk in trauma patients developing AKI, especially in those requiring renal replacement therapy, than in their counterparts without AKI. This risk appears to increase with worsening degree of kidney injury.[259]

In a prospective observational trial, risk factors for developing AKI in the trauma patient included advanced age, higher ISS values (greater than 17), the presence of hemoperitoneum, shock, hypotension or bone fractures, rhabdomyolysis with creatine phosphokinase greater than 10,000 IU/L, presence of respiratory failure requiring mechanical ventilation, and a GCS score less than 10.[260]

Pathophysiology of AKI in Trauma

In the trauma patient, renal function is affected by hypovolemia from hemorrhage, general anesthesia, intraoperative organ manipulation, postoperative fluid shifts, sepsis, rhabdomyolysis, and nephrotoxic agents. In hemorrhagic shock, the kidneys detect hypotension and respond by vasoconstriction of the efferent arterioles, which leads to an increase in renal vascular resistance with a concomitant decrease in renal blood flow.[257] The result is a stable glomerular filtration rate, which permits the excretion of toxins and byproducts. Some blood flow (400 mL/minute) is directed to core areas. The phenomenon is termed *autoregulation* and can be maintained with decreases in renal blood flow of up to 70% of the baseline.[261] Further decreases in blood pressure lead to vasoconstriction of both afferent and efferent arterioles, resulting in decreased glomerular filtration rate. Once systolic blood pressure falls below 70 mm Hg, all blood is shunted away from the kidneys to the systemic circulation, and glomerular filtration ceases, leading to acute renal injury.[257]

Acute kidney injury not only occurs right after massive hemorrhage, but can also occur during surgery after the initial injury. In this case, anesthesia induction leads to hypotension, taking away the compensatory vasoconstriction of the kidneys to maintain glomerular filtration. Combined with hypovolemia secondary to ongoing bleeding, it can lead to acute renal failure and a decrease in urine output that persist even after the operating room.[257] The main goal during surgery is to stabilize hemodynamics by expanding plasma volume with intravenous fluids and blood product transfusion.

After definitive bleeding management in the operating room, patients experience large fluid and electrolyte shifts during the extravascular fluid sequestration phase, which can again lead to decreased cardiac output, renal blood flow, glomerular filtration, and urine output.[257]

Diuresis with loop diuretics and the use of dopamine and fenoldopam as renal vasculature dilators have both fallen out of favor, given evidence of no benefit and potential harm.[262]

Table 43.8 Review of Studies Evaluating Somatostatin/Octreotide in the Management of SBS

Study Citation	Sample Size	Trial Design	Intervention	Result
Dharmsathaphorn K, et al.[236]	4	Open-label study of patients with SBS	Octreotide at 4 mcg/min for 24 hr IV	Reduced fecal weight from 1,892 to 1,236 g/day (p<0.05)
Cooper JC, et al.[237]	5	Double-blind study. Patients with SBS with severe diarrhea (4–7 L)	Octreotide administered at 25 mcg/hr or saline for 3 days	Significantly less ileostomy output in octreotide group (505 g vs. 948 g, p<0.05)
Shaffer JL, et al.[238]	6	Randomized, placebo-controlled, double-blind study. Patients with SBS with high stoma output (> 1.3 L/day)	Octreotide at 50, 100, and 150 mcg/day or placebo	Octreotide significantly reduced ostomy output (2.39 vs. 4.03; p<0.001)
Nightingale JMD, et al.[239]	6	Open-label study. Patients with SBS requiring 4–5 L of IV fluid replacement per day	Octreotide at 100–300 mcg/day	Reduction in stoma output (0.5–5 kg/day)
Rodrigues CA, et al.[240]	4	Open-label study of patients with SBS	Octreotide 50 mcg q6hr	Patients had reduction in transit time and increase in water reabsorption
Ladefoged K, et al.[241]	6	Double-blind placebo-controlled trial of patients with SBS with high stoma output (2–8 L/day)	Octreotide 25 mcg/hr IV short term and 50 mcg q6hr SC long term	Significantly reduced fecal mass (p<0.005) short term but not long term (> 4 mo)
Kusuhara K, et al.[242]	12	Randomized, placebo-controlled study of patients with SBS with high ileostomy output (> 1 L)	Octreotide 300 mcg/day divided SC or placebo for 5 days	Reduced ileostomy output from 997 mL to 736 mL (p<0.05)
O'Keefe SJD, et al.[243]	10	Open-label study of patients with SBS with high jejunostomy output (> 3 L/day)	Octreotide 300 mcg/day divided SC for 10 days	Reduced stoma output from 8.1 L to 4.8 L (p<0.03)
Nightingale JMD[244]	6	Open-label study of patients with SBS with high stoma output	Octreotide 50 mcg IV twice daily	Stoma output reduced in all patients

SBS = short bowel syndrome; SC = subcutaneously.

Table 43.9 Review of Studies Evaluating GH and Teduglutide in the Management of SBS

Study Citation	Sample Size	Trial Design	Intervention	Result
Ellegard L, et al.[245]	10	Randomized, double-blind, placebo-controlled crossover study of patients with SBS	0.17 mg/kg of GH per day or placebo for 8 wk	GH increased weight from 57.3 kg to 59.6 kg ($p<0.05$). No change in absorptive capacity
Byrne TA, et al.[246]	8	Open-label study of patients with SBS requiring some TPN support	0.14 mg/kg GH daily with glutamine supplementation for 3 wk	Significantly increased water, protein, carbohydrate, and calorie absorption. Decreased stool output (1.78 vs. 1.3 kg, $p<0.05$)
Scolapio JS, et al.[247]	8	Randomized, double-blind, placebo-controlled, crossover study of patients with SBS	0.14 mg/kg GH daily with glutamine supplementation and special diet (60% carbohydrates) for 6 wk	Increased weight (mean 3.02, $p<0.05$) and lean mass (3.96, $p<0.05$). Weight returned to normal when therapy stopped
Szkudlarek J, et al.[248]	8	Double-blind, crossover study of patients with SBS	0.14 mg/kg GH daily with glutamine supplementation for 28 days	GH did not increase absorption of nutrients or weight ($p>0.05$)
Seguy D, et al.[249]	12	Randomized, double-blind, placebo-controlled crossover study of patients with SBS on supplemental TPN	0.05 mg/kg GH daily with glutamine supplementation and high carbohydrates for 3 wk	Increased intestinal absorption of energy (15%, $p<0.002$). Body weight and lean mass also increase significantly
Weiming Z, et al.[250]	37	Open-label study of patients with SBS requiring some TPN support	0.05 mg/kg GH daily with glutamine, high carbohydrates for 3 wk	Significantly increased intestinal absorption capacity. 18 of the 23 patients followed for > 2 yr were weaned off TPN
Byrne TA, et al.[251]	41	Randomized, double-blind, placebo-controlled, study of patients with SBS. Three arms of study: glutamine, GH alone, and glutamine + GH	0.1 mg/kg GH daily with glutamine supplementation for 4 wk. 3-mo follow-up	Significant ($p<0.05$) reductions in TPN volume and calories in GH alone group (5.9 L/wk; 4,338 calories/week) and GH + glutamine (7.7 L/wk; 5,751 calories/wk) group compared with glutamine alone. Only group on both glutamine and GH maintained benefits at 3 mo
Jeppesen PB[252]	8	Unblended study of patients with SBS without terminal ileum or colon	Teduglutide 400 mcg SC twice daily for 35 days	Increased intestinal energy absorption (3.5%, $p=0.04$), weight (1.2 kg, $p=0.01$), and transit time (30 min, $p<0.05$)
Jeppesen PB, et al.[253]	19	Randomized unblinded study of three doses of teduglutide in patients with SBS with end jejunostomy	Teduglutide SC once or twice daily at 0.03, 0.1, and 0.15 mg/kg for 21 days	Pooled data show that teduglutide increased wet weight (743 g, $p<0.001$), reduced fecal weight (711 g, $p<0.001$), increased villi height (38%, $p=0.03$) and crypt depth (22%, $p=0.01$)
Jeppesen PB, et al.[254]	83	Randomized, double-blind, placebo-controlled study of patients with SBS	Placebo or teduglutide was administered SC once daily at 0.05 and 0.1 mg/kg for 24 wk	Graded response score based on TPN volume reduction was significant ($p=0.007$) for the 0.05-mg/kg group but not the 0.1 mg/kg group compared with placebo. The discrepancy could be a result of higher TPN volumes in the 0.1-mg/kg group
Jeppesen PB, et al.[255]	43	Randomized, double-blind, placebo-controlled study of patients with SBS requiring TPN supplementation	Placebo or teduglutide was administered SC once daily at 0.05 mg/kg for 24 wk	Significantly higher reduction in TPN weekly volume in the teduglutide group vs. placebo (4.4 L vs. 2.3 L, $p<0.001$)
Vipperla K, et al.[256]	76	Randomized, double-blind, placebo-controlled study of patients with SBS requiring TPN supplementation	Placebo or teduglutide was administered SC once daily at 0.05 mg/kg for 24 wk	Responder rate was 63% in teduglutide group vs. 30% in placebo ($p<0.002$). Responder defined at reduction in TPN volume by 20%–110% at week 24

GH = growth hormone.

Other mechanisms of AKI include crush injuries accompanied by rhabdomyolysis, contrast-induced nephropathy, abdominal hypertension, and use of nephrotoxic medications.

Types and Management

Although trauma patients experience AKI because of various etiologies, only those specific to the trauma population will be covered in this section. To learn about other causes of AKI, please see other chapters in the book.

Rhabdomyolysis-Associated AKI

Rhabdomyolysis is a condition of muscle damage in which there is leakage of muscle cell contents including electrolytes, myoglobin, and other proteins such as creatine phosphokinase into the circulation.[263] The clinical presentation of rhabdomyolysis includes limb weakness, myalgia, swelling, and gross pigmenturia without hematuria.[263] Rhabdomyolysis can be seen in the trauma patient secondary to a direct muscle injury (e.g., blunt trauma or burns) or hypoxic muscle injury (e.g., penetrating trauma, peripheral vascular disease) and accounts for up to 28% of cases of posttraumatic AKI requiring dialysis.[264] AKI is caused by intrarenal vasoconstriction, direct and ischemic injury to the tubules, and renal tubular obstruction by myoglobin.[263]

Renal vasoconstriction occurs as a result of intravascular fluid depletion secondary to fluid sequestration within the damaged muscle, decreased concentrations of the vasodilator nitric oxide, and increased mediators of vasoconstriction such as endothelin-1 and tumor necrosis factor α.[263] In addition, myoglobin is a heme protein containing ferrous oxide (Fe^{2+}). When it binds to oxygen, it forms ferric oxide (Fe^{3+}), a hydroxyl radical that causes injury to renal cells. A creatine phosphokinase concentration greater than 5,000 U/L, a serum creatinine concentration greater than 1.5 mg/dL, a base deficit of -4 or less, and myoglobinuria are predictive of AKI after an episode of rhabdomyolysis.

Management of rhabdomyolysis includes repleting intravascular volume through early, aggressive fluid resuscitation; administering intravenous fluids at 400 mL/hour; and producing a urine output of 3 mL/kg/hour until creatine phosphokinase concentrations are decreased.[265,266] Alkalinization of the urine has the theoretical benefits of decreasing the precipitation of protein-myoglobin complex, inhibiting redox cycling of myoglobin and reducing injury to the tubules, and decreasing vasoconstriction caused by metmyoglobin in the acidic urine.[266] Clinical evidence on the use of sodium bicarbonate has not firmly confirmed its theoretical benefits, but it is important to recognize that hyperchloremic metabolic acidosis can result with the administration of large volumes of 0.9% sodium chloride.[267] In patients who may be at risk of developing hyperchloremic metabolic acidosis, use of sodium bicarbonate may be a reasonable alternative.[263] The use of diuretic in rhabdomyolysis remains controversial. Mannitol, an osmotic diuretic, increases urinary flow by creating a fluid concentration gradient from the injured muscle into the vasculature as well as acting as a free-radical scavenger, but its use has yet to be validated, and higher doses of mannitol can cause renal vasoconstriction and tubular toxicity, leading to renal failure (osmotic nephrosis).[268,269] Diuretics should not be used in patients with hypovolemia.

Renal replacement therapy is indicated in the patient with rhabdomyolysis in whom there are indications for dialysis such as acidosis or volume overload.[270]

Increased Intraperitoneal Pressure–Associated AKI

Trauma patients with massive hemorrhage or late septic shock requiring large-volume resuscitation may develop abdominal compartment syndrome. The increased pressure leads to a reduction in renal blood flow and glomerular filtration rate. Once abdominal decompression has been achieved through celiotomy, renal blood flow is restored, provided interruption was not prolonged and intrinsic renal injury has not taken place.[263]

Extremities: Deep Venous Thrombosis Prophylaxis in Trauma

Epidemiology and Risk Factors

Venous thromboembolism (VTE) is unfortunately a common and potentially life-threatening complication of trauma. The incidence of VTE within the trauma population ranges from 5% to 63% depending on risk factors, mode of detection, and type of prophylaxis; however, a meta-analysis reported a pooled rate of 11.8% for deep venous thrombosis (DVT) and 1.5% for pulmonary embolism.[271-273] The trauma population is at a particularly higher risk than the general population for VTE because it tends to possess most, if not all, of Virchow triad, specifically coagulopathy, vascular injury, and immobility.[274] Vascular injury and immobility are obvious risk factors in the trauma population. The causes of DVT require a deeper understanding of the pathophysiologic changes related to traumatic injury. The data suggest that several changes in the clotting cascade occur, specifically decreases in antithrombin III, decreases in proteins C and S, suppression of fibrinolysis, increases in tissue factor release, and increases in thrombin generation.[275-281] A multivariate analysis in the prospective study by Geerts et al. established that the major clinical risk factors for VTE in trauma were age, blood transfusions, surgery, fractures of the femur or tibia, and injury to the spinal cord.[282] In addition, a study by Knudson et al. highlighted that patients with traumatic injuries who were immobile for more than 3 days or who had either pelvic or lower extremity fractures were also at high risk of VTE.[283]

Prevention

With trauma patients carrying several risk factors, pharmacologic prophylaxis for VTE prophylaxis is imperative. Table 43.10 summarizes these data. Of note, both studies by Knudson et al. had low DVT rates and were therefore underpowered to find a difference.[283,285] The landmark study that established enoxaparin as the drug of choice for DVT prophylaxis in the trauma population was conducted by Geerts et al. and compared heparin 5,000 units with enoxaparin 30 mg given subcutaneously twice daily.[286] Some have challenged the use of venography in this study as an oversensitive detector of clinically asymptomatic VTEs; however, venography was the gold standard at the time of this study. With respect to the significance of asymptomatic VTEs, practice dictates their detection, and the risk of pulmonary embolisms warrants management. Despite the lack of randomized controlled trials evaluating low-molecular-weight heparins in patients with trauma since the Geerts et al. study, the strength of recommendation for low-molecular-weight heparin fell from a 1A recommendation to a 2C in the most recent iteration of the CHEST guidelines.[287,288] The reason for this change is based on the redefining of a "significant event" from including any type of VTE to including only fatal pulmonary embolism, nonfatal pulmonary embolism, and symptomatic DVT or VTE.[287,288] Nonetheless, low-molecular-weight heparins continue to play a pivotal role in preventing VTE in trauma patients. Figure 43.1 is a suggested algorithm for evaluating a trauma patient for VTE prophylaxis given the data discussed in this chapter.

VTE Pharmacologic Prophylaxis Timing and Dosing

In addition to selecting the optimal agent, the time to initiate DVT prophylaxis in the critically ill trauma patient can be challenging. Injuries in which the consequences of bleeding are high include TBI, injuries to solid organ (liver, spleen, kidney), and injuries to the spinal cord, and the clinician may be hesitant to initiate early prophylactic therapy. Nathens et al. performed a retrospective analysis of concurrently collected data on 315 trauma patients who were divided into three groups as follows: patients with DVT prophylaxis initiated within 48 hours, patients who received no DVT prophylaxis, and patients who received DVT prophylaxis after at least 7 days of injury.[289] The data showed a 3-fold increased risk of DVT when therapy was delayed beyond 4 days (risk ratio -3; 95% CI, 1.4–6.5). A second study by Aito et al. of 275 patients with injury to the spinal cord also showed a trend toward fewer DVTs in patients who received DVT prophylaxis within 3 days than in those who received DVT prophylaxis 8–28 days later (2% vs. 26%).[290] A more recent prospective study by Stannard et al. of 224 patients showed that those who had early mechanical prophylaxis followed by delayed pharmacologic prophylaxis had DVT rates similar to those who had early pharmacologic prophylaxis. This study, however, excluded patients with severe TBI and SCIs who are known to be at high risk.[291] Two studies have evaluated the safety of early pharmacologic prophylaxis in high-risk DVT populations. Alejandro et al. evaluated bleeding risks in a retrospective analysis of 188 trauma patients who received low-molecular-weight heparin after blunt splenic injuries.[292] Patients who were initiated on DVT prophylaxis early (less than 48 hours) had similar nonoperative management failures (4% vs. 6%, p=0.593) and transfusion requirements (50 vs. 56.2%, p=0.507). A retrospective analysis by Eberle et al. of 312 trauma patients with blunt abdominal organ injuries who were treated nonoperatively showed that the patients who were initiated on DVT prophylaxis within 48 hours of injury had rates of failure of nonoperative management and bleeding rates similar to those who were initiated early.[293] Although the early initiation group had a lower ISS, they had risk factors for bleeding similar to those of the group

Table 43.10 Review of Studies Evaluating Pharmacologic DVT Prophylaxis in Trauma Patients

Study Citation	Sample Size	Trial Design	Intervention	Result
Dennis JW, et al.[284]	281	Prospective, randomized trial	Heparin 5,000 units q12hr vs. SCDs	DVT rate – 2.9% vs. 8.8%, respectively (p=0.02)
Knudson MM, et al.[283]	251	Prospective, randomized trial	Heparin 5,000 units q12hr vs. SCDs vs. control	No. of DVTs – 2 vs. 4 vs. 9, respectively (p=0.057)
Knudson MM, et al.[285]	372	Prospective, randomized trial	Enoxaparin 30 mg q12hr vs. SCD vs. atrioventricular impulse device	No. of DVTs – 1 vs. 5 vs. 3 (p=NS)
Geerts et al.[286]	344	Prospective, randomized, double-blind trial	Enoxaparin 30 mg q12hr vs. heparin 5,000 units q12hr	DVT rate – 31% vs. 44%, respectively (p=0.014)

DVT = deep venous thrombosis; SCD = sequential compression device.

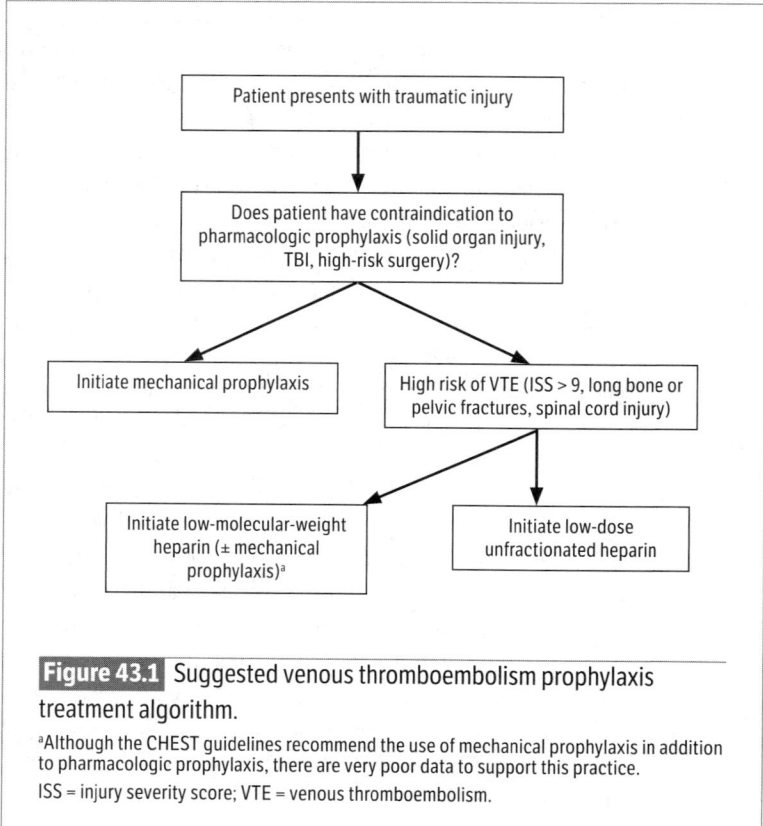

Figure 43.1 Suggested venous thromboembolism prophylaxis treatment algorithm.

aAlthough the CHEST guidelines recommend the use of mechanical prophylaxis in addition to pharmacologic prophylaxis, there are very poor data to support this practice.
ISS = injury severity score; VTE = venous thromboembolism.

with late initiation of prophylaxis. A prospective observational study by Norwood et al. of 525 patients with TBI (mean GCS score of 10 – moderate TBI) who were initiated on DVT prophylaxis with enoxaparin within 48 hours of injury showed that 3.4% (n=18) of patients developed progressive hemorrhage after the initiation of enoxaparin, although most (n=12) had no change in neurological status or outcome.[294] Of note, 10 of the 18 patients with further hemorrhage had protocol violations in which enoxaparin was initiated before the repeat CT of the brain at 24 hours (75 protocol violations for the entire study). If these were excluded, this would have reduced the rate further to 1.8%. Because of these findings, the authors concluded that early enoxaparin is a reasonable intervention in the population with TBI, although only after a stable repeat head CT at 24 hours. Because of the limited data, neither the Brain Trauma Foundation guidelines nor the Eastern Association for the Surgery of Trauma guidelines for the nonoperative management of blunt splenic or hepatic injury make a recommendation for the timing of VTE prophylaxis at this time.[295,296]

The final challenge with VTE prophylaxis is dosing. Although no clinical outcome data are currently associated with the dosing of VTE prophylaxis, an astute clinician should consider the following. In a pharmacokinetic study of trauma patients, Haas et al. showed that the antifactor Xa activity of 30 mg of subcutaneous enoxaparin is highly variable and drops below the therapeutic range of 0.1–0.2 IU/mL, especially in patients with profound edema (greater than 10 kg).[297] A pharmacokinetic study by Rutherford et al. that evaluated a subcutaneous injection of 40 mg once daily in trauma patients also showed that, although mean peak activity was therapeutic, mean trough concentrations were well below the therapeutic target range (mean 0.044 IU/mL). The authors recommended against this regimen for routine prophylaxis in the trauma population.[298] Most recently, a paper by Costantini et al. recommended a protocol for adjusting the enoxaparin dose to achieve therapeutic peak concentrations of 0.2–0.4 IU/mL and showed no increased bleeding with the higher doses (range 40–60 mg twice daily).[299] In summary, these papers highlight the pharmacokinetic derangements that occur in the critically ill trauma patient. Further study is warranted to assess whether an adjustment in the dose of enoxaparin reduces VTE rates without worsening the bleeding risk.

In conclusion, drug therapy plays a critical role in managing the various conditions that patients with traumatic injuries may experience. Knowledge of the complex interaction between the pathophysiologic changes that occur in trauma and drug therapy is essential for the pharmacist to provide optimal clinical care to these patients. This chapter is not all-inclusive because it pertains to drug therapy in trauma, but it is a primer for the major pharmacotherapy needs of this population and will assist the clinician in providing that optimal care.

REFERENCES

1. Centers for Disease Control and Prevention, National Center for Injury Prevention and Control. Web-Based Injury Statistics Query and Reporting System (WISQARS). Available at www.cdc.gov/injury/wisqars/. Accessed April 10, 2015.

2. Finkelstein EA, Corso PS, Miller TR. The Incidence and Economic Burden of Injuries in the United States. Oxford: Oxford University Press, 2006.

3. Codner PA, Brasel KJ. Initial assessment and management. In: Mattox KL, Moore EE, Feliciano DV, eds. Trauma, 7th ed. New York: McGraw-Hill, 2013.

4. American College of Surgeons Committee on Trauma. Advanced Trauma Life Support for Doctors, 8th ed. Chicago: American College of Surgeons Committee, 2008:1-18.

5. Jubran A. Pulse oximetry. Crit Care 1999;3:R11-R17.

6. Kragh JF, Walters TJ, Baer DG, et al. Survival with emergency tourniquet use to stop bleeding in major limb trauma. Ann Surg 2009;249:1-7.

7. Rozycki GS, Oschner MG, Jaffin JH, et al. Prospective evaluation of surgeons' use of ultrasound in the evaluation of trauma patients. J Trauma 1993;34:516-27.

8. Dolich MO, McKenney MG, Varela JE, et al. 2576 ultrasounds for blunt abdominal trauma. J Trauma 2001;50:108-12.

9. Rozycki GS, Feliciano DV, Ochsner MG, et al. The role of ultrasound in patients with possible penetrating cardiac wounds: a prospective multicenter study. J Trauma 1999;46:542-52.

10. Alarcon LH, Puyana JC, Peitzman AB. Management of shock: introduction. In: Mattox KL, Moore EE, Feliciano DV, eds. Trauma, 7th ed. New York: McGraw-Hill, 2013.

11. Gutierrez G, Reines HD, Wulf-Gutierrez ME. Clinical review: hemorrhagic shock. Crit Care 2004;8:373-81.

12. Lucas CE. The water of life: a century of confusion. J Am Coll Surg 2001;192:86-93.

13. American College of Surgeons Committee on Trauma. Advanced Trauma Life Support for Doctors. Chicago: American College of Surgeons, 2009.

14. Tisherman SA, Barie P, Bokhari F, et al. Clinical practice guidelines: endpoints of resuscitation. J Trauma 2004;57:898-912.

15. Finfer SR, Vincent JL. Resuscitation fluids. N Engl J Med 2013;369:1243-51.

16. Rizoli S. PlasmaLyte. J Trauma 2011;70:S17-18.

17. Young JB, Utter GH, Schermer CR, et al. Saline versus Plasma-Lyte A in initial resuscitation of trauma patients. A randomized trial. Ann Surg 2014;259:255-62.

18. Finfer S, Bellomo R, Boyce N, et al. A comparison of albumin and saline for fluid resuscitation in the intensive care unit. N Engl J Med 2004;350:2247-56.

19. SAFE Study Investigators. Saline or albumin for fluid resuscitation in patients with traumatic brain injury. N Engl J Med 2007;357:874-84.

20. Annane D, Siami S, Jaber S, et al. Effects of fluid resuscitation with colloids vs crystalloids on mortality in critically ill patients presenting with hypovolemic shock. The CRISTAL randomized trial. JAMA 2013;310:1809-17.

21. Busuito C, Ledgerwood AM, Lucas CE. Colloid with high fresh frozen plasma/red blood cell resuscitation does not reduce postoperative fluid needs. J Trauma Acute Care Surg 2014;76:1008-12.

22. Myburgh JA, Finfer S, Bellomo R, et al. Hydroxyethyl starch or saline for fluid resuscitation in intensive care. N Engl J Med 2012;367:1901-11.

23. Zarychanski R, Abou-Setta A, Turgeon A, et al. Association of hydroxyethyl starch administration with mortality and acute kidney injury in critically ill patients requiring volume resuscitation. A systematic review and meta-analysis. JAMA 2013;309:678-88.

24. Fraga GP, Bansal V, Coimbra R. Transfusion of blood products in trauma: an update. J Emerg Med 2010;39:253-60.

25. Cap A, Hunt B. The pathogenesis of traumatic coagulopathy. Anaesthesia 2015;70(suppl 1):96-101.

26. Kauvar DS, Lefering R, Wade CE. Impact of hemorrhage on trauma outcome: an overview of epidemiology, clinical presentations, and therapeutic considerations. J Trauma 2006;60(6 suppl):S3-11.

27. Tieu BH, Holcomb JB, Schreiber MA. Coagulopathy: its pathophysiology and treatment in the injured patient. World J Surg 2007;31:1055-64.

28. Valeri CR, Khuri S, Ragno G. Nonsurgical bleeding diathesis in anemic thrombocytopenic patients: role of temperature, red blood cells, platelets, and plasma-clotting proteins. Transfusion 2007;47:S206-48.

29. Wolberg AS, Meng ZH, Monroe DM III, et al. A systematic evaluation of the effect of temperature on coagulation enzyme activity and platelet function. J Trauma 2004;56:1221-8.

30. Martini WZ, Pusateri AE, Uscilowicz JM, et al. Independent contributions of hypothermia and acidosis to coagulopathy in swine. J Trauma 2005;58:1002-9.

31. Alam HB, Velmahos GC. New trends in resuscitation. Curr Probl Surg 2011;48:531-64.

32. Kobayashi L, Costantini TW, Coimbra R. Hypovolemic shock resuscitation. Surg Clin North Am 2012;92:1403-23.

33. ATLS Subcommittee. Advanced trauma life support (ATLS®): the ninth edition. J Trauma Acute Care Surg 2013;74:1363-6.

34. Bickell WH, Wall MJ, Pepe PE, et al. Immediate versus delayed fluid resuscitation for hypotensive patients with penetrating torso injuries. N Engl J Med 1994;331:1105-9.

35. Wang CH, Hsieh WH, Chou HC, et al. Liberal versus restricted fluid resuscitation strategies in trauma patients: a systematic review and meta-analysis of randomized controlled trials and observational studies. Crit Care Med 2014;42:954-61.

36. Borgman MA, Spinella PC, Perkins JG, et al. The ratio of blood products transfused affects mortality in patients receiving massive transfusions at a combat support hospital. J Trauma 2007;63:805-13.

37. Holcomb JB, Wade CE, Michalek JE, et al. Increased plasma and platelet to red blood cell ratios improves outcome in 466 massively transfused civilian trauma patients. Ann Surg 2008;248:447-58.

38. Holcomb JB, Tilley BC, Baraniuk S, et al. Transfusion of plasma, platelets, and red blood cells in a 1:1:1 vs. a 1:1:2 ratio and mortality in patients with severe trauma. JAMA 2015;313:471-82.

39. Kobayashi L, Costantini TW, Coimbra R. Hypovolemic shock. Surg Clin North Am 2012;92:1403-23.

40. Boffard KD, Riou B, Warren B, et al. Recombinant factor VIIa as adjunctive therapy for bleeding control in severely injured trauma patients: two parallel randomized, placebo-controlled, double-blind clinical trials. J Trauma 2005;59:8-15.

41. Rizoli SB, Boffard KD, Riou B, et al. Recombinant activated factor VII as an adjunctive therapy for bleeding control in severe trauma patients with coagulopathy: subgroup analysis from two randomized trials. Crit Care 2006;10:R178.

42. Hauser CJ, Boffard K, Dutton R, et al. Results of the CONTROL trial: efficacy and safety of recombinant activated factor VII in the management of refractory traumatic hemorrhage. J Trauma 2010;69:489-500.

43. Bebulin®. Available at www.baxter.com/downloads/healthcare_professionals/products/bebulin_pi.pdf. Accessed June 6, 2015.

44. Profilnine® SD. Available at www.fda.gov/ucm/groups/fdagov-public/@fdagov-biogen/documents/document/ucm261964.pdf. Accessed June 6, 2015.

45. Kcentra®. Available at www.labeling.cslbehring.com/PI/US/Kcentra/EN/Kcentra-Prescribing-Information.pdf. Accessed June 6, 2015.

46. Octaplex®. Available at www.octapharma.ca/fileadmin/user_upload/octapharma.ca/20120613_PM_Octaplex_approved.pdf. Accessed June 6, 2015.
47. Nienaber U, Innerhofer P, Westermann I, et al. The impact of fresh frozen plasma vs. coagulation factor concentrates on morbidity and mortality in trauma-associated haemorrhage and massive transfusion. Injury 2011;42:697-701.
48. CRASH-2 trial collaborators, Shakur H, Roberts I, et al. Effects of tranexamic acid on death, vascular occlusive events, and blood transfusion in trauma patients with significant haemorrhage (CRASH-2): a randomised, placebo-controlled trial. Lancet 2010;376:23-32.
49. CRASH-2 trial collaborators, Roberts I, Shakur H, et al. The importance of early treatment with tranexamic acid in bleeding trauma patients: an exploratory analysis of the CRASH-2 randomised controlled trial. Lancet 2011;377:1096-101.
50. Morrison JJ, Dubose JJ, Rasmussen TE, et al. Military application of tranexamic acid in trauma emergency resuscitation (MATTERs) study. Arch Surg 2012;147:113-9.
51. Morrison JJ, Ross JD, Dubose JJ, et al. Association of cryoprecipitate and tranexamic acid with improved survival following wartime injury. JAMA Surg 2013;148:218-25.
52. Harrigan MR, Falola MI, Shannon CN, et al. Incidence and trends in the diagnosis of traumatic extracranial cerebrovascular injury nationwide inpatient sample database, 2003-2010. J Neurotrauma 2014;31:1056-62.
53. Davis JW, Holbrook TL, Hoyt DB, et al. Blunt carotid artery dissection: incidence, associated injuries, screening and treatment. J Trauma 1990;30:1514-7.
54. Fusco MR, Harrigan MR. Cerebrovascular dissections: a review. Part II: blunt cerebrovascular injury. Neurosurgery 2011;68:517-30.
55. Biffl WL, Moore EE, Offner PJ, et al. Optimizing screening for blunt cerebrovascular injuries. Am J Surg 1991;178:517-22.
56. Singh RR, Barry MC, Ireland A, et al. Current diagnosis and management of blunt internal carotid artery injury. Eur J Vasc Endovasc Surg 2004;27:577-84.
57. Burlew CC, Biffl WL. Blunt cerebrovascular trauma. Curr Opin Crit Care 2010;16:587-95.
58. Cogbill TH, Moore EE, Meissner M, et al. The spectrum of blunt injury to the carotid canal: a multicenter perspective. J Trauma 1994;37:473-9.
59. Cothren CC, Moore EE, Biffl WL. Anticoagulation is the gold standard therapy for blunt carotid injuries to reduce stroke. Arch Surg 2004;139:540-5.
60. Bromberg WJ, Collier BC, Diebel LN, et al. Blunt cerebrovascular injury practice management guidelines: the Eastern Association for the Surgery of Trauma. J Trauma 2010;68:471-7.
61. Biffl WL, Moore EE, Offner PJ, et al. Blunt carotid arterial injuries: implications of a new grading scale. J Trauma 1999;47:845-53.
62. Troop BR, Carr SC, Hurley JJ, et al. Blunt carotid injuries. Contemp Surg 1996;48:280-4.
63. Perry MO, Snyder WH, Thal ER. Carotid artery injuries caused by blunt trauma. Ann Surg 1980;192:74-7.
64. Martin RF, Eldrup-Jorgensen J, Clark DE, et al. Blunt trauma to the carotid arteries. J Vasc Surg 1991;14:789-93.
65. Unger SW, Tucker WS Jr, Mrdeza MA, et al. Carotid arterial trauma. Surgery 1980;87:477-87.
66. Ramadan R, Rutledge R, Oller D, et al. Carotid artery trauma: a review of contemporary trauma center experiences. J Vasc Surg 1995;21:46-55.
67. Fabian TC, George SM, Croce MA, et al. Carotid artery trauma: management based on mechanism of injury. J Trauma 1990;30:953-61.
68. Cogbill TH, Ernst EE, Meissner M, et al. The spectrum of blunt injury to the carotid artery: a multi-center perspective. J Trauma 1994;37:473-9.
69. Fabian TC, Patton JH Jr, Croce MA, et al. Blunt carotid injury. Importance of early diagnosis and anticoagulant therapy. Ann Surg 1996;223:513-25.
70. Kraus RR, Bergstein JM, DeBord JR. Diagnosis, treatment and outcomes of blunt carotid arterial injuries. Am J Surg 1998;178:190-3.
71. Biffl WL, Moore EE, Ryu RK, et al. The unrecognized epidemic of blunt carotid arterial injuries: early diagnosis improves neurologic outcome. Ann Surg 1998;228:462-70.
72. Davis JW, Holbrook TL, Hoyt DB, et al. Blunt carotid artery dissection: incidence, associated injury, screening, and treatment. J Trauma 1990;30:1514-7.
73. Parikh AA, Luchette FA, Valente JF, et al. Blunt carotid artery injuries. J Am Coll Surg 1997;185:80-6.
74. Francis JL, Groce JB, and the Heparin Consensus Group. Challenges in variation and responsiveness of unfractionated heparin. Pharmacotherapy 2004;24:108S-19S.
75. Wahl WL, Brandt MM, Thompson BG, et al. Antiplatelet therapy: an alternative to heparin for blunt carotid injury. J Trauma 2002;52:896-901.
76. Cothren CC, Biffl WL, Moore EE, et al. Treatment for blunt cerebrovascular injuries: equivalence of anticoagulation and antiplatelet agents. Arch Surg 2009;144:685-90.
77. Morton RP, Hanak BW, Levitt MR, et al. Blunt traumatic occlusion of the internal carotid and vertebral arteries. J Neurosurg 2014;120:1446-50.
78. Biffl WL, Ray CE, Moore EE, et al. Treatment-related outcomes from blunt cerebrovascular injuries: importance of routine follow-up arteriography. Ann Surg 2002;235:699-707.
79. Edwards NM, Fabian TC, Claridge JA, et al. Antithrombotic therapy and endovascular stents are effective treatment for blunt carotid injuries: results from long-term follow up. J Am Coll Surg 2007;204:1007-15.
80. DiCocco JM, Fabian TC, Emmett KP, et al. Optimal outcomes for patients with blunt cerebrovascular injury (BCVI): tailoring treatment to the lesion. J Am Coll Surg 2011;212:549-59.
81. Cothren CC, Moore EE, Ray CE, et al. Carotid artery stents for blunt cerebrovascular injury: risks exceed benefits. Arch Surg 2005;140:480-5.
82. Post AF, Boro T, Ecklund JM, et al. Injury to the brain. In: Mattox KL, Moore EE, Feliciano DV, eds. Trauma, 7th ed. New York: McGraw-Hill, 2013:chap 19. Available at http://accesssurgery.mhmedical.com/content.aspx?bookid=529&Sectionid=41077259. Accessed May 29, 2015.

83. Clark RS, Bayir H, Chu CT, et al. Autophagy is increased in mice after traumatic brain injury and is detectable in human brain after trauma and critical illness. Autophagy 2008;4:88-90.
84. Lai Y, Hickey RW, Chen Y, et al. Autophagy is increased after traumatic brain injury in mice and is partially inhibited by the anti-oxidant gamma-glutamylcysteinyl ethyl ester. J Cereb Blood Flow Metab 2008;28:540-5.
85. Morganti-Kossmann MC, Rancan M, Stahel PF, et al. Inflammatory response in acute traumatic brain injury: a double edged sword. Curr Opin Crit Care 2002;8:101-5.
86. Kroemer G, Galluzzi L, Brennner C. Mitochondrial membrane permeabilization in cell death. Physiol Rev 2007;87:99-163.
87. Chesnut RM, Marshall LF, Klauber MR, et al. The role of secondary brain injury in determining outcome from severe head injury. J Trauma 1993;34:216-22.
88. CRASH Trial Collaborators. Effect of intravenous corticosteroids on death within 14 days in 10,008 adults with clinically significant head injury (MRC CRASH Trial): randomized placebo-controlled trial. Lancet 2004;364:1321-8.
89. Edwards P, Arango M, Balica L, et al. Final results of MRC CRASH, a randomised placebo-controlled trial of intravenous corticosteroid in adults with head injury-outcomes at 6 months. Lancet 2005;365:1957-9.
90. Maas AIR, Murray G, Henney H III, et al. Efficacy and safety of dexanabinol in severe traumatic brain injury: results of a phase III randomized, placebo-controlled clinical trial. Lancet Neurol 2006;5:38-45.
91. Temkin NR, Anderson GD, Winn HR, et al. Magnesium sulfate for neuroprotection after traumatic brain injury: a randomized controlled trial. Lancet Neurol 2007;6:29-38.
92. Skolnick BE, Maas AI, Narayan RK, et al. A clinical trial of progesterone for severe traumatic brain injury. N Engl J Med 2014;371:2467-76.
93. Wright DW, Yeatts SD, Silbergleit R, et al. Very early administration of progesterone for acute traumatic brain injury. N Engl J Med 2014;371:2457-66.
94. Narayan RK, Greenberg RP, Miller JD, et al. Improved confidence of outcome prediction in severe head injury. J Neurosurg 1981;54:751-62.
95. Vincent JL, Berre J. Primer on the medical management of severe traumatic brain injury. Crit Care Med 2005;33:1392-9.
96. Rothman SM, Olney JW. Glutamate and the patho-physiology of hypoxic-ischemic brain damage. Ann Neurol 1986;19:105-11.
97. Siesjo BK, Bengtsson F, Grampp W, et al. Calcium excitotoxins, and neuronal death in the brain. Ann N Y Acad Sci 1989;568:234-51.
98. Choi DW. Ionic dependence of glutamate neurotoxicity. J Neurosci 1987;7:369-79.
99. Xiao F. Bench to bedside: brain edema and cerebral resuscitation: the present and future. Acad Emerg Med 2002;9:933-46.
100. Marshall LF, Smith RW, Rauscher LA, et al. Mannitol dose requirements in brain-injured patients. J Neurosurg 1978;48:169-72.
101. James HE. Methodology for the control of intracranial pressure with hypertonic mannitol. Acta Neurochir (Wien) 1980;51:161-72.
102. Schwartz M, Tator C, Rowed D, et al. The University of Toronto head injury treatment study: a prospective, randomized comparison of pentobarbital and mannitol. Can J Neurol Sci 1984;11:434-40.
103. Muizelaar JP, Lutz HA, Becker DP. Effect of mannitol on ICP and CBF and correlation with pressure autoregulation in severely head injured patients. J Neurosurg 1984;61:100-6.
104. Mendelow AD, Teasdale GM, Russell T, et al. Effect of mannitol on cerebral blood flow and cerebral perfusion pressure in human head injury. J Neurosurg 1985;63:43-8.
105. Smith HP, Kelley DL, McWhorter JM, et al. Comparison of mannitol regimens in patients with severe head injury undergoing intracranial monitoring. J Neurosurg 1986;65:820-4.
106. Vialet R, Albanese J, Thomachot L, et al. Isovolume hypertonic solutes (sodium chloride or mannitol) in the treatment of refractory posttraumatic intracranial hypertension: 2 mL/kg 7.5% saline is more effective than 2 mL/kg 20% mannitol. Crit Care Med 2003;31:1683-7.
107. Qureshi AI, Suarez JI, Bhardwaj A, et al. Use of hypertonic (3%) saline/acetate infusion in the treatment of cerebral edema: effect on intracranial pressure and lateral displacement of the brain. Crit Care Med 1998;26:440-6.
108. Qureshi AI, Suarez JI, Castro A, et al. Use of hypertonic saline/acetate infusion in treatment of cerebral edema in patients with head trauma: experience at a single center. J Trauma 1999;47:659-65.
109. Horn P, Münch E, Vajkoczy P, et al. Hypertonic saline solution for control of elevated intracranial pressure in patients with exhausted response to mannitol and barbiturates. Neurol Res 1999;21:758-64.
110. Cooper DJ, Myles PS, McDermott FT, et al. Prehospital hypertonic saline resuscitation of patients with hypotension and severe traumatic brain injury: a randomized controlled trial. JAMA 2004;291:1350.
111. Ware ML, Nemani VM, Meeker M, et al. Effects of 23.4% sodium chloride solution in reducing intracranial pressure in patients with traumatic brain injury: a preliminary study. Neurosurgery 2005;57:727-36.
112. Kerwin AJ, Schinco MA, Tepas JJ III, et al. The use of 23.4% hypertonic saline for the management of elevated intracranial pressure in patients with severe traumatic brain injury: a pilot study. J Trauma 2009;67:277-82.
113. Doyle JA, Davis DP, Hoyt DB. The use of hypertonic saline in the treatment of traumatic brain injury. J Trauma 2001;50:367-83.
114. Holcroft J, Vassar M, Turner JE, et al. 3% NaCl and 7.5% NaCl dextran for resuscitation of severely injured patients. Ann Surg 1987;206:278-88.
115. Vassar MJ, Perry CA, Gannaway WL, et al. 7.5% sodium chloride/dextran for resuscitation of trauma patients undergoing helicopter transport. Arch Surg 1991;126:1065-72.
116. Vassar MJ, Perry CA, Holcroft JW. Prehospital resuscitation of hypotensive trauma patients with 7.5% sodium chloride versus 7.5% sodium chloride with added dextran: a controlled trial. J Trauma 1993;34:622-32.
117. Vassar MJ, Fischer RP, O'Brien PE. A multicenter trial for resuscitation for resuscitation of injured patients with 7.5% sodium chloride. The effect of added dextran 70. The Multicenter

118. Wade C, Grady J, Kramer G, et al. Individual patient cohort analysis of the efficacy of hypertonic saline/dextran in patients with traumatic brain injury and hypotension. J Trauma 1997;42:S61-5.
117. group for the study of hypertonic saline in trauma patients. Arch Surg 1993;128:1003-13.
119. Kamel H, Navi BB, Nakagawa K, et al. Hypertonic saline versus mannitol for the treatment of elevated intracranial pressure: a meta-analysis of randomized clinical trials. Crit Care Med 2011;39:554-9.
120. White H, Cook D, Venkatesh B. The use of hypertonic saline for treating intracranial hypertension after traumatic brain injury. Anesth Analg 2006;102:1836-46.
121. Forsyth LL, Liu-DeRyke X, Parker D Jr, et al. Role of hypertonic saline in the management of intracranial hypertension after stroke and traumatic brain injury. Pharmacotherapy 2008;28:469-84.
122. Qureshi AI, Suarez JI, Bhardwaj A. Malignant cerebral edema in patients with hypertensive intracerebral hemorrhage associated with hypertonic saline infusion: a rebound phenomenon? J Neurosurg Anesthesiol 1998;10:188-92.
123. Gross AK, Norman J, Cook AM. Contemporary pharmacologic issues in the management of traumatic brain injury. J Pharm Pract 2010;23:425-40.
124. Bratton S, Bullock MR, Carney N, et al. Guidelines for the management of severe head injury. Brain Trauma Foundation. J Neurotrauma 2007;24(suppl 1):S1-S106.
125. Lee MW, Deppe SA, Sipperly ME, et al. The efficacy of barbiturate coma in the management of uncontrolled intracranial hypertension following neurosurgical trauma. J Neurosurg 1994;11:325-31.
126. Cook AM, Weant KA. Pharmacological therapies for the treatment of elevated intracranial pressure: focus on metabolic suppression. Adv Emerg Nurs J 2007;29:309-18.
127. Eisenberg HM, Frankowski RF, Contant CF, et al. High-dose barbiturate control of elevated intracranial pressure in patients with severe head injury. J Neurosurg 1988;69:15-23.
128. Wermeling D, Blouin R, Porter W, et al. Pentobarbital pharmacokinetics in patients with severe head injury. Drug Intell Clin Pharm 1987;21:459-63.
129. Winer JW, Rosenwasser RH, Jimenez F. Electroencephalographic activity and serum and cerebrospinal fluid pentobarbital levels in determining the therapeutic end point during barbiturate coma. Neurosurgery 1991;29:739-42.
130. Cruz J. Adverse effects of pentobarbital on cerebral venous oxygenation of comatose patients with acute traumatic brain swelling: relationship to outcome. J Neurosurg 1996;85:758-61.
131. Yablon SA. Posttraumatic seizures. Arch Phys Med Rehabil 1993;74:983-1001.
132. Servit Z, Musil F. Prophylactic treatment of posttraumatic epilepsy: results of a long-term follow-up in Czechoslovakia. Epilepsia 1981;22:315-20.
133. Temkin NR. Risk factors for posttraumatic seizures in adults. Epilepsia 2003;44(suppl 10):18-20.
134. Chang BS, Lowenstein DH. Practice parameter: antiepileptic drug prophylaxis in severe traumatic brain injury. Report of the quality standards subcommittee of the American Academy of Neurology. Neurology 2003;60:10-6.
135. Lothman EW, Bertram EH III, Stringer JL. Functional anatomy of hippocampal seizures. Prog Neurobiol 1991;37:1-82.
136. McNamara JO. Development of new pharmacological agents for epilepsy: lessons from the kindling model. Epilepsia 1989;30:S13-8.
137. Lamar CD, Hurley RA, Rowland JA, et al. Post-traumatic epilepsy: review of risks, pathophysiology and potential biomarkers. J Neuropsychiatry Clin Neurosci 2014;26:108-13.
138. Bratton S, Bullock MR, Carney N, et al. Guidelines for the management of severe head injury. Brain Trauma Foundation. XIII. Antiseizure prophylaxis. J Neurotrauma 2007;24(suppl 1):S83-6.
139. Young B, Rapp RP, Norton JA, et al. Failure of prophylactically administered phenytoin to prevent early posttraumatic seizures. J Neurol 1983;58:231-5.
140. Temkin NR, Dikmen SS, Wilensky AJ, et al. A randomized, double-blind study of phenytoin for the prevention of post-traumatic seizures. N Engl J Med 1990;323:497-502.
141. Temkin NR, Dikmen SS, Anderson GD, et al. Valproate therapy for prevention of posttraumatic seizures: a randomized trial. J Neurosurg 1999;91:593-600.
142. Inaba K, Menaker J, Branco BC, et al. A prospective multicenter comparison of levetiracetam versus phenytoin for early posttraumatic seizure prophylaxis. J Trauma Acute Care Surg 2013;74:766-73.
143. Chiles BW, Cooper BW. Acute spinal injury. N Engl J Med 1996;334:514-20.
144. Bawa M, Fayssoux R. Vertebrae and spinal cord. In: Mattox KL, Moore EE, Feliciano DV, eds. Trauma, 7th ed. New York: McGraw-Hill, 2013.
145. Bracken MB, Shepard MJ, Collins WF, et al. A randomized, controlled trial of methylprednisolone of naloxone in the treatment of acute spinal-cord injury. N Engl J Med 1990;322:1405-11.
146. Bracken MB, Shepard MJ, Collins WF, et al. Methylprednisolone or naloxone treatment after acute spinal cord injury: 1-year follow-up data. J Neurosurg 1992;76:23-31.
147. Anderson DK, Braughler JM, Hall ED, et al. Effects of treatment with U-74006F on neurological outcome following experimental spinal cord injury. J Neurosurg 1988;69:562-7.
148. Bracken MB, Shepard MJ, Collins WF, et al. Spinal cord injury: a review of current therapy, future treatments and basic science frontiers. Neurochem Res 2013;38:895-905.
149. Hurlbert RJ. Methylprednisolone for acute spinal cord injury: an inappropriate standard of care. J Neurosurg 2000;93(1 suppl):1-7.
150. Coleman WP, Benzel D, Cahill DW, et al. A critical appraisal of the reporting of the National Acute Spinal Cord Injury Studies (II and III) of methylprednisolone in acute spinal cord injury. J Spinal Disord 2000;13:185-99.
151. Short DJ, El Masry WS, Jones PJ. High-dose methylprednisolone in the management of acute spinal cord injury: a systematic review from a clinical perspective. Spinal Cord 2000;38:273-86.
152. Pitts LH, Ross A, Chase GA, et al. Treatment with thyrotropin-releasing hormone (TRH) in patients with traumatic spinal cord injuries. J Neurotrauma 1995;12:235-43.
153. Fehlings MG, Baptiste DC. Current status of clinical trials for acute spinal cord injury. Injury 2005;36(suppl 2):B113-122.

154. Coleman WP, Benzel D, Cahill DW, et al. Pharmacological therapy of spinal cord injury during the acute phase. Spinal Cord 2000;38:71-6.
155. Chinnock P, Roberts I. Gangliosides for acute spinal cord injury. Cochrane Database Syst Rev 2005;2:CD004444.
156. Fox N, Schwartz D, Salazar JH, et al. Evaluation and management of blunt traumatic aortic injury: a practice management guideline from the Eastern Association for the Surgery of Trauma. J Trauma Acute Care Surg 2015;78:136-46.
157. Arthurs ZM, Starnes BW, Sohn VY, et al. Functional and survival outcomes in traumatic blunt thoracic aortic injuries: an analysis of the National Trauma Databank. J Vasc Surg 2009;49:988-94.
158. Wall MJ Jr, Tsai P, Mattox KL, et al. Heart and thoracic vascular injuries. In: Mattox KL, Moore EE, Feliciano DV, eds. Trauma, 7th ed. New York: McGraw-Hill, 2013:chap 26.
159. Mirvis SE, Shanmuganathan K. Diagnosis of blunt traumatic aortic injury 2007: still a nemesis. Eur J Radiol 2007;64:27-40.
160. Azizzadeh A, Keyhani K, Miller CC III, et al. Blunt traumatic aortic injury: initial experience with endovascular repair. J Vasc Surg 2009;49:1403-8.
161. Fabian TC, Davis KA, Gavant ML, et al. Prospective study of blunt aortic injury: helical CT is diagnostic and antihypertensive therapy reduces rupture. Ann Surg 1998;227:666-77.
162. Pate JW, Gaveant ML, Weiman DS, et al. Traumatic rupture of the aortic isthmus: program of selective management. World J Surg 1999;23:59-63.
163. Rabin J, Dubose J, Sliker CW, et al. Parameters for successful nonoperative management of traumatic aortic injury. J Thorac Cardiovasc Surg 2014;147:143-50.
164. Demetriades D, Velmahos GC, Scalea TM, et al. Diagnosis and treatment of blunt thoracic aortic injuries: changing perspectives. J Trauma 2008;64:1415-9.
165. Xenos ES, Abedi NN, Davenport DL, et al. Meta-analysis of endovascular vs open repair for traumatic descending thoracic aortic rupture. J Vasc Surg 2008;48:1343-51.
166. Fox N, Schwartz D, Salazar JH, et al. Evaluation and management of blunt traumatic aortic injury: a practice management guideline from the Eastern Association for the Surgery of Trauma. J Trauma 2015;78:136-46.
167. Demetriades D, Velmahos GC, Scalea TM, et al. Operative repair or endovascular stent graft in blunt traumatic thoracic aortic injuries: results of an American Association for the Surgery of Trauma Multicenter Study. J Trauma 2008:64;561-70.
168. Azizzadeh A, Ray HM, Dubose JJ, et al. Outcomes of endovascular repair for patients with blunt traumatic aortic injury. J Trauma Acute Care Surg 2014;76:510-6.
169. Demetriades D, Velmahos GC, Scalea TM, et al. Blunt traumatic thoracic aortic injuries: early or delayed repair—results of an American Association for the Surgery of Trauma Prospective Study. J Trauma 2009;66;967-73.
170. Stone HH, Strom PR, Mullins RJ. Management of the major coagulopathy with onset during laparotomy. Ann Surg 1983;197:532-5.
171. Rotondo MF, Schwab CW, McGonigal MD, et al. 'Damage control': an approach for improved survival in exsanguinating penetrating abdominal injury. J Trauma 1993;35:375-83.
172. Sugrue M, D'Amours SK, Joshipura M. Damage control surgery and the abdomen. Injury 2004;35:642-8.
173. McQuiggan MM, Marvin RG, McKinley BA, et al. Enteral feeding following major torso trauma: from theory to practice. New Horiz 1999;7:131-46.
174. Cerra FB. Hypermetabolism, organ failure and metabolic support. Surgery 1987;101:1-11.
175. Border JR, Chenier R, McMenamy RH, et al. Multiple systems organ failure: muscle fuel deficit with visceral protein malnutrition. Surg Clin North Am 1976;56:1147-59.
176. Gentile LF, Cuenca AG, Efron PA, et al. Persistent inflammation and immunosuppression: a common syndrome and new horizon for surgical intensive care. J Trauma Acute Care Surg 2012;72:1491-501.
177. Adams S, Dellinger EP, Wertz MJ, et al. Enteral versus parenteral nutritional support following laparotomy for trauma: a randomized prospective trial. J Trauma 1986;26:882-9.
178. Moore EE, Jones TN. Benefits of immediate jejunostomy feeding after major abdominal trauma—a prospective, randomized study. J Trauma 1986:26:874-81.
179. Moore FA, Moore EE, Jones TN, et al. TEN versus TPN following major abdominal trauma—reduced septic mortality. J Trauma 1989;29:916-23.
180. Kudsk KA, Croce MA, Fabian TC, et al. Enteral versus parenteral feeding: effects on septic morbidity after blunt and penetrating abdominal trauma. Ann Surg 1992;215:503-10.
181. Moore FA, Feliciano DV, Andrassy RJ, et al. Early enteral feeding, compared with parenteral, reduces postoperative septic complications. The results of a meta-analysis. Ann Surg 1992;216:172-83.
182. Eyer SD, Micon LT, Konstantinides FN, et al. Early enteral feeding does not attenuate metabolic response after blunt trauma. J Trauma 1993;34:639-44.
183. The National Heart, Lung, and Blood Institute Acute Respiratory Distress Syndrome (ARDS) Clinical Trials Network. Initial tropic vs full enteral feeding in patients with acute lung injury. JAMA 2012;307:795-803.
184. Kwon RS, Banerjee S, Desilets D, et al. Enteral nutrition access devices. Gastrointest Endosc 2010;72:236-48.
185. Nicholas JM, Cornelius MW, Tchorz KM, et al. A two institution experience with 226 endoscopically placed jejunal feeding tubes in critical ill surgical patients. Am J Surg 2003;186:583-90.
186. Kozar RA, McQuiggan MM, Moore EE, et al. Postinjury enteral tolerance is reliably achieved by a standardized protocol. J Surg Res 2002;104:70-5.
187. MacLeod JB, Lefton J, Houghton D, et al. Prospective randomized control trial of intermittent versus continuous gastric feeds for critically ill trauma patients. J Trauma 2007;63:57-61.
188. Doig GS, Simpson F, Sweetman EA, et al. Early parenteral nutrition in critically ill patients with short-term relative contraindications to early enteral nutrition. JAMA 2013;309:2130-8.
189. Schecter WP, Hirshberg A, Chang DS, et al. Enteric fistulas: principles of management. J Am Coll Surg 2009;209:484-91.
190. Edmunds LH Jr, Williams GM, Welch CE. External fistulas arising from the gastrointestinal tract. Ann Surg 1960;152:445-71.

191. Jamshidi R, Schecter WP. Biological dressings for the management of enteric fistulas in the open abdomen: a preliminary report. Arch Surg 2007;142:793-6.
192. Tsuei BJ, Skinner JC, Bernard AC, et al. The open peritoneal cavity: etiology correlates with the likelihood of fascial closure. Am Surg 2004;70:652-6.
193. Miller RS, Morris JA Jr, Diaz JJ Jr, et al. Complications after 344 damage-control open celiotomies. J Trauma 2005;59:1365-71.
194. Barker DE, Kaufman HJ, Smith LA, et al. Vacuum pack technique of temporary abdominal closure: a 7-year experience with 112 patients. J Trauma 2000;48:201-6.
195. Kirkpatrick AW, Baxter KA, Simons RK, et al. Intra-abdominal complications after surgical repair of small bowel injuries: an international review. J Trauma 2003;55:399-406.
196. Teixeira PG, Inaba K, Dubose J, et al. Enterocutaneous fistula complicating trauma laparotomy: a major resource burden. Am Surg 2009;75:30-2.
197. Bradley MJ, DuBose JJ, Scalea TM, et al. Independent predictors of enteric fistula and abdominal sepsis after damage control laparotomy: results from the prospective AAST open abdomen registry. JAMA Surg 2013;148:947-54.
198. Aguirre A, Fischer JE, Welch CE. The role of surgery and hyperalimentation in therapy of gastrointestinal-cutaneous fistulae. Ann Surg 1974;180:393-401.
199. Slater R. Nutritional management of enterocutaneous fistulas. Br J Nurs 2009;18:225-30.
200. Ham M, Horton K, Kaunitz J. Fistuloclysis: case report and literature review. Nutr Clin Pract 2007;22:553-7.
201. Patel YC. Somatostatin and its receptor family. Front Neuroendocrinol 1999;20:157-98.
202. Tulassay Z. Somatostatin and the gastrointestinal tract. Scand J Gastroenterol 1998;228:115-21.
203. De Herder WW, Lamberts SWJ. Somatostatin and analogues: diagnostic and therapeutic uses. Curr Opin Oncol 2002;14:53-7.
204. Isenmann R, Schielke DJ, Morl FK, et al. Adjuvant therapy with somatostatin iv in postoperative fistulae of the pancreas, gall bladder, and small intestine. A multicenter randomized study. Akt Chir 1994;29:96-9.
205. Torres AJ, Landa JI, Moreno-Azcoita M, et al. Somatostatin in the management of gastrointestinal fistulas: a multi-center study. Arch Surg 1992;127:97-9.
206. Leandros E, Antonakis PT, Albanopoulos K, et al. Somatostatin versus octreotide in the treatment of patients with gastrointestinal and pancreatic fistulas. Can J Gastroenterol 2004;18:303-6.
207. Hernandez-Aranda JC, Gallo-Chico B, Flores-Ramirez LA, et al. Treatment of enterocutaneous fistula with or without octreotide and parenteral nutrition. Nutr Hosp 1996;11:226-9.
208. Jamil M, Ahmed U, Sobia H. Role of somatostatin analogues in the management of enterocutaneous fistulae. J Coll Physicians Surg Pak 2004;14:237-40.
209. Sancho JJ, di Constanzo J, Nubiola P, et al. Randomized double-blind placebo-controlled trial of early octreotide in patients with postoperative enterocutaneous fistula. Br J Surg 1995;82:638-41.
210. Scott NA, Finnegan S, Irving MH. Octreotide and postoperative enterocutaneous fistulae: a controlled prospective study. Acta Gastroenterol Belg 1993;56:266-70.
211. Vanderhoof JA, Langnas AN. Short bowel syndrome in children and adults. Gastroenterology 1997;113:1767-78.
212. Allard JP, Jeejeebhoy KN. Nutrition support and therapy in short bowel syndrome. Gastroenterol Clin North Am 1989;18:589-601.
213. Dabney A, Thompson J, DiBaise J, et al. Short bowel syndrome after trauma. Am J Surg 2004;188:792-5.
214. Buchman AL, Scolapio J, Fryer J. AGA technical review on short bowel syndrome and intestinal transplantation. Gastroenterology 2003;124:1111-34.
215. Bryant J. Observations upon the growth and length of the human intestine. Am J Med Sci 1924;167:499-520.
216. Faucci A, Cerrro P, Fraracci L, et al. Small bowel length measured by radiology. Gastrointest Radiol 1984;9:349-51.
217. Borgstrom B, Dahlqvist A, Lundh G, et al. Studies of intestinal digestion and absorption in the human. J Clin Invest 1957;36:1521-36.
218. Jeejeebhoy KN. Short bowel syndrome: a nutritional and medical approach. Can Med Assoc J 2002;166:1297-302.
219. Parekh N, Seidner K, Steiger E. Managing short bowel syndrome; making the most of what the patient still has. Cleve Clin J Med 2005;72:833-8.
220. Clarke RM. Mucosal architecture and epithelial cell production rate in the small intestine of the albino rat. J Anat 1970;107:519-29.
221. Johansson C. Studies of gastrointestinal interactions. VII. Characteristics of the absorption pattern of sugar fat and protein from composite meals in man. A quantitative study. Scand J Gastroenterol 1975;10:33-42.
222. Nightingale JM, Lennard-Jones JE, Gertner DJ, et al. Colonic preservation reduces need for parenteral therapy, increases incidence of renal stones, but does not change high prevalence of gallstones in patients with a short bowel. Gut 1992;33:1493-7.
223. Woolf GM, Miller C, Kurian R, et al. Nutritional absorption in short bowel syndrome. Dig Dis Sci 1987;32:8-15.
224. Nightingale JMD. Management of patients with short bowel. World J Gastroenterol 2001;7:741-51.
225. Fordtran JS, Locklear TW. Ionic constituents and osmolality of gastric and small intestinal fluids after eating. Am J Dig Dis 1966;11:503-21.
226. Westergaard H, Spady DK. Short bowel syndrome. In: Sleisenger MH, Fordtran JS, eds. Gastrointestinal Diseases, 5th ed. Philadelphia: Saunders, 1993:1249-57.
227. Ammon HV, Philips SF. Inhibition of colonic water and electrolyte absorption by fatty acids in man. Gastroenterology 1973;65:744-9.
228. Earnest DL, Johnson G, Williams HE, et al. Hyperoxaluria in patients with ileal resection: an abnormality in dietary oxalate absorption. Gastroenterology 1974;66:1114-22.
229. Misiakos EP, Macheras A, Kapetanakis T, et al. Short bowel syndrome: current medical and surgical trends. J Clin Gastroenterol 2007;41:5-18.
230. Mokete B, De Cock R. Xerophthalmia and short bowel syndrome [letter]. Br J Gastroenterol 1998;82:1340-1.

231. Selby PL, Peackock M, Bambach CP. Hypomagnesemia after small bowel resection: treatment with 1a-hydroxylated vitamin D metabolites. Br J Surg 1984;71:334-7.

232. Howard L, Ovesen L, Sataya-Murti S, et al. Reversible neurological symptoms caused by vitamin E deficiency in a patient with short bowel syndrome. Am J Clin Nutr 1982;36:1243-9.

233. Conly JM, Stein K, Worobetz L, et al. The contribution of vitamin K2 (menaquinones) produced by the intestinal microflora to human nutritional requirements for vitamin K. Am J Gastroenterol 1994;89:915-23.

234. Matarese LE, O'Keefe SJ, Kandil HM, et al. Short bowel syndrome: clinical guidelines for nutrition management. Nutr Clin Pract 2005;20:493-502.

235. Nightingale JMD, Lennard-Jones JE, Walker ER. A patient with jejunostomy liberated from home intravenous therapy after 14 years. Contribution of balance studies. Clin Nutr 1992;11:101-5.

236. Dharmsathaphorn K, Gorelick FS, Sherwin RS, et al. Somatostatin decreases diarrhea in patients with the short bowel syndrome. J Clin Gastroenterol 1982;4:521-4.

237. Cooper JC, Williams NS, King RFGJ, et al. Effects of a long-acting somatostatin analogue in patients with severe ileostomy diarrhea. Br J Surg 1986;73:128-31.

238. Shaffer JL, O'Hanrahan T, Rowntree S. Does somatostatin analogue (201-995) reduce high output stoma effluent? A controlled trial. Gut 1998;29:A1432-3.

239. Nightingale JMD, Walker ER, Burnham WR, et al. Octreotide (a somatostatin analogue) improves the quality of life in some patients with a short intestine. Aliment Pharmacol Ther 1989;3:367-73.

240. Rodrigues CA, Lennard-Jones JE, Walker ER. The effects of octreotide soy polysaccharide, codeine and loperamide on nutrient, fluid and electrolyte absorption in the short bowel syndrome. Aliment Pharmacol Ther 1989;3:159-69.

241. Ladefoged K, Christensen KC, Hegnhoi J, et al. Effect of long acting somatostatin analogue SMS 201-995 on jejunostomy effluents in patients with severe short bowel syndrome. Gut 1989;30:943-9.

242. Kusuhara K, Kusunoki M, Okamoto T, et al. Reduction of effluent volume in high output ileostomy patients by a somatostatin analogue, SMS 201-995. Int J Colorect Dis 1992;7:202-5.

243. O'Keefe SJD, Peterson ME, Fleming R. Octreotide as an adjunct to home parenteral nutrition in the management of permanent end-jejunostomy syndrome. J Parenter Enteral Nutr 1994;18:26-34.

244. Nightingale JMD. The Sir David Cuthbertson Medal Lecture. Clinical problems of a short bowel and their treatment. Proc Nutr Soc 1994;53:373-91.

245. Ellegard L, Bosaeus I, Nordgren S, et al. Low-dose recombinant growth hormone increases body weight and lean body mass in patients with short bowel syndrome. Ann Surg 1997;225:88-96.

246. Byrne TA, Morrissey TB, Nattakom TV, et al. Growth hormone, glutamine and a modified diet enhances nutrient absorption in patients with severe short bowel syndrome. J Parenter Enteral Nutr 1995;19:296-302.

247. Scolapio JS, Camilleri M, Fleming CR, et al. Effect of growth hormone, glutamine and diet on adaption in short bowel syndrome: a randomized, controlled study. Gastroenterology 1997;113:1074-81.

248. Szkudlarek J, Jeppesen PB, Mortensen PB. Effect of high dose growth hormone with glutamine and no change in diet on intestinal absorption in short bowel patients: a randomized, double-blind, crossover, placebo-controlled study. Gut 2000;47:199-205.

249. Seguy D, Vahedi K, Kapel N, et al. Low-dose growth hormone in adult home parenteral nutrition-dependent short bowel syndrome patients: a positive study. Gastroenterology 2003;124:293-302.

250. Weiming Z, Ning L, Jieshou L. Effect of recombinant human growth hormone and enteral nutrition on short bowel syndrome. J Parenter Enteral Nutr 2004;28:377-81.

251. Byrne TA, Wilmore DW, Iyer K, et al. Growth hormone, glutamine, and an optimal diet reduces parenteral nutrition in patients with short bowel syndrome. Ann Surg 2005;242:655-61.

252. Jeppesen PB. Teduglutide, a novel glucagon like peptide 2 analog in the treatment of patients with short bowel syndrome. Ther Adv Gastroenterol 2012;5:159-71.

253. Jeppesen PB, Hartmann B, Thulesen J. Glucagon-like peptide 2 improves nutrient absorption and nutritional status in short bowel patients with no colon. Gastroenterology 2001;120:806-15.

254. Jeppesen PB, Sanguinetti EL, Buchman A. Teduglutide (ALX-0600) a dipeptidyl peptidase IV resistant glucagon like peptide 2 analogue improves intestinal function in short bowel syndrome patients. Gut 2005;54:1224-31.

255. Jeppesen PB, Pertkiewicz M, Messing B, et al. Teduglutide reduces need for parenteral support among patients with short bowel syndrome with intestinal failure. Gastroenterology 2012;143:1473-81.

256. Vipperla K, O'Keefe SJ. Study of teduglutide effectiveness in parenteral nutrition-dependent short bowel syndrome subjects. Expert Rev Gastroenterol Hepatol 2013;7:683-7.

257. Lucas CE, White MT, Ledgerwood AM. Renal failure. In: Mattox KL, Moore EE, Feliciano DV, eds. Trauma, 7th ed. New York: McGraw-Hill, 2013.

258. Brandt MM, Falvo AJ, Rubinfeld IS, et al. Renal dysfunction in trauma: even a little costs a lot. J Trauma 2007;62:1362-4.

259. Bihorac A, Delano M, Schold J, et al. Incidence, clinical predictors, genomics, and outcome of acute kidney injury among trauma patients. Ann Surg 2010;252:158-65.

260. Vivino G, Antonelli M, Moro M, et al. Risk factors for acute renal failure in trauma patients. Intensive Care Med 1998;24:808-14.

261. Hayes DF, Werner MH, Rosenberg IK, et al. Effects of traumatic hypovolemic shock on renal function. J Surg Res 1974;16:490-7.

262. Kidney Disease: Improving Global Outcomes (KDIGO) Acute Kidney Injury Work Group. KDIGO Clinical Practice Guideline for Acute Kidney Injury. Kidney Int Suppl 2012;2:1-138.

263. Bosch X, Poch E, Gray J. Rhabdomyolysis and acute kidney injury. N Engl J Med 2009;361:62-72.

264. Sharp L, Rozycki G, Feliciano D. Rhabdomyolysis and secondary renal failure in critically ill surgical patients. Am J Surg 2004;188:801-6.

265. Shimazu T, Yoshioka T, Nakata Y, et al. Fluid resuscitation and systemic complications in crush syndrome: 14 Hanshin-Awaji earthquake patients. J Trauma 1997;42:641-6.

266. Gunal AI, Celiker H, Dogukan A, et al. Early and vigorous fluid resuscitation prevents acute renal failure in the crush victims of catastrophic earthquakes. J Am Soc Nephrol 2004;15:1862-7.

267. Brown CV, Rhee P, Chan L, et al. Preventing renal failure in patients with rhabdomyolysis: do bicarbonate and mannitol make a difference? J Trauma 2004;56:1191-6.

268. Better OS, Rubinstein I, Winaver JM, et al. Mannitol therapy revisited (1940-1997). Kidney Int 1997;52:886-94.

269. Visweswaran P, Massin EK, Dubose TD Jr. Mannitol-induced acute renal failure. J Am Soc Nephrol 1997;8:1028-33.

270. Zhang L, Kang Y, Fu P, et al. Myoglobin clearance by continuous venous-venous haemofiltration in rhabdomyolysis with acute kidney injury: a case series. Injury 2012;43:619-23.

271. Bendinelli C, Balogh Z. Postinjury thromboprophylaxis. Curr Opin Crit Care 2008;14:673-8.

272. Chandler WL, Dunbar NM. Thrombin generation in trauma patients. Transfusion 2009;49:2652-60.

273. Velmahos GC, Kern J, Chan LS, et al. Prevention of venous thromboembolism after injury: an evidence based report. Part I: analysis of risk factors and evaluation of the role of vena caval filters. J Trauma 2000;49:132-9.

274. Hak DJ. Prevention of venous thromboembolism in trauma and long bone fractures. Curr Opin Pulm Med 2001;7:338-43.

275. Seyfer AE, Seaber AV, Dombrose FA, et al. Coagulation changes in elective surgery and trauma. Ann Surg 1981;193:210-3.

276. Owings JT, Bagley M, Gosselin R, et al. Effect of critical injury on plasma antithrombin activity: low antithrombin levels are associated with thromboembolic complications. J Trauma 1996;41:396-406.

277. Attar S, Boyd D, Layne E, et al. Alterations in coagulation and fibrinolytic mechanisms in acute trauma. J Trauma 1969;9:939-65.

278. Enderson BL, Chen JP, Robinson R, et al. Fibrinolysis in multisystem trauma patients. J Trauma 1991;31:1240-6.

279. Meissner MH, Chandler WL, Elliott JS. Venous thromboembolism in trauma: a local manifestation of systemic hypercoagulability. J Trauma 2003;54:2245-31.

280. Engelman DT, Gabram SGA, Allen L, et al. Hypercoagulability following multiple trauma. World J Surg 1996;20:5-10.

281. Dries DJ. Activation of the clotting system and complement after trauma. New Horiz 1996;4:276-88.

282. Geerts WH, Code KI, Jay RM, et al. A prospective study of venous thromboembolism after major trauma. N Engl J Med 1994;331:1601-6.

283. Knudson MM, Lewis FR, Clinton A, et al. Prevention of venous thromboembolism in trauma patients. J Trauma 1994;37:480-7.

284. Dennis JW, Menawat S, Thron JV, et al. Efficacy of deep venous thrombosis prophylaxis in trauma patients and identification of high-risk groups. J Trauma 1993;35:132-8.

285. Knudson MM, Morabito D, Paiement GD, et al. Use of low molecular weight heparin in preventing thromboembolism in trauma patients. J Trauma 1996;41:446-59.

286. Geerts WH, Jay RM, Code KI, et al. A comparison of low dose heparin with low-molecular-weight heparin as prophylaxis against venous thromboembolism after major trauma. N Engl J Med 1996;335:701-7.

287. Geerts WH, Bergqvist D, Pineo GF, et al. Prevention of venous thromboembolism: American College of Chest Physicians Evidence-Based Clinical Practice Guidelines, 8th ed. Chest 2008;133:381S-453S.

288. Gould MK, Garcia DA, Wren SM, et al. Prevention of VTE in Nonorthopedic Surgical Patients Antithrombotic Therapy and Prevention of Thrombosis, 9th ed: American College of Chest Physicians Evidence-Based Clinical Practice Guidelines. Chest 2012;141(suppl):e227S-e277S.

289. Nathens AB, McMurray MK, Cuschieri J, et al. The practice of venous thromboembolism prophylaxis in the major trauma patient. J Trauma 2007;62:557-63.

290. Aito S, Pieri A, D'Andrea M, et al. Primary prevention of deep venous thrombosis and pulmonary embolism in acute spinal cord injured patients. Spinal Cord 2002;40:300-3.

291. Stannard JP, Lopez-Ben RR, Volgas DA, et al. Prophylaxis against deep vein thrombosis following trauma: a prospective, randomized comparison of mechanical and pharmacologic prophylaxis. J Bone Joint Surg Am 2006;88:261-6.

292. Alejandro KV, Acosta JA, Rodriguez PA. Bleeding manifestations after early use of low-molecular-weight heparins in blunt splenic injuries. Am Surg 2003;69:1006-9.

293. Eberle BM, Schnuriger B, Inaba K, et al. Thromboembolic prophylaxis with low-molecular-weight heparin in patients with blunt solid abdominal organ injuries undergoing nonoperative management: current practice and outcomes. J Trauma 2011;70:141-7.

294. Norwood SH, Berne JD, Rowe SA, et al. Early venous thromboembolism prophylaxis with enoxaparin in patients with blunt traumatic brain injury. J Trauma 2008;65;1021-7.

295. Stassen NA, Bhullar I, Cheng JD, et al. Selective nonoperative management of blunt splenic injury: an Eastern Association for the Surgery of Trauma practice management guideline. J Trauma 2012;73:S294-S300.

296. Stassen NA, Bhullar I, Cheng JD, et al. Selective nonoperative management of blunt hepatic injury: an Eastern Association for the Surgery of Trauma practice management guideline. J Trauma 2012;73:S288-93.

297. Haas CE, Nelsen JL, Raghavendran K, et al. Pharmacokinetics and pharmacodynamics of enoxaparin in multiple trauma patients. J Trauma 2005;59:1336-44.

298. Rutherford EJ, Schooler WG, Sredzienski E, et al. Optimal dose of enoxaparin in critically ill trauma and surgical patients. J Trauma 2005;58:1167-70.

299. Constantini TW, Min E, Box K, et al. Dose adjusting enoxaparin is necessary to achieve adequate venous thromboembolism prophylaxis in trauma patients. J Trauma Acute Care Surg 2013;74:128-35.

Pediatric Critical Care

Elizabeth Farrington, Pharm.D., FCCP, FCCM, FPPAG, BCPS

LEARNING OBJECTIVES

1. Identify the most common cause of cardiac arrest in pediatric patients.
2. Know the different types of shock and those that occur most commonly in children.
3. Describe the initial treatment of all forms of pediatric shock, and understand why the treatment of shock in pediatric patients may differ from that in adults.
4. Understand why the incidence of septic shock is highest in the first year of life and the impact of underlying medical conditions on mortality rate.
5. Explain why the definitions of systemic inflammatory response syndrome are different between pediatric and adult patients.
6. Describe how the normal physiology of children causes them to respond to septic shock differently from adults.
7. Understand that developmental changes and immaturity of the respiratory system make respiratory distress the most common reason for hospital admission in the first year of life.
8. Develop a pharmacotherapy plan for a pediatric patient with status asthmaticus admitted to the PICU.
9. Describe why the different choices for the pharmacotherapy of intubation vary depending on the cardiovascular stability of the patient, the stomach being empty or full, and the underlying cause of the respiratory distress.
10. Understand how the anatomic differences of the child's brain render it more susceptible to certain types of injuries after head trauma.
11. Develop a pharmacotherapy plan for the treatment of traumatic brain injury in a pediatric patient, understanding that goals may differ according to the patient's age.
12. Understand why stress ulcer prophylaxis, a standard of care in the adult ICU, is less well defined in the PICU.
13. Explain differences in the risk of developing deep venous thrombosis (DVT) depending on age and possible sources of DVT in critically ill children.
14. Explain why infants are at a higher risk of hypoglycemia than are older children, discuss the importance of point-of-care glucose testing, and develop a pharmacotherapy plan for the treatment of hypoglycemia, if identified.

ABBREVIATIONS IN THIS CHAPTER

ABG	Arterial blood gas	MVC	Motor vehicle collision
CO	Cardiac output	NAT	Nonaccidental trauma
CPP	Cerebral perfusion pressure	PICU	Pediatric intensive care unit
CSF	Cerebrospinal fluid	RSV	Respiratory syncytial virus
CVP	Central venous pressure	SA	Status asthmaticus
DVT	Deep venous thrombosis	SIRS	Systemic inflammatory response syndrome
ED	Emergency department		
ICP	Intracranial pressure	Svo_2	Mixed venous oxygen saturation
GCS	Glasgow Coma Scale	SVR	Systemic vascular resistance
ICU	Intensive care unit	TBI	Traumatic brain injury
MAP	Mean arterial pressure		

INTRODUCTION

The epidemiology of patients admitted to either the pediatric emergency department (ED) or the pediatric intensive care unit (PICU) differs from that typically seen in adult critical care settings.[1,2] In an evaluation of 361 children presenting to an ED, the most common medical reasons for admission were cardiocirculatory causes (32%), neurological conditions (26%), and respiratory causes (23%).[1] Cardiocirculatory causes included hypovolemic, septic, cardiac, and anaphylactic shock. Neurological conditions consisted primarily of seizures, status epilepticus, and meningitis or encephalitis. The most common respiratory cause for admission was respiratory syncytial virus (RSV) bronchiolitis, followed by pneumonia, pleural effusions, and status asthmaticus (SA). Eighteen percent of the patients were admitted after trauma. Diabetic ketoacidosis accounted for 6% of the admissions. Other diagnoses included intoxications, near-drowning, snakebites, and burns. An assessment of the most common causes for PICU admission showed similar results. In a review of 1,149 children admitted during a 2-year period to the PICU of a university-affiliated children's hospital, most (38%) were given a diagnosis of cardiovascular diseases, followed by respiratory illnesses (28%), other medical causes (10%), neurologic illness (8%), and trauma (8%). Another 7% were admitted for postoperative care.[2] In the past 10 years, fewer children have been admitted to the PICU after accidents or with croup or epiglottitis.[2] These changes can be explained by the requirement for mandatory car seats for children, administration of dexamethasone in the ED to patients with croup, and universal administration of the conjugate *Haemophilus influenzae* type b immunization.

Much of pediatric practice is dedicated to helping the child make the transition from the intrauterine environment through infancy, childhood, and adolescence to adulthood. One of the greatest challenges in treating pediatric patients is recognizing the many developmental physiologic changes and understanding how they affect assessment and treatment of the patient. These differences are discussed in detail as they pertain to specific disease states and summarized in Table 44.1. The definition and presentation of many disease states encountered in the critical care setting, including respiratory depression, supraventricular tachycardia, hypotension, and shock, vary depending on the age of the patient because of physiologic variations. There are also newborn emergencies that are unique to the physiologic transitions that occur in the first month of life. Pediatric health care providers practicing in critical care settings such as the ED or the PICU must be adept at incorporating these physiologic differences into medication selection, dosing, and monitoring to optimize patient care.

Pediatric Cardiopulmonary Resuscitation

In marked contrast to studies of pediatric cardiac arrest, adult cardiac arrest studies have focused on the diagnosis and treatment of ventricular fibrillation (VF) in both inpatient and out-of-hospital cardiac arrest. Studies have shown that VF is the most common initial dysrhythmia in adults with sudden death; in some reports, the prevalence of VF was 60%–85%. Cardiac arrest caused by VF or pulseless ventricular tachycardia as the initial cardiac rhythm occurs in only 5%–15% of pediatric cases of in-hospital and out-of-hospital cardiac arrest.[3] In contrast to adults, cardiac arrest in infants and children does not usually result from a primary cardiac cause; more often, it is the terminal result of progressive respiratory failure or shock. Therefore, it is essential to recognize and aggressively treat pediatric patients admitted with respiratory distress, pneumonia, and shock to prevent the development of systemic hypoxemia, hypercapnia, and acidosis, which may then progress to bradycardia, hypotension, and eventually cardiorespiratory arrest.

The adult advanced cardiovascular life support guidelines recommend 40 units of vasopressin or epinephrine as the first or second dose of medication administered to adults with asystole,[3] with subsequent medication doses as epinephrine. Epinephrine is the drug of choice for managing pediatric asystole.[4] Subsequent doses of epinephrine can be administered every 3–5 minutes by the intravenous or intraosseous route, using the appropriate intravenous/intraosseous dose of 0.01 mg/kg using the 1:10,000 or 0.1-mg/mL concentration (maximum 0.1 mg/dose). Treatment of pediatric asystole does not include vasopressin administration because progressive respiratory failure and shock, not underlying cardiovascular disease, are the most common causes of asystole in pediatric patients.

Shock

Shock may be classified as hypovolemic, distributive, cardiogenic, or obstructive. Hypovolemic shock is the most common type of shock in pediatric patients, typically caused by acute gastroenteritis. Hypovolemic shock occurs when circulating intravascular volume decreases to a point at which adequate tissue perfusion can no longer be maintained. Hypovolemia causes a decrease in preload and adversely affects cardiac output (CO). Initially, hypovolemia activates the peripheral and central baroreceptors that cause catecholamine-mediated vasoconstriction and tachycardia. This initial response can maintain adequate circulation and blood pressure even after an acute loss of as much as 15% of the circulating blood volume. Shock is caused by inadequate blood flow and oxygen delivery to meet the metabolic demands of the tissues[4] and progresses from an initial compensated state to a decompensated

continued on page 899

Table 44.1 Physiologic Differences

System	Physiologic Difference	Clinical Significance
Cardiovascular	Infants have immature sarcomeres and are calcium-dependent for cardiac contractility	They are dependent on calcium influx for cardiac contractility. Therefore, a single dose of calcium chloride may significantly change an infant's BP
	Infants and children have decreased stroke volume and therefore a higher baseline HR	The definition of SVT in infants is an HR > 220 beats/min, whereas in children and adolescents, it is an HR > 160 beats/min
	Children normally have a lower BP than adults and can better preserve adequate BP by vasoconstriction and increasing HR	Tachycardia provides the most efficient method of increasing cardiac output in infants and children. BP by itself is not a reliable end point for evaluating the adequacy of resuscitation in children. Hypotension is the last thing to occur in pediatric shock states
	Infants and small children have only ~80 mL/kg of blood volume. Older children and adolescents have ~70 mL/kg	1. Clinical pharmacists need to carefully choose laboratory values; they recommend considering the value of the result versus the significance to the patient's hemoglobin
		2. Adding an extracorporeal circuit can significantly drop drug levels in an infant because the circuit volume may be close to the patient's own blood volume. Additional loading doses of sedation and analgesia may be required when support is initiated
	BP is defined in children on the basis of sex, age, and height percentile	A single number is not used to define normal BP in children. The definition of hypotension also varies: • < 60 mm Hg in term neonates (0–28 days) • 70 mm Hg in infants (1–12 mo) • 70 mm Hg + (2 × age in years) in children 1–10 yr of age • 90 mm Hg in children ≥ 10 yr • A MAP in a neonate should be approximately their gestational age
	Cardiac arrhythmias: Most are clinically insignificant (i.e., they do not compromise cardiac output of systemic perfusion)	Arrhythmias most commonly seen in children: Bradycardia SVT
Pulmonary	The nose provides almost half the total airway resistance in children. Infants < 2 mo are obligate nasal breathers, and their nose is short, soft, and small with almost circular nares. The nares will double in size from birth to 6 mo, but they can easily be occluded from edema, secretions, or external pressure	Simply clearing the nasal passageways with saline and bulb suctioning can significantly improve an infant's respiratory condition
	Although all the conducting airways are present at birth and the airway branching pattern is complete, the airways are small. The airways will increase in size and length throughout childhood	The most common reason for admission to the hospital in the first year of life is respiratory distress. As the airways increase in size, the incidence of respiratory distress will decrease
	Tidal volume in children is the same as in adults ~6–7 mL/kg	To have adequate gas exchange, respiratory rates are higher in infants and decrease with age. Therefore, the definition of respiratory distress will vary according to age
	Normal airway resistance is highest in infants because it is inversely proportional to 1/radius	Any airway narrowing from bronchospasm, edema, or mucus accumulation will significantly increase the airway resistance and increase the infant's work of breathing
	Not only are the airways smaller in an infant, but supporting airway cartilage and elastic tissue are not developed until school age	The child's airways are susceptible to collapse and may easily become obstructed as a result of laryngospasm, bronchospasm, and edema or mucus accumulation
	The cartilaginous ribs of the infant and young child are twice as compliant as the bony ribs of the older child or adult. During episodes of respiratory distress, the infant's chest wall will retract further than will that of a patient with a bony rib cage	This will reduce the patient's ability to maintain functional residual capacity (FRC) or increase tidal volume, thus further increasing the patient's work of breathing
	The alveolar epithelium and endothelial layers continue to develop until 10–12 yr of life	Discrete lung injury early in life may not impair lung development because compensatory alveolar growth may occur

Table 44.1 Physiologic Differences (continued)

System	Physiologic Difference	Clinical Significance
	The intercostal muscles are not fully developed until school age, so they act primarily to stabilize the chest wall during the first years of life. Because the intercostal muscles have neither the leverage nor the strength to lift the rib cage in the young child, the diaphragm is responsible for the generation of tidal volume	Anything that impedes diaphragm movement, such as a large stomach bubble, abdominal distension, or peritonitis, can result in respiratory failure in the young child
	The narrowest part of the pediatric airway is the cricoid cartilage, not the vocal cords	Treatment of postextubation stridor may be more difficult. Therefore, use of dexamethasone 0.25–0.5 mg/kg/dose (max 10 mg/dose) IV q 6 hr for four to eight doses has been used as preventive therapy in traumatic intubations or in patients with no leak pressure
Neurologic	1. Infants and young children have large, heavy heads. The head is unstable because of its relative size to the rest of the body 2. The infant's weak neck muscles also allow for greater movement when the head is acted on by acceleration/deceleration forces 3. The skull is thinner during infancy and early childhood, providing less protection for the brain and allowing forces to transfer more effectively across the shallow subarachnoid space 4. The base of the infant's skull is relatively flat, which also contributes to greater brain movement in response to acceleration/deceleration forces 5. The infant's brain has a higher water content (~88% vs. 77% in an adult), which makes the brain softer and more prone to acceleration/deceleration injury. The infant brain is typically fully myelinated by 1 yr of age	1. If an infant or young child falls a significant distance, is ejected during an MVC, or is thrown from a bicycle after colliding with an automobile, the head will tend to lead (i.e., the infant or child will fly head first), and severe head injuries will occur when the head ultimately strikes the ground or another object 2. Infants are at higher risk of acceleration/deceleration injuries 3. The brain water content is inversely related to the myelination process, and the higher percentage of unmyelinated brain in neonates and infants makes them more susceptible to sheer injuries 4. There are differences in the pathology after pediatric TBI by age group. In infants and young children, diffuse injury, such as diffuse cerebral swelling, and subdural hematomas are more common than focal injury, such as contusions, which are typically seen in older children and adults. The typical pattern of hypoxic-ischemic injury in infants and young children after NAT is rarely seen in older children and adults who are survivors of abuse
Endocrine	Neonates and infants have low glycogen stores and high metabolic demand	This makes them at high risk of hypoglycemia in times of stress, infection, or poor feeding
Renal	Neonates are born with the adult complement of nephrons; however, only 50% reach the renal cortex. Tubular length and glomerular size will increase with normal growth and development	Normal UOP: Infants and children = 1–2 mL/kg/hr Adolescents = 0.5 mL/kg/hr
	Development of GFR is linear as long as the neonate is born > 34 weeks' gestation. Children reach an adult GFR at ~12–19 mo. The Schwartz equation should be used to calculate creatinine clearance in children	In the first years of life, cannot use the absolute number calculated from the Schwartz equation to decide whether medication doses need to be adjusted, but must adjust when they drop below 50% of normal. At 1 yr, you may use the calculated number. Cannot use a Cockcroft-Gault equation to calculate creatinine clearance in infants, children, or adolescents. It will overestimate their clearance
Immune system	Passive immunity is normally conveyed from the mother to the fetus through transmission of immunoglobulins during the last trimester. As a result, premature neonates are immunoglobulin-deficient. Even the full-term neonate has decreased polymorphonuclear leukocyte function and small polymorphonuclear storage pools compared with older children and adults, as well as decreased ability to synthesize new antibodies. Finally, neonates cannot make and deliver adequate amounts of phagocytes to infection sites. Stores of maternal immunoglobulin are depleted at 2–5 mo of age. Adult levels of immunoglobulin are not typically achieved until 4–7 yr of age	Infants and children < 7 yr are particularly vulnerable to polysaccharide-carrying bacteria. Historically, *Haemophilus influenzae*, *Streptococcus pneumoniae*, and *Neisseria meningitidis* caused most of the significant infections in the age group. Low immunoglobulin levels also make the infant susceptible to viral infections 1. Neonates and infants < 3 mo with temperature ≥ 38°C should be evaluated with blood, urine, and possibly CSF cultures 2. Nosocomial infections in infants and children < 7 yr tend to be bacteremias and pneumonias (not UTIs and wound infections); therefore, empiric antibiotics until cultures are negative are appropriate

BP = blood pressure; GFR = glomerular filtration rate; HR = heart rate; IV = intravenous(ly); MVC = motor vehicle collision; NAT = nonaccidental trauma; q = every; SVT = supraventricular tachycardia; TBI = traumatic brain injury; UOP = urinary output; UTI = urinary tract infection.

shock. Typical signs of compensated shock include tachycardia, cool and pale distal extremities, prolonged (greater than 2 seconds) capillary refill, weak peripheral pulses compared with central pulses, and normal systolic blood pressure. As shock progresses, patients exhaust their ability to compensate. These patients will have signs of inadequate end organ perfusion, including depressed mental status and decreased urine output.

Initial volume resuscitation in all forms of shock is similar. It is recommended to push isotonic crystalloid fluid (i.e., normal saline or lactated Ringer solution) in 20-mL/kg boluses administered over 5 minutes. Immediately afterward, the patient should be assessed for signs of improved perfusion using clinical criteria such as reduction in heart rate, improvement in blood pressure, capillary refill, quality of pulses, and change in mental status. If the clinical signs of shock persist, another 20 mL/kg of isotonic fluid should be administered, reaching, if necessary, at least 60 mL/kg within the first 15–30 minutes of treatment.[4,5]

This aggressive resuscitation strategy was recently questioned after publication of the Fluid Expansion as Supportive Therapy (FEAST) study evaluating the efficacy of fluid boluses in African children with severe infection. This study enrolled about 3,150 patients from age 60 days to 12 years who presented with a severe febrile illness complicated by impaired consciousness, respiratory distress, or both and evidence of impaired perfusion. Patients were randomized to 20–40 mL/kg of albumin 5% or 0.9% saline solution versus no fluid bolus (control). The 48-hour mortality was 10.6% (albumin), 10.5% (saline), and 7.3% (control). The reported relative risk of death between groups was as follows: saline bolus versus control 1.44 (confidence interval [CI], 1.09–1.9; p=0.01), albumin bolus versus saline bolus 1.01 (CI, 0.78–1.29; p=0.96), and any bolus versus control 1.45 (CI, 1.13–1.86; p=0.003). It is unclear whether these data can be extrapolated to all patient groups. Fifty-seven percent of the patients enrolled had a diagnosis of malaria. Around 45% of the patients enrolled received a blood transfusion. These percentages are much higher than those reported in U.S. and European studies evaluating the choice of fluids for resuscitation in pediatric patients with severe infection and shock. Further studies will be required before a change is made in the current recommendations.[6]

The therapeutic end points of fluid resuscitation in patients with shock are capillary refill less than 2 seconds, normal pulses with no difference between central and peripheral pulses, warm limbs, urine output greater than 1 mL/kg/hour, normal mental status, decreased lactate as measured on arterial blood gases (ABGs), and increased base deficit. Children normally have a lower blood pressure than do adults and can better preserve adequate blood pressure by vasoconstriction and increasing heart rate. As a result, blood pressure by itself is not a reliable end point for evaluating the adequacy of resuscitation in children.

Hypotension is the last thing to occur in pediatric shock states. The definition of hypotension, stated as the 5% for systolic blood pressure for age in the 2015 pediatric advanced life support guidelines,[4] is as follows:

- less than 60 mm Hg in term neonates (0–28 days)
- less than 70 mm Hg in infants (1–12 months)
- less than 70 mm Hg + (2 × age in years) in children 1–10 years of age
- less than 90 mm Hg in children 10 years or older

Fluid resuscitation should be continued until there is clinical improvement or an apparent hypervolemic state, as evidenced by rales, a gallop rhythm, or hepatomegaly.

Septic Shock

In 1969, an analysis of gram-negative sepsis showed a 98% mortality rate in children when shock syndrome developed.[7] In a recent population-based study of U.S. children with severe sepsis (defined as bacterial or fungal infection with at least one acute organ dysfunction), Hartman et al. reported an increase in the incidence of severe sepsis in 2000–2005 as 0.56–0.89 cases, respectively, per 1,000 children. In addition, the increase reported in newborns was from 4.5 to 9.7 cases per 1,000, led by sepsis in very low birth weight neonates. In children 15–19 years of age, the reported increase was from 0.37 to 0.48 cases per 1,000.[8] The mortality rate in this study was 8.9%, unchanged from in 2000, but significantly lower than that reported for adult patients with severe sepsis and septic shock (about 30% and 50%, respectively). This dramatic improvement in outcome has been achieved through a better understanding of the physiology of shock. The use of aggressive fluid resuscitation and the implementation of time-sensitive goal-directed therapies, as well as the application of technologic advances in respiratory, cardiovascular, renal, and nutritional support and the improvement in antibacterial, antiviral, and antifungal therapy, have resulted in improved survival in infants and children with septic shock and the resultant multisystem organ failure.[4,9-14] Watson and colleagues[35] found that 49% of sepsis cases occurred in children who had underlying illnesses that might place them at risk of higher morbidity and mortality. In the Children's Hospital of Pittsburgh, the mortality rate from sepsis for children who were previously healthy was 2% compared with 12% in children with chronic illnesses.[15]

PHYSIOLOGIC DIFFERENCES

Infants and young children are at a higher risk of severe systemic illness after infection than are adults. Infants are particularly vulnerable to infections for several reasons.[14] Passive immunity is normally conveyed from the mother to the fetus through the transmission of immunoglobulins during the last trimester. As a result, premature neonates are immunoglobulin-deficient. Even the full-term neonate has decreased polymorphonuclear leukocyte function and small polymorphonuclear storage pools compared with older children and adults, as well as decreased ability to synthesize new antibodies. Finally, neonates cannot make and deliver adequate amounts of phagocytes to infection sites. This leaves them particularly vulnerable to polysaccharide-carrying bacteria and explains why, historically, *H. influenzae*, *Streptococcus pneumoniae*, and *Neisseria meningitidis* have caused most of the significant infections in the first years of life. Low immunoglobulin levels also make the infant susceptible to viral infections. Stores of maternal immunoglobulin are depleted at about 2–5 months of age. Adult immunoglobulin levels are not typically achieved until 4–7 years of age. Because of these physiologic differences, as well as differences in bacterial resistance patterns, the list of most likely pathogens in children with sepsis differs from that in adults. Table 44.2 lists common pediatric pathogens and appropriate empiric antibiotic coverage. Antibiotics should be administered within 1 hour of diagnosis, after the collection of appropriate cultures.[5]

DEFINITIONS

In an effort to develop a consensus definition of the pediatric sepsis continuum including systemic inflammatory response syndrome (SIRS), infection, sepsis, severe

Table 44.2 Causative Pathogens and Recommended Treatments

Age/Risk Factors	Microorganism	Empiric Antibiotic Coverage
Premature neonates	*Enterococcus faecalis*	Ampicillin + aminoglycoside OR
	Gram-negative enterics	Cefotaxime + aminoglycoside
	Methicillin-resistant *Staphylococcus aureus* (MRSA)	OR
		Vancomycin + aminoglycoside
	Staphylococcus epidermidis	
Neonate	*Listeria monocytogenes*	Ampicillin + aminoglycoside OR
	Escherichia coli	Ampicillin + cefotaxime
	Group B *Streptococcus*	Acyclovir (if patient presents with seizures, until HSV R/O)
	Gram-negative enterics	
1–3 mo	*L. monocytogenes*	Ampicillin + cefotaxime or Ceftriaxone ± vancomycin[a]
	E. coli	
	Group B *Streptococcus*	
	Haemophilus influenzae	
	Streptococcus pneumoniae	
	Neisseria meningitidis	
>3 mo	*H. influenzae*	Cefotaxime or ceftriaxone ± vancomycin[a]
	S. pneumoniae	
	N. meningitidis	
Immunocompromised	*Pseudomonas aeruginosa*	Ceftazidime or cefepime or piperacillin/tazobactam + vancomycin
	S. aureus	
	S. epidermidis	
Ventriculoperitoneal (VP) shunt	*S. aureus*	Cefotaxime or ceftriaxone ± vancomycin[a]
	S. epidermidis	
	Gram-negative enterics	
Associated with head trauma or chronic otitis media	*S. pneumoniae*	Cefotaxime or ceftriaxone ± vancomycin[a]

[a]Vancomycin trough level 15–20 mcg/mL.

sepsis, septic shock, and multisystem organ dysfunction syndrome, a group of international experts in the fields of adult and pediatric sepsis and clinical research gathered in 2002. A panel was chosen that consisted of published pediatric critical care physicians and scientists with clinical research experience in pediatric sepsis.[16]

Because the clinical variables used to define SIRS and organ dysfunction are greatly affected by the normal physiologic changes that occur as children age, the group first defined six age-specific clinical and physiologic categories for vital sign and laboratory variables to meet SIRS criteria (Table 44.3): newborn, neonate, infant, toddler and preschool, school-aged child, and adolescent and young adult. Premature infants were not included because their care occurs primarily in NICUs (neonatal intensive care units), not PICUs.

Before discussing treatment, practitioners should understand the terms used to define sepsis. In 1992, SIRS was proposed by the American College of Chest Physicians and the Society of Critical Care Medicine to describe the nonspecific inflammatory process occurring in adults after trauma, infection, burns, pancreatitis, and other diseases.[16,17] Sepsis was defined as SIRS associated with infection.[17,18] The SIRS criteria were developed for use in adults. Not until 2005 was a consensus definition published for SIRS in children; this definition is listed in Table 44.4. A separate pediatric definition for SIRS was essential. Tachycardia and tachypnea, pivotal to the adult definition of SIRS, are common presenting symptoms of many pediatric disease processes. Therefore, the pediatric definition also includes that temperature and leukocyte abnormalities be present. Finally, numeric values for each criterion were established to account for the different physiology in children. Table 44.5 gives the age-specific cutoffs for each criterion. These values were established

Table 44.3 Pediatric Age Groups for Severe Sepsis Definitions[a]

Age Category	Definition
Newborn	0 days to 1 wk
Neonate	1 wk to 1 mo
Infant	1 mo to 1 yr
Toddler and preschool	2–5 yr
School-aged child	6–12 yr
Adolescent and young adult	13 to < 18 yr

[a]Goldstein B, Giroir B, Randolph A, et al. International pediatric sepsis consensus conference: definitions for sepsis and organ dysfunction in pediatrics. Pediatr Crit Care Med 2005;6:2-8.

Table 44.4 Definitions of SIRS, Infection, Sepsis, Severe Sepsis, and Septic Shock[a]

SIRS	The presence of at least two of the following four criteria, one of which must be abnormal temperature or leukocyte count: - Core temperature of > 38°C or < 36°C (must be measured by rectal, bladder, oral, or central catheter probe) - Tachycardia defined as at least 2 SD above normal for age in the absence of external stimulus, chronic drugs, or painful stimuli; or otherwise persistent elevation over 0.5–4 hr OR for children < 1 yr old: bradycardia, defined as a mean HR < 10% percentile for age in the absence of external vagal stimulus, β-blocker drugs, or congenital heart disease; or otherwise unexplained depression over a 0.5-hr period - Mean respiratory rate > 2 SD above normal for age or mechanical ventilation for an acute process not related to underlying neuromuscular disease or receipt of general anesthesia - Leukocyte count elevated or depressed for age (not secondary to chemotherapy-induced neutropenia) or > 10% immature neutrophils
Infection	A suspected or proven (by positive culture, tissue stain, or polymerase chain reaction test) infection caused by any pathogen OR a clinical syndrome associated with a high probability of infection. Evidence of infection includes positive findings on clinical examination, imaging or laboratory tests (e.g., white blood cells in a normally sterile body fluid, perforated viscus, chest radiograph consistent with pneumonia, petechial or purpuric rash, or purpurea fulminans)
Sepsis	SIRS in the presence of or as a result of suspected or proven infection
Severe sepsis	Sepsis plus one of the following: cardiovascular organ dysfunction OR acute respiratory distress syndrome OR two or more other organ dysfunctions. Organ dysfunctions are defined in Table 44.5
Septic shock	Sepsis and cardiovascular organ dysfunction as defined in Table 44.5

[a]Goldstein B, Giroir B, Randolph A, et al. International pediatric sepsis consensus conference: definitions for sepsis and organ dysfunction in pediatrics. Pediatr Crit Care Med 2005;6:2-8.

SIRS = systemic inflammatory response syndrome.

Table 44.5 Age-Specific Vital Signs and Laboratory Variables[a,b]					
	Heart Rate (beats/minute)		Respiratory Rate (breaths/minute)	Leukocyte Count (leukocytes × 10^3/mm)	Systolic BP (mm Hg)
Age Group	Tachycardia	Bradycardia			
0 days to 1 wk	> 180	< 100	> 50	> 34	< 65
1 wk to 1 mo	> 180	< 100	> 40	> 19.5 or < 5	< 75
1 mo to 1 yr	> 180	< 90	> 34	> 17.5 or < 5	< 100
2–5 yr	> 140	N/A	> 22	> 15.5 or < 6	< 94
6–12 yr	> 130	N/A	> 18	> 13.5 or < 4.5	< 105
13 to < 18 yr	> 110	N/A	> 14	> 11 or < 4.5	< 117

[a]Goldstein B, Giroir B, Randolph A, et al. International pediatric sepsis consensus conference: definitions for sepsis and organ dysfunction in pediatrics. Pediatr Crit Care Med 2005;6:2-8.

[b]Lower values for HR, leukocyte count, and systolic BP are for the 5th percentile, and upper values for HR, respiratory rate, or leukocyte count are for the 95th percentile.
N/A = not applicable.

according to the expert opinion of the international panel on sepsis that was convened in 2002.

Temperature is one of the features of the pediatric SIRS definition. A core temperature of greater than 38.5°C or less than 36°C may indicate serious infection. A core temperature is one measured by rectal, bladder, oral, or central catheter probe. Hypothermia is more likely to occur in infants.[19,20] Temperatures measured by the tympanic, toe, or auxiliary route are not sufficiently accurate. Temperature may also be documented by a reliable source at home within 4 hours of presentation to the hospital or physician's office. If environmental overheating, such as that produced by over-bundling, is suspected, the child should be returned to a neutral temperature environment, unbundled, and the temperature measurement repeated in 15–30 minutes.[16]

In children, SIRS requires the presence of an abnormal temperature (hypothermia or hyperthermia) or an abnormal leukocyte count (low or high) in the presence of tachypnea and tachycardia. Sepsis is defined as the proven or suspected infection in the setting of SIRS.[16-18] Severe sepsis is defined as sepsis in the setting of acute respiratory distress syndrome, cardiovascular organ dysfunction, or two or more acute organ dysfunctions (respiratory, renal, hematologic, neurologic, or hepatic). Organ dysfunctions are modified for children and summarized in Table 44.6. Carcillo et al. defined septic shock in pediatric patients as the presence of tachycardia and poor perfusion, including decreased peripheral pulses compared with central pulses, altered alertness, capillary refill greater than 2 seconds, mottled or cool extremities, and decreased urine output.[10] The definition of septic shock in children does not include hypotension, as required in adults. This is because children often maintain their blood pressure until they are severely ill. Shock may occur long before hypotension occurs in children with septic shock (failure to improve with adequate fluid resuscitation), catecholamine-resistant septic shock (failure to improve with fluids and catecholamines), and refractory septic shock (failure to improve with fluids, catecholamines, and vasodilators). In addition, there are developmental differences in the hemodynamic response to sepsis between neonates, children, and adults. Practitioners in the PICU may encounter all age ranges and must thus be familiar with the clinical differences between age groups because this may affect therapy.

Adult and pediatric patients have different adaptive responses that must be considered when selecting therapeutic management. This is important for pediatric practitioners to understand because many adolescent patients may respond as an adult. Among adult patients, the most common hemodynamic alterations include diminished systemic vascular resistance (SVR) and elevated CO. Systemic vascular resistance is diminished because of decreased vascular responsiveness to catecholamines, alterations in α-adrenergic receptor signal transduction, and the elaboration of inducible nitric oxide synthase. Adults have myocardial dysfunction with a decreased ejection fraction; however, CO is maintained or increased by tachycardia and reduced SVR.

Pediatric septic shock is associated with severe hypovolemia, and children often respond well to aggressive fluid resuscitation. Pediatric patients have diverse hemodynamic profiles during fluid-refractory septic shock: 58% have low cardiac indexes responsive to inotropic medications with or without vasodilators, 20% have high cardiac indexes and low SVR responsive to vasopressor therapy, and 22% present with both vascular and cardiac dysfunctions, necessitating the use of vasopressors and inotropic support.[21] The pediatric patient is different from the adult patient with septic shock because low CO, not low SVR, is associated with mortality in pediatric septic shock. In fact, 78% of children show some degree of cardiac dysfunction on presentation after fluid resuscitation. Furthermore, about 50% of patients require a change in their vasopressor or inotropic management, or the addition of another agent, emphasizing that the hemodynamic status in children can change rapidly. Finally, a reduction in oxygen

Table 44.6 Organ Dysfunction Criteria

Cardiovascular Dysfunction
Despite administration of isotonic IV fluid bolus ≥ 40 mL/kg in 1 hr
- Decrease in BP (hypotension) < 5th percentile for age or systolic BP < 2 SD below normal for age[a] OR
- Need for vasoactive drug to maintain BP in normal range (dopamine > 5 mcg/kg/min or dobutamine, epinephrine, or norepinephrine at any dose) OR
- Two of the following:
- Unexplained metabolic acidosis: Base deficit > 5 mEq/L
- Increased arterial lactate > 2 times the upper limit of normal
- Oliguria: Urine output < 0.5 mL/kg/hr
- Prolonged capillary refill: > 5 s
- Core to peripheral temperature gap > 3°C

Respiratory[b]
- Pao_2/Fio_2 < 300 in absence of cyanotic heart disease or preexisting lung disease OR
- $Paco_2$ > 65 torr or 20 mm Hg over baseline $Paco_2$ OR
- Proven need[c] or > 50% Fio_2 to maintain saturations > 92% OR

Need for nonelective invasive or noninvasive mechanical ventilation[d]

Neurologic
- GCS < 11 OR
- Acute change in mental status with a decrease in GCS ≥ 3 points from abnormal baseline

Hematologic
- Platelet count < 80,000/mm³ or a decline of 50% in platelet count from highest value recorded during the past 3 days (for chronic hematology/oncology patients) OR
- International normalized ratio > 2

Renal
- Serum creatinine > 2 times the upper limit of normal for age or a 2-fold increase in baseline creatinine

Hepatic
- Total bilirubin ≥ 4 mg/dL (not applicable for newborn) OR
- ALT 2 times the upper limit of normal for age

[a]See Table 44.5.
[b]Acute respiratory distress syndrome must include a Pao_2/Fio_2 ratio < 200 mm Hg, bilateral infiltrates, acute onset, and no evidence of left heart failure. Acute lung injury is defined identically except that the Pao_2/Fio_2 ratio must be < 300 mm Hg.
[c]Proven need assumes oxygen requirement was tested by decreasing flow if required.
[d]In postoperative patients, this requirement can be met if the patient has developed an acute inflammatory or infectious process in the lungs that prevents him or her from being extubated.
ALT = alanine transaminase; GCS = Glasgow Coma Scale.

delivery rather than a defect in oxygen extraction can be the major determinant of oxygen consumption in children.[22]

The relative ability of infants and children to augment CO through increased heart rate, as seen in adults, is limited by their preexisting elevated heart rate, which precludes proportionate increases in heart rate without compromising diastolic filling time. In addition, in adults, ventricular dilation is a compensatory response used to maintain CO. However, the increased connective tissue content of the infant's heart and the diminished content of actin and myosin limit the potential for acute ventricular dilation.[23]

Neonatal septic shock can further be complicated by the physiologic transition from fetal to neonatal circulation. Sepsis-induced acidosis and hypoxia can increase pulmonary vascular resistance and thus arterial pressure, thereby maintaining the patency of the ductus arteriosus. This results in persistent pulmonary hypertension (PPHN) of the newborn and persistent fetal circulation. Neonatal septic shock with PPHN will increase the workload on the right ventricle, leading to right ventricular failure, tricuspid regurgitation, and hepatomegaly. Therefore, therapies directed at reversing right ventricular failure by reducing pulmonary artery pressures are commonly needed in neonates with fluid-refractory septic shock and PPHN. The treatment of PPHN will not be discussed in this chapter.

INITIAL MANAGEMENT

Since the landmark study by Rivers in 2001[9] showed a 33% reduction in mortality in adult patients with sepsis when patients were aggressively treated with early fluid resuscitation, early red cell transfusion, and early inotropic therapy within 6 hours of presentation, goal-directed therapy has been advocated for patients who present in septic shock. Although aggressive interventions to allow for optimization of oxygen delivery (e.g., placing central lines to measure central venous pressure [CVP] or mixed venous oxygen saturation [Svo$_2$]) are no longer recommended, the components of early goal-directed therapy include prompt resuscitation of poor perfusion through the administration of intravenous fluids and appropriately targeted inotropic and/or vasopressor therapy, early empiric antimicrobial therapy, drainage of infection, and appropriate and continuous monitoring of hemodynamic status.[5,9-12]

In addition to goal-directed therapy, support of the airway and breathing is essential to optimize oxygen delivery. Supplemental oxygen should be administered to all patients presenting with signs of septic shock, and endotracheal intubation may be necessary. Because goal-directed therapy includes aggressive fluid resuscitation, early and immediate vascular access is essential to the treatment of septic shock. Ideally, two peripheral intravenous catheters should be placed promptly. Intraosseous access should be considered in any patient for whom peripheral vascular access is not rapidly established. Although ideal, a central venous line is not required for initial fluid resuscitation.

All patients with septic shock have some degree of hypovolemia because of many factors, including increased insensible losses (i.e., excessive sweating, fever, and increased respiratory rate), excessive fluid losses from diarrhea or vomiting, third spacing of fluid caused by capillary leak, and diminished oral intake. Relative hypovolemia occurs because of systemic vasodilation.

With the exception of the FEAST trial in Africa discussed earlier, no data suggest a difference in the survival rates of pediatric patients after resuscitation with colloids (blood products) compared with crystalloid fluids.[24] The choice of fluid is less important than the volume administered. Adequate volume is necessary to sustain cardiac preload, increase stroke volume, and improve oxygen delivery. Crystalloids and colloids, specifically packed red blood cells, have equal effects on improving stroke volume. In addition, both restore tissue perfusion to the same degree if they are titrated to the same level of filling pressure.

The optimal hemoglobin for patients in septic shock has not been established. In the early management of sepsis in adults, maintaining hemoglobin concentrations of 7–9 g/dL to improve oxygen-carrying capacity has been documented to improve sepsis survival by improving tissue perfusion. Anemia in sepsis has been associated with increased mortality, but so has the administration of blood.[25] Therefore, according to the limited data available, the Society of Critical Care Medicine has recommended that hemoglobin concentrations be maintained at 8–10 g/dL with the understanding that data for this practice are limited.[5] Because pediatric data are limited, it is appropriate to extrapolate from the adult literature of maximizing tissue oxygen delivery if there is evidence of poor tissue perfusion. Once tissue hypoperfusion, acute hemorrhage, or lactic acidosis has resolved, red cell transfusion should be administered only when hemoglobin concentrations are less than 7 g/dL with a target goal of 8–10 g/dL.[5,26] Fresh frozen plasma may be infused to correct abnormal prothrombin time (PT) and partial thromboplastin time (PTT) values, but fresh frozen plasma should not be pushed because it may produce acute hypotensive effects because of vasoactive kinins and high citrate concentrations. Finally, there is no literature to suggest that 5% albumin administration improves outcome with respect to sepsis mortality. Albumin administration may be considered in patients who are hypoalbuminemic, but routine use of albumin is not recommended.[27]

As described previously for the management of hypovolemic shock, patients with septic shock should be reassessed for signs of improved perfusion using clinical criteria such as reduction in heart rate, improvement in blood pressure, capillary refill, quality of pulses, and mental status with each fluid bolus. If the clinical signs of shock persist, another 20 mL/kg of isotonic fluid should be administered, reaching, if necessary, 60 mL/kg within the first 15–30 minutes of treatment.[4,5] Some children with septic shock require as much as 200 mL/kg in the first hour.[11] The results of the FEAST trial have raised the question of whether certain patient populations with shock may be harmed by the administration of aggressive intravenous fluid.[6] This question remains to be answered.

Patients remaining in shock despite fluid resuscitation are given inotropic support to attain normal blood pressure for age and capillary refill time of less than 2 seconds. Every hour that goes by without implementing these therapies is associated with a 1.5-fold increased risk of mortality.[26] Patients who do not respond rapidly to initial fluid boluses or those with insufficient physiologic reserve should be considered for invasive hemodynamic monitoring. Invasive monitoring of CVP is instituted to ensure that the satisfactory right ventricular preload is present, typically using a goal of 10–12 mm Hg, and that oxygen-carrying capacity is optimized by packed red blood cell transfusion to correct anemia to a goal hemoglobin concentration greater than 7 g/dL.[5,11]

Fluid-refractory shock is defined as the persistence of signs of shock after sufficient fluids have been administered to achieve a CVP of 8–12 mm Hg and/or signs of fluid overload, as evidenced by new-onset rales, increased work of breathing and hypoxemia from pulmonary edema, hepatomegaly, or a diminished mean arterial pressure (MAP). Diuretics and peritoneal dialysis/continuous renal replacement therapy are indicated for patients who develop signs and symptoms of fluid overload.

Up to 40% of CO may be required to support the work of breathing; therefore, in the presence of respiratory distress, an elective tracheal intubation followed by mechanical ventilation will contribute to redistributing blood flow away from respiratory muscles toward other vital organs. Mechanical intubation, however, is not without adverse effects. It is imperative that the patient receive adequate fluid resuscitation before the intubation because the change from spontaneous breathing to positive pressure ventilation will decrease the effective preload to the heart. Ventilation may reduce the left ventricular afterload that may be beneficial in patients with low cardiac index and high SVR. In addition, ventilation may allow an alternative method to alter acid-base balance. If sedatives and analgesics are used for intubation, it is critical to choose agents that do not cause further vasodilation.

Although laboratory studies rarely affect the management of septic shock in the first hour of therapy, patients should have laboratory studies sent routinely, assessing for hematologic abnormalities, metabolic derangements, or electrolyte abnormalities that may contribute to morbidity. A peripheral white blood cell count may aid in the choice of broad-spectrum antibiotics, whereas hemoglobin and platelet count will help assess the need for early blood transfusion. A type and screen should be sent to the blood bank to prepare for any necessary transfusions. Electrolyte abnormalities are common in sepsis; recognition and treatment of metabolic abnormalities such as hypoglycemia and hypocalcemia will improve outcome. A disseminated intravascular coagulation panel, including PT, PTT, and fibrinogen, will aid in assessing the severity of illness. If abnormalities exist, they may need to be corrected before performing invasive procedures. Finally, an arterial or venous blood gas will determine the adequacy of ventilation and oxygenation and the severity of acidemia.

Unfortunately, clinical response to fluid resuscitation is a relatively insensitive indicator of the completeness of restoration of microvascular blood flow. The success of adequate fluid resuscitation can be guided by additional parameters: invasive blood pressure monitoring, CVP, measurement of Svo_2, measurement of blood lactate, and urine output. An elevated serum lactate concentration suggests that tissue is hypoperfused and undergoing anaerobic metabolism, even in patients who are not hypotensive. Because low CO is associated with increased O_2 extraction, Svo_2 can be used as an indirect indicator of whether CO is adequate to meet tissue metabolic demand. If tissue oxygen delivery is adequate, Svo_2 should be greater than 70%.[12] In the goal-directed study by Rivers,[9] the patients in whom maintaining an Svo_2 greater than 70% using blood transfusion to a hemoglobin concentration of 10 g/dL and inotropic support to increase CO had a 40% reduction in mortality compared with patients in whom only MAP and CVP were monitored. This finding in children with septic shock was reproduced by de Oliveira, reducing mortality from 39% to 12% when directing therapy to a goal Svo_2 greater than 70%.[13]

CARDIOVASCULAR DRUG THERAPY

Pharmacologic support in children with septic shock must be individualized because different hemodynamic abnormalities exist in pediatric patients, and the primary hemodynamic abnormalities may change with time and progression of the patient's disease. Twenty percent of children present with predominant vasodilatory shock, called "warm" shock. This form of shock is associated with vasodilation and capillary leak, but normal or elevated CO. The patients have strong pulses, warm extremities, good capillary refill, and tachycardia. In warm shock, using a vasopressor such as dopamine, norepinephrine, phenylephrine, or vasopressin to promote vasoconstriction would be of most benefit. Fifty-eight percent of children present with "cold shock," or predominantly a poor CO state. Clinically, this manifests as weak pulses, cool extremities, slow capillary refill, and hepatic and pulmonary congestion. Using an inotrope (e.g., dobutamine, epinephrine, or milrinone) with or without a vasodilator would be most beneficial in cold shock. Careful assessment of clinical response is critical because a combination of vasodilatory and cold shock with a low SVR and poor CO can occur in 22% of children.

Dopamine

In shock unresponsive to initial fluid resuscitation, the initial vasopressor of choice is dopamine, according to the pediatric advanced life support guidelines.[4] Dopamine has direct and indirect effects on dopamine receptors, α-receptors, and β-receptors on both the heart and the peripheral vasculature. One of the mechanisms of dopamine action is improvement in endogenous catecholamine release. In severe septic states, presynaptic vacuoles may be depleted of norepinephrine, which may explain why dopamine may have diminished activity. In addition, infants younger than 6 month may not have developed their component of sympathetic innervations; therefore, they have reduced releasable stores of epinephrine.[11]

Dopamine should be initiated at 5 mcg/kg/minute and titrated in increments of 2.5 mcg/kg/minute every 3–5 minutes until the goal of improved perfusion, blood pressure, or both is achieved.[4] The maximum recommended dopamine dose is 20 mcg/kg/minute; doses higher than 20 mcg/kg/minute may contribute to increased myocardial oxygen demand without much improvement in vasopressor activity. Dopamine-resistant shock is diagnosed after titrating dopamine to 20 mcg/kg/minute with the persistence of signs and symptoms of shock. At this point, the patient should be reassessed. Measure the patient's hemoglobin, and administer packed red blood cells to improve the hemoglobin to 8–10 g/dL. This may improve tissue oxygenation. Measure CVP to assess intravascular volume status with the goal of achieving a CVP of 8–12 mm Hg; Svo_2 can be used as a marker of CO (if the hemoglobin concentration is within the normal range), together with the clinical examination. Dopamine-resistant shock commonly responds to epinephrine or norepinephrine.

A recent double-blind, prospective, randomized controlled trial evaluated dopamine versus epinephrine as the initial vasoactive drug for pediatric septic shock in 120 pediatric patients (63 dopamine; 57 epinephrine). There were 17 deaths (14.2%): 13 (20.6%) in the dopamine group and 4 (7%) in the epinephrine group (p=0.033). Early administration of epinephrine appeared to be associated with increased survival in this population. However, dopamine was dosed at 5–10 mcg/kg/minute (the low end of the dosing range) and epinephrine at 0.1–0.3 mcg/kg/minute. The dosing of epinephrine could be considered more aggressive; thus, the two treatment arms are not comparable. More studies are needed before epinephrine is considered the drug of choice in children.[28]

Recent adult data analyses raise the concern of increased mortality with dopamine use. One possible explanation is dopamine's ability to reduce the release of hormones such as prolactin from the anterior pituitary gland through stimulation of the dopamine DA_2 receptor, thus reducing cell-mediated immunity and inhibiting thyrotropin-releasing hormone release, worsening the impaired thyroid function known to occur in critical illness. For these reasons, some clinicians prefer low-dose epinephrine or norepinephrine as a first-line agent for fluid-refractory hypotensive hyperdynamic shock.[10]

Epinephrine

Epinephrine is a direct agent that is naturally produced in the adrenal gland and is the principal stress hormone with widespread metabolic and hemodynamic effects. It has both inotropic and chronotropic effects. Epinephrine is a reasonable choice for the treatment of patients with low CO and poor peripheral perfusion because it increases heart rate and myocardial contractility.[25] Depending on the dose administered, epinephrine may exert variable effects on SVR. At low doses (less than 0.3 mcg/kg/minute), epinephrine exerts greater β_2-adrenergic receptor activation, resulting in vasodilation in skeletal muscle and cutaneous vascular beds, shunting blood flow away from the splanchnic circulation. At higher doses, α_1-adrenergic receptor activation becomes more prominent and may increase SVR and heart rate. For patients with markedly elevated SVR, epinephrine may be administered simultaneously with a vasodilator. Epinephrine increases glucogenesis and glycogenolysis, resulting in elevated serum blood glucose concentrations. Therefore, patients receiving epinephrine infusions should have their serum glucose concentration monitored closely. Epinephrine should be initiated at 0.1 mcg/kg/minute and titrated in increments of 0.1 mcg/kg/minute every 3–5 minutes until the goal of improved perfusion and/or blood pressure is achieved.

Norepinephrine

Norepinephrine is a direct agent and is naturally produced in the adrenal gland. It is a potent vasopressor that redirects blood low away from skeletal muscle to the splanchnic circulation, even in the presence of decreased CO. Norepinephrine has been used extensively to elevate SVR in adults and children with sepsis. If the patient's clinical state is characterized by low SVR (e.g., wide pulse pressure with diastolic blood pressure less than one-half the systolic blood pressure), norepinephrine is recommended. About 20% of children with volume-refractory septic shock have a low SVR.[20] In addition, in children who are intubated and receiving sedatives or analgesics, the incidence of low SVR may be higher. In patients with impaired contractility, the additional afterload imposed by norepinephrine may substantially compromise CO. In some patients with both impaired or marginal CO and decreased SVR, myocardial contractility may need to be supported by adding an agent such as dobutamine.

Dobutamine

Dobutamine is a nonselective β_2-adrenergic agonist that produces improved myocardial contractility, chronotropy, and some lusitropy and improved myocardial relaxation. Its β_2 activity can lead to peripheral vasodilation, which must be considered before using it in a patient who may already be hypotensive. If hypotension does exist, dobutamine should be used in combination with other vasopressor therapy. Thus, dobutamine should be considered in the patient who has signs and symptoms or laboratory values consistent with poor tissue perfusion, but with an adequate blood pressure to tolerate some degree of vasodilation. Dobutamine should be initiated at 2.5 mcg/kg/minute and titrated in increments of 2.5 mcg/kg/minute every 3–5 minutes, to a maximum infusion rate of 20 mcg/kg/minute. Careful attention to the patient's blood pressure is critical. Improved perfusion, decreased lactate, and increased Svo_2 will help determine appropriate dosing.

Vasopressin

Although not a recommendation in the 2015 pediatric advanced life support guidelines, vasopressin has been suggested as an alternative therapy for refractory cardiac arrest or hypotension caused by a low SVR in children whose epinephrine infusion exceeds 1 mcg/kg/minute.[4] Vasopressin exerts its hemodynamic effects by the V1α receptor, promoting an increase in intracellular calcium in the peripheral vasculature, thus enhancing vasoconstriction and restoring systemic vascular tone. In a preliminary case series, vasopressin at a dose of 0.3–2 milliunits/kg/

minute (18–120 milliunits/kg/hour) improved blood pressure and urine output in patients with catecholamine-refractory, vasodilatory shock and allowed weaning of catecholamines once treatment was initiated.[29] In a more recent analysis by the American Heart Association, however, vasopressin use was associated with a lower rate of return to spontaneous circulation.[30] The use of vasopressin in critically ill children remains controversial.[4,5,11]

Vasodilators

Vasodilator medications are occasionally required in the treatment of pediatric patients with sepsis having markedly elevated SVR and normal or decreased CO. Vasodilators decrease SVR and improve CO by decreasing ventricular afterload. Nitroglycerin or nitroprusside may be used for this indication. Each has a short half-life; therefore, if hypotension occurs, the agent can rapidly be reversed by stopping the infusion. Both drugs can be infused at an initial rate of 0.5 mcg/kg/minute and titrated in increments of 0.5 mcg/kg/minute to a maximum infusion rate of 5–10 mcg/kg/minute. If nitroprusside is used, it is necessary to observe for sodium thiocyanate accumulation in the setting of renal failure and cyanide toxicity with hepatic failure or with prolonged infusions (greater than 72 hours) of more than 3 mcg/kg/minute. If the patient has tolerated infusions of nitroglycerin or nitroprusside, switching to the longer-acting agent milrinone should be considered.

Milrinone is a phosphodiesterase type 3 inhibitor that produces its hemodynamic effects by inhibiting the degradation of cyclic AMP in smooth muscle cells and cardiac myocytes. Phosphodiesterase type 3 inhibitors work synergistically with catecholamines, which produce their hemodynamic effects by increasing the production of cyclic AMP. Milrinone is useful in the treatment of patients with diminished myocardial contractility and output and decreased systemic resistance.[5,31] The concern with milrinone is its long half-life (2–6 hours); milrinone takes several hours to reach steady state. To achieve rapid serum concentrations, a loading dose of 50 mcg/kg administered over 10–30 minutes is recommended. This must be done with caution in patients with sepsis and shock because it may precipitate hypotension, requiring volume infusion, vasopressor infusion, or both. Administering the loading dose over several hours may avoid this adverse effect.

Corticosteroids

Although adjunctive corticosteroid therapy in patients in septic shock has not made a significant difference in outcome in any of the studies published to date, replacement may be of benefit in some patients.[32-34] In a recent study, 77% of children with septic shock admitted to two PICUs for 6 months had adrenal insufficiency.[34] Because of the limited evidence of their efficacy and safety in children, corticosteroids should be reserved for children with catecholamine-resistant shock, severe septic shock, and purpura; those who have previously received steroid therapies for chronic illness; those with pituitary or adrenal abnormalities; and those who previously received etomidate.[7-9,32-35] Assessment of serum cortisol should be used to guide treatment. There are no strict definitions, but adrenal insufficiency in adults with catecholamine-resistant shock has been defined as a random cortisol concentration of less than 18 mcg/dL or an increase in cortisol of 9 mcg/dL or less at 30 or 60 minutes after an adrenocorticotropic hormone stimulation test.[32] Similar values have been recommended for assessing serum cortisol in children with septic shock.[35] Published guidelines for hemodynamic support of pediatric and neonatal patients with septic shock recommend hydrocortisone 0.5–1 mg/kg intravenously every 6 hours (maximum 50 mg per dose).[16] As an alternative, some clinicians use a hydrocortisone regimen of a 50-mg/m² loading dose, followed by the same dose (50 mg/m²) divided into four doses and given every 6 hours (maximum 50 mg per dose).[35]

SEPSIS SUMMARY

The outcome of sepsis and septic shock depends on implementing time-sensitive goal-directed therapies. Early recognition of septic shock is critical to initiating rapid aggressive fluid resuscitation. Concurrent with the administration of oxygen, diagnosis of the source of the infection should be attempted and appropriate antibiotics administered within 1 hour of presentation. Vasopressor administration should be initiated if signs of shock persist despite adequate volume administration. If signs of shock persist, packed red blood cells should be administered to maintain hemoglobin at 8–10 g/dL. Frequent assessment, both clinical and laboratory, needs to be performed to allow adjustments in vasopressor and/or inotropic therapy, depending on the clinical presentation and ongoing physiologic derangements. Using a central venous catheter for measuring CVP and Svo_2 can help guide therapy.

RESPIRATORY DISTRESS

Respiratory distress, related to problems at all levels of the respiratory tract from the nose to the lungs, is a common occurrence in children.[4] The nose provides almost half the total airway resistance in children. Infants younger than 2 months are obligate nasal breathers, and their nose is short, soft, and small with almost circular nares. The nares will double in size from birth to 6 months, but they can easily be occluded from edema, secretions, or external pressure. Simply clearing the nasal passageways with saline and bulb suctioning can significantly improve an infant's respiratory condition. Other physiologic reasons for a high incidence of respiratory failure in infants and children are small and collapsible airways, an unstable chest wall, inadequate collateral ventilation for alveoli, poor control (tone) of the upper airway (particularly during sleep), tendency for the respiratory muscles to fatigue, reactivity of the pulmonary vascular bed (increased sensitivity of the vasculature, particularly in young infants), inefficient immune system, genetic disorders or syndromes, and residual problems related to premature birth such as bronchopulmonary dysplasia.

The most common reason for hospital admission in the first year of life is respiratory distress. This can be explained by the many physiologic differences seen in an infant. Although all the conducting airways are present at birth and the airway branching pattern is complete, the airways are small.[36] The airways will increase in size and length throughout childhood. As the airways increase in size, the incidence of respiratory distress will decrease. Not only are the airways smaller in an infant, but also the supporting airway cartilage and elastic tissue are not developed until the child is of school age. For these reasons, the child's airways are susceptible to collapse and may easily become obstructed as a result of laryngospasm, bronchospasm, and edema or mucus accumulation. Normal airway resistance is highest in infants because it is inversely proportional to 1/radius.[32] Therefore, any airway narrowing from bronchospasm, edema, or mucus accumulation will significantly increase the airway resistance and the infant's work of breathing. The cartilaginous ribs of the infant and young child are twice as compliant as the bony ribs of the older child or adult. During episodes of respiratory distress, the infant's chest wall will retract further than will that of a patient with a bony rib cage. This will reduce the patient's ability to maintain functional residual capacity or increase tidal volume, thus further increasing the patient's work of breathing.

The respiratory muscles consist of muscles of the upper airway, lower airway, and diaphragm. They contribute to the expansion of the lung and the maintenance of airway patency. Lack of development of the small airway muscles may render young infants less responsive than older children to bronchodilator therapy. Finally, the intercostal muscles are not fully developed until school age, so they act primarily to stabilize the chest wall during the first years of life. Because the intercostal muscles have neither the ability nor the strength to lift the rib cage in the young child, the diaphragm is responsible for generating tidal volume. Therefore, anything that impedes diaphragm movement, such as a large stomach bubble, abdominal distension, or peritonitis, can result in respiratory failure in the young child.

To assess a patient for respiratory distress, four areas should be evaluated: respiratory rate and effort, work of breathing, quality and magnitude of breath sounds, and mental status. Normal respiratory rates and definitions of respiratory distress vary with age (Table 44.7). A respiratory rate greater than 60 breaths/minute is abnormal in a child of any age but is of greatest concern in an older child. An abnormally slow or decreasing respiratory rate

Table 44.7 Age-Normal Respiratory Rates

Age	Respiratory Rate (breaths/minute)	Respiratory Distress (breaths/minute)
Newborn	30–60	60
2–12 mo	25–40	50
1–5 yr	20–30	40
6–10 yr	18–25	30
>10 yr	15–20	20

may herald respiratory failure. Inter-, sub-, and supracostal retractions increase with increasing respiratory distress. Although increased retractions are seen in infants, the efficiency of respiratory muscle function is decreased during the first years of life; therefore, the benefit in infants is reduced. Decreasing respiratory rate and diminished retractions in a child with a history of distress may signal severe fatigue. Nasal flaring is an effort to increase airway diameter and is often seen with hypoxemia. In addition, some infants will have an expiratory grunting noise. This noise is produced by children's involuntary effort to counter the loss of functional residual capacity by closing their glottis on active exhalation. Grunting produces positive end-expiratory pressure in an effort to prevent airway collapse. An expiratory grunt is classically seen in the presence of extensive alveolar pathology and is considered a sign of serious disease.

Among the many causes of respiratory distress in infants and children, the most common are infectious diseases, asthma, malignancies, trauma (both accidental and nonaccidental), poisonings, foreign body aspiration, anatomic upper airway obstruction, cardiogenic shock, and untreated left-to-right intracardiac shunts. Respiratory syncytial virus is among the most common causes of respiratory distress in infants and young children, leading to an estimated 90,000 hospitalizations each year.[33] However, only 7%–10% of infants admitted to the hospital for RSV will be admitted to the PICU. Although RSV can occur at any age, it is severest in children younger than 2 years. Prematurity, as well as chronic respiratory disease and congenital heart disease, increases the risk of severe RSV bronchiolitis requiring hospitalization. Unfortunately, there is no pharmacologic treatment for RSV. Treatment in the intensive care unit (ICU) is supportive care and intubation and mechanical support when necessary.

Oxygen should be administered immediately in any patient when respiratory difficulty is suspected. Infants and children consume 2–3 times more oxygen per kilogram of body weight than do adults under normal conditions and even more when they are ill or distressed. The specific indications for intubation in infants and children are as follows:

- Apnea
- Acute respiratory failure (Pao_2 less than 50 mm Hg in patients with fraction of inspired oxygen [Fio_2] greater than 0.5 and $Paco_2$ greater than 55 mm Hg acutely)
- Need to control oxygen delivery, with institution of positive end-expiratory pressure or to provide accurate delivery of Fio_2 greater than 0.5
- Need to control ventilation to decrease work of breathing, control $Paco_2$, or administer neuromuscular blocking agents
- Inadequate chest wall function, as in patients with neuromuscular disorders such as Guillain-Barré syndrome, spinal muscular atrophy, or muscular dystrophy
- Upper airway obstruction
- Protection of the airway for patients whose protective reflexes are absent, such as those with head trauma

MEDICATIONS FOR INTUBATION AND MECHANICAL VENTILATION

After the decision is made to proceed with intubation, the next decision needs to be whether pharmacologic agents are appropriate. Most pediatric patients require sedation before laryngoscopy and intubation. The goal is to depress the infant's or child's level of consciousness sufficiently to produce appropriate conditions for intubation. Pharmacologic therapy is used to produce adequate sedation, analgesia, and amnesia plus a blunting of the physiologic response to airway manipulation. Intubation in the awake state can elicit protective reflexes that trigger tachycardia, bradycardia, and elevation in blood pressure; increased intracranial pressure (ICP), intraocular pressure; cough; and bronchospasm. Pharmacologic control promotes a smoother intubation with less physiologic stress for the patient who often is already in a compromised state. Ideally, this should be accomplished while producing minimal hemodynamic compromise.[34]

Many factors should be considered when choosing agents for intubation: the agent's onset of action, the patient's hemodynamic status, the need to prevent increased intraocular or intracranial pressure that may be caused by intubation, and whether the stomach is full or empty. A wide variety of medications may be used for pediatric sedation, each with its own risk and benefits (Table 44.8).[34] In general, agents that act rapidly and are eliminated quickly are ideal. Often, drug choices are made according to the clinician's experience with a particular drug and the immediate availability of the drug. More importantly, the drug regimen chosen must be according to the patient's physiologic state. Agents with adverse effects that would exacerbate any underlying medical conditions must be avoided. Narcotics used in combination with anxiolytics are commonly used.

Patients with inadequate relaxation despite adequate sedation may require neuromuscular blockade, although these agents are not without risk. In a patient with a partial airway obstruction, neuromuscular blockade may worsen pharyngeal collapse, potentially resulting in complete airway obstruction. Therefore, neuromuscular blocking agents should only be used if the clinician is certain that adequate ventilation can be provided or that the patient can be intubated. If adequate chest rise and oxygen saturation cannot readily be maintained with bag-mask ventilation, neuromuscular blockers should not be used. Infants and children younger than 5 years have a high vagal tone and are therefore more likely to have bradycardia when intubated. Instrumentation of the airway can directly stimulate vagal receptors and induce bradycardia. In these patients, it is prudent to administer atropine 0.02 mg/kg (minimum 0.1 mg) before intubation to blunt the autonomic response. Lidocaine (1–1.5 mg/kg per dose with a maximum dose of 100 mg) may be administered intravenously to blunt the airway protective reflexes elicited by instrumentation. This may be particularly useful in a patient with elevated ICP.

In the patient with asthma, drugs that release histamine (e.g., morphine or atracurium) and have the potential to produce laryngospasm or bronchospasm should be avoided. The beneficial bronchodilatory adverse effects of ketamine, however, make it a useful choice in these patients. In a child with increased ICP, the choice of pharmacologic agent depends on the patient's hemodynamic status. Pentobarbital is an excellent choice in the hemodynamically stable patient, whereas etomidate is preferred if the patient is unstable or hypovolemia is suspected. Etomidate should not be used routinely in pediatric patients because a single dose administered for intubation has the potential to produce adrenal inhibition.[37] In children and adults with septic shock, etomidate administration is associated with a higher mortality rate.[37-39]

For all intubation, preoxygenation is carried out to increase the available oxygen in the lungs during the procedure, thus giving the practitioner some buffer time to intubate the patient. However, in patients with an elevated ICP or pulmonary vascular hypertension, hyperventilation is recommended to produce hypocarbia also.

In an infant or child with a full stomach, the risk of aspirating gastric contents is high. Rapid sequence intubation is used when there is an aspiration risk, such as in the child with a full stomach, and there is no concern of a difficult intubation.[40] The goal of rapid sequence intubation is to gain airway control with an endotracheal tube (ETT) as quickly as possible to prevent aspiration. The patient is preoxygenated by facemask; bag-mask ventilation should not be used because it causes gastric distension. Once all necessary intubation equipment is ready, rapidly

continued on page 912

Table 44.8 Pharmacologic Agents Used for Intubation and Continuous Sedation

Drug	Route	Dose	Onset	Duration	Benefits	Adverse Effects
Narcotics						
Morphine	IV	0.1 mg/kg/dose (max initial dose 2 mg); may repeat to a maximum total dose of 15 mg Neonates: 0.05 mg/kg/dose Continuous infusion Children: 20–50 mcg/kg/hr Neonates: 15 mcg/kg/hr Premature neonates: 10 mcg/kg/hr	Peak: 20 min	2–4 hr in neonates	Reversible (naloxone)	Histamine release, respiratory depression, hypotension, peripheral vasodilatation, euphoria, dysphoria, itching, central nausea and vomiting, decreased response to hypercarbia
Fentanyl	IV	1–3 mcg/kg/dose (max initial dose 100 mcg; may repeat to a total dose of 5 mcg/kg or 250 mcg) Continuous infusion 1–3 mcg/kg/hr (max initial dose 50–100 mcg/hr) Patient with coronary heart disease with an open chest: 5 mcg/kg/hr	1–3 min	30–90 min	Rapid onset, short acting, reversible (naloxone), relatively stable hemodynamic profile	Bradycardia, respiratory depression, decreased response to hypercarbia, acute chest wall rigidity, itching
Fentanyl	IN	1–2 mcg/kg maximum dose 100 mcg	3–5 min	~30 min	Rapid onset, short acting, reversible (naloxone), relatively stable hemodynamic profile	
Benzodiazepines						
Diazepam	IV	0.05 mg/kg/dose (max 5 mg); may repeat in 0.05-mg/kg increments (max 1 mg) to a total maximum dose of 10 mg	0.5–2 min	3 hr	Reversible (flumazenil)	Respiratory depression, lacks analgesic properties, hypotension and bradycardia, local irritation, pain
Lorazepam	IV	0.05–0.15 mg/kg/dose (max 4 mg)	15–30 min	0.5–3 hr	Reversible (flumazenil)	Respiratory depression, lacks analgesic properties, hypotension and bradycardia
Midazolam	IV/IM	0.05–0.15 mg/kg/dose (max initial dose 2 mg; may repeat in 1-mg increments to a total dose of 5 mg) Continuous infusion 0.05–0.1 mg/kg/hr (max initial dose 2 mg/hr)	1–5 min	20–30 min	Rapid onset, short acting, provides amnesia, reversible (flumazenil)	Respiratory depression, lacks analgesic properties, hypotension and bradycardia
Midazolam	IN	0.1–0.3 mg/kg/dose (max 10 mg) Use the 5-mg/mL concentration	2–5 min	30–60 min	May burn slightly on administration	Respiratory depression, lacks analgesic properties, hypotension and bradycardia

Table 44.8	Pharmacologic Agents Used for Intubation and Continuous Sedation *(continued)*					
Drug	**Route**	**Dose**	**Onset**	**Duration**	**Benefits**	**Adverse Effects**
Midazolam	PO	0.5–0.75 mg/kg/dose (max 10–20 mg)	30 min	2–6 hr	May use IV form of medication mixed in a beverage with flavor; otherwise, bitter in taste	Respiratory depression, lacks analgesic properties, hypotension and bradycardia
Barbiturates						
Pentobarbital	IV	2 mg/kg/dose (max 100 mg). May repeat in 1-mg/kg/dose increments to a total dose of 7 mg/kg. Do not exceed 200 mg total dose Continuous infusion 0.5–1 mg/kg/hr	1 min	15 min	Decreases intracranial pressure	
Pentobarbital	IM/PO/PR	2–6 mg/kg/dose	IM: 10–15 min PR/PO: 15–60 min	1–4 hr		
Miscellaneous						
Ketamine	IV	1 mg/kg/dose q 5 min titrated to effect Continuous infusion 0.5–1 mg/kg/hr	1–2 min	10–30 min	Rapid onset, airway protective reflexes stay intact, no hypotension or bradycardia Bronchodilation, useful to intubate patients with asthma	Increases airway secretions and laryngospasm (blunted with atropine). Elevated intracranial and intraocular pressure. Emergence reactions (blunted with benzodiazepines)
Ketamine	IM	4–5 mg/kg/dose	3–5 min	10–15 min	Same as above	Same as above
Ketamine	PO	6–10 mg/kg/dose			Same as above	Same as above
Ketamine	IN	6–8 mg/kg/dose	3–10 min	20–60 min	Same as above	Same as above
Etomidate	IV	0.3 mg/kg/dose initially; then 0.1 mg/kg/dose q 5 min to titrate to effect	10–20 s	4–10 min	Rapid onset Short acting Stable hemodynamic profile, decreased ICP	Potential for adrenal inhibition, nausea and vomiting on emergence
Propofol	IV	1–2 mg/kg/dose initially; then 0.5–2 mg/kg/dose q 3–5 min to titrate to effect Continuous infusion Infants and children: 50–150 mcg/kg/min Adolescents: 10–50 mcg/kg/min	30–60 s	5–10 min	IV general anesthetic, rapid onset and recovery	Cardiovascular and respiratory depression, contraindicated in patients with egg allergy, pain on injection

Table 44.8 Pharmacologic Agents Used for Intubation and Continuous Sedation (continued)

Drug	Route	Dose	Onset	Duration	Benefits	Adverse Effects
Dexmedetomidine	IV	0.5–1 mg/kg/dose Continuous infusion 0.4–0.7 mcg/kg/hr Doses as high as 2.5 mcg/kg/hr have been used				Hypotension and bradycardia
Dexmedetomidine	IN	0.5–2 mcg/kg/dose				
Neuromuscular Blockers						
Succinylcholine	IV	1 mg/kg/dose	30–60 s	4–7 min	Rapid onset Short duration	Potentiates hyperkalemia. Contraindicated in head trauma (↑ ICP), crush injury, burns, hyperkalemia. May induce neuroleptic malignant syndrome
Vecuronium	IV	0.1 mg/kg/dose Continuous infusion: 0.1 mg/kg/hr; monitor with TOF q shift	1–3 min	30–40 min	Cardiovascular stable	Slower onset Longer duration of action
Rocuronium	IV/IM	0.6–1 mg/kg/dose	60–75 s	20–30 min	Cardiovascular stable	
Reversal Agents						
Naloxone	IV	Overdose: 0.1 mg/kg/dose (max 2 mg) Slight respiratory depression: 0.01–0.02 mg/kg/dose (max 0.4 mg); may repeat q 2–3 min	2 min	20–60 min	Rapid onset	Shorter duration than most opioids; therefore, repeated doses may be needed
Flumazenil	IV	0.01 mg/kg/dose (max 0.2 mg); may repeat 0.005 mg/kg/dose at 1-min intervals to a max total dose of 1 mg	1–3 min	6–10 min	Rapid onset	Shorter duration than most benzodiazepines; therefore, repeated doses may be needed

ICP = intracranial pressure; IM = intramuscular(ly); IN = intranasal(ly); PO = oral(ly); PR = rectal(ly); TOF = train-of-four.

continued from page 909

acting sedative, analgesic, and paralytic medications are administered simultaneously. An end-tidal CO_2 detector should be attached to the ETT after intubation to confirm proper placement in the trachea. Colorimetric end-tidal CO_2 devices change from purple to yellow to confirm the presence of exhaled CO_2 and tracheal placement.

Endotracheal intubation and mechanical ventilation can be painful, frightening, and anxiety provoking, especially in a young child. To improve patient comfort, relieve anxiety, and lessen the work of breathing, anxiolytics, sedatives, and analgesics are commonly administered once the patient is intubated and mechanically ventilated. Maintaining adequate sedation is essential. Selection of appropriate agents is based on the patient's physiology. Guidelines for using continuous infusions are outlined in Table 44.9. In the paralyzed patient, neuromuscular blockade neither alters consciousness nor provides analgesia; therefore, adequate sedation and analgesia are essential. Providing effective analgesia and sedation to the pediatric patient depends on accurate ongoing efforts to assess the intensity of the patient's pain or anxiety. Assessing pain and anxiety in infants and critically ill children who are unable to communicate relies heavily on physiologic and behavioral responses. Several pain and sedation tools have been developed and validated specifically for use in children.[41] No single standard measure gives a complete qualitative or quantitative measure. Selection of an appropriate tool is based on the child's age, underlying medical condition, and cognition level. It is essential that these tools be used to evaluate the adequacy of the ICU sedation. Policies and procedures need to be in place for the appropriate selection and use of each tool, in addition to the training of

Table 44.9 ICU Treatment of Status Asthmaticus

First-line Therapies	
Continuous albuterol inhalation	10–40 mg/hr[a]
Corticosteroids (prednisolone/prednisone or methylprednisolone)	2–4 mg/kg/24 hr divided q 6–12 hr
Supplemental oxygen	To maintain O_2 saturations > 92%
Early supplemental therapies	
IV magnesium	25–75 mg/kg/dose (max 2 g/dose) infused over 20 min
Second-line therapies	
Noninvasive positive pressure	Titrated to comfort and tidal volume
IV terbutaline	10–20 mcg/kg loading dose, followed by a continuous infusion of 0.1–10 mcg/kg/min
IV aminophylline	Load 6 mg/kg/dose, followed by a continuous infusion of
	1–9 yr = 0.85–1 mg/kg/hr
	Goal serum concentration: 1–20 mcg/mL
Rescue therapies	
Intubation	Pressure-limited ventilation or pressure-regulated volume control modes
Helium-oxygen	60%–80% helium/20%–40% oxygen
IV ketamine	Load of 2 mg/kg/dose (max 100 mg/dose) followed by 0.5–5 mg/kg/hr

[a]Higher doses have been used in some centers.

all health care professionals to use each tool appropriately. The goal is to use the minimum amount of sedation needed to adequately sedate the intubated child while minimizing adverse effects.

STATUS ASTHMATICUS

Status asthmaticus or severe asthma exacerbation is defined as an acute episode that does not respond to standard treatment with short-acting β_2-agonists and corticosteroids.[42] Status asthmaticus is a primary cause of acute illness in children and one of the top indications for PICU admission.[42,43] The indications for ICU admission vary between institutions and may be determined by respiratory care staffing on the pediatric floor. Bronchial smooth muscle spasm, airway inflammation, and increased mucus production are the key components of an acute asthma exacerbation.[42,43] These factors produce increased pulmonary resistance and small airway collapse leading to increased work of breathing. As the degree of airway obstruction progresses, expiration becomes prolonged, and inspiration starts before the termination of the previous expiration. This results in air trapping and the classic hyperinflation seen on chest radiography. Airway obstruction and premature airway closure lead to ventilation/perfusion mismatching[44] and hypoxemia.[45] Lung hyperinflation, progressive increase in lung volumes, and an increase in pulmonary vascular resistance contribute to a decrease in right ventricular preload. Pulmonary vasoconstriction caused by hypoxia and acidosis leads to an increase in right ventricular afterload, and the high negative pulmonary pressure generated during inspiration in spontaneously breathing patients with asthma causes an increase in left ventricular afterload. These changes can be observed clinically in pulsus paradoxus, which is a decrease in systolic blood pressure by more than 10 mm Hg during inspiration.[42,43,46] In addition, tachycardia caused by bronchodilators further reduces ventricular filling time and may further reduce CO. This is evidenced clinically as a widened pulse pressure or low diastolic blood pressure and the need for additional intravascular volume. Patients rarely require inotropic support for the cardiovascular changes observed in SA.

EVALUATION

Prompt and rapid evaluations of the clinical status of patients with SA are essential to determine the appropriate pharmacotherapy and levels of monitoring. A gold standard for assessing SA in children does not exist. An assessment of observed signs and symptoms can be helpful to classify the disease severity. Peak expiratory flow rates (PEFRs) or FEV_1 (forced expiratory volume in 1 second) is difficult to reliably perform in children with acute asthma, especially in those younger than 5 years. In children 6–18 years of age, only 64% could perform PEFRs adequately.[47] As a result, many clinical asthma scores have been developed to quantify the child's degree of respiratory distress. None of these clinical asthma scores has been shown to be superior to any other. However, clinical scores correlate with the need for hospitalization, need for prolonged bronchodilator therapy, and severity of the exacerbation.[48] Clinical asthma scores are not as helpful in predicting disease progression.[49] Scores can be used not only to choose level of care, but also to wean pharmacotherapy as the patient improves.

Measuring pulse oximetry (Sao_2) is an important tool to determine asthma severity combined with the patient's physical examination. An initial Sao_2 less than 91% on room air or an Sao_2 unresponsive to oxygen treatment has been associated with the need for hospital admission.[48] For most patients, chest radiographs are unhelpful in the emergency assessment of asthma. Children with SA often have an abnormal chest radiograph with a variety of findings: hyper/hypoinflation, atelectasis, or increased extravascular fluid. These findings rarely affect patient treatment. In a small subset of children, a chest radiograph may be helpful: children with a temperature greater than 39°C, focal abnormalities on examination, and no family history of asthma as well as those who respond less favorably than anticipated to bronchodilator therapy. In addition, chest radiography may be warranted when there is clinical suspicion for pneumothorax, pneumomediastinum, or foreign body aspiration or after intubation.

Previously, evaluation of children with SA routinely included ABG measurement. Less invasive means of assessing respiratory status are widely available by pulse oximetry (to evaluate oxygenation) and end-tidal CO_2 (for evaluating ventilation).[50,51] These are simple, noninvasive methods of evaluating oxygenation and ventilation. Routine ABG measurement has also fallen out of favor because no set values for pH, Pco_2, or Po_2 are diagnostic of respiratory failure.[52] Children with acute asthma commonly have mild to moderate hypoxemia and hypocarbia or normocarbia on their initial blood gas caused by hyperventilation and ventilation/perfusion mismatch. Arterial blood gas measurement may be helpful in patients with the severest SA when a rising Pco_2 is worrisome, and an ABG is often predictive of respiratory failure. Once a decision is made to intubate a patient with SA, frequent ABG assessment through an indwelling arterial line is useful to follow clinical progress.

SYMPTOMS

The presentation of SA varies by severity, asthmatic trigger, and patient age. Most children with severe acute asthma present with cough, tachypnea, and increased work of breathing; use of accessory muscles; nasal flaring; and anxiety. Wheezing is a common clinical finding; however, the degree of wheezing correlates poorly with the severity of disease.[42] A noisy chest is a reassuring sign because it represents sufficient airflow to cause turbulence and vibration leading to wheezing. The presence of a silent chest because of limited airflow is an ominous sign in a patient with SA and heralds respiratory failure. Agitation or dyspnea, especially in adolescents, should be recognized as severe respiratory compromise. Other findings of impending respiratory failure and the need for a PICU admission include disturbance in the level of consciousness, inability to speak, markedly diminished breath sounds, diaphoresis, and the inability to lie down.

TREATMENT

General

First-line treatment of acute severe asthma consists of supplemental oxygen for hypoxemia, aerosolized albuterol plus ipratropium for bronchodilation, and corticosteroids for airway inflammation and edema. Typically, these therapies are administered in the ED. Failure to improve with first-line pharmacotherapy defines the patient as having SA.

Oxygen

Oxygen (humidified) is the first drug of choice in all patients with acute severe asthma. Children with SA have a greater frequency of hypoxia from ventilation/perfusion mismatching than do adults because of age-related differences, including lower functional residual capacity/total lung capacity ratio, increased chest wall compliance, and higher peripheral airway resistance.[42] Oxygen therapy is monitored by pulse oximetry with a goal Sao_2 greater than 92%.

Fluids

The need for intravenous fluid boluses should not be overlooked in children presenting with SA. These patients are often dehydrated because of poor oral intake and increased insensible fluid losses from tachypnea. In addition, the increased intrathoracic pressure from air trapping can lead to decreased venous return, and the tachycardia from bronchodilator therapy can reduce filling time, leading to decreased CO. The key is to avoid overhydration because this may lead to transpulmonary edema.

β-Agonists

β-Agonists remain the mainstay of therapy in SA. They produce smooth-muscle relaxation by binding to $β_2$-adrenergic receptors in the smooth muscles of the airways. Albuterol is the most commonly used β-agonist in the United States. It is a 50:50 racemic mixture of R-albuterol and S-albuterol. The R-enantiomer is pharmacologically active, whereas the S-enantiomer is considered inactive.

Levalbuterol is the pure R-enantiomer and is a preservative-free solution. One in vitro study indicated that the S-enantiomer may exaggerate airway hyperresponsiveness and also may have a proinflammatory effect.[53] This has not been shown clinically. In a randomized controlled trial of albuterol versus levalbuterol in children with SA, Qureshi et al. found no difference in clinical asthma score or adverse effects in children presenting to the ED with moderate to severe asthma exacerbations.[54] Considering the increased cost and lack of clinical benefit in clinical trials, levalbuterol should not be recommended routinely for patients with SA.

Traditionally, albuterol is initially administered by intermittent nebulization at 2.5–5 mg per dose. However, administration by a metered dose inhaler (MDI) with spacer is as effective as nebulization (6 inhalations per 2.5 mg) in children who can use them correctly.[53] The results of these studies should be evaluated carefully. Although the outcome with using an MDI was shown to be equivalent to administration by nebulization, the study personnel coached patients with the MDI and spacer to ensure adequate technique. This is not always practical in the clinical setting. For children who need more frequent doses of β-agonist, continuous nebulization (e.g., initial doses of 10 mg/hour) appears to be superior to intermittent doses and results in more rapid improvement.[55] In addition, continuous albuterol nebulization is less labor-intensive than several intermittent doses and may be more cost-effective.[55] A drawback of continuous therapy is that patients may be assessed less often, and adverse effects such as tachycardia, jitteriness, and hypokalemia may be more common. The maximum dose of nebulized albuterol in most studies is 40 mg/hour.

Corticosteroids

Steroid administration is recommended for all patients who lack improvement clinically after standard asthma treatment of albuterol 2.5 mg/500 mcg of ipratropium aerosolized every 20 minutes for three doses. Steroids administered in the ED can reduce hospitalization rates,[56] return hospital visits, and relapses if continued on discharge. Steroids decrease the inflammatory response, up-regulate β_2-adrenergic receptors, and decrease microvascular permeability and mucus production. Short-term use is usually not associated with significant adverse effects. However, hypertension, hyperglycemia, and behavioral changes have been reported.[42] The National Heart, Lung, and Blood Institute (NHLBI) guidelines currently recommend administering corticosteroids systemically rather than by the inhalation route.[57] Oral administration can be used if the child can tolerate oral medication, but if not, intravenous medication is preferred. The NHLBI guidelines suggest that 1–2 mg/kg every 24 hours of systemic prednisone/prednisolone or methylprednisolone can be used for acute asthma (maximum 60 mg every 24 hours), but they offer no recommendations for impending respiratory failure.[57] In a recent survey of pediatric intensivists, 66% of respondents reported using a starting dose of 4 mg/kg every 24 hours in SA in the PICU.[58] Intensivists using 4 mg/kg every 24 hours cite clinical experience as their deciding factor. Future research is needed to determine the most appropriate corticosteroid dosage and therapy duration in this critically ill patient population.

SECOND-LINE TREATMENTS

Magnesium

For children who present with SA and lack response to initial therapies, intravenous magnesium sulfate may be considered. It works through smooth muscle relaxation secondary to the inhibition of calcium uptake leading to bronchodilation. Magnesium can also inhibit mast cell degranulation, possibly decreasing inflammation. The NHLBI guidelines suggest a magnesium sulfate dose in children of 25–75 mg/kg per dose (maximum 2 g per dose) infused for 20 minutes.[57] Some investigators have suggested continuous infusion to target a serum concentration of 4 mg/dL; however, well-designed clinical trials showing serum concentration–targeted therapy are lacking. Possible adverse effects are muscle weakness, hypotension, tachycardia, skin flushing, and fatigue; however, these are uncommon. If hypotension occurs, it responds to the administration of intravenous fluids.

Terbutaline

Intravenous β-agonists should be considered in patients unresponsive to treatment with continuous nebulization. In severe exacerbations, inspiratory flow may be too poor to allow for adequate drug delivery of albuterol to the small airways, and intravenous therapy may be necessary to effectively provide β-agonist therapy. Terbutaline is considered the drug of choice in the United States. Intravenous terbutaline, administered according to a severity-related dosing algorithm, acutely improves lung function and gas exchange and shortens hospital and ICU length of stay.[59] Carroll and colleagues[60] have linked β_2-adrenergic receptor genetic polymorphisms with either a quicker response to β_2-agonist therapy and a shorter ICU and hospital length of stay or a poor response to β_2-agonist therapy and a longer ICU and hospital length of stay. The children with the poor responder genotype were significantly more likely to be African American than the more rapid responder phenotypes. The genetic polymorphism of most patients admitted to the PICU is unknown. However, in African American children whose continuous albuterol nebulization fails, treatment with a bronchodilator having a different mechanism of action may be indicated.

Methylxanthines

Theophylline and aminophylline act through the nonselective inhibition of phosphodiesterase and antagonize adenosine receptors in smooth muscles and inflammatory cells. The end result is bronchodilation, improved mucociliary clearance, and down-regulation of inflammation. In critically ill children with SA admitted to the PICU with impending respiratory failure, theophylline was as effective as intravenous terbutaline.[61] In addition, treatment with theophylline was more cost-effective than treatment with terbutaline.[61] Therefore, theophylline should be considered for patients whose continuous albuterol therapy fails.

NONINVASIVE POSITIVE PRESSURE VENTILATION

Noninvasive positive pressure ventilation is increasingly used in the care of children with SA. In these patients, a low level of continuous positive airway pressure can maintain small airway patency, reduce premature airway closure, and reduce the work of breathing. Early intervention improves outcomes and potentially avoids intubation in this population.[62,63]

HELIUM-OXYGEN

Heliox is a mixture of 60%–80% helium with 20%–40% oxygen. Because of its lower density, heliox flows through small and obstructed airways with less turbulence and resistance, reducing the work of breathing and improving oxygen delivery to the lower airways. Heliox mixtures have a high helium faction and a relatively low oxygen fraction, making the therapy useless in patients with profound hypoxia.

RESCUE THERAPIES

Intubation should be a last-resort therapy for children with SA. Intubation may aggravate bronchospasm and precipitate circulatory collapse. Next to severe hypoxia, rapid deterioration in the child's mental status, progressive exhaustion, and cardiac and respiratory arrests are indications to intubate. Once the decision to intubate has been made, a fluid bolus should be given to prevent the hypotension associated with positive pressure ventilation. Ketamine, because of its bronchodilatory action, is the preferred induction agent. Children may require significant amounts of sedation to avoid tachypnea and ventilator dyssynchrony. Neuromuscular blockade should be reserved for patients in whom adequate ventilation cannot be achieved at acceptable inspiratory pressures.

Despite many recent advances in the understanding of the pathophysiology of asthma, β-agonists and steroids remain the mainstay of treatment for SA. Current literature supports the use of adjuvant therapies such as magnesium as well as a resurgence in the use of methylxanthines. Noninvasive positive pressure ventilation may prevent the need for intubation. The goal in asthma is to avoid intubation, if possible. A summary of drug dosing in asthma may be found in Table 44.9.

PEDIATRIC TRAUMATIC BRAIN INJURY

Among children, traumatic brain injury (TBI) is the leading cause of mortality and leads to significant morbidity among survivors. Each year, more than 400,000 U.S. children have a TBI requiring an ED visit, resulting in 30,000 hospitalizations and 3,000 deaths.[64] The most common mechanisms of injury differ by patient age. Children younger than 4 years usually have injuries because of child abuse, falls, and motor vehicle collisions (MVCs). Child abuse, or nonaccidental trauma (NAT), represents up to two-thirds of severe TBI cases in some series. Although it is difficult to obtain accurate data, the incidence of TBI caused by NAT in the first 2 years of life was 17 per 100,000 person-years in a population-based study from North Carolina.[65] According to the National Center on Shaken Baby Syndrome, this translates to around 1,300 children per year in the United States who have severe head trauma from child abuse. In school-aged children 5–12 years of age, pedestrian-MVC and bicycle-related injuries are among the more common causes of severe injuries. For adolescents, MVCs replace falls as the leading cause of all injuries, followed by assault and sports-related injuries.

The anatomic differences in the infant's brain render it more susceptible to certain types of injuries after head trauma.[66] Infants and young children have large, heavy heads. The head is unstable because of its relative size to the rest of the body. If an infant or young child falls a significant distance, is ejected during an MVC, or is thrown from a bicycle after colliding with an automobile, the head will tend to lead (i.e., the infant or child will fly head first), and severe head injuries will occur when the head ultimately strikes the ground or another object. The infant's weak neck muscles also allow for greater movement when the head is acted on by acceleration/deceleration forces. The skull is thinner during infancy and early childhood, providing less protection for the brain and allowing forces to transfer more effectively across the shallow subarachnoid space. The base of the infant's skull is relatively flat, which also contributes to greater brain movement in response to acceleration/deceleration forces. In addition, the infant's brain has a higher water content (about 88% vs. 77% in an adult), which makes the brain softer and more prone to acceleration/deceleration injury. The water content is also inversely related to the myelination process, and the higher percentage of unmyelinated brain makes it more susceptible to sheer injuries. The infant brain is typically fully myelinated by 1 year of age. As the result of these physiologic differences, there are differences in the pathology after pediatric TBI by age group. In infants and young children, diffuse injury (e.g., diffuse cerebral swelling) and subdural hematomas are more common than the focal injury (e.g., contusions) that is typically seen in older children and adults. The typical pattern of hypoxic-ischemic injury in infants and young children after NAT is rarely seen in older children and adult survivors of abuse.

Goldstein et al. have published risk factors for NAT according to data gathered from several earlier reports.[67] They found that individuals with inflicted head injury tended to be younger, were more often from families of poorer socioeconomic backgrounds, and were more likely to have parents who were younger than 18 years and who had never been married. In addition, a history inconsistent with physical findings was strongly associated with the presence of inflicted head injury. Additional risk factors reported as associated with NAT are alcohol or drug abuse, previous social service intervention, or a history of child abuse, in combination with either retinal hemorrhages or an inconsistent history or physical examination. These investigators found that a combination of these factors was 100% predictive of child abuse in children admitted to a PICU. Nonaccidental trauma should be suspected when the injury does not meet the story (e.g., a fall of about 3 ft is required to cause significant head injury to an infant or child; a standard couch is 18 inches from the floor).[68]

The ability to evaluate the severity of TBI is essential to appropriately direct care, predict outcomes, and compare results to evaluate and improve patient care. Initial symptoms on presentation have little or no correlation with injury severity after TBI. The Glasgow Coma Scale (GCS) is a widely accepted method for initially evaluating and characterizing trauma patients with head injuries (Table 44.10). The scale is composed of visual, motor, and verbal components, with lower scores representing more serious injuries. The severity of TBI may be characterized as mild (GCS 13–15), moderate (GCS 9–12), or severe (GCS 3–8) on presentation; however, continued evaluation of GCS scores is the best way to track the patient's clinical progress.[69]

The radiologic examination of choice for the immediate assessment of a child with severe TBI is a noncontrast cerebral computed tomography (CT) scan. Most children with severe TBI undergo immediate CT imaging

Table 44.10 Modified Glasgow Coma Scale

Eye Opening

Score	≥ 1 yr	0–1 yr
4	Opens eyes spontaneously	Opens eyes spontaneously
3	Opens eyes to verbal command	Opens eyes to shout
2	Opens eyes in response to pain	Opens eyes in response to pain
1	No response	No response

Best Motor Response

Score	≥ 1 yr	0–1 yr
6	Obeys command	N/A
5	Localizes pain	Localizes pain
4	Flexion withdrawal	Flexion withdrawal
3	Flexion abnormal (decorticate)	Flexion abnormal (decorticate)
2	Extension (decerebrate)	Extension (decerebrate)
1	No response	No response

Best Verbal Response

Score	> 5 yr	2–5 yr	0–2 yr
5	Oriented and able to converse	Uses appropriate words	Cries appropriately
4	Disoriented and able to converse	Uses inappropriate words	Cries
3	Uses inappropriate words	Cries and/or screams	Cries and/or screams inappropriately
2	Makes incomprehensible sounds	Grunts	Grunts
1	No response	No response	No response

to delineate their injuries as soon as they have been fully assessed and sufficiently stabilized to permit safe transport to the radiology suite. If the brain injury does not need immediate surgical intervention, the patient's care is continued in the PICU with the implementation of therapies designed to minimize secondary brain injury. In a retrospective review of 309 children presenting with TBI, Chung et al. found that GCS scores were more useful in predicting survival among pediatric patients with TBI than were CT findings and the presence of injuries to other organ systems.[69] In addition, they identified a GCS score of less than 5, rather than a score of less than 8 as used in adults, as the threshold at which the patient was more likely to have a poor outcome. The authors also found that head CT findings of swelling or edema and subdural and intracerebral hemorrhage were associated with worse outcomes than subarachnoid or epidural hemorrhage.

Retinal hemorrhages are often, although not always, observed in inflicted head injury in infants and young children. These hemorrhages are the result of sheer forces disrupting vulnerable tissue interfaces. The vitreous body is adherent to the retina in early childhood; shaking can cause retinal hemorrhaging throughout several tissue layers, extending to the periphery of the retina. This pattern is unique to "shaken baby syndrome." Although useful for diagnosis, the ocular examination is often deferred initially when evaluating an infant or child for TBI because the medications used to facilitate funduscopy will preclude the use of pupillary reactivity as a tool to monitor evolving intracranial events.

According to the American Academy of Pediatrics guidelines on imaging for NAT, a skeletal survey is strongly recommended in all cases of suspected physical abuse in children younger than 24 months.[70] A skeletal survey consists of films of the extremities, skull, and axial skeletal images. Follow-up radiographs of the ribs to assess for healing fractures not seen in the acute phase may be helpful 2–3 weeks after the skeletal survey. As with the eye examination, the skeletal survey is often delayed until the child is more stable.

The initial treatment of a child with a head injury should focus on the basics of resuscitation: assessing and securing the airway, ensuring adequate ventilation, and supporting circulation.[71] In addition, the treatment goals of TBI are directed toward protecting against secondary brain insults, which can exacerbate neuronal damage and brain injury. Secondary brain insults are often the result of systemic hypotension, hypoxia, hypercarbia, anemia, and hyperglycemia. Aggressive treatment strategies are needed to prevent or treat these conditions to decrease morbidity and improve neurologic outcome after TBI in children. The criteria for tracheal intubation include hypoxemia not resolved with supplemental oxygen, apnea, hypercarbia ($Paco_2$ greater than 45 mm Hg), a GCS score of 8 or less, a decrease in GCS greater than 3 compared with the initial score, cervical spine injury, loss of pharyngeal reflex, or any clinical evidence of herniation. All patients should be assumed to have a full stomach and cervical spine injury, so the intubation should be carried out with a rapid sequence intubation using appropriate short-acting sedatives and muscle relaxants.

After intubation, mechanical ventilation goals include 100% oxygen saturation, normocarbia (35–39 mm Hg), and no hyperventilation, as confirmed by ABGs, end-tidal CO_2 monitoring, and chest radiographs showing the tracheal tube in good position. Unless the patient has signs or symptoms of herniation, prophylactic hyperventilation ($Paco_2$ less than 35 mm Hg) should be avoided.[71] Hyperventilation causes cerebral vasoconstriction, which decreases cerebral blood flow and subsequent blood volume. Although it will lower ICP, hyperventilation may result in ischemia. Furthermore, respiratory alkalosis caused by hyperventilation makes it more difficult to release oxygen to the brain, shifting the oxygen-hemoglobin curve to the left. Short-term use of hyperventilation, however, may be useful in preventing herniation while other medical therapies are implemented. In addition to mechanical ventilation, the head of the bed should be kept in the neutral position, and jugular venous obstruction should be avoided to prevent ICP elevation. Elevating the head of the bed to 30 degrees usually decreases ICP.

Assessment and reassessment of the patient's circulatory status, including central and peripheral pulse quality, capillary refill, heart rate, and blood pressure, is critical. Hypotension after pediatric TBI is associated with increased morbidity and mortality.[71] Initial treatment of hypotension in the child with a head injury is similar to that described earlier for pediatric shock; however, the goal systolic blood pressure in the patient with TBI is typically higher: the 50th–75th percentile for age, sex, and height or greater. Systolic blood pressure less than the 75th percentile has been associated with a 4-fold increase in the risk of poor outcome after severe TBI, even when values were 90 mm Hg or greater.[72] This suggests the possible benefit of a higher blood pressure target until ICP or cerebral perfusion pressure (CPP) monitoring is in place to guide therapy. Because of the need for higher systolic blood pressure, norepinephrine and phenylephrine, agents with greater vasopressor effects, are more commonly used in this patient population.[73]

The solution of choice for intravenous maintenance fluids in children with TBI is normal saline for children older than 1 year and 5% dextrose with normal saline for infants. Because hyperglycemia is known to worsen secondary brain insults, initial intravenous fluids for children should not contain dextrose. Infants are an exception because their low glycogen stores make them prone to hypoglycemia, especially with poor oral intake. Hypoglycemia can also worsen neurologic outcome and should be avoided. Frequent assessment of blood glucose either by point-of-care testing or on an ABG is recommended.

Fever increases metabolic demands and is associated with worse outcomes after TBI. Treatment should include 15 mg/kg per dose of acetaminophen orally or rectally every 6 hours as needed and a cooling blanket, when necessary. Ibuprofen should be avoided because it may increase the risk of bleeding. Patients who are hypothermic on arrival should only be actively rewarmed if there is hemodynamic instability or bleeding thought to be exacerbated by hypothermia. Serum electrolytes and osmolarity should be monitored regularly, together with an accurate assessment of urine output. This is important to identify the development of either syndrome of inappropriate antidiuretic hormone or diabetes insipidus. Both have been reported to occur after pediatric TBI.[71]

One of the most significant consequences of TBI is the development of intracranial hypertension. The presence of an open fontanel or sutures in an infant with severe TBI does not preclude the development of intracranial hypertension or negate the usefulness of ICP monitoring. Intracranial pressure monitoring is recommended for any child presenting with a GCS of 8 or less.[73] When possible, placement of a ventriculostomy catheter provides accurate pressure monitoring and allows for acute drainage of cerebrospinal fluid (CSF) for treatment of elevated ICP and assessment of CPP. The CPP value is calculated by subtracting the ICP from the MAP: CPP = MAP − ICP.

This value is important as an indication of blood flow and oxygen that reaches the brain. Maintaining CPP requires the optimization of MAP with fluid therapy, and if necessary, vasoactive drugs. In ICP elevation, inotropic or vasopressor agents may be used to optimize CPP by increasing MAP, even to the point of relative systemic hypertension. In adults, a CPP of 60–70 mm Hg is usually targeted.

No data correlate CPP in infants with outcome. However, pediatric TBI studies show that CPP values of 40–70 mm Hg are associated with a favorable outcome and that a CPP less than 40 mm Hg is associated with poor outcomes.[74] Because infants and children normally have a lower MAP and ICP, the Society of Critical Care Medicine Pediatric Fundamental Critical Care Support course recommends the following CPP ranges: 40–50 mm Hg in infants, 50–60 mm Hg in children, and 60–70 mm Hg in adolescents.[75] This is more specific than the 2003 pediatric recommendations, which recommend maintaining a CPP greater than 40 mm Hg and an "age-related continuum" of CPP of 40–65 mm Hg in infants and adolescents.[71]

Uncontrolled increased ICP is deleterious and must be treated aggressively as soon as possible to reduce cerebral ischemia. In this setting, the goal of any therapy is to lower ICP enough to increase CPP and improve cerebral oxygenation. All initial treatments should be reassessed for efficacy, including treatment of fever, avoidance of jugular venous outflow tract obstruction, maintenance of normovolemia and normocarbia, and provision of sedation and analgesia. Providing sedation and analgesia is of considerable importance because anxiety and pain increase ICP. If a patient has a ventriculoscopy and an elevated ICP, CSF should be drained until an ICP value of 15 mm Hg is reached; it should never be drained to 0 mm Hg because edema and diffuse brain swelling could cause an obstruction in the lateral ventricles. When a ventriculostomy is in place and CSF is frequently drained, it is important to replace the CSF drained with an equal amount of normal saline. Draining of large amounts of CSF without intravenous normal saline replacement is associated with the development of hypochloremic metabolic alkalosis. In patients whose ICP drainage fails, the intervention recommended is either the addition of a vasopressor to increase systolic blood pressure or the institution of hyperosmolar therapy.

Hyperosmolar therapy may be useful in preventing the ICP from exceeding 20 mm Hg and in maintaining normal CPP. Mannitol has long been the standard of care for managing elevated ICP.[71] However, although extensively used since 1961 to control elevated ICP, mannitol has never been compared with placebo. Mannitol reduces ICP by reducing blood viscosity, which promotes reflex vasoconstriction of the arterioles by autoregulation, thus decreasing cerebral blood volume and ICP. This mechanism is rapid but transient, lasting about 75 minutes and requiring an intact autoregulation. It also produces an osmotic effect by increasing serum osmolarity, causing the shift of water from the brain cell to the intravascular space. Although this effect is slower in onset (15–30 minutes), the osmotic effect lasts up to 6 hours. Mannitol is a potent osmotic diuretic; osmotic diuresis should be anticipated and fluid resuscitation available to avoid hemodynamic compromise. A Foley catheter is recommended in these patients for accurate measurement of urine output. Mannitol is excreted unchanged in the urine; serum osmolarity should be maintained lower than 320 mOsm/L to avoid the development of mannitol-induced acute tubular necrosis. Mannitol is recommended at 0.25–1 g/kg per dose.

Although mannitol has traditionally been the drug of choice for reducing elevated ICP, hypertonic saline (3% sodium chloride) is gaining favor. The main mechanism of action of hypertonic saline is an osmotic effect similar to that of mannitol. Hypertonic saline has several other theoretical benefits such as restoration of normal cellular resting membrane potential and cell volume, inhibition of inflammation, stimulation of atrial natriuretic peptide release, and improvement in CO.[71] The theoretical advantage over mannitol is that hypertonic saline can be administered in a hemodynamically unstable patient without the risk of a subsequent osmotic diuresis. Continuous infusions of 0.1–1 mL/kg/hour of hypertonic saline titrated to maintain an ICP less than 20 mm Hg have been used successfully in children.[71] Bolus doses of 3–5 mL/kg of 3% sodium chloride have been administered over 20–30 minutes. Serum osmolarity and serum sodium increase when this regimen is used, but sustained hypernatremia and hyperosmolarity appear to be generally well tolerated. Hypertonic saline has been administered with a serum osmolarity reaching 360 mOsm/L without adverse effects in pediatric patients. Another potential concern with the use of hypertonic saline is central pontine myelinolysis, which has been reported with rapid changes in serum sodium. Clinical trials have shown no evidence of demyelinating disorders.

Two nonsurgical options are included in the TBI guideline: barbiturate coma and therapeutic hypothermia.[71] Barbiturates exert neuroprotective effects by reducing cerebral metabolism, lowering oxygen extraction and demand, and alternating vascular tone. Barbiturate serum concentrations correlate poorly with clinical efficacy; therefore, monitoring of electroencephalographic (EEG) patterns for burst suppression is recommended. Burst suppression also represents near-maximum reduction in cerebral metabolism and cerebral blood flow. A pentobarbital loading dose of 10 mg/kg per dose may be administered over 30 minutes, followed by a continuous infusion of 1 mg/kg/hour. Additional loading doses, in 5-mg/kg per dose increments, may be necessary to achieve burst suppression. The primary disadvantage of barbiturate coma is the risk of myocardial depression and hypotension. In addition, the long-term effect on neurologic outcome is unknown. The TBI guideline states that high-dose barbiturate therapy may be considered in hemodynamically stable patients with salvageable severe head injury and refractory intracranial hypertension.[71]

Posttraumatic hyperthermia is defined as a core body temperature greater than 38.5°C, and hypothermia is defined as a temperature of less than 35°C. Although most clinicians agree that hyperthermia should be avoided in children with TBI, the role of hypothermia is unclear. Potential complications associated with hypothermia are increased bleeding risk, arrhythmias, and increased susceptibility to infection. A multicenter, international study of children with severe TBI randomly assigned to hypothermia therapy initiated within 8 hours after injury (32.5°C for 24 hours) or to normothermia (37°C) was published in 2008.[76] The study reported a worsening trend with hypothermia therapy: 31% of the patients in the hypothermia group had an unfavorable outcome, compared with 22% in the normothermia group. However, this study had several methodological problems. Although the investigators screened patients within 8 hours, the mean time to initiation of cooling was 6.3 hours, with a range of 1.6–19.7 hours. In addition, the protocol included a rapid rewarming of 0.5°C every 2 hours so that the patients were normothermic by a mean of 19 hours or 48 hours postinjury. The investigators found that the ICP was significantly lower in the hypothermia group during the cooling period but significantly higher than in the normothermic group during rewarming. Another trial conducted in Australia and New Zealand evaluated strict normothermia (temperature 36°C–37°C) versus therapeutic hypothermia (temperature 32°C–33°C).[75] Patients were enrolled within 6 hours of injury, and therapeutic hypothermia or strict normothermia was maintained for 72 hours. The rewarming rate was at a maximum of 0.5°C every 3 hours or slower if needed to maintain normal CPP or ICP less than 20 mm Hg. Rewarming took a median of 21.5 hours (16–35 hours) and was without complications. However, there was no difference in pediatric cerebral performance category scores between the two groups at 12 months.[77] It is unclear whether therapeutic hypothermia lacks efficacy because patients are not cooled soon enough (median time to target temperature 9.3 hours) or because of the heterogeneous nature of TBI. The pediatric TBI guideline states that despite the lack of clinical data, hypothermia may be considered in the setting of refractory hypertension.[71]

Decompressive craniectomy, removal of a section of skull to allow room for brain swelling without herniation, is another option for treating pediatric patients with TBI who lack response to standard therapies. A randomized trial of early decompressive craniectomy in children with TBI and sustained intracranial hypertension showed that 54% of the surgically treated patients had a favorable outcome compared with only 14% of the medically treated group.[78] Additional case series have confirmed that patients who receive a decompressive craniectomy have improved survival and neurologic outcomes compared with patients undergoing medical management alone.[55] However, as with barbiturate coma and therapeutic hypothermia, decompressive craniectomy is not without risk. A recent study reported an increased risk of posttraumatic hydrocephalus, wound complications, and epilepsy in children with severe TBI.[79] Further studies are needed to establish the timing, efficacy, and safety of this management strategy. The pediatric TBI guideline states that decompressive craniectomy should be considered in pediatric patients with severe TBI, diffuse cerebral swelling, and intracranial hypertension refractory to intensive medical management.

POSTTRAUMATIC SEIZURES

Posttraumatic seizures are classified as early (occurring within 7 days after injury) or late (occurring after 7 days). In the immediate period after severe TBI, seizures increase the brain metabolic demands, increase ICP, and are associated with secondary brain insults. Therefore, it is prudent to prevent posttraumatic seizures when the patient is at the highest risk of secondary brain insults. Infants and children are reported to have a greater risk of early PTS than are adults. Children younger than 2 years have almost a 3-fold greater risk of early posttraumatic seizures after TBI than do children 2–12 years of age. In addition to age, a low GCS (8–11) has been linked with an increased risk of early posttraumatic seizures. The pediatric TBI guideline states that prophylactic antiseizure therapy may be considered as a treatment to prevent early posttraumatic seizures. No prophylactic anticonvulsant therapy is recommended to prevent late posttraumatic seizures.[71]

Most of the published studies of children have used phenytoin for posttraumatic seizure prophylaxis. Both phenytoin and carbamazepine have been reported to reduce the incidence of posttraumatic seizure in adults. A large (n=813) prospective multicenter trial evaluated the effectiveness of levetiracetam for seizure prophylaxis in adults with severe TBI.[80] Although the trial showed that levetiracetam was as effective as phenytoin in preventing posttraumatic seizures after TBI, the authors concluded that the significant cost difference between the two treatments makes phenytoin the preferred therapy. There are currently no studies of levetiracetam for posttraumatic seizure prophylaxis in children.

STRESS-RELATED MUCOSAL BLEEDING

The use of prophylaxis to prevent stress-related mucosal bleeding, although common in adult ICU patients, is not widely used in PICUs. Studies conducted to date have provided a wide range of gastrointestinal (GI) tract bleeding rates in children, 10%–50%, with rates of clinically significant bleeding of around 1%–4%.[81,82] Several investigators have identified thrombocytopenia, coagulopathy, organ failure, and mechanical ventilation as important risk factors for GI bleeding, similar to studies conducted in adults. A recent systematic review suggested that critically ill pediatric patients benefit from prophylaxis; however, the results were limited by the small number of controlled studies available.[79]

There are no clear recommendations in pediatric patients for the use of histamine-2 blockers (H_2-blockers) versus proton pump inhibitors (PPIs) for stress ulcer prophylaxis in the PICU. However, in 2015, a retrospective cohort analysis reviewed 336,010 PICU admissions in 42 freestanding children's hospitals. Results showed that administering gastric acid suppressant medications, prescribed on the first day of PICU hospitalization, was common, occurring in 60% of hospitalizations. Among those receiving treatment, H_2-blockers were used more often (70.4%) than PPIs (17.8%), and both types of agents were used in 11.8% of cases.[83]

THROMBOSIS PROPHYLAXIS

Patients admitted to the PICU can range from newborns to young adults. Unlike in adults, there are no data on the use of subcutaneous heparin or low-molecular-weight heparins as prophylaxis to prevent deep venous thrombosis (DVT) in children. However, when children reach puberty, the hormone changes that take place appear to increase children's risk of thrombosis compared with adults. Although no published guidelines or consensus papers currently exist to guide therapy, all pubescent adolescents should be considered for DVT prophylaxis. Most thrombosis cases in infants and young children are associated with the long-term use of central venous catheters. Additional risk factors that have been reported in children include active inflammatory bowel disease, obesity, and infection.[84,85]

Unfortunately, a study evaluating low-dose heparin infused at 10 units/kg/hour did not prevent catheter-related thrombosis in infants after cardiac surgery.[86] Of note, the heparin dose used in this study was less than the anticoagulant dose recommended for infants and children (15–25 units/kg/hour). The routine use of DVT prophylaxis in children remains controversial; however, it should be considered in pubescent children.

HYPOGLYCEMIA

Hypoglycemia often develops in infants during episodes of stress, including shock, seizures, and sepsis. Infants have high glucose needs and low glycogen stores, which makes hypoglycemia a risk in a critically ill infant, especially one with poor enteral intake. Point-of-care glucose testing should be performed in any critically ill infant with a history of poor oral intake. The clinician should not wait to obtain serum chemistries. The aggressive fluid resuscitation recommended for hypovolemia and shock will only exacerbate hypoglycemia. More importantly, hypoglycemia needs to be prevented during cardiopulmonary and trauma resuscitation because it may cause seizures and has been linked with poor neurologic outcome.[4,5] Hypoglycemia in pediatric patients must always be promptly identified and treated. After diagnosis, the patient should be treated with a bolus of 0.5–1 g/kg of glucose or 5–10 mL/kg of a 10% dextrose solution as required to achieve a serum glucose greater than 100 mg/dL. Neonates, especially premature neonates, are more prone to intraventricular hemorrhage with rapid changes in serum osmolarity than are older infants and children; therefore, 0.2 g/kg or 2 mL/kg of 10% dextrose is recommended in this population until the target serum glucose is achieved.

CONCLUSION

Common causes for admission to the PICU differ from causes for admission to adult ICUs. In addition, changes in physiology with normal growth and development can make the definitions of a disease differ between infants and children, as with supraventricular tachycardia, or predispose a specific age group to more severe disease. The clinician must recognize the many physiologic changes that take place during normal growth and development and understand how they affect the patient's assessment and treatment. Pediatric health care providers practicing in critical care settings such as the ED or PICU must be adept at incorporating these physiologic differences into medication selection, dosing, and monitoring to optimize patient care.

REFERENCES

1. Claudet I, Bounes V, Fédérici S, et al. Epidemiology of admissions in a pediatric resuscitation room. Pediatr Emerg Care 2009;25:312-6.
2. Namachivayam P, Shann F, Shekerdemian L, et al. Three decades of pediatric intensive care: who was admitted, what happened in intensive care, and what happened afterward. Pediatr Crit Care Med 2010;11:549-55.
3. Callaway CW, Soar J, Aibiki M, et al. Part 4: advanced life support. 2015 international consensus on cardiopulmonary resuscitation and emergency cardiovascular care science with treatment recommendations. Circulation 2015;132(suppl 1):S146-S176.
4. deCaen AR, Maconochie IK, Aickin R, et al. Part 6: pediatric basic life support and pediatric advanced life support: 2015 international consensus on cardiopulmonary resuscitation and emergency cardiovascular care science with treatment recommendations. Circulation 2015;132(suppl 1):S177-S203.
5. Dellinger RP, Levy MM, Rhodes A, et al. Surviving Sepsis Campaign: international guidelines for management of severe sepsis and septic shock 2012. Crit Care Med 2013;41:580-637.
6. Maitlans M, Kaguli S, Opoko RO, et al. Mortality after fluid bolus in African children with severe infection. N Engl J Med 2011;364:2483-95.
7. Dupont HL, Spink WW. Infections due to gram-negative organisms: an analysis of 860 patients with bacteremia in the University of Minnesota Medical Center, 1958-1966. Medicine 1969;48:307-32.
8. Hartman ME, Linde-Zwirble WT, Angis DC, et al. Trends in the epidemiology of severe sepsis. Pediatr Crit Care Med 2013;14:686-93.
9. Rivers E, Nguyen B, Havstad S, et al. Early goal-directed therapy in the treatment of severe sepsis and septic shock. N Engl J Med 2001;345:1368-77.
10. Carcillo JA, Fields AI; American College of Critical Care Medicine Task Force Committee Members. Clinical practice parameters for hemodynamic support of pediatric and neonatal patients in septic shock. Crit Care Med 2002;30:1365-78.
11. Brierley J, Carcillo JA, Choong K, et al. Clinical practice parameters for hemodynamic support of pediatric and neonatal septic shock: 2007 update from the American College of Critical Care Medicine [published correction appears in Crit Care Med 2009;37:1536]. Crit Care Med 2009;37:666-88.
12. de Oliveira CF, de Oliveira DS, Gottschald AF, et al. ACCM/PALS haemodynamic support guidelines for paediatric septic shock: an outcome comparison with and without monitoring central venous oxygen saturation. Intensive Care Med 2008;34:1065-75.
13. de Oliveira CF. Early goal-directed therapy in treatment of pediatric septic shock. Shock 2010;34(suppl 1):44-7.
14. Wynn JL, Wong HR. Pathophysiology and treatment of septic shock in neonates. Clin Perinatol 2010;37:439-79.
15. Carcillo JA. Pediatric septic shock and multiple organ failure. Crit Care Clin 2003;19:413-40.
16. Goldstein B, Giroir B, Randolph A, et al. International pediatric sepsis consensus conference: definitions for sepsis and organ dysfunction in pediatrics. Pediatr Crit Care Med 2005;6:2-8.
17. Boone RC, Sprung CL, Sibbald WJ. Definitions for sepsis and organ function. Crit Care Med 1992;20:724-6.
18. Boone RC, Balk RA, Cerra FB, et al. Definitions for sepsis and organ failure and guidelines for the use of innovative therapies in sepsis. The ACCP/SCCM Consensus Conference Committee. American College of Chest Physicians/Society of Critical Care Medicine. Chest 1992;101:1644-55.
19. Kline MW, Lorin MI. Bacteremia in children afebrile at presentation to an emergency department. Pediatr Infect Dis J 1989;6:197-8.
20. Bonadilo WA. Incidence of serious infections in afebrile neonates with a history of fever. Pediatr Infect Dis J 1987;6:911-4.
21. Ceneviva G, Paschall JA, Maffel F, et al. Hemodynamic support in fluid refractory pediatric septic shock. Pediatrics 1998;102:e19.
22. Pollack MM, Fields AI, Ruttimann UE. Distributions of cardiopulmonary variables in pediatric survivors and nonsurvivors of septic shock. Crit Care Med 1985;13:454-9.
23. Feltes T, Pignatelli R, Kleinert S, et al. Quantitated left ventricular systolic mechanisms in children with septic shock utilizing noninvasive wall stress analysis. Crit Care Med 1994;22:1647-58.
24. Akech S, Ledermann H, Maitland K. Choice of fluids for resuscitation in children with severe infection and shock: systematic review. BMJ 2010;341:c4416.
25. Zimmerman JL. Use of blood products in sepsis: an evidence based review. Crit Care Med 2004;32(11 suppl):S542.
26. Carcillo JA, Davis AI, Zaritsky A. Role of early fluid resuscitation in pediatric septic shock. JAMA 1991;266:1242-5.
27. Finfer S, Bellomo R, Boyce N, et al. A comparison of albumin and saline for fluid resuscitation in the intensive care unit. N Engl J Med 2004;350:2247-56.
28. Ventura AM, Sheih HH, Bousso A, et al. Double-blind prospective randomized controlled trial of dopamine versus epinephrine as first-line vasoactive drugs in pediatric septic shock. CCM 2015;43:2292-302.
29. Mann K, Berg RA, Nadkarni V. Beneficial effects of vasopressin in prolonged pediatric cardiac arrest: a case series. Resuscitation 2002;52:149-56.
30. Duncan JM, Meaney K, Simpson P, et al. Vasopressin for in-hospital pediatric cardiac arrest: results from the American Heart Association National Registry of Cardiopulmonary Resuscitation. Pediatr Crit Care Med 2009;10:191-5.
31. Hoffman TM, Wernovsky G, Atz AM, et al. Efficacy and safety of milrinone in preventing low cardiac output syndrome in infants and children after corrective surgery for congenital heart disease. Circulation 2003;107:996-1002.
32. Shott SR. The nose and paranasal sinuses. In: Rudolph CD, Rudolph AM, eds. Rudolph's Pediatrics, 21st ed. New York: McGraw-Hill, 2003:1258.
33. Dawson-Caswell M, Muncie HL Jr. Respiratory syncytial virus infection in children. Am Fam Physician 2011;83:141-6.
34. Kumar P, Denson SE, Mancuso TJ, et al. Premedication for nonemergency endotracheal intubation in the neonate. Pediatrics 2010;125:608-15.
35. Watson RS, Carcillo JA, Linde-Zwirble WT, et al. The epidemiology of severe sepsis in children in the United States. Am J Respir Crit Care Med 2003;63:695-701.

36. Perkett EA. Lung growth in infancy and childhood. In: Rudolph CD, Rudolph AM, eds. Rudolph's Pediatrics, 21st ed. New York: McGraw-Hill, 2003:1905.

37. den Brinker M, Hokken-Koelega AC, Hazelzet JA, et al. One single dose of etomidate negatively influences adrenocortical performance for at least 24h in children with meningococcal sepsis. Intensive Care Med 2008;34:163-8.

38. Cuthbertson BH, Sprung CL, Annane D, et al. The effects of etomidate on adrenal responsiveness and mortality in patients with septic shock. Intensive Care Med 2009;35:1868-76.

39. Jackson WL Jr. Should we use etomidate as an induction agent for endotracheal intubation in patients with septic shock? A critical appraisal. Chest 2005;127:1031-8.

40. Zelicof-Paul A, Smith-Lockridge A, Schnadower D, et al. Controversies in rapid sequence intubation in children. Curr Opin Pediatr 2005;17:355-62.

41. Johansson M, Kokinsky E. The COMFORT behavioural scale and the modified FLACC scale in paediatric intensive care. Nurs Crit Care 2009;14:122-30.

42. Werner HA. Status asthmaticus in children. Chest 2001;119:1913-29.

43. Mannix R, Bachur. Status asthmaticus in children. Curr Opin Pediatr 2007;19:281-7.

44. Roca J, Ramis L, Rodriguez-Roison R, et al. Serial relationship between ventilation-perfusion inequality and spirometry in acute severe asthma requiring hospitalization. Am Rev Respir Dis 1988;137:1055-61.

45. Rodriguez-Roison R, Ballister E, Roca J, et al. Mechanisms of hypoxemia in patients with status asthmaticus requiring mechanical ventilation. Am Rev Respir Dis 1989;139:732-9.

46. Jardin F, Farcot JC, Boisante LD. Development of paradoxic pulse in bronchial asthma. Circulation 1982;66:887-94.

47. Gorelick MH, Stevens MW, Schultz T, et al. Difficulty in obtaining peak expiratory flow measurements in children with acute asthma. Pediatr Emerg Care 2004;20:22-6.

48. Keogh KA, Macarthur C, Parkin PC, et al. Predictors of hospitalization in children with acute asthma. J Pediatr 2001;139:273-7.

49. Baker MD. Pitfalls in the use of clinical asthma scoring. Am J Dis Child 1988;142:183-5.

50. Langhan ML, Zonfrillo MR, Spiro DM. Quantitative end-tidal carbon dioxide in acute exacerbations of asthma. J Pediatr 2008;152:829-32.

51. Moses JM, Alexander JL, Aqus MS. The correlation and level of agreement between end-tidal and blood gas PCO2 in children with respiratory distress: a retrospective analysis. BMC Pediatr 2009;9:20.

52. Carruthers DM, Harrison BD. Arterial blood gas analysis or oxygen saturation in the assessment of acute asthma? Thorax 1995;50:186-8.

53. Johnson F, Rydberg I, Aberg G, et al. Effects of albuterol enantiomers on in vitro bronchial reactivity. Clin Rev Allergy Immunol 1996;14:57-64.

54. Qureshi F, Zaritsky A, Welch C, et al. Clinical efficacy of racemic albuterol versus levalbuterol for the treatment of acute pediatric asthma. Ann Emerg Med 2005;46:29-36.

55. Papo MC, Frank J, Thompson AE. A prospective randomized study of continuous versus intermittent nebulized albuterol for severe status asthmaticus in children. Crit Care Med 1993;21:1479-86.

56. Bhogal SK, McGillivray D, Bourbeau J, et al. Early administration of systemic corticosteroids reduced hospital admission rates for children with moderate and severe asthma exacerbation. Ann Emerg Med 2012;60:84-91.

57. U.S. Department of Health and Human Services National Heart, Lung and Blood Institute. National Asthma Education and Prevention Program Expert Panel Report 3: Guidelines for the Diagnosis and Management of Asthma. Publication 08-4051. Bethesda, MD: U.S. Department of Health and Human Services, 2007.

58. Giuliano JS Jr, Faustino EV, Li S, et al. Corticosteroid therapy in critically ill pediatric asthmatic patients. Pediatr Crit Care Med 2013;14:467-70.

59. Carroll CL, Schramm CM. Protocol-based titration of intravenous terbutaline decreases length of stay in pediatric status asthmaticus. Pediatr Pulmonol 2006;41:350-6.

60. Carroll CL, Sala KA, Zucker AR, et al. Beta-adrenergic receptor polymorphisms associated with length of ICU stay in pediatric status asthmaticus. Pediatr Pulmonol 2012;47:233-9.

61. Wheeler DS, Jacobs BR, Kenreigh CA, et al. Theophylline versus terbutaline in treating critically ill children with status asthmaticus: a prospective, randomized controlled trial. Pediatr Crit Care Med 2005;6:142-7.

62. Thill PJ, McGuire JK, Baden HP, et al. Noninvasive positive pressure ventilation in children with lower airway obstruction. Pediatr Crit Care Med 2004;5:337-42.

63. Carroll CL, Schramm CM. Noninvasive positive pressure ventilation for the treatment of status asthmaticus in children. Ann Allergy Asthma 2006;96:454-9.

64. Bishop NB. Traumatic brain injury: a primer for primary care physicians. Curr Probl Pediatr Adolesc Health Care 2006;36:318.

65. Keenan HT, Runyan DK, Marshall SW, et al. A population-based study of inflicted traumatic brain injury in young children. JAMA 2003;290:621-6.

66. DeMeyer W. Normal and abnormal development of the neuroaxis. In: Rudolph CD, Rudolph AM, eds. Rudolph's Pediatrics, 21st ed. New York: McGraw-Hill, 2003:2174.

67. Goldstein B, Kelly MM, Bruton D, et al. Inflicted versus accidental head injury in critically injured children. Crit Care Med 1993;21:1328-32.

68. Rorke-Adams L, Duhaime CA, Jenny C, et al. Head trauma. In: Reece RM, Christians CW, eds. Child Abuse: Medical Diagnosis and Management, 3rd ed. Elk Grove Village, IL: American Academy of Pediatrics, 2009:54.

69. Chung CY, Chen CL, Cheng PT, et al. Critical score of Glasgow Coma Scale for pediatric traumatic brain injury. Pediatr Neurol 2006;34:379-87.

70. American Academy of Pediatrics. Section on radiology: diagnostic imaging of child abuse. Pediatrics 2009;123:1430-5.

71. Adelson PD, Bratton SL, Carney NA, et al. Guidelines for the acute medical management of severe traumatic brain injury in infants, children, and adolescents. Pediatr Crit Care Med 2003;4(3 suppl):S72-5.

72. Vavilala MS, Bowen A, Lam AM, et al. Blood pressure and outcome after severe traumatic brain injury. J Trauma 2003;55:1039-44.

73. Di Gennaro JL, Mack CD, Malakouti A, et al. Use and effect of vasopressors after pediatric traumatic brain injury. Dev Neurosci 2010;32:420-30.

74. Catala-Temprano A, Claret Teruel G, Cambra Lasaosa FJ, et al. Intracranial pressure and cerebral perfusion pressure as risk factors in children with traumatic brain injuries. J Neurosurg 2007;106(6 suppl):463-6.

75. Mejia R, ed. Traumatic Brain Injury in Pediatric Fundamental Critical Care Support. Mount Prospect, IL: Society of Critical Care Medicine, 2008.

76. Hutchison JS, Ward RE, Lacroix J, et al. Hypothermia therapy after traumatic brain injury in children. N Engl J Med 2008;358:2447-56.

77. Beca J, McSharry B, Erickson S, et al. Hypothermia for traumatic brain injury in children – a phase II randomized controlled trial. Crit Care Med 2015;43:1458-66.

78. Taylor A, Butt W, Rosenfeld J, et al. A randomized trial of very early decompressive craniectomy in children with traumatic brain injury. Childs Nerv Syst 2001;17:154-62.

79. Jagannathan J, Okonkwo DO, Dumont AS, et al. Outcome following decompression craniectomy in children with severe traumatic brain injury: a 10-year single-center experience with long-term follow-up. J Neurosurg 2007;106(4 suppl):268-75.

80. Inaba K, Menaker J, Branco BC, et al. A prospective multicenter comparison of levetiracetam versus phenytoin for early posttraumatic seizure prophylaxis. J Trauma Acute Care Surg 2013;74:766-71.

81. Deerojanawong J, Peongsujarit D, Vivatvakin B, et al. Incidence and risk factors of upper gastrointestinal bleeding in mechanically ventilated children. Pediatr Crit Care Med 2009;10:91-5.

82. Reveiz L, Guerrero-Lazano R, Camacho A, et al. Stress ulcer, gastritis, and gastrointestinal bleeding prophylaxis in critically ill pediatric patients: a systematic review. Pediatr Crit Care Med 2010;11:124-32.

83. Costarino AT, Dai D, Feng R, et al. Gastric acid suppressant prophylaxis in pediatric intensive care: current practice as reflected in a large administrative database. Pediatr Crit Care Med 2015;16:605-12.

84. Higgerson RA, Lawson KA, Christie LM, et al. Incidence and risk factors associated with venous thrombotic events in pediatric intensive care unit patients. Pediatr Crit Care Med 2011;12:628-34.

85. Zitomersky NL, Levine AE, Atkinson BJ, et al. Risk factors, morbidity, and treatment of thrombosis in children and young adults with active inflammatory bowel disease. JPGN 2013;57:343-7.

86. Schroeder AR, Axelrod DM, Silverman NH, et al. A continuous heparin infusion does not prevent catheter-related thrombosis in infants after cardiac surgery. Pediatr Crit Care Med 2010;11:489-95.

Chapter 45

Drug Shortages: An Overview of Causes, Impact, and Management Strategies

Samuel E. Culli, Pharm.D., MPH; and John J. Lewin III, Pharm.D., MBA, FASHP, FCCM, FNCS

LEARNING OBJECTIVES

1. List several of the multifactorial causes of drug shortages.
2. Describe the impact of drug shortages on patients, health care providers, and health care systems.
3. Gather information on current drug shortages from the ASHP and FDA websites.
4. Explain the various options for management and communication of a drug shortage that health care systems use to help mitigate the associated potential negative impact.

ABBREVIATIONS IN THIS CHAPTER

ASHP	American Society of Health-System Pharmacists	FDASIA	Food and Drug Administration Safety and Innovation Act
FDA	Food and Drug Administration	ISPE	International Society of Pharmaceutical Engineering

INTRODUCTION: PREVALENCE AND CURRENT TRENDS

Drug shortages are a significant threat to the quality and safety of the medical care provided to critically ill patients. Despite new regulations signed into law in 2012 giving the U.S. Food and Drug Administration (FDA) more authority to help prevent shortages and enhancing collaboration between the FDA and manufacturers, shortages of commonly used medications persist. New drug shortages have decreased from their peak in 2011 (a 47%–80% decrease from 2011 to 2014, depending on the source) (Figure 45.1).[1] However, at this time, there were more than 215 current drug shortages being tracked (Figure 45.2).[2] About 44% of the shortages reported in 2011–2013 are of generic injectable medications, which are vital in the treatment of critically ill patients.[3] In addition, four of the top five drug classes accounting for most shortages currently represent medications vital in the care of critically ill patients, including anesthetics/central nervous system agents, anti-infective agents, electrolytes/nutrition, and cardiovascular drugs (Figure 45.3).[3] Some examples of generic injectable medications that have recently been on shortage include calcium gluconate, cefazolin, epinephrine, norepinephrine, piperacillin/tazobactam, and vecuronium.

Causes of Drug Shortages

The causes of drug shortages are complicated and multifactorial. Each shortage often has its own unique causes. According to the FDA, the main cause of drug shortages is quality problems with a product or manufacturing plant such as sterility issues or the presence of particulate matter. Both of these can lead to drug recalls.[4] The FDA cites other causative issues, including plant shutdowns to address quality issues, concentration of the drug market to a few firms, and a lack of redundancy in manufacturing.[4] However, the cause of an individual shortage is reported as unknown almost 50% of the time (Table 45.1).

The International Society for Pharmaceutical Engineering (ISPE) surveyed drug manufacturers in its 2013 Drug Shortages survey. Almost half of the respondents identified quality issues as a primary cause of shortages, echoing the FDA's reports. Many of these quality issues related to equipment systems and facilities dealing with aseptic processing equipment. The issues were often the result of a mix of aging equipment and improper use of that equipment. However, ISPE noted that the most significant issue preventing maintenance or modernization of facilities is the length of time it may take to obtain proper regulatory approvals (up to 3–7 years).[4]

Since drug shortages started increasing in 2004, the FDA has improved its ability to prevent and respond to drug shortages. The FDA reported that in 2013, it helped prevent almost 80% of impending shortages.[1] Some of the success at prevention is the result of new powers granted by the FDA Safety and Innovation Act of 2012, which, among other things, require manufacturers to report discontinuations of their products 6 months in advance and allow the FDA to expedite its review of new or abbreviated drug applications that would help mitigate a shortage.[4]

IMPACT ON PATIENT SAFETY AND QUALITY OF CARE

Drug shortages have a negative impact at all levels of the health care system, including at the patient, health care professional, and institution or system level. Drug shortages may lead to patients receiving suboptimal care, patients being at an increased risk for adverse events or medication errors, treatment delays, cancellation of procedures, and patient harm.

Two surveys of several groups of health care professionals done in 2010 and 2012 showed that drug shortages have a significant impact on patient care.[5,6] From 20% to 40% of respondents to each survey noted that at least one patient had experienced an adverse event at a health system because of a drug shortage. In addition, more than 50% of respondents reported that medication errors had occurred in their facilities in the past year that were directly related to shortages. Other reports have noted the more serious harms that have occurred related to drug shortages such as a greater relapse rate of patients with certain types of cancer. In 2011, 15 deaths were potentially caused by the use of substitute drugs because of a drug shortage.[7,8]

Specific examples of medication errors and adverse events reported in surveys that were caused by drug shortages include the following[5]:

- Because of conservation efforts, a patient received inadequate sedation with propofol during a procedure and woke up
- Patients could not be extubated or weaned off the ventilator because of excess sedation from use of less familiar drugs
- A patient received rocuronium at the infusion rate intended for cisatracurium
- A patient received a 10-fold overdose of epinephrine during a code when there was confusion from having to stock an unfamiliar concentration of the drug

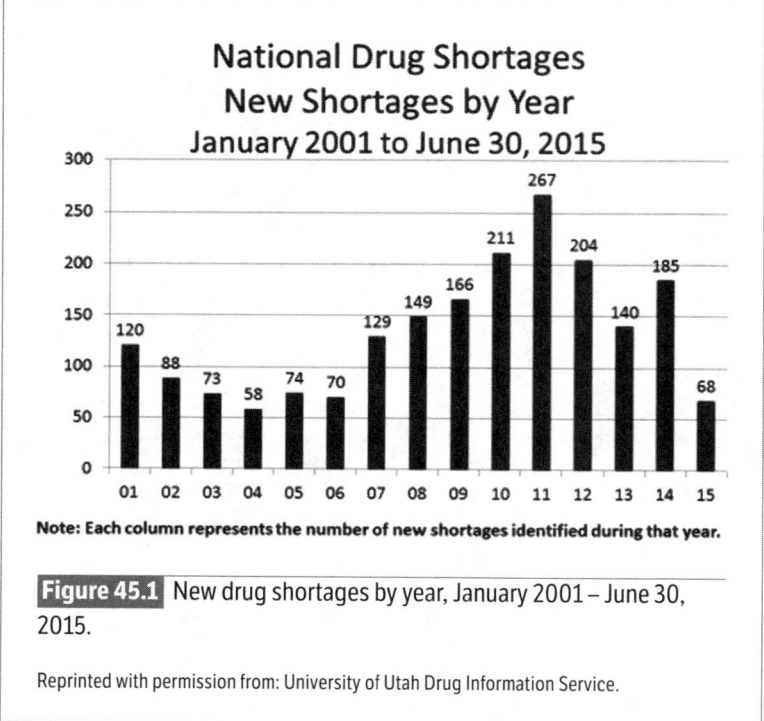

Figure 45.1 New drug shortages by year, January 2001 – June 30, 2015.

Reprinted with permission from: University of Utah Drug Information Service.

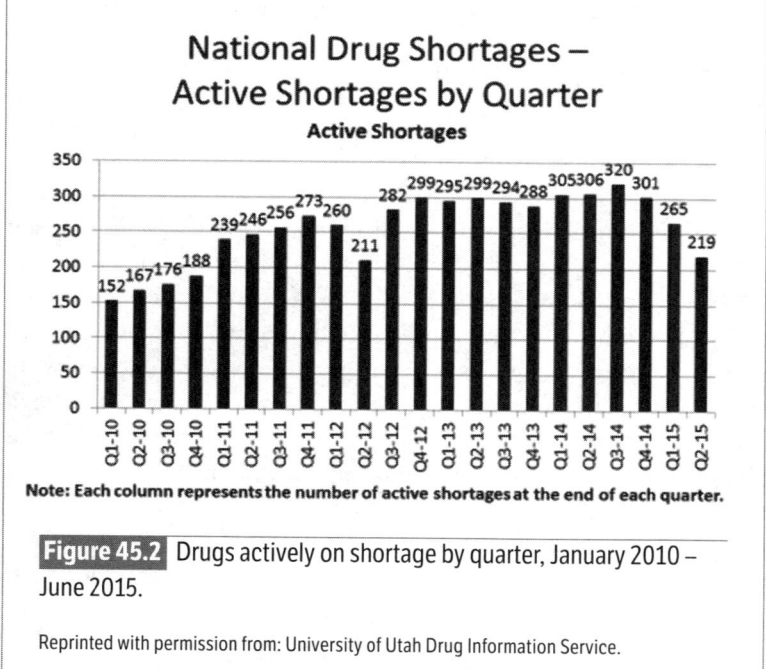

Figure 45.2 Drugs actively on shortage by quarter, January 2010 – June 2015.

Reprinted with permission from: University of Utah Drug Information Service.

- A patient died when the patient could not receive amikacin (which was the only medication the patient's infection was sensitive to)
- Two patients died after receiving intravenous hydromorphone that was prescribed and administered at the dose intended for intravenous morphine

In addition to direct harm to the patient, health care professionals are significantly affected by drug shortages. According to the same 2010 survey cited previously, the most common issue noted by health care professionals was the lack of timely information about a given shortage.[5] Drug shortages can lead to conflict and a tense work environment, which may be related to the lack of available information, the need to use nonoptimal therapies that providers are not used to using, and the need to make tough ethical decisions in order to conserve the dwindling supply of a drug.[9] There is speculation that shortages lead to changes in the training of prescribers and in prescribing patterns as prescribers become used to using a second- or third-line therapy when the first-line agent is on a long-term shortage.[10] The additional time required to manage shortages may add to the fatigue of a health care worker with an already full load of responsibilities, which could lead to errors and patient adverse effects. Drug shortages also force providers to take time away from other "high-impact, high-value" tasks such as patient care, education, and research.[9,11]

Finally, drug shortages have a significant financial impact. For example, the Premier Health Alliance estimated that an average of $230 million was spent annually from 2011 to 2013 across the country to purchase supplies of drugs on shortage from alternative suppliers.[7] In addition to the higher purchase price, the financial burden on institutions comes from ordering an increased quantity of a drug before or during an ongoing shortage. Also contributing to the financial burden are the additional personnel costs that may be required to manage shortages and potential lost revenue because of the delay or cancellation of procedures. A 2011 survey of pharmacy directors tried to quantify the impact of drug shortages on personnel time and costs.[11] The survey showed that an average of 17 hours was spent weekly on managing drug shortages. The survey also estimated that the personnel costs for managing shortages was $216 million annually in the United States, with the cost ranging from $25,000 to $48,000 per hospital, depending on the size of the hospital. However, this figure is likely an underestimate because some health systems have hired personnel solely to manage shortages, and at the time the survey was administered, the number of drug shortages was lower than it is now.

MANAGEMENT STRATEGIES FOR DEALING WITH DRUG SHORTAGES

It is vital for a hospital or health system to have a clearly defined plan and process for managing drug shortages to help mitigate the related risks and costs mentioned earlier (Figure 45.4). The strategic planning to manage drug shortages has been compared with the strategic planning for an emergency weather event or mass-casualty incident.[12] This planning and management is particularly vital for critically ill patients because generic injectables continue to be a significant portion of the drugs on shortage.

The first step in effectively managing drug shortages is to identify which medications are (or are likely to be) on shortage and gather information on the cause and expected duration of the shortage.[12,13]

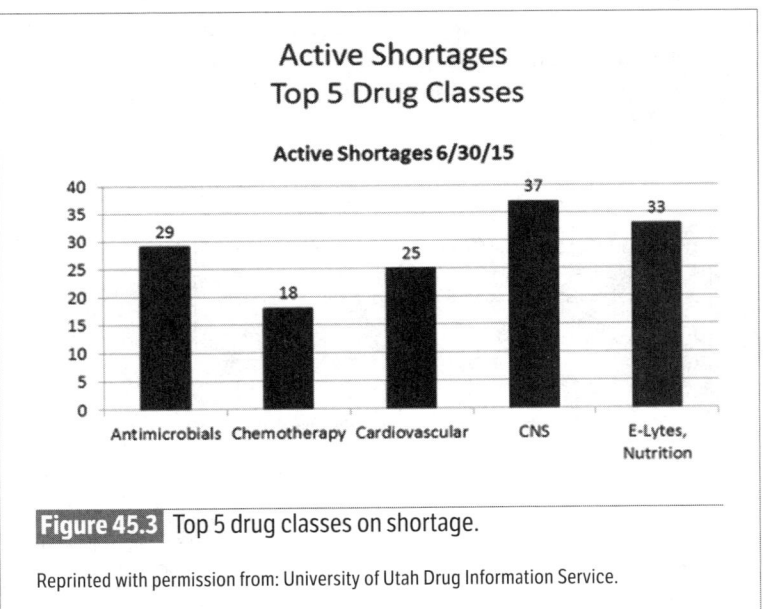

Figure 45.3 Top 5 drug classes on shortage.

Reprinted with permission from: University of Utah Drug Information Service.

Table 45.1 Reasons for Shortages as Determined by UUDIS During Investigation, 2014

Unknown 47%
Manufacturing 25%
Supply / Demand 17%
Raw Materials 2%
Business decision 9%

Having someone in charge of purchasing help to identify shortages by monitoring the issues with a product in the supply chain is one place for identification to occur. In addition, there are two main websites to find details about current drug shortages.[14,15] Both the American Society of Health-System Pharmacists (ASHP) and the FDA maintain online databases of current shortages together with pertinent information specific to each shortage (e.g., cause of shortage, alternative manufacturers). When researching a potential or actual shortage, it is helpful to visit both websites for details because the content may be different depending on the different ways each group defines a shortage and gathers its information. In general, the ASHP website will list more shortages and will include content directed more toward the health care professional.[1,16]

After the identification of an actual or potential shortage issue, the identified individual or group in charge of managing shortages should begin assessing the potential impact. The first task of assessment is to verify the current stock of the drug on hand and compare that with historic purchasing and drug use data to assess when the impact of the shortage may be felt. In addition, it is important to investigate and factor in the availability of the drug from any preapproved alternative sources, the availability and use of therapeutic alternatives, and the financial impact of ordering alternative agents. Ideally, at this point, the group in charge of managing shortages can analyze the threat to patients from a given shortage.[12,13]

A plan for best mitigating the impact of the shortage should be created according to the information initially gathered. There are several different means of mitigating risks of a drug shortage, and the mitigation plan for each shortage is unique. Often, alternative sizes or concentrations are available for a drug on shortage. In some instances, it may be possible to make background operational changes within the pharmacy such that providers prescribing or administering these agents are completely unaffected. If this is not possible, it may be necessary to decrease use of the drug by prioritizing patients, restricting the drug's use, and ordering and using alternative drugs. In these cases, it is important to engage the pharmacy and therapeutics committee or the ethics committee of an institution to help establish and communicate clear guidelines for the drug's use. One large academic medical center developed a policy around an ethically justifiable rationing approach for shortages.[17] Regardless of the plan, communication to any potential end users is vital to help ensure that a plan remains effective for as long as necessary. Regular communication through several different venues (electronic health and prescriber order entry systems, e-mail, postings on bulletin boards in applicable places, staff meetings, and any other means that your organization uses well) will help

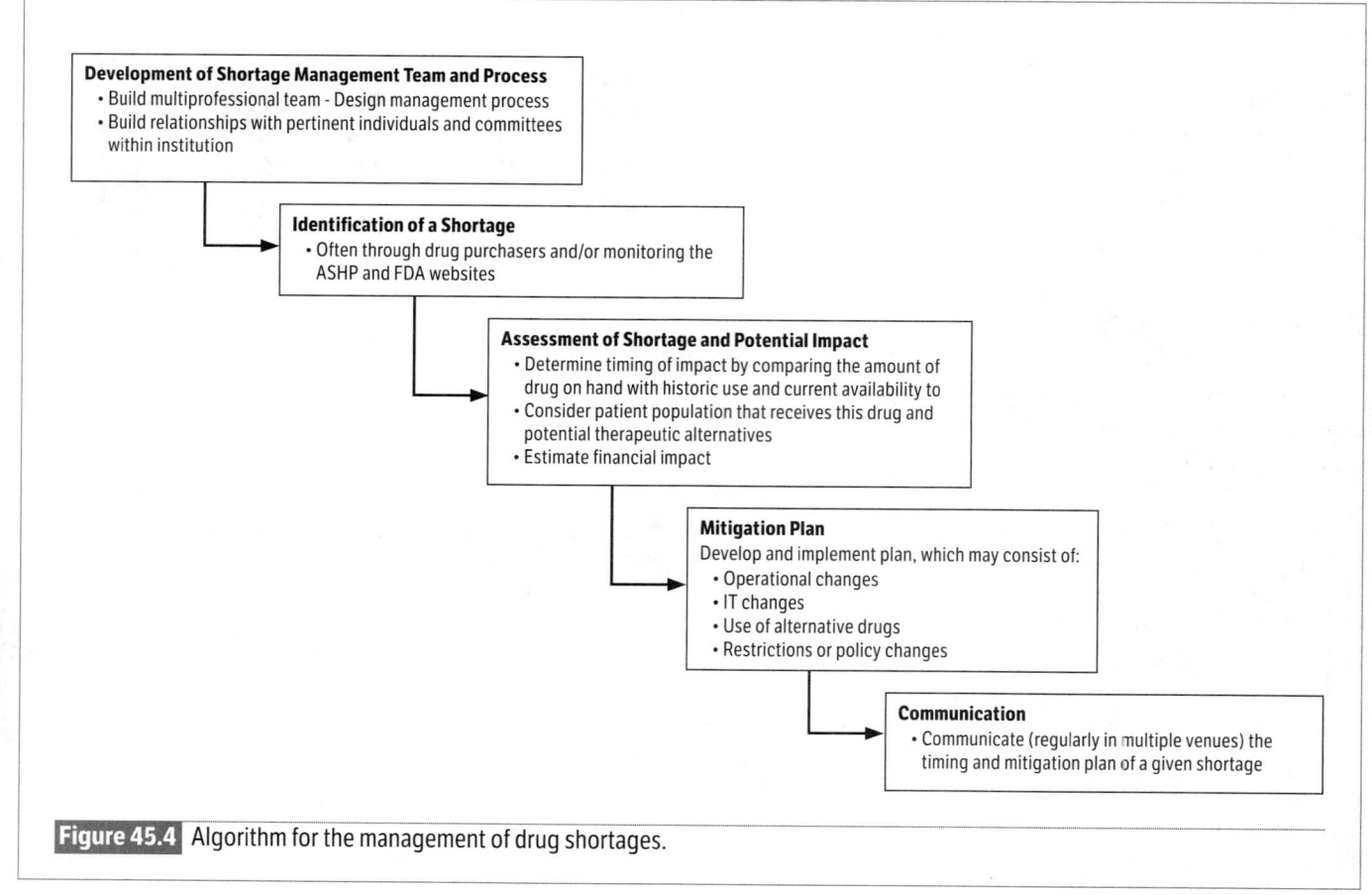

Figure 45.4 Algorithm for the management of drug shortages.

ensure that regular communication occurs.[12,13] Depending on the severity and potential ramifications of the shortage, senior medical and administrative leadership may need to be notified and engaged in supporting and disseminating any action plans.

Strong relationships and communication are vital to make the response to a drug shortage as safe and effective as possible. Although a pharmacy department may often take the lead, it is important to have relevant stakeholders, leaders, and committees from many different disciplines involved with planning and regularly providing feedback throughout the process. It may also be important to engage risk management and legal departments within an institution for a given shortage in order to help assess the impact of shortages that pose a larger threat to patient care so that they can plan accordingly. Finally, it may be helpful to build relationships with other hospitals to share information and emergency supplies.[12,13]

CONCLUSION

Although the number of new drug shortages per year has been declining since 2012, the ongoing drug shortage problem continues to place patients, health care teams, and health care institutions at risk of adverse outcomes. Drug shortages have several complex causes that are not quickly or easily fixed. Because of this, ongoing management with a team-based approach is necessary at the hospital level to mitigate these risks and prevent patient harm.

REFERENCES

1. Wosinka M, Fox E, Jensen V. Are shortages going down or not? Interpreting data from the FDA and the University of Utah drug information service. Health Affairs Blog. April 8, 2015. Available at http://healthaffairs.org/blog/2015/04/08/are-shortages-going-down-or-not-interpreting-data-from-the-fda-and-the-university-of-utah-drug-information-service/. Accessed May 15, 2015.

2. Loftus P. US drug shortages frustrate doctors, patients. Wall Street Journal. May 31, 2015. Available at www.wsj.com/articles/u-s-drug-shortages-frustrate-doctors-patients-1433125793. Accessed June 5, 2015.

3. U.S. Government Accountability Office. Drug Shortages: Public Health Threat Continues, Despite Efforts to Help Ensure Product Availability. GAO-14.-194. February 2014. Available at www.gao.gov/assets/670/660785.pdf. Accessed May 15, 2015.

4. American Hospital Association (AHA), American Society of Anesthesiologists (ASA), American Society of Clinical Oncology (ASCO), American Society of Health-System Pharmacists (ASHP), Institute for Safe Medication Practices (ISMP), and the Pew Charitable Trusts. 2014 Drug Shortages Summit Summary Report. August 1, 2014. Available at www.ismp.org/pressroom/2014-Drug-Shortages-Summit.pdf. Accessed May 15, 2015.

5. Institute for Safe Medication Practices. Drug shortages: national survey reveals high level of frustration, low level of safety. ISMP Med Saf Alert 2010;15:1-6. Available at www.ismp.org/newsletters/acutecare/articles/20100923.asp. Accessed May 15, 2015.

6. McLaughlin M, Kotis D, Thomson K, et al. Effects on patient care caused by drug shortages: a survey. J Manag Care Pharm 2013;19:783-8.

7. Johnson LJ. Hospitals coping better as drug shortages persist. Associated Press. February 28, 2014. Available at www.bostonglobe.com/business/2014/02/28/hospitals-coping-better-drug-shortages-persist/ri3StaN3qSfC2itCxVnHeN/story.html. Accessed June 5, 2015.

8. Koba M. The US has a drug shortage – and people are dying. Fortune Online. January 6, 2015. Available at http://fortune.com/2015/01/06/the-u-s-has-a-drug-shortage-and-people-are-dying/. Accessed June 5, 2015.

9. The Joint Commission. Health care worker fatigue and patient safety. Sentinel Event Alert. 2011;48:1-4. Available at www.jointcommission.org/assets/1/18/sea_48.pdf. Accessed June 5, 2015.

10. George A. A potential unexpected consequence of drug shortages on long-term prescribing patterns. Am J Health Syst Pharm 2015;72:916.

11. Kaakeh R, Sweet BV, Reilly C, et al. Impact of drug shortages on US health systems. Am J Health Syst Pharm 2011;68:1811-9.

12. Fox ER, Birt A, James KB, et al. ASHP guidelines on managing drug product shortages in hospitals and health systems. Am J Health Syst Pharm 2009;66:1399-406.

13. Institute for Safe Medication Practices. Weathering the storm: managing the drug shortage crisis. ISMP Med Saf Alert 2010;15:1-4. Available at www.ismp.org/newsletters/acutecare/arve meticles/20101007.asp. Accessed June 15, 2015.

14. U.S. Food and Drug Administration. Current Drug Shortages. Available at www.fda.gov/Drugs/DrugSafety/DrugShortages/. Accessed June 15, 2015.

15. American Society of Health-System Pharmacists. Drug Shortages: Current Drugs. Available at www.ashp.org/drugshortages/current/. Accessed June 15, 2015.

16. U.S. Food and Drug Administration Drug Shortage Staff, American Society of Health-System Pharmacists, and the University of Utah Drug Information Service. Contrasting the FDA (CDER) and ASHP Drug Shortage Websites: What's the Difference? August 2014. Available at www.ashp.org/DocLibrary/Policy/DrugShortages/FDA-versus-ASHP.pdf. Accessed August 5, 2015.

17. Rosoff PM, Patel, KR, Scates A, et al. Coping with critical drug shortages: an ethical approach for allocating scarce resources in hospitals. Arch Intern Med 2012;172:1494-9.

Chapter 46: Drug Interactions in the Intensive Care Unit

Cristian Merchan, Pharm.D.; and John Papadopoulos, Pharm.D., B.S., FCCM, BCNSP

LEARNING OBJECTIVES

1. Discuss the importance of recognizing drug interactions.
2. Differentiate between a pharmacokinetic and a pharmacodynamic drug-drug interaction (DDI).
3. Analyze specific examples of clinically significant DDIs relevant in the intensive care unit setting.
4. Explain the importance of drug-nutrient interactions.
5. Summarize an approach to evaluate the evidence of DDIs.

ABBREVIATIONS IN THIS CHAPTER

AUC	Area under the curve	MAO	Monoamine oxidase
DDI	Drug-drug interaction	P-gp	P-glycoprotein
DIPS	Drug Interaction Probability Scale	TdP	Torsades de pointes
H$_2$RA	Histamine-2 receptor antagonist	TOAC	Target-specific oral anticoagulant
ICU	Intensive care unit		

INTRODUCTION

The care of the critically ill patient is a complex process that requires clinicians to draw on their knowledge of pathophysiology, pharmacology, pharmacokinetics, clinical trials, and differential diagnoses. Patients cared for in an intensive care unit (ICU) environment receive several medications to treat a variety of acute and chronic ailments, as well as prophylactic medications to prevent complications such as stress-related mucosal damage and deep vein thrombosis. Each ICU clinician needs to understand the importance of drug interactions, given the complexity of pharmacologic interplay in the ICU environment, the common presence of organ dysfunction, and our heightened awareness for the need to provide optimal and safe care for our patients. Published data quantifying the magnitude of drug interactions and their effects on clinical outcomes in the ICU are limited. A single-center, prospective, observational study of 281 patients admitted to a medical ICU reported that drug interactions accounted for 4% of ICU admissions.[1] Additional data analyses report that the percentage of patients in the ICU with at least one drug interaction is 40%–73%.[2-6]

Several observational studies have been conducted to identify significant potential drug-drug interactions (DDIs) in a variety of ICU settings. Smithburger and colleagues conducted a prospective, observational study to identify DDIs in the cardiovascular and cardiothoracic ICUs.[2] Micromedex and Lexi-Interact interaction databases were used to screen each patient's medication profile and determine the severity of identified DDIs. Of the 400 patient medication profiles evaluated, 56% had one or more potential DDIs. The most significant DDIs were determined by assignment to the major interaction category by just one of the interaction databases. These included drugs that can prolong the corrected QT (QTc) interval, enhance antiplatelet or anticoagulant effects, and inhibit the cytochrome P450 (CYP) 3A4 enzyme. The most common drugs cited as involved in major interactions included amiodarone, aspirin, clopidogrel, heparin, warfarin, clonidine, and β-blockers. Smithburger and colleagues also conducted a similar evaluation in the medical ICU.[3] From the 240 patient medication profiles evaluated, 46% had one or more potential DDIs. The most significant DDIs involved medications that can enhance antiplatelet or anticoagulant effects, prolong the QTc interval, or inhibit

CYP3A4 or that can be classified as an antiepileptic. The most common drugs cited as involved in major interactions included aspirin, clopidogrel, selective serotonin reuptake inhibitors (SSRIs), β-blockers, valproic acid, and posaconazole. In addition, these studies highlight the importance of considering the differences between ICU populations when developing clinical decision support systems in order to reduce alert fatigue, and the studies provide enough information to determine an appropriate risk-benefit ratio for the patient receiving the interacting drugs. Nonetheless, further data are needed to adequately determine the impact of drug interactions in the ICU environment.

Drug interactions are generally classified as pharmacokinetic or pharmacodynamic, depending on the underlying mechanism. A pharmacokinetic interaction occurs when one drug alters the absorption, distribution, metabolism, or elimination of another agent. These interactions can be quantified by changes in area under the curve (AUC), half-life, or peak serum concentration. A pharmacodynamic interaction changes the pharmacologic response to a drug in an additive, synergistic, or antagonistic way. This review will focus on DDIs and drug-nutrient interactions that have high clinical relevance in the ICU setting.

PHARMACOKINETIC DDIS

Absorption

The small intestine is the primary site for enteral drug absorption, except for a few drugs that are absorbed in the stomach (e.g., aspirin). Patient and drug-specific factors influence enteral drug absorption and net bioavailability in the critically ill.[7,8] The clinical status of the patient is an important consideration when determining the intestine's ability to absorb enterally administered medications. Many factors contribute to intestinal ischemic damage in the critically ill, including acute hemorrhage, cardiac and abdominal surgery, inotropic and vasopressor therapy, various forms of shock, and abdominal compartment syndrome.[7,8] These factors redistribute blood flow away from the gastrointestinal (GI) tract and may prolong the time to reach peak concentrations and AUC of enterally administered medications. In addition, critically ill patients commonly receive stress ulcer prophylaxis with intravenous histamine-2 receptor antagonists (H_2RAs) or proton pump inhibitors (PPIs). Because many drugs are weak acids, the associated increase in gastric pH induced by the administration of gastric acid inhibitors can potentially alter the bioavailability of drugs normally absorbed through the GI tract that require an acidic medium for absorption (e.g., ketoconazole, itraconazole, dipyridamole).[7,8] Furthermore, delayed gastric emptying is commonly observed in patients who have postoperative ileus, mechanical ventilation, electrolyte abnormalities, splanchnic hypoperfusion, increased intracranial pressure, or opioid and sedative medication needs. Because these parameters delay the rate of gastric emptying, they may lead to a delay in the rate of drug absorption, time to peak concentration, and onset of drug action for enterally administered medications.[9] Another factor to consider in the critically ill is the effect of systemic inflammation on P-glycoprotein (P-gp) function. P-glycoprotein acts as an efflux pump that transports drugs back into the intestinal lumen after absorption. This efflux pump, in combination with any intestinal CYP3A4 inhibition, may substantially limit the bioavailability of drugs given enterally that are substrates for these systems. Systemic inflammation decreases the intestinal P-gp activity, which may lead to a consequential increase in the net oral bioavailability of enterally administered medications that are substrates for these systems.[10,11] Finally, the administration of enteral feeds, binders, or chelators can lead to a decrease in the AUC of select drugs. Table 46.1 provides specific examples of DDIs that affect the absorption of various medications prescribed in the ICU.

TARGETED TREATMENT STRATEGIES FOR DDIS INVOLVING ABSORPTION

Drug-drug interactions involving absorption can be handled in various ways. Therapeutic substitution (i.e., sucralfate or an H_2RA instead of a PPI) for drugs that require gastric acidity or appropriate administration spacing in the presence of a binder or chelator may mitigate an absorption-related interaction. Use of the intravenous route of medication administration should be considered in a critically ill patient when a medication need is critical.

P-glycoprotein (B)

P-glycoprotein acts as a drug efflux pump that is responsible for transporting drugs from the circulation into the lumen of the small intestine, bile duct, and proximal convoluted tubule (Table 46.2).[36-38] These pumps are located on the luminal membrane of the small intestine and blood-brain barrier and in the apical membranes of excretory cells such as hepatocytes and renal proximal tubule cells. The role of P-gp on the intestinal epithelial cells is to limit the cellular uptake and absorption into enterocytes, compared with its location in hepatocytes and renal tubular cells, where it enhances the elimination of drugs into the bile and urine, respectively.[36-38] In addition, P-gp provides enhanced opportunities for medications to be metabolized by intestinal CYP3A4. Subsequently, there is increased contact of medications to the CYP3A4 enzymes that contribute toward biotransformation and decreased overall systemic exposure.[36-38]

Targeted Treatment Strategies for DDI Involving P-gp

The role of P-gp in the realm of drug interactions may be limited (except for digoxin) unless there is concomitant CYP enzyme inhibition or induction (Table 46.3). If a concomitant P-gp/CYP enzyme interaction is identified,

Table 46.1 Clinically Relevant Drug Interactions of Absorption

Drug 1	Drug 2	Mechanism	Management
Increased gastric pH			
PPIs or H$_2$RAs	Atazanavir[12]	Lansoprazole decreased the AUC by 94%	PPIs should be avoided, when possible
PPIs raise gastric pH > 5 for up to 19 hr		Omeprazole 40 mg/day decreased the AUC by 65%–75%	Consider H$_2$RAs as alternatives, but need to space 12 hr apart
			In treatment-naive patients, if a PPI is warranted, the PPI dose should not exceed a dose comparable to omeprazole 20 mg and must be taken about 12 hr before atazanavir
	Mycophenolate mofetil[13,14]	Omeprazole 20 mg BID decreased the AUC by 20%	If coadministration is necessary, the dose of mycophenolate may need to be increased; can consider enteric-coated mycophenolate sodium to avoid interaction
	Posaconazole[15,16]	Decreased bioavailability with increase in gastric pH	Use DR tablets, if possible
			Avoid suspension formulation. If unavoidable, administer with a fatty meal or cola beverage
	Rilpivirine[17]	Omeprazole 20 mg/day decreased the AUC by 40%	PPIs are contraindicated in all patients taking rilpivirine
			Only H$_2$RAs that can be dosed once daily should be used. Administer at least 12 hr before or 4 hr after rilpivirine
Increased GI motility			
Metoclopramide	Cyclosporine[18]	Metoclopramide increased the peak and AUC of cyclosporine by 50% and 30%, respectively	Monitor and adjust cyclosporine concentrations as necessary.
			Monitor for signs and symptoms of cyclosporine toxicity, which may include acute kidney injury, cholestasis, or paresthesias
Presence of a binder or chelator			
Complex metals (calcium, aluminum, iron, magnesium)	Fluoroquinolones (ciprofloxacin and levofloxacin) and tetracyclines (doxycycline and minocycline)[19-22]	One randomized crossover study of 12 healthy volunteers reported that when either calcium carbonate or aluminum hydroxide tablets were taken 5 min before ciprofloxacin, the bioavailability was reduced by 40%–85% of the control value	Administer aluminum-, calcium-, or magnesium-containing products at least 2–4 hr before or 6 hr after the fluoroquinolone
			Administer iron at least 2 hr after the fluoroquinolone; avoid sustained-release iron
			Consider switching the fluoroquinolone to IV for severe infections in critically ill hospitalized patients
Bile acid sequestrates (cholestyramine)	Digoxin Levothyroxine Oral vancomycin Lipid-soluble vitamins Warfarin[23-25]	Bind to various drugs and decrease their oral bioavailability Much more likely to bind to acidic compounds than to basic compounds, but this is not an absolute because they can bind to basic medications as well (e.g., propranolol)	Separate the administration times of all oral medications by at least 2 hr before or 4 hr after the administration of bile acid sequestrants

Table 46.1	Clinically Relevant Drug Interactions of Absorption *(continued)*		
Drug 1	**Drug 2**	**Mechanism**	**Management**
Carbapenems	Valproic acid[26-28]	Carbapenems lower valproic acid concentrations through several mechanisms: -Inhibits intestinal absorption of valproic acid -Inhibits β-glucuronidase, which increases the systemic clearance of the parent drug by reducing the amount of drug available for recirculation -Improves glucuronidation of valproic acid Carbapenems reduce valproic acid plasma concentrations by 50%–80%; have led to breakthrough seizures in some patients	Recommend an alternative antibiotic or antiepileptic agent. If valproic acid must be coadministered with a carbapenem: -Increasing the valproic acid doses may not be sufficient to achieve therapeutic levels; monitor valproic acid plasma concentrations
Disruption of intestinal flora			
Ampicillin Macrolides Tetracyclines	Digoxin[29-32]	In about 10% of patients, digoxin is metabolized by *Eubacterium lentum* (a gram-positive anaerobic *Bacillus*). Coadministration of digoxin with these particular antibiotics may increase digoxin's bioavailability. Although not well delineated, P-gp inhibition may also play a role	Monitor digoxin concentrations, and monitor for signs and symptoms of toxicity. Less clinical relevance for patients taking Lanoxicaps® or digoxin elixir because of more complete absorption, with less unabsorbed drug available for metabolism in the colon
Antimicrobials	Warfarin[33-35]	Antimicrobials may reduce the synthesis of endogenously produced vitamin K by intestinal microflora. In addition, this phenomenon may be amplified by a cytokine-induced proinflammatory state that may inhibit CYP2C9, resulting in an increased risk of having INR elevations and bleeding events with warfarin Cefotetan and cefoperazone have an N-methylthiotetrazole (NMTT) side chain, and cefazolin has an N-methylthiadiazole (NMTD) side chain. Cleavage of the NMTT and NMTD side chains from the parent compounds mainly in the GI tract can inhibit vitamin K epoxide reductase and amplify the pharmacology of coadministered warfarin	Monitor INR, and titrate to goal therapeutic INR; monitor for signs and symptoms of bleeding Greatest INR elevations observed with the following medications because of concurrent CYP2C9 inhibition: Sulfamethoxazole Metronidazole Fluconazole Voriconazole Efavirenz

BID = twice daily; DR = delayed release; IV = intravenous(ly).

vigilance in therapeutic drug monitoring, indices of clinical end points, and signs and symptoms of toxicity needs to be used to determine the best clinical treatment course. Medication substitution, as described in the section on DDIs involving metabolism, may need to be used.

DDIS AND DISTRIBUTION: DISPLACEMENT FROM A CARRIER PROTEIN

Albumin and α_1-acid glycoprotein are the two most common plasma proteins that bind to acidic drugs (e.g., antiepileptics, benzodiazepines) and basic drugs (e.g., lidocaine, synthetic opioids, tricyclic antidepressants [TCAs]), respectively.[7,8,46] The extent of plasma protein binding depends on the concentration of plasma proteins, which may fluctuate in critical illness, and the affinity of the drug to the plasma protein. Albumin acts as a negative acute phase reactant, and the concentration decreases in the setting of sepsis, renal or liver failure, burns, surgery, and malnutrition. However, α_1-acid glycoprotein is a positive acute phase reactant in which increased concentrations are observed in inflammatory diseases, trauma, and acute myocardial infarctions.[7,8,46]

Displacement of one drug by another from plasma proteins can lead to an increase in the unbound free fraction of the displaced drug; the unbound free fraction is the pharmacologically active entity. For most drugs, displacement from plasma proteins results in only minor changes in free plasma drug concentrations and resultant enhanced distribution and elimination pharmacokinetics. Thus, the

Table 46.2 Major Substrates, Inhibitors, and Inducers of P-glycoproteins[39,40]

Substrate	Inhibitor	Inducer
Apixaban	Amiodarone	Carbamazepine
Colchicine	Atorvastatin	Dexamethasone
Cyclosporine	Cyclosporine	Phenobarbital
Dabigatran	Diltiazem	Phenytoin
Digoxin	Dronedarone	Rifampin
Linezolid	Erythromycin	Tenofovir
Methotrexate	Lopinavir	
Rivaroxaban	Ritonavir	
Ticagrelor	Tacrolimus	
	Verapamil	

Table 46.3 Clinically Relevant Drug Interactions Affected by P-glycoprotein

Drug 1	Drug 2	Mechanism	Management
P-glycoprotein inhibitors			
Amiodarone, Cyclosporine, Erythromycin, Itraconazole, Verapamil	Digoxin[41]	Results in increased serum digoxin concentrations. Affects enterally administered digoxin more than IV administered digoxin	Monitor digoxin concentrations and signs and symptoms of toxicity
Amiodarone	Apixaban[42,43]	Has not been studied, but potentially increases concentrations	Reduce apixaban dose to 2.5 mg orally BID
	Rivaroxaban[42,43]	Has marginal increases in rivaroxaban concentrations	Consider dose modifications only with concomitant renal impairment; avoid combination if the CrCl is < 30 mL/min
	Dabigatran[42,43]	Can increase dabigatran concentrations by up to 60%	
Any antifungal azole	Apixaban[42,43], Dabigatran[42,43], Rivaroxaban[42,43]	Apixaban, dabigatran, and rivaroxaban (TOACs) concentrations were increased by 100%–160%	Combination should be avoided, if possible. Consider dose reductions for each agent, but must evaluate the net risk vs. the net benefit. May need to consider warfarin as an alternative oral anticoagulant
P-glycoprotein inducers			
Rifampin	Linezolid[44,45]	In a pharmacokinetic study, linezolid 600 mg q12hr was given together with rifampin 600 mg q24hr. Concomitant administration led to a 21% decrease in linezolid Cmax and a 32% decrease in linezolid AUC. CYP3A has a small contribution (0.7%–10.5%) to linezolid clearance, which may be enhanced by rifampin	Evaluate the need for rifampin, and consider an alternative agent
	Apixaban[42,43], Dabigatran[42,43], Rivaroxaban[42,43]	Reduced concentration of all TOACs by greater than 50%. In addition, apixaban and rivaroxaban are CYP3A4 substrates, and enzyme induction may be a contributing factor	Combination should be avoided, if possible. May need to consider an alternative anticoagulant (e.g., low-molecular-weight heparin [because of concomitant enzyme induction, may need to avoid warfarin])

CrCl = creatinine clearance; q = every; TOAC = target-specific anticoagulant.

altered plasma binding would not be expected to clinically influence the pharmacologic response, and dose adjustments are not usually required.[7,8,46] Plasma binding displacement interactions become clinically important when the displaced medication has a narrow therapeutic index. In addition, the route of drug administration may be important for the clinical realization of displacement interactions. In theory, clinically important displacement interactions are most likely to occur shortly after an intravenous push administration of a highly protein bound drug. This interplay may be less clinically relevant with oral administration of the same medications given that the slow rate of enteral absorption may result in slow displacement and quick equilibration of plasma concentrations. Phenytoin and warfarin are two drug examples for which protein binding displacement interactions may be realized with the coadministration of higher-affinity albumin binders. Valproic acid, sulfamethoxazole, salicylates, and ceftriaxone are examples of medications that can potentially increase the free fraction of both phenytoin and warfarin.[46] However, the clinical significance of this interaction may be temporary and self-correcting. When the unbound concentration increases, the total clearance of either phenytoin or warfarin also increases as the liver metabolizes excess free drug, and steady state will return to the pre-displacement value.[7,8,46] One consideration with phenytoin specifically is that a marked increase in free drug could result in a reduction clearance because phenytoin follows nonlinear pharmacokinetics. Management of albumin displacement interactions includes therapeutic drug monitoring and monitoring for signs and symptoms of phenytoin or warfarin toxicity until a new steady state is achieved.

TARGETED TREATMENT STRATEGIES FOR DDI INVOLVING DISPLACEMENT FROM A CARRIER PROTEIN

Displacement interactions tend to be transient and are usually not clinically significant. If a carrier protein displacement interaction is identified, vigilance in therapeutic drug monitoring, monitoring for the indices of clinical end points, and monitoring the signs and symptoms of toxicity needs to be used to determine the best clinical treatment course.

CYP AND ITS ROLE IN METABOLISM

The liver is the primary organ responsible for drug metabolism, followed by the GI tract, kidney, lung, integument, and blood.[47-49] The liver has several sequential steps of drug elimination by metabolism and membrane transport. Phase 0 delivers drugs from the blood into the liver through a carrier-mediated uptake process.[48] Once inside the metabolizing hepatocyte, drug metabolism is divided into phase I (oxidation, hydrolysis, reduction) and phase II (glucuronide, sulfate, and glycine conjugation) enzymatic reactions. Phase I reactions are mediated by the CYP enzyme system and convert a parent drug to a more hydrophilic metabolite. Phase II metabolism, not mediated by CYP, produces an inactive water-soluble product that can be readily excreted by the kidneys. Finally, phase III metabolism involves the excretion of these newly formed metabolites by transporter pumps such as MRP2, MDR1/P-gp, and BCRP at the canalicular hepatocyte membrane.[48]

The most common and significant DDIs involve the CYP enzyme system. Cytochrome P450 is a family of heme-containing proteins located in the smooth endoplasmic reticulum of the hepatocytes. The CYP enzymes are also located, to a lesser extent, in the small intestine, kidneys, and lungs. The predominant CYP enzymes responsible for more than 90% of human drug metabolism are as follows: CYP3A4 (36%), CYP2D6 (19%), CYP2C9 (16%), CYP1A2 (11%), CYP2C19 (8%), and CYP2E1 (4%).[47-51] Other isoforms are minor contributors to total CYP activity and include CYP2B6 and CYP2J2. Individual CYP enzymes are specific to a substrate on the basis of a particular region of the drug molecule or enantiomer. Some substrates can be metabolized by more than one CYP enzyme, and these substrates can act as either an inducer or an inhibitor for these CYP enzymes.[47-51]

Enzyme inhibition is divided into reversible and irreversible inhibition.[8,47-51] Reversible inhibition (most common) is characterized as a dose-dependent interaction in which the substrate and inhibitor compete for the same site on the enzyme; the metabolism of the substrate is decreased. Irreversible inhibition is distinguished by the formation of reactive metabolites, which alter the conformation of the enzyme so that the active biotransformation site is no longer functional. This type of inhibition is both dose- and duration-dependent. The onset of inhibition typically occurs as soon as the inhibitor is in contact with the enzyme, and the maximal effect can be observed after steady state of the inhibitor and affected substrate has been reached.[8,47-51] Restoration of the CYP system after cessation of an enzyme inhibitor depends on several drug characteristics such as dose, half-life, presence of Michaelis-Menten pharmacokinetics, presence of genetic polymorphisms, and presence of organ dysfunction. Conversely, enzyme induction occurs when an inducer enhances the synthesis or reduces the breakdown of a CYP enzyme. The net effect observed is a decreased concentration or an increased biotransformation or prodrug activation of the affected substrate. The onset of induction will become apparent over several days to weeks as the amount of enzyme increases enough to change the drug clearance of the substrate; the offset occurs within a similar time interval. The maximum time of onset for enzyme induction depends on the half-life of the inducing agent and the time to steady state of the inducer. For example, when comparing rifampin and phenytoin, rifampin will reach steady-state serum concentrations quicker than phenytoin

Table 46.4 Major Substrates, Inhibitors, and Inducers of the CYP Enzyme System[40,47-51]

Substrate	Inhibitor	Inducer
CYP1A2		
Acetaminophen	Cimetidine	Carbamazepine
Lidocaine	Ciprofloxacin	Rifampin
	Erythromycin	
	Fluvoxamine	
CYP2B6		
Bupropion		
Prasugrel		
Propofol		
CYP2C9		
Ketamine	Amiodarone	Carbamazepine
Phenytoin	Fluconazole, voriconazole	Dexamethasone
Rosuvastatin	Isoniazid	Phenobarbital
S-warfarin	Metronidazole	Phenytoin
Valproic acid	Sulfamethoxazole	Rifampin
Voriconazole	Valproic acid	
CYP2C19		
Citalopram	Esomeprazole	
Clopidogrel	Fluconazole	Carbamazepine
Diazepam	Fluoxetine	Dexamethasone
Lacosamide	Omeprazole	Phenobarbital
Phenytoin	Oxcarbazepine	Phenytoin
Proton pump inhibitors	Voriconazole	Rifampin
R-warfarin		
Voriconazole		
CYP2D6		
Codeine	Amiodarone	
Carvedilol metoprolol propranolol	Bupropion	
Haloperidol	Fluoxetine, paroxetine, sertraline	
Ondansetron	Haloperidol	
Paroxetine	Quinidine	
Tramadol		
CYP2E1		
Acetaminophen		Isoniazid
CYP3A4		
Amlodipine, nifedipine, felodipine	Amiodarone	Carbamazepine
Apixaban, rivaroxaban	Amlodipine, nifedipine	Dexamethasone
Atorvastatin, simvastatin	Clarithromycin, erythromycin	Efavirenz
Boceprevir, telaprevir	Diltiazem, verapamil	Nevirapine
Carbamazepine	Fluconazole, itraconazole, posaconazole, voriconazole	Phenobarbital
Clarithromycin, erythromycin	Ritonavir	Phenytoin
Colchicine	Valproic acid	Rifabutin

Table 46.4 Major Substrates, Inhibitors, and Inducers of the CYP Enzyme System[40,47-51] (continued)

Substrate	Inhibitor	Inducer
Cyclophosphamide		Rifampin
Cyclosporine, tacrolimus		
Dexamethasone, hydrocortisone, methylprednisolone		
Diazepam, midazolam		
Diltiazem, verapamil		
Fentanyl		
Haloperidol		
Ketamine		
Nelfinavir, ritonavir, saquinavir		
Prasugrel, ticagrelor		
R-warfarin		
Sirolimus		

because of rifampin's shorter half-life. It will take longer for phenytoin to induce CYP enzymes compared with rifampin, and the induction will remain detectable for a greater length of time after discontinuation as a result of phenytoin's long half-life.[8,40,47-50] Table 46.4 provides a list of CYP isoenzymes and some common ICU medication substrates, inhibitors, and inducers. Table 46.5, Table 46.6, Table 46.7, and Table 46.8 review the effects of specific disease states and DDIs with the most common CYP metabolizing enzymes.

TARGETED TREATMENT STRATEGIES FOR DDI INVOLVING METABOLISM

Many medications that are used in the care of critically ill patients are cleared by CYP hepatic biotransformation. The bedside clinician must have a thorough understanding of the principles of enzyme induction and inhibition, including the onsets and offsets of such interactions. The astute clinician needs to evaluate the circumstances of an identified DDI and the relevance and potential downstream effects. The decision to adjust any medication dosages, implement alternative pharmacotherapy, and implement any monitoring strategy must be made on a case-by-case basis. Team communication is a vital component of these decisions, with a plan to modify a treatment plan if the desired end point is not met or if an adverse event is identified.

RENAL ELIMINATION

The kidneys, through a combination of passive glomerular filtration rate, active tubular secretion, and tubular reabsorption, are vital in the elimination of medications. Glomerular filtration is a passive process by which water and small-molecular-weight (less than 60 Da) ions and molecules diffuse across the glomerular-capillary membrane into the Bowman capsule and then enter the proximal tubule.[7,8] Tubular secretion is an active process that predominantly takes place in the proximal tubule and facilitates the removal of medications from plasma into the tubular lumen. Four distinct transporters mediate this secretory process: organic anion transporters (OATs), organic cation transporters (OCTs), nucleoside transporters, and P-gp transporters.[69,70] The OAT, OCT, and nucleoside transporters are uptake transporters that are located on the basolateral membrane of the proximal tubule and facilitate the entry of drugs into cells. Efflux transporters at the apical membrane of the proximal tubule enhance the removal of drugs from cells and into urine.

Renal uptake transporters are known to be associated with clinically relevant DDIs. Renal OAT1 and OAT3 are mainly involved in the secretion of acidic drugs.[69,70] In general, these substrates transport endogenous compounds such as prostaglandins, folate, and urate as well as several drugs that are listed in Table 46.9. This active process is mediated by the exchange of extracellular drug for intracellular α-ketoglutarate. The only well-established inhibitor of the OAT transport system is probenecid, which may result in a 30%–90% reduction in total renal clearance and a significant increase in plasma exposure of drugs subject to this transporter. The OCT2 transporter is mainly involved in the secretion of basic drugs as shown in Table 46.9.[69,70] This uptake process is facilitated by the proton gradient maintained at the apical membrane of proximal tubule cells, and efflux of drugs into the urine is mediated by the multidrug and toxin extrusion transporter 1 (MATE1).[69,70] Many drugs can inhibit the cationic tubular secretion pathways (mainly MATE1), and several

Table 46.5 Disease States and Effects of CYP Metabolism[40,47-52]

Disease/Predisposition	Mechanism	Effect on Drug Metabolism
Sepsis[53-58]	Lipopolysaccharide can cause the release of interleukin (IL)-1, IL-2, IL-6, and tumor necrosis factor (TNF)	Increased concentrations of circulating epinephrine and corticosteroids
	IL-2 inhibits CYP 1A2, 2C, 2E1, and 3A4 isoenzymes by around 63%, 55%, 40%, and 61%, respectively	Decreased clearance of drugs metabolized through these particular pathways
	TNFα inhibits 2C19	
	IL-6 inhibits 2C19, 1A2, and 3A4	
	Increased nitric oxide release during host-defense response inhibits drug metabolism by binding to the prosthetic heme of CYP	Decreased clearance of drugs metabolized through the CYP pathway
	Decrease in cardiac output during late sepsis • Results in a decrease in hepatic blood flow	Mainly affects drugs with high hepatic extraction ratios (e.g., opioids, lidocaine, TCAs)
Traumatic brain injury[59]	Induction of CYP3A4 enzymes increased by 27% and 91% at 24 hr and 2 wk, respectively	Increased metabolism of drug metabolized by CYP3A4
Hypothermia[60]	Decreased rate of redox reactions performed by CYP enzymes	Decreased clearance of drugs metabolized through the CYP pathway
Polymorphism[61]	Genetic polymorphism of the CYP2C9 enzyme: poor metabolizers contain a combination of *2 or *3 variant alleles (observed in 40% of the white population)	Dose reductions of warfarin, rosuvastatin, and phenytoin may be warranted
	Genetic polymorphism of the CYP2C19 enzyme: poor metabolizers contain a combination of *2 or *3 variant alleles (observed in 30% of the Asian population)	Poor metabolizers of 2C19 will have decreased conversion of clopidogrel (prodrug) to its active metabolite
	Genetic polymorphism of the CYP2D6 enzyme: poor metabolizers contain a combination of *3 or *4 variant alleles (observed in 20% of the African American population)	Higher risk of adverse effects from opioids and neuroleptics that are CYP2D6 substrates

are highlighted in Table 46.9. Renal transport inhibition DDIs usually result in a less than 50% increase in the AUC of the substrate drug. Of note, inhibition of renal transport would limit the effect on drug clearance to the fraction that is usually cleared by this route.

Tubular reabsorption of most medications occurs predominantly along the distal tubule and collecting duct. The extent of drug reabsorption is determined by urine flow rate, lipid solubility, and degree of ionization of the drug. For organic acids and bases, diffusion is inversely related to the extent of ionization because the non-ionized molecule is more lipid soluble and more likely to be reabsorbed.[7,8] For instance, the acidification of urine favors the excretion of weak organic bases, whereas the alkalinization of urine favors the elimination of weak organic acids.

Medications that can alkalinize the urine such as sodium bicarbonate and acetazolamide can enhance the elimination of weak acids such as salicylates, phenobarbital, chlorpropamide, diflunisal, and methotrexate. These principles of drug trapping may be useful in the toxicologic management of certain drug intoxications (i.e., salicylate overdose with sodium bicarbonate infusions).[69,70]

TARGETED TREATMENT STRATEGIES FOR DDI INVOLVING RENAL ELIMINATION

The clinical relevance of DDIs may be minimal. Possible explanations for this observation may be that few drugs mainly rely on tubular secretion for total body clearance, and the renal transport pathways are generally low-affinity

Table 46.6 Drug Interactions Involving CYP3A4[40,47-51]

Inhibitors/Inducers	Drug	Mechanism	Management
Azoles Macrolides (clarithromycin and erythromycin) Protease inhibitors	Midazolam	CYP3A4 inhibition; results in a 3- to 4-fold increase in the risk of prolonged sedation and respiratory depression	Titrate to goal RASS; may need to reduce the infusion rate
Phenytoin Rifampin		CYP3A4 induction; can decrease midazolam concentrations and therapeutic effect	Titrate to goal RASS May need to increase the infusion rate to achieve goal RASS. All drug interaction data reported with oral midazolam
Erythromycin	Cyclosporine	Increased GI absorption; CYP3A4, and P-gp inhibition. A 2- to 3-fold increase in cyclosporine concentrations. Resultant increased risk of acute kidney injury	Decrease the cyclosporine dose by 50% if coadministration is necessary. Monitor and adjust cyclosporine concentrations If erythromycin is used as a promotility agent, consider other GI motility agents such as metoclopramide. If erythromycin is used for *Legionella* pneumonia, consider either levofloxacin or azithromycin as an alternative agent
	Tacrolimus	CYP3A4 inhibition; resultant increased risk of acute kidney injury or QTc interval prolongation	See management strategies similar to those for cyclosporine
Voriconazole	Cyclosporine Tacrolimus	CYP3A4 inhibition; 2-fold increase in concentration of both agents. Potential for increased acute kidney injury, neurotoxicity, or QT interval prolongation	Reduce the dose of cyclosporine and tacrolimus by 50% if coadministration is necessary. Monitor both voriconazole and calcineurin inhibitor trough concentrations
Rifampin	Cyclosporine Tacrolimus	CYP3A4 induction; significantly decreased concentrations of both agents	Titrate cyclosporine and tacrolimus to goal trough concentrations. According to a review of the literature, doses of 2–5 times the normal value may be necessary

RASS = Richmond Agitation-Sedation Scale.

transporters.[69,70] Nonetheless, DDIs involving renal elimination pathways may have implications in patients who have renal impairment or who are receiving drugs with narrow therapeutic indices (i.e., methotrexate). Therapeutic drug monitoring and vigilance for detecting adverse drug events are warranted when a known renal transport inhibitor is used concomitantly with a renal transport substrate.

PHARMACODYNAMIC DDIS

Pharmacodynamic DDIs may occur in the ICU setting when two or more concomitant medications elicit a similar pharmacologic response. This additive or synergistic interplay may result in an exaggerated pharmacologic effect and possibly an adverse drug event. Several common examples are reviewed that may be observed by clinicians across a variety of ICU settings.

Serotonin Syndrome

Serotonin syndrome is a potentially serious adverse event that can result from excess serotonergic activity at central and peripheral serotonin-2A receptors. Symptoms develop rapidly within hours of medication administration and may include altered mental status, clonus (typically greater in the lower extremities), tremor, hyperthermia, diaphoresis, tachycardia, and mydriasis.[71-74]

The available literature on serotonin syndrome in the ICU is scarce and mostly limited to small case series and reviews.[71-74] Factors associated with a greater risk of serotonin syndrome include increased patient age, serotoninergic medication dosage, concomitant use of CYP inhibitors that can affect clearance of serotonergic medications, and renal or liver dysfunction.[71-74] Severe toxicity resulting in death has occurred with combinations of monoamine oxidase (MAO) inhibitors or amphetamines and SSRIs.[71-74] Table 46.10 highlights medications with clinically relevant serotonin-mediated effects.

A clinically relevant serotonergic DDI that can be seen in the ICU setting may occur with linezolid because it has weak reversible MAO-A and MAO-B inhibitory effects. The incidence of serotonin syndrome with concomitant linezolid and serotonergic agents is 0.24%–4% (e.g., SSRIs and serotonin-norepinephrine reuptake inhibitors [SNRIs]).[76] Linezolid should be avoided in patients taking concurrent SSRIs or SNRIs, if possible. If the serotonergic drug is to be discontinued, the physician must allow at least 5 half-lives of the parent drug and any active metabolites to clear before initiating linezolid, which may not be practical in the ICU setting.[76]

Targeted Treatment Strategies for Serotonergic Pharmacodynamic DDIs

Although serotonin syndrome is uncommon, it has the potential to complicate the administration of drugs commonly used in the ICU setting. When prescribing a serotonergic agent, it is important to obtain a clear history of the other drugs or herbal agents the patient has recently taken or recently discontinued. Life-threatening cases of serotonin syndrome may occur with the use of an irreversible

Table 46.7 Drug Interactions Involving CYP2C9 and CYP2C19[40,47-51]

Inhibitors/Inducers	Drug	Mechanism	Management
Phenytoin	Voriconazole	Phenytoin decreased the Cmax and AUC of voriconazole by 50% and 70%, respectively. A similar increase was observed in phenytoin concentrations owing to inhibition of CYP2C9 by voriconazole	Monitor voriconazole and phenytoin plasma concentrations. The maintenance dose of voriconazole should be increased from 4 mg/kg to 5 mg/kg IV every 12 hr or from 200 mg to 400 mg orally every 12 hr
Dexamethasone	Phenytoin[62,63]	A case report of phenytoin concentration showed an increase of almost 300% after dexamethasone was discontinued.	Monitor phenytoin concentrations, particularly on initiation and discontinuance of dexamethasone. Higher dose of dexamethasone may be needed if vasogenic cerebral edema is worsening with coadministration
		Phenytoin increases the metabolic clearance of corticosteroids; the extent depends on the dose and corticosteroid involved (dexamethasone > methylprednisolone, prednisolone > hydrocortisone)	
Fluconazole	Warfarin[64-67]	The S-enantiomer is metabolized by CYP2C9 and is 4–8 times more potent than the R-enantiomer (CYP3A4). Increased INR and warfarin concentrations; onset: 2–3 days and offset: 7–10 days	Monitor and titrate to a therapeutic goal INR
Metronidazole		Increased INR and warfarin concentrations; onset: 3–5 days and offset: 2 days	
Sulfamethoxazole		Increased INR and warfarin concentrations; onset: 2–5 days and offset: 2–14 days	
Amiodarone		Inhibited by amiodarone or its active metabolite, desethylamiodarone	

Table 46.8 Drug Interactions Involving CYP1A2

Inhibitors/Inducers	Drug	Mechanism	Management
Ciprofloxacin	Tizanidine[68]	CYP1A2 inhibition; increased peak concentrations of tizanidine 7-fold with resultant toxicity	Use an alternative antimicrobial

MAO inhibitor or with combinations of high dosages of serotonergic medications. In the example discussed, if linezolid and a serotonergic agent require concomitant administration and the benefits seem to outweigh any risks, clinicians should consider avoiding initiation of any additional serotonergic agents to the patient's medication regimen. It is then important to monitor for signs and symptoms of serotonin syndrome and to discontinue linezolid and other serotonergic agents if signs or symptoms develop.

Prolonged QT Interval Syndromes

Prolongation of the QT interval can predispose patients to a life-threatening polymorphic ventricular tachycardia called torsades de pointes (TdP).[77] A threshold of QTc interval prolongation at which TdP is certain to occur is not well defined. To highlight this point, a prospective, observational study of patients admitted to a cardiac critical care unit showed that 28% (n=251 of 900) of patients had a prolonged QT interval on admission, and 35% of these patients were administered a QT interval–prolonging medication during their ICU stay. Torsades de pointes did not occur throughout this study; the most common QT interval–prolonging medications administered were amiodarone, macrolides, and fluoroquinolones.[78]

Risk factors associated with a greater risk of QTc interval prolongation include age older than 65 years, female sex, hypokalemia, hypomagnesaemia, left ventricular systolic dysfunction, bradycardia, elevated plasma concentrations of QT interval–prolonging medications because of either a DDI or the absence of dose adjustment in the presence of organ dysfunction, and a history of QT interval prolongation.[77,79]

Drugs with the potential to precipitate TdP inhibit the rapid component of the delayed rectifier potassium current (IKr), which results in a reduction in the net repolarizing current and causes a prolongation of the ventricular action potential duration and a prolongation of the QT interval on the electrocardiogram (ECG).[77,79] Medications known to prolong the QT interval include class IA and III antiarrhythmic agents, tyrosine kinase inhibitors, macrolides, fluoroquinolones, azole antifungals, prokinetic agents, antipsychotics, TCAs, antidepressants, methadone, serotonin-3 antagonists, and certain nonsedating antihistamines.[79-81] However, not all QT interval–prolonging drugs (i.e., amiodarone) are associated with a risk of TdP. The low risk of TdP with amiodarone may be a result of minimized QTc dispersion, decreased early-after depolarization, and homogeneous prolongation of the action potential duration in all layers of the myocardial wall.[82,83] Ranolazine is another example of a medication that may prolong the QTc interval but not precipitate TdP, probably through inhibition of late sodium currents.[81]

Targeted Treatment Strategies to Minimize Adverse Events from QT Interval–Prolonging Medication

A thorough understanding of the risk factors for TdP and common medications that can prolong the QT interval is of paramount importance for all ICU clinicians. Care in understanding the influences of organ dysfunction and DDIs on prescribed medications is critical when these drugs are used in the ICU setting. If an identified DDI cannot be avoided, clinicians should obtain a baseline ECG and continue to monitor the effects of the drug combination with follow-up ECGs as necessary. The risk-benefit must be weighed and the patient evaluated for the potential of developing an arrhythmia when a decision is made to use QT interval–prolonging medications. Table 46.11 describes the most commonly encountered medication classes associated with QT interval prolongation and some possible management strategies.

Table 46.9 Drugs That Undergo Active Tubular Secretion[69,70]

Transporter	Substrate	Inhibitors
OAT1	Acyclovir	Furosemide
	Adefovir, cidofovir	Probenecid
	Methotrexate	
	Oseltamivir	
	Pravastatin	
OAT3	Cidofovir	Bumetanide
	Famotidine, ranitidine	Furosemide
	Oseltamivir	Probenecid
	Pravastatin	
	Valacyclovir	
OCT2	Amiodarone, dofetilide, procainamide	Cobicistat
	Cisplatin	Dolutegravir
	Digoxin	Quinolones
	Diltiazem, verapamil	Rilpivirine
	Levofloxacin	Ritonavir
	Metformin	Trimethoprim

Table 46.10 Medications with Clinically Relevant Serotonin-Mediated Effects[71-75]

Inhibitors of Serotonin Metabolism	Blockers of Serotonin Reuptake	Serotonin Precursors or Agonists	Enhancers of Serotonin Release	Drug Interactions Associated with Severe Serotonin Syndrome
Linezolid	Cocaine	LSD	Amphetamines	SSRIs + MAOIs
Methylene blue	Citalopram		Buspirone	Paroxetine + buspirone
MAOIs (e.g., isocarboxazid, tranylcypromine)	Clomipramine		Cocaine	Linezolid + citalopram
	Escitalopram		Lithium	Tramadol + venlafaxine + mirtazapine
	Fluoxetine		Mirtazapine	
	Fluvoxamine		Tramadol	
	Imipramine			
	Paroxetine			
	Phenylpiperidine opioids			
	Dextromethorphan			
	Fentanyl			
	Meperidine			
	Methadone			
	Tramadol			
	Sertraline			
	Venlafaxine			
	Ziprasidone			

MAOI = monoamine oxidase inhibitor.

Increased Risk of Bleeding

All anticoagulant and antiplatelet agents must be used cautiously in the ICU setting. Risk factors associated with an increased risk of bleeding include age older than 65 years, systolic blood pressure readings greater than 160 mm Hg, abnormal renal or liver function, previous stroke, a bleeding history, labile international normalized ratio (INR), use of antiplatelet agents or nonsteroidal anti-inflammatory drugs (NSAIDs), and recent alcohol use. Medications that can increase a patient's bleeding risk include any anticoagulant, P_2Y_{12} inhibitors, glycoprotein IIb-IIIa inhibitors, aspirin, NSAIDs, cilostazol, dipyridamole, tissue plasminogen activator, corticosteroids, and SSRIs.[84-86]

The SSRIs, and to a lesser extent the SNRIs, have been associated with an increased risk of GI bleeding, especially when used in combination with NSAIDs.[87-89] The proposed mechanism is by the blockade of platelet serotonin reuptake, leading to platelet serotonin depletion and impaired platelet aggregation. In addition, animal studies have shown a dose-dependent increase in gastric acid secretion with the administration of paroxetine, sertraline, and fluoxetine, which may increase aggressive factors that can lead to GI tract damage and hemorrhage.[86-89]

Furthermore, fluoxetine, fluvoxamine, and paroxetine inhibit several hepatic CYP enzymes (i.e., 1A2, 2D6, 3A4, and 2C9) and can significantly increase the serum concentrations of concomitant medications that may be associated with a bleeding risk (e.g., warfarin).[87-89] Because of the potential compounded platelet dysfunction associated with SSRIs or SNRIs, it is recommended to discontinue these agents in patients admitted to the ICU with GI bleeds; monitoring for SSRI or SNRI withdrawal is prudent during this time.[8]

Use of the target-specific oral anticoagulants (TOACs) with antiplatelet agents is another area for potential concern.[84] Published data are insufficient to guide clinical practice, and there is an element of uncertainty on how to safely use TOACs in combination with antiplatelet agents. It is highly recommended to formally assess the event and bleeding risk using the CHA2DS2-VASc and HAS-BLED scores, respectively.[85,86] Table 46.12 delineates the risk associated with the combination of TOACs and antiplatelet agents according to the available literature.

Targeted Treatment Strategies to Minimize Bleeding Risk in the ICU Setting

Bleeding diathesis can have a significant impact in the care of critically ill patients. Clinicians need to be cognizant of

Table 46.11 Management Strategies to Reduce the Risk of Torsades de Pointes[77,79-81]

General management strategies to prevent drug-induced TdP

1. Obtain a baseline ECG before initiation
2. Manually measure and calculate the QTc interval
3. Maintain serum potassium and magnesium concentrations within the normal range
4. Adjust doses of QT interval–prolonging drugs that rely on renal elimination or hepatic metabolism
5. Reduce dose or discontinue QT interval–prolonging drug if the QT interval increases > 60 msec from pretreatment value
6. Avoid concomitant administration of QT interval–prolonging drugs or CYP-mediated inhibition of these drugs
7. Discontinue QT interval–prolonging drugs if the QTc is > 500 msec

Specific drug classes that can prolong the QT interval	
Fluoroquinolones	Inhibition of potassium channels varies in potency among the listed agents (moxifloxacin > levofloxacin > ciprofloxacin)
	Overall, the risk of TdP is lowest with ciprofloxacin
Macrolides	Inhibition of potassium channels and strong inhibition of CYP3A4 metabolism with erythromycin or clarithromycin
	Lower risk of TdP with azithromycin than with erythromycin or clarithromycin
Antipsychotics	Ziprasidone, thioridazine, and haloperidol have the greatest potential for prolonging the QT interval, followed by risperidone, paliperidone, clozapine, olanzapine, quetiapine, and aripiprazole
Anti-nausea	QT interval prolongation of ondansetron is dose-dependent
	Single IV doses should not exceed 16 mg. Subsequent IV doses must not exceed 8 mg and must be given 4–8 hr after the initial dose. All IV doses must be infused over at least 15 min
Antifungals	QT interval prolongation may occur because of either a pharmacodynamic drug-drug interaction with other QT interval–prolonging drugs or a strong inhibition of CYP3A4 metabolism of the azole antifungal agents
	Compared with posaconazole and voriconazole, fluconazole has less risk of inducing TdP

TdP = torsades de pointes.

---

the role of each anticoagulant and antiplatelet agent used and how coadministration may positively or negatively affect clinical outcomes. Concomitant administration of these agents may be warranted, especially in the context of patients who have several disease states that may include the arterial and venous vascular systems. Prescribers need to be vigilant in monitoring for evidence of clinical efficacy as well as toxicity when these agents are used clinically. Continuously evaluating the need for coadministration, assessing for DDIs with the addition of any new medications, and providing good patient communication and follow-up are key elements for the safe use of these medication classes.

DRUG-NUTRIENT INTERACTIONS

Drug-nutrient interactions can negatively affect the care of a critically ill patient. Critical care clinicians can prevent possible complications, improve patient outcomes, and decrease cost simply by recognizing the severity and relevance of potential drug-nutrient interactions or interactions of medications with alimentary tract access devices. Several factors must be considered when analyzing for drug-nutrient interactions. First, various nutritional elements may interact with the drug and render the agent inactive or with altered efficacy. Second, the location of the enteral feeding tube may affect the absorption of a given medication. Finally, the different medication formulations and release mechanisms available add to the complexity of drug administration through the available feeding tube.[8,95] Table 46.13 describes several common interactions between select medications and enteral nutrition and possible actions that may minimize this effect.

Targeted Treatment Strategies to Minimize Drug-Nutrient Interactions

The management of drug-nutrient interactions must be individualized according to the drug, the patient's underlying medical conditions, the availability of alternative treatment options, and the feasibility of the intervention according to the clinical setting. The plan must be communicated with all health care providers involved in the care of the patient and may be subject to change, depending on the patient's clinical response. If enteral nutrition is held for the administration of a medication, the rate of enteral feeds must be adjusted to maintain the same 24-hour volume and administered calories. In addition, the total volume of flushes needs to be monitored and considered when assessing fluid intake and volume status.

EVALUATING THE PRESENCE OF DRUG INTERACTIONS AND DETERMINING THE CLINICAL SIGNIFICANCE

There are few controlled DDI clinical studies, and significant variability is reported among individual cases.[100-103] Databases such as Micromedex, LexiComp, Clinical

continued on page 946

Table 46.12 Bleeding Risk Associated with TOACs in Combination with Antiplatelet Agents[90-94]

Anticoagulant	Trial	TOAC + Antiplatelet Agent	Safety End Point
Dabigatran	RE-DEEM[90] Dabigatran 50–150 mg BID + ASA + clopidogrel	99% received dual antiplatelet therapy	The combination increased the rates of the primary composite outcome of major bleeding or clinically relevant minor bleeding with doses greater than 75 mg of dabigatran (7.8% vs. 2.2%, p≤0.001). Most commonly reported bleeding events with dabigatran doses > 75 mg were GI bleeding and epistaxis compared with placebo
Rivaroxaban	ATLAS ACS-TIMI 46[91] Rivaroxaban total daily dose of 5–20 mg either daily or BID + ASA or ASA + clopidogrel	22% received ASA monotherapy 78% received dual antiplatelet therapy	Increased the rates of TIMI major bleeding not related to CABG (2.2% vs. 0.6%, p≤0.001) and ICH (0.6% vs. 0.1%, p=0.015) No significant increase in fatal bleeding (0.2% vs. 0.1%, p=0.51)
	ATLAS ACS2-TIMI 51[92] Rivaroxaban 2.5–5 mg BID + ASA + clopidogrel	93% received dual antiplatelet therapy	Combination therapy with both rivaroxaban doses significantly increased the rate of TIMI major bleeding (2.1% vs. 0.6%, p≤0.001), as well as minor bleeding, bleeding requiring medical attention, and ICH (0.6% vs. 0.2%, p=0.009
Apixaban	APPRAISE[93] Apixaban 2.5–10 mg BID + ASA or ASA + clopidogrel	76% received dual antiplatelet therapy	Note: 10 mg BID + 20 mg daily arms were terminated early because of excessive bleeding The combination increased the rates of the primary composite outcome of major bleeding or clinically relevant minor bleeding with a total daily dose of apixaban 10 mg (5.6% vs. 0.8%, p=0.005) The most common types of bleeding were subcutaneous bruising and hematomas, epistaxis and gingival bleeding, hematuria, and GI bleeding. When major bleeding and reduction in ischemic events were considered, apixaban 10 mg daily resulted in an absolute net reduction of 1.6% in clinical events in the overall population. Therefore, apixaban 10 mg was reevaluated in the APPRAISE-2 trial
	APPRAISE-2[94] Apixaban 5 mg BID + ASA + clopidogrel or ASA	81% received dual antiplatelet therapy	Trial was terminated early because of excessive bleeding Combination therapy significantly increased TIMI major bleeding (2.4% vs. 0.9%, p≤0.001) and ICH (0.6% vs. 0.2%, p=0.03) No significant difference in net clinical outcome (CVD, death, MI, stroke, and fatal bleeding) in adding apixaban to regimen of patients on dual antiplatelet therapy (p=0.80)

ASA = aspirin; CVD = cardiovascular disease; ICH = intracranial hemorrhage; MI = myocardial infarction; TIMI = thrombolysis in myocardial infarction.

Table 46.13 Clinically Relevant Drug-Nutrient Interactions in the ICU[95-99]

Medication	Mechanism	Action
Carbamazepine	Adheres to polyvinyl chloride walls of feeding tubes	Dilute the suspension with equal amounts of sterile water or 0.9% sodium chloride injection
Fluoroquinolones (ciprofloxacin and levofloxacin)	Chelation of fluoroquinolones with the calcium, aluminum, magnesium, and zinc found in enteral nutrition results in decreased absorption. Absorption may also be decreased if administered by a jejunostomy tube	For severe infections, administer the fluoroquinolone intravenously. For mild to moderate infections or for prophylaxis: Hold enteral nutrition for 1 hr before and 2 hr after medication administration. Flush enteral feeding tube with 20 mL of water before and after medication administration. If the jejunostomy tube is the only enteral route available, consider administering the fluoroquinolone intravenously
Cyclosporine, tacrolimus	Grapefruit juice inhibits intestinal CYP3A4 and P-gp	Avoid grapefruit juice. Monitor concentrations of each respective medication
Diazepam solution	Adheres to polyvinyl chloride walls of feeding tubes	Avoid solution. Crush tablets or administer intravenously
Digoxin[99]	Poorly absorbed in presence of enteral feeding formulas that contain fiber. The largest reported change in plasma digoxin caused by the addition of 10–22 g of dietary fiber is < 15%	May not be clinically significant. Monitor concentrations, if warranted
Levodopa	Amino acids may compete with levodopa for absorption in the small intestine. Effects observed with protein intake > 1 g/kg/day	Enteral nutrition should be held for 2 hr before and after levodopa administration. Flush enteral feeding tube with 20 mL of water before and after medication administration. Monitor patients for Neuroleptic Malignant Syndrome (NMS)-like signs or symptoms or changes in Parkinson disease signs or symptoms
Levothyroxine	Coadministration with enteral nutrition may decrease absorption. May adhere to polyvinyl chloride walls of feeding tubes	Enteral nutrition should be held for 1–2 hr before and after levothyroxine administration. Flush enteral feeding tube with 20 mL of water before and after medication administration. Monitor thyroid function tests as needed
Phenytoin	Binds to protein calcium caseinates. May adhere to polyvinyl chloride or polyurethane walls of feeding tubes	Enteral nutrition should be held for 1–2 hr before and after phenytoin administration. Flush enteral feeding tube with 20 mL of water before and after medication administration. Monitor plasma concentrations as needed. If the nasogastric tube is the only available option and therapeutic plasma concentrations are not attained with holding enteral nutrition around medication dosing, can administer phenytoin sodium IV (diluted in normal saline) by the enteral feeding tube; phenytoin sodium IV has a pH of 11 and may avoid pH-dependent loss of drug to the polyurethane feeding tubing

Table 46.13 Clinically Relevant Drug-Nutrient Interactions in the ICU[95-99] (continued)

Medication	Mechanism	Action
Tetracyclines (e.g., minocycline)	Absorption is decreased by chelation with calcium in enteral nutrition formulas	Enteral nutrition should be held for 1–2 hr before and after minocycline administration
		Flush enteral feeding tube with 20 mL of water before and after medication administration
Warfarin	Current enteral nutrition formulations have minimal amounts of vitamin K; interaction with warfarin is minimal	Enteral nutrition should be held for 1 hr before and after warfarin administration
		Flush enteral feeding tube with 20 mL of water before and after medication administration
	Hydrolyzed proteins in enteral nutrition formulas may bind to warfarin and decrease its bioavailability	Monitor INR, and adjust the warfarin dose accordingly

continued from page 944

Pharmacology, Facts and Comparisons eAnswers, and Drug Interactions: Analysis and Management can assist in identifying DDIs. However, each of these drug databases uses different approaches to identify and evaluate the same body of literature. For instance, Micromedex uses a 5-item rating scale (i.e., major, moderate, minor, none, and not specified) to classify the severity of DDIs.[103] Drug Interactions: Analysis and Management uses a 5-item summary known as the ORCA (Operational Classification) system. The ORCA system is based on the severity of the interaction and the net benefit of administering the drug pair; ratings include avoid the combination, usually avoid the combination, minimize risk, no action needed, and no interaction.[104] Sometimes little agreement is found among these drug databases for what may be considered a serious and clinically relevant DDI. The overshadowing issue with these databases is that they are simply reporting DDIs that can occur.[101-103] This is a reflection of DDIs that are included in the U.S. Food and Drug Administration–approved product labeling; classification of DDIs by therapeutic class rather than by individual agent and blanket inclusion of all drug formulations.[102,103] From the prescriber's perspective, if these drug databases are linked to a computer prescriber order entry system, too many alerts to fire may be caused that prescribers may consider clinically irrelevant and may result in alert fatigue and oversight of clinically significant alerts.

Because this has become a growing and recognized problem, an expert workgroup funded by the Agency for Healthcare Research and Quality has developed guidelines for the systemic appraisal of DDIs and recommended principles for including and presenting DDIs into clinical decision support systems.[100] These guidelines define a clinically relevant DDI as one that is associated with either toxicity or loss of efficacy and that warrants the attention of health care professionals. The primary goal of the evidence workgroup in this consensus guideline is to identify the best approach for evaluating whether a DDI truly exists.[100] It is acknowledged that the evidence supporting a DDI may be derived from case reports or retrospective reviews or extrapolated from in vitro studies and a few controlled clinical studies. A standard approach is recommended in these guidelines in order to evaluate case reports; thus, the Drug Interaction Probability Scale (DIPS) and the Drug Interaction Evidence Evaluation (DRIVE) instrument were created to be used for a given body of literature.[100,105] The DIPS is a 10-item scale that was designed to assess the probability of a causal relationship between an event observed in a patient and a potential DDI.[105] The total score is used to estimate the probability that the observed event is causally related to the medications. Probability is assigned as doubtful, possible, probable, or highly probable. The DRIVE instrument establishes the existence of a DDI through the following methods: uses simple evidence categories, includes causality assessment with DDI case reports (by DIPS), applies reasonable extrapolation from the existing data, addresses evidence or statements provided in product labeling, and describes study quality criteria and interpretation in the context of DDIs.[100] If the evidence of a DDI has been appropriately analyzed using the DIPS and DRIVE instruments, clinicians must then determine the clinical relevance. The factors to consider include the clinical consequences to the patient, the incidence at which the DDI occurs, any risk factors or mitigating factors that determine the susceptibility to the DDI, and an assessment of the seriousness of the DDI.[100,102] This process seems methodologically sound; however, the DRIVE instrument must be formally evaluated and validated before used in the large drug databases previously discussed.

In addition, drugs that belong to the same pharmacologic class should be treated individually unless proven otherwise. Most class-based DDIs are pharmacodynamic in nature, whereas pharmacokinetic interactions can rarely be generalized and applied to all agents within a drug class.[100,102] Even if the DDI was classified as a class effect, the magnitude of the effect may vary among each agent. A primary example of this point is that azoles have different potencies for the inhibition of the CYP3A4 enzyme. For instance, itraconazole causes a 27-fold increase in the AUC of triazolam, and fluconazole causes a 4.4-fold increase in the AUC of triazolam; both are clinically relevant, but the magnitudes are very different. Therefore, the evidence workgroup recommends that, in the absence of drug-specific data, a class-based interaction be reasonably assumed if the mechanism of interaction is consistent with the known pharmacology of one or both drug classes involved.[100,102]

Additional work is needed to recognize, determine the significance of, and monitor clinically relevant DDIs. It is the responsibility of every clinician to be vigilant in identifying DDIs. Each member of the multidisciplinary team has a role in the prevention, identification, and resolution of DDIs in order to optimize patient care and ensure safe medication administration. Physicians should justify and review each drug regularly, screen for DDIs with each drug addition or deletion, and integrate the information that is discussed on multidisciplinary rounds.[8] Pharmacists should review each medication order for DDIs, assist in drug selection or substitution, and monitor for any adverse drug events.[8] Nurses should assess and monitor drug administration and document any adverse drug events or change in patient status.[8] The health system multidisciplinary team should work together to regularly reevaluate and update the list of DDIs identified within its clinical decision support system to remain current with the evolving scientific literature.

CONCLUSION

There are several factors to consider when identifying and determining the clinical significance of DDIs. Micromedex, LexiComp, Clinical Pharmacology, Facts and Comparisons eAnswers, and Drug Interactions: Analysis and Management can assist clinicians in identifying DDIs. The severity ratings may vary among these databases, and the clinical significance of the ratings used has not been fully established. The DDI alerting systems in every institution vary according to what is commonly observed as significant to that specific institution. Internal expert opinion and one of the mentioned drug information databases are commonly used to build an institution's electronic DDI alerting system. Once an internal identification system has been determined, a clinician's evaluation of an identified DDI should include understanding the mechanism and onset of the DDI, possible patient outcomes, and clinically appropriate alternative therapeutic options. This rationale and thought process may aid in the decision to either avoid or monitor a drug combination that is tailored to the pharmacotherapeutic need of an individual patient.

REFERENCES

1. Rivkin A. Admissions to a medical intensive care unit related to adverse drug reactions. Am J Health Syst Pharm 2007;64:1840-3.
2. Smithburger PL, Kane-Gill SL, Seybert AL. Drug-drug interactions in cardiac and cardiothoracic intensive care units. Drug Saf 2010;33:879-88.
3. Smithburger PL, Kane-Gill SL, Seybert AL. Drug-drug interactions in the medical intensive care unit: an assessment of frequency, severity and the medications involved. Int J Pharm Pract 2012;20:402-8.
4. Lima REF, Cassiani SHB. Potential drug interactions in intensive care patients at a teaching hospital. Rev Lat Am Enfermagem 2009;17:222-7.
5. Askari M, Eslami S, Louws M, et al. Frequency and nature of drug-drug interactions in the intensive care unit. Pharmacoepidemiol Drug Saf 2013;22:430-7.
6. Uijtendaal EV, Harssel LM, Hugenholtz GW, et al. Analysis of potential drug-drug interactions in medical intensive care unit patients. Pharmacotherapy 2014;34:213-9.
7. Roberts DJ, Hall RI. Drug absorption, distribution, metabolism and excretion considerations in critically ill adults. Expert Opin Drug Metab Toxicol 2013;9:1067-84.
8. Papadopoulos J, Smithburger PL. Common drug interactions leading to adverse drug events in the intensive care unit: management and pharmacokinetic considerations. Crit Care Med 2010;38(6 suppl):S126-35.
9. Nguyen NQ, Ng MP, Chapman M, et al. The impact of admission diagnosis on gastric emptying in critically ill patients. Crit Care 2007;11:R16.
10. Zhou SF. Structure, function and regulation of P-glycoprotein and its clinical relevance in drug disposition. Xenobiotica 2008;38:802-32.
11. Fernandez C, Buyse M, German-Fattal M, et al. Influence of the pro-inflammatory cytokines on P-glycoprotein expression and functionality. J Pharm Pharm Sci 2004;7:359-71.
12. Khanlou H, Farthing C. Co-administration of atazanavir with proton pump inhibitors and H2 blockers. J Acquir Immune Defic Syndr 2005;39:503.
13. Kofler S, Shvets N, Bigdeli AK, et al. Proton pump inhibitors reduce mycophenolate exposure in heart transplant recipients – a prospective case-controlled study. Am J Transplant 2009;9:1650-6.
14. Kees MG, Steinke T, Moritz S, et al. Omeprazole impairs the absorption of mycophenolate mofetil but not of enteric-coated mycophenolate sodium in healthy volunteers. J Clin Pharmacol 2012;52:1265-72.
15. NOXAFIL (posaconazole) oral suspension [product information]. Kenilworth, NJ: Schering, December 2008.
16. Kraft WK, Chang PS, Van Iersel M, et al. Posaconazole tablet pharmacokinetics: lack of effect of concomitant medications altering gastric pH and gastric motility in healthy subjects. Antimicrob Agents Chemother 2014;58:4020-5.
17. EDURANT (rilpivirine) oral tablets [product information]. Raritan, NJ: Tibotec Therapeutics, April 2011.
18. Wadhwa NK, Schroeder TJ, O'Flaherty E, et al. The effect of oral metoclopramide on the absorption of cyclosporine. Transplant Proc 1987;43:211-3.

19. Frost RW, Lasseter KC, Noe AJ, et al. Effects of aluminum hydroxide and calcium carbonate antacids on the bioavailability of ciprofloxacin. Antimicrob Agents Chemother 1992;36:830-2.

20. Li RC, Nix DE, Schentag JJ. Interaction between ciprofloxacin and metal cations: its influence on physicochemical characteristics and antibacterial activity. Pharm Res 1994;11:917-20.

21. Nix DE, Watson WA, Lener ME, et al. Effects of aluminum and magnesium antacids and ranitidine on the absorption of ciprofloxacin. Clin Pharmacol Ther 1989;46:700-5.

22. Nguyen VX, Nix DE, Gillikin S, et al. Effect of oral antacid administration on the pharmacokinetics of intravenous doxycycline. Antimicrob Agents Chemother 1989;33:434-6.

23. Harmon SM, Seifert CF. Levothyroxine cholestyramine interaction reemphasized. Ann Intern Med 1991;115:658-9.

24. Neuvonen PJ, Kivisto K, Hirvisalo EL. Effects of resins and activated charcoal on the absorption of digoxin, carbamazepine and furosemide. Br J Clin Pharmacol 1988;25:229-33.

25. Robinson DS, Benjamin DM, McCormick JJ. Interaction of warfarin and nonsystemic gastrointestinal drugs. Clin Pharmacol Ther 1971;12:491-5.

26. Spriet I, Goyens J, Meersseman W, et al. Interaction between valproate and meropenem: a retrospective study. Ann Pharmacother 2007;41:1130-6.

27. Tobin JK, Golightly LK, Kick SD, et al. Valproic acid-carbapenem interaction: report of six cases and a review of the literature. Drug Metabol Drug Interact 2009;24:153-82.

28. Mancl EE, Gidal BE. The effect of carbapenem antibiotics on plasma concentrations of valproic acid. Ann Pharmacother 2009;43:2082-7.

29. Ludden TM. Pharmacokinetic interactions of the macrolide antibiotics. Clin Pharmacokinet 1985;10:63-79.

30. Lindenbaum J, Rund DG, Butler VP, et al. Inactivation of digoxin by the gut flora: reversal by antibiotic therapy. N Engl J Med 1981;305:789-94.

31. Dobkin JF, Saha JR, Butler VP, et al. Inactivation of digoxin by Eubacterium lentum, an anaerobe of the human gut flora. Trans Assoc Am Physicians 1982;95:22-9.

32. Rund DG, Lindenbaum J, Butler VP, et al. Decreased digoxin cardioinactive-reduced metabolites after administration as an encapsulated liquid concentrate. Clin Pharmacol Ther 1983;34:738-43.

33. Baillargeon J, Holmes HM, Lin YL, et al. Concurrent use of warfarin and antibiotics and the risk of bleeding in older adults. Am J Med 2012;125:183-9.

34. Kawamoto K, Uchida K. Effect of N-methyltetrazolethiol on liver microsomal vitamin K reductase. Jpn J Pharmacol 1989;50:159-65.

35. Morgan ET. Regulation of cytochrome p450 by inflammatory mediators: why and how? Drug Metab Dispos 2001;29:207-12.

36. Thiebaut F, Tsuruo T, Hamada H, et al. Cellular localization of the multidrug resistance gene product P-glycoprotein in normal human tissues. Proc Natl Acad Sci USA 1987;84:7735-8.

37. Konig J, Muller F, Fromm MF. Transporters and drug-drug interactions: important determinants of drug disposition and effects. Pharmacol Rev 2013;65:944-66.

38. Lee CA, Cook JA, Reyner EL, et al. P-glycoprotein related drug interactions: clinical importance and a consideration of disease states. Expert Opin Drug Metab Toxicol 2010;6:603-19.

39. PL Detail-Document, P-glycoprotein Drug Interactions. Pharmacist's Letter/Prescriber's Letter. October 2013.4

40. U.S. Food and Drug Administration (FDA). Drug Development and Drug Interactions: Table of Substrates, Inhibitors and Inducers. October 27, 2014. Available at www.fda.gov/Drugs/DevelopmentApprovalProcess/DevelopmentResources/DrugInteractionsLabeling/ucm093664.htm.

41. Neuhoff S, Yeo KR, Barter Z, et al. Application of permeability-limited physiologically-based pharmacokinetic models: part I-digoxin pharmacokinetics incorporating P-glycoprotein-mediated efflux. J Pharm Sci 2013;102:3145-60.

42. Hellwig T, Gulseth M. Pharmacokinetic and pharmacodynamic drug interactions with new oral anticoagulants: what do they mean for patients with atrial fibrillation? Ann Pharmacother 2013;47:1478-87.

43. Heidbuchel H, Verhamme P, Alings M, et al. EHRA practical guide on the use of new oral anticoagulants in patients with non-valvular atrial fibrillation: executive summary. Eur Heart J 2013;34:2094-106.

44. Egle H, Tritler R, Kummerer K, et al. Linezolid and rifampin: drug interaction contrary to expectations? Clin Pharmacol Ther 2005;77:451-3.

45. Gebhart BC, Barker BC, Markewitz BA. Decreased serum linezolid levels in a critically ill patient receiving concomitant linezolid and rifampin. Pharmacotherapy 2007;27:476-9.

46. Sansom LN, Evans AM. What is the true clinical significance of plasma protein binding displacement interactions? Drug Saf 1995;12:227-33.

47. Mann HJ. Drug-associated disease: cytochrome P450 interactions. Crit Care Clin 2006;22:329-45.

48. Doring B, Petzinger E. Phase 0 and phase III transport in various organs: combined concept of phases in xenobiotic transport and metabolism. Drug Metab Rev 2014;46:261-82.

49. Michalets EL. Update: clinically significant cytochrome P-450 drug interactions. Pharmacotherapy 1998;18:84-112.

50. PL Detail-Document. Cytochrome P450 drug interactions. Pharmacist's Letter/Prescriber's Letter. October 2013.

51. Spriet I, Meersseman W, de Hoon J, et al. Mini-series: II. Clinical aspects. Clinically relevant CYP450-mediated drug interactions in the ICU. Intensive Care Med 2009;35:603-12.

52. Morgan ET. Impact of infectious and inflammatory disease on cytochrome P450-mediated drug metabolism and pharmacokinetics. Clin Pharmacol Ther 2009;85:434-8.

53. Renton KW. Cytochrome P450 regulation and drug biotransformation during inflammation and infection. Curr Drug Metab 2004;5:235-43.

54. Elkahwaji J, Robin MA, Berson A, et al. Decrease in hepatic cytochrome P450 after interleukin-2 immunotherapy. Biochem Pharmacol 1999;57:951-4.

55. Frye RF, Schneider VM, Frye CS, et al. Plasma levels of TNF-alpha and IL-6 are inversely related to cytochrome P450-dependent drug metabolism in patients with congestive heart failure. J Card Fail 2002;8:315-9.

56. Chen YL, Le Vraux V, Leneveu A, et al. Acute-phase response, interleukin-6, and alteration of cyclosporine pharmacokinetics. Clin Pharmacol Ther 1994;55:649-60.

57. Knupfer H, Schmidt R, Stanitz D, et al. CYP2C and IL-6 expression in breast cancer. Breast 2004;13:28-34.

58. Lee JK, Zhang L, Men AY, et al. CYP-mediated therapeutic protein-drug interactions clinical findings, proposed mechanisms and regulatory implications. Clin Pharmacokinet 2010;49:295-310.

59. Kalsotra A, Turman CM, Dash PK, et al. Differential effects of traumatic brain injury on the cytochrome p450 system: a perspective into hepatic and renal drug metabolism. J Neurotrauma 2003;20:1339-50.

60. Zhou J, Poloyac SM. The effect of therapeutic hypothermia on drug metabolism and drug response: cellular mechanisms to organ function. Expert Opin Drug Metab Toxicol 2011;7:803-16.

61. Hirota T, Eguchi S, Leiri I. Impact of genetic polymorphisms in CYP2C9 and CYP2C19 on the pharmacokinetics of clinically used drugs. Drug Metab Pharmacokinet 2013;28:28-37.

62. Lackner TE. Interaction of dexamethasone with phenytoin. Pharmacotherapy 1991;11:344-7.

63. Renaudin J, Fewer D, Wilson CB, et al. Dose dependency of Decadron(R) in patients with partially excised brain tumors. J Neurosurg 1973;39:302-5.

64. Gericke KR. Possible interaction between warfarin and fluconazole. Pharmacotherapy 1993;13:508-9.

65. Kazmier FJ. A significant interaction between metronidazole and warfarin. Mayo Clin Proc 1976;51:782-4.

66. Cook DE, Ponte CD. Suspected trimethoprim/sulfamethoxazole-induced hypoprothrombinemia. J Fam Pract 1994;39:589-91.

67. Kurnik D, Loebstein R, Farfel Z, et al. Complex drug–drug–disease interactions between amiodarone, warfarin and the thyroid gland. Medicine 2004;83:107-13.

68. Granfors MT, Backman JT, Neuvonen M, et al. Ciprofloxacin greatly increases concentrations and hypotensive effect of tizanidine by inhibiting its cytochrome P450 1A2-mediated presystemic metabolism. Clin Pharmacol Ther 2004;76:598-606.

69. Lepist EL, Ray AS. Renal drug-drug interactions: what we have learned and where we are going. Expert Opin Drug Metab Toxicol 2012;8:433-48.

70. Feng B, LaPerle JL, Chang G, et al. Renal clearance in drug discovery and development: molecular descriptors, drug transporters and disease state. Expert Opin Drug Metab Toxicol 2010;6:939-52.

71. Pedavally S, Fugate JE, Rabinstein AA. Serotonin syndrome in the intensive care unit: clinical presentations and precipitating medications. Neurocrit Care 2014;21:108-13.

72. Edelstein CS, Tepper S, Shapiro RE. Drug-induced serotonin syndrome: a review. Expert Opin Drug Saf 2008;7:587-96.

73. Gillman PK. A review of serotonin toxicity data: implications for the mechanisms of antidepressant drug action. Biol Psychiatry 2006;59:1046-51.

74. Tepper SJ. Serotonin syndrome: SSRIs, SNRIs, triptans, and current clinical practice. Headache 2012;52:195-7.

75. Barann M, Stamer UM, Lyutenska M, et al. Effects of opioids on human serotonin transporters. Naunyn Schmiedebergs Arch Pharmacol 2015;388:43-9.

76. Ramsey TD, Lau TT, Ensom MH. Serotonergic and adrenergic drug interactions associated with linezolid: a critical review and practical management approach. Ann Pharmacother 2013;47:543-60.

77. Trinkley KE, Page RL, Lien H, et al. QT interval prolongation and the risk of torsades de pointes: essentials for clinicians. Curr Med Res Opin 2013;29:1719-26.

78. Tisdale JE, Wroblewski HA, Overholser BR, et al. Prevalence of QT interval prolongation in patients admitted to cardiac care units and frequency of subsequent administration of QT-interval prolonging drugs. Drug Saf 2012;35:459-70.

79. Owens RC Jr. Risk assessment for antimicrobial agent-induced QTc interval prolongation and torsades de pointes. Pharmacotherapy 2001;21:301-19.

80. Harris S, Hilligoss DM, Colangelo PM, et al. Azithromycin and terfenadine: lack of drug interaction. Clin Pharmacol Ther 1995;58:310-5.

81. Drew BJ, Ackerman MJ, Funk M, et al. Prevention of torsade de pointes in hospital Settings: a scientific statement from the American Heart Association and the American College of Cardiology foundation endorsed by the American Association of Critical-Care Nurses and the International Society for Computerized Electrocardiology. J Am Coll Cardiol 2010;55:934-47.

82. Lazzara R. Amiodarone and torsade de pointes. Ann Intern Med 1989;111:549-51.

83. Frommeyer G, Millberg P, Witte P, et al. A new mechanism preventing proarrhythmia in chronic heart failure: rapid phase-III repolarization explains the low proarrhythmic potential of amiodarone in contrast to sotalol in a model of pacing-induced heart failure. Eur J Heart Fail 2011;13:1060-9.

84. Ahren I, Bode C. Direct oral anticoagulants in acute coronary syndrome. Semin Hematol 2014;51:147-51.

85. De Caterina R, Husted S, Wallentin L, et al. New oral anticoagulants in atrial fibrillation and acute coronary syndromes: ESC Working Group on Thrombosis-Task Force on Anticoagulants in Heart Disease position paper. J Am Coll Cardiol 2012;59:1413-25.

86. aber U, Mastoris I, Mehran R. Balancing ischemia and bleeding risks with novel oral anticoagulants. Nat Rev Cardiol 2014;11:693-703.

87. de Abajo FJ, Garcia-Rodriguez LA. Risk of upper gastrointestinal tract bleeding associated with selective serotonin reuptake inhibitors and venlafaxine therapy: interaction with nonsteroidal anti-inflammatory drugs and effect of acid-suppressing agents. Arch Gen Psychiatry 2008;65:795-803.

88. Li H, Cheng Y, Ahi J, et al. Observational study of upper gastrointestinal tract bleeding events in patients taking duloxetine and nonsteroidal anti-inflammatory drugs: a case-control analysis. Drug Healthc Patient Saf 2014;6:167-74.

89. Andrade C, Sandarsh S, Chethan KB, et al. Serotonin reuptake inhibitor antidepressants and abnormal bleeding: a review for clinicians and a reconsideration of mechanisms. J Clin Psychiatry 2010;71:1565-75.

90. Oldgren J, Budaj A, Granger CB, et al. Dabigatran vs. placebo in patients with acute coronary syndromes on dual antiplatelet therapy: a randomized, double-blind, phase II trial. Eur Heart J 2011;32:2781-9.

91. Mega JL, Braunwald E, Mohanavelu S, et al. Rivaroxaban versus placebo in patients with acute coronary syndromes (ATLAS ACS-TIMI 46): a randomized, double-blind, phase II trial. Lancet 2009;374:29-38.

92. Gibson CM, Mega JL, Burton P, et al. Rationale and design of the anti-Xa therapy to lower cardiovascular events in addition to standard therapy in subjects with acute coronary syndrome-thrombolysis in myocardial infarction 51 (ATLAS-ACS 2 TIMI 51) trial: a randomized, double-blind, placebo-controlled study to evaluate the efficacy and safety of rivaroxaban in subjects with acute coronary syndrome. Am Heart J 2011;161:815-21.

93. Alexander JH, Becker RC, Bhatt DL, et al. Apixaban, an oral, direct, selective factor Xa inhibitor, in combination with antiplatelet therapy after acute coronary syndrome: results of the Apixaban for Prevention of Acute Ischemic and Safety Events (APPRAISE) trial. Circulation 2009;119:2877-85.

94. Alexander JH, Lopes RD, James S, et al.; for the APPRAISE 2 Investigators. Apixaban with antiplatelet therapy after acute coronary syndrome. N Engl J Med 2011;365:699-708.

95. Otles S, Senturk A. Food and drug interactions: a general review. Acta Sci Pol Technol Aliment 2014;13:89-102.

96. Penrod LE, Allen JB, Cabacungan LR. Warfarin resistance and enteral feedings: 2 case reports and a supporting in vitro study. Arch Phys Med Rehabil 2001;82:1270-1.

97. Heldt T, Loss SH. Drug-nutrient interactions in the intensive care unit: literature review and current recommendations. Rev Bras Ter Intensiva 2013;25:162-7.

98. Wohlt PD, Zheng L, Gunderson S, et al. Recommendations for the use of medications with continuous enteral nutrition. Am J Health Syst Pharm 2009;66:1458-67.

99. Johnson BF, Rodin SM, Hoch K, et al. The effect of dietary fiber on the bioavailability of digoxin in capsules. J Clin Pharmacol 1987;27:487-90.

100. Scheife RT, Hines LE, Boyce RD, et al. Consensus recommendations for systematic evaluation of drug-drug interaction evidence for clinical decision support. Drug Saf 2015;38:197-206.

101. Phansalkar S, Desai A, Choksi A, et al. Criteria for assessing high-priority drug-drug interactions for clinical decision support in electronic health records. J Am Med Inform Assoc 2012;19:735-43.

102. Smithburger PL, Buckley MS, Bejian S, et al. A critical evaluation of clinical decision support for the detection of drug-drug interactions. Expert Opin Drug Saf 2011;10:871-82.

103. Smithburger PL, Kane-Gill SL, Benedict NJ, et al. Grading the severity of drug-drug interactions in the intensive care unit: a comparison between clinician assessment and proprietary database severity rankings. Ann Pharmacother 2010;44:1718-24.

104. Hansten PD, Horn JR, Hazlet TK. ORCA: OpeRational ClassificAtion of drug interactions. J Am Pharm Assoc (Wash) 2001;41:161-5.

105. Horn JR, Hansten PD, Chan LN. Proposal for a new tool to evaluate drug interaction cases. Ann Pharmacother 2007;41:674-80.

Chapter 47: Acute Illness Scoring Systems

Thomas J. Johnson, Pharm.D., MBA, FASHP, FCCM, BCPS

LEARNING OBJECTIVES

1. Describe the utility of acute illness scoring systems in the critically ill.
2. List the common acute illness scoring systems.
3. Describe the application and benefits of each system.

ABBREVIATIONS IN THIS CHAPTER

AKIN	Acute Kidney Injury Network	MELD	Model for end-stage liver disease
APACHE	Acute Physiology and Chronic Health Evaluation	MODS	Multiple Organ Dysfunction Score
		MPM	Mortality probability model
APS	Acute Physiology Score	PSI	Pneumonia Severity Index
CURB-65	Confusion, urea, respiratory, blood pressure, 65 (age)	RIFLE	Risk, injury, failure, loss, and end-stage renal disease
GCS	Glasgow Coma Scale	SAPS	Simplified Acute Physiology Score
ICU	Intensive care unit	SOFA	Sequential Organ Failure Assessment
ISS	Injury Severity Score	TISS	Therapeutic Intervention Scoring System

INTRODUCTION

Many scoring systems are used in acute hospital settings and particularly in the critical care areas. Patients are admitted to intensive care units (ICUs) with a variety of primary diagnoses, and each patient presents with his or her own set of underlying conditions. Furthermore, the type and acuity of patients in a particular ICU is affected by the organization of the hospital, the patient population of that hospital or area, and the types of physicians and subspecialists that are available. Patient populations need to be defined by objective and clear criteria and not simply by the unit to which they are admitted. A "critically ill patient" could be defined in several ways according to these and more variables. Acute illness scoring systems try to provide specific, objective measurements that are reproducible in many ICU environments.

Objective and reproducible measures are particularly necessary if research and quality improvement projects are to be successfully completed and the results applied to similar populations. Selecting an appropriate scoring system can be one of the key elements of developing a successful project. Scoring systems are often used to develop or identify risk stratification for a given patient population. By dividing patient populations into various risk groups, a researcher can better compare like patients and apply appropriate statistical tests and comparisons. Quality improvement projects effectively use scoring systems by selecting validated scoring systems that are commonly used by facilities with like patient populations. For example, if a particular ICU selects a scoring system that is not used by similar units or institutions with similar patient populations, that system will not allow for appropriate comparisons and may give data that are unreliable or may lead to projects that are not focused on the correct outcome.

In addition to research applications, clinicians are often faced with providing guidance to families or evaluating their own practices to help predict which patients will need continuing intensive care and which patients may benefit from lower acuity of care, or even withdrawal of care. Although most scoring systems are not intended for individual patient decision-making, they can help establish baseline statistics that can be used to better inform clinicians and families about the overall outcomes that may be expected given the available evidence.[1-5] For all of these reasons, many types of acute illness scoring systems have been developed to provide consistency in the reporting and evaluation of patients with critical illness for a variety of disease states and predicted outcomes.

OVERVIEW OF ACUTE SCORING SYSTEMS

Most scoring systems are developed by collecting data on many patients and comparing the available data with the patients' ultimate outcome.[1,2,5] Two key elements in the evaluation and use of scoring systems are calibration and discrimination.[1,5] Calibration evaluates the performance of a scoring system across patient populations, comparing the actual outcome with the predictive outcome. One of the more common statistical tests for assessing calibration is the Hosmer-Lemeshow test. Although this test provides better data as the size of the database increases, it should not be the sole test used to determine optimal test calibration for a particular patient population.[6] Discrimination describes the ability of a model to accurately discriminate between patients who die and those who do not. Statistical tests such as the area under the receiver operating characteristic (ROC) curve describe discrimination of a particular model.[5] An ROC of 0.5 represents a purely chance association, and discrimination of a particular score improves as the ROC nears 1.0.[1,6] Therefore, before using a given predictive scoring system in a quality improvement or research project, or before considering use in aiding a prognostic model for care decisions, the statistical reliability of the scoring system should be thoroughly investigated.

Scoring systems can be applicable to acutely ill patient populations in general or applicable only to specific disease states. Selecting the best scoring system for a research project or identifying the most appropriate criteria for optimizing patient care can be challenging for any critical care practitioner. The key elements are understanding the validated populations for a scoring system, selecting the appropriate data points for a particular disease state, and then correctly and consistently calculating scores.[7] In the past several years, the proliferation of online and application-based calculators has made the data entry and calculation components relatively easy. However, selecting the correct data for entry often depends on having a clear understanding of the score, the applicable populations, and how to accurately select the appropriate data points for entry into the system.[3] This chapter reviews many of the common scoring systems used in clinical practice, identifies the basic calculation approaches, and lists the primary patient populations and uses for each score.

APACHE Score

The Acute Physiology and Chronic Health Evaluation (APACHE; Cerner Corp., North Kansas City, MO) scoring system is one of the most well-known and commonly used scoring systems to assess severity of illness in critically ill patients.[1] The APACHE system was first developed in the late 1970s/early 1980s and is currently in the fourth revision of the system, although the APACHE II and III versions of the score remain in common use within practice.[8-12]

Clinicians should be trained on how to accurately calculate and use the score specific to the version in order to optimize inter- and intra-rater reliability.[1,13-15] Preferably, the required data points are automatically fed to the APACHE scoring system from the medical record to minimize variability, but manual data collection is also an option although usually much more time-consuming.[3] The APACHE II score consists of three domains that include the Acute Physiology Score (APS), the Age score, and the Chronic Health Score.[8] The APS component is determined by identifying the worst values recorded (high or low) within the previous 24 hours or within 24 hours of admission.[16] Because values may change, it is important to note the application of the scoring system and the ways in which data were reported in a quality project or research design. Those values are then converted to a score that is summed. Values not available result in a score of zero for that element. A similar methodology is used for the III and IV versions.

Many versions of the APACHE scoring systems are available on the web. However, the APACHE III and IV systems have additional data points compared with APACHE II, and calculating the score without specific training and significant practice can lead to incorrect results and significant variability.[13-15] By comparison, the APACHE II score is relatively easy to calculate by investigators or clinicians who lack full access to the APACHE IV data system. As with any scoring system, there is some intra- and interrater variation in calculating the scores with any of the APACHE versions, which can limit the usefulness of the score if strict attention to methodology is lacking.[17]

Two elements of the APACHE score can be especially prone to introducing variability into the scoring system. One of the most difficult data elements to determine is the Glasgow Coma Scale (GCS) score in patients who are mechanically ventilated and sedated. The GCS measures basic neurological function on the basis of response to pain (1–6 points), verbal response (1–5 points), and eye-opening response (1–4 points), with total scores ranging from 3 to 15. To avoid false elevation of the APS score within the APACHE system, the pre-sedation GCS level should be recorded whenever possible. Medications and other therapies will likely affect the level of response of the patient and therefore the GCS.[18] The Chronic Health Score component of the score is the second area that significantly affects reliability of the system. Although this component is clearly defined when using most online calculators, it may not be easily described when homemade calculators or shortened versions of the scoring tool are used. Of note, multiple chronic conditions are not additive for this score because the patient can only receive a maximum of 5 points within the Chronic Health Score.

The current version of the APACHE (APACHE IV) scoring system provides the most accurate information regarding the predicted mortality of a patient population as well as the predicted length of stay.[10,19] However, the APACHE II version still provides reasonable calibration and discrimination for some patient populations.[20] As an investigator or quality project leader chooses a tool, the resources available will often drive which version of APACHE is selected.

Several websites offer online calculation of the score with good explanations of how to proceed. The version (II, III, or IV) being used should be noted because the appropriate collection and recording of data differ, depending on the version. Furthermore, online calculators often offer a calculated mortality rate or probability, but the rates determined by these systems may not be as accurate as the data that would be obtained with the APACHE IV system in full use and, in general, should not be used to predict mortality or outcome for specific individual patients.

The APACHE scoring system remains one of the most common tools for comparing the outcomes of a particular unit with those of peers as well as a common risk stratification tool for research studies that need to quantify severity of illness for their study population(s). Critical care clinicians should have a functional knowledge of this system and understand how the reported results may affect quality outcomes or identify appropriate patient populations for applying research results.

SAPS Score

The Simplified Acute Physiology Score (SAPS) was initially described in 1984 and was then revised in 1993 as the SAPS II.[21,22] The SAPS II score identifies 17 variables to provide a predicted mortality rate. The original study evaluated data within the first 24 hours of ICU admission; however, some calculators and investigators have used worst values in the past 24 hours to calculate the score.[23] The mortality accuracy of the SAPS II score is somewhat questionable at this point because the data used to determine the mortality rates are now more than 20 years old.[24] The SAPS 3 score was developed to address some of the inconsistencies with the SAPS II score, used patients from several regions of the world, and improves on the predictability of the score and simplifying data collection.[1,24-26] The SAPS 3 score is an "admission score" because the data were collected within an hour before or after ICU admission.[25,26] Furthermore, SAPS II and SAPS 3 were developed with data from patients in several countries as opposed to the APACHE system, which primarily used patients from the United States.[1]

Mortality Probability Model

The mortality probability model (MPM) was originally developed in the 1980s, and the current revision (MPM_0-III) has been in use since 2007.[27,28] The MPM uses variables present on admission to the ICU such as comorbidities, acute diagnoses, and only three physiologic variables to provide mortality prediction. The current revision has a slightly lower level of discrimination than other models (e.g., APACHE).[27] A further limitation of this model is that it does not work as well for patients with rapid changes within the first 24–48 hours of ICU admission because it only uses admission variables. However, the level of data collection is less with the MPM_0-III model, and it does not require a diagnosis for use, so it may have advantages, depending on how data are collected within an EMR (electronic medical record).[27,28]

SOFA Score

The Sequential Organ Failure Assessment (SOFA) score is calculated on the basis of the function of six organ systems (pulmonary, cardiovascular, central nervous system, renal, coagulation, and hepatic).[29-32] Each organ system is scored on a 0–4 scale, and the SOFA has a maximum score of 24. In contrast to some of the other scoring tools, the SOFA score is intended to be tracked on a daily basis within the ICU, and the day-to-day change can be used as an objective measure to track the progress of an individual patient. Mortality rates have been correlated with both the peak SOFA score and the change in score from ICU admission.[29,31,33] The SOFA score was also combined with the APACHE score to try to improve the prediction of mortality rates in at least one study.[34] This score is particularly useful in research trials and quality projects where tracking and evaluating day-to-day progress of the patient is important to study outcome.

MODS Score

The Multiple Organ Dysfunction Score (MODS) is very similar to the SOFA score. Six organ systems are scored on a 0–4 scale with a maximum total score of 24.[35] The main difference between the MODS and SOFA scores is the scoring of the cardiovascular system. The MODS approach uses a computation with the heart rate and blood pressures, whereas the SOFA score uses an approach of recording both blood pressure readings and whether vasopressor support is necessary. The MODS score was specifically described as an outcomes measurement in the original publication.[35] However, a predictive component is available with associated mortality rates based on the calculated score and the number of ICU days for the patient. The MODS and SOFA scores have been compared in clinical practice and found to be similar in predicting and measuring outcomes.[30]

TISS Score

Not all scoring systems are focused on patient mortality. For example, the Therapeutic Intervention Scoring System (TISS) can be used to measure and help determine staffing needs (particularly nursing) by measuring specific nursing activities.[36-38] The score was initially developed in the 1970s, revised in the 1980s, and shortened to the TISS-28 score in the 1990s.[36] The areas measured in the score include basic measures, cardiovascular support, ventilator support, renal support, neurological support, metabolic support, and specific interventions. The TISS and TISS-28 scores have also been used to measure certain outcomes and costs.[39]

SCORING SYSTEMS IN SPECIFIC DISEASE STATES

Trauma

Several scores are used in measuring the severity of injury in trauma patients.[40-49] Many of the common scores described previously in this chapter can be applied to trauma patients, but many scores have also been developed to be used specifically in trauma patients.[50] Some scores do not require full knowledge of all injuries.[48,51] In addition, several scores are based on the anatomic location and type of injury to calculate the full score.[41,45,46] Trauma scores are used to provide triage assistance, to quantify injury patterns for registry database submission, or both. Three of the most common scores are described in the sections that follow.

ISS Score

The Injury Severity Score (ISS) has been used for more than 40 years to describe the initial injury in trauma patients.[46] The score is calculated on the basis of the sum of squares of the three most injured body areas, with a score range of 1–75. The ISS can help predict mortality, allow for data comparison for quality improvement for a trauma program, and be part of data submission to trauma registries. As with other scores, online calculators are readily available, but calculated scores should not be used as a sole method to predict mortality for individual patients.

A revision to the ISS has also been published.[52] The new ISS provides improved mortality accuracy over the original score using the worst injuries regardless of body region.[49,53] This better represents multiple injuries that may be more severe in one anatomic area.

Revised Trauma Score

The Revised Trauma Score is a calculation based on respiratory rate, systolic blood pressure, and the GCS.[44,45] Each value is then coded to a score of 0–4. The coded score is then entered into a calculation to obtain to a final score that provides a mortality estimate that can be readily found with online calculators. Of note, this calculation more heavily weights the GCS to better represent the impact of head injury on overall survival.

TRISS Score

The Trauma Score and Injury Severity Score (TRISS) is a combination of the Revised Trauma Score and the ISS and incorporates the patient's age.[41] This score is used in several areas including many registry databases, trauma outcomes research, and internal quality improvement programs. The TRISS calculation provides a probability of survival, but as with any scoring system, this should be used cautiously for any individual patient decisions.

Acute Kidney Injury

RIFLE Score

The RIFLE acronym stands for risk, injury, failure, loss, and end-stage renal disease and is a system used to stratify acute kidney injury.[54] The acute elements (risk, injury, and failure) are defined by a specific set of criteria listed in Table 47.1. Serum creatinine changes, glomerular filtration rate changes, and urine output concentrations are used to categorize the acute elements of the score. The use of urine output concentrations provides a more timely identification of kidney dysfunction than does the use of kidney injury definitions that rely solely on laboratory values. Before the RIFLE system was developed, acute kidney injury was not consistently defined,

Table 47.1 RIFLE Criteria for Acute Kidney Injury[54]

	SCr Changes	Urine Output
Risk	1.5 × increase in SCr from baseline or decrease in GFR by ≥ 25%	< 0.5 mL/kg/hr for at least 6 hr
Injury	2 × increase in SCr from baseline or decrease in GFR by ≥ 50%	< 0.5 mL/kg/hr for at least 12 hr
Failure	3 × increase in SCr from baseline or a SCr of ≥ 4 mg/dL or decrease in GFR by ≥ 75%	< 0.3 mL/kg/hr for at least 24 hr or anuria for 12 hr
Loss	Complete loss of kidney function for at least 4 weeks	
End-stage renal disease	Complete loss of kidney function for > 3 mo	

GFR = glomerular filtration rate; SCr = serum creatinine.

and many studies have been completed in the past decade that evaluate the ability to predict outcome and stratify patients with acute kidney injury.[55-61]

The RIFLE system is one example of a scoring tool that can be used to describe either a patient population or individual patients. In describing a patient population for a research study, an investigator may use the RIFLE system to describe the number of patients who met each of the various criteria. However, the bedside clinician may use the RIFLE system to determine the degree of organ dysfunction for an individual patient.[61] It is important to understand how a specific scoring tool is used in a particular context to understand the implications of the data that are presented.

AKIN Staging

The Acute Kidney Injury Network (AKIN) has suggested alterations to the RIFLE criteria by adjusting the changes in serum creatinine and urine output; this is described in Table 47.2.[55,62] However, the AKIN score has not shown demonstrable advantage over the RIFLE criteria with respect to discrimination or calibration.[55,57-59,63]

The RIFLE and AKIN criteria can be very important tools for the critical care pharmacist to remember and understand. Many medications used in the critically ill patient have the potential to induce damage to the kidney or are cleared by the kidneys and require dose adjustments with alteration in kidney function. Appropriate monitoring of both urine output and serum creatinine concentrations, using the RIFLE or AKIN criteria as a guide, is an important part of the overall patient care plan.

Although the RIFLE and AKIN criteria can be helpful in determining the degree of kidney injury or failure, they do not directly assist with medication dose adjustments. Typically, the Cockcroft-Gault equation is used for most medication dose adjustment. However, this equation was not developed with critically ill patients that have many changing variables in mind.[64]

Table 47.2 Acute Kidney Injury Network Score[62]

Stage	Serum Creatinine	Urine Output
1	Increase of ≥ 1.5–2 × baseline or increase of ≥ 0.3 mg/dL	< 0.5 mL/kg/hr for > 6 hr
2	Increase of > 2–3 × baseline	< 0.5 mL/kg/hr for > 12 hr
3	Increase of > 3 × baseline or SCr > 4.0 mg/dL with acute increase of at least 0.5 mg/dL	< 0.3 mL/kg/hr for > 24 hr or anuria for > 12 hr

Pancreatitis

Pancreatitis can be a difficult disease state to accurately describe expected or predicted outcome because patients can become extremely ill very quickly. Therefore, several scoring systems have been developed through the years to describe objective measures and to accurately describe the likely outcomes of the disease process and assist in identifying patients in whom rapid aggressive care is most beneficial. The Ranson criteria are the oldest and most widely known set of criteria.[65,66] However, in the 40+ years since these criteria were developed, other systems have been developed with increasing prognostic capabilities.[67-70]

The Ranson criteria use 11 variables scored as either 0 or 1.[65,66] Five of the variables (age, white blood cell count, glucose, aspartate aminotransferase, and lactate dehydrogenase) are scored at admission, and the remaining six are scored within 48 hours (serum calcium, change in hematocrit, hypoxemia, blood urea nitrogen [BUN] increase, base deficit, and fluid overload). The scoring breakpoints are different depending on whether the pancreatitis episode was caused by gallstones. Severe pancreatitis is defined by a score of 3 or greater. Although the Ranson criteria provide a reasonable predictive outcome, it takes a full 48 hours to complete the score and requires that specific laboratory variables be drawn within the specified period.

In contrast, the BISAP (Bedside Index of Severity in Acute Pancreatitis) is a simpler scoring system completed as soon as the variables are available after admission.[67,69] These variables include a BUN concentration greater than 25 mg/dL, impaired mental status, SIRS (systemic inflammatory response syndrome), age older than 60, and pleural effusions. Each variable receives a score of 0 or 1, and the total score of greater than 3 describes severe acute pancreatitis. Each point scored is correlated with an increase in mortality. Compared with the Ranson criteria, the BISAP score performs at a similar specificity but somewhat lower sensitivity.[67]

Scoring systems for pancreatitis severity have also been evaluated according to computed tomography (CT) results. Scores like the CT severity index (CTSI) and Balthazar grading system have been compared with clinical (non-radiographic) scoring systems, but with similar predictive results.[69,71]

The Atlanta classification (2012) is the standard consensus-driven tool for describing acute pancreatitis.[68] This classification describes acute pancreatitis and mild, moderate, or severe acute pancreatitis on the basis of both CT findings and organ dysfunction described by the modified Marshall score. The modified Marshall score evaluates renal, respiratory, cardiovascular, hematologic, and neurological systems.

Ultimately, several clinical- and radiologic-based scoring systems for acute pancreatitis perform at similar levels of sensitivity and specificity. Beyond the specific scores for pancreatitis, APACHE and other general critical illness scores have utility in pancreatitis scoring.[71,72] Some scores provide for mortality prognostication and resource use, whereas others serve to better describe patient populations for research purposes.

Pneumonia

Pneumonia scoring systems are not necessarily limited to ICU patients, but they are commonly used to describe the severity of illness of these patients in studies involving critically ill patients. Some of the most common pneumonia scores are the CURB-65 score and the Pneumonia Severity Index (PSI).[73,74] The CURB-65 score is calculated by giving a point for each of the variables listed in Box 47.1.[74] A score of 0 can likely be treated at home, whereas a score of 3 or more indicates a higher risk of death, and ICU admission should be considered particularly for a score of 4 or 5. The PSI uses a two-step process with a relatively simple yes/no algorithm to classify a patient into a low-risk score (category I) or into the higher-risk II–V scoring range.[73] The higher-risk calculation then assigns points from a variety of symptoms and comorbidities from five categories: age, place of residence, physical examination findings, comorbid conditions, and radiologic and laboratory findings.

Clinical application of the CURB-65 score and the PSI may include use in some decision support tools or be used for predicting or directing location of care.[75,76] The PSI has less discrimination for ICU care, and the many data points make it difficult to use in a prospective manner unless data are automatically taken from the medical record.[76] Although the CURB-65 score is fairly easy to calculate, it may underestimate the severity of illness in some patients, particularly older adult patients who are frail.[76,77]

Acute Liver Failure

Acute liver failure is another common condition in critically ill patients and there are several scoring systems associated with the disease process.[11,78-81] Patients appear very ill, and it is difficult to determine their prognosis and level of care. Furthermore, acute liver failure often occurs on top of underlying chronic liver failure. Therefore, scores such as the model for end-stage liver disease (MELD) score and the Child-Pugh score are commonly used, but they often show no greater predictive ability than the APACHE system or scores like the SOFA score.[11,73,80]

The Child-Pugh score ranges from 5 to 15 and is calculated with a score of 1–3 in each of these five categories: ascites, encephalopathy, international normalized ratio (INR), albumin, and bilirubin. The score then indicates class A (5–6), B (7–9), or C (10–15) depending on the score range. The MELD score uses the INR, serum creatinine concentration, and bilirubin concentrations as well as the cause of liver disease within an equation to provide a score and a predicted mortality rate.[82] Mortality increases with every 10 points in the MELD score. Prognostic scores for hepatic disease are sometimes used to prioritize patients for certain procedures or transplant selection on the basis of overall probability of survival.

SUMMARY

Many scoring systems are available to evaluate critically ill patients. Some are disease-specific, whereas others are predictive simply on the basis of the presenting condition of the patient or the patient's day-to-day progress. Some are a mix of disease-specific and physiologic values. Although scoring systems may at times be useful in predicting mortality and providing information to caregivers and families, most systems are primarily used to stratify patients for research purposes or to evaluate populations of patients to assist in quality improvement initiatives. With the advent of many mobile apps and decision support tools, many of these scores can be easily or even automatically calculated. An understanding of the use and application of such scoring systems is important for any clinician practicing in the ICU so that the most effective and accurate scoring system can be used appropriately and not misinterpreted or applied to patients or disease states for which that particular score was not intended. Pharmacists should be particularly aware of scoring systems that may affect the use of medications by accurately predicting patients or populations that are comparable with published literature. Furthermore, the interpretation of many studies of critically ill patients requires a knowledge of scoring systems so that patient populations can be matched appropriately.

REFERENCES

1. Breslow MJ, Badawi O. Severity scoring in the critically ill: part 1—interpretation and accuracy of outcome prediction scoring systems. Chest 2012;141:245-52.
2. Breslow MJ, Badawi O. Severity scoring in the critically ill: part 2: maximizing value from outcome prediction scoring systems. Chest 2012;141:518-27.
3. Salluh JI, Soares M. ICU severity of illness scores: APACHE, SAPS and MPM. Curr Opin Crit Care 2014;20:557-65.
4. Kareliusson F, De Geer L, Tibblin AO. Risk prediction of ICU readmission in a mixed surgical and medical population. J Intensive Care 2015;3:30.

Box 47.1. CURB-65 Score[74]

Confusion, new-onset
Urea > 7 mmol/L
Respiratory rate ≥ 30 breaths/minute
Blood pressure < 90 mm Hg systolic or ≤ 60 mm Hg diastolic
Age older than **65** years

5. Bouch DC, Thompson JP. Severity scoring systems in the critically ill. Contin Educ Anaesth Crit Care Pain 2008;8:181-5.
6. Kramer AA, Zimmerman JE. Assessing the calibration of mortality benchmarks in critical care: the Hosmer-Lemeshow test revisited. Crit Care Med 2007;35:2052-6.
7. Ferreira AM, Sakr Y. Organ dysfunction: general approach, epidemiology, and organ failure scores. Semin Respir Crit Care Med 2011;32:543-51.
8. Knaus WA, Draper EA, Wagner DP, et al. APACHE II: a severity of disease classification system. Crit Care Med 1985;13:818-29.
9. Knaus WA, Wagner DP, Draper EA, et al. The APACHE III prognostic system. Risk prediction of hospital mortality for critically ill hospitalized adults. Chest 1991;100:1619-36.
10. Zimmerman JE, Kramer AA, McNair DS, et al. Acute Physiology and Chronic Health Evaluation (APACHE) IV: hospital mortality assessment for today's critically ill patients. Crit Care Med 2006;34:1297-310.
11. Duseja A, Choudhary NS, Gupta S, et al. APACHE II score is superior to SOFA, CTP and MELD in predicting the short-term mortality in patients with acute-on-chronic liver failure (ACLF). J Dig Dis 2013;14:484-90.
12. Knaus WA, Zimmerman JE, Wagner DP, et al. APACHE-acute physiology and chronic health evaluation: a physiologically based classification system. Crit Care Med 1981;9:591-7.
13. Booth FV, Short M, Shorr AF, et al. Application of a population-based severity scoring system to individual patients results in frequent misclassification. Crit Care 2005;9:R522-529.
14. Greenwood B, Szumita PM, Levy H, et al. Error rates among clinical pharmacists in calculating the APACHE II score. Pharmacotherapy 2007;27:285-9.
15. Ledoux D, Finfer S, McKinley S. Impact of operator expertise on collection of the APACHE II score and on the derived risk of death and standardized mortality ratio. Anaesth Intensive Care 2005;33:585-0.
16. Ho KM, Dobb GJ, Knuiman M, et al. A comparison of admission and worst 24-hour Acute Physiology and Chronic Health Evaluation II scores in predicting hospital mortality: a retrospective cohort study. Crit Care 2006;10:R4.
17. Kho ME, McDonald E, Stratford PW, et al. Interrater reliability of APACHE II scores for medical-surgical intensive care patients: a prospective blinded study. Am J Crit Care 2007;16:378-83.
18. Livingston BM, Mackenzie SJ, MacKirdy FN, et al. Should the pre-sedation Glasgow Coma Scale value be used when calculating Acute Physiology and Chronic Health Evaluation scores for sedated patients? Scottish Intensive Care Society Audit Group. Crit Care Med 2000;28:389-94.
19. Zimmerman JE, Kramer AA, McNair DS, et al. Intensive care unit length of stay: benchmarking based on Acute Physiology and Chronic Health Evaluation (APACHE) IV. Crit Care Med 2006;34:2517-29.
20. Gilani MT, Razavi M, Azad AM. A comparison of Simplified Acute Physiology Score II, Acute Physiology and Chronic Health Evaluation II and Acute Physiology and Chronic Health Evaluation III scoring system in predicting mortality and length of stay at surgical intensive care unit. Niger Med J 2014;55:144-7.
21. Le Gall JR, Loirat P, Alperovitch A, et al. A simplified acute physiology score for ICU patients. Crit Care Med 1984;12:975-7.
22. Le Gall JR, Lemeshow S, Saulnier F. A new Simplified Acute Physiology Score (SAPS II) based on a European/North American multicenter study. JAMA 1993;270:2957-63.
23. Sakr Y, Krauss C, Amaral AC, et al. Comparison of the performance of SAPS II, SAPS 3, APACHE II, and their customized prognostic models in a surgical intensive care unit. Br J Anaesth 2008;101:798-803.
24. Nassar AP, Malbouisson LM, Moreno R. Evaluation of Simplified Acute Physiology Score 3 performance: a systematic review of external validation studies. Crit Care 2014;18:R117.
25. Metnitz PG, Moreno RP, Almeida E, et al. SAPS 3—from evaluation of the patient to evaluation of the intensive care unit. Part 1: objectives, methods and cohort description. Intensive Care Med 2005;31:1336-44.
26. Moreno RP, Metnitz PG, Almeida E, et al. SAPS 3—from evaluation of the patient to evaluation of the intensive care unit. Part 2: development of a prognostic model for hospital mortality at ICU admission. Intensive Care Med 2005;31:1345-55.
27. Higgins TL, Teres D, Copes WS, et al. Assessing contemporary intensive care unit outcome: an updated Mortality Probability Admission Model (MPM0-III). Crit Care Med 2007;35:827-35.
28. Higgins TL, Kramer AA, Nathanson BH, et al. Prospective validation of the intensive care unit admission Mortality Probability Model (MPM0-III). Crit Care Med 2009;37:1619-23.
29. Ferreira FL, Bota DP, Bross A, et al. Serial evaluation of the SOFA score to predict outcome in critically ill patients. JAMA 2001;286:1754-8.
30. Peres Bota D, Melot C, Lopes Ferreira F, et al. The Multiple Organ Dysfunction Score (MODS) versus the Sequential Organ Failure Assessment (SOFA) score in outcome prediction. Intensive Care Med 2002;28:1619-24.
31. Vincent JL, Ferreira F, Moreno R. Scoring systems for assessing organ dysfunction and survival. Crit Care Clin 2000;16:353-66.
32. Vincent JL, Moreno R, Takala J, et al. The SOFA (Sepsis-related Organ Failure Assessment) score to describe organ dysfunction/failure. On behalf of the Working Group on Sepsis-Related Problems of the European Society of Intensive Care Medicine. Intensive Care Med 1996;22:707-10.
33. Qiao Q, Lu G, Li M, et al. Prediction of outcome in critically ill elderly patients using APACHE II and SOFA scores. J Int Med Res 2012;40:1114-21.
34. Ho KM. Combining sequential organ failure assessment (SOFA) score with acute physiology and chronic health evaluation (APACHE) II score to predict hospital mortality of critically ill patients. Anaesth Intensive Care 2007;35:515-21.
35. Marshall JC, Cook DJ, Christou NV, et al. Multiple organ dysfunction score: a reliable descriptor of a complex clinical outcome. Crit Care Med 1995;23:1638-52.
36. Miranda DR, de Rijk A, Schaufeli W. Simplified Therapeutic Intervention Scoring System: the TISS-28 items—results from a multicenter study. Crit Care Med 1996;24:64-73.
37. Padilha KG, de Sousa RM, Queijo AF, et al. Nursing Activities Score in the intensive care unit: analysis of the related factors. Intensive Crit Care Nurs 2008;24:197-204.

38. Keene AR, Cullen DJ. Therapeutic Intervention Scoring System: update 1983. Crit Care Med 1983;11:1-3.
39. Vincent JL, Moreno R. Clinical review: scoring systems in the critically ill. Crit Care 2010;14:207.
40. Pohlman TH, Geibel J, Bjerke HS, et al. Trauma scoring systems. 2014. Available at http://emedicine.medscape.com/article/434076-overview. Accessed September 3, 2015.
41. Boyd CR, Tolson MA, Copes WS. Evaluating trauma care: the TRISS method. Trauma Score and the Injury Severity Score. J Trauma 1987;27:370-8.
42. Borgman MA, Maegele M, Wade CE, et al. Pediatric trauma BIG score: predicting mortality in children after military and civilian trauma. Pediatrics 2011;127:e892-897.
43. Brockamp T, Nienaber U, Mutschler M, et al. Predicting on-going hemorrhage and transfusion requirement after severe trauma: a validation of six scoring systems and algorithms on the TraumaRegister DGU. Crit Care 2012;16:R129.
44. Champion HR, Sacco WJ, Carnazzo AJ, et al. Trauma score. Crit Care Med 1981;9:672-6.
45. Champion HR, Sacco WJ, Copes WS, et al. A revision of the Trauma Score. J Trauma 1989;29:623-9.
46. Baker SP, O'Neill B, Haddon W, et al. The injury severity score: a method for describing patients with multiple injuries and evaluating emergency care. J Trauma 1974;14:187-96.
47. Lecky F, Woodford M, Edwards A, et al. Trauma scoring systems and databases. Br J Anaesth 2014;113:286-94.
48. Raum MR, Nijsten MW, Vogelzang M, et al. Emergency trauma score: an instrument for early estimation of trauma severity. Crit Care Med 2009;37:1972-7.
49. Smith BP, Goldberg AJ, Gaughan JP, et al. A comparison of Injury Severity Score and New Injury Severity Score after penetrating trauma: a prospective analysis. J Trauma Acute Care Surg 2015;79:269-74.
50. Hwang SY, Lee JH, Lee YH, et al. Comparison of the Sequential Organ Failure Assessment, Acute Physiology and Chronic Health Evaluation II scoring system, and Trauma and Injury Severity Score method for predicting the outcomes of intensive care unit trauma patients. Am J Emerg Med 2012;30:749-53.
51. Kondo Y, Abe T, Kohshi K, et al. Revised trauma scoring system to predict in-hospital mortality in the emergency department: Glasgow Coma Scale, Age, and Systolic Blood Pressure score. Crit Care 2011;15:R191.
52. Osler T, Baker SP, Long W. A modification of the injury severity score that both improves accuracy and simplifies scoring. J Trauma 1997;43:922-5; discussion 925-6.
53. Lavoie A, Moore L, LeSage N, et al. The New Injury Severity Score: a more accurate predictor of in-hospital mortality than the Injury Severity Score. J Trauma 2004;56:1312-20.
54. Bellomo R, Ronco C, Kellum JA, et al.; workgroup ADQI. Acute renal failure – definition, outcome measures, animal models, fluid therapy and information technology needs: the Second International Consensus Conference of the Acute Dialysis Quality Initiative (ADQI) Group. Crit Care 2004;8:R204-212.
55. Bagshaw SM, George C, Bellomo R, et al. A comparison of the RIFLE and AKIN criteria for acute kidney injury in critically ill patients. Nephrol Dial Transplant 2008;23:1569-74.
56. Bagshaw SM, George C, Dinu I, et al. A multi-centre evaluation of the RIFLE criteria for early acute kidney injury in critically ill patients. Nephrol Dial Transplant 2008;23:1203-10.
57. Lopes JA, Fernandes P, Jorge S, et al. Acute kidney injury in intensive care unit patients: a comparison between the RIFLE and the Acute Kidney Injury Network classifications. Crit Care 2008;12:R110.
58. Joannidis M, Metnitz B, Bauer P, et al. Acute kidney injury in critically ill patients classified by AKIN versus RIFLE using the SAPS 3 database. Intensive Care Med 2009;35:1692-702.
59. Haase M, Bellomo R, Matalanis G, et al. A comparison of the RIFLE and Acute Kidney Injury Network classifications for cardiac surgery-associated acute kidney injury: a prospective cohort study. J Thorac Cardiovasc Surg 2009;138:1370-6.
60. Englberger L, Suri RM, Li Z, et al. Clinical accuracy of RIFLE and Acute Kidney Injury Network (AKIN) criteria for acute kidney injury in patients undergoing cardiac surgery. Crit Care 2011;15:R16.
61. Colpaert K, Hoste EA, Steurbaut K, et al. Impact of real-time electronic alerting of acute kidney injury on therapeutic intervention and progression of RIFLE class. Crit Care Med 2012;40:1164-70.
62. Mehta RL, Kellum JA, Shah SV, et al. Acute Kidney Injury Network: report of an initiative to improve outcomes in acute kidney injury. Crit Care 2007;11:R31.
63. Chang CH, Lin CY, Tian YC, et al. Acute kidney injury classification: comparison of AKIN and RIFLE criteria. Shock 2010;33:247-52.
64. Cockcroft DW, Gault MH. Prediction of creatinine clearance from serum creatinine. Nephron 1976;16:31-41.
65. Ranson JH, Rifkind KM, Roses DF, et al. Prognostic signs and the role of operative management in acute pancreatitis. Surg Gynecol Obstet 1974;139:69-81.
66. Ranson JH, Rifkind KM, Roses DF, et al. Objective early identification of severe acute pancreatitis. Am J Gastroenterol 1974;61:443-51.
67. Papachristou GI, Muddana V, Yadav D, et al. Comparison of BISAP, Ranson's, APACHE-II, and CTSI scores in predicting organ failure, complications, and mortality in acute pancreatitis. Am J Gastroenterol 2010;105:435-41; quiz 442.
68. Banks PA, Bollen TL, Dervenis C, et al. Classification of acute pancreatitis—2012: revision of the Atlanta classification and definitions by international consensus. Gut 2013;62:102-11.
69. Bollen TL, Singh VK, Maurer R, et al. A comparative evaluation of radiologic and clinical scoring systems in the early prediction of severity in acute pancreatitis. Am J Gastroenterol 2012;107:612-9.
70. Bollen TL. Imaging of acute pancreatitis: update of the revised Atlanta classification. Radiol Clin North Am 2012;50:429-45.
71. Chatzicostas C, Roussomoustakaki M, Vardas E, et al. Balthazar computed tomography severity index is superior to Ranson criteria and APACHE II and III scoring systems in predicting acute pancreatitis outcome. J Clin Gastroenterol 2003;36:253-60.
72. Chatzicostas C, Roussomoustakaki M, Vlachonikolis IG, et al. Comparison of Ranson, APACHE II and APACHE III scoring systems in acute pancreatitis. Pancreas. 2002;25:331-5.

73. Fine MJ, Auble TE, Yealy DM, et al. A prediction rule to identify low-risk patients with community-acquired pneumonia. N Engl J Med 1997;336:243-50.

74. Lim WS, van der Eerden MM, Laing R, et al. Defining community acquired pneumonia severity on presentation to hospital: an international derivation and validation study. Thorax 2003;58:377-82.

75. Jones BE, Jones J, Bewick T, et al. CURB-65 pneumonia severity assessment adapted for electronic decision support. Chest 2011;140:156-63.

76. Sligl WI, Marrie TJ. Severe community-acquired pneumonia. Crit Care Clin 2013;29:563-601.

77. Richards G, Levy H, Laterre PF, et al. CURB-65, PSI, and APACHE II to assess mortality risk in patients with severe sepsis and community acquired pneumonia in PROWESS. J Intensive Care Med 2011;26:34-40.

78. Boone MD, Celi LA, Ho BG, et al. Model for End-Stage Liver Disease score predicts mortality in critically ill cirrhotic patients. J Crit Care 2014;29:881.e887-813.

79. Chatzicostas C, Roussomoustakaki M, Notas G, et al. A comparison of Child-Pugh, APACHE II and APACHE III scoring systems in predicting hospital mortality of patients with liver cirrhosis. BMC Gastroenterol 2003;3:7.

80. Karvellas CJ, Bagshaw SM. Advances in management and prognostication in critically ill cirrhotic patients. Curr Opin Crit Care 2014;20:210-7.

81. Seak CJ, Ng CJ, Yen DH, et al. Performance assessment of the Simplified Acute Physiology Score II, the Acute Physiology and Chronic Health Evaluation II score, and the Sequential Organ Failure Assessment score in predicting the outcomes of adult patients with hepatic portal venous gas in the ED. Am J Emerg Med 2014;32:1481-4.

82. Cholongitas E, Papatheodoridis GV, Vangeli M, et al. Systematic review: the model for end-stage liver disease—should it replace Child-Pugh's classification for assessing prognosis in cirrhosis? Aliment Pharmacol Ther 2005;22:1079-89.

Chapter 48: Leading and Managing Intensive Care Unit Pharmacy Services

Robert J. Weber, Pharm.D., M.S., FASHP, BCPS

LEARNING OBJECTIVES

1. Describe at least three ways that hospitals benefit from intensive care unit (ICU) pharmacy services.
2. Describe how a hospital's strategic goals affect designing and implementing ICU pharmacy services.
3. List at least three factors that justify ICU pharmacy services.
4. Describe at least two ways that pharmacist clinical credentialing and privileging enhances ICU pharmacy services.

ABBREVIATIONS IN THIS CHAPTER

ACCP	American College of Clinical Pharmacy	ME	Medication error
ASHP	American Society of Health-System Pharmacists	PGY2	Postgraduate year two
ICU	Intensive care unit	SCCM	Society of Critical Care Medicine

INTRODUCTION

Critical care medicine has grown from a small group of physicians participating in patient care rounds in surgical and medical intensive care units (ICUs) in the early 1980s to their integrated role on a high-technology multidisciplinary ICU team in 2015. The first published textbook chapter on critical care pharmacy services in 1981 notes only 12 physician training programs in critical care medicine, with about 500 physicians practicing the specialty with no board-certifying examination. In addition, the Society of Critical Care Medicine (SCCM) was only 10 years old at the chapter's publication.[1] The year 2015 marks the 45th year of SCCM, with almost 16,000 trained professionals engaged in the multidisciplinary critical care model.[2]

Pharmacy's growth in the area of critical care is as exponential. The first residency training programs for ICU pharmacists were designed by a few pioneers and at several institutions. Of note, in 1981, the Ohio State University recruited and trained one of the nation's first critical care residents; that same institution was selected in 1982 to conduct the first critical care fellowship program, sponsored by the American Society of Health-System Pharmacists (ASHP).[3] Similar to critical care physicians, pharmacists will be offered a board-certifying examination for the first time in October 2015.[4]

The role of the pharmacist in the ICU is to provide a broad-based approach to medication use through a *comprehensive pharmacy service*. For example, a pharmacist attending ICU patient care rounds may be able to recommend an appropriate drug for a specific critical condition—but may be unable to provide timely drug delivery because of the lack of a pharmacy distribution area (e.g., a pharmacy satellite) in the immediate vicinity of the ICU. The service provided by the pharmacist is not *comprehensive* because the pharmacist is unable to provide the medication in a timely manner. Or furthermore, the ICU nurse caring directly for a patient may be burdened with the responsibility of compounding an intravenous medication because of a lack of pharmacy intravenous admixture preparation services. Pharmacy-based services for preparing intravenous products have been shown to prevent errors and improve efficiencies; lacking this service in the ICU does not provide a comprehensive approach to care. The lack of comprehensive pharmacy services shown in these two scenarios may lead to inefficiencies, errors, or delays in treatment.

Today's ICU requires a comprehensive pharmaceutical service that includes both operational and clinical services to meet its medication needs. A position statement published some 15 years ago by thought leaders in critical care pharmacy is still applicable today—that optimal critical care pharmacy services involve clinical cognitive pharmacists' skills together with operational services such as a pharmacy satellite, preparation of intravenous admixtures, and an integrated electronic medical record supporting an automated medication administration record.[5] Table 48.1 lists the components of comprehensive ICU pharmaceutical services.

Critical care pharmacy specialists are uniquely positioned to provide comprehensive pharmacy services because of their cognitive skills and relationship with other members of the ICU team. However, establishing and maintaining operational services requires administrative skills not necessarily taught during postgraduate year two (PGY2) training. The administrative skills necessary to develop a comprehensive ICU pharmacy service such as pharmacy operations management, pharmacy practice model design, human resources management, and financial reporting are often not the focus of the training in residency or fellowship programs. Although ASHP's educational outcomes, goals, and objectives for PGY2 training in critical care require the review and evaluation of leadership and practice management skills, the degree to which they are covered is often variable and dependent on the pharmacy's organizational structure and residency resources.

The following case exemplifies how an ICU pharmacist uses leadership and management skills to be an effective ICU practitioner. Recently, an academic medical center reviewed the drug costs associated with patients on mechanical ventilation greater than 96 hours. The costs were so much outside the range compared with those of peers that the only suggested way to reduce expense was to significantly reduce the medication inventory or people. That review showed cost opportunities in the areas of extracorporeal membrane oxygenation (ECMO) therapy.

The pharmacist reviewed the patient cases and combined his clinical knowledge of ECMO and appropriate medication use to the institution's data. The ICU pharmacist then sorted the costs by various patient characteristics and developed a Pareto analysis for the senior management on the distribution of medication expenses in ECMO. The ICU pharmacist developed a presentation and executive summary for the chief of thoracic surgery, together with a plan for implementing a Plan-Do-Check-Act approach to decreasing costs. After 12 months, the medication costs for patients on ECMO were normalized to the 50th percentile for the compare group, preventing any other drastic reductions in staff or services for these patients. Without knowledge of some basic leadership and management skills, the ICU pharmacist would have been unable to effectively address a clinical problem that increased an organization's use of resources.

This chapter provides a primer to the critical care pharmacy specialist on leading and managing ICU pharmacy services. Specifically, this chapter describes the elements of a comprehensive ICU pharmacy service and its impact on a hospital organization, together with the skills necessary to lead and manage an ICU pharmacy service. This chapter also discusses the future role of pharmacists in the ICU and the impact of new technology on ICU pharmacy services. A large retrospective study showed that increased pharmacist staffing positively affects hospital mortality rates; however, the pharmacy services coverage is not consistent across hospitals.[6] As a result, every critical care specialist must now possess skills that focus not only on the clinical care of ICU patients, but also on the business and leadership acumen to develop an effective role for the critical care pharmacist in the interdisciplinary ICU model. With a focus on skills in practice leadership and management, together with clinical skills, critical care pharmacy services will continue to grow in this country.

Table 48.1 Components of a Comprehensive ICU Pharmacy Service

Component	Description
Facility	ICU pharmacy medication dispensing area separate from the traditional "med room." Contains all appropriate inventory, equipment, and space for pharmacy order review, preparation, and clinical consultation
Staffing and competency	Pharmacist "on site" in the ICU for hours meeting the needs of patients, staff. Pharmacy technician support for medication dispensing. Pharmacists and technicians are appropriately credentialed to ensure that basic competency is met in pharmaceutical dispensing, preparation, and monitoring. A clinical privileging process or peer-review system must be implemented to ensure ongoing professional practice competence
Quality and safety	Resources to identify and track MEs; implementing a system for staff to report MEs and adverse drug reactions. Training of ICU staff on new medications and equipment to prevent MEs should be done by a pharmacist or pharmacy technicians. Databases should be used that compare a specific ICU performance in quality and safety with others across a region or by a similar patient demographic
Financial management	Resources to track the use of medications and associated costs. Financial performance should also be compared with that of other institutions of a similar demographic or financial profile

ME = medication error; ICU = intensive care unit.

ICU PHARMACY SERVICES AND THE HOSPITAL

Comprehensive pharmaceutical services for ICU patients are based on the significant medication needs of these patients. In most ICUs, patients are admitted because of their need for intensive, one-on-one nursing care and the focused attention of the medical staff. Intensive care unit patients have multisystem and multiorgan failure, requiring very specific pharmacotherapy to manage these issues. The ICU pharmacy service also promotes quality and safety in health care by reducing the risk of adverse drug events and medication errors (MEs).

Medication Needs of ICU Patients

Intensive care unit patients require more medications than do non-ICU patients. An informal observational study in a university hospital showed that the ICU patient had on average 26 different medication orders, compared with 11 for the non-ICU patient. A large percentage (greater than 65%) of these medications are for intravenous formulations; ICU patients' ability to take oral medication may be compromised by their inability to swallow or because edema of the gastrointestinal (GI) tract limits drug absorption. In addition, ICU patients may require the use of tubes or catheters to access the GI tract, requiring that medications be available in the oral formulation or compounded as an oral liquid.

Intravenous medications are the primary dosage formulation administered to ICU patients—and many require extemporaneous compounding by hospital staff. Compounding of intravenous medications is most appropriately done under the proper conditions as required by the United States Pharmacopeia (USP). The USP sets the standards for drug product formulation and testing; USP chapter <797> details the requirements for the safe compounding of intravenous medications for both immediate use and batch preparation.[7] Most regulatory agencies, including the Joint Commission, state boards of pharmacy, and health departments, require hospitals to comply with USP guidelines for preparing intravenous admixtures.

A significant medication need of patients is the timely delivery of medications in urgent and emergent situations. Some hospitals use satellite pharmacy spaces in the ICU to place the pharmacy staff and the medication dispensing equipment closer to the patients, reducing the logistics of medication delivery from a central pharmacy area. Many pharmacy departments are located in the basement of a hospital, and often, pneumatic tube carrier systems are unavailable. As a result, delivering medication may require a technician to hand deliver the medication, using elevators, steps, and walkways to reach the ICU. Locating a pharmacy satellite area in or around the ICU eliminates these delivery issues and makes the medication available in a timely manner. The joint statement from SCCM and the American College of Clinical Pharmacy (ACCP) on critical care pharmacy services lists a satellite pharmacy with 24-hour, 7-day/week services as an optimal provision of pharmaceutical care services.[8]

Medication Costs and Quality in the ICU

The costs of medications for ICU patients exceed those for non-ICU patients. In a study of almost 23,000 ICU patients, researchers showed that ICU drug costs accounted for almost 38% of total drug costs and increased at a rate much greater than for non-ICU drug expenses.[9] Furthermore, pharmacy charges ranked as the fourth highest charge in an organization. These data emphasized the differences in the costs of ICU pharmacotherapy and the importance of developing evidence-based practices for drug use and disease state management in the ICU together with multidisciplinary collaborations.

Patients treated in an ICU have multiorgan failure, leading to a significant risk of adverse drug reactions and MEs because of the organ toxicity of antibiotics, intravenous medications, and anticoagulant and antiarrhythmic drugs. In addition to complex drug therapy and the rapidly changing condition of ICU patients, the environment may be chaotic and confusing, leading to errors caused by communication issues. Other factors include complex drug administration requirements and altered pharmacokinetics. The incidence of ICU MEs in general has been documented at a median value of 106 per 1,000 patient-days, or around 10%.[10] The severity of MEs in the ICU exceeds that in the non-ICU. The harm caused by an ME is usually an injury related to events such as hypotension from mistaken overdoses of medication, organ damage from overdosages of medication, and cardiac arrhythmias from rapid administration of cardiac medications. Because MEs have a greater incidence of harm, vigilance in monitoring patients and preventing MEs is essential.

LEADERSHIP SKILLS REQUIRED IN LEADING AND MANAGING ICU PHARMACY SERVICES

This chapter has reviewed important aspects of the impact of the comprehensive pharmaceutical service on the medication needs of ICU patients. Implementing ICU pharmaceutical services requires a broad knowledge of operational and clinical pharmacy services, specifically focused on the needs of ICU patients. This next section of the chapter discusses in some detail the important skills necessary to lead and manage ICU pharmacy services. These skills focus on basic leadership skills such as developing strategic planning, justifying pharmacy services, providing operational and clinical services management, managing personnel, and using alternative pharmacy practice models. In addition, resources for gaining these skills will be presented so that pharmacists can gain the necessary knowledge in a non-traditional manner (e.g., web resources, conference, home study programs).

These leadership skills are also important for managing the relationships that the ICU pharmacist may have with the network of individuals who coordinate the care of ICU patients (Figure 48.1). For example, interactions with several members of this network require variable leadership and management skills. Moreover, the pharmacy administrator requires the ICU pharmacist to be a clinical expert but also to have the ability to effectively plan for service growth and deal effectively with physician relationships. The nursing leadership of the ICU requires the ICU pharmacist to understand how nursing workflow and priorities intersect with pharmacy operations, resolving any issues that may interfere with those priorities.

Strategic Planning

Strategic planning is the skill of developing a work plan for a clinical service that is consistent with the strategic needs of an organization.[11] The ICU pharmacy service consistently meets the strategic plan of any hospital organization by addressing the specific impact of the pharmacy service previously discussed. Many organizations fail in their strategic plan because of a very simple shortfall—the plans are too detailed and complex. Simple plans are much more effective because it is easier for staff to remember and understand their applicability to the organization. A simple strategic planning framework focuses on three key elements: analysis, planning groups, and execution. These three areas, if given the proper attention, will result in an effective strategic plan for the ICU pharmacy service. Intensive care unit pharmacists must be involved in establishing the pharmacy's plan for this area because their understanding of patient needs and how pharmacy meets patient needs is central to any strategic plan for an ICU. Because strategic planning is not often taught in training, excellent resources are available. In particular, the National Council of Nonprofits offers an excellent guide for strategic planning.[12] An analysis of the ICU pharmacy service is usually conducted through interviews with key stakeholders, as well as examining essential ICU data on medication cost, quality, and safety metrics and staff and patient satisfaction. The stakeholders should include physicians, nurses, administrators, and patients. The interviews assess the stakeholders' thoughts on the strengths and weaknesses of the ICU pharmacy program and thoughts on the department's future directions. Additional analyses involve conducting a SWOT (strength, weakness, opportunity, and threat) analysis of the pharmacy services and surveying the pharmacy staff on their thoughts for future directions of the pharmacy service. The result of the analysis establishes strategic priorities and tactics for the ICU pharmacy services, examples of which are listed in Table 48.2 and Table 48.3. These priorities must match directly and contribute to the organization's goals.

The planning groups on the ICU pharmacy services address the priorities developed from the strategic planning process. For example, enhancing the ICU pharmacy practice model requires establishing a planning group that will develop guiding principles, conduct an assessment of the strengths and weaknesses of the model, and recommend a plan for practice model changes. Other planning groups may include an employee satisfaction group and a research focus group. Through these planning groups, tactics can be developed to increase the ICU pharmacy service's growth. A tactic is a careful action or plan to achieve a specific end.

The most important aspect of a successful strategic plan for a comprehensive ICU pharmacy service is executing the tactics design to meet the strategic plan. Successful execution requires skill in communication and project management. Most strategic plans are designed as a sophisticated "to-do" list that outlines the tactics together with a timeline and the responsible individual for implementing those tactics. Meaningful metrics for the success of an ICU pharmacy service strategic plan include, but are not limited to, patient satisfaction scores, clinical productivity, harmful MEs, order processing times, readmission rates, staff satisfaction, and financial performance (cost of drugs adjusted for patient acuity). A strategic plan is a fundamental and required tool for pharmacy departments that want to improve their overall performance. A good plan involves having an effective analysis, establishing venues for employee input, and executing and tracking its progress. Patient-centered

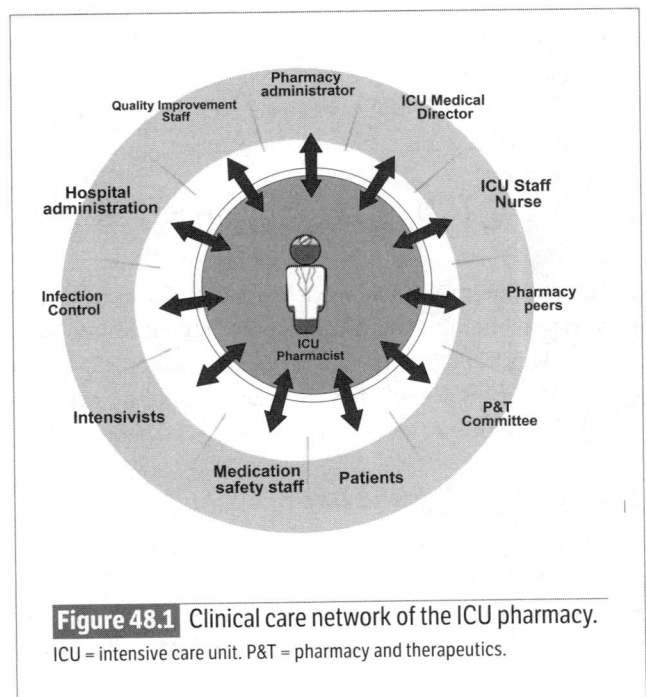

Figure 48.1 Clinical care network of the ICU pharmacy.
ICU = intensive care unit. P&T = pharmacy and therapeutics.

Table 48.2 Activities Necessary to Leading and Managing ICU Pharmacy Services

Activity	Examples of Activities
Strategic planning	Conduct a SWOT analysis and gather stakeholder feedback; develop a summary document of a strategic plan; develop a database to track outcomes of a strategic plan (e.g., scorecard); communicate the results of the plan to other disciplines
Cost justification of ICU services	Develop a business plan for ICU pharmacy services; conduct cost-benefit, cost-effectiveness, or cost-minimization analyses
Clinical service management	Develop standards for clinical practice related to patient assessment, management, and documentation; review and manage peer-review processes; identify and conduct interdisciplinary reviews of adverse events; design innovative and effective practice models; serve as a residency program director or preceptor in a PGY2 critical care specialty residency
Operations management	Prepare a staffing schedule to meet patient needs; provide a justification for new ICU pharmacy personnel or to maintain current ICU staffing; develop and implement a productivity and workload report; use Lean and other continuous quality improvement techniques to improve efficiency
Personnel management	Develop a recruitment and retention plan for ICU pharmacy staff; write an effective job description; conduct progressive discipline in accordance with fair labor standards

SWOT = strength, weakness, opportunity, and threat.

services for the ICU pharmacy can only be successful through a well-done and well-executed strategic plan.

The role of the ICU pharmacist in strategic planning is shown by the following example. A pharmacy director of a 300-bed hospital is moving the central pharmacy to another area of the hospital—far away from the ICU, which was previously serviced by the central pharmacy. As a result, the pharmacy director places developing an ICU pharmacy satellite as a key strategy in the department's goals, tasking the ICU pharmacy to develop the strategic plan for the pharmacy design and operation. The ICU pharmacist surveys stakeholders to determine the needs of the pharmacy satellite, establishes an inventory to meet the clinical needs of the patients, and designs the appropriate staffing. Finally, the ICU pharmacist supervises the execution of the construction and opening plans for the pharmacy.

Justifying ICU Pharmacy Services

The strategic plan sets the framework for establishing a comprehensive pharmaceutical service; often, the plan requires a justification through the administrative structure in a hospital organization. Justifying a new service or an expansion of an existing service requires a combination of information based on published literature and institutional data.

Institutional-Specific Data

There are very specific institutional data that are important to justifying pharmacy services. These data include staffing ratios for nurses and physicians, medication costs for ICU patients, reported harmful MEs, length of stay, readmission information, mortality, and patient and family satisfaction.

Most institutions require that the pharmacy department submit a return on investment (ROI) for new programs; this requirement would be no different if the pharmacy department were justifying a comprehensive pharmacy service. An ROI is the benefit to the investor resulting from an investment of some resource. A high ROI means that the investment gains compare favorably with investment cost. As a performance measure, the ROI is used to evaluate the efficiency of an investment or to compare the efficiency of many different investments.[13] The ROI for a pharmacy service is calculated by determining the costs of the ICU pharmacy service (facilities/space, people, inventory) compared with the benefits of the service. The benefits of the service may be measured by cost savings or avoidable hospital deaths. Pharmacy-specific services that contribute to avoided hospital deaths that can be used in the ICU by pharmacists include managing policies and protocols, providing informal educational services, conducting medication use evaluations, attending medical rounds, conducting medication histories, managing adverse drug events, and responding to resuscitation events.[13]

Published Data

Table 48.4 includes the fundamental, desirable, and optimal critical care pharmacy services. A 2013 report describes the role of the pharmacist as a member of the multidisciplinary team, including very specific clinical activities.[14] The cost implications and potential adverse events prevented by the interventions of a critical care pharmacist were studied in an academic medical center. Interventions for an almost 5-month period were analyzed in a retrospective manner, with almost 85% of the interventions determined to have prevented a potentially serious adverse event. The total cost impact of the pharmacist interventions annualized to around $600,000–$850,000 in cost avoidance.[15]

Another study shows the role of the critical care pharmacist in identifying significant drug-drug interactions. A prospective study showed that pharmacist involvement in a profile (medication regimen) review significantly reduced the incidence of drug-drug interactions compared with the control period (no pharmacist review of the medication regimen).[16] Finally, pharmacists and physicians were surveyed on the perception of their impact on the clinical and financial impact of pharmacy services in the ICU. Critical care pharmacy services were perceived to have beneficial clinical and financial outcomes—specifically, the services considered fundamental by SCCM and ACCP. The study also showed strong support for the funding of critical care pharmacy services and reimbursement for pharmacists practicing in the ICU.[17]

Operational and Clinical Services Management

Managing operational and clinical services requires knowledge of several areas. The clinical services coverage requires planning to ensure that pharmacists are available to participate in patient care activities. For example, understanding the clinical rounding scheduled of the team is critical—and pharmacists should be scheduled appropriately to participate in those rounds. Documenting and measuring clinical workload is a critical skill that establishes the appropriate time standards for various clinical activities. These standards should be used to develop the required number of hours for providing clinical services.

Managing operations also requires knowledge of Lean Six Sigma (Lean), a methodology that relies on a collaborative team effort to improve performance in the ICU pharmacy area (usually a satellite pharmacy, central pharmacy

Table 48.3 Tactics for Leading and Managing ICU Pharmacy Services

Strategic Priority	Examples of Tactics
Become a national leader in the ASHP Pharmacy Practice Model Initiative (PPMI) for the ICU	1. Finalize the framework of the ICU practice model that establishes all levels of staff working at the top of their license and in a coordinated way 2. Expand clinical privileges to 100% of ICU pharmacists 3. Complete implementing a computerized patient scoring system to prioritize ICU workflow 4. Define the framework and functions of pharmacy APPE students in the ICU 5. Develop a framework for collaboration with the college of pharmacy and obtain buy-in from all levels of the organization
Optimize operational and clinical efficiency	1. Maintain ICU staffing levels at greater than or less than the 50th percentile of Reuters Action OI comparator institutions 2. Achieve 100% of the cost-reduction goal for non-labor spending (medications) in the ICU
Exceed standards of medication safety in the ICU by maximizing technology and the roles of our staff	1. Reduce the number of harmful MEs by 5%–10% of FY 2015 baseline 2. Improve "smart pump" compliance in the ICU to national standards 3. Improve the effectiveness of the ICU Safety Solutions Committee
Retain qualified ICU pharmacists and technicians	1. Implement at least one to three initiatives that respond to issues addressed by the ICU pharmacy employees 2. Develop a committee to recommend ICU staff for local, state, and national pharmacy awards—and recommend at least one to three people for awards 3. Conduct at least one or two formal employee recognition ceremonies and one or two informal recognition ceremonies in the ICU pharmacy area
To contribute to the overall body of ICU pharmacy knowledge	1. Increase submitted peer-review publications and book chapters by 2%–5% from FY 2014 levels 2. Successfully complete our review with the ICU specialty residency program earning full accreditation 3. Publish a review of the success of the residency research program, with a focus on the ICU residency research projects

APPE = advanced pharmacy practice experience; FY = fiscal year.
Adapted from: The Ohio State University Wexner Medical Center Strategic Plan, executive summary 2014-2015.

Table 48.4 Fundamental, Desirable, and Optimal Critical Care Pharmacy Services[13]

Pharmacy Service	Fundamental	Desirable	Optimal
Clinical activities	• Conduct medication histories • Assess suspected drug-related ICU admissions for causality • Prospectively evaluate drug therapy • Provide pharmacokinetic monitoring • Monitor therapeutic regimen for efficacy and safety • Intervene to change therapy • Evaluate parenteral nutrition orders • Document recommendations in the medical record • Provide drug information and IV compatibility	• Determine need to continue maintenance drugs during the acute illness • Provide therapeutic management advice to patient or physician • Provide formal nutrition consultation • Respond to resuscitation events	• Assist physicians in discussions with patient and family members to help make informed decisions regarding treatment options
Educational activities	• Provide informational and educational services to pharmacists or other ICU health care professionals	• Provide didactic lectures to health care professionals, students, residents, and fellows in critical care pharmacology and therapeutics	• Coordinate or direct residency or fellowship programs • Implement pharmacist and pharmacy technician training programs for personnel working in the ICU • Teach advanced cardiac life support • Educate lay groups and medical personnel in the community about the role of pharmacists as part of the multidisciplinary team
Scholarly activities	• Supervise handling of investigational drugs	• Collect data • Screen patients for study enrollment • Aid in the study protocol design • Aid in data analyses • Coordinate research • Aid in manuscript preparation • Disseminate case reports and practice insights	• Procure funding • Perform laboratory analyses • Disseminate results of clinical research, outcome, and administrative research, or laboratory analyses
Administrative activities	• Document services provided to the ICU • Serve on ICU and pharmacy committees • Monitor and report adverse drug events to hospital committee • Conduct medication use evaluations	• Attach economic impact to services provided by the ICU • Develop and implement ICU policies and protocols	• Design new pharmacy programs for the ICU

IV = intravenous.
Reprinted with permission from the American College of Chest Physicians. Preslaski CR, Lat I, MacLaren R, et al. Pharmacist contributions as members of the Multidiscplinary ICU team. Chest 2013 Nov; 144(5).

service, or infusion service) by systematically removing waste to include expired medications, errors, overproduction, and inventory.[18] The elements of Lean include designing a process such that the defect-free rate is 99.99966%, or six sigma.

An important aspect of operational and clinical services management is the ability to understand and use institutional data. Specifically, these data include staffing ratios for nurses and physicians, medication costs for ICU patients, reported harmful MEs, length of stay, readmission information, mortality, and patient and family satisfaction. For example, the ICU pharmacy service would use statistics on patient volume to appropriately provide staffing to the ICU pharmacy; drug expense data can be used to focus interventions to include appropriateness or cost-savings projects.

Pharmacoeconomic Analytical Skills

The role of pharmacoeconomics in the ICU is important because ICU medications may be costly, but using these costly medications may be cost-effective in the treatment of a given ICU patient. The ICU pharmacist should understand the basic pharmacoeconomic terms and how to apply various analyses to drug use in the ICU. This is also important because many therapies in the ICU often lack the appropriate level of graded medical evidence. Table 48.5 lists the type of economic analyses and some examples in ICU patients.[19]

Personnel Management

People are the most valued asset in health care; organizations are successful if they have engaged satisfied and passionate employees. In addition, employees expect to be supervised and managed in a way that provides them with job satisfaction and upward career mobility. It is important that the critical care specialist have the skills to manage both professional and technical personnel to include developing clear job descriptions, tracking performance management, and providing effective feedback on performance. Intensive care unit pharmacists are being selected for jobs that are located in a pharmacy satellite—with responsibilities to help in managing pharmacists and technicians. This management requires providing feedback to staff on issues around clinical practice. In particular, the ICU pharmacist may also provide feedback to nursing staff on practice issues such as methods for administering and monitoring medications. There are several reasons to create clear job descriptions for the ICU pharmacy service; in general, job descriptions provide clear performance expectations, help with recruiting and hiring, and differentiate between various jobs within the pharmacy department. Job descriptions include the following: (1) the job or position title (and job code number, if applicable); (2) the reporting structure for the position; (3) a brief summary (one to three sentences) of the position and its overarching responsibility, function, or role within the organization and how it interrelates to other functions within the organization; (4) a list of the position's essential or key job duties; (5) the qualifications for the position (the specific knowledge, skills, employment, or other experiences, training, language, or aptitudes required for the job); (6) the educational requirements for the job, if any, such as degrees and licensing; and (7) the qualities or attributes that contribute to superior performance in the position. A well-written job description is a necessary component of effective personnel management because this document provides clarity on role function and performance expectations.

Clinical Privileging of ICU Pharmacists

In May 2012, the Centers for Medicare & Medicaid Services (CMS) modified its definition of medical staff to include non-physician practitioners.[20] Pharmacists practicing in the ICU are an example of non-physicians who can now be classified as part of the medical staff, which creates an opportunity to privilege pharmacists if state and federal regulations are observed. Institutional clinical pharmacists are still unable to bill for their patient care services, but this change in CMS policy provides additional strategies for pharmacists to generate revenue for clinical services.

Table 48.5 Economic Analyses with Examples for ICU Patients

Type of Study	Definition	ICU Examples
Cost minimization	Analyses that compares the cost per course of treatment when alternative therapies have demonstrably equivalent clinical effectiveness	• Formulary review of intravenous acetaminophen in managing febrile episodes in the ICU • Antibiotic therapy for ICU patients at low risk of nosocomial pneumonia
Cost benefit	Analysis in which benefits and costs are calculated in monetary terms	• Aminoglycoside dosing programs in burn patients • Control of endemic methicillin-resistant *Staphylococcus aureus*
Cost-effectiveness	Analysis that compares the relative costs and outcomes (effects) of two or more courses of action	• Thrombolysis in acute myocardial infarction • Length-of-stay analysis of ICU patients
Cost utility	Analysis that estimates the ratio between the cost of a health-related intervention and the benefit it produces with respect to the number of years lived in full health by the beneficiaries	• Prophylaxis against recurrence of peptic esophageal strictures • Mechanical ventilation in chronic obstructive pulmonary disease

Adapted from: McKenzie C, Borthwick M, Thakeer M, et al. Developing a process for credentialing advanced level practice in the pharmacy profession using a multi-source evaluation tool. Pharm J 2011;286:1-4.

Privileging Basics

Privileging is the process by which a health care organization authorizes an individual to perform a particular clinical service within a defined scope of practice.[21] Privileging is integral to the ability of physicians and mid-level practitioners (e.g., nurse practitioners, physician assistants) to provide independent clinical activities in a hospital or clinic. Privileging should not be confused with credentialing. Credentialing is the process by which an organization reviews and verifies an individual's credentials to ensure that they meet established standards. A brief case shows the differences between credentialing and privileging. A hospital's cardiac surgery department may require that physicians have the credentials of a medical degree, a state license, and specific residency training in interventional cardiology. That same hospital may only privilege specific physicians' valve replacements depending on the credentialed physician's specific case experience and outcomes.

For pharmacists, credentialing has been limited to verification by the health-system human resources department that pharmacists are graduates of an accredited school or college of pharmacy and that their license is in good standing. As an example, for a pharmacy department to credential and privilege pharmacists for administering immunizations, a pharmacist license as a credential and completion of a certificate program may be required. In addition, the department may require some competency assessment/review of knowledge on immunization indications, dosage, injection technique, and patient monitoring techniques.

Privileging pharmacists for ICU pharmacy activities can be a complicated process, and the pharmacy director must understand the basic steps of privileging and be able to apply them to privileging of the pharmacy staff. Because privileging is conducted by a hospital's medical staff, gaining the support of ICU physicians to privilege pharmacists is a key initial step in the process. The director of pharmacy must develop a strategy that shows the benefits and values of privileging pharmacists for medication-related clinical activities.

Once the pharmacy gains support for pharmacist privileging in the ICU, the necessary credentials for practicing pharmacists, specific scope of patient care service in the ICU, and initial and ongoing monitoring of quality performance in the patient care service must be determined. Although no official standards specify the credentials necessary for ICU pharmacists to become privileged, minimum requirements may include a pharmacy degree and a license to practice pharmacy. Expanded requirements can include residency training, board certification, number of years in practice, and level of specialization and competency examinations. As part of the privileging process, individuals will also need to undergo initial and ongoing quality monitoring. The institution must establish policies regarding which specific elements related to competency will need to be reviewed for ongoing evaluation and the frequency with which these reviews will need to occur. The scope of practice delineates the boundaries within which the pharmacist can provide clinical services and may differ depending on state pharmacy and medical laws and the bylaws of an organization's medical staff. Independent activities where pharmacists can be privileged in the ICU may include the following: anticoagulation management; medication reconciliation (adjusting medication on discharge or transfer from the ICU); modification of drug regimens according to a patient's renal, hepatic, and hematologic parameters; management of total parenteral nutrition therapy; conversion of intravenous medication to equivalent oral dosages; initiation of culture-directed antimicrobial therapy; *Clostridium difficile* management; and ventilator-associated prophylaxis management. Table 48.6 describes the specific activities involved with some privileges for ICU pharmacists.

Privileging Activities

Within each of these various clinical activities, specific procedures or tasks that fall within the scope of practice must be specified. For example, for pharmacists who are privileged to manage anticoagulation, specific procedures include selecting the medication and the proper dosage and frequency, ordering appropriate laboratories, and selecting the appropriate consultative help (e.g., dietitian consult to prevent food and drug interactions). The pharmacy department must also develop an internal process to approve pharmacists to be privileged for a specific ICU patient care service. This involves defining appropriate performance measures for specific clinical privileges.

The United Kingdom Clinical Pharmacy Association established a critical care group that designed a process for credentialing advanced-level practice in critical care; this framework may serve as a guide for the growth of critical care privileging in U.S. hospitals.[22] The group proposed a multipronged glossary of assessment tools for critical care proficiency: practice portfolio, case-based discussion, mini-clinical evaluations, and a 360-degree peer assessment. The practice portfolio contained documents to validate the experience of a practitioner in a specific area. Of importance, the portfolio should contain data to support the ACLF (advanced to consultant level framework), which is a UK-recognized framework describing the level of competency in pharmacy practice. Case-based discussions are designed to assess clinical decision-making and a candidate's ability to apply knowledge to resolving the issues presented in the patient case. The mini-clinical evaluation exercise is based on the American Board of Internal Medicine approach, and it involves a group discussion with candidates on a specific case, with a series of predetermined questions about the case. Finally, the 360-degree assessment seeks input from all practitioners who work with the pharmacist in the clinical arena; usually, the evaluators are members of the team in which the pharmacist is a member. This framework may serve as a guide to a comprehensive evaluation of the skills needed to determine the competency of a pharmacist independently practicing in an ICU as a member of a multidisciplinary team.[23]

Privileging Benefits

Privileging of pharmacists in the ICU has a variety of benefits. It improves the efficiency of pharmacists and physicians by avoiding the need for direct physician oversight of pharmacist activities. For example, pharmacists may modify a drug dosage for a patient and enter a verbal order change in the electronic medical record with a physician co-signature. Given the time to identify and sign verbal orders in an electronic system, eliminating this activity by privileging pharmacists to independently perform the activity allows physicians to increase their ability to care for more patients, increasing the organization's clinical revenue. Pharmacists also can more effectively use their time optimizing drug therapy and addressing medication-related problems without being limited by the availability of a physician.

CONCLUSION

Pharmacy services in the ICU are of great benefit to patients; in particular, comprehensive pharmacy services that use clinical and operational services to patients are the optimal pharmacy practice model. To establish comprehensive services, pharmacists must use both clinical and leadership skills. This chapter reviewed the leadership and management skills necessary for pharmacists to implement comprehensive ICU pharmacy services. Most pharmacists participating in PGY2 critical care pharmacy specialty training programs or pharmacists who have obtained their ICU pharmacy skills "on the job" have very little training in leadership and management. Lack of these skills may be a barrier to developing a comprehensive ICU pharmacy service.

Table 48.6 Examples of Clinical Privileges for ICU Pharmacists

Clinical Privilege	Description
Core privileges – basic privileges that can be applied to all patient care units, including the ICU	• Evaluate subjective and objective patient information • Coordinate appropriate referrals • Provide consultation in decision-making/planning for clinical services • Following prescriber medication initiation, order and adjust laboratory tests related to monitoring medication therapy as necessary • Following prescriber-determined enteral route (e.g., PO, NG, PEG), adjust medication route or dosage form of existing medication orders accordingly while maintaining the originally intended dose • Modify preoperative antimicrobial regimen on the basis of preoperative antimicrobial protocol • Delete duplicative medication therapy within the same therapeutic class when necessary
IV to PO transition	• Transition patients from intravenous to oral therapy according to the pharmacy and therapeutics committee's IV to PO policy
Pharmacokinetic and anticoagulant monitoring	• After prescriber initiation, monitor and adjust medications on the basis of renal, hepatic, antithrombotic indications and hematologic parameters
Total parenteral nutrition management	• Following prescriber initiation, modify and adjust TPN therapy and associated fluids and electrolytes in conjunction with a licensed dietitian
Clostridium difficile management	• After prescriber diagnosis of *C. difficile* and physician initiation, modify and adjust therapeutic management
ICU antimicrobial stewardship	• Following prescriber initiation, monitor and adjust culture-directed antimicrobial therapy with de-escalation of antimicrobials
Ventilator-associated pneumonia prophylaxis	• Following mechanical ventilation, assess need for chlorhexidine mouthwash
Stress ulcer prophylaxis	• After prescriber initiation of stress ulcer prophylaxis, assess, modify, or discontinue therapy as appropriate
Medication reconciliation on transition of patient care	• Assess and modify medication orders on the basis of the patient's level of care

NG = nasogastric; PEG = percutaneous endoscopic gastrostomy; PO = oral; TPN = total parenteral nutrition.

Adapted from: The Ohio State University Wexner Medical Center Credentialing and Privileging Program for Pharmacists.

Resources are available for pharmacists to develop their leadership and management skills. The ASHP Foundation's Center for Health-System Pharmacy Leadership, through the Leadership Resource Center (LRC), provides tools and opportunities for a variety of ICU practitioners who are experienced, emerging, or aspiring leaders. The LRC can provide teachings for those learning new skills or those honing existing leadership skills with the ultimate goal of enhancing their leadership knowledge and personal development. The LRC offers a Leadership Primer that provides foundational concepts for leading in a complex health care environment. A Leadership Self-Assessment also offers personal insights into individual strengths and development opportunities. In addition, a Leader's Tool Kit offers awareness, user tips, and access to worksheets for useful leadership tools that can be used in the ICU. Finally, the LRC's Focused Learning Modules offer in-depth self-study opportunities on key leadership topics, including (1) leading for influence and advocacy, (2) clinical microsystems: transformational framework for lean thinking, and (3) transformational change. Now, more than ever, the critical care specialist must possess skills that focus not only on the clinical care of ICU patients, but also on the business and leadership acumen needed to develop an effective role for the critical care pharmacist in the interdisciplinary ICU model. With a focus on the skills needed in practice leadership and management, together with clinical skills, critical care pharmacy services will continue to grow in this country.

REFERENCES

1. Angaran DM. Critical care pharmacy services. In: McLeod DC, Miller WA, eds. The Practice of Pharmacy. Cincinnati: Harvey Whitney, 1981:171-82.
2. Society of Critical Care Medicine. Critical Care Statistics. Available at www.sccm.org/Communications/Pages/CriticalCareStats.aspx. Accessed August 10, 2015.
3. The Ohio State University College of Pharmacy. Script News. Available at www.pharmacy.ohio-state.edu/sites/default/files/forms/alumni/publications/ScriptNews_WI2008.pdf. Accessed August 9, 2015.
4. Board of Pharmacy Specialties (BPS). Critical Care Pharmacy (First examination scheduled for Fall 2015). Available at https://www.bpsweb.org/specialties/criticalcarepharmacy.cfm. Accessed August 10, 2015.
5. Rudis MI, Brandl KM. Position paper on critical care pharmacy services. Crit Care Med 2000;11:3746-50.
6. Bond CA, Raehl CL, Francke T. Clinical pharmacy services, hospital pharmacy staffing, and medication errors in the United States hospitals. Pharmacotherapy 2002:22:134-47.
7. Pharmaceutical Compounding—Sterile Preparations. Available at www.doh.wa.gov/Portals/1/Documents/2300/USP797GC.pdf. Accessed October 6, 2015.
8. Erstad BL, Haas CE, O'Keefe T, et al. Interdisciplinary patient care in the intensive care unit: focus on the pharmacist. Pharmacotherapy 2011;31:128-37.
9. Weber RJ, Kane S, Oriolo VA, et al. The impact of ICU drug use on hospital costs: a descriptive analysis with recommendations for optimizing ICU pharmacotherapy. Crit Care Med 2003;31:S17-S24.
10. Kane-Gill S, Weber RJ. Principles and practices of medication safety in the intensive care unit. Crit Care Clin 2006;22:273-290.
11. Sanborn M. Developing a meaningful strategic plan. Hosp Pharm 2009;44:625-9.
12. National Council of Nonprofits. Strategic Planning for Nonprofits. Available at https://www.councilofnonprofits.org/tools-resources/strategic-planning-nonprofits. Accessed September 23, 2015.
13. Pokhrel S. Return on investment (ROI) in public health: strengths and limitations. Eur J Public Health 2015 Jul 29. [Epub ahead of print]
14. Preslaski C, Lat I, MacLaren R, et al. Pharmacist contributions as members of the multidisciplinary team. Chest 2013;144:1687-95.
15. Kopp BJ, Mrsan M, Erstad BL, et al. Cost implications of and potential adverse events by interventions of a critical care pharmacist. Am J Health Syst Pharm 2007;64:2483-7.
16. Rivkin A, Yin H. Evaluation of the role of the critical care pharmacist in identifying and avoiding or minimizing significant drug-drug interactions in medication intensive care patients. J Crit Care. 2011;26:104.1-104.e6.
17. MacLaren R, McQueen RB, Campbell J. Clinical and financial impact of pharmacy services in the intensive care unit: pharmacist and prescriber perceptions. Pharmacotherapy 2013;33:401-10.
18. Lamm MH, Eckel S, Daniels R, et al. Using lean principles to improve outpatient adult infusion clinic chemotherapy preparation turnaround times. Am J Health Syst Pharm 2015;72:1138-46.
19. Angus DC, Rubenfeld GD, Roberts MS, et al. Understanding costs and cost-effectiveness in critical care. Am J Respir Crit Care Med 2002;165:540-50.
20. Available at https://www.cms.gov/Regulations-and-Guidance/Legislation/CFCsAndCoPs/Downloads/CMS-3244-F.pdf. Accessed July 12, 2015.
21. Council on Credentialing in Pharmacy. Credentialing and privileging of pharmacists: a resource paper from the Council on credentialing in Pharmacy. Am J Health Syst Pharm 1014;71:1891-900.
22. Young K, Farrell J, McKenzie C, et al. New Ways of Working—Adult Critical Care Specialist Pharmacy Practice. London: Department of Health and Clinical Pharmacy Association, 2005.
23. McKenzie C, Borthwick M, Thakeer M, et al. Developing a process for credentialing advanced level practice in the pharmacy profession using a multi-source evaluation tool. Pharm J 2011;286:1-4.

Chapter 49: Medication Safety and Active Surveillance

Sandra L. Kane-Gill, Pharm.D., M.Sc., FCCP, FCCM; and
Mitchell S. Buckley, Pharm.D., FCCP, FASHP, FCCM, BCPS

LEARNING OBJECTIVES

1. State the incidence of medication errors (MEs) and adverse drug events (ADEs).
2. Discuss the relationship between MEs and ADEs.
3. Explain why the critically ill population is at greater risk of MEs and ADEs.
4. Describe the retrospective and prospective methods of ADE detection in a medication safety surveillance system.
5. Consider surveillance strategies that can be used to prevent ADEs.
6. State how to measure an effective surveillance system.

ABBREVIATIONS IN THIS CHAPTER

ADE	Adverse drug event	DRHC	Drug-related hazardous condition
ADR	Adverse drug reaction	ICU	Intensive care unit
AKI	Acute kidney injury	ME	Medication error
CDS	Clinical decision support	PPV	Positive predictive value

INTRODUCTION

Medication errors (MEs) and adverse drug events (ADEs) remain a significant concern in the critically ill population. Several factors have been identified in the intensive care unit (ICU) population as increasing the risk of experiencing a ME or ADE. Medication errors are concerning because they can result in ADEs. Unfortunately, ADEs have been associated with deleterious outcomes including an increased risk of hospitalization, costs, and mortality. Medication errors and ADEs can occur at any stage within the medication use process (prescribing, transcription, dispensing, and administration) with preventative strategies targeting each of these phases. A multifaceted approach involving both, prospective and retrospective, medication surveillance systems can detect events for systematic improvements, mitigate ADE progression and reduce preventable ADEs.

MEDICATION SAFETY

Terminology

Medication errors and *ADEs* are terms often used in medication safety (Table 49.1).[1,2] The National Coordinating Council for Medication Error Reporting and Prevention defines an ME as a preventable incident resulting in inappropriate drug use while the medication is in the control of the health care professional, patient, or consumer.[3] Medication errors may occur at any step in the medication use process regardless of whether patient harm occurred.[4,5] An ADE is an injury experienced by the patient as a direct result of medication use, but it is not necessarily the result of an ME.[4]

Confusion in the literature arises for ADEs because clinicians and researchers are not decisive with their definition of injury. Injury should be explained by the occurrence of end-organ damage, so an episode of asymptomatic drug-induced hyperkalemia (no end-organ damage) is not classified as an ADE, and an episode of drug-induced hyperkalemia that results in an arrhythmia (end-organ damage) is considered an ADE.[2] The elevated potassium concentration caused by a drug is considered a drug-related hazardous condition (DRHC) because high potassium concentrations from drugs are an antecedent to injury and the opportunity for a pharmacist to intervene, thus preventing injury—in this case, an arrhythmia.[2,5,6] The idea of an intermediate step or a DRHC, before an ADE occurs, can be applied to physiologic parameters as well as to laboratory values. This is shown in drug-induced hypotension that has not yet resulted in end-organ damage (i.e., acute kidney injury [AKI] or a myocardial infarction).[6]

Adverse events can be classified as "preventable" or "non-preventable" as well as "potential."[1,5] An ME occurring with no patient injury is simply an ME. An ME that results in injury is a preventable ADE. The occurrence of an ADE without an ME is a non-preventable ADE. Non-preventable ADEs are more common than preventable ADEs.[1,5,7] An ME that has the opportunity for injury is defined as a "potential ADE." The classic example is a patient with a penicillin allergy who receives a penicillin antibiotic but has no reaction; thus, there is the potential for injury, but none has occurred. Potential ADEs may be intercepted.

The inconsistency surrounding the definition of an ADE versus that of an adverse drug reaction (ADR) is challenging to interpret, making comparisons between studies difficult. For some clinicians, a non-preventable ADE is considered synonymous with an ADR.[1,5] For others, an ADR is thought to be any unexpected, unintended, undesired, or excessive response that requires medical attention.[6,8,9] The relationship among these various terms is shown in Figure 49.1.[2]

Table 49.1 Definitions of Common Medication Safety Terms

Term	Definition
ME	A preventable incident leading to the misuse of a drug at any stage within the medication use process, regardless of whether harm occurred
ADE	Any patient injury attributed to medications
Drug-related hazardous condition	Antecedent to drug-induced injury and the opportunity for a pharmacist to intervene, thus preventing injury
Preventable ADE	Injury caused by an ME that could have been avoided
Non-preventable ADE (i.e., adverse drug reaction)	Injury caused by a drug without an ME occurring

ADE = adverse drug event; ME = medication error.

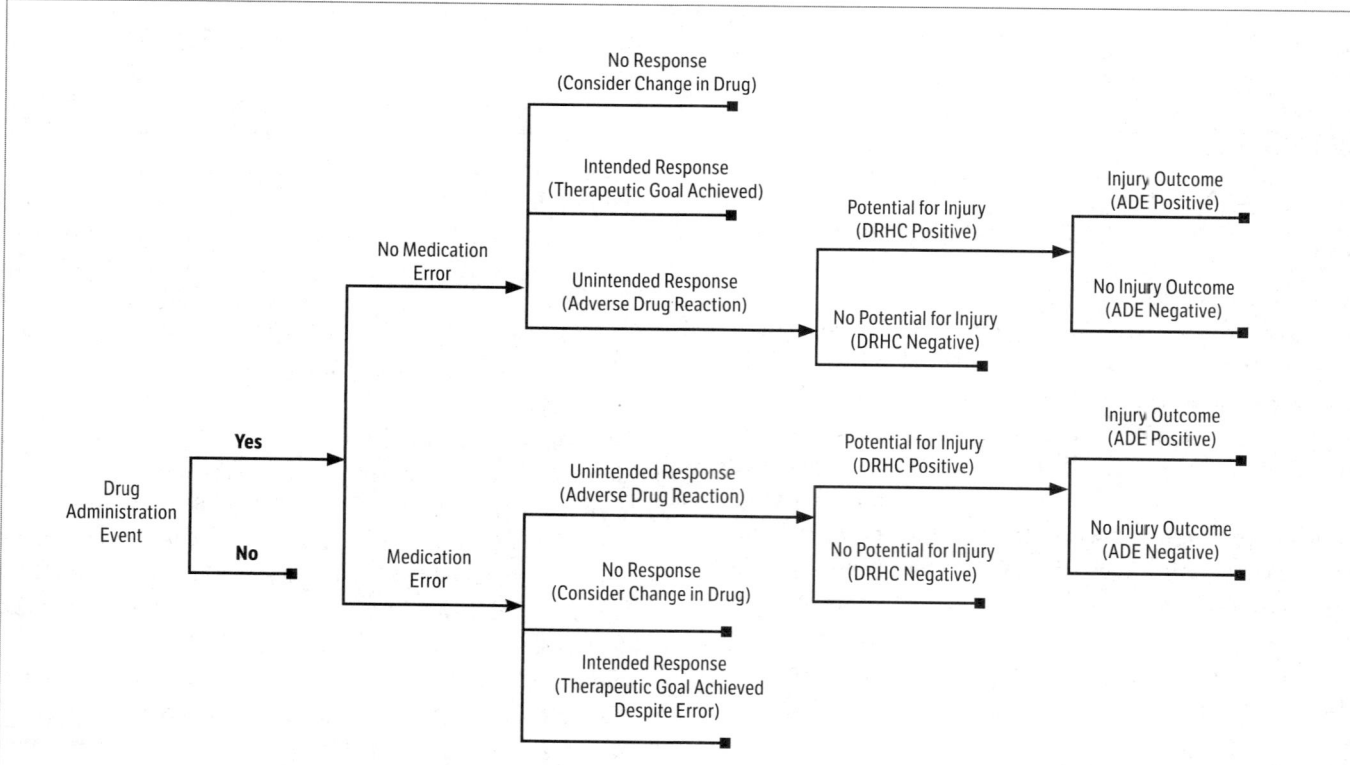

Figure 49.1 Relationship between medication errors and adverse drug events.
ADE = adverse drug event; DRHC = drug-related hazardous condition.
Reprinted by permission from Wolters Kluwer Health, Inc. Kane-Gill SL, Dasta JF, Schneider PJ, Cook CH. Monitoring abnormal laboratory values as antecedents to drug-induced injury. J Trauma 2005 Dec;59(6):1457-62.

Epidemiology of MEs and ADEs in the ICU

Medical errors and adverse events remain unacceptably high in the ICU, with drug therapy as one of the main causes.[7,10-12] Medication errors occur more commonly than ADEs. The reported rate of MEs in the critically ill population is highly variable, ranging from 1.2 to 947 events for every 1,000 patient-days, with a median rate of 105.9 errors for every 1,000 patient-days.[13] Differences in definitions, detection techniques, and specific ICU populations observed explain the wide variance in reported ME rates.[13] Medication errors are of concern because of the possibility of resultant injury, known as a preventable ADE.[1,2,13] The incidence of ADEs is about 2-fold higher in the ICU population than in the general ward population (19 vs. 10 events, respectively, for every 1,000 patient-days).[14] However, the rate of ADEs is no different after adjusting for the number of medications. Adverse drug event rates in the ICU have been reported to occur in about one-third of patients at a rate as high 87.5 events for every 1,000 patient-days.[15-17]

The severity of ADEs is greater in the ICU than in the general ward. Cullen et al. found a higher rate of "life-threatening" consequences of ADEs in ICU patients than in non-ICU patients (26% vs. 11%, $p<0.001$).[14] No significant differences in the severity between medical and surgical ICUs were found.[14] Other studies have corroborated these findings, reporting that the overall greater harm occurs in the ICU than in the general ward populations (odds ratio [OR] 1.89, 1.62–2.17).[18,19] Medication errors resulting in ADEs causing permanent harm (OR 2.45, 1.17–5.13), requiring life-sustaining intervention (OR 2.91, 1.86–4.56), or causing death (OR 2.48, 1.18–5.19) were more likely to occur in the critically ill population.[18] Kane-Gill et al. found that a higher rate of MEs in the ICU than in the general ward resulted in temporary harm requiring intervention (10% vs. 4.4%) and interventions necessary to sustain life (1.7% vs. 0.8%).[19]

Prolonged hospitalization, increased patient morbidity, and an increased risk of mortality are negative consequences of ADE occurrences. Adverse drug events result in prolonged hospitalization more commonly in critically ill patients than in general ward patients.[19] An average difference of 20 days was seen for patients who had an ADE in the ICU compared with patients who had an ADE in the general ward (37.5 vs. 17.3 days, respectively; $p<0.001$).[14] For patients in the ICU who had an ADE compared with those who did not, the hospital length of stay increased by 1.5–2 times, a finding that was consistent for medical and surgical ICU patients.[15,20,21] In addition, the ICU length of stay incrementally increased with the number of ADEs experienced by the patient.[22] In one report, the length of stay in the ICU for critically ill patients experiencing an ADE increased by about 3.5 days,[21] and in another report, the length of stay increased by 2.38 days for every ADE.[22] One meta-analysis found that the ICU length of stay for subjects with an ADE increased by 6.7 days compared with subjects without any ADEs.[10] Although the costs associated with ADEs specifically in the ICU are unknown, the estimated economic impact is substantial. One study evaluating ADEs associated with only intravenous medications in ICU patients at an academic hospital found an increased cost of $6,647.[23] Furthermore, total hospital expenditures after an ADE in the ICU compared with expenditures in the non-ICU have been shown to be similar ($36,204 vs. $26,391, respectively, $p=0.22$).[14] The crude mortality rate is significantly higher in hospitalized patients with an ADE than in hospitalized patients without an ADE (3.5% vs. 1.1%, $p<0.001$, respectively).[24] Fortunately, the risk of death attributed to MEs in ICU patients is reported to be less than 5%.[18,25-27]

Systems Analysis of ADEs in the ICU

The medication use process system has been divided into several nodes, including the ordering, transcribing/documenting, distributing, administering, and monitoring phases.[28] Implementing safe medication practices to avoid or minimize the risk of a patient's having a preventable ADE depends on understanding the proximal causes and system failures that occur at each of these phases.[13] Identifying all the factors leading to MEs and preventable ADEs at each of these phases enables institutions to develop strategies to improve safe medication use. Development of the technology used in health care today has evolved around an understanding of the system failures within the medication use process. In general, error reduction at the medication administration node has been a common target for improving patient safety because it is the final stage of the medication use process before the patient receives the medication and therefore lacks review by other health care professionals to potentially intercept the error. Smart pump infusion and barcode medication administration technologies focus on the administration phase to ensure that medications are delivered safely and accurately. Other technologies such as computerized physician order entry focus on the prescribing stage to eliminate errors associated with illegible handwriting and missing information (e.g., medication route). Unfortunately, use of technology alone does not eliminate all proximal causes and may in fact introduce different factors that lead to preventable ADEs such as workflow workarounds or not using the technology as intended. Therefore, institutions must evaluate each of the process nodes for continuous process improvement because solutions may target various process nodes.

Several studies have evaluated the MEs and ADEs occurring at each stage of the medication use process in ICU patients. One study using a direct observation technique found that the rate of preventable ADEs was highest in the prescribing phase (77%), followed by the administration phase (23%).[25] Although no ADEs were identified in the transcription and distribution stages, several potential ADEs were intercepted at the administration node. A prospective, multicenter study evaluated preventable ADEs identified by two methods. Pharmacists observed prescribing and transcription orders during patient care rounding, and a study physician coordinator solicited reports from health care professionals for all aspects of the medication use process. The investigators reported ADE events by the medication use process node: prescribing (62.5%), administration (33.3%), transcription (4.1%), and dispensing (0%).[27] By contrast, a subgroup analysis of ICU patients in the ADE Prevention Study, a prospective study that identified ADEs using solicited and self-reported incidents and chart review, found the most common node of ADEs and potential ADEs to be the administration phase (44%), followed by the prescribing phase (38%).[14] These studies show that although preventable ADEs may occur at any stage of the medication use process, medication ordering and administration remain the highest-risk stages. However, the rate of errors at each medication process node may vary depending on the technology (e.g., computerized physician order entry, smart infusion pumps) available at an institution; thus, contemporary rates may be different. The proximal causes leading to these MEs are different between these two stages. Lack of drug knowledge, lack of communication, and inadequate monitoring have been determined as the underlying causes contributing to MEs in the ordering phase, whereas memory lapses and inappropriate techniques are common during the administration phase.[25,27] An improvement strategy depends on the process node as well as on the factors identified as contributing to preventable ADEs. Therefore, it is imperative that health care institutions evaluate system failures at each of these process nodes to identify sustainable improvement strategies.

ICU Population at Greater Risk

Critically ill patients are at a higher risk of having an ADE than are non-ICU patients.[14] Factors contributing to this increased risk have been correlated with the complexity of the patients, medications, and environment in an ICU setting (Table 49.2).[20,29,30] Patient-specific characteristics such as advanced age or prolonged hospitalizations increase the risk of an ADE.[20,29,30] A cross-sectional study identified 230 ADEs in 79 ICU patients. Severity of illness was found to be a risk factor for patients having an ADE. The mean SOFA (Sequential Organ Failure Assessment) score for patients with an ADE was significantly higher than for patients without an ADE (10 vs. 8, respectively, p<0.001).[31] Other possible risk factors for an ADE were patients requiring mechanical ventilation and those with renal dysfunction, continuous sedation, or vasoactive support.[31] Furthermore, a retrospective case-control study of ICU patients at an academic medical institution found that the highest risk of an ADE was in patients with AKI (OR 16.2, 8.13–32.28), followed by thrombocytopenia (platelet count less than 100,000 mm^3) (OR 2.93, 1.56–5.48) and emergency admissions (OR 2.04, 1.04–4.00).[20]

The number and complexity of medications used in the ICU is also a major risk factor leading to increased MEs and ADEs. The Institute for Safe Medication Practices defines a "high-alert" medication as an agent carrying an increased risk of causing patient harm when used erroneously.[20] These are medications with complex dosing strategies, narrow therapeutic indices, and unique administration techniques and medications that require intense monitoring to ensure safe and effective use.[20] Therapeutic drug classes commonly associated with MEs and ADEs include cardiovascular agents, anticoagulants, sedatives, and antimicrobials.[20,27,29-31] High-risk medications are a risk factor for adverse event development, with as much as a 3 times greater odds of developing an ADE with each additional high-risk medication.[16,20] A multicenter, observational study of medical ICUs among three academic medical facilities did not observe that "off-label" medication use alone was a risk factor for an ADR.[16] However, the ADR rate increased by 8% for each additional medication used in an "off-label" manner.[16] Parenteral drugs and the number of high-risk medications administered are also independent risk factors for MEs and ADEs in the ICU.[20,26] Critically ill patients are more commonly exposed to intravenous medications and prescribed more drugs than are general ward patients.[14]

The fast-paced nature and complexity of critical care services provided are variables possibly leading to errors and adverse events. A potential relationship between nursing resources and adverse events exists.[31] Seynaeve et al. completed a retrospective chart review looking at specific drug triggers and found that patients with at least one ADE had a significantly higher nursing workload and activities than did those without an ADE (p=0.002).[31] Furthermore, any lack of communication among health care providers involved in the care of the ICU patient may pose the risk of an ME or ADE.[5,29] Several providers are often involved in the care of critically ill patients, which may be a challenge when integrating seamless care among all healthcare providers.[5,29] Physician staffing models and work hours in the ICU are another important factor that may increase the risk of errors.[32]

Common ADEs

Several medications are implicated in the development of ADEs commonly experienced by the critically ill patient. Thrombocytopenia may occur in more than 50% of ICU patients, and up to 25% of these cases are reported to have drug-induced causes.[33] Several medications are implicated in the development of thrombocytopenia (Table 49.3). Heparin is the most common agent associated with drug-induced thrombocytopenia in critically ill patients. About 10%–20% of patients on heparin may experience the nonimmune-mediated reaction of heparin with no significant clinical sequelae, despite therapy continuation. Although the incidence of immune-mediated heparin-induced thrombocytopenia is lower (1%), about 30%–80% of these patients develop a thromboembolic event.[33] Several antibiotics commonly used in ICU patients, including, but not limited to, -lactams, linezolid, and vancomycin, have been associated with thrombocytopenia. Linezolid, with an incidence of about 2%, potentially carries a higher risk than other antibiotics. In postmarketing surveillance, the incidence increases to 5% in patients receiving more than 14 days of therapy.[33] Of interest, one post hoc analysis from two prospective, randomized, multicenter studies evaluated the risk of thrombocytopenia in patients treated with linezolid for nosocomial pneumonia.[34] In this study, the incidence of thrombocytopenia in the linezolid group was low and not significantly different from that in the vancomycin group (2.8% and 3.6%, respectively).

Acute kidney injury is another common adverse event seen with commonly used medications in the ICU.[35] The incidence of drug-induced AKI is about 20%–30% in ICU patients and may be as high as 60% in older adult patients. An extensive list of medications is associated with AKI (Table 49.3). The incidence of aminoglycoside-induced AKI exceeds 50% in the ICU, although according to estimates that are more conservative, the incidence is 10%–20%.[36] Drug-induced AKI from amphotericin B is reported to be as high as 80%, although the true incidence may vary depending on the prevention strategies used.[35] Identifying drug-induced causes is difficult because most ICU patients have other factors possibly contributing to AKI. Moreover, the variability in definitions of AKI used in these reports may influence the true incidence.

Oversedation and hypotension associated with sedatives are also common in ICU patients. Several studies show that a high proportion of the ICU patients who require continuous sedation are oversedated. One observational study identified that about 41%–57% of ICU patients were sedated deeper than they should have been, depending on the day the sedation assessment was completed, and another investigation found that about 30% of ICU patients were unresponsive.[37-39] Several causes contribute to sedating an ICU patient deeper than the clinician's goal level. The lack of a sedation protocol targeting light sedation levels and the nonadherence to such protocols in institutions with already established sedation protocols may be reasons contributing to oversedation.[37] Another reason may be that the critical care clinician is not considering the pharmacokinetic/pharmacodynamic properties of these agents in patients with renal and/or hepatic dysfunction, as well as obesity. Another common ADE associated with sedation is hypotension.[6,40] The incidence is variable, depending on the specific agent evaluated and the definition used.

Drug-induced bleeding attributed to anticoagulants and thrombolytics remains a serious concern in the critically ill population. Prophylactic low-molecular-weight heparin has been shown to cause bleeding in 10%–25% medical-surgical ICU patients, with about 5% of the cases considered major bleeding.[41] A prospective, multicenter trial compared thromboprophylaxis with low-dose unfractionated heparin to dalteparin in 3,746 ICU patients.[42] Intention-to-treat analysis found no significant differences between heparin and dalteparin for any bleeding (13.2% vs. 13.0%, respectively; p=0.93) or major bleeding (5.6% vs. 5.5%, respectively; p=0.98). Major bleeding from prophylactic low-molecular-weight heparin in trauma patients is about 0.8%–3.5%, with up to 19% of patients having some type of bleeding when low-molecular-weight heparin is initiated within 48 hours after injury.[41] Therapeutic anticoagulation and its associated risk of bleeding is lacking specifically in the ICU population, although the rate of any bleeding has been estimated to be 5%–20%.[41] The incidence of major bleeding attributed to thrombolytic use for pulmonary embolism varies. Some randomized controlled trials showed no major bleeding events, whereas others found rates approaching 30%.[41] Analyses of pooled data from these trials found major bleeding rates from thrombolytics to be 9.1%, and some bleeding occurred in 22.7%.[43]

Table 49.2 Risk Factors Associated with Medication Errors and Adverse Drug Events in the ICU

Category	Potential Risk Factor
Patient related	Severity of illness
	Length of stay
	Advanced age
	Acute kidney injury
	Thrombocytopenia
	Type of admission
	Number of interventions/procedures
Medication related	"High-alert" drug use
	Number of drugs
	Type of medication used (e.g., cardiovascular, antimicrobial)
	Complexity of administration (e.g., intravenous, intrathecal)
	Requires intense monitoring
ICU environment related	Provider knowledge and training
	Sleep deprivation
	Inadequate staffing
	Lack of communication

ICU = intensive care unit.

Unfortunately, the true incidence of these common ADEs remains unknown. These ADEs are often multifactorial in complex ICU patients with several comorbidities, so pinpointing the cause to a specific medication remains a challenge. Furthermore, these rates may vary depending on the agent, dose, and definition used for these ADEs in published reports. Most studies evaluating the incidence of ADEs used expert evaluation of incidents to determine whether an ADE occurred. Use of pharmacovigilance algorithms (e.g., Naranjo, Kramer, Jones) may help improve the ability to determine the causality of a drug-induced ADE in critically ill patients.[44] Strategies used in managing the ADE beyond supportive care may largely depend on the severity of the ADE and the extent of complications experienced by the patient. The first step typically includes discontinuing the suspected medication, identifying an alternative drug, and determining the benefit-risk ratio of continuing the suspected agent. A reduction in the dose of the suspected or known medication may alleviate some ADEs as well.

ACTIVE SURVEILLANCE

As pharmacists, we need to be the leaders in the active surveillance of MEs and ADEs. The ideal surveillance system is multifaceted, including both retrospective and prospective approaches (Table 49.4).[45] Retrospective surveillance allows events to be detected after they have already occurred and often after the patient is discharged from the hospital. The advantage to retrospective surveillance is the compilation of data that allow for rigorous and structured evaluation (i.e., a root-cause analysis) to prevent future events. Prospective surveillance is completed in real time or as close to real time as possible, often affording the opportunity for intervention and prevention of an ADE or mitigation of ADE severity. Furthermore, retrospective and prospective surveillance can be categorized into targeted and non-targeted chart review. Non-targeted chart review requires a comprehensive review of the patient's medical record to investigate the details of an event. Targeted chart review entails a review of a targeted section of the patient's medical record or a review of a medical record for a targeted patient. Retrospective and prospective surveillance will be discussed in detail.

Retrospective Surveillance

Retrospective surveillance with non-targeted chart review is the most comprehensive approach to event detection with no selectivity or boundaries. Clearly, the disadvantage is the laborious nature of this approach and the resources necessary to execute such a project. More realistically, patients are randomly selected in a specified time interval (i.e., 20 charts each month) and are possibly representative of a specified patient population (i.e., ICU patients).[46] Another consideration is the need to adequately train those reviewing the charts so that the criteria for consistency can be established. The advantage to this comprehensive, non-targeted chart review is that it detects more events than do other methods of detection, and often, events are representative of those occurring at various stages of the medication use process.[47] A study comparing a comprehensive non-targeted chart review with a prospective trigger method identified 398 actual ADEs and 275 actual ADEs, respectively, and only 76 events overlapped between surveillance methods.[48]

Retrospective targeted chart review that is focused on a specific section of a chart is usually accomplished through triggers. Triggers commonly include antidote medications, abnormal laboratory values, and abnormal serum concentrations.[49] Systems to identify patients receiving antidote medications include reporting the financial records for patients who received an antidote medication using the pharmacy information technology system or tracking patients with a financial transaction for an antidote medication using automated dispensing cabinet reports. Abnormal laboratory data would be tracked using the institution's electronic medical record. The Institute for Healthcare Improvement (IHI) recommends 13 triggers for surveillance in its current medication module, and most triggers are used for detecting severe events.[50] Triggers can be used in a manual format (e.g., pharmacist review) or an automated format; both formats have been used with success.[51] The success of a retrospective chart

Table 49.3 Medications Associated with Common Adverse Drug Events

Adverse Drug Event	Medication and Drug Classes
Thrombocytopenia	Heparin and low-molecular-weight heparins
	Histamine-2 receptor antagonists
	Glycoprotein IIb/IIIa inhibitors
	Valproic acid
	Antibiotics (linezolid, β-lactams)
	β-Lactam
Acute kidney injury	Nonsteroidal anti-inflammatory drugs
	Angiotensin-converting enzyme inhibitors and angiotensin receptor blockers
	Calcineurin inhibitors
	Aminoglycosides
	Amphotericin B
	Radiocontrast media

Table 49.4 Description of the Methods of Detection for Prospective and Retrospective Surveillance

Methods of Detection	Description
Incidence reports	• Voluntary reports by health care professionals • Applied to retrospective and prospective surveillance, but real-time intervention with prospective surveillance is a challenge without a timely review and dedicated resources
Non-targeted chart review	• Comprehensive review of a patient's medical record to investigate the details of an event • Applied to retrospective and prospective surveillance, but real-time intervention with prospective surveillance is a challenge without a timely review and dedicated resources

Targeted chart review	• A review of a targeted section of the patient's medical record or a review of a medical record for a targeted patient
	• Applied to the both retrospective and prospective surveillance, but the approach may vary
	• Retrospective approaches include:
	  ○ Section of the chart (i.e., discharge summary)
	  ○ Administrative data
	  ○ Triggers
	• Prospective approach includes:
	  ○ Triggers

Direct observation	• View nurses' administration of medications with detailed documentation of the entire activity by a trained observer, and the data are later evaluated for medication errors • Applied as prospective surveillance because observed in real time but evaluated later for errors, so immediate patient intervention does not occur
Patient/family communication	• Patient and family engagement to report events • Application to prospective surveillance would be ideal and would allow an opportunity for intervention with sufficient resources
Pharmacist surveillance	• Pharmacist participation in and surveillance of drug ordering and monitoring • Applied to prospective surveillance and allows for real-time intervention

review surveillance method is measured by the number and type of events detected relative to other detection methods. Retrospective targeted chart review has consistently identified more ADEs in the ICU than have voluntary incident reports. For example, a retrospective targeted chart review of five antidote medications identified 77 events, none of which were voluntarily reported and only seven of which were identified with administrative data.[52] Although more events have been identified with a comprehensive chart review, a targeted approach identifies different events, and in fact, the overlap between targeted and non-targeted review is small, 11% for every one evaluation.[51] In addition, a retrospective targeted chart review using IHI triggers has shown utility in identifying ADEs in the ICU at 228 ADEs for every 1,000 patient-days or one ADE for every four admissions.[31,53]

To optimize the triggers used for a retrospective review, triggers should be evaluated for their performance. A performance characteristic quantifies how well the trigger performs at identifying an ADE. Performance characteristics are reported as the number needed to alert, positive predictive value (PPV), negative predictive value, sensitivity, and specificity.[49,54] The performance of five antidote triggers for detecting ADEs in a medical ICU was as low as a PPV of 0.02 for methylprednisolone and as high as a PPV of 0.52 for sodium polystyrene.[52] Of importance, performance characteristics of triggers may be expected to vary by patient care environment and should be tested for each. A trigger such as corticosteroids may be less specific for an ADE with a lower PPV in the ICU than in a non-ICU because there may be greater use for corticosteroids in the ICU. Little work has been done to compare performance characteristics of triggers between ICU and non-ICUs, and of the work done so far, no aberrant differences have been noted, but more triggers need to be considered.[55] Another consideration on trigger performance variation is the use of triggers for retrospective or prospective ADE detection because the retrospective approach may have more definitive objective data to analyze at the time of the trigger evaluation.[44]

Retrospective targeted chart reviews can be focused on specific patients or sections of the chart that are not prompted by a trigger. For example, there may be a need to target all ICU patients or to target patients receiving a specific drug or drug class (i.e., opioids). A priority patient population, such as older adults, may be of interest to your institution, thus generating the need for additional surveillance of these patients. Targeted chart review for specific populations could include tracking administrative data or ICD-9 codes for ADEs known as E-Codes.[56] In addition, surveillance could include a retrospective chart review for an evaluation of the section of the chart on the day of transfer from an ICU to a non-ICU; this would be a targeted population and a targeted section of the chart. A review of the transfer summary revealed many more ADEs that occurred in the ICU than in hospital discharge summaries.[57,58]

The type of surveillance that most institutions rely on are incident reports.[59] Unfortunately, only a small number of events are reported by hospital staff using incident reporting.[48,60] Incident reports can be a type of retrospective targeted chart review, but many institutions do not conduct a chart review for incident reports. Moreover, with minimal investigation performed, the reports are only taken at face value and therefore do not qualify as targeted chart review. However, incident reports are still considered retrospective surveillance. Ideally, to maximize the benefit of incident reports, some investigation for a root cause should be conducted. Federal regulations mandate the reporting of serious events to the state.[61] In addition, the Joint Commission has minimum requirements for incident reporting of sentinel events to this organization.[62] Incident reports can detect events across the gamut of the medication use process. This method of surveillance is one of the least expensive approaches; however, it consistently detects fewer events than other methods because of poor reporting by health care professionals.[45] Institutions that rely on incident reports for the sole source of event detection should try to maximize reporting. Make it as easy as possible by streamlining the process, using automation, providing feedback for reported events, using incentives, and ensuring a no-blame policy.

Prospective Surveillance

Prospective surveillance is usually done in a targeted manner using trigger alerts from clinical decision support (CDS) as the impetus for event investigation. Alerts can be applied manually, or they can be automated.[51] Clinical decision support is a type of health information technology that "provides clinicians, staff, patients or other individuals with knowledge and person-specific information, intelligently filtered or presented at appropriate times, to enhance health and health care."[63] Clinical decision support using alerts as a trigger to initiate a targeted chart review will be discussed by (1) CDS during the prescriber order entry, (2) CDS during order verification, and (3) CDS for monitoring.

Clinical decision support used to generate alerts during the order entry process are provided to the prescriber. Although these may be used as an impetus to initiate a targeted chart review of limited data (e.g., weight, other drug orders, laboratory values), they are also used as a prevention tool to reduce the number of MEs associated with inappropriate prescribing. Pharmacists are often engaged in developing alerts with a diverse team of health care professionals and information technology team members to determine the rules or signals for the alerts. Several examples of signals for alerts during the order entry process include ordering a total daily dose of morphine in a patient older than 65 years that exceeds the institution's limits, ordering a nephrotoxic agent in a patient with a rising serum creatinine concentration, or ordering an epidural medication in a patient receiving an anticoagulant. The alert can have a range of actions, from passive with a simple notification to a hard stop that will prevent the prescriber from continuing the order for possible impending patient harm. Clinical decision support of this type has been useful in reducing MEs from inappropriate prescribing, reducing the timeliness of medication therapy change or discontinuation, and reducing progression to ADEs.[51,64]

Clinical decision support used to generate alerts during the order verification process originates from homegrown systems and vendor systems. These alerts are still focused on the errors in the prescribing stage of the medication use process. The example most familiar to pharmacists is drug-drug interaction alerts. When pharmacists receive an alert for a possible drug-drug interaction, they are expected to investigate the patient's chart—at minimum, the patient's electronic medication administration record—to assess the need for an intervention to prevent an ADE.

Alerts occurring during order verification or prescribing run the risk of substantial alert fatigue. Alert fatigue occurs when a clinician is exposed to several alerts, both true positives and false negatives, and the clinician becomes desensitized to the alerts over time. Reduction in alert fatigue for drug-drug interactions has been tried by refining alerts to avoid signal-to-noise ratio, deploying only alerts that are considered serious events (i.e., a tiered approach), incorporating end-user opinion in developing alerts, and developing rules according to specific patient populations, such as those in the ICU.[55-67]

Clinical decision support used to generate alerts for drugs during the monitoring stage will be discussed in two categories: (1) alerts that use laboratory values and (2) alerts that use antidote medications as the signal. These alerts, when used for prospective surveillance, can prevent patient harm if identified quickly enough.[68,69] If a patient with moderate renal dysfunction has an elevated potassium of 5.7 mEq/L from using a potassium-sparing diuretic and the patient is asymptomatic, an alert can be generated at the intermediate step before the occurrence of patient harm (i.e., an arrhythmia). This CDS intermediate step is a DRHC. If the alert does not generate until this patient's potassium concentration is 6.8 mEq/L and the patient is having a cardiac arrhythmia, the opportunity to intervene and mitigate the progression of ADEs with prospective surveillance has been missed. At this point, the emphasis is on ADE management, not prevention. Several laboratory values have been used as the signal for alerts, including electrolytes, international normalized ratio, partial thromboplastin time, and drug concentrations. Alerts using laboratory values require some sophistication to optimize alert performance and reduction in alert fatigue. Laboratory-based alerts were initially designed using a specific value with a broad investigation for drug-related causes. Laboratory-based alerts have become more advanced, with signals/rules that generate the alert for a specified abnormal laboratory value only for a patient who is receiving a drug that is associated with the abnormal laboratory value.[48,70] In addition, laboratory rule performance can be improved by altering the criteria for the signal with drug-induced thrombocytopenia; this may mean changing the signal from a drop in the platelet count of less than 100,000/mm^3 to an absolute decrease in the platelet count of greater than 50%, hence changing the PPV from 0.36 to 0.83.[70] Of note, improving specificity can affect sensitivity. Using antidote medications for ADE prevention is a little more complicated because the antidote can be administered after patient harm has already occurred. Antidote medication alerts for prevention will require dedicated resources, allowing for prompt investigation and a rapid response team approach for timely interventions. Antidote medications that have been used include naloxone and dextrose 50%.[71]

Other types of monitoring alerts that have been studied relatively less commonly are errors of omission and drug-induced physiologic responses. Agents with narrow therapeutic ranges, including heparin and warfarin, require consistent monitoring; thus, infrequent monitoring or lack of timely monitoring may be an opportunity to generate an alert to ensure safe medication use. Monitoring of drug-associated physiologic abnormalities has been evaluated even less commonly. This requires a CDS that is integrated with the electronic medical record and that can capture the physiologic monitoring in real time. This CDS system can be applied to episodes of drug-induced hypotension in the ICU.[6]

The success of CDS for prospective surveillance can be measured by ME reduction, ADE reduction, number of interventions, and number of interventions that are considered clinically significant.[49,55,71] Consistency in measuring these outcomes will require precise and predetermined definitions. In addition, the performance characteristics of each alert can be measured with alert refinement that is applied accordingly for improvement. This evaluation process will likely require a committed quality improvement program.

In addition to categorizing surveillance by the type of chart review, prospective surveillance by other methods is possible, including direct observation; interviews of patients, families/caregivers, or health care professionals; and pharmacist participation in patient care (rounds and telemedicine). It is most challenging to identify errors during the administration stage in the medication use process. Surveillance requires direct observation to effectively identify errors. Direct observation is the viewing of nurses administering medications and the provision of detailed documentation of the entire activity by a trained observer. This documentation is later evaluated for MEs by comparing the nurse's activities with the prescriber's orders, the institution's policies, and drug information resources.[72,73] Therefore, direct observation allows for prospective surveillance because it is completed in real time, but the goal of this method is not to intervene in patient care at that moment. Direct observation has been effectively applied to the ICU.[25,74,75] Engaging patients and their families in patient care is highly encouraged. Asking the patient about the occurrence of ADEs is a surveillance method that has been effectively applied to settings other than the ICU.[76,77] Finally, pharmacist participation in ICU patient care for ME and ADE prevention has been evaluated in several studies. In one study, a critical care pharmacist reviewing medication orders for patients admitted to the ICU resulted in a significant reduction in prescribing errors and preventable ADEs.[78] Pharmacists' proactive medication recommendations often result in the addition of a drug if an error of omission occurs.[79] The classic and well-designed study by Leape and colleagues showed that a pharmacist's participation in patient care rounds reduced ADEs by 66%.[80]

Overall, the best surveillance system will include both retrospective and prospective evaluations, with the goal of preventing ADEs for prospective surveillance. The retrospective surveillance will require many methods for identifying the most events because different methods detect different events. Including automation, whenever possible, may more efficiently use resources. It is important to have a process in place that allows for the assessment of the retrospective surveillance data to make future systematic improvements. To ensure the optimal performance of the surveillance system, monitoring through a quality improvement program is essential.

REFERENCES

1. Morimoto T, Gandhi TK, Seger AC, et al. Adverse drug events and medication errors: detection and classification methods. Qual Saf Health Care 2004;13:306-14.

2. Kane-Gill SL, Dasta JF, Schneider PJ, et al. Monitoring abnormal laboratory values as antecedents to drug-induced injury. J Trauma 2005;59:1457-62.

3. National Coordinating Council for Medication Error Reporting and Prevention. 2015. What Is a Medication Error? Available at www.nccmerp.org/about-medication-errors. Accessed March 30, 2015.

4. Bates DW, Boyle DL, Vander Vliet MB, et al. Relationship between medication errors and adverse drug events. J Gen Intern Med 1995;10:199-205.

5. Kane-Gill SL, Jacobi J, Rothschild JM. Adverse drug events in intensive care units: risk factors, impact, and the role of team care. Crit Care Med 2010;38(suppl):S83-89.

6. Kane-Gill SL, LeBlanc JM, Dasta JF, et al.; Critical Care Pharmacotherapy Network. A multicenter study of the point prevalence of drug-induced hypotension in the ICU. Crit Care Med 2014;42:2197-203.

7. Rothschild JM, Landrigan CP, Cronin JW, et al. The Critical Care Study: the incidence and nature of adverse events and serious medical errors in intensive care. Crit Care Med 2005;33:1694-700.

8. American Society of Health-System Pharmacists. ASHP Guidelines on Adverse Drug Reaction Monitoring and Reporting. Available at www.ashp.org/DocLibrary/BestPractices/MedMisGdlADR.aspx. Accessed May 24, 2015.

9. World Health Organization. Definitions. Available at www.who.int/medicines/areas/quality_safety/safety_efficacy/trainingcourses/definitions.pdf. Accessed May 24, 2015.

10. Ahmed AH. Outcome of adverse events and medical errors in the intensive care unit: a systematic review and meta-analysis. Am J Med Qual 2015;30:23-30.

11. Valentin A, Capuzzo M, Guidet B, et al. Patient safety in intensive care: results from the multinational Sentinel Events Evaluation (SEE) study. Intensive Care Med 2006;32:1591-8.

12. Garrouste-Orgeas M, Timsit JF, Vesin A, et al. Selected medical errors in the intensive care unit: results of the IATROREF study: parts I and II. Am J Respir Crit Care Med 2010;181:134-42.

13. Kane-Gill SL, Weber RJ. Principles and practices of medication safety in the ICU. Crit Care Clin 2006;22:273-90.

14. Cullen DJ, Sweitzer BJ, Bates DW, et al. Preventable adverse drug events in hospitalized patients: a comparative study of intensive care and general care units. Crit Care Med 1997;25:1289-97.

15. Park S, In Y, Suh GY, et al. Evaluation of adverse drug reactions in medical intensive care units. Eur J Clin Pharmacol 2013;69:119-31.

16. Smithburger PL, Buckley MS, Culver MA, et al. A multicenter evaluation of off-label medication use and associated adverse drug reactions in adult medical ICUs. Crit Care Med 2015 Apr 8. [Epub ahead of print]

17. Colpaert K, Claus B, Somers A, et al. Impact of computerized physician order entry on medication prescription errors in the intensive care unit: a controlled cross-sectional trial. Crit Care 2006;10:R21.

18. Latif A, Rawat N, Pustavoitau A, et al. National study on the distribution, causes, and consequences of voluntary reported medication errors between the ICU and non-ICU settings. Crit Care Med 2013;41:389-98.

19. Kane-Gill SL, Kowiatek JG, Weber RJ. A comparison of voluntarily reported medication errors in intensive care and general care units. Qual Saf Health Care 2010;19:55-9.

20. Kane-Gill SL, Kirisci L, Verrico MM, et al. Analysis of risk factors for adverse drug events in critically ill patients. Crit Care Med 2012;40:823-8.

21. Vargas E, Terleira A, Hernando F, et al. Effect of adverse drug reactions on length of stay in surgical intensive care units. Crit Care Med 2003;31:694-8.

22. Vargas E, Simon J, Martin JC, et al. Effect of adverse drug reactions on length of stay in intensive care units. Clin Drug Invest 1998;15:353-60.

23. Nuckols TK, Paddock SM, Bower AG, et al. Costs of intravenous adverse drug events in academic and nonacademic intensive care units. Med Care 2008;46:17-24.

24. Classen DC, Pestotnik SL, Evans RS, et al. Adverse drug events in hospitalized patients. Excess length of stay, extra costs, and attributable mortality. JAMA 1997;277:301-6.

25. Kopp BJ, Erstad BL, Allen ME, et al. Medication errors and adverse events in an intensive care unit: direct observation approach for detection. Crit Care Med 2006;34:415-25.

26. Valentin A, Capuzzo M, Guidet B, et al. Errors in administration of parenteral drugs in intensive care units: multinational prospective study. BMJ 2009;338:b814.

27. Benkirane RR, R-Abouqal R, Haimeur CC, et al. Incidence of adverse drug events and medication errors in intensive care units: a prospective multicenter study. J Patient Saf 2009;5:16-22.

28. Leape LL, Bates DW, Cullen DJ, et al. Systems analysis of adverse drug events. ADE Prevention Study Group. JAMA 1995;274:35-43.

29. Moyen E, Camire E, Stelfox HT. Clinical review: medication errors in critical care. Crit Care 2008;12:208.

30. Camire E, Moyen E, Stelfox HT. Medication errors in critical care: risk factors, prevention and disclosure. CMAJ 2009;180:936-43.

31. Seynaeve S, Verbrugghe W, Claes B, et al. Adverse drug events in intensive care units: a cross-sectional study of prevalence and risk factors. Am J Crit Care 2011;20:e131-e140.

32. Landrigan CP, Rothschild JM, Cronin JW, et al. Effect of reducing interns' work hours on serious medical errors in intensive care units. N Engl J Med 2004;351:1838-48.

33. Priziola JL, Smythe MA, Dager WE. Drug-induced thrombocytopenia in critically ill patients. Crit Care Med 2010;38(suppl):S145-54.

34. Nasraway SA, Shorr AF, Kuter DJ, et al. Linezolid does not increase the risk of thrombocytopenia in patients with nosocomial pneumonia: comparative analysis of linezolid and vancomycin use. Clin Infect Dis 2003;11:1509-16.

35. Bentley ML, Corwin HL, Dasta J. Drug-induced acute kidney injury in the critically ill adult: recognition and prevention strategies. Crit Care Med 2010;38(suppl):S169-74.

36. Oliveira JF, Silva CA, Barbieri CD, et al. Prevalence and risk factors for aminoglycoside nephrotoxicity in intensive care units. Antimicrob Agents Chemother 2009;53:2887-91.

37. Devlin JW, Mallow-Corbett S, Riker RR. Adverse drug events associated with the use of analgesics, sedatives, and antipsychotics in the intensive care unit. Crit Care Med 2010;38(suppl):S231-43.

38. Payen JF, Chanques G, Mantz J, et al. Current practices in sedation and analgesia for mechanically ventilated critically ill patients: a prospective multicenter patient-based study. Anesthesiology 2007;106:687-95.

39. Weinert CR, Calvin AD. Epidemiology of sedation and sedation adequacy for mechanically ventilated patients in a medical and surgical intensive care unit. Crit Care Med 2007;35:393-401.

40. Jakob SM, Ruokonen E, Grounds M, et al. Dexmedetomidine vs midazolam or propofol for sedation during prolonged mechanical ventilation. JAMA 2013;307:1151-60.

41. Barletta JF, Cooper B, Ohlinger MJ. Adverse drug events associated with disorders of coagulation. Crit Care Med 2010;38(suppl):S198-S218.

42. Cook D, Meade M, Guyatt G, et al. Dalteparin versus unfractionated heparin in critically ill patients. N Engl J Med 2011;364:1305-14.

43. Wan S, Quinlan DJ, Agnelli G, et al. Thrombolysis compared with heparin for the initial treatment of pulmonary embolism: a meta-analysis of randomized controlled trials. Circulation 2004;110:744-9.

44. Kane-Gill SL, Forsberg EA, Verrico MM, et al. Comparison of three pharmacovigilance algorithms in the ICU setting: a retrospective and prospective evaluation of ADRs. Drug Saf 2013;35:645-53.

45. Stockwell DC, Kane-Gill SL. Developing a patient safety surveillance system to identify adverse events in the intensive care unit. Crit Care Med 2010;38(6 suppl):s117-25.

46. Rozich JD, Haraden CR, Resar RK. Adverse drug event trigger tool; a practical methodology for measuring medication related harm. Qual Saf Health Care 2003;12:194-200.

47. Olsen S, Neale G, Schwab K, et al. Hospital staff should use more than one method to detect adverse events and potential adverse events: incident reporting, pharmacist surveillance and local real-time record review may all have a place. Qual Saf Health Care 2007;16:40-4.

48. Jha AK, Kuperman GJ, Teich JM, et al. Identifying adverse drug events: development of computer-based monitor and comparison with chart review and stimulated voluntary report. J Am Med Inform Assoc 1998;5:305-14.

49. Handler SM, Altman RL Perera S, et al. A systematic review of the performance characteristics of clinical event monitor signals used to detect adverse drug events in the hospital setting. J Am Med Inform Assoc 2007;14:686.

50. Griffin FA, Resar RK. IHI Global Trigger Tool for Measuring Adverse Events (Second Edition). 2009. IHI Innovation Series White Paper. Cambridge, MA: Institute for Healthcare Improvement. Available at IHI.org. Accessed May 25, 2015.

51. Tawadrous D, Shariff SZ, Haynes RB, et al. Use of clinical decision support systems for kidney-related drug prescribing: a systematic review. Am J Kidney Dis 2011;58:903-14.

52. Kane-Gill SL, Bellamy CJ, Verrico MM, et al. Evaluating the positive predictive values of antidote signals to detect potential adverse drug reactions (ADRs) in the medical intensive care unit (ICU). Pharmacoepidemiol Drug Saf 2009;18:1185-91.

53. Carnevali L, Krug B, Amant F, et al. Performance of the adverse drug event trigger tool and the global trigger tool for identifying adverse drug events: experience in a Belgian hospital. Ann Pharmacother 2013;47:1414-9.

54. Moore C, Li J, Hung CC, et al. Predictive value of alert triggers for identification of developing adverse drug events. J Patient Saf 2009;5:223-8.

55. DiPoto JP, Buckley MS, Kane-Gill SL. Evaluation of an automated surveillance system using trigger alerts to prevent adverse drug events in the intensive care unit and general ward. Drug Saf 2015;38:311-7.

56. Kane-Gill SL, Van Den Bos J, Handler SM. Adverse drug reactions in the hospital and ambulatory care settings identified using a large administrative database. Ann Pharmacother 2010;44:983-93.

57. Anthes AM, Harinstein LM, Smithburger PL, et al. Improving adverse drug event detection in critically ill patients through screening intensive care unit transfer summaries. Pharmacoepidemiol Drug Saf 2013;22:510-6.

58. Murff HJ, Forster AJ, Petersen JF, et al. Electronically screening discharge summaries for adverse medical events. J Am Med Inform Assoc 2003;10:339-50.

59. Kane-Gill SL, Devlin JW. Adverse drug event reporting in the intensive care units: a survey of current practices. Ann Pharmacother 2006;40:1267-73.

60. Levinson DR. 2012. Hospital incident reporting systems do not capture most patient harm. Available at psnet.ahrq.gov/resource.aspx?resourceID=23842. Accessed August 11, 2015.

61. Patient Safety Authority. Pennsylvania Patient Safety Reporting System. 2015. Available at patientsafetyauthority.org/PA-PSRS/Pages/PAPSRS.aspx. Accessed June 1, 2015.

62. The Joint Commission. 2014. Sentinel Event Policy and Procedures. Available at www.jointcommission.org/Sentinel_Event_Policy_and_Procedures/default.aspx. Accessed June 1, 2015.

63. HealthIT.gov. Clinical Decision Support. 2013. Available at www.healthit.gov/policy-researchers-implementers/clinical-decision-support-cds. Accessed June 1, 2015.

64. Evans RS, Pestotnik SL, Classen DC, et al. Preventing adverse drug events in hospitalized patients. Ann Pharmacother 1994;28:523-7.

65. Hines LE, Malone DC, Murphy JE. Recommendations for generating, evaluating and implementing drug-drug interaction evidence. Pharmacotherapy 2012;32:304-13.

66. Paterno MD, Maviglia SM, Gorman PN, et al. Tiering drug-drug interaction alerts by severity increases compliance rates. J Am Med Inform Assoc 2009;16:40-6.

67. Smithburger PL, Buckley MS, Bejian S, et al. A critical evaluation of clinical decision support for the detection of drug-drug interactions. Expert Opin Drug Saf 2011;10:871-82.

68. Jha AK, Laguette J, Seger J, et al. Can surveillance systems identify and avert adverse drug events? A prospective evaluation of a commercial application. J Am Med Inform Assoc 2008;15:647-53.

69. Seger AC, Jha AK, Bates DW. Adverse drug event detection in a community hospital utilizing computerized medication and laboratory data. Drug Saf 2007;30:817-24.

70. Harinstein LM, Kane-Gill SL, Smithburger PL, et al. Use of an abnormal laboratory value-drug combination to detect drug-induced thrombocytopenia in critically ill patients. J Crit Care 2012;27:242-9.

71. Kane-Gill SL, Visweswaran S, Saul MI, et al. Computerized detection of adverse drug reactions in the medical intensive care unit. Int J Med Inform 2011;80:570-8.

72. Barker KN, Flynn EA, Pepper GA, et al. Medication errors observed in 36 health care facilities. Arch Intern Med 2002;162:1897-903.

73. Barker KN, Flynn EA, Pepper GA. Observation method of detecting medication errors. Am J Health Syst Pharm 2002;59:2314-6.

74. Ford DG, Seybert AL, Smithburger PL, et al. Impact of simulation-based learning on medication errors rates in critically ill patients. Intensive Care Med 2010;36;1526-31.

75. Buckley MS, Erstad BL, Kopp BJ, et al. Direct observation approach for detecting medication errors and adverse drug events in a pediatric intensive care unit. Pediatr Crit Care Med 2007;8:145-52.

76. Kaboli PJ, Glasgow JM, Jaipaul CK, et al. Identifying medication misadventures: poor agreement among medical record, physician, nurse, and patient reports. Pharmacotherapy 2010;30:529-38.

77. Van den Bemt PM, Egberts AC, Lenderink AW, et al. Adverse drug events in hospitalized patients. A comparison of doctors, nurses and patients as sources of reports. Eur J Clin Pharmacol 1999;55:155-8.

78. Klopotowska JE, Kupier R, vanKan HJ, et al. On-ward participation of a hospital pharmacist in a Dutch intensive care unit reduces prescribing errors and related patient harm: an intervention study. Crit Care 2010;14:R174.

79. Bourne RS, Choo CL. Pharmacist proactive medication recommendations using electronic documentation in a UK general care unit. Int J Clin Pharm 2012;34:351-7.

80. Leape LL, Cullen DJ, Clapp MD, et al. Pharmacist participation on physician rounds and adverse drug events in the intensive care unit. JAMA 1999;282:267-70.

Care of the Immunocompromised Patient

Heather Personett, Pharm.D., BCPS; and Simon W. Lam, Pharm.D., FCCM, BCPS

LEARNING OBJECTIVES

1. Design a plan for assessing and managing the prophylactic, empiric, and definitive use of antimicrobial regimens in patients with febrile neutropenia.
2. Identify risk factors for developing donor-derived infections, and determine appropriate antimicrobial therapy.
3. Recognize common reasons for intensive care unit admission and common medication issues among HIV-positive patients.
4. Devise a treatment strategy for managing treatment-experienced HIV-positive patients, including the management of common opportunistic infections.
5. Distinguish differences in the diagnosis and treatment of common noninfectious pulmonary complications occurring in immunocompromised patients.
6. Develop a therapeutic plan for tumor lysis syndrome prevention in a high-risk patient.
7. Recommend supportive care treatment for posterior reversible leukoencephalopathy associated with calcineurin inhibitors.

ABBREVIATIONS IN THIS CHAPTER

ANC	Absolute neutrophil count	NRTI	Nucleotide/nucleoside reverse transcriptase inhibitor
CNI	Calcineurin inhibitor		
DAH	Diffuse alveolar hemorrhage	OI	Opportunistic infection
FN	Febrile neutropenia	PCR	Polymerase chain reaction
GI	Gastrointestinal	PERDS	Peri-engraftment respiratory distress syndrome
HAART	Highly active antiretroviral therapy		
ICU	Intensive care unit	PJP	*Pneumocystis jiroveci* pneumonia
IgG	Immunoglobulin G	PRES	Posterior reversible leukoencephalopathy syndrome
IRIS	Immune reconstitution inflammatory syndrome		
		UA	Uric acid
MAC	*Mycobacterium avium* complex	TE	*Toxoplasma* encephalitis
		TLS	Tumor lysis syndrome

INTRODUCTION

Immune system suppression may occur as a result of the pathophysiology of illness or medications. Diseases such as hematologic malignancies, acute liver failure, or human immunodeficiency virus (HIV) leave hosts functionally immunocompromised, with both the adaptive and the innate immune systems unable to mount the same defensive response as in healthy individuals. Suppression of the immune system may lead to an increased incidence and severity of infections and malignancy. Conversely, a certain degree of immune system suppression may be desirable, in an effort to prevent the rejection of a transplanted organ by host defenses or end-organ damage in the setting of an autoimmune disorder. As both the mechanisms and the degrees of immunosuppression vary, so do the types of related complications. This chapter describes several common clinical challenges faced by pharmacists caring for the critically ill immunosuppressed patient.

INFECTIOUS COMPLICATIONS OF IMMUNOSUPPRESSION

Febrile Neutropenia

Febrile neutropenia (FN) is common, developing in upward of 50% of patients with solid tumors and 80% of patients with hematologic malignancy receiving myelosuppressive chemotherapy.[1] However, only 20%–30% of patients with FN episodes have clinically documented infections. In such patients, common sites of tissue-based infections include the gastrointestinal (GI) tract (enterocolitis, colorectal), lung, and skin and soft tissue. Bacteremia occurs in 10%–25% of patients.[2] Unexplained fevers are common and may arise from chemotherapy or medications commonly used in critically ill patients. In addition, receipt of blood products, withdrawal from opioids or other medications, and development of deep venous thrombosis may be reasons for fever among patients with FN. Even though most patients who develop FN have no identifiable site or microbiologic evidence of infection, all patients with FN, particularly those requiring intensive care, should receive empiric antimicrobials as soon as possible. The prompt initiation of antimicrobials for patients with FN has been correlated with improved patient outcomes.[3]

Definition

Despite the lack of studies evaluating the relative sensitivity and specificity of different definitions of FN, several guidelines provide general criteria as a starting point for identifying patients who may require antimicrobials. According to the Infectious Diseases Society of America and National Comprehensive Cancer Network guidelines, fever is defined as a single oral temperature of 101°F (38.3°C) or greater or a temperature of 100.4°F (38.0°C) or greater sustained for 1 hour. By the same guidelines, neutropenia is defined as an absolute neutrophil count (ANC) of less than 500 cells/mm^3 or an ANC that is less than 1,000 cells/mm^3 and expected to decrease to less than 500 cells/mm^3 during the next 48 hours.[2,4] The specific definitions for determining FN are general guidelines for clinicians. Therefore, given the considerable interpatient variability, clinical judgment is of paramount importance in identifying patients who may require antimicrobial treatment despite not meeting the traditional criteria for FN. For critically ill patients, particularly those with evidence of hemodynamic compromise, clinicians should be more liberal with the definitions of FN and have a higher inclination to provide early antimicrobial therapy. For instance, critically ill patients with neutropenia may be considered for antimicrobial therapy even when having low-grade temperatures that do not meet the traditional definitions of fever.

Risk Assessment

Because most patients with cancer admitted to an intensive care unit (ICU) are likely to have signs and symptoms of infection and require treatment, it is beyond the scope of this chapter to discuss the role of prophylaxis. Patients presenting with FN may have drastically different clinical courses, ranging from full recovery to life-threatening medical events. As such, characterizing a patient's risk of developing serious infectious complications has both prognostic and treatment implications. Those with the highest risk include individuals with significant medical comorbidity, clinical instability, profound neutropenia (ANC of 100 cells/mm^3 or less), anticipated prolonged neutropenia (7 days or more), evidence of organ dysfunctions, severe mucositis, or a Multinational Association for Supportive Care in Cancer Risk Index score less than 21 (see Table 50.1).

All patients requiring admission to the ICU likely fall within the high-risk category for developing serious complications. As such, these patients should be empirically treated with broad-spectrum intravenous antimicrobials and monitored closely. Laboratory tests should involve at least two sets of blood cultures, including one set from each existing lumen of a central venous catheter and peripheral vein site. Additional cultures should be sent if there is a suggestion of other sites of infection. Physical signs and symptoms of infections are usually diminished or absent in patients with FN; therefore, a heightened level of scrutiny and attention should be used when doing a physical examination to assess for different sites of infection.

Initial Empiric Antimicrobials

In high-risk patients, intravenous empiric antibacterial therapy with an antipseudomonal β-lactam such as cefepime, carbapenem (meropenem or imipenem/cilastatin), or piperacillin/tazobactam is recommended.[2,4] The dose and interval for these agents are often different from

Table 50.1 The MASCC Predictive Model for Risk of Complication in Patients with Febrile Neutropenia

Characteristics	Score
Burden of illness	
No symptoms or mild symptoms	5
Moderate symptoms	3
Severe symptoms	0
No hypotension (systolic blood pressure > 90 mm Hg)	5
No chronic obstructive pulmonary disease	4
Solid tumor or hematologic malignancy with no previous fungal infection	4
No dehydration requiring parenteral fluids	3
Outpatient status	3
Age < 60 yr	2

MASCC = Multinational Association of Supportive Care in Cancer.

Reproduced with permission from: Sylvester RK. Infections in patients with cancer. In: Schumock GT, Brundage DM, eds. Pharmacotherapy Self-Assessment Program, 5th ed. Book 10. Hematology/Oncology. Oncology I. Lenexa, KS: American College of Clinical Pharmacy, 2006:147-64.

those for non-neutropenic patients. See Table 50.2 for suggested doses of commonly used antimicrobials. For most hemodynamically stable patients, monotherapy with an antipseudomonal β-lactam is sufficient. However, for those with hemodynamic instability, consideration should be given to administering combination gram-negative therapy (e.g., aminoglycosides). In addition, an evaluation of local microbiologic epidemiology, resistance patterns, and patient history of colonization and prior infection should be done to determine whether additional or alternative therapies are necessary. Studies that have evaluated the addition of additional gram-negative agents to antipseudomonal β-lactams for the empiric treatment of FN have largely had equivocal results. In fact, a recent meta-analysis evaluating β-lactam monotherapy compared with the combination of aminoglycosides and β-lactams found higher rates of adverse events (nephrotoxicity), infection-related mortality, and fungal superinfections to be associated with combination therapy.[5] However, few of the studies within this meta-analysis specifically evaluated critically ill patients. Furthermore, in the non-neutropenic septic shock population, the receipt of combination therapy was associated with improved outcomes.[6] Taken together, it appears that combination gram-negative therapy should not be routinely recommended for patients with FN; however, it can be considered for patients with hemodynamic instability.

Vancomycin should also be considered as part of the initial empiric regimen for patients with FN having hemodynamic instability.[2] This is also true for patients with suspected serious catheter-related infection (e.g., chills, rigors, evidence of cellulitis around catheter site), soft tissue infection, and radiographic evidence of pneumonia. Similar to the studies evaluating aminoglycosides, adding additional gram-positive coverage to β-lactam monotherapy has not led to improved outcomes.[7] Hence, the routine use of vancomycin as part of the empiric regimen cannot be recommended. If vancomycin is initiated, therapy should be reassessed after 2 days and discontinued if a resistant gram-positive pathogen is not discovered.[2]

Table 50.2 Empiric Antibacterial Dosing for Febrile Neutropenia

Gram-Positive Agents	Dose	Comments/Precautions
Vancomycin	15 mg/kg IV q12hr[a]	• Dosing adjustments based on therapeutic drug monitoring
Daptomycin	6 mg/kg IV q24hr[a]	• Dose adjustments based on renal function
		• Not indicated for pneumonia (no lung penetration)
		• Weekly CPK monitoring
Linezolid	600 mg PO/IV q12hr	• May cause myelosuppression (usually after 2 weeks of therapy); therefore, not routinely used for neutropenic fever
Antipseudomonal β-lactams		
Cefepime	2 g IV q8hr[a]	
Ceftazidime	2 g IV q8hr[a]	• Minimal gram-positive activity
Imipenem/cilastatin	500 mg IV q6hr[a]	• May lower seizure threshold
Meropenem	2 g IV q8hr[a]	• Meropenem preferred to imipenem for CNS infection
Doripenem	500 mg IV q8hr[a]	• Doripenem has limited data in neutropenic fever
Piperacillin/tazobactam	4.5 g IV q6hr[a]	• Not recommended for suspected CNS infection
		• May result in false-positive galactomannan
Other Antibacterials		
Tobramycin	5–7 mg/kg q24hr[a]	• No gram-positive coverage
Gentamicin	5–7 mg/kg q24hr[a]	• To be used only in conjunction with β-lactams
Amikacin	15–20 mg/kg q24hr[a]	• Dosing adjustments based on therapeutic drug monitoring
Ciprofloxacin	400 mg IV q8hr	• To be used only in conjunction with β-lactams
Levofloxacin	750 mg IV q24hr	• Avoid use if patient used fluoroquinolone prophylaxis

[a]Dose adjustments for renal dysfunction may be needed.
CPK = creatinine phosphokinase; IV = intravenously; q = every.

Antimicrobial doses administered to patients with FN should be the maximum dose approved according to manufacturer labeling, after adjustments are made for baseline renal dysfunction. Optimizing pharmacodynamics is of critical importance in patients without their innate immune system to assist in combating an infection. There are suggestions in the literature that patients with FN may benefit from targeting pharmacodynamic goals that are more aggressive.[8] The importance of pharmacodynamic target attainment, implications of the lack of innate immune system, and known pharmacokinetic derangements seen in critically ill patients combine to warrant the use of aggressive antimicrobial dosing strategies (e.g., use of highest allowable dose, extended-interval aminoglycoside dosing). See the chapter on Pharmacokinetic/Pharmacodynamic Considerations for further discussions on this topic.

Modification and Therapy Duration

In general, modifications to the initial antibiotic regimen should be guided by clinical and microbiologic data. All critically ill patients with FN should be closely monitored for clinical response, adverse effects, and emergence of resistant infections. The median time to defervescence in patients with FN is usually about 5 days.[9] Hence, patients who are persistently febrile, but otherwise clinically stable, should not require alterations to the initial antimicrobial agents for the first 4–5 days. Specifically, adding vancomycin for persistently febrile patients within the first 3 days of their FN episode did not lead to a decreased time to defervescence.[10] In contrast, patients who develop clinical instability after receipt of initial empiric antibiotics should have their coverage broadened, potentially including a second gram-negative agent and vancomycin, if not initially started.

Patients who are persistently or recurrently febrile despite 4–7 days of broad-spectrum antibiotics should be considered for empiric antifungal therapy and should undergo further evaluation for the underlying cause of fever depending on patient symptoms (e.g., additional cultures, computed tomography [CT] scans, fungal antigen or serologic markers, *Clostridium difficile* toxin tests).[2] Empiric fungal coverage should use an agent with mold coverage (e.g., echinocandin, voriconazole, posaconazole, amphotericin). If a patient was previously receiving antifungal prophylaxis with one of those agents, an alternative with a different mechanism of action should be used. Of note, if patient was previously receiving a narrower-spectrum triazole (e.g., fluconazole), switching to a broader-spectrum triazole with mold coverage is appropriate. Although preemptive therapy, where antifungals are withheld until the patient has positive serologic assays, cultures, or radiographic findings, is an acceptable choice, it has never been evaluated in critically ill patients. Given the severity of illness in critically ill patients, it seems prudent to administer empiric antifungal therapy for those who are febrile for 4–7 days despite antibiotics. This is particularly true if the duration of neutropenia is anticipated to be prolonged (greater than 10 days).

Stable afebrile patients with microbiologically documented infection during their neutropenic episode should have their antimicrobial regimen narrowed to specifically cover the identified pathogen. The treatment duration for each type of infection is similar to what is recommended in non-neutropenic patients. However, therapy should be continued through the duration of neutropenia until the ANC recovers to greater than 500 cells/mm^3. For most patients without documented infections, the gram-negative therapy should continue until the resolution of both fevers and neutropenia, at minimum.[2]

Role of Hematopoietic Growth Factors

The use of hematopoietic growth factors, in conjunction with antimicrobials, for the treatment of FN is controversial. Studies have shown differences in surrogate outcomes (e.g., days of neutropenia, duration of fever, length of stay) with the use of hematopoietic growth factors; however, none has identified a mortality difference.[11,12] A recent meta-analysis of 14 randomized controlled studies evaluating the use of growth factors in patients with FN showed no improvements in overall mortality or infection-related mortality.[13] However, patients who received growth factors were less likely to require hospitalization beyond 10 days, recovered more quickly from fever, and had shorter durations of neutropenia and antimicrobial use. Of note, none of the studies included in this meta-analysis specifically evaluated critically ill patients. The interpretation of available data has led to varying recommendations from different guidelines. The current Infectious Diseases Society of America guidelines recommend against the use of growth factors in patients with established fever and neutropenia.[2] Similar recommendations are made by the American Society of Clinical Oncology guidelines; however, they suggest that growth factors can be considered for patients at high risk of infection-associated complications.[14] The high-risk criteria listed are similar to those provided earlier in the chapter (e.g., significant medical comorbidity, clinical instability, profound neutropenia, prolonged neutropenia, end-organ dysfunction, severe mucositis, Multinational Association for Supportive Care in Cancer Risk Index score less than 21). No grading of recommendations was provided in this guideline, and the authors acknowledge this as a consensus opinion. Given the considerable controversy and the lack of definitive data, it seems prudent that growth factors should not be routinely used for the treatment of FN. However, for patients with persistent FN at high risk of developing complications, they may be considered. Of note, a survey completed by the American Society of Clinical Oncology, before the publication of the latest iteration of the guidelines, showed a 60% growth factor usage rate for the treatment of FN.[15]

Donor-Derived Infection

Definition and Epidemiology

As the need for solid organ transplantation continues to exceed the available supply, criteria for organ donation are expanding. Although this leads to increased organ availability, the pool now includes more marginal specimens and organs from high-risk donors, which may result in increased infection risk in the recipient. Some donor-derived transmissions are expected, such as cytomegalovirus or hepatitis B, and routine postoperative care addresses these pathogens with prophylaxis or preemptive therapy. Others are unexpected and carry a high risk of morbidity and mortality.[16] Infection transmission is possible when a donor has active infection of any source, including blood, urine, or the central nervous system.[17-20] The likelihood that transmission resulted from the transplanted allograft is categorized as proven, probable, and possible.[21] Unfortunately, lack of infection recognition and underreporting may limit conclusions about the true incidence of this problem. However, current data suggest that rates of donor-derived infection are increasing. Although infection is likely transmitted in less than 1% of reported cases, the associated morbidity and mortality is significant, as evidenced by an attributable mortality rate of up to 30%.[16,22]

Recent evidence suggests bacterial pathogens are the most common source of donor-derived infection.[16] Although donor infection with gram-negative bacilli is associated with a greater risk of transmission and poorer patient outcomes,[22] case reports implicate both gram-negative and gram-positive organisms. These include several multidrug-resistant strains of *Pseudomonas* spp. and methicillin-resistant *Staphylococcus aureus*. Such transmissions have resulted in meningitis and bacteremia with complications including pneumonia, endocarditis, and septic arthritis.[19,20,23] In addition to bacterial infections, viral and fungal donor-derived infections have been reported.[16,22]

Risk Assessment

Pharmacists participating in the care of organ donors can assist the multidisciplinary team in recognizing individuals at high risk of transmitting infection. These include individuals with high-risk sexual contacts; those having received treatment for syphilis, gonorrhea, chlamydia, or genital ulcers within 12 months; inmates; intravenous drug users; and those having undergone dialysis within 12 months.[22] Heightened awareness of risk may prompt providers to do closer surveillance for clinical, serologic, and microbiologic signs of infection, thus increasing the likelihood of identifying an active infection at risk of transmission through donation. When practitioners caring for a recipient are made aware of the presence of infection in the donor, the pharmacist should help ensure prompt initiation of appropriate antimicrobial therapy and continued follow-up to ultimately determine organism speciation and susceptibilities.

Role of Antimicrobial Therapy

Guidelines address the treatment of infected organ donors as well as recipients of these allografts. It is recommended that individuals with bacterial meningitis or bacteremia at the time of donation be treated with targeted antimicrobial therapy for at least 24–48 hours before organ procurement, whenever possible. The organ recipients are recommended to receive antimicrobials to which the isolated organism is susceptible for 7–14 days.[22] Of note, expanding the spectrum of activity of perioperative antimicrobials to include coverage of organisms known to have been isolated in a donor has failed to prevent transmission in several reported cases. These events reinforce the need for continued targeted antimicrobial therapy beyond routine perioperative prophylaxis. In addition, several cases report the occurrence of donor-derived infections weeks outside the immediate peri-transplant period, after presumed eradication of active infection in the recipient. As such, this must be considered when evaluating transplant patients presenting with acute decompensation in clinical status.[19,20]

Human Immunodeficiency Virus

Critical Care Management

Since the initial diagnosis of the first case of HIV infection in 1981, there have been great changes to the epidemiology, management, and outcomes of these patients. In particular, the ICU treatment of patients with HIV has been revolutionized by the advent of highly active antiretroviral therapy (HAART) and routine use of opportunistic infection (OI) prophylaxis. Before this, admissions to the ICU were commonly associated with respiratory failure from pneumonia, which resulted in high short-term mortality.[24] However, the use of HAART has led to a decline in the morbidity and mortality associated with HIV, as well as the incidence of OI.[25] These improvements have led to new and different types of challenges for critical care practitioners. Besides familiarity with OIs, ICU practitioners must now be in tuned to the nuances, adverse effects, and drug interactions of HAART, in addition to the presentation and management of immune reconstitution syndrome.

Treatment-Naive Patients

Despite advances in screening and increased public attention to HIV, an estimated 20% of infected individuals are unaware of their diagnosis.[26] As such, clinicians should maintain a high level of vigilance to identify patients at risk of HIV. Patients with traditional risk factors for HIV

Table 50.3 AIDS-Defining Conditions

- Bacterial infections, multiple/recurrent
- Candidiasis: Esophageal; bronchi; trachea; or lungs
- Cervical cancer: Invasive
- Coccidioidomycosis: Disseminated or extrapulmonary
- Cryptococcosis: Extrapulmonary
- Cryptosporidiosis: Chronic intestinal (for > 1 mo)
- Cytomegalovirus disease
- Unexplained encephalopathy
- Herpes simplex: Chronic ulcer(s) (for > 1 mo); bronchitis; pneumonitis; or esophagitis
- Histoplasmosis: Disseminated or extrapulmonary
- Lymphoid interstitial pneumonia
- Lymphoma: Burkitt; immunoblastic; or brain
- *Mycobacterium avium* complex or *M. kansasii*: Disseminated or extrapulmonary
- *M. tuberculosis*: Any site (pulmonary or extrapulmonary)
- *Mycobacterium*: Other species or unidentified species; disseminated or extrapulmonary
- *Pneumocystis jiroveci* pneumonia
- Pneumonia: Recurrent
- Progressive multifocal leukoencephalopathy
- Salmonella septicemia (recurrent)
- Toxoplasmosis of brain
- Unexplained wasting syndrome

Reproduced with permission from: Lam SW, Bauer SR. HIV infection. In: Murphy JE, Wun-Len Lee M, eds. Pharmacotherapy Self-Assessment Program, 2015 Book 2. Infectious Diseases. Lenexa, KS: American College of Clinical Pharmacy, 2015.

---

or AIDS-defining diseases (Table 50.3) should receive additional serological testing.

For patients with newly diagnosed HIV who present to the ICU, the decision to initiate HAART is controversial. Studies of stable patients (non-critically ill) consistently show that early administration of HAART leads to better immunologic responses and clinical outcomes. However, the benefits of early HAART initiation must be weighed with the potential of adverse reactions and logistical issues associated with administration in the ICU. Some potential logistical concerns include the lack of oral access or appropriate formulations for feeding tube administration, the inability to access a patient's long-term commitment and adherence to the regimen, and the high probability of interruptions in therapy. Furthermore, patients in the ICU may have acute organ dysfunctions that increase the risk of potential adverse drug reactions. In general, if consistent therapy cannot be ensured, it is best deferred.

Patients recently initiated on HAART may also develop immune reconstitution inflammatory syndrome (IRIS). Immune reconstitution inflammatory syndrome is characterized by the unexpected worsening of existing OI or the unmasking of previously unrecognized disease when HAART has been recently initiated.[27] This can lead to several acute organ dysfunctions, including worsening respiratory failure requiring mechanical ventilation. The pathophysiology of IRIS is associated with the recovery of the immune system leading to proinflammatory cytokine storm. Risk factors associated with IRIS include the presence of disseminated disease or high antigen load, high baseline viral load, low baseline $CD4^+$ count, and rapid response to HAART. Although IRIS can be a severe consequence associated with the initiation of HAART, it is unlikely that treatment-naive patients will have IRIS during their ICU stay. The median onset of IRIS from the initiation of HAART is usually around 1 month; however, much earlier onset has been seen. For patients who present with OI, evidence does not suggest that early administration of HAART is associated with a higher incidence of IRIS, and HAART may decrease the risk of death or new AIDS-defining disease.[28]

In conclusion, when a patient with a new diagnosis is admitted to an ICU, HAART therapy should be initiated or continued, if possible. This is particularly true if the $CD4^+$ count is less than 500 cells/mm^3 or the patient presents with active OI. Data analyses consistently show that earlier treatment is associated with improved outcomes. However, if clinicians cannot ensure the consistent delivery of medications due to adverse reactions, drug interactions, drug formulation issues, and/or lack of gastric access, then HAART should be withheld.

Treatment-Experienced Patients

Patients admitted to the ICU already on HAART represent a different set of challenges. Once again, the decision to continue HAART largely depends on the ability to safely and consistently administer therapy. Route of administration, new renal or hepatic impairment, and the potential for treatment interruptions must be considered. If one of the antiretroviral therapies cannot be safely administered, all therapies should be discontinued to decrease the promotion of resistance.[29] The possible exception to this rule is for patients chronically on nonnucleoside reverse transcriptase inhibitors, which have long half-lives (about 3 weeks). In these patients, discontinuing all HAART may functionally equate to receiving nonnucleoside reverse transcriptase inhibitor monotherapy; therefore, clinicians should consider continuing to administer other antiretrovirals with shorter half-lives to minimize possible selection for nonnucleoside reverse transcriptase inhibitor resistance. In addition to these considerations, ICU clinicians caring for HIV-positive patients should be cognizant of the common interactions between antiretrovirals and medications commonly used in critically ill patients.[29] See Table 50.4 for examples.

Another cause for ICU admission among patients with HIV may be HAART-associated adverse reactions. Although newer generations of HAART are usually well tolerated, many patients remain on older antiretrovirals. Hence, clinicians should readily recognize the possible

Table 50.4 Common Interactions Between Antiretrovirals and Commonly Used Medications in Critically Ill Patients

Agent	Antiretroviral	Interactions
Stress ulcer prophylaxis (proton pump inhibitors, histamine-2 receptor antagonists)	Rilpivirine: Contraindicated with proton pump inhibitors	Decrease in antiretroviral concentrations
	Atazanavir: Relatively contraindicated with proton pump inhibitors (administer no more than the equivalent of omeprazole 20 mg/day, and separate administration by at least 12 hr)	
Triazole antifungals: voriconazole, posaconazole, itraconazole	Protease inhibitors	Increase in antiretroviral concentration
	Nonnucleoside reverse transcriptase inhibitors	Decrease in antifungal concentrations
Antibacterial		
Rifampin	Protease inhibitors	Decrease in antiretroviral concentration
	Nonnucleoside reverse transcriptase inhibitors	
Clarithromycin	Protease inhibitors	Increase in clarithromycin concentration
	Nonnucleoside reverse transcriptase inhibitors	
Metronidazole	Fosamprenavir, lopinavir, ritonavir	Disulfiram reaction
Antiarrhythmics		
Amiodarone	Indinavir, ritonavir, tipranavir	Increased antiarrhythmic concentrations
Flecainide, propafenone, quinidine	Lopinavir, ritonavir, tipranavir	Increased antiarrhythmic concentrations
Diltiazem	Atazanavir, fosamprenavir	Increased antiarrhythmic concentrations
Statins	Protease inhibitors	Increased concentrations of statins – in decreasing order of interaction potential (lovastatin, simvastatin, rosuvastatin, atorvastatin, pravastatin)
	Nonnucleoside reverse transcriptase Inhibitors	
Anticonvulsants: Carbamazepine, phenobarbital, phenytoin	Protease inhibitors	Increase in antiretroviral concentrations
	Nonnucleoside reverse transcriptase inhibitors	Decrease in anticonvulsant concentrations
Midazolam	Protease inhibitors	Increase in midazolam concentration
	Nonnucleoside reverse transcriptase inhibitors	
	Cobicistat/elvitegravir	
Methadone	Nonnucleoside reverse transcriptase inhibitors	Opioid withdrawal
	Fosamprenavir, ritonavir, lopinavir, nelfinavir, didanosine, saquinavir	
Sildenafil	Protease inhibitors	Increase in sildenafil concentration
	Delavirdine	
Warfarin	Delavirdine, efavirenz	Increase in warfarin concentration

Reproduced with permission from: Lam SW, Bauer SR. HIV infection. In: Murphy JE, Wun-Len Lee M, eds. Pharmacotherapy Self-Assessment Program, 2015 Book 2. Infectious Diseases. Lenexa, KS: American College of Clinical Pharmacy, 2015.

adverse effects associated with HAART. Furthermore, many of the HAART-associated adverse effects have no specific treatments; therefore, prompt discontinuation of the offending agent is crucial.

Despite advances in the management of HIV, a combination of two nucleotide/nucleoside reverse transcriptase inhibitors (NRTIs) remains the backbone of many HAART regimens.[29,33] Many NRTIs may cause lactic acidosis by disrupting mitochondrial replication through inhibition of DNA polymerase. Mild hyperlactatemia is common in patients receiving NRTIs; however, severe lactic acidosis can also occur and may be life threatening. Before the formulation of newer NRTIs, the rate of severe lactic acidosis occurred at a rate of 1.3 cases per 1,000 person-years of exposure.[30] The risk of developing severe lactic acidosis is highest among older NRTIs, particularly zidovudine, stavudine, and didanosine. The symptoms of severe lactic acidosis are nonspecific and include fatigue, malaise, nausea, vomiting, and abdominal pain. Hence, a high level of vigilance is needed to identify patients who are at risk. The treatment of severe lactic acidosis is largely supportive and entails prompt discontinuation of the possible offending agent.

Another adverse effect of concern commonly seen with older antiretroviral therapy is abacavir-associated hypersensitivity. Up to 3% of patients on abacavir may have such a reaction within a few weeks of initiating therapy.[31] The initial presenting symptoms include fever, rash, and GI symptoms. Treatment involves prompt discontinuation of therapy and supportive care. Patients with ongoing or worsening symptoms should be evaluated for other causes. Hypersensitivity is more prominent among patients with the presence of an *HLA-B*5701* allele, which has an 8% prevalence among whites in North America. Rechallenging patients with established hypersensitivity is strictly contraindicated because severe life-threatening hypersensitivity has been reported.[31] Other severe life-threatening adverse drug reactions among antiretrovirals include Stevens-Johnson syndrome and hepatic necrosis syndrome associated with nevirapine, rhabdomyolysis associated with raltegravir, and intracranial hemorrhage associated with tipranavir.

Opportunistic Infection: Prophylaxis and Treatment

The discussion of opportunistic infections (OIs) will cover *Pneumocystis jiroveci* pneumonia (PJP), *Toxoplasma gondii* encephalitis, and *Mycobacterium avium* complex (MAC). Other OIs such as candidiasis, cryptococcal meningitis, herpes simplex virus, and cytomegalovirus can be found in the Invasive Fungal Infections and Invasive Viral Infection chapters. Although the discussion of OIs will largely focus on HIV-positive patients, with the increasing number of critically ill immunocompromised patients with solid organ transplant and cancer, these infections are increasingly seen in HIV-negative patients. In general, management of OI in HIV-positive patients can be extrapolated to patients without HIV.

P. jiroveci Pneumonia

Pneumocystis pneumonia is caused by *P. jiroveci*, a ubiquitous fungal organism known to cause severe respiratory infections in immunocompromised host. The advent of HAART and prophylaxis has dramatically decreased the incidence of PJP, with most cases occurring in patients who are unaware of their HIV status or those not receiving or nonadherent to their HAART regimen.[32]

Patients with PJP commonly present to the ICU with respiratory distress that is characterized by progressive dyspnea and non-productive cough in the preceding days to weeks. Hypoxemia is common and can range from mild to severe. Patients with severe hypoxemia and large alveolar-arterial oxygen difference may require mechanical ventilation. Chest radiograph usually reveals diffuse, bilateral infiltrates.[33-37]

Because the presentation, laboratory findings, and radiographic characteristics of PJP are nonspecific, diagnosis requires histopathologic or cytopathologic identification of the organism from an induced sputum, bronchoalveolar lavage, or lung biopsy specimen. Traditionally, because the organism does not grow readily with routine microbiologic techniques, laboratories have relied on several different staining techniques. Recent development of a PJP polymerase chain reaction (PCR) test may provide an additional method for identifying PJP. The sensitivity of the PJP PCR is high; however, its specificity for distinguishing true PJP infection from colonization is low; hence, it should function as a rule-out test.[33,34]

Prophylaxis

Patients with HIV having a $CD4^+$ count less than 200 cells/mm^3 or a history of oropharyngeal candidiasis should receive chemoprophylaxis against PJP. Trimethoprim/sulfamethoxazole 1 double-strength tablet once daily is the preferred prophylactic regimen because this dose also confers prophylaxis against toxoplasmosis and other respiratory bacterial infections.[33-37] Because trimethoprim/sulfamethoxazole is such an effective agent against PJP, patients with a history of mild to moderate adverse drug reactions should be rechallenged or undergo desensitization. However, trimethoprim/sulfamethoxazole may also cause life-threatening reactions such as Stevens-Johnson syndrome or toxic epidermal necrolysis, which would necessitate discontinuation of therapy with no further exposure to the medication. For these patients, alternative prophylactic regimens such as dapsone or nebulized pentamidine may be considered. Patients with HIV admitted to the ICU should be assessed to ensure that prophylaxis is continued or initiated. Although there are criteria for discontinuing OI prophylaxis, they are usually not applicable in an ICU setting.

Treatment

The treatment of choice for critically patients with PJP is high-dose intravenous trimethoprim/sulfamethoxazole (15–20 mg/kg of trimethoprim divided every 6–8 hours), adjusted for renal function.[33-37] Intravenous pentamidine 4 mg/kg once daily may be used in patients with previous severe adverse effects or allergic reactions associated with trimethoprim/sulfamethoxazole; however, this drug is associated with significantly more adverse effects, including pancreatitis, GI discomfort, nephrotoxicity, and dysglycemia. Oral regimens, such as equivalent doses of oral trimethoprim/sulfamethoxazole or clindamycin/primaquine, should only be used in patients with no known drug absorption issues and those with clinical improvement. Treatment of PJP should be continued for a total of 21 days. Patients with moderate to severe disease complicated by hypoxemia (Pao_2 less than 70 mm Hg or alveolar-arterial oxygen gradient of 35 mm Hg or greater) should receive adjunctive corticosteroids. Ideally, prednisone should be initiated within 72 hours of initiating PJP treatment. Those meeting the criteria for severe hypoxemia should have the steroids tapered over the 21-day treatment course (prednisone 40 mg twice daily × 5 days, 40 mg daily × 5 days, 20 mg daily × 11 days). For those without enteral access, methylprednisolone may be used at 75% of the prednisone dose. Adjunctive corticosteroids have been correlated with the attenuation of worsening hypoxemia, which is caused by the rapid acceleration of inflammation from the initiation of anti-*Pneumocystis* therapy.[35]

T. gondii Encephalitis

T. gondii is a protozoan organism that may cause encephalitis in immunocompromised patients. Clinical disease is most common among patients with a $CD4^+$ count less than 50 cells/mm³. Infection is almost solely (95%) because of reactivation of latent tissue cysts.[36] Hence, patients who are immunoglobulin G (IgG) seropositive for antitoxoplasma antibodies are at the highest risk of developing disease. Among adults in North America, the rate of seroprevalence is about 11%. Developing primary disease is possible through exposure to undercooked meat or shellfish containing tissue cysts or oocysts shed from cat feces.

The most common symptoms in patients presenting to the ICU with *Toxoplasma* encephalitis (TE) are headache, confusion, and motor weakness. Brain imaging typically reveals many lesions within the cerebral cortex or ganglia. Definitive diagnosis requires detection of the organism through a CT-guided needle biopsy, although most clinicians rely on a combination of clinical symptoms, radiologic findings, serostatus, and response to treatment as an empiric diagnosis.[33-37]

Prophylaxis

Patients with HIV having a $CD4^+$ count less than 100 cells/mm³ should be initiated on a prophylactic regimen against TE. Because active disease is primarily from reactivation of latent cysts, patients who are not IgG seropositive do not require prophylactic therapy. However, if this strategy is used, patients should be retested for serostatus each time their $CD4^+$ counts drop below 100 cells/mm³. Trimethoprim/sulfamethoxazole 1 double-strength tablet once daily is the preferred prophylactic regimen. If patients cannot tolerate trimethoprim/sulfamethoxazole, the recommended alternative is dapsone/pyrimethamine plus leucovorin.

Treatment

The preferred treatment of TE is a combination of pyrimethamine, sulfadiazine, and leucovorin.[33-37] An alternative agent for patients who cannot tolerate sulfadiazine is clindamycin. Aside from the known adverse effects of the earlier regimen, such as hematologic toxicities, rash, and GI disturbances, administration in critically ill patients may be challenging because of the lack of availability of parenteral formulations of pyrimethamine and sulfadiazine. For patients without reliable gastric access, intravenous trimethoprim/sulfamethoxazole (10 mg/kg of trimethoprim divided twice daily) may be considered. In a small study, the use of intravenous or oral trimethoprim/sulfamethoxazole led to similar rates of complete response compared with the preferred therapy of pyrimethamine and sulfadiazine, plus leucovorin.[37] Patients with a history of seizure disorders may benefit from prophylactic anticonvulsants while receiving acute treatment.[38] The choice of anticonvulsants in patients with HIV having TE is poorly studied; however, phenytoin is the most widely used. Because of cytochrome P450 (CYP) 3A4 induction by phenytoin and the possible drug interactions leading to decreased concentrations of HAART therapy, some experts recommend the use of newer antiepileptics, such as levetiracetam.[39] In general, patients respond within 14 days of initiating therapy with improvements in mental status and radiologic assessment. Therapy for TE should be continued for at least 6 weeks, with longer courses indicated if patients have incomplete clinical or radiologic response. Completion of acute treatment should be followed by secondary prophylaxis, which usually entails reduced-dose pyrimethamine, sulfadiazine, and leucovorin, continuing for at least 6 months after recovery of $CD4^+$ counts to greater than 200 cells/mm³.

M. avium Complex

M. avium complex are ubiquitous organisms responsible for disseminated, multiorgan disease among patients with HIV. This infection is most commonly seen in patients with HIV having a $CD4^+$ count less than 50 cells/mm³. Symptoms, which include fever, weight loss, fatigue, night sweats, and diarrhea, are usually mild and nonspecific and slowly progress over weeks. Physical examination often reveals a combination of lymphadenopathy, hepatomegaly, and splenomegaly. Confirmatory diagnosis requires isolation of MAC from blood, tissue, or other sterile sites. Of note, routine evaluation of cultures for MAC is not indicated because treatment is not necessary in asymptomatic patients.

Prophylaxis

Patients with HIV having a CD4+ count less than 50 cells/mm³ should receive chemoprophylaxis against MAC.[33-37] Azithromycin and clarithromycin are considered first-line agents. Given the high propensity for drug interactions between clarithromycin, which inhibits CYP3A4, and commonly used ICU medications, azithromycin 1200 mg once weekly may be the preferred regimen. Intravenous therapy may be considered for critically ill patients who cannot tolerate oral therapy. No studies have evaluated the use of intravenous azithromycin for prophylaxis of MAC. Although unlikely to cause adverse reactions, intravenous azithromycin at the same dose will likely lead to supratherapeutic concentrations because oral azithromycin has a bioavailability of only around 35%. For patients at high risk of developing QT prolongation, an intravenous dose reduction may be prudent.

Treatment

Treatment of MAC should consist of at least two drugs because the development of resistance occurs more readily with monotherapy. The preferred regimen is a combination of macrolide (clarithromycin or azithromycin) and ethambutol 15 mg/kg/day, adjusted for renal function. Some clinicians may consider adding rifabutin as a third agent.[33-37] Macrolide resistance is increasingly reported among patients with MAC, estimated to be as high as 11% in those previously exposed to macrolides.[40] Hence, resistance testing should be implemented in all patients with MAC, particularly those who have previously received macrolide therapy. Improvements should be seen within 2–4 weeks of treatment initiation. Patients with persistently positive cultures after 4–8 weeks should be evaluated with repeated susceptibility testing, given the possibility for the development of resistance. New regimens should be tailored according to these results and, ideally, involve several agents not previously tried. Perhaps equally important to MAC treatment is the optimization of HAART to improve a patient's immune function. Therapy for MAC should continue for at least 12 months, though extending the treatment course may be necessary for those without adequate immune reconstitution.

NONINFECTIOUS COMPLICATIONS OF IMMUNOSUPPRESSION

Pulmonary Complications

Peri-engraftment Respiratory Distress Syndrome

Peri-engraftment respiratory distress syndrome (PERDS), also called engraftment syndrome, occurs in about 5% of patients immunosuppressed for blood and marrow transplantation. This complication is characterized by a temperature greater than 101°F (38.3°C), pulmonary infiltrates on chest radiograph, a widespread erythrodermatous rash, diarrhea, and hypoxia with oxygen saturations less than 90% on room air. When respiratory function is severely compromised, patients often require ICU admission. This constellation of symptoms typically occurs within 5 days of engraftment (ANC greater than $0.5 \times 10^3/mm^3$) and in patients without cardiac dysfunction or documented infection, though the latter is difficult to rule out in real time in most clinical situations.[41] Although its pathophysiology is poorly understood, PERDS is thought to result from complex interactions between lung endothelial tissue damaged from chemotherapy and radiation conditioning regimens and cytokines released at the time of neutrophil engraftment.[42] Attributable mortality may be as high as 21%.[41-43]

A diagnosis of PERDS is often made after ruling out other causes of respiratory decompensation, such as infectious pneumonia, transfusion reaction, or pulmonary edema arising from cardiac dysfunction. The relationship between PERDS and diffuse alveolar hemorrhage (DAH) is complex and discussed in detail later in this chapter. In addition to supportive care, steroids can be considered for treatment when respiratory distress is severe enough to require ICU admission. Although data are limited, several reports indicate successful prevention and treatment of this condition with steroid use. At one center, a decrease in the incidence of PERDS was seen when instituting routine prophylaxis with prednisone at 0.5 mg/kg/day on posttransplant days 4–14.[43] Another center retrospectively reported symptomatic improvement and decreased oxygen requirements with the use of methylprednisolone 1–2 g/day for 3 days. Response was usually seen within 1–4 days after treatment. The 3 days of high-dose steroids was followed by a rapid taper, though the exact strategy was not clearly outlined.[42]

Diffuse Alveolar Hemorrhage

Diffuse alveolar hemorrhage may occur in the setting of several diseases, including, but not limited to, connective tissue disease, antiphospholipid antibody syndrome, and as a complication of blood and marrow transplantation. This chapter will focus specifically on the clinical presentation and treatment of patients with DAH in the blood and marrow transplant setting.

Although the exact pathogenesis is unclear, it is thought that vascular damage and inflammation from chemotherapy and radiation, combined with host immune-mediated events, contribute to pulmonary microvasculature injury resulting in bleeding and alveolar damage. This occurs in 1%–7% of patients undergoing blood and marrow transplantation and most often manifests in the first month after transplantation, though case reports detail this phenomenon as far as 12 months from transplantation.[44,45] Widely accepted diagnostic criteria include diffuse pulmonary infiltrates present on imaging and progressively bloodier fluid returns during bronchoalveolar lavage, which have greater than 20% hemosiderin-laden macrophages on cellular analysis.[46] These macrophages can take 48–72 hours to develop and thus it is possible, though uncommon, for them to be absent if bronchoalveolar lavage is done early in the course of DAH. Conversely, clearance from respiratory secretions may take 2–4 weeks. Symptoms accompanying DAH also include a sudden onset of dyspnea, hypoxemia, fever, and non-productive cough. Hemoptysis is present in about 20% of cases. Confirmatory diagnosis is often difficult, given the similarity with which other pulmonary complications present, including PERDS, graft-vs.-host disease, and infectious and noninfectious pneumonias.

If DAH is suspected, the mainstay of treatment is supportive, maintaining adequate oxygenation and optimizing hemostasis. It has been theorized that steroids may be useful to suppress immune-mediated contributors to DAH; however, their role remains controversial.[46] A single retrospective cohort of autologous and allogeneic blood and marrow transplant patients compared 43 individuals receiving high-dose steroids (greater than 30 mg/day of methylprednisolone equivalent tapered over days to weeks) with 22 receiving low-dose steroids (30 mg/day of methylprednisolone equivalent or less) or no steroids.[47] Although those receiving high-dose steroids had an improved likelihood of survival to hospital discharge, the small sample size, extreme variability in steroid dosing regimens, and lack of rigorous methodology call into question the significance of these results. In addition, subsequent analyses failed to show any clear survival benefit.[45,48] Commonly reported dosing strategies provided 500–1,000 mg of methylprednisolone daily for 3 days with tapering strategies individualized to patient response or provider preference. Of note, studies do not report an increased incidence of new infection in the setting of steroid use[45-48]; however, when evaluating the true safety of steroids, patient-specific characteristics must be considered. In the absence of clinical response to steroid therapy, patients being treated for invasive fungal infection, experiencing significant delirium, and those with severe muscle atrophy or receiving neuromuscular blockade (all common complications in this patient population) may not be ideal candidates for an extended course of high-dose steroids. Although a paucity of data supporting steroid use leaves many practitioners with doubts about the effectiveness of this strategy, the high mortality rates associated with this condition (30%–100%) often result in steroid use as salvage therapy.[44-46]

Tumor Lysis Syndrome

Definition and Pathophysiology

Tumor lysis syndrome (TLS) is one of the most common emergencies encountered in the care of patients with hematologic malignancies.[49] Either spontaneously or after initiation of cytoreductive therapy, malignant cells rapidly release their contents, including electrolytes, proteins, and nucleic acids, into systemic circulation, potentially triggering many consequences. Patients may be given a diagnosis of TLS on the basis of laboratory findings or clinical developments according to the widely used Cairo-Bishop classification system (Table 50.5).[50] Given the potential severity of consequences and rapidly progressive nature of this condition, laboratory TLS should be immediately addressed, even in the absence of symptoms, to prevent deterioration in clinical status.

Risk Assessment

One of the keys to anticipating the potential for TLS and mitigating its consequences is a thorough patient risk assessment. This probability most closely relates to cancer type but is also affected by patient characteristics and supportive care. Patients with hematologic malignancies with a high tumor burden, notably acute myeloid and lymphoblastic leukemia, chronic lymphocytic and myeloid leukemia, and Burkitt and non-Hodgkin lymphoma, remain among the highest-risk populations for developing TLS.[51] It has also been reported, though uncommonly, in patients receiving treatment for bulky solid organ tumors.[52,53] Given that tumor burden is typically greatest at the outset of disease treatment, the probability of developing TLS is usually highest during the first cycle of chemotherapy for both hematologic and oncologic malignancies. Clinical status may elevate TLS risk in some cases. For example, patients with preexisting renal dysfunction, hypoperfusion, hypovolemia or those who are receiving nephrotoxic medications are at heightened risk of end-organ damage. Elevated baseline uric acid (UA) concentrations or receipt of exogenous electrolytes contributes to worsening laboratory abnormalities.[51] In addition, delayed implementation of preventive measures in those predisposed represents a missed opportunity for intervention. Risk recognition and prompt initiation of appropriate pharmacotherapy and supportive care is one area in which pharmacists play a pivotal role on the multidisciplinary care team.

Disease Manifestations

Rapid lysis of malignant cells often results in abrupt serum elevation of electrolytes, commonly phosphorous and potassium. The significance of hyperkalemia is underscored by its potential to cause significant arrhythmias and cardiac arrest. Excess serum phosphorus may lead to

Table 50.5 Cairo-Bishop Classification of Laboratory and Clinical Tumor Lysis Syndrome

Metabolic Abnormality	Criteria for Laboratory Tumor Lysis Syndrome[a,b]	Criteria for Clinical Tumor Lysis Syndrome[c]
Hyperuricemia	Uric acid > 8 mg/dL or 25% increase from baseline	
Hyperphosphatemia	Phosphorus > 4.5 mg/dL or 25% increase from baseline	
Hyperkalemia	Potassium > 6.0 mmol/L or 25% increase from baseline	Cardiac arrhythmia or sudden death likely related to hyperkalemia
Hypocalcemia	Corrected calcium < 7.0 mg/dL or ionized calcium < 1.12 mg/dL or 25% increase from baseline	Cardia arrhythmia, sudden death likely related to hypocalcemia, seizure, or neuromuscular toxicity
Acute kidney injury	Not applicable	Increase in serum creatinine of 0.3 mg/dL or oliguria for ≥ 6 hr

[a]Values diagnostic for adult patients only.
[b]Diagnosis requires two or more metabolic abnormalities to be present within same 24-hour period 3 days before or 7 days after initiation of cytotoxic therapy.
[c]Requires diagnosis of laboratory tumor lysis syndrome in addition to clinical symptoms.

precipitation of renal and extrarenal deposits of calcium phosphate crystals, representing one mechanism of acute kidney injury in TLS.[49,54] Another complication of hyperphosphatemia is secondary hypocalcemia, putting patients at risk of neurotoxicity, dysrhythmia, and seizure. Unfortunately, many of these laboratory abnormalities may be augmented in the setting of renal dysfunction, resulting in a greater likelihood of clinical sequelae.

The nucleic acids from the DNA released into the circulation from lysing cells are broken down into hypoxanthine. This is further metabolized to xanthine and then to UA by xanthine oxidase. Rapid accumulation of these products can contribute to acute kidney injury through formation of urate crystals in the distal renal tubules and collecting ducts, obstructing the tubular lumen.[55] The process is potentiated by both an acid environment, due to a decrease in UA solubility, and the presence of calcium phosphate crystals, which causes UA to precipitate more readily. Even in the absence of precipitation, UA activates the renin-angiotensin system, reducing available nitric oxide and resulting in renal vasoconstriction.[55] Rising xanthine concentrations may also cause nephropathy or urolithiasis, regardless of pH.[49]

Crystal-independent mechanisms play a role in acute kidney injury as well. Lysed malignant cells spill cytokines and chemokines into circulation, and these inflammatory mediators induce local vasoconstriction at the level of the kidney. Reduced renal perfusion and hypoxia add to the tubular injury caused by crystal precipitates.[55]

Prevention and Treatment

Risk assessment and proactive implementation of preventive measures in high-risk patients remain the keys to detecting TLS and mitigating the severity of sequelae. Aggressive hydration and brisk urine output enhance excretion of UA and phosphate through expansion of intravascular volume and improvement in renal blood flow. Maintaining renal perfusion is also important in protecting the kidneys from ischemic injury. If tolerated, consider administering crystalloid fluids at a rate of 2.5–3 L/m²/day. The choice of fluids should be individualized according to the patient's clinical status. For example, chloride-poor products such as Ringer lactate may more desirable than normal saline, given the latter's potential to perpetuate an acidic environment. However, in patients with preexisting severe hyperkalemia, Ringer lactate should be avoided in large volumes; goal urine output remains 3–5 mL/kg/hour.[49,56] After ruling out obstructive renal injury, loop diuretics may be used to maintain this goal urine output in the setting of adequate intravascular volume.[51] Of note, urinary alkalinization is no longer recommended for TLS prevention, given a lack of evidence supporting its efficacy. Although UA is more soluble in a basic environment, this increases the risk of precipitation of calcium phosphate crystals. Furthermore, xanthine, the precursor to UA, has low solubility, regardless of pH.[55]

By preventing the metabolism of nucleic acids via xanthine oxidase, allopurinol can help circumvent accumulation of UA and hypoxanthine and the resultant renal injury. Of note, doses for TLS prevention are typically higher than those used in the treatment of gout. Guidelines suggest initiating allopurinol at 50–100 mg/m² orally three times daily or at 10 mg/kg/day given in divided doses. The maximum recommended oral daily dose is 800 mg.[51] Although general dosing guidelines advocate for a 50% dose reduction in patients with significant renal impairment, the benefits of aggressive dosing in maintaining or recovering renal function must be considered. In the absence of clear allopurinol-related toxicity, data analyses do not support dose reduction in this population. Therapy should start 12–24 hours before cytoreductive treatment and continue until normalizations of UA concentrations, leukocyte count, and laboratory values occur and the tumor burden is significantly decreased.

Routine electrolyte monitoring and prompt management of derangements when identified reduce the risk of deleterious clinical effects.[54] Serum chemistries including UA, potassium, phosphate, and calcium should be monitored every 6 or 8 hours in patients at a high or moderate risk of TLS.[51] Electrolyte, UA, and creatinine abnormalities are most likely to be appreciated within 48 hours of cytoreductive treatment. It is also important to evaluate patients' medication profiles for external sources of these substrates, such as dietary intake, maintenance fluids, or multivitamins. Phosphate binders may be used in patients with hyperphosphatemia, though calcium-containing products should be avoided in the setting of hypercalcemia. In cases of severe electrolyte abnormalities or clinical manifestation thereof, emergent dialysis may be considered.[51,56]

Rasburicase is an intravenous medication that catalyzes the oxidation of UA to the inactive and soluble product, allantoin. It may be used for the prevention of hyperuricemia or, in the event of early detection, before the manifestation of renal injury. For patients already experiencing a decline in renal function, rapid metabolism of UA may mitigate further damage, with the ultimate goal being to avoid the need for dialysis.[51,57,58] Uric acid concentrations are noted to decrease as soon as 4 hours after a single administration of rasburicase and may continue declining for up to 72 hours.[57,59,60] Initial investigations studied treatment success with doses of 0.15–0.2 mg/kg given daily for up to 5 days.[57,58] However, studies that are more recent show equivalent efficacy with fixed doses of 3 or 6 mg, with an infrequent need for repeat dosing. This represents a significantly more cost-effective strategy, optimizing health care resources.[58-61] The drug properties of rasburicase are such that it is removed by dialysis; therefore, it may be prudent to avoid administration in patients for whom dialysis is imminent. When considering the use of rasburicase, note its contraindication in patients with G6PD (glucose-6-phosphate dehydrogenase) deficiency, given the potential for severe hemolysis in some patients.[57] Proactive identification of patients at highest risk of TLS who may benefit from rasburicase allows for appropriate testing before initiating cytoreductive therapy. In addition, proper technique is required for accurate laboratory monitoring of UA after an administered dose. To avoid enzymatic degradation of UA by rasburicase, blood samples must be stored in pre-chilled, heparin-containing tubes; kept refrigerated; and analyzed immediately by laboratory personnel.

Acute Calcineurin Inhibitor–Associated Neurotoxicity

Epidemiology and Pathophysiology

Although a valuable component of modern immunosuppression, calcineurin inhibitors (CNIs) carry a risk of several troublesome adverse effects. This class of immunosuppressants is commonly used for rejection prevention after solid organ transplantation, graft-vs.-host disease suppression after blood and marrow transplantation, and management of various other disease states that require immune modulation. In addition to nephrotoxicity, neurotoxicity is one of the most commonly encountered adverse effects of CNIs, with serious events reported in up to 43% of patients.[62-64] Arguably, the most severe of these is posterior reversible leukoencephalopathy syndrome (PRES).

There are two proposed mechanisms for the pathology behind PRES. The first describes T-cell activation, which initiates a cytokine response.[65,66] Resultant inflammation damages vascular brain endothelium, leading to vasogenic edema and ultimately tissue hypoperfusion. This process may be precipitated by several concomitant comorbidities such as infection, hypertension, preeclampsia, or organ rejection.[65] Second, severe systemic hypertension may lead to transient disruption of autoregulation, a consequence of which is cerebral vasodilation. This allows fluid and blood into brain parenchyma, causing cerebral edema.[64] Evidence of these events can be seen with CT or magnetic resonance imaging, which is considered the gold standard for syndrome diagnosis.[64,65]

Symptoms commonly associated with PRES include encephalopathy, elevated blood pressure, and seizure activity. Encephalopathy ranges from mild disruption of consciousness or lethargy to severe agitation or coma.[65,67] Reports describe seizures commonly preceded by vision changes or headache.[68] Hypertension is often considered a hallmark of the clinical presentation of PRES associated with any cause; however, reports clearly indicate it is not present in all cases. Mean arterial pressure can exceed 115–130 mm Hg in some cases, but epidemiologic data suggest that around 50% of cases present with normal or only slightly elevated blood pressure.[65,67] It is thought that the risk of PRES is highest within the first 30 days of CNI therapy,[62] although reports detail cases occurring as many as 10 months after drug initiation.[63,69,70] In some instances diagnosis is made when CNI blood levels are considered elevated beyond normal limits (greater than 12–15 ng/mL in most cases) or as a result of rapidly increasing concentrations. This is not universally the case, however, because literature reveals frequent occurrence with normal CNI blood concentrations. This can indicate that blood concentrations may not accurately reflect those present in the brain.[65]

Treatment

Practitioners must thoroughly evaluate patients for potential causes of PRES aside from CNI therapy. If a CNI is determined to be the cause or a contributor, syndromal reversal ultimately depends on adjustment of CNI therapy in the form of dose reduction or discontinuation. When

PRES is first recognized, providers commonly withdraw these medications. Pharmacists should assist in evaluating the appropriateness of an alternative treatment approach, if one is available for the underlying disorder. For patients in whom CNI therapy is overwhelmingly favorable, several case reports detail successful resolution of symptoms with a reduction in the target blood concentration or switching to a different medication within the same class.[66,68,70] If these strategies are chosen, the patient should be closely monitored for signs of PRES during the initial reintroduction of CNI therapy. Symptomatic management should include cessation of seizures, hemodynamic stabilization, and electrolyte optimization. Seizures should be managed initially with benzodiazepines or alternatively phenytoin, which may induce metabolism of CNIs. Other antiepileptics can be considered for refractory status epilepticus.[71] Blood pressure should ideally be maintained at the patient's premorbid baseline. Given the suspected role of cerebral hypoperfusion in the pathophysiology of PRES, rapid overcorrection and persistent hypotension should be avoided. Overall symptomatic improvement may lag behind normalization of CNI blood concentrations, given the slow transit of CNIs across the blood-brain barrier, but is typically seen within several days of treatment.[72] Resolution of radiographic evidence of PRES may be further delayed or occasionally persist, showing permanent cerebral volume loss.

CONCLUSION

Immune system suppression, whether as a result of disease or medication, is seen in a variety of patients, and pharmacists play a pivotal role in the optimization of their care. This may include prompt recognition of opportunistic and other infections, initiation and monitoring of antimicrobial therapy, assessment of indications for infection prophylaxis, maintenance of the balance between immunosuppressive medications and host defenses, and identification of possible adverse drug reactions associated with therapy. By familiarizing themselves with the unique complications seen in critically ill immunocompromised patients, pharmacists can continue to contribute to multidisciplinary health care in distinct and significant ways.

REFERENCES

1. Klastersky J. Management of fever in neutropenic patients with different risks of complications. Clin Infect Dis 2004;39(suppl 1):S32-37.
2. Freifeld AG, Bow EJ, Sepkowitz KA, et al. Clinical practice guideline for the use of antimicrobial agents in neutropenic patients with cancer: 2010 update by the Infectious Diseases Society of America. Clin Infect Dis 2011;52:e56-93.
3. Zuckermann J, Moreira LB, Stoll P, et al. Compliance with a critical pathway for the management of febrile neutropenia and impact on clinical outcomes. Ann Hematol 2008;87:139-45.
4. Baden LR, Bensinger W, Angarone M, et al. NCCN Guidelines, Version 2.2015. Prevention and Treatment of Cancer-Related Infections. 2015. Available at www.nccn.org/professionals/physician_gls/f_guidelines.asp. Accessed July 9, 2015.
5. Paul M, Dickstein Y, Schlesinger A, et al. Beta-lactam versus beta-lactam-aminoglycoside combination therapy in cancer patients with neutropenia. Cochrane Database Syst Rev 2013;6:CD003038.
6. Kumar A, Zarychanski R, Light B, et al. Early combination antibiotic therapy yields improved survival compared with monotherapy in septic shock: a propensity-matched analysis. Crit Care Med 2010;38:1773-85.
7. Paul M, Dickstein Y, Borok S, et al. Empirical antibiotics targeting gram-positive bacteria for the treatment of febrile neutropenic patients with cancer. Cochrane Database Syst Rev 2014;1:CD003914.
8. Ariano RE, Nyhlen A, Donnelly JP, et al. Pharmacokinetics and pharmacodynamics of meropenem in febrile neutropenic patients with bacteremia. Ann Pharmacother 2005;39:32-8.
9. Bow EJ, Rotstein C, Noskin GA, et al. A randomized, open-label, multicenter comparative study of the efficacy and safety of piperacillin-tazobactam and cefepime for the empirical treatment of febrile neutropenic episodes in patients with hematologic malignancies. Clin Infect Dis 2006;43:447-59.
10. Wade JC, Glasmacher A. Vancomycin does not benefit persistently febrile neutropenic people with cancer. Cancer Treat Rev 2004;30:119-26.
11. Clark OA, Lyman GH, Castro AA, et al. Colony-stimulating factors for chemotherapy-induced febrile neutropenia: a meta-analysis of randomized controlled trials. J Clin Oncol 2005;23:4198-214.
12. Garcia-Carbonero R, Mayordomo JI, Tornamira MV, et al. Granulocyte colony-stimulating factor in the treatment of high-risk febrile neutropenia: a multicenter randomized trial. J Natl Cancer Inst 2001;93:31-8.
13. Mhaskar R, Clark OA, Lyman G, et al. Colony-stimulating factors for chemotherapy-induced febrile neutropenia. Cochrane Database Syst Rev 2014;10:CD003039.
14. Smith TJ, Khatcheressian J, Lyman GH, et al. 2006 update of recommendations for the use of white blood cell growth factors: an evidence-based clinical practice guideline. J Clin Oncol 2006;24:3187-205.
15. Bennett CL, Weeks JA, Somerfield MR, et al. Use of hematopoietic colony-stimulating factors: comparison of the 1994 and 1997 American Society of Clinical Oncology surveys regarding ASCO clinical practice guidelines. Health Services Research Committee of the American Society of Clinical Oncology. J Clin Oncol 1999;17:3676-31.
16. Green M, Covington S, Taranto S, et al. Donor-derived transmission events in 2013: a report of the Organ Procurement Transplant Network Ad Hoc Disease Transmission Advisory Committee. Transplantation 2015;15:15.
17. Doucette KE, Al-Saif M, Kneteman N, et al. Donor-derived bacteremia in liver transplant recipients despite antibiotic prophylaxis. Am J Transplant 2013;13:1080-3.
18. Kaul DR, Covington S, Taranto S, et al. Solid organ transplant donors with central nervous system infection. Transplantation 2014;98:666-70.

19. Miceli MH, Gonulalan M, Perri MB, et al. Transmission of infection to liver transplant recipients from donors with infective endocarditis: lessons learned. Transpl Infect Dis 2015;17:140-6.
20. Wendt JM, Kaul D, Limbago BM, et al. Transmission of methicillin-resistant *Staphylococcus aureus* infection through solid organ transplantation: confirmation via whole genome sequencing. Am J Transplant 2014;14:2633-9.
21. Garzoni C, Ison MG. Uniform definitions for donor-derived infectious disease transmissions in solid organ transplantation. Transplantation 2011;92:1297-300.
22. Ison MG, Grossi P. Donor-derived infections in solid organ transplantation. Am J Transplant 2013;13(suppl 4):22-30.
23. Watkins AC, Vedula GV, Horan J, et al. The deceased organ donor with an "open abdomen": proceed with caution. Transpl Infect Dis 2012;14:311-5.
24. Rosen MJ, Clayton K, Schneider RF, et al. Intensive care of patients with HIV infection: utilization, critical illnesses, and outcomes. Pulmonary Complications of HIV Infection Study Group. Am J Respir Crit Care Med 1997;155:67-71.
25. Kaplan JE, Hanson D, Dworkin MS, et al. Epidemiology of human immunodeficiency virus-associated opportunistic infections in the United States in the era of highly active antiretroviral therapy. Clin Infect Dis 2000;30(suppl 1):S5-14.
26. HIV surveillance—United States, 1981-2008. MMWR Morb Mortal Wkly Rep 2011;60:689-93.
27. French MA. HIV/AIDS: immune reconstitution inflammatory syndrome: a reappraisal. Clin Infect Dis 2009;48:101-7.
28. Zolopa A, Andersen J, Powderly W, et al. Early antiretroviral therapy reduces AIDS progression/death in individuals with acute opportunistic infections: a multicenter randomized strategy trial. PLoS ONE 2009;4:e5575.
29. Panel on Antiretroviral Guidelines for Adults and Adolescents. Guidelines for the Use of Antiretroviral Agents in HIV-1-Infected Adults and Adolescents. Department of Health and Human Services. Available at http://aidsinfo.nih.gov/ContentFiles/AdultandAdolescentGL.pdf. Accessed July 9, 2015. 1-282.
30. Lonergan JT, Behling C, Pfander H, et al. Hyperlactatemia and hepatic abnormalities in 10 human immunodeficiency virus-infected patients receiving nucleoside analogue combination regimens. Clin Infect Dis 2000;31:162-6.
31. Escaut L, Liotier JY, Albengres E, et al. Abacavir rechallenge has to be avoided in case of hypersensitivity reaction. AIDS 1999;13:1419-20.
32. Rosen MJ, Narasimhan M. Critical care of immunocompromised patients: human immunodeficiency virus. Crit Care Med 2006;34(9 suppl):S245-250.
33. Fan LC, Lu HW, Cheng KB, et al. Evaluation of PCR in bronchoalveolar lavage fluid for diagnosis of *Pneumocystis jirovecii* pneumonia: a bivariate meta-analysis and systematic review. PLoS ONE 2013;8:e73099.
34. Onishi A, Sugiyama D, Kogata Y, et al. Diagnostic accuracy of serum 1,3-beta-D-glucan for *Pneumocystis jiroveci* pneumonia, invasive candidiasis, and invasive aspergillosis: systematic review and meta-analysis. J Clin Microbiol 2012;50:7-15.
35. Consensus statement on the use of corticosteroids as adjunctive therapy for pneumocystis pneumonia in the acquired immunodeficiency syndrome. The National Institutes of Health-University of California Expert Panel for Corticosteroids as Adjunctive Therapy for Pneumocystis Pneumonia. N Engl J Med 1990;323:1500-4.
36. Luft BJ, Remington JS. Toxoplasmic encephalitis in AIDS. Clin Infect Dis 1992;15:211-22.
37. Torre D, Casari S, Speranza F, et al. Randomized trial of trimethoprim-sulfamethoxazole versus pyrimethamine-sulfadiazine for therapy of toxoplasmic encephalitis in patients with AIDS. Italian Collaborative Study Group. Antimicrob Agents Chemother 1998;42:1346-9.
38. Panel on Opportunistic Infections in HIV-Infected Adults and Adolescents. Guidelines for the Prevention and Treatment of Opportunistic Infections in HIV-Infected Adults and Adolescents: Recommendations from the Centers for Disease Control and Prevention, the National Institutes of Health, and the HIV Medicine Association of the Infectious Diseases Society of America. Available at http://aidsinfo.nih.gov/contentfiles/lvguidelines/adult_oi.pdf. Accessed March 12, 2015. 1-407.
39. Satishchandra P, Sinha S. Seizures in HIV-seropositive individuals: NIMHANS experience and review. Epilepsia 2008;49(suppl 6):33-41.
40. Havlir DV, Dube MP, Sattler FR, et al. Prophylaxis against disseminated *Mycobacterium avium* complex with weekly azithromycin, daily rifabutin, or both. California Collaborative Treatment Group. N Engl J Med 1996;335:392-8.
41. Lee CK, Gingrich RD, Hohl RJ, et al. Engraftment syndrome in autologous bone marrow and peripheral stem cell transplantation. Bone Marrow Transplant 1995;16:175-82.
42. Capizzi SA, Kumar S, Huneke NE, et al. Peri-engraftment respiratory distress syndrome during autologous hematopoietic stem cell transplantation. Bone Marrow Transplant 2001;27:1299-303.
43. Mossad S, Kalaycio M, Sobecks R, et al. Steroids prevent engraftment syndrome after autologous hematopoietic stem cell transplantation without increasing the risk of infection. Bone Marrow Transplant 2005;35:375-81.
44. Afessa B, Abdulai RM, Kremers WK, et al. Risk factors and outcome of pulmonary complications after autologous hematopoietic stem cell transplant. Chest 2012;141:442-50.
45. Majhail NS, Parks K, Defor TE, et al. Diffuse alveolar hemorrhage and infection-associated alveolar hemorrhage following hematopoietic stem cell transplantation: related and high-risk clinical syndromes. Biol Blood Marrow Transplant 2006;12:1038-46.
46. Agusti C, Ramirez J, Picado C, et al. Diffuse alveolar hemorrhage in allogeneic bone marrow transplantation. A postmortem study. Am J Respir Crit Care Med 1995;151:1006-10.
47. Metcalf JP, Rennard SI, Reed EC, et al. Corticosteroids as adjunctive therapy for diffuse alveolar hemorrhage associated with bone marrow transplantation. University of Nebraska Medical Center Bone Marrow Transplant Group. Am J Med 1994;96:327-34.
48. Raptis A, Mavroudis D, Suffredini A, et al. High-dose corticosteroid therapy for diffuse alveolar hemorrhage in allogeneic bone marrow stem cell transplant recipients. Bone Marrow Transplant 1999;24:879-83.
49. Howard SC, Jones DP, Pui CH. The tumor lysis syndrome. N Engl J Med 2011;364:1844-54.

50. Cairo MS, Bishop M. Tumour lysis syndrome: new therapeutic strategies and classification. Br J Haematol 2004;127:3-11.

51. Coiffier B, Altman A, Pui CH, et al. Guidelines for the management of pediatric and adult tumor lysis syndrome: an evidence-based review. J Clin Oncol 2008;26:2767-78.

52. Krishnan G, D'Silva K, Al-Janadi A. Cetuximab-related tumor lysis syndrome in metastatic colon carcinoma. J Clin Oncol 2008;26:2406-8.

53. Noh GY, Choe DH, Kim CH, et al. Fatal tumor lysis syndrome during radiotherapy for non-small-cell lung cancer. J Clin Oncol 2008;26:6005-6.

54. Kraft MD, Btaiche IF, Sacks GS, et al. Treatment of electrolyte disorders in adult patients in the intensive care unit. Am J Health Syst Pharm 2005;62:1663-82.

55. Shimada M, Johnson RJ, May WS Jr, et al. A novel role for uric acid in acute kidney injury associated with tumour lysis syndrome. Nephrol Dial Transplant 2009;24:2960-4.

56. Abu-Alfa AK, Younes A. Tumor lysis syndrome and acute kidney injury: evaluation, prevention, and management. Am J Kidney Dis 2010;55(5 suppl 3):56.

57. Goldman SC, Holcenberg JS, Finklestein JZ, et al. A randomized comparison between rasburicase and allopurinol in children with lymphoma or leukemia at high risk for tumor lysis. Blood 2001;97:2998-3003.

58. Pui CH, Mahmoud HH, Wiley JM, et al. Recombinant urate oxidase for the prophylaxis or treatment of hyperuricemia in patients with leukemia or lymphoma. J Clin Oncol 2001;19:697-704.

59. Knoebel RW, Lo M, Crank CW. Evaluation of a low, weight-based dose of rasburicase in adult patients for the treatment or prophylaxis of tumor lysis syndrome. J Oncol Pharm Pract 2011;17:147-54.

60. Vines AN, Shanholtz CB, Thompson JL. Fixed-dose rasburicase 6 mg for hyperuricemia and tumor lysis syndrome in high-risk cancer patients. Ann Pharmacother 2010;44:1529-537.

61. Darmon M, Guichard I, Vincent F. Rasburicase and tumor lysis syndrome: lower dosage, consideration of indications, and hyperhydration. J Clin Oncol 2011;29:e67-68.

62. Zivkovic SA, Eidelman BH, Bond G, et al. The clinical spectrum of neurologic disorders after intestinal and multivisceral transplantation. Clin Transplant 2010;24:164-8.

63. Bartynski WS, Tan HP, Boardman JF, et al. Posterior reversible encephalopathy syndrome after solid organ transplantation. Am J Neuroradiol 2008;29:924-30.

64. Wu Q, Marescaux C, Wolff V, et al. Tacrolimus-associated posterior reversible encephalopathy syndrome after solid organ transplantation. Eur Neurol 2010;64:169-77.

65. Bartynski WS. Posterior reversible encephalopathy syndrome, part 2: controversies surrounding pathophysiology of vasogenic edema. Am J Neuroradiol 2008;29:1043-9.

66. Horbinski C, Bartynski WS, Carson-Walter E, et al. Reversible encephalopathy after cardiac transplantation: histologic evidence of endothelial activation, T-cell specific trafficking, and vascular endothelial growth factor expression. Am J Neuroradiol 2009;30:588-90.

67. Lee VH, Wijdicks EF, Manno EM, et al. Clinical spectrum of reversible posterior leukoencephalopathy syndrome. Arch Neurol 2008;65:205-10.

68. Kilinc M, Benli S, Can U, et al. FK 506-induced fulminant leukoencephalopathy after kidney transplantation: case report. Transplant Proc 2002;34:1182-4.

69. Heidenhain C, Puhl G, Neuhaus P. Late fulminant posterior reversible encephalopathy syndrome after liver transplant. Exp Clin Transplant 2009;7:180-3.

70. Thyagarajan GK, Cobanoglu A, Johnston W. FK506-induced fulminant leukoencephalopathy after single-lung transplantation. Ann Thorac Surg 1997;64:1461-4.

71. Staykov D, Schwab S. Posterior reversible encephalopathy syndrome. J Intensive Care Med 2012;27:11-24.

72. Eidelman BH, Abu-Elmagd K, Wilson J, et al. Neurologic complications of FK 506. Transplant Proc 1991;23:3175-8.

Chapter 51

Clinically Applied Pharmacogenomics in Critical Care Settings

Samuel G. Johnson, Pharm.D., FCCP; and Christina L. Aquilante, Pharm.D., FCCP

LEARNING OBJECTIVES

1. Recognize pharmacogenomic testing applications relevant to the intensive care unit.
2. Interpret a patient's genotype in the context of drug therapy selection and monitoring.
3. Construct an efficient pathway to provide clinical pharmacogenomic testing in the intensive care unit.

ABBREVIATIONS IN THIS CHAPTER

ADR	Adverse drug reaction	PD	Pharmacodynamic
CPIC	Clinical Pharmacogenetics Implementation Consortium	PK	Pharmacokinetic
		PM	Poor metabolizer
EM	Extensive metabolizer	SNP	Single nucleotide polymorphism
GWAS	Genome-wide association study	TNFα	Tumor necrosis factor alpha
ICU	Intensive care unit	UM	Ultrarapid metabolizer
IM	Intermediate metabolizer	VKOR	Vitamin K epoxide reductase

INTRODUCTION

Patients in critical care settings are highly susceptible to adverse drug reactions (ADRs), mainly because of pharmacokinetic (PK) and pharmacodynamic (PD) changes. Adverse drug reactions are a significant public health concern leading to increased mortality, hospital admissions, length of stay, and health care costs. Inadequate therapeutic response to many commonly used drugs is also a common occurrence because medications are often prescribed using a "trial-and-error" approach in the intensive care unit (ICU). The same is true for drug dosing in the critically ill, which largely remains a "one-size-fits-all" approach that is based on studies of healthy volunteers and less-complicated patient populations. Genetic variation contributes to interindividual differences in drug disposition, response, and toxicity, and as such, pharmacogenetic testing may reduce ADRs and increase therapeutic effectiveness. This chapter will review the available evidence for pertinent genetic variants that influence the PK, PD, and ADRs of drugs used in ICU patients. Current recommendations for pharmacogenetic testing in clinical practice and an exploration of drug, patient, regulatory, and practical issues that presently limit more widespread implementation of pharmacogenetic testing will also be discussed.

EMERGENCE OF CLINICAL PHARMACOGENOMICS

Pharmacogenetics is the study of the relationship between single gene variants (i.e., polymorphisms) and variability in drug disposition, response, and toxicity.[1] Pharmacogenomics represents an expansion of the field and includes the study of variants in a large collection of genes, up to the whole genome.[1] A summary of common genetic terms is provided in Box 51.1.

Pharmacogenetics and pharmacogenomics are both subsets of personalized (precision) medicine, with the goal of identifying patients who should not receive certain drugs or who should receive modified drug dosing because of inherited genetic variants. Interest in pharmacogenomics, as evidenced by the many publications in the field, has increased in the past 20 years. This growing body of literature provides many examples of significant alterations in drug metabolism, drug transport, and drug-gene interactions caused by variants in the respective genes.[3] Despite a common belief that the field represents a future innovation, pharmacogenetics has been detailed in the medical literature since the early 1950s. Historically, pharmacogenetic studies examined the association between single gene variants, PK parameters (e.g., excessive exposure), and ADRs. From a research perspective, most pharmacogenetic investigations have used a candidate gene approach whereby prespecified genetic variants and their association with a phenotypic trait of interest were evaluated. One notable feature of this approach is the need for prior knowledge of the most likely mechanisms underlying drug disposition, response, or toxicity. However, completion of the Human Genome Project in 2003 set the stage for a more exploratory or agnostic approach to uncover the genetic underpinnings of drug response. In this respect, genome-wide association studies (GWAS) are now used to interrogate variants that represent a large portion of variation across the human genome and to evaluate the association between these variants and variability in drug disposition, response, and toxicity. In contrast to the candidate gene approach, GWAS require no prior knowledge of drug action in the body. Landmark human genome sequencing and haplotype mapping efforts (e.g., the HapMap and 1000 Genomes projects) have further informed pharmacogenomic research endeavors. Along these lines, genomic technologies have evolved at a rapid pace. For example, next-generation sequencing technologies, whereby millions of DNA strands are sequenced in parallel, have resulted in substantially higher throughput than older sequencing methods. This has led to an interrogation of all nucleotide bases in the genome (i.e., whole-genome sequencing) and all nucleotide bases in the protein-coding regions of the genome (i.e., whole-exome sequencing). It is anticipated that whole-genome and whole-exome sequencing will foster the expansion of pharmacogenomic research and application by aiding in the discovery of rare and novel variants that are not captured by GWAS.

From a clinical perspective, the increasing affordability and availability of DNA microarrays provides a cost-effective mechanism for assessing thousands of variants simultaneously. This has ushered in the era of preemptive ("just in case") genetic testing whereby DNA microarrays are used to test many variants in relevant pharmacogenes, and this information is stored electronically for future use. However, although many pharmacogenomic associations have been discovered during the past decade, only a few examples are actively being implemented in the clinical setting. Several factors influence the application of pharmacogenetic testing in clinical practice, including analytic validity (the ability of a genetic test to accurately and reliably measure the genotype of interest), clinical validity (the accuracy with which a genetic test can predict the presence or absence of the phenotype of interest), and clinical utility (the likelihood that the genetic test will lead to an improved outcome) (www.cdc.gov/genomics/gtesting/ACCE/). With respect to clinical utility, the Clinical Pharmacogenetics Implementation Consortium (CPIC) was formed as a shared project between the NIH (National Institutes of Health)-sponsored Pharmacogenomics Research Network and the Pharmacogenomics Knowledgebase, with a goal of developing peer-reviewed guidelines for certain drug-gene pairs to help clinicians understand how available genetic test results should be used to optimize drug therapy.[4] The CPIC guideline development process uses systematic evidence review to rate the strength of recommendations and primarily assumes that clinical genotyping results are already available.[5] In addition to CPIC, the Dutch Pharmacogenetics Working Group of the Royal Dutch Pharmacists Association has developed clinical practice guidelines that are based on systematic evidence reviews.[6] Ultimately, critical care clinicians should include pharmacogenetic information in the therapeutic decision-making process with specific attention given to the strength of the available evidence, using available guidelines as a supportive framework. In the next sections, we will discuss key examples of genetic variants that influence the PK and/or PD of agents used in the ICU, together with factors that influence their clinical application (e.g., availability of evidence-based guidelines).

IMPACT ON PK

CYP2D6 Polymorphisms

Cytochrome P450 2D6 (CYP2D6) plays an important role in the metabolism and bioactivation of about one of every four drugs in clinical use, including many antidepressants (e.g., paroxetine, fluvoxamine, amitriptyline), antipsychotics (e.g., haloperidol, risperidone, clozapine), and opioids (e.g., codeine, tramadol).[7-9] The *CYP2D6* gene is highly polymorphic, with 120 allelic variants currently indexed by the CYP Allele Nomenclature Committee (The Human Cytochrome P450 [*CYP*] Allele Nomenclature Database; www.cypalleles.ki.se/). Variant *CYP2D6* alleles include gene deletions, single nucleotide polymorphisms (SNPs), and copy number variations (e.g., gene duplications), among others. These polymorphic alleles translate into differences in CYP2D6 metabolizing enzyme activity and are broadly characterized as functional (normal or increased enzyme activity), reduced-function (decreased enzyme activity), or nonfunctional (inactive or no enzyme) alleles.[10] According to the type and number of *CYP2D6* alleles, individuals are assigned a CYP2D6 phenotype classification (i.e., extensive metabolizer [EM], intermediate metabolizer [IM], poor metabolizer [PM], or ultrarapid metabolizer [UM]). Individuals with the CYP2D6 EM (i.e., "normal") phenotype carry two functional alleles, two reduced-function alleles, one functional allele and one nonfunctional allele, or one functional allele and one reduced-function allele.[10] Intermediate metabolizers carry one reduced-function allele and one nonfunctional allele.[10] Poor metabolizers carry two nonfunctional alleles.[9] Ultrarapid metabolizers carry several copies of a functional allele (e.g., as many as 13).[10] CYP2D6 phenotypes vary by race and ethnicity. For example, the CYP2D6 PM phenotype is found in 5%–10% of whites, 0%–19% of blacks, and less than 1% of Asians.[11] Although genotype analysis has become the method of choice to predict a person's CYP2D6 metabolic activity status, substantial differences exist in the number of genetic variants assayed as well as in the manner in which genetic tests are interpreted. The current process for translating *CYP2D6* genotype results to phenotype assignments is not universal; however, in this section, the traditional phenotype terminology (i.e., EM, IM, PM, and UM) is used.[12]

For many CYP2D6 substrates, variation in CYP2D6 metabolizing enzyme activity is the primary factor contributing to interindividual variability in drug response. Determining an individual's CYP2D6 metabolic activity status can help in the selection of individuals who require an alternative drug or dosage regimen. Patients with reduced-function or nonfunctional CYP2D6 enzyme (e.g., IMs or PMs) attain high parent drug concentrations with standard medication dosing and have less metabolite formation. Depending on which pharmacologic moiety is active, the outcome may be exaggerated efficacy/increased toxicity associated with the parent drug, or therapeutic failure (if it is a prodrug that must be converted to an active metabolite). In UMs, the converse can be expected (i.e., therapeutic failure if an active parent drug or exaggerated efficacy/increased toxicity if a prodrug).[13]

Even though CYP2D6 potentially influences response or toxicity to many drugs, clinical acceptance of *CYP2D6* genotyping in routine practice is currently rare outside of academic or specialty medical centers.[14] Furthermore, evidence to support specific clinical applications for ICU patients is even less developed. However, the Pharmacogenomics Knowledgebase (www.pharmgkb.org) currently lists 34 different CPIC guidelines to help manage drug-gene interactions for CYP2D6 (Table 51.1). In addition, a summary of commonly used drugs in the critical care setting with pharmacogentic associations is provided in Table 51.2.

Although no CPIC guideline currently exists, a gene-drug interaction of particular interest to critical care clinicians is *CYP2D6* and haloperidol, given the common use of this drug to treat delirium. Haloperidol clearance has been directly correlated with the number of functional *CYP2D6* genes in psychiatric patients. In general, studies have found that CYP2D6 PMs receiving haloperidol have

Box 51.1. Glossary of Genomics Terms[1,2]

Allele: One of two or more alternative forms of a gene that arise by inheritance and that are found at the same location on a chromosome. For most autosomal genes, an individual will have two alleles, one inherited from the mother and one inherited from the father.

Autosomal trait: A trait caused by a chromosome that is not a sex chromosome.

Candidate gene study: An evaluation of prespecified genetic variants and their association(s) with a phenotypic trait or disease. This approach requires prior knowledge of the likely mechanisms underlying drug disposition, response, or toxicity.

Diplotype: A pair of haplotypes, with one haplotype inherited from the mother and one haplotype inherited from the father.

DNA microarray: Solid support on which thousands of DNA sequences from different genes are attached. This technology is used to genotype many (e.g., thousands) variants at one time. DNA microarrays that are specifically designed to interrogate single nucleotide polymorphisms (SNPs) are known as SNP arrays.

Genetic variant: A difference in DNA sequence compared with a reference sequence.

Genome: Complete set of genetic material for an organism.

Genome-wide association study: An evaluation of variants that represent a large portion of variation across the human genome and their associations with a phenotypic trait or disease. This approach does not require prior knowledge of the mechanisms underlying drug disposition, response, or toxicity.

Genotype: Broadly defined, the genetic makeup of an organism with reference to a single trait or set of traits. This term is also used to describe the combination of alleles an individual inherits at a specific region of DNA.

Genotyping: Laboratory testing that reveals the specific alleles inherited by an individual at a particular region of DNA.

Haplotype: Set of closely linked alleles that are located on one chromosome and inherited together as a unit or "block."

Homozygous: The same alleles at a specific region of DNA.

Heterozygous: Different alleles at a specific region of DNA.

Linkage disequilibrium: Nonrandom association of alleles at different loci on the same chromosome.

Mutation: A genetic variant that is rare, often defined as occurring in less than 1% of the population. Mutations are often associated with genetic diseases, such as cystic fibrosis or sickle cell anemia.

Pharmacogenetics: Study of the relationship between single gene variants and variability in drug disposition, response, and toxicity.

Pharmacogenomics: Study of the relationship between variants in a large collection of genes, up to the whole genome, and variability in drug disposition, response, and toxicity.

Phenotype: The set of measurable characteristics of an individual caused by genotype, environment, or a combination of both.

Polymorphism: A genetic variant that is common, often defined as occurring in 1% or more of the population.

Single nucleotide polymorphism (SNP): Difference in one nucleotide (base pair) in a DNA sequence. SNPs are the most common type of polymorphism in the genome.

Wild type: A characteristic that refers to the typical form of a trait as it occurs in nature. Also called the most common allele in a population.

a greater incidence of ADRs, including pseudoparkinsonism (increased sum of extrapyramidal symptom scores; p=0.02), a prolonged elimination half-life (19.1 ± 3.6 vs. 12.9 ± 4.0 hours, p=0.04), and a lower apparent oral clearance (12.8 ± 4.1 vs. 27.0 ± 11.3 mL/minute/kg, p=0.02), than do EMs.[15,16] However, additional factors (i.e., smoking status and body weight) also contribute to the observed ADRs.[16]

Although haloperidol is a useful example, the prescribing of risperidone for psychosis and other behavioral disorders is increasingly common. In studies involving risperidone, the CYP2D6 PM phenotype was associated with a moderate-to-marked increase in drug discontinuation attributable to ADRs (namely pseudoparkinsonism).[28,29] Pharmacokinetic analyses support these observations, with evidence that PMs have a 63% decrease in the metabolism and fraction of the active metabolite.[30]

Studies exploring the impact of CYP2D6 polymorphisms on variability in toxicity or response to cardiovascular drugs (i.e., β-blockers) also suggest a need for individualized therapy. One large population-based study reported that CYP2D6 PMs receiving β-blockers metabolized by CYP2D6 (e.g., metoprolol, carvedilol, nebivolol, propranolol, and alprenolol) had a significantly lower heart rate and diastolic blood pressure than EMs,[31] which was not reproduced in patients receiving β-blockers not metabolized by CYP2D6 (e.g., atenolol).

Understanding opioid metabolism and disposition is essential for assessing the risk of toxicity and, in some cases, for providing additional information regarding the risk of therapeutic failure. Opioids significantly metabolized by the CYP enzyme system may be subject to drug-gene interactions. Codeine provides a good example of the potential clinical utility of CYP2D6 genotyping.[14] Codeine, a prodrug, is metabolized by CYP2D6 to form morphine. CYP2D6 PMs do not effectively convert codeine to morphine, resulting in decreased analgesic effects compared with EMs.[9] Conversely, CYP2D6 UMs have increased conversion of codeine to morphine compared with EMs, as well as an increased risk of morphine toxicity and a clinically significant risk of severe morbidity and mortality.[32]

Patient response to tramadol, an alternative opioid agent commonly used for pain management, is also affected by CYP2D6 genotype, with CYP2D6 PMs at risk of insufficient analgesia and UMs at risk of serious ADRs (e.g., respiratory depression).[6,33] The extent to which other opioids (e.g., hydrocodone, oxycodone) are affected by CYP2D6 variation is under investigation. Preliminary evidence suggests that CYP2D6 PMs have lower peak concentrations of hydromorphone after a dose of hydrocodone; however, CYP2D6 metabolizer status does not appear to affect response to hydrocodone therapy. Similarly, CYP2D6 PMs have lower peak concentrations of oxymorphone after a dose of oxycodone than do EMs.[34] However, discordant findings from prospective clinical studies currently suggest limited clinical utility of CYP2D6 genotyping for oxycodone therapy. In general, the CPIC guidelines recommend that opioids not metabolized by CYP2D6, including morphine, oxymorphone, buprenorphine, fentanyl, methadone, and hydromorphone,

Table 51.1 Available Evidence-Based Dosing Guidelines for Drugs According to *CYP2D6* and *CYP2C19* Genotypes

Clinical Pharmacogenetics Implementation Consortium (CPIC) Guidelines	Dutch Pharmacogenetics Working Group (DPWG) Guidelines
Amitriptyline and CYP2C19, CYP2D6	Amitriptyline and CYP2D6
Clomipramine and CYP2C19, CYP2D6	Aripiprazole and CYP2D6
Codeine and CYP2D6	Atomoxetine and CYP2D6
Desipramine and CYP2D6	Carvedilol and CYP2D6
Doxepin and CYP2C19, CYP2D6	Clomipramine and CYP2D6
Imipramine and CYP2C19, CYP2D6	Clozapine and CYP2D6
Nortriptyline and CYP2D6	Codeine and CYP2D6
Trimipramine and CYP2C19, CYP2D6	Doxepin and CYP2D6
	Duloxetine and CYP2D6
	Flecainide and CYP2D6
	Flupenthixol and CYP2D6
	Haloperidol and CYP2D6
	Imipramine and CYP2D6
	Metoprolol and CYP2D6
	Mirtazapine and CYP2D6
	Nortriptyline and CYP2D6
	Olanzapine and CYP2D6
	Oxycodone and CYP2D6
	Paroxetine and CYP2D6
	Propafenone and CYP2D6
	Risperidone and CYP2D6
	Tamoxifen and CYP2D6
	Tramadol and CYP2D6
	Venlafaxine and CYP2D6
	Zuclopenthixol and CYP2D6

From: the Pharmacogenomics Knowledge Base. Available at https://www.pharmgkb.org/gene/PA128. Accessed March 2, 2015.

Table 51.2 Commonly Used Drugs in Critical Care Settings with Pharmacogenetic Associations

Drug or Drug Class	Gene	Therapeutic Recommendations
Haloperidol	CYP2D6	PMs: Reduce dose by 50% or select alternative drug (e.g., pimozide, flupenthixol, fluphenazine, quetiapine, olanzapine, clozapine)[16]
Proton pump inhibitors (omeprazole, esomeprazole, lansoprazole, rabeprazole)	CYP2C19	UMs: *Helicobacter pylori* eradication: Increase dose by 100%–200%. Be alert to insufficient response.
Antifungals (voriconazole)	CYP2C19	PMs and IMs: Monitor serum concentrations to minimize toxicity (i.e., QTc prolongation)[20]
		UMs: Monitor serum concentrations to ensure effectiveness (especially for invasive fungal infections in immunocompromised patients)[21,22]
Opioids (codeine, tramadol, oxycodone)	CYP2D6	PMs and IMs: Analgesia: Select alternative drug (e.g., acetaminophen, NSAID, morphine—not tramadol or oxycodone), or be alert to symptoms of insufficient pain relief[9,14,23]
		UMs: Analgesia: Select alternative drug (e.g., acetaminophen, NSAID, morphine—not tramadol or oxycodone), or be alert to ADRs. Cough: Be extra alert to ADRs caused by increased morphine plasma concentrations[9,14,23-27]

IM = intermediate metabolizer; PM = poor metabolizer; QTc = corrected QT interval; UM = ultrarapid metabolizer.

From: the Pharmacogenomics Knowledge Base. Available at https://www.pharmgkb.org/gene/PA128. Accessed 2015 March 2, 2015.

together with nonopioid analgesics, be considered as alternatives for use in CYP2D6 PMs and UMs according to the type, severity, and chronicity of the pain being treated.[9]

Antiemetic therapy—particularly with ondansetron—is the last example for clinical utility of the *CYP2D6* genotype in critically ill patients. Patients having CYP2D6 EM, IM, or PM phenotypes are more likely to have an increased response to ondansetron than are patients having CYP2D6 UM phenotypes. This increased response leads to a reduced risk of vomiting after chemotherapy or anesthesia. However, no significant associations have been found for nausea.[35,36]

CYP2C9 Polymorphisms

Cytochrome P450 2C9 is another drug-metabolizing enzyme involved in the phase I metabolism of about 10% of drugs, including oral anticoagulants (e.g., warfarin), antiepileptics (e.g., phenytoin), oral antidiabetics (e.g., glyburide), NSAIDs (nonsteroidal anti-inflammatory drugs) (e.g., celecoxib), and anti-infectives (e.g., sulfamethoxazole).[37-39]

Several variants have been identified in the *CYP2C9* gene that influence CYP2C9 metabolizing enzyme function. *CYP2C9*1* is the normal-activity allele, and *CYP2C9*2* and *CYP2C9*3* are the most commonly studied decreased-function alleles. *CYP2C9*2* is present in about 13%, 0%, and 3% of whites, Asians, and blacks, respectively. *CYP2C9*3* is present in about 7%, 4%, and 2% of whites, Asians, and blacks, respectively.[39] An individual carrying two normal-activity alleles (i.e., *1/*1) is assigned the EM phenotype. An individual carrying one normal-activity allele and one decreased-function allele (i.e., *1/*2 or *1/*3) is assigned the IM phenotype. An individual carrying two decreased-function alleles (i.e., *2/*2, *2/*3, or *3/*3) is assigned the PM phenotype.[39]

To date, warfarin has been heavily studied with respect to *CYP2C9* genetics because of its frequent use and narrow therapeutic index. The FDA's Adverse Event Reporting System affirms that ADRs attributable to warfarin are common; in fact, warfarin is among the top 10 most commonly reported drugs during the past 20 years.[40] *CYP2C9* genotype accounts for 9%–12% of the observed variance in warfarin maintenance dose requirements.[41] In general, individuals carrying *CYP2C9*2* or *3 alleles have lower warfarin dose requirements and a longer time to achieve a therapeutic international normalized ratio (INR) than do EMs.[42] A recent retrospective study found that patients carrying variant *CYP2C9* alleles (e.g., *2, *3) had a significantly increased risk of serious or life-threatening bleeding events after warfarin therapy.[43] However, a prospective study revealed conflicting data showing no association between variant *CYP2C9* alleles and the risk of warfarin-associated bleeding.[44] Depending on the approach to initiating anticoagulation in clinical practice, *CYP2C9* genotype is a factor to consider for warfarin, in addition to *VKORC1* (drug target) genotype, drug-drug interactions, drug-disease interactions, and drug-diet interactions. The practicalities and controversies of warfarin genotyping in clinical practice are discussed in more detail in the *VKORC1* section.

A *CYP2C9* drug-gene interaction also exists for phenytoin, one of the most commonly used antiepileptics in the ICU. Phenytoin clearance through CYP2C9-mediated hydroxylation is a primary mechanism, although at high concentrations, CYP2C19 is also involved. Many studies have reported higher phenytoin plasma concentrations and lower phenytoin dose requirements in CYP2C9 variant allele carriers (i.e., IMs or PMs) than in EMs. In this respect, CYP2C9 genotype–guided dose adjustments have been recommended for phenytoin therapy (e.g., 25% dose reduction for IMs and 50% dose reduction for PMs).[39] Despite this information, data supporting the link between altered phenytoin plasma concentrations and ADRs are lacking, presumably because of the nonlinear, saturable PK, and auto-inductive effects of this drug.

CYP2C19 Polymorphisms

Cytochrome P450 2C19 is responsible for the metabolism of antiplatelet agents (e.g., clopidogrel), proton pump inhibitors (e.g., lansoprazole, omeprazole), antidepressants (e.g., amitriptyline, citalopram, sertraline), and antifungal agents (e.g., voriconazole).[45] The CYP2C19 gene is highly polymorphic, with SNPs that result in decreased or increased CYP2C19 metabolizing enzyme activity. CYP2C19*1 is the normal-activity allele, CYP2C19*2 and CYP2C19*3 are loss-of-function (i.e., decreased or no function) alleles, and CYP2C19*17 is an increased-function allele. An individual with two normal-function alleles (i.e., *1/*1) is assigned the EM phenotype. An individual with one normal-function allele and one loss-of-function allele (e.g., *1/*2 or *1/*3) is assigned the IM phenotype. An individual with two loss-of-function alleles (e.g., *2/*2 or *3/*3) is assigned the PM phenotype. An individual carrying two increased-function alleles (e.g., *17/*17) or one normal-function allele and one increased-function allele (e.g., *1/*17) is assigned the UM phenotype.[8,46] The frequency of the CYP2C19 PM phenotype is 2%–5% in whites, 2%–5% in African Americans, and 15% in Asians.[47] The frequency of the CYP2C19*17 allele is about 22% in whites, 19% in African Americans, and 17% in Asians (South/Central).[8] The impact of the CYP2C19 genotype on clinical outcomes associated with clopidogrel antiplatelet therapy has received much attention in patients with acute coronary syndromes. Clopidogrel undergoes a two-step bioactivation process to form an active thiol metabolite. The CYP2C19 enzyme is important in each step of this process. Clopidogrel response varies widely in the general population, and many studies have shown that CYP2C19*2 carriers (e.g., *1/*2 or *2/*2 genotypes) have lower concentrations of the clopidogrel active metabolite and higher on-treatment platelet aggregation than noncarriers.[46,48] In addition, several studies link CYP2C19 PM and IM status to an increased risk of major adverse cardiovascular events in clopidogrel-treated patients with acute coronary syndromes, likely because of reduced formation of the active clopidogrel metabolite.[46,49-52] Although the primary concern in this respect is loss of efficacy, CYP2C19 UMs may be at higher risk of ADRs (e.g., hemorrhage), likely because of increased formation of the active clopidogrel metabolite.[53,54] The primary takeaway is that variability in response to clopidogrel treatment associated with an increased risk of death or thrombotic recurrences is present in 5%–40% of patients treated with conventional doses of clopidogrel, with a multifactorial etiology that includes genetic polymorphisms and nongenetic factors (e.g., comorbidities, drug-drug interactions, age).[55]

Another relevant example of the application of CYP2C19 pharmacogenetics to critical care is in the use of proton pump inhibitors. The CYP2C19 genotype is responsible for 80% of the metabolism of omeprazole, lansoprazole, and pantoprazole.[17,56,57] Clinical data show that CYP2C19 PMs have 4- to 15-fold higher plasma concentrations of omeprazole and lansoprazole, and superior acid suppression, relative to EMs.[17] Having CYP2C19 IM or PM status may lead to enhanced proton pump inhibitor–mediated *Helicobacter pylori* eradication and ulcer healing; however, a consistent demonstration of improved outcomes relative to the CYP2C19 phenotype remains elusive. Future research endeavors are needed to firmly establish the clinical utility of CYP2C19 genotyping for the proton pump inhibitors; however, when preemptive testing is available, clinicians may consider relevant drug-gene interactions for individual patient management.

Voriconazole is a narrow therapeutic index antifungal agent with nonlinear PK whose plasma exposure is influenced, in part, by CYP2C19 metabolizer status.[21] For example, in healthy volunteers, CYP2C19 PMs had 4-fold higher voriconazole exposure than EMs.[58] Although CPIC has not yet developed guidelines for this drug, the Dutch Pharmacogenetics Working Group guidelines recommend the monitoring of voriconazole serum concentrations in CYP2C19 IMs and PMs. This will help minimize the risk of concentration-dependent ADRs. In addition, knowledge of CYP2C19 UM status may help prevent therapeutic failure caused by inadequate drug concentrations.[21] Given the high costs associated with hospitalization for treatment-resistant invasive fungal infections, health systems are increasingly considering CYP2C19 genotyping and therapeutic drug monitoring for voriconazole therapy to prevent avoidable health care use.[20,22]

CYP3A Polymorphisms

Tacrolimus is a calcineurin inhibitor immunosuppressant commonly used in solid organ and hematopoietic stem cell transplantation. Tacrolimus has a narrow therapeutic range and large interpatient variability in the dose required to achieve therapeutic trough concentrations.[59] Low tacrolimus exposure may increase the risk of graft rejection, whereas high tacrolimus exposure may increase the risk of ADRs (e.g., nephrotoxicity, neurotoxicity, hyperglycemia).[60]

Tacrolimus is predominantly metabolized by CYP3A5 and, to a lesser extent, by CYP3A4. The *CYP3A5* gene contains several variants, *3, *6, and *7, which result in loss of protein expression or nonfunctional protein.[61] Individuals carrying two copies of the *CYP3A5*1* allele (*CYP3A5 *1/*1*) are assigned the expresser (EM) phenotype. An individual carrying one functional allele and one nonfunctional allele (i.e., *1/*3, *1/*6, or *1/*7) is assigned the expresser (IM) phenotype. An individual carrying two nonfunctional alleles (e.g., *3/*3, *6/*6) is assigned the non-expresser (PM) phenotype.[59] Substantial differences in *CYP3A5* variant allele frequencies exist on the basis of race. For example, *CYP3A5*3 is present in 92% of whites, 32% of African Americans, and 74% of Asians.[59]

Therapeutic drug monitoring is routinely used to manage tacrolimus blood concentrations in clinical practice, but therapeutic drug monitoring does not identify the optimal starting dose of tacrolimus for an individual patient. Several studies, in various transplant populations, have shown that CYP3A5 expressers have lower dose-adjusted tacrolimus trough concentrations than do CYP3A5 non-expressers.[59] In this respect, a prospective study of kidney transplant recipients showed that *CYP3A5* genotype-guided tacrolimus dosing resulted in a significantly higher percentage of patients with tacrolimus in the target range 3 days after initiating therapy compared with the control arm (43.2% vs. 29.1%, respectively).[62] This study did not show a significant difference in clinical outcomes (e.g., acute rejection) between genotype-guided and standard tacrolimus dosing. However, a recent meta-analysis of kidney transplant recipients showed a modestly increased risk of acute rejection in CYP3A5 expressers (odds ratio 1.32, p=0.04).[63] According to the CPIC guidelines, no definitive evidence exists to indicate that *CYP3A5* genotype–guided tacrolimus dosing improves long-term clinical outcomes. However, the clinical utility of *CYP3A5* genotyping appears to be in the ability to more effectively achieve target trough tacrolimus concentrations, particularly at the initiation of therapy.[59] In this respect, CPIC guidelines recommend that CYP3A5 expressers (EMs or IMs) receive 1.5–2 times the recommended tacrolimus starting dose, not to exceed 0.3 mg/kg/day. In contrast, it is recommended that CYP3A5 non-expressers (PMs) start therapy with standard recommended doses. In both cases, therapeutic drug monitoring should be used to guide dose adjustments. These recommendations apply to the use of tacrolimus in patients with kidney, heart, lung, and hematopoietic stem cell transplants and in patients with liver transplants when the donor and recipient genotypes are identical. In sum, *CYP3A5* genotyping may be most helpful to guide initial tacrolimus dosing in the hopes of more rapidly achieving target trough concentrations.[59] Genetic testing does not preclude the need for therapeutic drug monitoring or the need to consider other patient-specific factors that may influence tacrolimus therapy (e.g., age, drug-drug interactions).

N-Acetyltransferase 2

N-acetyltransferase 2 is a phase II drug-metabolizing enzyme that acetylates several agents, including isoniazid, hydralazine, procainamide, phenelzine, dapsone, and sulfonamides. Observations that some patients receiving isoniazid were more prone to peripheral neuropathy led to identification of the slow acetylator phenotype. Across the general population, phenotype frequencies vary among different ethnic populations (e.g., about 50% of whites are slow acetylators, whereas the frequency is much lower in Asians). For critically ill patients, slow acetylators have an increased risk of immune-mediated toxicity (systemic lupus erythematosus) with specific agents used in the ICU (i.e., hydralazine, procainamide, and sulfamethoxazole). In addition, fast acetylators may carry a higher risk of preventable ADRs. For example, procainamide, which is bioactivated in vivo to a pharmacologically active class III antiarrhythmic metabolite, N-acetylprocainamide, increases the risk of torsades de pointes—especially in renally compromised patients. Because procainamide is still used in specific clinical scenarios (e.g., rate control for patients with Wolff-Parkinson-White syndrome and atrial fibrillation), N-acetyltransferase 2 phenotype remains important to evaluate as a clinical consideration.[64,65]

SLCO1B1 Genotype

Statins are widely used lipid-lowering agents with a proven record for reducing cardiovascular morbidity and mortality. Statins are associated with myalgias, myopathy, and, rarely, rhabdomyolysis. Mechanisms leading to increased risk of statin-induced myopathy have been incompletely characterized and are likely multifactorial—including comorbidities, presence of significant drug-drug interactions, and genetic variation. Several clinical factors are associated with statin-induced myopathy, including advanced age, slight body mass index, female sex, metabolic comorbidities, drug-drug interactions, hypothyroidism, and Asian ancestry.[66]

Statin dose remains perhaps the strongest predictor of statin-induced myopathy, with a reported incidence that is almost 10-fold higher in patients on high-dose statin therapy. Although this dose-dependent relationship appears to be a class effect for statins, evidence suggests that this effect is most clinically significant with respect to simvastatin.[67]

Of importance, statins are substrates of the organic anion transporting polypeptide 1B1 (OATP1B1), an uptake transporter located on the basolateral surface of hepatocytes. Variation in *SLCO1B1*, the gene that encodes OATP1B1, produces a defective transport protein, which increases systemic exposure and toxicity.[68-70] A GWAS identified a significant association between the functional *SLCO1B1* c.521T>C SNP and simvastatin-induced myopathy, showing a 4.5-fold increased risk in heterozygotes and a 16.9-fold increased risk in variant homozygotes.[71] The c.521 T>C SNP is contained in the *SLCO1B1*5* haplotype, which is carried in about 1%–3% of whites, up to 2% of Africans, and up to 1% of Asians, and also in the *SLCO1B1*15* haplotype, which is carried in about 14% of whites, 3% of Africans, and up to 13% of Asians.[67,72] CPIC guidelines exist for simvastatin dosing in relation to *SLCO1B1* c.521 T>C genotype.[72] Specifically, individuals with *SLCO1B1* c.521 T/T (normal function) genotype have a normal simvastatin-induced myopathy risk and may be prescribed the desired starting dose, with doses adjusted on the basis of disease-specific guidelines. Individuals with the *SLCO1B1* c.521 T/C (intermediate function) genotype have an intermediate simvastatin-induced myopathy risk. CPIC guidelines recommend a lower simvastatin dose or consideration of an alternative statin (e.g., pravastatin or rosuvastatin). Finally, individuals with the *SLCO1B1* c.521 C/C (low function) genotype have a high simvastatin-induced myopathy risk. It is recommended that these patients be prescribed a lower dose or that an alternative statin be considered (e.g., pravastatin or rosuvastatin). In each case presented, the FDA recommends against simvastatin 80 mg/day unless the dose has already been tolerated for 12 months.[72]

IMPACT ON PD

VKORC1 Polymorphisms

The vitamin K epoxide reductase (VKOR) enzyme catalyzes the recycling of reduced vitamin K, which is essential for the formation of clotting factors II (prothrombin), VII, IX, and X. Warfarin inhibits this enzyme, thereby producing anticoagulant effects. Many common SNPs exist in *VKORC1*, the gene encoding VKOR. The g.-1639G>A SNP is contained in a haplotype associated with reduced VKOR expression. Individuals with this SNP are more sensitive to warfarin, as evidenced by decreased therapeutic dose requirements (28% smaller per allele carried). In addition to *CYP2C9* polymorphisms, *VKORC1* genotype is an important consideration for predicting warfarin dose requirements and accounts for 25%–30% of observed dose variance in white populations. In addition, combining *VKORC1* and *CYP2C9* genotypes explains up to 59% of the variability in warfarin dose requirements. Two GWAS analyzing hundreds of thousands of SNPs across the human genome further confirmed that *VKORC1* and *CYP2C9* provide the greatest contributions to warfarin dose variability in whites. Although variation in both genes has been associated with excessive anticoagulation, *VKORC1* variants, unlike *CYP2C9*, have not been associated with an increased risk of hemorrhage.[73-76]

Two recent randomized trials evaluating the clinical impact of genotype-guided warfarin dosing are the European Pharmacogenetics of Anticoagulant Therapy (EU-PACT) trial and the Clarification of Optimal Anticoagulation Through Genetics (COAG) trial. Both trials examined the effects of genotype-guided warfarin dosing compared with empiric dosing strategies; however, only the EU-PACT study showed an overall improvement in time to achieve therapeutic INR, which was shorter in the genotyping arm (21 vs. 29 days; p<0.001).

The primary outcome of the COAG trial was to assess the percentage of time in therapeutic range within the first 4 weeks of therapy. Results indicated that 45% of patients in both arms reached therapeutic INR levels within 4 weeks, and there were no differences in bleeding or thromboembolic events. About one-third of the patients were African Americans, and the percentage of time in therapeutic range within the African American subgroup who received dosing on the basis of clinical variables was 43.5%, whereas in the genotyping arm, the percentage of time in therapeutic INR was 35%, favoring clinical-variable dosing versus genotyping dosing in African Americans (p=0.01). Of importance, 76% of African Americans (compared with 25% of non–African Americans) had no genetic variation in the SNPs assessed, and other variants known to predict dosing variability in African Americans (e.g., *CYP2C9 *5, *6, *8,* and **11*) were not assayed in the COAG trial.[77,78] Taken together, including the pharmacogenetic information for warfarin in a systematic approach to assessing and treating critically ill patients on the basis of available evidence and expert opinion could help avoid dosing errors that may adversely affect patient outcomes.

Human Leukocyte Antigens

Human leukocyte antigen class I and class II constitute the major human histocompatibility complex and assist in the initiation of the immune response by presenting antigens to T cells. Three different genes (*HLA-A, HLA-B,* and *HLA-C*) exist within class I. The *HLA-B* genes are highly polymorphic and have been strongly associated with ADRs.[71] Stevens-Johnson syndrome and toxic epidermal necrolysis caused by therapy with the antiepileptic drug carbamazepine have been linked to the *HLA-B*15:02* genotype—particularly in Han Chinese. Because of the relatively high prevalence of this allele in Han Chinese and other Asian populations, the FDA recommends *HLA-B*15:02* screening for all patients of Asian ancestry before initiating carbamazepine.[80-83]

Another strong link between *HLA* genotype and ADRs is shown by abacavir hypersensitivity associated with the *HLA-B*57:01* allele.[84] Although this anti-HIV medication is not commonly used in the ICU, it provides the clearest evidence to date of the clinical utility of a pharmacogenetic biomarker for preventing ADRs. About

5%–8% of patients have a limiting hypersensitivity reaction to abacavir within the first 6 weeks of therapy. The *HLA-B*57:01* variant is found in 8% of whites, but it is rare in African American and Asian populations. The Prospective Randomized Evaluation of DNA Screening in a Clinical Trial (PREDICT-1) was conducted in 1,956 patients across 19 countries to determine the effectiveness of *HLA-B*57:01* screening to prevent hypersensitivity. Results showed that prospective screening for the *HLA-B*57:01* allele in the predominantly white population prevented 100% of abacavir hypersensitivity reactions. These results and similar data from a case-control trial involving nonwhite populations led to the formal recommendation of pretreatment screening for *HLA-B*57:01* in the current HIV treatment guidelines.[85] Future research will likely elucidate additional *HLA* variants that underlie drug hypersensitivity reactions, which is a pertinent critical care issue.

KCNH2, Other Cardiac Ion Channels, and Associated Proteins

KCNH2, otherwise known as the human ether-a-go-go-related gene, encodes for a potassium voltage-gated ion channel responsible for the rapid component of the delayed rectifier current (IKr) in cardiac cells. Mutations in *KCNH2* reduce cardiac repolarizing current, prolong the action potential, and are a cause of congenital long-QT syndrome. Virtually all drugs that prolong the QT interval and cause the potentially fatal arrhythmia called *torsades de pointes* also block the IKr/human ether-a-go-go-related gene channel. The list of offending drugs is large and includes many drugs commonly prescribed in the ICU, such as antiarrhythmics (quinidine, disopyramide, procainamide, dofetilide, ibutilide, sotalol, and amiodarone), antibiotics (erythromycin, clarithromycin, sparfloxacin, and pentamidine), antiemetics (droperidol), antipsychotics (haloperidol, thioridazine, chlorpromazine, mesoridazine, and pimozide), bepridil, methadone, among others. The incidence of torsades de pointes in those receiving antiarrhythmics has been estimated to be as high as 5%, and although some clinical risk factors have been identified, the ADR remains unpredictable for individual patients. Several studies support the involvement of variation in *KCNH2* and other cardiac ion channel–associated genes. In one of the larger studies, Yang et al. screened 92 patients with drug-induced long-QT syndrome and found that 10%–15% of individuals carried a mutation in the coding region of at least one of a series of sodium or potassium channel genes (*KCNH2*, *KCNQ1*, *SCN5A*, *KCNE1*, or *KCNE2*). Similarly, *KCNE1*, *KCNE2*, and *KCNH2* variants were identified in 4 of 32 patients with drug-induced long-QT syndrome evaluated in another study. Two very large European ancestry GWAS further identified some of these ion channel genes as being important determinants of QT interval variability. Further studies are needed to define the relative importance of these genes and to determine the strength of the association of specific variants with an increased risk of drug-induced long-QT syndromes in critically ill patients.[86-91]

Tumor Necrosis Factor Alpha and Sepsis

Sepsis syndrome is one of the most common causes of morbidity, mortality, and resource expenditure in critically ill patients.[92] In this complex syndrome, invasive infection, trauma, or other insults elicit an abnormal host inflammatory response that, in a minority of patients, gives rise to profound hemodynamic instability (septic shock), organ failure, and death. The principal focus of clinical investigation in this area is based on attempts to understand the host inflammatory response and to develop interventions to modulate such response. Common variants present in genes encoding inflammatory mediators could affect the regulation of the inflammatory response. A SNP in the tumor necrosis factor alpha (*TNFA*) gene g.-308G>A has been among the most thoroughly studied in this context. Mira et al. reported that the g.-308A allele (also known as *TNF2*) was more common in patients with sepsis and was associated with a significantly increased risk of mortality compared with case-matched controls.[93] Similarly, O'Keefe et al. reported that the presence of *TNF2* was associated with an increased risk of the development of sepsis, but not mortality, after severe injury in a cohort of patients.[94] In contrast, Tang et al. reported that *TNF2* occurred with no greater frequency in patients with sepsis than in patients without sepsis. However, for the subset of patients who developed shock, this genetic variant was associated with an increased rate of mortality.[95] Inconsistent findings in studies examining the clinical significance of the *TNFA* g.-308G>A SNP in patients with sepsis or those at risk of this disease are representative of problems with gene-association studies in general. Systematic analyses of studies trying to link genetic variants to complex traits have shown that the significant results reported in the initial studies are often not replicated in subsequent experiments. Linkage-disequilibrium studies can be confounded because the effects of variants in a locus of interest (for example, the *TNFA* g.-308 SNP) may be influenced by the effects of adjacent variants (e.g., those present elsewhere in the *TNFA* gene), genetic variants present in independently segregating loci (e.g., those encoding other inflammatory mediators), and nongenetic factors. For the critically ill individual, these nongenetic factors include the nature and location of the inciting infection, the manner in which supportive care is provided, and the age and premorbid health status of the patient. In addition, populations studied in many trials are heterogeneous. In the reports cited, populations differed substantially with respect to geography as well as in their underlying clinical condition. The challenge for critical care investigators will be to design gene-association studies that are both appropriately controlled and of sufficient power so that the genetic determinants of disease susceptibility and drug effect can be measured accurately.[96-98]

INCORPORATING PHARMACOGENOMICS INTO PATIENT CARE

Despite the many established associations between genetic variants and drug response, pharmacogenomic testing and genotype- or phenotype-based prescribing have not been widely implemented in clinical practice. Drug, patient, research design, regulatory, and practical issues currently limit the integration of pharmacogenomics into the clinical setting, including the ICU. Regarding drug factors, knowledge that an enzyme is involved in the metabolism of a drug and that a genetic variant exists is not sufficient to recommend genetic testing. The functional consequences of the variant, the quantitative role of the gene product to the drug's overall PK and PD, and the agent's therapeutic index must be considered. Clopidogrel, for example, is metabolized by several CYP enzymes, yet only *CYP2C19* variants are important for the increased risk of major adverse cardiovascular events. Few examples currently exist in which a drug-ADR relationship can be predicted by variation at a single gene locus (e.g., abacavir and *HLA-B*57:01*). In contrast, most drug response and toxicity examples (e.g., torsades de pointes or warfarin dose-response) are polygenic. Drugs may also have a wide therapeutic index or a toxicity that is mild or easy to detect, suggesting that genotyping is not necessary, such as with *CYP2D6* polymorphisms and β-blockers. Drugs that are pharmacologically active themselves and that have active metabolites, such as some tricyclic antidepressants, also complicate efforts to associate genetic variants with ADRs. Many patient issues facing the critically ill are known to produce wide variability in drug response and ADR risk. In addition to considering genetic variation, multidisciplinary critical care teams must evaluate the impact of impaired organ function, comorbidities, polypharmacy, drug interactions, and many other factors when providing pharmacotherapy. The paucity of pharmacogenomic research involving critically ill patients undermines an appreciation of the potential role that genetics play in this population. Of the 107 pharmacogenomic studies currently listed as seeking volunteers in an online repository of human clinical studies being conducted globally, most involve oncology drugs.[99] Only one study specifically mentions recruiting in the ICU, and 14 studies involve drugs with relevance to critically ill patients.[100] Future investigations must determine the relative contribution of genetics to overall drug response and ADR risk in the critically ill in order to advance pharmacogenomics in the ICU setting.

Practical issues also hamper the widespread clinical adoption of genotyping. Medical education has not kept up with the rapid pace of pharmacogenomics. Citing this, recommendations for bolstering training in medical, pharmacy, and nursing schools globally have been advanced.[101] An urgent need also exists for reliable bedside genetic testing because the turnaround time for tests that must be sent to accredited laboratories is not ideal. For example, according to the manufacturer, AmpliChip[102] results can be generated in 8 hours, with the printed report received within several days. This time interval is problematic when appropriate drug dosing is needed immediately, such as with clopidogrel after myocardial infarction. It is less of an issue for long half-life drugs used for chronic therapy, such as warfarin, because algorithms have been created for dose modification once genetic information becomes available. Furthermore, alternative therapies with more favorable safety profiles and less monitoring than warfarin exist. As these issues are resolved, it is likely that more data from studies evaluating genetic predisposition to ADRs will be implemented in ICU clinical practice. Critical care practitioners should continue to be aware of new data and advances in the field of pharmacogenomics to appreciate the contribution that genetic variation makes to interindividual variation in drug disposition, response, and toxicity.

SUMMARY

Critically ill patients have an increased risk of ADRs. Although many factors contribute to the variation in patient response to pharmacotherapy, the impact of genetic variation on drug PK and PD is increasingly being appreciated. Clinical pharmacogenomics provides critical care practitioners with additional tools to optimize medication effectiveness and improve safety profiles for the armamentarium of medications used in the critical care setting.

REFERENCES

1. Roden DM, Altman RB, Benowitz NL, et al. Pharmacogenomics: challenges and opportunities. Ann Intern Med 2006;145:749-57.
2. Johnson SG, Aquilante CL. Clinical implementation of pharmacogenomics—evaluating the evidence. In: Johnson JA, Elingrod VL, Kroetz DL, et al., eds. Pharmacogenomics: Applications to Patient Care, 3rd ed. Lenexa, KS: American College of Clinical Pharmacy, 2015:19-31.
3. Beitelshees AL, McLeod HL. Applying pharmacogenomics to enhance the use of biomarkers for drug effect and drug safety. Trends Pharmacol Sci 2006;27:498-502.
4. Relling MV, Klein TE. CPIC: Clinical Pharmacogenetics Implementation Consortium of the Pharmacogenomics Research Network. Clin Pharmacol Ther 2011;89:464-7.
5. Caudle KE, Klein TE, Hoffman JM, et al. Incorporation of pharmacogenomics into routine clinical practice: the Clinical Pharmacogenetics Implementation Consortium (CPIC) guideline development process. Curr Drug Metab 2014;15:209-17.
6. Swen JJ, Nijenhuis M, de Boer A, et al. Pharmacogenetics: from bench to byte—an update of guidelines. Clin Pharmacol Ther 2011;89:662-73.

7. Hicks JK, Swen JJ, Thorn CF, et al. Clinical Pharmacogenetics Implementation Consortium guideline for CYP2D6 and CYP2C19 genotypes and dosing of tricyclic antidepressants. Clin Pharmacol Ther 2013;93:402-8.

8. Hicks JK, Bishop JR, Sangkuhl K, et al. Clinical Pharmacogenetics Implementation Consortium (CPIC) guideline for CYP2D6 and CYP2C19 genotypes and dosing of selective serotonin reuptake inhibitors. Clin Pharmacol Ther 2015;98:127-34.

9. Crews KR, Gaedigk A, Dunnenberger HM, et al. Clinical Pharmacogenetics Implementation Consortium guidelines for cytochrome P450 2D6 genotype and codeine therapy: 2014 update. Clin Pharmacol Ther 2014;95:376-82.

10. Crews KR, Gaedigk A, Dunnenberger HM, et al. Clinical Pharmacogenetics Implementation Consortium guidelines for cytochrome P450 2D6 genotype and codeine therapy: 2014 update. Clin Pharmacol Ther 2014;95:376-82.

11. Bertino JS Jr, Kashuba A, Ma JD, et al. Pharmacogenomics: An Introduction and Clinical Perspective. New York: McGraw-Hill, 2012.

12. Hicks JK, Swen JJ, Gaedigk A. Challenges in CYP2D6 phenotype assignment from genotype data: a critical assessment and call for standardization. Curr Drug Metab 2014;15:218-32.

13. de Leon J. The crucial role of the therapeutic window in understanding the clinical relevance of the poor versus the ultrarapid metabolizer phenotypes in subjects taking drugs metabolized by CYP2D6 or CYP2C19. J Clin Psychopharmacol 2007;27:241-5.

14. Crews KR, Caudle KE, Dunnenberger HM, et al. Considerations for the utility of the CPIC guideline for CYP2D6 genotype and codeine therapy. Clin Chem 2015;61:775-6.

15. Desai M, Tanus-Santos JE, Li L, et al. Pharmacokinetics and QT interval pharmacodynamics of oral haloperidol in poor and extensive metabolizers of CYP2D6. Pharmacogenomics J 2003;3:105-13.

16. Brockmoller J, Kirchheiner J, Schmider J, et al. The impact of the CYP2D6 polymorphism on haloperidol pharmacokinetics and on the outcome of haloperidol treatment. Clin Pharmacol Ther 2002;72:438-52.

17. Furuta T, Shirai N, Sugimoto M, et al. Influence of CYP2C19 pharmacogenetic polymorphism on proton pump inhibitor-based therapies. Drug Metab Pharmacokinet 2005;20:153-67.

18. Tamura T, Kurata M, Inoue S, et al. Improvements in Helicobacter pylori eradication rates through clinical CYP2C19 genotyping. Nagoya J Med Sci 2011;73:25-31.

19. Sapone A, Vaira D, Trespidi S, et al. The clinical role of cytochrome p450 genotypes in Helicobacter pylori management. Am J Gastroenterol 2003;98:1010-5.

20. Shi HY, Yan J, Zhu WH, et al. Effects of erythromycin on voriconazole pharmacokinetics and association with CYP2C19 polymorphism. Eur J Clin Pharmacol 2010;66:1131-6.

21. Owusu OA, Egelund EF, Alsultan A, et al. CYP2C19 polymorphisms and therapeutic drug monitoring of voriconazole: are we ready for clinical implementation of pharmacogenomics? Pharmacotherapy 2014;34:703-18.

22. Baddley JW, Andes DR, Marr KA, et al. Antifungal therapy and length of hospitalization in transplant patients with invasive aspergillosis. Med Mycol 2013;51:128-35.

23. Prows CA, Zhang X, Huth MM, et al. Codeine-related adverse drug reactions in children following tonsillectomy: a prospective study. Laryngoscope 2014;124:1242-50.

24. Andresen H, Augustin C, Streichert T. Toxicogenetics—cytochrome P450 microarray analysis in forensic cases focusing on morphine/codeine and diazepam. Int J Legal Med 2013;127:395-404.

25. Madadi P, Avard D, Koren G. Pharmacogenetics of opioids for the treatment of acute maternal pain during pregnancy and lactation. Curr Drug Metab 2012;13:721-7.

26. Shaw KD, Amstutz U, Jimenez-Mendez R, et al. Suspected opioid overdose case resolved by CYP2D6 genotyping. Ther Drug Monit 2012;34:121-3.

27. Eissing T, Lippert J, Willmann S. Pharmacogenomics of codeine, morphine, and morphine-6-glucuronide: model-based analysis of the influence of CYP2D6 activity, UGT2B7 activity, renal impairment, and CYP3A4 inhibition. Mol Diagn Ther 2012;16:43-53.

28. Leon J, Susce MT, Pan RM, et al. A study of genetic (CYP2D6 and ABCB1) and environmental (drug inhibitors and inducers) variables that may influence plasma risperidone levels. Pharmacopsychiatry 2007;40:93-102.

29. Gasso P, Mas S, Papagianni K, et al. Effect of CYP2D6 on risperidone pharmacokinetics and extrapyramidal symptoms in healthy volunteers: results from a pharmacogenetic clinical trial. Pharmacogenomics 2014;15:17-28.

30. Yoo HD, Cho HY, Lee SN, et al. Population pharmacokinetic analysis of risperidone and 9-hydroxyrisperidone with genetic polymorphisms of CYP2D6 and ABCB1. J Pharmacokinet Pharmacodyn 2012;39:329-41.

31. Bijl MJ, Visser LE, van Schaik RH, et al. Genetic variation in the CYP2D6 gene is associated with a lower heart rate and blood pressure in beta-blocker users. Clin Pharmacol Ther 2009;85:45-50.

32. Kelly LE, Madadi P. Is there a role for therapeutic drug monitoring with codeine? Ther Drug Monit 2012;34:249-56.

33. Orliaguet G, Hamza J, Couloigner V, et al. A case of respiratory depression in a child with ultrarapid CYP2D6 metabolism after tramadol. Pediatrics 2015;135:e753-e755.

34. Cleary J, Mikus G, Somogyi A, et al. The influence of pharmacogenetics on opioid analgesia: studies with codeine and oxycodone in the Sprague-Dawley/Dark Agouti rat model. J Pharmacol Exp Ther 1994;271:1528-34.

35. Perwitasari DA, Wessels JA, van der Straaten RJ, et al. Association of ABCB1, 5-HT3B receptor and CYP2D6 genetic polymorphisms with ondansetron and metoclopramide antiemetic response in Indonesian cancer patients treated with highly emetogenic chemotherapy. Jpn J Clin Oncol 2011;41:1168-76.

36. Stamer UM, Lee EH, Rauers NI, et al. CYP2D6 genotype dependent oxycodone metabolism in postoperative patients. Anesth Analg 2011;113:48-54.

37. Van BD, Marsh S, McLeod H, et al. Cytochrome P450 2C9-CYP2C9. Pharmacogenet Genomics 2010;20:277-81.

38. Johnson JA, Gong L, Whirl-Carrillo M, et al. Clinical Pharmacogenetics Implementation Consortium Guidelines for CYP2C9 and VKORC1 genotypes and warfarin dosing. Clin Pharmacol Ther 2011;90:625-9.

39. Caudle KE, Rettie AE, Whirl-Carrillo M, et al. Clinical pharmacogenetics implementation consortium guidelines for CYP2C9 and HLA-B genotypes and phenytoin dosing. Clin Pharmacol Ther 2014;96:542-8.

40. Sakaeda T, Tamon A, Kadoyama K, et al. Data mining of the public version of the FDA Adverse Event Reporting System. Int J Med Sci 2013;10:796-803.

41. Limdi NA, Beasley TM, Crowley MR, et al. VKORC1 polymorphisms, haplotypes and haplotype groups on warfarin dose among African-Americans and European-Americans. Pharmacogenomics 2008;9:1445-58.

42. Johnson JA, Gong L, Whirl-Carrillo M, et al. Clinical Pharmacogenetics Implementation Consortium guidelines for CYP2C9 and VKORC1 genotypes and warfarin dosing. Clin Pharmacol Ther 2011;90:625-9.

43. Kawai VK, Cunningham A, Vear SI, et al. Genotype and risk of major bleeding during warfarin treatment. Pharmacogenomics 2014;15:1973-83.

44. Kimmel SE, French B, Kasner SE, et al. A pharmacogenetic versus a clinical algorithm for warfarin dosing. N Engl J Med 2013;369:2283-93.

45. Weeke P, Roden DM. Applied pharmacogenomics in cardiovascular medicine. Annu Rev Med 2014;65:81-94.

46. Scott SA, Sangkuhl K, Stein CM, et al. Clinical Pharmacogenetics Implementation Consortium guidelines for CYP2C19 genotype and clopidogrel therapy: 2013 update. Clin Pharmacol Ther 2013;94:317-23.

47. Scott SA, Sangkuhl K, Shuldiner AR, et al. PharmGKB summary: very important pharmacogene information for cytochrome P450, family 2, subfamily C, polypeptide 19. Pharmacogenet Genomics 2012;22:159-65.

48. Mega JL, Hochholzer W, Frelinger AL III, et al. Dosing clopidogrel based on CYP2C19 genotype and the effect on platelet reactivity in patients with stable cardiovascular disease. JAMA 2011;306:2221-8.

49. Wallentin L, James S, Storey RF, et al. Effect of CYP2C19 and ABCB1 single nucleotide polymorphisms on outcomes of treatment with ticagrelor versus clopidogrel for acute coronary syndromes: a genetic substudy of the PLATO trial. Lancet 2010;376:1320-8.

50. Mega JL, Topol EJ, Sabatine MS. CYP2C19 genotype and cardiovascular events. JAMA 2012;307:1482-3.

51. Mega JL, Simon T, Collet JP, et al. Reduced-function CYP2C19 genotype and risk of adverse clinical outcomes among patients treated with clopidogrel predominantly for PCI: a meta-analysis. JAMA 2010;304:1821-30.

52. Mega JL, Close SL, Wiviott SD, et al. Genetic variants in ABCB1 and CYP2C19 and cardiovascular outcomes after treatment with clopidogrel and prasugrel in the TRITON-TIMI 38 trial: a pharmacogenetic analysis. Lancet 2010;376:1312-9.

53. Park MW, Her SH, Kim HS, et al. Impact of the CYP2C19*17 polymorphism on the clinical outcome of clopidogrel therapy in Asian patients undergoing percutaneous coronary intervention. Pharmacogenet Genomics 2013;23:558-62.

54. Grosdidier C, Quilici J, Loosveld M, et al. Effect of CYP2C19*2 and *17 genetic variants on platelet response to clopidogrel and prasugrel maintenance dose and relation to bleeding complications. Am J Cardiol 2013;111:985-90.

55. Karazniewicz-Lada M, Danielak D, Glowka F. Genetic and non-genetic factors affecting the response to clopidogrel therapy. Expert Opin Pharmacother 2012;13:663-83.

56. Furuta T, Shirai N, Sugimoto M, et al. Pharmacogenomics of proton pump inhibitors. Pharmacogenomics 2004;5:181-202.

57. Furuta T, Shirai N, Ohashi K, et al. Therapeutic impact of CYP2C19 pharmacogenetics on proton pump inhibitor-based eradication therapy for Helicobacter pylori. Methods Find Exp Clin Pharmacol 2003;25:131-43.

58. Ikeda Y, Umemura K, Kondo K, et al. Pharmacokinetics of voriconazole and cytochrome P450 2C19 genetic status. Clin Pharmacol Ther 2004;75:587-8.

59. Birdwell KA, Decker B, Barbarino JM, et al. Clinical pharmacogenetics implementation consortium (CPIC) guidelines for CYP3A5 genotype and tacrolimus dosing. Clin Pharmacol Ther 2015;98:19-24.

60. Kershner RP, Fitzsimmons WE. Relationship of FK506 whole blood concentrations and efficacy and toxicity after liver and kidney transplantation. Transplantation 1996;62:920-6.

61. Kuehl P, Zhang J, Lin Y, et al. Sequence diversity in CYP3A promoters and characterization of the genetic basis of polymorphic CYP3A5 expression. Nat Genet 2001;27:383-91.

62. Thervet E, Loriot MA, Barbier S, et al. Optimization of initial tacrolimus dose using pharmacogenetic testing. Clin Pharmacol Ther 2010;87:721-6.

63. Rojas L, Neumann I, Herrero MJ, et al. Effect of CYP3A5*3 on kidney transplant recipients treated with tacrolimus: a systematic review and meta-analysis of observational studies. Pharmacogenomics J 2015;15:38-48.

64. Andres HH, Weber WW. N-acetylation pharmacogenetics. Michaelis-Menten constants for arylamine drugs as predictors of their N-acetylation rates in vivo. Drug Metab Dispos 1986;14:382-5.

65. Dubbels R, Kattner E, Sell-Maurer D, et al. Sulfadimidine and isoniazid loading in man and laboratory rats. Pharmacokinetic and pharmacogenetic results on drug acetylation. Arzneimittelforschung 1980;30:1574-9.

66. Ramsey LB, Johnson SG, Caudle KE, et al. The clinical pharmacogenetics implementation consortium guideline for SLCO1B1 and simvastatin-induced myopathy: 2014 update. Clin Pharmacol Ther 2014;96:423-8.

67. Link E, Parish S, Armitage J, et al. SLCO1B1 variants and statin-induced myopathy—a genomewide study. N Engl J Med 2008;359:789-99.

68. Igel M, Arnold KA, Niemi M, et al. Impact of the SLCO1B1 polymorphism on the pharmacokinetics and lipid-lowering efficacy of multiple-dose pravastatin. Clin Pharmacol Ther 2006;79:419-26.

69. Maeda K, Ieiri I, Yasuda K, et al. Effects of organic anion transporting polypeptide 1B1 haplotype on pharmacokinetics of pravastatin, valsartan, and temocapril. Clin Pharmacol Ther 2006;79:427-39.

70. Niemi M, Schaeffeler E, Lang T, et al. High plasma pravastatin concentrations are associated with single nucleotide polymorphisms and haplotypes of organic anion transporting polypeptide-C (OATP-C, SLCO1B1). Pharmacogenetics 2004;14:429-40.

71. Link E, Parish S, Armitage J, et al. SLCO1B1 variants and statin-induced myopathy—a genomewide study. N Engl J Med 2008;359:789-99.

72. Ramsey LB, Johnson SG, Caudle KE, et al. The clinical pharmacogenetics implementation consortium guideline for SLCO1B1 and simvastatin-induced myopathy: 2014 update. Clin Pharmacol Ther 2014;96:423-8.

73. Li X, Liu R, Yan H, et al. Effect of CYP2C9-VKORC1 interaction on warfarin stable dosage and its predictive algorithm. J Clin Pharmacol 2014 Sep 4. [Epub ahead of print]

74. Nahar R, Saxena R, Deb R, et al. CYP2C9, VKORC1, CYP4F2, ABCB1 and F5 variants: influence on quality of long-term anticoagulation. Pharmacol Rep 2014;66:243-9.

75. Shaw K, Amstutz U, Hildebrand C, et al. VKORC1 and CYP2C9 genotypes are predictors of warfarin-related outcomes in children. Pediatr Blood Cancer 2014;61:1055-62.

76. Tatarunas V, Lesauskaite V, Veikutiene A, et al. The effect of CYP2C9, VKORC1 and CYP4F2 polymorphism and of clinical factors on warfarin dosage during initiation and long-term treatment after heart valve surgery. J Thromb Thrombolysis 2014;37:177-85.

77. Pirmohamed M, Burnside G, Eriksson N, et al. A randomized trial of genotype-guided dosing of warfarin. N Engl J Med 2013;369:2294-303.

78. Kimmel SE, French B, Kasner SE, et al. A pharmacogenetic versus a clinical algorithm for warfarin dosing. N Engl J Med 2013;369:2283-93.

79. Karlin E, Phillips E. Genotyping for severe drug hypersensitivity. Curr Allergy Asthma Rep 2014;14:418.

80. Chen P, Lin JJ, Lu CS, et al. Carbamazepine-induced toxic effects and HLA-B*1502 screening in Taiwan. N Engl J Med 2011;364:1126-33.

81. Chung WH, Hung SI, Chen YT. Genetic predisposition of life-threatening antiepileptic-induced skin reactions. Expert Opin Drug Saf 2010;9:15-21.

82. Chung WH, Hung SI, Chen YT. Human leukocyte antigens and drug hypersensitivity. Curr Opin Allergy Clin Immunol 2007;7:317-23.

83. Leckband SG, Kelsoe JR, Dunnenberger HM, et al. Clinical Pharmacogenetics Implementation Consortium guidelines for HLA-B genotype and carbamazepine dosing. Clin Pharmacol Ther 2013;94:324-8.

84. Martin MA, Hoffman JM, Freimuth RR, et al. Clinical Pharmacogenetics Implementation Consortium guidelines for HLA-B genotype and abacavir dosing: 2014 update. Clin Pharmacol Ther 2014;95:499-500.

85. Mallal S, Phillips E, Carosi G, et al. HLA-B*5701 screening for hypersensitivity to abacavir. N Engl J Med 2008;358:568-79.

86. Yang P, Kanki H, Drolet B,, et al. Allelic variants in long-QT disease genes in patients with drug-associated torsades de pointes. Circulation 2002;105(16):1943-8.

87. Tabata T, Yamaguchi Y, Hata Y, et al. Modification of KCNH2-encoded cardiac potassium channels by KCNE1 polymorphism. Circ J 2014;78:2331.

88. Liu L, Hayashi K, Kaneda T, et al. A novel mutation in the transmembrane nonpore region of the KCNH2 gene causes severe clinical manifestations of long QT syndrome. Heart Rhythm 2013;10:61-7.

89. Warner B. Genetic variation in KCNH2 and a unique hERG isoform in patients with schizophrenia: efficacy-safety link. Am J Psychiatry 2012;169:1318-9.

90. Winkel BG, Larsen MK, Berge KE, et al. The prevalence of mutations in KCNQ1, KCNH2, and SCN5A in an unselected national cohort of young sudden unexplained death cases. J Cardiovasc Electrophysiol 2012;23:1092-8.

91. Sato A, Chinushi M, Suzuki H, et al. Long QT syndrome with nocturnal cardiac events caused by a KCNH2 missense mutation (G604S). Intern Med 2012;51:1857-60.

92. Galen BT, Sankey C. Sepsis: an update in management. J Hosp Med 2015 July 28. [Epub ahead of print]

93. Mira JP, Charpentier J. [Can genetics guide or modify the management of severe sepsis?]. Ann Fr Anesth Reanim 2003;22 Spec No 1:48-52.

94. O'Keefe GE, Hybki DL, Munford RS. The G-->A single nucleotide polymorphism at the -308 position in the tumor necrosis factor-alpha promoter increases the risk for severe sepsis after trauma. J Trauma 2002;52:817-25.

95. Tang BM, Huang SJ, McLean AS. Genome-wide transcription profiling of human sepsis: a systematic review. Crit Care 2010;14:R237.

96. Azevedo ZM, Moore DB, Lima FC, et al. Tumor necrosis factor (TNF) and lymphotoxin-alpha (LTA) single nucleotide polymorphisms: importance in ARDS in septic pediatric critically ill patients. Hum Immunol 2012;73:661-7.

97. Paskulin DD, Fallavena PR, Paludo FJ, et al. TNF -308G > a promoter polymorphism (rs1800629) and outcome from critical illness. Braz J Infect Dis 2011;15:231-8.

98. Calvano JE, Um JY, Agnese DM, et al. Influence of the TNF-alpha and TNF-beta polymorphisms upon infectious risk and outcome in surgical intensive care patients. Surg Infect (Larchmt) 2003;4:163-9.

99. Rodriguez-Antona C, Taron M. Pharmacogenomic biomarkers for personalized cancer treatment. J Intern Med 2015;277:201-17.

100. Allen JM, Gelot S. Pharmacogenomics in the intensive care unit: focus on potential implications for clinical practice. Recent Pat Biotechnol 2014;8:116-22.

101. ASHP statement on the pharmacist's role in clinical pharmacogenomics. Am J Health Syst Pharm 2015;72:579-81.

102. Thomas RE, Chau SB. The AmpliChip: a review of its analytic and clinical validity and clinical utility. Curr Drug Saf 2015;2:113-24.

CONTRIBUTORS

Erik Abel, Pharm.D., BCPS
The Ohio State University Wexner
 Medical Center
Department of Pharmacy
Columbus, Ohio

Prasad Abraham, Pharm.D., FCCM, BCPS
Grady Health System
Department of Pharmacy and Drug
 Information
Atlanta, Georgia

Ohoud A. Aljuhani, Pharm.D.
University of Arizona
Department of Pharmacy Practice
Tucson, Arizona

Christina L. Aquilante, Pharm.D., FCCP
University of Colorado
Department of Pharmaceutical Sciences
Aurora, Colorado

Jeffrey F. Barletta, Pharm.D., FCCM
Midwestern University
Department of Pharmacy Practice
Glendale, Arizona

Seth R. Bauer, Pharm.D., FCCM, BCPS
Cleveland Clinic
Department of Pharmacy
Cleveland, Ohio

Laura Baumgartner, Pharm.D., BCPS, BCCCP
Touro University
Department of Clinical Sciences
Vallejo, California

Michael L. Bentley, Pharm.D., FCCP, FCCM, FNAP
Virginia Tech Carilion School of
 Medicine, Roanoke, Virginia
Director, Global Health Science,
 The Medical Affairs Company,
 Kennesaw, Georgia representing
 Global Health Science Center,
 The Medicines Company

Karen Berger, Pharm.D., BCPS
New York Presbyterian Hospital,
Weill Cornell Medical Center
Department of Pharmacy
New York, New York

Katherine Bidwell, Pharm.D., BCPS
University of Virginia Health System
Department of Pharmacy
Charlottesville, Virginia

P. Brandon Bookstaver, Pharm.D., FCCP, BCPS (AQ-ID), AAHIVP
University of South Carolina
Department of Clinical Pharmacy and
 Outcomes Sciences
Columbia, South Carolina

Bradley A. Boucher, Pharm.D., FCCP, MCCM, BCPS
University of Tennessee
Department of Clinical Pharmacy
Memphis, Tennessee

Gretchen M. Brophy, Pharm.D., FCCP, FCCM, FNCS, BCPS
Virginia Commonwealth University
Pharmacotherapy and Outcomes Science
 and Neurosurgery
Richmond, Virginia

Jeffrey J. Bruno, Pharm.D., BCPS, BCNSP
University of Texas MD Anderson
 Cancer Center
Department of Pharmacy
Houston, Texas

Mitchell S. Buckley, Pharm.D., FCCP, FASHP, FCCM, BCPS
Banner—University Medical Center
 Phoenix
Department of Pharmacy
Phoenix, Arizona

Todd W. Canada, Pharm.D., FASHP, FTSHP, BCNSP
University of Texas MD Anderson
 Cancer Center
Department of Pharmacy
Houston, Texas

Shanna Cole, Pharm.D.
Western Michigan University
Homer Stryker, MD School of Medicine
Kalamazoo, Michigan

Samuel E. Culli, Pharm.D., MPH
The Johns Hopkins Hospital
Department of Pharmacy
Baltimore, Maryland

William E. Dager, Pharm.D., FCCP, FCCM, FCSHP, FASHP, MCCM, BCPS-AQ Cardiology
University of California Davis
Department of Pharmacy
Sacramento, California

Joseph F. Dasta, M.S., FCCM, MCCM
The Ohio State University
Division of Pharmacy Practice and
 Science
Columbus, Ohio

Ashlee Dauenhauer, Pharm.D.
Banner University Medical Center
Tucson, Arizona

Caroline B. Derrick, Pharm.D., BCPS
University of South Carolina
Department of Internal Medicine
Columbia, South Carolina

John W. Devlin, Pharm.D., FCCP, FCCM
Northeastern University
Department of Pharmacy and Health
 System Sciences
Boston, Massachusetts

Paul P. Dobesh, Pharm.D., FCCP, BCPS-AQ Cardiology
University of Nebraska Medical Center
Department of Pharmacy Practice
Omaha, Nebraska

Thomas C. Dowling, Pharm.D., Ph.D., FCCP, FCP
Ferris State University
College of Pharmacy
Grand Rapids, Michigan

Amy L. Dzierba, Pharm.D., FCCM, BCPS
New York–Presbyterian Hospital
Columbia University Medical Center
Department of Pharmacy
New York, New York

Brian L. Erstad, Pharm.D., FCCP, MCCM, FASHP, BCPS
University of Arizona
Department of Pharmacy Practice and
 Science
Tucson, Arizona

Elizabeth Anne Farrington, Pharm.D., FCCP, FCCM, FPPAG, BCPS
New Hanover Regional Medical Center
Wilmington, North Carolina

David V. Feliciano, M.D., FACS
Indiana University Medical Center
Department of Surgery
Indianapolis, Indiana

Douglas N. Fish, PharmD, FCCP, FCCM, BCPS-AQ ID
University of Colorado
Department of Clinical Pharmacy
Aurora, Colorado

Jeremy Flynn, Pharm.D., FCCP, FCCM
University of Kentucky
College of Pharmacy
Lexington, Kentucky

David R. Foster, Pharm.D., FCCP
Purdue University
Department of Pharmacy Practice
Indianapolis, Indiana

Gilles L. Fraser, Pharm.D., MCCM
Maine Medical Center
Department of Pharmacy
Portland, Maine

Robert N. E. French, M.D., MPH
University of Arizona College of Medicine/Arizona Poison and Drug Information Center
Tucson, Arizona

Andrew C. Fritschle Hilliard, Pharm.D., BCPS, BCCCP
Eskenazi Health
Indianapolis, Indiana

David J. Gagnon, Pharm.D., BCCCP
Maine Medical Center
Department of Pharmacy
Portland, Maine

Rita Gayed, Pharm.D., BCCCP
Grady Health System
Department of Pharmacy and Clinical Nutrition
Atlanta, Georgia

James F. Gilmore, Pharm.D., BCCCP, BCPS
Brigham and Women's Hospital
Department of Pharmacy Services
Boston, Massachusetts

Katja M Gist, DO, MA, MSCS
University of Colorado, Department of Pediatrics
Children's Hospital Colorado
Aurora, Colorado

Curtis E. Haas, Pharm.D.
University of Rochester Medical Center
Department of Pharmacy
Rochester, New York

Martina C. Holder PharmD, BCPS
University of Florida Health Shands
Department of Pharmacy
Gainesville, Florida

Nicholas B. Hurst, M.D., M.S.
University of Arizona
College of Medicine
Tucson, Arizona

Judith Jacobi, Pharm.D., MCCM, FCCP, DPNAP, BCPS, ACCP President 2014–2015
Indiana University Health Methodist Hospital
Indianapolis, Indiana

Samuel G. Johnson, Pharm.D., BCPS, FCCP
University of Colorado
Department of Clinical Pharmacy
Aurora, Colorado

Thomas J. Johnson, Pharm.D., MBA, FASHP, FCCM, BCPS, BCCCP
Avera McKennan Hospital and University Health Center
Sioux Falls, South Dakota

J. Dedrick Jordan, M.D., Ph.D.
University of North Carolina School of Medicine
Department of Neurology
Chapel Hill, North Carolina

Melanie S. Joy, Pharm.D., Ph.D., FCCP, FASN
University of Colorado
Department of Pharmaceutical Sciences
Aurora, Colorado

Sandra L. Kane-Gill, Pharm.D., M.Sc., FCCP, FCCM
University of Pittsburgh
School of Pharmacy
Pittsburgh, Pennsylvania

Salmaan Kanji, Pharm.D.
Ottawa Hospital
Department of Pharmacy
Ottawa, Ontario

Stephen R. Karpen, Pharm.D.
University of Arizona
College of Pharmacy
Tucson, Arizona

David C. Kaufman, M.D.
University of Rochester Medical Center
Department of Surgery
Rochester, New York

Tyree H. Kiser, Pharm.D., FCCP, FCCM, BCPS
University of Colorado
Department of Clinical Pharmacy
Aurora, Colorado

Michael Klepser, Pharm.D.
Ferris State University
College of Pharmacy
Kalamazoo, Michigan

Marin H. Kollef, M.D.
Washington University School of Medicine
Division of Pulmonary and Critical Care Medicine
St. Louis, Missouri

Nicole L. Kovacic, Pharm.D.
Maine Medical Center
Department of Pharmacy
Portland, Maine

Simon W. Lam, Pharm.D., FCCM, BCPS, BCCCP
Cleveland Clinic
Department of Pharmacy
Cleveland, Ohio

Ishaq Lat, Pharm.D., FCCP, FCCM, BCPS
Rush University Medical Center
Department of Pharmacy
Chicago, Illinois

John J. Lewin III, Pharm.D., MBA, FASHP, FCCM, FNCS
The Johns Hopkins Hospital
Department of Pharmacy
Baltimore, Maryland

Robert MacLaren, Pharm.D., MPH, FCCP, FCCM
University of Colorado
Department of Clinical Pharmacy
Aurora, Colorado

Stephanie Mallow Corbett, Pharm.D, FCCM
University of Virginia Health System
Department of Pharmacy
Charlottesville, Virginia

Kali Martin, Pharm.D.
Ferris State University
College of Pharmacy
Grand Rapids, Michigan

Steven J. Martin, Pharm.D., BCPS, FCCP, FCCM
Ohio Northern University
Rudolph H. Raabe College of Pharmacy
Ada, Ohio

Kathryn R. Matthias, Pharm.D., BCPS-AQ ID
University of Arizona
Department of Pharmacy Practice and Science
Tucson, Arizona

Joseph E. Mazur, Pharm.D., BCPS
Medical University of South Carolina
Department of Pharmacy Services
Charleston, South Carolina

Ali McBride, Pharm.D., M.S., BCPS, BCOP
The University of Arizona Cancer Center
Department of Pharmacy
Tucson, Arizona

M. Claire McManus, Pharm.D.
St. Elizabeth's Medical Center
Department of Pharmacy
Boston, Massachusetts

Cristian Merchan, Pharm.D., BCCCP
NYU Langone Medical Center
Department of Pharmacy
New York, New York

Scott T. Micek, Pharm.D., FCCP, BCPS
St. Louis College of Pharmacy
Department of Pharmacy Practice
St. Louis, Missouri

Kathryn Morbitzer, Pharm.D.
UNC Eshelman School of Pharmacy
School of Pharmacy
Chapel Hill, North Carolina

Claire V. Murphy, Pharm.D., BCPS
Ohio State University Wexner Medical Center
Department of Pharmacy
Columbus, Ohio

Michelle Nadeau, Pharm.D., BCPS
Yale–New Haven Hospital
Department of Pharmacy
New Haven, Connecticut

Melissa Nestor, Pharm.D., BCPS
University of Kentucky HealthCare
College of Pharmacy
Lexington, Kentucky

Komal Pandya, Pharm.D., BCPS
University of Kentucky
College of Pharmacy
Lexington, Kentucky

John Papadopoulos, B.S., Pharm.D., FCCM, BCNSP, BCCCP
NYU Langone Medical Center
Department of Pharmacy
New York, New York

Keith M. Olsen, Pharm.D., FCCP, FCCM
University of Nebraska Medical Center
College of Pharmacy
Omaha, Nebraska

Kate Oltrogge Pape, Pharm.D., BCPS
University of Iowa Hospitals and Clinics
Department of Pharmaceutical Care
Iowa City, Iowa

Lance J. Oyen, Pharm.D., FCCM, FCCP, BCPS
Mayo Clinic
Department of Pharmacy
Rochester, Minnesota

Steven E. Pass, Pharm.D., FCCP, FCCM, FASHP, BCPS
Texas Tech University
HSC School of Pharmacy
Dallas, Texas

Asad E. Patanwala, Pharm.D.
University of Arizona
Department of Pharmacy Practice and Science
Tucson, Arizona

Sajni Patel, Pharm.D., BCPS
University of Chicago Medicine
Department of Pharmacy
Chicago, Illinois

Heather Personett, Pharm.D., BCPS
Mayo Clinic
Department of Pharmacy
Rochester, Minnesota

Gregory Peitz, Pharm.D., BCPS
University of Nebraska Medical Center
Department of Pharmaceutical and Nutrition Care
Omaha, Nebraska

Brent N. Reed, Pharm.D., FAHA, BCPS-AQ Cardiology
University of Maryland
Department of Pharmacy Practice and Science
Baltimore, Maryland

Denise H. Rhoney, Pharm.D., FCCP, FCCM, FNCS
UNC Eshelman School of Pharmacy
Department of Practice Advancement and Clinical Education
Chapel Hill, North Carolina

A. Josh Roberts, Pharm.D., BCPS-AQ Cardiology
University of California, Davis
Department of Pharmacy
Sacramento, California

Jo E. Rodgers, Pharm.D., FCCP, BCPS-AQ Cardiology
University of North Carolina School of Pharmacy
Division of Pharmacotherapy and Experimental Therapeutics
Chapel Hill, North Carolina

Andrew M. Roecker, Pharm.D., BCPS
Ohio Northern University
Rudolph H. Raabe College of Pharmacy
Ada, Ohio

Carol J. Rollins, M.S., RD, Pharm.D., FASHP, FASPEN, BCNSP
Banner University Medical Center Tucson and University of Arizona
Department of Pharmacy Practice and Science
Tucson, Arizona

A. Shaun Rowe, Pharm.D., BCPS
University of Tennessee
Department of Clinical Pharmacy
Knoxville, Tennessee

Curtis N. Sessler, M.D., FCCP, FCCM
Virginia Commonwealth University Health System
Department of Internal Medicine
Richmond, Virginia

Mazda Shirazi, M.D., Ph.D.
University of Arizona
Department of Emergency Medicine; Department of Pharmacy Practice
Tucson, Arizona

Colgan T. Sloan, Pharm.D., BCPS
University of Arizona
Department of Pharmacy Practice
Tucson, Arizona

Curtis L. Smith, Pharm.D., BCPS
Ferris State University
Department of Pharmacy Practice
Lansing, Michigan

Zachary A. Stacy, Pharm.D., M.S., FCCP, BCPS
St. Louis College of Pharmacy
Division of Acute Care; Department of Pharmacy Practice
St. Louis, Missouri

Paul M. Szumita, Pharm.D., FCCM, BCCCP, BCPS
Brigham and Women's Hospital
Department of Pharmacy
Boston, Massachusetts

Robert L. Talbert, Pharm.D.
University of Texas
Pharmacotherapy Education and Research Center
San Antonio, Texas

Eljim P. Tesoro, Pharm.D., BCPS
University of Illinois at Chicago
Department of Pharmacy Practice
Chicago, Illinois

James E. Tisdale, Pharm.D., FCCP, FAPhA, FAHA, BCPS
Purdue University
Department of Pharmacy Practice
Indianapolis, Indiana

Toby C. Trujillo, Pharm.D., FCCP, FAHA, BCPS-AQ Cardiology
University of Colorado Skaggs School of Pharmacy and Pharmaceutical Sciences
Department of Clinical Pharmacy
Aurora, Colorado

Cory M. Vela, Pharm.D.
Moffitt Cancer Center
Department of Pharmacy
Tampa, Florida

Amber Verdell, Pharm.D., BCPS, BCNSP
West Coast University
Department of Pharmacy Practice
Los Angeles, California

Stacy Voils, PharmD, M.Sc., BCPS
University of Florida
Department of Pharmacotherapy and Translational Research
Gainesville, Florida

Robert J. Weber, Pharm.D., M.S., FASHP, BCPS
The Ohio State University Wexner Medical Center
Department of Pharmacy
College of Pharmacy
Pharmacy Practice and Science
Columbus, Ohio

David Williamson, B. Pharm, M.Sc., Ph.D., BCPS
University of Montreal
Faculty of Pharmacy
Montreal, Quebec

Amanda Zomp, Pharm.D., BCPS
University of Virginia
Department of Pharmacy
Charlottesville, Virginia

REVIEWERS

The American College of Clinical Pharmacy, Dr. Erstad, and the authors would like to thank the following individuals for their careful chapter review.

Earnest Alexander, Pharm.D.
Tampa General Hospital
Department of Pharmacy
Tampa, Florida

William L. Baker, Pharm.D., FCCP, FACC, BCPS-AQ Cardiology
University of Connecticut
Department of Pharmacy Practice
Storrs, Connecticut

Elizabeth Beltz, Pharm.D.
University of Iowa
Department of Pharmacy
Iowa City, Iowa

Christopher Bland, Pharm.D., BCPS, FIDSA
University of Georgia
Department of Clinical and Administrative Pharmacy
Savannah, Georgia

Mary Beth Bobek, Pharm.D., CPP
New Hanover Regional Medical Center
Wilmington, North Carolina

Kevin Box, Pharm.D.
University of California, San Diego
Department of Pharmacy
San Diego, California

Trisha Branan, Pharm.D., BCCCP
University of Georgia
Department of Clinical and Administrative Pharmacy
Athens, Georgia

Lisa Burry, Pharm.D.
Mount Sinai Hospital
Department of Pharmacy and Medicine
Toronto, Ontario

Josh Caraccio, Pharm.D., BCPS
Utah Valley Regional Medical Center
Department of Pharmacy
Provo, Utah

Amber Castle, Pharm.D., BCPS, BCCCP
Yale–New Haven Hospital
Department of Pharmacy
New Haven, Connecticut

Alexandra Cheung, Pharm.D.
Mount Sinai Hospital
Department of Pharmacy
Toronto, Ontario

Henry Cohen, Pharm.D., FCCM, BCPP
Kingsbrook Jewish Medical Center
Department of Pharmacy Services
Brooklyn, New York

Aaron Cook, Pharm.D., BCPS
University of Kentucky
Department of Pharmacy Services
Lexington, Kentucky

Amanda Corbett, Pharm.D., BCPS, FCCP
University of North Carolina
Division of Pharmacotherapy and Experimental Therapeutics
Chapel Hill, North Carolina

Cheryl D. Cropp, Pharm.D., Ph.D.
University of Arizona
College of Pharmacy
Department of Pharmacy Practice/ Translational Genomics Research Institute (TGen)
Phoenix, Arizona

Roland Dickerson, Pharm.D., BCNSP, FCCP
University of Tennessee
Department of Clinical Pharmacy
Memphis, Tennessee

Jeremiah Duby, Pharm.D., BCPS
University of California, Davis, Medical Center
Department of Pharmacy Services
Davis, California

Sandy Estrada, Pharm.D., BCPS
Lee Memorial Hospital
Department of Pharmacy
Fort Myers, Florida

Stacey Folse, Pharm.D., MPH
Emory University Hospital
Department of Pharmaceutical Services
Atlanta, Georgia

Lisa L. Forsyth, Pharm.D., FCCM
Beaumont Hospital, Royal Oak
Department of Pharmaceutical Services
Royal Oak, Michigan

Erin R. Fox, Pharm.D., FASHP
University of Utah Health Care
Drug Information Service
Salt Lake City, Utah

Anthony T. Gerlach, PharmD, BCPS, FCCM, FCCP
The Ohio State University
Department of Pharmacy
Columbus, Ohio

Katherine Gharibian, Pharm.D.
University of Michigan
Department of Clinical Pharmacy
Ann Arbor, Michigan

Myke Green, Pharm.D., BCOP
University of Arizona
Department of Pharmacy Services
Tucson, Arizona

Bonnie C. Greenwood, Pharm.D.
University of Massachusetts Medical School
Clinical Pharmacy Services
Shrewsbury, Massachusetts

John Horn, Pharm.D., FCCP
University of Washington
Department of Pharmacy
Seattle, Washington

Yvonne Huckleberry, Pharm.D., BCPS
Banner University Medical Center
Medical Intensive Care Unit (Pharmacy)
Tucson, Arizona

Theresa Human, Pharm.D., BCPS
Barnes-Jewish Hospital, Washington University
Department of Pharmacy
St. Louis, Missouri

Brian Kopp, Pharm.D., BCPS, FCCM
Banner University Medical Center
Department of Pharmacy Services
Tucson, Arizona

Seung Joo Lee, Pharm.D.
University of Toronto
Department of Pharmacy
Toronto, Ontario

Courtney McKinney, Pharm.D., BCPS
Intermountain Medical Center
Department of Pharmacy Services
Salt Lake City, Utah

Charles Medico, Pharm.D., BCPS
Geisinger Medical Center
Department of Enterprise Pharmacy
Danville, Pennsylvania

Wenya Miao, Pharm.D.
Mount Sinai Hospital
Department of Pharmacy
Toronto, Ontario

John Murphy, Pharm.D., FCCP
University of Arizona
Department of Pharmacy Practice and Science
Tucson, Arizona

David Nix, Pharm.D.
University of Arizona
Department of Pharmacy Practice and Science
Tucson, Arizona

Erin M. Nystrom, Pharm.D., BCNSP
Mayo Clinic
Department of Pharmacy
Rochester, Minnesota

Christopher Paciullo, Pharm.D., BCCCP, FCCM
Emory University Hospital
Department of Pharmaceutical Services
Atlanta, Georgia

William Peppard, Pharm.D., BCPS
Froedtert and the Medical College of Wisconsin
Department of Pharmacy
Milwaukee, Wisconsin

Hanna Phan, Pharm.D., BCPS
University of Arizona
Department of Pharmacy Practice and Science; Department of Pediatrics
Tucson, Arizona

Asia N. Quan, Pharm.D., BCPS
Maricopa Integrated Healthcare System
The Arizona Burn Center
Phoenix, Arizona

John Radosevich, Pharm.D., BCCCP, BCPS
St. Joseph's Hospital and Medical Center
Department of Pharmacy
Phoenix, Arizona

Hal Richards, Pharm.D., BCNSP
St. Joseph's Candler Health System
Department of Pharmacy
Savannah, Georgia

Garrett Schramm, Pharm.D., BCPS
Mayo Clinic
Department of Pharmacy
Rochester, Minnesota

Susan Skledar, RPh, MPH, FASHP
University of Pittsburgh
Department of Pharmacy and Therapeutics
Pittsburgh, Pennsylvania

Maria Stubbs, RPh, BCPS
VA San Diego Healthcare System
Department of Pharmacy
Carlsbad, California

Scott Taylor, Pharm.D., M.Sc., BCPS
Via Christi Hospitals
Department of Pharmacy
Wichita, Kansas

Michael C. Thomas, Pharm.D., BCPS, FCCP
Western New England University
Department of Pharmacy Practice
Springfield, Massachusetts

Sarah Todd, Pharm.D., BCPS
Emory University Hospital
Department of Pharmacy
Atlanta, Georgia

Todd Sorensen, Pharm.D.
University of Minnesota
Department of Pharmaceutical Care and Health Systems
Minneapolis, Minnesota

Sara Stahle, Pharm.D., BCPS
The University of Chicago Medicine
Department of Pharmacy
Chicago, Illinois

Zachariah Thomas, Pharm.D.
Director, Global Health Science
The Medicines Company
New York, New York

Velliyur Viswesh, Pharm.D., BCPS
Roseman University of Health Sciences
Department of Pharmacy Practice
Henderson, Nevada

Sol Atienza Yoder, Pharm.D., BCOP
Aurora Health Care
Department of Pharmacy
Milwaukee, Wisconsin

Dinesh Yogaratnam, Pharm.D., BCPS, BCCCP
Massachusetts College of Pharmacy and Health Sciences University
Department of Pharmacy Practice
Worcester, Massachusetts

INDEX

Note: Page numbers followed by b, f, or t indicate material in boxes, figures, or tables, respectively.

A

AACE. *See* American Association of Clinical Endocrinologists
AAG. *See* α$_1$-acid glycoprotein
AANS. *See* American Association of Neurological Surgeons
AASLD. *See* American Association for the Study of Liver Diseases
AB5000 Circulatory Support System, 739
ABA. *See* American Burn Association
ABCDE, for trauma, 863
ABCDEF, for delirium, 195
abciximab, 475t, 667t, 673–674
abdominal compartment syndrome, 848, 868
ABG. *See* arterial blood gas
ABO compatibility, 486
absolute neutrophil count (ANC), 359, 984
absorption, 548, 552
    ALF and, 585–586
    DDIs and, 931–933, 932t–933t
AC. *See* adrenal crisis
Academy of Nutrition and Dietetics, 100
ACAG. *See* albumin-corrected AG
ACC. *See* American College of Cardiology
ACCM/SCCM. *See* American College of Critical Care Medicine/Society of Critical Care Medicine
ACE. *See* angiotensin-converting enzyme
ACEIs. *See* angiotensin-converting enzyme inhibitors
acetaminophen, 153t, 154, 575, 776, 796t, 936t
acetazolamide, 18–19
acetoacetate, 15
acetone, 15
acetylcholine, 200
acetylcholine inhibitors, 214–215
acetylcholinesterase inhibitors, 216
acetylcysteine, 578–581, 849
α$_1$-acid glycoprotein (AAG), 258
acid-base disorders, 3–26
    bicarbonate and, 6–7
    case studies for, 23–26
    clinical findings for, 11t
    clinical syndromes, 13–23
    intravenous fluids and, 21–23
    PEA and, 702
    potassium and, 69–70
    secondary responses to, 12t
    stepwise diagnosis of, 10–13, 10t
    Stewart model for, 7–10
acidemia, 4, 5
acidosis, 5. *See also* metabolic acidosis
    AF and, 717
    agitation and, 162
    ALF and, 575
    coagulopathy and, 473
    lactic, 14, 16, 228, 476, 764
    liver and, 7
    malignant hyperthermia and, 215
    potassium and, 69–70
    respiratory, 19–21, 20t, 339t, 628, 629, 634
    TIC and, 867

Acinetobacter spp., 247, 292, 308
ACLS. *See* advanced cardiac life support
ACOS. *See* asthma-COPD overlap syndrome
acquired immunodeficiency syndrome (AIDS). *See* HIV/AIDS
ACS. *See* acute coronary syndrome
ACT. *See* activated clotting time
ACTH. *See* adrenocorticotropic hormone
activated clotting time (ACT), 471, 508–509, 511f, 512f, 674, 682
activated partial thromboplastin time (aPTT), 470–471, 472, 499–500, 501, 502t, 503–506, 504f, 505f
    ACT and, 508–509
    anti-Xa and, 504–506, 505f
    for bivalirudin, 674
    for DTIs, 506, 506f
    inhalation injury and, 849
    MCS and, 746–747
    morbid obesity and, 826
    TEG and, 515
    VTE and, 455, 456
activated prothrombin complex concentrate (aPCC), 458
active surveillance, 976–979, 977t
Acute Catheterization and Urgent Intervention Triage Strategy (ACUITY), 677
acute coronary syndrome (ACS), 453, 660–682
    anticoagulants for, 668t, 674–675
    antithrombotics for, 666–675, 667t–669t
    β-blockers for, 665–666
    cardiac biomarkers for, 662–663, 662t
    CCB for, 666
    chest pain with, 662
    ECG for, 663–664, 663t
    GPIIb/IIIa inhibitors for, 667t, 673–674
    hypertensive crisis and, 768t, 775–776, 777f
    oxygen therapy for, 664–665
    P2Y inhibitors for, 667t, 669–673
    pathophysiology of, 660–664
    PCI for, 673, 674, 675, 677
    platelet transfusions and, 598
    risk scores for, 661–662, 661t
acute decompensated heart failure (ADHF), 645–657
    cardiac transplantation for, 656–657
    clinical presentation of, 646–648
    hemodynamic subsets for, 646–648, 647t
    hemodynamic support for, 651–654
    inotropes for, 652–654, 653t
    laboratory testing for, 647–648
    loop diuretics for, 648–649, 648t
    LVADs for, 656
    MCS for, 646, 654–656, 655t
    PCWP and, 649, 652
    thiazide diuretics for, 649, 649t
    vasodilators for, 649–652, 651t
    volume management for, 648–650
Acute Decompensated Heart Failure National Registry (ADHERE), 648, 652
Acute Dialysis Quality Initiative (ADQI), 526

acute ischemic stroke (AIS), 403–413
    classification, risk factors, and diagnosis for, 404
    hyperglycemia and, 409
    hypertension and, 407, 408t
    pathophysiology of, 404
    seizures and, 410
    treatment of, 404–409, 406f
acute kidney disease, vs. CKD, 548–553, 552t
acute kidney injury (AKI), 116, 523–533, 524t, 730, 994
    ADEs and, 975, 976t
    AF and, 717
    assessment of, 526–528
    biomarkers for, 528
    drug clearance and, 259
    drug dosing in, 538–564
    drug-induced, 530–533, 531t
    ECMO and, 742
    etiology of, 524
    hypomagnesemia and, 80
    incidence and prognosis for, 523–524
    intrarenal, 525–526
    laboratory testing for, 525t
    from normal saline, 41
    pathophysiology of, 524–526
    postrenal, 526
    prevention and treatment of, 528–533, 529t, 531t
    rhabdomyolysis and, 884
    RRT for, 524, 529, 530, 538–564
    scoring systems for, 954–955
    severity staging of, 527t
    sodium chloride solutions and, 34
    trauma and, 881–884
Acute Kidney Injury Network (AKIN), 527, 527t, 955, 955t
acute liver failure (ALF), 573–589
    absorption and, 585–586
    classifications of, 573t
    clinical presentation of, 578
    CTP for, 577, 586t, 587t, 588–589
    epidemiology of, 574
    etiology of, 575–576
    management of, 578–584
    nonpharmacologic therapy for, 584
    pathophysiology of, 574–575
    PK for, 585, 588t
    prognosis for, 576–578, 579t
    scoring systems for, 956
acute lung injury (ALI), 107, 116, 117–118, 118t
acute lymphoblastic leukemia, 803, 805
acute myocardial infarction (AMI), 70, 74, 664t, 712, 717, 776
    bradycardia and, 710
    hypertensive crisis and, 758, 759
    hypomagnesemia and, 80–81
    SCA and, 693t, 700
    shock and, 229
    VT and, 722, 723

Acute Physiology and Chronic Health
    Evaluation (APACHE II), 71–72,
    952–953
  ALF and, 578
  antimicrobials and, 242–243
  delirium and, 191
  GCS and, 952
  glucose management and, 130
  hypophosphatemia and, 83
  β-lactam antibiotics and, 268
  nutrition and, 100
  for pancreatitis, 955–956
  PN and, 105
Acute Physiology Score (APS), 952
acute postoperative hypertension (APH),
    769t, 772–774, 774f
acute respiratory distress syndrome (ARDS),
    34, 42, 45, 49, 559, 902
  histoplasmosis and, 327
  MCS for, 737t
  NMBAs for, 199, 206–207, 208,
    209t–211t
  omega-3 fatty acids for, 115, 116,
    117–118
Acute Study of Clinical Effectiveness of
    Nesiritide in Decompensated Heart
    Failure (ASCEND), 652
acute tubular necrosis (ATN), 524, 525
acyclovir, 192t, 333, 334t, 531t, 532
ADA. See American Diabetes Association
Addison disease, 81, 800–801, 800t
ADE Prevention Study, 974
adenosine, 204, 614, 672, 715t
adenosine diphosphate (ADP), 468, 474, 661
adenosine triphosphate (ATP), 82, 83, 468, 471
  ALF and, 574
  malignant hyperthermia and, 204
  ticagrelor and, 671
adenovirus, 576, 638
ADEs. See adverse drug events
ADH. See antidiuretic hormone
ADHERE. See Acute Decompensated Heart
    Failure National Registry
ADHF. See acute decompensated heart failure
adipose tissue, metabolic acidosis and, 14
adjusted body weight (AdjBW), 822, 823
ADP. See adenosine diphosphate
ADQI. See Acute Dialysis Quality Initiative
adrenal crisis (AC), 800
adrenal disorders, 800–802
adrenal insufficiency, 800–801, 800t
α_2-adrenergic agonists, 785, 788–789
adrenergic blockers, 851
β-adrenergic blockers, 628, 697
adrenergic-receptor antagonists, 766–767
adrenocorticotropic hormone (ACTH)
  adrenal insufficiency and, 800–801
  stress response and, 99
β_2-adrenoreceptors, 14
Adrogue-Madias equation, 64
advanced cardiac life support (ACLS), for
    SCA, 691–692
advanced trauma life support, for trauma,
    863–865
adverse drug events (ADEs), 971–979
  active surveillance for, 976–979, 977t
  defined, 972t
  epidemiology of, 973
  medication safety and, 971–976
  MEs and, 972f
  pharmacogenomics and, 999–1008
  systems analysis of, 973–974

Adverse Event Reporting System, of FDA,
    1003
AEDs. See automated external defibrillators
Aerosolized Iloprost Randomized Study
    (AIR), 617
AF. See atrial fibrillation
AG. See anion gap
Agency for Healthcare Research and Quality,
    946
agitation, 161–175
  clinical significance of, 163
  cocaine and, 777
  defined, 161
  delirium with, 187
  etiology of, 162–163
  incidence of, 161
  nonpharmacologic therapy for, 166
  opioids for, 166–168
  sedatives for
    alternative for, 170–173, 171t
    assessment of, 163–166
    traditional for, 168–170, 169t
α_2-agonists, 170
β-agonists, 629, 849, 914–915
AHA. See American Heart Association
AIR. See Aerosolized Iloprost Randomized
    Study
air leak syndromes, 737t
AIS. See acute ischemic stroke; ASIA
    Impairment Scale
AKI. See acute kidney injury
AKIN. See Acute Kidney Injury Network
alanine aminotransferase (ALT), 576
ALBIOS. See Albumin Italian Outcome
    Sepsis
albumin, 30–32, 36–37
  for aSAH, 432
  for burns, 848
  calcium and, 88
  cefotaxime and, 42
  DDIs and, 933
  for ECMO, 742
  for hemorrhagic shock, 866
  MAP and, 41
  nutrition and, 99
  for peritonitis, 42
  plasmapheresis and, 556
  for PPH, 834
  randomized trials for, 52t
  for sepsis, 44–45
  for shock, 310–312
  uses of, 43t
  Vss and, 256
albumin and lactate corrected AG (ALCAG),
    11, 15
Albumin in Subarachnoid Hemorrhage
    (ALISAH), 431
Albumin Italian Outcome Sepsis (ALBIOS),
    41
albumin-corrected AG (ACAG), 6, 12
albuterol, 631, 657, 849, 914–915
ALCAG. See albumin and lactate corrected
    AG
alcohol
  abuse
    acetaminophen-ALF and, 575
    agitation and, 162
  aSAH and, 417
  frostbite and, 856
  hypophosphatemia and, 83
  Mallory-Weiss tears from, 594
  withdrawal from
    hypertensive crisis and, 759

phenobarbital for, 172
alcoholic hepatitis, 580–581
aldosterone, 69, 800–801
ALF. See acute liver failure
ALF Study Group, 574, 575, 576
ALI. See acute lung injury
ALISAH. See Albumin in Subarachnoid
    Hemorrhage
ALIVE trial, 699–700
alkalemia, 4
alkalosis, 5
  metabolic, 4, 18–19
  overshoot, 17
  respiratory, 21
allergic rhinitis, 234
allopurinol, 577, 806, 806f
ALT. See alanine aminotransferase
alteplase, 455t, 475t
altered mental status
  ALF and, 573
  aSAH and, 427
  with encephalitis, 333
  hypothyroidism and, 794
  SVC and, 814
amantadine, 162, 192t
Ambrisentan in Pulmonary Arterial
    Hypertension, Randomized,
    Double-Blind, Placebo-Controlled,
    Multicenter, Efficacy (ARIES), 618
American Academy of Pediatrics, 918
American Association for the Study of Liver
    Diseases (AASLD), 357, 578, 582,
    583
American Association of Clinical
    Endocrinologists (AACE), 132
American Association of Neurological
    Surgeons (AANS), 396
American Burn Association (ABA), 41–42,
    845
American College of Cardiology (ACC), 663,
    681
American College of Chest Physicians, 456
American College of Critical Care Medicine/
    Society of Critical Care Medicine
    (ACCM/SCCM), 132–133
American College of Obstetricians and
    Gynecologists, 833
American College of Surgeons, 477
American Diabetes Association (ADA), 132
American Heart Association (AHA), 404,
    420, 657, 681, 690, 692, 695, 771
American Psychiatric Association, 186
American Society for Parenteral and Enteral
    Nutrition (ASPEN), 99, 100, 101,
    103, 114, 115, 116, 133
American Society of Health-System
    Pharmacists (ASHP), 362, 960
American Spinal Injury Association (ASIA),
    396
American Stroke Association (ASA), 420, 771
American Thoracic Society, 103, 629
AMI. See acute myocardial infarction
amikacin, 549t, 854t, 985t
α-amino-3-hydroxy-5-methyl-isoxazole-4-
    propionate (AMPA), 373, 389
γ-aminobutyric acid (GABA)
  baclofen and, 781–782, 782f
  benzodiazepines and, 782, 786–787
  delirium and, 191
  NMBAs and, 207
  propofol and, 169, 782
  SE and, 373
  treprostinil and, 617

volatile anesthetics and, 173
aminoglutethimide, 802, 802t
aminoglycosides
  AKI from, 525, 531, 531t, 975
  ECMO and, 563, 744
  extended-interval drug dosing for, 271–272
  hypomagnesemia and, 80
  for morbid obesity, 828–829
  NMBAs and, 214–215
  PD of, 827t
aminophylline, 633
aminorex, 613
amiodarone, 478t, 936t, 940t
  for AF, 718–719, 718t, 723f, 726t
  antiretrovirals and, 989t
  bradycardia from, 710
  delirium from, 192t
  myxedema coma and, 793
  P-glycoprotein and, 934t
  plasmapheresis for, 557t
  for PSVT, 716t
  for SCA, 699–700
  ticagrelor and, 672
  for VT, 724–725, 727t
amitriptyline, 1004
amlodipine, 618
ammonia, 7, 171, 578, 600
ammonium chloride, 19
amoxicillin, 577, 601t
amoxicillin/clavulanic acid, 638
AMPA. See α-amino-3-hydroxy-5-methyl-isoxazole-4-propionate
amphetamines, 162, 613, 940
amphotericin B, 326, 327
  AKI from, 526, 531t, 532, 975
  for *Aspergillus*, 325
  for *Candida*, 323
  for *Cryptococcus neoformans*, 323–324
  delirium from, 192t
  for FN, 986
  hypomagnesemia and, 80
  pregnancy and, 831, 832
  properties of, 320t
ampicillin, 557t, 933
amrinone, 549t
amyl nitrite, 852t
amyloidosis, 710
amyotrophic lateral sclerosis, 217
anal fissures, 592
analgesics, 147–158. *See also* opioids
  analgosedation approach to, 149–152, 150f
  delirium from, 192t
  ECMO and, 743
  multimodal, 153–156, 153t
  with non-opioids, 153–156, 153t
  nonpharmacologic therapy for, 155–156
  in pregnancy, 833
  for procedural pain, 156–157
  for respiratory alkalosis, 21
  therapeutic options in, 152–156
  in transition from ICU to ward, 157–158
analgosedation approach, to analgesia, 149–152, 150f
anaphylactic shock, 234–235
ANC. *See* absolute neutrophil count
andexanet, 597–598
androgens, 800–801
anemia, 479–480
  ADP and, 474
  aSAH and, 436

endothelin receptor antagonists and, 618
hypertensive crisis and, 759
MCS and, 745
riociguat and, 619
anesthetics
  ALF from, 577
  bradycardia from, 710
  NMBAs and, 214
  for SE, 381
  TdP from, 729t
aneurysmal subarachnoid hemorrhage (aSAH), 410, 416–438
  DCI and, 418–419, 420, 426, 427–434
  DVT and, 435–436
  early brain injury and, 418–419
  epidemiology of, 416
  fever and, 436–437
  grading scales for, 421, 421t
  hydrocephalus and, 427
  hypertensive crisis and, 769t, 772, 772f
  hyponatremia and, 434–436
  initial stabilization of, 420–421
  management and complication prevention for, 421, 422t, 425–426
  multidisciplinary team for, 420
  paroxysmal sympathetic hyperactivity and, 437–438
  pathophysiology of, 417–420, 419f
  pharmacotherapy for, 424t–425t
  rebleeding and, 417, 421, 425–426
  risk factors for, 417
  seizures and, 426–427
  subarachnoid spaces and, 431
  thermoregulation for, 436–437
  treatment of, 431–434
angioedema, 407
angiotensin II, 758, 764
angiotensin receptor blockers (ARBs), 526, 530–531, 531t, 831, 833
angiotensin-converting enzyme (ACE), 758
angiotensin-converting enzyme inhibitors (ACEIs), 530–531, 531t, 654, 690, 764, 831, 833
angiotensinogen, 758
anion gap (AG), 4, 5–6, 21
  metabolic acidosis and, 13t, 14–15, 16
antacids, 88, 594
α₁-antagonists, 799
anthropometry, 821
antiarrhythmics, 478t, 699–700, 726, 729t, 989t
antibacterials
  antiretrovirals and, 989t
  as concentration-dependent drugs, 265
  as time-dependent drugs, 263–265
antibiograms, 295, 729t
antibiotics. *See also* antimicrobials; β-lactam antibiotics
  agitation and, 162
  ALF from, 577
  for COPD, 637–638
  at endotracheal intubation, 363–364
  for MCS, 750
  MIC for, 555
  for morbid obesity, 826–8830, 827t
  for myxedema coma, 793
  NMBAs and, 214
  PD of, 827t
  resistance to, strategies to minimize, 295
  for respiratory acidosis, 20
  for SSIs, 353–356, 354t–355t
  TdP from, 726
anticancer drugs, 729t

anticholinergics, 162, 192t, 632, 639
anticoagulants
  for ACS, 668t, 674–675
  ADEs and, 975
  for AF, 720–721
  for BCVIs, 870–872
  complications with, 449–450
  DDIs with, 942–943, 944t
  for DIC, 473–474
  GI bleeding and, reintroduction of, 601–602
  hemorrhage with, 494–495
  for HIT, 464–465
  IHD and, 540
  for invasive procedures, 463–464
  in ischemia-driven strategy, 678
  laboratory testing for, 499–517
    ACT for, 508–509
    anti-Xa for, 506–507, 508f
    aPTT for, 501, 503–506, 504f, 505f
    chromogenic factor X and, 503
    D-dimer for, 515–516, 516t
    dTT for, 509
    ecarin clotting time for, 509–510
    Hemoclot thrombin inhibitor for, 511
    Heptest and Heptest-Stat for, 508
    methods for, 499–500
    PiCT for, 511
    platelet reactivity tests for, 516–517
    regulatory requirements for, 500
    reptilase time for, 512
    ROTEG for, 513–515
    samples for, 500–501
    TEG for, 512–515
    thrombin generation assays for, 511–512
  Mallory-Weiss tears from, 594
  MCS and, 745–750
  for morbid obesity, 825–826
  for NSTE, 677
  peptic ulcer disease from, 593
  in pregnancy, 833
  for respiratory acidosis, 20
  reversal of, 458, 462t, 462t–463t, 475t, 494–495
    for drug-induced coagulopathies, 475t
    for GI bleeding, 597–598
    for ICH, 411–412
    for STEMI, 680
  for VTE, 451–459, 451t, 452t, 454t
anticonvulsants, 192t, 376t–377t, 989t, 991
antidepressant discontinuation syndrome, 783
antidepressants, 192t, 726, 729t, 783–784, 783t, 812
antidiuretic hormone (ADH), 59, 230. *See also* syndrome of inappropriate antidiuretic hormone
antiemetics, 726, 729t, 1003
antiepileptics, 577, 991
antifibrinolytics, 426, 482t, 869–870
antifungals, 247
  ALF from, 577
  antiretrovirals and, 989t
  for burns, 854t
  for *Candida*, 322, 324t
  CYP and, 1004
  drug dosing of, 273–274
  ECMO and, 744
  for FN, 986
  liver drug clearance and, 258
  MIC for, 266
  for mucormycosis, 326
  PD and PK of, 265–266

P-glycoprotein and, 934t
prophylaxis with, 357–358
QT interval and, 943t
resistance to, 319–320, 322–323, 324t
TdP from, 729t
antihistamines, 192t, 235, 617
Antihypertensive Treatment in Acute Cerebral Hemorrhage (ATACH), 770
antihypertensives, 832–833
antimicrobial stewardship programs (ASPs), 247–248, 248f, 287, 331, 364
antimicrobials, 241–248
  ALF from, 576, 577
  ARC for, 244, 262
  ASPs for, 247–248, 248f
  biomarkers for, 246–247
  for burns, 853, 854t
  clinical decision support systems for, 242–243
  for COPD, 637–638
  CrCl for, 244
  DDIs with, 933
  de-escalation of, 245–246, 246f
  for donor-derived infections, 987
  drug dosing of, 243–244, 261–266
  drug shortages of, 927f
  duration of, 247
  ECMO and, 743–744
  for FN, 984–986, 985t
  for GNB, de-escalation of, 245–246, 246f
  for hepatic encephalopathy, 581
  MDR to, 242
  MIC for, 243, 244, 253
  for morbid obesity, 826–830
  PD of, 252–275
    for burns, 853
    drug dosing of, 263–266
    goals for, 263, 264t
    limitations of, 274–275
    for sepsis and septic shock, 308
  PK of, 244, 252–275
    alterations in critical illness, 254, 255t, 259t
    for burns, 853
    changes in drug absorption, 254
    drug clearance for, 256–260
    drug dosing of, 261–263
    half-life of, 261
    limitations of, 274–275
    protein binding and, 260–261
    Vss for, 255–256
  in pregnancy, 832
  prolonged infusions of, 244–245
  prophylaxis with, 351–364
    for CIEDs, 362
    drug dosing of, 355–356
    ECMO and, 361
    for HCT, 359
    ICP and, 363
    for MCS, 750
    at mechanical ventilation, 363–364
    for nasal packing, 364
    for neurosurgery, 362–363, 362t
    for neutropenia, 359–360
    principles of, 352
    for spontaneous bacterial peritonitis, 357
    for SSIs, 353–357, 354t–355t
    for subdural grids, 363
    for TAH, 361
    for VADs, 360–361

  for VAP, 363–364
  protocolized management of, 243
  rapid diagnostics for, 245
  resistance to
    to clarithromycin, 601
    to metronidazole, 601
    SSIs and, 352
  selection of, 241–242
  for severe sepsis and septic shock, 241–242, 307–309
  TDM for, 245
  timing of administration of, 243
  underdrug dosing of, 244t
  for VAP, 243
antioxidants, 115, 399, 581
antiplatelets
  for ACS, 666, 667t, 669
  CYP and, 1004
  DAPT, 670, 672, 674, 675
  DDIs with, 942–943, 944t
  GI bleeding and, reintroduction of, 601–602
  in ischemia-driven strategy, 678
  platelet transfusions for, 598
  reversal of, for ICH, 412
antiprotozoal, 266
antipsychotics, 172, 192t, 193, 726, 729t, 943t
antipyretics, 21
antipyrine, 587
antiretrovirals, 989t. See also highly active antiretroviral therapy
antithrombin (AT), 450, 558, 884
antithrombotics, 675–678
  for ACS, 666–675, 667t–669t
  for BCVIs, 870–872
  with fibrinolysis, 681–682
  MCS and, 745–750, 746t, 748t–749t
  for STEMI, 678–682
Antithrombotic Trialists' Collaboration, 669
α$_2$-antitrypsin, 417
antivirals, 266, 334t–335t, 576. See also highly active antiretroviral therapy
  for EBV, 337
  for influenza, 341
  for VHFs, 344
anti-Xa, 458, 460, 463, 471, 474, 500f, 504–506, 505f, 506–507, 508f
  for apixaban, 509f
  LMWH and, 833
  MCS and, 747
  morbid obesity and, 826
  for rivaroxaban, 509f
anxiety, 759, 799
ANZICS. See Australian and New Zealand Intensive Care Society
aortic dissection, 229, 758–759, 768t, 774–775, 774t, 775f, 776
aortic regurgitation/insufficiency, 736–737
APACHE II. See Acute Physiology and Chronic Health Evaluation
aPCC. See activated prothrombin complex concentrate
APH. See acute postoperative hypertension
apixaban, 451t, 452t, 454t, 463t, 475t, 495
  anti-Xa for, 509f
  for GI bleeding, 596, 597t, 598
  P-glycoprotein and, 934t
APOE. See apolipoprotein E
apolipoprotein E (APOE), 420
apoptosis, 574
APS. See Acute Physiology Score
aPTT. See activated partial thromboplastin time

arbovirus, 332t, 344–346, 345t
ARBs. See angiotensin receptor blockers
ARC. See augmented renal clearance
ARDS. See acute respiratory distress syndrome
area under the curve (AUC), 47, 273, 547, 931
area under the receiver operating characteristic curves (aROCs), 99
argatroban, 452t, 454t, 459, 462t, 475t, 745
arginine, 115
arginine vasopressin (AVP), 59, 313–314, 810–811, 812
ARIES. See Ambrisentan in Pulmonary Arterial Hypertension, Randomized, Double-Blind, Placebo-Controlled, Multicenter, Efficacy
ARISE. See Australasian Resuscitation in Sepsis Evaluation
Arizona Center for Education and Research on Therapeutics (AZCERT), 726
aROCs. See area under the receiver operating characteristic curves
ARREST trial, 699–700
arrhythmias. See cardiac arrhythmias
arterial blood gas (ABG), 4, 899, 914
ASA. See American Stroke Association
aSAH. See aneurysmal subarachnoid hemorrhage
ASCEND. See Acute Study of Clinical Effectiveness of Nesiritide in Decompensated Heart Failure
ascorbic acid. See vitamin C
ASHP. See American Society of Health-System Pharmacists
ASIA. See American Spinal Injury Association
ASIA Impairment Scale (AIS), 396
aspartate transaminase (AST), 574
ASPEN. See American Society for Parenteral and Enteral Nutrition
Aspergillus spp., 247, 266, 324–325
aspirin, 475t, 485, 557t, 666, 667t, 669
  asthma and, 628
  GI bleeding from, 595
  for NSTE, 676
  peptic ulcer disease from, 591, 593
ASPs. See antimicrobial stewardship programs
AST. See aspartate transaminase
asthma, 626–639
  anaphylactic shock and, 234
  clinical presentation of, 628–629
  epidemiology of, 626–627
  management of, 635t–636t
  NIV for, 630–631
  NMBAs for, 208, 209t–211t
  oxygen therapy for, 630
  in pregnancy, 634
  treatment for, 629f, 631–634
asthma-COPD overlap syndrome (ACOS), 626, 628, 639
asynchronous defibrillation, 730
asystole, 690, 701–702, 856, 896
AT. See antithrombin; atrial tachycardia
ATACH. See Antihypertensive Treatment in Acute Cerebral Hemorrhage
atherosclerosis, 404, 592
Atlanta classification, for pancreatitis, 955
ATN. See acute tubular necrosis
ATOLL. See STEMI Treated with Primary Angioplasty and Intravenous Lovenox or Unfractionated Heparin
atorvastatin, 430, 577, 726t
ATP. See adenosine triphosphate
atracurium, 202, 207, 549t

atrial fibrillation (AF), 70, 627, 714–721, 720*f*
   AT and, 713
   drugs for, 718*t*, 723*f*, 726*t*
   treatment algorithm for, 722*f*
atrial flutter, 70, 627
atrial tachycardia (AT), 712–714
atrioventricular node block (AV block), 708–712
   ECG for, 708, 708*f*, 709*f*, 710*f*
   pacemakers for, 712
atrioventricular node reciprocating tachycardia (AVNRT), 712–714, 712*f*
atrioventricular reciprocating tachycardia (AVRT), 712–714
atropine, 192*t*, 692, 702, 710–711
AUC. *See* area under the curve
AUC$_{0-24}$/MIC. *See* ratio of the 24-hour area under the serum concentration versus time curve to pathogen MIC
augmented renal clearance (ARC), 244, 260, 262, 267, 744
Australasian Resuscitation in Sepsis Evaluation (ARISE), 48, 304
Australian and New Zealand Intensive Care Society (ANZICS), 48
autoimmune hepatitis, 578
automated external defibrillators (AEDs), 691, 695
autoregulation, 404, 404*f*
AV block. *See* atrioventricular node block
average A-weighted energy-equivalent sound pressure in decibels (dBA LAeq), 163
AVNRT. *See* atrioventricular node reciprocating tachycardia
AVP. *See* arginine vasopressin
AVRT. *See* atrioventricular reciprocating tachycardia
AZCERT. *See* Arizona Center for Education and Research on Therapeutics
azithromycin, 992
azoles, 939*t*

B

B lymphocytes, 337
Bacille-Calmette-Guérin (BCG), 577
baclofen, 781–783, 782*f*, 782*t*
bacteremia, 716, 745, 984
BAL. *See* bronchoalveolar lavage
Balthazar grading system, for pancreatitis, 955
barbiturate coma, 582, 920
barbiturates, 172, 393, 911*t*
base excess (BE), 7, 18
basic life support, 691
Baux formula, 844
BCAAs. *See* branched-chain amino acids
BCG. *See* Bacille-Calmette-Guérin
BC-GN. *See* gram-negative blood culture test
BC-GP. *See* gram-positive blood culture test
B-CONVINCED. *See* Beta-Blocker Continuation versus Interruption in Patients with Congestive Heart Failure Hospitalized for a Decompensation Episode
BCVIs. *See* blunt cerebrovascular injuries
BE. *See* base excess
Bedside Index of Severity in Acute Pancreatitis (BISAP), 955
Behavioral Pain Scale (BPS), 149, 437
benfluorex, 613

benzodiazepines, 162, 168–169, 173, 191, 587, 786–788, 788*t*
   for endotracheal intubation in children, 910*t*–911*t*
   GABA and, 782, 786–787
   for hypertensive crisis, 761
   for nicotine withdrawal, 784
   pregnancy and, 833
   for SE, 373, 375
benzoylecgonine, 776
benztropine, 192*t*
benzyl alcohol, 833
Bernard-Soulier disease, 476
Beta-Blocker Continuation versus Interruption in Patients with Congestive Heart Failure Hospitalized for a Decompensation Episode (B-CONVINCED), 654
Better Bladder, 562
Bhaskar, E, 64
bicarbonate, 4, 6–7, 15. *See also* sodium bicarbonate
Bickell, WH, 868
Bickford, A, 826
Biffl, WL, 870, 871
bilirubin, 38, 578
biomarkers
   for ACS, 662–663, 662*t*
   for AKI, 528
   for antimicrobials, 246–247
   for PAH, 620
   for TBI, 389–390
BIS. *See* bispectral index
BISAP. *See* Bedside Index of Severity in Acute Pancreatitis
bismuth subsalicylate, 601*t*
bispectral index (BIS), 165–166, 166*f*
bisphosphonate, 810
bivalirudin, 452*t*, 454*t*, 459, 462*t*, 475*t*, 677–678
   for ACS, 668*t*, 674–675
   MCS and, 745
   for STEMI, 680–681
black cohosh, 577
blastomycosis, 326
Blatchford score, for rebleeding, 600, 601*t*
α-blockers, 192*t*, 618
β-blockers, 710, 931, 1002
   for ACS, 665–666, 775
   for ADHF, 654
   for AF, 718–719, 718*t*
   for aortic dissection, 774
   for burns, 852
   for HF, 690
   for pheochromocytoma, 799
   for PSVT, 715
   VT and, 724
blood glucose (BG). *See* glucose
blood pressure. *See also* diastolic blood pressure; hypertension; hypotension; systolic blood pressure
   aSAH and, 425
   COPD and, 629
   hypertensive crisis and, 758–759
   ICH and, 413
   pheochromocytoma, 797
   SCI and, 397
blood transfusions
   for anemia, 479–480
   aSAH and, 431–432
   DTIs and, 459
   for GI bleeding, 596
   for hypovolemic shock, 232

blood urea nitrogen (BUN), 46, 525, 578, 955
bloodstream infections, aSAH and, 437
bloody vicious triad, 867
blunt cerebrovascular injuries (BCVIs), 870–872
BMI. *See* body mass index
BNP. *See* brain natriuretic peptide
body mass index (BMI), 107, 822
   cefazolin and, 35
   fondaparinux and, 457–458
   hypertensive crisis and, 759
   morbid obesity and, 823–830
   nutrition and, 99–100
   UFH and, 455
   underweight patients and, 830
Bordetella pertussis, 284
Borg dyspnea score, 617
bortezomib, 657
bosentan, 618
BPS. *See* Behavioral Pain Scale
BPS-Non-intubated (BPS-NI), 149
Bradley, MJ, 880
bradycardia, 81, 173, 227, 708–712, 711*f*
   syncope and, 672
bradykinin, 764
brain natriuretic peptide (BNP), 647–648, 717
Brain Trauma Foundation (BTF), 390, 392, 395, 886
branched-chain amino acids (BCAAs), 119
breast cancer, 805, 807, 811, 814
BREATHE, 617
Brilinta. *See* cyclopentyltriazolopyrimidine
Brill-Edwards method, 747
bromfenac, 577
bromocriptine, 162, 192*t*
bronchoalveolar lavage (BAL), 247
bronchodilators, 20, 341–342, 631–632, 634, 637, 639
Brunkhorst, FM, 129
BTF. *See* Brain Trauma Foundation
Budd-Chiari syndrome, 576, 578
bumetanide (Bumex), 648, 648*t*
BUN. *See* blood urea nitrogen
bupropion, 784, 936*t*
Burke, JF, 353
Burkitt lymphoma, 803, 805, 993
burns, 842–857
   antimicrobials for, 853, 854*t*
   arginine and, 115
   ascorbic acid for, 848–849
   carbon monoxide and, 849–850, 850*t*
   chemical, 857
   crystalloids and colloids for, 41–42
   cyanide and, 849–850, 852*t*
   depth of, 845*t*
   from electrical injuries, 856
   fluid resuscitation for, 845–847, 846*t*, 847*t*
   glucose and, 843, 853–855
   hyperglycemia and, 843, 853–855
   hypovolemic shock and, 229
   inhalation injury with, 848–849
   mortality risk factors with, 844
   NMBAs and, 217
   nutrition and, 121–122
   nutrition for, 851–852
   renal failure from, 259
   sepsis and, 852–853
   severity assessment of, 843–844, 844*f*
   SIRS and, 852–853
   VTE and, 855–856

C

CABG. *See* coronary artery bypass graft
cachexia, 830
Cairo, MS, 805
calcineurin inhibitors (CNIs), 526, 531*t*, 533, 995–996
calcitonin, 89, 810, 811*t*
calcitriol, 88–89
calcium, 88–91, 89*f*. *See also* hypercalcemia; hypocalcemia
   HCM and, 808
   hemostasis and, 468
   respiratory alkalosis and, 21
   sodium bicarbonate and, 17
   TdP and, 730
   TLS, 995
calcium channel blockers (CCB), 614–615, 666, 761
   for aSAH, 429
   bradycardia from, 710
   NMBAs and, 214–215
   pregnancy and, 832
calcium chloride, 78, 81, 88, 90–91
calcium gluconate, 81, 88, 90–91, 92*t*, 712, 857
calcium phosphate, 806
CALORIES trial, 106
CAM. *See* complementary and alternative medicine
CAM-ICU. *See* confusion assessment method for the intensive care unit
cAMP. *See* cyclic adenosine monophosphate
Canadian Clinical Practice Guidelines, 101, 107, 114–115
cancer, 803–816. *See also specific organs and types*
   HCM and, 807–810, 809*f*
   MSCC and, 814–815
   SIADH and, 810–813, 813*t*
   SVC and, 813–814
   TLS and, 803–807
   underweight patients with, 830
   VTE and, 450
Candida albicans, 320–322
Candida spp., 242, 320–323, 327*t*
   ALF and, 583
   antibiotic de-escalation for, 245
   antifungals for, 266, 322, 324*t*, 358
   HCT and, 359
   MDR of, 292–293
   MIC for, 320
   PNA-FISH for, 286
   triazoles for, 322–323, 324*t*
   in vitro interpretative criteria for, 323*t*
cangrelor, 667*t*, 669–673
CAPD. *See* continuous ambulatory peritoneal dialysis
capillary leak syndrome, 256, 552
carbamazepine, 153*t*, 154, 577, 936*t*, 989*t*
carbapenem, 171–172, 268, 744, 827*t*, 828, 933
carbapenem-resistant Enterobacteriaceae (CRE), 292
carbon dioxide (CO_2), 6–8
   asthma and, 628
   COPD and, 628
   H. pylori and, 600
   metabolic acidosis and, 14
   respiratory acidosis and, 19
   sodium bicarbonate and, 17
carbon monoxide, 849–850, 850*t*
carbonic acid, 6–7
carboplatin, 812

carboprost, 834
carboxyhemoglobin, 849–850, 850*t*
cardiac arrest. *See* sudden cardiac arrest
Cardiac Arrhythmia Suppression Trial (CAST), 723
cardiac arrhythmias, 707–730. *See also specific types*
   asthma and, 629
   from electrical injuries, 856
   hypokalemia and, 70–71
   malignant hyperthermia and, 204
   metabolic acidosis and, 16
   respiratory alkalosis and, 21
   supraventricular, 708–721
   ventricular, 721–730
   VHFs and, 344
cardiac index (CI), 646
cardiac output (CO), 225, 649, 896, 899
   aSAH and, 433, 436
   burns and, 843
   in children, 902
   MCS and, 737*t*
   phenylephrine and, 312
cardiac tamponade, 229, 233, 693*t*
cardiac transplantation, 656–657, 710, 737*t*
cardiogenic shock, 259, 621, 654–655, 737*t*
cardiomyopathy, 722, 737*t*
cardiopulmonary bypass surgery, 42
cardiopulmonary resuscitation (CPR)
   for children, 896
   for SCA, 688, 690–691, 693–695, 697–699
Cardiorenal Rescue Study in Acute Decompensated Heart Failure (CARRESS-HF), 650
cardiovascular implantable electronic devices (CIEDs), 357, 362
β-carotene, 115
carotid sinus hypersensitivity, 710
CARRESS-HF. *See* Cardiorenal Rescue Study in Acute Decompensated Heart Failure
caspofungin, 326, 561, 587*t*, 854*t*
CAST. *See* Cardiac Arrhythmia Suppression Trial
catecholamines, 14, 69, 99
   burns and, 843
   pheochromocytoma, 797
   respiratory alkalosis and, 21
   for septic shock, 229–230, 313–314
   SRMD and, 592
catheter-related bloodstream infections, 291
CATIS. *See* China Antihypertensive Trial in Acute Ischemic Stroke
CCB. *See* calcium channel blockers
CCPD. *See* continuous cycler-assisted peritoneal dialysis
CD4, 337–338, 988
CDC. *See* Centers for Disease Control and Prevention
CDS. *See* clinical decision support
cefazolin, 356, 363
cefepime, 162, 192*t*, 244, 268, 549*t*, 577, 834, 985*t*
cefmetazole, 353
cefotaxime, 42
cefotiam, 549*t*
ceftazidime, 244, 268, 549*t*, 835, 854*t*, 985*t*
ceftobiprole, 244
ceftriaxone, 256, 357, 549*t*, 561, 835
cefuroxime, 549*t*
Centers for Disease Control and Prevention (CDC), 291–292, 335, 344, 626–627

Centers for Medicare & Medicaid Services (CMS), 351–352, 967
central cord syndrome, 396
central nervous system (CNS)
   cocaine and, 776
   hypercalcemia and, 91
   hypocalcemia and, 90
   hyponatremia and, 59
   hypothyroidism and, 794
   metabolic acidosis and, 16
   neurosurgical infections and, 362
   nitroprusside and, 764
   opioids and, 152
   respiratory acidosis and, 20
   respiratory alkalosis and, 21
   VTE and, 450
   VZV and, 336–337
central venous catheters (CVC), 226–227
central venous oxygen saturation ($Scvo_2$), 303–304, 305
central venous pressure (CVP), 45, 47, 226–227, 302–304, 307, 529
CentriMag, 655, 655*t*, 746*t*
cephalexin, 364
cephalosporin, 244, 268, 744, 827*t*, 828, 831, 834–835
cerebral blood flow, 21, 690, 759
cerebral edema, 59–60, 574, 575, 581, 582–583
cerebral perfusion pressure (CPP), 418–419, 427, 582, 913, 919
cerebral vasospasm, 427, 428–429
cerebrospinal fluid (CSF), 333, 419, 427
   shunting devices, 362, 363
cerivastatin, 577
cervical cancer, 811
cervical spine fractures, 870
CG. *See* Cockcroft-Gault equation
cGMP. *See* cyclic guanosine monophosphate
Chagas disease, 710
chain of survival, 690
CHAMPION PHOENIX, 673
Chan, AL, 634
Chawla LS, 4
chemical burns, 857
chemotherapy
   drug shortages of, 927*f*
   hypomagnesemia and, 80
   SIADH and, 811–812
   SVC and, 814
CHEST. *See* Crystalloid versus Hydroxyethyl Starch Trial
chest pain, 662, 775
chikungunya, 345*t*
child abuse. *See* nonaccidental trauma
Child-Pugh score (CTP), for ALF, 577, 586*t*, 587*t*, 588–589, 956
children, 895–922
   asystole in, 896
   CPR for, 896
   CRRT for, 555
   DVT in, 921
   endotracheal intubation for, 909, 910*t*–912*t*, 913
   Haemophilus influenzae in, 896
   hypoglycemia in, 921
   hypothermia in, 902
   hypovolemic shock in, 896, 899
   MV for, 909, 913
   organ dysfunction criteria for, 903*t*
   physiologic differences of, 897*t*–898*t*, 899–900
   respiratory distress in, 907–909
   retinal hemorrhages in, 918

RSV in, 896, 908
SA in, 913–916, 913t
SE in, 383
sepsis in, 900–907, 901t
septic shock in, 899, 900–907, 901t
severe sepsis in, 900–903, 901t
shock in, 896, 899
SIRS in, 900–903, 901t
SRMD in, 921
TBI in, 916–921
thrombosis in, 921
VF in, 896
vital signs for, 902t
China Antihypertensive Trial in Acute Ischemic Stroke (CATIS), 771
Chiu, HM, 747
Chlamydia pneumoniae, 638
Chlamydia trachomatis, 284
chloride, 15, 18–19, 530
chlorothiazide (Diuril), 649, 649t
chlorpromazine, 172
chlorthalidone (Hygroton), 649, 649t
cholestyramine, 932t
cholinesterase inhibitors, 193–194
chromogenic factor X, 503
chronic kidney disease (CKD), 116, 117, 730, 757
  vs. acute kidney disease, 548–553, 552t
chronic lymphocytic leukemia, 805, 811
chronic obstructive pulmonary disease (COPD), 626–639
  clinical presentation of, 628–629
  epidemiology of, 626–627
  management of, 634–639, 635t–636t
  MV for, 629, 631
  NIV for, 630–631
  oxygen therapy for, 630
  triggers of, 628
Chung, CY, 918
Chvostek sign, 90
CI. See cardiac index
cidofovir, 333, 334t, 336, 549t
CIEDs. See cardiovascular implantable electronic devices
cilastatin, 549t, 985t
cimetidine, 936t
CIP/M. See critical illness polyneuropathy and myopathy
ciprofloxacin, 273, 357, 549t, 577, 932t, 936t, 940t
  AKI from, 526
  for burns, 854t
  drug-nutrient interactions with, 945t
  ECMO and, 561
  for FN, 985t
  pregnancy and, 832
cirrhosis, 42, 357, 358t, 492–494, 586
cisatracurium, 202, 207
cisplatin, 531t, 532–533, 812
citalopram, 936t, 1004
CK. See creatine kinase
CK-BB, 662–663, 662t
CKD. See chronic kidney disease
CK-MM, 662–663, 662t
CL. See clot lysis
Clarification of Optimal Anticoagulation Through Genetics (COAG), 1006
clarithromycin, 577, 587t, 601, 601t, 939t, 989t, 992
CLARITY-TIMI. See Clopidogrel as Adjunctive Reperfusion Therapy-Thrombolysis in Myocardial Infarction

Classen, DC, 353
clavulanic acid, 549t
clazosentan, 431
Clazosentan to Overcome Neurological Ischemia and Infarct Occurring After Subarachnoid Hemorrhage (CONSCIOUS), 431
clevidipine, 761–763, 762t
CLIA. See Clinical Laboratory Improvement Amendments
Clichy's criteria, for ALF, 576–578, 579t
clindamycin, 258, 353, 363, 587t, 991
clindamycin/primaquine, 991
clinical decision support (CDS), 978
Clinical Laboratory Improvement Amendments (CLIA), 500
Clinical & Laboratory Standards Institute (CLSI), 501
Clinical Pharmacogenetics Implementation Consortium (CPIC), 1000
clonazepam, 173
clonidine, 170, 173, 710, 784, 785, 787f, 788–789, 799
clopidogrel (Plavix), 475t, 602, 667t, 669–673, 676–677, 680t, 936t, 1004
Clopidogrel and Aspirin Optimal Dose Usage to Reduce Recurrent Events–Seventh Organization to Assess Strategies in Ischemic Syndromes (CURRENT-OASIS), 669
Clopidogrel and Metoprolol in Myocardial Infarction Trial (COMMIT), 775
Clopidogrel as Adjunctive Reperfusion Therapy-Thrombolysis in Myocardial Infarction (CLARITY-TIMI), 670, 681
Clopidogrel for the Reduction of Events During Observation (CREDO), 677
Clopidogrel in Unstable Angina to Prevent Recurrent Events (CURE), 669
Clostridium difficile, 245, 284, 291, 594–595, 986
clot lysis (CL), 513
clotting factors
  acidosis and, 473
  fibrinogen and, 486
  hemostasis and, 468–470
  INR and, 470
  INR for, 502
  liver and, 474
  PT and, 470
  PTT and, 470
  TEG and, 515
CLSI. See Clinical & Laboratory Standards Institute
Cmax/MIC. See ratio of maximum serum drug concentration to MIC
CMS. See Centers for Medicare & Medicaid Services
CMV. See cytomegalovirus
CNIs. See calcineurin inhibitors
CNS. See central nervous system; Congress of Neurological Surgeons
CO. See cardiac output
CO_2. See carbon dioxide
COAG. See Clarification of Optimal Anticoagulation Through Genetics
coagulopathy, 472–474, 472t
  ALF and, 575, 583
  Dengue fever and, 346
  fluid resuscitation and, 473
  hypovolemic shock and, 232–233
  MCS and, 745–750

reversal or prevention of, 480–484, 481t, 482t
  TIC, 867–870
  trauma and, 490–491
cocaine, 428, 577, 613, 774
  hypertensive crisis and, 759, 777f, 77677
coccidioidomycosis, 327
Cochrane group, 39
Cockcroft-Gault equation (CG), 259–260
codeine, 936t
Cohn, Edwin, 36
colistin, 549t
College of American Pathologists, 456
colloids
  for AKI, 529–530
  for burns, 41–42
  for critically ill patients, 49, 52
  crystalloids and, equivalency chart for, 311t
  electrolyte composition of, 39t
  for hemorrhage, 477
  for hemorrhagic shock, 866
  oncotic pressure, osmolality, osmolarity, and tonicity and, 30–32
  overview of, 36–39
  for shock, 310–312
  studies in critical patients for, 39–42
  for trauma, 40–41
  Vss and, 256
Colloids versus Crystalloids for the Resuscitation of the Critically Ill (CRISTAL), 529, 866
colonoscopy, 598–600
colorectal cancer, 592, 814
coma, 68, 191, 333
  barbiturate, 582, 920
  hypermagnesemia and, 81
  myxedema, 793–795, 795t
  SVC and, 814
COMMIT. See Clopidogrel and Metoprolol in Myocardial Infarction Trial
compartment syndrome, 848, 868
  frostbite and, 857
complementary and alternative medicine (CAM), 577
complete blood count, 46, 578
comprehensive pharmacy service, 960, 961t
computed tomography (CT), 333, 395, 428, 747, 814
  for aortic dissection, 774
  for aSAH, 417, 420–421
  for hemorrhagic shock, 864
  for nutrition, 100
  for PN, 105
  for TBI, 917–918
  TPA and, 407
  for VZV, 336–337
confusion assessment method for the intensive care unit (CAM-ICU), 173–174, 188–189, 189f, 784
congenital heart disease, 613
congestive heart failure, 627, 808
Congress of Neurological Surgeons (CNS), 396
conivaptan, 67, 650, 812, 813t
conjugated estrogen, 482t
CONSCIOUS. See Clazosentan to Overcome Neurological Ischemia and Infarct Occurring After Subarachnoid Hemorrhage
CONSENSUS II. See Cooperative New Scandinavian Enalapril Survival Study II

Consensus Statement on Malnutrition, 100–101
continuous ambulatory peritoneal dialysis (CAPD), 539
continuous cycler-assisted peritoneal dialysis (CCPD), 539
continuous renal replacement therapy (CRRT), 116–117, 542, 549t–552t, 555
continuous venovenous hemodiafiltration (CVVHDF), 116, 539, 542, 543, 545f, 546f
continuous venovenous hemodialysis (CVVHD), 539, 544f
continuous venovenous hemofiltration (CVVH), 116, 539, 540, 543
CONTROL trial, 869
convection, in drug clearance, 547–548
Cooperative New Scandinavian Enalapril Survival Study II (CONSENSUS II), 776
COPD. See chronic obstructive pulmonary disease
copper, 122
Cori cycle, 14
coronary artery bypass graft (CABG), 154, 716, 717, 721
coronary artery disease, 627
coronary perfusion pressure (CPP), 690, 695
coronavirus, 342, 343t, 638
corrected QT interval (QTc), 158, 168, 195, 273, 727–728, 730, 930
correctional insulin, 139, 139t
Corticosteroid Randomisation After Significant Head Injury (CRASH), 394, 395, 869
Corticosteroid Therapy for Septic Shock (CORTICUS), 314–315
corticosteroids, 20, 343, 398–399, 632
  for ACOS, 639
  for ADHF cardiac transplantation, 657
  anaphylactic shock and, 235
  for COPD, 637
  delirium from, 192t
  for EBV, 337
  for HSV, 333
  for MSCC, 815
  for myxedema coma, 793
  peptic ulcer disease from, 593
  for PJP, 991
  in pregnancy, 634
  for RSV, 342
  for SA in children, 915
  for septic shock, 314–315, 907
  for TBI, 394
  treprostinil and, 617
  withdrawal from, 800
CORTICUS. See Corticosteroid Therapy for Septic Shock
cortisol, 99, 800–801
Costantini, TW, 886
Cothren, CC, 871
COX-1. See cyclooxygenase-1
COX-2. See cyclooxygenase-2
Cp. See plasma concentration
CPIC. See Clinical Pharmacogenetics Implementation Consortium
CPOT. See Critical-Care Pain Observation Tool
CPP. See cerebral perfusion pressure; coronary perfusion pressure
CPR. See cardiopulmonary resuscitation
Cpss. See plasma concentration at steady state

CRASH. See Corticosteroid Randomisation After Significant Head Injury
CrCl. See creatinine clearance
CRE. See carbapenem-resistant Enterobacteriaceae
C-reactive protein, 291, 759
creatine kinase (CK), 662–663, 662t, 776, 856
creatinine, 34, 46, 578, 995
creatinine clearance (CrCl), 244, 260, 618s, 619, 764
CREDO. See Clopidogrel for the Reduction of Events During Observation
Creon, 120
CRISTAL. See Colloids versus Crystalloids for the Resuscitation of the Critically Ill
critical illness polyneuropathy and myopathy (CIP/M), 205–207, 205f
Critical-Care Pain Observation Tool (CPOT), 149, 437
Crohn disease, 79, 592
CRRT. See continuous renal replacement therapy
crush injuries, 217
cryoprecipitate, 473, 486, 492, 583, 869
cryptococcosis, 338
Cryptococcus neoformans, 323–324
Crystalloid versus Hydroxyethyl Starch Trial (CHEST), 40, 867
crystalloids
  acid-base disorders and, 4
  adverse effects of, 35
  for AKI, 529–530
  for burns, 41–42
  colloids and, equivalency chart for, 311t
  for critically ill patients, 49, 52
  electrolyte composition of, 39t
  for hemorrhage, 477
  oncotic pressure, osmolality, osmolarity, and tonicity and, 30–32
  overview of, 30–35
  for severe sepsis and septic shock, 41, 302
  for shock, 309–310
  studies in critical patients for, 39–42
  for trauma, 40–41
  Vss and, 256
Crystalloids Morbidity Associated with Severe Sepsis (CRYSTMAS), 45
CS. See Cushing syndrome
CSF. See cerebrospinal fluid
CT. See computed tomography
CT angiography, 870
CT severity index (CTSI), 955
CTP. See Child-Pugh score
CTSI. See CT severity index
Cullen, DJ, 973
CURB-65, 956
CURE. See Clopidogrel in Unstable Angina to Prevent Recurrent Events
Curling ulcers, 593
CURRENT–OASIS. See Clopidogrel and Aspirin Optimal Dose Usage to Reduce Recurrent Events-Seventh Organization to Assess Strategies in Ischemic Syndromes
Cushing syndrome (CS), 801–802, 801t, 802t
Cushing ulcers, 593
CVC. See central venous catheters
CVP. See central venous pressure
CVVH. See continuous venovenous hemofiltration

CVVHD. See continuous venovenous hemodialysis
CVVHDF. See continuous venovenous hemodiafiltration
cyanide, 764–765, 849–850, 852t
cyanosis, 204, 814
cyclic adenosine monophosphate (cAMP), 811
cyclic guanosine monophosphate (cGMP), 610, 618, 665, 765
cyclooxygenase-1 (COX-1), 666, 668
cyclooxygenase-2 (COX-2), 389, 595
cyclopentyltriazolopyrimidine (Brilinta), 680t
cyclophosphamide, 812, 937t
cyclosporine, 557t, 932t, 934t, 937t, 939t, 945t
CYP. See cytochrome P450
cystatin C, 527
Cystic Fibrosis Foundation, 120
cytochrome P450 (CYP)
  AC and, 800
  acetaminophen and, 575
  antifungals and, 319
  carbamazepine and, 154
  cirrhosis and, 586
  clopidogrel and, 670
  DDIs and, 930–931, 935–937, 936t–937t, 939t, 940t
  disease states and, 938t
  drug clearance and, 258
  endothelin receptor antagonists and, 618
  hemodialysis and, 552–553
  nicardipine and, 761
  nimodipine and, 430
  P-glycoprotein and, 931–933
  phenytoin and, 378–379, 991
  PK and, 1000–1005, 1002t, 1003t
  PPIs and, 602
  TdP and, 730
  TE and, 991
  ticagrelor and, 672
  underweight patients and, 830
  valproic acid and, 172
cytokines, 99, 234, 299, 540, 994
  burns and, 843
  SRMD and, 592
cytomegalovirus (CMV), 332, 333–336, 338, 339, 360
cytotoxic T lymphocytes, 628

D

dabigatran, 451t, 452t, 454t, 934t
  anticoagulant reversal for, 475t, 495
  for GI bleeding, 596, 597t
DAD-HF. See Dopamine in Acute Decompensated Heart Failure
Dagan, O, 563
DAH. See diffuse alveolar hemorrhage
dalbavancin, 294
dalteparin, 451t, 452t, 454t, 475t, 596, 597t
damage control, 879
Danish Verapamil Infarction Trial (DAVIT-II), 666
dantrolene, 204, 215
DAPT. See dual antiplatelet therapy
daptomycin, 549t, 829, 854t, 985t
dasatinib, 613
DAVIT-II. See Danish Verapamil Infarction Trial
dBA LAeq. See average A-weighted energy-equivalent sound pressure in decibels

DBP. *See* diastolic blood pressure
DCC. *See* direct current cardioversion
DCI. *See* delayed cerebral ischemia
D-dimer (fibrin degradation product), 471
    for anticoagulant testing, 515–516, 516t
    hypertensive crisis and, 759
DDIs. *See* drug-drug interactions
De Orbe Novo (Martyr d'Anghiera), 198
decompressive craniectomy, for TBI in children, 920
decongestants, 759
deep venous thrombosis (DVT), 435–436, 449, 884–886, 885t, 921
delayed cerebral ischemia (DCI), 418–419, 420, 426, 427–434
delayed ischemic neurological deficit, 428
delayed PN, 103
delirium, 186–195
    ABCDEF for, 195
    agitation and, 162, 187
    assessment of, sedatives and, 173–174
    dexmedetomidine for, 194, 195t
    from drugs, 191–192, 192t
    I-C-U-D-E-L-I-R-I-U-M-S mnemonic for, 193, 194t
    pathophysiology of, 187, 188f
    risk factors for, 191–192
    TdP and, 726
    treatment for, 193–195
Demadex. *See* torsemide
demeclocycline, 812, 813t
demyelinating disease, 217
Dengue fever, 344–346, 345t
denosumab, 810, 811t
desmopressin, 482t, 485, 598
desmoteplase, 407
Devine, BJ, 822
dexamethasone, 192t, 333, 796t
    CYP and, 936t, 937t, 940t
    for MSCC, 815
dexfenfluramine, 613
dexmedetomidine, 170, 173, 710, 784, 785, 788–789, 912t
    for delirium, 194, 195t
    pregnancy and, 833
dextrans, 36
dextrose, 31, 49, 78–79, 140
(1,3)-β-d-glucan, 327
(1,3)-β-D-glucan, 247
diabetes
    aortic dissection and, 774
    CS and, 801
    diagnosis of, 134
    nutrition and, 120–121
diabetes insipidus, 67, 231
diabetes mellitus, 717, 757
diabetes with neuropathy, 627
diabetic ketoacidosis (DKA), 14–15, 16, 81, 140–143, 141t
Diagnostic and Statistical Manual of Mental Disorders, 186, 189, 785
dialysis
    with convection and ultrafiltration, 548
    for hyperphosphatemia, 88
DIAS-3, 407
diastolic blood pressure (DBP), 757, 759
diazepam, 375, 376t, 910t, 936t, 937t, 945t
DIC. *See* disseminated intravascular coagulation
diclofenac, 154, 577
DiCocco, JM, 871
didanosine, 577
dietary reference intakes (DRIs), 110

dietary supplements, 576
diffuse alveolar hemorrhage (DAH), 992–993
diffusion, in drug clearance, 547
digital subtraction angiography, 429
digitalis, 215
digoxin, 78, 557t, 835
    for ADHF, 654
    for AF, 718t, 719
    bradycardia from, 710
    DDIs with, 932t, 933
    drug-nutrient interactions with, 945t
    for PAH, 619
    for PSVT, 716t
    succinylcholine and, 207
    toxicity, 70
dihydropyridine, 666
DILI. *See* drug-induced liver injury
diltiazem, 666, 672, 710, 761
    for AF, 718, 718t, 726t
    antiretrovirals and, 989t
    for PSVT, 715t
diluted thrombin time (dTT), 506, 509, 512f
dimorphic fungi, 326–327
diphenhydramine, 162, 192t
DIPS. *See* Drug Interaction Probability Scale
dipyridamole, 475t, 485
direct current cardioversion (DCC), 714, 719–720, 721, 724
direct thrombin inhibitors (DTIs), 474, 501, 509–510, 512f, 745
    ACT for, 508
    activated clotting time for, 471
    aPTT for, 506, 506f
    chromogenic factor X and, 503
    for GI bleeding, 596, 597t
    for HIT, 464–465
    TEG for, 515
    for VTE, 458–459, 458t
direct-acting oral anticoagulants (DOACs), 507, 515
Disability Rating Score, for aSAH, 427
disaccharides, 581
disseminated intravascular coagulation (DIC), 344, 473–474
distribution volume, 552
distributive shock, 234–235
disulfiram, 577
Diuretic Optimization Strategies Evaluation (DOS), 648, 649
diuretics, 207, 215, 649. *See also* loop diuretics; thiazide diuretics
    nitroprusside and, 765
    for PAH, 619, 620
Diuril. *See* chlorothiazide
diverticulosis, 592
DKA. *See* diabetic ketoacidosis
D-lactate, 14
DO_2. *See* oxygen delivery
DOACs. *See* direct-acting oral anticoagulants
dobutamine (Dobutrex), 258
    for ADHF, 652–654, 653t
    for aSAH, 432
    for PAH, 619
    for septic shock, 306, 906
dofetilide, 719, 720, 723f
donor-derived infections, 987
dopamine, 101, 229, 230, 258
    for ADHF, 650, 654
    for AKI, 533, 882
    for aSAH, 433
    cocaine and, 776
    for PAH, 620
    for septic shock in children, 905–906

Dopamine in Acute Decompensated Heart Failure (DAD-HF), 650
dopaminergics, 162, 192t
doripenem, 268, 550t, 985t
DOS. *See* Diuretic Optimization Strategies Evaluation
doxapram, 639
doxycycline, 577, 932t
DRHC. *See* drug-related hazardous condition
DRIs. *See* dietary reference intakes
DRIVE. *See* Drug Interaction Evidence Evaluation
dronedarone, 710
drotrecogin alfa, 315
drug clearance
    antibiotics, 256–260
    of anticoagulants, 463
    in CRRT, 549t–552t
    with ECMO, 564
    ECMO and, 742
    liver and, 257, 584–585, 585t
    plasmapheresis and, 556–557, 556t
    with RRT, 543–548
drug dosing
    in AKI, 538–564
    in ALF, 584–589
    for aminoglycosides, 271–272
    of antifungals, 273–274
    of antimicrobials, 243–244, 261–266, 355–356
    of antivirals, 334t–335t
    for EN, 107
    for fluid resuscitation, 42–45
    MARS and, 835–836, 836f
    for morbid obesity, 823–830
    obesity and, 821–829
    PD for, 555
    PK for, 553–554
    for PPH, 834
    in pregnancy, 830–834, 831t
    in special populations, 821–836
    therapeutic plasma exchange and, 834–835
    for underweight patients, 830
Drug Interaction Evidence Evaluation (DRIVE), 946
Drug Interaction Probability Scale (DIPS), 946
drug shortages, 916t, 925–929
    causes of, 925–926, 927t
    impact of, 926–927
    management strategies for, 927–929, 928f
drug-drug interactions (DDIs), 930–947
    absorption and, 931–933, 932t–933t
    with anticoagulants, 942–943, 944t
    with antiplatelets, 942–943, 944t
    with antiretrovirals, 989t
    CYP and, 935–937, 936t–937t, 939t, 940t
    displacement in, 933–935
    evaluation of, 944–947
    PD and, 939–943
    P-glycoprotein and, 931–933, 934t
    PK of, 931
    protein binding and, 933–935
    QT interval and, 941
    renal system and, 937–939
drug-induced AKI, 530–533, 531t
drug-induced liver injury (DILI), 575–576
drug-nutrient interactions, 943–944, 945t–946t

drug-related hazardous condition (DRHC), 971, 972t
DTIs. See direct thrombin inhibitors
dTT. See diluted thrombin time
dual antiplatelet therapy (DAPT), 670, 672, 674, 675
dual mechanism block, 202
durable implantable VADs, 740–741
Dutch Pharmacogenetics Working Group, 1000
DVT. See deep venous thrombosis
dysoxia, 225–226
dyspepsia, 619
dysphagia, 595
dyspnea, 672, 814

E

Early Albumin Resuscitation in Septic Shock (EARSS), 41
early brain injury, 418–419
Early Glycoprotein IIb/IIIa Inhibition in Non-ST-segment Elevation Acute Coronary Syndrome (EARLY-ACS), 677
Early Goal-Directed Therapy (EGDT), 47–48
Early Parenteral Nutrition Completing Enteral Nutrition in Adult Critically Ill Patients (EPaNIC), 103–105
EARSS. See Early Albumin Resuscitation in Septic Shock
Eastern Association for Surgery of Trauma, 872
Ebola virus, 344
EBV. See Epstein-Barr virus
ecarin clotting time, 509–510
ECASS. See European Cooperative Acute Stroke Study
ECF. See enterocutaneous fistula; extracellular fluid
ECG. See electrocardiogram
echinocandins, 258, 322, 322t, 326, 831, 986
echocardiography
    for electrical injuries, 856
    for PAH, 613–614
    TEE, 721
    for thrombosis, 747
    TTE, 48
ECLIPSE. See Evaluation of Clevidipine in the Perioperative Treatment of Hypertension Assessing Safety Events
ECLS. See extracorporeal life support
ECMO. See extracorporeal membrane oxygenation
E-Codes, 978
ECPR. See extracorporeal cardiopulmonary resuscitation
ecstasy, 577
eczema, 234
ED95, 207
EDD. See extended daily hemodialysis
EDEN study, 110
edoxaban, 451t, 452t, 454t, 463, 495, 596, 597t
Edwards, NM, 871
EEG. See electroencephalography
efavirenz, 936t
effective SID, 8

Efficacy and Safety of Subcutaneous Enoxaparin in Non–Q wave Coronary Events (ESSENCE), 678, 826
Efficacy of Vasopressin Antagonism in Heart Failure Outcome Study with Tolvaptan (EVEREST), 650
Efficacy of Volume Substitution and Insulin Therapy in Severe Sepsis (VISEP), 41, 129
Effient. See thienopyridine
efflux pumps, 290, 291
EG-1962, 430
EGDT. See Early Goal-Directed Therapy
eicosanoids, 419
EKOS catheters, 409, 453
electrical injuries, 856
electrocardiogram (ECG)
    for ACS, 663–664, 663t
    for AF, 714
    for AV block, 708, 708f, 709f, 710f
    for electrical injuries, 856
    IABP and, 736
    for PAH, 613
    potassium and, 805
    for SCA, 702
electroencephalography (EEG)
    for cerebral vasospasm, 429
    for SE, 382–383
electrolyte disorders, 58–93. See also calcium; magnesium; phosphorus; potassium; sodium
    agitation and, 162
    asthma and, 629
    bradycardia and, 710
    Dengue fever and, 346
    malignant hyperthermia and, 204
    replacement protocols for, 73t, 92
    TLS and, 804
    VT and, 722
electroneutrality, 5
ELISA. See enzyme-linked immunoassay
Elsharnouby, NM, 849
emphysema, 628
EN. See enteral nutrition
enalaprilat, 762t, 764
encainide, 723
encephalitis, 162, 217, 331–332, 332t, 345–346
endocarditis, 716, 987
endocrine disorders, 793–802. See also pheochromocytoma
    adrenal disorders, 800–802
    thyroid, 793–797
endophthalmitis, 320
endoscopy, for GI bleeding, 598–600
endothelial growth factor, 611
endothelial nitric oxide synthase (eNOS), 420, 430
endothelin receptor antagonists, 617–618
endothelin type A (ETA), 610, 617
endothelin type B (ETB), 610, 617
endothelin-1, 610, 617
endothelin-1 antagonists, 431
endothelium, hypertensive crisis and, 758
endotracheal intubation
    antibiotics and, 363–364
    for children, 909, 910t–912t, 913
    for hypermagnesemia, 81
    for SA in children, 816
    for SCA, 692
    for trauma, 863
    VAP and, 363–364

Endovascular Treatment for Small Core and Proximal Occlusion Ischemic Stroke (ESCAPE), 773
energy expenditure, guidelines for, 108t–109t
eNOS. See endothelial nitric oxide synthase
enoxaparin, 451t, 452t, 454t, 463, 475t, 678, 886
    for ACS, 668t, 674–675
    for GI bleeding, 596, 597t
    for NSTE, 677
ENT-1. See equilibrative nucleoside transporter 1
enteral nutrition (EN), 101–106
    for burns, 851
    drug dosing for, 107
    glutamine in, 114
    pancreas and, 119–120
    RDA with, 110
    SRMD and, 593
    for TBI, 879
Enterobacter spp., 292, 359, 583
Enterobacteriaceae, 292–293
Enterococcus spp., 292–293, 352
    VRE, 290, 293
enterocutaneous fistula (ECF), 879–880, 880t
enterovirus, 284, 332t, 343
enzyme-linked immunoassay (ELISA), 291
EPaNIC. See Early Parenteral Nutrition Completing Enteral Nutrition in Adult Critically Ill Patients
EPIC II. See Extended Prevalence of Infection in Intensive Care
epinephrine, 14, 230, 258, 620, 701
    AMI and, 712
    for anaphylactic shock, 235
    for asthma, 632
    cocaine and, 776
    EN and, 101
    myocardial ischemia and, 712
    in pregnancy, 634
    ROSC and, 695
    for SCA, 692, 695–697
    for septic shock, 312–313, 906
epistaxis, 759
epoprostenol, 610, 614, 615–617, 616t, 620
Epstein-Barr virus (EBV), 332, 335, 337
eptifibatide, 475t, 667t, 673–674
equilibrative nucleoside transporter 1 (ENT-1), 672
ergot alkaloids, 834
ertapenem, 355
erythrocyte sedimentation rate, 759
erythromycin, 258, 934t, 936t, 939t
ESBL. See extended-spectrum beta lactamase
ESC. See European Society of Cardiology
ESCAPE. See Endovascular Treatment for Small Core and Proximal Occlusion Ischemic Stroke; Evaluation Study of Congestive Heart Failure and Pulmonary Artery Catheterization Effectiveness
Escherichia coli, 242, 292, 352, 357, 359, 583
esmolol, 763t, 766, 831
esomeprazole, 587t, 936t
esophageal varices, 119, 592
ESPEN. See European Society for Parenteral and Enteral Nutrition
ESSENCE. See Efficacy and Safety of Subcutaneous Enoxaparin in Non-Q wave Coronary Events
estrogen, 485
eszopiclone, 587t
ETA. See endothelin type A

ETB. *See* endothelin type B
ethylene glycol, 15, 525
etodolac, 577
EU-PACT. *See* European Pharmacogenetics of Anticoagulant Therapy
European Cooperative Acute Stroke Study (ECASS), 405, 406
European Medicines Agency, PH and, 612
European Pharmacogenetics of Anticoagulant Therapy (EU-PACT), 1006
European Society for Parenteral and Enteral Nutrition (ESPEN), 101, 103
European Society of Cardiology (ESC), 663, 832
euvolemia, 436
euvolemic hypernatremia, 68
Evaluation of Clevidipine in the Perioperative Treatment of Hypertension Assessing Safety Events (ECLIPSE), 773
Evaluation Study of Congestive Heart Failure and Pulmonary Artery Catheterization Effectiveness (ESCAPE), 646, 647
EVEREST. *See* Efficacy of Vasopressin Antagonism in Heart Failure Outcome Study with Tolvaptan
excretion, of drugs, 553
exercise testing, for PAH, 614
extended daily hemodialysis (EDD), 539
Extended Prevalence of Infection in Intensive Care (EPIC II), 60, 68
extended-spectrum beta lactamase (ESBL), 290, 292–293
extended-spectrum penicillins, 744
Extending the Time for Thrombolysis in Emergency Neurological Deficits–Intraarterial (EXTEND-IA), 409
extracellular fluid (ECF), 58, 59, 67, 69
   ECMO and, 562
   hyperphosphatemia and, 88
   hypophosphatemia and, 83
   sodium bicarbonate and, 17
extracorporeal cardiopulmonary resuscitation (ECPR), 735
extracorporeal life support (ECLS), 735–736, 741
extracorporeal membrane oxygenation (ECMO), 559–564, 560f, 561t, 741–744, 746t
   AKI and, 742
   analgesia and, 743
   antimicrobials and, 361, 743–744
   MCs and, 735
   for PAH, 620
   PK and, 559–560, 562f, 563t, 742, 742f
   RRT and, 564
   Vd and, 562–564, 742
extra-NMJ actions, of NMBAs, 202–203
extrinsic pathway, 469, 470f, 503f
ezetimibe, 577

F

fT>MIC. *See* time during which unbound/free drug concentration remains above the pathogen MIC
factor eight inhibitor bypassing inhibitor activity (FEIBA), 233, 233t, 412, 458
FACTT. *See* Fluids and Catheters Treatment Trial

FACTT Lite. *See* Fluid and Catheter Treatment Trial Lite
famotidine, 162
Fanconi syndrome, 87
Faraklas, I, 856
fasciculations, NMBAs and, 214
FAST. *See* focused assessment with sonography for trauma
fatty liver of pregnancy, 576
FDA. *See* Food and Drug Administration
FEAST. *See* Fluid Expansion as Supportive Therapy
febrile neutropenia (FN), 983–987, 984t, 985t
FEIBA. *See* factor eight inhibitor bypassing inhibitor activity
FENa. *See* fractional excretion of sodium
fenfluramine, 613
fenoldopam, 533, 763t, 767, 882
fentanyl, 151t, 156, 167, 167t, 910t, 937t
   delirium from, 192t
   ECMO and, 743
   in pregnancy, 833
FEV_1. *See* forced expiratory volume in 1 second
fever
   aSAH and, 436–437
   Dengue, 344–346, 345t
   Lassa, 344
   rheumatic, 710
   TBI in children and, 919
   VHFs, 343–344
   yellow, 345t
FFP. *See* fresh frozen plasma
fibrin degradation product. *See* D-dimer
fibrinogen, 32, 468, 482t, 485–486, 869
fibrinolysis, 407, 485–486, 495
   GPIIb/IIIa inhibitors and, 682
   ICH and, 681
   for PE, 234
   for STEMI, 681–682
Figge-Stewart approach, 10
Finsterer, U, 17
flecainide, 710, 715t, 719, 722–723, 723f, 989t
Flolan, 615
fluconazole, 273, 319, 327, 550t, 561, 986
   for burns, 854t
   for *Candida*, 322
   CYP and, 936t, 940t
   for neutropenia, 360
   pregnancy and, 831, 832
flucytosine, 323–324
fludrocortisone, 397
Fluid and Catheter Treatment Trial Lite (FACTT Lite), 45, 49
fluid creep, 847–848
Fluid Expansion as Supportive Therapy (FEAST), 43, 899, 904
fluid resuscitation, 29–53, 50f. *See also* colloids; crystalloids
   acid-base disorders and, 4, 21–23
   for AKI, 529–530
   for ARDS, 45
   for aSAH, 432
   for burns, 845–847, 846t, 847t
   coagulopathy and, 473
   CVP and, 47
   distribution by body compartment, 44t
   drug dosing for, 42–45
   future directions for, 49, 53
   for GI bleeding, 596
   for hemorrhage, 476–479
   for hemorrhagic shock, 864t, 865–867
   for hyperglycemic emergencies, 141

   for hypernatremia, 69
   for hypovolemic shock, 231–232
   for influenza, 341
   MAP and, 48
   for metabolic acidosis, 16
   monitoring of, 45–49, 46t
   for obstructive shock, 233
   peripheral line administration for, 32–34
   RCT for, 30, 37–40, 42, 45, 49
   reviews and guidelines for, 51t
   for rhabdomyolysis, 884
   for SA in children, 914
   for septic shock, 45–46, 300–307, 899
   for shock, 229, 309–312, 899
   for stroke, 409
   for TBI in children, 918–920
   for TIC, 867–870
   for TLS, 805–806
   TTE for, 48
   for underweight patients, 830
   vasopressors and, 43
   Vss and, 256
Fluids and Catheters Treatment Trial (FACTT), 45, 49, 530
flumazenil, 912t
fluoroquinolones, 162, 272–273, 827t, 943t, 945t
   DDIs with, 932t
   ECMO and, 563
   for morbid obesity, 828
   pregnancy and, 831, 832
   thrombocytopenia and, 478t
fluoxetine, 577, 936t
fluvoxamine, 936t
FN. *See* febrile neutropenia
focused assessment with sonography for trauma (FAST), 864–865
fondaparinux, 451t, 452t, 454t, 457–458, 464, 668t, 674–675, 678
   anticoagulant reversal for, 462t, 475t
   for STEMI, 681
Food and Drug Administration (FDA), 30, 39, 67
   acetylcysteine and, 579
   Adverse Event Reporting System of, 1003
   antibiotics and, 262
   anticoagulant testing and, 500
   antimicrobial drug dosing and, 262
   antipsychotics and, 172
   DDIs and, 946
   drug shortages, 925
   ecarin clotting time and, 510
   endothelin receptor antagonists and, 618
   epoprostenol and, 615
   ertapenem and, 355
   fondaparinux and, 457–458
   GHB and, 782
   glucose management and, 135
   hemodialysis and gentamicin and, 272
   hydroxycobalamin and, 765
   iloprost and, 617
   NephroCheck and, 528
   nimodipine and, 420, 429
   omega-3 fatty acids and, 116
   pancreatic enzymes and, 120
   PCR and, 285
   PH and, 612
   recombinant human activated protein and, 315
   on ribavirin, 342
   riociguat and, 619
   sildenafil and, 618

simvastatin and, 1006
teduglutide and, 881
TPA and, 407
VADs and, 739
forced expiratory volume in 1 second (FEV$_1$), 627, 628, 629, 633, 634, 913
forced vital capacity (FVC), 627, 628
foscarnet, 80, 333, 334t, 336, 337
fosfomycin, 550t
fosphenytoin, 333, 376t, 378–379
FOUR. *See* Full Outline of Unresponsiveness
fractional excretion of sodium (FENa), 527–528
frank hematemesis, 595
Frank-Starling curve, 227–228, 477, 646
free radicals, 290, 580
free thyroxine (FT4), 794
FREEDOM C, 616
fresh frozen plasma (FFP), 473, 481–483, 481t, 486, 556, 834
    for ALF, 583
    for anticoagulant reversal, 495
    for cirrhosis, 492
    DTIs and, 459
    for GI bleeding, 596
    for hemorrhagic shock, 867
    in MTP, 868, 869
    VKA and, 411–412
frostbite, 856
FT4. *See* free thyroxine
Full Outline of Unresponsiveness (FOUR), 388, 389t
fungal infections, 247, 319–327
    AF and, 716
    dimorphic, 326–327
    fusariosis, 326
    molds, 324–325
    mucormycosis, 325–326
    rapid diagnostic tools for, 325t
    scedosporiosis, 326
    yeasts, 320–323
furosemide (Lasix), 78–79, 648, 648t, 811t
fusariosis, 326
FVC. *See* forced vital capacity

G

GABA. *See* γ-aminobutyric acid
gabapentin, 153t, 154–155
galactomannan, 247
galactomannan antigen detection assays, 327
ganciclovir, 334t, 336, 550t
ganglionic blockade, with NMBAs, 203
gangliosides, 399
Garnacho-Montero, J, 206
gastroesophageal reflux, 619
gastrointestinal system (GI)
    acid-base disorders and, 4
    antibiotic drug absorption and, 254
    antifungals and, 319
    bleeding, 591–602
        anticoagulant reversal for, 597–598
        anticoagulants and, reintroduction of, 601–602
        antiplatelets and, reintroduction of, 601–602
        with clopidogrel, 602
        colonoscopy for, 598–600
        diagnosis of, 595–596
        endoscopy for, 598–600
        hemostatic agents for, 598, 599t
        with hypovolemic shock, 229
        initial management for, 596–600
        lower, 592, 593, 596
        Mallory-Weiss tears and, 592, 593, 594
        NSAIDs and, 154, 601–602
        from peptic ulcer disease, 591, 592, 593
        prevention of, 594–595
        rebleeding with, 599t, 600–601
        spontaneous bacterial peritonitis and, 357
        SRMd and, 592, 593
        stress ulcer prophylaxis for, 594–595
        upper, 591–592, 595–596
    CRE and, 292
    FN and, 984
    hypercalcemia and, 91
    hypokalemia and, 70
    hypomagnesemia and, 79
    hypophosphatemia and, 83
    hypothyroidism and, 794
    metabolic alkalosis and, 18
    mixed acid-base disorders and, 21
    nutrition and, 99
    opioids and, 152
    SCI and, 398
    TBI and, 879
gate control theory, 155–156
GBS. *See* Guillain-Barré syndrome
GCS. *See* Glasgow Coma Scale
GDMT. *See* guideline-directed medical therapy
Geerts, WH, 884, 885
gemtuzumab, 577
genetics
    ACOS and, 628
    aSAH and, 417
    coagulopathy and, 474
    MDR and, 291
    pheochromocytoma, 797
    SE and, 385
    TdP and, 726
GeneXpert, for methicillin-susceptible *Staphylococcus aureus*, 245
genome-wide association studies (GWAS), 1000, 1006
gentamicin, 272, 550t, 985t
GFR. *See* glomerular filtration rate
GH. *See* growth hormone
GHB. *See* γ-hydroxybutyrate
GI. *See* gastrointestinal system
Gibbon, J., Jr., 735
GINA. *See* Global Initiative for Asthma
GLA. *See* γ-linolenic acid
Glanzmann disease, 476
Glasgow Coma Scale (GCS), 388, 389t, 794, 863, 917t, 952
    for aSAH, 421
    BCVIs and, 870
    for ICH, 411
    for TBI, 917–918
Glasgow Outcomes Scale-Extended, 427
Global Initiative for Asthma (GINA), 627, 631, 639
Global Initiative for Chronic Obstructive Lung Disease (GOLD), 627, 629, 639
Global Registry of Acute Coronary Events (GRACE), 661t, 662
Global Utilization of Streptokinase and Tissue Plasminogen Activator for Occluded Coronary Arteries (GUSTO), 678, 681
glomerular filtration rate (GFR), 15, 82–83, 262, 523, 524
GLP. *See* glucagon-like peptide; Good Laboratory Practices
glucagon, 140, 712, 843
glucagon-like peptide (GLP), 881
glucocorticosteroids, 162, 632, 795, 801, 814
Glucontrol study, 129–130
glucose. *See also* hyperglycemia; hypoglycemia
    aSAH and, 435
    burns and, 843, 853–855
    hypernatremia and, 68
    ICH and, 413
    management of, 128–145
        clinical management team in, 144
        guidelines for, 131–133, 133t
        hyperglycemic emergency management, 140–143
        insulin for, 136–140, 136t, 137t, 138t, 139t
        medications for, 136–140
        monitoring in, 135
        multidisciplinary steering committee in, 143–144
        primary literature summary for, 130–131
        RCT for, 131t
        future, 134–136
        team approach to, 143–144
    metabolic acidosis and, 14
    nutrition and, 120–121
    shock and, 46
    stress response and, 99
    stroke and, 409
GLUT-4, 843
glutamate, 373
glutamine, 7, 114–115
glutathione, 115, 575
glycemic variability, 134
glycine, 169
glycoprotein (GP), 468
glycoprotein IIb/IIIa (GPIIb/IIIa), 468, 471, 485
    ACS and, 660–661
    ACT and, 509
    inhibitors of, 667t, 673–674, 677, 680, 682
    thrombocytopenia and, 478t
GNB. *See* gram-negative bacilli
GOLD. *See* Global Initiative for Chronic Obstructive Lung Disease
Goldstein, B, 917
Good Laboratory Practices (GLP), 287
Goodpasture syndrome, 834
GP. *See* glycoprotein
GPIIb/IIIa. *See* glycoprotein IIb/IIIa
GRACE. *See* Global Registry of Acute Coronary Events
gram stains, 283–284, 287
gram-negative bacilli (GNB)
    antimicrobials for, 245–246, 246f, 247
    as donor-derived infection, 987
    neurosurgical infections and, 362
    peptic ulcer disease from, 592
    vancomycin and, 290–291
    VAP from, 244
gram-negative blood culture test (BC-GN), 284, 320
gram-positive bacteria, 359, 716
gram-positive blood culture test (BC-GP), 284t
Griffith, Harold, 198

growth hormone (GH), 99, 843, 881, 883t
  rhGH, 851, 852
guanfacine, 788–789
guanylate cyclase, 665
guideline-directed medical therapy (GDMT), 646, 657
Guillain-Barré syndrome (GBS), 154, 834
Gunnerson, KJ, 14
GUSTO. *See* Global Utilization of Streptokinase and Tissue Plasminogen Activator for Occluded Coronary Arteries
GWAS. *See* genome-wide association studies

H

H1N1, 339, 559, 736
H$_2$RBs. *See* histamine-2 receptor antagonists
HAART. *See* highly active antiretroviral therapy
habitus, 821
Haemophilus influenzae, 638, 896
hairy leukoplakia (HLP), 337
HAIs. *See* health-care associated infections
haloperidol, 172, 726
  CYP and, 936t, 937t, 1002
  delirium and, 192t, 193
halothane, 577, 710
Hamburger, Hartog, 34
HAP. *See* hospital-acquired pneumonia
haptoglobin, 745
Harris-Benedict equations, 107, 119
Hartford nomogram, 271
Hartman, ME, 899
Hartmann, Alexis, 35
Hartmann's solution, 35
HBO. *See* hyperbaric oxygen
HCAP. *See* health care-associated pneumonia
HCM. *See* hypercalcemia of malignancy
HCT. *See* hematopoietic cell transplantation
headache
  with aSAH, 437
  endothelin receptor antagonists and, 618
  hypertensive crisis and, 759
  pheochromocytoma, 797
  riociguat and, 619
health care-associated pneumonia (HCAP), 242
health-care associated infections (HAIs), 291–292
heart block, 70
heart failure (HF), 610, 738f. *See also* acute decompensated heart failure
  AF and, 717
  bradycardia and, 710
  congestive, 627, 808
  hypertensive crisis and, 759
  metabolic acidosis and, 16
  renal failure from, 259
  SCA and, 690
  succinylcholine and, 207
  VT and, 722
  VTE and, 450
heart failure with reduced ejection fraction (HFrEF), 645, 719, 725, 728
heart-lung transplantation, 620
HeartMate II, 656, 740–741, 746t
HeartWare, 656, 740–741, 746t
Helicobacter pylori, 591, 592, 593, 600–601, 601t, 1004
heliox, 633, 638, 816

HELLP syndrome. *See* hemolysis, elevated liver enzymes, low platelets
hematochezia, 595
hematopoietic cell transplantation (HCT), 359, 360
hematopoietic growth factors, 986–987
hemochromatosis, 710
Hemoclot thrombin inhibitor, 511
hemodialysis, 117, 231, 272
  CYP and, 552–553
  for HCM, 811t
  for hyperkalemia, 78–79
  for TdP, 730
hemodilution, for aSAH, 431
hemoglobinuria, 745
hemolysis, elevated liver enzymes, low platelets (HELLP syndrome), 576
hemorrhage. *See also specific types*
  with anticoagulants, 494–495
  with cirrhosis, 492–494
  fluid resuscitation for, 476–479
  hemostatic agents for, 468–495
  in pregnancy, 494
  with surgery, 486–490, 487t, 489t
  trauma and, 489t, 492
hemorrhagic conversion, 406
hemorrhagic shock, 490, 863–867, 864t
hemorrhagic stroke, 410–413
hemorrhoids, 592
hemostasis, 469–471
  measuring, 470–471
hemostatic agents
  for GI bleeding, 598, 599t
  for hemorrhage, 468–495
hemothorax, 863
Henderson-Hasselbalch equation, 6–7
heparin, 557t, 597. *See also* low-molecular weight-heparin; unfractionated heparin
  for BCVIs, 870–872
  for inhalation injury, 849
  MCS and, 746–747
heparin-induced thrombocytopenia (HIT), 450, 464–465, 476, 674, 975–976
  DTIs for, 458–459
  IHD and, 540
  in pregnancy, 833
hepatic encephalopathy, 573–574, 575, 580t, 581–582
hepatic insufficiency, 474, 492–493
hepatic system. *See* liver
hepatitis A virus, 575, 576
hepatitis B virus, 574, 575, 576, 987
hepatitis C virus, 284, 476
hepatitis E virus, 574, 575, 576
hepatocytes, 574
Heptest, 508
Heptest-Stat, 508
herbal preparations, 577
Herget-Rosenthal, S, 527
herpes simplex virus (HSV), 284, 331–333, 332t, 339, 576
herpes zoster, 338
HES. *See* hydroxyethyl starch
Heshmati, F, 633
Hespan, 38
Hessels, L, 71
Hextend, 38
HF. *See* heart failure
HFrEF. *See* heart failure with reduced ejection fraction
HHS. *See* hyperglycemic hyperosmolar state
hiatal hernia, Mallory-Weiss tears from, 594

HIE. *See* hyperinsulinemia-euglycemia
highly active antiretroviral therapy (HAART), 335–336, 338, 987–990, 992
His-Purkinje system, 710
histamine, 203, 204–205, 419, 843
histamine-2 receptor antagonists (H$_2$RAs), 162, 478t, 594–595, 598, 931
  for SRMD in children, 921
histoplasmosis, 327
HIT. *See* heparin-induced thrombocytopenia
HIV/AIDS, 331–332, 337–338, 987–992
  CMV and, 335
  Cryptococcus neoformans and, 323–324
  defining conditions of, 988t
  EBV and, 337
  HAART for, 335–336
  HSV and, 332
  immunosuppression in, 983
  MAC and, 991–992
  PAH and, 613
  PJP and, 990–991
  prophylaxis for, 990–992
  TE and, 991
  thrombocytopenia and, 476
  underweight patients with, 830
  VZV and, 336
HLA. *See* human leucocyte antigens
HLA-B*1502, 385
HLA-B*5701, 990
HLP. *See* hairy leukoplakia
Hodgkin lymphoma, 710, 805
homocysteine, 759
horny goat weed, 577
hospital-acquired pneumonia (HAP), 244, 295
HSV. *See* herpes simplex virus
Human Genome Project, 1000
human immunodeficiency virus (HIV). *See* HIV/AIDS
human leucocyte antigens (HLA), 1006–1007
Hunt and Hess score, for aSAH, 421, 421t, 437
hydralazine, 577, 762t, 766, 831, 832
hydrocephalus, 427
hydrochloric acid, 19
hydrochlorothiazide (Microzide), 649, 649t
hydrocortisone, 192t, 315, 795, 796t, 937t
hydrogen ion acidosis, 693t
hydromorphone, 151t, 167–168, 167t, 192t
hydrophilic drugs, 256, 262, 543–546, 563, 742, 744
hydrophobia, 346, 543–546
hydroxocobalamin, 850, 852t
β-hydroxybutyrate, 15
γ-hydroxybutyrate (GHB), 782
hydroxycobalamin. *See* vitamin B$_{12}$
hydroxycut, 577
hydroxyethyl starch (HES), 36, 38–39, 311, 867
hydroxymethylglutaryl coenzyme A reductase, 430
hydroxyzine, 173
Hygroton. *See* chlorthalidone
hyperaldosteronism, 759
hyperammonemia, 171–172, 581
hyperbaric oxygen (HBO), 850
hypercalcemia, 87, 91
hypercalcemia of malignancy (HCM), 807–810, 809f, 810t, 811t
hypercapnia, 628–629, 634
hypercarbia, 794
hyperchloremic metabolic acidosis, 15, 16, 21
hyperglycemia

AIS and, 409
aSAH and, 417, 435
burns and, 843, 853–855
causes of, 128
hypernatremia and, 67
hypomagnesemia and, 80
ICH and, 413
metabolic acidosis and, 14
nutrition and, 120–121
SSIs and, 357
stress response and, 99
hyperglycemic emergencies, 140–143, 142t, 143t
hyperglycemic hyperosmolar state (HHS), 140–143, 141t
hyperinsulinemia-euglycemia (HIE), 712
hyperkalemia, 71t, 74–79
bradycardia and, 710
lactated Ringer and, 476
management of, 77–79, 78f
MCS and, 745
SCA and, 693t
from succinylcholine, 217–218
succinylcholine and, 207
TLS and, 804, 807, 993
treatment for, 76t–77t
hyperlactatemia, 14
hypermagnesemia, 80t, 81–82
hypernatremia, 17, 64t, 67–69
hyperosmolarity, 17, 392–393, 392t
hyperparathyroidism, 91
hyperphosphatemia, 87–88, 90, 804, 807, 994
hypertension. *See also* pulmonary arterial hypertension
AF and, 716, 717
AIS and, 407, 408t
APH, 769t, 772–774, 774f
aSAH and, 428, 431–433
cocaine and, 776
CS and, 801
intra-abdominal, 212–213
PH, 16, 610, 612–613, 612t, 737t
portal, 575, 613
PPHN, 903
hypertensive crisis, 757–777
aSAH and, 769t, 772, 772f
blood pressure and, 758–759
clinical presentation of, 758–759
diagnosis of, 759–760
end-organ damage from, 758t
epidemiology of, 757
ICH and, 758, 768t, 770f
laboratory testing for, 759
pathophysiology of, 758
in pregnancy, 767–769, 770f
pregnancy and, 768t
retinopathy and, 759
special considerations with, 767–777, 768t–769t
treatment for, 760–767, 762t–763t
hypertensive encephalopathy, 758, 759
hyperthermia
baclofen withdrawal and, 782
malignant, 172, 203–204, 215
SCI and, 397–398
hypertonic, 31
hypertonic hyponatremia, 59
hypertonic saline, 231–232, 427
for SIADH, 812, 813t
for TBI ICP, 392
in children, 919–920
hypertonic sodium chloride, 32–33, 34, 35, 582

hypertriglyceridemia, 170
hyperuricemia, 804
hyperventilation, 389–392, 411, 582
hypervolemia, 431–433
hypoalbuminemia, 5, 7, 38, 256
hypoaldosteronism, 15
hypocalcemia, 87, 90–91, 92t, 728, 804, 807
hypocaloric feeding, 107
hypoglycemia, 130–131, 140
ALF and, 575
aSAH and, 435
in children, 921
cocaine and, 776
ICH and, 413
myxedema coma and, 793–795
SCA and, 693t
stroke and, 409
hypokalemia, 70–74, 71t, 173, 728, 759
SCA and, 693t
VT and, 722
hypomagnesemia, 74, 79–81, 80t, 81t, 90, 173, 430, 728
hyponatremia, 59–67, 64t, 794
aSAH and, 434–436
assessment of, 60–61
clinical manifestations of, 59–60
etiology of, 66–67
management of, 61–67, 62t
ODS and, 60, 61–62, 64
overcorrection of, 65–66
severely symptomatic, 62–64
SIADH and, 60, 66, 67, 810
vasopressin receptor antagonists in, 67
hypoparathyroidism, 88, 90
hypophosphatemia, 83, 87
hypotension
ADEs and, 975
AF and, 717
ALF and, 575
anaphylactic shock and, 234
Dengue fever and, 346
DKA and, 15
hypermagnesemia and, 81
hypocalcemia and, 90
malignant hyperthermia and, 204
metabolic acidosis and, 16
nitroglycerin and, 765
propofol and, 169
refractory, 30
riociguat and, 619
SCI and, 396
severe sepsis and septic shock and, 299
shock and, 225
SRMD and, 593
TBI in children and, 918
VHFs and, 344
hypothermia. *See also* therapeutic hypothermia
bradycardia and, 710
in children, 902
coagulopathy and, 472
CYP and, 938t
with hypovolemic shock, 232
for ICH, 582–583
malignant hyperthermia and, 215
myxedema coma and, 795
SCA and, 693t
SCI and, 397–398
TBI in children and, 919
TIC and, 867
hypothyroidism, 81
hypotonic, 31
hypotonic hyponatremia, 59, 61f, 66

hypovolemia, 409, 529–530, 693t, 896, 899
hypovolemic hypernatremia, 68
hypovolemic shock, 46–47, 229, 230–233, 865
in children, 896, 899
plasmapheresis and, 556
renal failure from, 259
hypoxanthine, 806, 994
hypoxemia, 20, 21, 162, 991
COPD and, 629
hypothyroidism and, 794
influenza and, 340
SCI and, 396
succinylcholine and, 218
hypoxia, 634, 693t, 722, 737t

I

IABP. *See* intra-aortic balloon pump
IABP-SHOCK II. *See* Intraaortic Balloon Pump in Cardiogenic Shock
Ibrahim, RB, 556, 559
ibuprofen, 153t
ibutilide, 715t, 719, 720, 723f
IBW. *See* ideal body weight
ICDSC. *See* Intensive Care Delirium Screening Checklist
ICF. *See* intracellular fluid
ICH. *See* intracranial hemorrhage
ICP. *See* intracranial pressure
ICS. *See* inhaled corticosteroids
ICUAW. *See* intensive care unit-acquired weakness
I-C-U-D-E-L-I-R-I-U-M-S mnemonic, 193, 194t
idarucizumab, 597
ID/AST system, 245
ideal body weight (IBW), 822–823, 824
IDSA. *See* Infectious Diseases Society of America
IgA. *See* immunoglobulin A
IgE. *See* immunoglobulin E
IGFBP-7. *See* insulin-like growth factor binding protein 7
IgG. *See* immunoglobulin G
IgM. *See* immunoglobulin M
IHD. *See* intermittent hemodialysis
IHI. *See* Institute for Healthcare Improvement
IL. *See* interleukins
iloprost, 617
imipenem, 268, 550t, 854t, 985t
immune reconstitution inflammatory syndrome (IRIS), 338, 988
immunoglobulin A (IgA), 315
immunoglobulin E (IgE), 204, 234, 627
immunoglobulin G (IgG), 315, 346, 657
immunoglobulin M (IgM), 315, 335, 346
immunosuppression, 983–996. *See also* HIV/AIDS; tumor lysis syndrome
CNI neurotoxicity and, 995–996
in DAH, 992–993
donor-derived infections and, 987
in FN, 983–987, 984t
in HIV, 983
in PERDS, 992
IMPACT-HF. *See* Initiation Management Predischarge Process for Assessment of Carvedilol Therapy in Heart Failure
Impella, 655, 655t, 737–739, 746t

IMPROVE. *See* International Medical Prevention Registry on Venous Thromboembolism
Infectious Diseases Society of America (IDSA), 322, 358, 359
inferior vena cava (IVC), filters, 451, 461
inflammatory bowel disease, 592
influenza, 339–341, 340*t*, 559
inhalation injury, 848–849
inhaled corticosteroids (ICS), 632
inhaled nitric oxide, 614, 620
Initiation Management Predischarge Process for Assessment of Carvedilol Therapy in Heart Failure (IMPACT-HF), 654
Injury Severity Score (ISS), 954
innate immune system, 575
inodilators, 306
inotropes, 229–230, 306, 314, 652–654, 653*t*, 717, 737*t*
INR. *See* international normalized ratio
Institute for Healthcare Improvement (IHI), 976
insulin, 136–140, 136*t*, 137*t*, 138*t*, 139*t*, 142–143, 142*t*, 143*t*
　for burns, 121
　DKA and, 15, 16
　potassium and, 69
　resistance, stress response and, 99
insulin-like growth factor binding protein 7 (IGFBP-7), 528
Intensive Blood Pressure Reduction in Acute Cerebral Hemorrhage Trial (INTERACT), 770
Intensive Care Delirium Screening Checklist (ICDSC), 173, 189, 190*t*
intensive care unit–acquired weakness (ICUAW), 205
INTERACT. *See* Intensive Blood Pressure Reduction in Acute Cerebral Hemorrhage Trial
Interagency Registry for Mechanically Assisted Circulatory Support (INTERMACS), 736
interferon-α, 613
interferon-β, 577, 613
interferon-γ, 327
interleukins (IL)
　IL-1, 574
　IL-1b, 301, 389, 490
　IL-6, 301, 389, 574
　IL-10, 390
INTERMACS. *See* Interagency Registry for Mechanically Assisted Circulatory Support
intermittent hemodialysis (IHD), 529–530, 539, 540, 541, 541*t*, 542, 544*f*
International Medical Prevention Registry on Venous Thromboembolism (IMPROVE), 453
international normalized ratio (INR)
　ALF and, 573, 574, 578, 956
　for anticoagulant testing, 501, 502–503
　chromogenic factor X and, 503
　clotting factors and, 470
　coagulopathy and, 472
　for DTIs, 459
　PAH and, 619
　PCCs and, 495
　for TIC, 867
　VKA and, 411
　for warfarin, 463, 1003
International SCI Pain Basic Data Set, 398

international sensitivity index (ISI), 502
International Society for Heart & Lung Transplantation (ISHLT), 360, 745–746
International Society for Pharmaceutical Engineering (ISPE), 925–926
International Subarachnoid Aneurysm Trial (ISAT), 426
intra-abdominal hypertension, 212–213
intra-aortic balloon pump (IABP), 655, 655*t*, 717, 735, 736–737, 746*t*
Intraaortic Balloon Pump in Cardiogenic Shock (IABP-SHOCK II), 655
intra-arterial catheters, 226
intracellular fluid (ICF), 58, 59, 69, 83, 88, 843
Intracoronary Stenting and Antithrombotic Regimen: Rapid Early Action for Coronary Treatment (ISAR-REACT), 674, 678
intracranial hemorrhage (ICH), 410–413, 411*t*
　ALF and, 581, 582–583
　anticoagulant reversal for, 411–412
　antiplatelet reversal for, 412
　blood pressure and, 413
　DAPT and, 670
　fibrinolysis and, 681
　hypernatremia and, 68
　hypertensive crisis and, 758, 768*t*, 769–770, 770*f*
　seizures and, 413
　thermoregulation for, 413
　TPA and, 406–407
　VKA for, 411–412
　VTE and, 395, 413
intracranial pressure (ICP)
　ALF and, 574
　antimicrobial prophylaxis and, 363
　aSAH and, 418–419, 427
　bradycardia and, 710
　CSF shunting devices and, 363
　ICH and, 410, 582
　NMBAs for, 208–209
　respiratory alkalosis and, 21
　TBI and, 390–393, 390*f*–391*f*
　　in children and, 918, 919
　　hyperosmolarity and, 392–393, 392*t*
intrarenal (intrinsic) AKI, 525–526
intravenous immunoglobulins (IVIG), 315, 335*t*, 342, 343, 345
Intravenous Nimodipine West European Stroke Trial (INWEST), 771
intrinsic pathway, 469, 470–471, 470*f*, 503*f*
intrinsic positive end-expiratory pressure (PEEPi), 628, 638
invasive fungal infections (IFIs). *See* fungal infections
INWEST. *See* Intravenous Nimodipine West European Stroke Trial
IRIS. *See* immune reconstitution inflammatory syndrome
iron, antioxidants and, 115
ISAR-REACT. *See* Intracoronary Stenting and Antithrombotic Regimen: Rapid Early Action for Coronary Treatment
ISAT. *See* International Subarachnoid Aneurysm Trial
isavuconazole, 326
ischemia-driven strategy, 675, 678
ischemic colitis, 592
ischemic penumbra, 404
ISHLT. *See* International Society for Heart & Lung Transplantation

ISI. *See* international sensitivity index
isoflurane, 577
isoniazid, 577, 936*t*
isotonic, 31
isotonic hyponatremia, 59
ISPE. *See* International Society for Pharmaceutical Engineering
ISS. *See* Injury Severity Score
itraconazole, 326, 577, 934*t*, 989*t*
IVC. *See* inferior vena cava
IVIG. *See* intravenous immunoglobulins

J

James equation, 822–823
Janmahasatian, S, 822, 823
Japanese encephalitis, 345, 345*t*
Joint National Committee on Prevention, Detection, Evaluation, and Treatment of High Blood Pressure (JNC-7), 757, 759
Joint Section on Disorders of the Spine and Peripheral Nerves, 396

K

Kahn, SA, 849
Kane-Gill, SL, 973
Kcentra, 233, 233*t*, 597, 869
KCH. *See* King's College Hospital criteria
KCNH2, 1006
KDIGO. *See* Kidney Disease Improving Global Outcomes
ketamine, 153*t*, 155, 162, 172, 192*t*, 633, 816, 911*t*
　bradycardia from, 710
　CYP and, 936*t*, 937*t*
　for SE, 377*t*, 380–381
ketoacidosis, 14
ketoconazole, 577, 802, 802*t*
ketones, 14, 16
ketorolac, 153*t*, 157
Kew, KM, 633
kidney. *See also* acute kidney injury; chronic kidney disease
　ALF and, 587
　ammonium and, 7
　cirrhosis and, 492
　drug clearance and, 258–260
　hyperphosphatemia and, 88
　respiratory acidosis and, 20
　volatile anesthetics and, 173
Kidney Disease Improving Global Outcomes (KDIGO), 527, 527*t*
kidney failure, 162, 384–385, 450, 474
King's College Hospital (KCH) criteria, for ALF, 576–578, 579*t*
Kiser, TH, 637
Klebsiella pneumoniae, 290, 292
Klebsiella spp., 357, 359
Korotkoff sounds, 226
Kress, JP, 633
Kruse, JA, 72
Kuf. *See* ultrafiltration coefficient
Kurtz, I, 10
Kussmaul respirations, 15

L

LABAs. *See* long-acting β-agonists
labetalol, 763*t*, 766–767, 831, 832
laboratory testing, 283–287
    for ADHF, 647–648
    for AKI, 525*t*
    for anticoagulants, 499–517
        chromogenic factor X and, 503
        Heptest and Heptest-Stat for, 508
        methods for, 499–500
        regulatory requirements for, 500
        samples for, 500–501
    ASPs for, 287
    for hypertensive crisis, 759
    for SE, 382–383
laboratory TLS (LTLS), 804, 804*t*
lacosamide, 333, 376*t*, 379, 936*t*
β-lactam antibiotics, 244–245, 256, 263–264, 267–270, 269*t*–270*t*, 563
    for burns, 854*t*
    ESBL, 290, 292–293
    for morbid obesity, 828
    PBPs and, 291
    pregnancy and, 831, 832
    TDM for, 262
    thrombocytopenia and, 478*t*, 975
lactate, 4, 68, 301, 578
    metabolic acidosis and, 14, 16
    shock and, 46, 228–229
lactate dehydrogenase (LDH), 342, 745
lactated Ringer, 21–22, 35, 69, 344, 476, 596
    for burns, 845–847
    for hyperchloremic metabolic acidosis, 16
    for hypovolemic shock, 231
lactic acidosis, 14, 16, 228, 476, 764
lactulose, 581
LAMB. *See* liquid formulations of amphotericin B
lamivudine, 577
lansoprazole, 1004
Lasix. *See* furosemide
Lassa fever, 344
laudanosine, 207
Lazarus-Barlow, WS, 36
LBBB. *See* left bundle branch block
LBW. *See* lean body weight
LDH. *See* lactate dehydrogenase
lean body weight (LBW), 822–823, 824
left bundle branch block (LBBB), 664
left ventricle (LV)
    failure, 758
    hypertrophy, 759
left ventricular assist devices (LVADs), 360–361, 646, 656, 746*t*, 747
Legionella pneumophila, 291
length of stay (LOS), 99, 163, 174, 175
    AF and, 717
    arginine and, 115
    aSAH and, 437
    methadone and, 168
    omega-3 fatty acids and, 115
    PN and, 103
lethal triad, 867
leucovorin, 991
leukemia, 323, 360, 803, 993
leukopenia, 342, 346, 420
leukotriene inhibitors, 577
leukotriene receptor antagonists, 633–634
Leuven MICU trial, 129
Leuven SICU trial, 129

levalbuterol, 631, 915
levetiracetam, 192*t*, 333, 376*t*, 378–379, 394–395, 427, 831
levocarnitine, 171–172
levodopa, 945*t*
levofloxacin, 273, 359, 854*t*, 932*t*, 945*t*, 985*t*
levosimendan, 306
levothyroxine, 932*t*, 945*t*
Leykin, Y, 217
lidocaine, 215, 617, 936*t*
    for SCA, 692, 699
    for VT, 723, 724, 727*t*
ligament of Treitz, 592
LightCycler SeptiFast Test, 245
Lillehei, C. Walton, 735
LiMAx test, 587
Lin, H, 856
linezolid, 192*t*, 244–245, 271, 550*t*, 827*t*
    for burns, 854*t*
    ECMO and, 561, 744
    for FN, 985*t*
    for morbid obesity, 829
    for MRSA, 294
    P-glycoprotein and, 934*t*
    for serotonin syndrome, 940
    thrombocytopenia and, 478*t*, 975
γ-linolenic acid (GLA), 117–118
lipophilic drugs, 256, 543–546, 561, 561*t*, 563
liquid formulations of amphotericin B (LAMB), 266
LIS. *See* lung injury score
lithium carbonate, 550*t*
liver
    acid-base disorders and, 4
    anticoagulants and, 463
    cirrhosis and, 492–493
    coagulopathy and, 474
    drug clearance and, 257, 584–585, 585*t*
    nitrogen and, 7
    NMBAs and, 207
    nutrition and, 118–119
    potassium in, 69
    stress response and, 99
    volatile anesthetics and, 173
    warfarin and, 463
liver failure. *See also* acute liver failure
    agitation and, 162
    SE and, 384–385
    SRMD and, 593
    VTE and, 450
liver transplantation. *See* orthotopic liver transplantation
LMWH. *See* low-molecular weight-heparin
lofexidine, 785
log P, 543, 561, 561*t*, 742
lomefloxacin, 550*t*
long QT syndrome (LQTS), 725–726, 729–730, 1007
long-acting β-agonists (LABAs), 632, 637
loop diuretics, 18, 66, 67, 72, 78–79, 526, 808, 882
    for ADHF, 648–649, 648*t*
    pregnancy and, 833
loop of Henle, 18, 80, 524
lopinavir/ritonavir, 342
lorazepam, 169, 192*t*, 375, 376*t*, 587, 910*t*
LOS. *See* length of stay
lovastatin, 672
low-molecular weight-heparin (LMWH), 464, 474, 507, 515, 558, 677, 721
    for ACS, 674–675
    coagulant reversal for, 458, 462*t*, 495, 597
    for GI bleeding, 596, 597*t*

    INR for, 502
    for morbid obesity, 826
    in pregnancy, 831, 833
    for underweight patients, 830
    for VTE, 395, 398, 413, 455, 456–457, 830, 833
LQTS. *See* long QT syndrome
LTLS. *See* laboratory TLS
L-tryptophan, 613
Ludwig, KP, 826
Lugol solution, 796*t*
lung
    ALI, 107, 116, 117–118, 118*t*
    cancer, 627, 805, 807, 814
    transplantation, 620
lung injury score (LIS), 849
LV. *See* left ventricle
LVADs. *See* left ventricular assist devices
lymphoma, 323, 803, 808
lymphopenia, 342

M

MA. *See* maximum amplitude
MAC. *See Mycobacterium avium* complex
macitentan, 618
macrolides, 563, 831, 832, 933, 939*t*, 943*t*
macronutrients, 106–110
macrophages, 628
magnesium, 79–82, 215, 700, 730. *See also* hypermagnesemia; hypomagnesemia
    for aSAH, 430–431
    for SA in children, 815
Magnesium for Aneurysmal Subarachnoid Hemorrhage (MASH-2), 430
magnesium sulfate, 80–81, 632–633, 638–639, 726*t*, 857
magnetic resonance imaging (MRI)
    for aortic dissection, 774
    for aSAH, 420
    for cerebral vasospasm, 428
    for HSV, 333
    for ICH, 411
    for MSCC, 815
    for SVC, 814
    for VZV, 336–337
Ma-Huang, 577
maintenance fluid administration, 48–49
MALDI-TOF MS. *See* matrix-assisted laser desorption ionization time of flight mass spectrometry
malignant hyperthermia, 172, 203–204, 215
malignant spinal cord compression (MSCC), 814–815
Mallory-Weiss tears, 592, 593, 594
malnutrition, 98–106, 575, 710, 765
manganese, 115
mannitol, 67, 392, 427, 582, 884, 919
MAOIs. *See* monoamine oxidase inhibitors
MAP. *See* mean arterial pressure
Maquet Bioline, 560
Maquet Cardiopulmonary AG, 560
Maquet Safeline, 560
Maquet Softline, 560
Marburg virus, 343–344
Marfan syndrome, 774
MARS. *See* molecular adsorbent recirculating system
Martyr d'Anghiera, Peter, 198
MASH-2. *See* Magnesium for Aneurysmal Subarachnoid Hemorrhage

massage, 156
massive transfusion protocols (MTPs), 473
    for PPH, 494
    for TIC, 867–870
    for trauma, 490–492
MATE1. *See* multidrug and toxin extrusion transporter 1
matrix-assisted laser desorption ionization time of flight mass spectrometry (MALDI-TOF MS), 245, 286–287
MATTERs. *See* Military Application of Tranexamic Acid in Trauma Emergency Resuscitation
maximum amplitude (MA), 513
maximum clot firmness (MCF), 513
MCA. *See* middle cerebral artery
McDonald, M, 353
MCF. *See* maximum clot firmness
McGill Pain Questionnaire, 148
MCS. *See* mechanical circulatory support
MDI. *See* metered dose inhaler
MDR. *See* multidrug-resistant bacteria
MDRD. *See* Modified Diet in Renal Disease
mean arterial pressure (MAP), 41, 48, 225, 226, 301, 302, 304, 305–306, 759
    aSAH and, 427
    EN and, 102
    IABP for, 736
    phenylephrine and, 312
    stroke and, 404
    TBI in children and, 919
    vasopressors and, 305
mean pulmonary artery pressure (mPAP), 610, 614
measles, 332*t*
mechanical circulatory support (MCS), 735–751
    for ADHF, 646, 654–656, 655*t*
    anticoagulants and, 745–750
    antithrombotics and, 745–750, 746*t*, 748*t*–749*t*
    coagulopathy and, 745–750
    comorbidities and, 739*t*
    complications of, 739*t*, 744–750
    devices, 740*t*
    hemolysis and, 747*f*, 748, 749*f*, 750
    indications for, 736, 737*t*
    infection treatment and prevention for, 750, 750*t*
    landmarks in, 736*t*
    pharmacological challenges with, 741–744
    PK of, 741*f*
    thrombosis and, 747, 747*f*, 749*f*, 750
mechanical ventilation (MV)
    acid-base disorders and, 4
    AF and, 716, 717
    agitation and, 162
    antibiotic drug clearance and, 258
    antimicrobial prophylaxis at, 363–364
    for aSAH, 437
    for asthma, 631
    for children, 909, 913
    CMV and, 339
    for COPD, 629, 631, 638
    for coronavirus, 342
    CVP and, 47
    delirium and, 191
    for hypovolemic shock, 46–47
    iloprost and, 617
    for myxedema coma, 793, 795
    NMBAs and, 205–206
    nutrition and, 109
    in pregnancy, 634
    for respiratory acidosis, 20
    for SCI, 396–397
    TPA and, 407
medical intensive care unit (MICU), 129
medication errors (MEs), 962, 971–979, 972*f*
    active surveillance for, 976–979, 977*t*
    epidemiology of, 973
    medication safety and, 971–976
    systems analysis of, 973–974
medication withdrawal. *See* withdrawal
Medtronic Carmeda, 560
Medtronic Trillium, 560
melanoma, 805
MELD. *See* Model for End-Stage Liver Disease
melphalan, 577, 812
MELT. *See* middle cerebral artery embolism
Melzack, R, 155
MEN 2. *See* multiple endocrine neoplasia type 2
meningitis, 162, 437, 987
meperidine, 154
meropenem, 262–263, 268, 550*t*, 854*t*, 985*t*
MERS. *See* Middle East respiratory syndrome
MEs. *See* medication errors
mesenchymal stem cell transplantation, 399
mesenteric ischemia, 592
meta-analysis, 130
metabolic acidosis, 13–18
    AG and, 13*t*, 14–15, 16
        respiratory alkalosis and, 21
    delirium and, 191
    hyperkalemia and, 78–79
    hypertensive crisis and, 759
    hypoalbuminemia and, 7
    nitroprusside and, 764–765
    Plasma-Lyte for, 22
    rhabdomyolysis and, 884
    SBE and, 7
    secondary responses to, 15–16
    serum bicarbonate and, 4
metabolic alkalosis, 4, 18–19
metanephrines, for pheochromocytoma, 799
METAPLUS trials, 114
metered dose inhaler (MDI), 631, 634, 637, 915
methadone, 167*t*, 168, 173, 785, 786*t*, 989*t*
methamphetamines, 613
methanol, 15
methemoglobinemia, 765
methicillin-resistant *Staphylococcus aureus* (MRSA), 242, 244, 284, 291, 294, 351, 363
    antimicrobials resistance and, 290
    as donor-derived infection, 987
    HCT and, 359
    SSIs and, 352, 353, 357
methicillin-susceptible *Staphylococcus aureus* (MSSA), 242, 245, 284, 352
methimazole, 796*t*
methotrexate, 531*t*, 532
methoxamine, 695
methyldopa, 577
methylergonovine, 834
methylprednisolone, 192*t*, 342, 796*t*, 937*t*
    for COPD, 637
    for DAC, 993
    for PERDS, 992
    in pregnancy, 634
    for SCI, 398–399
methylxanthines, 633, 639, 816
metoclopramide, 192*t*, 932*t*
metolazone (Zaroxolyn), 649, 649*t*
metronidazole, 258, 587*t*, 601
    antiretrovirals and, 989*t*
    CYP and, 936*t*, 940*t*
    for *H. pylori*, 601
    for hepatic encephalopathy, 581
metyrapone, 802, 802*t*
Meyhoff, CS, 217
MIC. *See* minimum inhibitory concentration
micafungin, 326, 551*t*
Micrococcus spp., 615
microdialysis, 429
micronutrients, 110–116
Microzide. *See* hydrochlorothiazide
MICU. *See* medical intensive care unit
midazolam, 38, 168–169, 192*t*, 551*t*, 937*t*, 939*t*
    antiretrovirals and, 989*t*
    ECMO and, 743
    for endotracheal intubation in children, 910*t*, 911*t*
    for rabies, 347
    for SE, 375, 376*t*, 377*t*, 380
middle cerebral artery (MCA), 408
middle cerebral artery embolism (MELT), 408
Middle East respiratory syndrome (MERS), 342, 343*t*
midodrine, 397
mifepristone, 802, 802*t*
Mifflin equations, 106–107
Military Application of Tranexamic Acid in Trauma Emergency Resuscitation (MATTERs), 870
Miller, JT, 849
milrinone (Primacor), 101, 619–620, 652–654, 653*t*, 907
miltefosine, 326
Milwaukee protocol, for rabies, 347
minimum inhibitory concentration (MIC), 326
    for aminoglycosides, 271–272
    for antibacterials, 263–264
    for antibiotics, 555
    for antifungals, 266, 273, 320
    for antimicrobials, 243, 244, 253
    for fluoroquinolones, 272
    for β-lactam antibiotics, 263–264, 267
    for vancomycin, 270–271
mini-stroke. *See* transient ischemic stroke
minocycline, 294, 932*t*
mitotane, 802, 802*t*
mitral regurgitation, 759
mivacurium, 199, 202, 217
mixed acid-base disorders, 21, 204
Mobidiag Prove-It Sepsis, 285
modafinil, 162
Model for End-Stage Liver Disease (MELD), 576–578, 579*t*, 956
Modified Diet in Renal Disease (MDRD), 259–260
MODS. *See* Multiple Organ Dysfunction Score
molds, 324–325
molecular adsorbent recirculating system (MARS), 821, 835–836, 836*f*
molecular weight, 543
monamine oxidase inhibitors (MAOIs), 939–941
Moraxella catarrhalis, 638
morbid obesity
    antibiotics for, 826–8830, 827*t*
    anticoagulants for, 825–826

antimicrobials for, 826–8830
drug dosing for, 823–830
NMBAs for, 825
sedatives for, 825
moricizine, 723
morphine, 151t, 155, 156, 168, 192t, 910t
for ACS, 666
ECMO and, 743
pharmacologic properties of, 167t
in pregnancy, 833
Morrison, JJ, 870
mortality probability model (MPM), 953
Morton, RP, 871
motor vehicle collisions (MVCs), 916
Moviat, M, 18–19
moxifloxacin, 273, 551t
mPAP. *See* mean pulmonary artery pressure
MPM. *See* mortality probability model
MR CLEAN, 409
MRI. *See* magnetic resonance imaging
MRSA. *See* methicillin-resistant *Staphylococcus aureus*
MSCC. *See* malignant spinal cord compression
MSSA. *See* methicillin-susceptible *Staphylococcus aureus*
MTPs. *See* massive transfusion protocols
mucormycosis, 325–326
Multidisciplinary Consensus Conference, 420
multidrug and toxin extrusion transporter 1 (MATE1), 937
multidrug-resistant bacteria (MDR), 289–295
to antimicrobials, 242
mechanisms of, 290–291
mutations and, 291
P. aeruginosa as, 267
threats of, 292–294
multimodal analgesia, 153–156, 153t
multiple endocrine neoplasia type 2 (MEN 2), 797
multiple myeloma, 710, 805, 807, 811, 814
Multiple Organ Dysfunction Score (MODS), 953
multiple organ failure syndrome, 259
mumps, 332t
mupirocin, 359
Murphy, GS, 216
muscarinic receptors, 169, 202–203
muscle relaxation techniques, 156
muscular dystrophy, 207, 217
mushroom poisoning, 578
music therapy, 156
MV. *See* mechanical ventilation
MVCs. *See* motor vehicle collisions
Mycobacterium avium complex (MAC), 338, 991–992
Mycobacterium tuberculosis, 284
mycophenolic acid, 551t
Mycoplasma pneumoniae, 638
myocardial infarction. *See* acute myocardial infarction; ST-segment elevation myocardial infarction
myocardial ischemia, 710, 712
myocarditis, 710, 737t
myoglobin, 663
myotonic muscular dystrophy, 710
myxedema coma, 793–795, 795t

N

NABIS:H II. *See* National Acute Brain Injury Study: Hypothermia II
N-acetyl-*p*-benzoquinone imine (NAPQI), 575
N-acetyltransferase, 1005
nAChR. *See* nicotinic cholinergic receptor
nafcillin, 258
Na-K-ATPase pump, 69
naloxone, 666, 692, 785, 912t
NAPQI. *See* *N*-acetyl-*p*-benzoquinone imine
Narcotrend Index, 165
Narotam, PK, 362, 362t
nasal packing, 364
NASCIS. *See* National Acute Spinal Cord Injury Study
nasogastric tube (NG), 60
NAT. *See* nonaccidental trauma
National Acute Brain Injury Study: Hypothermia II (NABIS: H II), 394
National Acute Spinal Cord Injury Study (NASCIS), 398–399
National Center for Shake Baby Syndrome, 916
National Comprehensive Cancer Network (NCCN), 359, 984
National Confidential Enquiry into Patient Outcome and Death (NCEPOD), 514
National Coordinating Council for Medication Error Reporting and Prevention, 971
National Healthcare Safety Network, 352
National Heart, Lung, and Blood Institute (NHLBI), 815
National Institute for Health and Care Excellence (NICE), 48–49, 51f
National Institute of Neurological Disorders and Stroke (NINDS), 398, 404
National Institutes of Health Stroke Scale (NIHSS), 405
National Quality Forum (NQF), 306
National Spinal Cord Injury Statistical Center, 395
National Stroke Association, 410
National Traumatic Coma Data Bank, 208–209
Natrecor. *See* nesiritide
natriuretic peptides, 620
NCCN. *See* National Comprehensive Cancer Network
NCEPOD. *See* National Confidential Enquiry into Patient Outcome and Death
NCS. *See* Neurocritical Care Society
NCSE. *See* non-convulsive status epilepticus
necrosis
ALF and, 574
retinal hemorrhages and, 759
nefazodone, 577
nelfinavir, 577, 937t
neomycin, 581
neostigmine, 216–217
NephroCheck, 528
nephrosis, 42
nephrotoxins, 525–526
nesiritide (Natrecor), 651–652, 651t
neuraminidase inhibitors, 341
neurocardiac syncope, 710
Neurocritical Care Society (NCS), 420, 427, 432

neurofibromatosis (NF), 797
neuromuscular blocking agents (NMBAs), 198–218
for ARDS, 199, 206–207, 208, 209t–211t
for asthma, 208, 209t–211t
CIP/M and, 205–207, 205f
cross-reactivity of, 202–203
for DAC, 993
depolarizing, 202
for endotracheal intubation in children, 912t
extra-NMJ actions of, 202–203
fasciculations and, 214
ganglionic blockade with, 203
histamine and, 203, 204–205
hypersensitivity and, 204–205
for ICP, 208–209
ICUAW from, 205
interactions with, 214–215
for intra-abdominal hypertension, 212–213
malignant hyperthermia and, 203–204, 215
mechanism of action of, 201–202
monitoring of, 215–216
for morbid obesity, 825
muscarinic receptors and, 202–203
ND, 201–202, 214
NMJ and, 199, 200f
obesity and, 217
pharmacologic effects of, 202–207, 202t
PK of, 207
pregnancy and, 832
priming of, 214
rapid sequence intubation and, 213–214
RCT for, 206–207
reversal of, 216–217
for SA, 208
in children, 816
for sepsis, 209t–211t, 213
for surgical procedures, 213–214
sympathetic stimulation by, 203
for TBI ICP, 393
for temperature management after cardiac arrest, 211–212
vagolytic actions of, 203
neuromuscular junction (NMJ), 199, 200f
neuropathic pain, 154–155, 398
neuropeptide Y, 373
neurosurgery, antimicrobial prophylaxis for, 362–363, 362t
neutral protamine Hagedorn (NPH), 138
neutropenia, 359–360
neutrophils, 34, 628, 632
nevirapine, 936t
New York Heart Association (NYHA), 612, 615, 617
NEWTON. *See* Nimodipine Microparticles to Enhance Recovery While Reducing Toxicity After Subarachnoid Hemorrhage
NF. *See* neurofibromatosis
NF-κB. *See* nuclear factor kappa B
NG. *See* nasogastric tube
NHLBI. *See* National Heart, Lung, and Blood Institute
nicardipine, 430, 761, 762t, 774–775, 831, 832
NICE. *See* National Institute for Health and Care Excellence
NICE-SUGAR. *See* Normoglycemia in Intensive Care Evaluation and Surviving Using Glucose Algorithm Regulation

nicotine, 162, 784–785
nicotine replacement therapy (NRT), 784
nicotinic cholinergic receptor (nAChR), 784
nicotinic receptors, 169, 200–201
nifedipine, 831, 832
NIHSS. *See* National Institutes of Health Stroke Scale
nimodipine, 420, 429–430
Nimodipine Microparticles to Enhance Recovery While Reducing Toxicity After Subarachnoid Hemorrhage (NEWTON), 430
NINDS. *See* National Institute of Neurological Disorders and Stroke
Nipride. *See* nitroprusside
nitrates, 618, 665
nitric oxide, 580, 849, 994
   cGMP and, 610, 618
   eNOS, 420, 430
   inhaled, 614, 620
   nitroglycerin and, 665
nitrofurantoin, 577
nitrogen, 7
nitroglycerin, 258, 651–652, 651t, 665, 762t, 765
nitroprusside (Nipride)
   for ADHF, 651–652, 651t
   for aortic dissection, 774–775
   DKA and, 15
   for hypertensive crisis, 762t, 764–766
   pregnancy and, 831, 833
   for septic shock in children, 907
nitrous oxide, aSAH and, 419–420
NIV. *See* noninvasive ventilation
NKCC. *See* sodium-potassium-chloride cotransporter
NMBAs. *See* neuromuscular blocking agents
N-methyl-d-aspartate (NMDA), 155, 168, 373, 389
NMJ. *See* neuromuscular junction
NOACs. *See* nonvitamin K antagonist oral anticoagulants
Nogo-A, 399
nonaccidental trauma (NAT), 916–918
non-convulsive status epilepticus (NCSE), 373, 375f
non-Hodgkin lymphoma, 805, 811, 814, 993
noninvasive positive pressure ventilation, 816
noninvasive ventilation (NIV), 630–631
non-opioids, 153–156, 153t
nonpharmacologic therapy
   for agitation, 166
   for ALF, 584
   for analgesia, 155–156
   for delirium prevention, 192–193
   for SCA, 701
   for SE, 381
non-preventable ADE, 972, 972t
nonresponsiveness, 670
non-small cell lung cancer, 805
nonsteroidal anti-inflammatory drugs (NSAIDs), 153–154
   AKI from, 526
   ALF from, 576, 577
   for aSAH, 436
   asthma and, 628
   CYP and, 1003
   delirium from, 192t
   GI bleeding from, 595, 601–602
   Mallory-Weiss tears from, 594
   peptic ulcer disease from, 591, 592
   for procedural pain, 157
   SIADH and, 812

non-ST-segment elevation (NSTE), 664, 676t
   antithrombotics for, 675–678
nonvitamin K antagonist oral anticoagulants (NOACs), 411, 412
norepinephrine, 101, 258, 695
   for aSAH, 427, 433
   cocaine and, 776
   for PAH, 620
   for septic shock in children, 906
   for shock, 230, 312–313
   for underweight patients, 830
norfloxacin, 357
normal saline, 34–35, 41, 692, 810, 918
Normoglycemia in Intensive Care Evaluation and Surviving Using Glucose Algorithm Regulation (NICE-SUGAR), 129, 130, 854
NOR-TEST, 407
Norwood, SH, 886
NPH. *See* neutral protamine Hagedorn
NQF. *See* National Quality Forum
NRS. *See* numeric rating scale
NRT. *See* nicotine replacement therapy
NRTIs. *See* nucleotide/nucleoside reverse transcriptase inhibitors
NSAIDs. *See* nonsteroidal anti-inflammatory drugs
NSTE. *See* non-ST-segment elevation
nuclear factor kappa B (NF-κB), 299, 314
nucleic acid testing, 284–285
nucleotide/nucleoside reverse transcriptase inhibitors (NRTIs), 990
numeric rating scale (NRS), for pain assessment, 148–149
NUTRIC. *See* Nutrition Risk in the Critically Ill
nutrition, 97–122
   assessment of, 99–101
   for burns, 851–852
   burns and, 121–122
   diabetes and, 120–121
   drug-nutrient interactions, 943–944, 945t–946t
   glucose and, 120–121
   hyperglycemia and, 120–121
   liver and, 118–119
   macronutrients and, 106–110
   malnutrition and, 98–106
   micronutrients and, 110–116
   MV and, 109
   pancreas and, 119–120
   renal system and, 116–117
   respiratory system and, 117–118
   for SCI, 398
   stress response and, 99
   for TBI, 879
   timing and route of support for, 101–106
   underfeeding vs. full nutrition, 110t
Nutrition Risk in the Critically Ill (NUTRIC), 100–101
NYHA. *See* New York Heart Association

O

OASIS. *See* Organization to Assess Strategies in Acute Ischemic Syndromes
OATP1B1. *See* organic anion transporting polypeptide 1B1
OATs. *See* organic anion transporters

obesity, 106–107. *See also* morbid obesity
   AF and, 716
   antimicrobials and, 356
   CS and, 801
   drug dosing and, 821–829
   fondaparinux and, 457–458
   NMBAs and, 217
   PK and, 823
   SE and, 384
   UHF and, 453–454
   Vss and, 256
   VTE and, 450
obstructive shock, 229, 233–234
Octaplex, 597, 869
octreotide, 598, 880, 880t, 882t
OCTs. *See* organic cation transporters
ODS. *See* osmotic demyelination syndrome
odynophagia, 595
ofloxacin, 551t
OI. *See* opportunistic infection
oliguria, 575
OLT. *See* orthotopic liver transplantation
omega-3 fatty acids, 115, 116–118, 118t
omeprazole, 936t, 1004
oncotic pressure, 30–32, 38
ondansetron, 936t
Operational Classification (ORCA), 946
opiate antagonists, 20
opioids, 151t, 152–153, 152f, 157
   for ACS, 666
   for agitation, 166–168
   agitation and, 162
   in analgosedation approach to analgesia, 150
   CYP and, 1002–1003
   NMBAs and, 215
   pharmacologic properties of, 167t
   in pregnancy, 833
   SIADH and, 812
   withdrawal from, 785–786, 785f, 785t, 786t, 787f
opportunistic infection (OI), 987, 988
   dimorphic fungi, 326–327
OPTIMIZE-HF. *See* Organized Program to Initiate Lifesaving Treatment in Hospitalized Patients with Heart Failure
oral antidiabetic medications, 136
oral contraceptives, 450
ORCA. *See* Operational Classification
Orenitram. *See* treprostinil
organic anion transporters (OATs), 937
organic anion transporting polypeptide 1B1 (OATP1B1), 1005
organic cation transporters (OCTs), 937
Organization to Assess Strategies in Acute Ischemic Syndromes (OASIS), 677, 681, 682
Organized Program to Initiate Lifesaving Treatment in Hospitalized Patients with Heart Failure (OPTIMIZE-HF), 648
oritavancin, 294
Orrell equation, 89
orthostatic hypotension, 595
orthotopic liver transplantation (OLT), 574, 576, 583, 584
oseltamivir, 334t, 341
osmolality, 30–32
osmolarity, 30–32, 32–33, 32–34, 33, 57
osmotic demyelination syndrome (ODS), 60, 61–62, 64, 68
osteoporosis, 801

ovarian cancer, 808
overshoot alkalosis, 17
oxandrolone, 851–852
oxazepam, 587
oxcarbazepine, 936t
Oxepa, 117, 1154
oxygen consumption (VO$_2$), 225, 228
oxygen delivery (DO$_2$), 225, 228, 231, 234
oxygen therapy
  for ACS, 664–665
  for asthma and COPD, 630
  for respiratory acidosis, 20
  for respiratory distress in children, 908
  for SA in children, 914
oxyhemoglobin, 419
oxyiminoalkanoic acid, 577
oxytocin, 834

P

P selectin, 468
P waves, 74, 710, 713
P2Y inhibitors, 515, 516, 667t, 669–673, 675, 680t
PAC. *See* pulmonary arterial catheters
pacemakers, 712, 736
packed red blood cells (PRBCs), 432, 479–480, 867, 868–869
Paco$_2$, 6–8, 633
  DKA and, 16
  metabolic acidosis and, 15
  metabolic alkalosis and, 18
  respiratory acidosis and, 19–20
  respiratory alkalosis and, 21
PAD. *See* pain, agitation, and delirium
Paget disease, 91
PAH. *See* pulmonary arterial hypertension
PAI-1. *See* plasminogen activator inhibitor-1
pain
  with ACS, 662
  with aSAH, 437
  assessment of, 148–152, 149f
    for communicative patients, 148–149
    for noncommunicative patients, 149
  gate control theory of, 155–156
  hypertensive crisis and, 759
  with SCI, 398
pain characteristics in low back pain syndrome (PQRST), 662
pain, agitation, and delirium (PAD), 163
palivizumab, 335t, 342
pamidronate, 808–810, 811t
pancreas, 119–120, 121t
pancreatic cancer, 808
pancreatitis, 170, 171, 955–956
Pancreaze, 120
pancuronium, 202, 207
pantoprazole, 1004
papilledema, 759
paradoxical breathing, 629
paradoxical worsening, 338
parasympathetic nervous system, 710
parathyroid hormone (PTH), 80, 82, 88–89, 90
  HCM and, 808
parenteral nutrition (PN), 18, 32, 101–106, 104t, 114, 119–120
Parikh, AA, 871
Parkland formula, 845, 846t, 847t
paroxetine, 936t
paroxysmal supraventricular tachycardia (PSVT), 712–714, 715t–716t, 720f

paroxysmal sympathetic hyperactivity, 437–438
partial thromboplastin time (PTT), 470, 501, 904
parvovirus B19, 576
Patient Registry for Primary Pulmonary Hypertension, 610
Patients Hospitalized for Acute Decompensated Congestive Heart Failure (UNLOAD), 650
PBP2a transpeptidase, 294
PBPs. *See* penicillin-binding proteins
PCCs. *See* prothrombin complex concentrates
PCI. *See* percutaneous coronary intervention
PCR. *See* polymerase chain reaction
PCT. *See* procalcitonin
PCWP. *See* pulmonary capillary wedge pressure
PD. *See* pharmacodynamics
PDE-5. *See* phosphodiesterase type 5
PE. *See* pulmonary embolism
PEA. *See* pulseless electrical activity
peak expiratory flow rate (PEFR), 628, 629, 632, 633, 637, 913–914
pediatrics. *See* children
PEEP. *See* positive end-expiratory pressure
PEEPi. *See* intrinsic positive end-expiratory pressure
PEFR. *See* peak expiratory flow rate
penicillin, 744, 827t, 828
  extended-spectrum, 744
penicillin-binding proteins (PBPs), 291
Penn State equations, 106–107
pentobarbital, 377t, 380, 582, 911t
peptic ulcer disease, 591, 592, 593, 600–601
peptide nucleic acid fluorescence in situ hybridization (PNA-FISH), 245, 286
peramivir, 334t, 341
percutaneous coronary intervention (PCI), 673, 674, 675, 677, 680–681, 682
PERDS. *See* peri-engraftment respiratory distress syndrome
pericarditis, 229, 233, 710
peri-engraftment respiratory distress syndrome (PERDS), 992
peripheral line administration, 32–34
peripheral nerve stimulation/train-of-four (PNS/TOF), 206, 216
peripherally inserted central catheter (PICC), 623
peristalsis, 398
peritoneal dialysis, 117, 542, 730
peritonitis, 42
permanent AF, 714
permanent pacemaker devices (PPDs), 362
perphenazine, 172
persistent inflammation-immunosuppression catabolism syndrome (PICS), 879
persistent pulmonary hypertension (PPHN), 903
personal protective equipment (PPE), 344
Pertzye, 120
PGI$_2$. *See* prostaglandin I$_2$
P-glycoprotein, 672, 931–933, 934t
PH. *See* pulmonary hypertension
Pharmacist in Heart Failure Assessment Recommendation and Monitoring (PHARM), 657
pharmacodynamics (PD)
  in ADHF, 649
  of aminoglycosides, 271–272
  of antibacterials, 263–264
  of antibiotics, 827t

of antifungals, 265–266, 272–273
of antimicrobials, 252–275
  for burns, 853
  drug dosing of, 263–266
  goals for, 263, 264t
  limitations of, 274–275
  for sepsis and septic shock, 308
of antiprotozoal, 266
of antivirals, 266
basic principles of, 253–254
of clopidogrel, 671
DDIs and, 939–943
for drug dosing, 555
of fluoroquinolones, 272–273
of β-lactam antibiotics, prolonged and continuous infusions of, 267–270, 269t–270t
of linezolid, 271
pharmacogenomics and, 999–1008
with plasmapheresis, 558–559
of vancomycin, 270–271
pharmacoeconomics, 967, 967t
pharmacogenomics, 999–1008
  CYP polymorphisms and, 1000–1005
  HLA and, 1006–1007
  incorporating into patient care, 1008
  KCNH2 and, 1006
  N-acetyltransferase and, 1005
  PK and, 1000–1006
  SLCO1B1 genotype and, 1005–1006
  TNF-α and, 1007–1008
  VKOR and, 1006
Pharmacogenomics Knowledgebase, 1000
Pharmacogenomics Research Network, 1000
pharmacokinetics (PK)
  in ADHF, 649
  in ALF, 585, 588t
  of aminoglycosides, 271–272
  of antibacterials, 263–264
  of antifungals, 265–266, 272–273
  of antimicrobials, 244, 252–275
    alterations in critical illness, 254, 255t, 259t
    of antimicrobials, changes in drug absorption, 254
    for burns, 853
    drug clearance for, 256–260
    drug dosing of, 261–263
    half-life of, 261
    limitations of, 274–275
    protein binding and, 260–261
    for sepsis and septic shock, 308
    Vss for, 255–256
  of antiprotozoal, 266
  of antivirals, 266
  of cefazolin, 35
  for chronic kidney disease, 543–553
  CYP polymorphisms and, 1000–1005, 1002t, 1003t
  of DDIs, 931
  for drug dosing, 553–554
  ECMO and, 559–560, 562f, 563t, 742, 742f
  of fluoroquinolones, 272–273
  of linezolid, 271
  of MCS, 741f
  of NMBAs, 207
  obesity and, 823
  pharmacogenomics and, 1000–1006
  for SCA, 692
  underweight patients and, 830
  of vancomycin, 270–271

1038

pharmacy services management, 960–970
  hospital and, 962
  justification for, 964–965
  leadership in, 962–963, 964t
  medication costs and, 962
  optimization of, 966t
  personnel management in, 967–969
  pharmacoeconomics in, 967, 967t
  privileging in, 967–969, 969t
  strategic planning in, 963–964, 965t
phencyclidine, 172, 936t
phenelzine, 215
phenobarbital, 172, 347, 376t, 378, 936t, 989t
phenoxybenzamine, 799
phentolamine, 763t, 767, 799
phenylalkylamines, 761
phenylephrine, 101, 230, 258, 313
  for aSAH, 427, 432, 433
  for HSV, 333
  for PAH, 620
  for SCA, 695
phenylpropanolamine, 613
phenytoin, 38, 551t, 583, 989t
  ALF from, 577
  for aSAH, 427
  CYP and, 936t, 939t, 940t, 991, 1003–1004
  DDIs with, 935
  drug-nutrient interactions with, 945t
  for SE, 376t, 378–379
  therapeutic plasma exchange and, 835
  thrombocytopenia and, 478t
pheochromocytoma, 768t, 773–774, 797–800
phosphate, 82, 83, 84t–87t, 87, 995
phosphodiesterase type 5 (PDE-5), 610, 775
  inhibitors of, 618, 619–620
phosphorus, 82–88, 82f, 993–994.
    See also hyperphosphatemia;
    hypophosphatemia
Physician Quality Reporting System (PQRS), 351–352
PI. See pulsatility index
PICC. See peripherally inserted central catheter
PICS. See persistent inflammation-immunosuppression catabolism syndrome
PiCT. See prothrombinase-induced clotting time
piperacillin, 551t
piperacillin/tazobactam, 262–263, 268, 985t
pirbuterol, 631
pituitary adenoma, 801
PJP. See Pneumocystis jiroveci pneumonia
PK. See pharmacokinetics
Plan-Do-Check-Act, 961
plasma. See also fresh frozen plasma
  therapeutic plasma exchange, drug dosing and, 834–835
plasma concentration (Cp), 554
plasma concentration at steady state (Cpss), 554
Plasma-Lyte, 16, 18, 22, 866–867
plasmapheresis, 556–557, 556t, 558–559
plasminogen activator inhibitor-1 (PAI-1), 407, 611
Platelet Glycoprotein IIb-IIIa in Unstable Angina: Receptor Suppression Using Integrilin Therapy (PURSUIT), 661t, 662
Platelet Inhibition and Patient Outcomes (PLATO), 672, 673, 678, 680
platelet reactivity tests, 516–517

Platelet Receptor Inhibition in Ischemic Syndrome Management in Patients Limited by Unstable Signs and Symptoms (PRISM-PLUS), 678
platelet-derived growth factor, 611
platelets
  ALF and, 575
  for cirrhosis, 492
  enhancing function of, 485
  function measurement of, 471
  mapping of, TEG for, 515
  MCS and, 745
  in MTP, 869
  optimization of, 485
  thrombocytopenia and, 476
  transfusions of, 596, 598
PLATO. See Platelet Inhibition and Patient Outcomes
Plavix. See clopidogrel
PN. See parenteral nutrition
PNA-FISH. See peptide nucleic acid fluorescence in situ hybridization
Pneumocystis jiroveci, HIV and, 338
Pneumocystis jiroveci pneumonia (PJP), 990–991
pneumomediastinum, 629
pneumonia. See also ventilator-associated pneumonia
  aSAH and, 437
  asthma and COPD and, 628
  from Candida, 320
  as donor-derived infection, 987
  HAP, 244, 295
  HCAP, 242
  HSV and, 339
  from inhalation injury, 849
  PERDS and, 992
  PJP, 990–991
  SCI and, 398
  scoring systems for, 956
  from VZV, 337
Pneumonia Severity Index (PSI), 956
pneumothorax, 629
  tension, 229, 233, 693t
PNS/TOF. See peripheral nerve stimulation/train-of-four
POCT. See point-of-care testing
point-of-care testing (POCT), 135–136, 140
POISE-2, 533
polycystic kidney disease, 417
polymerase chain reaction (PCR), 284–285, 291, 335, 339, 344
  for Dengue fever, 346
  for HSV, 333
  for PJP, 990
  for VZV, 337
polyvinyl chloride (PVC), 742
portal hypertension, 575, 613
posaconazole, 258, 319, 326, 931, 986, 989t
positive end-expiratory pressure (PEEP), 258
positive predictive value (PPV), 285
posterior reversible leukoencephalopathy syndrome (PRES), 995–996
postpartum hemorrhage (PPH), 494, 834
postrenal AKI, 526
potassium, 17, 18, 69–79. See also hyperkalemia; hypokalemia
  supplementation of, 74f
  TdP and, 728, 730
  TLS and, 804, 995
potassium chloride, 49, 72
PPDs. See permanent pacemaker devices
PPE. See personal protective equipment

PPH. See postpartum hemorrhage
PPHN. See persistent pulmonary hypertension
PPIs. See proton pump inhibitors
PPV. See positive predictive value
PQRS. See Physician Quality Reporting System
PQRST. See pain characteristics in low back pain syndrome
PR interval, 74, 80, 710
Pragmatic Randomized Optimal Platelet and Plasma Ratios (PROPPR), 491
prasugrel, 475t, 667t, 669–673, 936t, 937t
PRBCs. See packed red blood cells
PREDICT-1. See Prospective Randomized Evaluation of DNA Screening in a Clinical Trial
prednisone, 557t, 634, 796t, 811t, 992
pregnancy
  aortic dissection and, 774
  asthma in, 634
  drug dosing in, 830–834, 831t
  hemorrhage in, 494
  hypertensive crisis in, 767–769, 768t, 770f
  SE in, 384
  VTE and, 450
prekallikrein, 471
PRES. See posterior reversible leukoencephalopathy syndrome
Present Pain Index, 148
preventable ADE, 972, 972t
Primacore. See milrinone
priming thrombin, 469–471
PRIS. See propofol-related infusion syndrome
PRISM-PLUS. See Platelet Receptor Inhibition in Ischemic Syndrome Management in Patients Limited by Unstable Signs and Symptoms
privileging, in pharmacy services management, 967–969, 969t
PROACT II. See Prolyse in Acute Cerebral Thromboembolism II
probiotics, 116
procainamide, 715t, 719, 723f, 725, 727t, 1005
procaine, 215
procalcitonin (PCT), 246–247, 291, 299–300, 308–309, 310f
procedural pain, 156–157
ProCESS. See Protocolized Care for Early Septic Shock
prochlorperazine, 172
progesterone, 394, 399
Progesterone for the Treatment of Traumatic Brain Injury (ProTECT), 394
progressive multifocal leukoencephalopathy, 338
prokinetics, 192t
Prolyse in Acute Cerebral Thromboembolism II (PROACT II), 408
ProMISe. See Protocolised Management in Sepsis
PROMMTT. See Prospective, Observational, Multicenter, Major Trauma Transfusion
propafenone, 710, 719, 722, 723, 723f, 989t
propofol, 162, 169–170, 192t, 782
  bradycardia from, 710
  CYP and, 936t
  for endotracheal intubation in children, 911t
  pregnancy and, 833
  for SE, 377t, 379–380

1039

propofol-related infusion syndrome (PRIS), 170
PROPPR. *See* Pragmatic Randomized Optimal Platelet and Plasma Ratios
propranolol, 557t, 796t, 852
propylene glycol, 14, 169, 375
propylthiouracil, 577, 796t
Prospective, Observational, Multicenter, Major Trauma Transfusion (PROMMTT), 491
Prospective Randomized Evaluation of DNA Screening in a Clinical Trial (PREDICT-1), 1006
prostacyclin, 610, 620, 666
prostaglandin E, 117
prostaglandin I_2 (PGI_2), 610, 615
prostate cancer, 811, 814
protease inhibitors, 939t
ProTECT. *See* Progesterone for the Treatment of Traumatic Brain Injury
protein binding, 258, 543, 546, 552
    ALF and, 587
    antimicrobials and, 260–261
    DDIs and, 933–935
    ECMO and, 560, 742
    plasmapheresis and, 557
protein C, 315, 490
proteins
    burns and, 122
    stress response and, 99
proteinuria, 759
prothrombin, 468, 1006
prothrombin complex concentrates (PCCs), 233, 233t, 483–484, 495
    for GI bleeding, 596–597, 598
    in MTP, 869
    VKA and, 411–412
    warfarin and, 461
prothrombin time (PT), 470, 472, 500, 502–503, 502t
    for ALF, 578
    for apixaban, 509f
prothrombinase-induced clotting time (PiCT), 511
Protocolised Management in Sepsis (ProMISe), 48, 304
Protocolized Care for Early Septic Shock (ProCESS), 48
proton pump inhibitors (PPIs), 593, 594–595, 670
    CYP and, 602, 936t, 1004
    DDIs with, 931, 932t
    for GI bleeding, 598
        rebleeding with, 600
    for SRMD in children, 921
pseudoephedrine, 397
Pseudomonas aeruginosa, 247, 267, 293–294, 308, 362, 638
PSI. *See* Pneumonia Severity Index
PSVT. *See* paroxysmal supraventricular tachycardia
psychotropics, 577
PT. *See* prothrombin time
PTH. *See* parathyroid hormone
PTT. *See* partial thromboplastin time
Puhringer, FK, 217
pulmonary arterial catheters (PAC, Swan-Ganz catheter), 227–228, 615, 646, 647
pulmonary arterial hypertension (PAH), 609–623
    diagnosis of, 613–614
    epidemiology of, 610

monitoring of, 620, 621t
obstructive shock and, 233
pathophysiology of, 610–612, 611f
treatment for, 614–620, 620f
vasodilators for, 622
WHO and, 612, 613t
pulmonary capillary wedge pressure (PCWP), 227–228, 646, 649, 652
pulmonary edema, 436, 617, 619, 758, 759, 992
pulmonary embolism (PE), 229, 233–234, 449, 461
    fibrinolysis for, 234
    hypertensive crisis and, 769t, 777
    MCS for, 737t
    SCA and, 693t, 700
pulmonary function tests, 614, 632
pulmonary hypertension (PH), 16, 610, 612–613, 612t, 737t. *See also* pulmonary arterial hypertension
pulmonary vascular resistance (PVR), 611
pulsatility index (PI), 656
pulse oximetry, 863, 914
pulseless electrical activity (PEA), 688, 689, 690, 700, 701–702
pulseless ventricular tachycardia (PVT), 689, 690, 693–701
pulsus paradoxus, 628–629
PURSUIT. *See* Platelet Glycoprotein IIb-IIIa in Unstable Angina: Receptor Suppression Using Integrilin Therapy
PVC. *See* polyvinyl chloride
PVR. *See* pulmonary vascular resistance
PVT. *See* pulseless ventricular tachycardia
pyrazinamide, 577
pyridostigmine, 216
pyrimethamine, 991
pyruvate, 14
pyruvate dehydrogenase, 301

Q

QRS complex, 74, 80, 710, 721, 776, 804
QT interval, 173, 726, 785, 941, 943t
QTc. *See* corrected QT interval
Quadrox D oxygenator, 742
quetiapine, 577
QuickFISH, 286
quinidine, 215, 936t, 989t
quinine, 551t
quinolones, 192t

R

RAAS. *See* renin-angiotensin-aldosterone system
rabies, 332t, 346–347
radiation enteritis, 79
radiation therapy
    for MSCC, 815
    for SVC, 814
radiographic contrast media, 526, 531t, 533
Ralib, AM, 523
Ramsay sedation scale, 164, 164t
randomized controlled trials (RCTs)
    for fluid resuscitation, 30, 37–40, 42, 45, 49
    for glucose management, 131t, 134–136
    for HSV, 333
    for NMBAs, 206–207

Randomized Evaluation of Mechanical Assistance for the Treatment of Congestive Heart Failure (REMATCH), 361
ranitidine, 162, 593, 601t
RANK. *See* receptor activator of nuclear factor-κB
RANKL. *See* receptor activator of nuclear factor-κB ligand
Ranson criteria, for pancreatitis, 955
rapeseed oil, 613
rapid sequence intubation (RSI)
    ketamine for, 633
    NMBAs and, 213–214
    for trauma, 863
RAS. *See* reticular activating system
rasburicase, 806–807, 806t, 995
RASS. *See* Richmond Agitation-Sedation Scale
ratio of maximum serum drug concentration to MIC (C_{max}/MIC), 253, 262, 266, 271–272, 273
ratio of the 24-hour area under the serum concentration versus time curve to pathogen MIC (AUC_{0-24}/MIC), 253, 262, 266, 270–271
RBCs. *See* red blood cells
RCTs. *See* randomized controlled trials
RDA. *See* recommended dietary allowance
real-time PCR, 284–285
rebleeding
    aSAH and, 417, 421, 425–426
    with GI bleeding, 599t, 600–601
receiver operating characteristic (ROC), 952
receptor activator of nuclear factor-κB (RANK), 810
receptor activator of nuclear factor-κB ligand (RANKL), 810
recombinant activated factor VIIa (rFVIIa), 233, 458, 482t, 484, 492
    for ALF, 583
    for cirrhosis, 492–493
    in MTP, 869
    for PPH, 494, 834
recombinant human activated protein C, 315
recombinant human growth hormone (rhGH), 851, 852
recommended dietary allowance (RDA)
    with EN, 110
    for potassium, 70
red blood cells (RBCs), 69, 485
    for anemia, 479–480
    for hemorrhagic shock, 867
    for PPH, 494
    PRBCs, 432, 479–480, 867, 868–869
REDOXs trials, 114
REE. *See* resting energy expenditure
refeeding syndrome, 83
refractory hypotension, 30
refractory seizures, 172
refractory status epilepticus (RSE), 371, 377t, 379–381, 383f
Registry to Evaluate Early- and Long-term Pulmonary Arterial Hypertension Disease Management (REVEAL), 610
Rehm, M, 17
Reinelt, P, 722
Reiter syndrome, 710
REMATCH. *See* Randomized Evaluation of Mechanical Assistance for the Treatment of Congestive Heart Failure

remifentanil, 150, 151t, 167t, 168
Remodulin. See treprostinil
REMS. See Risk Evaluation and Mitigation Strategies
renal cell carcinoma, 808, 814
renal failure, 81, 575
   AF and, 716
   electrical injuries and, 856
   hypertensive crisis and, 759
   metabolic acidosis and, 15
   from NSAIDs, 154
   from septic shock, 259
   from severe sepsis, 259
   SRMD and, 593
renal insufficiency, 808
Renal Optimization Strategies Evaluation (ROSE), 650
renal replacement therapy (RRT)
   advantages and disadvantages of, 542
   for AKI, 523, 524, 529, 530, 538–564
   drug clearance with, 543–548
   ECMO and, 564
   for metabolic acidosis, 16
   outcomes of, 539
   for rhabdomyolysis, 884
   for TLS, 807
   types of, 540–543
   typical conditions in, 541t
renal system. See also kidney
   anticoagulants and, 463
   DDIs and, 937–939
   nutrition and, 116–117
   opioids and, 152
renal tubular acidosis (RTA), 12–13
renin-angiotensin-aldosterone system (RAAS), 231, 524, 758, 764
   ACS and, 775, 776
reptilase time, 512
respiratory acidosis, 19–21, 20t, 339t, 628, 629, 634
respiratory alkalosis, 21
respiratory failure, 162, 342, 575, 716, 743
respiratory quotient (RQ), 117
respiratory syncytial virus (RSV), 339, 341–342, 638, 896, 908
respiratory system. See also lung
   acid-base disorders and, 4
   metabolic acidosis and, 15
   nutrition and, 117–118
   viral infections, 339–343
respiratory tract infections, 716
resting energy expenditure (REE), 843, 851
Resuscitation Outcomes Consortium (ROC), 33
reteplase, 455t
reticular activating system (RAS), 333
retinal hemorrhages, 759, 918
retinitis, 336, 338
retinopathy, 759
return of spontaneous circulation (ROSC), 690, 695
Revatio. See sildenafil
REVEAL. See Registry to Evaluate Early- and Long-term Pulmonary Arterial Hypertension Disease Management
Revised Trauma Score, 954
rFVIIa. See recombinant activated factor VIIa
rhabdomyolysis, 88, 204, 207, 856, 884
RHC. See right heart catheterization
rheumatic fever, 710
rheumatoid arthritis, 710
rhGH. See recombinant human growth hormone

rhinovirus, 638
ribavirin, 334t, 342, 344
ribosomal RNA (rRNA), 286
Richmond Agitation-Sedation Scale (RASS), 163, 165, 165t, 784
rifampin, 577, 587t, 989t
   CYP and, 936t, 939t
   P-glycoprotein and, 934t
   thrombocytopenia and, 478t
rifaximin, 581–582
RIFLE. See risk, injury, failure, loss of kidney function, and end-stage kidney disease
right heart catheterization (RHC), 610, 614
right ventricle (RV)
   ADHF and, 654
   afterload, PVR and, 611
   PAH and, 610, 619
Ringer, Sydney, 35
riociguat, 619
risk, injury, failure, loss of kidney function, and end-stage kidney disease (RIFLE), 34, 526–527, 527t, 954–955, 954t
Risk Evaluation and Mitigation Strategies (REMS), 782
risperidone, 1002
ritonavir, 937t
rituximab, 557t, 657
rivaroxaban, 451t, 452t, 454t, 463t, 475t, 495
   anti-Xa for, 509f
   for GI bleeding, 596, 597, 597t, 598
   P-glycoprotein and, 934t
Rivers, E, 304–305, 904–905
ROC. See receiver operating characteristic; Resuscitation Outcomes Consortium
Rockall score, for rebleeding, 600, 600t
rocuronium, 202, 912t
Rodrigo, G, 633
ROSC. See return of spontaneous circulation
ROSE. See Renal Optimization Strategies Evaluation
Rosenberg, RS, 338
rosuvastatin, 936t
rotational TEG (ROTEG), 492, 513–515
Rotondo, MF, 879
Royal Dutch Pharmacists Association, 1000
RQ. See respiratory quotient
rRNA. See ribosomal RNA
RRT. See renal replacement therapy
RSE. See refractory status epilepticus
RSI. See rapid sequence intubation
RSV. See respiratory syncytial virus
RTA. See renal tubular acidosis
Rumack-Matthew nomogram, 580, 580f
RV. See right ventricle

S

SA. See status asthmaticus
SABA. See short-acting β-agonist
SAFE. See Saline versus Albumin Fluid Evaluation
salbutamol, 637
salicylate, 15, 776, 935
Saline versus Albumin Fluid Evaluation (SAFE), 40, 41, 529, 866
SAPS. See Simplified Acute Physiology Score
saquinavir, 937t
sarcoidosis, 710
sarcoma, 814
SARS. See severe acute respiratory syndrome

SAS. See sedation-agitation scale
SBE. See standard base excess
SBP. See spontaneous bacterial peritonitis; systolic blood pressure
SBS. See short bowel syndrome
SCA. See sudden cardiac arrest
SCCM. See Society of Critical Care Medicine
scedosporiosis, 326
schistosomiasis, 613
SCI. See spinal cord injury
SCIP. See Surgical Care Improvement Project
scleroderma, 710
SCr. See serum creatinine
SCUF. See slow continuous ultrafiltration
Scvo$_2$. See central venous oxygen saturation
SE. See status epilepticus
sedation-agitation scale (SAS), 164–165, 164t
sedatives, 162, 163–166, 170–173, 171t, 437
   delirium and, 173–174, 192t
   interruption of, 175
   for morbid obesity, 825
   for nicotine withdrawal, 784
   NMBAs and, 206
   in pregnancy, 833
   for respiratory alkalosis, 21
   strategies for, 174–175
   traditional, 168–170, 169t
   withdrawal from, 173
seizures. See also status epilepticus
   AIS and, 410
   aSAH and, 426–427
   hypernatremia and, 68
   hypertensive crisis and, 759
   hypomagnesemia and, 80
   hyponatremia and, 59
   ICH and, 413, 583
   refractory, 172
   SVC and, 814
   TBI and, 394–395, 920–921
selective serotonin reuptake inhibitors (SSRIs), 593, 613, 783–784, 783t, 931, 940
selenium, 113–114, 115, 122
self-extubation, 163
sepsis. See also severe sepsis; systemic inflammatory response syndrome
   AF and, 714
   agitation and, 162
   AKI and, 525
   albumin for, 44–45
   antioxidants and, 115
   arginine and, 115
   burns and, 852–853
   in children, 900–907, 901t
   CYP and, 938t
   delirium and, 191
   glucose and, 133
   MCS and, 745
   metabolic acidosis and, 16
   mixed acid-base disorders and, 21
   NMBAs for, 206, 209t–211t, 213
   PCT for, 299–300
   procalcitonin for, 247
   SRMD and, 593
   TNF-α and, 1007–1008
   underweight patients with, 830
septic arthritis, 987
septic shock, 234, 298–316
   AF and, 714
   antibiotic de-escalation for, 246
   antimicrobials for, 241–242, 307–309
   burns and, 852–853
   in children, 899, 900–907, 901t

crystalloids and colloids for, 41
diagnosis of, 299–301
fluid resuscitation for, 45–46, 300–307
host response in, 302f
management bundle for, 306–307
PAH and, 621
pathophysiology of, 299
PCT for, 299–300, 308–309, 310f
procalcitonin for, 247
renal failure from, 259
supportive therapies for, 315
tissue perfusion impairment in, 303f
treatment pathways for, 315
underweight patients with, 830
Sequential Organ Failure Assessment (SOFA), 100, 114, 244, 246, 845, 953
SERAPHIN. See Study with an Endothelin Receptor Antagonist in Pulmonary Arterial Hypertension to Improve Clinical Outcome
serotonergics, 162
serotonin, 776
serotonin and norepinephrine reuptake inhibitors (SNRIs), 783–784, 783t, 940
serotonin syndrome, 939–941
sertraline, 1004
serum bicarbonate, 4
serum creatinine (SCr), 4, 526, 528, 576, 759
severe acute respiratory syndrome (SARS), 342, 343t
severe sepsis, 298–316
  AF and, 714, 716, 717
  antibiotic de-escalation for, 246
  antimicrobials for, 241–242, 307–309
  ARDS and, 902
  burns and, 852–853
  in children, 900–903, 901t
  crystalloids and colloids for, 41
  diagnosis of, 299–301
  fluid resuscitation for, 300–307
  host response in, 302f
  management bundle for, 306–307
  pathophysiology of, 299
  PCT for, 299–300, 308–309, 310f
  procalcitonin for, 247
  renal failure from, 259
  supportive therapies for, 315
  tissue perfusion impairment in, 303f
  treatment pathways for, 315
severely symptomatic hyponatremia, 62–64
sexually transmitted infections (STIs), 338
SGA. See subjective global assessment
sGC. See soluble guanylate cyclase
shaken baby syndrome, 916
SHEA. See Society for Healthcare Epidemiology of America
Shekar, K, 560
shock, 225–235. See also specific types
  albumin for, 310–312
  assessment of, 46
  catecholamines for, 229–230, 313–314
  in children, 896, 899
  colloids for, 310–312
  crystalloids for, 309–310
  CVC for, 226–227
  differentiation of states of, 229–232
  dopamine and, 230
  epinephrine for, 230
  fluid resuscitation for, 30, 229, 309–312
  hemodynamic markers and perfusion for, 226–229, 227t
  influenza and, 340

inotropes for, 229–230
intra-arterial catheters for, 226
metabolic acidosis and, 16
mixed acid-base disorders and, 21
norepinephrine for, 230
PAC for, 227–228
phenylephrine for, 230
vasopressors for, 229–230, 231f, 313–314
shock liver, 576
short bowel syndrome (SBS), 880–881, 882t, 883t
short-acting β-agonist (SABA), 628, 631–632, 634, 637, 639
shortness of breath, 717, 759, 797
SIADH. See syndrome of inappropriate antidiuretic hormone
sick sinus syndrome, 709–710, 712
sickle cell disease, 417
SICU. See surgical intensive care unit
SID. See strong ion difference
SIG. See strong ion gap
sildenafil (Revatio, Viagra), 618, 621, 989t
Silverman, RA, 632–633
Simplified Acute Physiology Score (SAPS), 953
simvastatin, 106, 430, 577, 672
Simvastatin in Aneurysmal Subarachnoid Hemorrhage (STASH), 430
single nucleotide polymorphisms (SNPs), 1000, 1006
sinus bradycardia, 708, 708f
sinusitis, 618
sirolimus, 587t, 937t
SIRS. See systemic inflammatory response syndrome
skin
  infections of, testing for, 291
  normal structure and function of, 843
SLCO1B1 genotype, 1005–1006
SLCO1B1 genotype and, 1005–1006
SLEAP study, 191
SLED. See sustained low-efficiency hemodialysis
sleep apnea, 710
slow continuous ultrafiltration (SCUF), 539, 542, 543f
small cell lung cancer, 805
smoking. See also nicotine
  aSAH and, 428
  asthma and, 627
  COPD and, 628
SNPs. See single nucleotide polymorphisms
SNRIs. See serotonin and norepinephrine reuptake inhibitors
Society for Healthcare Epidemiology of America (SHEA), 362, 363
Society of Critical Care Medicine (SCCM), 101, 103, 437, 960
  arginine and, 115
  delirium and, 193, 194, 196
  glutamine and, 114
  PAD and, 163
  on pain assessment, 148
  probiotics and, 116
  TBI in children and, 919
Society of Thoracic Surgeons (STS), 131–132
sodium. See hypernatremia; hyponatremia
sodium acetate, 18
sodium bicarbonate, 16–17, 18, 700–701, 702, 805–806, 884
sodium chloride, 34, 49, 63–65, 66, 617, 884
sodium homeostasis, 58–59
sodium iodide, 796t

sodium nitrite, 850, 852t
sodium nitroprusside. See nitroprusside
sodium oxybate (Xyrem), 782
sodium thiosulfate, 850, 852t
sodium-potassium-chloride cotransporter (NKCC), 18
SOFA. See Sequential Organ Failure Assessment
soluble guanylate cyclase (sGC), 610, 619
somatostatin, 598, 880, 880t, 882t
somnolence, 81
Sort, P, 42
sotalol, 710, 727t, 730
spinal cord injury (SCI), 395–399
  blood pressure and, 397
  epidemiology and pathophysiology of, 395–396
  management of, 396–398, 397t
  MV for, 396–397
  neuroprotective therapy for, 398–399
  NMBAs and, 217
  succinylcholine and, 207
  thermoregulation for, 397–398
  VTE and, 398
splenomegaly, 476
spontaneous bacterial peritonitis (SBP), 357
SRMD. See stress-related mucosal disease
SSC. See Surviving Sepsis Campaign
SSIs. See surgical site infections
SSRIs. See selective serotonin reuptake inhibitors
St. John's wort, 613
standard base excess (SBE), 4, 7, 10
Staphylococcus aureus. See also methicillin-resistant Staphylococcus aureus; methicillin-susceptible Staphylococcus aureus
  CIEDs and, 362
  COPD and, 628
  influenza and, 351
  nasal packing and, 364
  neurosurgical infections and, 362
  PAC and, 615
  SSIs from, 352
Staphylococcus epidermidis, 352
Staphylococcus spp., 286, 583
Starling, EH, 36
STASH. See Simvastatin in Aneurysmal Subarachnoid Hemorrhage
statins
  ALF from, 577
  antiretrovirals and, 989t
  for aSAH, 430
  SLCO1B1 genotype and, 1005–1006
status asthmaticus (SA), 208, 913–916, 913t
status epilepticus (SE), 371–385, 373t
  children with, 383
  diagnosis of, 373–374
  EEG for, 382–383
  emergent treatment for, 375, 376t
  epidemiology of, 371–372
  etiology of, 372–373, 372t
  genetics and, 385
  HSV and, 333
  kidney failure and, 384–385
  laboratory testing for, 382–383
  liver failure and, 384–385
  obesity and, 384
  pathophysiology of, 373
  in pregnancy, 384
  prophylaxis for, 374
  RSE, 371, 377t, 379–381, 383f
  treatment for, 374–382, 376t–377t, 382t

urgent treatment for, 375–379, 376t
stavudine, 577
STEMI. *See* ST-segment elevation myocardial infarction
STEMI Treated with Primary Angioplasty and Intravenous Lovenox or Unfractionated Heparin (ATOLL), 681
steroids, 450
    for DAC, 993
    for PERDS, 992
    for PJP, 991
    for TBI, 394
Stevens-Johnson syndrome, 171, 990
Stewart model, for acid-base disorders, 7–10
STIs. *See* sexually transmitted infections
Streptococcus pneumoniae, 291, 351, 638
Streptococcus pyogenes, 351
Streptococcus spp., 583
stress response, 99
stress ulcers, 594–595
stress-related mucosal disease (SRMD), 592, 593, 921
stroke, 403–413. *See also* acute ischemic stroke
    AF and, 716
    assessment of, 405t
    BCVIs and, 870
    classification, risk factors, and diagnosis for, 404
    clinical presentation of, 505
    epidemiology of, 403–404
    fluid resuscitation for, 409
    glucose and, 409
    hemorrhagic, 410–413
    hypertensive crisis and, 768t
    hypoglycemia and, 409
    hypomagnesemia and, 80–81
    hypovolemia and, 409
    NMBAs and, 217
    pathophysiology of, 404
    TIA, 403–410
    TPA for, 404–407
    treatment of, 404–409
stroke volume, 312
strong ion difference (SID), 7–10, 14, 16
    intravenous fluids and, 21–22
    metabolic alkalosis and, 18, 19
    respiratory acidosis and, 20
    THAM and, 17
strong ion gap (SIG), 4, 8, 14, 15, 17
strong ions, 5
STS. *See* Society of Thoracic Surgeons
ST-segment depression, 70
ST-segment elevation myocardial infarction (STEMI), 664, 670, 678–682, 679f, 692, 776
Study of the Neuroprotective Activity of Progesterone in Severe Traumatic Brain Injuries (SYNAPSE), 394
Study with an Endothelin Receptor Antagonist in Pulmonary Arterial Hypertension to Improve Clinical Outcome (SERAPHIN), 617–618
subarachnoid hemorrhage. *See* aneurysmal subarachnoid hemorrhage
subarachnoid spaces, 431
subdural grids, 363
subjective global assessment (SGA), 100–101
substance abuse
    agitation and, 162
    ALF from, 577
    frostbite and, 856
substance P, 764

succinylcholine, 202, 203, 207, 217–218, 912t
sucralfate, 594
sudden cardiac arrest (SCA), 688–703
    ACLS for, 691–692
    algorithm for, 694f
    antiarrhythmics for, 699–700
    asystole and, 690, 701–702
    basic life support for, 691
    causes and interventions for, 693t
    CPR for, 688, 690–691, 693–695, 697–699
    drug administration in, 692
    ECG for, 702
    epidemiology of, 689, 689t
    etiology and clinical presentation of, 689–690
    evidence-based recommendations for, 696t
    general management of, 690–692
    magnesium for, 700
    nonpharmacologic therapy for, 701
    PEA and, 688, 701–702
    PVT and, 689, 690, 693–701
    sodium bicarbonate for, 700–701
    TH for, 702–703
    thrombolysis for, 700
    vasopressin for, 692, 697–699, 698t
    vasopressors for, 695–697
    VF and, 688, 690, 693–701
sudden cardiac death (SCD). *See* sudden cardiac arrest
sulfadiazine, 991
sulfamethoxazole/trimethoprim. *See* trimethoprim/sulfamethoxazole
sulfonamides, 526, 531t, 532
superior vena cava syndrome (SVC), 813–814
Superior Yield of the New Strategy of Enoxaparin, Revascularization and Glycoprotein IIb/IIIa Inhibitors (SYNERGY), 677
superoxide dismutase, 115
support stockings, 451
supraventricular arrhythmias, 708–721
supraventricular tachyarrhythmias, 595
Surgical Care Improvement Project (SCIP), 131–132, 351
surgical intensive care unit (SICU), 129
surgical site infections (SSIs), 351
    antimicrobial prophylaxis for, 353–357, 354t–355t
    neurosurgical infections and, 362
    risks for, 356–357
Surviving Sepsis Campaign (SSC), 133, 242, 299, 300, 301t, 315
    on catecholamines, 312–313
    management bundle of, 306–307
    underweight patients and, 830
sustained low-efficiency hemodialysis (SLED), 539, 541–542
SVC. *See* superior vena cava syndrome
SVO_2. *See* venous oxygen saturation
SVR. *See* systemic vascular resistance
Swan-Ganz catheters. *See* pulmonary arterial catheters
sympathetic nervous system, 99, 420
sympathomimetics, 759
SYNAPSE. *See* Study of the Neuroprotective Activity of Progesterone in Severe Traumatic Brain Injuries
syncope
    AF and, 717
    bradycardia and, 672
    respiratory alkalosis and, 21

syndrome of inappropriate antidiuretic hormone (SIADH), 60, 66, 67, 810–813, 813t
SYNERGY. *See* Superior Yield of the New Strategy of Enoxaparin, Revascularization and Glycoprotein IIb/IIIa Inhibitors
systemic inflammatory response syndrome (SIRS), 247, 562, 575
    burns and, 852–853
    in children, 900–903, 901t
systemic lupus erythematosus, 710
systemic vascular resistance (SVR), 227, 231, 902
systolic blood pressure (SBP)
    aSAH and, 417, 431
    cirrhosis and, 357, 358t
    hypertensive crisis and, 757, 759
    IABP for, 736
    iloprost and, 617
    sepsis and, 301
    severe sepsis and septic shock and, 305
    shock and, 225, 226
    VT and, 723

T

T cell-mediated immune response, 335, 337–338
T waves, 70, 74, 80
T3. *See* triiodothyronine
T4. *See* thyroxine
tachycardia
    AT, 712–714
    aSAH and, 420
    AVRT, 712–714
    cocaine and, 776
    COPD and, 629
    DKA and, 15
    GI bleeding and, 595
    malignant hyperthermia and, 204
    nitroglycerin and, 765
    PSVT, 712–714, 715t–716t, 720f
    PVT, 689, 690, 693–701
    SIRS and, 900
    VT, 70, 689, 721–725, 727f, 728f
tachyphylaxis, 764
tachypnea, 420, 628, 629, 900
TACO. *See* transfusion-associated cardiac overload
tacrolimus, 557t, 937t, 939t, 945t, 1004–1005
TAH. *See* total artificial heart
takotsubo cardiomyopathy, 420
TandemHeart, 655, 655t, 737, 746t
TARGET. *See* Treatment Approaches in Renal Cancer Global Evaluation Trial
Targeted Platelet Inhibition to Clarify the Optimal Strategy to Medically Manage Acute Coronary Syndromes (TRILOGY-ACS), 678
target-specific oral anticoagulants (TOACs), 942, 944t
tazobactam, 551t
TBI. *See* traumatic brain injury
TBSA. *See* total body surface area
TBW. *See* total body water; total body weight
TCD. *See* transcranial Doppler
TDM. *See* therapeutic drug monitoring
TdP. *See* torsades de pointes
TE. *See* thromboembolism; *Toxoplasma* encephalitis

tedizolid, 294
teduglutide, 881, 883t
TEE. *See* transesophageal echocardiogram
TEG. *See* thromboelastography
telavancin, 294
temazepam, 587
tenecteplase, 407, 455t, 475t
tension pneumothorax, 229, 233, 693t
terbinafine, 326, 577
terbutaline, 632, 815
terlipressin, 598
Terumo Cardiovascular Systems, 560
Terumo X Coating, 560
tetracycline, 601t, 831, 832, 932t, 933, 946t
TH. *See* therapeutic hypothermia
THAM. *See* tris-hydroxymethyl aminomethane; tromethamine
theophylline, 633, 657
therapeutic drug monitoring (TDM)
    for aminoglycosides, 263
    for antifungals, 273–274
    for antimicrobials, 245
    for β-lactam antibiotics, 262
    for tacrolimus, 1005
    for vancomycin, 263
therapeutic hypothermia (TH), 381, 399, 472, 702–703
Therapeutic Intervention Scoring System (TISS), 954
therapeutic plasma exchange, drug dosing and, 834–835
thermoregulation
    for AIS, 409
    for aSAH, 436–437
    for ICH, 413
    for SCI, 397–398
thermoslim, 577
thiazide diuretics, 18, 72, 649, 649t, 808
thienopyridine (Effient), 671, 680t
thiocyanate, 765
thiopentone, 561
thiosulfate, 765
thrombin generation assays, 511–512
thrombin time (TT), 509
thrombocytopenia, 474–476, 477t, 478t. *See also* heparin-induced thrombocytopenia
    ADEs and, 975–976, 976t
    coronavirus and, 342
    Dengue fever and, 346
    hypertensive crisis and, 759
    IABP and, 655
    valproic acid and, 171
thromboelastography (TEG), 489t, 490f, 492, 512–515, 513t, 514f, 516t
thromboembolism (TE), 449, 455, 619, 717
Thrombolysis in Myocardial Infarction (TIMI), 661–662, 661t, 681, 826
thrombolytics, 20, 431, 455t, 692, 700
thrombophlebitis, 32
thrombosis. *See also* deep venous thrombosis; venous thromboembolism
    in children, 921
    MCS and, 747, 747f, 749f, 750
    SVC and, 814
thromboxane A_2 (TXA$_2$), 611, 661, 666, 668
thyroid disorders, 793–797
thyroid function tests, 794f
thyroid storm (thyroid crisis), 795–797, 796t, 797t, 798t
thyroid-stimulating hormone (TSH), 99, 794
thyroxine (T4), 793–797
TIA. *See* transient ischemic stroke

TIC. *See* trauma-induced coagulopathy
ticagrelor, 475t, 667t, 669–673, 937t
ticarcillin, 551t
tigecycline, 243, 244, 294, 587t, 744
time during which unbound/free drug concentration remains above the pathogen MIC (*f*T>MIC), 253, 260, 262, 263, 266, 267–270, 273
TIMI. *See* Thrombolysis in Myocardial Infarction
TIMP-2. *See* tissue inhibitor of metalloproteinase 2
tinzaparin, 596, 597t
TIPS. *See* transjugular intrahepatic portosystemic shunts
tirilazad mesylate, 399
tirofiban, 475t, 667t, 673–674
TISS. *See* Therapeutic Intervention Scoring System
tissue inhibitor of metalloproteinase 2 (TIMP-2), 528
tissue plasminogen activator (tPA), 404–407, 700, 857
tizanidine, 788–789
TLS. *See* tumor lysis syndrome
T-lymphocytes, 115
TNF-α. *See* tumor necrosis factor-α
TOACs. *See* target-specific oral anticoagulants
tobacco. *See* smoking
tobramycin, 551t, 557t, 835, 854t, 985t
TOF. *See* train-of-four
tolvaptan, 67, 650, 812, 813t
Tomlinson, BE, 62
tonic-clonic seizures, 373, 375f, 384
tonicity, 30–32
topiramate, 377t, 381
torsades de pointes (TdP), 725–730, 728f, 729t, 730f
    dofetilide and, 720
    KCNH2 and, 1007
    QT interval and, 726, 941, 943t
torsemide (Demadex), 648, 648t
total artificial heart (TAH), 361, 740–741
total body surface area (TBSA), 843
total body water (TBW), 58, 67, 68
total body weight (TBW), 822–823, 824, 830
total parenteral nutrition (TPN), 4, 130, 138–139, 881
toxic shock syndrome (TSS), 364
Toxoplasma encephalitis (TE), 991
tPA. *See* tissue plasminogen activator
TPN. *See* total parenteral nutrition
train-of-four (TOF), 201
TRALI. *See* transfusion-related acute lung injury
tranexamic acid, 233, 395, 492, 834, 869–870
transcranial Doppler (TCD), 428
transcutaneous pacing, 81
transesophageal echocardiogram (TEE), 721
transferrin, 99
transforming growth factor β, 390, 611
transfusion. *See* blood transfusions; massive transfusion protocols
transfusion-associated cardiac overload (TACO), 480, 483, 485, 486, 493
transfusion-related acute lung injury (TRALI), 479–480, 485, 486
transfusion-related immunomodulation (TRIM), 479–480, 485, 486
transient ischemic stroke (TIA), 403–410
transjugular intrahepatic portosystemic shunts (TIPS), 578
transthoracic echocardiography (TTE), 48

transthyretin, 99
trauma, 861–886
    ABCDE for, 863
    advanced trauma life support for, 863–865
    airway maintenance for, 863
    AKI and, 881–884
    antioxidants and, 115
    arginine and, 115
    BCVIs, 870–872
    coagulopathy and, 490–491
    crystalloids and colloids for, 40–41
    DVT and, 884–886, 885t
    hemorrhage and, 489t, 492
    hemorrhagic shock and, 490, 863–865, 864t
    NMBAs and, 217
    renal failure from, 259
    scoring systems for, 954
    VTE and, 450, 884–886, 886f
Trauma Score and Injury Severity Score (TRISS), 954
trauma-induced coagulopathy (TIC), 867–870
traumatic brain injury (TBI), 388–395, 872–879
    aSAH and, 427
    biomarkers for, 389–390
    in children, 916–921
    CYP and, 938t
    ECF and, 879–880, 880t
    epidemiology and pathophysiology of, 388–390
    hyperventilation and, 389–392
    ICP and, 390–393, 390f–391f
    hyperosmolarity and, 392–393, 392t
    nutrition for, 879
    SAFE and, 866
    SBS and, 880–881
    seizures from, prophylaxis for, 394–395
    VTE and, 395, 886
Treatment Approaches in Renal Cancer Global Evaluation Trial (TARGET), 674
treprostinil (Orenitram, Remodulin, Tyvaso), 616–617, 616t
Trial to Assess Improvement in Therapeutic Outcomes by Optimizing Platelet Inhibition with Prasugrel Thrombolysis In Myocardial Infarction 38 (TRITON-TIMI 38), 671, 680
triamterene, 526
triazoles, 321t, 322–323, 324t, 989t
triiodothyronine (T3), 793–797
TRILOGY-ACS. *See* Targeted Platelet Inhibition to Clarify the Optimal Strategy to Medically Manage Acute Coronary Syndromes
TRIM. *See* transfusion-related immunomodulation
trimethoprim/sulfamethoxazole, 575, 935, 940t
    ALF from, 577
    for PJP, 990, 991
    pregnancy and, 831
    for TE, 991
    thrombocytopenia and, 478t
triple-H therapy, 431–433
tris-hydroxymethyl aminomethane (THAM), 17–18, 33
TRISS. *See* Trauma Score and Injury Severity Score

TRITON-TIMI 38. *See* Trial to Assess Improvement in Therapeutic Outcomes by Optimizing Platelet Inhibition with Prasugrel Thrombolysis In Myocardial Infarction 38
troglitazone, 577
tromethamine (THAM), 702
troponin, 620, 663
Trousseau sign, 90
TSH. *See* thyroid-stimulating hormone
TSS. *See* toxic shock syndrome
TT. *See* thrombin time
TTE. *See* transthoracic echocardiography
tuberculosis, 91, 338
tubocurarine, 198–199
tumor lysis syndrome (TLS), 803–807, 805t, 993–995, 994t
    hyperphosphatemia and, 88
    management of, 805–807, 806t
    risk factors for, 804t, 805
tumor necrosis factor-α (TNF-α)
    ALF and, 574
    sepsis and, 1007–1008
    TBI and, 389–390
    trauma and, 490
TXA_2. *See* thromboxane A_2
Tyvaso. *See* treprostinil

U

UA. *See* uric acid
UAG. *See* urinary anion gap
UCr. *See* urine creatinine
UFH. *See* unfractionated heparin
ulcerative colitis, 79, 592
ultrafiltration, 547–548, 650–651
ultrafiltration coefficient (Kuf), 540
ultrasonography, for AKI, 528
Ultresa, 120
UNa. *See* urine sodium concentration
underweight patients, drug dosing for, 830
unfractionated heparin (UFH), 458, 462t, 474, 475t, 501
    for ACS, 668t, 674–675
    ACT for, 508–509
    activated clotting time for, 471
    for AF, 721
    anti-Xa for, 507
    aPTT for, 504
    fibrinolysis and, 682
    INR for, 502
    in ischemia-driven strategy, 678
    for NSTE, 677
    in pregnancy, 833
    for STEMI, 680–681
    TT for, 510
    for VTE, 395, 413, 451t, 452t, 453–456, 454t
United States Pharmacopeia (USP), 962
UNLOAD. *See* Patients Hospitalized for Acute Decompensated Congestive Heart Failure
unmasking, 338
unstable angina, 664, 758
urea, 7
uric acid (UA), 806, 807, 993–995
urinary anion gap (UAG), 12–13, 15
urinary tract infections (UTIs), 162, 291, 437, 618, 717
urine antigen testing, 291
urine creatinine (UCr), 528
urine microscopy, 528
urine output, 526, 805–806, 994
urine sodium concentration (UNa), 528
USP. *See* United States Pharmacopeia
UTIs. *See* urinary tract infections

V

VADs. *See* ventricular assist devices
valacyclovir, 334t, 337
valganciclovir, 334t, 336
valproate, 38, 333, 831, 933, 936t
valproic acid, 170–172, 376t, 378, 577, 931, 935
Van den Berghe, G, 129, 130, 853–855
vancomycin, 244–245, 270–271, 827t, 835, 932t
    AKI from, 531t, 532
    for burns, 854t
    for CSF shunting devices, 363
    drug clearance of, 551t
    ECMO and, 743–744
    for FN, 985t
    GNB and, 290–291
    for hepatic encephalopathy, 581
    for morbid obesity, 829
    for MRSA, 294, 353
    pregnancy and, 832
    TDM for, 263
    thrombocytopenia and, 478t, 975
vancomycin-resistant *Enterococcus* (VRE), 290, 293
VAP. *See* ventilator-associated pneumonia
varenicline, 784
varicella zoster virus (VZV), 332, 332t, 336–337, 576
VAS. *See* Visual Analog Scale
vasoconstrictors, 620
Vasodilation in the Management of Acute CHF (VMAC), 652
vasodilators, 622t, 774–775
    for ADHF, 649–652, 651t
    for hypertensive crisis, 764–766
    for septic shock in children, 907
vasopressin, 258
    EN and, 101
    for GI bleeding, 598
    for PAH, 620
    for PEA, 701
    for SCA, 692, 697–699, 698t
    for septic shock in children, 906–907
vasopressin receptor antagonists, 67, 650
vasopressin receptors. *See* antidiuretic hormone
vasopressors, 14, 43, 101, 695–697
    for ADHF cardiac transplantation, 657
    for aSAH, 427, 433
    for hypermagnesemia, 81
    MAP and, 305
    for myxedema coma, 793
    for PAH, 620
    for PEA, 701
    for shock, 229–230, 231f, 313–314
    for underweight patients, 830
    VTE and, 450
vasoreactivity challenge, 614
Vd. *See* volume of distribution
vecuronium, 202, 207, 912t
Veletri, 615
venlafaxine, 577, 587t
venous oxygen saturation (SVO_2), 646
    shock and, 228
venous thromboembolism (VTE), 449–465
    AIS and, 410
    anticoagulants for, 451–459, 451t, 452t, 454t
    aPTT and, 504
    burns and, 855–856
    DTIs for, 458–459, 458t
    ICH and, 413
    prevention of, 450–451
    SCI and, 398
    TBI and, 395, 886
    thrombolytics for, 455t
    trauma and, 884–886, 886f
    in underweight patients, 830
ventilator-associated pneumonia (VAP)
    antibiotic de-escalation for, 246
    antimicrobials for, 243, 247, 363–364
    resistance to, 290
    endotracheal intubation and, 363–364
    from GNB, 244
    minimizing, 295
    testing for, 291
    tigecycline for, 243
ventricular arrhythmias, 721–730
ventricular assist devices (VADs)
    antimicrobial prophylaxis for, 360–361
    classification of, 738t
    durable implantable, 740–741
    extracorporeal or paracorporeal, 739
    MCS and, 655, 735
    percutaneous, 737–739
    SSIs and, 357
ventricular fibrillation (VF), 74, 688, 690, 693–701, 896
ventricular tachycardia (VT), 70, 689, 721–725, 727f, 728f. *See also* pulseless ventricular tachycardia
verapamil, 666, 710, 715t, 718t, 761, 934t, 937t
Verigene test, 284
VF. *See* ventricular fibrillation
VHFs. *See* viral hemorrhagic fevers
VHL. *See* von Hippel-Lindau syndrome
Viagra. *See* sildenafil
vinblastine, 812
Vincent, JL, 47, 91
vincristine, 811
Viokace, 120
viral hemorrhagic fevers (VHFs), 343–344
viral infections, 331–347. *See also specific infections*
    ALF from, 576
    COPD and, 637–638
    in respiratory acidosis, 339t
    of respiratory system, 339–343
Virchow triad, 884
VISEP. *See* Efficacy of Volume Substitution and Insulin Therapy in Severe Sepsis
Visual Analog Scale (VAS), 148–149
vitamin B_{12} (hydroxycobalamin), 765
vitamin C (ascorbic acid), 113, 115, 122, 525, 848–849
vitamin D, 88, 90, 91, 110, 113
    burns and, 122
    HCM and, 808
    hypophosphatemia and, 83
    PTH and, 82
vitamin E, 113, 115
vitamin K, 480–481, 482t, 492, 495
    ALF and, 583
    DTIs and, 459

vitamin K antagonists (VKA), 411–412, 412t, 495, 596–597
vitamin K epoxide reductase (VKOR), 1006
vitamin K–dependent factor, 510
VKA. *See* vitamin K antagonists
VKOR. *See* vitamin K epoxide reductase
VMAC. *See* Vasodilation in the Management of Acute CHF
VO_2. *See* oxygen consumption
volatile anesthetics, 162, 172–173
volume of distribution (Vd), 543, 557
    ECMO and, 562–564, 742
volume of distribution at steady state (Vss), 255–256
    antimicrobial half-life and, 261
    of fluconazole, 273
    of hydrophilic drugs, 256, 262
    for β-lactam antibiotics, 266–267
Voluven, 38
von Hippel-Lindau syndrome (VHL), 797
von Willebrand disease, 474, 745
von Willebrand factor (vWF), 468, 474, 485, 486, 598, 611
voriconazole, 192t, 258, 319, 552t, 557, 587t, 936t, 989t
    for *Aspergillus*, 325
    CYP and, 936t, 939t, 940t, 1004
    for FN, 986
    for fusariosis, 326
    pregnancy and, 831, 832
    for scedosporiosis, 326
VRE. *See* vancomycin-resistant *Enterococcus*
Vss. *See* volume of distribution at steady state
VT. *See* ventricular tachycardia
VTE. *See* venous thromboembolism
vWF. *See* von Willebrand factor
VZV. *See* varicella zoster virus

W

Wahl, WL, 871
Wall, PD, 155
warfarin, 451t, 452t, 454t, 459, 462t, 474, 475t, 495, 989t
    for BCVIs, 870–871
    CYP and, 936t, 937t, 940t, 1003
    DDIs with, 932t, 933, 935
    drug-nutrient interactions with, 946t
    for GI bleeding, 596, 597t
    for HIT, 465
    INR for, 463
    liver and, 463
    for PAH, 619
    pregnancy and, 831
    VKORC and, 1006
water homeostasis, 58–59
weak ions, 5
Weil, MH, 47
West, Ranyard, 198
West Nile virus (WNV), 344–346, 345t
white blood cells, 575
WHO. *See* World Health Organization
Wilson disease, 578
withdrawal, 781–789
    from α_2-adrenergic agonists, 788–789
    from alcohol
        hypertensive crisis and, 759
        phenobarbital for, 172
    from antidepressants, 783–784, 783t
    from baclofen, 781–783, 782t
    from corticosteroids, 800
    from nicotine, 784–785
    from opioids, 785–786, 785f, 785t, 786t, 787f
    from sedatives, 173
    from SNRIs, 783–784, 783t
    from SSRIs, 783–784, 783t
WNV. *See* West Nile virus
Wolff-Parkinson-White syndrome (WPW), 712–714, 1005
Women's Health Initiative, 689
World Federation of Neurological Surgeons, 421
World Health Organization (WHO), 100, 163
    on aSAH, 416
    BMI and, 822
    endothelin receptor antagonists and, 618
    epoprostenol and, 615
    iloprost and, 617
    on influenza, 339
    PAH and, 612, 613t
    riociguat and, 619
WPW. *See* Wolff-Parkinson-White syndrome
Wright, Lewis H., 198

X

Xa inhibitors, 495, 596, 597t
xanthine, 806, 994
Xyrem. *See* sodium oxybate

Y

yeasts, 320–323
yellow fever virus, 345t
Yunos, NM, 22, 530

Z

zafirlukast, 577
zanamivir, 341
Zaroxolyn. *See* metolazone
Zenpep, 120
zinc, 115, 122
zoledronic acid, 808–810, 811t

DISCLOSURE OF POTENTIAL CONFLICTS OF INTEREST

Consultancies: Erik Abel (Revo Biologics); Jeffrey Barletta (Hospira; Cubist); Christopher Bland (Theravance Pharmaceuticals; Cubist Pharmaceuticals); Kevin Box (Dignity Health Care); Amanda Corbett (Food and Drug Administration); Joseph Dasta (Abbvie; AcelRx; Hospira; Jannsen Scientific Affairs; Mallinckrodt Pharmaceuticals; Medicines Company; Otsuka America Pharmaceuticals; Pacira Pharmaceuticals; Phillips Visicu); John Devlin (Society of Critical Care Medicine); Roland Dickerson (Fresenius Kabi Global); Paul Dobesh (AstraZeneca; The Medicines Company; Daiichi Sankyo, Inc.); Brian Erstad (Critical Path Institute); Elizabeth Farrington (BPS Pediatric Specialty Council); Douglas Fish (Bayer Healthcare; Cempra, Inc.); Curtis Haas (Excellus Blue Cross/Blue Shield; KJT Group); Martina Holder (CMS); Theresa Human (Cumberland Pharmaceutical; UCB Pharma); Thomas Johnson (American Society of Health-System Pharmacists; Society of Critical Care Medicine); Melanie Joy (Boehringer Ingelheim Pharmaceuticals, Inc.; Eli Lilly; Janssen Pharmaceuticals); Sandra Kane-Gill (Agency for Healthcare Research and Quality); David Kaufman (Vital Therapies, Inc.); Marin Kollef (Accelerate; Cubist; Merck); Robert MacLaren (GSK); Stephanie Mallow Corbett (American College of Critical Care Medicine; Center for Academic Partnerships for Interprofessional Research and Education; Thomas Jefferson Medical Reserve Corps Advisory Board); Ali McBride (Sanofi); David Nix (Critical Path Institute); Hanna Phan (Vertex Pharmaceuticals; Pediatric Pharmacy Advocacy Group; Cystic Fibrosis Foundation Data Safety Monitoring Board); Hal Richards (Board of Pharmacy Specialties); Jo Rodgers (Amgen; Novartis); Carol Rollins (American Society of Health-System Pharmacists; American Society for Parenteral and Enteral Nutrition; National Home Infusion Association); Todd Sorensen (Board of Pharmacy Specialties); Zachary Stacy (Janssen Pharmaceuticals); Robert Talbert (U.S. Pharmacopeial Convention; Expert Exchange; McGraw-Hill); Eljim Tesoro (Philips VISICU); James Tisdale (National Institutes of Health; American College of Clinical Pharmacy; American Heart Association; American College of Cardiology)

Grants: Erik Abel (Extracorporeal Life Support Organization; American Society of Health-Systems Pharmacists); Kevin Box (American Society of Health-System Pharmacists Foundation); Lisa Burry (Technology Evolution in the Elderly); Amanda Corbett (Gilead; NIH); John Devlin (AstraZeneca; NHLBI-NIH); Paul Dobesh (AstraZenekaDaiichi Sankyo); Thomas Dowling (MediBeacon, LLC); Brian Erstad (Mallinckrodt; American Society of Health-System Pharmacists); Douglas Fish (Merck Pharmaceuticals); Katherine Gharibian (Astellas Pharma Inc.; Theravance Biopharma Inc.; NxStage Medical Inc.); Katja Gist (American Heart Association; Children's Hospital Colorado Research Institute); Theresa Human (Astellas); Stephanie Mallow Corbett (Health Resources and Services Administration; University of Virginia Colligan Quality Improvement Grant; Paragon Biomedical; NIH ROI); Steven Martin (Health Resources and Services Administration); Kathryn Matthias (ASHP Foundation; University of Arizona Foundation; ADVANCE Grant, University of Arizona); Ali McBride (Sanofi); Courtney McKinney (American Society of Health-System Pharmacists); Scott Micek (Pfizer, Cubist, Forest, Astellas, Optimer, Astra Zeneca, and Merck); David Nix (Valley Fever Solutions); Asad Patanwala (American College of Clinical Pharmacy; Mallinckrodt Pharmaceuticals); Hanna Phan (American Society of Health-System Pharmacists Research and Education Foundation; Cystic Fibrosis Foundation); Denise Rhoney (Otsuka); James Tisdale (Indiana Clinical and Translational Sciences Institute; American Health Association Midwest Affiliate); David Williamson (Hospira)

Lecture Services: Christopher Bland (Cubist Pharmaceuticals; Merck Pharmaceuticals); Bradley Boucher (The Medicines Company); John Devlin (AstraZeneca); Erin Fox (University of Illinois College of Pharmacy; American Society of Health-System Pharmacists; Association of Surgical Technologists; National Association of EMS Physicians; American Medical Association; National Association of State EMS Officials; American Bar Association; International Pharmaceutical Federation; St. Jude Hospital; Healthcare Supply Chain Association; American College of Clinical Pharmacy); Myke Green (Merck); Melanie Joy (Pri-Med); Sandra Kane-Gill (SCCM and CRRT meeting); Marin Kollef (Cubist; Merck); Stephanie Mallow Corbett (Society of Critical Care Medicine; Virginia Society of Health-System Pharmacists; University Health System Consortium); Zachary Stacy (AstraZeneca; Janssen Pharmaceuticals); James Tisdale (Indiana Chapter of the American College of Cardiology; American Heart Association; American Society of Health-System Pharmacists; American College of Cardiology; American College of Clinical Pharmacy; University of Manitoba; Canadian Society of Hospital Pharmacists; Nova Southeastern University); David Williamson (Pfizer)

Stock Ownership; Relationships with Companies or Vendors: Joseph Dasta (Abbott; Bristol Meyer Squibb; Eli Lilly; Express Scripts ; Merck Pharmaceuticals; Pfizer); David Feliciano (McGraw-Hill); Thomas Johnson (Jones and Bartlett Learning); Melanie Joy (Katharos, Inc.); Zachariah Thomas (The Medicines Company); James Tisdale (American Society of Health-System Pharmacists)